New Generation Vaccines

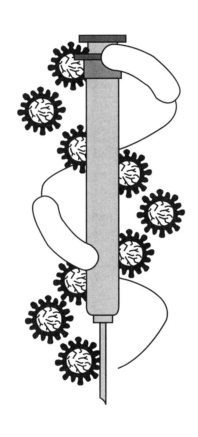

New Generation Vaccines

Third Edition, Revised and Expanded

edited by

Myron M. Levine
University of Maryland School of Medicine
Baltimore, Maryland, U.S.A.

James B. Kaper
University of Maryland School of Medicine
Baltimore, Maryland, U.S.A.

Rino Rappuoli
Chiron Vaccines
Siena, Italy

Margaret A. Liu
Transgene, S.A.
Strasbourg, France
and Karolinska Institute
Stockholm, Sweden

Michael F. Good
Queensland Institute of Medical Research
Brisbane, Queensland, Australia

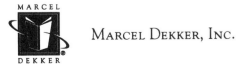

MARCEL DEKKER, INC.

NEW YORK · BASEL

The previous edition was published as *New Generation Vaccines: Second Edition, Revised and Expanded*
Myron M. Levine, Graeme C. Woodrow, James B. Kaper, Gary S. Cobon, eds., 1997

Although great care has been taken to provide accurate and current information, neither the author(s) nor the publisher, nor anyone else associated with this publication, shall be liable for any loss, damage, or liability directly or indirectly caused or alleged to be caused by this book. The material contained herein is not intended to provide specific advice or recommendations for any specific situation.

Trademark notice: Product or corporate names may be trademarks or registered trademarks and are used only for identification and explanation without intent to infringe.

Library of Congress Cataloging-in-Publication Data
A catalog record for this book is available from the Library of Congress.

ISBN: 0-8247-4071-8

This book is printed on acid-free paper.

Headquarters
Marcel Dekker, Inc.
270 Madison Avenue, New York, NY 10016, U.S.A.
tel: 212-696-9000; fax: 212-685-4540

Distribution and Customer Service
Marcel Dekker, Inc.
Cimarron Road, Monticello, New York 12701, U.S.A.
tel: 800-228-1160; fax: 845-796-1772

Eastern Hemisphere Distribution
Marcel Dekker AG
Hutgasse 4, Postfach 812, CH-4001 Basel, Switzerland
tel: 41-61-260-6300; fax: 41-61-260-6333

World Wide Web
http://www.dekker.com

The publisher offers discounts on this book when ordered in bulk quantities. For more information, write to Special Sales/ Professional Marketing at the headquarters address above.

Current printing (last digit):

10 9 8 7 6 5 4 3 2 1

PRINTED IN THE UNITED STATES OF AMERICA

Foreword

The fact that this welcome third edition of *New Generation Vaccines* comes so hard on the heels of the second edition is just one sign of the great vigor and momentum of vaccinology, now universally acknowledged as a discipline in its own right. During the first golden age of immunology, the era of Louis Pasteur, Robert Koch, Emil von Behring, and Paul Ehrlich, the nexus between medical microbiology and immunology was very close: vaccines were the practical goal of nearly all investigations of the immune system. But before the end of the 19th century, Ehrlich was to show that one could produce antibodies to the plant toxin ricin, derived from the castor bean, and Bordet discovered antibodies to red blood cells. The observation that nonmicrobial materials could act as antigens was vastly extended by Landsteiner, who showed that specific antibodies could be made against small organic chemicals that had never before existed in nature. Suddenly immunology had burst out of the confines of medical microbiology. Scientists became fascinated with the puzzle of antibody diversity—how one animal could make such a vast array of different antibodies—and the medical side of the discipline soon encountered clinical problems such as autoimmunity, allergy, transplant rejection, and even cancer control. During the second golden age of immunology, around 1955–1975, when nature's broad strategy was revealed, the divorce between immunology and vaccinology was almost complete.

Several forces fostered a remarriage. HIV/AIDS clearly demanded new thinking for an effective vaccine. Also, from the mid-'70s on, the efforts of the World Health Organization and of private foundations such as the Rockefeller Foundation, the Wellcome Trust, and the MacArthur Foundation tempted more academics into vaccinology by a combination of persuasion (publicizing the parlous state of research into vaccines chiefly of interest to developing nations) and substantial grants. Gene cloning was a major catalyst, as in so many other fields, and soon candidate antigens aplenty were produced by recombinant DNA technology. This in turn showed most subunit vaccines to be only weakly immunogenic, and immunologists interested in immune regulation entered the fray, exploring both the nature of adjuvanticity and the possible role of cytokines in enhancing and guiding responses to vaccines. As a result, this third edition carries many contributions from card-carrying immunologists. At the same time, the editors have realized that scientific breakthroughs alone cannot lead to the protection of the 130 million infants born each year worldwide. Therefore, economic, logistic, regulatory, financial, ethical, and political aspects of global vaccinology are also addressed.

The volume begins with a brief historical perspective and then introduces the many high technologies involved in the creation of the new generation of vaccines. These include not only the most advanced platform technologies of the biotechnology revolution but also the equally elaborate methods of assessment: toxicological studies, phased clinical trials, preliminary and definitive evaluation of efficacy, cataloguing of adverse events, and measurement of eventual impact. Some of the major international programs supporting more widespread use of vaccines are also described and the central, not sufficiently appreciated, role of regulatory authorities is outlined.

Eradication of smallpox was a true public health triumph and global eradication of wild poliomyelitis virus is within sight as a fitting encore. It is therefore particularly valuable and timely to get an "insider's" view of the status of the global polio eradication initiative.

The way that basic immunology can impinge on vaccinology is explored next. Then, a very important series of chapters examines the once arcane but now increasingly scientific field of adjuvants, construing that term in the widest sense to include not only physicochemical immunopotentiation but also novel delivery systems. A special category of the latter is described in depth, namely, live viruses or bacteria as vectors for genetic vaccine constructs, a field that appears promising for the very difficult vaccines such as for HIV/AIDS and malaria. The surprising delivery potential of the mucosal and transcutaneous routes is also reviewed. DNA vaccines and "prime-boost" strategies receive chapters of their own.

Following these chapters, which deal with generic issues, we come to a series of sections dealing with specific diseases. These are grouped in a logical progression. A first set of chapters looks at diseases for which licensed vaccines are in place, exploring issues such as impact, future potential, and, where appropriate, reasons for the need for further improvements, citing relevant examples.

Next come chapters concerning diseases for which licensed vaccines do not yet exist, or, in the case of rotavirus, for which a licensed vaccine was withdrawn. This extraordinary series of examples shows how far the subject has come, even since the second edition. Nevertheless, the chapters do not attempt to hide what a distance there is still to travel. At the same time, it is hard to contain a sense of excitement when contemplating the long-range potential here. Should the next 10 to 20 years prove as successful as they appear from our present perspective, increased attention will have to be given to combinations and alternative delivery systems lest our babies become pincushions! Equally, serious thought will have to be given to financing, even in the industrialized countries. Currently, vaccines account for 2–3% of the sales of the pharmaceutical industry, and public health taken as an ensemble for about 5% of all health expenditures. Surely both figures will have to rise substantially if the full promise of vaccinology is to be realized.

Peering a little further into the future, it is not unreasonable to suggest that vaccines will extend their power into areas of medicine beyond communicable diseases, and multiple chapters explore this issue. Anticancer vaccines have been the subject of research for several decades, although the most clear-cut success area is that of vaccines against infections that can cause cancer. The next probable "cab off the rank" here—a vaccine against human papilloma virus for the prevention of cervical cancer—bids fair to become as important as the prototype, namely, the hepatitis B vaccine. Vaccines against autoimmune diseases, atherosclerosis, Alzheimer's disease, and drug addiction are more speculative, but the relevant chapters make fascinating reading.

It is saddening to record that vaccines against agents of bioterrorism now constitute a new, but obligate, area of study and concern. It is reassuring to note that the very large budget that has been made available in the United States for such research will also benefit vaccinology more broadly as the National Institutes of Health is looking for bright ideas as well as developmental research.

Can a work be monumental on the one hand and accessible on the other? Can it be both theoretically satisfying and practically useful? Can it contribute meaningfully to the described remarriage of immunology and infectious disease science? The answer is that it can if the editors have an Olympian overview of the field and the authors chosen are authoritative and committed experts in their specialty. This comprehensive third edition of *New Generation Vaccines* is a rare triumph, a vindication of the dedication of all concerned, a "must have" acquisition for any library, institutional or personal, purporting to be serious about supporting vaccine science.

We are living in exciting times in global vaccinology. The Global Alliance for Vaccines and Immunization is spearheading a new global thrust. Individual countries (or groupings like the European Union) are investing more heavily than ever before in research. Vaccine manufacturers in both industrialized and developing countries are raising their game as far as Third World diseases are concerned. Very new initiatives such as the Global Fund to fight HIV/AIDS, tuberculosis, and malaria constitute potential sources for the mass-purchase of vaccines, should effective ones become available. A multitude of public sector–private sector partnerships are springing up as if a post–September 11, 2001, world is at last recognizing that the gross global inequities must be addressed, and that health is not a bad place to begin. As the 21st century unfolds, *New Generation Vaccines* will be a precious guide to many seeking to create a better world.

Gustav J.V. Nossal, Ph.D, Hon. M.D., Hon. Dr.Sc.
Honorary Governor and Patron
Walter and Eliza Hall Institute of Medical Research
Professor Emeritus
The University of Melbourne
Melbourne, Victoria, Australia

Preface to the Third Edition

In the intervening years since the publication of the second edition of *New Generation Vaccines,* extraordinary advances have occurred in the field of vaccines and immunization. These encompass not only breakthroughs in research and development but also advances in assuring vaccine safety, standardizing the way clinical trials are performed (and how data are monitored and validated), manufacture of vaccines, and the public health use of vaccines. The third edition of *New Generation Vaccines* highlights these and many other relevant changes in the field of vaccinology and puts them in a historical perspective.

At the time of publication of the last edition, clinical trials with DNA vaccines were just beginning and there was great expectation that this technology might revolutionize vaccinology. The results of these clinical trials, now available, reveal that DNA vaccines used alone do not meet expectations. On the other hand, fundamental improvements in DNA vaccines and the advent of "heterologous prime-boost" strategies have rekindled interest in their use in focused ways. DNA vaccines appear able to prime subjects so that they can respond to the same antigens when presented in another formulation as a boosting regimen, for example, by means of a viral live vector.

Since the last edition, the Bill and Melinda Gates Foundation has completely revolutionized the funding of research and development and the performance of clinical trials of candidate vaccines against neglected diseases, such as malaria, AIDS, tuberculosis, leishmaniasis, Dengue fever, Group A *Neisseria menigitidis*, and shigellosis.

Another seminal event since the publication of the second edition has been the formation of the Global Alliance for Vaccines and Immunization (GAVI) and its financial instrument, the Vaccine Fund. Working in unison through GAVI, major global partners in immunization (e.g., the World Health Organization, UNICEF, the World Bank, the Gates Foundation, etc.) are raising immunization coverage and introducing new vaccines to infants residing in the world's 74 poorest countries. A chapter in this edition describes GAVI and the Vaccine Fund, including their research objectives.

Since the last edition, two new conjugate vaccines have been licensed, including a seven-valent pneumococcal conjugate that is now used widely in the United States and a Group C meningococcal conjugate that is used extensively in the United Kingdom. Programmatic use of these vaccines has had a profound impact in diminishing the respective disease burdens.

Since the last edition was published, a major dichotomy has appeared between the industrialized world and developing countries with respect to the vaccines administered to infants and children, their site of manufacture, the formulations and combinations of vaccine antigens, and immunization schedules. A vibrant vaccine industry is emerging in developing countries (e.g., India, Indonesia, Brazil, Cuba) that now supplies most of the vaccine utilized in developing countries; these vaccines are becoming increasingly distinct from those used in industrialized countries. Vaccine safety is increasingly becoming a focus of public concern in industrialized countries, where many pediatric infectious diseases (e.g., diphtheria, measles, pertussis) have largely disappeared and populations do not feel threatened by these infections. In industrialized countries, the switch from live oral polio vaccine to inactivated polio vaccine, the introduction of less reactogenic acellular pertussis vaccine, the discontinuation of use of thimerosal as a preservative in multidose vials, and the withdrawal of a live rotavirus vaccine after it was incriminated as a rare cause of intussusception within one week following immunization of infants are all examples of this trend as regulatory and public health actions are taken to enhance vaccine safety. These topics are all covered in a series of chapters on regulatory issues and vaccine safety. In contrast, in developing countries where infections such as measles, pertussis, and diphtheria still pose notable risks of severe disease and death, and financial resources are constrained, the emphasis is to achieve the highest coverage possible with the most potent vaccines, even at the cost of some reactogenicity.

Another trend in industrialized countries is the search for vaccines to prevent or treat ("vaccine therapy") various chronic infections that afflict these populations and create an enormous economic burden. Accordingly, chapters that describe strategies to develop vaccines against Alzheimer's disease, rheumatoid arthritis, insulin-dependent diabetes, multiple sclerosis, and various forms of cancer are included in this edition.

The science of immunology continues to blaze new trails for vaccinology, and multiple chapters in this edition review this work. Practical ways of immunizing without the use of needles are also covered, including mucosal immunization, transcutaneous immunization, and the use of needle-free injection devices.

The tragedy of September 11, 2001, when terrorists hijacked airliners and flew them into the World Trade Center towers in New York City resulting in thousands of deaths, and the bioterrorist dissemination of anthrax spores through the postal system that followed shortly thereafter and resulted in two dozen cases and six deaths (and in major disruption of civil society) had a perceptible impact on vaccinology. Following these events, governments in the United States and many other countries encouraged the development of new or improved vaccines against several potential bioterror agents and diverted resources toward that end. Chapters covering this subject are also found in this edition.

The pace and extent of modern vaccine development make it impossible to include within a single volume all the notable research advances on all vaccines. Accordingly, as before, there are gaps. For example, progress on the development of vaccines to prevent *Pseudomonas aeruginosa* pulmonary disease in cystic fibrosis patients is omitted, as are updates on progress in administering attenuated measles vaccine by aerosol and the development of new measles vaccines that aim to immunize infants in the developing world who are too young to get the current parenteral vaccine.

Assembling the third edition of *New Generation Vaccines* has been a formidable undertaking that required input and help from many individuals. We heartily thank all the authors who contributed the diverse chapters that comprise the fundamental strength of the volume. We also express our indebtedness to Sandra Beberman and Barbara Mathieu of Marcel Dekker, Inc., who provided invaluable assistance and guidance. Special thanks and appreciation go to our families and friends who gave encouragement and showed patience during the many evening and weekend hours consumed in the preparation and editing of the book. Finally, this volume could not have been completed without the organizational prowess, fastidious attention to detail, tenacity, technical competence, and diplomatic skills of Mrs. Dottie Small, Assistant to Myron M. Levine.

Myron M. Levine
James B. Kaper
Rino Rappuoli
Margaret A. Liu
Michael F. Good

Preface to the Second Edition

The second edition of *New Generation Vaccines* appears at a propitious time, two centuries after Edward Jenner initiated the dawn of vaccination in 1796 by demonstrating that inoculation with material from cowpox lesions induced protection against smallpox. Indeed, as the 20th century comes to an end, vaccines are now recognized as among the most cost-effective preventive measures available in modern medicine's armamentarium. With aggressive use of vaccines, smallpox has been eradicated globally, poliomyelitis regionally, and measles has been brought under control worldwide. Moreover, the tools of modern biotechnology make it within the realm of possibility to prepare candidate vaccines against almost any infectious disease, as long as sufficient resources are committed. In this second edition, we acknowledge the arrival of vaccinology as a discipline that has come of age.

A global picture of public health interventions with vaccines is depicted in two chapters in this second edition, one documenting the triumphs of the Expanded Programme on Immunization and the other describing international disease eradication and disease control efforts. In other chapters, the painstaking stepwise process by which candidate vaccines move progressively from Phase 1 and 2 clinical trials to Phase 3 and 4 trials is discussed.

We have attempted to provide reviews of the fundamentals advances in immunology and biotechnology that constitute the underpinnings to vaccine development. Many chapters offer illustrative examples of vaccine candidates representing the application of state-of-the-art biotechnology. However, it is also clear that technologies gain and lose popularity, with some succeeding and others disappearing. For instance, notably absent are examples based on the use of antiidiotypic antibodies, and there are few examples of synthetic peptide vaccines, indicating how enthusiasm for these technologies has dissipated since the first edition. In contrast, live-vector vaccine technology has matured, and therefore considerable attention is paid to the use of vaccinia and attenuated *Salmonella* live vectors. Multiple examples of antigen delivery systems such as polylactide/poly-glycolide microspheres, liposomes, cochleates, and viruslike particles are contained in this edition, A very popular new technology, "DNA vaccines," did not exist in 1990, when the first edition was published; this revolutionary approach has gained extraordinary momentum in the time between the planning of this edition and its publication. Results of clinical trials being carried out with DNA vaccines in the late 1990s should indicate whether this approach will flourish.

In many chapters, considerable attention is paid to mucosal immunization, not only to achieve SIgA responses to protect mucosal surfaces but as a way of eliciting serum antibodies and cell-mediated immune responses. An ultimate form of mucosal immunization might be with "edible vaccines," as explained in the chapter that describes the engineering of transgenic plants expressing vaccine antigens.

With contributions from leaders in their respective fields, we have tried to provide many examples of improves vaccines for diseases against which licensed vaccines already exist and of new vaccines against diseases that were previously unassailable by immunoprophylaxis. Unfortunately, it was impossible to be completely inclusive. Examples of specific material not covered in this edition include the excellent recent progress made by teams in Vienna, Boston, and Berne working on vaccines against *Pseudomonas aeruginosa*, and update on maternal immunization, and progress in vaccines against leprosy, cytomegalovirus, and group B streptococcal infections.

Several new vaccines have become licensed in many countries since the first edition. *Haemophilus influenzae* type b conjugate vaccines, for example, have had an extraordinary impact in industrialized countries where they have been used in a programmatic way. These vaccines have been found to interfere with respiratory tract colonization by *H. influenzae* type b. As a consequence, there has been an interruption of transmission, and a herd immunity effect has been observed. Vaccines against hepatitis A, varicella, typhoid fever (Ty21a and Vi polysaccharide), cholera (CVD 103-HgR live vaccine and B subunit-killed whole-cell combination vaccine) and Japanese B encephalitis, and acellular pertussis vaccines have been licensed in various countries since the first edition. The development of vaccines against several infectious diseases of importance solely (or mainly) in developing countries, such as malaria, has been lagging, compared to the extraordinary progress made in vaccines considered to be priorities for the industrialized countries (e.g., *H. Influenzae* type b conjugates and accellular pertussis vaccines). Moreover, where new vaccines against infections important in developing countries have become licensed (e.g., Ty21a, Vi polysaccharide, and the live and nonliving oral cholera vaccines), they have not been introduced for routine use; rather, these are largely vaccines used by travelers from industrialized countries who visit developing countries. Finding ways to help developing countries introduce programmatic use of new vaccines poses a challenge that must be addressed by the vaccinology and public health communities.

Even as the technology for vaccine development has burgeoned and clinical vaccine testing has become more sophisticated, so have public perceptions and the views of regulatory agencies changed with time, For this reason, chapters on regulatory issues have been included to further broaden the perspective of the book.

The editors would like to thank the many contributors who have provided outstanding chapters for this edition. Special thanks go to family and friends whose support and patience sustained us during the many evening and weekend hours required to plan and edit this edition. This book could not have been completed without the competent assistance of Dottie Small and Brenda Lown at the Center for Vaccine Development and Henry Boehm at Marcel Dekker, Inc.

Myron M. Levine
Graeme C. Woodrow
James B. Kaper
Gary S. Cobon

Contents

**Vaccines Against Cancer and Other Chronic Diseases
and Vaccine Therapy**

1

Vaccines and Vaccination in Historical Perspective

Myron M. Levine
University of Maryland School of Medicine, Baltimore, Maryland, U.S.A

Rosanna Lagos
Centro para Vacunas en Desarrollo-Chile, Santiago, Chile

I. INTRODUCTION

The history of immunization, from the earliest attempts to modern, genetically engineered vaccine candidates, represents a long road marked with many milestones. Extensive historical reviews document many of the cardinal achievements [1–4]; however, it is not the purpose of this chapter to recapitulate these events in any depth. Rather, a few of the most pivotal milestones will be mentioned briefly, such as variolation, Jenner's experiments of inoculating subjects with cowpox to prevent smallpox, and the earliest live and inactivated bacterial and viral vaccines and toxoids. This chapter will emphasize the historical accounts of several aspects of vaccinology that heretofore have not generally been well described. These include some early attempts at eliciting local immunity via oral vaccines, attempts over the centuries at grappling with the problem of how to assess the safety and efficacy of candidate vaccines before their widespread use, and the evolution of controlled field trial methodology.

II. THE DAWN OF IMMUNOPROPHYLAXIS

The first attempts to prevent an infectious disease via immunoprophylaxis involved the process of "variolation," wherein the contents of smallpox vesicles, pustules, or scabs were used to inoculate individuals who had not previously experienced the disease [4]. Records of this procedure date back to about 1000 A.D. in China [4]. Scabs from mildly affected smallpox patients were stored for approximately 1 month (longer in winter), ground up in a ratio of 4:1 with the plant *Uvularia grandiflora*, and then inoculated intranasally. A slight fever was expected 6 days thereafter, which rose markedly on the seventh day, to be followed by the onset of the rash on the ninth or tenth days following inoculation. Fatalities were reportedly uncommon in comparison with victims of natural smallpox infection. It was stated that [4] "Not one in 10, not one in 100 does not recover."

Parenteral variolation was practiced in the Indian subcontinent, southwest Asia, and North Africa in the sixteenth and seventeenth centuries. Reports of variolation reached England as early as 1698–1700, through the letters of Joseph Lister, an Englishman working in China with the East India Company [5]. Over the next 15 years, further reports came from many sources. Many references credit Lady Mary Wortley Montagu with having "introduced" the practice of variolation into Great Britain in 1721. Lady Mary herself suffered from smallpox in 1715, leaving her pockmarked. While living in Constantinople as the wife of the British ambassador, she became aware of variolation as it was practiced every autumn by skilled Turkish women. In 1717, Lady Montagu had her 6-year-old son inoculated with smallpox under the supervision of Charles Maitland, the surgeon to the British Embassy [5,6].

Lady Montagu wrote to a friend in England, Sarah Chiswell, extolling the practice of variolation and vowed to make the procedure fashionable in England upon her return. In 1721, 3 years after she returned to England, an epidemic of smallpox raged in London. Lady Mary contacted Maitland, who was also in Great Britain at that time, and convinced him to variolate her 3-year-old daughter. Maitland agreed, but demanded that there be two witnesses, one of whom was Dr. James Keith [6]. Keith was so impressed with the outcome that he had his 6-year-old son variolated. Because these first inoculations were carried out in the face of considerable attention by the College of Physicians as well as the Royal Court, Lady Mary, whose insistence led to the first inoculation, has been widely credited with having introduced the practice into Great Britain. However, Miller [6] argues that Lady Mary's contribution to variolation becoming an accepted and widespread practice in England was, in fact, quite minimal and that the real driving force for the introduction of variolation into the British Isles was Hans Sloane, physician to the king of England and president of the Royal Society.

III. THE ORIGIN OF VACCINATION

During the last decades of the eighteenth century, smallpox was rampant in Europe, despite the increasing use of variolation as a preventive measure. Among rural folk during this period, it was increasingly appreciated that milkmaids were selectively spared the ravages of smallpox and that this was somehow related to the mild pox infection they often acquired from the cows they milked [2,4]. Although several scholars and physicians in the period 1765–1791 acknowledged this association and some, like Benjamin Justy, even inoculated family members with cowpox [2], appropriate credit must be given to Edward Jenner for his pioneering achievements (Fig. 1). In 1796, he undertook to rigorously test the putative protective effect of a prior cowpox infection against smallpox by actively immunizing an 8-year-old boy with cowpox, and later challenging the child with smallpox (i.e., by variolation). Other vaccinations of additional children, followed by challenge, were carried out thereafter.

Jenner had the foresight and perseverance to publish his results and, for the rest of his professional life, promulgated the practice of "vaccine inoculation" [7,8].

During the nineteenth century, smallpox vaccination became increasingly popular and accepted in other areas, including Europe and North America [4]. It is fitting that smallpox became the first (and so far, the only) communicable disease to be actively eradicated, an accomplishment achieved in the decade 1967–1977. An enigma that remains unresolved after the eradication of smallpox concerns the origin of vaccinia, the smallpox vaccine virus. Whatever its origin, vaccinia is a separate species within *Orthopoxvirus*, genetically distinct from both cowpox and variola viruses. Hypotheses that have been promulgated include the theory that it represents a hybrid between cowpox and variola virus, that it derives from cowpox virus, or that it is a descendant of a virus (perhaps of equine hosts) that no longer exists in nature.

As Jenner demonstrated with cowpox and smallpox, there are instances among viruses where, because of the host specificity of virulence, an animal virus gives aborted and attenuated infection in the human host, sometimes leading to an acceptable level of protection. Examples include influenza viruses, rotaviruses and parainfluenza viruses. Remarkable

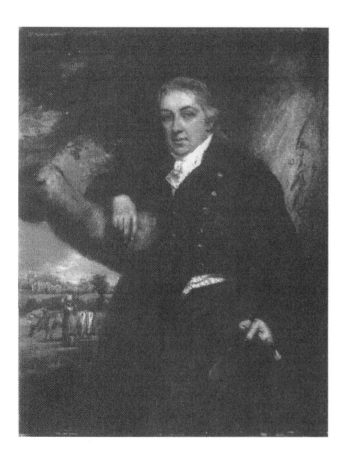

Figure 1   Edward Jenner (1749–1823), father of vaccinology. (An 1800 pastel portrait of Edward Jenner by J. R. Smith, courtesy of The Wellcome Institute Library, London, UK.)

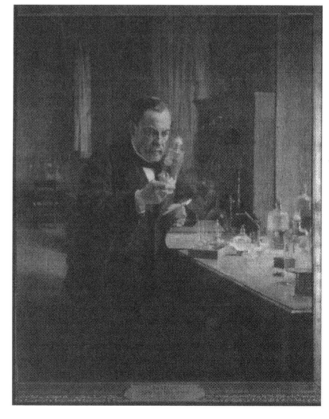

Figure 2   Louis Pasteur (1822–1895), a nineteenth century pioneer of vaccinology. (Print courtesy of Institut Pasteur, Paris, France.)

is the fact that the Jennerian approach to immunoprophylaxis remains valid in modern vaccine development, as the reader will see in the chapter "Live Vaccines Strategies to Prevent Rotavirus Disease." Finally, it is worth noting that Louis Pasteur, himself one of the most influential pioneers of vaccinology, coined the term *vaccine*, in honor of Jenner, to refer generically to immunizing agents (Fig. 2).

IV. THE FIRST USES OF ATTENUATED BACTERIA AS PARENTERAL AND ORAL IMMUNIZING AGENTS

In the last quarter of the nineteenth century, bacteriology became a burgeoning science. One after another, bacteria came to be revealed as etiological agents of important human and veterinary diseases such as cholera, typhoid fever, anthrax, plague, diphtheria, and tuberculosis. The ability to obtain pure cultures of the causative bacteria paved the way for the development of vaccines.

Pasteur observed that cultures of *Pasteurella septica*, which causes the lethal disease fowl cholera in chickens, lost their virulence when the cultures were allowed to sit for 2 weeks [9]. He found that chickens inoculated with the old cultures did not develop illness and, furthermore, were protected when subsequently inoculated with highly virulent fresh cultures. Pasteur concluded that in old cultures the bacteria undergo certain changes that result in attenuation but not in loss of immunogenicity.

Pasteur applied his theory in an attempt to attenuate *Bacillus anthracis*, the cause of anthrax, an infection of cows, sheep, and goats (and occasionally humans) that is often fatal. Pasteur found that maintaining shallow cultures of *B. anthracis* at a temperature of 42–43 °C for 2 weeks resulted in a loss of virulence (furthermore, spores did not form at this temperature). In these early experiments, Pasteur established an approach that was followed in multiple later attempts at immunoprophylaxis: the first inoculations given in the immunization schedule were highly attenuated in order to maximize safety, whereas subsequent inoculations were somewhat less attenuated to increase antigenicity.

On May 5, 1881, Pasteur and his colleagues Emile Roux and Charles Chamberland carried out a historic public experiment in Pouilly-le-Fort, France [10]. They inoculated one set of farm animals (24 sheep, 1 goat, and 6 cows) with an initial highly attenuated vaccine; a second inoculation with a less-attenuated vaccine preparation was given on May 17, 1881. On May 31, these immunized animals and a set of uninoculated controls (24 sheep, 1 goat, 4 cows) were challenged with virulent *B. anthracis*. Over the next 4 days, spectacular results documented the efficacy of the vaccine: in the control group, the 24 sheep and the goat died and the 4 cows became overtly ill, whereas there was only one death (a sheep) among the vaccinated animals. Within a short time, the anthrax vaccine became widely used in France. As early as 1882, Pasteur was able to report excellent results from the use of the vaccine in more than 79,000 sheep in France [11].

The first bacterial vaccine used in humans was administered in 1884, barely 1 year after the initial isolation of

Vibrio cholerae by Robert Koch [12], when Jaime Ferran inoculated live, putatively weakened *V. cholerae* parenterally [13]. Ferran's vaccine, which consisted of broth cultures containing "attenuated" vibrios, was administered to about 30,000 individuals who eagerly sought protection during the 1884 epidemic of cholera in Spain. This experience generated much interest internationally, and commissions from several countries came to inspect and evaluate Ferran's work. The most influential committee, sponsored by the Pasteur Institute, Paris, criticized Ferran's vaccine and argued that no convincing proof was provided to support claims for a prophylactic effect [41]. Furthermore, it was reported that Ferran's live vaccine was heavily contaminated with other microorganisms and that only a small proportion of the bacteria were *V. cholerae* [14]; contamination may have accounted for the severe adverse reactions associated with this vaccine and its apparent lack of efficacy [14].

In 1891, only 1 year after Waldermar Haffkine had joined the Pasteur Institute in Paris, Pasteur asked him to carry out research to develop an immunizing agent against cholera [15]. Following Pasteur's general principle that live vaccines confer protection superior to vaccines consisting of killed microorganisms, Haffkine prepared two modified *V. cholerae* strains for use as live vaccines. The first strain was attenuated by culture at 39° C with continuous aeration, whereas the second strain underwent multiple intraperitoneal passages in guinea pigs in an attempt to increase its virulence. Haffkine utilized these strains sequentially as parenteral immunizing agents; the attenuated strain was inoculated first, followed 6 days later by the strain of supposedly enhanced virulence [16]. Typical side reactions following vaccination included fever, malaise, and headache, as well as pain and swelling at the injection site. In later evaluations of the vaccine, Haffkine abandoned the initial inoculation with the attenuated vibrio and administered to humans only the pathogenic strain without an increase in adverse reactions. Statistical analysis of several clinical trials of Haffkine's live cholera vaccine in India suggested that it was efficacious [17]. Nevertheless, further use of the vaccine was abandoned because of difficulty in standardizing it and producing it in large quantities.

The other early success in attenuated bacterial vaccines was the bacille Calmette–Guérin (BCG) vaccine against tuberculosis. Camille Calmette and Alphonse Guérin obtained a stable, attenuated strain incapable of causing tuberculosis in the highly susceptible guinea pig [18]. It was achieved by repeatedly subculturing (213 times over 13 years), in the presence of ox bile, a tubercle bacillus originally isolated from a cow by Edmond Nocard in 1902 [18]. The first administration of BCG vaccine to a human occurred in 1921, when a newborn infant, whose mother had died of tuberculosis, was given an oral dose without adverse effects. Calmette initially advised that the vaccine be administered orally to young infants; accordingly, by the late 1920s, approximately 50,000 French infants had received the apparently well-tolerated BCG vaccine [19]. By the late 1920s, the intradermal route of inoculation rapidly began to replace the oral route of vaccination. It was not until the 1950s that controlled field trials confirmed the efficacy of at least one strain of BCG [20].

V. EARLY INACTIVATED WHOLE-CELL BACTERIAL VACCINES

Three parenteral inactivated whole-cell bacterial vaccines to protect humans against cholera, typhoid fever, and plague, originally developed at the end of the nineteenth century, were used with little modification for three-quarters of a century thereafter. In each instance, the isolation of the causative agent in pure culture was followed shortly thereafter by vaccine candidates.

A. Cholera Vaccines

In 1896, Wilhelm Kolle [21] recommended the use of agar-grown, heat-inactivated whole *V. cholerae* organisms as a parenteral immunizing agent. This nonliving vaccine was markedly simpler to prepare and to standardize than Haffkine's live parenteral vaccine. By 1911, Haffkine was also utilizing inactivated vibrios as a vaccine with 0.5% phenol as a preservative [22]. Kolle-type vaccines were first used on a large scale during the 1902 cholera epidemic in Japan [23]. In the 1960s and early 1970s, randomized, controlled field trials carried out in Bangladesh [24–26], the Philippines [27], Indonesia [28], and India [29] documented that killed whole-cell cholera vaccines can confer significant short-term protection in older children and adults.

B. Typhoid Vaccines

In 1896, Richard Pfeiffer [30] and Almoth Wright [31] independently reported that a vaccine against typhoid fever could be prepared by inactivating cultures of typhoid bacilli with heat and preserving them in phenol [32]. By 1915, killed whole-cell parenteral typhoid vaccines had become widely used by the military in Europe and in the United States. Systematic use of the vaccine in the U.S. Army, in 1912, was followed by a diminution of approximately 90% in the incidence of typhoid fever [33]. Thus epidemiological data suggested that the vaccine was protective [34], although rigorous controlled field trials of efficacy of the parenteral heat-phenol typhoid vaccine were not carried out until the 1950s [35]. Controlled field trials sponsored by the World Health Organization (WHO) in the 1950s and 1960s demonstrated that the heat-phenolized vaccine conferred about 50–75% protection against typhoid fever [34,36–38].

VI. LIVE VIRUS VACCINES

Following their success with the development of a vaccine against anthrax, Pasteur and coworkers turned their attention toward the problem of rabies [39,40]. Although unable to cultivate the virus as they could a bacterium, they nevertheless established that the infectious agent resided within the spinal cord and brain of infected animals. Pasteur and his team inoculated nerve tissue from a rabid animal submeningeally into rabbits and removed the spinal cord after the rabbits died; they were able to pass the infection from rabbit to rabbit in this manner. Roux discovered that if the spinal cords were desiccated for 15 days, they lost their ability to induce rabies. Spinal cords dried for less than 2 weeks were less attenuated, whereas minimally dried spinal cord clearly contained virulent virus. Pasteur's group prepared a vaccine that consisted of dried spinal cord suspended in saline. Their immunization schedule involved daily inoculations for 14 days, commencing with material from spinal cord that had been dried for 14 days and progressing on the successive days to the use of cord dried for less and less time. This was continued until, after 2 weeks, the final inoculation was carried out with minimally dried cord, which contained virulent virus. Needless to say, this vaccination procedure was quite controversial, even among the members of Pasteur's group. What is extraordinary is how Pasteur and colleagues identified the tissues where the rabies virus resides and how they managed to achieve attenuation yet retain immunogenicity.

In the late 1920s and early 1930s [41,42], Max Theiler and colleagues developed an attenuated strain of yellow fever virus by repeated passage of the wild-type Asibi strain in minced chick embryo tissue, from which the head and spinal cord had been selectively removed to minimize the amount of nerve tissue. Somewhere between the 89th and 114th passages, the virus lost its neurotoxicity. Theiler adapted this attenuated virus, strain 17D, to grow in chick embryos. In the 1930s and 1940s, this attenuated virus vaccine set a standard for safety, immunogenicity, and efficacy that continues to draw admiration even today. Strain 17D remains one of the best all-around vaccines ever developed. It has been safely given to hundreds of millions of adults and children and provides long-term protection. This is an amazing feat, but particularly so when one considers that the vaccine was developed in an era before modern tissue culture techniques and concepts of viral genetics had evolved.

VII. "SUBUNIT" AND "EXTRACT" VACCINES

The early diphtheria and tetanus toxoids should be regarded as the pioneer subunit vaccines. In each instance, their development followed a similar course. Discovery of the etiological agents of diphtheria by Edwin Klebs [43] and Frederick Loeffler [44], and of tetanus by Shibasaburo Kitasato [45] was followed by the demonstration that *Corynebacterium diphtheriae* and *Clostridium tetani* were elaborate potent exotoxins. Inoculation of broth cultures of these bacteria through porcelain filters resulted in sterile filtrates that were toxic for animals, leading to syndromes characteristic of human disease [46]. The production of specific antitoxins for passive protection came next, and this was followed by the use of toxin/antitoxin mixtures to achieve active immunization [47]. As will be reviewed later, mistakes in the preparation of such mixtures sometimes led to disastrous consequences. Ultimately, it was found that through treatment with formalin, diphtheria and tetanus toxins could be rendered biologically innocuous and yet retain their ability to stimulate neutralizing antitoxin [48,49]. Alexander Glenny [49] claims to have prepared formalinized diphtheria toxoid as early as 1904. In a personal communication to Henry Parish [1], Glenny related that his first toxoid was prepared by accident! He observed that a batch of diphtheria toxin lacked toxic activity yet elicited antitoxin in animals as efficiently as fully active toxin. The *C. diphtheriae* cultures used to produce the toxin had been grown in large earthenware containers which could not be readily sterilized. One of the steps in sterilizing the containers for the next batch involved washing them with formalin. Glenny hypothesized that residual formalin had apparently inactivated the toxin. He subsequently proved that formalin could, indeed, alter diphtheria toxin to toxoid, rendering it innocuous yet preserving its antigenicity.

VIII. STIMULATION OF LOCAL IMMUNITY

Many infectious agents interact with the mucosa of the gastrointestinal tract, the respiratory tract, or the urinary tract, as a site of colonization or as a preliminary step before invasion. Recognition of the mucosal immune system as a unique component of the overall immune system of the mammalian host underlies extensive current research to develop oral or intranasal vaccines to prevent enteric infections such as cholera, typhoid fever, rotavirus diarrhea and shigellosis, and respiratory infections such as influenza and respiratory syncytial virus (RSV) bronchiolitis. The leading pioneer in the concept of local immunization was Alexandre Besredka [50], who was generations ahead of his time in his approach and his concepts. However, Besredka did not believe that antibodies were involved in mediating the local immunity that he stimulated. Albert B. Sabin's pioneering work, which resulted in a practical and effective live oral vaccine against poliomyelitis, set a paradigm for other oral and nasal vaccines (Fig. 3).

The parts of this book describing vaccines against cholera show that the modern approach to prevent this disease involves oral immunization with either inactivated antigens or attenuated bacteria. However, these modern oral cholera vaccines are descendants of a long tradition. For example, the first report of nonliving whole *V. cholerae* used as an oral vaccine in humans was published in 1893 [51]; it related the lack of adverse reactions following the ingestion of multiple doses containing billions of inactivated vibrios.

In the 1920s and 1930s, field trials of Besredka's killed oral *V. cholerae* vaccine, combined with bile (the so-called bilivaccine), were carried out in India [52–54] and Indochina [55]. Significant protection was apparently achieved. In the Indian trials, the oral vaccine was also compared with a killed parenteral whole-cell vaccine. However, it is not certain if the vaccine and control (nonvaccinated) groups were fairly randomized, such that the risk of infection was equal. Nevertheless, the oral bilivaccine provided 82% protection and the parenteral vaccine 80% protection during the period of surveillance [52–54]. The bilivaccine was administered in a total of three doses on consecutive days; the subject to be vaccinated first ingested a bile tablet, followed 15 min thereafter by a bilivaccine tablet containing 70 billion dried vibrios. Because of the bile component, the bilivaccine commonly caused adverse reactions, including nausea, vomiting, and acute diarrhea; it appears that, in large part as a consequence of these reactions, further work with the bilivaccine was abandoned.

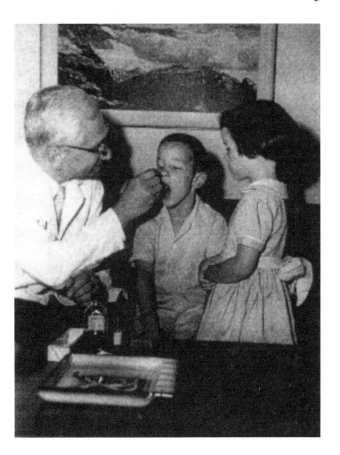

Figure 3 Albert B. Sabin (1906–1993), a twentieth century pioneer of vaccinology, administering oral polio vaccine—1959. (Print courtesy of Heloisa Sabin.)

Early investigators who pursued the concept of coproantibodies in the gut and local antibodies on other mucosal surfaces include Arthur Davies in the 1920s [56]; R. Torikata and M. Imaizuma [57] and Theodore Walsh and Paul Cannon in the 1930s [58], and William Burrows [59] in the 1940s.

IX. CLINICAL EVALUATION OF THE SAFETY AND EFFICACY OF VACCINE CANDIDATES

When a vaccine candidate appears, its safety must first be demonstrated in a series of small clinical trials before the large-scale use of the vaccine can be considered. The need for such studies was recognized as early as the introduction of variolation into England in 1722, when royal permission was given to variolate six condemned prisoners in an effort to determine the safety of that procedure [5,6]. The prisoners were offered pardon in exchange for their participation—if they survived. In November 1721, it was announced in the London newspapers that some orphan children of St. James parish, Westminster, would be inoculated as an experiment to assess the effect of variolation in children [5,6]. The use of prisoners and institutionalized children for vaccine safety studies in the 1720s established a precedent that continued until the mid-1970s. For example, in the United States in the 1950s, the attenuated poliovirus vaccine was initially tested for safety and immunogenicity in adult prison volunteers [60], whereas the inactivated poliomyelitis vaccine was evaluated early on in institutionalized children [61]. In the early 1970s, the ethics of experimentation in such populations, particularly prisoners, underwent reevaluation [62]. There emerged a new consensus that considered prisons to be inherently coercive environments in which it was difficult to guarantee informed consent [63]. As a consequence, by the mid-1970s, the use of prison volunteers for Phase I studies to assess the safety and immunogenicity of vaccines had virtually disappeared.

There also exists a long history of evaluating the efficacy of candidate vaccines in experimental challenge studies. In the first of Jenner's famous experiments, James Phipps, an 8-year-old boy was inoculated on the arm with cowpox. Jenner wrote [8]:

> Not withstanding the resemblance which the pustule, thus excited on the boy's arm, bore to variolous inoculation, yet as the indisposition attending it was barely perceptible, I could scarcely persuade myself the patient was secure from the Small Pox. However, on his being inoculated some months afterwards, it proved that he was secure. This case inspired me with confidence; and as soon as I could again furnish myself with Virus from the Cow, I made an arrangement for a series of inoculations. A number of children were inoculated in succession, one from the other; and after several months had elapsed, they were exposed to the infection of the Small Pox; some by Inoculation, others by variolous effluvia, and some in both ways; but they all resisted it.

To put Jenner's challenge of cowpox-vaccinated children with smallpox virus into proper perspective, one must appreciate that variolation was a widespread practice in England in the last quarter of the eighteenth century.

In Berlin, Germany, during the Great Depression, Wolfgang Casper, a physician who worked in the gonococcal wards of the Rudolf Virchow Hospital, developed a gonococcal vaccine consisting of a polysaccharide extract of gonococci [64]. In 1930, he carried out an unusual clinical experiment to test its efficacy. Casper recruited 10 destitute individuals whom he had previously seen with gonorrhea and who had recovered [3]. These 10 volunteers were moved into a ward at the hospital and provided with room and board. Five received his gonococcal vaccine and five were injected with a placebo. At a later point, a female volunteer, a prostitute, was brought onto the ward to spend one night with the 10 male volunteers, all of whom had sexual intercourse with the prostitute. Within 1 week, 4 of the 5 placebo recipients had developed gonorrhea vs. none of the 5 recipients of Casper's vaccine [3].

Preliminary, small-scale clinical studies to assess the safety and immunogenicity of new candidate vaccines (Phase I studies) constitute a critical first step in the evaluation of any vaccine, as is discussed in the chapter in this book by Carol O. Tacket, Karen Kotloff, and Margaret Rennels. Similarly, experimental challenge studies to assess vaccine efficacy represent an important step in the development of

vaccines for those infectious agents that readily respond to antimicrobial therapy or those that cause self-limited illness and for which well-established models of experimental infection exist. Data from these safety, immunogenicity, and challenge studies serve to identify vaccine candidates worthy of further evaluation in large-scale field trials. In recent years, this evaluation process has been applied to vaccines against cholera [65,66], shigellosis [67], malaria [68], and influenza [69]. In the modern era, there exist strict ethical guidelines to recruit the volunteers who participate in such clinical trials and to obtain their informed consent, assuring that they understand the potential risks involved and the procedures to which they will be exposed. Under the sponsorship of the World Health Organization, the Vaccine Trial Centre was established at the Faculty of Tropical Medicine of Mahidol University in Bangkok, Thailand, in the mid-1980s. This represents the first unit in a developing country where challenge studies with various pathogenic organisms could be undertaken to assess vaccine efficacy following rigorous ethical and technical local review of protocols according to international standards [70].

The relative importance of experimental challenge studies that assess vaccine efficacy in volunteers increased in 1993, when the Vaccines and Related Biologic Products Advisory Committee to the Center for Biologics Evaluation and Research of the Food and Drug Administration (FDA) voted that the results of such studies should constitute sufficient evidence of the vaccine's efficacy for submission of a Product Licensure Application. The case in point considered by the committee was the efficacy of a new live oral cholera vaccine for use in adult U.S. travelers [71]. The conclusion was that the challenge studies provided a better measure of the efficacy of the vaccine for U.S. adults than would the results of a field trial in an endemic area involving a population repeatedly exposed to cholera antigens. Previously, the efficacy of live oral cholera vaccine CVD 103-HgR, as demonstrated in volunteer challenge studies, was sufficient to allow the licensure of that vaccine in Switzerland and Canada.

X. LARGE-SCALE FIELD TRIALS TO ASSESS VACCINE EFFICACY

In modern times, the prospective randomized, double-blind, controlled field trial under conditions of natural challenge is the definitive "gold standard" test of the efficacy of a vaccine. In general, the result of at least one such trial is required for the licensure of a vaccine in most countries. One exception to this general rule is cited above.

Historically, the development of epidemiological methods for conducting field trials to evaluate the efficacy of vaccines represented an obvious and necessary offspring of the development of new vaccines themselves. According to Cvjetanovic [17], the first attempts to determine vaccine efficacy by controlled field trials were the tests of Haffkine's live cholera vaccine in India. Initially, uncontrolled trials were carried out by Haffkine throughout India, in 1893 and 1894, involving 42,197 individuals, and, from 1895 through 1896, involving an additional 30,000 persons [72–74]. However, the historic testing of his vaccine, from an epidemiological perspective, involved relatively small groups of individuals residing in prisons and on tea plantations [72–74]. As reviewed by Cvjetanovic [17], Haffkine concluded that to properly assess the efficacy of his cholera vaccine, equal-sized groups of individuals should be compared, who were randomly allocated to receive vaccine or to serve as unimmunized controls, and who faced essentially identical risk of exposure to natural infection.

Many consider that the first large-scale vaccine field trial that was rigorously designed and executed according to modern standards was the trial initiated by Macleod et al. [75] of a multivalent pneumococcal vaccine, which was carried out among recruits at a training base during World War II. In this double-blind study in a high-risk population, 7730 persons were allocated to receive vaccine or saline placebo, and surveillance was maintained for pneumococcal disease with bacteriological confirmation of clinical cases. In this book, the chapter authored by John Clemens, Abdollah Naficy, Malla Rao, and Hye-won Koo ("Long-term Evaluation of Vaccine Protection: Methodological Issues for Phase II and IV Studies") shows how much field trial methodology has evolved since Macleod and coworkers carried out their trial in the early 1940s.

A decade after Macleod's field trial on pneumococcal vaccine, the famous Francis field trial of inactivated Salk poliovirus vaccine was undertaken in the United States, involving the inoculation of more than 650,000 children [76].

XI. VACCINE CALAMITIES

An occasional byproduct of the development of new vaccines has been the inadvertent occurrence of severe adverse reactions or fatalities because of contamination, incomplete attenuation, inadequate detoxification, or idiosyncrasy. Such untoward events were obviously more common with the early vaccines. They led to an awareness of the importance of maintaining strict procedures for manufacture, testing of safety, potency, purity, and (where relevant) sterility. These events also gave rise to the formation of regulatory agencies to oversee the control of biological products. Sir Graham Wilson devoted an entire book, *The Hazards of Immunization*, to this topic [77]; it contains information on relevant materials up to the mid-1960s. Some of the more prominent disasters and incidents related to vaccines, culled from various sources, are briefly summarized below.

A. The Mulkowal Disaster

In October 1902, in Mulkowal, India, 19 persons died from tetanus after being inoculated with Haffkine's inactivated parenteral whole-cell plague vaccine drawn from the same bottle. An investigative commission concluded that contamination had occurred during the manufacture of the vaccine in Haffkine's laboratory in Bombay, India [15]. Initially, Haffkine was held personally responsible and was suspended as director of the government laboratory at Bombay. Sir Ronald Ross was instrumental in releasing the report of a

board of inquiry, showing that Haffkine and his laboratory were blameless [15]. Under further pressure from Sir Ronald Ross, Haffkine was officially exonerated and offered the directorship of a laboratory in a government hospital in Calcutta. In a final vindication, in 1925, the Plague Research Laboratory of Bombay was renamed the Haffkine Institute.

B. The Lubeck Disaster

During its initial introduction, the BCG vaccine was administered via the oral route and was given primarily to young infants. In Lubeck, Germany, approximately 250 infants were inadvertently fed virulent *Mycobacterium tuberculosis* instead of attenuated BCG [78,79]; 72 of these infants died of tuberculosis, all but 1 within 12 months. The virulent strain of human tubercle bacillus had been kept in the same laboratory as the stock for the BCG vaccine and had inadvertently been used instead of the vaccine strain. Investigation of the incident vindicated the safety of the BCG vaccine and initiated regulatory measures to assure proper laboratory conditions, training of personnel, and procedures in laboratories where vaccines are manufactured.

C. Disasters Following Diphtheria Immunization

As noted above, the earliest active immunization against diphtheria consisted of the concomitant administration of mixtures of diphtheria toxin and antitoxin. Tragedies caused by efforts in the manufacture stage were recorded in Dallas, TX; Concord and Bridgewater, MA; Baden, Austria [77,80]; Russia [81]; and China [82]. In another instance, in Bundaburg, Australia, a diphtheria toxin–antitoxin mixture became contaminated with *Staphylococcus aureus* during the manufacture of a product that contained no preservative [77,83]. Of 21 children inoculated from the same bottle, 12 died of sepsis, 6 became seriously ill but survived, while only 3 children remained healthy. *S. aureus* was isolated from abscesses in the ill but surviving children.

D. Typhoid Fever Following Immunization with a Heat-Treated Oral Typhoid Vaccine

In 1904, U.S. Army bacteriologists proposed to administer killed typhoid bacilli as an oral vaccine against typhoid fever. The bacterial culture was intended to be inactivated by heating at 56°C for 1 hr. Initial cultures of the heated vaccine were sterile. Of 13 men who ingested the vaccine, 7 developed clinical typhoid fever and 3 others suffered "febrile illness," with onset at 6–16 days after ingestion of the first dose of vaccine [84]. Repeat bacteriological examination of the vaccine demonstrated that a few viable typhoid bacilli were recoverable (2–3 organisms/mL).

E. Hepatitis Following Vaccination Against Yellow Fever

The attenuated yellow fever virus vaccine strain 17D developed by Theiler remains as one of the safest and most effective vaccines ever developed. However, during World War II, it was administered to U.S. servicemen along with human immune serum. Among approximately 2.5 million troops vaccinated, 28,600 cases of icteric hepatitis occurred, leading to 62 deaths [85]. Through careful epidemiological investigations and volunteer studies, it was discovered that some lots of immune serum used were contaminated with a hepatitis virus [86]. When human serum ceased to be given along with the yellow fever vaccine, the problem disappeared.

F. The Cutter Incident

Shortly after the favorable results of the Francis field trial of Salk inactivated poliovirus vaccine were publicized in April 1955, the FDA licensed Salk-type vaccine prepared by several manufacturers. During a 10-day period in April 1955, a total of 120,000 children were immunized with two lots of inactivated vaccine manufactured by Cutter Laboratories of Berkeley, CA [87–89]. Cases of poliomyelitis occurred among 60 recipients of these vaccine lots and 89 of their family members. The median incubation period for vaccinees was 8 days, whereas the median incubation was 24 days for the family contacts. During faulty production, wild poliovirus did not have sufficient contact with formalin to inactivate all the virus present.

G. Swine Influenza Vaccine and Guillain–Barré Syndrome

In the United States in the spring of 1976, fatal influenza occurred in two individuals (one of whom was a healthy young adult) from whom a "swine" influenza virus (Hsw1N1) was cultured. Through serological studies, it was determined that the virus antigenically resembled that of the great influenza epidemic of 1918–1919, which was characterized by high case fatality even in young adults. Accordingly, the Public Health Service, fearing a possible large-scale outbreak of Hsw1N1 disease in the coming winter, undertook a national program to prepare a swine flu vaccine and to initiate a nationwide immunization campaign. The intention was to have the vaccine prepared and safety-tested and mass vaccination under way before the onset of the winter influenza season. Between October 1 and mid-December 1976, approximately 45 million doses of swine flu vaccine were administered. However, beginning in late November and early December, reports began to appear about the occurrence of Guillain–Barré polyneuritis syndrome among recent recipients of vaccine. By December 16, the findings of a preliminary investigation corroborating this association led to a discontinuation of further immunizations with the vaccine. An extensive and detailed investigation carried out by prominent epidemiologists led by Alexander Langmuir [90] concluded that the administration of the swine flu vaccine during the national campaign resulted in a 3.96- to 7.75-fold increase in risk of developing Guillain–Barré syndrome during the first 6 weeks postvaccination compared with the normal, expected, endemic incidence.

XII. SUMMARY COMMENT

We find ourselves entering a particularly promising era in the history of vaccinology, spurred on by the application of tools of modern biotechnology, resulting in a new generation of novel vaccines. And yet, even as we look ahead with great anticipation at this unfolding "golden era" of vaccinology, we glance back with admiration at the legacy of pioneering achievements left by our scientific forefathers, who developed the first vaccines, provided our initial understanding of immune mechanisms, and forged the early methods to assess the safety, immunogenicity, and efficacy of vaccines in clinical and field trials.

REFERENCES

1. Parish HJ. A History of Immunization. Edinburgh: Livingstone, 1965:1–356.
2. Stern BI. Should we be vaccinated? A Survey of the Controversy in its Historical and Scientific Aspects. New York: Harper, 1927:1–146.
3. Chase A. Magic Shots: A Human and Scientific Account of the Long and Continuing Struggle to Eradicate Infectious Diseases by Vaccination. New York: Morrow, 1982:1–576.
4. Fenner F, Henderson DA, Arita L, Jezek Z, Ladnyi ID. Smallpox and its Eradication. Geneva: World Health Organization, 1988.
5. Steams RP, Pasti G Jr. Remarks upon the introduction of inoculation for smallpox in England. Bull Hist Med 1950; 24:103–122.
6. Miller G. Putting Lady Mary in her place: a discussion of historical causation. Bull Hist Med 1981; 55:2–16.
7. Jenner E. An inquiry into the causes and effects of the variolae vaccinae, a disease discovered in some of the western counties of England, particularly Gloucestershire, and known by the name of the cow pox. London, 1798. Reprinted in Camac CNB, ed. Classics of Medicine and Surgery. New York: Dover, 1959:213–240.
8. Jenner E. The Origin of the Vaccine Inoculation. London: Shury, 1801:1–12.
9. Pasteur L. De l'attenuation du virus du choléra des poules. CR Acad Sci Paris 1880; 91:673–680.
10. Pasteur L, et al. Sur la vaccination charbonneuse. CR Acad Sci Paris 1881; 92:1378–1383.
11. Pasteur L. Une statistique au sujet de la vaccination préventive contre le charbon, portant sur quatre vingt–cinq-mille animaux. CR Acad Sci Paris 1882; 95:1250–1252.
12. Koch R. Der zweite Bericht der deutschen Cholera Commission. Dtsch Med Wochenschr 1883; 9:743–747.
13. Ferran J. Sur la prophylaxie du choléra au moyen d'injections hypodermiques de cultures pures du bacille-virgule. CR Acad Sci Paris 1885; 101:147–149.
14. Bornside GH. Jaime Ferran and preventive inoculation against cholera. Bull Hist Med 1981; 55:516–532.
15. Bomside GH. Waldemar Haffkine's cholera vaccines and the Ferran–Haffkine priority dispute. J Hist Med Allied Sci 1982; 37:399–422.
16. Haffkine WM. Inoculation de vaccins anticholériques à l'homme. CR Seances Soc Biol 1892; 44:740–746.
17. Cvjetanovic B. Contribution of Haffkine to the concept and practice of controlled field trials. Prog Drug Res 1975; 19:481–489.
18. Calmette A, et al. Essais d'immunisation contre l'infection tuberculeuse. Bull Acad Med 1924; 91:787.
19. Calmette A. La Vaccination Preventive Contre la Tuberculose par le BCG. Paris: Masson, 1927:1–250.

20. Great Britain Medical Research Council. BCG and vole bacillus vaccines in the prevention of tuberculosis in adolescence and early life. Br Med J 1956; 1:413–427.

21. Kolle W. Zur aktiven Immunisierung des Menschen gegen Cholera. Zentralbl Bakteriol 1 Abt Orig 1896; 19:97–104.

22. Manifold CC. Report of a case of inoculation with carbolized anti-choleraic vaccine (Haffkine). Indian Med Gaz 1893; 28: 101–103.

23. Murata N. Uber die Schutzimpfung gegen Cholera. Zentralbl Bakteriol 1 Abt Orig 1904; 35:605.

24. Benenson AS, et al. Cholera vaccine field trials in East Pakistan: 2. Effectiveness in the field. Bull WHO 1968; 38:359–372.

25. Mosley WH, et al. The 1968–1969 cholera vaccine field trial in rural East Pakistan: effectiveness of monovalent Ogawa and Inaba vaccines and a purified Inaba antigen, with comparative results of serological and animal protection tests. J Infect Dis 1970; 121(suppl):SI–S9.

26. Mosley WH, et al. Field trials of monovalent Ogawa and Inaba cholera vaccines in rural Bangladesh—Three years of observation. Bull WHO 1973; 49:381–387.

27. Philippines Cholera Committee. A controlled field trial of the effectiveness of cholera and cholera El Tor vaccines in the Philippines. Bull WHO 1965; 32:603–625.

28. Saroso JS, et al. A controlled field trial of plain and aluminum hydroxide adsorbed cholera vaccines in Surabaya, Indonesia, during 1973–75. Bull WHO 1978; 56:619–627.

29. Das Gupta A, et al. Controlled field trial of the effectiveness of cholera and cholera El Tor vaccines in Calcutta. Bull WHO 1967; 37:371–385.

30. Pfeiffer R, Kolle W. Experimentelle Untersuchungen zur Frage der Schutzimpfung des Menschen gegen Typhus abdominalis. Dtsch Med Wochenschr 1896; 22:735–737.

31. Wright AK. On the association of serous hemorrhages with conditions and defective blood coagulability. Lancet 1896; 2:807–809.

32. Groschel DHM, Hornick RB. Who introduced typhoid vaccination: Almoth Wright or Richard Pfeiffer? Rev Infect Dis 1981; 3:1251–1254.

33. Kuhns DM, Learnard DL. Typhoid and paratyphoid fevers. In: Hays SB, Coates JB Jr, Hoff EC, Hoff PM, eds. Preventive Medicine in World War II: Vol 4. Communicable diseases transmitted chiefly through respiratory and alimentary tracts. Washington, DC: Office of the Surgeon General, Department of the Army, 1958, chap. 22.

34. Levine MM. Typhoid fever vaccines. In: Plotkin S, Mortimer E, eds. Vaccines. 2d ed. Philadelphia: Saunders, 1994:597–633.

35. Yugoslav Typhoid Commission. Field and laboratory studies with typhoid vaccines. Bull WHO 1957; 16:897–910.

36. Levine MM, et al. Progress in vaccines against typhoid fever. Rev Infect Dis 1989; 11(suppl 3):S552–S567.

37. Ashcroft MT, et al. A seven-year field trial of two typhoid vaccines in Guiana. Lancet 1967; 2:1056–1060.

38. Yugoslav Typhoid Commission. A controlled field trial of the effectiveness of acetone-dried and inactivated and heat-phenol-inactivated typhoid vaccines in Yugoslavia. Bull WHO 1964; 30:623–630.

39. Pasteur L. Méthode pour prévenir la rage après morsure. CR Acad Sci Paris 1885; 101:765–772.

40. Pasteur L, et al. Nouvelle communication sur la rage, avec la collaboraton de MM Chamberland et Roux. CR Acad Sci Paris 1884; 98:457–463.

41. Theiler M, Smith HH. The effect of prolonged cultivation in vitro upon the pathogenicity of yellow fever virus. J Exp Med 1937; 65:767–786.

42. Theiler M, Smith HH. The use of yellow fever virus modified by in vitro cultivation for human immunization. J Exp Med 1937; 65:787–800.

43. Klebs E. Ueber Diphtherie. Verh Dtsch Kans Inn Med 1883; 2:139–154.

44. Loeffler F. Untersuchungen uber die Bedeutung de Mikrorganismen fur die Entstehung der Diphtherie beim Menschen, bei der Taube und beim Kalbe. Mitt Klin Gesund Berlin 1884; 2:421.

45. Kitasato S. Ueber den Tetanusbacillus. Z Hyg 1889; 7:225–234.

46. Roux E, Yersin A. Contribution a l'étude de la diphthérie. Ann Inst Pasteur 1888; 2:629–661.

47. Park WH. Toxin–antitoxin immunization against diphtheria. JAMA 1922; 79:1584–1591.

48. Ramon G. L'anatoxine diphthérique. Ses propriétés—Ses applications. Ann Inst Pasteur 1928; 42:959–1009.

49. Glenny AT, Hopkins BE. Diphtheria toxoid as an immunizing agent. Br J Exp Pathol 1923; 4:283–288.

50. Besredka A. Local Immunization (translated by Plotz H). Baltimore: Williams & Wilkins, 1927:1–181.

51. Sawtschenko J, Sabolotny DK. Versuch einer Immunisation des Menschen gegen Cholera. Zentralbl Allg Pathol Pathol Anat 1893; 4:625–636.

52. Russell AJH. Besredka's cholera bilivaccin versus anti-cholera vaccine: a comparative field test. Vol 1. In: Transactions of the Seventh Congress of the Far Eastern Association of Tropical Medicine, Calcutta, 1927:523–530.

53. Russell AJH. Le bilivaccin anticholérique et le vaccin anticholérique ordinaire. Essai de comparaison pratique. In: Graham JD ed. Recherches sur le Choléra et la Vaccination Anticholérique dans l'Inde Brittanique. Bull Off Int Hyg Publ 1928; 20:703–709.

54. Russell AJH. Cholera in India. Vol. 1. In: Transactions of the Ninth Congress of the Far Eastern Association of Tropical Medicine, Nanking, 1934:398.

55. Sarramon. Sur l'emploi du vaccin anticholérique par vole buccale. Bull Soc Med-Chir Indoch 1930; 8:180–183.

56. Davies A. An investigation into the serological properties of dysentery stools. Lancet 1922; 2:1009–1112.

57. Torikata R, Imaizuma M. Zum Unterschiede zwischen der Injektions- Und der oralen Immunisierung. Z Immunitätsforsch 1938; 94:342–351.

58. Walsh TE, Cannon PR. Immunization of respiratory tract: a comparative study of the antibody content of the respiratory and other tissues following active, passive, and regional immunization. J Immunol 1938; 35:3131.

59. Burrows W, et al. Studies on immunity to cholera: IV. The excretion of coproantibody in experimental enteric cholera in the guinea pig. J Infect Dis 1947; 81:261–281.

60. Sabin AB. Behaviour of chimpanzee—avirulent poliomyelitis viruses in experimentally infected human volunteers. Am J Med Sci 1955; 230:1–8.

61. Salk JE, et al. Studies in human subjects on active immunization against poliomyelitis: 1. A preliminary report of experiments in progress. J Am Med Assoc 1953; 151:1081–1098.

62. Academy Forum. Experiments and Research with Humans: Values in Conflict. Washington, DC: National Academy of Sciences, 1975:1–234.

63. National Commission for the Protection of Human Subjects of Biomedical and Behavioral Research. Research involving prisoners. Appendix to report and recommendations. DHEW Publ (OS) 76-132, 1976.

64. Casper WA. Spezifische cutieaktionen an Gonorrhoikern mit Spezifischen, Eiwess-Freien Substanzen aus Gonokokken. Klin Wochenschr 1930; 9:2154–2158.

65. Levine MM, et al. Safety, immunogenicity and efficacy of recombinant live oral cholera vaccines, CVD 103 and CVD 103HgR. Lancet 1988; 2:467–470.

66. Black RE, et al. Protective efficacy in humans of killed whole-Vibrio oral cholera vaccine with and without the B subunit of cholera toxin. Infect Immun 1987; 55:1116–1120.

67. Herrington D. Studies in volunteers to evaluate candidate Shigella vaccines: further experience with a bivalent *Salmonella typhi–Shigella sonnei* vaccine and protection conferred by previous *Shigella sonnei* disease. Vaccine 1990; 8:353–357.

68. Herrington D, et al. Safety and immunogenicity in man of a synthetic peptide malaria vaccine against *Plasmodium falciparum* sporozoites. Nature 1987; 328:257–259.

69. Clements ML, et al. Advantage of live attenuated cold-adapted influenza virus over inactivated vaccine for A/Washington/80 (H3N2) wild-type infection. Lancet 1984; 1:705–708.

70. Sunthurasamai P, et al. Clinical and bacteriological studies of El Tor cholera after ingestion of known inocula in Thai volunteers. Vaccine 1992; 10:502–505.

71. Minutes of the January 26, 1993 Meeting of the Vaccines and Related Biologic Products Advisory Committee to the Center for Biologics Evaluation and Research of the U.S. Food and Drug Administration, Bethesda, MD. Use of challenge studies in evaluation of cholera vaccines.

72. Haffkine WM. Les vaccinations anticholériques aux Indes. Bull Inst Pasteur 1906; 4:697–737.

73. Haffkine WM. Protective inoculation against cholera. Calcutta, 1913:38–39.

74. Powell A. Further results of Haffkine's anticholera inoculation. J Trop Med Hyg 1899; 2:115.

75. MacLeod CM, et al. Prevention of pneumococcal pneumonia by immunization with specific capsular polysaccharides. J Exp Med 1945; 82:445–465.

76. Francis T Jr, et al. An evaluation of the 1954 poliomyelitis vaccine trials. Summary report. Am J Public Health, 1955; 45(5, part 2).

77. Wilson GS. The Hazards of Immunization. London: University of London, Athlone Press, 1967:1–324.

78. Berlin Correspondent. The Lübeck trial. Lancet 1932; 1:259–260.

79. Berlin Correspondent. The Lübeck trial. Lancet 1932; 1:365.

80. Anonymous. The Vienna antitoxin controversy. Lancet 1926; 2:1074–1075.

81. Jakovleva JL. Polyneurite diphthérique consecutive à l'injection de toxine diphthérique. Excerpted in: Bull Inst Pasteur 1927; 25:312.

82. Ten Broeck C, et al. Diphtheria toxin–antitoxin mixture. China Med J 1927; 41:414–423.

83. Annotation. The Bundaberg tragedy. Med J Aust 1928; 2:31–32.

84. Tigertt WD. The initial effort to immunize American soldier volunteers with typhoid vaccine. Mil Med 1959; 134:342.

85. Editorial. Jaundice following yellow fever vaccination. J Am Med Assoc 1942; 73:1110.

86. Findlay GM, Martin NH. Jaundice following yellow fever immunization: transmission by intranasal installation. Lancet 1943; 1:678.

87. Nathanson N, Langmuir AD. The Cutter incident. Poliomyelitis following formaldehyde-inactivated poliovirus vaccination in the United States during the spring of 1955: I. Background. Am J Hyg 1963; 78:16–28.

88. Nathanson N, Langmuir AD. The Cutter incident: poliomyelitis following formaldehyde-inactivated poliovirus vaccination in the United States during the spring of 1955: II. Relationship of poliomyelitis to Cutter vaccine. Am J Hyg 1963; 78:29–60.

89. Nathanson N, Langmuir AD. The Cutter incident. Poliomyelitis following formaldehyde-inactivated poliovirus vaccination in the United States during the spring of 1955: III. Comparison of the clinical character of vaccinated and contact cases occurring after use of high rate lots of Cutter vaccine. Am J Hyg 1963; 78:61–81.

90. Langmuir AD, et al. An epidemiologic and clinical evaluation of Guillain–Barré syndrome reported in association with the administration of swine influenza vaccines. Am J Epidemiol 1984; 119:841–889.

2

An Overview of Biotechnology in Vaccine Development

James B. Kaper
University of Maryland School of Medicine, Baltimore, Maryland, U.S.A.

Rino Rappuoli
Chiron S.r.l., Siena, Italy

The current era of vaccine development is unprecedented in terms of the broad range of technologies that are being applied in this area. The technological revolution consisting of recombinant DNA, genomics, proteomics, and progress in understanding the immune system has removed most of the technical barriers that formerly limited vaccine developers and has presented amazing new opportunities to use vaccination approaches to prevent and treat not only infectious diseases but also cancer, allergies, and many chronic diseases. As surely as Jenner's use of cowpox pustules more than 200 years or Pasteur's use of cultured microorganisms more than 100 years ago mark revolutions in the history of vaccine development, the use of biotechnology in the current era of vaccine development has enabled totally unprecedented advancements in the development of vaccines.

This chapter will present a broad overview of the use of biotechnology in vaccine development organized into four broad areas. The first area, initially applied more than 20 years ago in the development of the recombinant hepatitis B vaccine, is the use of recombinant DNA technology to produce antigens for subunit vaccines and to create defined mutations for attenuated vaccines. The second area is the development of novel antigen delivery systems including vector vaccines, transgenic plants, and DNA vaccines. The third area includes the use of genomics to discover novel antigens for vaccine development. The most revolutionary approach in this area is "reverse vaccinology," but techniques that characterize in vivo gene expression also utilize genomic approaches for antigen discovery. The final area is the application of biotechnology to understand the immune system and enhance antigen presentation and processing. The range of techniques in this area include the development of transgenic animals to study fundamental issues of immune response and the use of recombinant cytokines, chemokines, and novel adjuvants to stimulate the appropriate immune response. Selected aspects of these four areas will be briefly reviewed in this chapter with an emphasis on genomic techniques for antigen discovery, as this topic is not specifically covered elsewhere in this volume. For most of the topics, primary references will not be given but can be found in other chapters that deal specifically and extensively with the topics.

I. ANTIGEN PRODUCTION

A. Subunit Vaccines

The first human vaccine developed using recombinant DNA technology was the hepatitis B vaccine, which was licensed in the United States in 1987. The recombinant vaccine replaced a vaccine consisting of 22-nm particles of the S antigen that were obtained from the plasma of hepatitis B carriers. Although the plasma-derived vaccine was safe and effective, the extensive viral inactivation procedures involved in producing it required up to 65 weeks for production of a lot, thus making it a very expensive vaccine. The S antigen was cloned in yeast cells and the resulting 22 nm-particulate antigens were much easier, quicker, and cheaper to produce than those derived from plasma. Since this initial success, production of protein antigens using recombinant DNA techniques has become standard practice for subunit vaccine development.

A noteworthy variation of the cloned antigen subunit vaccine can be found in a recombinant acellular pertussis vaccine. After the initial cloning and sequencing of the *ptx* genes encoding pertussis toxin (PT), detailed structure-function analysis identified amino acid residues in the S1 subunit that were critical for the ADP-ribosyl transferase activity of the holotoxin. A double mutation of two key residues produced a toxin that lacked toxicity yet maintained an unaltered antigenic conformation. This genetically detoxified toxin was combined with purified filamentous hemagglutinin and pertactin to make an acellular vaccine that was safer and more immunogenic than the traditional killed whole cell vaccine [1]. This vaccine, which is now licensed and widely used in many countries, illustrates that not only can naturally occurring antigens be cloned and efficiently purified by recombinant techniques, but also antigens that do not exist in nature can be engineered and produced for use in subunit vaccines. An extension of this approach can be seen with epitope-based vaccines (see "Epitope-Based Vaccine"), which combine multiple epitopes from different antigens from the same pathogen or even from different pathogens into a single protein using synthesized genes.

B. Live Attenuated Vaccines

The inverse of using recombinant DNA techniques to produce subunit vaccines by cloning or more antigens is using these techniques to develop live attenuated vaccines by deleting genes encoding one or more virulence or metabolic factors from wild-type pathogens. Whereas traditional live attenuated bacterial or viral vaccines were derived by serial in vitro passage or random chemical mutagenesis, with unknown secondary effects and the risk of reversion, recombinant attenuated vaccines are specifically engineered to inactivate targeted functions with nonreverting mutations.

Two broad categories of mutations are used to construct live attenuated vaccine strains. The first category includes mutations in genes encoding a critical virulence factor, for example, deleting the *ctx* genes encoding cholera toxin in *Vibrio cholerae* (see Chapter 44) . The second category includes mutations in genes encoding critical metabolic factors, such as the *aro* genes encoding the metabolic pathway responsible for synthesis of aromatic amino acids in *Salmonella* and other intracellular pathogens (see Chapter 41). The large deletions constructed in these genes eliminate the possibility of reversion to virulence, which was the most serious disadvantage of the live Salk polio vaccine. (New attenuated polio vaccine strains with nonreverting mutations have been developed but the impending global eradication of polio using the Salk vaccine means that these newer vaccines will not be tested for efficacy.) Although the construction of mutations in pathogenic bacteria and viruses is relatively straightforward, the earliest versions of the attenuated *V. cholerae* and *Salmonella* strains proved to be unacceptably reactogenic in human subjects and so additional mutations were required (see Chapters 44 and 41). The unexpected reactogenicity seen with the first recombinant live attenuated vaccines illustrates a common problem in the molecular vaccine era in that technical issues are rarely the limiting factor in vaccine development but instead the limiting factors are deficiencies in our understanding of the disease pathogenesis or protective immune response.

II. ANTIGEN DELIVERY

There are numerous antigen delivery systems currently being investigated such as liposomes, proteosomes, immunostimulatory complexes (ISCOMS), immunostimulating reconstituted influenza virosomes (IRIVs), virus-like particles (VLPs), microencapsulation, and other technologies. These systems, which are reviewed in Chapters 22 through 25 in this volume, largely do not utilize recombinant DNA technology. In this section, we will briefly highlight novel antigen delivery systems that could not have existed in the prerecombinant DNA era.

A. Vector Vaccines

Vector vaccines employ live attenuated bacterial or viral strains to carry protective antigens of foreign, unrelated antigens and deliver these heterologous antigens to the immune system. One of the most successful vector vaccines yet developed is a vaccinia virus vector that expresses rabies glycoprotein. This vaccine, administered orally to animals via live recombinant vaccine-impregnated bait scattered in rabies-endemic areas, has already been credited with substantial reductions in rabies in wildlife populations in various countries (see Chapter 27). Numerous foreign antigens have been expressed in a wide variety of bacterial and viral vectors, leading to hundreds if not thousands of possible antigen/vector combinations. Fusion of antigen genes to different targeting sequences can direct the antigens to different bacterial/viral compartments, e.g., surface vs. internal locations and/or to different host cell compartments, e.g., endoplasmic-reticulum or lysosome. Vector vaccines can also be engineered to express cytokines or other mediators to increase immune response or to shift the balance between Th1 or Th2 responses. Bacterial species that have been employed as vector vaccines include attenuated strains of *Salmonella enterica* serovar Typhi and serovar Typhimurium, *Shigella*, *Vibrio cholerae*, *Listeria monocytogenes*, *Mycobacterium bovis* (BCG), and *Yersinia enterocolica* (reviewed in Chapter 30). Other bacterial vectors have included nonpathogenic strains derived from normal flora such as *Streptococcus gordonii* (reviewed in Chapter 57), *Lactobacillus casei*, and *Lactobacillus lactis*. Some of the intracellular pathogens, particularly attenuated *Salmonella* and *Shigella*, have been further exploited to deliver DNA vaccine plasmids to host cells, particularly antigen presenting cells such as dendritic cells, macrophages, etc., whereby the foreign antigen is expressed via a promoter active in eukaryotic cells (see Chapter 30). These bacterial DNA vector strains offer the additional advantage of being delivered by the oral route rather than the parenteral route. A variety of attenuated viruses have also been employed as vectors including vaccinia and other poxviruses (see Chapter 27), adenovirus (see Chapter 28), and single-stranded RNA virus replicon vectors such as alphaviruses, coronaviruses, picornaviruses, flaviviruses, influenza viruses, rhabdoviruses, and paramyxoviruses (see Chapter 29). Depending on the virus, the route of administration of these vectors could be parenteral, oral, or intranasal, and engineered changes in viral tropism offer the potential to target these vectors to specific cell types such as dendritic cells (see Chapter 28).

B. Transgenic Plants

Transgenic plants expressing antigens of infectious agents offer tremendous potential for the expression of protein antigens. Such antigens can be delivered orally to the mucosal immune system, giving rise to the term "edible vaccines" to describe these transgenic plants (see Chapter 26). A variety of plants have been exploited for this purpose including tobacco, potatoes, tomatoes, and corn. The amount of foreign antigen produced varies according to the plant species and the integration site of the gene encoding the antigen. For insertion into the nucleus, antigen levels of 0.01–2% of total soluble plant protein have been reported (Chapter 26). One recent report utilized a chloroplast insertion site, which resulted in foreign protein expression levels of up to 45% of total soluble plant protein [2]. Thus, transgenic plants can potentially produce large amounts of protein antigens very efficiently on an industrial agricultural scale. Numerous antigens have been expressed in plants including proteins from rabies, respiratory syncytial virus (RSV), measles, norovirus, rotavirus, hepatitis B and C, HIV, *V. cholerae*, enterotoxigenic *E. coli*, *Staphylococcus aureus*, *Pseudomonas aeruginosa*, and protective immunity against challenge has been shown in animals for several of these vaccines. Initial clinical trials have studied transgenic plants expressing antigens from enterotoxigenic *E. coli*, norovirus, and hepatitis B, and all have been found to be safe and immunogenic, although no protection data have yet been gathered in humans. Although important questions remain to be completely addressed, e.g., protective efficacy, potential for oral tolerance, public acceptance of genetically modified plants, etc., transgenic plants expressing vaccine antigens offer the potential for efficient and inexpensive production of vaccines that could be produced in developing countries.

C. DNA Vaccines/Genetic Immunization

An antigen delivery system first described a decade ago does not actually deliver antigens per se. Instead, this system delivers the gene encoding a specific antigen under the control of a strong eukaryotic or viral promoter (e.g., a CMV promoter) into mammalian cells where the antigen is transcribed, translated, and expressed. This technology, called DNA vaccines (Chapter 31) or genetic immunization [3], has been utilized in more than 1000 publications since it was first described [3]. The DNA is delivered on coated gold particles administered via a gene gun or by i.m. injection and the expressed protein is processed and presented to the immune system by the MHC class 1-restricted pathway, resulting in cytotoxic T lymphocyte (CTL) induction, the MHC class-II restricted pathway resulting in helper T cell responses, and to B cells resulting in the induction of antibodies. Numerous viral, bacterial, and parasite antigens have been delivered by DNA vaccines and striking humoral and cellular responses and protective immunity from challenge have been reported for many of these systems (see Chapter 31). In addition to infectious diseases, this technology has also been utilized in animal models of allergy, asthma, and cancer. Most applications of DNA vaccines/genetic immunization have delivered one or two antigens that were chosen on the basis of immunogenicity data obtained with other systems. However, this approach can also be used on a genomic scale to inoculate expression libraries of entire bacterial or viral genomes into animals

that are subsequently challenged to determine what pools of clones confer protection (see Section III.D).

The spectacular results obtained in mice with DNA vaccines have not been readily extended to trials involving primates and humans, where limited effectiveness has been shown (reviewed in Chapter 31). A variety of genetic constructs, delivery methods, and adjuvants are being studied to improve responses in humans. One of the most promising approaches is a prime-boost strategy where a DNA vaccine is used to prime and another technology, e.g., vaccinia expressing the same antigen, is used to boost (see Chapters 31, 32, and 71). The prime–boost strategy is being used not only for DNA vaccines but also with the entire spectrum of immunization approaches resulting from the application of biotechnology to vaccine development.

III. ANTIGEN DISCOVERY THROUGH GENOMICS

The science of genomics is revolutionizing all areas of biomedical research and vaccine development is no exception. Conventional subunit vaccine development focused on one or more protective antigens discovered by growing the pathogen in laboratory conditions and dissecting it into individual components. Each candidate component is then tested for its ability to induce immunity. Limitations of this approach include the fact that only those antigens that can be purified in quantities suitable for vaccine testing can be studied, the fact that critical protective antigens may only be expressed in vivo and not in vitro, and the time-consuming nature of identifying, purifying, and testing the individual components of the pathogen. While obviously successful in many cases, this approach took a long time to yield vaccines against those pathogens for which the solution was easy and failed to produce vaccines for those bacteria and parasites that did not have obvious immunodominant protective antigens. And when dealing with non-cultivable microorganisms, the limitations of this approach are obvious.

The ability to examine potential antigens on a genome-wide scale is significantly changing the field of antigen discovery. Advances in DNA sequencing technology now allow the determination of the complete genome sequence of a bacterium in a few months at a relatively low cost. Complete genome sequences are available for more than 80 bacteria, most of which are pathogens, with an additional 100 bacterial genomes in progress. The availability of the genome of large parasites such as *Plasmodium falciparum*, together with that of the vector *Anopheles gambiae*, and the human host, provides for the first time the entire genomic information of the three living organisms whose interaction is responsible for malaria, the disease which affects one third of the human population. The availability of complete genome sequences and recent advances in recombinant DNA technology mean that every possible antigen of a pathogen can be tested for its ability to induce a protective immune response. Furthermore, these approaches allow the examination of potential protective antigens without the bias that can result from focusing on antigens that are highly expressed under in vitro laboratory growth conditions.

A. Reverse Vaccinology

Rather than starting with the pathogenic organism grown in vitro and fractionated into individual components that are then tested for immunogenicity, the technology known as reverse vaccinology starts with the genome sequence of a pathogen [4]. In silico (computer) analysis is applied to the predicted protein products of every potential open reading frame in the genome to predict those antigens that are most likely to be vaccine candidates. Potential vaccine candidates are chosen using a variety of criteria including predicted localization on the bacterial surface, outer membrane or secreted proteins, lipoproteins, inner membrane proteins, periplasmic proteins, and proteins with homology to known virulence factors of other microorganisms. The selected proteins are then expressed as recombinant proteins by using PCR primers containing appropriate restriction sites to amplify and clone the gene into expression vectors. The expression vectors contain sequences encoding a 6xHis tag or glutathione-*S*-transferase, thereby allowing rapid purification of the recombinant protein by simple column chromatography. The use of robotics greatly enhances the high throughput cloning and purification steps.

The purified recombinant proteins are then tested for their potential to engender a protective immune response. The tests employed differ according to the pathogen, but a rapid test that can give some indication of protective immunity potential is most preferable when screening a large number of recombinant proteins. At one end of the spectrum of tests is the use of the recombinant proteins to raise immune serum in mice, which is then employed in ELISA or flow cytometry techniques to demonstrate the ability of the immune serum to recognize the native antigen on the surface of the bacteria. At the other end of the spectrum, animal challenge models may be the only screening method for protective immunity. In between these two extremes are other assays such as complement-mediated lysis of Gram-negative bacteria in the presence of specific antibody or an opsonophagocytosis assay measuring antibody and complement-dependent bacterial killing in the presence of neutrophils isolated from fresh blood. Usually, a series of tests are performed involving simple, rapid tests for the initial screen to decrease the number of candidates and animal challenge studies for those proteins that successfully complete the initial screen.

Reverse vaccinology was first applied to the identification of vaccine candidates against serogroup B meningococcus [5]. Of the 2158 putative open reading frames (ORFs) annotated for this pathogen, 600 ORFs were selected as candidate antigens and cloned into *E. coli* for expression as a fusion protein. Three hundred fifty of the 600 ORFs were successfully expressed, purified, and used to immunize mice and screened for potential protective immune response. Ninety-one proteins were found to be surface-exposed and antisera raised against 29 of these included bactericidal antibodies. The genetic diversity of the most promising antigens was examined by sequencing the genes for these proteins from 31 meningococcal strains isolated in different parts of the world; candidates showing substantial sequence variation were discarded from further consideration. These

studies, discussed in further detail in Chapter 36, have resulted in 15 very promising antigens that are being further developed as vaccine candidates [1].

Reverse vaccinology identifies novel antigens not previously identified by conventional approaches and has a number of advantages. The hazards of growing large volumes of pathogenic organisms are avoided and the process can be readily applied to nonculturable organisms. Candidate antigens can be examined without the need to first establish the abundance of the antigen, determine whether it is expressed in vivo or not, develop the optimal cultural conditions for expression of the antigen, etc. The rate-limiting step is the availability and convenience of good correlates of protection, a limitation that also applies to conventional vaccine development efforts. The other limitation of reverse vaccinology is the inability to identify nonprotein antigens such as polysaccharides and the identification of CD1-restricted antigens such as glycolipids. Since the initial application of this technique to group B meningococcus, reverse vaccinology has also been successfully applied to other pathogens such as *Streptococcus pneumoniae*, *Chlamydia pneumoniae*, and *Staphylococcus aureus* (reviewed in Ref. 4). The application of reverse vaccinology to viruses could lead to the discovery of novel viral antigens other than structural proteins that are typically the target of conventional vaccine development. For example, two decades have been spent expressing every possible form of the HIV envelope protein (gp120, gp140, or gp160, etc.) or subdomains of this protein. A genomic approach would identify potential antigens that are either not part of the final viral particle or present in such low quantities that they could not be purified and used in a conventional vaccine approach. Recent promising results using Tat, Nef, Rev, and Pol antigens in HIV vaccines suggest that development of vaccines against viruses such as HIV or HCV using a reverse vaccinology approach would be a productive approach to pursue (reviewed in Ref. 4).

B. Epitope-Based Vaccines

Another example of in silico vaccine design on a genomic scale is a new generation of immunogens based on predictions of T-cell epitopes. The concept of using epitopes for the design of immunogens is not novel, having been the basis of vaccine candidates since the 1980s. But what is novel today is the availability in public databases of the genome sequence of most human pathogens and of the sequence of the human genome itself. This unprecedented amount of information makes possible the computational design of new immunogens based on the combination of epitopes deriving from different antigens from the same pathogen or even from different pathogens. The epitopes can be selected by a number of available algorithms that form the basis of modern computational immunology. (See Chapter 15 for a discussion of these algorithms and applications of epitope-based vaccines.) The selection not only allows the inclusion of epitopes that are predicted to be most immunogenic and to bind to most HLA haplotypes, but also allows the exclusion of those epitopes that may have some common sequence with human sequences and that may be potential causes of autoimmunity and side effects. This powerful bioinformatics approach has been used to predict and prioritize epitopes within the genomes of several viruses, including HIV, HCV, and HBV, and even an entire bacterial genome, *Mycobacterium tuberculosis* (see Chapter 15). In those cases when helper or cytotoxic cellular immunity mediates protection (for instance, in many viral infections and cancer), epitope vaccines, delivered via synthetic peptides, recombinant proteins, or by DNA vaccination, may find practical application.

C. In Vivo Gene Analysis

Several genomic approaches have been developed to identify genes and proteins that are expressed in vivo during the course of infection. The mere fact that a gene is expressed in vivo does not guarantee that the gene product will engender protective immunity. But the identification of in vivo-expressed genes, particularly those that are not expressed under in vitro conditions, provides novel candidate proteins that could form the basis of new vaccines or therapeutic interventions. A number of techniques have been developed to detect in vivo gene expression including STM, IVET, and others (reviewed in Ref. 6).

Signature-tagged mutagenesis (STM) was developed to overcome the burden of screening single transposon mutants of a bacterial pathogen individually in an animal model. In STM, a collection of transposons, each tagged with a unique 40-bp nucleotide sequence, are generated and used to mutagenize a bacterial pathogen. The transposon-tagged mutants can be distinguished from one another using DNA probes based on the unique 40-bp sequences. The mutants are then pooled and inoculated into animals. Those mutants with insertions in genes critical for in vivo growth or for withstanding host defenses will not be recovered from the animal after the course of infection. The output pool of mutants is hybridized to the unique 40-bp tags present in the input pool to identify those mutants that did not survive the infection. In an application of STM to *N. meningitidis*, a library of 2850 insertional mutants was tested in an infant rat model and 73 genes that are essential for bacteremic disease were identified [7]. Eight insertions were in genes encoding known virulence factors but the remaining 65 genes had not been previously implicated in the pathogenesis of disease because of this organism. Several of the gene products identified in this way are now being developed as vaccine candidates for *N. meningitidis*.

The in vivo expression technology (IVET) approach utilizes a library of gene fusions containing pathogen promoters fused to a reporter gene. The library is inoculated into animals, and activation of the reporter gene indicates activation of the promoter to which it is fused (reviewed in Ref. 6). The original description of IVET involved creating transcriptional fusions of random fragments of the *S. typhimurium* chromosome with a promoterless *purA* gene, a gene essential for the synthesis of purines. The library was introduced into a *S. typhimurium purA* mutant, which cannot survive in mice, and pools of the fusion strains are inoculated

into mice. Those strains that contain the *purA* reporter gene fused to a promoter that is active in vivo will survive mouse passage. After 3 days, the surviving strains were recovered and screened on laboratory media for clones with low promoter activity in vitro. The sequences of the in vivo-activated promoters were compared to the genomic sequence, and structural genes transcribed by these promoters were further characterized for their role in pathogenesis and as a potential immunogens. A further derivative of IVET, called RIVET or resolvase IVET, utilizes a promoterless *tnpR* gene encoding a site-specific recombinase (resolvase) as a reporter gene. Activation of a promoter fused to the *tnpR* gene results in excision of a fragment of DNA located between two copies of the *res* sequence, the site on which the TnpR resolvase acts. By testing for loss of a selective or differential marker encoded on the excisable fragment, in vivo-activated genes can be identified, even if the genes are only active early in the course of infection and repressed later during the course of infection.

Additional technologies to detect in vivo-expressed genes are available that do not require any genetic manipulation of strains. Microarray technology involves the extraction of mRNA from pathogens grown in vivo or under other specific conditions and the hybridization of the resulting cDNA to an array containing all predicted open reading frames of an organism. Those genes that are specifically expressed in vivo can be readily identified and further investigated as potential immunogens. Proteomics involves the separation of proteins expressed under specific in vivo or in vitro conditions using 2-D gel electrophoresis. The precise molecular mass of an isolated protein of interest is determined using mass spectroscopy (MALD-TOF), a technology suitable for rapidly analyzing large numbers of proteins. By comparing the experimentally determined mass to the predicted masses of proteins potentially encoded on a pathogen's genome, the isolated protein can be identified. Microarrays and proteomics are powerful technologies that can rapidly examine thousands of genes and proteins for in vivo expression or expression within a certain cell type, e.g., macrophages. However, limitations of these techniques include the difficulty of isolating sufficient quantities of mRNA or proteins in a form free from contaminating mRNA or proteins of host cells or other organisms.

D. Expression Library Immunization

A genomic approach to the identification of protective antigens is called "expression library immunization" (ELI) (reviewed in Ref. 3). An expression library of a pathogen's genomic DNA is constructed under control of a promoter active in eukaryotic cells in a plasmid vector capable of replication within host cells. Portions of the DNA library containing 10^3–10^4 clones ("sibs") are used to immunize animals via gene gun or other methods used for DNA immunization, and the immunized animals are challenged with a virulent strain of the pathogenic organism. Those library portions that confer partial or complete protection from challenge are then retested with smaller numbers of clones, e.g., 500 sibs, to see which pool of clones confers protection. By reducing the complexity of the expression library and testing for protective efficacy in a step-wise fashion, individual clones are eventually isolated that can confer immunity. Expression library immunization allows the entire genome to be tested for vaccine potential by using the animal to select the immunogenic clones. This approach allows all of the proteins encoded in a genome to be tested for protective efficacy in a systematic fashion without pre-existing bias as to which genes may encode protective antigens.

IV. ADVANCES IN IMMUNOLOGY

The application of biotechnology and molecular techniques has resulted in dramatic advances in our understanding of the immune system and in our ability to manipulate this system to enhance antigen presentation and processing, thereby enhancing the efficacy of vaccines. One of the most striking advances has been the development of transgenic animals with single and multiple knockout mutations in genes encoding important immune system components. A genomic approach that is producing important insights into the immune system is gene expression profiling using DNA microarrays, which allows the simultaneous determination of the expression of thousands of individual genes in response to infectious agents and vaccines. Biotechnology companies now produce a plethora of recombinant cytokines, chemokines, monoclonal and polyclonal antibodies, and other reagents that are essential components of modern immunology research. Many of these recombinant proteins and/or the genes encoding them are being exploited to enhance and direct the immune responses to antigens. Only a few major advances in this area will be discussed here, but additional details will be found in Chapter 14 and other chapters in this volume.

A. The Linkage of Innate to Acquired Immunity

The past few years have seen an explosion of research in the field of innate immunity. It is now widely recognized that innate immunity and the resulting inflammatory process play a key role in initiating the adaptive immune response and determining the nature of this response (see Chapter 14 [Sztein]). An adaptive immune response is initiated after cells considered to be part of the innate immune response, e.g., dendritic cells (DC) and other antigen presenting cells (APC), take up, process, and present antigens to naïve recirculating lymphocytes in secondary lymphoid tissue (e.g., regional lymph nodes). The findings on innate immunity are turning out to be instrumental in the understanding of the mechanisms of action of several adjuvants, mainly those derived from bacterial components. Cells of the innate immune system recognize a wide range of microorganisms through surface receptors (pattern recognition receptors or PRRs) that recognize invariant molecules present in diverse microbes (pathogen-associated molecular patterns or PAMPs), but not in the host. An important family of PRRs is the Toll-like receptors (TLR), which are emerging as key players in the delivery of initial signals to the immune system. Several PAMPs have been useful as vaccine adjuvants, for example, bacterial lipopolysaccharide (LPS) interacts with TLR4 on APCs, thereby initiating the expression of inflammatory cytokines and costimulatory molecules. In addition to LPS, TLR4 is also implicated in the recognition of the heat shock protein of 60 kDa (hsp60) and of lipoteichoic acid, which have long been known for their adjuvant activity. Nucleic acids containing unmethylated CpG dinucleotides commonly found in bacteria interact with TLR9 and stimulate the innate and ultimately the adaptive immune system in a variety of ways. TLR2 recognizes several microbial components, such as peptidoglycan, bacterial lipoproteins, and zymosan. It is likely that the strong adjuvant activity of complete Freund's adjuvant, which contains mycobacteria, and of monophosphoryl lipid A (MPL), derived from the bacterial cell wall, may be at least partly explained by the interaction with TLR2.

It is now recognized that activation of PRRs profoundly affects the behavior of many cells types, modulates the type of adaptive immune response induced, and recruits macrophages, neutrophils, lymphocytes, and other cells to the inflammatory site (see Chapter 14).

TLR–PAMP interactions on the surface of DCs play a critical role in the induction of adaptive immunity by upregulating the expression of costimulatory molecules required for the activation of naïve T cells specific for antigenic peptides expressed on the same DCs in conjunction with MHC molecules. The new information resulting from research in this area plus the numerous recombinant cytokines and other reagents now available allows a more "tailor-made" approach to generating immune responses to vaccines.

B. Lymphokines and Other Immunomodulators

Numerous cytokines, chemokines, and other immunomodulatory factors have been produced in large amounts using recombinant DNA techniques and co-administered with antigens to improve or modulate the immune response at various points in the generation and maintenance of the immune response. A complementary approach is to couple or otherwise co-administer genes encoding these proteins with genes encoding the desired antigens to modulate the response (see Chapter 20). These genes can be introduced via DNA immunization or incorporated into bacterial or viral vector vaccines. For example, a key branch point in the immune response is the Th1 vs. Th2 response. Co-administration of IFN-γ, IL-12, or IL-18-encoding plasmids has been shown to enhance the induction of Th1 responses while co-administration of IL-4, IL-5, IL-10, and IL-13 enhances aTh2 response. When cytotoxic T lymphocyte (CTL) responses are desirable, administration of a broad array of cytokines, including IL-2, IL-12, IL-15, IL-18, and GM-CSF, has been shown to enhance this outcome. A number of costimulatory and adhesion molecules, including CD80 (B7-1), CD86 (B7-2), CD40 ligand, ICMA-1 (CD54), and LFA-3, have also been shown to increase CTL responses. Co-immunization with a variety of CCR7 ligands such as IL-8, IP-10, MIP-2, RANTES, MCP-1, MIP-1α, MIP-1β, and others can yield a variety of results including increased antibody production, enhanced T-cell-mediated immunity, and increased numbers of DC in secondary lymphoid tissues. Further discussion of the ability of these and other factors to modulate the immune response is presented in Chapter 20.

Numerous adjuvants are now under study to enhance immune responses (see Chapters 18, 19, 20, and 21). The currently licensed adjuvants and the vast majority of those under investigation are used for parenteral administration. Because of intrinsic anatomical characteristics and by serving as the portal of entry of most pathogens, mucosal surfaces represent ideal sites for vaccine delivery. Several live-attenuated vaccines (e.g. polio, *Salmonella* and *V. cholerae* vaccines) are given orally. However, nonreplicating, purified antigens are poorly immunogenic when delivered mucosally and may even induce a state of tolerance. The best mucosal immunogens are those with an inherent ability to attach to epithelial cells, e.g., *Escherichia coli* heat-labile enterotoxin (LT), cholera toxin (CT), bacterial fimbriae, etc. Heat-labile enterotoxin and cholera toxin have been shown to be potent mucosal adjuvants but are unsafe to use as oral adjuvants. Mutants of LT and CT have been engineered to "genetically detoxify" the A subunit, which is responsible for the ADP-ribosylation activity of the holotoxin ultimately leading to diarrhea, while retaining the intact B subunit, which is responsible for binding of the holotoxin. Mutant toxins such as LTK63, LTR72, and R192G retain adjuvant activity and are currently being evaluated with a variety of antigens (see Chapter 21). Interestingly, wild-type CT and LT toxins have potent adjuvant activity when administered by transcutaneous immunization and are currently being clinically evaluated (see Chapter 34).

C. Improved Responses to T-Independent Antigens Via Conjugate Vaccines

Production of antibodies to most nonprotein antigens, such as glycolipids, nucleic acids, and polymeric polysaccharides, does not require help by cognate T cells and are therefore referred to as thymus-independent (TI) antigens (reviewed in Chapter 14). Bacterial capsular polysaccharides are important TI antigens and for several invasive pathogens, such as *Haemophilus influenzae*, *N. meningitidis*, *Streptococcus pneumoniae*, the surface polysaccharides are crucial protective antigens. Initial vaccines containing the polysaccharide from *H. influenzae* b (Hib) were effective in older children but were poorly immunogenic in infants, a critical target population for vaccines against. Research into this discrepancy revealed that TI antigens could be subdivided depending on whether they are able (TI-1) or not able (TI-2) to induce immune response in neonates. It was further determined that by coupling polysaccharides, which are TI-2 antigens, to T-cell-dependent protein antigens such as diphtheria toxoid or tetanus toxoid, strong anti-polysaccharide antibodies could be elicited in infants. This realization led to the development of polysaccharide-protein conjugate vaccines that have resulted in dramatic decreases in Hib disease, as reviewed in Chapter 37. Conjugate vaccines have also been developed and are now licensed for *N. meningitidis* (see Chapters 36 and 37), *S. pneumoniae* (see Chapter 38), and *Salmonella* Typhi (see Chapter 40). The breakthrough in understanding how TI-2 antigens can be manipulated to improve immunogenicity is one of the most important advances in recent bacterial vaccine development.

V. CONCLUSION

There have been tremendous technical advances in vaccine development over the last two decades, particularly in molecular aspects. Indeed, current limitations and problems in vaccine development are rarely due to technical constraints but are usually due to an incomplete understanding of the biological system, including aspects of both the host and the pathogen. The major limitations in the development of many vaccines are the lack of suitable animal models and immune correlates that accurately predict protection in humans, limitations that have plagued us for decades. Indeed, vaccines have been developed that can protect mice against nearly any infectious disease but translation of the successes in mice into human protection has been problematic for many vaccines. Here, too, technology will play an important role in the development of transgenic animals that may more accurately predict efficacy in humans. With continued improvements in our understanding of the immune system and the pathogenesis of disease due to infectious agents, the current "golden era" of vaccine development will continue for the foreseeable future.

REFERENCES

1. Greco D, et al. A controlled trial of two acellular vaccines and one whole-cell vaccine against pertussis. Progetto Pertosse Working Group. N Engl J Med 1996; 334:341–348.
2. De Cosa B, et al. Overexpression of the Bt *cry2Aa2* operon in chloroplasts leads to formation of insecticidal crystals. Nat Biotechnol 2001; 19:71–74.
3. Johnston SA, et al. Genetic immunization: what's in a name? Arch Med Res 2002; 33:325–329.
4. Rappuoli R. Reverse vaccinology, a genome-based approach to vaccine development. Vaccine 2001; 19:2688–2691.
5. Pizza M, et al. Identification of vaccine candidates against serogroup B meningococcus by whole-genome sequencing. Science 2000; 287:1816–1820.
6. Chiang SL, et al. In vivo genetic analysis of bacterial virulence. Annu Rev Microbiol 1999; 53:129–154.
7. Sun YH, et al. Functional genomics of *Neisseria meningitidis* pathogenesis. Nat Med 2000; 6:1269–1273.

3

Initial Clinical Evaluation of New Vaccine Candidates: Investigators' Perspective of Phase I and Phase II Clinical Trials of Safety, Immunogenicity, and Preliminary Efficacy

Carol O. Tacket, Karen L. Kotloff, and Margaret B. Rennels
University of Maryland School of Medicine, Baltimore, Maryland, U.S.A.

I. INTRODUCTION

Among the tools available to control infectious diseases, vaccines rank high in effectiveness and economic feasibility. Vaccines once consisted of either live whole virus analogs or killed virus preparations. Now new viral, bacterial, and parasitic vaccines are frequently defined by gene sequences or amino acid epitopes. Likewise, vaccine testing has progressed to become a discipline of its own, which includes scientific, epidemiological, ethical, and feasibility aspects. This chapter deals with some of these issues related to Phases I and II vaccine testing.

II. SELECTION OF VACCINE CANDIDATES

Creative and innovative vaccine candidates emerge from research laboratories in academic institutions, government agencies, and private pharmaceutical and biotechnological companies all over the world. The decision to begin human testing of a candidate vaccine depends on a number of criteria.

First, the vaccine candidate must address a public health need and be a logical means of control for the disease of interest. For example, in the United States, outbreaks of *Cryptosporidium parvum* may be best prevented by improved water treatment rather than by vaccination. Similarly, infections with Shiga toxin producing *Escherichia coli* can be best prevented by improved meat inspection and consumer education about cooking practices, rather than by mass vaccination of children.

Second, the vaccine candidate must have been designed with a sound scientific rationale. There are two mirror-image principles commonly used to develop vaccines. On the one hand, the vaccine may consist of a known or suspected protective antigen, for example, purified hepatitis B surface antigen or *Hemophilus influenzae* type b polysac-

charide. Alternatively, the vaccine may be a live strain of a pathogen attenuated by genetic deletion of known virulence factors, for example, live oral cholera vaccine CVD 103-HgR.

Third, there must be an expectation of safety. The risk/benefit ratio for vaccines against most infectious diseases must be very low since such vaccines are designed for use in healthy individuals who may be at low risk of disease. In contrast, in the development of therapeutic agents, a larger risk may be acceptable since there is the opportunity for therapeutic benefit. Safety of the vaccine candidate, therefore, must be formally demonstrated in an appropriate animal model using a dose and route of administration which is proposed for clinical studies.

Fourth, there must be animal studies demonstrating the immunogenicity of the product when given in the appropriate dose and by the appropriate route and, if possible, a demonstration of efficacy against challenge with the wild-type pathogen in animals. Animal models to demonstrate immunogenicity and efficacy against challenge have been developed for a number of vaccines, e.g., cotton rats for respiratory syncytial virus and mice for *Salmonella*.

Fifth, it is desirable that the vaccine be prepared in a practical formulation at the onset of Phase I studies. This is not an absolute requirement since it is often necessary to first establish the safety and immunogenicity of a prototype vaccine in a preliminary formulation. However, changes in responses to vaccine can be observed when scale-up manufacturing is done or practical formulations are produced [1,2].

Finally, the last consideration is one of commercial development. In a free market, public health need and scientific rationale supporting the likelihood of success of a candidate vaccine will increase the chances that a new vaccine will attract the financial resources needed for its development to licensure and use as a public health tool.

III. GENERAL DESCRIPTION: PHASES OF CLINICAL TRIALS

The clinical investigation of a new candidate vaccine progresses in three phases. Although these phases are usually conducted sequentially, they may overlap. A Phase I trial is the first human use of the vaccine candidate in healthy volunteers. Participants in Phase I studies are typically closely monitored. These studies are designed to determine the frequently occurring, short-term side effects and the dose response to a candidate vaccine. In a Phase I vaccine study, the immune response to the vaccine is measured; the analogous information in a similar study of a drug would be its pharmacological characteristics in a small number of subjects. The information generated in Phase I about the vaccine's safety profile and immunogenicity should be sufficient to design expanded studies of safety and immunogenicity in Phase II.

Phase II studies are controlled, closely monitored studies of safety and immune response in an expanded number of subjects, perhaps several hundred. Some individuals who participate in Phase II studies may represent the target population for which the test vaccine is intended. For example, infants or elderly subjects may be enrolled if the vaccine candidate is intended for ultimate use in these populations. Multiple Phase II studies are often conducted to develop a database to direct the design of Phase III studies.

The development of a vaccine candidate can be accelerated if there is a human challenge model for the disease against which the vaccine is directed. This allows a preliminary assessment of vaccine efficacy (so-called Phase IIb) by comparing disease attack rates in vaccinees and unvaccinated control volunteers. These challenge studies can be ethically justified if they are conducted by qualified investigators with rigorous adherence to a scientifically valid protocol with clear safeguards for the volunteers [3,4]. It should be recognized that such challenge studies represent experimental models and may not exactly reproduce the disease as it occurs in an endemic area. For example, the inoculum used for challenge for diarrheal illnesses such as cholera and enterotoxigenic *E. coli* is probably higher than what occurs commonly in nature. This is to ensure that the attack rate among challenged volunteers is high enough to achieve statistical differences when comparing small numbers of vaccinated and unvaccinated individuals. However, the experimental challenge model is designed so that the challenge is not so rigorous as to overcome immunity; often the model has been tested by establishing that immunity induced by primary challenge-induced infection is not overwhelmed by a second challenge with the same pathogen [5]. This level of immunity, i.e., immunity after primary infection, is often the gold standard for immunity induced by vaccination. At the Center for Vaccine Development, University of Maryland, challenge models have been applied to testing vaccines against cholera, diarrheagenic *E. coli*, *Shigella*, Rocky Mountain spotted fever, malaria, influenza, and typhoid fever.

If acceptable safety and immunogenicity are observed during Phase II, Phase III studies are planned to evaluate efficacy. Generally, a Phase III study is a double-blind, controlled study of the new vaccine in a more heterogeneous population, under conditions more closely resembling those under which the vaccine may eventually be used. The study may include as a control group either a true placebo, a licensed vaccine against another disease, or another licensed or experimental vaccine against the same disease. In a Phase III study, the rate of occurrence of side effects that occur infrequently may be measured more accurately. Defined endpoints must be chosen and a hypothesis must be stated. A sample size should be chosen based on assumptions of the expected incidence of disease and the reduction in disease incidence that is anticipated in vaccinees. A pivotal study is a Phase III study which provides the most convincing data supporting the licensure of the vaccine. The pivotal protocol must be rigorously designed and analyzed with impeccable statistical considerations.

After Phase III studies demonstrating the safety and efficacy of the vaccine candidate, the sponsor of the vaccine who will market the product in the United States submits a Biologic Licensing Application (BLA) to the Food and Drug Administration (FDA). Approval requires that the safety and efficacy be demonstrated in well-designed, controlled studies. Once the application is approved, the vaccine may be sold commercially for the specific indication. After the BLA is approved, FDA requires that the holder of the BLA conduct postmarketing surveillance and submit periodic reports including incidence of adverse reactions and follow-up of ongoing Phase III studies. These data are generally descriptive in nature. After marketing approval, additional formal studies may also be designed to continue to measure efficacy and side effects. These studies, termed Phase IV studies, may detect previously unknown, rare adverse reactions among recipients of the marketed vaccine.

IV. FACILITIES

In general, facilities for vaccine testing include clinical office space for interviews for screening, obtaining consent, and conducting follow-up procedures, facilities for specimen collection and storage, and emergency equipment for treating anaphylactic reactions. The majority of studies can be conducted in an outpatient facility. In Phases I and II studies of vaccines, unlike drug studies, participants usually take only one to three doses of the experimental agent. Many early studies of new vaccines require that signs and symptoms be recorded for a relatively short period after vaccination and that a limited number of blood tests be obtained to measure immune response over a period of weeks to months.

The intensity of surveillance depends on the type of vaccine and the anticipated nature and incidence of side effects. Phase I studies of live vaccines in adults are usually conducted in an inpatient facility to collect preliminary safety data and to determine the excretion of vaccine and potential for person-to-person transmission. For example, the degree of attenuation of some live enteric vaccines is unknown; these must be given under close inpatient supervision [6,7]. Live vaccine studies may require frequent collection of stool samples or respiratory secretions for culture. In addition, for studies requiring very intense surveillance or frequent collection of specimens, inpatient studies may be required to ensure that every event (e.g., fever) is detected and recorded and to ensure compliance with collection of every specimen. For example, live oral *Salmonella enterica* serovar Typhi vaccine strain CVD 906 was found to be insufficiently attenuated and to cause symptoms of typhoid fever in some inpatient volunteers [8]. Concerns about the release of genetically engineered organisms into the environment before their preliminary safety and potential for person-to-person transmission have been established require that some studies be conducted on a closed isolation ward with strict contact isolation measures.

In the United States, the National Institute of Allergy and Infectious Diseases supports several Vaccine Treatment and Evaluation Units at academic institutions. Some of these centers have access to inpatient units where volunteers can be housed for intensive surveillance and specimen collection.

In studies of experimental vaccines in children and infants, surveillance for adverse effects and collection of specimens is carried out in an outpatient setting. Telephone interviews with parents or guardians, collection of questionnaires filled out by parents, and review of medical records are means utilized to collect safety information. Children return to the clinic or physician's office for blood drawing or collection of respiratory secretions. Collection of stools can be accomplished either by instructing the caretaker to bring in soiled diapers or by sending a messenger to the home. Day-care settings can be arranged for studies in which it is necessary to collect extensive clinical data or multiple specimens. The children are observed during the day by nursing staff, and they return home in the evening where the parents continue surveillance. This arrangement is sometimes optimal for Phase I studies of live, attenuated vaccines.

V. REGULATORY ISSUES

A. History of the Regulation of Vaccine Development

The ancient Egyptians and Hebrews had strict meat handling laws, and later, ancient Greeks and Romans had regulations prohibiting the addition of water to wine. In the Middle Ages, grocers and druggists had trade guilds which prohibited adulteration of drugs and spices. In the United States, there have been laws governing the size of a loaf of bread and prohibiting the adulteration of bread; in 1785, the first comprehensive food adulteration law was enacted in the United States.

In 1938, the Federal Food, Drug, and Cosmetic (FD&C) Act was enacted in response to a number of deaths caused by the use of diethylene glycol (antifreeze) as the vehicle for an elixir of sulfanilamide. This act required sponsors of Investigational New Drugs (IND) to submit safety data about the candidate product before premarket approval. The turning point for modern regulatory affairs was the passage in 1962 of the Kefauver–Harris Amend-

ments to the FD&C Act. The 1962 amendments required that efficacy data, as well as safety data, be submitted to support IND applications. These amendments followed shortly after the discovery that thalidomide caused birth defects. Although thalidomide was never approved in the United States, it was being used extensively in research. Before the 1962 amendments, there was no requirement that FDA be notified of the use of investigational drugs or regulate their use. Today, sponsors of new vaccines must submit both safety and effectiveness data to support the application. Since these data are gathered through clinical investigations, all sponsors must prepare an IND application and follow a set of principles known as Good Clinical Practice (GCP).

In the United States, when Congress passes a law, the regulatory agency involved writes the regulation and is responsible for enforcing the law. The Code of Federal Regulations (CFR) contains these regulations. Title 21 of the CFR deals with food and drugs, and Title 45 Part 46 deals with protection of human subjects. These regulations give specific directions for all individuals—sponsors, monitors, and investigators—involved in a vaccine trial. The following parts of Title 21 are relevant to clinical investigations of vaccines:

> Part 50 (informed consent).
> Part 56 [Institutional Review Boards (IRBs)].
> Part 312 (Investigational New Drug applications).
> Part 601 (licensing).
> Part 814 (premarket approvals).

B. Good Clinical Practice

Good Clinical Practice is the set of federal regulations and guidelines for clinical trials which will support an eventual application for licensure of a new vaccine or drug. Good Clinical Practice is designed to ensure the quality and integrity of clinical data and to protect the rights and safety of volunteers. Good Clinical Practice guidelines are described in detail in numerous internet sites from various agencies, including the U.S. Department of Health and Human Services Office for Human Research Protection (OHRP), U.S. Food and Drug Administration (FDA), U.S. Army, U.S. Centers for Disease Control and Prevention, the International Conference on Harmonization (IHC), and others. These websites are listed in Table 1. These regulations are comprehensive, including protocol design and development, informed consent guidelines, record keeping, data reporting, adverse event reporting, etc.

C. Elements of an Investigational New Drug Application

The components of an IND application are described in 21 CFR Part 312. An IND is filed for a vaccine that has never been approved in the United States, for a new dose, route, or schedule of administration of an approved vaccine, or for a new indication of an approved vaccine. The application includes a completed and signed form FDA 1571, which is

Table 1 Useful Internet Sites

Organizations
National Institutes of Health (NIH)
   http://www.nih.gov/
DHHS Office for Human Research Protections (OHRP)
   http://ohrp.osophs.dhhs.gov/polasur.htm
U.S. Food and Drug Administration (FDA)
   http://www.fda.gov/default.htm
FDA Information for Health Professionals
   http://www.fda.gov/oc/oha/default.htm
FDA Center for Biologics Evaluation and Research (CBER) Regulatory Page
   http://www.fda.gov/cber/index.html
International Conference on Harmonization of Technical Requirements
      for Registration of Pharmaceuticals for Human Use (ICH) Topics and Guidelines
   http://www.ifpma.org/ich1.html
U.S. Army Medical Research and Materiel Command HomePage Human
      Subjects Protection and Regulatory Divisions-Regulatory Compliance and Quality
   http://mrmc-www.army.mil/
Centers for Disease Control and Prevention Human Subjects Requirements
   http://www.cdc.gov/od/ads/hsr2.htm
European Forum for Good Clinical Practice
   http://www.efgcp.org
Protection of Human Subjects
Belmont Report
   http://www.fda.gov/oc/ohrt/irbs/belmont.html
Declaration of Helsinki
   http://www.wma.net/e/approvedhelsinki.html
45CFR46-Human Subjects Protection
   http://ohrp.osophs.dhhs.gov/humansubjects/guidance/45cfr46.htm
NIH Policy and Guidelines on the Inclusion of Children as Participants
      in Research Involving Human Subjects
   http://ohrp.osophs.dhhs.gov/humansubjects/guidance/hsdc98-03.htm
National Institutes of Health (NIH) Guidelines on the Inclusion of Women
      and Minorities as Subjects in Clinical Research
   http://ohrp.osophs.dhhs.gov/humansubjects/guidance/hsdc94-01.htm
FDA Information Sheets: Guidance for Institutional Review Boards and
      Clinical Investigators
   http://www.fda/gov/oc/oha/IRB/toc.html
Clinical Research
FDA Good Clinical Practice (ICH E6)
   http://www.fda.gov/cder/guidance/959fnl.pdf
CBER Guidances/Guidelines/Points to Consider
   http://www.fda.gov/cber/guidelines.htm
FDA Investigational New Drug Application (IND)
21CFR312-Investigational New Drug Application
   http://www.fda.gov/cber/ind.htm

a master administrative document with a table of contents that serves as a check list for the elements of the application. The signature of the sponsor indicates that that sponsor agrees to conduct the investigation in accordance with all applicable regulatory requirements, specifically, to wait 30 days after the FDA receives the IND before beginning the study, not to conduct the study if the study is placed on clinical hold, and that an Institutional Review Board (IRB) will review and approve the study.

After the form 1571, there is an introductory statement about the vaccine's characteristics, a general investigational plan, an investigator's brochure, and the clinical protocol. Form FDA 1572 and the curricula vitae of the investigators are included. The form 1572 is a contract between the clinical investigator and the federal government to assure one's compliance with 21 CFR 312, involving adherence to protocol, use of informed consent, record keeping, reporting, etc. Next are sections on chemistry, manufacturing and control information, pharmacology and toxicology information, and previous human experience. As the development of the vaccine progresses, the IND application is supplemented with protocol amendments, new protocols, new investigators, safety reports, information about microbiology or toxicology, and annual reports.

D. Obligations of Sponsors

The sponsor of a clinical investigation is the person who has assumed responsibility for compliance with the FD&C Act and FDA regulations and guidelines. The sponsor submits and maintains the IND application. Not until the IND has been prepared can the investigational product be shipped for the purpose of conducting clinical trials. A sponsor who both initiates and conducts a clinical investigation is called a "sponsor-investigator." The specific legal responsibilities of the sponsor, contained in 21 CFR, include selecting investigators, providing adequate information to investigators, monitoring investigations, ensuring compliance with proper IND procedures, and informing FDA and the investigators of any adverse effects or risks of the product being studied. Sponsors may transfer all or part of their obligations to a contract research organization.

E. Obligations of Monitors

The monitor of a clinical investigation confirms that the study is conducted according to the protocol developed by the investigator and sponsor and according to the FDA regulations. This is accomplished by meeting with the investigator and the research staff before a study begins and confirming the adequacy of the investigator's facilities. The monitor makes periodic reviews of the investigator's source documents, case report forms, and required reports. Problems with the study must be documented and corrective actions must be taken.

F. Obligations of Investigators

Similarly, an investigator's responsibilities are contained in the FDA regulations. An investigator's agreement to conduct an investigation in accordance with regulations and with the clinical protocol is documented when the investigator signs a form FDA 1572 which is filed with the IND application. In summary, the investigator must obtain IRB approval for the protocol, the consent document, and recruiting materials used to identify volunteers. The investigator must obtain approval for study amendments and file regular reports with the IRB. The investigator must keep immaculate records and must report serious and unexpected adverse events to the sponsor and the IRB. The investigator must administer the vaccine and maintain records accounting for the product disposition. The investigator is responsible for educating the volunteers and obtaining written informed consent before volunteers become involved in the study. The investigator is obligated to store records and allow FDA representatives to inspect the study records.

In 2000, the U.S. National Institutes of Health (NIH) issued a directive requiring that federally funded clinical researchers provide evidence of training on the protection of human research participants and on Good Clinical Practice. An online tutorial for NIH intramural investigators was offered as an example (http://ohsr.od.nih.gov).

G. Institutional Review Boards

An Institutional Review Board is a group designated by an institution to review and approve biomedical research involving humans. IRBs are responsible for the well being of subjects involved in clinical trials. The board includes at least five members, at least one who is not a scientist and one who is not affiliated with the institution. The IRB reviews protocols, investigator's brochures, consent forms, recruiting materials, and additional safety information. The membership of an IRB, standard operating procedures, review of research, voting, and quorums are defined in Part 56 of 21 CFR.

H. Record Keeping and Product Accountability for Clinical Trials

Compulsive record keeping is an important component of Good Clinical Practice. Recently, the need for privacy and protection of medical records has led to new regulations under the Health Insurance Portability and Accountability Act of 1996. Under these new complex regulations, restraints on the use of medical information for research were imposed in 2003. The new privacy rules are under debate as regulators attempt to balance the public interest in research with the public interest in privacy [9,10].

Both investigators and sponsors should retain the same records. Case report forms are uniform at all the sites conducting the study and allow the sponsor to look at the same information in the same format from different sites. The case report forms may be used for data entry and analysis and should be designed to efficiently capture the data points that precisely correspond to the aims and endpoints of the protocol. "Source documents," those records on which the information about a participant is first recorded, may be used for some studies. The type of information to be collected may vary with the protocol, but, in general, it would include subject identification, protocol name and number, sponsor's name, date of participant's visit, procedures and tests completed, concomitant medications, occurrence of adverse experiences, and the name of the person entering the information and the date. Corrections to the study records must be initialed and dated.

In 1997, the U.S. FDA established regulations about the use of electronic records in clinical trials (21 CFR Part 11). The regulations permit use of electronic signatures. Investigators now have the option of maintaining records as paper or electronic files. The electronic record must provide an audit trail, i.e., a record of who enters or changes data and when [11]. Teleforms for electronic database entry and on-line case report forms are likely to replace paper forms in the future. The FDA guidelines can be found at http://www.fda.gov/ora/compliance_ref/part11/.

Investigators usually develop a protocol-specific quality management plan to ensure the correctness of the data collected. A sponsor should have a policy about monitoring case report forms which indicates how frequently forms are to be monitored and how intensively. Monitors compare source documents with case report forms, looking for inconsistencies, errors, and appropriate signatures.

In addition to maintaining clinical records, investigators are required to maintain records for the receipt and disposition of all the experimental product. The records should include the name of the material, its IND number, its condition, the lot number, date, and source. Records should show the name of persons who received the study vaccine and what was done with extra doses. Each dose must be accounted for. To assure that the experimental product is not tampered with, vaccine materials should be stored in a secure refrigerator, freezer, or cabinet.

I. Reporting Adverse Experiences

The NIH has recently developed policies for safety monitoring of all studies that evaluate investigational drugs and biologics. This policy on Data and Safety Monitoring can be found at http://grants.nih.gov/grants/guide/notice-files/ not98-084.html released in 1998 and Further Guidance on Data and Safety Monitoring for Phase I and Phase II Trials issued in 2000 at http://grants.nih.gov/grants/guide/notice-files/NOT-OD-00-038.html. These policies require that there is a system for oversight and monitoring of clinical trials. The mechanism of oversight depends on the risk and complexity of the trial and may be a full Data and Safety Monitoring Board, a safety committee, or an individual independent safety monitor.

Food and Drug Administration regulations require investigators to report all adverse experiences to the sponsor of a study. If the experience is serious or unexpected, the event must be reported promptly to both the sponsor and responsible IRB. A serious adverse experience is "any experience that is fatal or life-threatening, is permanently disabling, requires or extends inpatient hospitalization, or is a congenital anomaly, cancer, or overdose." An unexpected adverse experience is "any adverse experience that is not identified in nature, severity, or frequency in the current investigator brochure; or, if an investigator brochure is not required, that is not identified in nature, severity, or frequency in the risk information described in the general investigational plan or elsewhere in the current application" (21 CFR 312.32). As a general rule, many sponsors require investigators to report all adverse experiences even if the event is not apparently related to the vaccine. The investigator must keep a record to indicate the treatment and outcome of the adverse experience.

J. Regulatory Considerations in International Trials

International trials are of particular significance in vaccine development, in which the ultimate target population may be individuals in a country other than that in which the vaccine was manufactured. Such trials may reveal differences in safety, immunogenicity, and efficacy when the vaccine is studied in a new population. For example, a live oral cholera vaccine was less immunogenic when given to Thai adults than to U.S. adults [1], and oral polio vaccine was less immunogenic in children in a developing country [12]. The experimental vaccine may or may not be studied under U.S. IND. If not, the vaccine must be manufactured outside the United States. Several provisions must be met for the U.S. FDA to accept data from an international trial. These include the following: (i) the data must be applicable to U.S. populations; (ii) international investigators must be competent; (iii) the protocol must be reviewed for ethical considerations; and (iv) the site must be available for FDA inspection.

In studies in foreign countries, the same standards that apply to studies in the United States should be used [13]. The research should be developed in close collaboration with local investigators and other authorities in the country in which it will be performed [14]. The FDA does not require that case report forms or source documents be completed in English, but a translator may be required if the site or records are inspected. Local customs may affect several aspects of the trial, such as the means of obtaining and documenting informed consent and the recognition and reporting of the types of experiences that are considered adverse events.

VI. PROTOCOL DEVELOPMENT

A. General Considerations

The success of a vaccine trial in Phase I or Phase II is largely predicted by the quality of the protocol. According to the CFR, a protocol must contain the following components: (i) a statement of the purpose and objectives of the study; (ii) the name and address of the investigator, the name and address of the research facilities, and the name and address of the reviewing IRB; (iii) a statement of the number of participants and the inclusion and exclusion criteria for participating; (iv) the study design, including the type of control group, if any; (v) the dose to be given and the method for determining the dose; (vi) a description of the outcomes to be measured; (vii) a description of the measures to be taken to monitor the participants and to reduce risks.

In addition, many protocols contain a discussion of the scientific background and rationale to place the study in context. It is important to include information about the disease, its clinical nature and epidemiological importance, and whatever is known about the elements of protective immunity. This is useful in justifying the need for the study and risk to volunteers.

The type of study, e.g., controlled, double- or single-blinded, and the method of randomization, if any, should be included. Outcomes to be observed need to be clearly described; objective definitions of outcomes are highly desirable. Definitions of safety (e.g., degree of temperature that defines fever) and immunogenicity (e.g., definition of sero-conversion) need to be clearly decided and documented during protocol development. A justification for the dosage should be provided. The means of monitoring patients and contingencies for handling side effects should be described.

Protocols include a section describing the statistical tests to be used to analyze the results and a section to justify the sample size chosen. In Phase I studies, however, it is not always possible to detect statistically significant differences between groups because of the small numbers of participants.

B. Considerations for Studies Involving Children and Infants

In designing a protocol to be carried out in children, additional considerations are required. In 1998, NIH issued a Policy and Guidelines on the Inclusion of Children as Participants in Research Involving Human Subjects, providing guidance on inclusion of children and justification for exclusion of children in research funded by NIH. In considering the inclusion of children in vaccine studies, the first decision to be addressed is the age group to be vaccinated. The answer depends upon the age at which children are at risk for the infection the vaccine is designed to prevent. For most pathogens, it is optimal to provide protection as early in life as possible. However, the presence of small amounts of maternal neutralizing antibody may inactivate some live viral vaccines, such as measles vaccine, requiring that immunization be postponed to a later age. Usually, pediatric vaccine development proceeds in older children and progresses stepwise to younger children until the target age group is reached.

Early infancy is a time when children receive multiple routine vaccinations. An important issue is whether or not to give an experimental vaccine at the same visit with licensed vaccines. Frequently, Phase I studies will dictate a 4-week separation between the study vaccine and any other vaccinations to avoid either confounding the safety data or inducing immune interference with simultaneously administered vaccines. To be logistically practical and economically feasible, new vaccines should eventually be incorporated into the routine vaccination schedule of infancy. Therefore the effects on safety and immunogenicity of concurrent immunization should be evaluated in Phase II studies. The number of doses of vaccine to be administered must also be determined. Two or more doses are often necessary to overcome maternal antibody or to induce priming. This issue is most commonly addressed by giving two or three doses and measuring antibody levels before and after each immunization. The necessity, practicality, and ethics of including a placebo group should also be carefully weighed.

In designing a protocol for pediatric studies, one must carefully balance the need to be minimally invasive but to collect all necessary data. This sometimes requires compromises. The most difficult aspect of carrying out a successful pediatric vaccine trial is the recruitment of sufficient numbers of children. Parents are protective of their children and will refuse to enroll their child or continue to participate in a study that they perceive is too invasive or requires undue discomfort for their child. The number of times that specimens are sampled, therefore, should be kept to a minimum.

C. Considerations for Vaccines Prepared by Recombinant DNA Technology or Containing Recombinant DNA

The development of attenuated viral and bacterial strains for use as vaccines was one of the obvious applications of the techniques for recombining DNA discovered in the 1970s. Before this time, live viral [15] and bacterial [16] vaccine strains were developed by repeated in vitro passage or by chemical mutagenesis, techniques that resulted in undefined mutations. Nevertheless, live vaccines against diseases such as measles, mumps, rubella, and typhoid fever were developed and licensed. Recombinant DNA technology offered the means to develop attenuated vaccines in which the precise molecular mechanism of attenuation could be known.

Despite the precision of molecular DNA techniques, vaccines developed using recombinant DNA were thought by some to be threatening to the natural environment. To document the potential for environmental consequences of vaccinating humans with such vaccines, sponsors are required to include an environmental analysis (21 CFR 312.23) which includes justification for a claim for categorical exclusion or an environmental assessment. Such justification might include data showing the survivability of the vaccine strain in various natural environments such as local water, soil, and food, especially in comparison with the wild-type pathogen [17]. Phase I protocols to study the safety of recombinant vaccines generally contain provisions for studying the potential for person-to-person transmission of these strains.

D. Considerations for Vaccines that Can Be Transmitted Person-to-Person

Many of the currently used live bacterial and viral vaccines are shed in respiratory secretions (e.g., live attenuated influenza vaccine) or stool (e.g., polio vaccine) and are potentially transmitted person to person [18]. Transmission of oral polio vaccine was considered desirable in the early years of its use since such transmission led to herd immunity [19]. Transmission to pregnant women or immunocompromised individuals is now recognized as a risk of the use of live vaccines which can be spread from person to person, e.g., transmission of vaccinia virus or its recombinant virus to an individual with eczema can result in severe vaccinia infection [20].

As a result of this concern, many Phase I and Phase II clinical protocols include preliminary measurements of the potential for person-to-person spread of live vaccine candidates. Initially, this may require that the vaccine strain be studied in isolation until a gross assessment of its transmissibility is established, for example, among unvaccinated adults residing with vaccinees on a research isolation ward. Examples of such studies to assess person-to-person transmission include studies of *Salmonella typhi* vaccine strain CVD 908-*htr*A [21] and of a recombinant vaccinia virus expressing gp160 of HIV [22]. In Phase II, volunteers who reside with infants, pregnant women, or immunocompromised individuals may be excluded because of the possibility of transmission of a vaccine strain whose safety is not completely established. Phase II studies of transmissibility might include cultures of the stool or respiratory secretions of household contacts of vaccinees and, in later phases, attempts at vaccine isolation from environmental reservoirs such as sewage.

The testing of live oral cholera vaccine strain CVD 103-HgR (Mutacol®, Orochol®, Berna Biotech) is a good example of how such testing is executed. This *V. cholerae*

O1 strain is deleted in 94% of the toxic A subunit of cholera toxin [23]. In Phase II clinical studies, the possibility of transmission of this strain to contacts of vaccinees and to the environment around the households of vaccinees was investigated [24,25]. In brief, this strain was shed for a short period by only a small proportion of vaccinees, was minimally transmitted to contacts of vaccinees, and was not recovered from the natural environment near vaccinees.

VII. SELECTION OF VOLUNTEERS

A. General Considerations

Initial Phase I studies of candidate vaccines generally involve healthy adult volunteers, i.e., those who have no abnormality that would confound the interpretation of the safety of the product or increase the likelihood of their having an adverse event. Healthy volunteers may be recruited from the community at large or from interested students or employees at research institutions. Students and employees can be a vulnerable population, however, and care must be taken to ensure that there is no element of pressure or coercion to participate. In addition, some protocols may have a seroeligibility requirement, usually the absence of serum antibody to a particular antigen. Rarely, a protocol may specify that only individuals of a certain HLA type may participate, when preclinical data indicate that immune responses will be restricted to a certain genotype [26]. The protocol generally indicates what tests must be performed to establish the volunteers' health. For example, some or all of the following may be done: medical history, physical examination, complete blood count, serum chemistries, urinalysis, HIV serology, and pregnancy test. Formerly, women of childbearing potential were sometimes precluded from participation. However, in 1993, Guidelines for the Study and Evaluation of Gender Differences in the Clinical Evaluation of Drugs were issued stating that women be included provided that appropriate precautions against becoming pregnant are taken and that women are counseled about the importance of these precautions. Efforts should be made to ensure that women participants are not pregnant at the time of enrollment and that women are informed about animal reproduction studies and teratogenic potential of the vaccine. Generally, however, such data are not available for experimental vaccines. In 2000, NIH issued Guidelines on the Inclusion of Women and Minorities as Subjects in Clinical Research http://grants.nih.gov/grants/funding/women_min/guidelines_update.htm). In 2001, the U.S. Department of Health and Human Services released additional protections pertaining to research in pregnant women http://ohrp.osophs.dhhs.gov/humansubjects/guidance/45cfr46.htm). In these additional regulations, there must be direct benefit to the woman or fetus as a result of the research or there must be only minimal risk to the fetus, and the new information learned in the research cannot be obtained in any other way.

Phase II vaccine studies also involve healthy adults. Once preliminary safety has been established in the Phase I study, the screening to demonstrate the health of volunteers may be less rigorous. For example, the following may be done: medical history, complete blood count, HIV serology, and pregnancy test.

B. Considerations for Studies Involving Children and Infants

Pediatric vaccine trials are carried out in healthy children who have no personal or family history of immune deficiency. The exception to this would be a vaccine targeted for a particular population, such as a *Pseudomonas* vaccine for children with cystic fibrosis. Screening of healthy children generally involves only medical history and physical examination. Specific baseline data may be collected if there is specific concern about the potential vaccine side effects; for example, liver function tests are performed if a live viral vaccine might cause hepatitis.

Transmission of live viral vaccine strains to contacts through the stools or respiratory secretions is a particular concern in studies involving young children. Until it is demonstrated that the vaccine virus is not transmitted, initial live viral vaccine studies should not include children attending group day care or children residing in a household with an immunosuppressed individual.

Recruitment of children into vaccine trials is usually carried out through outpatient settings providing well child care, such as private practices, hospital clinics, and health maintenance organizations. The optimal method of approaching families varies depending upon the population served and the setting. In many centers, a study nurse and/or investigator approach the parent or guardian on the day they wish to enroll the child. Sending literature to the parents before the vaccine visit provides an important opportunity for the family to discuss the study and to contact the study personnel by telephone for further information before they must make the decision whether or not to participate.

VIII. CONSENT

A. General Considerations

The FDA regulations concerning informed consent are contained in 21 CFR Part 50. Consent is not an endpoint but a continuing communication between participant and investigator during which the participant receives all the information needed to participate in the study. The process should include ample opportunities for the free exchange of information and for the participant to ask questions. Consent should be obtained under circumstances that give the potential participant the opportunity to carefully consider the decision to participate with no coercion or undue influence. Such features as the place, the time, and the person who provides the information may affect a subject's ability to make an informed judgment.

The principles of informed consent include the following: (i) the purposes, procedures, and experimental nature of the protocol are described fairly; (ii) the discomforts and risks to be expected are described; (iii) information about appropriate alternative procedures (for vaccine studies, this might be information about the existence of a licensed vaccine for the same disease); (iv) information about whom to ask for further information; and (v) the statement that an individual is free to withdraw his consent and discontinue participation without prejudice.

It is important that the information provided be understandable to the participants. This means that the information must be presented in the participant's language and that technical and medical terms must be explained or replaced with lay terms appropriate to the participant's level of education. Often a consent form can be simplified by using short, declarative sentences. In addition, the consent document should not include statements that release the investigator from responsibility or that waive the volunteer's rights. Consent must be documented in writing.

The FDA requires that the IRB review and approve the advertisements and other materials used to recruit participants. Recruiting materials are considered an extension of the consent process. These materials, such as advertisements and fliers, should not be misleading. The FDA recommends that the advertisement include only the following: (i) name and address of the investigator; (ii) purpose of the research and a summary of eligibility criteria; (iii) a description of the benefits (including payment); and (iv) the location of the research and person to contact for more information (FDA Information Sheet, "Advertising for Study Subjects," February 1989). It is important to avoid making claims about the vaccine.

It is also important that the payment of volunteers not be so much as to affect the ability of the volunteer to assess risks and benefits appropriately. Few research groups or organizations have specific standards [27–29]. Volunteer compensation scales should be carefully conceived to ensure that economically disadvantaged individuals are not unduly influenced by the financial compensation offered. This concern applies not only to economically disadvantaged individuals, but students and middle class populations as well. Dickert and Grady [30] describe three approaches related to volunteer payments. The first approach is the Market Model, which is grounded in the free-market principle that supply (availability of interested and eligible volunteers) and demand (the investigator's desire to complete a trial with a specified number of subjects within a defined time frame) determine how much subjects should be paid for participation. A second model is the Reimbursement Model, in which payment is provided simply to cover volunteers' expenses (travel, meals, parking, child care), similar to jury duty payments, such that the volunteers accrue no profit, thereby minimizing financial inducement. The third and most accepted model is the Wage Payment Model. This model purports that participating in research is similar to many other forms of unskilled labor in that it requires little skill and training but may involve some risk. In this model, subjects are paid for work that is valuable to society, based on a standard wage for unskilled labor. In general, volunteers should have characteristics that make them suitable for other jobs in the community, particularly entry-level jobs, to ensure that the decision to participate in research is truly optional.

Investigators who have conflicts of interest should make these known to volunteers in the consent form. A conflict of interest exists when an investigator has financial or personal

relationships that inappropriately influence the investigator's actions or judgment [31].

B. Considerations for Studies Involving Children and Infants

Children are not empowered to grant informed consent until they have reached the legal age of majority or have been deemed emancipated. The degree of involvement of a child in the decision to participate in a vaccine trial depends upon the child's intellectual capacity and stage of development. Assent to participate usually should be obtained from children with an intellectual age of 7 years. In trials involving children, a parent or guardian assumes responsibility for the child and grants consent by proxy. This places an increased responsibility on the sponsor, the investigator, and the IRB to assure that risk is minimized, the study is fully understood by the parent, and that there is no coercion to participate. It is essential that the parent understands that participation is entirely voluntary and that the parent may withdraw the child from the study at any time. An investigator who also serves as the child's primary care physician has the additional burden to assure that the parent does not feel compelled to enroll the children to please the physician.

Remuneration for participation is a more sensitive issue in trials involving children than adults. Rewards must be only a token of appreciation and not of a magnitude to induce parents to enroll the child into the study. Generally acceptable compensation includes a small savings bond, free routine vaccinations, or payment for costs incurred by the trial, such as travel.

IX. SUMMARY

Vaccine testing enters the twenty-first century using methods based on sound epidemiological and ethical principles by which the safety and efficacy of future vaccines will be established. Although vaccine development may be an empirical science, the methodological framework for clinical testing to determine safety and efficacy has been largely codified. Precedents have been set for the study of vaccines containing recombinant DNA and for methods to study the transmissibility of live vaccines. We anticipate that clinical vaccine testing will continue to be a productive and exciting area of clinical research as vaccines against infectious diseases, such as malaria, tuberculosis, HIV, and agents of bioterror, are developed.

REFERENCES

1. Su-Arehawaratana P, Singharaj P, Taylor DN, Hoge C, Trofa A, Kuvanont K, Migasena S, Pitisuttitham P, Lim YL, Losonsky G, Kaper JB, Wasserman SS, Cryz S, Echeverria P, Levine MM. Safety and immunogenicity of different immunization regimens of CVD 103-HgR live oral cholera vaccine in soldiers and civilians in Thailand. J Infect Dis 1992; 165:1042–1048.
2. Levine MM, DuPont HL, Hornick RB, Snyder MJ, Woodward W, Gilman RH, Libonati JP. Attenuated, streptomycin-dependent *Salmonella typhi* oral vaccine: potential

deleterious effects of lyophilization. J Infect Dis 1976; 133: 424–429.

3. Miller FG, Grady C. The ethical challenge of infection-inducing challenge experiments. Clin Infect Dis 2001; 33:1028–1033.

4. Rosenbaum JR, Sepkowitz KA. Infectious disease experimentation involving human volunteers. Clin Infect Dis 2002; 34:963–971.

5. Kotloff KL, Nataro JP, Losonsky GA, Wasserman SS, Hale TL, Taylor DN, Sadoff JC, Levine MM. A modified *Shigella* volunteer challenge model in which the inoculum is administered with bicarbonate buffer: clinical experience and implications for *Shigella* infectivity. Vaccine 1995; 13:1488–1494.

6. Levine MM, Kaper JB, Herrington D, Ketley J, Losonsky G, Tacket CO, Tall B, Cryz S. Safety, immunogenicity and efficacy of recombinant live oral cholera vaccines, CVD 103 and CVD 103-HgR. Lancet 1988; ii:467–470.

7. Hohmann EL, Oletta CA, Killeen KP, Miller SI. *phoP/phoQ*-deleted *Salmonella typhi* (Ty800) is a safe and immunogenic single dose typhoid fever vaccine in human volunteers. J Infect Dis 1996; 173:1408–1414.

8. Hone DM, Tacket CO, Harris A, Bay B, Losonsky G, Levine MM. Evaluation of a double *aro* mutant of *Salmonella typhi* ISP1820 in volunteers and in U937 human macrophage-like cells. J Clin Invest 1992; 90:412–420.

9. Kulynych J, Korn D. The effect of the new federal medical-privacy rule on research. N Engl J Med 2002; 346:201–204.

10. Annas GJ. Medical privacy and medical research-judging the new federal regulations. N Engl J Med 2002; 346:216–220.

11. DeMarinis AJ, Tandy MK. 21 CFR Part 11: electronic records and signatures—the shock of it! Res Pract 2000; 1:157–182.

12. Patriarca PA, Wright PF, John TJ. Factors affecting the immunogenicity of oral poliovirus vaccine in developing countries: review. Rev Infect Dis 1991; 13:926–939.

13. Shapiro HT, Meslin EM. Ethical issues in the design and conduct of clinical trials in developing countries. N Engl J Med 2001; 345:139–142.

14. Varmus H, Satcher D. Ethical complexities of conducting research in developing countries. N Engl J Med 1997; 337: 1003–1005.

15. Lavergne B, Frappier-Davignon L, Quevillon M, Hours C. Clinical trial of Trivirix for measles, mumps, and rubella immunization. Can Dis Wkly Rep 1986; 12:85–88.

16. Germanier R, Furёr E. Isolation and characterization of *galE* mutant Ty21a of *Salmonella typhi*: a candidate strain for a live oral typhoid vaccine. J Infect Dis 1975; 141:553–558.

17. Cryz SJ Jr, Kaper J, Tacket C, Nataro J, Levine MM. *Vibrio cholerae* CVD 103-HgR live oral attenuated vaccine: construction, safety, immunogenicity, excretion and non-target effects. In: Non-Target Effects of Live Vaccines. Vol 84. Dev Biol Stand, Karger, 1995:237–244.

18. Levine MM. Non-target effects of live vaccines: myth, reality and demagoguery. Non-Target Effects of Live Vaccines. Vol. 84. Dev Biol Stand, Karger, 1995:33–38.

19. Sabin AB. Oral poliovirus vaccine: history of its development and prospects for eradication of poliomyelitis. J Am Med Assoc 1965; 194:130–134.

20. Lane JM, Ruben FL, Neff JM, Millar JD. Complications of smallpox vaccination, 1968. N Engl J Med 1969; 281:1201–1208.

21. Tacket CO, Sztein MB, Losonsky GA, Wasserman SS, Nataro JP, Edelman R, Galen JE, Pickard D, Dougan G, Chatfield SN, Levine MM. Safety and immune response in humans of live oral *Salmonella typhi* vaccine strains deleted in *htrA* and *aroC aroD*. Infect Immun 1997; 65:452–456.

22. Cooney EL, Collier AC, Greenberg PD, Coombs RW, Zarling J, Arditti DE, Hoffman MC, Hu S-L, Corey L. Safety of and immunological response to a recombinant vaccinia virus vaccine expressing HIV envelope glycoprotein. Lancet 1991; 337: 567–572.

23. Kaper JB, Lockman H, Baldini MM, Levine MM. Recombinant nontoxinogenic *Vibrio cholerae* strains as attenuated cholera vaccine candidates. Nature 1984; 308:655–658.

24. Simanjuntak CH, O'Hanley P, Punjabi NH, Noriega F, Pazzaglia G, Dykstra P, Kay B, Suharyono, Budiarsno A, Rifai A, Wasserman SS, Losonsky GA, Kaper J, Cryz S, Levine MM. The safety, immunogenicity and transmissibility of single-dose live oral cholera vaccine CVD 103-HgR in 24 to 59 month old Indonesian children. J Infect Dis 1993; 168: 1169–1176.

25. Gotuzzo E, Butron B, Seas C, Penny M, Ruiz R, Losonsky G, Lanata CF, Wasserman SS, Salazar E, Kaper JB, Cryz S, Levine MM. Safety, immunogenicity, and excretion pattern of single-dose live oral cholera vaccine CVD 103-HgR in Peruvian adults of high and low socioeconomic levels. Infect Immun 1993; 61:3994–3997.

26. Hart MK, Weinhold KJ, Scearce RM, Washburn EM, Clark CA, Palker TJ, Haynes BF. Priming of anti-human immunodeficiency virus (HIV) CD8 + cytotoxic T cells in vivo by carrier-free HIV synthetic peptides. Proc Natl Acad Sci USA 1991; 88:9448–9452.

27. Dickert N, Ezekiel E, Grady C. Paying research subjects: an analysis of current policies. Ann Intern Med 2002; 136:368–373.

28. Newton L. Inducement, due and otherwise. IRB 1982; 4:4–6.

29. Macklin R. On paying money to research subjects. IRB 1981; 3.

30. Dickert N, Grady C. What's the price of a research subject? Approaches to payment for research participation. N Engl J Med 1999; 341, 198–203.

31. Davidoff F, DeAngelis CD, Drazen JM, Hoey J, Højgaard L, Horton R, Kotzin S, Nicholls MG, Nylenna M, Overbeke AJPM, Sox HC, van der Weyden MB, Wilkes MS. Sponsorship, authorship, and accountability. N Engl J Med 2001; 345:825–827.

4

Long-Term Evaluation of Vaccine Protection: Methodological Issues for Phase III and Phase IV Studies

John D. Clemens
International Vaccine Institute, Seoul, South Korea, and National Institute of Child Health and Human Development, National Institutes of Health, Bethesda, Maryland, U.S.A.

Abdollah Naficy and Malla R. Rao
National Institute of Allergy and Infectious Disease, National Institutes of Health, Bethesda, Maryland, U.S.A.

Hye-won Koo
International Vaccine Institute, Seoul, South Korea

Remarkable advances in biotechnology have enabled the rapid identification of antigens that elicit protective immune responses against infectious agents and are promising candidates as human vaccines. The profusion of new candidate vaccines has itself created challenges for the proper evaluation of these agents. Rigorous and meticulous scientific evaluations are required before the introduction of a vaccine into public health practice. In this chapter, we provide an overview of several methodological considerations which are relevant to field evaluations of the clinical protection conferred by vaccine candidates that have proved suitably safe and immunogenic in earlier animal and human studies.

I. TYPES OF EVALUATIONS

Evaluations of the protection conferred by vaccines against clinical infections occur both before and after vaccine licensure. Before licensure, vaccines are conventionally tested in an orderly sequence of "phases." In the Code of Federal Regulations, the phases of clinical trials are described by using Arabic numerals (Phase 1, Phase 2, Phase 3), whereas in World Health Organization publications Roman numeration is generally used (e.g., Phase I, Phase II, Phase III). Because of the international dissemination of this book, in this chapter we will utilize the latter. Phase I and II studies

evaluate the safety, immunogenicity, and transmissibility of vaccine candidates in relatively small numbers of subjects. For the relatively few diseases in which volunteer challenge models have been established, such as cholera, Phase II studies may also evaluate the protection conferred by vaccination against an experimental challenge of volunteers with the target pathogen. For vaccines found to be suitably safe and immunogenic in Phase I–II studies, Phase III studies are conducted to provide rigorous evidence about vaccine efficacy. Phase III studies are constructed as experiments with clear hypotheses and are conducted in a population that normally experiences the disease against which the vaccine is targeted.

After licensure, clinical protection may be monitored in several ways with Phase IV studies. Sometimes protection is assessed by evaluating postimmunization immune responses to vaccines administered in routine practice. When such studies are conducted in an area endemic for the target infection for the vaccine, it is necessary to evaluate immune responses in both vaccinees and nonvaccinees, so that immune responses attributable to vaccination can be distinguished from responses to natural infections. Examples of such studies include measurement of serum hemagglutination inhibition antibodies after measles vaccination and assessments of cutaneous delayed hypersensitivity to tuberculin after bacille Calmette–Guérin (BCG) vaccination [1,2].

Such studies may provide useful information about the immunogenicity of vaccines, and for those vaccines for which immunological correlates of clinical protection are well established, they can serve as appropriate methods for monitoring the protection conferred by vaccines that have been deployed in public health practice.

However, because immunological correlates of protection are not known for many vaccines, direct clinical assessments of vaccinees vs. nonvaccinees are often required to determine whether a vaccine, as routinely administered in public health practice, is suitably safe and protective. Recent examples of such postmarketing surveillance studies include assessments of the clinical effectiveness of *Haemophilus influenzae* type b polysaccharide vaccine in children [3], and of pneumococcal polysaccharide vaccine in subgroups of individuals who are at high risk for serious pneumococcal disease [4]. Because of ethical considerations, such studies are usually designed in an observational rather than an experimental fashion, often as cohort or case-control studies [5].

In this chapter, we primarily focus on the use of randomized clinical trials (RCTs) for Phase III vaccine evaluations. We also briefly discuss the approaches to evaluating the vaccine protection and safety in Phase IV studies.

II. RANDOMIZED CLINICAL TRIALS OF VACCINES

A. Overview

The RCT has become recognized as the most powerful research design for providing scientifically credible evidence about therapeutic efficacy [6,7], leading many national drug regulatory agencies to require evidence of efficacy from properly conducted RCTs before licensure of a new vaccine. Indeed, it may be anticipated that most, if not all, field evaluations of efficacy of experimental vaccines conducted in the future will be designed to conform to the RCT paradigm.

Figure 1 provides a diagrammatic outline of a simple, two-group RCT of an experimental vaccine. Individuals recruited from a target population are enrolled for the study after the acquisition of informed consent and ascertainment of eligibility. Study participants are then randomized to the experimental vaccine group or to a comparison (control) group. After randomization, study participants are followed concurrently to detect target infections with onsets during a defined period of follow-up. The incidence of the target infection in the different groups is then compared, to assess whether or not protection occurred in the group receiving the experimental vaccine, relative to the comparison group. Incidence may be expressed as a rate, the number of detected infections divided by the cumulative person–time at risk; or as a risk, the number of infected persons detected over some specified period of time, divided by the number of persons at risk.

It we take group B as the comparison group, such contrasts are typically expressed as rate ratios or risk ratios (RR), both based on the occurrence in group A divided by that in group B. The conventional index of protection, protective efficacy (PE), is then calculated as PE = (1− RR) × 100% [8]. PE reflects the proportionate reduction of the incidence of the target infection in the experimental vaccine group relative to the comparison group. A value of 0% denotes no protection, that of 100% corresponds to complete protection, and negative values indicate a lower incidence in the comparison group than in the experimental vaccine group.

B. Target Population

In any trial, it is first necessary to choose an appropriate target population for the evaluation. Clearly, it will be necessary to select a population in which the target infection occurs predictably and with a sufficient frequency to evaluate whether vaccination reduces the incidence of the target infection. Such populations may be defined on the

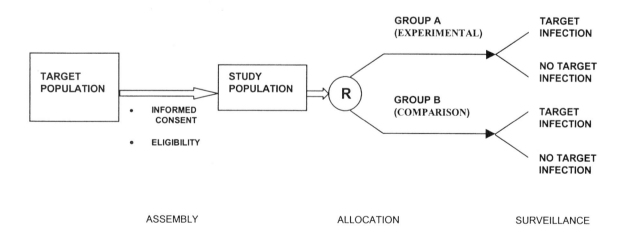

Figure 1 A schematic of the sequence of events in a two-group, randomized, controlled vaccine trial. In this sequence, the study population is assembled from a target population and is then randomized to receive an experimental vaccine or a comparison agent. The experimental and comparison groups are then followed longitudinally and concurrently to detect target infections.

basis of geographic location as well as age, gender, and a variety of additional characteristics. For example, a classic trial of plasma-derived hepatitis B vaccine was conducted in homosexual men who resided in New York [9], and trials of newer generation vaccines against leprosy have focused on family contacts of known patients with leprosy [10]. Regardless of the target population chosen for the trial, it is necessary to enumerate and characterize the population before the trial to enable later assessment of whether or not the final group for the study was representative of the intended target population.

C. Recruitment

After defining the target population for study, investigators must next recruit participants from this population. An important element of recruitment is informed consent. The specific requirements for obtaining informed consent may vary according to the age of the subject and the subject's legal capacity to give informed consent as well as the particular *milieu* for the trial. In general, acquisition of informed consent indicates that subjects have agreed to participate after understanding the purposes and elements of the trial, as well as the possible benefits and risks of participation, and after being guaranteed that their decision to participate and to continue participating are completely voluntary [11].

D. Eligibility

Usually, consenting individuals must fulfill additional eligibility criteria before enrollment in a trial. At a minimum, these eligibility criteria should exclude any persons with absolute indications for, or contraindications to, any of the agents under evaluation [12]. Such exclusions are ethically necessary if the trial is to use an impartial allocation procedure, such as randomization, that assigns compared agents without reference to the individual needs or desires of the participants.

Additional eligibility criteria may be imposed to further restrict the characteristics of the population under evaluation. Persons with serious underlying illnesses, who may not respond to vaccination, may be excluded in some trials. Investigators may also choose to focus on immunologically "pure" individuals, who have not previously experienced the target infection and have not been immunized before with a vaccine against this infection. A trial may also limit participants to persons who are at very high risk of acquiring the target infection by virtue of a history of exposure or of relevant host characteristics. Although such restrictions are commonly imposed to increase the detectability of vaccine protection, they may also substantially modify the research question that the trial addresses.

E. Allocation and Administration

Depending on the purpose of the trial, a group receiving an experimental vaccine may be compared with a group assigned to a different vaccine against the target infection, to an agent not anticipated to affect the risk of the target infection, or to no agent at al [13]. Postponement of alloca-

tion of the compared agents until after acquisition of informed consent and ascertainment of eligibility helps to ensure that decisions about recruitment, participation, and eligibility do not depend on which of the agents has been assigned [14,15]. Moreover, because this sequence ensures that only enrolled subjects are assigned to the compared agents, it minimizes irregularities created by persons who drop out of the study after assignment but before receipt of an agent under study. A powerful mechanism to prevent such biases in the intake of participants is to conceal the identities of the compared agents from both participants and investigators (*double blinding*) [16]. Double-blinded administration of agents also safeguards against a bias that can occur if participants are given the opportunity to choose additional measures to prevent the target infection on the basis of knowledge about which of the compared agents has been received.

It is important that the compared agents be allocated with a nondiscretionary method that, as far as possible, creates groups with equivalent baseline risks for the target infection under evaluation. The most powerful technique for accomplishing this goal is to allocate eligible subjects to different agents in a formally randomized fashion [17–19]. Formally randomized allocation, a prerequisite for modern trials of new vaccines, has the additional desirable property of providing a theoretical basis for statistical appraisals of differences in the occurrence of outcome events as well as other characteristics in the compared groups [20].

F. Surveillance

Vaccine field trials typically conduct surveillance for at least four types of events. First, systematic surveillance must be instituted for the target infection that the vaccine is intended to prevent. Arrangements must be made for systematic collection of data relevant to the diagnosis of the target infection, and the study must be designed to ensure that members of the compared groups have an equivalent probability of receiving relevant diagnostic procedures when they develop the target infection [16]. It is also mandatory that the diagnostic evidence be interpreted in an objective manner that is not influenced by knowledge of which agent has been received. Double-blinded surveillance constitutes the most powerful method to safeguard against biased detection and ascertainment of outcomes, although alternative strategies are available when double blinding is not possible [21].

A second important goal of surveillance is to detect adverse reactions after vaccination. Preliminary studies before the trial will usually have identified likely candidate side effects as well as the time frame of development for these side effects, which is usually a period of a few days after vaccination. Participants should be monitored for these anticipated events as well as for the possibility of less likely reactions that may occur with longer latency periods after vaccination.

Immune responses to vaccination constitute a third category of events to be monitored. Evidence of expected levels of immune responses to vaccination document that the vaccine lots under evaluation were properly prepared, stored, and administered. If a vaccine proves effective in preventing the target disease, the trial may permit assessment of the relationship between levels of response and the degree of protection.

A fourth category of events under surveillance, competing events, are outcomes other than occurrence of the target infection that terminate a participant's period of follow-up [14,15]. Follow-up arbitrarily stops at the end of a study but may also be prematurely terminated by loss from the study for such reasons as death, refusal to continue participation, and migration away from the study area. Such events are important for several reasons. Deaths, in addition to terminating follow-up, may themselves be important outcome events. Moreover, all of these events create the opportunity for unequal periods of follow-up among participants and therefore must be considered in calculating periods at risk for expressing the incidence of the target infection. Finally, if the tendency to become lost to follow-up differs in the compared groups, the losses themselves may create a differential opportunity to detect the target infection in the groups and may thereby influence estimates of the comparative occurrence of the target infection. As with surveillance for the target infection, suitably objective methods, such as double blinding, are necessary to prevent biased detection and ascertainment of side effects, immune responses, and competing events.

III. ADDITIONAL ISSUES FOR PHASE III RANDOMIZED CLINICAL TRIALS OF VACCINES

Although the basic paradigm of a controlled vaccine field trial may seem reasonably straightforward, additional issues require consideration in both the design and the analysis of a vaccine trial. In the following sections, we outline several of these issues.

A. Posing Research Questions for the Trial

Posing the research questions for the trial appropriately and with adequate specificity is crucial to the success of a Phase III trial, because research questions guide the design, conduct, and analysis of the trial. Modern vaccine trials are designed to address primary research questions, evidence bearing on which will be considered by regulatory agencies in deliberations about vaccine licensure, and secondary questions, which address additional scientific issues of interest. Adequate formulation of primary research questions demands clear specification of the target population for the study; the formulation and constituents of the vaccine, together with its mode and schedule of administration; the comparison agent to be used as a control agent; the target infections whose occurrence will serve as the basis for estimating vaccine protection; the adverse event outcomes whose occurrence will serve as the basis for evaluating vaccine safety; and the immune outcomes whose occurrence will serve as a basis for assessing vaccine immunogenicity. Each of these features needs to be articulated in a way that accurately reflects how a vaccine will be used in practice, to

ensure that a trial's results will meet regulatory expectations for vaccine licensure.

B. Demarcating the Type of Vaccine Protection to be Measured

When we administer a vaccine to a subject, our hope is that the vaccine will elicit relevant forms of immunity that will make that subject less susceptible to becoming infected when exposed to the target pathogen. This protection, which reflects the effects of the vaccine on the individual independently of whether or not other individuals in the same population are also vaccinated, is called *direct protection* [22]. However, for most vaccines, we attempt to immunize populations rather than individuals. For pathogens that are transmitted from person to person, targeting a population rather than an individual for vaccination may have the added effect of reducing the intensity of transmission of the pathogen in the population. One possible result of this *indirect protection* is that nonimmunized, susceptible individuals may be protected because they are less likely to come into contact with the pathogen [22,23]. An additional possible result is that the protection of vaccines may be augmented, because the immunity conferred by many vaccines is greater against a small challenge inoculum of a pathogen than against a heavy challenge inoculum.

A Phase III trial of a vaccine can measure either direct protection per se or direct and indirect protection combined. To accomplish the former, allocation of subjects to vaccine and the comparison agents must not create high concentrations of vaccinees within the geographical units within which the pathogen is transmitted. This is usually accomplished by randomizing individuals rather than groups and by randomizing within blocks that balance the numbers of vaccines and controls within epidemiologically relevant groups of individuals. To permit the estimation of combined direct and indirect protection, an opposite strategy must be used: groups, rather than individuals, must be the units of allocation [24]. If we imagine a trial in which an agent with no activity against the target pathogen (e.g., a placebo) is randomly allocated to other groups, we can see that several subgroups of subjects are formed (Fig. 2): vaccinated and nonvaccinated subjects within the groups allocated to the vaccine, and recipients of the control agent and nonrecipients of the control agent within the groups allocated to receive the control agent. Comparison of the incidence of the target infection in vaccinees vs. that in recipients of the control agent estimates *total protection*, a combined measure of direct protection and of indirect protection of vaccines owing to any reduction of transmission. Comparison of nonvaccinees with nonrecipients of the control agent allows estimation of indirect protection of nonvaccinated members of vaccinated groups ("herd immunity"). Finally, overall comparison of the incidence of infection in groups allocated to the vaccine vs. groups allocated to the control agent, regardless of the agent actually received, permits estimation of the *overall protection* of vaccination in the entire group targeted for the vaccine [25].

Most regulatory agencies require that Phase III trials be individually randomized, presumably because of a prefer-

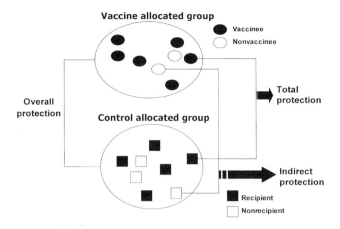

Figure 2 A diagram of measurement of vaccine protection in a cluster-randomized vaccine trial. Two hypothetical clusters are shown, and the types of individuals to be contrasted for measurement of different types of vaccine protection are identified.

ence for estimation of direct vaccine protection per se, because direct vaccine protection reflects the "intrinsic" protection of the vaccinated individual, irrespective of the vaccine coverage of other persons in contact with that individual. However, a recently completed Phase III trial of pneumococcal polysaccharide–protein conjugate vaccines in Native American infants in the United States employed cluster randomization specifically because it was anticipated that this vaccine would induce a indirect protection, which could be a major determinant of the vaccine's public health value [26].

C. Clarification of the Perspective of the Trial

To ensure the scientific credibility of the results, vaccine trials must be designed to safeguard against bias. However, even after a trial has been suitably designed to prevent bias, an additional fundamental decision remains: Should the trial be designed to measure the intrinsic effects of vaccination when it is given under ideal conditions, or should the design ensure that the results can be used to predict how well the vaccine will perform in public health practice? Trials designed to accomplish the former goal are often termed *efficacy trials*, and trials constructed to accomplish the latter objective are frequently referred to as *effectiveness trials* [24,27].

Each type of trial has different requirements for the selection of study subjects, choice of the compared agents, units of allocation, selection and definition of outcome events, and demarcation of the participants to be analyzed [24,28–30]. An efficacy trial may attempt to restrict study subjects to persons who are likely to respond to vaccination and are at sufficiently high risk for the target infection that protection will be readily detectable. For example, early studies of pneumococcal polysaccharide vaccine examined vaccine efficacy in otherwise healthy South African gold miners, who were documented to be at very high risk of

serious pneumococcal infections [31]. On the other hand, an effectiveness trial would study groups who are anticipated to be target groups for vaccination after licensure. For pneumococcal vaccine utilized in developed countries, the target group is composed of the elderly and others at high risk because of underlying disorders [32]. That the results of these two selection strategies are not necessarily interchangeable is illustrated by the controversy that arose when several post-marketing surveillance studies suggested that the high levels of efficacy of pneumococcal vaccine observed in healthy individuals were not exhibited by the debilitated groups targeted for public health application [33].

To enhance the detectability of vaccine protection, an efficacy trial tests vaccines whose formulations and regimens are designed to yield optimal protection and whose proper administration is assured by idealized experimental conditions. If ethically permissible, an efficacy trial will often contrast the group that receives the new vaccine with a comparison group that receives an agent not anticipated to protect against the target infection. In contrast, an effectiveness trial will test vaccines formulated in a manner that is most suitable for application in public health practice, conduct the evaluation in the realistic environment of a public health program, and, where appropriate, compare the performance of a new vaccine against that of a standard vaccine directed toward the same disease.

Past evaluation of Ty21a oral vaccine against typhoid fever illustrates these differences. An early efficacy trial conducted in Alexandria, Egypt, evaluated a preparation of high potency but with little applicability to public health practice because of its inconvenient formulation [34]. After demonstration of high efficacy in this early trial, later trials, conducted in Chile, evaluated more convenient enteric-coated capsule and reconstituted lyophilized "liquid" formulations [35,36,36a]. Whereas the early trials of this vaccine were placebo-controlled, a later trial, designed to answer practical questions relevant to public health implementation, compared only different regimens of active vaccine [36,36b].

To measure the intrinsic effects of vaccination, efficacy trials typically seek to measure only direct vaccine protection, because indirect effects are not intrinsic to the vaccine but depend on the pattern and extent of vaccine coverage of a population. Accordingly, the unit of allocation in an efficacy trial is typically an individual, rather than a group of individuals, and additional measures, such as blocked randomization, are often used to balance vaccinees and non-vaccinees within the groups in which transmission occurs. For live vaccines that can be excreted and transmitted to contacts, such as the Sabin oral polio vaccine, efforts are made to physically isolate vaccinees from controls to prevent "contamination" of the control group by inadvertent vaccination. In contrast, the pragmatic goals of an effectiveness trial are often best met by allocation of groups rather than individuals, because the goal is to capture the overall benefit of vaccinating a target population and because these benefits include direct as well as indirect protection of both vaccinees and nonvaccinees residing in the target population.

Trials of capsular polysaccharide–tetanus toxoid (PRP–T) conjugate vaccine against *H. influenzae* type b (Hib) in

Chile [37] and England [38] illustrate the use of group allocation in effectiveness trials. In the former, community clinics in metropolitan Santiago were randomized either to receive this vaccine mixed with diphtheria–pertussis–tetanus (DTP) vaccine at 2, 4, and 6 months of age or to receive DTP alone. In the latter, districts near Oxford were allocated to receive or not to receive PRP–T in conjunction with DTP at 2, 3, and 4 months of age. In both studies, all infants in the groups allocated to vaccine or no vaccine were followed for the occurrence of invasive Hib disease, regardless of whether or not they had received PRP–T.

The definition of the target infection for an efficacy trial aims to demarcate the biological events that are anticipated to be responsive to vaccine-induced immunity but that may be too narrow in scope to permit judgments about the usefulness of the vaccine in public health practice. For example, it was anticipated from North American volunteer challenge studies that the primary effect of ingestion of an oral B subunit-killed, whole-cell cholera vaccine would be to reduce the occurrence of clinically severe cholera [39]. An efficacy trial of this vaccine in Bangladesh was therefore designed with the primary goal of assessing vaccine efficacy against clinically severe infections [40]. Although prevention of life-threatening cholera is certainly an important public health goal, an effectiveness study might be concerned with the overall impact of vaccination against all diarrheal episodes associated with *Vibrio cholerae* 01 as well as the effect of vaccination on all episodes of clinically severe diarrhea and on diarrheal deaths.

Analyses of efficacy trials commonly consider only participants who have received a complete course of a properly administered agent. Among these analyzed participants, evaluations of such trials commonly restrict target infections to events that begin after a window of time during which it is anticipated that participants will have had an opportunity to manifest fully developed immune responses to vaccination. To minimize the possibility of bias caused by such temporal restrictions, they must be applied equally to each of the compared groups [30]. In contrast, effectiveness trials, which are concerned with the effects of a policy to administer a vaccine, would analyze all participants originally randomized to the compared agents and would include all events occurring after randomization. If groups constituted the units of allocation, all targeted members of the allocated groups would constitute the most relevant denominators. Although such an "intent to treat" analytical strategy can be justified based on the effectiveness perspective of a trial, it was also argued that this strategy for defining outcomes and populations at risk is necessary to avoid bias from distortion of the original groups created by randomized allocation [41].

The restricted populations, idealized regimens, responsive outcomes, and analytical strategies of efficacy trials will almost always reduce the sample size requirements of such studies and may also reduce associated costs and logistical demands. An efficacy trial thus constitutes a logical first step in the field evaluation of the protection conferred by a new vaccine [42]. Such efficacy trials typically form the basis for regulatory decisions about vaccine licensure. However, if a vaccine yields promising results in an efficacy study but doubts still remain about the practical utility of a new vaccine for public health practice, it may then be appropriate to mount one or more effectiveness trials before decisions are made about the application of the vaccine in public health programs. Because of this complementarity of efficacy and effectiveness trials, it has been suggested that efficacy trials be termed "Phase IIIA" trials, and effectiveness trials be termed "Phase IIIB" trials [24].

D. Sample Size Estimation and Interpretation of Background Information

Methods for calculating sample sizes required for RCTs are described in detail elsewhere [43]. One formula [44] commonly employed for two-group trials in which equal-sized groups are desired gives the size per group (N) as:

$$N = \frac{(Z_a + Z_b)^2}{d^2}[P_1(1 - P_1) + P_2(1 - P_2)]$$

In this formula, p_1 is the expected incidence of the target infection in the comparison group; p_2 is the expected incidence in the group receiving the experimental vaccine; Z_a is the Z score taken as the threshold for declaring the $[p_1-p_2]$ differences as "statistically significant" (e.g., 1.96 for a two-tailed P value of 0.05); Z_b is the Z score for beta error, the maximum tolerated probability of missing a significant difference when one really exists (e.g., 0.84 for a probability of 0.20). Because enrollment of a suitably large sample is a prerequisite for any trial, the variables and parameters specified by this formula provide useful information that must be known or about which decisions must be made in planning a vaccine trial.

To estimate p_1, it is necessary to inspect earlier surveillance data for the target infection in the population contemplated for the trial. Predicting p_1 can be particularly challenging for several reasons. First, for most infectious illnesses, a single year of surveillance will not be sufficient to estimate the expected incidence with confidence, as substantial year-to-year variation in incidence is common. For example, in Matlab, Bangladesh, where surveillance for cholera has been maintained for over 20 years, variations in annual incidence have been over 25-fold [45]. Because it is ethically imperative that trials be designed to maximize the likelihood of yielding statistically meaningful results, it is always desirable to be conservative in projecting the likely incidence of the target infection in the comparison group [46]. Second, because the expected incidence may differ dramatically, depending on demographic and other characteristics, it is important that estimates for the calculation be made for the group meeting the eligibility criteria for the trial. Third, investigators planning a trial must usually rely on earlier incidence data from routine public health surveillance, rather than from the special, prospective surveillance system that is usually instituted for a trial. Relatively loose clinical and microbiological criteria for defining infections are usually used in routine surveillance, tending to elevate the observed incidence in relation to that detected with the much stricter diagnostic criteria employed in the prospective surveillance of a trial. Conversely, during a clinical trial, efforts are usually made to evaluate all patients who might have the target infection, many of whom would have been missed in routine surveillance, and to systematically deploy diagnostic tests on all such patients. This feature of surveillance during Phase III trials would tend to elevate the observed incidence in relation to that observed with routine surveillance. Because of the unpredictability of the net balance between the factors that would inflate and factors that would diminish the incidence in a Phase III trial, in relation to antecedent routine surveillance, conservatism is required in projecting incidence rates derived from earlier routine surveillance to be expected in a Phase III trial.

Yet, a fourth consideration in estimating p_1 is that volunteers enrolled for a trial usually are not representative of, and often have lower rates of infection than, the population from which they are drawn. In a field trial of killed, oral cholera vaccines in Bangladesh, placebo recipients had a nearly 20% lower incidence of cholera than age- and gender-eligible persons who did not participate in the trial [47].

Fifth, projections about p_1 for a trial must account for anticipated subanalyses. Many trials are designed not merely to estimate vaccine protection in the entire study population, but in subgroups of the population, such as those defined by age or other demographic variables. If such subgroups are of interest, the expected incidence of the target infection in each subgroup must be considered in designing a trial. Moreover, many pathogens have different phenotypes that may affect vaccine protection. For example, a field trial of killed, oral cholera vaccines found that the biotype of *V. cholerae* 01 (El Tor vs. classical) was an important modifier of vaccine protection [48]. If different phenotypes of a target pathogen circulate in the population for a trial and if phenotype-specific vaccine protection is to be measured, p_1 must be estimated separately for each of the different phenotypes of interest in designing the trial and estimating sample size requirements.

As soon as the incidence for the comparison group has been estimated, p_2 is readily calculable from the formula for protective efficacy. Therefore, investigators must determine what minimum level of protective efficacy should be detectable in the trial. Depending on the perspective of the trial, either of two strategies can be adopted. In a biologically oriented efficacy trial, evidence from earlier studies can be marshaled to arrive at a best guess about the likely level of protection. In a more pragmatically oriented effectiveness trial, the decision rests more on a minimum level of protection and a minimum duration of this protection that would be required to justify introducing a vaccine into public health practice. Such decisions must rely on quantitative analysis of numerous factors, such as the burden and costs of the target infection, the costs and side effects of the new vaccine, and the costs, benefits, and risks of alternative methods of prevention and treatment [49].

The minimum level of protective efficacy to be detected must also take into account the planned strategy of analysis, as described earlier. If only persons who receive a complete course of appropriately administered vaccine are to be analyzed, as is often carried out in efficacy trials, estimates

of protection can be desirable in efficacy trials, and estimates of protection can be based on the expected intrinsic potency of the vaccine. Conversely, if an intent-to-treat strategy is employed, whereby persons are analyzed according to their assigned agent regardless of whether the assigned agent was administered as intended, estimates of anticipated protection will have to account for the vagaries of incomplete and improper dosing that will inevitably occur in a proportion of participants.

Decisions about Z_a address what P value will be considered as the threshold of statistical significance for rejecting the overall hypothesis of no protective efficacy. These decisions must also address whether statistical tests used to estimate P values will be interpreted in a one- or two-tailed fashion. A P value of 0.05 is the traditional, if somewhat arbitrary, threshold for declaring that a difference in incidence between compared groups in unlikely to have arisen by chance. However, as described in more detail in Section III.H, a more conservative P value threshold may be desirable for a trial in which multiple analyses are planned [50,51]. One-tailed tests may be appropriate when differences in the occurrence of the target infection are of interest only if they occur in one direction (e.g., with a higher incidence in one group vs. another group), and if a difference in the other direction would be of so little interest that it would not be statistically appraised. For a one-tailed P value, Z_a will be substantially lower than that for the same probability interpreted in a two-tailed fashion, so this decision has important consequences for required sample sizes. A decision must also be formed about Z_b, or the Z score corresponding to the maximum tolerated probability of missing a significant difference if one really exists [52]. Probabilities for beta error are always interpreted in a one-tailed fashion; by convention, a beta error ≤ 0.20 ($Z \geq 0.84$) is usually considered acceptable.

Although a complete discussion of sample size calculations is beyond the scope of this chapter, several additional points should be mentioned. The sample size must reflect the finally analyzed denominators. If these consist only of persons who receive a complete regimen of an assigned agent, it will also be important to consider the source population from whom this final sample is assembled. From individuals who meet the age and gender restrictions for the trial, some will be considered ineligible as a result of other exclusionary criteria, some will refuse, some will be absent at the time of vaccination, and some will receive the assigned agents in an incomplete or erroneous fashion. In addition, after initial assembly of participants, subjects may be lost to follow-up or may otherwise have their follow-up terminated, as described earlier. These events yield a population effectively under follow-up that is much lower than the source population, necessitating careful and conservative planning in the selection of the source population [43]. For example, in the field trial of killed oral cholera vaccines in Bangladesh, only 32% of the source population ultimately received a complete course of vaccine or placebo and were followed for the first year after dosing [46].

If vaccine efficacy is to be estimated for subgroups, it will be necessary to estimate the proportion of participants who are likely to be included in each subgroup, and to calculate an overall sample size large enough that a statistically meaningful comparison will be possible for each subgroup of interest. If differences in vaccine efficacy between subgroups are to be evaluated, sample sizes substantially larger than those required for assessments of subgroup-specific efficacy will usually be required [53].

Because the calculated sample size requirements reflect the group of subjects successfully recruited for a trial, the size of the source population for recruitment must be considered. Investigators sometimes fail to realize that the finally analyzed subjects for trial occasionally represent a very small fraction of the population. In a field trial of killed, oral cholera vaccines conducted in rural Bangladesh, for example [54], in relation to the overall population of Matlab, Bangladesh, where the trial was conducted and where the entire population was assessed for eligibility and approached for informed consent, if deemed eligible, only about one-third of persons were fully dosed and followed for the first year of surveillance. If this latter group were to constitute the final group under analysis, the source population for recruiting these participants would therefore have to be three times as large.

Finally, sometimes merely rejecting the null hypothesis of no vaccine efficacy does not provide an adequate assurance that a good vaccine is good enough. For example, in response to the troublesome side effects of conventional whole-cell pertussis vaccine, acellular pertussis vaccines have been developed and tested. To be considered suitable for licensure, these vaccines must, in addition to being safe, be as protective as conventional vaccines. Sample size considerations of trials comparing acellular vaccines with conventional vaccines therefore had to demonstrate that the protective efficacy of acellular vaccines was not substantially inferior to that of conventional pertussis vaccines [55]. Demonstration of noninferiority of one agent in comparison to another requires a different approach to the calculation of sample size requirements. Instead of seeking to reject the null hypothesis of no difference between the agents with adequate power, this approach seeks to assure that the confidence interval for the difference in outcomes between the agents excludes values suggesting that the new agent (e.g., acellular pertussis vaccine) is unacceptably inferior to the standard agent (e.g., conventional pertussis vaccine).

E. Issues in Allocation of the Compared Agents

Randomized allocation is such an important safeguard against bias that it should be regarded as essential in field evaluations of new vaccines. However, even if randomized allocation is planned, several issues still require attention.

An obvious decision to be made is whether the allocation procedure is to yield groups with similar or intentionally unequal numbers of subjects. Whereas groups of similar size are usually preferred in two-group trials, the decision is less straightforward for trials with more than two groups, particularly when a single nonvaccinated group is to be compared with multiple vaccinated groups. For such multiple-group trials, there is disagreement about whether equal or unequal sample sizes provide optimal statistical efficiency

[56]. Moreover, on ethical grounds, there may be compelling reasons to minimize the number of participants in the group that will not be vaccinated. If unequal sizes per group are desired, randomization procedures can easily be adapted to yield the desired allocation ratio.

Stratified allocation—in which subjects are randomly allocated to different agents within subgroups defined by relevant risk factors for the target infection, typically in a balanced fashion (with use of "blocking") within these strata—has been advocated as a method to improve the similarity of baseline characteristics of compared groups [57]. This technique is helpful in safeguarding against bias in trials involving small numbers of participants, particularly when these participants differ greatly in their risks for the outcome under study. Such conditions commonly apply to clinical trials of therapy for ill persons who have substantially different prognostic expectations. This technique may also be relevant to vaccine trials with small sample sizes, but it is unlikely to confer great advantage over the use of simple randomization in assigning compared agents for large-scale field trials [58].

Blocked allocation is also commonly employed in small trials in which there is concern that simple randomization may not yield groups of the desired size. For example, in a two-celled trial of vaccine vs. placebo intended to compare groups of equal sizes, randomization might take place within blocks of every four consecutively assigned subjects to ensure that two subjects receive vaccine and two receive placebo [58].

As described earlier, it is conventionally recommended that randomization of subjects should occur only after enrollment procedures for participation have been completed. However, in practice, this prescribed sequence may be a difficult requirement to fulfill, particularly in less-developed settings, where communications may be inadequate to permit a vaccination team to contact a central randomization unit and where it may not be desirable to involve field teams in the task of allocation [21]. In such circumstances, it may be preferable to allocate the agents in a randomized fashion before recruitment and ascertainment of eligibility and to safeguard against biases in the enrollment of participants by administration of the compared agents in a double-blinded fashion. With this strategy, each member of an already characterized population can be randomly preassigned an agent, as in a field trial of oral cholera vaccines in Bangladesh [40], or doses of agents can be randomly ordered, either physically within storage containers or via a coded assignment list, and the doses can be given consecutively as participants are enrolled into the study.

Another issue requiring consideration is the unit of participants to be allocated to the compared agents. From a statistical viewpoint, it is most efficient to consider the individual participant as the unit to be allocated [43]. However, allocation of individuals may be difficult for vaccines that are excreted and transmitted from a vaccinated individual to nonvaccinated contacts, and it may not be applicable when an effectiveness rather than an efficacy perspective is selected. To evaluate the protection conferred by a transmissible vaccine, it is necessary to demarcate as units for allocation the groups of individuals between whom transmission of the vaccine is unlikely. For example, in a trial of orally administered, live Ty2a typhoid vaccine in Chile, classrooms of students were allocated to the compared agents, in part to safeguard against the possibility of "contamination" of nonvaccinated controls by transmission of the vaccine organism [35,36a].

When calculating sample sizes in trials in which a group is the unit of allocation, it is important to account for the degree of clustering of the target infection within the groups to be allocated. Cholera, for example, occurs in highly focal outbreaks within a community, even in endemic area [45]. In general, the greater the magnitude of such clustering, the larger will be the number of subjects required for the evaluation. In addition, when groups rather than individuals serve as units of allocation, statistical techniques appropriate for this allocation strategy will be required in analyzing the results of the trial [59].

Finally, in addition to providing safeguards against biased allocation, it is necessary to measure whether the allocation created groups that were comparable in baseline characteristics which might affect the occurrence of the target infection [17–19]. Documentation of equivalent distributions in the compared groups reassures that the randomization procedure was appropriately executed, although some imbalances in the distributions of baseline features may be expected by chance [20]. Adjustment of estimates of vaccine protective efficacy for unequally distributed variables can be undertaken with stratified analyses or multivariate models. Comparison of these adjusted estimates with the crude estimates provides an indication as to whether distortions of vaccine protection could have arisen because of unequal baseline susceptibility to infection in the compared groups [20]. In addition to baseline characterization of participants, it also is important to document reasons for nonparticipation and baseline characteristics of the nonparticipants. Such data permit the assessment of whether participants were representative of the target population; if subjects were preassigned to different agents, these data can be analyzed to evaluate whether differential participation of those assigned to the compared groups was a likely source of bias.

F. Issues in the Administration of the Compared Agents

Several questions routinely arise about how the agents should be packaged and labeled, as well as about what data should be collected concerning the process of administration. Agents can be packaged as single doses or as containers with multiple doses. In general, it will be advantageous to package the agents in single doses, both to minimize vaccine deterioration in the field and also to circumvent human errors in measuring doses. If the agents are to be coded, as is necessary to maintain double blinding, several factors must be considered: simplicity, avoidance of errors in administration, and prevention of discovery of the identities of the agents. Whereas a unique code for each dose, usually with a number, provides the greatest protection against the unblinding of a trial, this strategy may increase the complexity of administering agents and of

recording what was administered, and it may also create logistical difficulties if the same agent is to be given on multiple occasions. Use of fewer codes may alleviate these problems but may make it easier for participants or investigators to detect the identities of the codes. Whatever system of coding is employed, letter or number codes are substantially simpler to work with than color codes. Because of the inevitable tendency of research workers to be inquisitive about the identities of the coded agents and in view of the difficulties in making truly identical agents for comparison in vaccine trials, it is also useful at the end of a trial to conduct a survey of investigators and other workers in the trial to assess opinions about the identities of the different codes. This exercise, which will permit an empirical estimate of the likelihood that the trial was indeed conducted in a double-blinded fashion, is particularly valuable if only a few different codes are used for the compared agents.

Several additional aspects of the administration of the agents require documentation. First, even if the agents are preassigned, it is important that vaccination teams record the code of what was actually given. If single-unit doses are administered, it is useful to employ self-adhesive stickers that give the code and that can be removed from each dose and affixed to a vaccination record book. This documentation is important, because errors in administration are inevitable. For example, in a trial of oral cholera vaccines in Bangladesh [40], 573 of 234,032 (0.2%) doses were not given as assigned, despite the use of a simple A–B–C coding system for the three compared agents. Second, it is desirable to record observations about the completeness of dosing. Incomplete dosing can occur with any route of administration, but it may be a particular problem for noninjectable agents. In the Bangladesh oral cholera vaccine trial, 6367 (3%) doses were not completely ingested, in part because of the large volumes (50–160 mL, depending on age) of the doses [40]. Although analytical strategies for handling participants who received erroneous or incomplete doses may vary according to the perspective of the trial, documentation of the frequency of such vagaries is always helpful in interpreting the apparent degree of vaccine protection.

If the agents under investigation require a cold chain to preserve potency, it will be desirable at each step in the itinerary, from the manufacturer to the recipient, to document that necessary thermal conditions were maintained. A variety of thermal monitors are available for this purpose. If a particular level of an immune response to vaccination is known to occur after proper administration of fully potent vaccine, assessment of immune responses in representative samples of the vaccinated and comparison groups may provide a useful indication of the adequacy of the manufacture, storage, and administration of the vaccine. Finally, samples of the batches of vaccine delivered to the field site for use in the trial should be preserved for evaluation of potency. All of these tactics are of particular interest for trials in which protection by vaccination is lower than expected, and it is necessary to distinguish deficiencies in the intrinsic potency of a vaccine from problems in manufacture, storage, and administration.

G. Issues in Surveillance

The scope of surveillance activities in a trial may include detection of the target infection and other clinical events relevant to the assessment of vaccine protection, observations of side effects, assessment of immune responses, and recording of competing events. For each of these outcomes, decisions must be made about the approach to detecting events, the time frame for surveillance, as well as the methods to be employed to safeguard against biased detection of the events.

1. Scope

The range of detected events for assessment of vaccine protection may vary substantially with the method of detection. Passive surveillance of illnesses through monitoring of routine visits by patients to health facilities provides a logistically simple approach to detecting outcomes. However, with passive surveillance, only those illnesses that are severe enough to prompt solicitation of medical care will be detected, and persons who have more ready access to treatment facilities or who are more "medicalized" in their use of health care facilities may be overrepresented. Moreover, the type of events detected may be affected by the focus of the treatment facility under surveillance. For example, a trial that uses infectious disease hospitals to detect outcome events may miss the neurological or cardiovascular side effects of vaccination. With an active surveillance strategy, the investigator maintains a schedule of contacts with each participant, regardless of whether the participant is ill or not, and thereby has the opportunity to detect illnesses that span a wide spectrum of severity and characteristics. In addition, with active surveillance, it may be possible to detect asymptomatic infections, whose interruption may be relevant to preventing transmission of disease. The salient disadvantage of active surveillance, however, is the considerable expense and logistical complexity of maintaining regular, active contact with an entire study population, particularly in studies that are large or that entail a prolonged period of follow-up.

For certain types of target infections, active surveillance will yield a greater apparent incidence than that noted by passive surveillance, thereby reducing sample size requirements for evaluation of vaccine protection. For example, in Matlab, Bangladesh, which has been a site for several cholera vaccine field trials, comparison of active and passive surveillance data for children aged under 2 years demonstrated that only about 6% of diarrheal illnesses detected by active surveillance were brought to treatment facilities for care [60]. However, investigators specifically interested in the effect of vaccination on clinically severe disease should remember that the overall incidence rates based on active surveillance may reflect primarily nonsevere infections. This difference in clinical spectrum may substantially affect the magnitude of vaccine protective efficacy if a vaccine acts to diminish the severity of the clinical manifestations of an infection, as has been noted for whole-cell pertussis vaccines [61] and inactivated oral vaccines against cholera [62]. For such vaccines, estimates of vaccine efficacy based on passive surveillance are likely to be higher than estimates based on

active surveillance. Thus choices between active and passive surveillance in a trial should not be based merely on trade-offs between logistical ease and disease incidence but should consider the possible impact of the surveillance technique on the magnitude of vaccine protection. Depending on the nature of the events to be detected, passive surveillance, active surveillance, or a combination of the two may be appropriate for detection of target infections.

Detection of adverse events following dosing, and comparing rates of specific adverse events in the groups under study are essential components of a Phase III trial. Indeed, Phase III trials, because of their large size, offer a unique opportunity for evaluating vaccine safety before a vaccine is licensed. In past years, the approach taken by Phase III trials was often to focus on documentation of frequent and expected adverse events, occurring only during the first few days after dosing. The focus was primarily on documenting common side effects, generally of mild severity. Often, these trials measured adverse events in only a small subsample of the trial population, as large sample sizes were not required to document frequent side effects, such as the occurrence of pain or erythema at an injection site. Some trials failed to conduct surveillance for adverse events altogether.

Several changes have occurred during the past several years in the approach to documenting vaccine safety in Phase III trials. First, it is now well recognized that not all adverse effects of vaccination are easily predicted. For example, intussusception following oral receipt of live rhesus rotavirus-reassortant vaccine, an event that is now well documented, was not an expected side effect of this vaccine, at least at the time that Phase III trials were undertaken [63]. Therefore, it is inappropriate in Phase III trials to constrain the focus of surveillance to adverse events that can readily be predicted. Second, it is no longer acceptable to target surveillance only to adverse events that occur quite commonly, nor to place only a subsample of participants under surveillance for adverse events. Newer-generation live oral rotavirus vaccines, for example, will be tested in Phase III trials that, in aggregate, will be large enough to detect an attributable incidence of intussusception of approximately 1 case in 10,000 vaccine recipients. Expanding the scope of surveillance in this fashion will have a major effect in increasing the size, cost, and complexity of future Phase III trials.

Surveillance for immune responses will almost always require actively scheduled tests, although immune testing of vaccinated participants who develop target infections and are detected in ordinary treatment settings may offer the opportunity to evaluate whether poor immune responses accounted for the illness in these vaccines [64]. If the goal of these immune assessments is merely to confirm that the vaccines under study elicited expected levels of immune responses, it may be necessary only to evaluate a sample of the trial population. However, Phase III trials also commonly attempt to evaluate the relationship between the magnitude of induced responses and the level of vaccine-induced protection. To achieve this latter objective, responses in vaccinees who ultimately developed the target infection are compared with responses of vaccinees who did not. Because breakthrough infections are usually small in number in a trial of a protective vaccine, it will often be necessary to obtain postdosing specimens for immunological evaluation from most or all subjects in a trial to enable a statistically satisfactory evaluation of immunologic correlates of protection.

Detection of deaths and outmigrations is important to enable the calculation of the person–time at risk during follow-up of trial participants. Detection of these events may be possible by consulting vital event data routinely collected for the population under study, but detection of losses for other reasons (e.g., refusal to continue participation) as well as adequate characterization of the reasons for losses to follow-up will usually require an active strategy. Because the assessment of cause-specific mortality should constitute an element of surveillance for side effects in any Phase III trial, arrangements must be made to obtain clinical records for illness leading up to all deaths in trial participants or, lacking such data, it is important that relatives of decedents be interviewed to obtain "verbal autopsies."

2. Time Frame

The time frame for surveillance must be planned to address the questions posed by the trial. Because field trials provide the best opportunity to evaluate the duration of protection conferred by vaccination, it will usually be desirable to plan for the possibility of long-term surveillance. However, investigators should not be lulled into the intellectual trap of extending the period of surveillance merely as a mechanism to raise the cumulative incidence of the target infection and thereby to reduce sample size requirements. If short-term efficacy is of interest, sample size requirements should be calculated on the basis of the expected incidence for the shortest duration of follow-up to be analyzed [46].

It is now appreciated that vaccine side effects can occur long after vaccine dosing. For example, quite unexpectedly, mortality rates during the third year of life were found to be elevated in female infants who received high-titered measles vaccines at 6 months of age [65]. As a result, national regulatory authorities are increasingly demanding that Phase III trials be designed to capture adverse events of any grade of severity; those that are predictable as well as those that are not; those that occur at any point during the follow-up of subjects in the trial, not just the first several days after dosing; and those that occur infrequently.

Similarly, although short-term immune responses are often measured to gauge whether the vaccine induced the expected levels of immune responses and to assess immune correlates of vaccine protection, serial surveys of immune responses may estimate the kinetics of decay of immunity over time.

The duration of a trial may be truncated if severe side effects are noted during vaccination, contraindicating further dosing, or if a large health benefit occurs in a group that receives an active agent, so that ethical considerations demand that participants randomized to other agents have the opportunity to receive the beneficial agent. This latter consideration is likely to be a major factor in the design of future trials of vaccines against human immunodeficiency virus, particularly if a vaccine that reduces the rate of

infection is identified [66]. Because investigators may have a vested interest in prolonging a trial in order to obtain estimates of long-term protection, it is desirable to place such decisions in the hands of monitoring committees of scientific peers who are not in any way involved in the trial and who can make decisions purely on behalf of the subjects in the trial [67]. Modern Phase III trials are usually monitored by at least two bodies external to the investigative team: a Data and Safety Monitoring Board (DSMB) and an Institutional Review Board (IRB). The DSMB is typically composed of professionals with expertise in disciplines relevant to the trial, such as biostatistics, epidemiology, and clinical infectious diseases. These individuals cannot have any role as investigators in the trial. Typically, a DSMB has the authority to review and approve the final protocol for the trial. It also serves to monitor the trial periodically by assessing both the performance of the trial in meeting its process goals, such as subject enrollment, and by evaluating the adverse events and study endpoints that are observed among trial participants. In the last activity, they are responsible for recommending early termination of a trial to the sponsor.

3. Detection Bias

Detection bias distorts estimates of vaccine efficacy via unequal surveillance of vaccines vs. controls for the target outcome. This bias can occur in at least three ways. First, if there are unequal losses to follow-up of study participants in the compared groups, there may be an unequal opportunity to detect outcome events [21]. Although analytical techniques, such as life-table analyses, are designed to adjust estimates of protection for unequal periods of follow-up in compared groups, such techniques may not adequately correct for a bias that may occur if the reasons for the losses and the characteristics of the lost subjects differ in the compared groups [14,15]. Losses to follow-up are less likely to create a bias if they are few in number and if decisions to drop out of the study are not based on knowledge of which agent has been received. Therefore, protection against this bias is best accomplished by choosing a study population that is likely to comply with the study protocol and to have a low rate of migration, by vigilant efforts to maintain contact with the study population, and by double blinding of the trial. Moreover, it is essential that the numbers and characteristics of subjects who are lost to follow-up, as well as the reasons for the losses, be analyzed for each group to permit judgments about whether or not unequal losses in the compared groups were likely to have created a bias.

Second, if subjects in the compared groups have an unequal probability of receiving diagnostic procedures that are necessary to detect outcome events, the comparative occurrence of the events in the groups may be distorted [21]. Double-blinded surveillance provides the most effective safeguard against this possibility. However, effective use of this safeguard will not always be possible in vaccine field trials. For example, in trials of BCG vaccination against tuberculosis and leprosy, it was not ethically permissible to employ a comparative agent whose side effects, including creation of a cutaneous scar, were similar to those of BCG [68,69]. For trials that are not conducted in a double-blinded fashion, it is important that investigators employ alternative safeguards against biased diagnostic evaluations or at least that they evaluate whether a differential intensity of diagnostic testing of subjects in the compared groups was likely to have distorted estimates of vaccine protection [21]. For example, in field trials of BCG against tuberculosis, use of mass radiographic screening for pulmonary disease, irrespective of the presence of symptoms and of solicitation of clinical care, provided an important safeguard against biased application of diagnostic tests [68].

Third, even if bias has not resulted from differential losses to follow-up or from differential diagnostic surveillance, biased detection of outcomes can still occur if the evidence collected during diagnostic evaluations has not been interpreted in an objective fashion. In a truly double-blinded trial, bias caused by differential diagnostic ascertainment is not a major risk. In a trial in which double-blinded surveillance is not possible, alternative arrangements must be made to ensure objective diagnoses. For example, to prevent biased diagnoses in trials of BCG vaccination against leprosy, a useful tactic was to cover the injection sites of both vaccinees and nonvaccinees during physical examinations [69]. Similarly, in trials of BCG against tuberculosis in which mass chest radiography was used to detect potential cases of tuberculosis, an additional safeguard against biased diagnoses was provided by blinding radiologists to the vaccination status of subjects whose chest films were under evaluation [21]. In addition to such tactics for preventing biased diagnoses, it is also necessary to maximize the accuracy of diagnoses by ensuring that the diagnostic data have been collected in a systematic and accurate fashion and that appropriate and explicit diagnostic criteria have been uniformly applied to the collected data. Diagnostic inaccuracies, even if they occur in a random fashion, may substantially distort measures of the comparative occurrence of events in the groups under study [70].

Finally, in evaluating the possible role of detection bias in distorting estimates of vaccine protective efficacy, it may be helpful to inspect vaccine protection against an *indicator condition*—a disease whose diagnostic evaluation is similar to that for the target infection but against which no vaccine efficacy can logically be anticipated. If the vaccine under evaluation fails to protect against such a condition, the likelihood of detection bias is diminished. For example, in the trial of inactivated oral cholera vaccines in Bangladesh, it was demonstrated that neither vaccine conferred protection against bloody diarrheas, as had been predicted by expectations that protection would primarily occur against diarrhea due to *V. cholerae* 01 and enterotoxigenic *Escherichia coli*, but not against invasive enteropathogens [71].

H. Issues in Analyzing Data

Although a detailed discussion of statistical strategies for analyzing data in vaccine field trials is beyond the scope of this chapter, a few general comments deserve emphasis. It is important that groups under analysis be assessed for their comparability at baseline (e.g., at allocation), and that the comparability of losses to follow-up be evaluated after baseline. If imbalances are detected, appropriate analytical techniques should be used to check if the results might have been distorted by baseline and postbaseline imbalances and to correct denomination for losses to follow-up [20].

It is also important that analyses be planned in advance of the study. Before inspection of the data, explicit criteria should be developed for determining which participants will constitute the groups under analysis, and detailed criteria should be formulated for defining outcome events in these analyzed participants. Because the design and interpretation of analyses may be distorted by biases of the data analyst, it has also been recommended that analyses be undertaken and interpreted without knowledge of the agents received by the compared groups [16].

It is unwise for investigators to continuously inspect the occurrence of outcome events in the different groups as the data accumulate because such action poses several dangers. First, if the comparison group for the study receives an agent that is known to be inactive against the target infection and if vaccinated groups are protected, the observed differences in rates of the target infection may "unblind" the investigation and jeopardize the scientific quality of data as surveillance continues. Second, the apparent degree of protection by a vaccine may fluctuate widely with time. For example, during the initial years of follow-up in a trial of oral Ty21a vaccine against typhoid in Area Norte of Santiago, Chile, efficacy fluctuated from 0% to 100% during various 3-month intervals, although there was no consistent trend over time [36]. If investigators use accumulating surveillance data to determine intervals for evaluating "short-term" and "long-term" protection, such fluctuations may lead to the choice of intervals that severely distort estimates of protection. Of course, these considerations do not argue against ongoing inspection of data by an independent scientific committee, for ethical reasons outlined earlier. However, because of the danger of spurious conclusions that can be drawn during multiple scrutiny of the data [67], it is important that such committees employ suitably conservative statistical strategies in evaluating the data and that investigators be kept unaware of these analyses unless it is necessary to terminate the trial.

Multiple analyses of accumulating data constitute one facet of the more general multiple-comparisons problem, alluded to earlier [20,50,51,67,72]. The multiple comparisons problem arises when investigators undertake inter-group comparisons of several outcomes or if the inter-group occurrence of an outcome is compared between several pairs of agents (if more than two are under study), within several subgroups of participants, or at multiple points in time during follow-up. As more analyses are conducted, the overall probability of finding at least one "statistically significant" difference when no true difference exists also increases. For example, if $P < 0.05$ is the threshold for declaring a difference significant, this means that the investigator is willing to tolerate a 1:20 chance of finding a statistically significant difference arising from chance fluctuations when, in fact, there is no difference between the groups under analysis. If 20 independent comparisons are evaluated, the overall probability that at least one will be statistically significant at $P < 0.05$, even if no difference exists, will be 0.64, not 0.05.

To compensate for this problem, several statistical techniques have been developed for reducing the P value chosen as the threshold for declaring an individual comparison as statistically significant [50,72]. However, because such techniques create progressively smaller P-value thresholds as the total number of comparison increases, the application of these methods in trials with numerous analyses would make it difficult or impossible to detect statistically significant differences. Application of these techniques is proper only for analyses that are anticipated in advance rather than being suggested after inspection of data [50,51]. These and other dilemmas have created controversy about the proper approach for dealing with multiple comparisons in the analysis of RCTs [51]. Although many strategies are possible, one approach would be to pose primary analyses, addressing the major questions of the trials, and secondary analyses, evaluating other topics of interest. Adjustments of P-values for multiple comparisons would be made only for the primary analyses, and the results of these analyses would be considered as rigorous hypothesis-testing assessments. Secondary analyses would employ ordinary (e.g., $P < 0.05$) P-value thresholds but would be conducted as hypothesis-generating exercises requiring conservative interpretation [40].

Finally, an increasing emphasis is being placed on the use of confidence intervals in statistical evaluations of vaccine efficacy, rather than merely declaring protective efficacy as "statistically significant" at some arbitrary threshold (e.g., $P < 0.05$) [73]. This is because a statistically significant result for vaccine protection merely implies that the results for protective efficacy reject the null hypothesis of no vaccine protection; declaration of statistically significant protective efficacy provides no information about the range of values for protection that are statistically compatible with the observed level of efficacy. For the latter, the confidence internal surrounding the estimate of efficacy at a desired level of precision (e.g., 95%) must be calculated. In trials aimed at detecting whether or not the vaccine is protective, the lower boundary of the confidence interval portrays not only whether the results reject the null hypothesis (e.g., do not include 0% efficacy) but also how low protective efficacy might really be, allowing for the play of chance in the trial's results. For trials designed to determine whether the efficacy of a tested vaccine is at or above some predetermined level, the lower boundary tells whether or not the tested vaccine's true efficacy is likely to be at or above the desired level [55].

I. Good Clinical Practice

In recent years, regulatory agencies have placed much emphasis on the concept of conducting vaccine trials leading to vaccine licensure with designs and procedures that conform to "Good Clinical Practice" (GCP) [74]. The essential elements of Good Clinical Practice are outlined in Table 1. In essence, these elements are designed as basic criteria to ensure that trials are conducted in an ethically justifiable fashion, are scientifically sound, and are verifiable. The last feature refers to the need to create sufficient documentation during a trial so that an independent auditor could verify that the findings of a trial accurately reflect the data actually collected.

Table 1 The Principles of Good Clinical Practice[a]

1. Clinical trials should be conducted in accordance with the ethical principles that have their origin in the Declaration of Helsinki, and are consistent with GCP and the applicable regulatory requirement(s).
2. Before a trial is initiated, foreseeable risks and inconveniences should be weighed against the anticipated benefit for the individual trial subject and society. A trial should be initiated and continued only if the anticipated benefits justify the risks.
3. The rights, safety, and well-being of the trial subjects are the most important considerations and should prevail over interests of science and society.
4. The available nonclinical and clinical information on an investigational product should be adequate to support the proposed clinical trial.
5. Clinical trials should be scientifically sound, and described in a clear, detailed protocol.
6. A trial should be conducted in compliance with the protocol that has received prior Institutional Review Board (IRB)/Independent Ethics Committee (IEC) approval/favorable opinion.
7. The medical care given to, and medical decisions made on behalf of, subjects should always be the responsibility of a qualified physician or, when appropriate, of a qualified dentist.
8. Each individual involved in conducting a trial should be qualified by education, training, and experience to perform his or her respective task(s).
9. Freely given informed consent should be obtained from every subject prior to clinical trial participation.
10. All clinical trial information should be recorded, handled, and stored in a way that allows its accurate reporting, interpretation, and verification.
11. The confidentiality of records that could identify subjects should be protected, respecting the privacy and confidentiality rules in accordance with the applicable regulatory requirement(s).
12. Investigational products should be manufactured, handled, and stored in accordance with applicable good manufacturing practice (GMP). They should be used in accordance with the approved protocol.
13. Systems with procedures that assure the quality of every aspect of the trial should be implemented.

[a] From Ref. 74.

IV. POSTLICENSURE OBSERVATIONAL STUDIES

After a vaccine has been licensed, it is still necessary to monitor its safety and the protection it confers in practice. Various types of studies are commonly used to evaluate new vaccines once they have been introduced into practice. These include serological assessments of vaccine-induced immunity, evaluations of the levels of vaccine coverage of the intended target population, and assessments of the safety of new vaccines and their protection against clinical disease. A detailed consideration of all of these studies is beyond the scope of this chapter. Here we consider why it is necessary to conduct postlicensure studies of vaccine safety and clinical protection and briefly consider several of the more common designs for clinical studies of these issues.

A. Reasons for Conducting Postlicensure Studies of Safety and Protection

The are several reasons for continued vigilance in monitoring clinical safety and protection [75]. The spectrum of vaccine recipients in practice may expand beyond that studied in Phase III trials, and this expansion may lead to a decline in vaccine protection. For example, this phenomenon has been noted for conventional influenza vaccines, which often perform better in young, healthy subjects frequently used for testing than in elderly patients, who constitute one of the primary targets for these vaccines [76]. Alternatively, the target population may not change but may later be found to be less than optimally focused. For example, long after conventional measles vaccine was put into practice in the United States, it was discovered that administration of this vaccine at 12 months of age accounted for some vaccine failures, leading to a later recommendation that the vaccine be given at 15 months [77].

The vagaries of manufacturing practice may lead to the inadvertent release of lots of vaccine that are not fully protective, or are harmful. The former was recently illustrated by problems with the immunogenicity of certain postlicensure lots of PRP-OMP, a Hib capsular polysaccharide—*Neisseria meningitidis* outer membrane protein conjugate vaccine [78], while the latter was perhaps most dramatically illustrated by the Cutter incident, in which inadequately inactivated lots of Salk polio vaccine caused paralytic polio among U.S. vaccine recipients in the 1950s [79].

Even without manufacturing errors, the formulation or dosing regimen of a vaccine may ultimately prove unsuitable when the vaccine is administered on a large scale. Sabin oral polio vaccine is less immunogenic when given to infants residing in less developed settings. This observation has led to the conclusion that more doses of this vaccine may be required to protect infants and children in these settings [80]. Similarly, the titers of the three serotypes contained in the Sabin vaccine had to be modified when postlicensure studies found that the vaccine failed to confer suitable protection against type-3 infections in certain developing countries [81].

Appropriately manufactured vaccines may be responsible for rare or long-latency adverse effects that are not detectable with prelicensure Phase III trials and only appear when the vaccine has been administered to larger numbers of persons over long intervals of time. Although prelicensure studies showed an inactivated vaccine against swine influenza to be safe, a putative association between vaccination and the rare development of Guillain–Barré syndrome emerged when the vaccine was applied on a mass scale [82].

The vagaries of public health practice may lead to errors in vaccine storage or administration that may vitiate vaccine protection. This phenomenon was noted for earlier generations of conventional measles vaccine, for which storage at unacceptably high temperatures led to reduction of vaccine potency [83].

Agents coadministered with vaccine in practice may cause unexpected reductions of vaccine potency. This problem was noted for human diploid cell rabies vaccine, whose immunogenicity is reduced by concomitantly administered chloroquine, explaining an unexpected vaccine failure in a Peace Corps volunteer who took both agents [84].

Finally, the mass administration of a vaccine may lead to higher levels of vaccine protection than were expected on the basis of Phase III trials, owing to the indirect effects of vaccination in reducing transmission of the target pathogen. This phenomenon was recently noted for PRP-conjugate vaccines against invasive Hib disease; despite moderate levels of coverage of targeted children in several industrialized countries, mass administration of these vaccines has virtually eliminated invasive Hib disease in these settings [85]. Although this cannot be classified as a postlicensure "problem," it is important to document these indirect vaccine effects.

B. Methodological Approaches

After licensure, it is sometimes appropriate to evaluate new vaccines with RCTs. For example, it may be of interest to compare the performance of different licensed vaccines with one another or different regimens of such vaccines. Such an evaluation was recently reported in the "mix and match" study of different licensed PRP-conjugate vaccines, in which vaccine safety and immunogenicity were assessed in subjects randomized to various multidose regimens of the same vaccine or to different vaccines interchanged with one another within a given regimen [86].

Often, however, it will not be ethically permissible, logistically feasible, or scientifically appropriate to use RCTs to evaluate a vaccine after it has been licensed [11,12]. Ethical problems arise in any such design in which an indicated vaccine is withheld from study subjects who are experimentally allocated to an inert control agent. In addition, because of the expense of RCTs, it is not possible to consider performing a new trial for each question that arises about a vaccine after its introduction into practice. Scientifically, the questions posed after licensure usually address the performance of the vaccine as it is actually given in practice, and it may be difficult to fully replicate practice with a trial, even using the effectiveness trial approach outlined in Section III.B.

For these reasons, observational study designs are most commonly used to evaluate the safety and protection of a vaccine used in practice. These studies are called observational rather than experimental because the investigator does not allocate subjects to receive alternative agents according to some deliberate plan, such as randomization, but assesses the outcomes of receipt or nonreceipt of vaccine as occurs during routine clinical care [87]. Because clinical outcomes under study can be either adverse events or the target illnesses to be prevented by vaccination, these allow assessment of both vaccine safety and vaccine protection.

1. Indirect Approaches: Before-and-After Studies

Perhaps, the simplest way to evaluate a vaccine applied in practice to a population is simply to monitor the incidence of the outcome—a side effect or the disease to which the vaccine is directed—before and after the vaccine is introduced. Such evaluations have, for example, provided convincing evidence about the effectiveness of PRP–protein conjugate and measles–mumps–rubella (MMR) vaccines as well as oral polio vaccines, for which mass immunization has nearly or completely eliminated the target diseases [85,88,89]. When the overall incidence of the disease outcome before and after initiation of a vaccine program is assessed, the study is an indirect evaluation of vaccine performance, because vaccinees are not directly compared with nonvaccinees to evaluate the vaccine. Instead, the evaluation of the vaccine relies on the temporal trend of disease in the entire target population, regardless of the proportion of its members who became vaccinated.

Apart from situations in which there are dramatic vaccine effects upon diseases that, in lieu of vaccination, occur predictably year after year and in which disease surveillance is reliable and constant over time, such studies are difficult to interpret. This is because, without comparison of the experience of vaccinees with concurrently followed nonvaccinees, it is usually difficult to know whether temporal changes in the occurrence of disease outcomes reflect the effect of the vaccine, changes in disease epidemiology unrelated to the vaccine, changes in intensity or accuracy of surveillance for the disease, changes in other interventions that may modify the occurrence of the disease, or changes in diagnostic definitions or reporting of disease [87].

2. Direct Approaches

Controlled, Cohort Studies. If we consider the alternative approach of directly comparing concurrently assembled vaccinees and nonvaccinees for disease outcomes, the most straightforward design is a controlled cohort study [5,75,87,90]. In such a study, the compared groups are then assessed for the incidence of the studied outcome, determined through longitudinal surveillance after assembly. These compared cohorts can be assembled historically, in present time, or a mixture of the two. Similarly, the follow-up of the compared cohorts can occur during an interval prior to the investigation, pari passu with the investigation, or both. A major advantage of controlled cohort evaluations is that they allow comparisons of the cohorts for multiple disease outcomes within a single study. As a result, if properly designed, a single controlled cohort study can evaluate multiple potential side effects and multiple potential protective effects of vaccination. Another advantage over simple before-and-after comparisons is that cohort studies enable direct estimation of vaccine protection by the same expression, $PE = (1-RR) \times 100\%$, cited earlier for RCTs. This is because RCTs are themselves controlled cohort studies.

However, controlled cohort studies have several limitations. For adequate statistical power to detect vaccine effects, such studies must detect a suitable number of disease outcome events. These studies are thus best reserved for situations in which the studied outcomes frequently occur, thus ensuring adequate statistical power to detect intergroup differences. These investigations are also better suited for evaluations of outcomes that occur relatively shortly after vaccination, so as to minimize the logistical complexities and financial expense of prolonged follow-up of a study population. Examples of research questions well suited to cohort studies include evaluations of vaccine protection against common childhood diseases, such as measles [91], and assessments of vaccine protection during defined outbreaks of the target disease, in which the study population experiences a high attack rate of disease. Because most postlicensure assessments of putative vaccine side effects focus on long-latency or rare events, cohort designs are not commonly used for such evaluations.

Case-Control Studies. When the disease outcome under study is rare or occurs long after vaccination, it is usually more feasible to evaluate the vaccine by using the case-control study design [5,75,92]. With this design, groups are assembled not on the basis of being vaccinated or not, as in a cohort study, but on the basis of having developed the disease outcome ("cases") or not ("controls"). Cases and controls are then contrasted for earlier receipt of vaccination. In a case-control study, cases and controls can be assembled with use of historical records, prospective surveillance, or a mixture of the two. However, histories of vaccination in these studies always rely on historical information.

Case-control assessments have several advantages. Because cases are directly sampled with these designs, case-control studies are well suited for studying rare disease outcomes of vaccination as well as outcomes that may occur with long-latency periods after vaccination. Moreover, because the investigator can arbitrarily select a statistically optimal number of controls for each case and can often enroll the required sample of cases and controls over a relatively brief period of time, the case-control design maximizes statistical power to detect outcomes associated with vaccination, minimizes sample size requirements, and substantially reduces the logistical complexity and financial expense of the investigation.

The case-control design does not provide an estimate of disease incidence in vaccinees and nonvaccinees; therefore, the RR component of the protective efficacy formula is not directly calculable. However, when the disease outcome for the study is rare or when suitable sampling strategies are used for selecting cases and controls [93], the RR from a controlled cohort design is approximated by the odds ratio (OR) of vaccination in cases vs. controls, where OR = (odds of vaccination in cases)/(odds of vaccination in controls) and PE = $(1-OR) \times 100\%$.

A major disadvantage of this approach is that, because cases are defined only on the basis of one disease outcome, a case-control study can evaluate only one outcome of vaccination. However, with a well-focused research hypothesis, case-control studies can enable powerful assessments of vaccine performance in practice. For example, recent case-control studies have provided useful postlicensure evaluations of vaccine protection against such rare diseases as invasive Hib [94] and pneumococcal [4] infections. In addition, this design has proved extremely helpful in evaluating rare but serious potential adverse effects, such as Guillain–Barré syndrome following vaccination with swine influenza vaccine and serious pediatric neurological syndromes following vaccination with conventional whole-cell pertussis vaccine [82,95].

Variant Designs. It has been proposed that vaccine performance can sometimes be assessed in the context of prevalence surveys designed primarily to assess vaccine coverage of a target population [75]. At the time of the survey, respondents are asked about the date of past vaccination as well as the date of intervening disease, and vaccine protection is calculated as if a conventional controlled cohort study had been carried out on vaccinees vs. non-vaccinees. This design differs from a conventional controlled cohort study in that it evaluates only those members of the original cohorts of vaccinees and nonvaccinees who are still present at the time of the survey. It thereby ignores cohort members who have migrated out or died during the interval before the survey. Consequently, this design is sometimes referred to as a "residue cohort." An interesting hybrid design was developed to assess pneumococcal polysaccharide vaccine protection [96]. In this design, isolates from cases of invasive pneumococcal disease sent to a referral center were typed, and histories of antecedent vaccination were obtained without knowledge of these types. Considering that conventional pneumococcal polysaccharide vaccine contains only a fraction of pneumococcal serotypes encountered in infected patients and because serotypes contained in the vaccine are not expected to protect against infections caused by other serotypes, the nonvaccine serotype infections can be considered a suitable control group for the vaccine serotype "cases," and the expression $(1-OR) \times 100\%$ estimates vaccine protective efficacy.

Finally, because it is sometimes necessary to evaluate putative vaccine side effects in situations in which vaccine coverage is very high, leaving very few unvaccinated subjects for comparison, an innovative design, termed "case-series," has been used. In this design, the incidence of the side effect of interest is compared within two windows of time for the same subject: a window of vulnerability, the postdosing interval in which the side effect is postulated to occur; and a window of invulnerability, another postdosing interval, reasonably proximate in time to the window of invulnerability, in which the side effect is postulated not to occur. This is analogous to cross-over designs used in RCTs, in which the essential comparison is the within-subject occurrence of the target outcome before and after the cross-over from one agent to another. Interestingly, this design was used very successfully in the evaluation of intussusception following oral receipt of live rhesus rotavirus-reassortant vaccine, an event that is now well documented, was not an expected side effect of this vaccine, at least at the time that Phase III trials were undertaken [63]. Case-series analysis produced estimates of the relative risk of this outcome in vaccinees that were quite similar to estimates from case-control studies [97].

3. Increasing Importance of Population-Based Databases

Recent years have witnessed an explosion of allegations about putative serious side effects associated with receipt of vaccines. Some of these alleged associations, such as the occurrence of intussusception following oral receipt of live rhesus rotavirus-reassortant vaccine, have been verified by credible scientific studies [97,98]. Others, such as the alleged occurrence of inflammatory bowel disease or autism following MMR vaccine, have not been substantiated [99,100]. Because assertions about vaccine safety can threaten public confidence in vaccines used in routine practice, it has proved essential that credible, suitably controlled studies be undertaken and completed rapidly when such assertions arise. In the past, public health systems relied principally on side effects voluntarily reported by individual physicians. An example of such a system is the Vaccine Adverse Event Reporting System (VAERS) managed by the Public Health Service [101]. Because of the selective and incomplete reporting of side effects inherent in these systems, as well as uncertainties about the occurrence of denominators of vaccinees at risk and the occurrence of target side effects in nonvaccinees, special large-linked, computerized databases were created, such as the Vaccine Safety Datalink (VSD), which was established by the Centers for Disease Control [102]. These databases link histories of receipt or nonreceipt of vaccines in a defined population with comprehensive records of treatment encounters and hospitalizations for specific outcome conditions in the same population. In addition, information about demographic and socioeconomic variables for each subject are collected, to permit control for possible confounders in analyses of vaccine–side effect associations. If maintained for a suitably large cohort of the target population, these databases enable rapid, controlled analyses and provide the public health community with the evidence necessary for proper regulation of the usage of licensed vaccines. Unfortunately, although such databases are becoming increasingly common in industrialized countries, they are virtually nonexistent in developing countries, where there is an urgent need for postlicensure surveillance of vaccines [103].

4. Methodological Limitations of Observational Vaccine Evaluations

Postlicensure observational studies are indispensable tools for providing information about the safety of vaccines and the protection they confer as they are routinely given in practice. Nevertheless, it is important that investigators be aware of certain general limitations of these studies. As already mentioned, the absence of concurrent controls and the indirect focus on populations rather than a direct focus on individuals constitute weaknesses of indirect before-and-after studies which can severely limit the inferences that can be drawn from these studies. However, even direct study designs can be limited by problems with the quality of information used, by bias, and by intrinsic difficulties in estimating the total protective impact upon the target disease, including both direct and indirect protection.

Most observational assessments of vaccines rely on retrospective information, either documented or recalled, to ascertain histories of vaccination and the occurrence of disease outcomes. The accuracy of this information can be reduced, sometimes significantly, by imperfect recall, inaccurate routine diagnoses, inaccurate records, and incomplete records. These issues are not major problems for RCTs of vaccines, because vaccination is assigned in such trials and surveillance for disease outcomes is prospective, usually incorporating uniform diagnostic procedures and criteria as well as systematic recording of outcomes.

Bias in observational studies, which distorts the relationship between vaccination and disease outcomes, can arise either because of the way that a vaccine is given and outcomes are detected in practice, or because of the way the investigators choose groups for comparisons and collect information about individuals in these groups. Bias can arise when persons who are vaccinated in practice do not represent the target population for vaccination with respect to their risks of disease outcomes and when vaccinated and nonvaccinated persons do not receive equally intense and accurate diagnostic surveillance for disease outcomes. Moreover, in selecting vaccinees and nonvaccinees for a controlled, cohort study or cases and controls for a case-control study, there is the potential for biased choices to be made that can alter vaccine–disease outcome relationships. Finally, biases can occur in classifying the vaccination and disease status of study subjects if decisions about vaccination status are not made without knowledge of disease status and vice versa. As noted earlier, the randomization, double blinding, comprehensive follow-up, and systematic and accurate diagnostic procedures employed in an RCT of a vaccine provide the best available safeguards against these biases.

As noted earlier, for infections transmitted from person to person, attainment of a sufficiently high level of vaccine coverage of the target population has the potential not only to reduce the susceptibility to infection directly, via induction of protective immunity, but also to augment this protection indirectly by interrupting transmission of the pathogen in the community. However, because postlicensure observational assessments typically compare disease outcomes among vaccinees vs. nonvaccinees sampled from the same population, and because the benefits of reduced transmission within a population are shared by both vaccinees and nonvaccinees, these studies will usually fail to fully measure the indirect protective effects of vaccination in vaccines and will totally miss the herd immune benefits of vaccination that accrue to nonvaccinees [23–25].

Finally, despite past successes of the case-crossover design in evaluating the associations between vaccines and side effects, it must be realized that use of the design is limited to the relatively uncommon situations in which clear-cut windows of vulnerability and invulnerability can be defined in advance of the study. Moreover, because the serial order of windows of vulnerability and invulnerability are typically defined in the same way for each subject in a case-crossover study, and is not randomized as in a cross-over clinical trial, these studies are potentially vulnerable to biases which can occur if the incidence of side effects is confounded by ordered effects.

Citation of these limitations is not meant to denigrate the value or utility of postlicensure observational studies. Nor is it meant to detract from available tactics in the design, execution, and analysis of these studies that can minimize these potential problems [104]. However, it should be clear from this discussion that the double-blinded RCT serves as the gold-standard design for ensuring the validity of a vaccine evaluation and that postlicensure observational assessments can only strive to approach the assurance of validity provided by properly executed trials.

V. COMMENT

In this chapter, we have attempted to outline the basic paradigm for the design of modern field trials to evaluate new vaccines. The broad outlines of the RCT paradigm are relatively simple and, in principle, are identical with well-established guidelines for designing trials of clinical therapies [87]. Despite this apparent overall simplicity, however, numerous subtle issues arise when the general principles are applied to the specific questions raised in a particular trial. The perspective of the research question must be clarified, and the design of the trial must be carefully adapted so that the study population, compared agents, and outcomes address this question. Wherever possible, strategies must be formulated to minimize the opportunity for distortion of results by bias while, at the same time, yielding estimates of vaccine protection, safety, and immunogenicity with acceptable statistical precision and generalizability. Extensive background data are required to plan a trial with these features, and great care is required to document the performance of the trial and the absence of bias at every stage of its execution.

We have not included any discussion of the additional complexities that occur when RCTs are conducted in a multicenter fashion or in less developed settings, nor have we addressed the many issues which are important in executing a field trial [105]. A minimum list of these issues would include scrupulous attention to fulfilling contemporary ethical requirements, which are rapidly changing [105–108]; the development and maintenance of productive relationships between the research project and the participating community as well as between scientific collaborators in the project; recruitment, training, and supervision of personnel; procurement and maintenance of supplies and equipment; supervision, coordination, and quality control of field and laboratory procedures; and proper collection and management of data. Even with an excellently designed study, suitable attention to these issues will be required for the achievement of a successful trial.

Finally, we have attempted to underscore the importance of continued evaluation of the performance of a vaccine, even after it has been deployed in practice. Because such assessments must usually rely on observational study designs, they will be considerably more vulnerable to biases than Phase III RCTs. Nevertheless, when conducted with attention to safeguards against these biases, such studies provide critical information to public health workers in their attempt to ensure not merely that vaccines are delivered to a high fraction of the targeted population but also that recipients of the vaccine are being protected as expected and are not experiencing unacceptable vaccine side effects.

REFERENCES

1. Lepow M, Nankervis G. Eight-year serologic evaluation of Edmonston live measles vaccine. J Pediatr 1969; 75:407–411.
2. Dam HG, et al. Present knowledge of immunization against tuberculosis. Bull WHO 1976; 54:255–269.
3. Murphy T. Haemophilus b polysaccharide vaccine: need for continuing assessment. Pediatr Infect Dis 1987; 6:701–703.
4. Shapiro E, et al. The protective efficacy of polyvalent pneumococcal polysaccharide vaccine. N Engl J Med 1991; 325: 1453–1460.
5. Orenstein WA, et al. Field evaluation of vaccine efficacy. Bull WHO 1985; 63:1055–1068.
6. Byar DP, et al. Randomized clinical trials: perspectives on some recent ideas. N Engl J Med 1976; 295:74–80.
7. Bailar J. Introduction. In: Shapiro SH, Louis TA, eds. Clinical Trials: Issues and Approaches. New York: Marcel Dekker, 1983:1.
8. Greenwood M, Yule G. The statistics of anti-typhoid and anti-cholera inoculations. Proc R Soc Med 1915; 8:113.
9. Szmuness W, et al. Hepatitis B vaccine: demonstration of efficacy in a controlled clinical trial in a high risk population in the United States. N Engl J Med 1980; 303:833–841.
10. Institute of Medicine. New vaccine development. Establishing Priorities: Vol. 2. Diseases of Importance in Developing Countries. Washington, DC: National Academy Press, 1986: 241.
11. Levine RJ, Lebacqz K. Ethical considerations in clinical trials. Clin Pharm Ther 1979; 25:728–749.
12. Clemens J, Horwitz R. Longitudinal methods for evaluating therapy. Biomed Pharmacother 1984; 38:440–443.
13. Feinstein AR. Clinical biostatistics—III: The architecture of clinical research. Clin Pharmacol Ther 1970; 11:432–441.
14. Peto R, et al. Design and analysis of randomized clinical trials requiring prolonged observation of each patient: I. Introduction and design. Br J Cancer 1976; 34:585–612.
15. Peto R, et al. Design and analysis of randomized clinical trials requiring prolonged observation of each patient: II. Analysis and examples. Br J Cancer 1977; 35:1–39.
16. Chalmers TC. The control of bias in clinical trials. In: Shapiro SH, Louis TA, eds. Clinical Trials: Issues and Approaches. New York: Marcel Dekker, 1983:115.
17. Feinstein AR. Clinical biostatistics: XXII. The role of randomization in sampling, testing, allocation, and credulous idolatry (part 1). Clin Pharmacol Ther 1973; 14:601–615.
18. Feinstein AR. Clinical biostatistics: XXIII. The role of randomization in sampling, testing, allocation, and credulous idolatry (part 2). Clin Pharmacol Ther 1973; 14:898–915.
19. Feinstein AR. Clinical biostatistics: XXIV. The role of randomization in sampling, testing, allocation, and credulous idolatry (conclusion). Clin Pharmacol Ther 1973; 14:1035–1051.
20. Meier P. Statistical analysis of clinical trials. In: Shapiro SH, Louis TA, eds. Clinical Trials: Issues and Approaches. New York: Marcel Dekker, 1983:115.
21. Clemens JD, et al. The BCG controversy: a methodological and statistical reappraisal. J Am Med Assoc 1983; 249: 2362–2469.
22. Halloran M, et al. Direct and indirect effects in vaccine efficacy and effectiveness. Am J Epidemiol 1991; 133:323–331.
23. Fine P. Herd immunity: history, theory, practice. Epidemiol Rev 1993; 15:265–302.
24. Clemens J, et al. Evaluating new vaccines for developing countries: efficacy or effectiveness? J Am Med Assoc 1996; 275:390–397.
25. Struchiner C, et al. The behaviour of common measure of association used to assess a vaccination programme under complex disease transmission patterns—a computer simulation study of malaria vaccines. Int J Epidemiol 1990; 19: 187–196.
26. Moulton L, et al. Design of a group-randomized Streptococcus pneumoniae vaccine trial. Control Clin Trials 2001; 22:438–452.
27. Cochrane AL. Effectiveness and Efficiency. London: Nuffield Provincial Hospitals Trust, 1972.
28. Schwartz D, Lellouch J. Explanatory and pragmatic attitudes in therapeutic trials. J Chronic Dis 1967; 20:637–648.
29. Sackett DL. The competing objectives of randomized trials. N Engl J Med 1980; 303:1059–1060.
30. Sackett D, Gent M. Controversy in counting and attributing events in clinical trials. N Engl J Med 1979; 301:1410–1412.
31. Smit P, et al. Protective efficacy of pneumococcal polysaccharide vaccines. J Am Med Assoc 1977; 238:2613–2616.
32. Schwartz JS. Pneumococcal vaccine: clinical efficacy and effectiveness. Ann Intern Med 1982; 96:208–220.
33. Fraser DW, Broome CV. Pneumococcal vaccine: to use or not. J Am Med Assoc 1981; 245:498–499.
34. Wahdan MH, et al. A controlled trial of live Salmonella typhi Ty21a oral vaccine against typhoid: three year results. J Infect Dis 1982; 145:292–295.
35. Levine MM, et al. Large-scale field trial of Ty21a live oral typhoid vaccine in enteric-coated capsule formulation. Lancet 1987; 1:1049–1052.
36. Levine MM, et al. The efficacy of attenuated Salmonella typhi oral vaccine strain Ty21a evaluated in controlled field trials. In: Holmgren J, Lindberg A, Molby R, eds. Development of Vaccines and Drugs Against Diarrhoea. Lund, Sweden: Student Litteratur, 1986:90.
36a. Levine MM, et al. Comparison of enteric-coated capsules and liquid formulation of Ty21a typhoid vaccine in randomised controlled field trial. Lancet 1990; 336:891–894.
36b. Ferreccio C, et al. Comparative efficacy of two, three, or four doses of Ty21a live oral typhoid vaccine in enteric-coated capsules: a field trial in an endemic area. J Infect Dis 1989; 159:766–769.
37. Lagos R, et al. Large-scale, postlicensure, selective vaccination of Chilean infants with PRP–T conjugate vaccine: practicality and effectiveness in preventing invasive Haemophilus influenzae type b infections. Pediatr Infect Dis 1996; 15:216–222.
38. Booy R, et al. Efficacy of Haemophilus influenzae type b conjugate vaccine PRP-T. Lancet 1994; 344:362–366.
39. Black RE, et al. Protective efficacy in humans of killed whole Vibrio oral cholera vaccine with and without the B subunit of cholera toxin. Infect Immun 1987; 55:1116–1120.

40. Clemens JD, et al. Field trial of oral cholera vaccines in Bangladesh. Lancet 1986; 2:124–127.

41. Armitage P. Exclusions, losses to follow-up, and withdrawals from clinical trials. In: Shapiro SH, Louis TA, eds. Clinical Trials: Issues and Approaches. New York: Marcel Dekker, 1983:99.

42. Sackett D. On some prerequisites for a successful clinical trial. In: Shapiro SH, Louis TA, eds. Clinical Trials: Issues and Approaches. New York: Marcel Dekker, 1983:65.

43. Donner A. Approaches to sample size estimation in the design of clinical trials—a review. Stat Med 1984; 3:199–214.

44. Armitage P. Statistical Methods in Medical Research. Oxford, England: Blackwell, 1971:183.

45. Glass RI, et al. Endemic cholera in rural Bangladesh, 1966–80. Am J Epidemiol 1977; 116:959–970.

46. Clemens J, et al. The design and analysis of cholera vaccine trials: recent lessons from Bangladesh. Int J Epidemiol 1993; 22:724–730.

47. Clemens JD, et al. Nonparticipation as a determinant of adverse health outcomes in a field trial of oral cholera vaccines. Am J Epidemiol 1992; 135:865–874.

48. Clemens J, et al. Field trial of oral cholera vaccines in Bangladesh: results from three-year follow-up. Lancet 1990; 335:270–273.

49. Drummond M. Guidelines for health technology assessment: economic evaluation. In: Feeny D, Guyatt G, Tugwell P, eds. Health Care Technology: Effectiveness, Efficiency, and Public Policy. Vol. 18. Montreal: The Institute for Research on Public Policy, 1986:107–128.

50. Mosteller F. Controversies in design and analysis of clinical trials. In: Shapiro SH, Louis TA, eds. Clinical Trials: Issues and Approaches. New York: Marcel Dekker, 1983:13.

51. Smith D, et al. Impact of multiple comparisons in randomized clinical trials. Am J Med 1987; 83:545–550.

52. Freiman J, et al. The importance of beta, the type II error, and the sample size in the design and interpretation of the randomized control trial. Survey of 71 "negative" trials. N Engl J Med 1978; 299:690–694.

53. Smith PG, Day NE. The design of case-control studies: the influence of confounding and interaction effects. Int J Epidemiol 1984; 13:356–365.

54. Clemens J, et al. Field trial of oral cholera vaccines in Bangladesh: results of one year of follow-up. J Infect Dis 1998; 158:60–69.

55. Blackwelder W. Similarity/equivalence trials for combination vaccines. Ann NY Acad Sci 1995; 754:321–328.

56. Lachin J. Statistical elements of the randomized clinical trial. In: Tygstrup N, Lachin J, Juhl E, eds. The Randomized Clinical Trial and Therapeutic Decisions. New York: Marcel Dekker, 1982:82.

57. Feinstein AR, Landis JR. The role of prognostic stratification in preventing bias permitted by random allocation of treatment. J Chronic Dis 1976; 29:277–284.

58. Pocock S. Clinical Trials: A Practical Approach. Chichester, England: Wiley, 1983:80–81.

59. Donner A, Donald A. Analysis of data arising from a stratified design with the cluster as the unit of randomization. Stat Med 1987; 6:43–52.

60. Black RE, et al. Incidence and severity of rotavirus and *Escherichia coli* diarrhoea in rural Bangladesh: implications for vaccine development. Lancet 1981; 1:141–143.

61. Grob P, et al. Effect of vaccination on the severity and dissemination of whooping cough. Br Med J 1981; 2:1925–1928.

62. Clemens J, et al. Evidence that inactivated oral cholera vaccines both prevents and mitigates *Vibrio cholerae* 01 infections in a cholera-endemic area. J Infect Dis 1992; 166:1029–1034.

63. Jacobsen R, et al. Adverse events and vaccination—the lack of power and predictability of infrequent events in a pre-licensure study. Vaccine 2001; 19:2428–2433.

64. Granoff DM, et al. *Haemophilus influenzae* type b disease in children vaccinated with type b polysaccharide vaccine. N Engl J Med 1986; 315:1584–1590.

65. Expanded Programme on Immunization. Safety of high titre measles vaccine. Weekly Epidemiol Rec 1992; 67:357–362.

66. Frances DP, Petricciana JC. The prospects and pathways toward a vaccine for AIDS. N Engl J Med 1985; 313:1586–1590.

67. Meinert C. Clinical Trials: Design, Conduct, and Analysis. Oxford, England: Oxford University Press, 1986:208–216.

68. Great Britain Medical Research Council. BCG and vole bacillus vaccines in the prevention of tuberculosis in adolescence and early life. Br Med J 1956; 1:413.

69. Brown JA, et al. BCG vaccination of children against leprosy: first results of a trial in Uganda. Br Med J 1966; 1:7–14.

70. Fleiss J. Statistics for Rates and Proportions. 2d ed. New York: Wiley, 1981:193.

71. Clemens JD, et al. Impact of B subunit killed whole-cell and killed whole-cell only oral vaccines against cholera upon treated diarrhoeal illness and mortality in an area endemic for cholera. Lancet 1988; 1:1375–1379.

72. Miller R. Simultaneous Statistical Inference. New York: McGraw-Hill, 1966:10–12.

73. Rothman K. A show of confidence. N Engl J Med 1978; 299:1362–1363.

74. International Conference on Harmonisation. E6: Guideline for Good Clinical Practice, 1996.

75. Orenstein W, et al. Assessing vaccine efficacy in the field: further observations. Epidemiol Rev 1988; 10:212–241.

76. Patriarca P, et al. Efficacy of influenza vaccine in nursing homes: reduction in illness and complications during an influenza A (H_3N_2) epidemic. J Am Med Assoc 1985; 253:1136–1139.

77. Marks J, et al. Methodological issues in the evaluation of vaccine effectiveness: measles vaccine al 12 vs. 15 months. Am J Epidemiol 1982; 116:510–523.

78. Egan W, et al. Lot-release criteria, post-licensure quality control, and the *Haemophilus influenzae* type b conjugate vaccines. J Am Med Assoc 1995; 273:888–889.

79. Nathanson N, Langmuir A. The Cutter incident: poliomyelitis following formaldehyde-inactivated poliovirus vaccination in the United States during spring of 1995: II. Relationship of poliomyelitis to Cutter vaccine. Am J Hyg 1963; 78:29–60.

80. Patriarca P, et al. Factors affecting the immunogenicity of oral polio vaccine in developing countries: a review. Rev Infect Dis 1991; 13:926–939.

81. Patriarca P, et al. Randomised trial of alternative formulations of oral polio vaccine in Brazil. Lancet 1988; 1:429–433.

82. Schonberger L, et al. Guillian–Barré syndrome following vaccination in the national influenza immunization program, United States, 1976–77. Am J Epidemiol 1979; 110:105–111.

83. Lerman S, Gold E. Measles in children previously vaccinated against measles. J Am Med Assoc 1971; 216:1311–1314.

84. Pappaioanou M, et al. Antibody response to preexposure human diploid-cell rabies vaccine given concurrently with chloroquine. N Engl J Med 1986; 314:280–284.

85. Peltola H, et al. Rapid disappearance of *Haemophilus influenzae* type b meningitis after routine childhood immunization with conjugate vaccines. Lancet 1992; 340:592–594.

86. Anderson E, et al. Interchangeability of conjugate *Haemophilus influenzae* type b vaccines in infants. J Am Med Assoc 1995; 273:849–853.

87. Feinstein AR. Clinical Epidemiology: The Architecture of Clinical Research. Philadelphia: Saunders, 1985:17–18.

88. Peltola H, et al. Rapid effect on endemic measles, mumps, and rubella of nation-wide vaccination programme in Finland. Lancet 1986; 1:137–139.

89. De Quadros C, et al. Eradication of poliomyelitis: progress in the Americas. Pediatr Infect Dis J 1991; 10:222–229.

90. Smith P, et al. Assessment of protective efficacy of vaccines against common diseases using case-control and cohort studies. Int J Epidemiol 1984; 13:87–93.

91. Hull H, et al. Measles mortality and vaccine efficacy in rural West Africa. Lancet 1983; 1:972–975.

92. Comstock G. Evaluating vaccination effectiveness and vaccine efficacy by means of case-control studies. Epidemiol Rev 1994; 16:77–89.

93. Rodrigues L, Kirkwood B. Case-control designs in the study of common diseases: updates on the demise of the rare disease assumption and the choice of sampling scheme for controls. Int J Epidemiol 1990; 19:205–213.

94. Shapiro ET, et al. The protective efficacy of Haemophilus b vaccine polysaccharide vaccine. J Am Med Assoc 1988; 260:1419–1422.

95. Alderslade R, et al. The National Childhood Encephalopathy Study. Whooping Cough: Reports from the Committee on the Safety of Medicines and the Joint Committee on Vaccination and Immunisation. London: Department of Health and Social Security, Her Majesty's Stationary Office, 1981:79–154.

96. Bolan G, et al. Pneumococcal vaccine efficacy in selected populations in the United States. Ann Intern Med 1986; 104:1–6.

97. Murphy TV, et al. Intussusception among infants given an oral rotavirus vaccine. N Engl J Med 2001; 344:564–572.

98. Kramarz P, et al. Population-based study of rotavirus vaccination and intussusception. Pediatr Infect Dis 2001; 20:410–416.

99. Wakefield AJ, et al. Ileal–lymphoid–nodular hyperplasia, non-specific colitis, and pervasive developmental disorder in children. Lancet 1998; 351:637–641.

100. Taylor B, et al. Autism and measles, mumps, and rubella vaccine: no epidemiological evidence for a causal association. Lancet 1999; 53:2026–2029.

101. Chen RT, et al. The Vaccine Adverse Event Reporting System (VAERS). Vaccine 1994; 12:542–550.

102. Chen RT, et al. Vaccine Safety Datalink project: a new tool for improving vaccine safety monitoring in the United States. Pediatrics 1997; 99:765–773.

103. Hall A, Clemens J. Adverse reactions to vaccines in the tropics. Trop Med Int Health 2000; 5:229–230.

104. Horwitz R, Feinstein A. The application of therapeutic-trial principles to improve the design of epidemiologic research: a case-control study suggesting that anticoagulants reduce mortality in patients with acute myocardial infarction. J Chronic Dis 1981; 34:575–583.

105. Smith P, Morrow R. Field Trials of Health Interventions in Developing Countries: A tool box. 2d ed. London: Macmillan Education Ltd, 1966:72–81.

106. World Medical Association. Declaration of Helsinki: recommendations guiding medical doctors in biomedical research involving human subjects. Helsinki: World Medical Association, 1964 (Revised 1975, 1983, 1989 and 2000).

107. Council for International Organizations of Medical Sciences (CIOMS). International Ethical Guidelines for Biomedical Research Involving Human Subjects. Geneva, 1993.

108. Piantadosi S. Ethical consideration. Clinical Trial. A Methodologic Perspective. New York: John Wiley & Sons, 1997: 41.

5

Ethical Considerations in the Conduct of Vaccine Trials in Developing Countries

Charles Weijer
Dalhousie University, Halifax, Nova Scotia, Canada

Claudio F. Lanata
Instituto de Investigacion Nutricional, Lima, Peru

No single issue in the last two decades of the ethics of research has evoked as much controversy as the conduct of clinical trials in developing countries. Facets of the controversy include the following questions: Is there a single international standard for informed consent? Is there a role for community consultation and consent? Where should clinical trials first be conducted? Which standard of care, that of the host or that of the sponsor country, is the right standard? What is owed to research participants at the conclusion of the study? How to manage review of research by multiple ethics committees? Each of these questions ultimately emanates from global cultural diversity and inequities in the distribution of healthcare resources.

The debate was sparked by a 1997 article in the *New England Journal of Medicine* challenging the use of placebo in clinical trials testing short-course zidovudine for the prevention of perinatal transmission of HIV [1]. At the time of the trials, the ACTG 076 regimen was widely used in developed countries and was known to be effective in reducing the rate of perinatal transmission of HIV by approximately two-thirds. Thus, the authors argue, the use of placebo rather than the ACTG 076 regimen as a control treatment in these trials deprived research participants access to effective treatment. Permitting such trials to go forward would in effect, they believe, sanction a double standard for research in developed and developing countries.

Defenders of the short-course zidovudine trials point out that the call for these trials came from developing countries themselves [2]. Important differences relevant to perinatal transmission of HIV exist between developing and developed countries: Antenatal care is not widely accessible in developing countries; facilities for the intravenous administration of zidovudine required by the ACTG 076 regimen do not exist; mothers who are infected with HIV are none-theless advised to breast feed; and the ACTG 076 regimen is simply unaffordable. Thus the relevant question to physicians and their patients in developing countries is not how the short-course regimen compares to an inaccessible treatment, rather how it compares to the best-available care locally, namely, nothing [3].

Vaccine research in developing countries has not been immune to controversy. A series of clinical trials in the United States and Finland demonstrated that the tetravalent rhesus rotavirus (RRV-TV) vaccine prevents serious rotavirus diarrhea in developed countries [4–7] as well as in developing countries [8,9]. After being approved by the Food and Drug Administration (FDA), it was recommended for universal use in the United States. However, once widespread vaccination in the United States was underway and 1.5 million doses were given, a transient association between RRV-TV vaccination and intussusception was observed. In October 1999, while the definitive studies to prove this association were under way, the vaccine manufacturer voluntarily withdrew the RRV-TV vaccine from the U.S. market. This led to dispute as to whether research with the vaccine should (or could) continue in developing countries [10].

The purpose of this chapter is to provide the vaccine researcher working in developing countries with an understanding of the basic ethical principles of research, international regulations, and current ethical controversies when conducting research with human subjects in developing countries.

I. ETHICAL PRINCIPLES

The conduct of clinical research is guided by three ethical principles, first articulated in the *Belmont Report*: respect for persons, beneficence, and justice [11]. The principle of respect for persons requires that researchers seriously take the choices of people who are capable of deciding for themselves. Furthermore, those who cannot decide for themselves are entitled to protection. The principle of respect for persons maps onto the moral rule of informed consent. It is the source of the researcher's obligation to obtain agreement from each research subject for study participation. For informed consent to be valid, the research subject must have the capacity to make the choice, to be able to make a free choice, to be adequately informed, and to understand the information with which the subject has been presented.

The principle of beneficence is typically expressed in terms of two complementary rules. First, do no harm; second, maximize potential benefits while minimizing risks. The complexity of risk analysis in research belies simplistic expressions, such as an "acceptable harm–benefit ratio" or "balance of benefits to harms." The first step in unpacking these metaphors is the recognition that clinical research may contain a mixture of procedures, some offering potential benefit to research subjects (therapeutic procedures), while others are solely administered to answer the study question (nontherapeutic procedures) [12].

Therapeutic procedures in clinical research are justified if there exists a state of honest, professional disagreement in the community of expert practitioners as to the preferred treatment [13]. This so-called state of clinical equipoise ensures that the medical treatment of a patient is not diminished by virtue of study participation. Nontherapeutic procedures, by definition, do not offer the prospect of benefit to individual study participants, and hence a harm–benefit calculus is inappropriate. Rather, nontherapeutic procedures are acceptable if the risks associated with them are minimized, and are reasonable in relation to the knowledge to be gained [12]. For a study to be allowed to proceed, the moral tests for both therapeutic and nontherapeutic procedures must be passed.

The principle of justice may be defined as an ethical obligation to fairly treat people. Researchers must neither exploit the vulnerable, nor exclude without good reason those who stand to benefit from study participation [14]. For proposed eligibility criteria to be evaluated, each criterion must be accompanied by a clear justification in the study protocol. The inclusion of a vulnerable population in research must also be justified. Research subjects may be vulnerable in one or more of three ways: they are unduly susceptible to harm (e.g., pregnant women); they are incapable of providing informed consent (e.g., children); or they are so situated as to cast the voluntariness of consent in doubt (e.g., prisoners) [15]. Finally, in so far as is possible and practicable, the study population ought to mirror the target clinical population.

II. INTERNATIONAL REGULATION

International codes of ethics for research are a response to a history of abuses in research involving human subjects.

During the Nuremberg war-crime trials, an influential set of principles for research was drawn up in 1947, which were later known as the Nuremberg Code. Subsequently, the United Nations General Assembly signed in 1948 the Universal Declaration of Human Rights, which includes a right not to be experimented upon without informed consent. The World Medical Association (WMA) began drafting a code specifically for physicians conducting research in 1953. However, it was not until 1964 that the recommendations were adopted as the *Declaration of Helsinki*. The *Declaration of Helsinki* has been revised five times, most recently in 2000 [16]. The Council for International Organizations of Medical Sciences (CIOMS) published lengthy and detailed commentary on the *Declaration of Helsinki* with a special emphasis on research conducted in developing countries in 1993 called the *International Ethical Guidelines for Biomedical Research Involving Human Subjects*. This document was revised in 2002 [17]. In 1996, the International Conference on Harmonization published its *Guidance on Good Clinical Practice*. The document provides unified technical standards for clinical trials, so data generated in one country would be mutually acceptable by regulatory authorities the United States, Japan, and the European Union. Finally, in 2000, Joint United Nations Program on HIV/AIDS published *Ethical Considerations in HIV Preventive Vaccine Research* to provide guidance to HIV vaccine researchers [18].

Clearly researchers conducting vaccine trials in developing countries face a complex web of international regulations (Table 1). What guidance can be distilled for researchers?

The most relevant international documents to vaccine researchers are the WMA *Declaration of Helsinki*, CIOMS *International Ethical Guidelines for Biomedical Research Involving Human Subjects* (Table 2), and the UNAIDS *Ethical Considerations in HIV Preventive Vaccine Research*. As we shall discuss below, each of the documents contains controversial provisions. The documents also possess important elements in common. As each document is guided by the same moral principles, it is not surprising that there is considerable convergence among these documents. All of the documents require that proposals to conduct clinical research be submitted to an independent committee to ensure ethical acceptability (WMA 13; CIOMS 2; UNAIDS 6). Informed consent must be obtained from study participants (WMA 22; CIOMS 4; UNAIDS 12). If a research subject is incapable of providing consent, then the consent to study participation must be sought from the subject's legally authorized representative (WMA 24; CIOMS 4; UNAIDS 18). The potential benefits and harms of study participation must be carefully evaluated (WMA 16; CIOMS 8; UNAIDS 9,10). Finally, vulnerable populations in research are entitled to special protection (WMA 8; CIOMS 13; UNAIDS 7).

While this general guidance is of use to all researchers, those conducting vaccine trials in the international setting require more specific guidance, especially on issues of current controversy. The following guidance is based on provisions in one or more of the relevant international guide-

Table 1 Chronology of International Ethics Guidelines for Biomedical Research

Year	Document	Issuing authority
1947	Nuremberg Code	
1948	Universal Declaration of Human Rights	United Nations General Assembly
1964	Declaration of Helsinki (1)	World Medical Association
1966	International Covenant on Civil and Political Rights	United Nations General Assembly
1975	Declaration of Helsinki (2nd revision—Tokyo)	World Medical Association
1983	Declaration of Helsinki (3rd revision—Venice)	World Medical Association
1989	Declaration of Helsinki (4th revision—Hong Kong)	World Medical Association
1989	Convention on the Rights of Children	United Nations General Assembly
1991	International Guidelines for Ethical Review of Epidemiological Studies	Council for International Organizations of Medical Sciences -CIOMS /World Health Organization -WHO
1993	International Ethical Guidelines for Biomedical Research Involving Human Subjects	Council for International Organizations of Medical Sciences—CIOMS/World Health Organization (WHO)
1995	Guidelines for Good Clinical Practice for Trials on Pharmaceutical Products	World Health Organization (WHO)
1996	Declaration of Helsinki (5th revision—South Africa)	World Medical Association
1996[a]	International Conference on Harmonization (ICH) Guidance on Good Clinical Practice	International Conference on Harmonization/ Committee for Proprietary Medical Products for the Pharmaceutical Industry
2000[a]	Declaration of Helsinki (6th revision—Scotland)	World Medical Association
2000[a]	Ethical Considerations in HIV Preventive Vaccine Research	Joint United Nations Program on HIV/AIDS
2000	Operational Guidelines for Ethics Committees that Review Biomedical Research	World Health Organization
2002	Surveying and Evaluating Ethical Review Practices	World Health Organization
2002[a]	International Ethical Guidelines for Biomedical Research Involving Human Subjects (draft revision)	Council for International Organizations of Medical Sciences—CIOMS/World Health Organization (WHO)

[a] The four most-quoted guidelines for the conduct of biomedical research with human subjects in developing countries include:

The Declaration of Helsinki, in its last revision, contains a terse articulation of 32 principles to guide the conduct of research.

The Guidance on Good Clinical Practice of the International Conference on Harmonization of 1996 provide unified technical standards for clinical trials, so data generated in one country would be mutually acceptable by regulatory authorities the United States, Japan, and the European Union.

Ethical Considerations in HIV Preventive Vaccine Research of the Joint United Nations Program on HIV/AIDS of 2000, which were created to help the conduct of this type of research as a response to the current controversies. It contains 18 guidance points and is unique in its focus on international vaccine research.

The International Ethical Guidelines for Biomedical Research Involving Human Subjects (draft revision) of CIOMS/WHO 2002 are a lengthy and detailed commentary on the Declaration of Helsinki with a special emphasis on research conducted in developing countries. It is intended to help WHO country members to develop their own national ethical policies for clinical research, guiding them how to adapt international ethical principles to their local realities, and to establish adequate procedures for the ethical review of research protocols of studies with human subjects participation. These guidelines contain 23 major recommendations.

lines as interpreted through the lens of grounding moral principles.

III. CURRENT CONTROVERSIES

A. Is There One International Standard for Informed Consent?

The obligation to obtain informed consent from research participants is well established. Precisely how informed consent is sought may reasonably differ from one context to another. The principle of respect for persons requires that

researchers be sensitive to beliefs and values of the group to which prospective study participants belong. If, as all of the documents require, study participants are to be adequately informed, the informed consent process must ensure that details of the research project are expressed in a way that is locally comprehensible. Thus the disclosure process must take into account local beliefs, literacy, and education.

Must research subjects sign a consent document? This concern flows, in part, from the requirement in U.S. regulation to document the consent process. However, from a moral rather than regulatory perspective, what matters is the quality of the disclosure process, and not whether a form is

Table 2 The International Ethical Guidelines for Biomedical Research Involving Human Subjects (CIOMS, 2002)

Section	Guideline	Subject
A. Prerequisities of biomedical research	1	Ethical justification and scientific validity of biomedical research involving human subjects
	2	Ethical review committees
	3	Ethical review of externally sponsored research
B. Informed consent of subjects	4	Individual informed consent
	5	Obtaining informed consent: essential information for prospective research subjects
	6	Obtaining informed consent: obligations of sponsors and investigators
	7	Inducement to participate
C. Assessment of risks and benefits	8	Benefits and risks of study participation
	9	Special limitations on risk when research involves individuals who are not capable of giving informed consent
	10	Research in populations or communities with limited resources
	11	Choice of control in clinical trials
D. Selection of research subjects	12	Equitable distribution of burdens and benefits in the selection of groups of subjects in research
	13	Research involving vulnerable persons
E. Biomedical research in special groups	14	Research involving children
	15	Research involving individuals who by reason of mental or behavioral disorders are not capable of giving adequately informed consent
	16	Women as research subjects
	17	Pregnant women as research subjects
F. Confidentiality of participation and research data	18	Safeguarding confidentiality
G. Compensation of research subjects for injury	19	Right of injured subjects to treatment and compensation
H. Capacity building	20	Strengthening capacity for ethical and scientific review and biomedical research
I. International collaborative research	21	Ethical obligation of external sponsor to provide health-care services

signed. In some cultural and political contexts, signing an official form may be associated with different meanings than in the United States, and hence may be an inappropriate requirement. Thus the CIOMS guidelines observe: "Consent may be indicated in a number of ways. The subject may imply consent by voluntary actions, express consent orally, or sign a consent form (CIOMS 4)." In other cases, documentation of consent may pose a substantial risk to subjects if their medical condition is stigmatized. Thus a waiver of documentation of consent "may also be approved when existence of a signed consent form would be an unjustified threat to the subjects' confidentiality (CIOMS 4)."

B. Is There a Role for Community Consultation and Consent?

The ethical principles in the *Belmont Report* have been criticized for being unduly individualistic and for failing to take into account the interests of communities [19]. As a result, a novel principle of respect for communities has been

proposed. However, the new principle's implementation poses difficult challenges for the researcher working with communities. When research is carried out in resource-poor communities, CIOMS guidelines require that research be "responsive to the health needs and the priorities of the population or community in which it is to be carried out (CIOMS 10)." Ensuring that research is responsive to a particular community's health needs requires a dialogue between community and researcher. Thus "community representatives should be involved in an early and sustained manner in the design, development, implementation, and distribution of results of . . . research (UNAIDS 5)."

In some communities, for instance aboriginal communities, the burden of decision making may traditionally rest more with community leaders than with individual community members [19]. As the CIOMS guidelines point out: "In some cultures an investigator may enter a community to conduct research or approach prospective subjects for their individual consent only after obtaining permission from a community leader, a council of elders, or another designated authority. Such customs must be respected (CIOMS 4)." The moral obligation to show respect for communities must be tempered with the simultaneous duty to demonstrate respect for persons. Thus community consent and individual consent have an asymmetrical relationship. The community's refusal may preclude a researcher's ability to approach community members for consent. "In no case, however, may the permission of a community leader or other authority substitute for individual informed consent (CIOMS 4)."

C. Where Should Clinical Trials First Be Conducted?

For the outsider, one of the curious things about the rotavirus vaccine story, described above, is the fact that clinical trials of the vaccine were first conducted in developed countries, while the majority of mortality from the disease occurs in developing countries. A policy decision to test vaccines of interest to developing countries first in developed countries will predictably lead to two consequences. First, the adoption of useful vaccines in developing countries will be delayed as testing goes on elsewhere. Second, the practice has the unintended effect of setting the bar for adoption of a vaccine too high. A country with a low burden of disease will (appropriately) be less likely to accept even small risks associated with a vaccine than a country with a high burden of disease. A 1 in 10,000 risk of intussusception associated with RRV-TV vaccine is rightly interpreted differently in a country with a mortality rate of 1 in 200,000 from the disease and a country with a mortality rate of 1 in 200 from the disease [10]. Thus any absolute requirement to test a new vaccine in developed countries before testing in developing countries is morally problematic.

In other areas of clinical research, it is generally accepted that clinical trials first need be conducted in high-risk populations, for if a new treatment fails, it is unlikely to be of use to any population. The same follows for vaccine clinical trials. It is important to recognize that there is no insuperable ethical obstacle to conducting early clinical trials in developing countries. The statement found in the UNAIDS document might well be generalized to all vaccine clinical trials. Generally, earlier clinical phases of HIV vaccine research should be conducted in communities that are less vulnerable to harm or exploitation, usually within the sponsor country. However, "countries may choose, for valid scientific and public health reasons, to conduct any study phase within their populations, if they are able to ensure sufficient scientific infrastructure and sufficient ethical safeguards (UNAIDS 8)." Differential burdens of disease or important biological differences, e.g., pattern of disease, between developed and developing country would satisfy the requirement for "valid scientific and public health reasons."

D. Which Standard of Care, that of the Host or Sponsor Country, Is the Right Standard?

The perinatal HIV prevention trials, described above, highlight a deep divide in research ethics regarding the nature of the researcher's obligation to research subjects [20]. A core concept in research ethics is that the medical care of the research subject ought not be disadvantaged by virtue of study participation. In the *Declaration of Helsinki*, this requirement is expressed as: "The benefits, risks, burdens, and effectiveness of a new method should be tested against those of the best current prophylactic, diagnostic, and therapeutic methods (WMA 29)." As there are inequities globally with respect to the distribution of healthcare resources, one might well ask: "Best current . . . therapeutic methods" where?

One might answer that the requisite standard should be that in a developed country or, alternatively, one might answer that it ought to be that in a developing country. Each possibility has its proponents; each set of proponents can point to international ethics documents to support its case. While the text of the *Declaration of Helsinki* is ambiguous on this issue, the intention of its authors is not. In a press release, the World Medical Association states: "The WMA opposes the notion that the nonavailability of drugs should be used as a justification to conduct placebo-controlled trials. Dr. Human [WMA Secretary General] said that 'this would lead to poor countries of the world being used as the laboratory of research institutions of the developed world' [21]." Adopting a local standard of care in isolation would surely present just such a risk to developing countries. However, no one to our knowledge is suggesting such a move.

Proponents of a local standard of care point out that other protections will prevent exploitation. Central to these protections is the requirement that research "responsive to the health needs and the priorities of the population or community in which it is to be carried out (CIOMS 10)." It is difficult to imagine an exploitative study of the sort Dr. Human is worried about that would both pass a local standard of care threshold and meet the health needs and priorities of the community in the developing country. Furthermore, the adoption of a local standard of care threshold also must not be allowed to take advantage of inefficiencies in a developing country's healthcare system. One may morally distinguish between the stated policies and objectives of a healthcare system (de jure local standard of care) and its implementation in the field (de facto local standard of care). The former, and not the latter, should guide the choice of a control treatment for a clinical trial [20]. The UNAIDS document sets a similar standard calling for the "highest level of care attainable in the host country (UNAIDS 16)."

E. What Is Owed to Research Participants at the Conclusion of the Study?

A further protection for research subjects and the communities in which they live is afforded by the obligation to share research benefits with study participants. However, the precise scope of this obligation is a matter of controversy. In the very least, researchers have an obligation to persons who actually participated in the trial. Thus the *Declaration of Helsinki* requires that: "At the conclusion of the study, every patient entered into the study should be assured of access to the best proven prophylactic, diagnostic and therapeutic methods identified by the study (WMA 30)." But might obligation be reasonably construed as broader than this? Some have argued that it may be.

The UNAIDS document places a larger responsibility on researchers to not only provide treatment to those who participated in the study, but also to those "other populations at high risk of HIV infection (UNAIDS 2)." The CIOMS guidelines agree with this position stating that the researcher and sponsor have an obligation to ensure that "any intervention or product developed, or knowledge generated, will be made reasonably available for the benefit of that population or community (CIOMS 10)." The CIOMS document takes the further step in suggesting that researchers and sponsors have an obligation to "ensure that biomedical research projects for which they are responsible in such countries contribute effectively to national or local capacity to design and conduct biomedical research, and to provide scientific and ethical review and monitoring of such research (CIOMS 20)."

The feasibility of these recommendations for the provision of treatment to entire community, population, or country may be questioned. For instance, it would have been very difficult, or even economically impossible, after completing the rotavirus vaccine trials in peri-urban Lima where 800 infants participated to provide the vaccine broadly [22]. The cost of the vaccine when introduced in the U.S. market was $27 per dose [23]. If the scope of the obligation were limited to infants in Lima (the community), this would require the vaccination, for free or at a substantially reduced price, of 150,000 children each year at a cost of $12,000,000. If the scope were broader yet (the country), it would require the vaccination of the 600,000 infants that are born each year in the whole of Peru at a cost of $48,000,000. And then ask the question for how long: One year? Five years? In perpetuity? Clearly, the obligation cannot be interpreted so broadly as to render impossible clinical trials designed to develop important vaccines for developing countries.

F. How to Manage Review of Research by Multiple Ethics Committees?

The review of research by multiple ethics committees poses numerous challenges to all researchers conducting multi-institutional research. Submissions to multiple committees inevitably result in lengthy delays. Worse yet, investigators are likely to encounter divergent responses from differing committees, and required changes from one committee may actually contradict required changes from another. As difficult as these problems are, they are commonplace and well recognized.

Researchers conducting vaccine trials in developing countries face what we believe is an even more difficult problem when research must be approved by ethics committees in both host and sponsor country. The commentary on CIOMS guideline 3 states, "Committees in both the country of the sponsor and the host country have responsibility for conducting both scientific and ethical review, as well as the authority to withhold approval of research proposals that fail to meet their scientific or ethical standards (CIOMS 3)." Conflict predictably ensues from the question: Whose ethical standards shall be followed?

The U.S. government now requires that any foreign institution conducting U.S. funded research sign a document affirming that it will comply with U.S. ethics standards (Assurance of Compliance). One result of this is that rigid criteria are applied to the consent forms used in developing countries. As a result, the length and complexity of information in consent forms has significantly increased over time, perhaps making it more difficult for prospective subjects to understand. When efforts are undertaken in the host country to simplify forms, ethics committees in the sponsoring developed countries often resist even the most reasonable changes.

Two solutions to this situation present themselves. First, the CIOMS guidelines allow for a separation of activities between ethics committees, although responsibility remains joint. CIOMS says, "When a sponsor or investigator in one country proposes to carry out research in another, the ethical review committees in the two countries may, by agreement, undertake to review different aspects of the research protocol (CIOMS 3)." Thus, by agreement, the ethics committee in the sponsoring country could have responsibility to assure the adequacy of the proposed scientific methods and the study's capacity to answer the objectives of the study. On the other hand, the ethics committee in the host country could then focus on ensuring that the study responds to the needs of the country, selection of study participants is equitable, and informed consent will be appropriately obtained.

Second, the United States must utilize the so-called protections at least equivalent clause. Research funded by the U.S. government generally must abide by provisions set out in the U.S. federal *Common Rule* as well as applicable international regulation [24]. Recognizing that international standards may not be identical to U.S. regulations, the *Common Rule* has a provision allowing for other regulations to be followed. It states that:

> [if] a Department or Agency head determines that the procedures prescribed by the institution afford protections that are at least equivalent to those provided in this policy, the Department or Agency head may approve the substitution of the foreign procedures in lieu of the procedural requirements provided in this policy [45 CFR 46.101(h)].

U.S. regulators have yet to specify exactly which international regulations fulfill the protections at least equivalent clause, thereby limiting its application.

IV. CONCLUSION

There can be little question that many challenges face the vaccine researcher in planning and conducting research in a developing country. The task is made more difficult by divergence among ethics guidelines. We hope that future revisions of current guidelines will provide guidance on current controversies and will aim to minimize divergence among documents. It is encouraging that separate bodies in developed countries, such as the U.S. National Bioethics Advisory Commission or the Nuffield Council on Bioethics in the United Kingdom, have indicated that solution to these controversies are not to be found in increased regulations, but in closer ties with developing countries and their institutions and researchers [25].

We agree with this approach. Dialogue and investment are required to join the divide between developed and developing countries in the context of research. There is an urgent need for investment in local capacity for research in developing countries. Only with funds and training from developed countries will researchers in developing countries be able to design and implement their own clinical trials addressing local health priorities. Investment is also required in the development of infrastructure and training for the ethical review of research. The Nuffield Council on Bioethics correctly observes "the guidelines and the *Declaration [of Helsinki]* will not be effective unless they are accompanied by training and the necessary resources to allow its adequate implementation in developing countries [26]."

REFERENCES

1. Lurie P, Wolfe SM. Unethical trials of interventions to reduce perinatal transmission of the human immunodeficiency virus in developing countries. N Engl J Med 1997; 337:853–856.
2. Varmus H, Satcher D. Ethical complexities of conducting research in developing countries. N Engl J Med 1997; 337:1003–1005.
3. Crouch RA, Arras JD. AZT trials and tribulations. Hastings Center Report 1998; 28(6):26–34.
4. Bernstein DI, et al. for the US Rotavirus Vaccine Efficacy Group. Evaluation of rhesus rotavirus monovalent and tetravalent reassortant vaccines in US children. JAMA 1995; 273:1191–1196.
5. Rennels MB, et al. Safety and efficacy of high-dose rhesus–human reassortant rotavirus vaccines report of the National Multicenter Trial. Pediatrics 1996; 97:7–13.
6. Joensuu J, et al. Randomized placebo-controlled trial of rhesus–human reassortant rotavirus vaccine for prevention of severe rotavirus gastroenteritis. Lancet 1997; 350:1205–1209.
7. Santosham M, et al. Efficacy and safety of high-dose rhesus–human reassortant rotavirus vaccine in Native American populations. J Pediatr 1997; 131:632–638.
8. Pérez-Schael I, et al. Efficacy of the rhesus rotavirus-based quadrivalent vaccine in young children in Venezuela. N Engl J Med 1997; 337:1181–1187.
9. Linhares AC, et al. Reappraisal of the Peruvian and Brazilian lower titer tetravalent rhesus–human reassortant rotavirus vaccine efficacy trials: analysis by severity of diarrhea. Pediatr Infect Dis J 1999; 18:1001–1006.
10. Weijer C. The future of research into rotavirus vaccine. Br Med J 2000; 321:525–526.
11. National Commission for the Protection of Human Subjects of Biomedical and Behavioral Research. The Belmont Report: ethical principles and guidelines for the protection of human subjects of research. OPRR [Office for Protection from Research Risks] Reports; 1979 (Apr 18):1–8.
12. Weijer C. The ethical analysis of risk. J Law Med Ethics 2000; 28:344–361.
13. Freedman B. Equipoise and the ethics of clinical research. N Engl J Med 1987; 317:141–145.
14. Weijer C. Selecting subjects for participation in clinical research: one sphere of justice. J Med Ethics 1999; 25:31–36.
15. Weijer C. Research involving the vulnerable sick. Account Res 1999; 7:21–36.
16. World Medical Association. *Declaration of Helsinki*, 2000. Website: *http://www.wma.net/e/policy/63.htm*. Date accessed: July 9, 2003.
17. Council for International Organizations of Medical Sciences (CIOMS). CIOMS International Ethical Guidelines for Biomedical Research Involving Human Subjects, 2002. Website: *http://www.cioms.ch/frame_ guidelines_nov_2002.htm*. Date accessed: July 9, 2003.
18. Joint United Nations Programme on HIV/AIDS (UNAIDS). Ethical considerations in HIV preventive vaccine research. Geneva: UNAIDS, 2000. Website: *http://www.unaids.org/ publications/documents/vaccines/vaccines/ethicsresearch.pdf*. Date accessed: July 9, 2003.
19. Weijer C, et al. Protecting communities in research: current guidelines and limits of extrapolation. Nat Genet 1999; 23: 275–280.
20. London AJ. The ambiguity and the exigency: clarifying 'standard of care' arguments in international research. J Med Philos 2000; 25:379–397.
21. World Medical Association. Media Release, When are placebo controlled trials ethically acceptable? November 28, 2001. Website: *http://www.wma.net/e/press/2001_1.htm*. Date accessed: July 9, 2003.
22. Lanata CF, et al. Safety, immunogenicity and protective efficacy of one or three doses of the *Rhesus* tetravalent rotavirus vaccine in infants from Lima, Peru. J Infect Dis 1996; 174:268–275.
23. Ehrenkranz P, et al. A policy decision for Peru: should rotavirus vaccine be included in the national immunization program? Rev Panam Salud Publica 2001; 10:240–248.
24. Department of Health and Human Services. Protection of human subjects. 45 Code of Federal Regulations 46, 2001. Website: *http://ohrp.osophs.dhhs.gov/humansubjects/guidance/ 45cfr46.htm*. Date accessed: July 9, 2003.
25. National Bioethics Advisory Commission. Ethical and Policy Issues in International Research: Clinical Trials in Developing Countries, 2001. Website: *http://www.georgetown. edu/research/nrcbl/nbac/pubs.html*. Date accessed: July 9, 2003.
26. Nuffield Council on Bioethics. Report: The Ethics of Research Related to Healthcare in Developing Countries, 2002. Website: *http://www.nuffieldbioethics.org/publications/ pp_0000000013.asp*. Date accessed: July 9, 2003.

6

Vaccine Economics: From Candidates to Commercialized Products in the Developing World

Amie Batson and Sarah Glass*
The World Bank, Washington, D.C., U.S.A.

Piers Whitehead
VaxGen Inc., Brisbane, California, U.S.A.

I. INTRODUCTION: THE IMPORTANCE OF ECONOMICS

The development and commercialization of vaccines depends not only on the scientific knowledge underpinning a candidate but also on the economic costs, risks, and returns associated with the required investments. Ultimately, assuring the best use of limited resources, or economics, is an important factor in all vaccine decisions, whether it is which candidates to develop, which vaccine to scale up, what presentation to select, or which vaccine to purchase for use in national immunization programs. Every step of the development process, from vaccine concept to marketable product, is gated by investment decisions. Understanding the economics guiding these decisions will help scientists and public health experts to achieve the objectives of accelerating the development and availability of priority vaccines, particularly for the developing world.

The private sector's[†] current investment in developing and manufacturing vaccines benefiting developing countries is not as large as would be desirable from the public sector[‡] perspective. In 1992, only 4% of the $55.8 billion spent globally on healthcare Research and Development (R&D) focused on diseases that account for most of the disease burden in the low- and middle-income countries [1]. This imbalance persisted in 2000, when a study by the Global Forum for Health Research found that only 10% of global research funds were dedicated to the 90% of disease burden that affects the world's poorest people [2]. More specifically, research and development of vaccines against leading infectious killers, such as human immunodeficiency virus (HIV), malaria, and tuberculosis, remained critically underresourced. For example, in 1999, only $350 million were spent by the public and private sectors on the development of prophylactic acquired immune deficiency syndrome (AIDS) vaccines and nearly two-thirds of this amount was disbursed by the National Institutes of Health (NIH) [3,4].

This mismatch between disease burden and investment demonstrates that product development is not determined solely, or even largely, by public health need or scientific knowledge. To illustrate this point, consider that industry has invested hundreds of millions to develop vaccines against Lyme disease and drugs against baldness, but very little in vaccines against high mortality infections such as dengue fever, meningococcal A disease, or malaria.

Understanding the economic factors encouraging or inhibiting investment in priority products allows public agencies to work with the vaccine industry in both industrial and developing countries in new ways such as public–private partnerships designed to share risks and returns. These partnerships will enable the public sector to play a more active role in shaping the economics governing critical investment decisions.

In this chapter, the role economics plays in vaccine development and commercialization is discussed, with a focus on the developing world. We describe the characteristics of the vaccine market and the costs to develop and produce a product and explore the economic bottlenecks impacting investment in vaccines, illustrating the issues with a case study of an HIV/AIDS vaccine. Finally, we discuss a series of options for addressing the economic challenges, categorized as "push" and "pull" approaches, and the types of public–private partnerships needed to implement them.

---

* *Current affiliation*: Stanford University, Stanford, California, U.S.A.
† Private sector defined as commercial vaccine manufacturers.
‡ Public sector defined as governments, academia, foundations, United Nations (UN) agencies, development banks, and other nongovernmental organizations.

II. THE MARKET: VACCINE DEMAND, SUPPLY, AND PRICING

The global vaccine market grew at an annual rate of approximately 9% from 1992 to 2000 from $3 to $6 billion [5]. In a study in early 2002, Mercer Management Consulting analyzed the market, segmenting by both product and customer groups. Mercer identified four product groups—basic pediatric [e.g., oral polio vaccine (OPV), measles, diphtheria–pertussis–tetanus (DPT), tetanus toxoid (TT)]; enhanced pediatrics [e.g., hepatitis B-containing and/or *Haemophilus* influenzae type b (Hib)-containing combinations, acellular pertussis]; proprietary pediatric (e.g., pneumococcal conjugate vaccine); and adult/travel—and four customer groups—low-, middle- and high-income buyers of pediatric vaccines and of adult/travel vaccines.

As shown in Figure 1, all of these product segments have grown except the basic pediatric category. Most of this growth has come from the high-income countries purchasing enhanced and new proprietary pediatric products. The proprietary products, including the most recently introduced product, Prevnar (a pneumococcal conjugate vaccine manufactured by Wyeth), is by far the fastest growing segment. In 2000, the year of its introduction, sales of Prevnar reached nearly $500 million and in 2001, roughly $900 million [6].

Revenues from basic pediatric vaccines, the core of the expanded program on immunization (EPI), have declined significantly since 1992. This decline reflects reduced use of the basic products in Organization for Economic Cooperation and Development (OECD) countries as they are replaced by enhanced pediatrics products. However, despite their relatively small contribution to revenues (13%), basic pediatric vaccines account for over 80% of the total vaccine doses produced globally as shown in Figure 2. In contrast, three proprietary pediatric products, pneumococcal conjugate, meningococcal conjugate, and varicella, represent $1.7 billion (i.e., nearly 30% of total vaccine revenues in 2000),

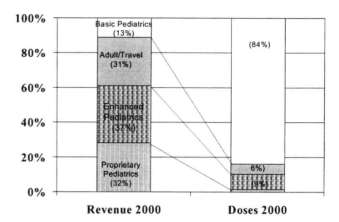

Figure 2 Value–volume skew in the vaccine market. (*Source*: Mercer analysis.)

but account for only 1% of the total market volume [5]. This illustrates one of the unusual characteristics of the vaccine market—its strong value-volume skew—by which large volumes of vaccines account for a small percentage of the global revenue.

The success of a few new proprietary products has been an important signal to vaccine firms that substantial revenues and profits can be made from the development of new vaccine products targeted at high-income countries. This strategy is comparable to the "blockbuster drug" strategy that has driven the pharmaceutical firms over the last decade.

A. Vaccine Pricing

The low prices charged for vaccines in developing countries relative to prices charged in industrial markets is the result of differential pricing (also called tiered pricing, equity pricing,

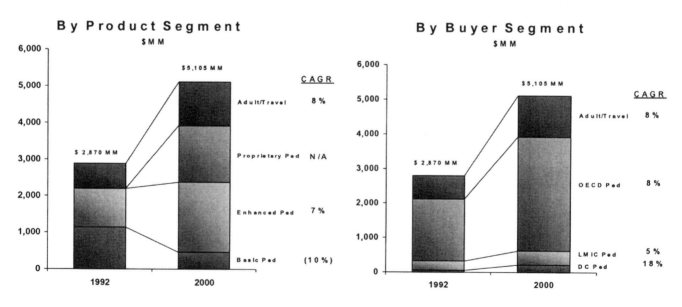

Figure 1 Vaccine market by product and buyer segment. (*Source*: Mercer analysis, 1992 Vaccine Report.)

and price discrimination), whereby different prices are charged for the same products in different markets. Using differential pricing, manufacturers can charge a low price in the poorest developing country markets, allowing these countries access to the product, and charge higher prices in the industrialized markets, allowing the manufacturer to recoup their research and development expenditures. This is a common business strategy, practiced in many industries including airlines which target the business traveler with higher prices by differentiating the product (e.g., open, changeable tickets, no weekend restrictions) and the sales channels (e.g., purchased through a travel agent). Arguably the result of historical accident more than planned strategy, the vaccine market has a segment with the lowest tier price for governments purchasing through international agencies, such as United Nations Children's Fund (UNICEF) or Pan American Health Organization (PAHO), and using multi-dose rather than monodose vials. Oral polio vaccine offers one compelling example of tiered pricing: In a given year, the highest price at which polio vaccine was offered was, on average, 30× the lowest price (Figure 3)* [7].

Figure 3 illustrates the distortion in manufacturer's product portfolios created by differential pricing; a few products have very high unit prices and very small volumes, while others have enormous volumes and low prices. Vaccine manufacturers must manage the perception of this price–volume imbalance both within and outside their company. Parent pharmaceutical firms often question the value of supplying the high-volume–low-price market, especially as the price differential between old and new vaccines grows. As shown in Figure 4,* the proprietary pediatric vaccines are priced significantly higher than basic pediatric vaccines. In 1990, Hib conjugate vaccines established new price points for routine childhood vaccines at roughly $5/dose for the U.S. public sector and $15/dose for the U.S. private sector. In just over 10 years, price points for new introduction vaccines in the United States have escalated to $46–60/dose. From industry's perspective, the introduction of higher margin products, such as Prevnar, makes investment in low-margin vaccines for the developing world even less attractive.

The magnitude of price tiering seen in the vaccine market has been facilitated by a number of factors. First, both high- and low-income markets have historically purchased the same product, allowing manufacturers to recoup their fixed cost investments through higher prices in high-income countries while enabling them to charge lower prices covering only direct costs to low- and middle-income countries second. Tiered pricing was enabled by excess production capacity that existed for several "mature" vaccines. The excess capacity allowed the manufacturer to serve more marginal markets, thus improving utilization of existing facilities, but without requiring any additional investment. Third, the fact that the majority of costs incurred in vaccine manufacture are relatively fixed (i.e., not related to volume)

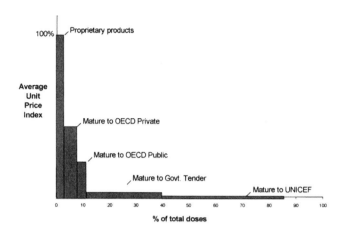

Figure 3 Typical vaccine market profile for a supplier. (*Source*: UNICEF, Mercer analysis.)

has allowed manufacturers to offer widely differing prices once the core fixed costs are covered. Finally, the acceptance by both suppliers and governments of different prices for different segments of the market has been critical.

Pooled procurement has helped facilitate differential pricing. UNICEF and PAHO purchase large quantities of basic pediatric vaccines at very low prices. The ability of the international procurement agencies to negotiate low prices, the willingness of governments to accept radically different prices depending on national wealth, and the willingness of various manufacturers to supply vaccine at these prices have all been important factors in the success of national immunization programs. As important as pooled procurement has been, it should be noted that the objectives of regional procurement—striving for the lowest price for a region rather than the poorest countries—threaten the equity notion underpinning tiered pricing.

Tiered pricing, however, has also some less desirable consequences. In comparison to other products and markets, the UNICEF and PAHO market generates little revenue and even less profit for many manufacturers—two key factors driving a company's decision to maintain production lines and to invest in R&D and new capacity. This places a burden on companies to justify internally their continued involve-

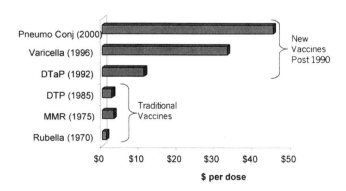

Figure 4 Price of traditional and new vaccines.

* From Economics of vaccines: From vaccine candidate to commercialized product. In: Bloom B, Lambert P-H, eds. The Vaccine Book. New York: Elsevier Science, 2003:345–370.

ment in this "marginal" market. The result is low levels of investment in vaccine R&D and production capacity for the products needed by the poorest countries and little incentive to improve manufacturing processes. The growing divergence between products used in high- and low-income countries and the switch by many developing countries to newer products, such as combinations, which have limited production capacity, reduce the potential for tiered pricing [8].

B. Diverging Products

The decline of basic pediatric vaccines and the growth of enhanced and proprietary vaccines illustrate the increasing divergence between industrial and developing country markets [9]. The divergence of products is the result of new vaccines targeting regional rather than "global" priorities, whether disease- or safety/efficacy-driven and second-generation vaccines substituting for older products that were once used globally.

In the past, a disease was typically controlled by one vaccine used in both industrial and developing countries. However, today, the same diseases are being controlled with different vaccines, depending on geography and cost. For example, in the 1990s, the majority of industrialized countries adopted diptheria–tetanus–acellular pertussis (DTaP), containing a purified acellular pertussis, as the vaccine of choice over diptheria–tetanus–whole cell pertussis (DTwP), containing whole cell pertussis [9]. Although more expensive and, as some believe, not as efficacious as DTwP, DTaP vaccine has fewer moderate adverse events associated with it and has enjoyed a greater acceptance among parents in industrialized countries [10]. The divergence in the number and the type of vaccines used in developing and industrial markets is illustrated in Table 1.

C. Demand

The six antigens that comprise the basic pediatric vaccines in most developing countries [measles, bacille Calmette–Gué-

rin (BCG), DPT, TT, OPV] are mature, off-patent products that have been available for decades. These vaccines are widely used around the world and reach between 50% and 80% of infants in developing countries each year. Due in part to increasingly efficient production resulting from both learning over time and economies of scale (i.e., cost per dose declines as volume increases because of increased spreading of fixed costs) and the influence of competition, these vaccines have been sold at very low prices and have provided low marginal rates of return to producers [11].

The introduction of newer vaccines, such as Hepatitis B and Hib conjugate, into developing countries has been very slow, notwithstanding that they have been available in industrial countries for many years. As shown in Figure 5, by the year 2000, 18 years after its introduction in the United States, hepatitis B vaccine had been introduced in less than 15% of sub-Saharan African countries. While these vaccines were provided to developing countries at prices well below those charged in industrial markets, the prices were still much higher than those of basic pediatric products. For example, as demand has shifted from diphtheria, tetanus, and pertussis (DTP) toward DTP combination products containing hepatitis B and/or Hib antigens, the prices being offered to countries through UNICEF and PAHO have increased from around $0.10/dose to between $0.90 and $3.50/dose [12]. In addition to the deterrent effect of these prices, various other barriers have prevented rapid introduction of cost-effective, life-saving vaccines. These include weak delivery systems, inadequate national disease burden data, and unwillingness of governments and donors to increase investments in immunization [13].

D. Low-Income Market: Need Does Not Equal Demand

The slow introduction of priority new vaccines in developing countries has created costly confusion between the public and the private sectors. Typically, when public health organ-

Table 1 Diverging Products Used in Developing and Industrial Markets

Disease target	Developing country product/formulation	Industrial country product/formulation
Measles	Measles	MMR
Diphtheria, pertussis, tetanus	Diptheria–tetanus–whole cell pertussis (DTwP)	Diptheria–tetanus–acellular pertussis (DTaP)
Polio	Oral polio vaccine (OPV)	Inactivated polio vaccine (IPV)
Tetanus	Tetanus toxoid (TT) (Td in some areas)	Tetanus–diphtheria
Hepatitis B	Monovalent, combined with DtwP	Monovalent, combined with DTaP, IPV, HepA
Hemophilous influenzae type b	Monovalent, combined with DTwP, HepB	Monovalent, combined with DTaP, IPV, HepB
Meningococcal	Meningitis A/C conjuagate (wanted)	Meningitis C conjugate, (Meningitis BC conjugate)
Pneumococcal	11-valent conjugate-wanted	7-valent conjugate-licensed; 11-valent under development
Product presentations	Multidose, thimerosal	Single dose, no thimerosal

(*Source*: Milstien J. WHO/V&B.)

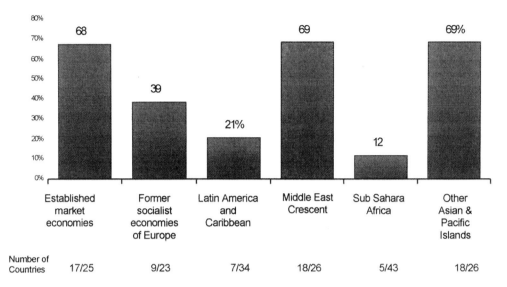

Figure 5 Countries who have introduced hepatitis B vaccine by 2000. (*Source*: Miller MA, Flanders WD. A Model to Estimate the Probability of Hepatitis B- and Haemophilus Influenzae Type B-vaccine Uptake into National Vaccination Programs.)

izations and vaccine manufacturers each refer to "developing country demand," they are defining demand differently. Public health organizations have often defined "the market" as those countries where there is a need for the vaccine (i.e., high-incidence countries). Annually, 64 million infants are born in low-income countries, and another 48 million are born in middle-income countries [14]. However, the *actual* market is the portion of this need that translates into revenue or demand for a given quantity of a vaccine at a given price. Thus while the need for a vaccine may be large given the number of individuals who would benefit from it, the actual demand is much smaller because many of those who need the vaccine are least able to pay for it. Despite 85% of the global population living in low- and middle-income countries [14], the vaccine market in the developing world is estimated to be only 10% of the global vaccine market of $6 billion and less than 0.2% of the global pharmaceutical market ($340 billion annually) [5,15].

Historically, the public health community's estimates of vaccine need (confusingly called demand) have been far larger than actual national or international willingness to pay for the vaccine (Table 2). The resulting gap between expected demand, based on public health need, and real de-

mand, based on willingness and capacity to pay, has had expensive implications for manufacturers. Several manufacturers have, in the past, built production capacity and planned their production runs to meet these inaccurate forecasts. Given the long lead times required to produce and to control batches of vaccines, these decisions were made 12–18 months in advance of expected uptake. When actual uptake was much lower than anticipated, manufacturers had to manage excess inventory and sudden changes in production schedules—both of which are inefficient and costly. The poor quality of forecasting has increased the risk (and cost) of serving the developing country market. It has also undermined the credibility of public sector agencies urgently calling for investment in new vaccines "needed" to combat such diseases as diarrheal diseases (e.g., rotavirus, *Shigella*) or malaria.

E. Vaccine Supply

The vaccine industry is currently dominated by a small number of multinational firms (Figure 6): GlaxoSmithKline, Aventis Pasteur, Wyeth, and Merck. These firms have seen their share of the vaccine market (measured by revenues) rise

Table 2 Who Uses and Who Buys Vaccines?

Children are the main recipients of vaccines; receiving between 8 and 12 different vaccines protect children from deadly and debilitating diseases such as measles, hepatitis, and diphtheria. In most countries, however, families do not purchase vaccines. As a preventive intervention that protects not only the individual child but also all who come in contact with the child, immunization has "positive externalities" and is primarily financed by governments and public health agencies including bilateral donors, multilateral institutions, development banks, and foundations. Each country relies on a different mix of funding sources for their immunization program; however, typically, the government finances the majority of the program's costs [16].

The decision by governments, donors, and bilaterals to purchase vaccines depends on the absolute resources available and how these resources are allocated given other needs. Disease burden, the potential impact of the vaccine, the vaccine's price, and the cost to deliver the vaccine to each child are all important considerations in deciding the amount of scarce resources to allocate to immunization [13].

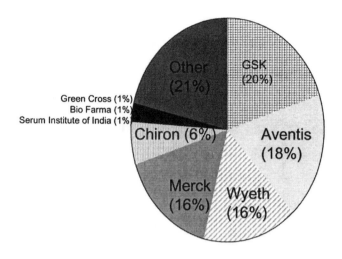

Figure 6   The vaccine players in the vaccine market.

from approximately 50% in 1988 to about 70% today. Small- to medium-sized companies, notably Chiron, and emerging companies in Korea, India, and Indonesia comprise an additional 10%, with the remaining revenues attributable to local OECD and developing country producers [5,15].

Until recently, uncertainty about market growth and profitability, combined with rising costs and growing fears of liability, resulted in a dramatic decline in the number of industrial country vaccine manufacturers. Many manufacturers merged, sold, or shut down their vaccine business. Of the 20 internationally active companies in the 1960s, fewer than 12 remained by the early 1990s [17]. However, the vaccine market is now looking much stronger. Even before the interest in vaccines stimulated by bioterrorism concerns, new product opportunities were creating revenue growth expectations in double digits for the years ahead [15]. Many of the new entrants to the vaccine-manufacturing field are smaller and based in middle- and low-income countries.

Since 1992, there has been an increase in not only the number of these emerging and local suppliers but also their overall production capacity and product range. However, most of the vaccines produced by local and emerging suppliers are still licensed and used primarily within the home market. The World Health Organization (WHO) conducted a series of studies on behalf of the Children's Vaccine Initiative (CVI) evaluating domestic vaccine production in 10 countries from 1993 to 1995 [18–24]. These studies found that while local producers were important supply sources, many faced significant structural, legal, and economic challenges. For example, vaccine prices, or worse, fixed budgets were often set by the government and, in many cases, did not cover the full costs of production, making it difficult for these publicly owned suppliers to maintain the facilities, to train staff, to expand production, or to invest in new vaccine R&D. In addition, many manufacturers did not have the authority to hire or to fire staff or to set competitive salaries. A few emerging suppliers have overcome these difficulties and represent an attractive low-price supply source for basic pediatric vaccines. However, these suppliers do not have a strong track record in new product development.

Given the quickly evolving vaccine market, both multinational and emerging suppliers will be important supply sources for the world. Multinational firms are likely to be the primary source of newly developed products for the short to the medium terms, while emerging suppliers may become the low-price supply source over the long term for the developing country markets.

III.   BRINGING A VACCINE TO MARKET: COSTS, RISKS, AND CONSTRAINTS

Each firm has a portfolio of R&D projects within which it allocates investments. While the public sector supports a great deal of basic research, private manufacturers usually finance most of the product development, production scale-up, and sales costs. Assessing and financing the risk associated with these investments is a major part of the pharmaceutical business. These risks span all the stages in bringing a vaccine to market and include not only the scientific and technical risks but also political and market-based factors. This combination of known costs and benefits plus possible risks determines a company's decision to invest in a product or not. Firms continually compare investments across the products in their portfolio. Products with high potential profits and low risk are more attractive investments than those with limited expected earnings and/or high risk. The expected profits, often measured as a percent of investment or "return on investment" (ROI), are a function of expected costs, risks, probable demand, and thus expected profit. Firms must not only ensure each project is viable but also that the total product revenues cover the R&D costs of ongoing and new projects. Given the relatively lower prices available in developing country markets, manufacturers are, not surprisingly, less willing to accept all the risk associated with vaccine investments for these markets. Understanding the risk–return trade-off, and possible areas over which the public sector has influence, provides the public sector with an opportunity to intervene in a manner that may diminish risks. Table 3 (footnote a) illustrates the average number of candidates, the time of development, and the cost of development for one successful product. On average, one successful product is registered for every five candidates supported in preclinical trials.

A.   Baseline Development Costs in a Perfect World

There is a set of defined costs which constitutes the investment needed to develop, to scale up, and to sell a vaccine in the absence of any failures, complications, or delays in a perfect world. These baseline costs include basic preclinical research, clinical trials, production scale-up, licensing fees, ongoing production, quality control, and marketing. The costs vary based on the particular characteristics of the disease, the vaccine, and the production technology. For example, because the incidence rate is lower, trials of an HIV/AIDS vaccine need to be larger and thus more expensive than trials of a vaccine to prevent pneumococcal ear infection.

The baseline costs associated with product development correspond to four distinct stages: (1) basic, preclinical

Table 3 Average Vaccine Development Costs per Product

	Pre-clinical	Phase 1	Phase 2	Phase 3	Pre-registration	Registration	Launch
Time	2.4	2.0	1.8	1.4	1.1	1.3	Total 10 years
Market entrance probabilities %	22%	39%	54%	68%		98%	
No. candidates in pipeline*	4.6	2.5	1.9	1.5		1***	
Cost drug development/candidate**($ MM)	8.5	12.0	33.0	39.0			
Cost of vaccine development/candidate Year 2000 ($ MM)	5–7	6–9	37–68	46–48		30–40***	

* n= 591 candidates between 1993 and 1994
** For large pharmaceutical firms $>360 million sales
*** Additional post marketing trials has increased regulatory and licensing costs in line with Phase 3 trials

research; (2) identifying a promising vaccine candidate through early clinical studies in humans; (3) developing and testing a candidate for a target market; and (4) scaling up manufacturing capacity for that market. Based on an analysis of the cost to develop an HIV/AIDS vaccine [25], Figure 7 shows the relative magnitude of these investments—turning each new stage into a decision gate initiating a reevaluation of the investment given the product's risks and potential return.

Assuring a vaccine for global use requires two additional stages of investment: (5) "relevance"—adapting and testing a vaccine to ensure safety and efficacy in additional populations; and (6) "supply"—ensuring adequate manufacturing capacity and funding/pricing structures to enable broad developing country access. To make a new vaccine broadly available at the earliest possible technical and regulatory opportunity, a manufacturer must make development and capital investments explicitly to support supply to the developing world markets. To have a business case for such incremental investments, a return must be available either directly from the developing world market or through other special financing interventions. In the case of vaccines for which no significant industrial market exists such as malaria, it follows that the developing country market and the associated financing must fund, and provide a return on, the entire investment.

B. Vaccine Production

Vaccine production has two primary stages: (1) bulk production consisting of activities such as growing or fermenting the active ingredients harvesting, and potentially attenuating the live virus or bacteria; and (2) fill/finish consisting of activities such as blending, filling vials, lyophilizing, labeling, and packaging. All firms require Good Manufacturing Practice (GMP) production facilities with appropriate quality control and quality assurance.

The costs associated with vaccine production can be categorized as variable (unit cost is constant for each vial), semivariable or batch fixed (unit costs associated with each batch), and fixed (unit costs are independent of volume and are fixed at the site level). Vaccine production is a "fixed cost business," in that roughly 85% of costs are fixed at either the batch or site level (plant, equipment, animals, labor), leaving only 15% truly variable (vials, stoppers, raw materials). As a result, unit costs fall rapidly with increases in volume. Importantly, however, the capacity for a given vaccine is largely determined at scale-up and is thereafter expensive and time-consuming to increase.

The cost to produce vaccine varies significantly from product to product. The primary factors affecting the cost are outlined in detail below and include the presentation, the scale of operations, the vaccine inputs, the supply location, the batch size, and certain vaccine production characteristics. Understanding the economics of production can guide public sector in its choice of suppliers, its policy decisions such as the optimal presentation of the vaccine and its strategy options such as the timing of commitment to purchase.

1. Presentation: Presentation (e.g., the number of doses per vial, labeling) is determined by the buyer rather than the supplier and so must be carefully considered when there are limited resources. As shown in Figure 8, single-dose presentations are significantly more expensive to produce than multidose presentations because of their impact on

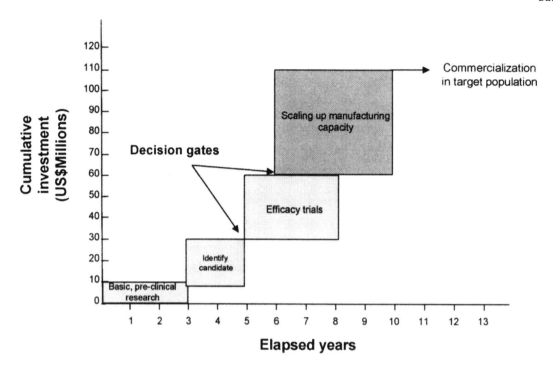

Figure 7 Baseline investments and decision gates in developing an HIV/AIDS vaccine for one target population. (*Source*: Batson, Ainsworth. Bull WHO, 2001.)

filling lot size. Lots of single-dose vials require almost the same labor and equipment as multidose vials, but with far smaller output. For an industrial country supplier, it was estimated that single-dose presentations added approximately $0.50/dose to the cost of a liquid vaccine and $1.00 to the cost of a lyophilized vaccine [5].

2. Scale of operations: Given the manufacturer's cost is a function of the number of doses produced, vaccine production is a very fixed cost business, which means that almost the same level of investment is needed whether 50 or 200 million doses are produced. However, obviously the per dose cost drops as volume increases. The importance of scale

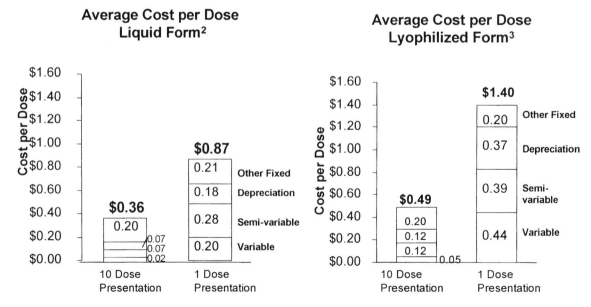

¹ **Multinational producers only;** ² **Includes TT, DTP, Hep :** 3 **Includes MEA, MMR, Hib.**

Figure 8 Average cost per dose across vaccines to produce liquid and lyophilized 1 and 10 dose vials. (*Source*: Mercer Management analysis.)

is best illustrated by comparing suppliers from the United States and Europe. U.S. vaccine firms are higher-cost producers relative to European firms because of the former's overall lower volume levels (fewer than 100 million doses annually vs. over 1 billion doses for certain European multinationals). The cost impact of this "scale effect" is estimated to add as much as $0.65/dose in cost for U.S. firms [5].

3. Reliance on inputs for vaccines: Having to purchase certain expensive inputs for a vaccine rather than producing them within the firm can dramatically impact the costs. As the demand for combination and conjugated vaccines has grown, almost all firms have been forced to purchase either antigens or protein carriers from outside firms. The increase in outsourced components significantly impacts the economics of vaccine production. First, outsourcing increases variable cost so the *marginal* cost of vaccines with significant outsourced components will likely be higher than those produced entirely in-house. Second, although it is not known, it is likely that these arrangements increase the *absolute* cost of the vaccine in question because the overhead costs and profit margin of the component supplier must also be factored in.

4. Supply base location: All else being equal, industrial country suppliers are higher-cost producers than large emerging suppliers because wage rates for pharmaceutical labor in lower-income countries, such as India and Indonesia, are less than 10% of comparable wage rates in high-income countries. This wage rate impact is estimated to give emerging suppliers as much as a $0.12/dose advantage over industrial country suppliers.

5. Vaccine batch size: The size of bulk batches is an important cost factor as shown in Figure 9.* Because the cost to manufacture and to test a batch is largely fixed, an increase in batch size results in lower per dose costs. Batch size is largely determined at the time of manufacturing scale-up. Once a plant is in place, there are two ways to increase batch size. The first is to add capacity, a process that requires additional capital, may disrupt production, and certainly requires regulatory approval and GMP certification. The second is to wait and to allow the experience effect to drive yield improvements and consequent increases in effective batch size. Although some vaccines, such as recombinant hepatitis B, appear to have experienced very rapid and dramatic improvements in yield, the available data suggests that for most vaccines, it takes years before batches are large enough to serve the developing country market. Given the difficulties of increasing batch size once a plant is built, the optimal strategy to assure capacity and relative affordability is to influence batch size at the time of scale-up, perhaps through early commitment to purchase.

6. Vaccine production characteristics: Different vaccines have differing testing and labor requirements, antigen combinations, and production process cycle times, each of which has impact on the cost of production. However, these differences have been estimated to have a relatively minor impact on total costs [5]. As an example, the most expensive

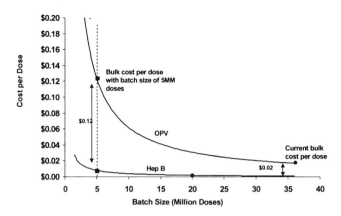

Figure 9 Batch size effect on bulk production costs (based on a representative sample of multinational suppliers). (*Source*: Mercer Management analysis.)

vaccine to produce at the bulk stage is OPV. However, the fact that this vaccine is manufactured by high-scale producers in large batches of multidose presentations results in one of the lowest per dose production costs of any vaccine.

C. Risks

In addition to the expected R&D and production costs, every product faces a range of semipredictable and unpredictable risks. Should they become real, any one of these risks can necessitate significant additional investment or—if the product fails entirely—result in wasted investment. Figure 10 illustrates some of the risks that exist at each stage of the product's life from earliest research to final sales. These risks build on the expected development, production, and sales costs and, ultimately, impact the estimated total or risk-adjusted costs of the product. For example, for a certain vaccine, a planned $50-million investment would result in a cost of $0.20/dose; however, if there is an unexpected 1-year delay in launching the clinical trial (costing $4 million) plus an unexpected problem with validating the new plant (adding another $10 million) and unexpectedly slow introduction of the product resulting in both extra inventory costs and lost revenues, a number of unplanned costs must be factored in. Added together, these unexpected events could increase the total costs to roughly $70 million, resulting in a unit cost of $0.30/dose, significantly over original expectations. Obviously, not all the things that could go wrong do go wrong. However, cost expectations should reflect the more realistic risk-adjusted estimate.

The following are more detailed descriptions of the different types of risks that contribute to the full costs of developing and producing a vaccine.

1. Research and development: Faced with finite human and financial resources to support R&D projects in the pipeline, the decision to invest in one candidate will absorb resources that could have been used for other products. The opportunity cost of supporting one project vs. another has real costs to the firm and must be factored into decisions.

Given the cost of efficacy trials, companies seek to minimize the risks of a trial failing or being delayed. How-

---

* From Economics of vaccines: From vaccine candidate to commercialized product. In: Bloom B, Lambert P-H, eds. The Vaccine Book. New York: Elsevier Science, 2003:345–370.

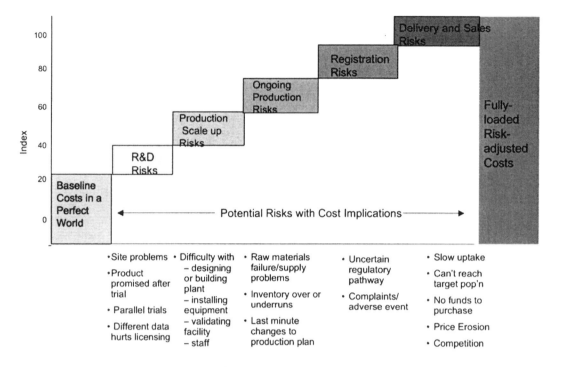

Figure 10 Potential risk with cost implications over product's life cycle.

ever, if there are not good animal models or correlates of immunity to help predict the probability of the product successfully protecting humans, such as, e.g., with HIV/AIDS vaccines, then investments in expensive Phase III trials for a vaccine candidate are even riskier. In addition, each additional trial to test efficacy in a different epidemiological region can add between $10 and $30 million to the product's development cost. Moreover, clinical trials conducted in developing countries with different epidemiological conditions may present risks to licensure in industrialized countries that outweigh the potential revenues from the developing country market.

Each product may also have unique risks. For example, as the number of antigens in a combination increases, so does the risk that at least one of the antigens will have reduced immunogenicity or efficacy or that an adverse event associated with one antigen will reduce demand for the combined product.

2. Production scale-up: Companies most often invest in the production scale-up before the final data from the Phase III trials is available. This early investment is for two reasons. First, it is a condition of licensure for any biologic that the company demonstrates that it can make its product in a repeatable fashion at commercial scale. Second, to assure timely availability of new products, a production facility must be fully operational as soon as the product is proven to be efficacious. However, if the product fails at a late stage, the firm risks losing most or all of its investment. Investment in production capacity is particularly difficult because many firms face growing internal competition for these resources. The opportunity cost and risks of building or using a facility for one product vs. another must be considered.

Sizing a facility appropriately, given uncertainties about future demand, is also difficult and risky. On one hand, a larger facility requires greater investment, but, because of economies of scale, can result in more efficient, lower-cost production in the long run if large volumes of the product are demanded. However, if demand is lower than expected, the facility will be underutilized, a costly waste of resources. On the other hand, a smaller facility requires less total investment, but the firm is less able to take advantage of economies of scale, thus the long-term cost per dose may be higher. If demand is greater than expected, then the company not only loses the market to a competitor but must also invest in resizing its facility, a costly and time-consuming mistake.

3. Regulatory and licensing issues: Regulatory requirements have become increasingly stringent and preparation of applications for marketing authorization is hampered by the differing requirements across countries. Obtaining separate authorizations for each market in which a manufacturer proposes to sell a vaccine is a long, costly, and uncertain process.

In addition, the growing difficulty in finding appropriate regulatory pathways for developing country vaccines produced in the United States and Europe increases the risk to licensure. Most new vaccines are produced in either the United States or European countries. The Food and Drug Administration (FDA) and the European Agency for the Evaluation of Medicinal Products (EMEA) each have a responsibility to regulate products for their home markets. However, these agencies are also called upon to regulate products intended for developing countries, which are developed and produced by manufacturers situated within their borders. If these agencies decline to or are prevented from applying their regulatory expertise for products that will not be marketed within their borders, the risks and costs to the companies will increase significantly.

Even once licensed, unexpected adverse events identified through postmarketing surveillance may result in a decline in demand for the product such as in the case of Wyeth's Rotashield. The millions of dollars invested in developing and scaling up production for this vaccine were lost once the product was associated with the risk of intussusception, a rare but severe complication.

Finally, intellectual property rights (IPR) are intended to safeguard returns on new products, enabling manufacturers to recoup their investment. Weak IPR protection increases the risk (in the eyes of the firm that made the initial investment) of multiple suppliers competing for the same market—without having invested in the R&D. This risk may be so significant that it reduces a firm's interest in developing a high-priority vaccine. Concern for IPRs has been less of a problem for vaccines than drugs because vaccines are, in large part, also protected by technical "know-how," the knowledge of how to scale up and consistently produce a biological product, as well as stricter import controls.

4. Ongoing production: Once a product is fully developed, licensed, and ready for production, firms face production risks that can occur at any time. A component of the close regulatory oversight around vaccine manufacture is that every batch is tested before being released. Seemingly inconsequential changes to the production materials or process, such as a change in brands of cleaning fluid used to wash out a fermenter, can cause a batch to fail and hence the investment in the batch to be lost. These failures can be particularly costly, given the relatively lengthy period required to produce a batch of vaccine (9–15 months). Batch failures and unexpected changes in demand can be costly to manufacturers as they may result in excess inventory, market shortages, or last-minute changes to the production schedule.

5. Delivery and sales: All of the investments will be meaningless if no market for the product materializes. A market may "disappear" if there is a change in the perceived risk of a disease or the national immunization priorities, the immunization delivery systems within a country is not able to reach the target population, or there is limited funding.

While public–private partnerships, such as the Global Alliance for Vaccines and Immunization (GAVI), provide support to strengthen immunization infrastructure and purchase new vaccines, in many countries, less than half the target population is immunized [26] and decisions to introduce the vaccine still depend on national decision makers having the necessary national data at hand.

The potential future market (e.g., demand at a given price) needs to offset all of the costs on a risk-adjusted basis and to provide a return, if private sector investment is to be attracted. However, for the developing country market, there is a great deal of uncertainty about not only which vaccines will be demanded and financed by governments and partners but also when these vaccines will be demanded and introduced. The slow and uncertain uptake discussed earlier in the chapter has greatly increased uncertainties,

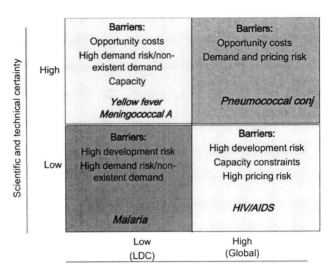

Figure 11 Barriers given degree of scientific certainty and potential market revenue.

and therefore perceived risk, in serving the developing country market.

D. Each Vaccine Is Different

The relative importance of different risks varies from vaccine to vaccine. Each vaccine faces a unique mix of obstacles that may be best overcome by different types of interventions. Figure 11 shows two key factors that influence how attractive or risky a vaccine is perceived to be—the potential market revenue and the degree of scientific certainty. For instance, a vaccine against a disease like malaria, which has low scientific certainty [27] and low-revenue potential, faces both high development and demand risk. By contrast, a meningococcal A conjugate vaccine intended primarily for Africa has high scientific and technical certainty, but a very limited revenue opportunity. In such a case, the primary barriers are the opportunity costs, the constraints on capacity, and the high demand risk. HIV vaccines, for which the revenue opportunity is high but the scientific and technical certainty is low, represent a tantalizing, often frustrating, opportunity for manufacturers. Accelerating its development may require incremental investments to tailor a vaccine to the needs of developing countries once a successful approach is discovered as well as innovative ways to ensure affordable pricing.

IV. A CASE STUDY OF THE RISKS, COSTS, AND CONSTRAINTS TO BRINGING A VACCINE TO MARKET: HIV/AIDS VACCINES

Despite the obvious need for an HIV vaccine, and the rhetoric endorsing this view, investment in both the public and the private sectors in HIV vaccine research and development has significantly lagged both need and rhetoric. Worldwide, combined public and private expenditure on R&D for preventive HIV vaccines was estimated to be only $350 million in 1999 [4]. While the public sector, most notably the NIH, has more than tripled its investment in HIV vaccine research from $100 million in 1995 to an estimated $360 million in 2002, the private sector has, for many of the reasons discussed in the preceding sections, proceeded cautiously with investment in the development of an HIV/AIDS vaccine for the developing world. Estimated industry investment in HIV vaccine development was in the range of $50–124 million in 1999 [4].

Hundreds of millions, even billions, of people around the world would benefit from an HIV vaccine. So why is the commercial sector so cognizant of market size, proceeding with such modest effort? In 1998, the World Bank AIDS Vaccine Task Force commissioned a study, cosponsored by the International AIDS Vaccine Initiative (IAVI), to understand the low levels of private investment [25]. Through interviews with various experts from vaccine manufacturing, biotechnology firms, and academia, the study concluded that while scientific obstacles remained a short-term impediment to AIDS vaccine development, a low expectation about the probable return on the investment was also a significant deterrent.

A. Barriers to Increased Investment

In 1998, the low levels of investment in an HIV vaccine could be partially explained by the inability of companies to foresee a realistic commercial return. At that time, companies feared that the industrial country market would consist only of high-risk individuals and, of course, the developing country markets were not expected to generate significant revenues. However, companies also cited the scientific risks as an equally important barrier. Respondents to the study stressed that it was the combination of scientific and economic risks including unpredictable industrial country uptake, questionable developing country market, perceived low probability of success of any existing candidates, and the high profile of some failures that in combination created corporate reluctance to increase investment.

The scientific barriers arise from a number of factors. First, two of the three approaches most commonly used for existing human vaccines (i.e., live attenuated strains of the virus and whole virus inactivated) have not been considered appropriate for an HIV/AIDS vaccine. Given the nature of the virus, safety concerns have prevented the testing of candidates based on these approaches. Inactivated vaccine candidates have also been hampered by concerns about potential manufacturing difficulties. The failure to neutralize primary isolates in preclinical testing has prevented most first-generation subunit candidates from entering efficacy trials although one improved recombinant subunit product started such trials in 1998 [28]. As a result, the bulk of current efforts are focused on approaches that have few or no current vaccine analogues and hence involve greater scientific uncertainty.

This scientific uncertainty is further compounded by the limited understanding of the virus, not knowing the corre-

lates of immunity, and the lack of relevant animal models— all of which contribute to a much higher degree of uncertainty about the potential efficacy of a vaccine candidate than is typical when industry considers investing in large and expensive Phase III efficacy trials. Study respondents noted that Phase III trials are normally supported only once there is relatively solid evidence that the product is viable and highly likely to be efficacious. In the case of an HIV/AIDS vaccine, firms would have to finance expensive trials to explore the product's efficacy without an early success predictor based on surrogates of efficacy.

The costs of these trials represent a significant investment: $30 million/trial was a frequently quoted figure. Respondents pointed out that while trials could be conducted in both industrial and developing countries, each had its own costs. A relatively low incidence of new HIV infections in industrial countries makes for large, expensive trials of uncertain statistical outcome. In developing countries, where the incidence is often much higher, allowing for more reasonably sized studies, significant political and infrastructure barriers were feared to raise costs. A further barrier noted by the respondents was the investment in process development and manufacturing capacity that must accompany efficacy trials if timely licensure of the product is desired. Investments in limited production capacity for an unproven product may be on the order of tens of millions of dollars; significant additional investment would be needed to scale up manufacturing capacity to meet global, rather than just industrial country, demand. All or most of this investment is lost if a viable commercial product does not result from the efficacy trials, or if demand does not materialize as predicted.

The firms interviewed noted the dilemma between scientific and business objectives created by the high risk of investment in development and production capacity (Figure 12).* The scientific uncertainty that makes it hard to predict what type of approach will likely protect against HIV makes industry reluctant to take on the costs of Phase III trials. However, without the knowledge learned from these trials, it will be difficult to identify the most promising approach. The result is a vicious cycle in which the failure to undertake Phase III trials perpetuates the lack of scientific knowledge that underlies industry's reluctance to invest in the trials in the first place.

Not surprisingly, the uncertainty surrounding the science and the future markets for an HIV vaccine translated into difficulty in raising private funds for vaccine development. Nearly all the smaller biotechnology companies cited difficulty in raising capital as a major barrier. Most smaller companies either limited their HIV vaccine activities to those covered by public sector grants or pursued HIV vaccine research in a low-profile fashion, often as part of a larger "platform" research effort. The difficulties faced by the small companies in raising finance were, in all probability, symp-

---

* From Economics of vaccines: From vaccine candidate to commercialized product. In: Bloom B, Lambert P-H, eds. The Vaccine Book. New York: Elsevier Science, 2003:345–370.

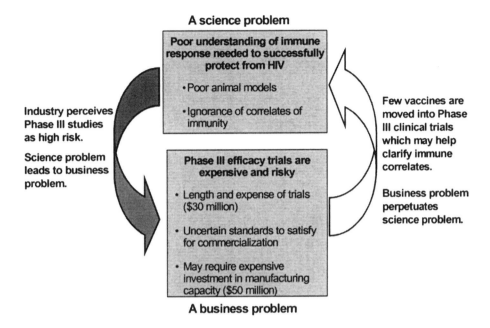

A science problem

Poor understanding of immune response needed to successfully protect from HIV

• Poor animal models

• Ignorance of correlates of immunity

Industry perceives Phase III studies as high risk.

Science problem leads to business problem.

Phase III efficacy trials are expensive and risky

• Length and expense of trials ($30 million)

• Uncertain standards to satisfy for commercialization

• May require expensive investment in manufacturing capacity ($50 million)

A business problem

Few vaccines are moved into Phase III clinical trials which may help clarify immune correlates.

Business problem perpetuates science problem.

Figure 12 A vicious cycle: Scientific barriers make industry reluctant to invest in the Phase III studies that may be required to solve the scientific barriers.

tomatic of the lack of confidence of the larger companies who are typically a major source of investment in smaller companies and arguably give a lead to the venture capital markets.

HIV/AIDS vaccine illustrates the importance of having a market with credible demand, i.e., the willingness and the ability to pay for a product. While there may be a large *potential* market for HIV vaccines, those who would most want and need a vaccine are those least able to afford one. Taking into account that over 95% of all new HIV infections occur in developing countries [29] and that the average annual per-capita total health expenditure in low-income countries was estimated to be less than U.S. \$20 in 1998, it is clear why industry would be concerned about its ability to recoup R&D and other costs and earn a return [30].

The public health agencies who are dedicated to improving health can influence the investment decisions of private vaccine firms. Detailed analyses, such as the study conducted on HIV/AIDS vaccine, help to identify the specific barriers limiting investment in a vaccine and, through this, the most appropriate solutions.

V. PUSH AND PULL MECHANISMS: CHANGING THE ECONOMIC EQUATION

The decisions to invest in the development and commercialization of vaccine, while tied to and influenced by scientific progress, are based largely on an evaluation of economic factors: the costs, risks, and timing of investments and the expected return on future sales. To influence these economic factors, the public sector is seeking new ways to assess and to share risk.

There is no "silver bullet" solution. Not only do the issues vary between vaccines, but public and private entities, while both seeking to promote widespread use of priority vaccines, do so with different objectives and incentives.

The public sector would ideally avoid all risk, only buying a product once it is developed, widely demanded, and available at a very low price. In contrast, the private sector would ideally only invest once there were solid market commitments, e.g., guarantees to purchase the product at a given, likely higher, price. Furthermore, neither the public nor the private sector wants to make investments if the risks of failure are high. Creative public–private partnerships that share specific risks and costs and protect the interests of all partners are essential for these high-risk products and markets.

There are two categories of strategies to accelerate the development and introduction of priority vaccines: push and pull mechanisms. Push mechanisms are those which reduce the risks and costs of investments, while pull mechanisms assure a future return in the event that a product is produced. While the merits of push and pull interventions have been debated extensively [31–33], much work remains to translate the two concepts into action. Historically, the public sector has invested substantially in early stage push mechanisms, particularly basic research and some early product development. There are fewer examples of pull mechanisms. However, the Global Alliance for Vaccines and Immunization (GAVI) and its sister entity, the Vaccine Fund, are a recent example, providing 5-year commitments to purchase newer vaccines for the poorest developing countries.

It is unlikely that the global immunization community will ever have the resources either to finance all the costs of

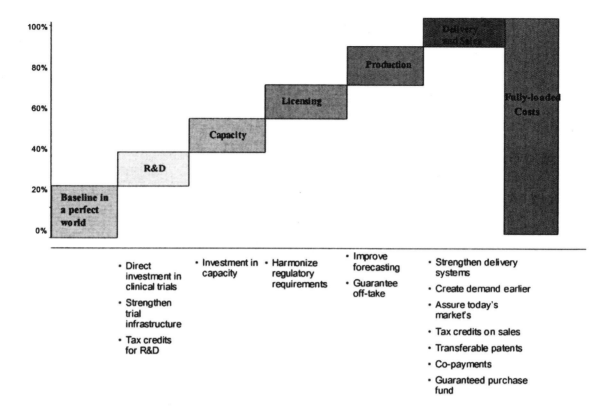

Figure 13 Approaches tailored to address specific risks.

vaccine development and production (100% push) or to purchase vaccines at prices equivalent to those paid in the United States or Europe (100% pull). The public sector must therefore leverage its resources by targeting its actions and its funds as directly as possible to the particular obstacles inhibiting a vaccine's progress. If the risks are linked to uncertainty about the science, such as in the case of an HIV/AIDS vaccine, then push mechanisms may prove more valuable than pull mechanisms which are too far in the future and too low probability to have much impact [25]. If the risks stem from the market despite the technical ability to produce the vaccine, such as in the case of the meningococcal A conjugate vaccine, then pull mechanisms become more important. As shown in Figure 13, different mechanisms can be tailored to best address risks occurring at different stages of the life cycle.

A. Push Mechanisms

Push options offer a number of benefits, the most important of which is that they reduce risk and thereby encourage investment where it might not otherwise occur (e.g., by funding a clinical trial in a geography that a manufacturer has little incentive to choose). Another important benefit is the familiarity with, and proven track record of, certain push interventions, which have been successfully used in the past. When structured to support broad objectives, such as the development of animal models, field studies of the natural

exposure, and resistance to disease, this mechanism can also help advance the development of all products targeted against a given disease.

However, certain types of push mechanisms, such as financing a clinical trial of a vaccine, necessitate specifying or picking one candidate or project. It is possible that better options may emerge at a later date, or that unsupported manufacturers will drop promising candidates. Product "failures" must also be expected, when one product is selected early in the process. Finally, push options do not promise a successful outcome. When projects or products do fail, the money will already have been spent and, in most cases, will be unrecoverable. The following are several possible push strategies that are or could be applied to vaccines.

1. Direct financing: Direct financing is used to fund or directly implement activities necessary to develop a vaccine. The main goal of this type of intervention is to increase the number of candidate vaccines and to generate data needed to assess a vaccine and to recommend its use. Public sector funds may go toward financing either platform activities or product-specific activities. In the category of platform activities, the public sector might fund research on geographical disease burden, diagnostics, impact of different vaccine presentations, correlates of immunity, animal models, or reagents. The public sector could also play a role in helping the private sector to navigate regulatory requirements and to establish clinical trial infrastructure. For specific products, the public sector can support clinical trials, particularly the

expensive Phase III efficacy trials. While the private sector expects to fund trials relevant for licensing the vaccine in industrialized countries, it has fewer incentives to finance trials in developing countries. Not only are developing country trials primarily of value to introduce the vaccine into this "uncertain, weak" market but also there is a risk that they can generate data or negative publicity that can threaten licensing in the industrial market.

The public sector could also help finance production scale-up. For some vaccines, the incremental costs of scaling up production to meet developing country demand may be too high, given the expected market return. Without public sector help, the private sector may be unwilling to incur these costs.

2. Facilitating research: Aside from providing money, there is an important role for the public sector in two other areas of clinical trial work: facilitation of the trials and adherence to ethics. Potential activities for the public sector include: working with local officials to inform and to educate country participants of the need for, and importance of, clinical trials and assisting in managing any problems that arise during the trial. Education is extremely important, particularly for diseases such as HIV/AIDS and malaria. Enrollees must understand that participating in the trial will not necessarily protect them against the disease and, equally important, that if they do contract the disease, their participation in the trial is not the cause. The public sector could also help manufacturers to clarify expectations and mechanisms for post-trial access to the vaccine. It is not uncommon for clinical trial participants to assume that their community will have guaranteed and continued access to a vaccine being tested. However, as the time between a clinical trial and a licensure of a vaccine is often lengthy and the introduction of a vaccine into developing countries even longer, this expectation needs to be addressed. In cases where the private sector is already ambivalent about conducting a trial in a developing country, demands for post-trial vaccine access may further reduce interest.

3. Harmonizing regulatory requirements: The development and ultimate use of biological products, such as vaccines, are carefully regulated to ensure their safety, immunogenecity, and efficacy. This regulatory function is carried out by the National Regulatory Authority (NRA) which is responsible for licensing and controlling the quality of all biological products used within the country. Currently, many NRAs have their own unique licensing requirements, compelling manufacturers to prepare and to submit separate licensing applications, an expensive, time-consuming, and, many argue, inefficient process. Efforts are underway to harmonize requirements in order to ensure product safety, but minimize the time and the cost of making a vaccine available to populations [10].

4. Tax credits for vaccine research: Structuring tax credits to encourage vaccine R&D is another push intervention under consideration. Like direct financing, tax credits have the benefit of being a familiar policy tool with a proven track record. The tax code of the United States currently contains an allowance for a 20% credit on R&D expenditures; although it must be renewed on an annual basis, it is noncontroversial and nearly unanimously supported by members of Congress and the industry. There remain two issues with using tax credits for vaccine R&D as a push mechanism. First, like other push mechanisms, the existence of the credit does not guarantee results. Second, tax credits can be difficult to implement and monitor.

B. Pull Mechanisms

At the other end of the spectrum, pull mechanisms can also help to reduce the risks of investing in priority products. For the public sector, pull mechanisms may be less risky as they can be structured so that money is committed only if a desirable and affordable vaccine becomes available. However, if financial commitments to specific products must be made early, it will be very difficult to determine the desired outcomes and prices far in advance of having an actual product. If a "winner" is chosen and a price is agreed, the public sector runs the risk of being "locked in" to an outcome that may prove not to be the best. Finally, the fact that these mechanisms have not been tested and so will only prove themselves well into the future increases their risks. For example, a future purchase commitment might be subject to political "changes of heart." For manufacturers who must invest early and heavily, changes of heart have serious financial implications. The following are a number of examples of different types of pull strategies.

1. Accelerating the uptake of existing vaccines: Increasing the uptake of existing vaccines sends a clear, credible signal to industry that the public sector is committed to purchasing and introducing new vaccines. The immediate allocation of hard cash is the best way to strengthen the market. However, while strengthening the market is the most credible way to assure industry of public support for vaccines in the long term, it is likely to be inadequate on its own to overcome the immediate financial risks and costs inhibiting development.

2. Prizes and tournaments: In this context, prizes are offered to whoever achieves a prespecified goal or product, while tournaments offer a reward to whoever has progressed farthest toward the target by a given date. The size of the prize usually corresponds to the level of investment required to win. While structured slightly differently, prizes and tournaments have similar advantages and risks. Both mechanisms encourage competition and therefore increase the number of potential vaccine candidates. They are also relatively easy for the public sector to implement. For the private sector, good public relations may be a valuable side effect of winning a prize or a tournament. Industry's lack of enthusiasm for this strategy, however, may limit the effectiveness of the prizes or the tournament model. Industry representatives have commented that they are "in the business of making vaccines, not winning prizes" [25]. Another serious drawback to prizes and tournaments is they do not guarantee that a viable, affordable vaccine will result. Nonetheless, the prize or tournament prize must be awarded to the winner regardless.

3. Co-payments: A co-payment—probably some amount not equal to the full price of the vaccine—is guaranteed to manufacturers in lieu of trying to lock in to a particular price for a vaccine. Co-payments are attractive to

industry because they are viewed as a commitment today, which is more credible than a promise for future payment. They are attractive to the public sector because they delay negotiations on the full price for a vaccine. However, it is unclear how the "correct" co-pay amount should be derived, and if the co-payment amount, which could end up being a fraction of the vaccine price, would offer enough of an incentive to industry.

4. Differential [tiered] pricing: In order for differential pricing to work, there must be a segmented market, minimal risk of parallel imports, and a willingness to accept and enforce differential prices, particularly in the markets with the higher prices. Differential pricing is currently the only mechanism that allows affordable access to a vaccine in developing and industrialized countries while still allowing industry to recoup its investment on a vaccine. In many cases, the time lag before the product is fully mature and has a significantly lower tiered price is 15 to 20 years. However, allowing industry to charge "what the market will bear" in industrial countries provides a significant incentive for investment, an incentive that would not exist if the price was set by the purchasing ability of sub-Saharan Africa. Finally, differential pricing is a familiar mechanism because it has been used in nearly every other sector from toothpaste to batteries and is often integral to wide spread use of products. Differential pricing, however, is difficult to implement. Safeguards must be instituted to prevent lower-tier prices from becoming the index down to which wealthy countries negotiate. The risk of products flowing back into wealthy markets either between countries or in the same country, while small to date, must also be managed. Finally, for differential pricing to be successful, government procurement agencies, politicians, and the public in industrialized nations must be willing to pay more for vaccines than the poorest developing countries, an idea that is often at odds with political agendas.

5. Market assurances: Market assurances are a type of "guaranteed" takeoff. The assurance may be structured as a commitment to an individual manufacturer or as a commitment to purchase a product from any manufacturer. Three variables may be part of a guarantee between the public to buy and the private sector to supply a given vaccine (1) the specific product, (2) the number of doses, and/or (3) the time frame. The contract or agreement may be backed by either "soft" or "hard" money guarantees, depending on the trade-off between opportunity cost and credibility: Money put aside now is the most credible to industry, but it carries the highest opportunity cost. Although the credibility of market assurances for future products can theoretically be increased through legally binding commitments, in reality, it is difficult to imagine how they would be enforced against public institutions such as WHO, UNICEF, or the World Bank. More credible is the development and implementation of contracts for today's products, a strategy being explored by GAVI and the Vaccine Fund. Industry's interest is likely to vary by vaccine as the commercial return promised by a market assurance may be extremely attractive for some vaccines, but be deemed too distant and uncertain for others.

6. Intellectual property right (IPR) enforcement/protection: IPRs are the foundation upon which the profit of pharmaceutical companies is based. When IPRs are violated, the incentives for industry to invest in vaccine R&D are greatly diminished. The public sector has already taken steps in this direction [e.g., setting up the World Trade Organization (WTO) to enforce the agreement on Trade-Related Aspects of Intellectual Property Rights (TRIPS)], but improvements remain to be made. However, simply put, IPRs provide continuing incentives for industry to invest in vaccine R&D, development, and distribution. IPRs, however, are difficult to implement, difficult to enforce, and politically unpopular with those who contend that cheap drugs need to be made available to bridge the gap between the "haves" and the "have nots." Questions remain about whether or not it will be possible to enforce TRIPS, and whether this mechanism provides enough of an incentive to ensure adequate investments.

7. Tax credits for vaccine sales: Like tax credits for vaccine R&D, tax credits for vaccine sales are perceived as a credible and familiar policy tool. From the standpoint of the public sector, tax credits are attractive because money is only spent once a product has been developed and sold. However, industry has not expressed much interest in this mechanism, possibly because tax credits on vaccine sales are too far in the future to justify investment that may not even result in a successful vaccine. In the event that a tax credit is enacted, it may be difficult to determine the appropriate level of credit. Finally, it is unclear how priorities will be set in the event that a number of these vaccines become available simultaneously, all competing within the same authorized cap.

C. Implementing Push–Pull Mechanisms: Public–Private Partnerships

The push and pull mechanisms discussed in the previous section are potential solutions to the economic challenges inhibiting rapid development and scale-up of priority vaccines. However, many of these ideas have yet to be tested. Public–private partnerships that allow the sectors to share the risks and costs of developing and introducing priority vaccines in novel ways may be a solution. However, both sectors have concerns about entering partnerships. A history of low uptake of vaccines and changing public priorities reduces industry's incentive to partner closely with many public sector entities. Conversely, concerns about industry's motives, the risk of failure, and the perceptions of the popular press are disincentives for the public sector to work with industry.

Despite these fears, partners on the GAVI Board believe that by harnessing the strengths of both private industry and public partners, they can achieve the ambitious goal of developing and making accessible priority vaccines for developing countries. To move forward with credible partnerships, two basic conditions must be met. First, both public and private partners must understand the costs, risks, and benefits driving the partnership. With this knowledge, partners can identify those costs and risks that are important and sensitive to public sector support—those with the highest "leverage." Second, both public and private partners must be confident that the mechanisms or agreements that define the partnership protect each of their interests. For the public sector, this means ensuring public investments result in more rapid development, expanded capacity, and/or lower prices. For the private sector, it means public "promises" translate into real financial commitments that cover investments.

VI. NEXT STEPS AND NEW APPROACHES

Daunting as the science is, the risks and uncertainties of vaccine development are amplified by the economic implications of each investment decision. By understanding the current vaccine market and its suppliers and the investment decisions occurring along the pathway from candidate to commercialized product, the reader can understand the role played by economics in shaping the vaccine world. Public sector partners are increasingly using this growing knowledge to explore possible solutions—push and pull mechanisms—that might change the economics of high-priority products for the developing world.

New mechanisms and partnerships will provide concrete evidence about both the critical obstacles inhibiting progress on specific vaccines and the value and feasibility of particular push and pull mechanisms. This evidence will increase the immunization community's understanding of the economic forces influencing the development of and access to the highest-priority vaccines.

The successful development and introduction of vaccines against the great plagues of our time will be the ultimate test of the immunization community's scientific knowledge and economic acumen. No one mechanism, either push or pull, and no one partner, either public or private, will single-handedly resolve all the issues relating to vaccine availability and access. By working together, public and private partners can identify the most feasible, high-impact solutions to jointly tackle some of the most formidable challenges facing the world, i.e., the development and the implementation of vaccines that can prevent HIV/AIDS, malaria, and tuberculosis.

REFERENCES

1. Kettler HE. Narrowing the Gap Between Provision and Need for Medicines in Developing Countries. London: Office of Health Economics, February 2000.
2. Creating Global Markets for Neglected Drugs and Vaccines: A Challenge for Public–Private Partnership. Global Health Forum I: Consensus Statement. San Francisco, February 2000.
3. Scientific Blueprint 2000. Accelerating Global Efforts in AIDS Vaccine Development, International AIDS Vaccine Initiative. New York, July 2000.
4. Ainsworth M, Batson A. Accelerating an AIDS Vaccine for Developing Countries: Recommendations for the World Bank, http://iaen.org/vacc/accelerateb.pdf, February 2000.
5. Mercer Management Consulting. Lessons Learned: New Procurement Strategies for Vaccines. Final Report to the GAVI Board, http://www.gaviftf.org/docs_activities/pdf/lessons_learned_draft_final.pdf, June 6, 2002.
6. American Home Products Corporation Annual Report, 2000.
7. Mercer Management Consulting. Presentation on the "Eco-

nomic Framework for Global Vaccine Supply: Optimal Methods to Meet Global Demand." Presented at the CVI/Rockefeller Conference on Global Supply of New Vaccines. Bellagio, Italy, February 3–7, 1997.
8. Whitehead P. Global Alliance Board Discussion Paper: Public Sector Vaccine Procurement Approaches. NY. USA, October 28, 1999.
9. Milstien J, et. al. Divergence of Products for Public Sector Immunization Programs. Presentation to the WHO Scientific Advisory Group of Experts (SAGE), June 2001.
10. CVI Forum. Combination Vaccines—Juggling with the Options. Geneva, Switzerland, Number 16, July 1998.
11. Batson A. Win–win interactions between the public and private sectors. Nat Med Vaccine Suppl May 1998; 4(5):487–491.
12. www.supply.unicef.org/publications/index_442.html, January 24, 2002.
13. Brugha R, Starling M, Walt G. GAVI, the first steps: lessons for the Global Fund. Lancet 2002; 359:435–438.
14. World Bank Population Projections 1994–1995. Baltimore, MD: Johns Hopkins University Press, 1994.
15. Siwolop S. Big Steps for the Vaccine Industry. New York Times, July 25, 2001, Section C1, C17.
16. Kaddar M, et al. Costs and Financing of Immunization Programs: Findings of Four Case Studies. Special Initiatives Report 26. Bethesda, MD: Partnerships for Health Reform Project Abt, Associates, Inc., May 2000.
17. CVI Forum, Special Vaccine Industry Issue. Geneva, Switzerland, Number 11, June 1996.
18. CVI Mission to the Brazil. Task Force on Situation Analysis Report. Geneva, Switzerland, 1994.
19. CVI Mission to Iran. Task Force on Situation Analysis Report. Geneva, Switzerland, 1993.
20. CVI Mission to Bangladesh. Task Force on Situation Analysis Report. Geneva, Switzerland, 1992.
21. CVI Mission to Nigeria. Task Force on Situation Analysis Report. Geneva, Switzerland, 1996.
22. CVI Mission to Pakistan. Task Force on Situation Analysis Report. Geneva, Switzerland, 1993.
23. CVI Mission to Egypt. Task Force on Situation Analysis Report. Geneva, Switzerland, 1993.
24. CVI Mission to Republic of South Africa. Task Force on Situation Analysis Report. Geneva, Switzerland, 1993.
25. Batson A, Ainsworth M. Obstacles and solutions: Understanding private investment in HIV/AIDS vaccine development. WHO Bull (Geneva) 2001; 79(8):721–728.
26. Revised Guidelines and Forms for Countries to Use in Submitting Proposals to GAVI and the Vaccine Fund, August 2001.
27. "Vaccine Challenges: Why is Developing a Malaria Vaccine Difficult?" found at www.malariavaccine.org/mal-vac2-challenge.htm, January 25, 2002.
28. State of Current Vaccine Research Page, International AIDS Vaccine Initiative, http://www.iavi.org/, January 16, 2002.
29. Need for Vaccine Page, International AIDS Vaccine Initiative. http://www.iavi.org/, January 24, 2002.
30. World Development Indicators. Washington, DC: World Bank, 1998.
31. Kremer M. Creating Markets for New Vaccines: Part II. Design Issues. Cambridge: National Bureau of Economic Research, May 12, 2000.
32. Madrid Y. A New Access Paradigm: Public Sector Actions to Assure Swift, Global Access to AIDS Vaccines. New York: International AIDS Vaccine Initiative, June 2001.
33. Tackling the Diseases of Poverty. A Report by the Performance Innovation Unit (PIU), UK Cabinet, May 2001, http://www.number-10.gov.uk/su/health/default.htm on January 16, 2001.

7

Development and Supply of Vaccines: An Industry Perspective

Michel Greco
Aventis Pasteur, Lyon, France

I. THE WORLD VACCINE MARKET, PRESENT AND FUTURE

The notion that vaccines are a market is fairly recent. Apart from Smallpox (Jenner), Rabies (Pasteur), and inactivated whole-cell parenteral typhoid vaccine (Wright and Pfeiffer) (see Chapter 1 "Vaccines and Vaccination in the Historical Perspective"), all vaccines have been discovered in the twentieth century, and most in the second half of the century. Also, within the pharmaceutical industry, vaccines have long been set apart, closer to public health authorities, and basically viewed as not-for-profit activities [1,2]. As a result, as recently as in the late 1980s, most pharmaceutical companies were leaving the field of vaccines [3]. Through a number of factors that shall be examined in more detail, the tide was reversed in the last decade of the twentieth century so that today vaccines are a much more competitive area [4]. Nevertheless, the field remains at best a "qualified" market that is strongly regulated and has high entry barriers and supply constraints, is largely "monopsonistic" in nature, and must adjust to specific price setting mechanisms [5].

The vaccine "market" actually comprises three major subsets:

- *Closed markets* where local producers supply the local needs with mostly Expanded Program on Immunization (EPI) monovalent vaccines, which generally cannot be exported, mainly for regulatory reasons, and which value can hardly be assessed [6,7].
- *Donor markets* managed by international organizations [World Health Organization (WHO), United Nations Children's Fund (UNICEF), Pan American Health Organization (PAHO), Global Alliance for Vaccines and Immunization (GAVI)...] who buy mostly EPI vaccines for routine or mass immunization in poor or developing countries, generally in multidose presentations and at tiered prices [8–10]. Although the value of this segment

has increased in the past, it remains a minor part of the overall vaccine market in value, if not in doses.
- *Commercial markets* are those markets, strongly regulated—public or private—where competition does exist and where pricing is implemented in a more classical way so that companies can fund their research and development activities, invest in state-of-the-art industrial facilities, and return a profit to the companies' shareholders. This is by far the largest part in monetary value of the global vaccine market [1,2,4,5], which will be analyzed in more detail in this chapter.

The commercial market is a small, fast-growing, concentrated market. As recently as the late 1980s, the market was worth less than $1 billion worldwide. At that time, it was mostly spread among basic bacterial vaccines and some viral vaccines, among many small national public institutes or companies and generally sold at low prices. In the course of the last 10 years, this market has increased around sixfold to reach $7 billion. But even at $7 billion, it must be emphasized that vaccines represent less than 2% of the global pharmaceutical market (Figure 1) around the same figure as a single lead pharmaceutical product. Looking to the future, it is expected that the market will continue to grow at double-digit rates throughout the decade to reach at least $15 billion (risk adjusted) by 2010 (Figure 2) [1]. Linked to the generally higher prices in North America, this part of the world represents 40% of the market value with Western Europe and the "rest of the world" representing 30% each (Figure 3). It is noteworthy that although the value of the Japanese market is significant (more than $400 million), the number and type of vaccines used there is more limited than in most developed markets. It appears likely that this situation will substantially change in the coming years.

In this chapter, the main reasons for growth of the vaccine industry, past and future [1,11], will be analyzed in some detail.

Vaccines $ 6.9 Billion = 1.8 %

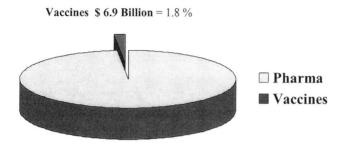

☐ **Pharma**
■ **Vaccines**

TOTAL Pharma : $ 380 Billion

Figure 1 Vaccines market share in the global pharmaceutical market 2001.

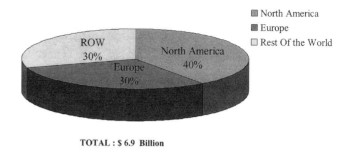

■ North America
■ Europe
☐ Rest Of the World

TOTAL : $ 6.9 Billion

Figure 3 Global vaccine market geographical breakdown 2001.

A. Innovation

Innovation has been and will remain the key driver of growth. What clearly drove the growth in the last 10–15 years was primarily the introduction of major new vaccines such as recombinant Hepatitis B, *Haemophilus influenzae* type b conjugate, Hepatitis A and, more recently, attenuated varicella, and meningocotal and pneumoccocal conjugate vaccines.

Another contributor to growth of the market is the array of innovative combination vaccines for pediatric and adult use, both for primary immunization and for booster use (Figure 4). The future should witness an acceleration of innovation, despite increasing risks. Indeed, currently there are approximately 400 new vaccine projects under study around the world. Obviously, many will not make it to the end [3,12–14]. Nevertheless, never before has there been so much research activity in this field.

Some of the reasons responsible for stimulating this research include:

1. Vaccines remain primarily directed to the prevention of infectious diseases, including bacterial infections that antibiotics are supposed to cure. The widespread use of antibiotics has led to increasing resistance of microorganisms to these compounds. Thus, in some instances, overuse of antibiotics "opens the way" for vaccines. This was true in the development of vaccines against *H. influenzae* type b and is even truer for pneumoccocal vaccines. This is likely to extend to other bacteria such as group A *Streptococcus pyogenes*, *Staphylococcus aureus*, and many others for which vaccines would provide both appropriate medical and economic answers.

2. The progress of medical science and the improved understanding of the immune system have led to a better knowledge of the etiology and pathogenesis of infectious diseases. For example, it has been

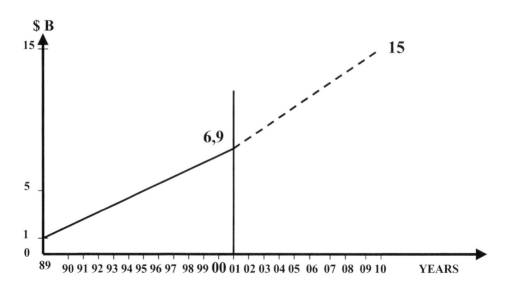

Figure 2 Global vaccine market evolution from a "nonmarket" to a sizable one.

Millions of $

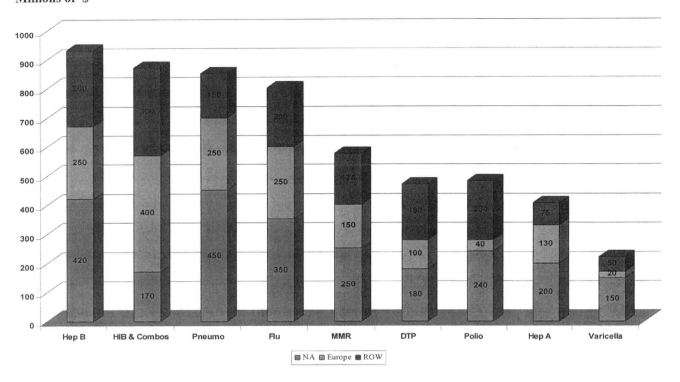

Figure 4 The top nine vaccine families represent 90% of the market in 2001.

shown that many chronic diseases could have an infectious origin, such as ulcers (*Helicobacter pylori*), coronary heart disease (*Chlamydia pneumoniae*), and some cancers (e.g., papillomavirus in cervix cancer, Epstein–Barr virus in nasopharyngeal carcinoma, and Hepatitis B virus in hepatocellular carcinoma).

3. Also, vaccines, which heretofore have been used mostly as preventative agents, are now being considered as possible therapeutic ones linked to scientific developments, and to economic or ethical reasons [15].

4. The emergence of biotechnology and molecular biology has led to the development of new tools allowing the more rational design of new products. New developments such as the sequencing of the human genome will further broaden the field of development and use of potential new vaccines.

5. Other aspects such as the development of new immunization systems also contribute to this innovation process: combined vaccines, safe syringes, needleless injections, transcutaneous administration, mucosal delivery, transgenic animals and plants, DNA immunization, and many more developments will, over time, completely change the approaches to immunization.

6. The development of information technology, including bioinformatics, allows an accelerated review of a much larger number of approaches.

All these and other reasons explain why innovation should remain a key driver in the expansion of the vaccine area generating many new projects (Figure 5; Table 1)

B. Demography

Demography is another key growth driver for the vaccine field, in many different ways.

1. Volume-wise, immunization is primarily driven by the continuing growth of the population in less-developed countries. More than 80% of the vaccine doses produced in the world are currently directed to those markets.

2. In industrialized countries, apart from innovation, the growth of immunization is largely driven by the "senior citizen" segment of the population that is continually expanding. Already, with vaccines directed at the prevention of influenza, pneumococcal infections, and soon zoster, in addition to the expanding use of booster immunization, this segment has a large growth potential. In a more general trend, immunization, which used to be directed mostly to infants, is extending to all stages of life.

3. Travel and migrations (whether voluntary or not) constitute another major potential source of clinical infectious diseases, which are quite often vaccine preventable. This includes specific "at-risk" populations such as deployed military contingents.

Innovation Drivers

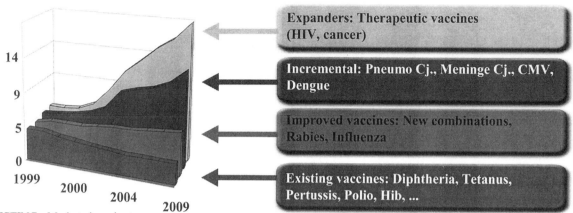

Billions $

Expanders: Therapeutic vaccines (HIV, cancer)

Incremental: Pneumo Cj., Meninge Cj., CMV, Dengue

Improved vaccines: New combinations, Rabies, Influenza

Existing vaccines: Diphtheria, Tetanus, Pertussis, Polio, Hib, ...

EXISTING : Marketed products

IMPROVED : New presentations of existing antigens

INCREMENTAL : Existing technologies / new disease targets

EXPANDERS : New technologies / new disease targets

Figure 5 The future of vaccines: an industrial perspective.

The overall consequence of these demographic trends is an ever-expanding demand for existing and new vaccines and a market structure where the balance of sales is progressively turning to adult/senior immunization as opposed to infants' vaccination (Figure 6).

C. Prevention

Among other key factors impacting the demand for vaccines is the realization that *prevention* makes sense both from a

medical standpoint (avoiding disease, resistance to therapy, side effects of drugs, etc.) and from an economic standpoint (pay a little now to reduce the public health bill down the road both in terms of direct and indirect costs). In this respect, a better recognition of the "value" of vaccines both in the developing and developed world will contribute to better vaccination coverage and to further increased efforts for the research of new vaccines. It is anticipated that the ever-greater use of pharmaco-economic studies will increasingly support the expansion of immunization.

D. Equity

In a global world, it is becoming increasingly unacceptable to see children in the poor countries continue to die from

Table 1 More than 400 New Vaccine Projects Worldwide

Main future vaccines	
–New Combos (DtaP, MMR, Hep, meninge, others	–Pneumo-conjugate
–Rotavirus	–Meningo conjugate
–Lyme	–*H. pylori*
–ETEC	–New flu
–HSV	–JEV
–RSV	–Dengue
–Zoster	–CMV
–EBV	–HPV
–Hep C	–Meningo B
–Gonococcus	–Tuberculosis
–Hep E	–Schistosomiasis
–NT HIB	–Strep A
–Malaria	–Strep B
–Urinary tract	–HIV prevent/therapeutic
–Otitis media	–Haemorrhagic fevers
–*Staphylococcus*	–Chlamydia

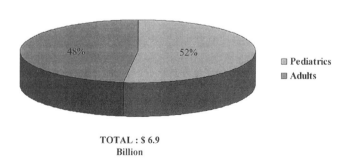

TOTAL : $ 6.9 Billion

Figure 6 Global vaccine market age segmentation in 2001. In 2010, adolescent and adult vaccines will likely represent 60% of market value.

• Partnership in support of immunization

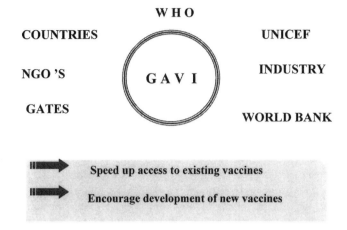

Figure 7 The future of vaccines: an industrial perspective.

vaccine-preventable diseases when the needed vaccines exist and can often be obtained at reduced prices [16,17]. This has led to a major initiative by the international community, including WHO, UNICEF, and a number of public or private organizations such as the Gates Foundation, and Industry, culminating in formation of the Global Alliance for Vaccines and Immunization (GAVI) [12,18,19]. Industry believes that, for the first time, such an initiative has a good chance of succeeding because all the actors are present (Figure 7), and a methodology exists to plan and implement activities and to guarantee that the results are monitored. Also, funding has been available from the onset and should be sustainable, driven by the Vaccine Fund.

E. Bioterrorism

Last but not least, the emergence of *bioterrorism* in the late 1990s and the cataclysmic event that will go down in history

as "September 11" has reignited demand for vaccines against bacteria or viruses that can be used as agents in biological warfare, including smallpox and anthrax [20]. This has led many authorities to question whether immunization could ever be stopped for diseases such as polio where final eradication is in sight, not to mention more exotic diseases. All these factors clearly indicate that the demand for existing and new vaccines will remain strong for the foreseeable future.

II. THE VACCINE INDUSTRY

The vaccine industry is fairly young. It finds its origin in national public institutes or companies that were set up to ensure that the basic health needs would be provided to the population, mostly for the prevention of diphtheria, tetanus, pertussis, and poliomyelitis.

With the development of additional new bacterial and viral vaccines, recombinant vaccines, and, more recently, of new technologies, and with the need to scale up production and heavily invest in capacity and compliance, a number of local producers—whether in developed or less-developed countries—have disappeared or been acquired; as a consequence, the vaccine industry has become increasingly concentrated with a few key players [1,2,10,21,22] (Figure 8).

–Aventis Pasteur is probably the oldest one among the major actors, with the broadest vaccine range and geographical coverage. It results from the merger in the late 1980s of Institut Mérieux, Pasteur Vaccins, and Connaught Laboratories Limited.

–GSK Biologicals originated in a small Belgian operation called RIT, which was acquired by Smith-Kline and French, and, subsequently, though mergers, became SmithKline Beecham (SB Biologicals), and, finally, Glaxo SmithKline Biologicals. A small operation until the mid-1980s, the company extensively grew based on its Hepatitis vaccine franchise (recombinant Hepatitis B and Hepatitis A). It then broadened its product range to include infant combination vaccines and expanded its international distribution.

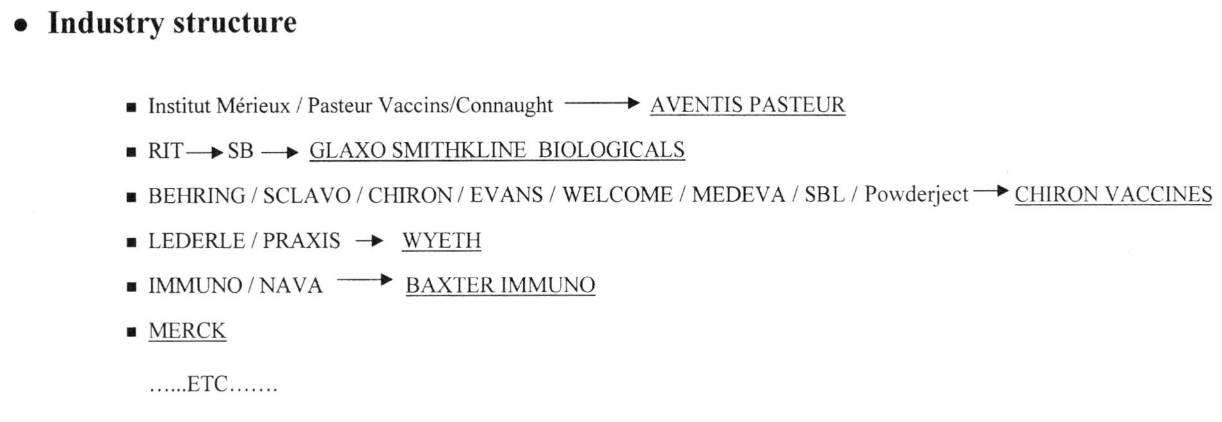

• Industry structure

■ Institut Mérieux / Pasteur Vaccins/Connaught ⟶ AVENTIS PASTEUR

■ RIT⟶ SB ⟶ GLAXO SMITHKLINE BIOLOGICALS

■ BEHRING / SCLAVO / CHIRON / EVANS / WELCOME / MEDEVA / SBL / Powderject ⟶ CHIRON VACCINES

■ LEDERLE / PRAXIS ⟶ WYETH

■ IMMUNO / NAVA ⟶ BAXTER IMMUNO

■ MERCK

……ETC…….

Figure 8 The future of vaccines: an industrial perspective.

–Merck Vaccines is a specialized division of Merck and Co. that has long been the U.S. market leader. It expanded in Europe through a joint venture with Aventis Pasteur but otherwise still has a limited activity in international markets.

These three players each represent between 20% and 25% of the world market.

–A fourth company, Wyeth, long a market leader in the United States, actually stopped distributing some basic pediatric vaccines before staging a resurgence at the end of the century with a pneumococcal conjugate vaccine (from a market perspective, possibly the first "blockbuster vaccine"), as well as a meningococcal C conjugate vaccine.
These four companies encompass approximately 80% of the world commercial vaccine market (Figure 9).
–Other less-dominant actors have resulted from the concentration of smaller companies, such as:

–Chiron Vaccines (Chiron, Behring, Sclavo, Evans, Welcome, SBL...)
–Baxter Vaccines (Immuno, Nava...)
–Berna (including Rheinbiotech)
–Etc...

–The remaining manufacturers in developed countries are mostly dependent on major manufacturers for supplying their needs and are generally meaningful only in their home markets (Australia, Japan, Korea, Netherlands...).

One can expect the future to bring even more amalgamation of vaccine manufacturers and the likelihood that the relative positions may well change again linked to the pace of innovation in the various companies and the success of the development projects that they have chosen to support. Apart from these already established companies, new actors should appear:

–Some major pharma companies may become involved in a selective manner in a particular therapeutic field, acting as "cherry pickers."
–Biotech companies are increasingly becoming involved in the innovation process as major companies outsource an increasing share of their R&D. In the future, some will try to develop into fully integrated operations.
–Also, producers from major less-developed countries (such as Serum Institute of India, Biopharma in Indonesia, Chinese producers, Brazilian companies, Cuban manufacturers, etc.) should become more prominent, especially as developed country manufacturers rationalize their product ranges, particularly with respect to "monovalent" vaccines such as measles, BCG, DTP, etc. It can be expected that as a result, over time, the developing country manufacturers will increasingly gain expertise and become more competitive with the main actors.

III. THE ENVIRONMENT OF VACCINES

Despite all the positive factors described above, the field of vaccines remains at best a "qualified" market, with many specific constraints or features, among which some deserve to be highlighted.

–Many vaccines are designed for populations everywhere, regardless of where they live or their income level, and it is increasingly argued that immunization is a fundamental right and that vaccines are "Public Goods" rather than "for profit" pharmaceuticals. This raises issues of equal access to vaccines, dual pricing, etc.
–Vaccines are given to healthy individuals to prevent disease. This leads to some interesting consequences: total efficacy is generally expected, side effects are viewed as unacceptable (a situation quite different from pharmaceuticals which are mostly used to cure sick people).
–Also, linked to the fact that some vaccine-preventable diseases have almost disappeared from many industrialized countries and to the trends in modern society (individual rights, access to information, etc.), more and more constituencies, particularly in industrialized countries, are arguing that personal decision should determine whether they or their family members should be immunized [23]. As vaccine-preventable diseases disappear, such attitudes become increasingly more prevalent because the fear of the vaccine sometimes becomes more important than the fear of the disease (Figure 10) [24].

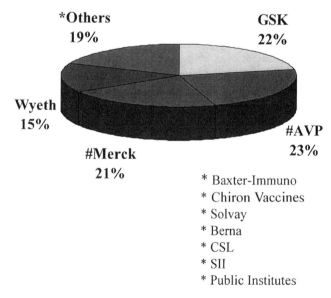

Figure 9 Manufacturers' market shares 2001. #The sales of Aventis Pasteur MSD, a European joint venture between Merck and Aventis Pasteur are split 50/50 between the two companies.

–As a corollary to these emerging concerns on safety, individual rights, information, the "principle of precaution" is increasingly taking precedence over that of protection of Public Health. In turn, this is raising major issues in terms of liabilities and Public Health policies [5].

–Even as the vaccine market is concentrated on the supply side, it is quite often equally concentrated on the buyers' side, whether at the world level (UNICEF), in global regions (PAHO), or in specific countries (industrialized as well as developing) where large public institutions acquire vaccines. This makes for a "monopsonistic" seller/buyer relationship, in which availability of supply plays an increasing role.

–Both for historical reasons and because vaccines are potentially directed to the total population, they have long been treated as commodities trading at low prices. In view of the increasing levels of investments in R&D, scale up, production, quality, and regulatory areas, this is no longer sustainable both for existing and new vaccines.

All these points make for a paradoxical market that is at the same time somewhat protected (the barriers to entry are high) and quite attractive (with demand constantly outpacing supply), but also very constrained by ever-increasing regulations and by its stakeholders and the environment at large. This is true both for the Research and Development Process and for the Supply Process.

IV. DEVELOPMENT AND SUPPLY OF VACCINES: MAJOR ISSUES FACING THE INDUSTRY

A large demand—present and future—and a limited number of existing or potential suppliers are facing a complex process of researching, developing, manufacturing, and supplying vaccines to the world at large. Without elaborating on each step of the process, some of the key issues or hurdles for the industry will be highlighted.

A. The Research and Development Process

Although the different stages of the Research and Development process (Figure 11) may look quite similar for vaccines as for pharmaceuticals, in general they are very specific in a number of ways and have substantially changed over the past few years.

1. Lead Generation

Lead generation used to be somewhat limited but fairly predictable. A vaccine in development would have a chance of success ranging from 10% to 100%, whereas figures for the Pharma Industry were running in a 1/10,000 range.

The "easy" vaccines have already been made. Paradoxically in some respects, the advent of biotechnology tools has resulted in more than 400 vaccine projects worldwide and many more at preclinical stage [1,11]. Moreover, they are more rationally designed and avoid, in principle, a number of pitfalls of traditional vaccines. Yet in practice, one finds a much higher failure rate and an increasing difficulty to determine early correlates of efficacy, therefore leading to a delayed proof of concept (Figure 12) [3,12–14,22]. In many cases, the proof of concept is only reached at the end of large efficacy trials, thereby leading to skyrocketing R&D costs.

2. Clinical Development

In the clinical field, linked to regulatory, safety, and quality requirements, time and costs have escalated. Especially, the need to detect very rare side effects for diseases that are themselves becoming less prevalent has led to huge increases in the number of clinical cases requested for safety and protection trials. Where a few hundred cases were needed a decade ago, the numbers have climbed to the thousands to reach sometimes 20,000 in the mid- to late 1990s. More recently, following the withdrawal of Wyeth's Rotavirus vaccine, a new candidate vaccine had to plan a 67,000-subject study. It is widely expected that in the not too distant future, studies requiring 100,000 subjects could be required. One can easily imagine the impact on timing, costs, and

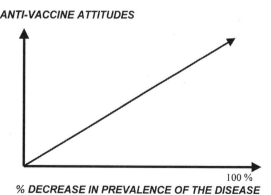

- 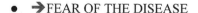 FEAR OF THE DISEASE

- VS

- FEAR OF THE VACCINES

ANTI-VACCINE ATTITUDES

100 %

% DECREASE IN PREVALENCE OF THE DISEASE

Figure 10 Evolution of vaccine perception.

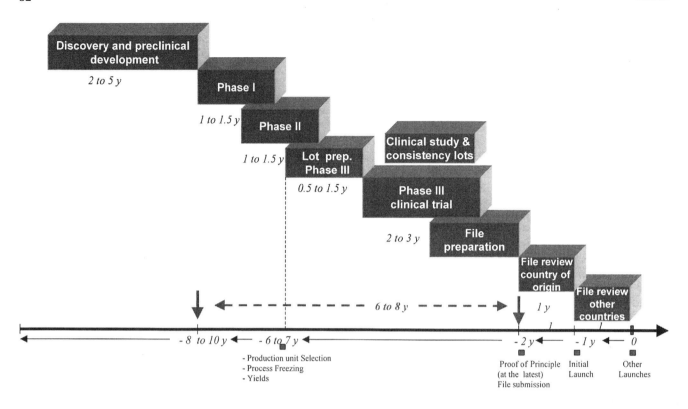

Figure 11 General concept of development phases.

pricing of such requirements. For timing, 10 years is now considered as a minimum, as shown in Figure 11, assuming a good initial understanding of the immune mechanism for the disease. It can only be much more when the virus is elusive or when the disease mechanisms are not always well understood (such as in HIV, malaria, tuberculosis, etc.).

For costs, where vaccines used to be quite cheap to develop compared to pharmaceuticals, the costs easily run in the hundreds of millions of dollars and clinical trials can sometimes only be conducted with the support of large public institutions, especially for the more costly late development phase [2]. The example in Figure 13 shows a typical distribution of costs among the various phases. These costs are based on an average size project and a fairly straightforward process with no major difficulties and do not include the now much more significant amounts to be spent on the regulatory process and on postmarketing surveillance. For

these reasons and others, proper planning that allows as many activities as possible to be run in parallel is a key to the competitiveness of companies in terms of time-to-market (Figure 14).

3. Formulation Development

Again, in relation to the ever-increasing safety concerns and improved quality standards, new vaccines have to avoid a number of agents that have long been shown to be useful and sometimes indispensable for vaccine formulation [25].

—*Bovine material* (mostly fetal calf serum) has been used in most vaccines as a growth medium. Following the Bovine Spongiform Encephalopathy (BSE) scare, this material had to be sourced from the so-called BSE-free countries. For new vaccines, avoiding bovine material has become the rule.
—*Human albumin* has long been used in the formulation of a number of vaccines to improve their stability. For similar reasons, the trend is to replace it by recombinant substances or other materials deemed more acceptable.
—It has long been shown that to optimize vaccine immunogenicity, adjuvantation was needed and that aluminum salts (hydroxide or phosphate) provided the best results. Now questions are being asked on the appropriateness of using these adjuvants, when no proof has been provided to show that alum has noxious properties. Many companies are involved

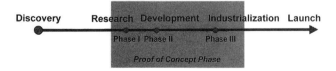

Figure 12 Research-to-Launch Process is a long process: spanning over 8–12 years.

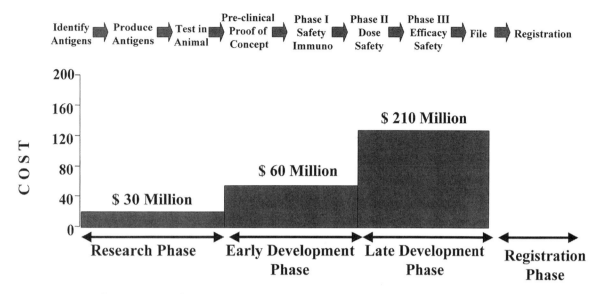

Figure 13 Vaccine development costs: Typical profile for a $300 million project.

in the development of new adjuvants. In most cases, these candidates seem to yield positive results in animals. But in moving from mice to men, none has yet matched results obtained with alum.

—In the same manner, preservatives have been used for many years to protect vaccines from bacterial contamination during the manufacturing process or downstream during product handling. This has proved necessary especially for multidose vaccines or to support WHO's "open vial" policy. In the year 2000, the American Academy of Pediatrics ruled that the use of mercury salts in vaccines was to be avoided [26], while not establishing a causal relationship between the presence of these compounds and specific undesirable or toxic effects in man. In developed countries, this has led to an overall move to single-dose vials that contain no preservatives but has also resulted in a strengthening of manufacturing procedures. Although feasible, it has led to major disruptions in the supply of vaccines to these markets as well as substantial price

increases. Should these decisions be enforced across the world, this would imply huge shortfalls in the supply of vaccines to less-developed countries, with the disappearance of a number of multidose vaccines, a resulting shortage in manufacturing capacity for monodose vaccines, and a steep increase in prices.

—Among other sensitive points, contrary to the general pharmaceutical industry, the vaccine industry still has to make extensive use of animals for its toxicity studies and for control of vaccines [27]. While it has been working hard to develop alternative cell-culture-based solutions, Industry still has to use mice, rabbits, and monkeys. Linked to pressures from lobbying groups, this is becoming increasingly sensitive and difficult and could also negatively impact the supply of vaccines.

—More generally, in relation to the pressures from regulatory authorities, in particular the Food and Drug administration (FDA), companies have had to reinforce the quality and compliance of their processes [28]. This has meant very large financial and human investments to perform the needed experiments and develop the requested documentation, adding to the cost, slowing down the overall process, and sometimes resulting in technical improvements that are difficult to implement.

B. The Manufacturing Process

Many issues relevant to vaccine research and development are equally applicable to manufacturing, with the additional need to scale up from the bench level to the pilot stage and the industrial stage, all the while ensuring consistency [2,3,14,27–31]. This raises scientific and technical issues, including validation, testing, and quality assurance. It also

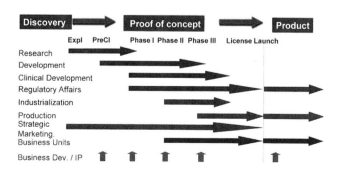

Figure 14 The Research-to-Launch Process involves many functions.

raises capacity and financing issues linked to heavy investments in buildings, facilities, equipment, and headcount.

In this respect, vaccines are clearly much more labor-intensive than pharmaceuticals. It is quite common to have 50% of the total headcount of vaccine companies in the industrial area. Also, apart from direct production, many more competencies are needed. The rule of thumb is that for two persons employed in production, at least one is needed in Quality Control. Quality and Compliance are enforced both internally by ever more stringent procedures Good Manufacturing Practices (GMP) and externally through inspections by public health authorities that can result in "remarks," "warnings," "consent decrees," or even to outright closures of plants [28]. This has now affected all major manufacturers one way or another and is adding to the issues relevant to costs, supply, and productivity.

In vaccine manufacturing, time is crucial, both short and long term. This highlights the necessity for good forecasting and good planning while always keeping in mind the uncertainties linked to biological production.

Short term, moving from the bulk to the distribution of the vaccine, is no simple operation and it takes anywhere from 9 to 22 months (with the exception of the influenza vaccine) to manufacture and release a vaccine (Figure 15). This practically means that an inaccurate forecast, poor production planning, a batch failure, a change in recommendations by the health authorities, delays in batch releases, etc. will almost automatically translate into delays of several months to a year at market level.

Longer term, investing in new manufacturing equipment or facilities, is also no simple exercise and can take anywhere between 2 years for a new packaging line (studying, ordering, installing, validating) to 5 years for a new facility and 7 years for a new site, assuming no major complications (Figure 16). In practical terms for the vaccine manufacturer, this means having to take a major financial risk without knowing whether the development project will be successful and will yield an actual product. These time and cost elements have become even more critical given the fact that manufacturing capacities have been saturated for the last few years and therefore new investments have to be assessed on the basis of dedicated capacities, using the lowest market prices to establish the payback and the Net Present Value of the investments. The relevant resulting product costs then have to be computed on a "full-cost" basis, not

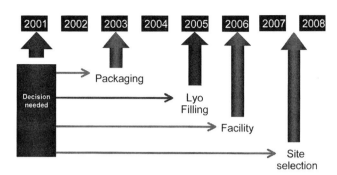

Figure 16 Decision timeline for capacity increase.

just on marginal costs as could be the case when capacities were not saturated.

C. The Supply Process

Having researched, developed, and manufactured vaccines, industry must supply them to the markets. Indeed, there is no such thing as a unified vaccine market, but rather several markets, each with their own specific features, as already mentioned: poor vs. developed countries; public vs. private markets; countries with different climates, epidemiologic patterns, infrastructure, etc.; and as a result, countries with different immunization schedules, vaccination coverage, and logistical requirements. Therefore supplying vaccines means being able to supply the right products with the appropriate presentation maintained in the cold chain—another vaccine specificity—in the right quantities and specifications, locally licensed and batch released, at a price.

Obviously, for the reasons already described above, there is no substitute to proper forecasting and planning to face an ever-increasing demand. Even in developed countries where normal market mechanisms operate, supplying the needs remains a challenge and often requires a real partnership between public authorities and industry. The challenge is even greater for less-developed countries, where the logistical infrastructure is often inadequate (whether for the physical distribution of the products or for an appropriate administration of the vaccination) and the buying power low.

V. SOCIETAL ISSUES

In a world where the "right to healthcare" is becoming an increasing concern, this situation raises issues of access, which some companies have addressed for a long time already, as well as issues of perception of vaccines [21].

A. Access to Immunization

1. Intellectual Property

Intellectual property (IP) is key to the survival of companies and to the pursuit of innovation [2,3,22]. It guarantees them an acceptable return on their research activities (which include both successful and unsuccessful projects). It trans-

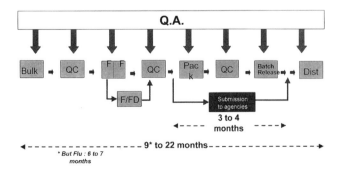

Figure 15 Main manufacturing steps.

lates into pricing policies that will provide such a return for a time. Now this may lead to the situation where vaccines—mostly recent ones—may prove too expensive for the health needs of less-developed countries.

This may be true in principle, albeit not necessarily in practice. All EPI vaccines except Hepatitis B have lost their patent protection a long time ago and these vaccines (including Hepatitis B) have been sold at very low prices to public buyers of less-developed countries. Still, quite often, supply is not sufficient because of the limited production capacity and the very low prices, not of patents.

The situation is obviously quite different for new patented products where the originating companies have to be guaranteed a fair return. Maintaining or even reinforcing patent laws is a must in developed countries. This has taken place to some extent with the extension of patent laws in some countries, for new indications and for orphan products, where the very limited size of the potential market is a strong deterrent to industry's interest.

At the same time, patents have also been weakened in a number of ways: the early introduction of generics (through such mechanisms as "Bolar" in the United States), the large number of countries still not enforcing patent laws, the threat of compulsory licensing, not only in less-developed countries but also in major markets such as the United States, linked to the bioterrorism scare. More generally, in the post-Seattle (antiglobalization movement), post-Pretoria (South African judicial ruling overriding patent), post-DOHA circumstances, society at large has been applying strong pressures to make pharmaceuticals and vaccines more readily available to the poorest countries. Industry, while fully aware of these changes, needs to understand where this is taking such things as Intellectual Property protection, which remains the main stimulus to innovation. Creative thinking is needed at this time to develop new ideas to ensure compatibility between these apparently conflicting goals. It will probably take time and a mix of different steps from all parties to reach a satisfactory solution.

2. Technology Transfers

One of the ways to improve access for the less-developed countries has sometimes been seen in Transfers of Technology (ToTs). These transfers may look like an easy solution. This is certainly not the case. As previously discussed, setting up a state-of-the-art manufacturing facility is not an easy task. It requires money, adequately trained people, an adequate local environment (especially for controls), and support from other partners. It also requires a large-enough guaranteed market. . . and time.

As a result, a technology transfer can only succeed if it is very well planned, through a stepwise approach and a learning process. An ill-planned/ill-conceived ToT will only result in failure, frustration, and resentment. Also, such transfers will have to be financially successful. Obviously, if prices are too low, this will prove detrimental for local companies who need to heavily invest to catch up with their counterparts in developed countries.

Now with the emergence of significant local manufacturers in the major less-developed countries, such as China,

India, Indonesia, Brazil, etc., the developed countries' manufacturers also have to decide for themselves whether to delocalize some productions or enter in partnerships, joint ventures or outright ToTs, as an element of their long-term strategy. This has already taken place in a number of countries and will certainly further develop over the years.

3. Dual Track

Because of the vast needs and to the strong downward pressures on vaccine prices for the poorest countries, practical solutions have had to be identified to ensure supply. Overtime, this has developed into a situation where a "dual track" exists between developed and developing countries for many vaccines:

> —Acellular pertussis vs. whole cell pertussis vaccines.
> —Jeryl-Lynn-based measles/mumps/rubella (MMR) vs. Urabe-based MMR or monovalent measles.
> —Inactivated polio vaccine (IPV) vs. oral polio vaccine (OPV).
> —Combined vaccines vs. monovalent vaccines.
> —Monodose vs. multidose vaccines.
> —Thiomersal-free vs. thiomersal-containing vaccines.
> —Wide access vs. limited access to new vaccines.

Obviously, dual-track has been closely related to dual pricing. Although ethically arguable in principle, such a situation is a pragmatic answer to a difficult situation. Taking a purely ideological stance would be counterproductive. What is probably a better answer is to make sure that any solution addresses epidemiological needs, is efficacious and safe, implemented with quality standards at the same level as for developed countries, and is price competitive.

4. Tiered Pricing

The practice of differential prices between affluent and poor countries has existed for a long time, especially for vaccines, and mostly for companies of European origin. This is linked to many factors, including Europe's historical relationship with these countries and different legal as well as cultural backgrounds between Europe and North America. This practice has been mostly applied to basic EPI vaccines for international tenders or local public markets (the most important ones) but much less for local private markets. Tiered pricing policies are only possible if limited to certain countries and if "normal" prices are implemented in developed markets, allowing not just paying for R&D, investments, margins, etc. but also—in a way—subsidizing these lower-priced markets. Such a strategy cannot be just the responsibility of industry [10,32]. Public authorities and international institutions and nongovernmental organizations (NGOs) also have to be involved, recognizing some basic rules and guaranteeing, among other things, that no reimportation will occur into developed markets, both for economical and technical reasons.

5. Access to New or Specific Vaccines

As already mentioned, one can readily understand that if achieving high coverage for EPI vaccines in the poorest countries is a challenge, introducing newer, more expensive

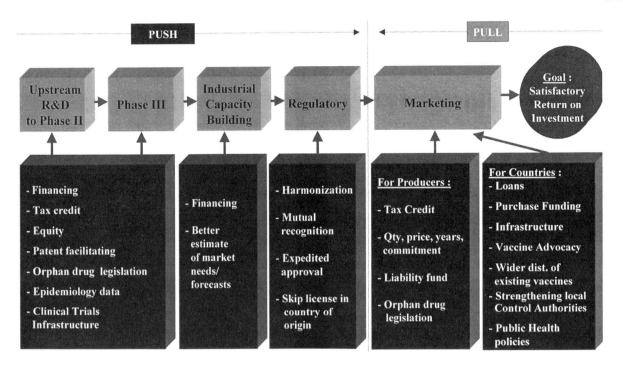

Figure 17   Typical Push/Pull mechanisms.

vaccines (not to mention future even higher-priced ones) is proving much more difficult. Pure market mechanisms have proved insufficient to tackle this situation. Only the joint effort of all stakeholders will have a chance to bring forward the beginning of a solution. As shown in Figure 7 above, the GAVI initiative has been the first such global approach with a chance of success. But sustaining initial results will require creativity and efforts on the part of all parties: countries, international institutions, nongovernmental organizations (NGOs), industry, etc. The priority will be to build local infrastructures able to implement consistent immunization strategies and to ensure long-term funding and ownership of these strategies. Focus will also certainly be a keyword. The creation of the Vaccine Fund is a clear step in this direction. Industry can and should be a full partner in this task. It should be encouraged to contribute, either through PUSH or PULL incentives (Figure 17) [33]. PUSH to help fund the development of vaccine solutions for the poorest countries; PULL to help create viable markets downstream.

B.   Perception of Vaccines

Along with ACCESS, PERCEPTION of vaccines is one of the other important issues facing immunization policies and policy makers. The paradox lies in the fact that it is simultaneously claimed that immunization is a "human right" but that getting immunized should result from an individual decision, thereby respecting "individual rights." This is especially tricky for vaccines because only a high-enough coverage can ensure effective "herd immunity", and, for some diseases, allow regional elimination or even global eradication (e.g., polio). At a time when vaccines have led to the

quasi disappearance of a number of diseases in many countries, the need to immunize is less strongly perceived and the side effects are more visible and more widely discussed.

Rare safety issues—sometimes based only on theory—can severely impact the success of immunization policies or campaigns in developed and less-developed countries [24]. In an era of instant and global communication [23], isolated incidents, pushed by strong antivaccine lobbies, can have devastating effects on public health. All parties, including industry, should accept that the paradigm has changed. Whereas in the past the producer used to call the shots, now the buyer and the regulator have assumed dominance and the power is now largely in the hands of the consumer and the media [23]. Also, recent developments such as the "principle of precaution" are here to stay, whether we like it or not. In such a situation, new attitudes need to be developed, accepting that all parties are accountable. We cannot just assume that vaccines are good for mankind and advocate their increased use. We also have to be more transparent, more informative, more open to challenge; we have to implement active "vaccine-vigilance" tools [24,34–36]. We have to anticipate, better coordinate efforts, and be prepared to stand by scientific data, while accepting that they may not always be the only answer to society's concerns in today's world.

REFERENCES

1.   Greco M. Key drivers behind the development of global vaccine market. Vaccine 2001; 19:1606–1610.
2.   Gregerson J-P. Vaccine development: the long road from initial idea to product licensure. In: Levine MM, Woodrow

GC, Kaper JB, Cobon GS, eds. New Generation Vaccines. New York: Marcel Dekker, 1997:1165–1178.

3. Douglas RG JR. How vaccines are developed. Curr Clin Top Infect Dis 1994; 14:192–204.

4. Dove A. Report predicts burgeoning vaccine markets. Nat Med 2001; 7:877.

5. Vandersmissen W. Business perspectives of a European vaccine manufacturer. Vaccine 2001; 20(suppl 1):S104–S106.

6. Milstien JB, et al. Global DTP manufacturing capacity and capability. Status report: January 1995. Vaccine 1996; 14:313–320.

7. Batson A, et al. The crisis in vaccine supply: a framework for action. Vaccine 1994; 12:963–965.

8. Woodle D. Vaccine procurement and self-sufficiency in developing countries. Health Policy Plan 2000; 15:121–129.

9. Vandersmissen W. WHO expectation and industry goals. Vaccine 2001; 19:1611–1615.

10. Batson A. Win–win interactions between the public and private sectors. Nat Med 1998; 4:487–491.

11. Greco M. The future of vaccines: an industrial perspective. Vaccine 2001; 20(suppl 1):S101–S103.

12. Levine MM, et al. Overview of vaccines and immunisation. Br Med Bull 2002; 62:1–13.

13. Levine MM. The legacy of Edward Jenner. BMJ 1996; 312:1177–1178.

14. Peter G, et al. Lessons learned from a review of the development of selected vaccines. National Vaccine Advisory Committee. Pediatrics 1999; 104:942–950.

15. Committee to Study Priorities for Vaccine Development DoHPaDP, Institute of Medicine. Vaccines for the 21st Century: A Tool for Decision making. In: Stratton KR, Durch JS, Lawrence RS, eds. Washington, DC: National Academy Press, 1999 (Ref Type: Report).

16. Jha P, et al. Improving the health of the global poor. Science 2002; 295:2036–2039.

17. Feachem RG. Poverty and inequity: a proper focus for the new century. Bull WHO 2000; 78:1–2.

18. Godal T. Viewpoint: immunization against poverty. Trop Med Int Health 2000; 5:160–166.

19. Nossal GJ. The Global Alliance for Vaccines and Immunization—a millennial challenge. Nat Immunol 2000; 1: 5–8.

20. Frey SE, et al. Clinical responses to undiluted and diluted smallpox vaccine. N Engl J Med 2002; 346:1265–1274.

21. Rappuoli R, et al. Medicine. The intangible value of vaccination. Science 2002; 297:937–939.

22. National Vaccine Advisory Committee. United States vaccine research: a delicate fabric of public and private collaboration. Pediatrics 1997; 100:1015–1020.

23. Cookson C. Benefit and risk of vaccination as seen by the general public and the media. Vaccine 2001; 20(suppl 1):S85–S88.

24. Chen RT. Vaccine risks: real, perceived and unknown. Vaccine 1999; 17(suppl 3):S41–S46.

25. Haase M. Regulating vaccines involving new technologies to ensure safety and timely licensure—the challenge. Vaccine 2001; 20(suppl 1):S68–S69.

26. Summary of the joint statement on thimerosal in vaccines. American Academy of Family Physicians, American Academy of Pediatrics, Advisory Committee on Immunization Practices, Public Health Service. MMWR Morb Mortal Wkly Rep 2000; 49:622,631.

27. Van Hoof J. Manufacturing issues related to combining different antigens: an industry perspective. Clin Infect Dis 2001; 33(suppl 4):S346–S350.

28. Monahan TR. Vaccine industry perspective of current issues of good manufacturing practices regarding product inspections and stability testing. Clin Infect Dis 2001; 33(suppl 4):S356–S361.

29. Vose JR. Perspectives on the manufacture of combination vaccines. Clin Infect Dis 2001; 33(suppl 4):S334–S339.

30. Falk LA, Ball LK. Current status and future trends in vaccine regulation—USA. Vaccine 2001; 19:1567–1572.

31. Falk LA, Arciniega J, McVittie L. Manufacturing issues with combining different antigens: a regulatory perspective. Clin Infect Dis 2001; 33(suppl 4):S351–S355.

32. Widdus R. Public–private partnerships for health: their main targets, their diversity, and their future directions. Bull WHO 2001; 79:713–720.

33. Batson A, Ainsworth M. Private investment in AIDS vaccine development: obstacles and solutions. Bull WHO 2001; 79: 721–727.

34. Singleton JA, et al. An overview of the vaccine adverse event reporting system (VAERS) as a surveillance system. VAERS Working Group. Vaccine 1999; 17:2908–2917.

35. Andrews NJ. Statistical assessment of the association between vaccination and rare adverse events post-licensure. Vaccine 2001; 20(suppl 1):S49–S53.

36. Murphy TV, et al. Intussusception among infants given an oral rotavirus vaccine. N Engl J Med 2001; 344:564–572.

8

Reaching Every Child—Achieving Equity in Global Immunization

R. Bruce Aylward and M. Birmingham
World Health Organization, Geneva, Switzerland

J. Lloyd
Program for Appropriate Technology in Health (PATH), Ferney-Voltaire, Switzerland

B. Melgaard[*]
World Health Organization Representative, Bangkok, Thailand

I. INTRODUCTION

Since the early 1960s, high-quality vaccines have been available to counter many of the most common infectious diseases that kill or severely harm children, such as measles, diphtheria, pertussis, polio, and tetanus [1]. Until as recently as 1975, however, less than 5% of the world's children had access to these vaccines, despite immunization being the most cost-effective of health interventions [2,3].

That extraordinary progress has been made in rectifying the gap in childhood immunization coverage between rich and poor countries is primarily the result of one of the largest and most successful public health initiatives ever—the Expanded Programme on Immunization (EPI). Through this program, a global network of national immunization services was developed, such that within 15 years, routine coverage of children had risen to nearly 75% worldwide [4], and world leaders were backing new and ambitious global immunization goals such as the eradication of poliomyelitis [5].

Although extraordinary progress has been made toward reaching all children with immunization services, as the last millennium closed on 31 December 1999, more than 25% of the children in the world were still not routinely receiving the basic childhood vaccines. Of more concern, in the first year of this new millennium nearly two million children died of vaccine-preventable diseases, with the majority of these deaths occurring in developing countries [6].

This chapter outlines the history and accomplishments of the global EPI effort and summarizes the challenges that must be overcome, particularly in developing countries, if every child is to be safely immunized with effective and appropriate vaccines as early as possible in life.

II. 1974–1984: THE EPI IDEA AND THE EPI TOOLS

A. Origins

The success of the global smallpox eradication initiative was perhaps the most importance stimulus for a World Health Organization (WHO) program to support the development of routine immunization services in developing countries [2]. By the end of 1973, smallpox had been restricted to only five countries in Asia and Africa [7], and it was widely agreed that the momentum of the Intensified Smallpox Eradication Programme should be exploited to control other vaccine-preventable diseases [8].

This consensus led WHO to establish the EPI in 1974, with the objective of raising childhood immunization coverage with an *expanded* number of antigens in an increasing number of countries [2]. While the Intensified Smallpox Eradication Programme remained WHO's highest immunization priority through the late 1970s, this period was used to develop the basic EPI principles such as the optimum vaccines and delivery strategies for developing countries.

Although the EPI initiative arose out of the smallpox program, many important elements were to differ substantially, perhaps none more so than the strategic approach.

---

[*] Previous affiliation: World Health Organization, Geneva, Switzerland.

For example, by the mid-1970s the smallpox eradication program had demonstrated the utility of wide-scale mass immunization campaigns to control other important vaccine-preventable diseases in developing countries, such as measles [9]. Following a large EPI feasibility study begun in Ghana in 1976, however, the founders of EPI opted to promote the delivery of vaccines through routine immunization services rather than large-scale campaigns.

The original EPI vaccines were determined largely by the global relevance of the target disease and the cost-effectiveness of its control through immunization [10]. Initially, antigens against six diseases were included: BCG (against tuberculosis), DPT (against diphtheria, pertussis, tetanus), polio and measles for infants with tetanus toxoid for pregnant women to prevent neonatal tetanus (NT) (Table 1) [11]. Specific immunization schedules and policies, often quite different from those of industrialized countries (i.e., younger ages of administration), were established to optimize the uptake and impact of these vaccines in the developing country setting [12–14]. It was in 1977, the year of the last case of smallpox [7], that the World Health Assembly (WHA) formally declared the EPI goal of delivering these six antigens to the world's children by 1990 [15].

It is difficult to overstate the obstacles that existed in the late 1970s between the manufacture of a vaccine, usually in an industrialized country, and its safe administration under field conditions in a developing country, thousands of miles away [16]. Despite the tremendous diversity of the countries and cultures targeted by the EPI, in these early years a standardized approach to overcoming the huge operational and technical barriers to universal childhood immunization was to prove feasible. The first EPI operations manual was developed by 1977, with seminars conducted in most of the six WHO regions to introduce the program to senior public health officials [2]. These seminars established agreement on many critical issues including the standard EPI immunization schedule, a global EPI position on contraindications to specific vaccines, and the first standardized "global" reporting system for immunization.

B. Equipment

Essential to moving from guidelines to actual immunization was the development and distribution of a range of cold-chain equipment that could maintain the potency of the EPI vaccines while withstanding the rigorous environment and

demanding conditions of developing-country use, particularly in rural tropical areas. Although the stability of the EPI-recommended vaccines varied depending on the antigen, the thermolability of OPV and the sensitivity to freezing of DTP dictated the parameters for the cold chain (originally set at 0° to 8°C, these were raised to 2° to 8°C in the year 2000 as newer more expensive and more freeze-sensitive vaccines were added) [17,18].

Because very little equipment was available that could guarantee these conditions amid the high ambient temperatures and unreliable electricity supply in many developing countries, by the late 1970s WHO's EPI had begun working with manufacturers to produce low-cost equipment for storing and transporting vaccines [19]. The technological solutions that were found included ice-lined refrigerators designed to protect vaccines against interruptions in the electricity supply and small, robust refrigerators for remote health centers operating on kerosene, gas, and solar energy [20,21] (Figure 1). By 1979, WHO had established a network of laboratories to evaluate new equipment and had published the first edition of the WHO/UNICEF Product Information Sheets (PIS), detailing the immunization equipment that met WHO specifications and could be recommended for use in developing countries. The PIS continues to be an essential resource for developing country immunization programs, covering a wide range of cold-chain, injection, disposal, and other equipment [22].

At the same time that this capacity to deliver potent vaccines to the field was being established it was also critical to minimize the risk of infectious complications due to unsterile EPI injections [23]. This has required the continuous development and evaluation of new injection, sterilization, and disposal equipment, and strategies [24,25]. In 1984, for example, the original glass syringes and open-boiling equipment of EPI were replaced with sterilizable plastic syringes and portable steam sterilizers, which had been developed specifically for WHO. As understanding of the risks posed by injections and injection equipment accumulated, EPI policy shifted toward the use of disposable injection equipment. To protect against the potential reuse of this equipment WHO facilitated the development of the "autodisable syringe" that could not be used more than once. This type of syringe, first used in mass vaccination campaigns, is now an essential component of a universal policy of WHO and UNICEF to use only autodestruct equipment for all immunizations by 2003 [26,27] (Figure 2).

C. Implementation, Evaluation, and Oversight

To extend immunization services beyond urban centers it was necessary to teach immunization techniques, injection safety, cold-chain maintenance, and program management from the national to village levels. By the end of 1977, the original EPI operations manual had been expanded into a training course for senior-level immunization program managers and the first course held in Kuala Lumpur, with participants from 19 countries. These materials were soon supplemented with training courses for cold chain and logistics (1978) and training and supervision (1979) [28]. By 1982, over 9500 people from 83 countries had been trained in one or more of these courses [2]. These standard

Table 1   WHO-Recommended EPI Schedule[a]

Contact	Age of child	Intervention
1	Birth	BCG, OPV, hepatitis B[b]
2	6 weeks	DPT, OPV, Hib, hepatitis B
3	10 weeks	DPT, OPV, Hib
4	14 weeks	DPT, OPV, Hib, hepatitis B
5	9 months	Measles, yellow fever, vitamin A

[a] The EPI also recommends that all pregnant women receive five appropriately spaced doses of tetanus toxoid for the prevention of neonatal tetanus.

[b] Alternatively, hepatitis B vaccine may be given at 6, 10, and 14 weeks of age in areas of low perinatal transmission.

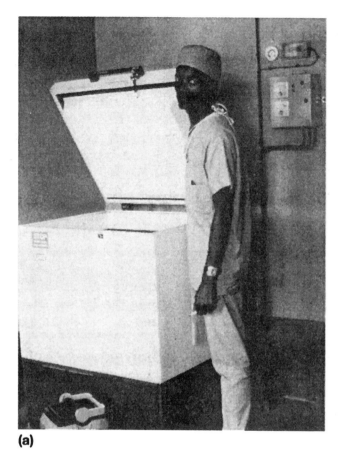

(a)

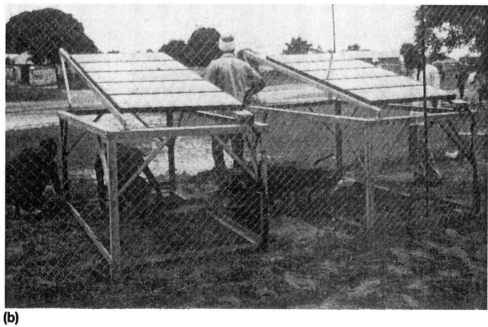

(b)

Figure 1 (a) Solar refrigerator in a Zaire clinic. (b) The solar panels are located outside the center, either on the roof or on the ground.

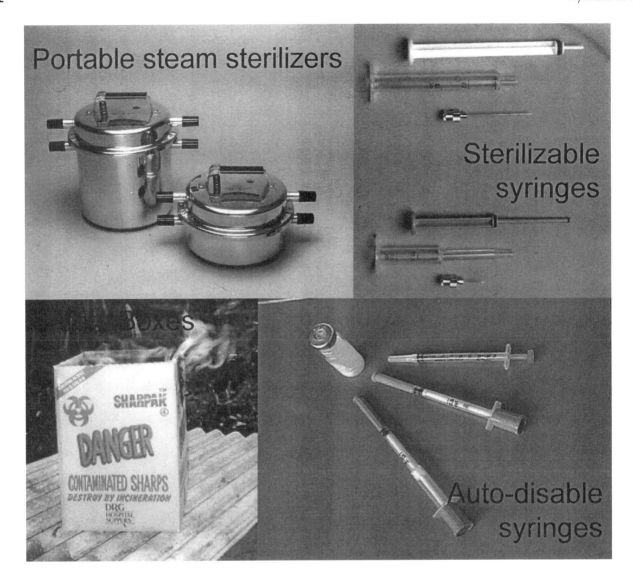

Figure 2 Selected equipment from the evolution of EPI injection equipment: steam sterilizers, plastic reusable syringes and needles, burn boxes, and autodisable syringes.

training materials have continuously been updated and expanded to include topics that now range from refrigerator repair to instruction on motorcycle maintenance.

The routine monitoring of global immunization performance by the WHO began in 1977. A central EPI information system was developed, with computer software for monitoring, at the national and regional levels, immunization coverage, surveillance data, and cold-chain equipment. The data generated permitted the first systematic estimates of developing country immunization coverage, thus facilitating the targeting of international technical and donor assistance. National immunization programs now annually report routine immunization coverage, surveillance, and other program data to WHO and UNICEF through a standardized reporting process [29].

In 1978, national EPI program reviews were introduced using a soon-to-be standardized methodology and joint national/international teams to evaluate all aspects of the im-

munization operations from the central to peripheral levels. Three hundred such reviews were conducted by 1994, often including a "30-Cluster EPI Coverage Survey" using the methodology that WHO had developed to corroborate reported immunization coverage [30,31]. These reviews played an important role in the development of national programs by motivating staff, identifying key areas for improvement, and raising political support by formally presenting the recommendations to national health authorities.

III. 1985–2000: OPTIMIZING THE IMPACT OF EPI

A. Expanding Access

Although the necessary EPI policies, strategic approaches and equipment were largely in place by 1984, less than 50%

of the world's children were being "fully immunized" at that time [2]. Achieving the goal of universal childhood immunization (UCI) by 1990, defined as 80% coverage in the WHA Resolution of 1977, would require a massive acceleration of activities.

Recognizing this, the Rockefeller Foundation hosted a high-level meeting of potential EPI supporters and partners, cosponsored by WHO, UNICEF, the World Bank, and the United Nations Development Program (UNDP) in 1984 in Bellagio, Italy [32]. The 34 leaders in attendance—from developing countries, public health institutions, and international agencies—strongly endorsed the EPI concept and committed to its further expansion. To facilitate the coordination of international assistance to national immunization efforts, the cosponsors of the meeting established the Task Force for Child Survival and Development.

UNICEF played a particularly critical role in the acceleration of immunization activities. Its charismatic leader adopted the goal of universal childhood immunization and vigorously promoted it with national leaders [33]. UNICEF further helped support national immunization programs by operationalizing the EPI program through its regional and country offices. In addition to UNICEF's early role in the international procurement of WHO-approved vaccines and equipment, the organization also played a major role in the national social mobilization efforts that were to improve community awareness of, and demand for, routine immunization services.

With the expansion of immunization activities, new technical issues arose and often threatened to undermine the optimal implementation of the programs. Ongoing operational and epidemiological research was essential to resolve vaccine or immunization issues that were often unique to developing countries [2]. For example, although the epidemiology of the EPI target diseases was well understood in industrialized nations, the burden of disease due to poliomyelitis and neonatal tetanus was often grossly underestimated in developing countries, frequently holding up the introduction of one of those vaccines in a particular country. These hurdles were only overcome after the development and implementation of standardized lameness and neonatal mortality surveys, demonstrating the importance of these diseases in the developing country setting [34,35]. Similarly, specific policies were needed to counter misconceptions about contraindications to EPI vaccines and reflect the safety of their simultaneous administration [36–38].

As the technical, financial, political, and logistical challenges to reaching all children with the EPI vaccines were systematically addressed, the period 1985–1990 saw a tremendous rise in routine immunization activities worldwide. By 1990, vaccines were protecting nearly 75% of the world's children from measles, tetanus, polio, diphtheria, and pertussis (Figure 3).

B. Accelerating Disease Control

As national immunization services were established or strengthened in developing countries, from the late 1980s onward WHO's technical oversight body for EPI turned its attention to the accelerated control of key EPI target diseases. In doing so, EPI was in fact returning to its original mandate in that "the primary concern of EPI is not immunization but disease control, using immunization as the strategy" [39]. This shift in emphasis was motivated by several

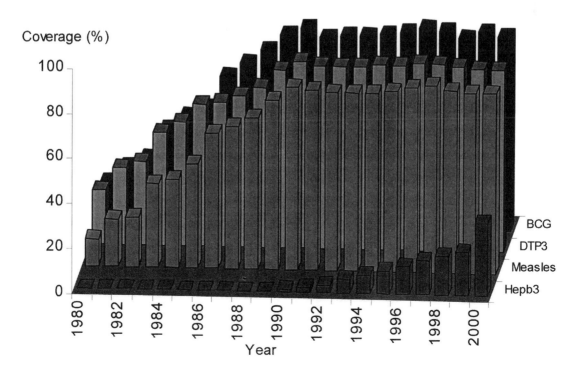

Figure 3 Global immunization coverage of selected antigens based on official reports from countries to WHO, 1980–2000.

other factors, not the least of which was the need to maintain donor and political support for what had become a very successful public health program.

Consequently, in 1989 new EPI goals were established that went beyond the raising of routine immunization coverage to include the eradication of poliomyelitis, the elimination of neonatal tetanus and the reduction of measles mortality and morbidity by 90% and 95%, respectively [40]. The international political importance of these ambitious goals increased substantially in 1990 when they were endorsed at the World Summit for Children, the largest ever gathering of heads of states [5].

Despite this early attention, outside of the Americas there was limited progress toward any of these goals before the mid-1990s. The main reason for this was the widespread deterioration in the quality, coverage, and commitment to routine immunization that had begun in the early 1990s due to several factors [41]. Of particular importance, the rapid gains of the EPI expansion in the late 1980s appears to have fuelled among donors a false sense of the robustness of the program leading to a rapid contraction of international financial support, usually before other more sustainable funding had been secured [42–44]. Around the same time, structural adjustment programs began to markedly affect national budgets and staffing patterns in many developing countries. These problems were further compounded by health sector reform processes, which frequently led to a stagnation of EPI performance as the highly centralized EPI

structures were integrated with other child health services and/or critical functions and staff were devolved to the subnational level [45]. Even within the UN agencies, the growing demands of other priorities and programs limited the time, attention, and resources that staff of all levels could devote to immunization.

By 1995, however, efforts to achieve the specific disease-control goals of EPI had stimulated the development of new strategic approaches for reaching every child, including close collaboration with many new partners. In particular, the goal of global polio eradication had a massive impact as it grew into the largest public health initiative ever. Spearheaded by WHO, Rotary International, UNICEF, and the U.S. Centers for Disease Control and Prevention (CDC), the goal of polio eradication brought together a broad coalition of donor and technical partners to support national efforts to improve the reach of immunization services and establish effective surveillance. Through a combination of routine immunization, National Immunization Days, surveillance for acute flaccid paralysis (AFP), and house-to-house mop-up activities [46,47], polio fell from an estimated 350,000 cases (35,000 reported) in over 125 countries in 1988 to an estimated 550 cases (480 reported) in 10 countries at the end of 2001 [48] (Figure 4).

Substantial progress toward the measles control goals was first made in the Americas by building on the infrastructure and strategic approaches that had been established for polio eradication. In 1985, the WHO Region of the Americas

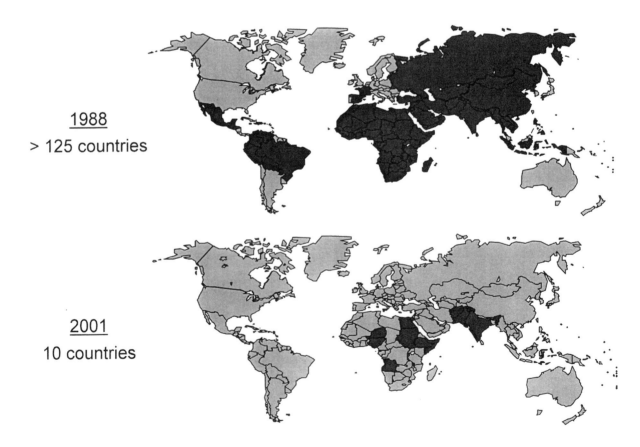

Figure 4 Distribution of endemic poliomyelitis in 1988 and at the end of 2001.

went beyond the original goal, adopting a resolution to eliminate measles in all member states. By conducting massive "catch-up" campaigns, raising routine immunization coverage, introducing case-based measles surveillance, and establishing regular "follow-up" campaigns, indigenous measles was virtually eliminated from the region [49,50] (Figure 5). By the end of 2000, a global action plan for accelerated measles control had been developed, three WHO regions had established measles elimination goals and a wide variety of countries in all regions had implemented the Pan American Health Organization (PAHO) strategic approach [51].

Perhaps the most challenging of these goals was NT elimination, defined as < 1 case per 1000 live births in every district of every country. The disease had little visibility, as onset occurred very early in life and predominantly in rural areas among underprivileged populations. Furthermore, prevention required the immunization of women, rather than children, with multiple doses of tetanus toxoid during antenatal visits. Although NT deaths fell by 51% between 1990 and 1999, an estimated 200,000 NT deaths still occurred in 2000 [52]. Consequently, in November 2000 a new 5-year strategic plan was launched to achieve the goal by 2005, through routine and supplemental tetanus toxoid vaccination, strengthening of clean delivery services, and surveillance to detect and target areas and populations at high risk [53]. By the end of 2001, 20 of the 57 targeted countries had plans of action and 13 were already implementing activities.

The pursuit of these accelerated disease control goals has helped raise the political visibility and attention to childhood immunization, particularly as national leaders personally launched the massive immunization campaigns.

These initiatives also greatly enhanced the international investment in global disease surveillance and developing country immunization programs. By the year 2000, for example, WHO alone had deployed over 3000 national and international personnel through the polio initiative to provide technical and administrative support to national immunization programs worldwide. New, efficient partnerships for immunization were also established through these initiatives, governed by cross-agency strategic plans and coordinated through national or regional level Interagency Coordinating Committees (ICCs). Perhaps most importantly, these efforts resulted in regular access to previously unreached geographic areas and populations, particularly through the strategic approaches and community engagement of the polio eradication initiative. In 2001 alone, an estimated 10 million health workers and volunteers immunized 575 million children with oral polio vaccine, even reaching areas affected by conflict [48].

C. Introducing New Antigens and Interventions

As the expansion of the global EPI network significantly enhanced access to children worldwide in the late 1980s, increasing attention was given to the feasibility of systematically using the EPI infrastructure to deliver other antigens and, potentially, other health interventions (Table 2). Despite the logic and cost-effectiveness of many such proposals, it was not until 1999 that substantial progress was made in this regard.

The first additional antigen to be formally recommended for inclusion in EPI since 1974 was the yellow fever

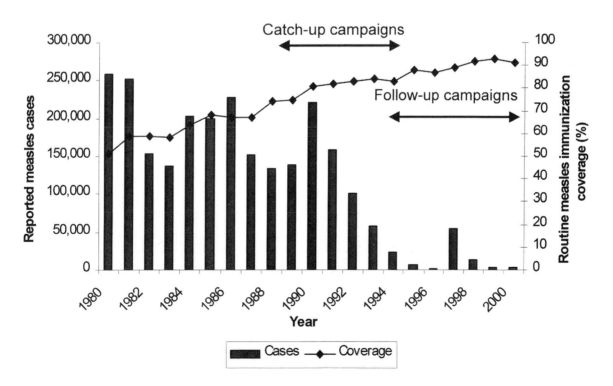

Figure 5   Measles immunization coverage and reported measles cases in the Americas, 1980–2000.

Table 2 Current EPI Interventions, Year of Recommendation, and Principle Reasons for Recommendation

Intervention	Year of recommendation	Major considerations leading to recommendation
BCG, DPT, OPV, measles, tetanus toxoid vaccines	1974	Target diseases were global health problems. Effective vaccines were available. Immunization was feasible and cost-effective.
Vitamin A (micronutrient)	1987	Substantial impact on childhood mortality in vitamin A deficient areas. Compatible with EPI logistics.
Yellow fever vaccine[a]	1989	Resurgence of the disease in Africa in the late 1980s. Morbidity and mortality were highest in children.
Hepatitis B vaccine	1992	Universal childhood immunization is the most effective strategy. Lower cost permitted public sector use.
Hib vaccine[b]	1998	Major cause of bacterial meningitis and pneumonia in children. Safe and effective vaccine.

[a] Recommended for use in 33 African countries.

[b] As appropriate to national capacities and priorities.

vaccine in 1989. Recognizing the resurgence of yellow fever as a public health problem in Africa in the late 1980s, WHO's EPI technical oversight body in 1989 recommended that 33 countries on the African continent include this vaccine in their infant-immunization programs. By 1999, however, reported yellow fever vaccine coverage in these countries was only 19%, compared with 80% for measles, which is given at the same age (9 months). The reasons for this poor uptake varied by country, ranging from a lack of resources for vaccine purchase to a failure to appropriately modify or implement national immunization policies.

The first "new" vaccine to be included in EPI was the hepatitis B vaccine. Although licensed in 1981, its very high cost initially prohibited wide-scale use, even within industrialized countries. Even when the cost began to decline, however, there was limited support for universal childhood immunization against hepatitis B in some international health circles because the disease did not cause substantial childhood morbidity, even though it was a leading cause of liver cancer and early death among males in developing countries. By the late 1980s, the price of the vaccine began to decline as new producers emerged and the market expanded. In 1992, further declines in the vaccine price, combined with increasing cost-effectiveness data and the failure of targeted hepatitis B immunization strategies, warranted WHO's recommendation for universal childhood immunization [54,55]. By 1999, 117 countries, primarily high and middle income, had implemented the recommendation, but the vaccine remained unavailable in most of the poorest countries that harbored the highest burden of the disease [56].

Despite compelling data as to the appropriateness of including yellow fever and hepatitis B vaccines in EPI, it was only after 1999 that there was the opportunity to substantially improve the uptake of both vaccines in the world's poorest countries. In one of the most important developments in the history of EPI, the Global Alliance for Vaccines and Immunization (GAVI) was established in that year, bringing new cooperation, resources, and tools to the strengthening of routine immunization programs and introduction of new vaccines. GAVI has mobilized old and new

partners around a set of objectives and goals that ensures coordination of international and national immunization and vaccine research efforts. Among the most important of the tools available to GAVI is the Vaccine Fund, established with a $750 million donation by the Bill and Melinda Gates Foundation and since augmented by other foundations and donor governments such that by the end of 2001 its assets had grown to over $1.1 billion [57,58].

As of March 2002, the Vaccine Fund had already provided over 40 countries with the financing necessary to introduce hepatitis B into their routine immunization services and six countries had received support for yellow fever vaccine purchase [58]. The Fund had also facilitated the purchase of *Haemophilus influenzae* type b (Hib) vaccine for 11 countries. In addition to this support for new vaccines, the creation of the GAVI alliance has had an enormous impact on national and international efforts to revitalize immunization services through its high-level political advocacy, interagency coordination and, through the Vaccine Fund, routine immunization financing [57].

Of the nonvaccine interventions promoted for inclusion in routine immunization services, the most important has been vitamin A. Since the discovery in the 1970s and 1980s that regular supplementation with that micronutrient could reduce all-cause childhood mortality by as much as 23% [59], there has been substantial interest in administering it during routine immunization contacts, particularly with measles at 9 months of age [60]. Although the logistical implications of including vitamin A are relatively minor, as it is heat stable and administered by mouth, 10 years later only a limited number of countries had implemented the policy. In the late 1990s, however, the linking of vitamin A and immunization contacts took a major step forward when countries began including the micronutrient in polio National Immunization Days (NIDs) [61]. By 2000, there were compelling data to further promote the use of vitamin A during routine immunization contacts—inclusion of the micronutrient in polio NIDs in 61 countries in the period 1998–1999 had averted over 400,000 childhood deaths [62]. By the end of 2000, 49 of the 136 countries with known vitamin A deficiency had begun distributing the micronutrient through routine immunization services.

Recognizing the opportunity that the EPI infrastructure provided, and building on the experience gained through the introduction of the yellow fever and hepatitis B vaccines and vitamin A, in the early 1990s WHO developed a framework to facilitate the introduction of new interventions [13]. This framework is intended to accelerate the evaluation of an intervention and, if necessary and feasible, modify its characteristics to streamline its integration into EPI programs.

IV. A NEW MILLENNIUM—NEW OPPORTUNITIES

In the year 2000, ambitious Millenium Development Goals were underwritten by all nations. These goals include a two-thirds reduction in child mortality by 2015. For this to be achieved, the full potential of the global EPI network must be exploited to prevent the three million vaccine-preventable deaths that continue to occur every year (Figure 6). Preventing these deaths requires extending the reach of immunization services to the more than 25% of the world's children who are yet to have regular access to immunization, the most cost-effective of health interventions. Particular attention must be given to increasing coverage among the world's poorest children who are disproportionately affected by vaccine-preventable and infectious diseases. That reaching all children with immunization is a feasible goal is abundantly evident in the progress achieved and experience gained over the past 25 years. The challenge will be to exploit the opportunities that exist to establish true equity in global childhood immunization.

One of the first challenges will be to ensure that there are accurate data with which to identify areas of low immunization coverage, particularly at the subnational level, so that corrective actions can be focused most effectively. During the last decade of the twentieth century, attention to coverage monitoring had declined as increased

emphasis was placed on the use of disease surveillance data to monitor the impact of immunization. Consequently, an extensive review of national data from 1980 to 1999 found that immunization coverage levels were actually lower than had been reported. In fact, global DTP3 coverage at the time of the World Summit for Children in 1990 was estimated to have been only 73% rather than 80%, with little improvement throughout the 1990s [29,56]. Moreover, global coverage figures masked important differences between and within countries. Most importantly, in sub-Saharan Africa less than 50% of children born in 2000 were fully immunized [56].

Using accurate data, the capacity, tools and processes must be established to develop multiyear plans that address access constraints for countries and areas with coverage of less than 80%. Such plans must accurately identify and map currently unreached children or geographic areas, identify the underlying causes, and plan for their resolution. Particular attention will need to be given to separating those low coverage areas due to poor management of existing services (e.g., with high "drop-out rates") from those where services are just not present or poorly attended. Tackling the management problem requires a much overdue revision and implementation of the basic EPI immunization management guidelines to adapt them to the realities of the much changed, often decentralized health systems that have evolved since the mid-1980s [63].

The "access" problem will require reestablishing the outreach services and infrastructure that were so important to the immunization gains of the late 1980s. To ensure the sustainability of such services, however, they will need to be more closely integrated into the delivery of other health services and tailored to the size and needs of the communities that they are serving. Recognizing this, the United Nations Foundation has supported the work of WHO and UNICEF to pioneer and pilot-test an initiative known as Sustainable Outreach Services (SOS). The SOS approach draws heavily on the lessons learned from the polio NIDs, using periodic contacts to reach people with limited or no access to health services. The delivery of immunization is combined with other interventions such as impregnated bed nets and micronutrient supplementation. SOS is based heavily on community participation in selecting the interventions and facilitating their delivery [64].

To assist countries in these efforts, the UN agencies and immunization partners will need to provide technical and financial support at least equal to that which it has provided in the ongoing effort to eradicate polio. WHO and UNICEF have already detailed the major elements of the polio eradication infrastructure and begun planning the systematic transition of the institutional arrangements (e.g., ICCs, laboratory networks, technical oversight groups), physical infrastructure (e.g., cold chain, communications and transportation equipment) and human resources to support broader immunization goals. In 2001, UNICEF also established "Immunization-Plus" as one of its five health priorities, signaling its intention to substantially increase its support to national immunization services [65].

Insufficient financing remains a major barrier toward equity in immunization, and the search for sustainable EPI funding remains a chronic challenge for the world's poorest

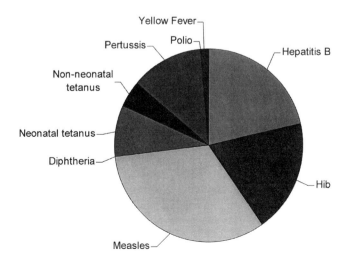

Figure 6 Distribution of the estimated three million annual deaths from diseases that are preventable by routine childhood vaccination, 2000.

countries. However, at no point in the history of EPI has there been as much attention to this area and as many promising initiatives [58,63]. For example, the Vaccine Fund of GAVI is requiring the development of national financial sustainability plans in countries receiving its resources. Meanwhile, most countries are expanding the scope of the Interagency Coordinating Committee that was established to coordinate polio eradication partner inputs, to encompass all immunization activities. Also at the country level, the decentralization of health services, with the devolution of planning functions and budget allocations, provides opportunities to improve coordination with other sectors and more effectively use resources to reach more children. Although the debt relief initiative for the highly indebted poor countries (HIPC) has yet to promote highly cost-effective health interventions such as immunization to the degree anticipated, this remains a potential mechanism for substantially enhancing financial support to immunization. At the international level, a GAVI Task Force is specifically addressing the issue of sustainable immunization financing with a particular emphasis on understanding and exploiting the many opportunities that exist. Finally, there is now concrete planning to extend the Vaccine Fund, which has become one of the most important new immunization financing instruments for poor countries, to beyond 2005.

In addition to the obvious logistical and managerial challenges to reach every child and ensure sustainable financing, the maturation of EPI has brought other extremely important although much less visible concerns. The importance of ensuring the safety of all immunizations led WHO to establish in 1999 a "priority project" in this area [66,67]. This has brought together the broad range of ongoing work in this area from ensuring "vaccines of assured quality" [including functioning national regulatory authorities (NRAs) worldwide], to improving injection safety and the monitoring and management of adverse events following immunization [68,69]. One of the most important developments in this project was the establishment of a WHO Vaccine Safety Advisory Committee to ensure the capacity to respond promptly, objectively, and with scientific rigor to vaccine safety issues anywhere in the world [70].

One of the more insidious threats to achieving and sustaining equity in global immunization is the growing challenge of "vaccine security." Ironically, the growth in global immunization activity and coverage has recently been accompanied by a contraction in both the number of manufacturers producing vaccines for the developing country market and the amount of vaccine they produce [71]. The principal causes of this problem have been the consolidation of the pharmaceutical industry in the mid-1990s and the divergence of developing and industrialized country vaccine markets [71]. Although UNICEF procured vaccines for 40% of the world's children in over 100 countries in 2001, it is operating in an increasingly challenging market where the gap between demand and supply has narrowed substantially. To manage this challenge and stabilize the market, UNICEF has substantially enhanced its long-term vaccine demand forecasting capacity in collaboration with WHO, increased its dialogue with manufacturers, and explored mechanisms to establish longer-term funding and contracts for vaccines.

V. CONCLUSION

The last millennium closed with great achievements in the delivery of routine immunization services in developing countries. Within a 25-year period, global immunization coverage rose from less than 5% to nearly 75%. Early in that period a whole range of cold-chain and injection equipment was developed specifically for the tropical developing country setting and has now become the standard in most. A global network of national immunization programs was established, standardized approaches were developed, monitoring systems introduced, and legions of health workers trained.

As the reach of this global immunization network expanded, ambitious new disease control objectives have brought polio to the brink of eradication and demonstrated that the interruption of measles, one of the leading killers of children, is feasible. The pursuit of these goals has led to a massive expansion of the technical support provided by UN agencies to national immunization programs and demonstrated that with the appropriate mix of planning, partnerships, resources, and community engagement, all children everywhere can be regularly accessed with immunization services. The launch of GAVI in the year 2000 provided a mechanism to effectively tackle the financing gap that had become one of the greatest barriers to achieving equity in the introduction of new vaccines and expanding services to the hardest to reach children. Finally, the wide-scale delivery of vitamin A during immunization contacts has begun to demonstrate that the broader promise of the global EPI infrastructure to facilitate the delivery of other interventions can be realized.

Although a new millennium has brought new challenges for EPI, the commitment, concepts, and capacity needed to achieve equity in the delivery of childhood immunization services on a global scale has never been stronger. However, reaching all children with even the most basic of vaccines will require a level of sustained financing, national ownership, and international donor interest that has thus far proven elusive.

ACKNOWLEDGMENTS

The authors are extremely grateful to Ms. Joan Hawe of the World Health Organization for her assistance with the references for this article, as well as Dr. Mark Kane of the Children's Vaccine Programme, Dr. Jay Wenger of the World Health Organization, and Dr. Yves Bergevin, Dr. Okwo Bele, Ms. Maryanne Neill, and Ms. Shanelle Hall of UNICEF for their comments on specific sections of the manuscript.

REFERENCES

1. Plotkin SL, Plotkin SA. A short history of vaccination. In: Plotkin SA, Mortimer EA, eds. Vaccines. 2d rev ed. Philadelphia: Saunders, 1994:1–11.
2. Henderson RH, et al. Reaping the benefits: getting vaccines

to those who need them. In: Woodrow GC, Levine MM, eds. New Generation Vaccines. New York: Marcel Dekker, 1990: 69–82.

3. World Bank. World Development Report 1993: Investing in health. Oxford: Oxford University Press, 1993.

4. World Health Organization. Expanded Programme on Immunization. Global Advisory Group—Part I. Wkly Epidemiol Rec 1992; 3:11–15.

5. World Summit for Children. World Declaration on the Survival, Protection and Development of Children. New York: United Nations, 1990.

6. World Health Report 2001. Mental Health: New Understanding, New Hope. Geneva: World Health Organization, 2001.

7. Fenner F, et al. The intensified smallpox eradication programme, 1967–1980. In: Smallpox and Its Eradication. Geneva: World Health Organization, 1988:421–538.

8. Bland J, Clements J. Protecting the world's children: the story of WHO's immunization programme. World Health Forum 1998; 19:162–173.

9. Foege WH. Measles vaccination in Africa. Measles Vaccination in Africa. Proceedings of the International Conference on Application of Vaccines Against Viral, Rickettsial, and Bacterial Diseases of Man. Washington, DC: Pan American Health Organization, 1971 (Scientific Publ. No. 226).

10. Henderson RH. Providing immunization: The state of the art. Protecting the World's Children: Vaccine and Immunization Within Primary Health Care. Proceedings of the Bellagio Conference. New York: The Rockefeller Foundation, 1984:18–37.

11. World Health Organization. Expanded Programme on Immunization. Wkly Epidemiol Rec 1977; 7:74–75.

12. Halsey N. The optimal age for administering measles vaccine in developing countries. In: Halsey N, de Quadros C, eds. Recent Advances in Immunization. Washington, DC: Pan American Health Organization, 1983:4–17.

13. Aylward B, et al. A framework for the evaluation of vaccines for use in the Expanded Programme on Immunization. Vaccine 1994; 12:1155–1159.

14. World Health Organization. Expanded Programme on Immunization. Immunization policy. Geneva: World Health Organization, 1995 (WHO Document No. WHO/EPI/GEN/95.3).

15. World Health Assembly. Expanded Programme on Immunization. Geneva: World Health Organization, 1977 (Resolution WHA30.53).

16. Lloyd JS. Improving the cold chain for vaccines. WHO Chron 1977; 31:13–18.

17. World Health Organization. Expanded Programme on Immunization. Heat stability of vaccines. Wkly Epidemiol Rec 1980; 55:252–254.

18. World Health Organization. Proper handling and reconstitution of vaccines avoids programme errors. Vaccines and Biologicals Update Dec 2000; Vol. 34. Geneva: World Health Organization, Dec 2000.

19. Lundbeck H, et al. A cold box for the transport and storage of vaccines. Bull WHO 1978;56), 427–432.

20. World Health Organization. Expanded Programme on Immunization. Ice lined refrigerators (ILR). Wkly Epidemiol Rec 1984; 59:63–64.

21. The cold chain for vaccine conservation: recent improvements. WHO Chron 1979; 33:383–386.

22. Expanded Programme on Immunization. Product Information Sheets. Geneva: World Health Organization, 2000 (WHO Document No. WHO/V&B/00.13).

23. Expanded Programme on Immunization. Safety of Injections in Immunization Programmes: WHO Recommended Policy-Geneva: World Health Organization, 1994 (WHO Document No. WHO/EPI/LHIS/94.1).

24. Aylward B, et al. Reducing the risk of unsafe injections in immunization programmes: the financial and operational implications of various injection technologies. Bull WHO 1995; 73:531–540.

25. Dicko M, et al. Safety of immunization injections in Africa: not simply a problem of logistics. Bull WHO 2000; 78(2): 163–169.

26. Marmor M, Hartsock P. Self-destructing (nonreusable) syringes. Lancet 1991; 338:438–439.

27. Expanded Programme on Immunization. Safety of injections: WHO–UNICEF–UNFPA Joint Statement on the Use of Auto-disable Syringes in Immunization Services. Geneva: World Health Organization, 1999 (WHO Document No. WHO/V&B/99.25).

28. Training the trainers in cold chain operation. WHO Chron 1980; 34:182–185.

29. World Health Organization. Vaccine-Preventable Diseases: Monitoring System—2001 Global Summary. Geneva: World Health Organization, 2002 (WHO Document No. WHO/V&B/01.34).

30. Expanded Programme on Immunization. Training for Mid-level Managers—The EPI Coverage SurveyGeneva: World Health Organization, 1991 (WHO Document No. WHO/EPI/MLM/91.10).

31. Henderson RH, Sundaresan T. Cluster sampling to assess immunization coverage: a review of experience with a simplified sampling method. Bull WHO 1982; 60:253–260.

32. Rockefeller Foundation. Protecting the World's Children: Vaccines and Immunization Within Primary Health Care. Proceedings of the Bellagio Conference. New York: Rockefeller Foundation, 1984.

33. Grant JP. The State of the World's Children in 1991. Oxford: Oxford University Press, 1991.

34. Bernier RH. Some observations on poliomyelitis lameness surveys. Rev Infect Dis 1984; 6(suppl 2):S371–S375.

35. Whitman C, et al. Progress towards the global elimination of neonatal tetanus. World Health Stat Q 1992; 45:248–256.

36. Galazka AM, et al. Indications and contraindications for vaccines used in the Expanded Programme on Immunization. Bull WHO 1984; 62:357–366.

37. American Academy of Pediatrics. Simultaneous Administration of Multiple Vaccines. Report of the Committee on Infectious Disease. Red Book, 1986, 10.

38. Clements CJ, et al. HIV infection and routine childhood immunization: a review. Bull WHO 1987; 65:905–911.

39. Henderson RH, et al. Immunizing the children of the world: progress and prospects. Bull WHO 1988; 66:535–543.

40. World Health Organization. World Health Assembly Resolution 42.32. In: Handbook of Resolutions and Decisions of the World Health Assembly and the Executive Board. Vol. 3 2d ed. (1985–1989). Geneva: World Health Organization, 1990:56–57.

41. Zoffman H. Changing the decreasing trend in immunization coverage. Sixteenth Meeting of the Global Advisory Group (Expanded Programme on Immunization), Washington, DC, Oct 11–15, 1993. Geneva: World Health Organization, 1993 (WHO Document No. EPI/GAG/93/WP.8).

42. Taylor ME, et al. Sustainability of Achievements: Lessons Learned from Universal Childhood Immunization. Report of a Steering Committee. New York, NY: UNICEF, 1996 (unpublished).

43. DeRoeck D. Immunization Financing in Developing Countries and the International Vaccine Market: Trends and Issues. Manila: Asian Development Bank, 2001 (ISBN: 971-561-349-7).

44. United States General Accounting Office Report to Congressional Requesters. Global Health: Factors Contributing to Low Vaccination Rates in Developing Countries. October 1999. GAO/NSIAD-00-4.

45. Feilden R, Nielsen OF. Immunization and Health Reforms: Making Reforms Work for Immunization. A Reference Guide. Geneva: World Health Organization, 2001 (WHO Document No. WHO/V&B/01.44).

46. Hull HF, et al. Paralytic poliomyelitis: seasoned strategies, disappearing disease. Lancet 1994; 343:1331–1337.

47. Tangermann R, et al. Current status of the global eradication of poliomyelitis. World Health Stat Q 1997; 50(3/4):188–194.

48. World Health Organization. Progress towards the global eradication of poliomyelitis, 2001. Wkly Epidemiol Rec 2002; 77(13):97–108.

49. de Quadros CA, et al. Measles elimination in the Americas: evolving strategies. JAMA 1996; 275:224–229.

50. World Health Organization. Progress towards interrupting indigenous measles transmission in the Western Hemisphere. Wkly Epidemiol Rec 2000; 75(40):354–358.

51. World Health Organization and the United Nations Children's Fund. Measles: Mortality reduction and regional elimination—strategic plan 2001–2005. Geneva: World Health Organization, 2001 (WHO Document No. WHO/V&B/01.13).

52. Birmingham M, Stein C. Burden of Vaccine-Preventable Disease. In: Bloom B, Lambert P-H, eds. The Vaccine Book. Academic Press, 2002.

53. United Nations Children's Fund, World Health Organization, United Nations Population Fund (UNFPA). Maternal and Neonatal Tetanus Elimination by 2005—Strategies for Achieving and Maintaining Elimination. New York: UNICEF, 2000.

54. World Health Assembly. Immunization and Vaccine Quality. Geneva: World Health Organization, 2000, 1992 (WHA Resolution No. WHA45.17).

55. Vryheid RE, et al. Infant and adolescent hepatitis B immunization up to 1999: a global overview. Vaccine 2000; 19(9–10):1026–1037.

56. World Health Organization. Vaccine-preventable diseases: monitoring system—2000 global summary. Geneva: World Health Organization, 2000 (WHO Document No. WHO/V&B/00.32).

57. Jacobs L, et al. A paradigm for international cooperation: the Global Alliance for Vaccines and Immunization (GAVI) and the Vaccine Fund. In: Levine MM, Kaper JB, Rappuoli R, Liu MA, Good MF, eds. New Generation Vaccines. New York: Marcel Dekker, 2004:101–106.

58. World Health Organization. State of the World's Vaccines and Immunization. Geneva: World Health Organization, 2002 (In press).

59. Beaton GH, et al. Effectiveness of Vitamin A Supplementation in the Control of Young Child Morbidity and Mortality in Developing Countries. New York, NY: United Nations, December 1993 (ACC/SCN State-of-the-Art Series, Nutrition Discussion Paper No. 13).

60. Expanded Programme on Immunization. Global Advisory Group. Wkly Epidemiol Rec 1987; 62:5–12.

61. Goodman T, et al. Polio as a platform: using national immunization days to deliver vitamin A supplements. Bull WHO 2000; 78(3):305–314.

62. Ching P, et al. The impact of vitamin A supplements delivered with immunization campaigns. Am J Public Health 2000; 90:1526–1529.

63. Melgaard B. Immunization in the 21st century—the way forward. Acta Trop 2001; 80:119–124.

64. World Health Organization. Sustainable Outreach Services (SOS): A Strategy for Reaching the Unreached with Immunization and other Services. Geneva: World Health Organization, 2000 (WHO Document No. WHO/V&B/00.37).

65. United Nations Children's Fund. Medium-term strategic plan for the period 2002–2005. New York: United Nations Children's Fund, 2001 (UNICEF Document No. E/ICEF/2001/13).

66. Scholtz M, Duclos P. Immunization safety: a global priority. Bull WHO 2000; 78(2):153–154.

67. Duclos P, Hofmann C-A. Immunization safety: a priority of the World Health Organization's Department of Vaccines and Biologicals. Drug Saf 2001; 24(15):1105–1112.

68. Milstien J, et al. Vaccine quality—can a single standard be defined? Vaccine 2001; 2956:1–4.

69. Mehta U, et al. Developing a national system for dealing with adverse events following immunization. Bull WHO 2000; 78(2):170–177.

70. World Health Organization. Vaccine safety—Vaccine Safety Advisory Committee. Wkly Epidemiol Rec 1999; 74:337–340.

71. United Nations Children's Fund. Vaccine security: ensuring a sustained, uninterrupted supply of affordable vaccines. New York: United Nations Children's Fund, 2001 (UNICEF Document No. E/ICEF/2002/6).

9

A Paradigm for International Cooperation: The Global Alliance for Vaccines and Immunization (GAVI) and the Vaccine Fund

Lisa Jacobs and Tore Godal
GAVI Secretariat, Geneva, Switzerland

Jacques-François Martin
The Vaccine Fund, Lyon, France

I. BACKGROUND

For more than a century, scientists and public health leaders have known that preventing infectious diseases is the most efficient form of health intervention. During the twentieth century, medical research led to the development of vaccines that prevent several crippling, often fatal, childhood diseases.

In fact, vaccines helped to reduce the health gap between rich and poor countries. Up until the 1970s, outside of the world's richest countries most children were not vaccinated against even a single disease. Following the successful eradication of smallpox in 1977, public health advocates and experts around the world collaborated to help build systems in developing countries to routinely provide infants with vaccination against six diseases: measles, diphtheria, pertussis, tetanus, poliomyelitis, and tuberculosis (using BCG vaccine).

By 1990, 75% of the world's children received these "basic six" vaccines. In the history of international public health, there has been no other routine health intervention that has received such high coverage as vaccination.

However, as a new century begins, the world falls short of realizing the full benefit of childhood immunization. By the end of the 1990s, approximately 34 million children were born every year that would not become immunized. In sub-Saharan Africa, fewer than half of the children were being immunized. As a result, every year, approximately three million additional lives could be saved from easily prevented infectious diseases if vaccines could reach their target populations.

Moreover, vaccines such as those against hepatitis B and *Haemophilus influenzae* type b (Hib) have not been introduced quickly enough in the poorest countries. New vaccines at late stages of development, such as those being created against pneumococcal pneumonia, meningococcal meningitis, and rotavirus diarrhea—diseases that kill millions of children every year in the developing world—are at risk of not reaching those who most need them. Finally, the search for vaccines against several of the most critical infectious disease threats of our time—HIV/AIDS, malaria, and tuberculosis—must be intensified, and effective health delivery systems must be strengthened to ensure that once these vaccines are successfully developed, all those in need can access them.

II. THE GLOBAL ALLIANCE FOR VACCINES AND IMMUNIZATION COMES ON THE SCENE

The Global Alliance for Vaccines and Immunization (GAVI) was launched in 2000 as a coalition committed to reinvigorating and sustaining the promise of widespread immunization (see Table 1). A partnership that includes national governments, UNICEF, WHO, The World Bank Group, the Bill & Melinda Gates Foundation and other foundations, nongovernmental organizations (NGOs), the vaccine industry, and research and technical health institutions, GAVI exists as a mechanism for coordinating and revitalizing immunization programs at international, regional, and national levels.

By significantly expanding the reach and effectiveness of immunization programs country by country, the GAVI partners hope to decrease the burden of disease globally. GAVI reaffirms that immunization is a cornerstone for

Table 1 GAVI Mission Statement

To save children's lives and protect people's health through the widespread use of vaccines.

GAVI strategic objectives:
Improve access to sustainable immunization services.
Expand the use of all existing, safe, and cost-effective vaccines where they address public health problems.
Accelerate the development and introduction of new vaccines and technologies.
Accelerate R&D efforts for vaccines needed primarily in developing countries.
Make immunization coverage a centerpiece in international development efforts.
Support national and international disease control targets for vaccine preventable diseases.

GAVI milestones include:
By 2005, 80% of developing countries will have routine immunization coverage of at least 80% in all districts.
By 2002, 80% of countries with adequate delivery system will introduce hepatitis B vaccine, and all countries by 2007.
By 2005, 50% of the poorest countries with high burden of disease and adequate delivery systems will have introduced Hib vaccine.
By 2005, the vaccine efficacy and burden-of-disease will be known for all regions for rotavirus and pneumococcal vaccines, and mechanisms identified to make the vaccines available to the poorest countries.

---

health, a key component of the broader framework of economic development and poverty reduction, and an essential step to protecting children's health and allowing each child to reach his or her greatest physical and intellectual potential.

A. The Vaccine Fund

The Vaccine Fund is a financing mechanism designed to help the GAVI alliance achieve its objectives by raising new resources and swiftly channeling them to developing countries. Because the partners of the Alliance provide direction and support in policy development and the processing of countries' proposals, administrative costs are kept low—almost all of Vaccine Fund resources go directly to countries.

The Vaccine Fund has received commitments from the governments of Norway, the United Kingdom, the United States, the Netherlands, Canada, Denmark, and Sweden and from the private sector, adding to its start-up grant from the Bill & Melinda Gates Foundation, pushing its total resources to above $1 billion for 2001–2005.

Although initially conceived as primarily a commodity-based vaccine purchase fund, the GAVI partners quickly responded to the overwhelming demand for funds to help repair fragile and faltering immunization and health systems in developing countries. Thus, in addition to supporting countries to introduce vaccines against hepatitis B (hepB), Hib, and yellow fever into their routine systems, a performance-based grant system was developed to provide addi-

tional resources for countries to use to strengthen their immunization services based on their own national priorities and needs. In the future, Vaccine Fund resources may be used to accelerate the development and introduction of vaccines needed in the developing world.

Although the Vaccine Fund does not procure the six "traditional" vaccines for countries, Fund resources aimed at strengthening immunization systems ensure that more children receive those lifesaving vaccines as well.

Funding decisions are made based on proposals received from countries. Following are the main conditions that a country must meet to receive support:

An Interagency Coordination Committee (ICC) must exist led by government and including representatives of local agencies involved with immunization. The ICC helps guide the application process and assists government with program management.
A recent review (within 3 years) of immunization services must have been carried out.
A multiyear plan outlining improvement and expansion of immunization services and mechanisms for sustainable financing must be available.

The GAVI partners designed the Vaccine Fund not to supplant other sources of funding but as a catalyst for additional funding. In fact, this has happened in many countries, with partners stepping in to provide needed support—from training to new refrigerators, and governments stepping in with more of their own budgets dedicated to immunization (Table 2).

1. The Proposal Review Process

The country proposals for support from GAVI and The Vaccine Fund are reviewed by the Independent Review Committee (IRC), an independent committee of experts whose members have been selected by the Executive Secretary after consultation with the Working Group. Panel members are selected for their broad expertise in health with specific knowledge of vaccines and immunization, independence from the partners of GAVI, and integrity. Due regard is paid to the importance of selecting experts on as wide a geographic basis as possible. Primarily, these experts have been selected from low- and middle-income countries.

The proposals must be received at the Secretariat by specific dates set annually, about which the eligible countries are notified. Prior to their review, proposals are screened by the Secretariat for completeness and basic eligibility. Each proposal is then preassessed by a group of relevant experts from WHO and other GAVI partners. The group looks for consistency of information, validity of data provided, coordination with polio eradication, and injection safety efforts. Their feedback is provided in written form to the IRC for their use during deliberations on the proposals.

Proposals are reviewed by the IRC at the GAVI Secretariat in Geneva at set times throughout the year. The IRC reviews the proposals in accordance with the policies laid down by the GAVI Board, following the criteria for eligibility and assessment as expressed in the guidelines prepared by the Working Group.

Table 2 Status of GAVI Support to Countries

At the World Health Assembly in May of 2000, the first call for proposals from GAVI and The Vaccine Fund was distributed to all eligible countries—the 74 countries with less than $1000 per capita.

As of early 2002:
Sixty-six countries have submitted proposals and 54 have been approved for support.
More than $800 million has been committed to these countries over the next 5 years.
The first cash support was disbursed in December 2000; vaccines started to reach countries in April 2001.
If countries achieve their plans, basic immunization rates in funded countries could increase by 17 percentage points and coverage of hepatitis B vaccine could increase from 18% to 65% by 2007, ultimately saving more than two million lives.

The recommendations of the IRC are communicated to the GAVI and Vaccine Fund Boards for final decision. Once the decisions are made, the GAVI Secretariat is responsible for communicating the decisions to the country ICCs, to partners at the regional and field levels, and to UNICEF Supply Division to trigger procurement of the necessary vaccines and supplies.

Committee members must sign a confidentiality and conflict of interest statement. Committee members who recently have been involved in any capacity in the immunization programmes in countries under review are not present during the deliberations of the review committee, and do not participate in the decisions for those countries.

B. GAVI Governance and Structure (see Fig. 1)

1. The GAVI Board

Sets the policies and review progress of the Alliance.

The GAVI Board is comprised of the highest-level representation from the partners, there are four renewable members—WHO, UNICEF, The World Bank, and the Bill & Melinda Gates Foundation. Eleven additional, rotating members responsible for representing the collective expertise and perspective of their constituencies. The current (May 2002) rotating members are:

> Foundation: United Nations Foundation.
> Government—developing countries (two): India and Mali.
> Government—industrialized countries (three): Norway, the United Kingdom, the United States.
> Nongovernmental organization (NGO): Children's Vaccine Program at PATH.
> Pharmaceutical industry—industrialized country: Wyeth-Lederle Vaccines.
> Pharmaceutical industry—developing country: Center for Genetic Engineering and Biotechnology (Cuba).
> Research institute: Institut Pasteur (Paris).
> Technical health institute: U.S. Centers for Disease Control (CDC).

Carol Bellamy, Executive Director of UNICEF, started her 2-year term as GAVI Chair in July 2001, taking over from WHO Director-General Gro Harlem Brundtland who served as GAVI's first chair. The Board meets on average twice a year and schedules periodic teleconferences as needed to review progress and policies.

2. The Vaccine Fund Board and Staff

Responsible for raising the world's awareness about the GAVI immunization goals and securing the funds needed to support those goals.

The Board of the Vaccine Fund is composed of high-profile individuals with wide experience in philanthropy and business. Its first Chairman is former South African President Nelson Mandela.

3. The GAVI Working Group

Supports the Board in policy development and implementation.

Composed of managers in the GAVI partner institutions, these staff are able to translate GAVI priorities into their respective agency work plans. The Working Group currently includes 10 members, representing WHO; UNICEF; the World Bank; the GAVI Secretariat; the Vaccine Fund; the Children's Vaccine Program at PATH, the Government of Tanzania, the University of Maryland School of Medicine, USAID; and GlaxoSmithkline Biologicals.

4. The GAVI Secretariat

Facilitates coordination between the partners and manages the review of country proposals to the Vaccine Fund.

The Secretariat is small—five professional staff and three administrative staff, housed in the European regional office of UNICEF in Geneva. The Secretariat's budget is financed by membership fees paid by the GAVI Board members and the Executive Secretary reports to the GAVI Board.

5. Task Forces

Established to address specific issues of concern to the Board.

Task forces are managed by their respective lead agencies, and include representatives of the relevant partner agencies. The Advocacy Task Force is chaired by UNICEF; the Task Force for Country Coordination is chaired by WHO; the Financing Task Force is co-chaired by the World Bank and USAID; and the Research and Development Task Force is co-chaired by WHO, the University of Maryland, and Chiron Vaccines.

6. Regional Working Groups

Coordinate technical support and information sharing between the national and international levels.

The regional working groups (RWGs) were established by partners with a technical presence at the regional level—in most cases WHO and UNICEF—in response to the need to more quickly identify and address the technical assistance requirements of countries, improve communication, and streamline efforts, in support of the GAVI and Vaccine Fund processes.

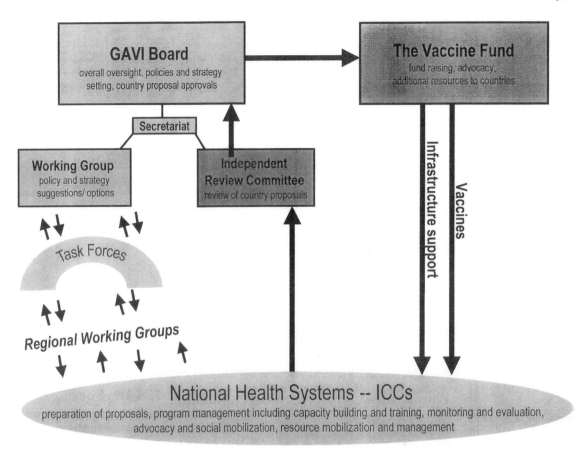

Figure 1 GAVI organogram.

7. National International Agency Committees

Critical to the GAVI partnership.

National ICCs represent the leadership and commitment of the national governments and analogous in their operations to the GAVI Board, i.e., enhancing partner roles through coordinated action. ICC decisions do not overrule governance of partners.

The roles and functions of ICCs vary considerably from country to country, depending on size, strength of the government, and the presence of other health system coordinating groups such as sector-wide groups.

ICCs increasingly are composed of both external donors and agencies and national/internal partners involved in local action. Thus, coordination does not only encompass technical and financial support for government action, but also coordination of implementers—such as NGOs—that may bring their own international or national resources.

III. R&D IN THE CONTEXT OF THE GAVI ALLIANCE

The global vaccine research community includes many diverse players, each contributing in different ways with vastly heterogeneous resources and distinct agendas. Much can be gained by coordinating agendas and goals to render

efforts complementary, avoid duplication, and maximize the use of limited resources.

The many partners involved in vaccine research and development activities and epidemiological studies in both industrialized and developing countries are represented in the Alliance in a truly synergistic effort. Partners include governmental research institutes, academic research programs, large vaccine manufacturers, biotechnology companies, units within Ministries of Health, etc. There are also partners that are not primarily engaged in research but who, as implementers of immunization, will provide critical input to researchers to advise them on what is needed, feasible, and desired at the front lines of primary care, and in contrast, what cannot be readily incorporated into primary care regimens.

With all of the current activity in vaccine R&D, it is important that in the context of GAVI, efforts focus on identifying those gaps where an alliance can have a strategic advantage. Thus, while the GAVI partners recognize that a high priority lies in HIV/AIDS and malaria, given the massive global effort to these projects worldwide, the Alliance decided to prioritize other vaccines that are receiving less attention.

In addition, even if these vaccines become available, many of the poorest countries lack the infrastructure to put these vaccines into public health use efficiently. Therefore, initially, GAVI partners decided to initially place their R&D focus on vaccines that have a lower technical risk and a greater potential for more near-term development and introduction.

In order to identify these priority vaccines, members of the GAVI Task Force on Research and Development (R&D TF) conducted wide consultation with the R&D community to develop consensus.

The criteria for choosing the disease specific projects was based upon several considerations:

> Either no currently registered vaccine or for which the existing vaccines have notable drawbacks that severely limit their public health usefulness (e.g., the existing vaccines are not immunogenic in infants, yet that age group is an epidemiological target for vaccination).
> High potential impact in terms of disease mortality rate and disability-adjusted life years (DALYs).
> Nonavailability of alternative solutions to managing the disease.
> Good potential for changing/improving the immunization system for the future in terms of capacity building and promoting behavioral or system change.
> High degree of feasibility with available tools and infrastructure; political commitment.

The consultation process led to a consensus that the three vaccines that should receive high priority in the context of GAVI are *Streptococcus pneumoniae*, rotavirus, and *Neisseria meningitidis* group A (which may be approached either as a monovalent group A, a bivalent group A/C, or a quadrivalent group A/C/Y/W135 vaccine). Success with these vaccines will alleviate the burden of important diseases in developing countries but will also build the infrastructures for efficient testing and delivery of vaccines that will come later, such as HIV, TB, and malaria.

GAVI partners are also focused on seeking out and developing new technologies that will improve safety, effectiveness, utility, or performance of immunization systems in developing countries. The same broad criteria for evaluating vaccine candidates were used for new technologies, and priority areas were identified to be the following:

> Decreased dependence upon and streamlining of the cold chain.
> Improved tools to measure immunization services performance.
> Reducing infectious wastes and ultimately eliminating the use of sharps (needles and syringes).

Preference will be given to research and development on new technologies being conducted in developing countries.

IV. LOOKING TO THE FUTURE: ISSUES AND CHALLENGES

A. Safety and Waste Management

Worldwide, each year, the overuse of injections and unsafe injection practices combine to cause an estimated 22.5 million hepatitis B virus infections, 2.7 million hepatitis C virus infections, and 98,000 HIV infections. Although injections given as a part of immunization programs account for a very limited proportion (approximately 5%) of the injections delivered and are widely considered the safest of all delivered, there is a growing body of data demonstrating the safety of immunization programs throughout the world need to be improved.

Based on the principle of "do no harm," the GAVI partners acknowledge the importance of improving the safety of immunization programs and have focused special attention on safety in relation to the other elements of immunization programs.

Appropriate disposal of medical waste is an important element of efforts to improve the safety of national immunization programs and should be based on the principle that the "polluter pays." Although at present there are very limited environmentally sound options for safely eliminating waste, the Alliance is committed to supporting countries in their immediate action, using the best practices available to minimize the risk of exposure to medical wastes for staff and the community. GAVI partners encourage further investment in the development of new environmentally sound, reasonably priced methods for disposing of medical wastes.

B. Vaccine Supply

The relatively small size of the developing country vaccine market has resulted in reduced private sector investment in relevant vaccines and thus reduced production capacity. GAVI, with private sector involvement and a 5-year perspective, lends a much-needed stability to delivery systems, demand creation, and vaccine supply. GAVI partners believe that if the public sector can work to help make the developing country vaccine market more attractive to vaccine manufacturers, children living in the poorest countries will live healthier lives by having access to better and more effective vaccines.

C. Sustainability

Financial sustainability is crucial to the success of immunization programs in countries and will be the measure of GAVI's success in the long term. However, the challenge of creating systems that are sustainable beyond the initial time of investment is one of the most critical issues facing all areas of development—not just GAVI.

To clarify the aim of strategies developed to enhance the sustainability of programs, the GAVI Board adopted a new definition of financial sustainability: "Although self-sufficiency is the ultimate goal, in the nearer term sustainable financing is the ability of a country to mobilize and efficiently use domestic and supplementary external resources on a reliable basis to achieve target levels of immunization performance."

In this way GAVI partners recognize that for the foreseeable future, maintaining high-quality immunization programs in the health systems of the poorest countries will require continued external support—from donor governments, NGOs, the private sector, and individuals—

support that has flagged in too many countries in recent years.

D. The Vaccine Fund: Future Needs

The Vaccine Fund was created to provide resources to countries to fill critical gaps in funding for immunization services. The GAVI Board identified that the most critical gaps at present are the weak health service infrastructure in many countries, the delay in introducing new life-saving vaccines as they become available, and the need to improve safety of immunization programs.

As the country programs progress, new gaps are likely to become apparent, and new vaccines now on the horizon will need to be introduced into routine immunization systems. Therefore, the Vaccine Fund will need to continually attract new resources.

E. Maintaining a Robust Learning Curve

It is important to retain the perspective of GAVI as an experiment. By joining in this public-private alliance the GAVI partners have committed to working together in new ways. As new hurdles arise, the Alliance has been able to reexamine and revise its policies and directions. For exam-

ple, The Vaccine Fund expanded its early focus on vaccines to include support for health system infrastructure. The critical issue of immunization safety has emerged so the GAVI Board adopted a new policy so that The Vaccine Fund now provides countries with safe injection devices for all routine immunizations.

Much of the early work of the Alliance has been dedicated to the development of policies and the proposal process for The Vaccine Fund, and providing the eligible countries the technical support they need to apply for support. Now that nearly all eligible countries have applied to The Vaccine Fund, with many of them approved, the GAVI partners are shifting emphasis to supporting implementation of improved immunization programs and issues of sustainability. Looking ahead, GAVI partners will need to continually monitor their impact to assess whether their efforts, and support from The Vaccine Fund, have in fact helped countries meet their targets.

The role of the partners—most of which have worked in immunization long before GAVI came together—cannot be stressed enough. With so much attention focused on GAVI and The Vaccine Fund as new contributors to the global immunization community, it must be remembered that all of the progress logged over the past 2 years has resulted from partner commitments—staff, resources, and financial support—in countries, regions, and at the global levels.

10

Economic Analyses of Vaccines and Vaccination Programs

Benjamin Schwartz and Ismael Ortega-Sanchez
Centers for Disease Control and Prevention, Atlanta, Georgia, U.S.A.

I. INTRODUCTION

Economic analysis has been used to assess a wide range of issues related to vaccines and vaccination programs. Vaccine development priorities for the United States have been assessed by the Institute of Medicine (IOM), categorizing prospective vaccines based on their development and implementation costs compared with the projected health benefits achieved by their use [1]. Manufacturers may use economic analyses to determine allocation of resources among candidate vaccines and to establish vaccine price. After a vaccine is licensed in the United States, cost effectiveness is one of the factors considered by the U.S. Advisory Committee on Immunization Practices in making recommendations for its use [2]. Once a vaccine is recommended, economic analysis may, in part, provide the basis for modifications, recommending new settings or populations in which the vaccine should be used. Economic evaluation of programmatic issues, such as approaches to increasing vaccination coverage, have also been assessed. Although balancing the economic value of immunization against other health programs has not been a key issue in some industrialized countries, for the developing world, the cost of vaccines and the economic analyses of immunization compared with other programs have been important [3].

In the industrialized world, vaccination programs have been characterized by rapid change. Advances in immunology, molecular biology, and technology have markedly accelerated the rate of new vaccine development. Between 1985 and 2000, new vaccines recommended in the United States have included DTaP, enhanced potency inactivated polio vaccine (IPV), *Haemophilus influenzae* type b (Hib) conjugate, hepatitis A and B, varicella, Lyme disease, rotavirus, and pneumococcal conjugate vaccines. Combination vaccines have been developed; however, as their development and licensure have lagged behind other new vaccines, as many as five injections at a single visit are now required to fully vaccinate an infant under the U.S. schedule. Vaccination costs have increased disproportionately to the number of antigens administered. In 1990, the cost of fully vaccinat-ing a child through 5 years of age in the United States was $243.90 which provided protection against nine diseases; in 2000, the cost of recommended vaccines was $605.85 to protect against 11 diseases, or $665.31 to protect against 12 diseases, in some geographic areas. Finally, the types and severity of outcomes prevented by vaccination may also be changing. New vaccines to prevent varicella, hepatitis A, Lyme disease, rotavirus, and pneumococcal infections prevent few deaths in industrialized countries compared with older products. Each of these changes—the increasing number of vaccines and injections, the increasing costs, and the lesser severity of the diseases being prevented—has resulted in greater scrutiny of recommendations for new vaccines and greater importance of the economic rationale for their use.

In the developing world, the Global Alliance for Vaccines and Immunizations and the increased availability of funding have catalyzed changes in vaccination programs. Virtually all countries have received increased support for program infrastructure and the introduction of new vaccines. Although external funding has overcome many barriers, the expectation that countries will assume a greater share of the burden over time makes economic analysis increasingly important for decision makers throughout the world.

The purpose of this chapter is to describe the types of economic analysis commonly used, their components, and the advantages, disadvantages, and controversies that exist with each approach. In addition, some of the limitations and inconsistencies of vaccine economic analyses published in the medical literature will be highlighted, emphasizing the importance of critical analyses of this body of work.

II. TYPES OF ECONOMIC ANALYSES

A. Cost–Benefit Analyses

Three types of analyses are commonly used to assess the economic rationale for immunization or other health-related programs: cost–benefit, cost-effectiveness, and cost–utility analyses (Table 1) [4]. *Cost–benefit analyses* (CBAs) compare the monetary benefits from implementation of a health program with its monetary costs. All inputs in a CBA, including health outcomes, are converted to monetary units, resulting in an outcome that is expressed as money saved or spent. The results of a CBA are typically presented either as the *net present value* (NPV) of the program or the *cost–benefit (CB) ratio*. NPV is defined as the difference between the discounted benefits and the discounted costs of the intervention, or $\text{NPV} = \sum_{t=0}^{N} \delta^t (B - C)_t$, where $\delta^t = 1/(1 + r)^t$, r = the discount rate as a decimal, and t = number of years analyzed (between $t = 0$ and N). Equivalently, results of the analysis can be expressed by the CB ratio, which is the ratio between the discounted costs and the benefits of the intervention, or

$$\text{CB} = \frac{\sum_{t=0}^{N} \delta^t C_t}{\sum_{t=0}^{N} \delta^t B_t}.$$

For new vaccines, where the price per dose has not yet been set, a "break-even" price can be calculated, where the net costs and benefits are equal (NPV = 0).

The CBA is useful to compare the economic value to society of programs with different impacts such as a health program with another (nonhealth) type of program. The NPV of an immunization program can be compared with the NPV of an early childhood education program or a program to encourage aquaculture. Another advantage of this approach is that the results are expressed in a way that is easily understood by policymakers and the public.

An important shortcoming of CBA is the need to quantify all the impacts of a program in monetary terms. Assigning a monetary value to health outcomes for a disability or death is problematic. While one approach is to assign a monetary value based on the net present value of the expected future earnings lost [4], this results in the ethical dilemma of valuing life differently based on country or, possibly, by gender or ethnic group within a country. While a number of different methods have been proposed to estimate the economic value of a life, no method is accepted universally. It is also difficult to assign a monetary value to the pain and suffering that occurs with an illness. The *willingness-to-pay* (WTP) or *contingent valuation* method has become a common strategy to define these values. WTP measures the

value placed on avoiding an outcome. Several approaches may be used to define WTP. One common approach involves surveying a population for the maximum they would spend to avert or decrease the risk of a specific hypothetical outcome [4]. Drawbacks with this approach include results being sensitive to how the outcome is presented; differences in valuation between those with different socioeconomic status or levels of education; difficulties setting values for very rare events such as severe adverse events following vaccination; and disparities between what people say and what they do. An alternative method taken, in part, from product development and marketing is *conjoint analysis*. Using this method, preferences are expressed for programs or products that have a range of defined attributes jointly as a "product profile" [5]. Although this approach has not been used for analyses of vaccines or vaccination programs, it may be a useful strategy to better value a product or program.

B. Cost-Effectiveness Analyses

Cost-effectiveness analysis (CEA) assesses the value of a program by calculating the expenditure per health outcome achieved (net cost/net health effect). Some common examples include cost per case prevented and cost per death averted. Average cost effectiveness (ACE) is used to describe costs and outcomes for an independent program, $\text{ACE} = C_A/E_A$, where A is a program or strategy. Incremental cost effectiveness (ICE) describes the ratio between costs and outcomes for programs that are being compared, $\text{ICE} = (C_A - C_B)/(E_A - E_B)$, where A and B are competing programs or strategies. Finally, marginal cost effectiveness (MCE) describes the costs and outcomes within a single program to show cost of expanding, $\text{MCE} = (C_{A^1} - C_A)/(E_{A^1} - E_A)$, where A^1 is an extension of A.

Because the denominator is a specific health event, CEA is used to choose between alternative interventions that are aimed at achieving a similar outcome. For example, CEA has been used to determine whether cholera vaccination in conjunction with rehydration therapy in refugee settings is cost-effective in preventing morbidity and mortality compared with rehydration therapy alone [6]. An advantage of CEA compared with CBA is that by comparing similar outcomes, it is unnecessary to convert health outcomes into monetary values.

A limitation of this approach, however, is that CEA can be used only if the interventions being compared share a

Table 1 Comparison of Characteristics of Cost–Benefit, Cost-Effectiveness, and Cost–Utility Analyses

	Cost–benefit analyses	Cost-effectiveness analyses	Cost–utility analyses
Outcome measure	Net present value	Cost per health outcome averted (or gained)	Cost per health utility (e.g., QALY) gained
Calculation of outcome measure	Benefits–costs	$\dfrac{\text{Net costs}}{\text{Net benefits}}$	$\dfrac{\text{Net costs}}{\text{Health utilities gained}}$
Useful for comparing	Health programs vs. nonhealth programs	Health program A vs. health program B (with same health outcome)	Health program A vs. health program B (with different health outcome)

common outcome measure. For many new vaccines in the United States, where the impact on morbidity far outweighs that on mortality, CEA is of little use in comparing value (e.g., for prevention of varicella, rotavirus gastroenteritis, and pneumococcal otitis media). In addition, the results of CEA are more difficult to apply in policymaking. For example, infant pneumococcal conjugate vaccination at a cost of $58 per dose would cost society $160 per episode of otitis media prevented, and $3200 per episode of pneumonia prevented [7]. Is the cost reasonable to achieve the specified health outcomes? Although one could compare directly the costs of preventing otitis media or pneumonia with those of treatment, such an approach would ignore the benefit of prevention compared with cure.

C. Cost–Utility Analyses

Cost–utility analysis (CUA) is a subset of cost-effectiveness analysis where a common outcome measure is developed to take into account different types of health impacts. The calculation of cost and impact in CUA is identical to that for CEA except that the denominator is expressed as health utilities gained. The CUA is most useful in three settings: (1) when comparing health programs that have different disease impacts; (2) when summarizing the overall impact of a program that affects both morbidity and mortality outcomes; and (3) when comparing a program that primarily affects mortality with one that primarily affects morbidity. Because results of CUA are expressed as cost per health benefit, this method could not be used to compare a health program with a nonhealth program.

One strength of CUA is that as with CEA, outcomes are expressed as cost per change in health status; thus, health outcomes do not need to be converted into monetary equivalents. However, a common metric does need to be established that allows comparison of qualitatively different health outcomes. *Years of potential life lost* (YPLL), *quality-adjusted life years* (QALYs), and *disability-adjusted life years* (DALYs) are examples of widely used utilities [4,8–11].

One common utility used in CUA, the QALY, provides a method to compare health outcomes, where both the quality and the duration of life are affected by a disease. QALYs represent the sum of each year of life multiplied by the quality of each of those years. Quality is expressed on a scale ranging from 1 (perfect health) to 0 (death). Several approaches have been used to establish quality values for morbid conditions. Using the *standard gamble* approach, respondents are asked to state a preference between living with a disability and an alternative that includes a risk of death (p) or of perfect health ($1-p$). The probability at which the respondent considers the two options equivalent represents the health utility. With the *time trade-off* method, respondents are asked how much perfect life they would trade to avoid life with a defined health condition [4]. Several utility scales are available, and recommended methods to derive health utilities have been published by the Panel on Cost Effectiveness in Health and Medicine, established by the Public Health Service [12].

Although CUA has been used more frequently in recent years to evaluate and compare health programs, there are several limitations of this method. Most importantly, the results of a CUA depend on the utilities assigned to acute and chronic morbid states. Preferences expressed using standard gamble or time trade-off methods are affected by the description of the health condition and the characteristics of the respondents. Generally, those who suffer a chronic condition score their health-related quality of life differently than the general population [4]. Developing health utilities may also be more difficult for acute conditions or when the respondent is not the one who would suffer the illness. For example, to derive health utilities for influenza vaccination of children one approach would be to interview parents to determine how much of their healthy life they would choose to trade in order to decrease the probability that their child develops influenza during a given year. By contrast, assessing health utilities would be easier when considering the potential value of therapeutic vaccines for chronic illnesses. For policymakers, understanding the meaning of a health utility is more difficult than evaluating a positive or negative value in a CBA or a cost per health outcome in a CEA. Therefore, presenting a comparison between programs or developing a scale to define what is a "good buy" for a QALY or other health utility may be important for those interpreting CUA results.

D. Examples of Economic Analysis Used to Evaluate Vaccines and Vaccination Programs

Each type of economic analysis has been used in assessing vaccines and vaccination programs. CUA has been used to compare and determine priorities among clinical preventive services. Eight studies of vaccination, including 33 cost–utility ratios published between 1976 and 1997, were evaluated along with 42 studies assessing other preventive services (e.g., chemoprophylaxis, screening tests, and counseling). Overall, vaccines were the most "cost-effective" interventions with a median cost per QALY of $1500 and a range from being cost saving to a cost of $140,000 per QALY [13]. Moreover, among 30 preventive services recommended by the U.S. Preventive Services Task Force, childhood vaccination was valued as the highest, based on the clinically preventable burden and the cost per QALY saved [14]. CUA was also used by the IOM to compare vaccine development priorities with priority categories defined by the cost per QALY saved [1]. By contrast, CEA and CBA have been employed more often to assess the impact of a new vaccine or a change in the vaccination schedule [7,15–17]. Programmatic issues, such as the use of reminder-recall or other interventions to increase vaccination coverage, have been assessed by CEA with the outcome measured as cost per person vaccinated [18]. Willingness-to-pay methods have been used to define preferences for safer or combination vaccines [19,20].

III. COMPONENTS OF ECONOMIC ANALYSES

Whatever economic analysis method is used, the quality of the analysis depends on including all important costs and benefits—as appropriate to the method selected and the perspective being taken (see Section 3.5. Distribution of Costs and Benefits)—and on being able to obtain accurate estimates for each of the components of the model. While it is often difficult to predict the health effects of a program, an economic analysis must also identify direct and indirect costs associated with program inputs and impacts. In instances where the accuracy of cost or impact data is unclear, sensitivity analyses that vary the uncertain components are a useful method to determine which parameters in the model are driving the results of the analysis.

A.   Developing the Model

The evaluation of a vaccine or vaccination program using CBA, CEA, or CUA begins with creating a conceptual model indicating expected costs and health impacts. A decision tree (Fig. 1) is a useful way to present the different program impacts and their estimated probability of occurrence. Many of the computer software programs for conducting economic analyses begin with the creation of a decision tree; however, this graphical representation is not required to conduct an economic analysis and many investigators prefer to use spreadsheet software. The key to an economic analysis, regardless of the software used, is to develop a comprehensive model that includes as many of the expected impacts and costs as possible.

In a decision tree, the range of possible outcomes and the probability that the outcome will occur are represented graphically. Typically, a decision tree begins with a "decision node" (presented as a box), where the alternative interventions are distinguished from one another (e.g., implement or not implement an immunization program). The next levels of the decision tree describe the consequence of the previous decision and its probability. Examples include vaccinated/ not vaccinated, adverse event/no adverse event, and disease/ no disease. The probability or each of these events is represented by a "probability node" (presented as a circle). Probability nodes may have several different possible outcomes. However, the alternative outcomes of a probability node must be mutually exclusive and exhaustive; consequently, the sum of the probabilities of a probability node will always equal 1. The final level of the decision tree, called the "outcome node" (presented as a triangle), represents the ultimate health outcome of the sequence of events along a branch of the decision tree. Different adverse events and types of disease should be specified separately along with the consequences of each (e.g., no sequelae, sequelae, or death).

B.   Estimating Impacts

Determining the impacts of a new vaccine and the probabilities of their occurrence is not easy. Although disease out-

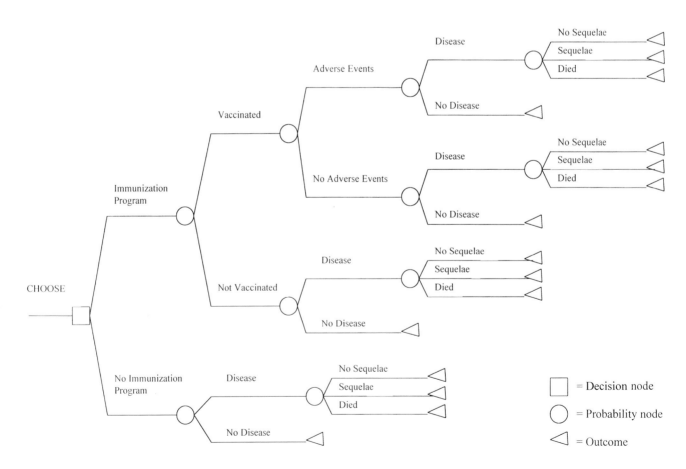

Figure 1   Example of a decision tree.

comes prevented can be defined simply as the product of the disease burden times the vaccine efficacy, accurately defining these parameters may be complex. An infection may result in several disease outcomes; some of these (e.g., pneumonia or otitis media) may seldom be etiologically diagnosed and disease burden may vary by age, population group, and by year. Health outcomes of an illness are also likely to differ by age and may change over time with the development of new therapies; the long-term impact of sequelae may be poorly defined. Results of randomized vaccine efficacy trials pre-licensure, where enrollees generally are healthy and vaccine is administered in controlled settings, may differ from those obtained when a vaccine is used broadly in the population. In addition, some impacts of vaccines cannot be determined until the vaccine is in widespread use. Herd immunity can substantially increase the benefits of vaccination, but cannot be measured from clinical trials in which the unit of randomization is the individual subject. Uncommon adverse events will also not be detected until after a vaccine is recommended and widely used.

C. Estimating Costs

Direct and indirect costs typically are considered in economic analyses of vaccination programs (Table 2). Direct costs include the costs related to health events that would occur with and without the program and the costs of the vaccination program itself. The direct costs of health events include costs of medical care visits, diagnosis and of acute and long-term treatment. The costs of transportation to the doctor's office or hospital and of housekeeping or childcare services during a period of illness are also direct costs. The direct costs of the vaccination program include the cost of vaccine, the administration, and the medical care visit including travel costs. Other program costs that may be less obvious include the costs of storing and transporting vaccine, of maintaining the cold chain, and of training health care workers to administer the new vaccine. The impact of these costs will be minimal and often is not included in analyses of vaccines delivered in industrialized countries; however, it may be important for vaccines administered through the public sector in developing countries where the incremental costs would be more substantial. Treatment of adverse events following immunization must be added to costs although for most vaccines, the magnitude of these costs will be small relative to other components of the model. Other costs may be considered in certain settings, depending on the purpose of the analysis. Vaccine development costs may be relevant if the analysis focuses on priorities for developing new vaccines. For a new vaccine to be used in developing countries, it may be reasonable to consider foreign exchange costs, discounting costs borne in local currency.

The largest category of indirect costs is typically described as losses in productivity due to time away from work, disability, or premature death as a consequence of the illness. Some analyses also include the costs of pain and suffering from illness, of adverse events, or an additional injection as indirect costs, with data derived using methods such as willingness to pay. For many recently recommended

Table 2 Examples of Direct and Indirect Costs Often Considered in Economic Analyses of an Immunization Program

Direct costs
Medical care costs associated with disease
 Inpatient services
 Outpatient services
 Long-term care (e.g., home health services, rehabilitation, equipment)
 Diagnostic tests and procedures
 Medications
 Other therapy
Vaccination program costs
 Vaccine
 Vaccine administration
 Medical care visit(s) for vaccination
 Medical care visit(s) for adverse events (inpatient/outpatient)
 Medication for therapy of adverse events
Transportation to and from medical services
Child care
Housekeeping
Vaccine research and development
Indirect costs
Change in productivity from illness or vaccine adverse event
 Time lost from death and illness
 Time lost for medical care visits
 Decreased productivity while at work due to illness or sequelae
 Time lost while caring for an ill family member
Foregone leisure time while ill or caring for an ill family member
Intangible costs (e.g., pain and suffering)

Source: Ref. 4.
Specific costs included will depend on the type of economic analysis and the perspective taken.

vaccines in the United States, inclusion of indirect costs has a substantial impact on the results of the analysis; this impact often is highlighted when the value of a new vaccine is described from the health care payer's perspective, where only direct costs are considered, as compared with the societal perspective, where both direct and indirect costs are included. For example, the break-even cost of vaccine in the United States for an infant rotavirus vaccination program was estimated at $9 from the health care payer's perspective compared with $51 from the societal perspective [16]. For vaccination of infants with pneumococcal conjugate vaccine, the costs were estimated at $18 and $46, respectively [7]. Routine varicella vaccination of U.S. children has been estimated to save $5 for every dollar invested from a societal perspective, but, from the payer's perspective, would cost about $2 for each case of chickenpox prevented [15]. Although indirect costs are routinely included in economic analyses and are recommended to be used by the Panel on Cost Effectiveness in Health and Medicine [12], there is no solid evidence supporting the assumption that in the absence of illness, national productivity would increase by the magnitude estimated. If workers use vacation or sick leave days when ill or when caring for a sick child, if they trade work shifts with a coworker when they make a medical care visit, or if industries would cut their workforce rather than increase output if worker absences were eliminated, then it would be incorrect to assume that societal productivity would increase if illness were prevented. Some economists respond to this by equating the value of "productivity" and leisure time, suggesting that lost leisure when ill or caring for a sick child has the same societal value.

Once decisions have been made regarding what costs to include in an economic analysis, the next step is to assign monetary values. For medical care and treatment, the use of costs, rather than price or charge, is recommended because the cost more closely reflects the true value placed on that service. Several databases, including Medicare payments or the payments made by large managed care organizations, are available to estimate costs of medical care. Charge data can be converted to costs by using published cost-to-charge ratios [4].

Indirect costs generally have been calculated from the number of days lost due to illness multiplied by the value of a work day. Approaches to valuing work differ: Some studies perform separate calculations for men and women; some consider the proportion who are employed full time, part time, or are unemployed; some distinguish between work days and weekends; and some assign a monetary value to "housekeeping" for persons not in the workforce. I am aware of no studies that assign lower indirect costs when the population affected by a disease is disproportionately in a lower socioeconomic group.

Because indirect costs of recently licensed vaccines have outweighed direct costs and because methods for defining indirect costs vary, public health personnel and policymakers must scrutinize the methods in economic evaluations and understand the choices made and estimates used. In four recent analyses of influenza vaccine [21–24], the number of work-loss days estimated for an ill adult ranged from 0.52 to 2 and the value of a work day ranged from $93.40 to $120 per day. In addition, one study [21] estimated the cost of influenza vaccine and its administration at $4 based on data published five years previously.

Estimates of the value of human life also vary between studies and may account for some of the variability in results. The human capital approach values life in a manner similar to capital equipment, whose productive output is lost or diminished due to premature death or disability. The value of the death is equivalent to the net present value of his/her expected future earnings. This approach is consistent with methods for calculating indirect (productivity) costs and often is used in CEA and CUA. Critiques of this approach are that it undervalues persons who are older or not in the workforce and that the value of life will differ between countries so that international comparisons of health states would tend to favor conditions that affect the populations of industrialized countries. Values obtained using the willingness-to-pay approach tend to be higher than using the human capital approach and may vary considerably between studies [25]. For diseases where mortality is a common

outcome, these differences may be important to the overall results of the analysis.

D. Discounting Costs and Health Effects

Quite often, the costs and benefits of a vaccination program accrue at some point in the future, long after the vaccination itself. Because society values accruing benefits early and delaying costs until later, a method called *discounting* is used to adjust all costs and benefits to their present value. It is important to note that discounting is not strictly an attempt to adjust for inflation because even with no inflation, individuals will prefer benefits that occur now compared with sometime in the future. Although no single discount rate is used universally, the Panel on Cost Effectiveness in Health and Medicine recommends using a rate of 3% [12]. Other rates may be chosen to facilitate comparison with other studies and in sensitivity analyses. The importance of discounting will vary for a vaccine, where the impact is acute and long-term consequences of infection are rare (e.g., influenza), and one where the health impacts occur long after the vaccine was administered (e.g., hepatitis B). A cost-effectiveness analysis for the use of hepatitis B vaccine in the Gambia provides an example of the impact of the discount rate used on results of the analysis (Fig. 2) [26]. In this CEA, the authors assume that the vaccine will be used as a routine infant immunization and that the efficacy is 85%. Because the costs for the vaccination program accrue now but the benefits associated with the prevention of hepatocellular carcinoma occur a median of 35 years in the future, discounting those future costs and benefits has a substantial impact on the results, demonstrated by the eightfold difference in cost per liver cancer death averted, depending on whether discounting is included. Note that use of a 3% discount rate would decrease the magnitude of this difference.

E. Distribution of Costs and Benefits

Economic analyses may assess costs and benefits using a family, a health care payer, or a societal perspective. Although vaccination recommendations in the United States have relied primarily on societal-level analyses, the decisions that are made may not be considered optimal at other analysis levels. For example, U.S. recommendations for routine childhood use of varicella, rotavirus, and pneumococcal conjugate vaccines are cost-neutral or cost-saving to society at current vaccine prices, but represent a net cost to health care payers, who do not benefit from the productivity cost savings accruing to society. Even when only direct costs are considered, the benefits of vaccination may not accrue to the party bearing the costs. For example, because of the high annual turnover in the client population of a managed care organization, the costs of a prevention program for hepatitis B or invasive pneumococcal disease among older adults may be borne by one organization, while another reaps the benefits of disease prevented years into the future. In many developing countries, the Ministry of Health bears the majority of the burden for the direct costs of a vaccination

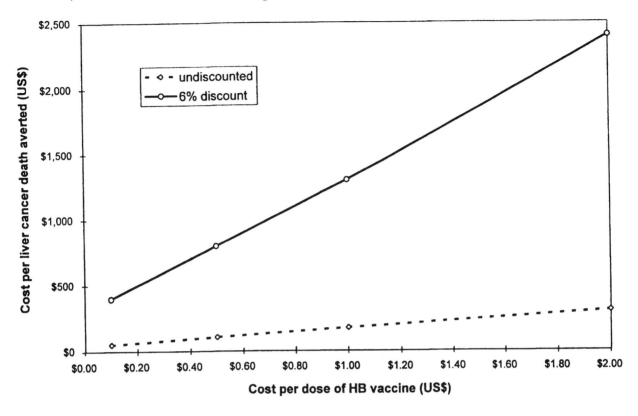

Figure 2 Impact of discounting on cost effectiveness of hepatitis B vaccination in The Gambia. (From Ref. 26.)

program, while the benefits of indirect costs averted are distributed throughout the population.

IV. SENSITIVITY ANALYSES

Parameter estimates in economic analyses are inherently uncertain, in part, because data on disease and its prevention are limited by the populations studied and because future events (e.g., the rate of inflation) cannot be known. Because of the uncertainty surrounding many of the estimates in economic models, sensitivity analyses are important to assess whether the results are robust—that is, the conclusions are valid across the range of reasonable estimates—or whether little confidence can be placed in the overall result and more data need to be collected to better quantify key parameters. In conducting a sensitivity analysis, one approach is for the investigator to define a plausible range across which the true value of each parameter may vary. The impact of changing each parameter between plausible extremes can be determined one by one in univariate sensitivity analyses. This type of analysis is useful in identifying the parameter(s) to which the overall result is most sensitive [7]. However, a univariate sensitivity analysis cannot determine the true range in possible outcomes or a confidence interval around the baseline result. Bivariate analyses or best-case and worst-case analyses that select extreme values for each parameter are also of limited value. Several statistical modeling techniques are available and are included in

standard cost-effectiveness software [12]. Multiple simulations, using Markov or Monte Carlo analyses, randomly varying the parameters across the reasonable range according to an assumed distribution, can approximate a confidence interval for a cost-effectiveness ratio [24].

V. INTERPRETING AND COMPARING ECONOMIC ANALYSES

As the results of economic analyses are more often being used to support recommendations for use of new vaccines, the importance of their results to vaccine manufacturers and health officials increases. Manufacturer support or disease prevention goals of academic and public health scientists may exert subtle influences on analytic methods and results. While neither manufacturer support nor disease prevention goals invalidate the results of a well-done study, it is important to assess economic analyses with careful attention to the methods used and a cautious (perhaps even skeptical) perspective when assessing the results. Key elements that should be included in a published economic analysis are shown in Table 3 [12]. Special care should be taken in evaluating the parameters to which the model is most sensitive. For example, when considering disease burden, what data are available (including, perhaps, data not presented in the manuscript) and are they generalizable? If data from multiple studies were available, how were they summarized and a base-case estimate selected? For a disease

Table 3 Key Items to Include in a Published Report of an Economic Analysis

---

(1) Approach
    General design of the analysis
    Target population for intervention
    Program description (e.g., case setting, model of delivery, timing of intervention)
    Description of comparison program
    Time horizon
    Perspective of the analysis
(2) Data and methods
    Identification of outcomes of interest
    Definition of outcome measures
    Description of model
    Modeling assumptions
    Diagram of event pathway or model
    Software used
    Sources for and data on model parameters (e.g., disease burden, program effectiveness, cost data)
    Strategy for summarizing data to develop base-case estimates when multiple data points are available
    Statement of methods for obtaining expert opinion, where it is used to estimate parameters
    Method to define preferences and preference weights
    Critique of data quality
    Statement of year of costs
    Statement of method used to adjust costs for inflation
    Statement of type of currency
    Statement of discount rate
(3) Results
    Results of model validation
    Aggregate cost and impact of the program
    Results of base-case analysis
    Results of sensitivity analysis
    Statistical estimates describing uncertainty, if possible
    Graphical representation of results and sensitivity analysis
(4) Discussion
    Summary of results
    Summary of sensitivity of results to assumptions and uncertainties in the analysis
    Robustness of the analysis
    Limitations of the study
    Relevance of the results to specific policy questions or decisions
    Results of related economic analyses

Source: Ref. 12.
Specific items included may differ based on the type of economic analysis undertaken.

that results in significant morbidity but in little mortality, what data are used to determine rates of work loss among adult caretakers of sick children and what economic values are assigned to their productivity? Based on the results of the sensitivity analysis, can the results of the study be considered robust across the range of plausible inputs or should the analysis be deemed noncontributory to decision making? Finally, as additional studies are done or as a vaccine is used postlicensure, are new data that result in changes in the assumptions or parameters available? In conducting economic analyses, adhering to standards rec-

ommended by the Panel on Cost Effectiveness in Health and Medicine may help eliminate potential biases and improve uniformity and, therefore, comparability between studies.

VI. SUMMARY

Economic analyses are an important element in setting priorities for health interventions, vaccine development, and vaccine recommendation. Results can provide the economic rationale for the use of scarce health resources on vaccines and vaccination programs and can provide guidance on the most effective ways to implement new and current vaccines. The type of economic analysis performed and the components included in the analysis will differ based on the questions addressed. Attention to the issues outlined in this chapter can help to provide the basis for well-designed economic analyses that will be useful to decision makers faced with many alternative health interventions, but limited economic resources.

REFERENCES

1. Stratton KR, et al. Vaccines for the 21st century: A tool for decisionmaking. Washington, DC: Institute of Medicine, National Academy Press, 1999:1–460.
2. CDC Advisory Committee on Immunization Practices Policies and Procedures. http://www.cdc.gov/nip/acip.
3. The World Bank. World Development Report 1993: Investing in Health. Oxford, England: Oxford University Press, 1993:1–330.
4. Haddix AC, et al. Prevention Effectiveness: A Guide to Decision Analysis and Economic Evaluation. New York: Oxford University Press, 1996:1–227.
5. Johnson FR, Bingham MF. Measuring Stated Preferences for Pharmaceuticals: A Brief Introduction. Triangle Economic Research, General working paper G-0002, June 13, 2000, http://www.ter/com/general.html.
6. Naficy A, et al. Treatment and vaccination strategies to control cholera in sub-Saharan refugee settings. JAMA 1998; 279: 521–525.
7. Lieu TA, et al. Projected cost effectiveness of pneumococcal conjugate vaccination of healthy infants and young children. JAMA 2000; 283:1460–1468.
8. Morrow RH, Bryant JH. Health policy approaches to measuring and valuing human life: conceptual and ethical issues. Am J Public Health 1995; 85:1356–1360.
9. Loomes G, McKenzie L. The use of QALYs in health care decision making. Soc Sci Med 1989; 28:299–308.
10. Murray CJL. Quantifying the burden of disease: the technical basis for disability adjusted life years. Bull WHO 1994; 72:429–445.
11. Nord E. Methods for quality adjustment of life years. Soc Sci Med 1992; 34:559–569.
12. Gold MR, et al. Cost Effectiveness in Health and Medicine. New York: Oxford University Press, 1996:3–425.
13. Stone PW, et al. Cost utility analyses of clinical preventive services: Published ratios, 1976–1997. Am J Prev Med 2000; 19:15–23.
14. Coffield AB, et al. Priorities among recommended clinical preventive services. Am J Prev Med 2001; 21:1–9.
15. Lieu TA, et al. Cost effectiveness of a routine varicella vaccination program for U.S. children. JAMA 1994; 271:375–381.

16. Tucker AW, et al. Cost effectiveness analysis of a rotavirus immunization program in the United States. JAMA 1998; 279:1371–1376.
17. Miller MA, et al. Cost effectiveness of incorporating inactivated poliovirus vaccine into the routine childhood immunization schedule. JAMA 1996; 276:967–971.
18. Lieu TA, et al. Effectiveness and cost effectiveness of letters, automated telephone messages, or both for underimmunized children in a health maintenance organization. Pediatrics 1998; 101:E3.
19. Lieu TA, et al. The hidden costs of infant vaccination. Vaccine 2001; 19, 33–41.
20. Sansom SL, et al. Rotavirus vaccine and intussusception: how much risk will parents in the United States accept to ontain vaccine benefits? Am J Epidemiol 2001; 154:1077–1085.
21. White T, et al. Potential cost savings attributable to influenza vaccination of school-aged children. Pediatrics 1999; 103: E73.
22. Cohen GM, Nettleman MD. Economic impact of influenza vaccination in preschool children. Pediatrics 2000; 106, 973–976.
23. Luce BR, et al. Cost effectiveness analysis of an intranasal influenza vaccine for the prevention of influenza in healthy children. Pediatrics 2001; 109:E24.
24. Nichol KM. Cost benefit analysis of a strategy to vaccinate healthy working adults against influenza. Arch Intern Med 2001; 161, 749–759.
25. Moore MJ, Vixcusi WK. Doubling the estimated value of life: results using new occupational fatality data. J Policy Anal Manage 1988; 7:476–490.
26. Hall AJ, et al. Cost-effectiveness of hepatitis B vaccine in the Gambia. Trans R Soc Trop Med Hyg 1993; 87:333–336.

11

The Role of the Food and Drug Administration in Vaccine Testing and Licensure

Norman Baylor and Karen Midthun
U.S. Food and Drug Administration, Rockville, Maryland, U.S.A.

Lydia A. Falk
National Institute of Allergy and Infectious Diseases, National Institutes of Health, Bethesda, Maryland, U.S.A.

I. INTRODUCTION

This chapter will provide a detailed overview of the roles and responsibilities of the Food and Drug Administration (FDA) in testing and licensing of vaccines. Moreover, this chapter will describe the FDA's role in the clinical evaluation of preventive vaccines, with a focus on the Investigational New Drug (IND) application process, the Biologics License Application (BLA) review and approval process, and postlicensure requirements. Finally, some of the regulatory and scientific challenges of newer vaccines using advanced genomic techniques will be addressed.

The Center for Biologics Evaluation and Research (CBER), Office of Vaccines Research and Review (OVRR) of the FDA is responsible for regulating vaccines produced by manufacturers licensed in the United States. Current authority for the regulation of vaccines resides in Section 351 of the Public Health Service Act (PHS Act) and specific sections of the Food, Drug, and Cosmetic Act (FD&C Act) [1]. A single set of basic regulatory approval criteria apply to vaccines, regardless of the technology used to produce the vaccine. In the United States, vaccines are regulated as biological products. The regulations used in implementing these Acts are contained in Title 21 of the Code of Federal Regulations (21CFR). The regulations in the CFR cover general requirements such as current good manufacturing practices, labeling, licensing procedures, and conduct of clinical trials. The CFR also covers methods to be used in, and the facilities or controls to be used for the manufacture, testing, processing, packaging, and holding of vaccines to assure that these products meet the requirements of the FD&C Act as to safety, strength, and purity.

The regulations detail the minimum requirements for the preparation of vaccines (Figure 1). It is worth noting that certain regulations have been changed or eliminated as a result of the FDA's constant challenge to develop standards for assessing the safety and efficacy of vaccines using more state-of-the-art technologies. For example, 21 CFR 620, Additional Standards for Bacterial Products, and 21 CFR 630, Additional Standards for Viral Vaccines, were revoked in August 1996. Instead of incorporating new standards into the regulations, the BLA itself contains all the appropriate testing methods for in-process and release testing for each specific new vaccine. This approach allows for flexibility in responding to scientific advances and new technologies as they emerge in vaccine development. The FDA also publishes guidances and other regulatory documents on specific topics to assist manufacturers and clinical investigators in developing new products (Table 1).

Prior to discussing the procedures for the regulation of vaccines, it would be useful to review certain definitions codified in the regulations. As further defined in 21 CFR Part 600, safety is "the relative freedom from harmful effect to persons affected, directly or indirectly, by a product when prudently administered, taking into consideration the characteristics of the product in relation to the condition of the recipient at the time." Purity is the "relative freedom from extraneous matter in the finished product, whether or not harmful to the recipient or deleterious to the product." Potency is "the specific ability or capacity of the product, as indicated by appropriate laboratory tests or by adequately controlled clinical data obtained through the administration of the product in the manner intended, to effect a given result." Simply put, to be licensed, a vaccine must be a preparation of known characterization and purity that has been demonstrated to be safe and effective. The exact standards required to meet these criteria for a particular vaccine are

❏ 21 CFR 25   Environmental impact considerations

❏ 21 CFR 50   Protection of human subjects

❏ 21 CFR 56   Institutional Review Boards

❏ 21 CFR 58   Good laboratory practice for nonclinical laboratory studies

❏ 21 CFR 201   Labeling

❏ 21 CFR 202   Prescription drug advertising (promotional labeling)

❏ 21 CFR 210   Current good manufacturing practice in manufacturing, processing, packing, or holding of drugs; general

❏ 21 CFR 211   Current good manufacturing practice for finished pharmaceuticals

❏ 21 CFR 312   Investigational new drug application (IND)

❏ 21 CFR 314.126   Adequate and well-controlled trials

❏ 21 CFR 600   Biological products: general

❏ 21 CFR 601   Licensing

❏ 21 CFR 610   General biological products standards

Figure 1 Food and Drug Administration regulations relevant to the manufacture, product quality, and clinical testing of vaccines. Regulations covering the Food and Drug Administration are located in Title 21 of the Code of Federation Regulations (CFR). The CFR can be accessed on-line and directly searched from http://www.access.gpo.gov/nara/cfr/. These may also be directly obtained from the Government Printing Office, Washington, D.C., 20402–9328.

dependent on the specific vaccine and the technology used to produce it.

Regulatory issues should be considered as early in the development process as possible, because ultimately, regulatory compliance is an essential basis for licensure, regardless of the quality of the safety and efficacy data. The first regulatory requirements that must be considered are purity and preclinical safety, the two prerequisites to move a vaccine from the laboratory to the clinic. Both must be demonstrated prior to beginning clinical trials. In addition to requirements for product quality, the quality of data generated in clinical studies is of the utmost importance because

Table 1 Guidance Documents

Points to consider in the characterization of cell lines to produce biologics (1993)
ICH guidance on quality of biotechnological/biological products: derivation and characterization of cell substrates used for production of biotechnological/biological products, Q5D (1998)
Points to consider in the manufacture and testing of monoclonal antibody products for human use (1997)
ICH guidance on viral safety evaluation of biotechnology products derived from cell lines of human or animal origin, Q5A (1995)
Points to consider on plasmid DNA vaccines for preventive infectious disease indications (1996)
Guidance for industry for the evaluation of combination vaccines for preventable diseases: production, testing, and clinical studies (1997)
Content and format of chemistry, manufacturing, and controls (CMC) information and establishment description information for a vaccine or related product (1999)
Guidance to industry on considerations for reprotoxicity studies for preventive vaccines for infectious disease indications (2000)
Guidance for industry—formal meetings with sponsors and applicants for PDUFA products (2000)
IND meetings for human drugs and biologics—chemistry, manufacturing, and controls information (2001)

safety and efficacy data from studies that do not or cannot meet regulatory requirements for adequate, well-controlled studies cannot lead to approval.

II. GENERAL CONSIDERATIONS FOR VACCINE TESTING

A. Vaccine Testing

The requirements for testing of licensed products are described in 21 CFR. Some of these requirements are generally applicable to all products, whereas others are tailored to the specific vaccine. Examples of tests that are generally applicable to all products include those for bacterial and fungal sterility, general safety, purity, identity, suitability of constituent materials, and potency [2]. Additional product-specific tests designed to provide additional assurance of safety or purity may be required; for example, testing of viral seeds and cell cultures for extraneous viruses is especially relevant for live viral vaccines. Although not all necessary tests for assessing safety, purity, and manufacturing consistency are prescribed in the regulations or guidance documents developed by the FDA, all production steps, as well as control and lot release testing must be described in the IND and in greater detail in the manufacturer's biologics license application. Once the product is licensed, testing is conducted according to the exact specifications in the manufacturer's license application.

When considering the issue of release testing, a general rule is that testing should be performed at the latest manufacturing step compatible with adequate assay performance. Specifically, the CFR provides a list of tests that should be completed on product that is in final container (e.g., identity, sterility, and general safety). In contrast, other release testing may be performed upstream prior to final fill of the product. Potency testing is an example where the test may be performed on either the product in final container or formulated bulk products; however, characteristics associated with potency (protein to polysaccharide ratio for conjugate vaccines) may be measured at earlier steps in the manufacturing process [3]. Consideration of such approaches should be discussed early on with the FDA and be based on sound scientific rationale. Although final container testing requirements are specified in the CFR, the importance of adequate in-process tests should not be minimized. The inclusion of critical in-process tests and specification may provide valuable information regarding consistency of manufacture and provide a mechanism for detection of early manufacturing or product deviations.

With regard to the required testing for licensed biologic products, the FDA is reevaluating the appropriateness of selected requirements and/or the test method cited in the CFR. For example, the general safety test is required by the FDA for all products, including vaccines. The general safety test, performed using guinea pigs and mice, is for the detection of extraneous toxic contaminants that may have been introduced during the manufacture or filling process. However, in the case of certain vaccine types, the relevance of the general safety test has been questioned. For example, the

relevance of evaluating an orally delivered vaccine by intraperitoneal injection of animals is questionable. In addition, the question of the utility of such a test for a product with inherent toxicity that interferes with the interpretation of the test, e.g., live bacterial vaccines, has been raised. Currently, the FDA is discussing whether to eliminate the requirement for the general safety test. Another example of where the FDA is revisiting the CFR requirements is in regard to the testing for pyrogenic substances by intravenous injection into rabbits. Because of the variability of in vivo tests such as the rabbit pyrogenicity test, consideration is given to alternative methods such as the limulus amoebocyte lysate (LAL) assay for endotoxins. Following discussions with the FDA, the LAL assay may be substituted for the rabbit pyrogenicity test and may provide a more quantitative assessment of endotoxin content in a product. The ability to assess endotoxin levels in vaccine lots may also provide a measure of manufacturing and process control from lot to lot.

Although guidelines exist for the general principles in developing and testing biologics, additional standards of purity, potency, and preclinical safety are most often developed for each specific product. The importance of additional in-process and manufacturing consistency controls should not be minimized. For example, additional controls are applied to characterizing purified antigen products and biotechnology products compared to those tests applied to relatively crude, killed, whole-cell bacterial vaccines. In the latter case, the manufacturing process applied to killed whole-cell bacterial vaccines should strive to eliminate cell-associated impurities. Control assays must demonstrate the absence of such impurities, to the highest degree of sensitivity that is possible. For these vaccines, demonstration of the absence of toxicity becomes a critical purity parameter and validation studies to demonstrate the safety of the final preparations become the cornerstone in safety and manufacturing control testing.

As touched upon earlier, well-defined manufacturing methods and controls are critical components in assessing the safety and purity of biologics. These parameters are also important in demonstrating consistency of manufacture from lot to lot. One important step in manufacturing consistency is the demonstration of process validation, which includes the appropriate selection of potency, purity, and identity tests to assure control over the manufacturing process. These tests should be identified early in the product development to ensure that the product is of defined quality and consistency and allows for "bridging" of products and the respective clinical responses induced during all phases of clinical evaluation. Further, all steps taken toward the adoption of a testing procedure, including the rationale, scope, and specifications, should be documented in the BLA.

In general, the manufacturer or sponsor develops manufacturing and control tests; however, there may be involvement of the regulatory agency as well. The CBER is particularly likely to become involved if the product is new or represents a novel problem in testing. As the product moves toward licensure, the sponsor develops the testing program in greater detail. The final testing methods must be established prior to conducting any major clinical trials that are designed to demonstrate efficacy and safety, as well as before production of manufacturing consistency lots. During the prelicensing phase, assay performance is evaluated to determine whether a test under development will be appropriate for lot release of every batch of product.

B. Good Manufacturing Practices

When a potential candidate vaccine is ready to move toward the licensing pathway, two parallel activities take place. The process for manufacturing the vaccine at a research scale must be developed into a process that is appropriate for the manufacture of large-scale clinical material. For example, purification procedures used in the manufacture must be amenable to scale-up and to regulatory approval. Modification of facilities may also be required to accommodate scale-up changes. In addition, facility and process validation must meet the needs of the clinical program and ultimately, the requirements for licensure. Manufacturing, quality (assurance and control), and regulatory input should be incorporated early in the development process to facilitate a more seamless transition from pilot to full-scale production.

To facilitate the transition beyond research scale, one should consult the requirements for current Good Manufacturing Practices (GMP), 21 CFR 211. Good Manufacturing Practices are regulations, guidelines, or advice published by a recognized body (governmental or nongovernmental) outlining minimum manufacturing, quality control, and quality assurance requirements for the preparation of a drug or biological for commercial distribution. Further, they address the manufacturing methods, facilities, controls, packaging, storage, and installations for pharmaceutical operations. Good Manufacturing Practice is that part of Quality Assurance which ensures that products are consistently produced and controlled to the quality standards appropriate to their intended use and as required by marketing authorization. Good Manufacturing Practice encompasses both production and quality control.

Quality Assurance (QA) encompasses all activities necessary to assure and verify confidence in the quality of a process used to manufacture a finished drug or biologic. Quality Assurance is a wide-ranging concept, which covers all matters that individually or collectively influence the quality of a product. It is the sum total of the organized "arrangements" made with the object of ensuring that medicinal products are of the quality required for their intended use. Therefore quality assurance incorporates Good Manufacturing Practice.

Quality Control (QC) involves test and inspection activities employed to determine the level of conformance of an item to its specification. Quality Control is that part of Good Manufacturing Practice which is concerned with sampling, specifications, and testing, and with the organization, documentation and release procedures which ensure that the necessary and relevant tests are actually carried out and that materials are not released for use, nor product released for sale or supply, until their quality has been judged to be satisfactory.

The basic concepts of QA, QC, and GMP are interrelated. Production operations must follow clearly defined procedures. They must comply with the principles of GMP to obtain products of requisite quality. Quality Control is not confined to laboratory operations, but must be involved in all decisions that may concern the quality of the product. The independence of QC from production is considered fundamental to the satisfactory operation of QC.

III. CLINICAL TESTING (INVESTIGATIONAL NEW DRUG PROCESS)

A. Overview of Clinical Evaluation

The clinical development of vaccines is carried out in four phases, as is the case for any drug or biologic (note that the FDA uses Arabic numerals in referring to the different phases). Initial Phase 1 studies are intended to evaluate safety; Phase 2 studies usually include dose-ranging studies that may provide an early indication of efficacy. Phase 1 and 2 studies provide clinical research information that directs the development of the final formulation and dosing schedule to be used in Phase 3. Phase 3 studies provide the pivotal efficacy and safety data that are required for licensure, and are generally large trials conducted in populations that represent the target population for the marketed product. The FDA strongly recommends that clinical trials designed to evaluate the safety, immunogenicity, and efficacy of vaccines be randomized and well controlled, especially in Phase 2 and 3 of clinical development. Choices of control groups and study design, as well as information on "adequate and well-controlled studies" can be found in 21 CFR 314.126. Phase 4 studies are generally large-scale postmarketing studies conducted to obtain additional data on adverse events focusing primarily on events that may occur at a very low frequency.

The clinical development of a product usually starts with a sponsor approaching the FDA for permission to conduct a clinical study with an investigational product through submission of an IND application. The FDA has a maximum of 30 days to review the IND application and determine whether study participants will be exposed to any unacceptable risks. To assist in the assessment of risk to subjects in the clinical study, the IND application must include information on the composition, source, and method of manufacture of the product; the methods used in testing the product's safety, purity, and potency; preclinical studies demonstrating safety and activity; and previous human experience. The focus in this section will be on Phase 1, 2, and 3 clinical trials for vaccines. If the clinical data support the safety and effectiveness of the new vaccine, these results may be submitted in a BLA to support approval for marketing the vaccine in the United States.

B. Phases of Clinical Development

1. Phase 1

Phase 1 vaccine trials are primarily intended to provide a preliminary evaluation of safety and immunogenicity. Initial Phase 1 trials for new vaccines are typically conducted in a small number, e.g., 20, of closely monitored healthy adult volunteers who are at low risk for infection. Additional Phase

1 studies are conducted, as necessary, to provide safety data for evaluating the vaccine in additional populations. Depending on the vaccine and the initial clinical data obtained, pediatric trials may begin after an initial Phase 1 trial in adults. Early clinical development in infants will often have a stepwise progression from older to younger age groups.

The Phase 1 study may include the evaluation of more than one vaccine dose, usually in a stepwise fashion of increasing dose by group. Dose-ranging groups may be studied concurrently or sequentially, depending on factors such as the reactogenicity detected in preclinical models or clinical studies of similar products.

2. Phase 2

Differentiation between a Phase 1 and Phase 2 vaccine trial is not always clear. The objectives of Phase 1 and 2 studies tend to merge together, with the distinction often being the size of the study. Phase 2 trials enroll more subjects, e.g., up to hundreds, and are often randomized and controlled. Evaluation of dose and schedule in a target population may begin in Phase 1 and continue into Phase 2. In general, the objective of Phase 2 vaccine trials is to determine the optimum dose and schedule required to maximize the immune response generated. Moreover, Phase 2 clinical development includes trials designed to provide more definitive immunogenicity data (i.e., more precise estimates of effect) regarding vaccine formulation, dose, schedule, and route of administration. In some cases, Phase 2 data may also provide information regarding specific adverse events that should be more carefully evaluated in a larger Phase 3 trial(s).

When designing the Phase 2 study, there are several considerations that should be incorporated into the study plan to allow for gathering optimal information in preparation of a pivotal Phase 3 study. These considerations include: (1) the evaluation of immune responses in the context of simultaneous administration of the investigational vaccine and already licensed vaccines that would likely be administered concurrently (e.g., during infancy or to travelers); (2) the concurrent administration of vaccines with other products normally expected to be administered simultaneously, e.g., immune globulins and drugs; (3) the development of laboratory assays that may be used for the case definition for an efficacy trial (e.g., serological tests used to distinguish the immune response in study participants elicited by vaccination from that elicited by wild-type infection); (4) immunogenicity (and efficacy) differences between populations that may result from differences in factors such as genetics, nutritional status, background infections, and prior exposure of vaccinees to the infectious agent; (5) background epidemiological data for the disease or infection under study, including seroincidence data; and (6) the determination of geographic strain specificity where appropriate, so that the vaccine will include antigen(s) that will be relevant to the infectious organisms occurring in the intended efficacy trial population.

3. Phase 3

Phase 3 studies enroll large numbers of individuals, and in most cases, include the pivotal efficacy trials as well as expanded safety studies. The FDA highly recommends that plans for Phase 3 studies be discussed with the Agency after Phase 2 data have been obtained and prior to initiation of the Phase 3 study to ensure that studies are adequately designed to meet intended goals, including support of product licensure.

The size and duration of a Phase 3 efficacy trial are determined by many factors, including the incidence of the infectious disease that the study vaccine is intended to prevent and the plans to assess the duration of protection afforded by the study vaccine. A small Phase 3 study may involve hundreds to several thousand participants; a large trial may involve tens of thousands of participants. By the start of Phase 3, there should be data from hundreds of vaccinees for whom detailed observations have been made and rates determined for common, nonserious events. Therefore for subsequent larger trials, a simplified design may be acceptable in which only a subset of subjects in each group is assessed in detail for the more common events while the focus on expanded safety data incorporates active monitoring of all participants to capture less frequent and serious adverse events. Extended follow-up of participants, e.g., following completion of an efficacy trial, may be required as part of a postmarketing commitment and, therefore, advanced planning for such follow-up should be considered.

Phase 3 efficacy studies should be carefully designed to allow a valid estimate of efficacy, and the 95% confidence limits on the efficacy estimate should be considered in calculating sample size [4,5]. In a trial where multiple immunizations may be necessary to attain optimal immune responses, maximum efficacy might not be attained until after the final immunization. Thus the sample size calculation should be adjusted to account for study participants who are lost to follow-up or incompletely immunized. Most efficacy trials employ a double-blind, randomized, and controlled study design. Factors that should be considered in the selection of a control include: (1) no vaccine is licensed for the indication being sought by the study vaccine and thus the use of a placebo is not precluded; (2) no vaccine is licensed for the indication being sought by the study vaccine but another vaccine appropriate for the study population could be used as the control (individuals randomized to the placebo group would receive the benefit of the vaccine utilized as the control); or (3) a vaccine licensed for the indication being sought by the study vaccine exists and should be used in comparison with the experimental vaccine. The FDA has published a guidance to industry that discusses the type of efficacy evidence needed to support licensure [6].

Study designs without a randomized control group, such as case-control studies, have been proposed; however, these designs pose many potential problems with regard to issues such as the comparability of study groups. Historical rather than concurrent randomized controls have also been considered. However, because of the many possible variations in subject baseline characteristics, changing standards of healthcare, and altering epidemiology of disease, historical controls have not usually been acceptable for establishing vaccine efficacy for licensure. Nonrandomized studies have significant limitations for interpreting safety data as well.

A vaccine efficacy trial should have a formally established independent Data Monitoring Committee (DMC) [7].

[The term Data and Safety Monitoring Board (DSMB) is also used to describe this type of committee.] Data Monitoring Committee members should have relevant multidisciplinary representation (e.g., clinicians and biostatisticians with relevant training and experience, bioethicists) and be independent of the sponsor and investigators. If the DMC will conduct a review of the interim data, the following information should be prospectively provided in the protocol: the conditions (e.g., specific schedule, number of events, etc.) that must be met before performing the interim analysis; the criteria for early termination of the study; and a list of the individuals who will have access to the interim data. A statistical plan for any interim analysis should be included with the original submission of the protocol. Any unmasked review of the data, including any review of the data by treatment group (regardless of whether the identity of the treatment is revealed) would be considered an interim analysis [8–13].

C. Use of Serological Endpoints to Support Efficacy

Evidence of safety and efficacy must be available prior to the licensing of any product. For new vaccines, efficacy is usually assessed in trials designed to demonstrate prevention of the targeted infectious disease, as discussed above. However, serological endpoints may be adequate to substantiate effectiveness for the purpose of licensure when a previously accepted correlation between such serological endpoints and clinical effectiveness already exists [see discussion in 21 CFR 601.25(d)(2)]. A serological correlate of protection for vaccine efficacy may be identified from a prior successful clinical efficacy trial with clinical disease endpoints, or may be inferred from sources such as population-based studies of immunized persons. Detailed information about each assay intended to assess immune response should be provided to the IND *in advance* of using the assay.

Evaluation of the validity of serological endpoints for a particular setting frequently includes assessments of both functional antibody levels and quantitative antibody levels, often by enzyme-linked immunosorbent assay (ELISA). The relevance of the ELISA antibody levels may depend on correlation with the functional antibody levels, especially for situations in which the strongest link to efficacy is the functional antibody levels. In some instances, such a serological correlate of protection may provide adequate efficacy data to support licensure of a new vaccine, e.g., a new tetanus and diphtheria vaccine. Serological endpoints have also been used to provide the efficacy data for new combination vaccines with components consisting of previously licensed products and/or antigens with efficacy already demonstrated in clinical trials. Extensive discussions of the clinical studies used to support licensure of combination vaccines are available [4,5,14].

IV. LICENSING REQUIREMENTS (REVIEW AND APPROVAL PROCESS)

Once all three phases of clinical development are successfully completed, a biologics license application (BLA) may be submitted to the FDA for review. To be considered, the license application must provide the multidisciplinary FDA reviewer team (medical officers, microbiologists, chemists, biostatisticians, etc.) with complete manufacturing and testing information, as well as efficacy and safety data. This information is necessary to make a risk/benefit assessment that results in a determination to recommend or reject the licensure of a vaccine. The CBER has published a guidance document for vaccine manufacturers that provides an overview of the chemistry, manufacturing, and control information that should be submitted in a BLA [15]. Vaccine approval also requires the provision of adequate product labeling to allow healthcare providers to understand the vaccine's proper use and indications, including its potential benefits and risks, to communicate with patients and parents, and to safely deliver the vaccine to the public. In addition, the proposed manufacturing facility undergoes a prelicensing inspection by CBER product and facility experts. During this inspection, the entire production process is reviewed in detail along with a review of all production equipment, utility systems, personnel, and batch records.

A. FDA Advisory Committee Deliberations

Prior to licensure of a new vaccine or the approval of a significant new indication for a currently licensed vaccine, the FDA will often request manufacturers to present their data to the Vaccines and Related Biological Products Advisory Committee (VRBPAC). This expert committee, which consists of non-FDA scientists, physicians, biostatisticians, and a consumer representative, provides advice to the Agency regarding the production, testing, safety, and efficacy of the vaccine for a proposed indication.

The FDA staff formulates relevant questions for the Committee and may also make presentations at the meeting. Consultation by the VRBPAC or other appropriate FDA advisory committees is not limited to the immediate prelicensure stage; clinical data and questions, as well as related preclinical issues, may be referred to an FDA advisory committees *at any time* during drug development. Review of transcripts from previous related advisory committee meetings may be informative to sponsors, and can be obtained from the CBER Freedom of Information (FOI) staff. Recent committee transcripts and documents may also be available on CBER's WWW site. Sponsors should review CBER guidance with regard to submitting materials for advisory committee meetings, especially with regard to due dates [16].

B. Postlicensure Activities

The FDA continues to oversee the production and performance of vaccines after licensure to ensure continuing safety and efficacy of the vaccine. After licensure, monitoring of the product and of production activities, including periodic facility inspections, continues as long as the manufacturer holds a license for the product. If requested by the FDA, manufacturers are required to submit to the FDA the results of their own tests for potency, safety, and purity for each vaccine lot. They may also be required to submit samples of each vaccine lot to the FDA for testing. However, if the sponsor requests an alternative procedure that provides continued assurance of safety, purity, and potency, the CBER may determine that routine submission of lot release protocols (showing results of applicable tests) and samples is not necessary.

Until a vaccine is given to a large population, all potential adverse events cannot be anticipated and therefore, CBER uses both active and passive methods for assessing safety. One method for expanding safety information is by conducting Phase 4 studies, i.e., formal studies on a vaccine once it is on the market. For any new approval (BLA or BLA supplement), manufacturers may be asked to perform specific postmarketing studies, for example, to provide additional assessments of less common or rare adverse events or to further assess the duration of vaccine-induced protection. The CBER's Office of Vaccines Research and Review usually requests that such protocol(s) be provided for FDA review and comment prior to application approval. As required by 506B of the FDAMA, in 2001, regulations went into effect that add requirements to submit status reports for certain postmarketing studies, i.e., studies in the areas of clinical safety, efficacy, and pharmacokinetic and nonclinical toxicology [17].

V. REGULATORY CHALLENGES WITH NEW VACCINE APPROACHES

The framework and guidances provided for regulation of vaccines are often "challenged" with the development of novel vaccine approaches. The following select examples of novel technologies will underscore the challenges facing vaccine developers and regulators alike in establishing testing methods that achieve the goals of demonstrating purity, potency, and safety.

A. Vectored Vaccines

The advances in molecular biology and the genomic revolution in organism sequencing has allowed for the generation of highly targeted vaccine approaches using a number of delivery mechanisms. Use of live replicating bacterial organisms such as *Bacillus* Calmette-Guerin (BCG) or *Salmonella* to express foreign genes has been the focus of much effort over the past few years [18]. The approach of using vectored vaccines to deliver antigens is of interest because this approach may allow for expression of antigens that could stimulate mucosal immunity or allow for a more persistent gene expression. The advances in genomics and immunology have allowed for the identification of gene sequences that may be important in providing protection from disease and critical elements involved in mounting both humoral and cellular responses.

When considering such an approach, early discussion with the FDA regarding manufacturing and testing, as well as clinical development, is recommended. For example, if the vectored vaccine contains sequences for generating a cell-mediated immune (CMI) response, the development of an appropriate potency test for the vectored vaccine should include an evaluation of the ability of the vaccine to induce such a response. Also, the sophistication of molecular biol-

ogy allows for creating vaccines expressing multiple antigens in the form of polypeptide sequences for generating cytotoxic lymphocyte responses or for generating responses to multiple serotypes/subgroups of the organisms. In this case, the product development and testing will need to address the control and release testing for detection of each of these epitopes. Of note, the preclinical safety testing of vectored vaccines eliciting humoral and/or CMI responses should be carefully addressed to ensure that the toxicity study is adequate to evaluate the possible direct and indirect toxicity of constitutive expression of transgenes and the possible generation of tissue cross-reactive immune responses. Additional testing to evaluate the persistence of the vectored vaccine and stability of the construct expression should also be addressed using an appropriate animal model. The choice of the animal model and design of such studies will require frequent and detailed discussions with the FDA.

Vectored vaccines may also pose a challenge with regard to the clinical development path. The example of a BCG-vectored HIV vaccine expressing neutralizing antibody and cell-mediated immune response epitopes illustrates several of the challenges facing this vaccine approach. Several aspects of developing such a vaccine were discussed at a World Health Organization (WHO) workshop [18]. One major area of concern identified was the need to establish appropriate assay methodologies to measure the immune response to both the humoral and cellular components of the vaccine. The clinical development path should include early discussions and efforts in establishing appropriate assays for measuring immune responses generated during the clinical study. Robust assays to measure clinical parameters that could reflect protection were viewed as essential prior to Phase 3 field trials.

Vectored vaccines can also present challenges as to the determination of an appropriate study design and illustrate the complexity of evaluating these vaccines clinically. For example, the BCG-vectored HIV vaccine may be viewed as a combination vaccine where the vaccine may impact disease conditions caused by more than one organism. In this case, the combination vaccine may include a preventive vaccine for tuberculosis and HIV. Guidance on the regulatory framework for evaluating combination vaccines [4–6,19] should be considered. Using a vaccine with proven efficacy or previously licensed as a vector poses a challenge to regulatory agencies. In the case of a recombinant BCG product, the issue of how to design a study to demonstrate that there is no negative effect on the efficacy of the BCG component may be difficult to address. The demonstration of bridging efficacy of the recombinant BCG back to the parental strain will require extensive discussions with the FDA. As with many combination vaccines, critical issues in clinical development are the ability to demonstrate no adverse effects on safety, immunogenicity, or efficacy of the parental individual vaccine components [19,20].

B. Plant-Based Vaccine Development

Another exciting new approach is plant-based vaccines. Recent advances in plant technology have allowed for the expression and correct processing of viral epitopes and bacterial toxin subunit proteins [21,22]. Plant-based approaches take advantage of the recent advances in genomics and understanding of plant biology, and offer the advantages of being relatively inexpensive to produce and store, easy to scale-up for mass production and allows for versatility of delivery [22,23]. Plant-based technology can be either the use of the plant as a "bioreactor" for the production and subsequent purification of proteins or as a production or "delivery" system. In this latter case, the vaccine is usually delivered as an edible product. The focus of this section will be on edible vaccines and the complexity of product development.

The use of plant-based technologies poses a challenge to the appropriate application of the regulatory framework for assessing vaccine safety, purity, and potency. With regard to manufacturing and testing, the questions of how to determine potency and consistency of manufacture are difficult to answer. Depending on the plant delivery system used, the purification of the expressed protein from the plant may be possible and allow for an assessment of potency based on quantity of gene expression extracted from a fixed amount of starting material [23]. Even if this approach is used, it is still difficult to assess the consistency of expression from plant to plant. The evaluation of gene expression on an individual plant basis is difficult and therefore also makes the determination of manufacturing consistency difficult to demonstrate. Also, agricultural facilities that produce plant-derived biologics provoke interesting discussions as to the requirements for manufacturing under conditions consistent with cGMP. A number of issues relative to the plant propagation should be considered and addressed as early as possible with the FDA. For example, discussion such as the containment of the transgenic plants to prevent possible spread of the transgenes to other plants; the use of pesticides/herbicides in the growth and as contaminants in the product; the water and soil conditions used in the propagation of the plant; and the evaluation of contaminating organisms or toxins in the product are critical to address early on with FDA and may require additional consults with other Federal agencies such as the United States Department of Agriculture (USDA) or the Environmental Protection Agency (EPA).

As with "traditional" vaccine production, the product developer using this approach should devise ways to establish and characterize master and working seed stocks and address the storage and stability of the seed stocks to be maintained over time in storage. As a part of characterization of the seed stocks, the genetic and product stability should be examined.

The use of plant-based technologies also involves additional safety concerns that are unique to this novel approach. For example, the use of plant-derived materials raises the concern that plant toxins may be present. The absence of such toxins should be determined as part of the characterization and selection of seed stocks and expression systems. In addition, the oral delivery of vaccines in plants raises the issue of whether such a delivery system would result in the generation of immune tolerance. If possible, these unique concerns should be addressed using appropriate animal models, if available, and be carefully examined in the clinical setting as part of clinical safety monitoring or follow-up.

In summary, the expanded application of molecular biology and genomics in vaccine technology has raised the possibility of creating novel genetically engineered organisms and plants whose mode of delivery involve novel routes of administration and immune stimulation mechanisms. With these advances in science come the challenges of how to best manufacture, test, and regulate these novel products. As these approaches move forward, it is essential that vaccine developers and the FDA enter into frequent discussions on the appropriateness of product and clinical testing.

ACKNOWLEDGMENTS

The authors wish to thank Ms. Linda Rosendorf and Karen Chaitkin for their thoughtful review of the manuscript. We would also like to thank Dr. Karen Goldenthal for her contributions to the clinical section of this manuscript.

This chapter reflects the authors' assessment of the approach to clinical trials and product development for preventive vaccines and is not intended to represent the official position of the FDA or the NIH.

REFERENCES

1. Public Health Service Act, Chapter 373, Title III, section 352.58, Stat 702, currently codified at 42 U.S.C. Section 262, 1 July 1944. Washington DC: U.S. Government Printing Office.
2. U.S. Code of Federal Regulations. Title 21, Part 600. Washington DC: U.S. Government Printing Office, 2000.
3. Falk LA, et al. Manufacturing issues with combining different antigens: a regulatory perspective. Clin Infect Dis 2001; 33(suppl 4):S351–S355.
4. U.S. Food and Drug Administration, Center for Biologics Evaluation and Research. Guidance for Industry for the Evaluation of Combination Vaccines for Preventable Diseases: Production, Testing and Clinical Studies (1997). [To obtain this document, connect to http://www.fda.gov/cber/guidelines.htm or call the Office of Communication, Training and Manufacturers Assistance at 1-800-835-4709.]
5. Goldenthal KL, et al. Prelicensure evaluation of combination vaccines. Clin Infect Dis 2001; 33(suppl 4):S267–S273.
6. U.S. Food and Drug Administration. Guidance for Industry—Providing Clinical Evidence of Effectiveness for Human Drug and Biological Products. 1997. [To obtain this document, connect to http://www.fda.gov/cber/guidelines.htm or call the Office of Communication, Training and Manufacturers Assistance at 1-800-835-4709.]
7. Food and Drug Administration. Draft Guidance for Clinical Trial Sponsors On the Establishment and Operation of Clinical Trial Data Monitoring Committees (2001). [To obtain this document, connect to http://www.fda.gov/cber/guidelines.htm or call the Office of Communication, Training and Manufacturers Assistance at 1-800-835-4709.]
8. O'Brien PC, Fleming TR. A multiple testing procedure for clinical trials. Biometrics 1979; 35:549–556.
9. Geller NL, Pocock SJ. Interim analyses in randomized clinical trials: ramifications and guidelines for practitioners. Biometrics 1987; 43:213–223.
10. Fleming TR. Design considerations for clinical trials. In: Kimura K, et al, ed. Cancer Chemotherapy: Challenges for the Future. Vol. 3. Tokyo: Excerpta Medica, 1988.
11. Emerson SS, Fleming TR. Interim analyses in clinical trials. Oncology 1990; 4:126–133.

12. Center for Drug Evaluation and Research/FDA, "Guideline for the Format and Content of the Clinical and Statistical Sections of an Application." July 1988. (Note: This 125-page guideline was prepared for drug approvals, but is still useful reading because many of the format, content, and statistical aspects of preparing a protocol, and collecting, analyzing, and presenting data are, in principle, very similar for drugs and biological products.)

13. Proceedings of "Practical Issues in Data Monitoring of Clinical Trials" meeting on 27–28 January 1992. Stat Med 1993; 12:419–616.

14. Horne AD, et al. Analysis of studies to evaluate immune response to combination vaccines. Clin Infect Dis 2001; 33(suppl 4):S306–S311.

15. U.S. Food and Drug Administration, Center for Biologics Evaluation and Research. Guidance for Industry: Content and Format of Chemistry, Manufacturing and Controls Information and Establishment Description Information for a Vaccine or Related Product. 1999. [To obtain this document, connect to http://www.fda.gov/cber/guidelines.htm or call the Office of Communication, Training and Manufacturers Assistance at 1-800-835-4709.]

16. U.S. Food and Drug Administration, Center for Biologics Evaluation and Research. Draft Guidance for Industry: Disclosing Information Provided to Advisory Committees in Connection with Open Advisory Committee Meetings Related to the Testing or Approval of Biologic Products and Convened by the Center for Biologics Evaluation and Research (2001). [To obtain this document, connect to http://www.fda.gov/cber/guidelines.htm or call the Office of Communication, Training and Manufacturers Assistance at 1-800-835-4709.]

17. Food and Drug Administration. Postmarketing Studies for Approved Human Drugs and Licensed Biologicals Products: Status reports. Federal Register 2000; 65:64607–64616.

18. Falk LA, et al. Recombinant Bacillus Calmette–Guerin as a potential vector for preventive HIV Type 1 vaccines. AIDS Res Hum Retrovir 2000; 16:91–98.

19. Falk LA, et al. Testing and licensure of combination vaccines for the prevention of infectious diseases. In: Ellis RW, ed. Combination Vaccines: Development, Clinical Research and Approval. Totowa: Humana Press Inc., 1999:233–248.

20. Falk LA, Ball LK. Current status and future trends in vaccine regulation—USA. Vaccine 2001; 19:1567–1572.

21. Belanger H, et al. Human respiratory syncytial virus vaccine antigen produced in plants. FASEB J 2000; 14:2323–2328.

22. Streatfield SJ, et al. Plant-based vaccines: unique advantages. Vaccine 2001; 19:2741–2748.

23. Daniell H, et al. Trends Plant Sci 2001; 6:219–226.

12
Developing Safe Vaccines

Leslie K. Ball
Office for Human Research Protections, Department of Health and Human Services, Rockville, Maryland, U.S.A.

Robert Ball
Center for Biologics Evaluation and Research, Food and Drug Administration, Rockville, Maryland, U.S.A.

Bruce G. Gellin
Vanderbilt University School of Medicine, Nashville, Tennessee, U.S.A.

*There is no insurance without a premium. Our business is to provide a greater and more comprehensive insurance and to diminish the size of the premium.**

I. INTRODUCTION

The tremendous benefits of immunization in reducing the morbidity and mortality of infectious diseases are well recognized, both from a public health perspective as well as from an individual perspective. Widespread use of vaccines in the past century has led to improved control of many infectious diseases including diphtheria, pertussis, and measles, and eradication or near eradication of diseases, i.e., smallpox and polio [1]. However, this public health triumph comes with the implicit understanding that effective health interventions such as immunizations are not completely free of risk. Vaccines are held to the highest standards of safety because they are usually given to healthy individuals (often children) to prevent an infectious disease to which they might be exposed in the future rather than treat an established disease or condition. Yet vaccines, like all pharmaceutical products, can have adverse effects ranging from transient common local reactions to rare but serious and irreversible events. Successful immunization strategies incorporate rigorous scientific assessments to ensure the safety of vaccines both pre- and postlicensure, and effectively communicate the benefits and risks to the public.

In this chapter, which will primarily focus on preventive vaccines for infectious disease indications, we present a practical approach for planning the safety evaluation of new vaccines by offering a framework for integrating safety into vaccine development. We develop the rationale for this framework by reviewing lessons learned from historical events and recent controversies, examining scientific methods for evaluating the safety of vaccines, and applying principles of risk management and risk communication to immunization safety.

II. EVOLUTION OF THE VACCINE SAFETY SYSTEM IN THE UNITED STATES

A. Past Experiences

Concerns over the safety of vaccines can affect public acceptance of immunizations, with consequent increases in rates of infectious diseases, as has been described in countries where whole-cell pertussis-containing vaccines were abandoned because of the alleged association with encephalopathy [2]. While vaccine safety controversies have sometimes garnered public and media attention on the basis of limited scientific information, significant advances have resulted from lessons learned when real vaccine safety problems emerged.

1. Immunization Against Smallpox: Variolation and Vaccination

The recognition that immunizations can cause adverse effects dates back several centuries, to the practice of "variolation," or the controlled inoculation of healthy individu-

---

* Sir Graham Wilson. The Hazards of Immunization. The Athlone Press, London; 1967.
The views represented here are those of the authors and not intended to represent those of their respective organizations.

als with infectious material obtained from individuals suffering from smallpox (Variola major) or previously inoculated with smallpox (Figure 1). When this practice was introduced in England from the Orient during the eighteenth century, it was observed that those inoculated occasionally developed disseminated lesions and even fatal smallpox infections. Mortality of variolated individuals was reported at rates of 1 in 50 during the earlier years of the practice to 1 in 2800 during the 1760s [3].

Jenner's smallpox vaccine, developed in 1796 from cowpox (Vaccinia virus) lesions, was associated with fewer serious reactions. Despite the improved safety profile, opposition to vaccination arose shortly thereafter, coalescing into organized resistance after an 1867 British law mandated smallpox vaccination [4]. Similar political opposition was seen in the United States when a compulsory vaccination program was initiated in response to a smallpox epidemic in 1901–1903 in Boston [5]. Those opposed to vaccination questioned the safety and efficacy of smallpox vaccination, and argued for individual liberty, i.e., the right to decide whether to be vaccinated. The debate against mandatory vaccination in Boston resulted in a landmark case, *Jacobson v. Massachusetts*, decided by the U.S. Supreme Court in 1905, which ruled that the state could pass laws mandating vaccination to protect the public from dangerous communicable diseases [5]. This intersection of individual rights with public health policy has resurfaced in subsequent immunization debates such as state mandates for routine childhood immunizations [6].

2. Bacterial Contamination of Biological Products

Several unfortunate episodes documented the critical importance of quality control, both in the manufacturing of vaccines and in their handling at the time of administration. As demand increased for vaccines and antitoxins, new processes were needed to increase the supply. The recognition that person-to-person inoculation as described above could transmit infectious diseases such as syphilis provided impetus for the commercial production of smallpox vaccine on "vaccine farms" where Vaccinia virus was propagated on the skin of cows [7]. But the production of biological products remained unregulated, and the lack of adequate quality control measures led to inevitable mishaps. In St.

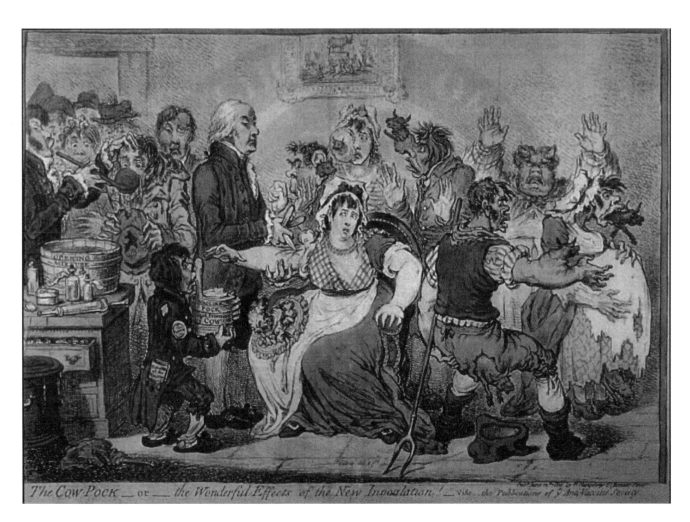

Figure 1 "The Cow Pock—or—the Wonderful Effects of the New Inoculation!" (From the Publications of the Anti-Vaccine Society/J. Gillray, 1802.)

Louis in 1901, 20 children became ill and 14 died following receipt of an equine diphtheria antitoxin contaminated with tetanus toxin. This event led to the passage of the Biologics Control Act of 1902 (The Virus, Serum, and Toxin Law), which contained several notable provisions, including license requirements for biological products and their manufacturing facilities, authority to conduct unannounced inspections, the requirement for accurate product labels, and penalties for noncompliance including revocation of license [8]. In 1928, 12 children died of staphylococcal sepsis in Queensland, Australia, following contamination of a multidose container of diphtheria toxin–antitoxin mixture, prompting the investigating committee to recommend that biological products should not be formulated in containers for multiple use unless a sufficient concentration of antiseptic was added to inhibit microbial growth [9].

3. Viral Contamination of Yellow Fever Vaccine

The need for careful quality control of all materials used in the manufacturing process was demonstrated when an investigational yellow fever vaccine was implicated as the cause of an estimated 50,000 cases of jaundice observed in 2 to 2.5 million U.S. soldiers immunized in 1942, with a case fatality rate of 2–3 per 1000. Investigation at the time pinpointed the cause as contamination of the human serum used as a stabilizing agent; serological testing decades later confirmed the etiology as hepatitis B [10–12]. Removing human serum from the manufacture of yellow fever vaccine halted the outbreak.

4. The Cutter Incident

Perhaps one of the most widely publicized problems with quality control was the so-called "Cutter Incident." Rapid scale-up of inactivated polio vaccine (IPV) production was required to meet projected demand for IPV during the initial U.S. polio immunization campaign, following public announcement of the results of the Francis Field Trial in 1955. Following observations of a temporal association between receipt of IPV and cases of paralytic polio, a meticulous epidemiological evaluation traced the source to certain lots of the Cutter vaccine in which scaled-up production resulted in aggregates of poliovirus incompletely inactivated by formalin. Affected lots were associated with 60 cases of paralytic polio in vaccine recipients, and 89 cases in family contacts [13]. This incident highlighted the importance of quality control for every change in the manufacturing process and careful epidemiological assessment to evaluate the association between a vaccine and an adverse event.

5. Vaccine-Associated Paralytic Polio

The critical role of epidemiological evaluation of very rare adverse events was further highlighted in the painstaking investigation that connected oral polio vaccine with the rare occurrence of paralytic poliomyelitis. In 1964, the Public Health Service commissioned a special advisory committee that met at the Communicable Diseases Center, now known as the Centers for Disease Control and Prevention (CDC), to evaluate whether a small number of cases of paralytic polio

observed in vaccinated individuals living in nonepidemic areas could be attributed to receipt of oral polio vaccine (OPV). Because no laboratory techniques were available at that time to distinguish vaccine from wild-type polio strains, the committee relied on epidemiological surveillance data between 1962 and 1964. While the committee acknowledged that the current state of the art of virology was unable to determine whether any individual case of paralysis could be directly attributed to the vaccine, they concluded that epidemiological evidence pointed to a causal link with OPV for at least some of the 57 cases deemed "compatible" or possibly because of vaccination [14]. The committee estimated the incidence of vaccine-associated paralytic polio to be 1 in 6 million doses for type 1, 1 in 2.5 million doses for type 3, and 1 in 50 million doses for type 2, but concluded that the benefits of routine immunization with OPV relative to the risks of naturally occurring disease outweighed the potential rare risk of paralytic polio following OPV [14]. That the committee's epidemiological assessment has been supported by subsequent laboratory data linking vaccine-associated cases with OPV strains [15] underscores the value of integrating surveillance data, clinical information, and scientific methods in the evaluation of adverse events.

6. Formalin-Inactivated Respiratory Syncytial Virus and Measles Vaccines

Adverse events following immunization have occurred in unpredictable ways. Examples include an enhanced lower respiratory illness observed in naive infant recipients of an investigational formalin-inactivated respiratory syncytial virus (RSV) vaccine following exposure to natural RSV disease [16,17]; and an atypical and often more severe clinical presentation of measles in individuals who had received a licensed inactivated measles vaccine and were subsequently exposed to wild measles virus, sometimes many years following immunization [18–20]. The condition of atypical measles has all but disappeared in the United States following the elimination of endemic measles disease and reliance on the live attenuated measles vaccine. However, the early experience with formalin-inactivated RSV vaccine has continued to hamper RSV vaccine development, due, at least in part, to limited understanding of enhanced RSV disease pathogenesis [21]. These experiences reinforced the need for improved laboratory methods evaluating adverse event immunopathology, careful monitoring for adverse events during clinical studies, the importance of maintaining an index of suspicion for events that may occur years following immunization, and introduced the potential for "enhanced" disease as an adverse event following vaccination.

7. Expert Panel Reviews of Vaccine Efficacy and Safety

In 1972, responsibility for regulating biological products in the United States was transferred from the National Institutes of Health (NIH) to the Food and Drug Administration (FDA). At that time, many biological products had been licensed and in widespread use for decades; however, some products lacked adequate documentation of efficacy and safety, in light of evolving standards for quality control and clinical trial design. In 1973, the FDA commissioned a series of panels consisting of outside experts to evaluate available data on safety and efficacy of licensed vaccines. For example, the panel review of bacterial vaccines and toxoids did not find evidence that any licensed vaccines were unsafe, but did find that several products lacked sufficient evidence to make a determination [22]. Many products so classified had not been produced or marketed in decades. Faced with having to provide additional data on manufacturing processes or from clinical trials, several manufacturers requested their licenses be voluntarily revoked [22]. While this review did result in a winnowing of the number vaccine manufacturers and vaccines licensed in the United States, the net effect was to ensure that all U.S. licensed vaccines met applicable standards at the time of review for quality control of manufacturing and clinical demonstration of safety and efficacy.

8. Pertussis Vaccine Controversy and the National Childhood Vaccine Injury Act

The political leverage of advocacy groups has affected a wide range of immunization activities, from vaccine research and development to immunization delivery, yet has been most profound regarding issues of vaccine safety, highlighting the fragile interrelationship among vaccine supply, coverage rates, and public confidence and acceptance of vaccines. This became vividly apparent during the 1970s and 1980s, when concerns were raised over a possible association between diphtheria and tetanus toxoids and whole-cell pertussis vaccines (DTP) with encephalopathy, first in Japan and Europe and later in the United States [23,24]. A consumer advocacy group, Dissatisfied Parents Together (DPT), was established in the United States [25], spurring public debate on this issue. Increased litigation against vaccine manufacturers led some to withdraw from the marketplace, further reducing the number of manufacturers, and prompting the CDC to stockpile vaccines in the event of critical shortages.

In response, a coalition of health professional organizations, consumer advocacy groups, and others pressed for the passage of the National Childhood Vaccine Injury Act of 1986 [26, as amended 1989]. The Act created the Vaccine Injury Compensation Program (VICP) and called for a unified national reporting system for vaccine-associated adverse events leading to the creation of the Vaccine Adverse Event Reporting System (VAERS), mandated comprehensive reviews of vaccine-related adverse events by the Institute of Medicine (IOM), provided for improved record keeping of vaccine administration, and mandated the development and distribution of vaccine information materials. Responding to the legislative mandate under the Act for comprehensive reviews of vaccine safety, the IOM performed extensive reviews in 1991 (pertussis and rubella vaccines) [24] and 1994 (diphtheria and tetanus toxoids, measles and mumps, polio, hepatitis B, and *Haemophilus influenzae* type b vaccines) [27]. Of note, the IOM concluded that there was either no evidence or there is insufficient evidence to establish a causal relationship for approximately two-thirds of the conditions studied, highlighting areas needing further research.

9. Shift in Benefit–Risk Assessment

The U.S. whole-cell pertussis vaccine controversy of the 1980s also focused attention and resources on development and use of vaccines with improved safety profiles, such as the acellular pertussis and enhanced inactivated polio vaccines. The widespread use of vaccines has led to dramatic decline in the incidence of infectious diseases and simultaneously dimmed the public's collective memory of the contagiousness, severity, and long-term sequelae of many infections that were once common in childhood. Consequently, a shift has occurred in the benefit-to-risk ratio of vaccines, both actual (i.e., the true risk of an individual experiencing a vaccine-preventable disease has declined) and perceived (i.e., the individual no longer views the disease as a threat), resulting in diminished acceptance of adverse effects, even those rarely occurring. Recognition of the improved local and systemic reactogenicity profile of acellular pertussis vaccines led U.S. immunization advisory bodies to replace whole-cell pertussis vaccines in the recommended schedule [28,29]. Similarly, the occurrence of eight to nine cases a year of paralytic polio in the United States associated with use of OPV, coupled with certification of polio eradication in the western hemisphere by the World Health Organization (WHO) in 1994, prompted the ACIP to recommend first a sequential IPV/OPV schedule [30], and later an IPV-only schedule [29].

B. Recent Events

1. Rhesus Rotavirus Vaccine and Intussusception

The recent experience with RRV in the U.S. illustrates the methodological difficulties in detecting rare adverse events and the public policy dilemma of balancing a vaccine's benefits with an infrequent but potentially life-threatening risk. Intussusception, or telescoping of the bowel causing acute obstruction, is a rare condition often of unknown etiology that occurs in infants. This condition was observed during prelicensure clinical studies in 5 of 10,054 infants receiving RRV (0.05%) and 1 of 4633 receiving placebo (0.02%), with the difference in RRV recipients versus controls not statistically significant ($P > 0.45$) [31]. Analysis of surveillance data did not suggest an association between wild-type rotavirus vaccine and this adverse event, and thus did not provide support for a biological mechanism [30]. However, the finding of intussusception in RRV recipients during prelicensure studies was noted in the product label, without attributing causality to the vaccine. Following U.S. licensure, reports to VAERS of intussusception following RRV led to the temporary suspension of vaccine use [32] and triggered epidemiological investigations including case-control/case-series [33] and retrospective cohort [34] studies. Analyses of these studies showed the association between RRV and intussusception to be strong, temporal, and specific, with the attributable risk estimated to be approximately 1 in 11,000 vaccine recipients [34].

Given strong evidence of an association (albeit rare), the potentially life-threatening nature of intussusception, and limited mortality due to rotavirus disease in the United States, the ACIP rescinded its recommendation for RRV in October 1999, and the manufacturer withdrew the vaccine from the market and ceased production [35]. The benefit–risk assessment for rotavirus vaccines is considerably different in developing countries, where the incidence of rotavirus infection is comparable to the United States but results in significantly higher morbidity and mortality. However, the U.S. risk management decision regarding RRV has had worldwide ramifications, with other countries reluctant to use a product withdrawn from the U.S. market [36]. Developers of new candidate rotavirus vaccines already in clinical studies have had to carefully consider what level of clinical safety data would be required for licensure, in light of the rarity of intussusception and the lack of an animal model to aid preclinical testing. As a consequence, clinical trials designed for a more robust assessment of rare adverse events are likely to be substantially larger and more costly than the prelicensure trials of RRV.

2. Immunization and Chronic Conditions

Alleged links between immunizations and chronic conditions such as MMR (measles, mumps, and rubella) vaccine and autism [37,38], thimerosal (used as a preservative in some vaccines) and various neurodevelopmental disorders including autism [39], the OspA Lyme vaccine and rheumatoid arthritis [40], immunizations and insulin-dependent diabetes [41], hepatitis B vaccine and multiple sclerosis [42], and the "antigen overload" hypothesis [43] have provided additional challenges in assessing the safety of vaccines. Assessment of a causal association between immunization and chronic conditions is complicated by the multifactorial etiology of many of these illnesses, the often imprecise onset of symptoms, and the difficulty of proving a negative (i.e., that the adverse event is not caused by the vaccine). However, such vaccine safety concerns may have an impact on vaccine acceptance and use, as illustrated by declines in MMR uptake in Great Britain [44] and the decision by the manufacturer of the U.S. licensed Lyme vaccine to cease production and distribution [45]. The complexity of these issues points to the need for a comprehensive and systematic approach to evaluate data on vaccine safety, which is to be discussed later in this chapter.

3. Vaccine Supply, Quality Control, and Liability

Recent vaccine shortages in the United States have highlighted the precarious interrelationship between vaccine supply, quality control requirements, and liability concerns. Inadequate supplies to meet the high demand for influenza, tetanus and diphtheria toxoid, pneumococcal conjugate, MMR, and other vaccines have forced immunization advisory bodies such as the ACIP and the American Academy of Pediatrics (AAP) Committee on Infectious Diseases to develop interim recommendations for a number of vaccines in response to shortages [46–50]. No single explanation appears to explain the insufficient supply of multiple vaccines from different manufacturers, but vaccine safety issues may play a role. Frequently cited reasons for the reluctance of pharmaceutical manufacturers to develop and market vaccines include the complexity of vaccine manufacturing procedures, liability concerns due to vaccine adverse events, and

small profit margins for vaccines compared with other pharmaceutical products [51]. As previously cited examples have illustrated, controlling manufacturing processes is an essential element of vaccine production. The need to overhaul production facilities to meet current good manufacturing practices (cGMP) and the difficulty in predicting demand for newly licensed vaccines, which depends in part on perceived safety, are additional factors mentioned for shortages of some vaccines [51]. The net result is little redundancy in vaccine supply, so a shortage of one product can have a ripple effect on the entire U.S. immunization program.

4. Vaccines and Biological Terrorism

The benefit–risk assessment for immunizations is not a fixed entity, as has been demonstrated by renewed interest in smallpox and anthrax vaccines generated by terrorist attacks on September 11, 2001, and the mailing of letters containing anthrax spores to public officials and media representatives [52]. Routine smallpox vaccination ended in the United States in 1972 when the pending global eradication of smallpox had essentially reduced the threat of smallpox in the United States to zero. In this setting, the risks of the vaccine—rare serious reactions such as encephalitis and eczema vaccinatum, which caused approximately seven to nine deaths per year—greatly outweighed the risks of the disease [53,54]. In recent years, a mandatory anthrax vaccination program by the U.S. military met with resistance by some military members concerned with the safety of the vaccine [55]. However, a thorough review of anthrax vaccine's safety profile [56], coupled with recognition of the benefits of immunization that have become more visible in light of recent terrorist activities, may shift perceptions and acceptance of this vaccine. At the same time, there are renewed efforts to develop new and safer vaccines against smallpox, anthrax, and other potential threats of bioterrorism [57,58].

III. SCIENTIFIC METHODOLOGY FOR DETERMINING VACCINE SAFETY

Establishing the safety of a particular vaccine requires a multiprong approach: preclinical research and testing, clinical studies, and postlicensure assessments including epidemiologic evaluations. Responsibility for evaluating vaccine safety begins with vaccine researchers and/or manufacturers, and later extends to regulatory authorities, other government and international agencies, immunization advisory bodies, and others. Much attention has been devoted to immunization safety efforts in the last decade in the United States and worldwide. The WHO with its vital role in worldwide immunization programs has made immunization safety, from quality control to vaccine delivery and effective response to vaccine safety concerns, a global priority [59,60]. The International Conference on Harmonization (ICH), a collaborative effort of regulatory authorities and pharmaceutical companies in Europe, Japan, and the United States, to harmonize requirements for registering pharmaceutical products, has developed recommendations on a range of preclinical, clinical, and postlicensure safety evaluations [61]. The role of the FDA for vaccine development is discussed elsewhere in this volume [Baylor, Falk, Midthun, this volume]. This section will review the scientific methodology underlying vaccine development as it pertains to safety.

In evaluating a vaccine's safety, it is important to recognize that safety is not an "all or nothing" phenomenon. This is acknowledged in the FDA definition of safety; that is, "the relative freedom from harmful effect to persons affected directly or indirectly by a product when prudently administered, taking into consideration the character of the product in relation to the condition of the recipient at the time [62]." Thus the property of safety is *relative* and *relational*; it depends upon the benefit–risk assessment at a particular point in time, the specific indication, and the intended recipient or population.

A. Laboratory Methods

The diversity of biological products necessitates some individualization of the preclinical evaluation; however, certain general principles should be kept in mind. Prior to introduction of an investigational vaccine in human volunteers, the investigator should provide evidence supporting the scientific rationale for a vaccine candidate (e.g., immunogenicity), data demonstrating the quality of the product, and preclinical safety information on the vaccine.

The development of appropriate animal models may be useful in evaluating disease pathogenesis, immune response, toxicity, and in some cases, efficacy against challenge with the infectious disease that the vaccine is intended to prevent. Product quality is assessed by evaluating the manufacturing process, the materials used during production, and the final product. Specific descriptions of the manufacturing process, documentation of the source and quality of the materials used in manufacture, and in-process testing help to characterize the safety of the product [63]. In addition, ICH has developed a wide range of guidance documents on quality assurance and in vitro and in vivo preclinical studies [61]. Recent concerns about transmissible spongiform encephalopathies have highlighted the need to document the sources of bovine-derived materials and have led the United States to exclude materials for vaccine manufacture from countries in which Bovine Spongiform Encephalopathy (BSE) or BSE risk exists [64–66].

Careful attention should be given to the design of preclinical toxicity studies, particularly when the investigational product consists of components not previously studied in humans such as new antigen delivery systems and novel adjuvants [67]. Vaccines intended for administration to pregnant women or women of childbearing potential should be evaluated for developmental toxicity; the specific timing of these studies in relation to the vaccine clinical development process depends on the population in such trials [68].

Additional laboratory testing of vaccines may be warranted depending on the particular product, e.g., adventitious agent testing for vaccines produced in animal or human cell substrates [69], preclinical studies evaluating the potential for integration of plasmid DNA into the host genome for DNA vaccines [70,71], and demonstration of adequate attenuation for live attenuated vaccines [72]. Attention

should be devoted to developing tests for sterility, general safety, identity, potency, and demonstrating purity of the vaccine, as these elements will be required for licensure [73]. Continued vigilance is necessary, particularly for novel vaccine technologies that require the development and standardization of new quality control measures. Laboratory evaluation of vaccine safety does not end when clinical studies begin or when a vaccine is licensed. Changes in the manufacturing process or components, the development of enhanced testing techniques, as well as new safety concerns identified in clinical studies or in postmarketing surveillance of a vaccine or one closely related, should prompt the investigator and/or manufacturer to consider whether re-evaluation of the product's preclinical safety is warranted.

B. Clinical Studies

1. Vaccine Clinical Studies and Human Subject Protections

Intrinsic to the design and conduct of clinical studies is compliance with accepted ethical principles guiding human participation in clinical trials, such as informed consent, equitable selection of subjects, and appropriate scientific and ethical review of the proposed study. Evolutions in thought regarding elements of ethical research, as well as the use of new vaccine technologies with uncertain risks, present new challenges for ensuring participant safety in clinical trials. Human subject protections are guided by ethical principles formalized in consensus documents such as the Belmont Report [74], various iterations of the Declaration of Helsinki [75], and the International Ethical Guidelines for Biomedical Research Involving Human Subjects [76]. Similar concepts are codified in Department of Health and Human Services (DHHS) Regulations as the "Common Rule" [77] adopted by 17 federal agencies that support or conduct research with human subjects, and FDA regulations that govern drug, biological, and device research [78].

2. Phases of Clinical Studies

The stages of human clinical studies are divided into *phases* for regulatory purposes [79]. In the United States, when a new vaccine is first tested in humans, a sponsor (a vaccine manufacturer, academic investigator, government agency, or other individual or organization) must first submit an Investigational New Drug (IND) application to the FDA [80]. During each phase, clinical studies should be designed and conducted under conditions that optimize human subject protections and provide sufficient data to proceed to the next phase.

Phase I. Phase I studies represent initial testing in humans. These studies are designed to evaluate safety and typically enroll small numbers of subjects, generally between 10 and 100. Because of the small sample size, these studies can identify only very common adverse effects and are descriptive in nature. These studies may also include a limited dose-ranging design to provide preliminary information on immune responses and the corresponding safety profile at particular doses. The recording of adverse events is facilitated by case report forms designed to capture expected adverse events, based on previous experience with the investigational product or one closely related, as well as the route of administration. For example, for a vaccine that is intramuscularly administered, investigators should monitor local reactions such as redness, swelling, and pain, and systemic complaints such as fever, accompanied by a grading scale to quantify severity. The case report form should also collect information on unanticipated adverse events.

Appropriate duration of active follow up will depend on the investigational product, generally a minimum of 3 days postvaccination for killed or subunit vaccines, and 2–3 weeks postvaccination or until the vaccine strain is no longer detectable for live attenuated products. In addition, further active follow up of all vaccines at the time of blood draw for serology, e.g., at 1 month postimmunization, is appropriate. Collection of data on local and systemic events can make use of diary cards, clinic visits, or telephone calls. The use of clinical criteria defined a priori for halting further administration to subjects (i.e., "stopping rules") may be an important safety feature to considered for products being tested in humans for the first time, especially when indicated by preclinical testing, or when the properties inherent to the vaccine suggest the potential for serious adverse effects (e.g., live attenuated vaccines). If the intended population is infants and no previous studies have been conducted in infants with the vaccine under study or one closely related, a stepwise approach is often used with initial studies conducted in adults before use in children.

Phase II. Phase II studies may include up to several hundred individuals and are designed to evaluate the general safety profile of the vaccine, including local reactions such as redness and swelling at the injection site as well as general side effects such as fever and malaise. These studies also include immunogenicity evaluations and often include dose ranging. The design of Phase II studies may be more elaborate and include blinding, randomization, and placebo controls. During Phase II, the safety of a vaccine may be assessed with other immunizations routinely administered at the same time to evaluate for the possibility of altered immune responses. These studies, although larger than in Phase I, will still be able to evaluate only the most common types of adverse events.

Phase III. Phase III studies are designed to gather additional information regarding efficacy and safety that is needed to assess the overall benefit–risk relationship of the vaccine for licensure. In this regard, they are sometimes referred to as "pivotal" studies because they are designed to include adequate data in the target population and proposed schedule of administration to support the intended use. Such studies are generally randomized and controlled.

For *Phase III* studies, the sample size is usually determined by the number required to establish efficacy of the new vaccine, and may range from a few hundred to tens of thousands of subjects. For some new vaccines, e.g., combination vaccines with components having well-accepted immune correlates of protection, it may be possible to provide evidence for efficacy based on immunogenicity rather than clinical efficacy endpoints; the sample sizes of such pivotal immunogenicity studies may be significantly less than that required to demonstrate clinical efficacy. In such cases, the sample sizes of pivotal safety studies should be adequate to evaluate less-common adverse events, such as those occurring at rates of 1 in 100, with careful consideration of the relevant adverse events to be monitored and the expected background incidence in the target population. Phase III vaccine studies usually have limited ability to detect rare adverse events (Table 1). To detect a doubling of less-common adverse events, such as those occurring at background rates of 1 in 100, requires approximately 5000 subjects. Clinical trials involving 50,000 individuals would be needed to detect doubling of an adverse event with a background incidence of 1/1000 [81,82].

Phase IV. Phase IV or *postmarketing* studies are usually conducted postlicensure to further investigate rare events. Some have advocated the use of expanded "simple" trials prelicensure to provide more precise data on risks of uncommon adverse events (see discussion below) [82].

The use of automated databases, such as those administered by health maintenance organizations, in Phase III studies may facilitate collection of data on less-common adverse events. Detailed information on common local and systemic adverse events may be collected in a subset of individuals enrolled in these studies using diary cards or via telephone or clinic follow-up. If data at any stage of clinical development raise significant concerns regarding the safety of the product, the FDA may request additional information or may halt ongoing or planned studies through a "clinical hold" [83].

Independent scrutiny with respect to the safety of human subjects during clinical trials is afforded by institutional review boards (IRBs), committees designated by institutions to approve the initiation and conduct of clinical studies. The IRB review and approval of clinical studies of new vaccines is required both by FDA and DHHS regulations. In designing clinical studies, investigators or sponsors should consider the use of Data Monitoring Committees (DMCs), also known as Data and Safety Monitoring Boards (DSMBs). Data Monitoring Committees consist of individuals with relevant expertise who provide ongoing review of data accumulated

Table 1 Sample Sizes Needed to Detect Increased Rates of Rare Adverse Events After Immunization

Rates (%)	Sample size[a]	Number of potentially affected individuals per million vaccine recipients
1.0 vs. 2.0	5,000	10,000
1.0 vs. 3.0	1,750	20,000
0.1 vs. 0.2	50,000	1,000
0.1 vs. 0.3	17,500	2,000
0.05 vs. 0.1	100,000	500
0.01 vs. 0.02	500,000	100
0.01 vs. 0.03	175,000	200

[a] Two-arm trial, power = 80%, alpha (2-sided) = 5%.
Source: Refs. 81 and 82.

during clinical studies. The role of the DMC is to advise the sponsor on the safety of current study participants and the continuing validity and scientific merit of the study [84]. Draft guidance is available from the FDA to help determine when a DMC is needed and how such committees should operate [84].

Ethical and practical issues facing investigators with respect to pivotal studies include the choice of research design, including the use of placebo controls when evaluating the efficacy of a vaccine against a disease for which a licensed vaccine already exists [85,86]. This issue is particularly relevant for clinical studies conducted in developing countries. Conducting clinical studies in international settings presents additional challenges such as ensuring adequate local review and oversight, the need for studies to be relevant to the health needs of the host country, and the sustaining newly introduced health interventions once the trial is completed [87–89]. Challenge studies of vaccine efficacy, i.e., inducing infection in subjects to study the efficacy of an experimental vaccine, can present issues for subject safety [90]. When planning challenge studies, investigators should carefully consider the reversibility of the infectious disease and its sequelae. Demonstrating efficacy when field efficacy trials or human challenge studies are not feasible or are unethical, e.g., vaccines against agents of bioterrorism, presents another potential hurdle. For products that reduce or prevent serious or life-threatening conditions where the product is expected to provide meaningful benefit over existing approaches, the FDA has recently finalized a new regulation describing how animal efficacy data can be used to support licensure [91]. In this setting, human clinical data on safety and immunogenicity would still be required.

3. Limitations of Prelicensure Vaccine Safety Assessments

The process outlined above for the development of vaccines prior to licensure and marketing has resulted in very safe vaccines. Regulations mandate strong controls on manufacturing processes, a staged approach to clinical development to systematically assess the benefits and risks of a vaccine, and rigorous controlled studies, usually randomized and blinded, to limit the effect of confounding and bias on outcome and thereby increase the likelihood of valid conclusions about safety and efficacy. However, prelicensure testing of vaccine safety cannot address all issues of concern. First, incomplete understanding of the immunopathophysiology of vaccine adverse effects has generally precluded the design of safer vaccines from "first principles," e.g., deleting a short peptide chain from a vaccine antigen to prevent the possibility of autoimmunity due to molecular mimicry. Second, in many instances, the safety database prior to licensure may include a relatively small number of vaccine recipients (~10,000) compared with the number who might ultimately receive the vaccine (e.g. ~4,000,000 infants in U.S. birth cohort per year for a routinely recommended childhood vaccine), so adverse effects occurring at a rate of 1/1000 or lower are unlikely to be distinguishable from expected background. Third, clinical trials often exclude subgroups of the general population such as the immunocompromised,

preterm infants, and individuals with chronic or self-limited illnesses, and may have limited data from different racial or ethnic groups or geographic locations. Thus prelicensure clinical studies may not address the variation in susceptibility to adverse effects that exists in the general population.

4. Vaccine Licensure

If efficacy and safety are demonstrated during preclinical and clinical development, a license application can then be submitted to regulatory authorities for evaluation, including data on the benefits and risks of the new product. In the United States, the sponsor and the FDA present their findings to the Vaccines and Related Biological Products Advisory Committee (VRBPAC), an external committee of experts, in an open public meeting for comment and advice on interpretation of the submitted data and other issues related to the acceptability of the new vaccine. The approval process also entails the provision of adequate information to healthcare providers and the public in the form of a product label that describes the vaccine's proper use, including its potential benefits and risks, and any contraindications.

C. Postlicensure Assessment of Vaccine Safety

The above mentioned limitations of clinical trials and the need to understand if observed adverse events are due to vaccines have led to the use of other approaches to detect and evaluate the causal connection between vaccines and rare adverse events after the vaccine has been licensed. These include additional clinical studies agreed to by the sponsor as a condition of licensure (sometimes called Phase IV studies), active and passive surveillance for unexpected adverse events after licensure, and targeted clinical, epidemiological, and laboratory studies to evaluate safety concerns that arise after the vaccine is in widespread use.

1. Phase IV Studies

Phase IV studies generally are designed to focus on issues that might have arisen during prelicensure testing, as well as to identify unexpected adverse events not observed prelicensure. These studies typically take place in the first few years after licensure with information expected to be presented in a timely fashion to regulatory agencies and immunization advisory groups. One example of how safety concerns arising during prelicensure development might necessitate Phase IV studies is provided by the theoretical association between arthritis and Lyme vaccine. During the development of Lyme vaccine, licensed in the United States in 1998, laboratory findings suggested that treatment-resistant Lyme arthritis might be caused by molecular mimicry between outer surface protein A (OspA) of *Borrelia burgdorferi* and the human protein LFA-1, in people with certain Human Leukocyte Antigen (HLA) genes [92]. Because the Lyme vaccine antigen consists of OspA, there was a theoretical concern that the vaccine might cause arthritis in susceptible individuals. Although increased risk of arthritis was not observed in approximately 5000 vaccine recipients in a randomized, blinded, placebo-controlled prelicensure trial

[93], a much larger Phase IV study was initiated to evaluate the risk of inflammatory arthritis in the general population. To date, no evidence of increased risk has been identified in this study [Chan, personal communication]. Nevertheless, the manufacturer withdrew the vaccine from the market in 2002, citing poor sales [95].

2. Vaccine Safety Surveillance

In addition to Phase IV studies planned prior to licensure, postmarketing monitoring of vaccine safety also involves identification of possible adverse effects of vaccination through surveillance of spontaneous adverse event reports made to vaccine manufacturers or directly to the FDA, followed by evaluation of these "signals" for a possible causal link to the vaccine.

Vaccine Adverse Event Reporting System. In the United States, systematic surveillance of adverse events after vaccination is undertaken using the Vaccine Adverse Event Surveillance System, jointly managed by the FDA and CDC [94,95]. The VAERS receives between 10,000 and 15,000 adverse event reports annually; approximately 10–15% are reported as serious (defined as life-threatening, hospitalization or prolongation of hospitalization, a persistent or significant disability/incapacity or a congenital anomaly/ birth defect, or a medical event that may require intervention to prevent one of the above situations [96]). Information on VAERS and vaccine safety including the VAERS database, the VAERS form, and access to on-line reporting, is available on the internet (www.vaers.org; www.fda.gov/cber/ vaers/vaers.htm; or www.cdc.gov/nip).

Utility of Passive Surveillance Systems. Passive surveillance systems such as VAERS do not actively track adverse events after vaccination, but rely on reports from healthcare providers, patients and their parents, and other interested parties. The VAERS is useful for detecting unrecognized adverse events, monitoring known reactions, identifying possible risk factors, and vaccine lot surveillance [94,95,97]. Priorities in analyzing VAERS data include adverse events reported after recently licensed vaccines, issues that have been identified to be of particular concern to the public, and rare adverse events not likely to be identified in clinical trials or controlled postmarketing safety studies (e.g., alopecia [98], and Stevens Johnson Syndrome [99]). Other priorities for VAERS analysis include those adverse events causally linked with immunization, to describe the range of clinical signs and symptoms, investigate potential risk factors, and pathophysiology (e.g., thrombocytopenia [100], syncope [101], and hypotonic–hyporesponsive episodes in infants (HHE) [102]). In addition, all reports of serious adverse events and death following vaccination are reviewed by FDA medical officers as they are received. Periodically, vaccine-specific surveillance summaries are prepared to describe reported adverse events and to look for unexpected patterns in clinical conditions that might suggest a causal link between the vaccine and the clinical condition [103–111].

Limitations of Passive Surveillance Systems. Limitations of surveillance systems dependent on spontaneously reported adverse events include lack of verification of reported diagnoses, lack of consistent diagnostic criteria for all cases with a given diagnosis, wide range in data quality, underreporting, inadequate denominator data, and lack of an unvaccinated control group [94,95,112,113]. The validity of reported diagnoses and completeness of information in VAERS reports has only been formally studied for a few conditions. In one study evaluating reports of encephalopathy, encephalitis, and multiple sclerosis [114], between 26% and 51% of reports for these conditions lacked sufficient information to make a diagnosis. Enhanced follow-up is sometimes conducted to systematically collect information as the first stage in the signal evaluation process [99,100,102].

Standardized Case Definitions. The absence of consistent definitions for adverse events has hampered analysis of VAERS data. Application of case definitions for HHE [115], encephalopathy, encephalitis, and multiple sclerosis [114] to VAERS reports has shown the value of case definition development. The Brighton Collaboration is an international effort to extend these efforts by developing standardized case definitions of adverse events following vaccination for additional conditions [116]. These definitions might be used as guidelines for reporting adverse events to VAERS or applied to prelicensure trials.

Passive Surveillance and Assessing Causality. The limitations of passive surveillance systems mean that it is usually not possible to assess whether a vaccine caused the reported adverse event. Individual case causality assessment has been employed to evaluate reports using Bayesian probability [117] and a standardized algorithm in Canada [118]. This latter method was adapted by the Anthrax Vaccine Expert Committee to evaluate reports of adverse events following anthrax vaccine for the Department of Defense [119]. This approach involves systematic review of individual cases to make a diagnosis, search for known etiologies, and assess the biological plausibility of the adverse event's being caused by the vaccine using expert opinion. Similar approaches have been considered for use in drug adverse event causality assessment, but their use has remained controversial when applied to unexpected adverse events [120–122]. As a result of the limitations of VAERS and individual case causality assessment, analysis of VAERS data focuses on describing clinical and demographic characteristics of reports and looking for patterns to detect "signals" of adverse events plausibly linked to a vaccine, thereby helping to define a hypothesis that can subsequently be examined in proper epidemiological studies. Even this limited and structured approach to analysis of VAERS data has proven controversial [123,124].

In addition to the approach described above combining descriptive epidemiology with medical judgment, several quantitative approaches have been proposed. These approaches all involve trying to identify conditions that are more commonly reported after a certain vaccine or combination of vaccines than after others. These methods are often collectively referred to as "data mining" and include older approaches such as proportional reporting ratios [125] as well as newer techniques [126,127]. Signals generated through such quantitative analysis are usually subject to clinical and descriptive epidemiological analysis to focus on the most interesting findings. These semiautomated approaches should help to improve the efficiency of screening tens of thousands of adverse events reported annually [128], although their utility in replacing traditional case series evaluations remains to be seen [129].

International Surveillance Systems. The vaccine safety efforts of the World Health Organization (WHO) include the development of national systems to deal with adverse events [130]. The WHO has also established a Global Advisory Committee on Vaccine Safety to make independent assessments of vaccine safety issues [59]. Many countries have surveillance systems and these data are aggregated by the WHO Collaborating Center for International Drug Monitoring at Uppsala, Sweden, including some data from vaccine adverse event surveillance systems. This center has developed a data mining technique for routine monitoring of this database and routinely publicizes possible signals. The United Kingdom's Medicine Control Agency (MCA) enhances their surveillance for new products with the "yellow card" system. New products are distributed with a reporting form (the "yellow card") to highlight the need for clinicians and pharmacists to be alert for and report adverse events. If an adverse event occurs, the reporter sends the form to the MCA and Committee on Safety of Medicine so that the adverse event can be evaluated.

3. Targeted Evaluations of Vaccine Safety Signals

Evaluation of signals usually requires epidemiological methods, sometimes combined with clinical and laboratory analysis. The CDC established the Vaccine Safety Datalink (VSD) as a resource for conducting cohort studies using large administrative databases maintained by health maintenance organizations to evaluate specific hypotheses [131,132]. Studies from the VSD have found increased risk of intussusception after rotavirus vaccine [34], and febrile but not nonfebrile seizures after DTP or MMR vaccines [133]. Analyses of VSD data have also produced important negative studies. For example, no difference was found in adverse events by brand of hepatitis B vaccine [134] and no association was found between rubella vaccine and chronic arthropathy in women [135], childhood vaccination and type 1 diabetes [136], and measles-containing vaccines and inflammatory bowel disease [137].

Other countries have also used population-based databases to study vaccine safety concerns. Among the best known is the General Practice Research Database (GPRD) in the United Kingdom [138]. Recent examples of the use of the GPRD include studies showing no association between MMR vaccine and increased incidence of autism [139] and oral polio vaccine and intussusception [140].

Ad hoc studies are sometimes needed to study rare adverse events if the vaccine or adverse event of concern is not sufficiently represented in even large databases such as the VSD, or if confirmation of a study outcome is sought in a different population. Such an approach was used to demonstrate that there was not an increased risk of multiple sclerosis or exacerbation of multiple sclerosis following

hepatitis B vaccine using the Nurses Health Study database and the European Database for Multiple Sclerosis [141–143]. An ad hoc case-control study was conducted to demonstrate an association between intussusception and the rhesus rotavirus vaccine (RRV) [33]. Similarly, a special study was conducted to estimate an excess risk of 1 case of Guillain–Barre syndrome (GBS) per million people administered flu vaccine in the 1992–1993 and 1993–1994 flu seasons [144].

The small relative and attributable risks identified by epidemiological investigations, such as the influenza vaccine—the GBS study mentioned above, push the limits of current population-based observational cohort methods in evaluating associations between vaccines and adverse events. Structured clinical and laboratory evaluations of individual cases as part of case-control studies of rare adverse events are needed to fill the gap between surveillance and population-based cohort studies. To provide a systematic resource for case-based evaluations, the CDC has organized the Centers for Immunization Safety Assessment (CISA) [47]. These centers will serve as referral sites for clinical vaccine safety questions; develop clinical protocols for the evaluation and management of adverse events possibly related to immunization; systematically evaluate patients with similar adverse events to identify mechanisms of action and risk factors; and develop and test protocols for revaccination of people who have experienced adverse events, as has been recently carried out in Australia [145].

One area of investigation that might be particularly fruitful for case-based approaches is evaluation of the hypothesis that genetic variability is a source of increased risk for rare adverse events. At present, only a few small studies have attempted to address this issue, primarily focusing on HLA genes. One study found higher frequencies of HLA-DR2 and DR5 in women who developed joint symptoms following rubella vaccination as compared to placebo recipients with joint symptoms [146]. Another study found an increased frequency of HLA-DR9 (DRB1*0901) and HLA-DR17 (DRB1*0301) in Thai patients who developed autoimmune encephalomyelitis following Semple rabies vaccine [147]. Studies evaluating polymorphisms in other genes influencing immune and inflammatory responses, such as T cell receptors [147] and cytokines [148,149], might also prove to be a productive approach. Additional research in this area may help determine if certain individuals should be excluded from receiving selected immunizations or if vaccines could be designed to reduce the risk of rare adverse effects based on knowledge of genetic susceptibility.

IV. COMPREHENSIVE ASSESSMENT, RICK MANAGEMENT, AND COMMUNICATION OF VACCINE SAFETY CONCERNS

Because data on vaccine safety come from many different sources, making an overall assessment, developing a risk management plan, and communicating the plan to healthcare professionals and the public should be carried out as part of an integrated process involving vaccine developers, government agencies, regulatory authorities, and immunization recommending bodies. Systematic methods for approaching this stage of the vaccine safety process are presented in this section.

A. Causality Assessment

Evaluating the causal link between a vaccine and an adverse event often requires integration of different levels of information because conclusive biological evidence or data from sufficiently powered and properly conducted clinical trials are usually not available. Several general considerations, patterned after those proposed by Hill in 1965 [150] and adapted by others [151], have been generally accepted in the field of epidemiology for causal inference. The IOM used the following criteria for assessing whether evidence indicates the presence of an association between an adverse event and vaccine exposure [24].

Strength of Association—The strength of an association refers to the magnitude of the measure of effect of an exposure, usually the relative risk or odds ratio, in a study comparing an exposed and an unexposed group. The larger the magnitude of the effect, the less likely any observed effect is due to chance, bias, or confounding. In general, in observational studies, relative risks of 2 or less are considered to be evidence of a weak association, because the likelihood the effect is due to chance, bias, or confounding is greater than if the effect is larger [152,153]. Ecological studies alone are not generally accepted as strong evidence of causality, because they do not link individual exposure to individual outcome, and can be subject to confounding by unknown or uncontrollable factors.

Dose–Response Relation—A dose–response relation is defined as an increased strength of association with increased magnitude of exposure. The existence of a dose–response relation strengthens an inference that an association is causal.

Temporally Correct Association—Exposure must precede the event by at least the duration of disease induction. This consideration may be limited by the fact that knowledge of the pathogenesis and natural history of an adverse event may be insufficient.

Consistency of Association—This consideration requires that an association be found regularly in a variety of studies, using different study populations and study methods.

Specificity of an Association—Uniqueness of an association between an exposure and an outcome provides a stronger justification for a causal interpretation than when the association is nonspecific. However, perfect specificity between an exposure and an effect cannot be expected in all cases because of the multifactorial etiology of many disorders.

Biological Plausibility—The existence of a possible mechanism of action that fits existing biological or medical knowledge is thought to increase the likelihood that an association is causal. Because little is known about the details of immunopathological effects of vaccination, it is easy to generate a

theory as to how a vaccine might cause an effect. Moreover, unexpected adverse effects are unexpected because they do not have a biological explanation for their occurrence. For these reasons, biological plausibility is often considered to be a major factor only if it favors causality.

Hill also included "experimental evidence," "analogy," and "coherence" as additional considerations in his original discussion of causal inference [150,151]. As noted earlier, experimental evidence from clinical trials is seldom available for very rare adverse events. "Analogy" has not been accepted as strong evidence of causality because analogies between exposure and a particular condition often can be drawn, even when causal relationships do not exist. Coherence "implies that a cause and effect interpretation for an association does not conflict with what is known of the natural history and biology of the disease [151]." This guideline has been interpreted as being similar to biological plausibility, but it might also be relevant to the process of balancing among the strength of the considerations supporting a causal interpretation against the strength of alternative explanations.

B. Risk Assessment

A complementary approach to evaluating vaccine safety concerns is the use of formal risk assessment methods, patterned after methods used for environmental exposures. The National Academy of Sciences approach involves hazard identification, dose–response analysis, exposure assessment, and risk characterization [154]. Hazard identification refers to the qualitative identification of the adverse effects in animals or humans. Dose–response analysis seeks to establish the relationship between the magnitude of the exposure and the incidence of the adverse event. Exposure assessment determines the magnitude, time, duration, and route of exposure. Risk characterization integrates the three prior steps into an assessment of causality and when adequate data are available, a quantitative estimate of risk.

Risk assessment has been most well developed for linkage of environmental chemical exposures to cancer risk, but has also been applied to neurological and other disorders. In these settings, risk assessments might involve development of complex mathematical models of disease pathogenesis linked to human risk through detailed exposure analysis that might include pharmacokinetic models, with human epidemiological studies providing empirical validation of model predictions. Complete information on human exposure and outcomes is often unavailable, so risk assessments have sometimes extrapolated outcomes in animals to humans, and from high dose to low dose exposures. In such scenarios, risk assessment serves a more qualitative purpose of identifying data gaps and framing the range of possible risk, to aid with policy making and prioritization of research. Therefore structured risk assessments may be useful in determining the scope of a potential problem, under a range of plausible assumptions.

Risk assessment methods have been applied to evaluate the possible effects of thimerosal in vaccines [155,156], as well as the risk of Bovine Spongiform Encephalopathy (BSE) from using bovine-derived products in vaccine manufacture [64]. The risk assessment of thimerosal was primarily qualitative and identified important gaps in knowledge. In contrast, the risk assessment of BSE from vaccines resulted in a quantitative estimate of the risk that was extremely low. In these examples, the risk assessments served an important role because of limited information and the need to make decisions under uncertainty. Risk assessment is likely to be used more often as mechanistic knowledge of adverse event pathophysiology improves and can be mathematically modeled, especially for rare exposures and outcomes that might be extremely difficult to study empirically, but for which quantitative estimates of risk are desired.

C. Benefit–Risk Analysis

As discussed throughout this chapter, vaccine approval and usage recommendations rely on benefit–risk analysis, on both a societal and individual basis. Historically, the benefit–risk analysis has been informal, primarily relying on expert opinion to integrate data [22]. Formal methods of benefit–risk analysis [157], including cost–benefit calculations, have been developed and have begun to be incorporated into vaccine decision making. Cost–benefit analyses of several vaccines have been published and strongly support the benefit of routine childhood immunizations [158,159]. Adverse events have not been widely integrated into these analyses, both because limited information on the cost of adverse events has been available and the existing data have not suggested cost is high relative to other costs in vaccination programs [160]. This might suggest that safety concerns are overemphasized relative to vaccine benefit, or that there is a different threshold for what constitutes an acceptable benefit–risk ratio between public health experts and the general public [161–163]. Better understanding and quantification of how benefits and risks are perceived and valued will be important for making informed benefit–risk evaluations and communicating and managing vaccine safety concerns [164].

D. Comprehensive Assessment in Practice: Institute of Medicine Safety Review Committee

Previously, we discussed the role of the IOM in reviewing vaccines safety concerns in response to the National Childhood Vaccine Injury Act of 1986. Recognizing the continued need for comprehensive analyses of vaccine safety, the CDC and NIH asked the IOM to establish an independent Immunization Safety Review Committee. The committee has been chartered to meet three times per year over the 3-year study period (2001–2003) to review immunization safety issues by examining the current biologic and epidemiologic evidence of causality, the biological mechanisms of adverse events, and the larger societal context. To date, the committee has evaluated and released reports on MMR and autism [165], thimerosal-containing vaccines and neurodevelopmental disorders [166], multiple immunizations and immune dysfunction [167], and hepatitis B vaccine and neurological

disorders [168]. In addition, a separate committee to evaluate the safety and efficacy of anthrax vaccine was convened at the request of the Department of Defense because of concerns from within and outside of the military [56]. With regard to MMR and autism, the IOM concluded that the evidence favors rejection of a causal relationship at the population level between MMR vaccine and autism spectrum disorders (ASD) [165]. The committee found inadequate evidence to accept or reject a causal relationship between thimerosal-containing vaccines and neurodevelopmental disorders [166]. The IOM committee evaluating anthrax vaccine concluded that the anthrax vaccine is an effective vaccine to protect humans against anthrax and that it was "reasonably safe" [56]. For each of the above immunization safety concerns, the IOM recommended additional research to clarify any possible connections and to improve the way the government communicates benefits and risks of vaccination to vaccine recipients.

E. Risk Management and Communication

Risk management in the context of immunizations is the process of maximizing the benefits of vaccines while minimizing associated risks when considered in the context of the population as well as the individual [169]. Risk management occurs at all stages of product development and use, as has been outlined in this chapter. Participants in risk management decisions include scientists developing vaccines, manufacturers, regulatory agencies, immunization advisory bodies (e.g., the Advisory Committee on Immunization Practices and AAP's Committee on Infectious Diseases), other government public health agencies (e.g., CDC, NIH, VICP), federal and state legislators, vaccine providers and patients. A vaccine is licensed when regulatory authorities judge that the benefits of using the vaccine outweigh the risks for the intended population and use. A major goal of the prelicensure studies and review is to ensure that accurate information about benefits and risks of vaccination is available to those participating in risk management decisions following licensure.

Once a vaccine is licensed, responsibility for risk management expands from regulatory authorities to include others making decisions on appropriate use of the product, including immunization advisory bodies, other government agencies monitoring and assessing vaccine safety, immunization providers, and individuals receiving vaccinations. However, the decision making capacity of individuals and healthcare providers regarding immunizations may be limited by school entry laws or by service in the military. In this context, delineating the benefits and risks is only the first step. Successful immunization strategies require an understanding of the ethical underpinnings of immunization policy [170], the role of risk perception in vaccination decisions [164], and optimal risk communication strategies [171,172]. At the heart of ethical immunization policies is the equitable allocation of benefits and risks between individuals and society. A systematic approach for developing immunization policy, integrating epidemiologic, economic and ethical concerns, may help focus risk management decisions and sustain societal consensus on immunizations [170].

Because science does not speak for itself, dissemination of accurate and meaningful information on the benefits and risks of immunization is essential to maintain public confidence in immunizations. Given the complexity of vaccine science and the many factors entering vaccine policy, there is concern that misinformation can adversely impact informed decision making, with consequences for the individual and the community [2,173–175]. The field of risk communication has developed from the need to find effective ways to communicate health risks. Researchers in this field have recognized the discrepancy between how scientists explained health risks and what the public believed [176], and have drawn upon scientific facts, ethical principles, cognitive and social psychology, and behavioral decision theory to improve approaches for conveying risk information [177,178]. In this context, communication begins by identifying the information of most relevance to individuals making immunization decisions, determining what these individuals know and filling in the gaps, recognizing that different populations are likely to have different information needs [171, 178–180].

Many factors influence the acceptability of risks to individuals; risks that are voluntary and controllable, considered natural (as opposed to man-made), and memorable are more likely to be accepted [181]. Risk communication research has demonstrated that individuals are unlikely to undertake a risk control measure, such as immunization, unless they perceive both a serious threat and some control over it [182], emphasizing the importance of involving individuals in immunization decisions.

In our contemporary society, individuals seek and receive immunization information from a variety of sources, complicating the task of public health officials and healthcare providers seeking to promote immunizations. The internet provides a wealth of relevant information but can serve as an unfiltered stream of anecdotes and allegations regarding adverse events following vaccination [183]. The media plays a critical role in shaping public perceptions on vaccine benefits and risks. The development and dissemination of accurate and balanced information at the time of vaccine licensure, and the prompt evaluation of new safety concerns arising postlicensure, may prevent an "early idealization–sudden condemnation" portrayal of a vaccine in the media that can affect public opinion and undermine immunization programs [184].

V. INTEGRATING SAFETY CONSIDERATIONS INTO NEW VACCINE DEVELOPMENT

In the preceding sections of this chapter, we have presented an overview of vaccine safety with important lessons learned from historical examples and reviewed the methods currently employed for evaluating and communicating safety concerns. Several themes emerge that are important for new vaccine developers. First, vaccines have real risks that may include serious adverse effects. Second, despite the favorable benefit-to-risk ratio in favor of vaccination, public concern about vaccine safety is legitimate and is best dealt with through the application of sound scientific methods to

vaccine evaluation, with clear communication of findings to the public. Third, the perceived risk of a vaccine is as vital to its success or failure as the efficacy and safety profiles. Fourth, we can learn from history, because public concerns about vaccine safety have demonstrated recurring themes, such as the need for quality control of production, philosophical beliefs about individual choice, and changing benefit-to-risk ratios.

The best way to prepare for vaccine safety issues is to build them into the product development cycle by "reverse engineering" potential safety concerns. This can be carried out by focusing on the target population and the product. At the earliest phases of development, vaccine researchers should bear in mind the product's ultimate indication and intended target population to be reflected in the product label, and apply this information in a development plan to acquire necessary data on safety and efficacy. Considering the "the label as the product" gives the vaccine developer the perspective needed to make judgments as to the type and quantity of safety data required to support licensure, including preclinical toxicity testing and sample size of clinical studies. For example, the required data might differ for a vaccine intended for universal use in children compared with one to be used in more niche populations such as adult travelers.

Depending on the product class, some potential safety concerns are known a priori or can be predicted from the historical experience of development of vaccines from the same class. Examples of particular concerns include the potential association of group A streptococcal vaccines with rheumatic heart disease due to cross reaction between the M proteins of vaccines with human tissues [185] inactivated RSV vaccines and enhanced RSV disease [17], and OPV and vaccine-associated paralytic polio. Even for product classes for which there is limited human experience, e.g., DNA vaccines, theoretical concerns or those generated from laboratory experience can guide the vaccine developer through the first steps of safety testing. Specific preclinical testing and clinical evaluations depend on the type of product under development, e.g., adventitious agent testing in vaccines produced in animal or human cell substrates, and monitoring for clinical symptoms and evaluating persistence of vaccine strains in studies of live attenuated vaccines.

Understanding the background incidence of illness occurring in the target population and anticipating risks that might be perceived as related to vaccination may be as important as understanding the product-related risks, because ultimately the intended population will need to be convinced that the vaccine is safe enough to use. The developer can begin this process by identifying the diseases in the target population that might be suspected to be related to the vaccine because onset or diagnosis may coincide with the timing of immunizations. History is a good guide in this arena. Neurological, rheumatological, and other immune-mediated disorders have been attributed to vaccines when other etiologies could not be established. In addition, disorders that are not well understood but have occurred with some temporal relation to immunization, such as Sudden Infant Death Syndrome or Gulf War syndrome, have also been linked with immunization in the minds of the public.

To deal with such concerns, researchers should decide whether it is necessary, based on benefit–risk considerations and incidence in the target population, to develop evidence that the vaccine does not cause a particular condition. Considerations should take into account risk perception in addition to actual risk, and whether such perceptions may affect public acceptance of the vaccine. For example, vaccine developers may choose to evaluate a possible association between a new rotavirus vaccine and intussusception. For concerns that warrant further evaluation, the next step is to decide where in the development cycle it can and should it be evaluated, e.g., preclinical testing, prelicensure clinical trials, or Phase IV studies. Ultimately, the aim of safety assessments should be to provide adequate data to support licensure and recommendations for use as well as communicating the benefits and risks of the vaccines to health care providers and the public.

VI. CONCLUSION

The current system of vaccine development and monitoring has resulted in vaccines with very low risk of serious adverse effects. However, continued vigilance regarding immunization safety is necessary based on lessons from the past, as well the need to ensure the safety of new vaccines and new immunization technologies. Perceptions of vaccine risks can affect public acceptance of immunizations and the success of immunization strategies. Immunization safety requires careful application of preclinical evaluation and quality control testing, well-designed clinical studies, and postlicensure assessments including surveillance for adverse events. The challenge remains to apply the best scientific methods to the task, and effectively communicate that science to the public.

ACKNOWLEDGMENTS

We are grateful for the comments of Susan S. Ellenberg, Ph.D., M. Miles Braun, M.D., M.P.H., Karen Goldenthal, M.D., Norman Baylor, Ph.D., and the editorial assistance of Jan Kelliher.

REFERENCES

1. Centers for Disease Control and Prevention. Achievements in Public Health 1900–1999: Control of Infectious Diseases. MMWR Morb Mort Wkly Rep 1999; 48:621–628.
2. Gangarosa EJ, et al. Impact of anti-vaccine movements on pertussis control: the untold story. Lancet 1998; 351:356–361.
3. White PJ, Shackelford PG. Edward Jenner and the scourge that was. Am J Dis Child 1983; 137:864–869.
4. Swales JD. The Leicester anti-vaccination movement. Lancet 1992; 340:1019–1021.
5. Albert MR, et al. The last smallpox epidemic in Boston and the vaccination controversy, 1901–1903. N Engl J Med 2001; 344:375–379.
6. Edwards KM. State mandates and childhood immunization. JAMA 2000; 284:3171–3173.
7. Nelson CT. Jonathan Hutchison on vaccination syphilis. Arch Derm 1969; 99:529–535.
8. Public Law: The Virus, Serum and Toxin Law of 1902, Pub. L. No. 57–244, 32 Stat. 728 (July 1, 1902).
9. Wilson, GS. The Hazards of Immunization. London: The Athlone Press, 1967.
10. Sawyer WA, et al. Jaundice in Army personnel in western region of United States and its relation to vaccination against yellow fever. Am J Hyg 1944; 40:35–107.
11. Seeff LB, et al. A serologic follow-up of the 1942 epidemic of post-vaccination hepatitis in the United States Army. N Engl J Med 1987; 316(16):965–970.
12. Furmanski M. Unlicensed vaccines and bioweapon defense in World War II. JAMA 1999; 282:822.
13. Nathanson N, Langmuir AD. The Cutter incident. Poliomyelitis following formaldehyde inactivated poliovirus vaccination in the United States during the spring of 1955. II. Relationship of poliomyelitis to Cutter vaccine. Am J Hyg 1963; 78:29–60.
14. Henderson DA, et al. Paralytic disease associated with oral polio vaccines. JAMA 1964; 190:41–48.
15. Sutter RW. A new epidemiologic and laboratory classification system for paralytic polio cases. Am J Public Health 1989; 79:495–498.
16. Fulginiti VA, et al. Respiratory virus immunization: I. A field trial of two inactivated respiratory virus vaccines; an aqueous trivalent parainfluenza virus vaccine and an alum-precipitated respiratory syncytial virus vaccine. Am J Epidemiol 1969; 89:435–448.
17. Kapikian AZ, et al. An epidemiologic study of altered clinical reactivity to respiratory syncytial virus (RSV) infection in children previously vaccinated with an inactivated RS virus vaccine. Am J Epidemiol 1969; 89:405–421.
18. Rauh LW, Schmidt R. Measles immunization with killed virus vaccine, serum antibody titers and experience with exposure to measles epidemic. Am J Dis Child 1965; 109:232.
19. Fulginiti VA, et al. Altered reactivity to measles virus. A typical measles in children previously immunized with inactivated measles virus vaccines. JAMA 1967; 202:1075–1080.
20. Annunziato D, et al. Atypical measles syndrome: pathologic and serologic findings. Pediatrics 1982; 70:203–209.
21. Simoes EAF, et al. Respiratory syncytial virus vaccine: a systematic overview with emphasis on respiratory syncytial virus subunit vaccines. Vaccine 2002; 20:954–960.
22. Food and Drug Administration. Biological products; Bacterial vaccines and toxoids; Implementation of efficacy review; Proposed rule. Fed Regul 1985; 50:51002–51117.
23. Thompson L, Nuell D. DPT: Vaccine Roulette [video recording]. Washington, DC: WRC-TV (NBC), 1982.
24. Howson CP, et al, eds. Adverse Effects of Pertussis and Rubella Vaccines. Report from the Institute of Medicine. Washington, DC: National Academy Press, 1991.
25. Coulter HL, Fisher BL. DPT: A Shot in the Dark; The Concerned Parents' Guide to the Risks of Diphtheria, Pertussis (Whooping Cough), and Tetanus Vaccination. New York, NY: Warner Books, 1986.
26. Public Law: The National Childhood Vaccine Injury Act of 1986, Pub. L. No. 99-660, §§311 et seq., 100 Stat. 3755, codified at 42 U.S.C.A. §§300aa-1 et seq. 1989.
27. Stratton KR, et al, eds. Adverse Events Associated with Childhood Vaccines: Evidence Bearing on Causality. Report from the Institute of Medicine. Washington, DC: National Academy Press, 1994.
28. Centers for Disease Control and PreventionPertussis vaccination: use of acellular pertussis vaccines among infants and young children. Recommendations of the Advisory Committee on Immunization Practices. MMWR Morb Mort Wkly Rep 1997; 46:RR-7.
29. Centers for Disease Control and PreventionNotice to Readers: Recommended Childhood Immunization Schedule—

United States, 2000. MMWR Morb Mort Wkly Rep 2000; 49:3535.

30. Centers for Disease Control and PreventionPoliomyelitis prevention in the US: introduction of a sequential vaccination schedule of IPV followed by OPV. Recommendations of the Advisory Committee on Immunization Practices. MMWR Morb Mort Wkly Rep 1997; 46:RR-3.

31. Rennels MB, et al. Lack of an apparent association between intussusception and wild or vaccine rotavirus infection. Pediatr Infect Dis J 1998; 17:924–925.

32. Centers for Disease Control and Prevention. Intussusception among recipients of rotavirus vaccine—United States, 1998–1999. MMWR Morb Mort Wkly Rep 1999; 48:577–581.

33. Murphy TV, et al. Intussusception among infants given an oral rotavirus vaccine. N Engl J Med 2001; 344:564–572.

34. Kramarz P, et al. Population-based study of rotavirus vaccination and intussusception. Pediatr Infect Dis J 2001; 20:410–416.

35. Centers for Disease Control and Prevention. Withdrawal of rotavirus vaccine recommendation. MMWR Morb Mort Wkly Rep 1999; 48:1007.

36. Cohen J. Rethinking a vaccine's risk. Science 2001; 293:1576.

37. Wakefield AJ, et al. Ileal-lymphoid hyperplasia, non-specific colitis, and pervasive developmental disorder in children. Lancet 1998; 351:637–641.

38. Wakefield AJ. MMR vaccination and autism. Lancet 1999; 354:949–950.

39. Bernard S, et al. A novel form of mercury poisoning. Med Hypotheses 2001; 56:462–471.

40. Trollmo C, et al. Molecular mimcry in Lyme arthritis demonstrated at the single cell level: LFA-1 alpha L is a partial agonist for outer surface protein A-reactive T cells. J Immunol 2001; 1966:5286–5291.

41. Classen JB, Classen DC. *Haemophilus* vaccine associated with increased risk of diabetes: causality likely. Diabetes Care 2001; 23:872–873.

42. Marshall E. A shadow falls on hepatitis B vaccination effort. Science 1998; 281:630–631.

43. Offit PA, et al. Addressing parents' concerns: do multiple vaccines overwhelm or weaken the infant's immune system? Pediatrics 2002; 109:124–129.

44. Kmietowicz Z. Government launches intensive media campaign on MMR. BMJ 2002; 324:383.

45. No author. Sole Lyme Vaccine is pulled off market. The New York Times 2002 February 28;Section A:5.

46. Centers for Disease Control and Prevention. Updated recommendations from the Advisory Committee on Immunization Practices in response to delays in supply of influenza vaccine for the 2000–01 season. MMWR Morb Mort Wkly Rep 2000; 49:888–892.

47. Centers for Disease Control and Prevention. Notices–grants and cooperative agreements: Clinical Immunization Safety and Assessment Centers. Fed Regul, 2001, 66.

48. Centers for Disease Control and Prevention. Notice to readers: Decreased availability of pneumococcal conjugate vaccine. MMWR Morb Mort Wkly Rep 2001; 50:783–784.

49. Centers for Disease Control and PreventionNotice to readers: Update: Supply of diphtheria and tetanus toxoids and aceullar pertussis vaccine. MMWR Morb Mort Wkly Rep 2002; 50:1159.

50. Centers for Disease Control and Prevention. Shortage of varicella and measles, mumps and rubella vaccines and interim recommendations from the Advisory Committee on Immunization Practices. MMWR Morb Mortal Wkly Rep 2002; 51:190–191.

51. Cohen J. U.S. vaccine supply falls seriously short. Science 2002; 295:1998–2001.

52. Stolberg SG. Anthrax threats point to limits in health systems. NY Times October 14, 2001; 1.

53. Centers for Disease Control and Prevention. Smallpox vaccine no longer available for civilians-United States. MMWR Morb Mort Wkly Rep 1983; 32:387.

54. Lane JM, et al. Deaths attributable to smallpox vaccination, 1959 to 1966, and 1968. JAMA 1970;21441–444.

55. Morris K. US military face punishment for refusing anthrax vaccine. Lancet 1999; 353:130.

56. Joellenbeck LM, et al, eds. The Anthrax Vaccine: Is it Safe? Does it Work? Report from the Institute of Medicine. Washington, DC: National Academy Press, 2002.

57. Rosenthal SR, et al., Developing new smallpox vaccine. Emerg Infect Dis 2001; 7:920–926.

58. Larkin M. Can vaccines thwart the consequences of a bioterrorist attack? Lancet Infect Dis 2002; 2:70.

59. Duclos P, Hofmann CA. Immunisation safety: a priority of the World Health Organization's Department of Vaccines and Biologicals. Drug Safety 2001; 24:1106–1112.

60. Dittmann S. Vaccine safety: risk communication—a global perspective. Vaccine 2001; 19:2446–2456.

61. International Conference on Harmonization. Available from: URL: http://www.ifpma.org/ich1.html. Accessed May 20, 2002.

62. U.S. Code of Federal Regulations. Title 21, Part 600.3(p). Washington, DC: U.S. Government Printing Office, 2001.

63. Food and Drug Administration. Guidance for industry: Content and format of chemistry, manufacturing and controls information and establishment description information for a vaccine or related product. FDA, Center for Biologics Evaluation and Research, Office of Vaccine Research and Review. Fed Regul 64 (1999) 518. Available from: URL: http://www.fda.gov/cber/gdlns/cmcvacc.pdf. Accessed May 6, 2002.

64. Food and Drug Administration. Bovine-derived materials: agency letters to manufacturers of FDA-regulated products. Fed Regul 1994; 59:44591–44594.

65. Food and Drug Administration. Letter to manufacturers of biological products—Recommendations regarding Bovine Spongiform Encephalopathy (BSE). April 19, 2000. Available from URL: http://www.fda.gov/cber/ltr/BSE041900.htm. Accessed May 6, 2002

66. Centers for Disease Control and Prevention. Notice to readers: Public Health Service recommendations for use of vaccines manufactured with bovine-derived materials. MMWR Morb Mort Wkly Rep 2000; 49:1137–1178.

67. Goldenthal KL, et al. Safety evaluation of vaccine adjuvants. AIDS Res Hum Retrovir 1999; 9:S47–51.

68. Food and Drug Administration. Draft guidance for industry: considerations for reproductive toxicity studies for preventative vaccines for infectious disease indications. FDA, Center for Biologics Evaluation and Research, Office of Vaccines Research and Review 2000b. Available from URL: http://www. fda.gov/cber/gdlns/reprotox.htm. Accessed May 6, 2002.

69. Lewis A, et al. A defined-risks approach to the regulatory assessment of the use of neoplastic cells as substrates for viral vaccine manufacture. Dev Biol 2001; 106:513–535.

70. Smith HA, Klinman DM. The regulation of DNA vaccines. Curr Opin Biotechnol 2001; 12:299–303.

71. Food and Drug Administration. Points to consider on plasmid DNA vaccines for preventive infectious disease indications. FDA, Center for Biologics Evaluation and Research, Office of Vaccines Research and Review 1996; Docket No. 96-N-0400. Available from URL: http://www.fda.gov/cber/gdlns/plasmid.pdf. Accessed May 6, 2002.

72. Falk LA, et al. Review of current preclinical testing strategies for bacterial vaccines. Dev Biol Stand 1998; 95:25–29.

73. U.S. Code of Federal Regulations. Title 21, Part 610. Washington, DC: US Government Printing Office, 2001.

74. National Commission for the Protection of Human

Subjects of Biomedical and Behavioral Research (National Commission). Belmont Report: ethical principles and guidelines for the protection of human subjects of research. Washington, DC: Department of Health and Human Services, 1979.

75. World Medical Association (WMA) Declaration of Helsinki: Ethical principles for medical research involving human subjects (adopted 18th WMA General Assembly, Helsinki, Finland, June 1964; amended: 29th WMA General Assembly, Tokyo, Japan, October 1975; 35th WMA General Assembly, Venice, Italy, October 1983; 41st WMA General Assembly, Hong Kong, September 1989; 48th WMA General Assembly, Somerset West, Republic of South Africa, October 1996; and 52nd WMA General Assembly, Edinburgh, Scotland, October 2000). Ferney-Voltaire, France. Available at URL: http://www.wma.net/e/policy/17-c_e.html. Accessed May 6, 2002.

76. Council for International Organizations of Medical Sciences (CIOMS). International Ethical Guidelines for Biomedical Research Involving Human Subjects. Geneva: CIOMS, 1993.

77. U.S. Code of Federal Regulations. Title 45, Part 46, Subpart A. Washington, DC: US Government Printing Office, 2001.

78. U.S. Code of Federal Regulations. Title 21, Part 50. Washington, DC: US Government Printing Office, 2001.

79. U.S. Code of Federal Regulations. Title 21, Part 312.21. Washington, DC: US Government Printing Office, 2001.

80. U.S. Code of Federal Regulations. Title 21, Part 312.20. Washington, DC: US Government Printing Office, 2001.

81. Ellenberg SS. Evaluating the safety of combination vaccines. Clin Infect Dis 2001; 33(Suppl 4):S319–322.

82. Ellenberg SS. Safety considerations for new vaccine development. Pharmacoepidemiol Drug Saf 2001; 10:411–415.

83. US Code of Federal Regulations Title 21, Part 312.42. Washington, DC: US Government Printing Office, 2001.

84. Food and Drug Administration. Draft guidance for clinical trial sponsors on the establishment and operation of clinical trial data monitoring committees. Fed Regul 2001; 66:58151–58153. Available from URL: http://fda.gov.dockets/98fr/112001.htm.

85. Simon R. Are placebo-controlled clinical trials ethical or needed when alternative treatment exists? Ann Intern Med 2000; 133:474–475.

86. Temple R, Ellenberg SS. Placebo-controlled trials and active-control trials in the evaluation of new treatments. Part 1: ethical and scientific issues. Ann Intern Med 2000; 133:455–463.

87. National Bioethics Advisory Commission (NBAC). Ethical and Policy Issues in International Research. Vol. 2. Rockville, MD: US Government Printing Office, 2001.

88. Shapiro HT, Meslin EM. Ethical issues in the design and conduct of clinical trials in developing countries. N Engl J Med 2001; 345:139–142.

89. Koski G, Nightengale SL. Research involving human subjects in developing countries. N Engl J Med 2001; 345:136–138.

90. Miller FG, Grady C. The ethical challenge of infection-inducing challenge experiments. Clin Infect Dis 2001 Oct 1; 33(7):1028–1033.

91. Food and Drug Administration. New drug and biological drug products; Evidence needed to demonstrate effectiveness of new drugs when human efficacy studies are not ethical or feasible. Fed Reg 2002; 67:37988–37998. Available from URL: http://www.fda.gov/cber/rules/humeffic.pdf. Accessed June 30, 2002.

92. Gross DM, et al. Identification of LFA-1 as a candidate autoantigen in treatment-resistant Lyme arthritis. Science 1998; 281:703–706.

93. Steere SL, et al. Vaccination against Lyme disease with recombinant *Borrelia burgdorferi* outer-surface lipoprotein with adjuvant. N Engl J Med 1998; 339:209–215.

94. Chen RT, et al. The Vaccine Adverse Event .Reporting System (VAERS). Vaccine 1994; 12:542–550.

95. Ellenberg SS, Chen RT. The complicated task of monitoring vaccine safety. Pub Health Rep 1997; 112:10–20.

96. US Code of Federal Regulations Title 21, Part 600.80. Washington, DC: US Government Printing Office, 2001.

97. Ellenberg SS, Braun MM. Monitoring the safety of vaccines: assessing the risks. Drug Saf 2002; 25:145–152.

98. Wise RP, et al. Hair loss following routine immunizations. JAMA 1997; 287:1176–1178.

99. Ball R, et al. Stevens Johnson syndrome after vaccination: reports to the Vaccine Adverse Event Reporting System. Pediatr Infect Dis J 2001; 20:219–223.

100. Beeler J, et al. Thrombocytopenia after immunization with measles vaccines: Review of the Vaccine Adverse Events Reporting System (1990 to 1994). Pediatr Infect Dis J 1996; 15:88–90.

101. Braun MM, et al. Syncope after immunization. Arch Pediatr Adolesc Med 1997; 151:255–259.

102. DuVernoy TS, Braun MM. Hypotonic Hyporesponsive Episodes Reported to the Vaccine Adverse Event Reporting System (VAERS), 1996–1998. Pediatrics 2000; 106:e52.

103. Niu MT, et al. Recombinant hepatitis B vaccination of neonates and infants: Emerging safety data from the Vaccine Adverse Event Reporting System. Pediatr Infect Dis J 1996; 15:771–776.

104. Wattigney WA, et al. Surveillance for poliovirus vaccine adverse events, 1991–1999: Impact of a sequential vaccination schedule of inactivated poliovirus vaccine followed by oral poliovirus vaccine. Pediatrics 2000; 107:e83.

105. Wise RP, et al. Postlicensure safety surveillance for varicella vaccine. JAMA 2000; 284:1271–1279.

106. Braun MM, et al, the VAERS Working Group. Infant immunization with acellular pertussis vaccines in the US: assessment of the first two years' data from the Vaccine Adverse Event Reporting System (VAERS). Pediatrics 2000; 106:e51. Available from: URL: http://www.pediatrics.org/.

107. Martin MM, et al. Advanced age a risk factor for illness temporally associated with yellow fever vaccination. Emerg Infect Dis 2001; 7:945–951.

108. Ball R, et al. Safety data on meningococcal polysaccharide vaccine from the Vaccine Adverse Event Reporting System. Clin Infect Dis 2001; 32:1273–1280.

109. Lathrop S, et al. Adverse event reports following vaccination for Lyme disease: December 1998–2000. Vaccine 2002; 20:1603–1608.

110. Silvers LE, et al. The epidemiology of fatalities reported to the Vaccine Adverse Event Reporting System, 1990–1997. Pharmacoepidemiol Drug Saf 2001; 10:279–285.

111. Zanardi L, et al. Intussusception among recipients of rotavirus vaccine: reports to the Vaccine Adverse Event Reporting System. Pediatrics 2001; 107:e97.

112. Rosenthal S, Chen R. The reporting sensitivities of two passive surveillance systems for vaccine adverse events. Am J Public Health 1995; 85:1706–1709.

113. Singleton JA, et al. An overview of the Vaccine Adverse Event Reporting System (VAERS) as a surveillance system. Vaccine 1999; 17:2908–2917.

114. Ball R, et al. Development of Case Definitions for Acute Encephalopathy, Encephalitis, and Multiple Sclerosis Reports to the Vaccine Adverse Event Reporting System. J Clin Epidemiol. In press.

115. Braun MM, et al. Report of a US Public Health Service Workshop on Hypotonic–Hyporesponsive Episode (HHE) Following Pertussis Immunization. Pediatrics 1998; 102:e52. Available from: URL: http://www.pediatrics.org/.

116. Brighton Collaboration. Available from: URL: http// www.brightoncollaboration.org/. Accessed May 20, 2002.

117. Fenichel GM, et al. Adverse events following immunization: assessing probability of causation. Pediatr Neurol 1989; 5:287–290.

118. Collet JP, et al. the advisory committee on causality assessment. Monitoring signals for vaccine safety: the assessment of individual adverse event reports by an expert advisory committee. Bull WHO 2000; 78:178–185.

119. Sever JL, et al. Safety of anthrax vaccine: a review by the anthrax vaccine expert committee (AVEC) of adverse events reported to the vaccine adverse event reporting system (VAERS). Pharmacoepidemiol Drug Saf 2002; 11:189–202.

120. Halsey NA. Anthrax vaccine and causality assessment from individual case reports. Pharmacoepidemiol Drug Saf 2002; 11:185–187.

121. Sever JL, et al. Response to editorial by Dr. Neal Halsey. Pharmacoepidemiol Drug Saf 2002; 11:189–202.

122. Jones JK. Determining causation form case reports. In: Strom BL, ed. Pharmacoepidemiology. 3rd edition. John Wiley and Sons, 2000.

123. Mortimer E. Stevens Johnson Syndrome after vaccination. Pediatr Infect Dis J 2001; 20:818–819.

124. Ball R, et al. Stevens Johnson Syndrome after vaccination. Pediatr Infect Dis J 2001; 20:819.

125. Evans SW, et al. Use of proportional reporting ratios for signal generation from spontaneous adverse drug reaction reports. Pharmacoepidemiol Drug Saf 2001; 10, 483–486.

126. Dumouchel W. Bayesian data mining in large frequency tables, with an application to the FDA spontaneous reporting system. Am Stat 1999; 53:177–190.

127. Niu MT, et al. Data mining in the US Vaccine Adverse Event Reporting System (VAERS): early detection of intussusception and other events after rotavirus vaccination. Vaccine 2001; 19:4627–4634.

128. Bortnichak EA, et al. Proactive safety surveillance. Pharmacoepidemiol Drug Saf 2001; 10:191–196.

129. Walker AM, Wise RP. Precautions for Proactive Surveillance. Pharmacoepidemiol Drug Saf. In press.

130. Mehta U, et al. Developing a national system for dealing with adverse events following immunization. Bull WHO 2000; 78:170–177.

131. Chen RT, et al. Vaccine Safety Datalink Project: a new tool for improving vaccine safety monitoring in the United States. Pediatrics 1997; 99:765–773.

132. DeStefano F. The Vaccine Safety Datalink project. Pharmacoepidemiol Drug Saf 2001; 10:403–406.

133. Barlow WE, et al. The risk of seizures after receipt of whole-cell pertussis or measles, mumps, and rubella vaccine. N Engl J Med 2001; 345:656–661.

134. Niu MT, et al. Comparative safety of two recombinant hepatitis B vaccines in children: data from the Vaccine Adverse Event Reporting System (VAERS) and Vaccine Safety Datalink (VSD). J Clin Epidemiol 1998; 151:503–510.

135. Ray P, et al. Risk of chronic arthropathy among women after rubella vaccination. Vaccine Safety Datalink Team. JAMA 1997; 278:551–556.

136. DeStefano F, et al. Childhood vaccinations, vaccination timing, and risk of type 1 diabetes mellitus. Pediatrics 2001; 108:e112.

137. Davis RL, et al. Measles–mumps–rubella and other measles-containing vaccines do not increase the risk for inflammatory bowel disease: a case-control study from the Vaccine Safety Datalink project. Arch Pediatr Adolesc Med 2001; 155:354–359.

138. Laurenson R, et al. Clinical information for research; the use of general practice databases. J Public Health Med 1999; 21:299–304.

139. Kaye JA, et al. Measles and rubella vaccine and the incidence of autism recorded by general practitioners: a time trend analysis. BMJ 2001; 322:460–463.

140. Jick H, et al. Live attenuated polio vaccine and the risk of intussusception. Br J Clin Pharmacol 2001; 52:451–453.

141. Ascherio A, et al. Hepatitis B vaccination and the risk of multiple sclerosis. N Engl J Med 2001; 344:327–332.

142. Confavreux C, et al. Vaccinations and the risk of relapse in multiple sclerosis study group. N Engl J Med 2001; 344:319–326.

143. Gellin BG, Schaffner W. The risk of vaccination—the importance of "negative" studies. N Engl J Med 2001; 344:372–373.

144. Lasky T, et al. The Guillain–Barre syndrome and the 1992–1993 and 1993–1994 influenza vaccines. N Engl J Med 1998; 339:1797–1802.

145. Gold M, et al. Re-vaccination of 421 children with a past history of an adverse vaccine reaction in a special immunisation service. Arch Dis Child 2000; 83:128–131.

146. Mitchel LA, et al. HLA-DR class II associations with rubella vaccine-induced joint manifestations. J Infect Dis 1998; 177:5–12.

147. Piyasirisilp S, et al. Association of HLA and T-cell receptor gene polymorphisms with Semple rabies vaccine-induced autoimmune encephalomyelitis. Ann Neurol 1999; 45:595–600.

148. Hacker UT, et al. In vivo synthesis of tumor necrosis factor alpha in healthy humans after live yellow fever vaccination. J Infect Dis 1998; 177:774–778.

149. Pourcyrous M, et al. Interleukin-6, C-reactive protein, and abnormal cardiorespiratory response to immunization in premature infants. Pediatrics 1998; 101:e3. Available from: URL: http://www.pediatrics.org.

150. Hill AB. The environment and disease: association or causation? Proc R Soc Med 1965; 58:295–300.

151. Rothman KJ. Modern Epidemiology. Boston: Little Brown & Co, 1986.

152. Wydner EL. Epidemiological issues in weak associations. Int J Epidemiol 1990; 19:S5–S7.

153. Monson RR. The interpretation of epidemiological data. Occupational Epidemiology. Boca Raton, FL: CRC Press, 1980.

154. National Research Council, Committee on the Institutional Means for Assessment of the Risks to Public Health. Risk Assessment in the Federal Government: Managing the Process. Washington, DC: National Academy Press, 1983.

155. Ball LK, et al. Assessment of thimerosal use in childhood vaccines. Pediatrics 2001; 107:1147–1154.

156. Clements CJ, et al. Thiomersal in vaccines (letter). Lancet 2000; 355:1279–1280.

157. Petitti DB. Meta-analysis, Decision Analysis, and Cost Effectiveness Analysis. New York: Oxford University Press, 1994.

158. Miller MA, Hinman AR. Cost–benefit and cost-effectiveness analysis of vaccine policy. In: Plotkin SA, Orenstein WA, eds. Vaccines. 3rd ed. Philadelphia, PA: WB Saunders Co, 1999.

159. Lieu TA, et al. Projected cost-effectiveness of pneumococcal conjugate vaccination of healthy infants and young children. JAMA 2000; 283:1460–1468.

160. Lieu TA, et al. The hidden costs of infant vaccines. Vaccine 2000; 19:33–41.

161. Zimmerman RK, et al. A national survey to understand why physicians defer childhood immunizations. Arch Pediatr Adolesc Med 1997; 15:657–664.

162. Sansom SL, et al. Rotavirus vaccine and intussusception: how much risk will parents in the United States accept to obtain vaccine benefits? Am J Epidemiol 2001; 154:1077–1085.

163. Abramson JS, Pickering LK. US immunization policy. JAMA 2002; 287:505–509.

164. Gellin BG, et al. Do parents understand immunizations? A national telephone survey. Pediatrics 2000; 106:1097–1102.

165. Stratton K, et al, eds. Immunization Safety Review: Measles–Mumps–Rubella Vaccine and Autism. Washington DC: National Academy Press, 2001a.

166. Stratton K, et al, eds. Immunization Safety Review: Thimerosal-containing Vaccines and Neurodevelopmental Disorders. Washington, DC: National Academy Press, 2001b.

167. Stratton K, et al, eds. Immunization Safety Review: Multiple Immunizations and Immune Dysfunction. Washington, DC: National Academy Press, 2002.

168. Stratton K, McCormick M, eds. Immunization Safety Review: Hepatitis B Vaccine and Demyelinating Neurological Disorders. Washington, DC: National Academy Press, 2002.

169. Food and Drug Administration. Managing the risks from medical product use: Creating a risk management framework. Report to the FDA Commissioner from the Task Force on Risk Management. May 1999a. Available from URL: http://www.fda.gov/oc/tfrm/riskmanagement.html. Accessed May 6, 2002.

170. Feudtner C, Marcuse EK. Ethics and immunization policy: promoting dialogue to sustain consensus. Pediatrics 2001; 107:1158–1164.

171. Evans G, et al. Risk Communication and Vaccination: Workshop Summary. Washington, DC: National Academy Press, 1997.

172. Ball LK, et al. Risky Business: Challenges in vaccine risk communication. Pediatrics 1998; 101:453–458.

173. Breiman RF, Zanca JA. Of floors and ceilings—defining, assuring, and communicating vaccine safety. Am J Public Health 1997; 87:1919–1920.

174. Feikin DR, et al. Individual and community risks of measles and pertussis associated with personal exemptions to immunization. JAMA 2000; 284:3145–3150.

175. Salmon DA, et al. Health consequences of religious and philosophical exemptions from immunization laws: individual and societal risk of measles. JAMA 1999; 282:47–53.

176. Cohen V. Vaccines and risks: the responsibility of the media, scientists, and clinicians. JAMA 1996; 276:1917–1918.

177. Slovic P. Perception of Risk. Science 1987; 236:282.

178. Slovic P. The Perception of Risk: Risk Science and Society Series. In: Lofsted RE, ed. London: Earthscan Publications Ltd, 2000.

179. Coussens CM, Fischoff B. Science and Risk Communication: A Mini-Symposium Sponsored By the Roundtable on Environmental Health Sciences, Research, and Medicine. Institute of Medicine. National Academy Press, 2002. Available from: URL: http://books.nap.edu/books/NI000368/html/. Accessed May 6, 2002.

180. Bennett P. Understanding Responses to Risk. In: Bennett P, Calman K, eds. Risk Communication and Public Health. New York, NY: Oxford University Press, 1999.

181. Covello VT, et al. Guidelines for communicating information about chemical risks prospectively and responsively. In: Mayo DG, Hollander D, eds. Acceptable Evidence: Science and Values in Risk Management. New York, NY: Oxford University Press, 1991:66–90.

182. Witte K. Putting the fear back in fear appeals: the extended parallel process model. Commun Monogr 1992; 59:329–349.

183. Wolfe RM, et al. Content and design attributes of anti-vaccination web sites. JAMA 2002; 281:3245–3248.

184. Danovaro-Holliday MC, et al. Rotavirus vaccine and the news media. JAMA 2002; 287:1455–1462.

185. Massell BF, et al. Rheumatic fever following streptococcal vaccination. JAMA 1969; 207:1115–1119.

13

Polio Eradication: Capturing the Full Potential of a Vaccine

R. Bruce Aylward, Rudolph Tangermann, and Roland Sutter
World Health Organization, Geneva, Switzerland

Stephen L. Cochi
Centers for Disease Control and Prevention, Atlanta, Georgia, U.S.A.

I. INTRODUCTION

In 1980, certification of the eradication of smallpox finally confirmed that certain diseases could not only be successfully controlled at very low incidence, but actually eradicated such that the control measures could be stopped, potentially for all time [1]. That a vaccine was the tool behind this first successful eradication initiative reaffirmed the promise and the potential of immunization in achieving this "ultimate goal of public health" [2]. The eradication of smallpox is frequently cited as the most important international public health achievement in the 20th century, and for many years has stood as a unique testament to humankind's capacity to completely eliminate a significant cause of morbidity and mortality [3].

It is now increasingly certain, however, that the early years of the 21st century will see the successful eradication of another important pathogen, in this case poliomyelitis, and again with immunization as the core strategy [4]. Despite having been launched in an environment that was rather hostile to targeted programs in the years following smallpox eradication [5], the global polio eradication initiative has grown to become the largest international health initiative ever, with the capacity to not only eliminate one of the leading causes of permanent disability, but to substantially enhance the capacity to control other important diseases, particularly those that are vaccine-preventable [6,7].

This chapter outlines the rationale for launching an eradication initiative against polio in 1988, the progress that has been made as of end-2001, and the challenges that remain to certify the world as polio-free, to achieve containment of wild poliovirus stocks, and to develop international consensus on postcertification polio immunization policy.

II. RATIONALE FOR POLIO ERADICATION

Building on the lessons of nearly 100 years of disease eradication, two international conferences in the late 1990s proposed three major criteria that should be met prior to undertaking the eradication of a specific disease [8,9]. These criteria provide a useful framework for explaining the rationale for launching the global polio eradication initiative: (1) biological and technical feasibility, (2) a positive benefit:cost ratio, and (3) sufficient societal and political support (Table 1).

A. Technical Feasibility

The issues that are central to evaluating the biological and technical feasibility of eradicating a disease [10] can be summarized as follows:

> An effective intervention and delivery strategy that can interrupt transmission
> Practical diagnostic tools with sufficient sensitivity and specificity
> Absence of a nonhuman reservoir.

There must also be "proof of concept," with the application of these interventions, strategies, and tools having been proven to interrupt the transmission of the target organism in a large geographical area [9]. By 1988, these issues had been largely resolved for polio through a combination of the available scientific background information and the progress toward regional eradication in the western hemisphere (WHO Region of the Americas) [11,12].

In terms of an effective intervention and delivery strategy, health authorities in Cuba had demonstrated as early as 1962 that the intermittent pulsing of the child population with oral poliovirus vaccine (OPV) in mass campaigns could

Table 1 Poliomyelitis and the 1997 Dahlem Eradication
Criteria

Criteria for targeting a disease for eradication	Poliomyelitis
Biological and technical feasibility	
Etiologic agent	Virus
Nonhuman reservoir	No
Effective intervention tool	OPV
Effective delivery strategy	NIDs
Simple/practical diagnostic	Stool culture
Sensitive surveillance	Facility-based active surveillance
Field-proven strategies	Western hemisphere
Costs and benefits	
Cases averted per year	> 350 000
Coincident benefits	Improved immunization and surveillance capacity
Intangible benefits	Culture of prevention and social equity
Estimated annual direct global savings	US$1.5 billion
Estimated total external financing	US$2.75 billion
Societal and political considerations	
Political commitment (endemic/industrial countries)	Variable/variable
Societal support (endemic/industrial countries)	Strong/strong
Disease burden in politically unstable areas (% cases from war-torn countries)	10–20% (estimated)
Core partnerships and advocates	WHO, Rotary, CDC, UNICEF
Technical consensus	World Health Assembly
Donor base (number of donors of US$1 million or more in 1998–1999)	26

WHO = World Health Organization; CDC = U.S. Centers for Disease
Control and Prevention.

rapidly interrupt the transmission of wild poliovirus [13,14].
By the 1980s, this strategy was having a similar impact in
Brazil [15], leading the Regional Director of the Pan American Health Organization (PAHO) to launch a regional
elimination campaign in 1985 [16].

The eradication initiative relied on the use of OPV in
countries where polio was endemic or had recently been
endemic, because inactivated poliovirus vaccine (IPV) had
only interrupted transmission in three industrialized
countries, all in northern Europe and all with very high
routine immunization coverage (Finland, the Netherlands,
and Sweden). Not only had OPV been found capable of
stopping transmission in tropical climates, it also induced

secretory intestinal immunity superior to that of IPV and
protected some close contacts of vaccinees [17,18]. Furthermore, the low cost and oral administration route of OPV
made it much more suited to the mass delivery strategy
required for eradication. Although there has been substantial opposition to the use of this campaign strategy, routine
immunization alone was proven to be insufficient to stop
wild poliovirus transmission in most developing countries
[19], even as coverage increased steadily after the establishment of the Expanded Program on Immunization (EPI) in
1974 [20].

Establishing a sensitive and specific system for polio
diagnosis was as demanding as the challenges of implementing mass OPV campaigns. Unlike the characteristic rash and
consequent scarring caused by smallpox, the majority of wild
poliovirus infections (> 99%) are subclinical [21] and cannot
be definitively confirmed clinically, even when there is paralysis [22,23]. Serological testing was inadequate for polio
diagnosis because it could not reliably distinguish antibodies
due to wild polioviruses from those produced by the vaccine.
Consequently, viral culture from stool specimens became the
preferred method for diagnosing polio in the eradication
initiative [24].

To practically apply this tool, PAHO developed a strategy of acute flaccid paralysis (AFP) surveillance, whereby all
cases of AFP in persons aged less than 15 years were to be
investigated, with the collection of two stool specimens
within 14 days of paralysis onset [25]. Because AFP cases
occur in the absence of polio, a standard of >1 case of nonpolio AFP per 100,000 population aged less than 15 years
was established as the principal indicator of surveillance
sensitivity for eradication [26–28]. Combined with indicators
for the completeness of specimen collection (target > 80%)
and their processing in a World Health Organization (WHO)-
accredited laboratory (target 100%), this allowed international comparisons of surveillance performance [29] and the
demonstration that surveillance was sufficient for certification [30]. A global network of enterovirus laboratories, with
a detailed accreditation system, was developed to ensure
reliable isolation, identification, and genomic characterization of poliovirus from the stool specimens of AFP cases
[31,32] (Fig. 1).

Finally, polio eradication is biologically feasible because humans are essential for the life cycle of the virus,
which has no other reservoir and does not amplify in the
environment. Although polio has been described among
orangutans, chimpanzees, gorillas in captivity, and chimpanzees in the wild, these species appear to be incidental
hosts with populations too small to sustain transmission
[33]. Similarly, viable viruses cannot be found in sewage or
surface water for more than several weeks after circulation
ceases among humans [33].

B. Benefit:Cost Ratio of Eradication

The direct humanitarian benefits of ensuring that polio will
never again be experienced by any person in perpetuity are
substantial. In the absence of vaccination, 0.5% of children
(i.e., 650,000) in every annual birth cohort of ca. 130 million
infants would become paralyzed as a result of poliovirus

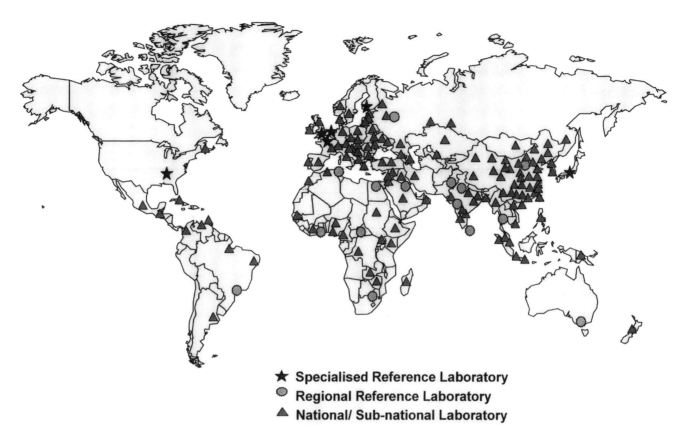

★ **Specialised Reference Laboratory**
◎ **Regional Reference Laboratory**
▲ **National/ Sub-national Laboratory**

Figure 1   Network of enterovirus laboratories that comprise the Global Polio Laboratory Network as of June 2002.

infection [34]. As recently as 1988, the year the eradication goal was adopted, an estimated 350,000 cases of paralytic polio were still occurring [35]. Because the majority of victims survive the acute illness, the prevalence of paralytic cases may be as high as 20 million. Lameness surveys in the 1970s revealed polio to be a leading cause of permanent disability in developing countries [36,37]. In the 1990s, surveys in Afghanistan and Cambodia demonstrated that polio continued to be a leading cause of permanent disability even in war-torn countries [38].

Economic analyses of disease eradication are problematic and somewhat controversial because of the lack of consensus on how to value benefits that accrue in perpetuity [39]. Despite these limitations, several attempts have been made to estimate the economic costs and benefits of poliomyelitis eradication [40–42]. The most comprehensive analysis estimated annual global savings of US$1.5 billion per year once polio has been eradicated and all control measures have been stopped [40]. A more recent analysis suggests that even in a "worst case scenario" in which a universal IPV strategy was implemented following global certification, the cost per DALY saved would still be quite low at less than US$50 [42].

Although these direct benefits of polio eradication are substantial, it was the indirect or consequent benefits that formed the basis for launching the initiative in the Americas [43] and were central to the World Health Assembly resolu-

tion that endorsed the global eradication target [44]. The "indirect benefits" included the potential for boosting immunization programs and for establishing sensitive surveillance systems, and were as important as the eradication of the disease itself [45].

C.   Societal and Political Support for Eradication

Perhaps the least understood determinant of the feasibility of eradicating an organism is the need for sufficient societal and political commitment to launch and to sustain such an initiative through the 15–20 years that will be required to implement the necessary strategies [46]. Although the successful conclusion of the smallpox eradication campaign in 1977 created some momentum for new eradication efforts, this enthusiasm was countered by concerns that pursuing targeted objectives could compromise efforts to develop strong primary health care systems [5]. Within the scientific community, substantial doubts as to the technical feasibility of polio eradication [47] were increasingly resolved with the progress in the Americas by the mid-1980s.

The event that is considered to have been pivotal in transforming the regional PAHO elimination goal into a global effort was a March 1988 meeting convened by the Task Force for Child Survival and Development [48]. During this meeting, the Director-General of WHO was convinced of the merit of a global eradication effort and, only 2 months later, put the matter to a vote at the World Health Assembly. In May 1988, the World Health Assembly, consisting of the Ministers of Health of all member states, unanimously endorsed the polio eradication resolution [44]. The eradication goal was subsequently reviewed and endorsed by the World Summit for Children in 1990, the largest ever gathering of Heads of State [49]. Health and political leaders from low-income, middle-income, and high-income countries have continued to reconfirm their commitment through resolutions adopted in forums such as the Organization of African Unity (OAU), the South Asian Association for Regional Cooperation (SAARC), and the 2002 G8 summit [50,51]. These leaders have repeatedly reinforced and publicly demonstrated their leadership role by participating in highly visible events such as the launching of National Immunization Days (NIDs).

III. PROGRESS TOWARD GLOBAL POLIO ERADICATION

A. Implementation of the Eradication Strategies

The principal strategies employed by the global polio eradication initiative were developed in the WHO Region of the Americas during the 1980s [43] and consist of: (1) achieving and maintaining high coverage with at least three doses of oral polio vaccine (OPV3); (2) providing supplementary doses of OPV to all children aged < 5 years during NIDs; (3) surveillance for all cases of AFP in children aged under 15 years of age, with the virological examination of stool specimens from each case; and (4) house-to-house OPV "mop-up" campaigns, targeting areas with persisting wild poliovirus transmission.

Reaching and maintaining high OPV3 coverage is the foundation of polio eradication. In a number of temperate, industrialized countries, high OPV3 alone has been sufficient to interrupt the transmission of wild poliovirus [52]. In developing countries, however, polio transmission usually persists, even with good OPV3 coverage, due to suboptimal sanitation, high population density, and lower levels of seroconversion compared with temperate climates [53]. Furthermore, global OPV3 coverage was only 67% in 1988, the year the global initiative began, and never reached more than 80% in the subsequent years [54], with substantial differences between WHO regions. As recently as 1999, the African Region had coverage of less than 50%.

The use of supplementary OPV campaigns for polio eradication is based on the work of Sabin et al. [55] and Grachev [56], who first used mass immunization to control polio epidemics in Hungary [57] and the Soviet Union. The PAHO refined the strategy prior to recommending NIDs for all endemic countries in the Americas in 1985. The effectiveness and global applicability of the NID strategy were further established in China and other countries of the Western Pacific Region [58,59] in the mid-1990s. National Immunization Days are conducted during the low season of poliovirus transmission in two rounds, 4–6 weeks apart [60]. During each round, OPV is administered to all children < 5 years of age, regardless of previous immunization status. By

rapidly increasing the systemic and intestinal immunity in this group, NIDs raise the overall level of immunity of the population, decreasing further spread of the virus [61]. As of 1999, NIDs had been introduced in all countries endemic for wild poliovirus, with subnational rounds added where appropriate.

Even with high-quality NIDs in individual countries, however, people crossing borders could transmit polio in the interval between the NIDs in one country and its neighbor, thus reestablishing virus circulation and reducing impact. Recognizing this, many countries decided to synchronize their NIDs (Fig. 2). In "Operation MECACAR," for example, 18 countries of the MEditerranean, CAucasus, Central Asian Republics, and Russia immunized 56 million children in each of two rounds in April and May 1995 [62]. Similar activities followed in South Asia and West Africa [63,64]. In July 2001, the conflict-affected countries of the Democratic Republic of the Congo, Angola, Congo, and Gabon began three rounds of synchronized NIDs, reaching 15 million children [4,64]. In most countries, NIDs were the largest public health activities ever conducted. China repeatedly immunized > 80 million children during NIDs, whereas up to 150 million children continue to be targeted during NID rounds in India [63,65]. In 2001 alone, NIDs or sub-NIDs reached over 575 million children in 94 countries [4].

Although process indicators and coverage estimates help evaluate the quality of NIDs, surveillance outcomes have been the real measure of their effectiveness [66]. By 2001, all WHO regions were approaching "certification quality" AFP surveillance, as measured by the three key AFP performance indicators (Table 2) [4]. Through a massive investment in human resources, equipment, and training, certification standard AFP reporting had been achieved or was imminent in countries as challenging as Afghanistan, Angola, the Democratic Republic of the Congo, Somalia, and southern Sudan. In the year 2001, every one of the 63,392 diagnostic specimens from 31,429 AFP cases in the world were processed in 1 of 145 WHO-accredited "polio" laboratories worldwide, with results for 91% of cases reported within 28 days after receiving the specimens [32].

Once surveillance has identified a final reservoir of wild poliovirus, mop-up campaigns are conducted on a house-to-house basis to ensure that every child in the area is found and immunized [12,17,43]. Massive mop-up campaigns were first used to interrupt the last foci of transmission in the Americas in Colombia in 1991 (850,000 children) and in Peru in 1992 (1.9 million children) [43]. During 1995–1997, mop-up campaigns targeting 3 million children eliminated the last polio reservoir of the WHO Western Pacific Region in the Mekong River delta area [67]. A two-region, four-country mop-up operation across Turkey, Syria, Iran, and Iraq interrupted the last chains of transmission in the WHO Region of Europe [68].

B. The Polio Eradication Infrastructure

Although polio eradication activities have been led, coordinated, and implemented by the governments of the polio-infected countries themselves, the support of an extraordinary partnership has been essential. This public–

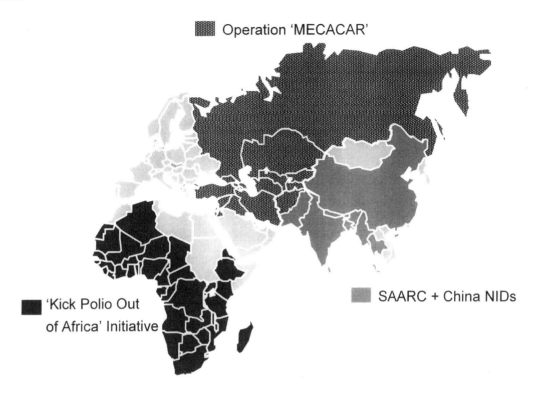

Figure 2 Selected examples of coordinated NIDs for the purpose of polio eradication (see text).

Table 2 Status and Results of Surveillance for Wild Poliovirus as Measured by Standard Performance Indicators, by WHO Region, 2001[a]

Region/country[b]	AFP cases reported	Annualized nonpolio AFP rate[c]	AFP cases with adequate specimens[d] (%)	Wild poliovirus confirmed cases
Africa	8,542	2.96	72	69
Angola	149	2.40	66	1
Ethiopia	553	1.90	47	1
Niger	229	4.40	80	6
Nigeria	1,937	3.80	67	56
Americas	2,192	1.15	90	0
Eastern Mediterranean	3,865	1.9	83	140
Afghanistan	214	1.69	74	11
Egypt	257	1.19	91	5
Pakistan	1,573	2.32	84	119
Somalia	129	4.09	59	7
Sudan	303	2.15	74	1
Europe	1,764	1.17	81	3[e]
Southeast Asia	10,612	1.85	83	268
India	7,470	1.86	83	268
Western Pacific	6,529	1.40	88	0
Global	33,504	1.62	82	483

[a] Data for 2001 as of August 10, 2002.

[b] Country totals reflect endemic countries and do not add up to regional and global totals.

[c] Annualized nonpoliomyelitis AFP rate per 100,000 persons aged <15 years.

[d] Two stool specimens collected within 14 days of onset of paralysis.

[e] Importations.

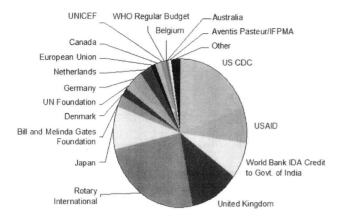

Figure 3 International contributions to the global polio eradication initiative, 1988–2001 (US$1870 million).

private partnership, spearheaded by the WHO, Rotary International, the U.S. Centers for Disease Control and Prevention (CDC), and the United Nations Children's Fund (UNICEF) has facilitated the inputs of donor governments (e.g., bilateral development agencies), other international organizations (e.g., UN funds, agencies, and programs), foundations, corporations, nongovernmental organizations (NGOs), and humanitarian organizations. The most remarkable of these partners is Rotary International, the private sector service organization which, through its Polio-Plus Program and 1.2 million members worldwide, will have contributed nearly US$600 million by end-2005 (Fig. 3).

Nongovernmental and humanitarian organizations such as the International Red Cross and Red Crescent Movement, Medecins Sans Frontieres (MSF), Save the

Children Fund, World Vision, and CARE have collaborated, particularly in conflict-affected areas. United Nations agencies have facilitated activities through the provision of transport, human resources, security, and communications. The WHO alone has deployed 2000 national and international staff to assist the implementation of eradication activities worldwide (Fig. 4).

A variety of mechanisms were established at the global, regional, and country levels to coordinate this partnership. Strategical planning, policy development, and priority setting are discussed and agreed through technical oversight bodies convened by WHO every 6–12 months at the global and regional levels. Resource mobilization and financing is managed through Interagency Coordinating Committee (ICC) meetings, at the regional and country levels. Similar mechanisms have been established to manage the core partnership and the global laboratory network.

C. Impact on Polio Transmission

When the global polio eradication initiative was launched in 1988, over 125 countries on five continents were known or suspected to have had indigenous transmission of wild poliovirus (Fig. 5). Wild poliovirus transmission was confirmed in all six of the WHO geopolitical regional groupings. Although only 35,031 cases were reported worldwide in 1988 [69], it is estimated that over 350,000 children were actually paralyzed in that year, with over 90% having gone unreported [3,35]. Fully half of these cases occurred on the Asian subcontinent, with the majority in India. Outside of the Americas, which had launched its regional eradication initiative in 1985, only a handful of areas, mainly industrialized countries and small island nations, were free of polio at that time.

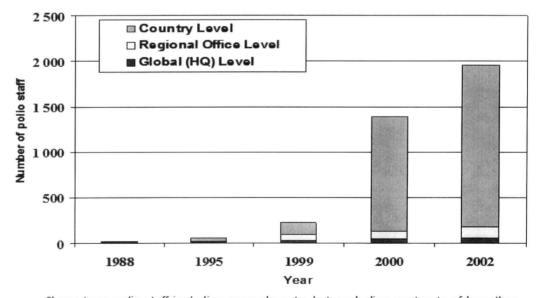

*Long term polio staff including secondments, but excluding contracts of less than six months and drivers. (year 2002 total including drivers = 2 515).

Figure 4 Growth of WHO national and international staff deployed through the polio eradication initiative, as of June 2002.

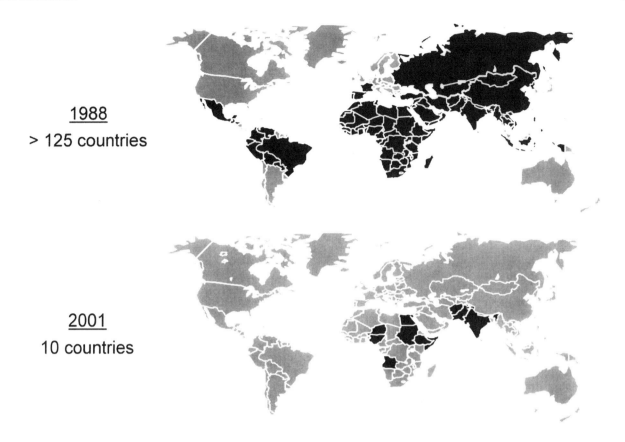

1988

> 125 countries

2001

10 countries

Figure 5   Known and suspected distribution of indigenous wild poliovirus in 1988, the year the global polio eradication initiative was launched, and at end-2001.

Following the WHA resolution to eradicate polio, progress was most rapid in the Americas, with the last case occurring in Peru in August 1991 [43]. In fact, it was only in the early to mid-1990s that strategy implementation began in earnest in other areas, most notably the Western Pacific, Eastern Mediterranean, and European Regions of WHO. Of the 28 countries of the Western Pacific, only six were still endemic by 1993: China, Cambodia, the Lao People's Democratic Republic (Lao PDR), the Philippines, and Vietnam [67]. As NIDs and mop-up campaigns were introduced by the mid-1990s, transmission was rapidly interrupted, with the last case occurring in Cambodia in March 1997 [67]. In the European Region, progress accelerated when NIDs were synchronized with the Eastern Mediterranean in Operation MECACAR, beginning in March–April 1995 [62]. Although repeated importations continued to plague the European Region, by 1998, the only focus of indigenous transmission was in southeast Turkey, where the last case occurred in November of that year [68].

In the Southeast Asian Region of WHO, one of the most important milestones was the launching of NIDs in India in 1995 [51]. By 2001, transmission had stopped in 9 of 10 countries in this most densely populated of WHO regions [4]. The exception was India, where indigenous polio was restricted to only 2 of 30 states by late 2000. The cessation of transmission in Indonesia (last case in 1995) and Bangladesh

(last case in 2000) reinforced the effectiveness of the eradication strategies in even the most highly populated areas [4]. Many of the 23 countries of the Eastern Mediterranean Region introduced the strategies in the early 1990s and stopped transmission soon thereafter, particularly in north Africa, the countries of the Levant, and the Arab Gulf States [70]. By end-2001, intense transmission was limited to Pakistan, with less than 10 virus-confirmed cases from each of Afghanistan, Somalia, the Sudan, and Egypt in that year [4]. In the WHO Region of Africa, which comprises 46 countries mostly in sub-Saharan Africa, eradication really began with the 1996 "Polio-free Africa" declaration at the OAU, championed by Mr. Nelson Mandela [50]. Within 2 years, transmission had been interrupted in all countries of southern and eastern Africa, with the exception of Angola [71]. By end-2001, the intensity and quality of NIDs had increased in the region such that indigenous polio was restricted to Nigeria, Niger, and Angola [4]. Even the Democratic Republic of the Congo appeared to be polio-free by the end of that year.

By end-2001, polio was on the brink of eradication, with only 10 countries still endemic for the wild virus (Fig. 5) and just 480 virologically confirmed cases worldwide in that year [4]. The 10 remaining endemic countries constituted three "high-transmission" zones (north India, Pakistan/Afghanistan, and Nigeria/Niger) and three "low-transmission" zones (Horn of Africa—consisting of Ethiopia, Sudan, Somalia; Angola; and Egypt). India was of particular concern, with 56% of all cases worldwide, even though there had been a 50% reduction in the number of infected districts and a two-thirds decline in the number of lineages of circulating type 1 wild poliovirus compared with 2000. Of particular note, type 2 wild poliovirus has not been isolated anywhere in the world since October 1999 [72].

During 2001, the rapid containment of wild poliovirus importations into four previously polio-free areas reaffirmed the robustness of the progress that has been made. In Bulgaria, Georgia, Algeria, and Zambia, virus importations from other countries were successfully eliminated with large-scale surveillance and immunization response activities.

D. Impact on Other Health Services

Although there is widespread consensus that progress has been made in eradicating polioviruses [4], there is substantial controversy as to whether this has strengthened the delivery of other health services [6,73]. Some observers have felt that polio eradication has been detrimental to a sound, integrated approach to health systems development, whereas others have argued that any untoward effects of the initiative have been relatively minor and have been outweighed by the benefits [74–76]. A number of studies have attempted to reconcile these positions through evaluations of the relationship between polio eradication and routine immunization service delivery, disease surveillance, the delivery of other preventive services, health systems development, broader social and societal benefits, or a combination of the above.

Irrefutable benefits in the delivery of other health services include a marked expansion of vitamin A supplementation, enhanced global disease surveillance capacity, improved cooperation among enterovirus laboratories worldwide, and stronger partner coordinating mechanisms [7,77]. Including vitamin A supplements in polio NIDs averted an estimated 400,000 childhood deaths in 1998–1999 alone, and strengthened the links between EPI contacts and micronutrient supplementation [78,79]. The surveillance capacity developed for polio has now been used to detect and respond to outbreaks of important diseases such as measles, meningitis, cholera, and yellow fever [80]. The international consensus on the value of this "indirect benefit" is reflected in widespread support for plans to expand and sustain this capacity to enhance the control of other important public health problems. In most WHO regions and in many countries, the mandate of the ICC that was established for the coordination of polio eradication partner inputs has now been expanded to facilitate the broader immunization goals of the Global Alliance on Vaccines and Immunization (GAVI) [81,82].

More controversial has been the impact of eradication on the delivery of routine immunizations [75,83,84]. That the polio initiative has made a huge investment in the physical and human resources for routine immunization is incontrovertible; the cold chain, communications, and transport capacity have been largely replaced or refurbished in many low-income countries, particularly in sub-Saharan Africa, and tens of thousands of vaccinators have been trained or

retrained worldwide. The question remains as to whether the disruptions caused by polio NIDs will have only short-term effects or long-term impacts on routine services [6].

Despite the many studies that have been undertaken to evaluate the broader impact of polio eradication on health systems, most were hampered by a lack of credible baseline data, the absence of "control groups," and the concurrent implementation of major health system reforms, such as decentralization and sectorwide approaches [6,85]. Most commentators do agree that positive synergies exist between polio eradication and health systems development but that these opportunities must be better exploited [7,85,86].

IV. THE "POSTERADICATION" ERA

As was the case with smallpox, substantial work is required in the areas of certification, containment, and postcertification polio immunization policy to realize the full benefits of the polio eradication initiative.

A. Certification of Global Polio Eradication

In 1995, an independent 13-member Global Certification Commission (GCC) was established to develop the criteria for, and oversee the process of, certification of eradication of wild poliovirus transmission [87]. A formal process has now been developed, which focuses on epidemiological blocks of countries, the length of polio-free time, and the quality of surveillance (Fig. 6) [30]. The GCC has stated that the key criterion for global certification will be the absence of wild poliovirus transmission throughout the world for three consecutive years in the presence of excellent surveillance [87, 88]. Surveillance for cases of AFP will provide the most important information, with the quality demonstrated by the standard AFP indicators now in use by the eradication initiative [29,88]. Of particular importance will be the investigation of at least one case of nonpolio AFP per 100,000 children aged less than 15 years, with the collection of adequate stool specimens from at least 80% of cases. Such quality surveillance has now proven to be a key indicator of whether a surveillance system could detect polio if the virus was present.

The GCC also decided in 1995 that certification would be on a region-by-region basis, with commissions estab-

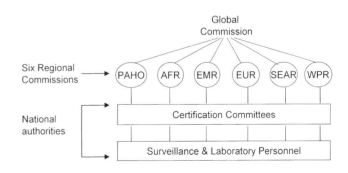

Figure 6 Structure of the process for global certification of the interruption of wild poliovirus transmission.

lished for each of the six WHO regions [87,88]. No region could be certified until every country had achieved the abovementioned criteria, with the data submitted and verified by a National Certification Committee. In 1997, the GCC stated that global certification would also require laboratory containment of wild poliovirus stocks and potentially infectious materials [88] as detailed in the *WHO Global Action Plan for the Containment of Wild Polioviruses* [89]. When two polio outbreaks were caused by circulating vaccine-derived polioviruses (cVDPVs) in 2000–2001 (see below), the GCC reviewed the implications for certification, deciding that it would be premature to include the absence of such events as a precondition for global certification [90].

The experience in three WHO regions (the Americas, Western Pacific, and Europe certified in 1994, 2000, and 2002, respectively), which comprises a total of 115 countries and over 3 billion people, has now demonstrated that the process and the criteria for certifying eradication of indigenous wild poliovirus transmission are sound [91].

B. Containment of Wild Polioviruses

That the last case of smallpox occurred as a result of a laboratory containment failure in Birmingham, England in 1978, 1 year after the global eradication of smallpox [92], serves as an important reminder of the need for effective containment of wild polioviruses. Consequently, the WHO began work on a global action plan for laboratory containment of wild polioviruses in 1997 to identify and to inventory laboratories worldwide that store wild poliovirus and potentially infectious materials, and to ensure that those materials are handled under appropriate biosafety conditions in the postcertification era. The goal of the containment plan is to reduce the risk of an accidental or intentional reintroduction of wild poliovirus into the community from a laboratory or vaccine production site.

The process of laboratory containment was developed through international consultation with a draft action plan widely distributed for comment in 1998, prior to publication of the WHO global action plan for laboratory containment of wild polioviruses in 1999 [89]. In mid-1999, the World Health Assembly unanimously passed resolution WHA52.22, urging all Member States "to begin the process leading to the laboratory containment of wild poliovirus" [93].

Implementation of the global action plan is a tremendous logistical challenge due to the large number of biomedical laboratories worldwide that need to be contacted. However, progress in the WHO European and Western Pacific Regions demonstrates that effective laboratory containment is feasible [94] (Table 3). As of mid-2002, 129 of 216 (60%) countries and territories had appointed a National Coordinator for containment and 122 (56%) had created a National Plan of Action. One hundred thirteen (52%) had begun listing biomedical laboratories, including several large industrialized countries such as Japan, Australia, Canada, and the United States [94,95]. Worldwide, over 80,000 laboratories had been identified for surveying. Over 50 countries (25%) had completed the precertification activities and had finalized an inventory of laboratories storing wild poliovirus materials. Finally, in collaboration with IPV manufacturers and regulatory authorities, WHO has also produced guidelines for the safe production and quality control of IPV manufactured from wild polioviruses [96].

C. Postcertification Polio Immunization Policy

Although the goal of all eradication initiatives is the elimination of the target organism such that control measures may be stopped [2], the ongoing debate as to the future of polio immunization policy demonstrates the complexity of this goal [91,97,98]. Although the economic benefits of stopping all polio immunization are an estimated US$1.5 billion per year, leading public health experts have expressed opposing views as to whether OPV cessation is feasible [97,98]. Consequently, the WHO has developed a framework to assess the risks of paralytic poliomyelitis in the postcertification era, and the potential options for managing those risks (Table 4). In summary, there are risks due to the continued use of the OPV and risks associated with the handling of wild polioviruses in IPV production sites and laboratories. In both categories, the risks are increasingly understood and quantifiable.

First and foremost is the well-defined risk of vaccine-associated paralytic poliomyelitis (VAPP). Vaccine-associated paralytic poliomyelitis will occur at a rate of approximately one case per million children receiving their first dose of OPV [99,100] in all areas where that vaccine continues to be used, with nearly the same number of cases associated with subsequent doses and among vaccinee contacts. Less well understood is the risk of polio outbreaks due to

Table 3 Status of Laboratory Containment Activities, as Measured by Key Indicators, by WHO Region, June 2002

Region (number of countries)	Coordinator appointed	Plan of action drafted	Laboratory list compiled	Survey conducted	Inventory completed
AMRO (47)	19	10	10	9	0
EURO (51)	51	51	51	51	20
WPRO (36)	36	36	36	36	32
EMRO (24)	18	18	12	12	2
SEARO (10)	7	7	4	4	0
AFRO (48)	0	0	0	0	0
Global (216)	129 (60%)	122 (56%)	113 (52%)	111 (51%)	54 (25%)

Table 4 Potential Risks of Paralytic Poliomyelitis in the Era After Global Certification of the Interruption of Wild Poliovirus Transmission (i.e., the "Postcertification" Era)

Risk factor	Potential risks
Continued use of OPV	(1) VAPP
	(2) cVDPV
	(3) Immunodeficiency syndrome with long-term excretion of a vaccine-derived poliovirus (iVDPV)
Continued handling of wild polioviruses	(1) Inadvertent release of a wild poliovirus from IPV production site
	(2) Inadvertent release of a wild poliovirus from a laboratory setting
	(3) Intentional release of a wild poliovirus

cVDPVs. Although the risk of such events had been postulated for some time [101], it was only in the year 2000 that the first cVDPV outbreak was identified when 22 children were paralyzed over a 12-month period on the Caribbean island of Hispaniola [102]. A second such outbreak occurred in the Philippines in 2001, paralyzing three children [103]. A third was under investigation in Madagascar as of mid-2002 [104]. Retrospective analyses of viruses from Egypt suggest that a VDPV also circulated in that country and paralyzed children between 1982 and 1993 [105]. Although cVDPVs appear to be much rarer than VAPP, their potential to reestablish widespread paralytic polio in the postcertification era is substantially greater.

The third risk of paralytic polio due to continued use of OPV is the potential for long-term carriers of VDPVs identified among immunodeficient persons to reseed the general population in a postimmunization era. Such carriers are extremely rare, however, with only 14 identified in the 40 years of widespread use of the vaccine. Of these, only two are known to be continuing to excrete a VDPV. An analysis of the risks posed by such persons suggests that it is minimal [91].

The risks of paralytic polio due to wild poliovirus handling in the postcertification era are three: (1) inadvertent release from an IPV production site; (2) inadvertent release from a laboratory; and (3) intentional release. The risks associated with the first two situations can be minimized through high-quality containment work to promote the safe handling and use of wild poliovirus stocks (described above). Experience with the containment guidelines in a number of large industrialized countries has now demonstrated that this is a manageable task [94,95]. Although the potential for intentional reintroduction of polio into the human community cannot be eliminated through containment efforts alone, it can be substantially reduced. Furthermore, standard assessments of potential biological agents suggest that poliovirus would not be a biowarfare candidate organism and would be an unlikely agent for bioterrorism [91,106].

The WHO's technical oversight body for polio eradication has outlined the following potential options for discontinuing OPV in the postcertification era [107]: (1) discontinue OPV after a mass campaign with OPV, with the option to continue IPV; (2) switch to universal IPV immunization; and (3) develop new vaccines that would not cause VAPP or cVDPV. Coordinated discontinuation of OPV would have the major advantage of stopping OPV at a time when population immunity will be very high, thus minimizing the risk of cVDPV. Although all countries would have the option of continuing to vaccinate with IPV, the continued use of IPV in industrialized countries as some experts advocate would protect against virus escaping from IPV manufacturing sites, deter the use of poliovirus as a biological weapon in these countries, and further minimize the risk of spread of a cVDPV from a long-term VDPV carrier.

Universal IPV would ensure that populations have at least some level of protection against cVDPV and would decrease the consideration of polio as a bioterrorism agent. However, this strategy would incur substantial costs, for relatively low population immunity, given the low seroconversion rates for IPV (type 1, ~60%; type 2, ~60%; and type 3, ~90%) when given at the usual EPI contact ages in developing countries [108]. In addition, manufacturers would need to greatly increase production capacity. Although the development of new live vaccines has been promoted, this may not be feasible based on current scientific knowledge and regulatory concerns. Furthermore, the costs of developing, testing, and seeking regulatory approval for a new vaccine would be enormous. Thus, it is unlikely that a new vaccine could be available during the timeframe of the eradication initiative unless huge public sector investments were made [106].

Although the first option described above is the most attractive in terms of programmatic feasibility and costs, it would be premature to endorse any strategy until there is a better understanding of the risks of cVDVP and iVDPV, the costs and benefits of alternate strategies, and how the perception of some risks may affect long-term policy decisions (including the risk of intentional release of wild poliovirus) [109]. Recognizing the need to establish international consensus on the future use of OPV, the WHO is coordinating a program of scientific research and country consultation that such decisions might be taken as early as 2004–2005. Regardless of the strategy selected, it will be necessary to establish a global stockpile of, and a production capacity for, OPV in case wild polioviruses are detected in the postimmunization era [91,110,111].

V. CONCLUSION

By end-2001, progress toward the interruption of wild poliovirus transmission worldwide had established the technical and operational feasibility of polio eradication. Ironically, with only 10 countries remaining endemic for the virus as of June 2002, a financing gap of US$275 million for the period 2003–2005 is the single greatest risk to achieving this goal [110]. Consequently, the first priority of the polio eradication initiative is to secure sufficient resources and commitment to achieve the quality of supplementary immunization needed to interrupt the final chains of transmission worldwide. During this period, increasing attention will also be given to the processes of certification, laboratory containment, and postcertification policy development so that the economic and humanitarian benefits of this initiative can be fully exploited. The final challenge facing this global initiative is to ensure that the legacy of polio eradication includes the adaptation of this infrastructure to successfully tackle other important public health problems.

ACKNOWLEDGMENTS

The authors are extremely grateful to Ms. Joan Hawe of the WHO for her assistance with the references for this article, as well as to Mr. Chris Wolff for his input on specific sections of the manuscript.

REFERENCES

1. Fenner F, et al. The intensified smallpox eradication programme, 1967–1980. Smallpox and Its Eradication. Geneva: World Health Organization, 1988:421–538.
2. Dowdle WR. The principles of disease elimination and eradication. In: Goodman RA, Foster KL, Throwbridge FL, Figueroa JP, eds. Global Disease Elimination and Eradication as Public Health Strategies. Proceedings of a conference held in Atlanta, GA, USA, February 23–25, 1998. Bull 1998; 76(suppl 2):22–25.
3. Aylward B, et al. When is a disease eradicable? 100 years of lessons learned. Am J Public Health 2000; 90:1515–1520.
4. Expanded Programme on Immunization. Progress towards the global eradication of poliomyelitis, 2001. Wkly Epidemiol Rec 2002; 77(13):97–108.
5. Dowdle RW, Cochi SL. Global eradication of poliovirus: history and rationale. In: Semler LB, Wimmer E, eds. The Picornaviruses. Washington, DC: ASM Press, 2002.
6. World Health Organization. Meeting on the impact of targeted programmes on health systems: a case study of the Polio Eradication Initiative (WHO document no. WHO/V&B/00.29). Geneva: World Health Organization, 2000.
7. Loevinsohn B, et al. Commentary: impact of targeted programmes on health systems—a case study of the Polio Eradication Initiative. Am J Public Health 2000; 92(1):19–23.
8. Dowdle WR, Hopkins DR, eds. The Eradication of Infectious Diseases: Dahlem Workshop Reports. Chichester: John Wiley, 1998.
9. Goodman RA, et al. Global disease elimination and eradication as public health strategies. Proceedings of a conference held in Atlanta, Georgia, USA, February 23–25, 1998. Bull WHO 1998; 76(suppl 2):1–162.
10. Ottesen EA, et al. Group report: how is eradication to be defined and what are the biological criteria? In: Dowdle WR, Hopkins DR, eds. The Eradication of Infectious Diseases: Dahlem Workshop Reports. Chichester: John Wiley, 1998:47–59.
11. Horstmann MD, et al. eds. International Symposium on Poliomyelitis Control. Rev Infect Dis 1984; 6(suppl 1):S301–S601.
12. de Quadros CA, et al. Eradication of poliomyelitis: progress in the Americas. Pediatr Infect Dis J 1991; 10:222–229.
13. Mas Lago P. Eradication of poliomyelitis in Cuba: a historical perspective. Bull WHO 1999; 77:681–687.
14. Cruz PR. Cuba: mass polio vaccination program, 1962–1982. Rev Infect Dis 1984; 6(suppl):S408–S412.
15. Risi JB. The control of poliomyelitis in Brazil. Rev Infect Dis 1984; 6(suppl 2):S391–S396.
16. Pan American Health Organization. Director announces campaign to eradicate poliomyelitis from the Americas by 1990. Bull Pan Am Health Organ 1985; 19:213–215.
17. Ghendon Y, Robertson SE. Interrupting the transmission of wild polioviruses with vaccines: immunologic considerations. Bull WHO 1994; 72:973–983.
18. Fox PJ, et al. Spread of a vaccine strain of poliovirus in southern Louisiana communities. In: Live Poliovirus Vaccines, Second International Conference (scientific publication no. 50). Washington, DC: Pan American Sanitary Bureau, 1960: 144–155.
19. Sabin AB. Strategies for elimination of poliomyelitis in different parts of the world with use of oral poliovirus vaccine. Rev Infect Dis 1984; 6(suppl 2):S391–S396.
20. Aylward BR, et al. Reaching every child-achieving equity in global immunization. In: Levine MM, Kaper BJ, Rappuoli R, Liu AM, Good FM, eds. New Generation Vaccines. New York: Marcel Dekker, 2004:89–100.
21. Cherry JD. Enteroviruses: coxsackieviruses, echoviruses and polioviruses. In: Feigin DR, Cherry DJ, eds. Textbook of Pediatric Infectious Diseases. 4th ed. Philadelphia, PA: WB Saunders, 1998:1819–1827.
22. Gear JHS. Nonpolio causes of polio-like paralytic syndromes. Rev Infect Dis 1984; 6(suppl 2):S379–S384.
23. Marx A, et al. Differential diagnosis of acute flaccid paralysis and its role in poliomyelitis surveillance. Epidemiol Rev 2000; 22:298–316.
24. Pinheiro PF, et al. Eradication of wild polioviruses from the Americas: wild poliovirus surveillance-laboratory issues. J Infect Dis 1997; 175(suppl 1):S43–S49.
25. de Quadros CA, et al. Eradication of wild poliovirus from the Americas: acute flaccid paralysis surveillance, 1988–1995. J Infect Dis 1997; 175(suppl 1):S37–S42.
26. McLean M, et al. Incidence of Guillain–Barré syndrome in Ontario and Quebec, 1983–1989. Epidemiology 1994; 5:443–448.
27. Prevots DR, Sutter RW. Assessment of Guillain–Barré syndrome mortality and morbidity in the United States: implications for acute flaccid paralysis surveillance. J Infect Dis 1997; 175(suppl 1):S151–S155.
28. World Health Organization Division of Mental Health and Expanded Programme on Immunization/Association Internationale pour la Recherche et l'Enseignement en Neurosciences. Acute Onset Flaccid Paralysis (unpublished document no. WHO/MNH/EPI/93.3). Geneva: World Health Organization, 1993.
29. Expanded Programme on Immunization. Acute flaccid paralysis (AFP) surveillance: the strategy for poliomyelitis eradication. Wkly Epidemiol Rec 1998; 73:113–117.
30. Smith J, et al. Certifying the elimination of poliomyelitis from Europe: advancing toward global eradication. Eur J Epidemiol 1998; 14:769–773.
31. Expanded Programme on Immunization. Poliomyelitis eradication: the WHO Global Laboratory Network. Wkly Epidemiol Rec 1997; 72:245–252.
32. Department of Vaccines and Biologicals. Expanding contributions of the global laboratory network for poliomyelitis eradication. Wkly Epidemiol Rec 2002; 77:133–137.
33. Dowdle RW, Birmingham ME. The biologic principles of poliovirus eradication. J Infect Dis 1997; 175(suppl 1):S286–S292.
34. Bernier R. Some observations on poliomyelitis lameness surveys. Rev Infect Dis 1984; 6(suppl 2):S371–S375.
35. Hull FH, et al. Paralytic poliomyelitis: seasoned strategies, disappearing disease. Lancet 1994; 343:1331–1337.

36. Ofosu-Amaah S, et al. Is poliomyelitis a serious problem in developing countries? Lameness in Ghanaian schools. Br Med J 1977; i:1012–1014.

37. Nicholas DD, et al. Is poliomyelitis a serious problem in developing countries? The Danfa experience. Br Med J 1977; i:1009–1012.

38. Francois I, et al. Causes of locomotor disability and need for orthopaedic devices in a heavily mined Taliban-controlled province of Afghanistan: issues and challenges for public health managers. Trop Med Int Health 1998; 3:391–396.

39. Acharya KA, Murray CJL. Economic appraisal of eradication programs: the question of infinite benefits. In: Dowdle RW, Hopkins RD, eds. The Eradication of Infectious Diseases: Dahlem Workshop Reports. Chichester: John Wiley and Sons, 1998:75–90.

40. Bart JK, et al. Global eradication of poliomyelitis: benefit–cost analysis. Bull WHO 1996; 74:35–45.

41. Musgrove P. Is polio eradication in the Americas economically justified? Bull Pan Am Health Organ 1988; 22(1):1–16.

42. Aylward BR, et al. Producing a global public good: polio eradication. In: Beaglehole R, Smith R, eds. Global Public Goods for Health. Oxford: Oxford University Press, 2003: 33–53.

43. de Quadros AC, et al. Polio eradication from the western hemisphere. Annu Rev Public Health 1992; 13:239–252.

44. Global Eradication of Poliomyelitis by the Year 2000. (World Health Assembly resolution WHA41.28). Geneva: World Health Organization, 1988.

45. Henderson DA. Eradication: lessons from the past. Bull WHO 1998; 76(suppl 2):17–21.

46. Cochi LS, et al. Group report: what are the societal and political criteria for eradication? In: Dowdle RW, Hopkins RD, eds. The Eradication of Infectious Diseases: Dahlem Workshop Reports. Chichester: John Wiley and Sons, 1998: 157–175.

47. Anonymous. Report on the International Conference on the Eradication of Infectious Diseases. Can infectious diseases be eradicated? Rev Infect Dis 1982; 4:912–984.

48. Task Force for Child Survival and Development. Protecting the World's Children: an Agenda for the 1990s. Talloires, France: Tufts University European Center, 1988.

49. World Summit for Children. World Declaration on the Survival, Protection and Development of Children. New York: United Nations, 1990.

50. Assembly of Heads of States and Government. Yaounde Declaration on Polio Eradication in Africa (Resolution AHG/Decl. 1; XXXII). Yaounde, Cameroon: Organization of African Unity, 1996.

51. Andrus KJ, et al. A new paradigm for international disease control: lessons learned from polio eradication in Southeast Asia. Am J Public Health 2001; 91:146–150.

52. McBean MA, et al. Serologic response to oral polio vaccine and enhanced-potency inactivated polio vaccines. Am J Epidemiol 1988; 128:615–628.

53. Patriarca AP, et al. Factors affecting the immunogenicity of oral polio vaccines in developing countries: a review. Rev Infect Dis 1991; 13:926–939.

54. World Health Organization. WHO Vaccine-Preventable Diseases: Monitoring System. 2001 Global Summary (WHO document no. WHO/V&B/01.34). Geneva: World Health Organization, 2002.

55. Sabin BA, et al. Oral poliovirus vaccine: effects of rapid mass immunization on population under conditions of massive enteric infections with other virus. JAMA 1960; 173:1521–1626.

56. Grachev VP. Long-term use of oral poliovirus vaccine from SABIN strain in the Soviet Union. Rev Infect Dis 1984; 6(suppl):S321–S322.

57. Domok I. Experiences associated with the use of live polio-

58. virus vaccine in Hungary, 1959–1962. Rev Infect Dis 1984; 6(suppl):S413–S418.

Expanded Programme on Immunization. Progress towards poliomyelitis eradication 1990–1994. China. Wkly Epidemiol Rec 1994; 69:377–379.

59. Expanded Programme on Immunization. Progress towards poliomyelitis eradication, 1994. Wkly Epidemiol Rec 1995; 70:97–101.

60. Birmingham EM, et al. National immunization days: state of the art. J Infect Dis 1997; 175(suppl):S183–S188.

61. Bodian D, Paffenbarger RS. Poliomyelitis infection in households: frequency of viremia and specific antibody response. Am J Hyg 1954; 60:83–98.

62. Expanded Programme on Immunization. Update: mass vaccination with oral poliovirus vaccine—Asia and Europe, 1996. Wkly Epidemiol Rec 1996; 71:329–332.

63. Expanded Programme on Immunization. Progress towards poliomyelitis eradication, Southeast Asia, 1998–1999. Wkly Epidemiol Rec 2000; 75:213–216.

64. Expanded Programme on Immunization. Progress towards poliomyelitis eradication, West and Central Africa, 1999–2000. Wkly Epidemiol Rec 2001; 76:158–162.

65. Expanded Programme on Immunization. Progress towards poliomyelitis eradication, 1990–1996: China. Wkly Epidemiol Rec 1996; 71:377–379.

66. Birmingham EM, et al. Poliomyelitis surveillance: the compass for eradication. J Infect Dis 1997; 175(suppl 1):S146–S150.

67. Expanded Programme for Vaccines and Immunization. Final stages of polio eradication, WHO Western Pacific Region, 1997–1998. Wkly Epidemiol Rec 1997; 74:20–24.

68. World Health Organization. Progress towards poliomyelitis eradication, WHO European Region, June 1998–2000. Wkly Epidemiol Rec 2000; 75:241–246.

69. Expanded Programme for Vaccines and Immunization. EPI Information System. Global Summary, September 1998 (WHO document no. WHO/EPI/GEN/98.10). Geneva: World Health Organization, 1998.

70. World Health Organization. Expanded Programme on Immunization (EPI). Update: mass vaccination with oral poliovirus vaccine, Asia and Europe, 1996. Wkly Epidemiol Rec 1996; 71:329–332.

71. Biellik RJ. Current status of polio eradication in Southern Africa. J Infect Dis 1997; 175(suppl 1):S20–23.

72. World Health Organization. Transmission of wild poliovirus type 2—apparent global interruption. Wkly Epidemiol Rec 2001; 76:95–97.

73. Hall GR, et al. Group report: what are the criteria for estimating the costs and benefits of disease eradication. In: Dowdle RW, Hopkins RD, eds. The Eradication of Infectious Diseases: Dahlem Workshop Reports. Chichester: John Wiley and Sons, 1998:107–115.

74. Taylor EC, Waldman RJ. Designing eradication programs to strengthen primary health care. In: Dowdle RW, Hopkins RD, eds. The Eradication of Infectious Diseases: Dahlem Workshop Reports. Chichester: John Wiley and Sons, 1998:145–155.

75. Taylor C, et al. Ethical dilemmas in current planning for polio eradication. Am J Public Health 1997; 87:922–925.

76. Aylward BR, et al. Disease eradication initiatives and general health services: ensuring common principles lead to mutual benefits. In: Dowdle RW, Hopkins RD, eds. The Eradication of Infectious Diseases: Dahlem Workshop Reports. Chichester: John Wiley and Sons, 1998:61–74.

77. MacAulay C, Verma M. Global Polio Laboratory Network: A Model for Good Laboratory Practice—A Study of the Quality Principles Within the Global Polio Laboratory Network. Bethesda: Quality Assurance Project, University Research Co., 1999.

78. Ching P, et al. The impact of vitamin A supplements delivered with immunization campaigns. Am J Public Health 2000; 90:1526–1529.

79. Goodman T, et al. Polio as a platform: using national immunization days to deliver vitamin A supplements. Bull WHO 2000; 78(3):305–314.

80. Nsubuga P, et al. Impact of Acute Flaccid Paralysis Surveillance on the Surveillance of Other Infectious Diseases in Africa. Paper presented at the 49th Annual Epidemic Intelligence Service (EIS) Conference, Centers for Disease Control and Prevention, Atlanta, USA, April 10–14, 2000.

81. World Health Organization. State of the World's Vaccines and Immunization. Geneva: World Health Organization, 2002 .

82. Jacobs L, et al. A Paradigm for International Cooperation: The Global Alliance for Vaccines and Immunization (GAVI) and the Vaccine Fund. In: Levine MM, Kaper BJ, Rappuoli R, Liu AM, Good FM, eds. New Generation Vaccines. New York: Marcel Dekker. In press.

83. Taylor Commission. The impact of the Expanded Program on Immunization and the polio eradication initiative on health systems in the Americas (PAHO report no. 1995-000003). Washington, DC: Pan American Health Organization, 1995.

84. Aylward BR, et al. Strengthening routine immunization services in the Western Pacific through eradication of poliomyelitis. J Infect Dis 1997; 175(suppl 1):S268–S271.

85. Mogedal S, Stenson B. Disease eradication: friend or foe to the health system? Synthesis report from field studies in Tanzania, Nepal and Lao PDR Paper presented at the Meeting on the Impact of Targeted Programmes on Health Systems: A Case-Study of the Polio Eradication Initiative (PEI). Geneva: World Health Organization, December 16–17, 1999.

86. Arora KN, et al. Pulse Polio Immunization Program Evaluation 1997–98. New Delhi: All India Institute of Medical Sciences, 1999.

87. Expanded Programme on Immunization. Report of the First Meeting of the Global Commission for the Certification of the Eradication of Poliomyelitis (WHO document no. WHO/EPI/GEN/95.6). Geneva: World Health Organization, 1995.

88. Global Programme for Vaccines and Immunization. Report of the Second Meeting of the Global Commission for the Certification of the Eradication of Poliomyelitis, Geneva, May 1, 1997 (WHO document no. WHO/EPI/GEN 98.03). Geneva: World Health Organization, 2001.

89. World Health Organization. WHO Global Action Plan for Laboratory Containment of Wild Polioviruses (WHO document no. WHO/V&B/99.32). Geneva: World Health Organization, 1999.

90. Department of Vaccines and Biologicals. Certification of the Eradication of Poliomyelitis. Report of the Sixth Meeting of the Global Commission for the Certification of the Eradication of Poliomyelitis, Washington, DC, March 28–29, 2001 (WHO document no. WHO/V&B/01.15). Geneva: World Health Organization, 2001.

91. Technical Consultative Group to the World Health Organization on the Global Eradication of Poliomyelitis. "Endgame" issues for the global polio eradication initiative. Clin Infect Dis 2002; 34:72–77.

92. Fenner F, et al. Smallpox and Its Eradication: Chapter 23. Smallpox in Non-Endemic Countries. Vol. 23. Geneva: World Health Organization, 1988:1069–1101.

93. World Health Assembly. Poliomyelitis Eradication (resolution 52.22). Geneva: World Health Organization, 1999.

94. Centers for Disease Control and Prevention. Global progress toward laboratory containment of wild polioviruses, June 2001. Morb Mortal Wkly Rep 2001; 50:620–623.

95. Centers for Disease Control and Prevention. National laboratory inventory as part of he global poliovirus containment. Morb Mortal Wkly Rep 2002; 51:646–647.

96. World Health Organization. Guidelines for the safe production and quality control of IPV manufactured from wild polioviruses. Addendum to the WHO Recommendations for Poliomyelitis Vaccine (Inactivated). Geneva: World Health Organization, 2003. In press.

97. Dove WA, Racaniello VR. The polio eradication effort: should vaccine eradication be next? Science 1997; 277:779–780.

98. Henderson DA. Countering the post eradication threat of smallpox and poliomyelitis. Clin Infect Dis 2002; 34:79–83.

99. Strebel MP, et al. Epidemiology of poliomyelitis in the United States: one decade after the last reported case of indigenous wild virus-associated disease. Clin Infect Dis 1992; 14:568–579.

100. Andrus KJ, et al. Risk of vaccine-associated paralytic poliomyelitis in Latin America, 1989–91. Bull WHO 1995; 73:33–40.

101. Fine EMP, Carneiro IAM. Transmissibility and persistence of oral polio vaccine viruses: implications for the global poliomyelitis eradication initiative. Am J Epidemiol 1999; 150:1001–1021.

102. Kew O, et al. Outbreak of poliomyelitis in Hispaniola associated with circulating type 1 vaccine-derived poliovirus. Science 2002; 296:356–359.

103. Expanded Programme on Immunization. Acute flaccid paralysis associated with circulating vaccine-derived poliovirus, Philippines 2001. Wkly Epidemiol Rec 2001; 76:319–320.

104. Department of Vaccines and Biologicals. Paralytic poliomyelitis in Madagascar, 2002. Wkly Epidemiol Rec 2002; 77:241–242.

105. Centers for Disease Control and Prevention. Circulation of a type 2 vaccine-derived poliovirus—Egypt, 1982–1993. Morb Mortal Wkly Rep 2001; 50(51):41–42.

106. Vaccines and Biologicals. New Polio Vaccines for the Post-Eradication Era, Geneva, 19–20 January 2000. Geneva, World Health Organization, 2000 (WHO document no. WHO/V&B/00.20).

107. Wood JD, et al. Stopping poliovirus vaccination after eradication: issues and challenges. Bull WHO 2001; 78: 347–363.

108. WHO Collaborative Study Group on Oral and Inactivated Poliovirus Vaccines. Combined immunization of infants with oral and inactivated poliovirus vaccines: results of a randomized trial in the Gambia, Oman, and Thailand. J Infect Dis 1997; 175(suppl 1):S215–S227.

109. Andrus KJ, et al. Polio immunization policy in the postcertification era. Criteria for policy development. In: Institute for Global Health & Taskforce for Child Survival and Development. Global health forum III. Post-certification polio immunization policy. San Francisco: Institute for Global Health, 2002.

110. Department of Vaccines and Biologicals. Global Eradication of Poliomyelitis. Report of the Seventh Meeting of the Global Technical Consultative Group for Poliomyelitis Eradication, Geneva, April 9–11, 2002. Geneva: World Health Organization, 2002.

111. Fine EMP, et al. Stopping a polio outbreak in the posteradication era. Brown F ed. Progress in Polio Eradication: Vaccine Strategies for the End Game. Vol. 105. Basel: Karger, 2001:129–147.

14

Recent Advances in Immunology that Impact Vaccine Development

Marcelo B. Sztein
University of Maryland School of Medicine, Baltimore, Maryland, U.S.A.

I. INTRODUCTION

The last decade witnessed an explosion in information concerning the mechanisms underlying the host's immune response to invading microorganisms, as well as during pathological conditions such as autoimmune diseases and cancer. This was largely a result of impressive technological advances, which include: (1) engineering of a multitude of single and multiple gene-knockout and transgenic animals (and more recently, "conditional knockout" and "knock-in" mutants); (2) the ability to track specific T cells by using fluorochrome-labeled peptide-major histocompatibility complex (MHC) tetramers; (3) sophisticated multicolor and flow cytometric sorting techniques that allow the identification and functional characterization of cell subpopulations based on the concomitant expression of multiple surface and intracellular molecules; (4) the availability of many cytokines, chemokines, and other immunoregulatory molecules produced by recombinant techniques; (5) gene expression profiling using DNA microarrays that allows one to simultaneously determine the expression of thousands of individuals genes in response to infection; and (6) the advent of proteomics (i.e., the large-scale analysis of proteins and their interactions). Moreover, the disclosure of the DNA sequence of entire genomes, not only of humans, but also from an ever-increasing number of other eukaryotic (e.g., yeasts, worm, and fly) and prokaryotic (currently over 20) organisms, is allowing the identification of large numbers of potential novel target antigens (Ag) for vaccine development.

In spite of the knowledge gained in recent years, there is no existing consensus on a general set of critical immunologic principles that should guide the development of new vaccines. Based on the information available to date, it is likely that the desired immunological response that must be elicited by effective vaccines will have to be tailored to each individual pathogen. This is due, in no short measure, to the complexity of the immune response, the diversity of patho-genic microorganisms, the various routes of entry into the host, and the ability of some invading pathogens to subvert the generation of protective immune responses. Consequently, it is difficult to select "a priori" among the many factors that influence the development of a successful vaccine, such as the choice of the appropriate "protective" Ag, route of administration, dose, schedule of immunization, adjuvants, and/or carriers used in the formulation. It is also difficult to accurately predict how the immunological status of the recipient will affect responses to the vaccine.

This review is intended to highlight, rather than to discuss in depth, recent advances in understanding the mechanisms underlying the generation of immune responses and immunological memory. Emphasis will be placed on those mechanisms that have directly advanced (or can potentially advance) the development of new vaccines or can improve existing vaccines. This chapter will succinctly review novel concepts on the integrated nature of innate and adaptive immunity and focus on recent findings in the areas of Ag processing and presentation, including costimulatory molecules, the role of cytokines and chemokines in linking adaptive and innate immunity, the molecular determinants underlying lymphoid cell trafficking, and the generation of memory lymphocytes. Because of space limitations, the reader will be referred, throughout this chapter, to excellent recent reviews for additional information.

II. AN INTEGRATED VIEW OF THE IMMUNE RESPONSE

The host's immune defense mechanisms against infectious agents can be divided into two main components: innate (i.e., native immunity) and adaptive (i.e., acquired immunity). Both of these complementary and highly interrelated components of the immune system are essential to protect the host from disease-causing viruses, bacteria, fungi, and parasites.

A. Innate Immunity

This component of the immune response plays a critical role immediately after a pathogen enters the host, providing a first line of defense against invading microorganisms. Innate immunity is primarily responsible for the elimination, or at least the control, of the invading microbe during the 4–7 days required for the establishment of an early adaptive immune response [1,2]. Moreover, it is now widely recognized that innate immunity and the resulting inflammatory process play a key role in initiating the adaptive immune response and determining its nature. A distinctive feature of innate immunity is that the response does not increase with successive exposures to the microbes.

Many cells are involved in innate immunity, including phagocytes (e.g., neutrophils, macrophages), dendritic cells (DC), natural killer (NK) cells, and eosinophils. A key characteristic of the cells that form part of the innate immune system is their ability to recognize a wide range of microorganisms through surface receptors [pattern recognition receptors (PRRs)] that recognize invariant molecules present in a wide range of microbes [pathogen-associated molecular patterns (PAMPs)], but not in the host [1]. This important area of research has received a remarkable degree of attention over the past few years [2–4]. Examples of PAMPs, which are present in both pathogenic and nonpathogenic microorganisms, include bacterial cell wall peptidoglycans of Gram-positive bacteria and lipopolysaccharide (LPS) of Gram-negative bacteria.

Pattern recognition receptors can be expressed on the cell membrane, in intracellular compartments or secreted [2]. Examples of PRRs expressed on the cell surface include the macrophage scavenger receptor (MSR), which recognizes polyanionic ligands [e.g., double-stranded RNA (dsRNA), LPS], lectin-like binding receptors on NK cells, and macrophage mannose receptors (MMR), which recognize carbohydrate structures present in bacteria and fungal pathogens. Intracellular PRRs include the protein kinase PKR and the $2'$-$5'$-oligoadenylate synthase which binds dsRNA (present in viruses), as well as the nucleotide-binding oligomerization domain (NOD) family of proteins, which appears to respond to LPS. Secreted PRRs (e.g., C-reactive protein, mannan-binding lectin, etc.) function by binding to microbes, leading to their elimination by complement-mediated mechanisms or phagocytosis. Toll-like receptors (TLRs) are an important family of PRRs that play a pivotal role in innate immune recognition. TLRs are characterized by extracellular domains that contain leucine-rich repeats and cytplasmic portions, responsible for intracellular signaling, similar to the intracellular domain of the type-1 IL-1 receptor. Ten TLRs which recognize a variety of different PAMPs have been described to date in mice and humans (Table 1). Of note, TLRs sometimes require other molecules to participate in the recognition of PAMPs. For example, TLR4 has to be coordinately associated with MD-2 and CD14, as well as CD11b/CD18 heterodimers, to enable optimal LPS-signaling leading to nuclear translocation of nuclear factor κB (NF-κB), and TLR2 has to dimerize with other TLRs, such as TLR1 or TLR6, to detect ligands and induce signaling [3–8]. To add to the complexity

of PAMP recognition, a CD14-independent LPS receptor cluster on the cell surface, composed of several proteins (i.e., hsp70, hsp90, CXCR4, and growth differentiation factor 5 [GDF5]), as well as the possible existence of intracellular receptors for LPS and invasive bacteria have recently been reported [3].

Recognition of "microbial nonself" through PRR recognition of PAMPs triggers signaling pathways that result in activated phagocytes, which are better equipped to engulf and destroy the offending pathogen, as well as to secrete many molecules responsible for the initiation of an inflammatory process. Molecules secreted following TLR-PAMP interactions include inflammatory cytokines (e.g., interferon (IFN)-α, IFN-β, interleukin-1α (IL-1α), IL-1β, IL-6, IL-12, and tumor necrosis factor (TNF)-α), chemokines (e.g., CXCL8 [IL-8], CCL20 [MIP-3α], CXCL10 [IP-10] and CCL2 [MCP-1]), and other moieties that directly or indirectly participate in the destruction of the microbe. As discussed in more detail below, these molecules profoundly affect the behavior of many cell types, modulate the type of adaptive immune response induced, and recruit macrophages, neutrophils, DC, lymphocytes and other cells to the inflammatory site. Of note, TLR–PAMP interactions on the surface of DC, a key Ag-presenting cell (APC), play a critical role in the induction of adaptive immunity by upregulating the expression of costimulatory molecules required for the activation of naive T cells specific for antigenic peptides expressed on the same DC in conjunction with MHC molecules [1]. It is also important to emphasize that cytokines and other molecules secreted by cells of the adaptive immune system (e.g., IFN-γ secreted by activated T lymphocytes), in turn, have marked effects on the innate immune response through activation of macrophages and other cells that ultimately participate directly in the destruction of the microbe.

B. Adaptive Immunity

In contrast to innate immunity, the effector mechanisms of adaptive immunity that include, among others, antibodies (Ab) and cell-mediated immune responses (CMI) [e.g., cytotoxic T lymphocytes (CTL) and cytokines such as interferon-γ (IFN-γ) and interleukin-4 IL-4)] are induced following exposure to antigens (Ag) or infections agents and increase in magnitude with successive exposures to the specific Ag. This ability to "recall" previous exposures to Ag and respond rapidly with immunological effector responses of increased magnitude (immunologic memory) constitutes the foundation for immunoprophylactic vaccination against infectious agents. Therefore this chapter will focus on some of the most significant recent advances in understanding the mechanisms which underlie the development of adaptive immune responses and immunologic memory. The main cell types involved in adaptive immune responses, responsible for the recognition of specific Ag, are T and B lymphocytes. However, it is very important to emphasize that an adaptive immune response can only be initiated after cells typically considered part of the innate immune response (e.g., DC and other APC) uptake, process, and present Ag to naive recir-

Table 1 Toll-Like Receptors

TLR	Cell location	Major ligands/agonists	Microbes	References
TLR1 [+ TLR2]	Surface	Phenol-soluble modulin (*S. epidermidis*)	Gram(+) bacteria	[121]
TLR2	Surface	Peptidoglycan (PGN)	Gram(+) and	[3,4,122–124]
		Heat shock protein HSP60	Gram(−) bacteria	
		Bacterial lipoproteins/lipopeptides	Mycobacteria	
		GPI anchor (*T. cruzi*)	Mycoplasma	
		Glycolipids	Protozoa	
		Zymosan (*S. cerevisiae*)	Fungi	
		LPS from *P. Gingivalis* and *L. interrogans*		
TLR3	Intracellular?	dsRNA	Viruses	[125]
		Poly I:C		
TLR4	Surface	Enterobacterial LPS	Gram(−) and	[3,4,6,7,123,124,126]
		Lipoteichoic acid (LTA)	Gram(+) Bacteria	
		Heat shock protein HSP60	Chlamydia	
		Respiratory syncytial virus F protein	Viruses	
		Teichuronic acid (*Micrococcus luteous*)		
		Bacterial fimbriae (*E. coli*).		
		Taxol		
		Extra domain A (EDA) of fibronectin		
		Fibrinogen		
TLR5	Surface	Flagellin	Bacteria	[127]
TLR6 [+ TLR2]	Surface	Phenol-soluble modulin (*S. epidermidis*)	Gram(+) bacteria	[4,121]
		Lipoproteins	Mycoplasma	
TLR7	Surface	Antiviral drugs (imidazoquinoline)	Unknown	[128,129]
TLR8	Surface	Antiviral drugs (imidazoquinoline)	Unknown	[128,129]
TLR9	Intracellular?	Unmethylated CpG DNA motifs	Bacteria	[130]

culating lymphocytes in secondary lymphoid tissues [e.g., regional lymph nodes (LN)].

1. Immune Responses Mediated by B Lymphocytes

B cells, derived from the bone marrow, are the precursors of Ab secreting cells [plasma cells (PC)]. B cells recognize Ag (proteins, carbohydrates, or simple chemical groups) through immunoglobulin (Ig) receptors on the cell membrane [9–11]. Following Ag recognition, they clonally expand and switch their expression of Ab isotype (e.g., IgM to IgG, IgE, or IgA) under the influence of cytokines derived from T cells, macrophages, and other cell types. Somatically mutated, high-affinity B cells are generated and selected by Ag in and around the germinal centers that are formed in LN, spleen, Peyers' patches (PP), and more disorganized lymphatic aggregates of the peripheral lymphoid system [9–12]. This process gives rise to two types of B cells: nonsecreting, long-lived memory B cells and Ab-secreting plasmablasts. Terminally differentiated, end-stage PC then migrate to other locations, such as bone marrow, through the differential expression of chemokine receptors (e.g., CXCR4), where they continue to secrete high-affinity Ab for many months [9]. Memory B cells also leave the germinal centers, homing to draining areas of LN and spleen, as well as extra lymphoid tissues such as the intestinal lamina propria. Following secondary exposure to Ag, a rapid and massive clonal expansion of memory B cell occurs, generating several-fold more PC than the level following the primary stimulation [9–12].

Antibodies are particularly effective against extracellular microbes and in neutralizing microbial toxins through several mechanisms, which differ depending on the particular Ig isotype. For example, IgG binding to specific antigenic determinants (epitopes) present in the infectious organisms leads to opsonization and increased phagocytosis by macrophages and neutrophils, which, in turn, leads to intracellular killing of the microbes. Furthermore, Ab binding to microbes might also result in bacterial cell lysis through a mechanism known as Ab-dependent cell-mediated cytotoxicity (ADCC). In ADCC, recognition of pathogens coated with IgG or IgA via Fc receptors present on the effector cells (e.g., neutrophils, macrophages, and particularly NK cells; eosinophils in the case of IgE) results in destruction of the microbes by several mechanisms, such as the release of lytic proteins stored in the granules of the effector cells. Binding of human IgG1, IgG3, and IgM to microbes also activates the complement pathway, which leads to lysis of the pathogenic organisms and promotes opsonization and enhanced phagocytosis. Another critical role of Ab is to neutralize potentially lethal Ag (e.g., bacterial toxins), through the formation of Ag–Ab complexes. In contrast to the epitopes being recognized by T cells (which are composed of aminoacid (aa) sequences that are continuous in the primary protein structure), B cells and Ab bind to epitopes that consist of aa that are either continuous or discontinuous (usually associated with lipids or carbohydrates) in the primary protein structure, but that are brought together during protein folding. Epitopes composed of continuous and discontinuous aa sequences are referred to as linear and conformational epitopes, respectively. Most Ab recognize conformational epitopes in native proteins. Production of Ab to most nonprotein Ag, such as glycolipids, nucleic acids, and polymeric polysaccharides, does not require help by cognate T cells and are, therefore, referred to as thymus-independent (TI) Ag [13–16]. In contrast to T-dependent Ag, TI Ag induce mostly IgM Ab of low affinity and, in the majority of cases, do not show significant heavy chain class switching, affinity maturation, or memory [13,15]. Thymus-independent Ag have been further subdivided into types 1 and 2, depending on whether they are able (type 1) or unable (type 2) to induce immune responses in neonates [15]. Examples of TI-1 Ag include LPS and *N. meningitidis* outer membrane protein, while most bacterial capsular polysaccharides and carbohydrates are TI-2 Ag. The fact that Ab responses to TI-2 Ag develop later in life is demonstrated by the limited responses observed in small infants immunized with, for example, polysaccharide vaccines. In contrast, it is now well established that immunization with conjugate vaccines composed of polysaccharides from, for example, *Haemophilus influenzae* type b or *Salmonella enterica* serovar Typhi coupled to T cell-dependent protein Ag elicit strong antipolysaccharide Ab responses, which can be increased with repeated immunization and which are very effective in protecting small infants from invasive *H. influenzae* type b or preschool children from *Salmonella enterica* serovar Typhi infection [14,17,18]. It is unclear what mechanisms underlie these responses and to what extent cytokines derived from APC or small numbers of nonspecific T cells are required to provide a second signal for B cell triggering after exposure to TI-2 Ag. Because of its importance in vaccine development, this remains an area of intense investigation.

2. Immune Responses Mediated by T Lymphocytes

T lymphocytes, in contrast to B cells, recognize peptides (short continuous aa sequences) derived from protein Ag that are presented on the surface of APC in conjunction with class I or class II MHC molecules (pMHC) in the presence of costimulatory molecules [19–21]. These Ag may originate from bacteria, viruses, or parasites that have infected host cells and reside intracellularly, or from the extracellular environment following internalization by endocytosis. Spectacular advances in the ability to track in vivo T cells of known specificity have led to the widely accepted view that naive T cells expressing TCR of appropriate specificity are activated, almost exclusively, by pMHC complexes presented by DC that have acquired the Ag at the site it entered the host and that, in the presence of the appropriate inflammatory stimuli, migrated to the T cell areas of secondary lymphoid tissues (e.g., LN, spleen, and PP). Following Ag presentation and activation in the presence of inflammatory stimuli (e.g., IL-1), T cells undergo an explosive clonal expansion (later to be followed by a contraction phase), mature into effector cells, and migrate to effector sites [22,23]. Some Ag-specific T cell clones remain for long periods of time as memory T cells (T_m) that, upon subsequent exposures to Ag, provide a stronger, rapid, and sometimes qualitatively different specific immune response. Induction of effective T_m

cells is critical for successful vaccination. Recent evidence from several laboratories indicates that there are at least two pools of T_m cells: (1) central memory T cells (T_{cm}), which recirculate through LN and quickly acquire the capacity to produce effector cytokines upon Ag stimulation, and (2) effector memory T cells (T_{em}), which recirculate through nonlymphoid tissues and are capable of immediate effector function (see Section 8) [23–25].

There are two main populations of T cells, those expressing CD4 molecules and those expressing CD8 molecules. CD4 and CD8 molecules are T-cell surface glycoproteins that serve as important accessory molecules (coreceptors) during Ag presentation by binding to class II and class I MHC molecules, respectively [19,21]. Consequently, CD4 and CD8 molecules, whose original use was primarily as markers to identify T-cell populations with different functional characteristics, play a major role in class II and I MHC-restricted T-cell activation. CD4$^+$ cells [T helper (Th)] are mainly involved in inflammatory responses and in providing help for Ab production by B cells, while CD8$^+$ cells, in addition to secreting cytokines, compose the majority of cytotoxic T lymphocytes (CTL) primarily involved in class I MHC-restricted killing of target cells infected by pathogenic organisms, including bacteria, viruses, and parasites [26–28].

T-cell activation triggered by cross-linking of TCR by pMHC complexes, aided by costimulatory molecules, results in the production of a multitude of molecules with strong immunoregulatory properties collectively known as cytokines and chemokines. Acting in concert, cytokines not only modulate the growth, maturation, and differentiation of all cells involved in the generation of adaptive immunity [19], but also strongly regulate innate immunity. An important finding in understanding the mechanisms of protection against infectious diseases was the realization, first reported by Mossman et al. in 1986 [29], of the existence of distinct Th cell populations that exhibit polarized patterns of cytokine production. These cell subsets, designated type 1 (Th1) and type 2 (Th2) CD4$^+$ T cells, are characterized by the production of IFN-γ and TNF-β, or IL-4, IL-5, IL-9, IL-10, and IL-13, respectively [26,27,29,30]. As discussed in more detail below, the predominance of these polarized patterns of cytokine production plays a pivotal role in determining the type and characteristics of the effector immune responses generated upon antigenic stimulation, e.g., whether the predominant responses will be Ab production (and of which isotypes), enhanced intracellular killing by macrophages, generation of effector CTL, etc. [26,27,29–32].

III. ANTIGEN PROCESSING AND PRESENTATION BY ANTIGEN PRESENTING CELLS

The presentation of Ag to T cells involves a series of intracellular events within the APC, including the generation of antigenic peptide fragments, binding of these peptides to MHC molecules to form stable peptide–MHC complexes, and transport of these complexes to the cell surface where they can be recognized by T-cell receptors (TCR) in the surface of T cells. Two main pathways of Ag processing and presentation ("classical pathways"), i.e., cytosolic and endosomic, have been described. The "cytosolic pathway" is predominantly used for presentation of peptides produced endogenously in the APC, such as viral proteins, tumor Ag, and self-peptides, associated with class I MHC molecules [33]. The presentation of large numbers of self-peptides complexed to class I MHC molecules results from the inability of APC to differentiate between self and nonself. Under normal conditions, most T cells selected to recognize self-peptides were eliminated during T-cell differentiation, or are actively downregulated, and consequently cannot be activated by self-peptide–class I MHC complexes. The second "classical pathway" of Ag processing and presentation, "endosomal pathway," which is predominantly used for presentation of soluble exogenous Ag bound to class II MHC molecules, involves the capture of Ag by APC, either by binding to a specific receptor or by uptake in the fluid phase by macropinocytosis [34–37]. Triggering of T cells through the TCR has been shown with as few as 200–600 pMHC complexes in the case of influenza nucleoproteins [38]. In most immune responses, antigenic fragments (epitopes) associated with class I MHC molecules trigger the activation of CD8$^+$ CTL responses, while epitopes derived from soluble proteins complexed to class II MHC molecules are recognized by CD4$^+$ Th cells. The existence of "alternative pathways" have also been recently described. The in-depth understanding of the mechanisms involved in these early stages of immune activation is critical for the development of successful vaccines.

A. Antigen Processing and Presentation by Class I MHC Molecules

This is the most commonly used pathway for processing of cellular proteins present in most, if not all, cellular compartments, including the cytosol, nucleus, and mitochondria, that, in association with class I MHC molecules, are available for recognition by CD8$^+$ T cells [33,38,39]. Class I molecules, whose expression is regulated by cytokines (e.g., IFN-γ), are expressed at high levels in T cells and APC (e.g., B cells, DC, and macrophages), and at moderate levels in most nucleated cells (e.g., neutrophils, hepatocytes).

1. Binding of Peptides to Class I MHC Molecules

Class I MHC molecules are composed of two separate, noncovalently linked polypeptide chains. The heavy chain (α chain) is an MHC-encoded, transmembrane polypeptide of 44 kDa (325 aa), and β2-microglobulin is a non-MHC encoded polypeptide of 12 kDa (100 aa), which is not attached to the cell, but that binds noncovalently to the extracellular portion of the α chain [39]. Class I MHC molecules bind peptides within a defined region, one per MHC molecule, called the "cleft," formed by aa of the α1 and α2 segments of the α chain, and is located on the surface of the MHC molecule. These epitope-binding clefts, which contain a high concentration of polymorphic aa, consist of a β-pleated sheet floor and α-helical sides. Peptides that are able to successfully trigger T-cell activation should not only contain aa that bind class I molecules by forming noncovalent bonds with both

the β-pleated sheet floor and α-helical sides of the cleft, but also contain some aa whose side chains point away from the cleft and are therefore available for recognition by T cells.

Epitope binding clefts of class I molecules have "closed" ends and one or more pockets in the β-pleated sheet floor to fit side chains of certain aa. Thus only peptides of the appropriate length that can fit inside the groove (typically 8–10 aa, although in some cases they can be up to 11 aa in length), and that usually contain 2 aa whose side chains bind noncovalently to the pockets, can bind class I MHC molecules with high affinity. One of these two rather invariant aa for a defined allele, called "anchor residues," is usually located in the carboxyl terminal position of the 9 aa sequence of the epitope. In most cases, it consists of a hydrophobic aa and binds to the F pocket of the MHC peptide-binding site. The second anchor residue is usually located in position 2 from the N-terminus of the peptide and binds to the B pocket of the MHC peptide-binding site. The remaining aa of the antigenic peptides do not bind or bind to a lower extent to the cleft, and their side chains are therefore available for recognition by T cells. In addition to recognition of MHC-bound peptides, the direct interaction of polymorphic aa of MHC molecules with TCR also contributes to T-cell activation [39,40].

Although MHC molecules bind peptides somewhat promiscuously, it is clear that defined peptide binding motifs bind defined MHC alleles. The existence of specific anchor residues in the majority of octa- or nonameric epitopes that bind to specific class I alleles led to the identification of "allele-specific consensus-motifs." Moreover, aa located near the "anchor residues," inside and outside the epitope, have also been shown to influence, either positively or negatively, the formation of stable MHC–peptide complexes [39,40]. The existence of "allele-specific consensus-motifs" has provided researchers with a powerful tool to assist them in the identification of potentially immunogenic (although not necessarily "protective") epitopes based on the primary aa sequence of the protein being targeted as a potential Ag to form part of subunit candidate vaccines [41,42].

Over the past few years, the number of consensus-motifs has increased, and continues to expand dramatically. However, the existing tools fall short in accurately predicting immunogenic epitopes because of several factors, including (1) differences in the precursor protein expression, (2) stability and rate of peptide transport into the ER, and (3) post-translational modifications present in a sizable proportion of naturally occurring epitopes [33]. Several MHC ligand databases that list some of the known human leukocyte antigen (HLA)-binding motifs and predictive algorithms are available over the Internet (e.g., http://bimas.dcrt.nih.gov/molbio/hla_bind/; http:hlaligand.ouhsc.edu/; etc.). Following the recommendations of a panel of experts recently convened by the National Institutes of Health (June 5, 2001), a comprehensive, unified, publicly accessible, searchable, centralized database of all known MHC-binding motifs and analysis/prediction tools, as well as standards to determine peptide binding affinity, is being established. The widespread availability of such information and computational tools will, without a doubt, greatly accelerate the pace of discovery of epitopes that can be of importance in the development of novel and more effective vaccines. A detailed description of the most current methods available for the prediction of immunogenic epitopes and the use of bioinformatics to process the vast amounts of information generated by these techniques is presented elsewhere in this book.

Based on their broad peptide-binding specificities, many HLA-A and -B alleles in humans can be grouped into major supertypes that bind defined class I HLA molecules. Among them are the HLA-A2 supertype, which includes A*0201–0207, A*6802, and A*6901 HLA molecules; the HLA-A3 supertype, which includes A*03, A*11, A*3101, A*3301, and A*6801 HLA molecules; and the HLA-B7 supertype, which includes B*0702, B*3501–03, B*51, B*5301, and B*5401 HLA molecules [43]. If confirmed, these observations can be of extraordinary importance for vaccine development, because the use of vaccines including a "cocktail" of only a few epitopes containing those supermotifs, in theory, could successfully trigger protective immune responses in the vast majority of individuals, regardless of the ethnicity of origin [43].

The use of defined epitopes is an attractive vaccine strategy, offering the following advantages: (1) the selection of epitopes from conserved regions of various proteins from the microorganism, i.e., avoiding variable antigenic epitopes which can lead to immune evasion; (b) increased safety; (c) the ability to select only those epitopes which are likely to play key roles in host-defense, or that tilt the immune response toward desired effector mechanism(s); and (4) the fact that multiple epitopes can be incorporated in a single vaccine. However, it is unlikely that a vaccine solely consisting of CTL epitopes will be successful. Accumulating evidence indicates that successful subunit peptide vaccines might require the use of the appropriate CTL epitopes in combination with "universal T helper epitopes" (i.e., able to bind to a large number of MHC class II molecules) and powerful adjuvants [44]. Moreover, significant efforts are being directed toward enhancing the immunogenicity of subunit vaccines by rationally modifying antigenic determinants (i.e., creating "agonist peptides") to enhance the host's immune response through upregulation of Ag recognition [45].

2. Cytosolic Pathway for Antigen Processing and Presentation by Class I MHC Molecules

It is generally accepted that class I MHC-associated peptides represent samples of the whole cellular protein content [33,38,46]. In general, the more abundant the protein of origin, the higher the frequency of MHC–peptide complexes, although some proteins present in low amounts have also been found to represent a significant percentage of MHC–peptide complexes [33,38,46]. Chief among the factors influencing the frequency of the MHC–peptide complexes is the stability of the class I–MHC complexes, which depends, to a large extent, on the aa sequence of the ligand (presence of appropriate anchor residues, etc.) and that can last from a few hours to several days or, in some cases, weeks.

Proteins synthesized intracellularly are degraded to peptide fragments of 8–11 aa in length by proteasomes, which consist of large (650 kDa), multicatalytic proteases

of 16–24 protein subunits that form a cylindrical organelle present in the cytoplasm of APC. Proteins probably have to be covalently linked to ubiquitin before they can be targeted for proteolytic degradation by proteasomes. Peptide fragments originating in this way can either be of the correct size or can be extended in their amino-termini [46]. In the latter case, they are subsequently trimmed by aminopeptidases into peptides of the correct length. Small peptide fragments are then transferred across the membrane of the endoplasmic reticulum (ER) by an adenosine-5-triphosphate (ATP)-dependent heterodimeric complex of two proteins encoded by the "transporter in Ag processing" (TAP) 1 and TAP 2 genes. Within the lumen of the ER, antigenic fragments bind to newly synthesized class I MHC α chains (bound to tapasin and calreticulin), stabilizing the association of α chains with newly synthesized β2-microglobulin chains to form stable trimeric complexes and preventing continued association with both tapasin and calreticulin. These class I MHC-peptide trimeric complexes are then transported to the Golgi apparatus. From there, class I MHC–Ag complexes reach the cell surface and become available for recognition by TCR.

Peptides that can optimally stabilize the trimer constitute the majority of the overall class I expression. Those peptides that can only weakly stabilize the trimer will be less represented because they may fail to reach the cell surface or, if they do, they will be prone to peptide dissociation, giving rise to most of the free class I-binding sites that allow exogenous peptide to sensitize target cells [33].

3. Cross-Presentation and Alternative Pathways for Antigen Processing and Presentation by Class I MHC Molecules

Cross-presentation was originally described as a process by which Ag was capable of being transferred from cells expressing the Ag to host APC [47–49]. Historically, this term has been associated with class I-restricted Ag, although cross-presentation can involve class I- or class II-restricted Ag [49]. T-cell activation resulting from cross-presentation can lead to T-cell priming (cross-priming) or T-cell tolerance (cross-tolerance) [49]. Cross-priming of naive T cells, largely a function of DC rather than macrophages, has been described for many Ag, including minor histocompatibility Ag, graft tissue Ag, self Ag, tumor Ag, viral proteins (e.g., Epstein–Barr virus, poliovirus, cytomegalovirus, influenza), ovoalbumin, etc. Although the Ag has no obvious mechanism for accessing the cytoplasmic processing and transport machinery of the APC, depending on the individual system, cross-priming has been shown to be dependent, or not, on proteasome- and TAP processing.

Several alternative routes have been proposed to explain this "exogenous pathway" in cross-presentation: (1) an endosome-only route in which Ag is loaded into class I molecules in the endosomes by using previously occupied (by peptide exchange) or unoccupied class I MHC molecules, or on the cell surface following the "regurgitation" of peptides processed in vacuolar phagocytic compartments to the cell membrane where they bind surface class I MHC molecules, and (2) a cytosolic route in which Ag are transported from the endosome to the cytosol, allowing them to follow the "classical" pathway. The latter mechanism might also be involved in allowing the escape into the cytosol of proteins synthesized by bacteria or protozoa (e.g., *Salmonella enterica* serovar Typhimurium, *Salmonella enterica* serovar Typhi, *Mycobacterium tuberculosis*) confined to the phagolysosomal compartment, which can then become available for processing through the cytosolic pathway [50–53]. Several hypotheses have been proposed to explain why cross-priming is a function of DC and not of macrophages, including (1) the fact that the uptake of apoptotic cells is mediated by different receptors in DC and macrophages, (2) the existence of an endosome-to-cytosol transport mechanism present in DC but not in macrophages, and (3) DC are much more efficient in stimulating primary CD8[+] CTL responses than macrophages. Whatever the mechanisms involved, an active cross-priming pathway in which DC can process Ag from apoptotic and/or necrotic cells is critical, in that it endows these potent APC with the capacity to capture and present Ag from (1) virus-infected, malignant, and transplanted cells that typically lack the accessory functions to be efficient APC and (2) from pathogens that either do not directly infect APC, or that suppress their Ag processing and presentation ability following infection.

B. Antigen Processing and Presentation by Class II MHC Molecules

The "endosomal or endocytic pathway" is predominantly used for the processing and presentation of exogenous Ag, such as proteins produced by extracellular bacteria and other infectious microorganisms that, in association with class II MHC molecules, can be presented to CD4[+] T cells. Class II molecules, whose expression is also regulated by cytokines (e.g., IFN-γ), are expressed at high levels on APC (e.g., B cells, DC, and macrophages) and thymic epithelial cells, and at moderate levels on T cells, but are absent from most other nucleated cells.

1. Binding of Peptides to Class II MHC Molecules

Class II MHC molecules consist of noncovalently associated α/β heterodimers. Both α chains (33 kDa) and β chains (29 kDa) are polymorphic, transmembrane polypeptide chains that are encoded by two separate MHC genes. Similar to class I, class II MHC molecules bind peptides within a defined peptide-binding region, one per MHC molecule and consisting of a β-stranded sheet floor and α-helical sides, formed by aa of the α1 and β1 segments of the α and β chains, respectively [37]. However, in contrast to class I MHC molecules, the binding cleft of class II molecules is open at both ends, allowing bound peptides to extend beyond the cleft. This characteristic results in the lack among class II-associated peptides of the strict aa length restriction and the presence of certain aa at either end observed for peptides associated with class I. In fact, although peptides isolated from class II molecules are typically 12–24 aa in length, peptides of more than 30 aa have also been recovered [37,54]. These characteristics have delayed the identification of a large number of peptide binding motifs for class II MHC

alleles. However, it has been possible to identify some binding motifs that involve two or three anchor positions from among a core region of 7–9 aa, which are presumed to occupy polymorphic pockets similar to those described for class I molecules [39,55]. However, these "anchor-like" positions are not as stringent in occupancy requirements as with class I motifs.

2. Endosomal Pathway for Antigen Processing and Presentation by Class II MHC Molecules

The first step in the "endocytic" Ag processing and presentation pathway involves the capture and uptake of native Ag by APC. The main mechanisms involved in the internalization of exogenous Ag include binding to nonspecific (e.g., mannose receptors) or specific (e.g., specific membrane Ig on B cells and receptors for the Fc portion of Ig and complement in macrophages and DC) receptors, or uptake from the fluid phase by macropinocytosis [34]. Ag bound to membrane receptors usually enter the cells by receptor-mediated endocytosis in clathrin-coated vesicles, while other soluble Ag in fluid phase are taken up by pinocytosis. These internalized Ag become localized in membrane-bound vesicles involved in intracellular transport and degradation of Ag called endosomes. It is unclear how the endosomal compartment associates with the lysosomal compartment, which contains a large number of proteolytic and other catalytic enzymes. However, it is well established that Ag processing occurs in both the endosomal and lysosomal compartments. Cleavage of native proteins into peptide fragments of 12–24 aa in length that can then bind to the peptide-binding region of class II MHC molecules, is mostly performed by cellular proteases that function optimally in the acidic environment of the endosomal and lysosomal compartments [37,56].

Class II α and β chains synthesized in the ER bind noncovalently with the non-polymorphic invariant chain (Ii)-associated peptide (CLIP) to form a stable trimeric complex, which promotes the proper folding of class II molecules, precludes the binding of antigenic fragments to the peptide-binding groove within the ER, and targets the movement of nonameric complexes, composed of three α chains, three β chains, and three Ii chains through the Golgi apparatus, to the trans-Golgi network and into the endosomal pathway. It is widely believed that, while some trimers might lose the Ii and bind peptide in the early endosomes, most of the degradation of Ii chains takes place in the more acidic and proteolytically active late endosomal/prelysosomal compartments. CLIP remains associated to the class II binding site throughout the proteolytic process involved in Ii degradation (which includes cathepsins S and L) until it is exchanged for other ligands, a process facilitated, in humans, by HLA-DM and HLA-DO molecules [54,56]. These ligands appear to be primarily unfolded, partially degraded proteins, rather than short peptides [37]. This binding preference explains the need for the ends of the class II binding site to be open to ensure continued degradation by exoproteases, leading to the eventual formation of bound peptides with differing N and C termini.

It is believed that loading of processed Ag to newly synthesized or recycled class II MHC molecules transpires in two compartments. The major compartment (called MIIC) contains newly synthesized class II molecules that are targeted by the Ii [54,56]. The second compartment consists of early endosomes containing mature class II MHC molecules that are internalized from the cell surface and recycled back [36,54,56]. The existence of these two compartments suggests that internalized Ag are processed all along the endocytic pathway and generate different epitopes, while encountering increasingly denaturing and proteolytic conditions [37,56]. Peptides generated at an early stage may bind recycling class II MHC molecules, whereas peptides generated later might be loaded into newly synthesized class II MHC molecules. Class II–peptide complexes within the endosomes are then transported to the cell surface and become available for recognition by TCR [37,39].

3. Alternative Pathways for Antigen Processing and Presentation to Class II MHC Molecules

In addition to exogenous Ag, peptides derived from endogenously synthesized proteins have also been shown to be processed through the endosomal pathway, bind to class II MHC molecules and those complexes expressed on the cell membrane. Autologous proteins can gain access to the endosomal pathway through "alternative" pathways, including: (1) the entrapment of cytosolic proteins in autophagosomes, which then fuse with vesicles of the lysosomal and endosomal compartments; (2) endogenous proteins expressed on the cell membrane that gain access to the cytoplasm employing the same pathway used by exogenous proteins; (3) the transport of cytosolic proteins into the endocytic compartment by molecules such as Hsc70; and/ or (4) endogenously synthesized peptides present in the ER and Golgi compartments that bind through still unknown mechanisms to class II molecules in those compartments [39]. As discussed above with regard to the alternative pathways of Ag processing and presentation by class I molecules, the significance and processes involved in endogenous Ag presentation by class II in the presentation of self Ag and in immunity to pathogenic organisms have not been fully elucidated [39]. Understanding the mechanisms of these alternative pathways of Ag presentation might prove to be of great importance in the design of novel vaccine strategies.

C. Nonclassical MHC Class I and Other Molecules Involved in Antigen Presentation

In addition to class I and II MHC molecules, a number of other molecules, characterized by their limited polymorphism and lower surface expression, have also been shown to participate in Ag presentation. These include nonclassical MHC class Ib molecules, as well as non-MHC-encoded proteins, such as CD1 and the neonatal Fc receptor (FcRn) [57].

1. Class Ib Molecules

Class Ib molecules are nonclassical, nonpolymorphic MHC-like molecules that include, in humans, HLA-E, -F, -G, and -H (also known as HFE), and MIC (MHC class I chain related) A and MICB [57]. Probably the best characterized of

these molecules is HLA-E, which plays an important role in NK function. The HLA-E molecules bind nonamers derived from the leader sequences of most classical class I molecules, as well as HLA-G, in a TAP-dependent process. HLA-E binds the inhibitory and activating forms of the CD94/NKG2 receptor (CD94/NKG2A and CD94/NKG2C, respectively) present in NK and some T cells. Binding of HLA-E to NK expressing CD94/NKG2A inhibits NK activity, while binding to NK expressing CD94/NKG2C, enhances NK killing of target cells. This system provides NK with a mechanism to monitor the expression of class I molecules in host cells by using a single receptor. In this way, cells that have downregulated class I molecules, as is frequently the case in tumor cells or virus-infected cells, will become susceptible to killing by NK [57]. Similar mechanisms might be operative in a subset of T cells. HLA-G expression at the maternal/fetal interface has rendered this molecule the subject of considerable attention. Although its function remains controversial, investigators have proposed that HLA-G might be responsible for the inhibition of maternal NK that may otherwise attack the trophoblast. Both MICA and MICB have been predominantly found in epithelial cells of the gastrointestinal tract and thymus, suggesting that they may play a role in Ag presentation to γδT cells, as well as in the selection of the T cell repertoire. In contrast to other nonclassical MHC molecules, HFE plays a role in iron metabolism. No information is available on the role of HLA-F.

2. CD1 Molecules

CD1 comprises a family of nonclassical, nonpolymorphic MHC molecules, preferentially expressed by DC and other APC that, based on sequence similarities, have been subdivided into two groups, i.e., group 1 (CD1a, CD1b, and CD1c) and group 2 (CD1d) [58–60]. Although these molecules are remarkably conserved in mammalian species, group 1 CD1 molecules are not present in rodents. A large body of evidence indicates that CD1-restricted T cells play an important role in protection from microbial infection by responding rapidly following recognition of defined microbial Ag. Ag presented by CD1 molecules include microbial lipid, glycolipid, and other nonprotein Ag, such as those present in *M. tuberculosis* and *M. leprae*. Both CD4[+] and CD8[+] T cells have been shown to recognize Ag restricted by group 1 CD1 molecules, suggesting that they may comprise a sizable proportion of T cells. A particular lymphocyte subset, NKT cells, has been shown to be CD1d-restricted. The canonically rearranged TCRα in these cells creates a semi-invariant TCR that may represent a novel "adaptive" PRR, which recognizes common glycolipid structural motifs [58]. CD1-mediated Ag processing and presentation takes place via the endosomal processing pathway and does not depend on products encoded by either TAP genes or the Ii for intracellular Ag transport [58–60].

D. Antigen Presenting Cells

The ability of cells to function as effective APC depends on their ability to process Ag for class I MHC-restricted CTL responses and/or class II MHC-restricted Th responses. As most of the cells of the body express class I MHC molecules and have the ability to express on the cell surface endogenously produced peptide complexes to class I MHC molecules, they have the potential to function as APC for $CD8^+$ CTL. In fact, cells which are endogenously producing viral, parasitic, or bacterial proteins or tumor Ag that gain access to the cytosol can be recognized and destroyed in a class I MHC-restricted fashion by specific CTL. In contrast, the main characteristics of APC required for presentation to Th cells in a class II-restricted fashion are the ability to take up soluble Ag from the extracellular compartment and process them to produce appropriate peptides that will then be complexed to class II MHC molecules and expressed on the cell membrane for recognition by Th cells. The cells that most efficiently present Ag to Th lymphocytes, the so-called "professional APC," include DC, macrophages, and B lymphocytes. Most professional APC express moderate to high levels of class II MHC molecules constitutively, and their expression can be upregulated upon activation by cytokines such as IFN-γ. Moreover, professional APC express many constimulatory and adhesion molecules, which are very important during the early stages of T-cell activation. In contrast, "nonprofessional APC," such as endothelial, epithelial, and mesenchymal cells, typically do not express class II MHC molecules constitutively, but can be induced to express them following exposure to T cell-derived cytokines, such as IFN-γ. Their role as APC in vivo is still unclear.

1. Dendritic Cells

A large body of evidence accumulated over the past few years clearly demonstrates that DC are the most effective APC involved in the activation of naive T cells [61–63]. Because of their key role in the induction of immunity, a thorough understanding of DC biology is of paramount importance in vaccine development. Dendritic cells comprise a heterogeneous cell population that originates in the bone marrow from hematopoietic stem cells and that reside, as immature DC, largely in peripheral tissues exposed to the environment, i.e., the sites of Ag entry. In the absence of ongoing inflammation and immune responses, DC's main function is to be vigilant for invading microbes in both lymphoid and nonlymphoid tissues (e.g., secondary lymphoid tissues, skin, blood, lymph, and mucosal surfaces). Immature DC express receptors for inflammatory chemokines that direct their migration to sites on inflammation. Upon recognition of microorganisms expressing PAMPs through PRRs, receptors for the Fc portion of Ig and other receptors (see Section II.A), exposure to cytokines, chemokines, and other inflammatory stimuli, and, under certain circumstances, self-Ag, DC quickly mature into efficient APC and migrate into draining LN where they initiate primary T cell responses. The maturation process involves the upregulation of MHC molecules, as well as costimulatory molecules (e.g., CD40, CD54, CD58, CD80, CC86), chemokine receptors (e.g., CCR7), and adhesion molecules which drive their migration into the lymphatic vessels and the T cell areas of the draining LN. To reiterate, in addition to presenting Ag, based on the type of cytokines they release and their expression of distinct

adhesion/costimulatory molecules, DC play a key role in determining the type of adaptive immunity elicited (e.g., polarized Th1 vs. Th2 responses).

Two main subsets of functionally distinct DC have been described in human peripheral blood, i.e., myeloid DC (mDC), also called "DC1," and lymphoid or plasmacytoid DC (pDC), also called "DC2," which can be differentiated based on the surface expression of molecules which determine their function [61,64–66]. Both populations of immature DC isolated from human peripheral blood lack lineage differentiation markers, including CD14, CD16, CD19, CD3, and CD56. mDC are lineage-negative, $CD11_C^+$, $CD123^{-/low}$, $CD4^+$, $CD80^{hi}$, $CD86^+$, $CD45RO^+$, $CD45RA^{low}$, $CD33^+$, $CD13^+$, $CD54^+$, $CD58^+$, $CD62L^{-/low}$, $CD36^{low}$, $CD83^+$ (small subset, most negative), HLA-DR^{hi}, CD206 [mannose receptor]$^+$, $CCR7^-$, $TLR2^+$, $TLR4^+$, $TLR7^-$,$TLR9^-$, $CD1a^+$, $CD1b^+$, $CD1c^+$, and $CD1d^+$ cells. Functionally, they exhibit high phagocytic potential and are likely to be rapidly recruited to the site of Ag entry (e.g., mucosal surfaces, skin). They are specialized to be the first to respond to microbial invasion via body surfaces. mDC produce large amounts of IL-12, IL-6, and TNF-α in response to TLR2 and TLR4 ligands, favoring the induction of Th1 responses [26,62]. However, the presence of other immunoregulatory molecules, such as prostaglandin E_2, may favor mDC priming of Th2 cells.

On the other hand, pDC are lineage-negative, $CD11c^-$, $CD123^{hi}$, $CD4^+$, $CD80^+$, $CD86^+$, $CD45RO^-$, $CD45RA^{hi}$, $CD13^-$, $CD62L^{hi}$, $CD33^-$, $CD83^-$, HLA-DR^{hi}, $CD206^-$, $CCR7^+$, $TLR2^-$, $TLR4^-$, $TLR7^+$, $TLR9^+$, $CD1a^-$, $CD1b^-$, $CD1c^-$, and $CD1d^-$ cells. These DC exhibit plasma cell-like morphology, and are functionally characterized by producing large amounts of IFN-α and IFN-β in response to TLR9 ligation. These are poorly phagocytic, are located mainly in T cell areas of lymphoid tissues, and are likely to be specialized to recognize self-Ag or blood-borne pathogens. They also play an important role in antiviral innate immunity through production of IFN-α and IFN-β. In general, pDC are believed to favor Th2 development, although this view has recently been challenged [26,62]. Because blood DC2s do not migrate to inflammatory cytokines, they probably reach the LN by responding to SDF-1 (a chemokine expressed in LN) using CXCR4, and CD62L interaction with ʟ-selectin ligands expressed in endothelial venules. This interaction may provide a maturational signal that couples CCR7 with migration, allowing the proper positioning of pDC in LN in response to secondary lymphoid tissue chemokines. To add to the complexity of the function of DC in Ag presentation, mDC and pDC regulate each other through the cytokines they release [61,62]. For example, IL-10 has been shown to induce apoptosis in developing DC, a process that can be overcome by the addition of tumor necrosis factor (TNF-α) or CD40L. Moreover, DC exhibit immunoregulatory effects on B cell proliferation, differentiation, and isotype switching [67].

Based on the extraordinary capabilities of DC to prime the immune system, a number of clinical trials have recently explored the use of DC in immunotherapy for cancer based on the injection of Ag-pulsed DC [61]. These studies showed that this approach is safe and yielded promising preliminary results, but definitive proof of efficacy is still pending. Further understanding of DC biology is undoubtedly one of the primary areas that, in the coming years, will provide critical information to advance novel vaccination strategies.

2. Other Antigen Presenting Cells

In contrast to DC, the main role of macrophages is to phagocytose, following recognition through PRRs and other receptors such as Ig Fc receptors, and destroy invading microbes. Ag peptides from the pathogens then become available for binding to MHC molecules for presentation to T cells. Once activated, they upregulate their expression of MHC and costimulatory molecules and can become rather effective APC. Nevertheless, macrophages are considerably less efficient than DC at activating naive T cells. Macrophages are a major source of proinflammatory cytokines, including IL-1α, IL-1β, IL-6, IL-8, IL-12, TNF-α, and TNF-β, that exert potent immunoregulatory activities on T cell responses. B cells can also function as professional APCs by presenting to Th cells peptides derived from soluble Ag following internalization and processing of Ag bound to the B cell receptor complex, which consists of the specific membrane Ig and associated invariant Igα (CD79β) and Igα (CD79β) polypeptides [68].

IV. APC–T CELL INTERACTIONS AND T-CELL ACTIVATION

A. Antigen Recognition by α/β TCR–CD3 Complexes

The receptor on the surface of the majority of T cells which recognizes MHC–Ag complexes on the APC is a heterodimer composed of an α ($\sim$ 40–60 kDa) and a β chain ($\sim$ 40–50 kDa) covalently linked by disulfide bonds [69]. Both α and β chains are transmembrane glycoproteins, members of the Ig superfamily, that contain variable and constant regions. Amino acid residues in the hypervariable regions of both chains contribute to binding to the MHC molecules and the peptide fragment aa side chains extending out from the peptide-binding groove [69]. While the TCR α/β heterodimer is responsible for recognition and binding to the MHC–peptide complexes, their ability to transduce signals inside the cells and trigger cell activation depends on several associated proteins, including the γ, δ, ε, and ζ CD3 proteins, which associate noncovalently with the α/β heterodimer to form the TCR–CD3 complex [70]. It appears that each TCR complex includes two TCR α/β heterodimers per CD3 cluster [69]. All CD3 molecules contain, in their cytoplasmic tails, tyrosine phosphorylation motifs, named immunoreceptor tyrosine-based activation motifs (ITAMs), which are critical for TCR-mediated T-cell activation. However, it should be emphasized that the signals generated by the TCR–CD3 complex are not sufficient to trigger T-cell activation. As will be discussed later in more detail, the presence of costimulatory signals is critical for successful T-cell activation. It should also be noted that TCR molecules and all CD3-associated proteins are the same in CD4$^+$ Th and CD8$^+$ CTL. In addition to signal transduction, CD3

proteins also play a vital role in the assembly and transport of α/β heterodimers to the cell surface [69].

B. Antigen Recognition by γ/δ TCR–CD3 Complexes

In addition to α/β heterodimers, a second type of TCR, consisting of evolutionarily conserved γ/δ heterodimers, is expressed in a small proportion of peripheral blood T lymphocytes (1–5%) and in more substantial numbers in regional sites, such as in mucosal surfaces of the gastrointestinal tract (10% in humans and up to 50% of intraepithelial lymphocytes in mice) [71,72]. These γ/δ TCR T cells seem to originate from a different lineage than T cells expressing α/β TCR and the majority of them are double negative for CD4 and CD8 molecules, although minor subpopulations of γ/δ TCR T cells have been shown to express CD8 consisting of α/α homodimers or the CD4$^+$ CD8$^+$ phenotype [71,72]. The biochemical structure of TCR γ and δ transmembrane glycoproteins, containing variable and constant regions, resembles that of TCR α and β chains [69]. These γ/δ TCR are also expressed in association with CD3 proteins and depend upon them for expression on the cell surface and signal transduction inside the cells. It is not entirely known at present how and which Ag are recognized by γ/δ TCR T cells, but it appears that these cells are activated by superantigens or Ag associated with nonpolymorphic MHC-like molecules (e.g., those encoded by the HLA-E, -F, and -G regions) or by CD1; only a small minority recognizes peptides presented in the context of classical class I and II MHC molecules [69,71,72]. Recognition by γ/δ TCR T cells of proteins and small phosphoantigens (phosphate-containing nonpeptide Ag) isolated from mycobacterial extracts does not require Ag processing, i.e., Ag are recognized directly [71,72]. These differences between the way in which γ/δ and α/β T cells recognize Ag suggest that specialized APC might not be required for the activation of γ/δ T cells, providing additional flexibility for the generation of effector CMI against infectious agents. T cells expressing the γ/δ TCR–CD3 complex have been shown to play a significant role in protection against infectious organisms (e.g., *Leishmania*, *Mycobacteria*, *Plasmodium*, *Salmonella*), particularly in the gastrointestinal tract and other mucosal surfaces, by mediating a number of effector immune responses, including cytokine production and CTL activity [71,72].

C. The Immunological Synapse

Studies conducted in the last decade have established that T-cell activation is a complex process that requires at least two signals, one provided by the interaction of the TCR complex ($\alpha\beta$ TCR and associated CD3 molecules) with pMHC on APC and a second, complementary signal provided by binding of CD28 (a costimulatory molecule on T cells) to members of the B7 family (e.g., CD80 [B7-1]) on APC [19,20]. Many additional molecules have also been shown to play important roles in T-cell activation. The term "immunological synapse" (IS) was recently coined to describe the organized molecular complex that is assembled at the interface between the T cell and the APC where the interaction between the TCR complex and pMHC molecules takes place [19–21,73,74]. Formation of IS has been described not only for CD4$^+$ and CD8$^+$ T cells, but also for NK cells, suggesting that they may be a common feature of lymphocyte activation. The IS has been found to have a remarkable level of organization, characterized by a "bull's eye" arrangement of supramolecular activation clusters (SMAC), which form within 30–60 min of T cell–APC contact [20]. The central portion of the IS (cSMAC) is enriched for TCR and pMHC complexes, as well as coreceptors CD4 or CD8 and CD28 and its ligand, CD80. The ring around the core (pSMAC) includes other costimulatory molecules [e.g., CD11a/CD18 (LFA-1) and its ligand, CD54 (ICAM-1), and CD2 and its ligands CD48 and CD58 (ICAM-3)], as well as signaling molecules in the cytoplasmic side of the T cell (e.g., protein kinase C θ and the src family kinase lck [19,20]). Interactions among adhesion molecules in the pSMAC, including LFA-1, CD54, CD2, CD48, and CD58, play key roles in maintaining small distances (~15 nm) between apposing T cell and APC membranes and in providing additional signaling [19,73,75].

Important findings derived from the study of the IS include the observations that an intact cystokeleton is an absolute requirement for the T cell but not for the APC, and that the formation of a stable IS for at least 1 hr is required for full T-cell activation. Several temporal stages have been described in T-cell activation, including T-cell polarization, initial adhesion, IS formation (initial signaling), and IS maturation (sustained signaling) [20]. Exposure of naive recirculating T cells to chemokines/cytokines (e.g., signaling from the innate system) and the resulting T-cell polarization, which includes cytoskeletal rearrangements, are the required steps preceding the initial APC–T cell interaction and the subsequent IS formation. The precise functions of the mature IS remain controversial. For example, recent evidence showing that the very early events of TCR signaling occur before the formation of the mature IS suggest that this phenomenon is not a requirement for TCR triggering [76]. However, IS appears to play important roles in amplifying weak TCR signaling through concomitant CD28 engagement in the cSMAC and in allowing polarized secretion by T cells [73]. Functional synapses (characterized by the induction of calcium signaling, movement of surface molecules, etc.) between the majority of T cells and DC are formed in the absence of specific Ag, highlighting the uniqueness of T cell–DC interactions [77]. Novel findings in the burgeoning field of IS formation in T-cell activation and signaling will undoubtedly lead to new approaches to enhance and/or modulate the type of immune responses induced by vaccination.

D. Brief Summary of Signal Transduction Events Following Activation Through the TCR–CD3 Complex

Intense research efforts over the past decade have greatly advanced our understanding of the complex biochemical events triggered by the TCR complexes following Ag recognition that ultimately result in the activation of genes in the nucleus leading to the production of cytokines and other important molecules involved in effector CMI responses.

However, a detailed description of these events is beyond the scope of this review. Instead, we will provide a brief summary of these phenomena and refer the reader to numerous excellent reviews that summarize in great detail current understanding of these phenomena [20,78–81].

The first event detected following TCR–CD3 ligation is the lck-mediated phosporylation of tyrosine residues within the ITAMs of the invariant CD3 and TCR ζ-chain dimers, and the recruitment and activation of ZAP-70. In turn, ZAP-70 phosphorylates a number of adapter proteins, i.e., proteins lacking enzymatic activities, but that, upon activation, change their conformation allowing other enzymes or adapters to bind resulting in the formation of multiprotein complexes. Phosphorylation of these adapter proteins, including LAT (linker for activation of T cells) and SLP-76, leads to the recruitment and activation of phospholypase Cγ1 [PLC-γ1], PI-3K, Itk, and GEFs to the activated TCR complex. Activation of these molecules initiates important signaling pathways. For example, PLC-γ1 cleaves phosphatidylinositol biphosphate (PIP$_2$) to yield diacylglycerol (DAG) and inositol triphosphate (IP$_3$). DAG, together with increased Ca^{2+}, activates protein kinase C, which, in turn, activates the transcription factor NfκB. On the other hand, IP$_3$ increases intracellular Ca^{2+}, leading to activation of calcineurin, which, in turn, activates the transcription factor NFAT. Other key molecules, guanine-nucleotide exchange factors (GEFs), activate Ras which, in turn, activates a mitogen-activated protein (MAP) kinase cascade, leading to the activation of Fos (a component of the AP-1 transcription factor). Together, NFκB, nuclear factor of activated T-cells (NFAT), and AP-1 induce specific gene transcription by binding to regulatory sites in the DNA (including the IL-2, IL-2Rα, and IFN-γ genes) [20,78–81]. The coordinated expression of genes which encode cytokines and other molecules, such as cyclins, ultimately results in T-cell proliferation and differentiation. Activation of these "early genes," is also followed by the appearance of a number of cell surface molecules that play critical roles in T-cell activation, differentiation, and proliferation, including CD69, CD25 (IL-2Rα), class II MHC molecules, etc. Notably, tyrosine phosphorylation, calcium flux, and the generation of inositol phospholipids reach maximum levels within 30 sec to 5 min following activation, coinciding with the early stages of IS formation [81]. However, elevation of intracellular Ca^{2+} ion levels, PI turnover, and transcription factors (e.g., NFAT) in the nucleus should be sustained for 60–120 min for effective signal transduction leading to cell proliferation, which coincides with the "commitment period" during the initial stages of T-cell activation and formation of the mature IS [74]. Naive T cells need 20 hr or longer of sustained stimulation to increase their size and become committed to proliferation [74].

E. Activation of T Cells by Superantigens

Superantigens consist of certain bacterial and viral proteins that, without processing, trigger activation of up to 20% of T cells, including CD4$^+$ and CD8$^+$ cells. This activation is triggered by high-affinity binding of these superantigens to the lateral sides of class II MHC molecules on APC and to the β chain (V_β) of α/β TCR T cells [69,82,83]. The recognition between T cells and superantigens is specific and clonally variable, because superantigens activate T cells bearing particular V_β regions. Triggering of T cells by superantigens requires the complete TCR–CD3 complex and accessory molecules, including CD4, CD8, CD2, and LFA-1 ($\alpha_L\beta_2$ integrin) [69,82,83]. Instead of priming an adaptive immune response to the pathogen, T-cell activation by superantigens causes a massive cytokine production, mainly by $CD4^+$ T cells. The cytokine response not only causes systemic toxicity, but also downregulates the host's adaptive immunity and might be involved in the triggering of autoimmune diseases. In addition, superantigens induce the activation of APC, leading to the production of proinflammatory cytokines, such as IL-1β and TNF-α. The high levels of APC and T-cell activation, and the ensuing release of cytokines triggered by superantigens, play a significant role in the generation of toxic shock syndrome and food poisoning associated with some bacterial infections. Superantigens include products of bacterial and viral origin. Bacterial superantigens include staphylococcal enterotoxins (SE)-A, SE-B, SE-C, SE-D, SE-E, the toxic shock syndrome toxin-1 (TSST-1), and those produced by streptococci, *Yersinia*, and *Mycoplasma arthritidis*. Viral superantigens include retroviral glycoproteins, such as the minor lymphocyte stimulating Ag (MIs) produced by the mouse mammary tumor viruses, and products of rabies and moloney leukemia viruses [69, 82,83].

V. ROLE OF CD28, CD40, 4-1BB, AND OTHER COSTIMULATORY MOLECULES IN LYMPHOCYTE ACTIVATION

From the discussion of the formation of the "immunological synapse," it is apparent that many molecules, in addition to the TCR/CD3 complex interacting with pMHC, are involved in the induction of lymphocyte activation. Chief among them are coreceptors CD4 or CD8 and costimulatory molecules CD28 and its B7 family ligands, CD80 and CD86, CD40 and its ligand, CD154 [CD40L] and 4-1BB and its ligand, 4-1BBL [84–87]. Interactions among these molecules are complex. Some of them, such as coreceptors CD4 and CD8, have a dual role by contributing to T cell–APC cell–cell adhesion and by actively participating in the signal transduction processes triggered following TCR–CD3 complex–pMHC interactions. Moreover, recent data indicate that $CD4^+$ and $CD8^+$ T cells exhibit different requirements for optimal stimulation [88]. For example, $CD4^+$ T-cell activation depends on CD154 (expressed predominantly in activated $CD4^+$ T cells) interacting with CD40 (expressed in B cells, DC, and macrophages) and on CD28 (in $CD4^+$ T cells) interacting with CD80 and CD86 in APC. Regarding $CD8^+$ T cell responses, two types have been described, i.e., those that are relatively independent (e.g., Sendai virus, influenza virus) or those that are relatively dependent (e.g., adenovirus, herpes simplex virus, tumor Ag) on Th cells. Th-independent $CD8^+$ T cell responses are less dependent on CD40/CD154 interactions than Th-dependent responses. In contrast, both types of $CD8^+$ T cell responses are dependent, to a considerable extent, on CD28/CD80–CD86 and 4-1BB (in $CD8^+$ T cells)/4-1BBL (in APC) interactions [88]. In addition to $CD8^+$ T cells, 4-1BB is expressed in many other cells, including $CD4^+$ T cells, NK, and APC, and 4-1BBL is expressed in APC and other cells. These observations suggest that these costimulatory molecules could also be involved in linking innate and adaptive immunity [84].

Some costimulatory molecules, such as CD28, are constitutively expressed in naive cells and their expression increases following activation, while others (such as CD152 [CTLA-4]) are only expressed after activation. CD152, despite binding the same receptors as CD28 (i.e., CD80 and CD86), is expressed later after activation and is involved in downregulating, rather than favoring, lymphocyte stimulation [85–87]. Furthermore, CD28 appears to play a key role in regulating the differentiation of Th1 and Th2 T cell subsets, favoring polarization toward Th2 responses [26]. The number of costimulatory molecules shown to be involved in lymphocyte activation is dramatically increasing, as is the complexity of their interactions. For example, new members of the B7 family were recently described [86]. These include ICOS, a receptor homologous to CD28 and CD152 (in activated T cells) that interacts with the ICOS-L (constitutively expressed in APC) providing positive costimulatory signals, and PD-1 (in activated T cells, B cells, and macrophages) interacting with PD-L1 and PD-L2 receptors (in activated DC, B cells, and macrophages) that downregulates lymphocyte activation [86]. A thorough understanding of the complex interactions among costimulatory molecules, which result in either enhancement or suppression of T-cell activation, will remain an important area of investigation in the coming years.

VI. CYTOKINES AND CHEMOKINES: LINKING ADAPTIVE AND INNATE IMMUNITY

As discussed above, it has become apparent that particular patterns of cytokines and chemokines secreted following pathogen invasion, as well as the temporal sequence of their production, play a dominant role in determining the outcome of the host's immune response and its ability to control infection. Because of space limitations, it is not possible to describe the many roles and interactions among cytokines and chemokines and their receptors. Thus for detailed descriptions of individual cytokines and chemokines, the reader is referred to a number of excellent books and reviews that have been recently published [89–98]. Instead, we will concentrate in briefly describing our current understanding on how the coordinated induction of chemokines and polarized cytokine patterns play a role in resistance to disease by invading pathogens, as well as their role in downregulating immune responses, and provide some examples on the intricate interactions among these potent mediators in cross-regulating innate and adaptive immunity.

A. Cytokines

These immunoregulatory molecules, secreted by immune, as well as other cells, play key roles in the clonal expansion of lymphocytes, in mediating the action of effector cells, and in regulating innate immunity. In spite of their diversity, most cytokines share the following characteristics: (1) they are produced by more than one cell type and act on many different cells (pleiotropism), sometimes exerting more than one effect on a single target cell; (2) their production follows cell activation, requires de novo RNA and protein synthesis, and is transient; (3) similar activities are typically performed by more than one cytokine (redundancy); (4) production of individual cytokines follows the release of other cytokines producing a "cascading effect"; (5) they regulate each other, either positively or negatively, sometimes synergizing or exhibiting additive effects; (6) they exert their functions by interacting with high-affinity specific receptors on the target cells (10^{-9} to 10^{-12} K_d) that they help regulate; (7) they can exert their activities locally, systemically, or both by acting in an autocrine (i.e., on the cells that produce them), paracrine (i.e., on adjacent cells), or endocrine (i.e., on distant cells) fashion; and, (8) their actions on the target cells usually involve regulation of proliferation and state of differentiation [89,90,93–98].

The diversity of cell sources and targets, overlapping biological functions, and disparate biochemical structures have rendered cytokines difficult to classify into defined categories. Nevertheless, based on their dominant biological activities, cytokines can be divided into three main classes: (1) those involved primarily in regulation of hematopoiesis [e.g., granulocyte-macrophage colony stimulating factor (GM-CSF), monocyte-macrophage-CSF (M-CSF), granulocyte-CSF (G-CSF), IL-3 (or multi-CSF), IL-7, IL-9, IL-11]; (2) those involved in proinflammatory activities typically associated with innate immunity (e.g., IL-1α, IL-1β, IL-6, IFN-α, IFN-β, TNF-α, chemokines); and (3) those predominantly involved in regulating activation, differentiation, and function of lymphocytes and other cells during inflammatory responses associated with adaptive immunity [e.g., IL-2, IL-4, IL-5, IL-10, IL-12, IFN-γ, TNF-β (lymphotoxin), transforming growth factor-β (TGF-β)].

B. The Th1/Th2 Paradigm

Distinct Th cell populations exhibit discrete or overlapping patterns of cytokine production that designate Th1 and Th2 CD4$^+$ T cells [26,27,29–32,99,100]. Th1 cells are characterized by the production of IFN-γ and TNF-β, while Th2 cells are characterized by the production of IL-4, IL-5, IL-9, IL-10, and IL-13. Cells producing a combination of these cytokines were named Th0. CD8$^+$ cells also exhibit type 1 (Tc1) and type 2 (Tc2) cytokine profiles [31,99]. The existence of CD4$^+$ T populations with strong downregulatory activity, characterized by the secretion of defined cytokine patterns (e.g., TGF-β), was reported recently [30]. Many Th cells exhibit "mixed" cytokine production (e.g., IL-2, IL-4, IL-5, and IFN-γ), which does not allow them to be classified into Th1 or Th2 cells, even within populations that are polarized toward Th1 or Th2 patterns [100]. Moreover, there is a certain plasticity by which Th1 cells can revert to a Th2 phenotype, although reversion in the opposite direction is more difficult [100].

Typically, Th1 responses promote CMI, such as CTL activity, delayed-type hypersensitivity (DTH), ADCC, macrophage activation, and provide help for the production of certain Ig isotypes (IgG2a in mice, probably IgG2 in humans). Consequently, Th1 responses have been associated with beneficial responses (or found to predominate) in infections caused by protozoa (e.g., *Leishmania major*, *Trypanosoma cruzi*), viruses (e.g., influenza), bacteria (e.g., *M. tuberculosis*, *M. leprae*, *S. enterica* serovar Typhi, *Bordetella pertussis*, *Chlamydia*, *Listeria monocytogenes*), and fungi (e.g., *Candida*) [31,101,102]. In contrast, Th1 responses have been associated with detrimental responses in helminthic infections and in pathological conditions, such as autoimmune disorders (e.g., experimental autoimmune encephalomyelitis, multiple sclerosis, and rheumatoid arthritis), chronic inflammation, transplant rejection, and pregnancy [31,32,101]. On the other hand, Th2 responses provide help for Ig production by B-cells, including IgE, IgG (IgG1 in mice, IgG4 in humans), and IgA, and promote mast cell and eosinophil growth and differentiation. Accordingly, Th2 responses were found to be associated with beneficial responses in infections caused by helminths (e.g., *Trichuris muris*, *Nippostrongylus brasiliensis*, *Brugia malayi*) and some bacteria (e.g., *Borrelia burgdorferi*), and with detrimental responses in infections caused by protozoans (e.g., *L. major*) and viruses (e.g., vaccinia, herpes simplex virus), and in pathological conditions such as allergy and atopic asthma [31,32,100,101].

To a considerable extent, Th1 and Th2 responses are mutually inhibitory phenotypes, leading to the predominance of either Th1 or Th2 responses. As soon as a T cell response progresses along a Th1 or Th2 pathway, it tends to become polarized in that particular direction [100], largely because of the inhibitory effects of Th1 cytokines on Th2 responses and vice versa. For example, IL-10 inhibits cytokine synthesis by Th1 cells and downregulates macrophage activation, while IFN-γ inhibits Th2 cell proliferation. In many experimental systems in animals, the resistance or susceptibility to infection in vivo can be altered by modulating the type of cytokine patterns by injection of exogenous cytokines (e.g., IFN-γ, TGF-β, IL-12, IL-4) and/or neutralizing monoclonal Ab to cytokines (e.g., anti-IFN-γ, anti-IL-4), during the early phases of the immune response. Many factors, including the nature and dose of Ag, the route of entry, the nature and maturation stages of the participating DC, the host's genetic make-up, and the cytokines and chemokines present in the microenvironment during the early stages of lymphocyte activation, are believed to play key roles in determining the predominant polarized cytokine patterns elicited by the invading pathogen [26,27,29–32,99,100]. For example, it has been suggested that the Th1-promoting capabilities of DC correlate with their ability to produce certain cytokines and chemokines, particularly IL-12, while the absence of these mediators might favor the generation of predominantly Th2 responses [26]. An in-depth understanding of the mechanisms involved in the generation of polarized Th1/Th2 responses has the potential, like few other areas in immunology, to dramatically impact vaccine development.

C. Regulatory T Cells and Cytokines Involved in the Downregulation of Immune Responses

In recent years, the existence of several subsets of regulatory T cells (Tr, formerly known as "suppressor" T cells) exhibiting defined phenotypes and patterns of cytokine production, distinct from Th1 and Th2 cells, has been firmly established [30]. Tr cells are believed not only to play a key role in maintaining self-tolerance by downregulating immunity to self Ag, but also to be intimately involved in the regulation of immunity to pathogens by suppressing pathogen-induced immunopathology or prolonging the persistence of microorganisms by downregulating protective Th1 immunity [30]. At least four distinct populations of Tr cells have been described to date: (1) Tr1 cells, which secrete high amounts of IL-10 and moderate levels of TGF-β, but not IL-2, IL-4, or IFN-γ; (2) Th3 cells, which secrete high levels of TGF-β; (3) CD4$^+$CD25$^+$ cells, shown to inhibit immunity through undefined mechanisms requiring cell–cell contact; and (4) CD8$^+$ Tr cells, which can secrete either IL-10 or TGF-β. Recent evidence showing that Tr1 cells suppress protective Th1 responses against *B. pertussis*, and the immunoregulatory properties of CD4$^+$CD25$^+$ cells in a model of *P. carini* infection, highlights the importance of Tr cells in the host's immune response to microorganisms [30]. IL-10-secreting DC ("DCr") apparently direct naive T cells toward a Tr1 subtype. Because of their predominantly downregulatory properties, production of IL-10 and/or TGF-β are the likely mediators of Tr activity. IL-10 suppresses adaptive immune responses and inflammation, while promoting the survival and differentiation of B cells [103]. Similarly, TGF-β inhibits the differentiation of both CD4$^+$ and CD8$^+$ naive T cells into effectors, blocks Th1 and Th2 development by inhibiting transcriptional activators, and downregulates macrophage activation, class II MHC expression, cytokine synthesis, NK cytolytic activities, and activation of neutrophils and endothelial cells by proinflammatory cytokines, while promoting IgA production [89,104]. Because of these powerful biological activities, IL-10 and TGF-β are likely to play a dominant role in preventing inappropriate responses to certain self- or environmental Ag.

Other cytokines have also been shown to play a role in downregulating immunity and inflammation. For example, the IL-1R antagonist (IL-1RA), mainly produced by macrophages, neutrophils, keratinocytes, and epithelial cells, acts as a competitive inhibitor of IL-1 by binding to the same receptors as IL-1 without triggering biological function [89]. In this way, IL-1RA acts as an antiinflammatory molecule by blocking IL-1-mediated proinflammatory activities. Soluble cytokine receptors for IL-1, IL-2, and many other cytokines have also been described and they are postulated to act as antiinflammatory mediators by binding to the corresponding cytokine in the microenvironment, thereby precluding them from binding to the corresponding cytokine receptor on the surface of the target cells. The understanding of the mechanisms underlying the induction and maintenance of Tr cells, as well as the release of other antiinflammatory cytokines, might lead to the development of novel vaccines against autoimmune diseases, as well as therapies to control graft rejection, inflammation, and allergy.

D. Chemokines

Chemokines are a distinct class of cytokines that exhibit chemoattractant properties, i.e., they cause cells with the appropriate receptors to migrate toward the chemokine source [91,92,105–107]. Moreover, recent data indicates that chemokines might also regulate the polarity and magnitude of T-cell cytokine responses [92]. More than 50 chemokines have been identified to date. Most chemokines fall into two main families, cys–X–cys (also called C–X–C; α-chemokines or inflammatory chemokines) and cys–cys (also called C–C or β-chemokines), depending on whether the two N-terminal cystein residues are adjacent or have an additional aa between them. The nomenclature of the ever growing number of chemokines and their receptors has been revised recently [108]. C–X–C chemokines (e.g., CXCL1–CXCL14) are mainly produced by macrophages, neutrophils, fibroblasts, endothelial cells, etc. and attract neutrophils predominantly. In contrast, C–C chemokines (e.g., CCL1-5, CCL7, CCL8, CCL11, and CCL13-27) are mostly produced by activated lymphocytes and attract monocytes, basophils, eosinophils, and lymphocytes [108]. Chemokine receptors have also been renamed, based on the chemokine subclass specificity of the receptor (e.g., CXCR1-5, CCR1-11) [108]. Chemokines and their receptors are now considered to be the most important regulators of leukocyte trafficking. They have been shown to play key roles in many fundamental immunological processes, including, among others: (1) leukocyte binding to endothelium leading to extravasation (together with selectins and other adhesion molecules); (2) control the traffic of developing B and T cells (through expression of defined sets of chemokine receptors at various maturational stages, e.g., naive T-cell activation, effector T cell differentiation and memory cell development; see below); (3) migration of DC to tissues and from tissues to LN (critical for immune surveillance, priming, and tolerance); (4) migration of monocytes to tissues in response to inflammatory stimuli; (5) interactions between naive T cells and DC and between T and B cells in secondary lymphoid organs; (6) Th2 attraction of eosinophils (through production of CCL11 [eotaxin-1], CCL24, CCL26, and others that bind CCR3 in eosinophils); (7) recruitment of Th1 cells to sites of inflammation (through CCR5 and CXCR3 expression); (8) migration of memory and effector CD4$^+$ and CD8$^+$ T cells to effector sites, such as the gut mucosa (through CCR9) or the skin (through CCR4 and CCR10) in conjunction with other adhesion molecules (e.g., integrin $\alpha_4\beta_7$ for gut homing and CLA for skin homing; see Section VII.C); and (9) PMN migration and degranulation [through CXCR1 and CXCR2 binding CXCL8 (IL-8)] [91,92,105–107].

Many chemokines are spontaneously produced at specific sites. For example, CCL21 (SLC) and CCL19 (MIP-3β, ELC) produced in the T cell area of LN, attract DC, T cells, and other leukocytes expressing their ligand, CCR7. However, these chemokines are also released by other cells, such as DC, to attract naive T cells. Because of the key role of chemokines in inflammation, several therapeutic modalities directed to control their activity in diseases associated with tissue destruction resulting from inflammatory responses (e.g., allergies, asthma, rheumatoid arthritis, pneumonia) are being vigorously explored.

E. Cytokines and Chemokines Linking Innate and Adaptive Immunity

Cytokines and chemokines are the major mediators between APC, lymphocytes, and other cells, and are central to the innate immune system's capacity to dramatically influence the type and magnitude of adaptive immunity and in the ability of the adaptive immune response to markedly affect inflammatory responses [109,110]. For example, cells of the innate immune system (e.g., macrophages, DC) secrete type I interferons (IFN-α, IFN-β), GM-CSF, IL-1, and TNF-α, which promote the activation and differentiation of DC (a major cell type linking innate and adaptive immunity), as well as IL-12, IL-15, and IL-18, which dramatically affect the adaptive immunity induced. Of note, IL-12 has been recently shown to induce DC and macrophages to secrete IFN-γ, a cytokine traditionally considered to be produced by cells of the adaptive immune response [94]. In turn, IFN-γ markedly affects the activation of cells of innate immunity, for example, by (1) stimulating the cytolytic activity of NK cells, (2) increasing the expression of class I and II MHC molecules and the production of an array of proinflammatory mediators including IL-1α, IL-1β, TNF-α, IL-6, and IL-8 by APC, and (3) directly promoting nonspecific killing of bacterial organisms by enhancing the microbicidal activity of macrophages through induction of nitric oxide synthase and protease activity [109,110]. Because of the central role that cytokines, chemokines, and their receptors play at virtually all levels during the generation of immune responses and as major players in linking innate and adaptive immunity, continued studies on their functions and complex interactions will provide invaluable information to help in the development of novel vaccine strategies.

VII. INTEGRINS, SELECTINS, AND CHEMOKINES IN CELL–CELL INTERACTIONS AND LYMPHOCYTE TRAFFICKING

A highly interrelated network of molecules and their receptors belonging to three separate families has been shown to play a leading role in directing the trafficking of immune cells to sites of inflammation and secondary lymphoid tissues. These include chemokines (see Section VI.D), integrins, and selectins.

A. Integrins

Integrins are a superfamily of heterodimers consisting of noncovalently associated α and β subunits that, by mediating cell–cell (e.g., endothelial cells) and cell–matrix (e.g., collagen, fibronectin) adhesion, play a major role in T-cell activation and homing to secondary immunological organs and sites of inflammation [111–113]. The fact that most members of the integrin family involve a common β subunit associating with specific α subunits lead to the original classification of integrins into the so-called β-integrin families. A total of 8 β subunits and 21 α subunits have been identified to date [111]. In some cases, a particular α chain subunit can bind to more than one β chain. Among the key integrin families involved in lymphocyte homing are members of the β_1 (CD29) family, which consists of at least nine members (heterodimers composed of β_1 and α_1–α_8 or α_v), the β_2 (CD18) family (heterodimers composed of β_2 and α_L, α_M, or α_x) and the β_7 family (heterodimers composed of β_7 and α_4 or α_{HML}).

The family of β_2 integrins, which is expressed on all leukocytes and has been shown to mediate transmembrane signal transduction, includes three homologous heterodimers composed of a common β_2 chain (CD18): complement receptor 3 (CR3, CD11b/CD18, found predominantly in monocytes, NK, and neutrophils, as well as in some lymphocytes), CR4 (CD11c/CD18, found in macrophages, granulocytes, and some T cells) and the $\alpha_L\beta_2$ integrin (LFA-1, CD11a/CD18) that is expressed in lymphocytes, monocytes, NK, and other leukocytes) [114]. For example, CR3 recognizes the iC3b complement component, the intercellular adhesion molecule-1 (ICAM-1), fibrinogen, and other ligands and relays this "proinflammatory information" to the cytoplasm via exodomain interactions [114].

B. Selectins

Selectins comprise a family of three carbohydrate-binding molecules involved in leukocyte–endothelial cell adhesion: L-selectin (CD62L; present in T and B lymphocytes, monocytes, NK, neutrophils, and other cells), E-selectin (CD62-E, ELAM-1; present in endothelial cells), and P-selectin (CD62-P; present in platelets, activated endothelial cells, and megakaryocytes). CD62L (peripheral lymph node homing receptor) is expressed at high levels in most naive $CD45RA^{hi}CD45RO^{lo}$ T cells, and its expression declines after activation. Thus CD62L is expressed at low levels in most T_m cells. CD62L plays a key role in the interaction of lymphocytes with high endothelial venules (HEV) by recognizing carbohydrate moieties in the surface glycoproteins of endothelial cells, including the glycosylation-dependent cell adhesion molecule-1 (GlyCAM-1), CD34, and the peripheral-node addressin (PNAd) in LN [112,115].

C. Role of Integrins, Selectins, and Chemokines: An Integrated View of Lymphocyte Tracking

Because the first step in lymphocyte migration to peripheral tissues involves leukocyte adhesion to the vascular endothelium, the capacity of integrins to bind to vascular addressins plays a critical role in lymphocyte homing. For example, integrins belonging to the β_7 integrin family, such as α_4/β_7 (LPAM-1, lymphocyte Peyer's patch adhesion molecule 1) and α_E/β_7 (HML-1), appear to be critical for lymphocyte homing to mucosal tissues [107,115–117]. The α_4/β_7 integrin binds to the mucosal addressin cell adhesion molecule-1 (MadCAM-1) present in endothelial cells of HEV [107, 117]. HEV, present in LN, PP in the intestine, tonsils, adenoids, appendix, and aggregates of lymphoid tissues in the gut mucosa, as well as in chronically inflamed nonlymphoid tissues but not in spleen, are critical target sites for lymphocyte recirculation [115]. The α_E/β_7 (HML-1) integrin, which binds to the E-cadherin chain expressed by mucosal epithelial cells, appears to be important in lymphocyte homing to the gut epithelium [107,117].

Another integrin, α_4/β_1 (CD49d/CD29, very late antigen-4 [VLA-4], LPAM-2), which binds to the vascular ligand vascular cell adhesion molecule-1 (VCAM-1) that is primarily expressed on the endothelium of nonmucosal sites of inflammation, appears to play a key role in homing of activated T cells to nonmucosal sites [117]. Similarly, LFA-

1 ($\alpha_L\beta_2$ integrin) is also involved in homing of activated lymphocyte to peripheral tissues by binding to the intercellular cell adhesion molecule-1 (ICAM-1) and ICAM-2 present in HEV [115]. Differential expression of integrins (e.g., $\alpha_6\beta_1$ in Th1 cells) can also contribute to the distinct homing behavior of Th1 and Th2 cells [112].

Taken together, the information discussed above on the role of chemokines, integrins, and selectins in lymphocyte trafficking clearly demonstrates that the homing potential of immune cells depends on the coordinated production of multiple molecules and expression of the appropriate receptors. For example, the fact that CD62L expression declines markedly after lymphocyte activation, which occurs concomitantly with the increased expression and affinity of adhesion molecules such as α_4/β_7 integrin, α_4/β_1 integrin and LFA-1 ($\alpha_L\beta_2$ integrin), promotes activated T cells to leave the LN and migrate to sites of inflammation in peripheral tissues, including the gut associated mucosa. In addition, concomitant expression of other receptors (e.g., CCR9 in $\alpha_4\beta_7^{hi}$ cells), might help direct their homing to particular areas of the mucosa, e.g., the intestinal mucosa, which has been shown to produce TECK, a CCR9 ligand [107]. TECK is absent or weakly expressed in other segments of the gastrointestinal tract (e.g., stomach and colon) and only a portion of lymphocytes in the colon express CCR9. Another example of the complexity of the signals involved in lymphocyte homing is trafficking to the skin. Lymphocytes with skin homing potential express the cutaneous lymphoma Ag (CLA) but do not express integrin $\alpha_4\beta_7$. These lymphocytes concomitantly express CCR4 (the ligand for CCL17, produced by cutaneous endothelium) and/or CCR10 (the ligand for CCL27, produced by keratinocytes) [107].

Elucidation of the molecular basis of lymphocyte homing will undoubtedly have an enormous impact on the vaccine development field in years to come. This knowledge will help determine the most appropriate routes of immunization or means to target Ag to the correct site for optimal presentation depending on the desired effector immune response. It will also help predict the most likely site and type of effector immunity elicited by immunization.

VIII. GENERATION OF MEMORY T AND B LYMPHOCYTES

Because the ultimate goal of vaccination is to elicit long-term immune protection, a thorough understanding of the mechanisms involved in the generation and maintenance of long-lived memory T and B cells, as well as plasma cells, is of paramount importance. However, in spite of great progress over the past few years in understanding the mechanisms involved in the generation and maintenance of memory cells, significant gaps still remain. Many factors, such as site and length of Ag exposure, Ag concentration, cytokines, and other inflammatory stimuli present in the milieu, and duration of TCR stimulation, are now known to be important in the generation of effector and memory T cells.

Based on their expression of homing molecules CD62L and CCR7, recent evidence supports the existence of two main populations of T_m cells: central memory T cells (T_{cm}) and effector memory T cells (T_{em}) [23–25,74]. T_{cm} are CD62L^{hi}CCR7$^+$, while T_{em} are CD62L^{dim}CCR7$^-$. Several studies have shown that T_{cm} migrate to peripheral LN, while T_{em} recirculate through nonlymphoid tissues, such as liver and lungs. This is likely due to the fact that CD62L interacts with PNAd in HEV of LN, and that CCR7 binds to chemokines CCL19 and CCL21 present in the luminal surface of endothelial cells in LN. Evidence indicates that T cells that downregulate CCR7 and CD62L expression concomitantly upregulate the expression of CCR2 and CCR5, which favors migration to inflamed tissues. T_{cm} and T_{em} populations have been reported to be functionally distinct. Following Ag stimulation, CD4$^+$ T_{cm} rapidly secrete mainly IL-2 and little IL-4, IL-5, or IFN-γ, while the reverse was observed to be true for T_{em} cells. Similarly, only the CD8$^+$ T_{em} population reportedly contains intracellular perforin, an important CTL effector molecule. Thus, because of their homing potential to peripheral sites and cytokine-secretion readiness, only the T_{em} populations appear to be ready for immediate effector action. On the other hand, T_{cm} cells would be available in secondary lymphoid tissues to stimulate DC, provide B cell help, and participate in the generation of a new wave of effector T cells. If confirmed, this model can be of great importance in guiding vaccine development.

Two key issues that remain largely unresolved focus on how memory T cells are generated and whether their long-term survival depends on continued Ag stimulation. The two leading theories to explain how memory cells are generated include: (1) T_m and effector cells are generated along separate pathways (as B memory cells do), e.g., depending on the cytokines and other stimuli present in the milieu, some cells become effector and some memory (divergent pathway), and (2) upon stimulation, T cells become effectors and following the active phase of the immune response, some develop into T_m cells (linear differentiation pathway), e.g., memory cells are directly derived from effector cells. A third model is a variation of the linear differentiation pathway in which the length of Ag stimulation determines whether T_{cm} (short stimulation) or T_{em} (long stimulation) populations are elicited. A fourth model, known as the "decreasing potential hypothesis," suggests that the duration and level of Ag to which naive T cells are exposed determines whether effector T cells die (e.g., this mechanism may dominate during chronic infections) or differentiate into T_m cells [24].

Equally controversial is the issue of whether Ag is required to maintain T_m cells. Most recent evidence indicates that both CD4$^+$ and CD8$^+$ T_m cells can persist in the absence of Ag for months or even years [25]. However, it is unclear whether, to persist for such long periods of time, these T_m cells must be periodically "restimulated" by nonspecific mechanisms. Such mechanisms include responding to cytokines (e.g., IL-15), activation by cross-reactive Ag, or as bystanders in unrelated immune responses because of their "increased readiness state" resulting from the increased expression of adhesion/accessory molecules and/or cytokine receptors [25]. Reports that Ag can remain in follicular dendritic cells (FDC) for long periods of time has led some investigators to propose that APC can pick up these Ag for presentation to T_m cells in a predominantly MHC class II-restricted fashion, suggesting that small amounts of Ag might be involved, at least to some extent, in maintaining $CD4^+$ T_m cells and B memory cells [118,119].

More information is known on the generation of B memory cells. To some extent, this is attributed to the fact that secondary and subsequent Ig responses can be easily differentiated from primary responses based on a more rapid response (because of increased numbers of Ag-specific cells), the predominance of IgG, IgA and/or IgE isotypes over IgM and the increased affinity of the Ig produced. It is generally accepted that the generation of memory B cells takes place in germinal centers, where clonal expansion, somatic hypermutation of Ig V regions, affinity selection, and class switching also take place [9–12,120]. Consensus has emerged that memory B cells differentiate along a separate pathway than plasma cells. In fact, some of the signals driving these different pathways are already known. For example, signaling through CD40 appears to be crucial for differentiation into B memory cells, while the presence of IL-2 and IL-10 in the absence of CD40L favors the generation of plasma cells [9–12,120]. It is also known that memory B cells leave the germinal center, and via the circulation, become localized in the draining areas of LN, or in the marginal zone of the spleen, or recirculate among the secondary lymphoid tissues. Clearly, further studies are needed before information on the critical events leading to the generation of T and B cell memory can be rationally applied to the development of vaccines.

IX. FUTURE DIRECTIONS

Throughout this chapter, owing largely to space constraints, I focused only on a handful of key areas during the generation of effector and memory cells that hold great potential to advance the development of safe, effective vaccines. These topics are, by no means, exclusive of many others (e.g., Ag–Ab interactions, B- and T-cell development and differentiation, Ig class switching, organizational structure of lymphoid organs and tissues, immunological tolerance, immunosenescence, etc.) that are undoubtedly of great importance in vaccine development.

In the coming years, the continued use of the novel technologies described above (e.g., genomics, proteomics) should bring spectacular advances in our understanding of the mechanisms underlying the induction, effector, and memory phases of the immune response. This information will continue to dramatically change our thinking of the strategies and molecular processes utilized by the immune system to protect the host against infectious microorganisms. The areas most likely to continue to be pivotal in further advancing the development of vaccines include: (1) the in-depth understanding of the pathways and antigenic epitopes involved in class I and class II MHC-restricted immune responses; (2) the further delineation of the function of DC cell subsets in linking the innate and immune system; (3) the precise role of costimulatory and adhesion molecules in Ag presentation and homing of effector and memory lymphocytes; (4) a better understanding of the rules governing the generation of cells secreting polarized cytokine profiles; (5) novel cytokine- and chemokine-mediated immunoregulatory mechanisms; and (6) the generation and maintenance of large pools of memory lymphocytes. These advances should create new opportunities to modify antigen structure, vaccine formulations, and targeting, leading to more efficient immune induction, more persistent immune responses and enhanced memory. For example, high hopes are held for targeting Ag to APC in conjunction with immunoregulatory cytokines and on the effective use of adjuvants. This information might also play a key role in advancing the development of attenuated live vector vaccines directly expressing foreign antigens or carrying DNA vaccine plasmids encoding foreign Ag. It is conceivable that eventually we will be able to develop vaccines that are "better than nature" in the sense that they may induce immune responses that are superior to natural infections in generating protective immunity. Finally, the information to be gained from sequencing the entire genomes of additional microorganisms holds great promise for the identification of large numbers of novel Ag that could be exploited as potential targets for vaccine development.

ACKNOWLEDGMENTS

This work was supported in part by Grant R01-AI36525 and Research Contracts N01-AI25461 and N01-AI65299 from the National Institutes of Health.

REFERENCES

1. Medzhitov R, Janeway CA Jr. Decoding the patterns of self and nonself by the innate immune system. Science 2002; 296:298–300.
2. Janeway CA Jr, Medzhitov R. Innate immune recognition. Annu Rev Immunol 2002; 20:197–216.
3. Dobrovolskaia MA, Vogel SN. Toll receptors, CD14, and macrophage activation and deactivation by LPS. Microbes Infect 2002; 4:903–914.
4. Underhill DM, Ozinsky A. Toll-like receptors: key mediators of microbe detection. Curr Opin Immunol 2002; 14:103–110.
5. Perera PY, et al. CD11b/CD18 acts in concert with CD14 and Toll-like receptor (TLR) 4 to elicit full lipopolysaccharide and taxol-inducible gene expression. J Immunol 2001; 166:574–581.
6. Shimazu R, et al. MD-2, a molecule that confers lipopolysaccharide responsiveness on Toll-like receptor 4. J Exp Med 1999; 189:1777–1782.
7. Medzhitov R, et al. A human homologue of the Drosophila Toll protein signals activation of adaptive immunity. Nature 1997; 388:394–397.
8. Jiang Q, et al. Lipopolysaccharide induces physical proximity between CD14 and toll-like receptor 4 (TLR4) prior to nuclear translocation of NF-kappa B. J Immunol 2000; 165:3541–3544.
9. Calame KL. Plasma cells: finding new light at the end of B cell development. Nat Immunol 2001; 2:1103–1108.
10. MacLennan I, Chan E. The dynamic relationship between B-cell populations in adults. Immunol Today 1993; 14:29–34.
11. Hardy RR, Hayakawa K. B cell development pathways. Annu Rev Immunol 2001; 19:595–621.

12. Lane P. Development of B cell memory and effector function. Curr Opinion Immunol 1996; 8:331–335.

13. Pike BL, et al. T-independent activation of single B cells: an orderly analysis of overlapping stages in the activation pathway. Immunol Rev 1987; 99:119–152.

14. Robbins JB, Schneerson R. Polysaccharide–protein conjugates: a new generation of vaccines. JID 1990; 161:821–832.

15. Bondada S. Accessory cell defect in unresponsiveness of neonates and aged to polysaccharide vaccines. Vaccine 2000; 19:557–565.

16. Zinkernagel RM. Neutralizing antiviral antibody responses. Adv Immunol 2001; 79:1–53.

17. Eskola J, et al. A randomized, prospective field trial of a conjugate vaccine in the protection of infants and young children against invasive Haemophilus influenzae type b disease. N Engl J Med 1990; 323:1381–1387.

18. Lin FY, et al. The efficacy of a Salmonella typhi Vi conjugate vaccine in two- to-five-year-old children. N Engl J Med 2001; 344:1263–1269.

19. Gao GF, et al. Molecular coordination of alphabeta T-cell receptors and coreceptors CD8 and CD4 in their recognition of peptide-MHC ligands. Trends Immunol 2002; 23:408–413.

20. Bromley SK, et al. The immunological synapse. Annu Rev Immunol 2001; 19:375–396.

21. Konig R. Interactions between MHC molecules and co-receptors of the TCR. Curr Opin Immunol 2002; 14:75–83.

22. Maini MK, et al. T-cell clonality in immune responses. Immunol Today 1999; 20:262–266.

23. Jenkins MK, et al. In vivo activation of antigen-specific CD4 T cells. Annu Rev Immunol 2001; 19:23–45.

24. Kaech SM, et al. Effector and memory T-cell differentiation: implications for vaccine development. Nat Rev Immunol 2002; 2:251–262.

25. Sprent J, Surh CD. T cell memory. Annu Rev Immunol 2002; 20:551–579.

26. Jankovic D, et al. Th1- and Th2-cell commitment during infectious disease: asymmetry in divergent pathways. Trends Immunol 2001; 22:450–457.

27. Abbas AK, et al. Functional diversity of helper T lymphocytes. Nature 1996; 383:787–793.

28. Harty JT, et al. CD8 + T cell effector mechanisms in resistance to infection. Annu Rev Immunol 2000; 18:275–308.

29. Mosmann TR, et al. Two types of murine helper T cell clone: I. Definition according to profiles of lymphokine activities and secreted proteins. J Immunol 1986; 136:2348–2357.

30. McGuirk P, Mills K. Pathogen-specific regulatory T cells provoke a shift in the Th1/Th2 paradigm in immunity to infectious diseases. Trends Immunol 2002; 23:450.

31. Mosmann TR, Sad S. The expanding universe of T-cell subsets: Th1, Th2 and more. Immunol Today 1996; 17:138–146.

32. Romagnani S. T-cell subsets (Th1 versus Th2). Ann Allergy Asthma Immunol 2000; 85:9–18.

33. Engelhard V, et al. Insights into antigen processing gained by direct analysis of the naturally processed class I MHC associated peptide repertoire. Mol Immunol 2002; 39:127.

34. Lanzavecchia A. Mechanisms of antigen uptake for presentation. Curr Opinion Immunol 1996; 8:348–354.

35. Watts C. Antigen processing in the endocytic compartment. Curr Opin Immunol 2001; 13:26–31.

36. Lennon-Dumenil AM, et al. A closer look at proteolysis and MHC-class-II-restricted antigen presentation. Curr Opin Immunol 2002; 14:15–21.

37. Castellino F, et al. Antigen presentation by MHC class II molecules: invariant chain function, protein trafficking, and the molecular basis of diverse determinant capture. Hum Immunol 1997; 54:159–169.

38. Falk K, Rotzschke O. Consensus motifs and peptide ligands of MHC class I molecules [Review]. Semin Immunol 1993; 5:81–94.

39. Germain RN. Antigen processing and presentation. In: Paul WE, ed. Fundamental Immunology. Philadelphia: Lippincott-Raven Publishers, 1999:287–340.

40. York IA, Rock KL. Antigen processing and presentation by the Class I major histocompatibility complex. Annu Rev Immunol 1996; 14:369–396.

41. Sourdive DJ, et al. Conserved T cell receptor repertoire in primary and memory CD8 T cell responses to an acute viral infection. J Exp Med 1998; 188:71–82.

42. De Groot AS, et al. Immuno-informatics: mining genomes for vaccine components. Immunol Cell Biol 2002; 80:255–269.

43. Sette A, Sidney J. Nine major HLA class I supertypes account for the vast preponderance of HLA-A and -B polymorphism. Immunogenetics 1999; 50:201–212.

44. Engler OB. Peptide vaccines against hepatitis B virus: from animal model to human studies. Mol Immunol 2001; 38:457–465.

45. Abrams SI, Schlom J. Rational antigen modification as a strategy to upregulate or downregulate antigen recognition. Curr Opin Immunol 2000; 12:85–91.

46. Rock KL, et al. Protein degradation and the generation of MHC class I-presented peptides. Adv Immunol 2002; 80:1–70.

47. den Haan JM, Bevan MJ. Antigen presentation to CD8 + T cells: cross-priming in infectious diseases. Curr Opin Immunol 2001; 13:437–441.

48. Blankenstein T, Schuler T. Cross-priming versus cross-tolerance: are two signals enough? Trends Immunol 2002; 23:171–173.

49. Heath WR, Carbone FR. Cross-presentation, dendritic cells, tolerance and immunity. Annu Rev Immunol 2001; 19:47–64.

50. Gao XM, et al. Recombinant Salmonella typhimurium strains that invade nonphagocytic cells are resistant to recognition by antigen-specific cytotoxic T lymphocytes. Infect Immun 1992; 60:3780–3789.

51. Pfeifer JD, et al. Phagocytic processing of bacterial antigens for class I MHC presentation to T cells. Nature 1993; 361:359–362.

52. Salerno-Goncalves R, et al. Characterization of CD8(+) effector T cell responses in volunteers immunized with Salmonella enterica serovar Typhi strain Ty21a typhoid vaccine. J Immunol 2002; 169:2196–2203.

53. Sztein MB. Cytotoxic T lymphocytes after oral immunization with attenuated vaccine strains of Salmonella typhi in humans. J Immunol 1995; 155:3987–3993.

54. Busch R, et al. Accessory molecules for MHC class II peptide loading. Curr Opin Immunol 2000; 12:99–106.

55. Schirle M, et al. Combining computer algorithms with experimental approaches permits the rapid and accurate identification of T cell epitopes from defined antigens. J Immunol Methods 2001; 257:1–16.

56. Ramachandra L, et al. Phagocytic processing of antigens for presentation by class II major histocompatibility complex molecules. Cell Microbiol 1999; 1:205–214.

57. Braud VM, et al. Functions of nonclassical MHC and non-MHC-encoded class I molecules. Curr Opin Immunol 1999; 11:100–108.

58. Gumperz JE, Brenner MB. CD1-specific T cells in microbial immunity. Curr Opin Immunol 2001; 13:471–478.

59. Burdin N, Kronenberg M. CD1-mediated immune responses to glycolipids. Curr Opin Immunol 1999; 11:326–331.

60. Moody DB, et al. The molecular basis of CD1-mediated presentation of lipid antigens. Immunol Rev 1999; 172:285–296.

61. Guermonprez P, et al. Antigen presentation and T cell stimulation by dendritic cells. Annu Rev Immunol 2002; 20:621–667.
62. Moser M, Murphy KM. Dendritic cell regulation of TH1–TH2 development. Nat Immunol 2000; 1:199–205.
63. Palucka K, Banchereau J. How dendritic cells and microbes interact to elicit or subvert protective immune responses. Curr Opin Immunol 2002; 14:420–431.
64. Reid SD, et al. The control of T cell responses by dendritic cell subsets. Curr Opin Immunol 2000; 12:114–121.
65. Liu YJ, et al. Dendritic cell lineage, plasticity and cross-regulation. Nat Immunol 2001; 2:585–589.
66. Penna G, et al. Cutting edge: selective usage of chemokine receptors by plasmacytoid dendritic cells. J Immunol 2001; 167:1862–1866.
67. MacPherson G, et al. Dendritic cells, B cells and the regulation of antibody synthesis. Immunol Rev 1999; 172:325–334.
68. Gold MR. To make antibodies or not: signaling by the B-cell antigen receptor. Trends Pharmacol Sci 2002; 23:316–324.
69. Davis MM, Chien Y. T-cell antigen receptors. In: Paul WE, ed. Fundamental Immunology. Philadelphia: Lippincott-Raven Publishers, 1999:341–366.
70. Cantrell D. T cell antigen receptor signal transduction pathways. Annu Rev Immunol 1996; 14:259–274.
71. Chien Y, et al. Recognition by gamma/delta T cells. Annu Rev Immunol 1996; 14:511–532.
72. Hayday AC. [gamma][delta] cells: a right time and a right place for a conserved third way of protection. Annu Rev Immunol 2000; 18:975–1026.
73. van der Merwe PA. Formation and function of the immunological synapse. Curr Opin Immunol 2002; 14:293–298.
74. Lanzavecchia A, Sallusto F. From synapses to immunological memory: the role of sustained T cell stimulation. Curr Opin Immunol 2000; 12:92–98.
75. Krummel MF, Davis MM. Dynamics of the immunological synapse: finding, establishing and solidifying a connection. Curr Opin Immunol 2002; 14:66–74.
76. Lee KH, et al. T cell receptor signaling precedes immunological synapse formation. Science 2002; 295:1539–1542.
77. Revy P, et al. Functional antigen-independent synapses formed between T cells and dendritic cells. Nat Immunol 2001; 2:925–931.
78. Werlen G, Palmer E. The T-cell receptor signalosome: a dynamic structure with expanding complexity. Curr Opin Immunol 2002; 14:299–305.
79. Kane LP, et al. Signal transduction by the TCR for antigen. Curr Opin Immunol 2000; 12:242–249.
80. Samelson LE. Signal transduction mediated by the T cell antigen receptor: the role of adapter proteins. Annu Rev Immunol 2002; 20:371–394.
81. Lewis RS. Calcium signaling mechanisms in T lymphocytes. Annu Rev Immunol 2001; 19:497–521.
82. Levinson AI, et al. B-cell superantigens: definition and potential impact on the immune response. J Clin Immunol 1995; 15:26S–36S.
83. Kotb M. Bacterial pyrogenic exotoxins as superantigens [Review]. Clin Microbiol Rev 1995; 8:411–426.
84. Kwon B, et al. New insights into the role of 4-1BB in immune responses: beyond CD8+ T cells. Trends Immunol 2002; 23:378–380.
85. Chambers CA, et al. CTLA-4-mediated inhibition in regulation of T cell responses: mechanisms and manipulation in tumor immunotherapy. Annu Rev Immunol 2001; 19:565–594.
86. Carreno BM, Collins M. The B7 family of ligands and its receptors: new pathways for costimulation and inhibition of immune responses. Annu Rev Immunol 2002; 20:29–53.
87. Salomon B, Bluestone JA. Complexities of CD28/B7: CTLA-4 costimulatory pathways in autoimmunity and transplantation. Annu Rev Immunol 2001; 19:225–252.
88. Whitmire JK, Ahmed R. Costimulation in antiviral immunity: differential requirements for CD4(+) and CD8(+) T cell responses. Curr Opin Immunol 2000; 12:448–455.
89. Krakauer T, et al. TNF and IL-1 Families, Chemokines, TGF-β, and others. In: Paul WE, ed. Fundamental Immunology. Philadelphia: Lippincott-Raven Publishers, 1999: 775–811.
90. Thomson A. The Cytokine Handbook. 3rd ed. San Diego: Academic Press, 1998.
91. Sallusto F, et al. The role of chemokine receptors in primary, effector, and memory immune responses. Annu Rev Immunol 2000; 18:593–620.
92. Luther SA, Cyster JG. Chemokines as regulators of T cell differentiation. Nat Immunol 2001; 2:102–107.
93. Colonna M, et al. Interferon-producing cells: on the front line in immune responses against pathogens. Curr Opin Immunol 2002; 14:373–379.
94. Frucht DM. IFN-gamma production by antigen-presenting cells: mechanisms emerge. Trends Immunol 2001; 22:556–560.
95. Fickenscher H, et al. The interleukin-10 family of cytokines. Trends Immunol 2002; 23:89–96.
96. Hamilton JA. GM-CSF in inflammation and autoimmunity. Trends Immunol 2002; 23:403–408.
97. Sims JE. IL-1 and IL-18 receptors, and their extended family. Curr Opin Immunol 2002; 14:117–122.
98. Fry TJ, Mackall CL. Interleukin-7: master regulator of peripheral T-cell homeostasis? Trends Immunol 2001; 22:564–571.
99. Romagnani S. Lymphokine production by human T cells in disease states. Annu Rev Immunol 1994; 12:227–257.
100. London CA, et al. Helper T cell subsets: heterogeneity, functions and development. Vet Immunol Immunopathol 1998; 63:37–44.
101. Carter LL, Dutton RW. Type 1 and type 2: a fundamental dichotomy for all T cell subsets. Curr Opinion Immunol 1996; 8:336–342.
102. Fearon DT, Locksley RM. The instructive role of innate immunity in the acquired immune response. Science 1996; 272:50–53.
103. Moore KW, et al. Interleukin-10 and the interleukin-10 receptor. Annu Rev Immunol 2001; 19:683–765.
104. Gorelik L, Flavell RA. Transforming growth factor-beta in T-cell biology. Nat Rev Immunol 2002; 2:46–53.
105. Mackay CR. Chemokines: immunology's high impact factors. Nat Immunol 2001; 2:95–101.
106. Moser B, Loetscher P. Lymphocyte traffic control by chemokines. Nat Immunol 2001; 2:123–128.
107. Kunkel EJ, Butcher EC. Chemokines and the tissue-specific migration of lymphocytes. Immunity 2002; 16:1–4.
108. Murphy PM, et al. International union of pharmacology: XXII. Nomenclature for chemokine receptors. Pharmacol Rev 2000; 52:145–176.
109. Luster AD. The role of chemokines in linking innate and adaptive immunity. Curr Opin Immunol 2002; 14:129–135.
110. Belardelli F, Ferrantini M. Cytokines as a link between innate and adaptive antitumor immunity. Trends Immunol 2002; 23:201–208.
111. Johnston B, Kubes P. The alpha4-integrin: an alternative pathway for neutrophil recruitment? Immunol Today 1999; 20:545–550.
112. D'Ambrosio D, et al. Localization of Th-cell subsets in inflammation: differential thresholds for extravasation of Th1 and Th2 cells. Immunol Today 2000; 21:183–186.
113. Shevach EM. Accessory molecules. In: Paul WE, ed. Fundamental Immunology. New York: Raven Press, 1993: 531–576.

114. Petty HR, Todd RF. Integrins as promiscuous signal transduction devices. Immunol Today 1996; 17:209–212.

115. Girard JP, Springer TA. High endothelial venules (HEVs): specialized endothelium for lymphocyte migration [Review]. Immunol Today 1995; 16:449–457.

116. Campbell JJ, Butcher EC. Chemokines in tissue-specific and microenvironment-specific lymphocyte homing. Curr Opin Immunol 2000; 12:336–341.

117. Butcher EC, et al. Lymphocyte trafficking and regional immunity. Adv Immunol 1999; 72:209–253.

118. Gray D. A role for antigen in the maintenance of immunological memory. Nat Rev Immunol 2002; 2:60–65.

119. Zinkernagel RM. On differences between immunity and immunological memory. Curr Opin Immunol 2002; 14:523–536.

120. McHeyzer-Williams MG, Ahmed R. B cell memory and the long-lived plasma cell. Curr Opin Immunol 1999; 11:172–179.

121. Hajjar AM, et al. Cutting edge: functional interactions between toll-like receptor (TLR) 2 and TLR1 or TLR6 in response to phenol-soluble modulin. J Immunol 2001; 166:15–19.

122. Kirschning CJ, et al. Human toll-like receptor 2 confers responsiveness to bacterial lipopolysaccharide. J Exp Med 1998; 188:2091–2097.

123. Vabulas RM, et al. Endocytosed HSP60s use toll-like receptor 2 (TLR2) and TLR4 to activate the toll/interleukin-1 receptor signaling pathway in innate immune cells. J Biol Chem 2001; 276:31332–31339.

124. Takeuchi O, et al. Differential roles of TLR2 and TLR4 in recognition of Gram-negative and Gram-positive bacterial cell wall components. Immunity 1999; 11:443–451.

125. Alexopoulou L, et al. Recognition of double-stranded RNA and activation of NF-kappaB by Toll-like receptor 3. Nature 2001; 413:732–738.

126. Ohashi K, et al. Cutting edge: heat shock protein 60 is a putative endogenous ligand of the toll-like receptor-4 complex. J Immunol 2000; 164:558–561.

127. Hayashi F, et al. The innate immune response to bacterial flagellin is mediated by Toll-like receptor 5. Nature 2001; 410:1099–1103.

128. Jurk M, et al. Human TLR7 or TLR8 independently confer responsiveness to the antiviral compound R-848. Nat Immunol 2002; 3:499.

129. Hemmi H, et al. Small anti-viral compounds activate immune cells via the TLR7 MyD88-dependent signaling pathway. Nat Immunol 2002; 3:196–200.

130. Hemmi H, et al. A Toll-like receptor recognizes bacterial DNA. Nature 2000; 408:740–745.

15

High-Throughput Informatics and In Vitro Assays for T-Cell Epitope Determination: Application to the Design of Epitope-Driven Vaccines

Anne S. De Groot[*,†] **and Hakima Sbai**
Brown University, Providence, Rhode Island, U.S.A.

William Martin[*]
EpiVax, Inc., Providence, Rhode Island, U.S.A.

John Sidney[‡] **and Alessandro Sette**[‡]
Epimmune Corporation, San Diego, California, U.S.A.

Jay A. Berzofsky
National Cancer Institute, National Institutes of Health, Bethesda, Maryland, U.S.A.

I. INTRODUCTION

Induction of epitope-specific T-cell responses may provide an effective means of protecting against diseases for which no conventional vaccines exist. Unlike B cells, which only recognize epitopes directly on the surface of free antigens, T lymphocytes recognize peptide fragments bound to class I or class II molecules encoded by the major histocompatibility complex (MHC). A peptide that binds MHC and is recognized by the T-cell receptor (TCR) constitutes a T-cell epitope. In humans, MHC class I molecules include HLA-A, HLA-B, and HLA-C. The MHC class II molecules include HLA-DR, HLA-DP, and HLA-DQ.

In general, MHC class I molecules present peptides 8-10 amino acids in length and these MHC-peptide complexes are predominately recognized by $CD8^+$ cytotoxic T lymphocytes (CTLs). Class I peptides usually contain an MHC I allele-specific motif sequence of two main anchor residues, usually located at position 2 and at the carboxy-terminus of the peptide ligand [1,2]. The MHC class II molecules bind peptides of 11-25 amino acids and are predominantly recognized by $CD4^+$ T helper (Th) cells. Peptides presented by class II molecules are longer and more variable in size than those presented by class I molecules, and usually contain three main anchors located at relative positions 1, 6, and 9 [3–8].

T-cell epitopes are derived from foreign protein antigens via two different pathways of protein degradation. The MHC class I molecules present peptides obtained from proteolytic digestion of endogenously synthesized proteins. Host-derived or pathogen-derived intracellular proteins are cleaved by a complex of proteases in the proteasome [9–20].

Small peptide fragments are then transported by ATP-dependent transporters associated with antigen processing

---

[*]Two of the contributing authors, William Martin and Anne S. De Groot, are senior officers and majority shareholders at EpiVax, a privately owned vaccine design company located in Providence, RI. These authors acknowledge that there is a potential conflict on interest related to their relationship with EpiVax and attest that the work contained in this research report is free of any bias that might be associated with the commercial goals of the company.

[†]Anne S. De Groot is also founder and scientific advisor to GAIA Vaccine Foundation, a not-for-profit organization that supports the development of a globally relevant, globally accessible AIDS vaccine. EpiVax and the TB/HIV Research Laboratory declared the "World Clade" vaccine project described in this manuscipt to be a not-for-profit project in August 2000. The World Clade vaccine project is now directed by GAIA Vaccine Foundation.

[‡]Alessandro Sette is now with La Jolla Institute for Allergy and Immunology, San Diego, California, U.S.A. John Sidney is a shareholder of Epimmune.

(TAPs) into the endoplasmic reticulum (ER), where they form complexes with nascent MHC class I heavy chains and β₂-microglobulin [21–24]. The peptide-MHC class I complexes are transported to the cell surface for presentation to the receptors of CD8⁺ T cells [25].

The MHC class II molecules generally bind peptides derived from the cell membrane or from extracellular proteins that have been internalized by antigen-presenting cells (APCs). The proteins are processed in an endosomal compartment called MHC class II compartment (MIIC), and the generated peptides are sorted by empty MHC class II molecules based on their affinity. The HLA-DM then catalyzes peptide exchange [26–31]. Class II molecules bound to peptide fragments are transported to the surface of APCs for presentation to CD4⁺ helper T cells.

From these different antigen processing and presentation pathways, two different T-cell responses are generated: a CD4⁺ Th immune response and a CD8⁺ CTL immune response. These two types of responses are relevant for different mechanisms of immunity. Prophylactic and therapeutic intervention in different disease settings may require induction of CD4⁺ response, CD8⁺ response, or both. For this reason, strategies to elicit both types of responses are of interest.

In the past decade, several research groups have applied bioinformatics tools and biochemical assays, in conjunction with various types of T-cell assays, to identify T-cell epitopes from several pathogens. These strategies will accelerate the development of new-generation T-cell epitope-based vaccines against cancers, viral pathogens such as hepatitis B virus (HBV), hepatitis C virus (HCV), and HIV, bacteria such as *Mycobacterium tuberculosis* (Mtb), and parasites such as *Plasmodium falciparum*.

II. APPROACHES FOR IDENTIFYING T-CELL EPITOPES FROM PROTEIN SEQUENCES

The first step in the development of an epitope-driven vaccine is the identification of allele-specific or promiscuous (presented by multiple HLA molecules) peptides that can be recognized by T cells in association with MHC class I or class II molecules. There are two different basic categories of approaches for identifying T-cell epitopes: the standard overlapping peptide approach and the bioinformatics approach.

The overlapping peptide approach identifies T-cell epitopes by constructing partially overlapping peptides covering the entire amino acid sequence of the protein of interest, and then by screening each of these peptides for their ability to bind HLA molecules or to induce a T-cell response. Although many T-cell epitopes have been identified using this method, the approach is laborious and expensive. Some investigators use 10- to 15-amino-acid-long peptides overlapping by five to eight amino acids, or variations on this theme. However, T-cell epitopes that fall in between the overlapping regions can be overlooked. This method also relies on peptide proteolysis, which may or may not occur in vitro when assays are being performed. For class I, the "exhaustive" overlapping approach involves making every possible overlapping peptide (often including 8-mer, 9-mer,

and 10-mer versions of the same potential epitope), covering the entire protein sequence. Although this approach is comprehensive, it is prohibitively expensive, labor-intensive for most laboratories, and unnecessary, given the precision of current epitope mapping tools.

With the rapid accumulation of accurate sequence information for a wide array of pathogens, the development of accurate informatics approaches to predicting antigenic sites from primary structure is particularly appealing. The decade spanning 1991-2001 saw the development of a large number of computer-driven algorithms that used the alphabetical representation of protein sequence information to search for T-cell epitopes.

DeLisi and Berzofsky [32] and Rothbard and Taylor [33] were the first research teams to suggest searching for a pattern of amino acids as a possible predictive tool for antigenicity, based on empirical observations of the periodicity of amino acid residues in T-cell epitopes. Predictions based on periodicity were a clear improvement over the overlapping method of epitope mapping, but they did not predict binding in an allele-specific manner. Consequently, the predictive value of these early algorithms was a limited improvement over previous methods [34], a mere first step. Allele specific motifs were first described in the late 1980s, as a result of the development of quantitative peptide-MHC binding assays [6,35–37].

Further development of improved computer-driven algorithms was made possible by three major technological advances: crystallographical studies of MHC molecules in complex with peptides, the sequencing of naturally occurring MHC-peptide ligands by Edman degradation, and the use of tandem mass spectrometry. The use of allele-specific "anchor-based" MHC binding motifs to prospectively identify T-cell epitopes [38] was described by Falk et al. [2] in 1991; Romero et al. [39] in 1991; Jardetzky [40] in 1991; Hunt et al. [8] in 1992; Leighton et al. [41], Geluk et al. [42], Wall et al. [43], Sidney et al. [44,47], Sette et al. [45], Ruppert et al. [46], O'Sullivan et al. [48], and Kondo et al. [49] beginning in the late 1980s; Chicz et al. [4] in 1993; Lipford et al. [50] in 1993; Parker et al. [51] in 1994; Hammer et al. [52] in 1994; and Meister et al. [34] in 1995.

Matrix-based approaches to mapping T-cell epitopes have also been developed by a number of different research teams. Matrix methods assign a positive or negative coefficient to each possible amino acid that could occupy each position in a peptide, based either on empirical data from many known epitopes binding that MHC molecule, or on computational estimates of the free energy of binding. The resulting 20×9 matrix of coefficients can be used to calculate a linear score for any given peptide sequence. Matrix-based algorithms were described by Sette et al. [53] in 1989 and have also been described by Parker et al. [54], Davenport et al. [55], Jesdale et al. [56], De Groot et al. [57], and Hammer et al. [52]. The crucial assumption that the matrix-based method relies on is that the contribution of each position along the peptide sequence is essentially independent of the other positions. This assumption appears to be quite accurate in most cases. There are, however, exceptions, which have shown the importance of pairwise interactions between neighboring residues in influencing peptide binding to MHC molecules, exist [58]. The matrix method also allows the assessment of the contribution of secondary anchor residues, engaging secondary binding pockets of the MHC molecule as well as short-range secondary and conformational effects [46].

The issue of secondary anchors and secondary effects on MHC binding has been addressed by Ruppert et al. [46,59] who have demonstrated that predictions based on the main anchors alone were not very effective. These authors determined that the presence of the main anchor residues was necessary but not sufficient for binding to occur. Specifically, only about 20-30% of anchor motif containing peptides bound to MHC, whereas the predictive efficacy of a motif-based algorithm increased to 70-80% when the predictive effect of secondary anchors was considered.

In general, a matrix-based computer algorithm searches for putative T-cell epitopes by scanning the entire protein of interest in increments of 8-mers, 9-mers, 10-mers, or 11-mers. EpiMatrix is one of several such tools, which scores each 8-mer to 10-mer overlapping frame in a protein sequence based on the estimated probability of its binding (EBP) to a selected MHC molecule [60]. Studies have demonstrated that EpiMatrix, among other matrix-based programs, accurately predicts MHC ligands (in both retrospective and prospective studies).

A number of additional approaches to epitope mapping have been developed. These include predictive strategies based on neural nets, threading algorithms, and nonlinear functions [35,37,61–66]. In some cases, it has been reported that these more complex strategies might increase accuracy or effectiveness of prediction. In side-by-side comparisons, however, different methods have been found to be essentially equivalent [67], thus providing powerful support to the "independent side chain contribution hypothesis" on which the matrix methods are based. In the experience of the Epimmune and EpiVax groups, the most important determinant of the accuracy of the prediction is the actual quality and quantity of the binding data utilized to derive the predictive method. To predict the binding capacity of a 10-mer sequence, in which every position can be occupied by any one of 20 different amino acids, one needs to solve an equation with $10 \times 20 = 200$ unknowns. It is intuitive that, if less than 200 data points are used, the results are probably questionable regardless of the method utilized. The more binding data points that are utilized to compose the matrix train, the neural network, or so on, the better. Epimmune's peptide database contains actual binding constants that have been measured for more than 6×10^4 different peptide molecules. Researchers at the Kent Ridge Digital Laboratories (Vladimir Brusic) [68] who are engaged in the design of epitope mapping algorithms have also compiled databases of MHC binding peptides.

Most recently, the teams of Sturniolo et al. [69], Zhang et al. [70], and Sette and Sidney [71,72] have proposed that unknown motifs might be predicted by mixing and matching MHC binding pocket characteristics. In the hands of a number of epitope mapping researchers, this new means of developing epitope prediction tools is proving extremely useful.

Several independent studies have been performed to address the question of how effective MHC binding motifs may be for the prediction of class I binding peptides. Specifically, in 1994 Kast et al. [73] synthesized all possible 9-mer peptides derived from the E6 and E7 proteins of Human Papilloma Virus (HPV)-18 and tested them for binding to HLA-A1, HLA-A2.1, HLA-A3, HLA-A11, and HLA-A24. They found that of 1200 peptide/HLA affinities measured, binding affinities of 500 nM or less were detected in only 22 cases (1.8%). In seven cases (0.6%), the affinity was high: 50 nM or less. Of the 22 peptides binding at the 500 nM level, 20 (91%) contained HLA-specific binding motifs. Most impressively, 7/7 (100%) of the peptides binding at the 50 nM level contained HLA-specific binding motifs. Thus, it was concluded that essentially all peptides binding to the HLA contained HLA-specific motifs. Although a total of 1200 HLA/peptide combinations were studied, the analysis of only 111 HLA/peptide combinations would have been required if the predictive power of HLA-specific motifs had been exploited. In other words, motif analysis could have reduced by more than 10-fold the number of peptides that needed to be considered for HLA binding analysis [73].

A number of different approaches have been used to demonstrate that class I MHC binding to HLA is predictive of a peptide's ability to induce CTL responses. First, in a series of studies by Van der Most et al. [74–76] and Vitiello et al. [77] where murine models of viral infection were used, all MHC binding peptides were tested for immunogenicity. Of 39 peptides that bound at the 500 nM level, 30 were tested for immunogenicity by direct peptide immunization, and at least 20 of them (67%) were immunogenic. It was also shown that at least 10/39 of the 500 nM binding peptides (26%) induced CTL capable of conferring protection from viral challenge, and/or recognized infected cells in vitro.

Second, the finding that HLA transgenic mice can mount an HLA-restricted T-cell response to approximately 85% of the peptide epitopes that are recognized by human T cells [78] provides strong support for the idea that the ability to bind to the HLA molecule plays the major role in determining peptide immunogenicity [79,80]. Similarly, it has been reported that HLA-A11 transgenic mice mounted responses to at least 75% and 54% of the peptides binding at the < 50 and 50-500 nM levels, respectively [81].

Binding affinity for HLA class I molecules and immunogenicity have been further characterized using HLA-A*0201 transgenic mice [67] and T cells derived from hepatitis B-infected human patients. In both cases, an affinity threshold of approximately 500 nM (and preferably 50 nM or less) appeared to determine the capacity of a peptide epitope to elicit a CTL response. These data correlated well with additional class I binding affinity measurements made using either naturally processed peptides or previously described T-cell epitopes [82].

An independent series of studies by DiBrino et al. [83] have examined similar issues. These authors suggest that endogenous and antigenic peptides may be primarily selected (rather than using peptide processing) to form stable HLA-A2 complexes [54]. HLA-A1-, HLA-A3-, and HLA-B44-specific motifs were utilized to predict potential epitopes derived from various proteins of the influenza A virus and of 18 peptides synthesized, eight bound and six of them

protein

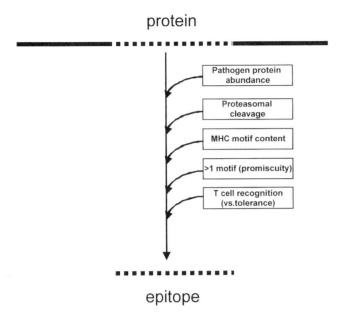

epitope

Figure 1 Aspects of antigen processing that determine whether an epitope is immunogenic in vitro and in vivo.

(75%) were recognized by CTL derived from individuals, presumably naturally exposed to infection with the influenza virus [83].

The affinity for the MHC molecule has the greatest impact on immunogenicity and immunodominance. Additionally, both the specificity of proteasomal cleavage, which is needed to create the appropriate peptide but could also destroy it [14,17,20,84,85], and the specificity of the TAP transporter, which selectively delivers peptides from the cytosol to the ER for loading onto class I MHC molecules [22,24,86–88], play critical roles in determining which epitopes are presented and which become immunodominant [89]. Indeed, the ability to induce an immune response can often be correlated to the relative amounts of peptide epitope that are processed and presented on the surface of the APC [90]. The abundance of a particular protein in intracellular compartments and the presence of proteolytic cleavage sites proximal and distal to the epitope are just two of many factors that determine whether an epitope is presented (Fig. 1) [12,91]. In this context, it is important to appreciate that generation of a given epitope as a result of antigen processing is not an all-or-none phenomenon. A number of studies have indeed shown that different epitopes are generated with different efficiencies [12,91], and efforts to estimate the efficiency of different steps involved in antigen processing have begun [16,92]. It appears that variation in epitope yield can modulate immunodominance and apparent immunogenicity [17,93]. It would also seem that the threshold number of peptide-MHC complexes necessary to stimulate a given T-cell is different between naïve and differentiated T cells. Accordingly, the thresholds necessary for induction of immune responses appear to be significantly higher than those necessary for triggering effec-

tor functions [94,95]. Thus, whether an epitope is scored as "being generated by antigen processing" or not is crucially dependent on the sensitivity of the assay method utilized. Indeed, it has been shown that vaccine optimization can increase the yield of a given epitope, and may allow elicitation of responses specific for such suboptimal "subdominant" epitopes [96].

However, the major determining factor for immunogenicity remains affinity for the MHC molecule. Thus, the ability to predict immunogenic peptides based on motif analysis and HLA binding measurements is quite high, in the range of 30-75%. Taken together, these data formally support the crucial role of determinant selection in the shaping of T-cell responses. Because high-affinity peptides seem to be immunogenic in most cases, these data further demonstrate that if holes exist in the functional T-cell repertoire, they remain relatively rare.

III. IMMUNODOMINANT, CRYPTIC, AND SUBDOMINANT T-CELL EPITOPES

In general, natural immune responses (defined as the immune responses produced following infection or disease) do not exploit the full range of epitope possibilities, meaning that only a small fraction of all possible peptides derived from a given pathogen actually induces a T-cell response (Table 1). This phenomenon is known as immunodominance [97–99]. According to common definitions [75,77,100], a dominant epitope induces a response on immunization with whole native antigens. Such a response is cross-reactive in vitro with the peptide epitope. By contrast, in the case of cryptic epitopes, the response elicited by peptide immunization is not cross-reactive in vitro with intact native antigens. Finally, a subdominant epitope evokes little or no response on immunization with whole antigens, but the response obtained by peptide immunization is cross-reactive with whole antigen in vitro (unlike the case of cryptic epitopes).

The main cause of immunodominance is that only a small fraction of all possible peptides binds to a given MHC [98,101]. This phenomenon was called "determinant selection" and was predicted by Rosenthal [102] in the mid-1970s, before peptide–MHC interactions were actually demonstrated.

Induction of a cellular immune response requires that peptide binding to MHC molecules is of sufficient affinity to produce enough peptide-class I complexes to activate naïve CTL. The binding affinity of a particular peptide for a given HLA molecule is a chemical attribute, can be quantified, and

Table 1 Variables Determining Immunodominance and Multispecificity in T-Cell Responses

Capacity to bind MHC (determinant selection)
T-cell responsiveness (holes in the repertoire)
Processing yield
Efficiency of transport
Clonal competition, antigen levels, duration of antigen
  exposure

is invariant in a given set of conditions. By contrast, the ability to detect T-cell activation is susceptible to many factors that can ultimately affect the apparent immunogenicity of an epitope. As a result, immunodominance and immunogenicity are not properties inherent to a peptide, they depend, rather, on a given immunological set of circumstances, i.e., a variety of factors, described in more detail below.

Not all epitopes that bind with good affinity to MHC are actually recognized during the "natural" course of immunity. In some cases, T-cell responses are not detected ("holes in the repertoire" [103]) because of immunoregulatory phenomena, thymic deletion, or peripheral tolerance. In other cases, the apparent lack of recognition occurs because during the natural processing of pathogen-derived proteins within host cells, the epitope is not efficiently generated [17] or properly transported into the ER [87]. Other factors related to antigen structure, route of administration, and differences of T-cell growth during immune activation can also influence immunodominance.

Whatever the reason for lack of prominent recognition of a given epitope in the course of natural infection, immunization with isolated or optimal epitopes can often induce a T-cell response that can actually recognize infected or cancerous cells. In these cases, the response is referred to as a subdominant response, and the epitope is correspondingly identified as a subdominant epitope [75,77]. These subdominant epitopes, along with the dominant epitopes, can play an important role in the development of effective epitope-based vaccines.

IV. HLA SUPERTYPE EPITOPES AND POPULATION COVERAGE

As mentioned above, T cells recognize a complex between a specific MHC type and a particular pathogen-derived epitope and, thus, a given epitope will elicit a response only in individuals that express an MHC molecule capable of binding that particular epitope. The MHC molecules are extremely polymorphic (several hundred different variants are known in humans). Therefore, selecting multiple peptides with different MHC binding specificities will afford increased coverage of the patient population targeted as vaccine recipients. The issue of population coverage in relation to MHC polymorphism is further complicated by the fact that different MHC types are expressed at dramatically different frequencies in different ethnicities. Thus, a failure to consider these matters may result in a vaccine with ethnically-biased population coverage. In any given population, however, it is possible to find five HLA class I molecules that are sufficient to cover at least 90% of the population [63].

One means of circumventing the problem of MHC restriction relies on the selection of epitopes restricted by MHC types that can be grouped in broad families or supertypes. These supertypes are characterized by largely overlapping peptide repertoires and are expressed at high frequencies in all major ethnicities [106–111] (see Refs. 71 and 72 and references therein for review). By targeting only three supertypes, population coverage in the 80-90% range can be achieved, regardless of the ethnicity of the target

population. Five supertypes allow coverage of virtually 100% of the population.

The HLA supertypes are not limited to human class I molecules. Recent studies have shown that nonhuman primates, such as chimpanzee [112,113], gorilla [114], and macaques [115–117], also express class I molecules that are functionally analogous to molecules of the human class I supertypes. These observations raise the possibility that the immunogenicity of epitope-based vaccines destined for human use might be tested in nonhuman primates. Furthermore, several studies have also demonstrated the existence of HLA-DR supertypes [118–120]. Two main DR supertypes seem to account for the vast majority of HLA-DR binding specificities.

A number of studies have shown that 85-100% of high-affinity binding peptides, which bind multiple HLA molecules, are recognized by recall responses detected in peripheral blood mononuclear cells (PBMCs) from immune or infected individuals [118,119,121–128]. Recognition by memory recall responses demonstrates that the epitope is not only generated in vivo in the course of natural infection, but also that a TCR repertoire, which is capable of recognizing that particular epitope, exists. Thus, CTL directed against that epitope should be expected to have potential clinical benefit.

Several reasons could contribute to the high frequency by which HLA supertype epitopes are antigenic. First, it has been shown that HLA supertype epitopes tend to bind with high affinity [106]. High-affinity epitopes could be intrinsically more immunogenic, and efficient capture of high-affinity epitopes by HLA molecules could also compensate for suboptimal epitope yield as a result of natural processing. It has also been suggested that components of the cell's processing machinery have specificities that coordinate with HLA supertypes, thus giving an additional potential advantage to HLA supertype epitopes. In particular, coordinate specificities have been reported for human HLA supertypes and the human TAP complex [22].

Different approaches can be utilized to identify supertype epitopes. One approach is computational. For example, ClustiMer (EpiVax) is a computer algorithm that searches for clustered T-cell epitopes. It estimates the MHC binding potential of each 9-mer to 10-mer frame to a number of different HLA alleles, and thus identifies "clustered" or promiscuous epitopes. In work performed by the TB/HIV Research Laboratory in collaboration with EpiVax, it was confirmed that EpiMatrix and ClustiMer effectively predicted cross-MHC binding. As with any computer-driven epitope selection, the "clustered" and supertype predictions delivered by ClustiMer analysis have to be confirmed in vitro. Sette et al. [71] used a more direct approach, synthesizing and testing candidate supertype epitopes for their binding capacity to the most common members of a given supertype.

Additional tools developed by EpiVax and Epimmune permit the evaluation of HLA coverage. The tool developed by the Epimmune group is called Epicover. This program is based on actual frequencies of different HLA molecules and actual or calculated binding constants. It allows, for given a set of epitopes, to calculate the population coverage and the number of epitopes recognized on average by a given population of vaccine recipients. It has been a useful tool to project population coverage in different ethnic groups, and to select sets of epitopes affording maximal, nonethnically-biased population coverage.

V. PATHOGEN HETEROGENEITY IN VACCINE DEVELOPMENT

Although all pathogens are heterogeneous to a certain extent, in some cases, pathogen diversity can be extreme. Diversity within different Human Immunodeficiency Virus (HIV) isolates is described by grouping HIV isolates within more than eight separate clades, and a high degree of diversity exists even within a given clade. Similarly, several different genotypes of HCV exist. Just as with HIV, multiple variants of HCV are usually encountered even within the HCV viruses infecting a given individual. The extent of variation encountered has suggested the use of the term "quasi-species" to describe different primary viral isolates. Extensive variability has been documented in many important parasites (such as *P. falciparum*) responsible for malaria, and bacteria (such as *Pneumococcus*) responsible for infections in the young and the elderly.

Such a high level of variability poses an interesting challenge for vaccine development. One approach to address such variability relies on developing "customized" vaccines, directed against one particular pathogen strain or cancer isolate. Vaccines based on this approach are under investigation for HIV and several cancer types. However, it is obvious that such a vaccine concept poses formidable practical complications in terms of manufacturing, cost, and efficacy evaluations. Another approach is to combine antigens from all, or most, of the important strains of a pathogen. This approach has been pursued in the case of the multivalent polysaccharide vaccines currently in use for infant vaccination. A similar vaccine, based on 23 different polysaccharide antigens, is currently used for adults. This situation exemplifies how, even when a monospecific response may be adequate to prevent infection from a single strain, a multispecific response might be highly desirable to counteract pathogen variability existing at the population level (Table 2).

In an epitope-based vaccine setting, focusing on conserved epitopes allows for targeting responses around pathogen variability, whether it exists prior to infection, or develops in the natural course of disease. The use of conserved epitopes would be expected to focus the immune response on sequences crucial for retaining the biological function of the pathogen proteins, and thus with intrinsically lower variability, even under immune pressure. However, conservation is often not absolute; thus, epitopes that are totally invariant in 70-80% of different HCV or HIV strains are usually considered "conserved" epitopes. In these cases, the use of multiple epitopes will allow us to address pathogen variability more adequately.

For example, if epitope A is conserved in 70% of the pathogen strain and epitope B is also conserved in 70% of

Table 2 Reasons for Higher Effectiveness of Multispecific Responses

Recruitment of higher number of precursors
Higher magnitude response
More rapid response

Counterbalance pathogen variation
Preexisting infection or tumor establishment (coverage)
Originating during the course of disease (pathogen escape)

Addressing heterogeneity of MHC molecules
Overall patient coverage
Ethnically balanced coverage

the cases, provided that the epitope variants occur in different specific strains or isolates, the probability of finding a strain that is not addressed by either epitope would be $[(1-0.7)(1-0.7)] = 0.09$, corresponding to coverage of 91% of the strains. Addition of a third or fourth epitope also conserved in 70% of isolates would obtain 97% and 99% coverage of the different pathogen strains, respectively.

Various bioinformatic tools are available to address the issue of variability (or conservation) of epitopes, and to assist in the selection of epitopes with the desired pattern of conservation. One of the first programs to assess epitope conservancy quantitatively was developed by Chisari and Brown in 1994 and was utilized to identify conserved HBV-derived epitopes [121,129], and was also applied to identify HCV-derived *P. falciparum*-derived, and HIV-derived epitopes [118,119,122,123,125,127,130]. Conservatrix, developed at the TB/HIV Research Laboratory, is a computer algorithm that searches any large database of sequences, such as the Los Alamos National Library (LANL) database, for highly conserved regions across all the isolates of a given pathogen. The TB/HIV Research Laboratory has used Conservatrix to identify T-cell epitopes that are conserved across HIV isolates [131] and is currently applying this search engine to evaluating HCV and HPV. Conservatrix has also been used to evaluate the genomes of similar viruses such as HIV type 1 (HIV-1) and HIV type 2 (HIV-2) for cross-reactive epitopes (De Groot et al., submitted for publication) and to evaluate the potential efficacy of vaccines developed for one virus against a related virus (De Groot et al., submitted for publication).

VI. EPITOPE IDENTIFICATION UTILIZING BIOINFORMATIC TOOLS

Since the description of MHC-specific motifs, hundreds of different studies have been performed, identifying epitopes from several different cancer, viral, bacterial, and parasitic targets. As of November 2001, a MEDLINE search using the key words [(MHC or HLA) AND motif* AND epitope*] yielded 575 hits. A few specific examples are described in more detail below. We wish to emphasize here that the list of papers referenced in this chapter is not exhaustive, and we apologize in advance to the colleagues of many important contributions that may not be described or referenced herein.

A. Identifying Hepatitis B Virus-Derived and Hepatitis C Virus-Derived T-Cell Epitopes

Chisari and Ferrari [132] were pioneers in the identification of HBV-derived epitopes. Some of their early studies have already been referred to above [67]; they have been seminal in establishing on a firm experimental basis the relationship between binding affinity and immunogenicity and antigenicity for T cells. Utilizing in vitro stimulation of PBMCs with HBV-derived synthetic peptides containing HLA-A2.1, HLA-A31, and HLA-Aw68 binding motifs, they originally described CTL responses to several epitopes within the HBV nucleocapsid and envelope antigens in patients with acute hepatitis [133]. In a subsequent study, six HLA-A2-restricted CTL epitopes located in the highly conserved reverse transcriptase and RNase H domains of the viral polymerase protein were also mapped. In that study, it was shown that the CTL response to polymerase is polyclonal, multispecific, and mediated by $CD8^+$ T cells in patients with acute viral hepatitis, but that it is not detectable in patients with chronic HBV infection or uninfected healthy blood donors. This study also demonstrated that these peptides represent naturally processed viral epitopes, and that nonresponsiveness at the CTL level was not due to infection by viral variants. Furthermore, CTL responses were detectable for more than a year after complete clinical recovery and seroconversion, reflecting either the persistence of trace amounts of virus or long-lived memory CTL in the absence of viral antigen [134].

A subsequent study was designed to identify highly conserved HBV-derived peptides that bind multiple HLA class I alleles with high affinity and are recognized as CTL epitopes in acutely infected patients [121]. The PBMCs from 67 patients with acute hepatitis B and 12 patients convalescent from acute hepatitis B were stimulated with panels of peptides, binding with high affinity to several class I alleles from the HLA-A2, HLA-A3, or HLA-B7 supertypes. Eight of the 19 peptides tested were recognized by two or more alleles in each supertype, and at the same time, sets of nested peptides were recognized in the context of alleles with unrelated peptide binding specificities. This was the first demonstration of the functional relevance of the supertype grouping of HLA class I molecules in a human viral disease setting. The data also represented a significant advance in the development of a totally synthetic vaccine to terminate chronic HBV infection. This study supported the notion that it was indeed feasible to use combined bioinformatic and biochemical methods, systematically, in the development of similar vaccines for the prevention and treatment of other chronic viral infections.

In the case of HCV, several laboratories have mapped epitopes presented by HLA-A2.1 molecules and capable of inducing CTL in patients and/or HLA-A2 transgenic mice [80,135–139]. Epimmune's group has focused on conserved

regions of the HCV genome to identify viral peptides that contain HLA class I binding motifs and bind with high affinity to the corresponding purified HLA molecules [130]. A total of 31 HLA-A1, HLA-A2.1, HLA-A3, HLA-A11, or HLA-A24 binding peptides were identified. Twelve conserved peptides that bind HLA-A2.1 with high or intermediate affinity were tested for immunogenicity in vitro in human primary CTL cultures and in vivo by direct immunization of HLA-A2.1/Kb transgenic mice. Six HLA-A2.1-restricted CTL epitopes were immunogenic in both systems. At least three of these peptide epitopes were endogenously processed and presented for CTL recognition. Using tetramers of HLA-A2.1 and an NS3 peptide of HCV, CTL frequencies in peripheral blood and liver could be quantitated, and shown to be at least 30-fold higher in liver than in peripheral blood [140].

A subsequent study was designed to identify CTL epitopes restricted by HLA types other than HLA-A2, to expand the epitope repertoire available for T cell-mediated therapeutic vaccine development [123]. Scanning of 14 different HCV genome sequences for the presence of conserved peptides containing the HLA-A3 and HLA-B7 motifs revealed 9-mer to 10-mer peptides. Peptides with good HLA binding affinities, which cross-reacted with at least three of five of the most common molecules of each supertype, were tested for the ability to stimulate a memory CTL response in the peripheral blood from selected HCV-infected patients and normal seronegative donors in vitro. Eight HLA-A3 supertype-restricted and one HLA-B7 supertype-restricted CTL epitopes, which were recognized by infected patients but not by healthy seronegative donors, were identified. In conclusion, these studies defined a set of CTL epitopes, which should enable the design of an ethnically unbiased therapeutic CTL vaccine for the treatment of patients with chronic HCV infection. The potential value of these epitopes was further underlined by a study that utilized the same set of supertype epitopes [124]. The CTL responses against multiple HCV epitopes were detected in 7 of 29 (24.1%) healthy family members (HFM) persistently exposed to chronically HCV-infected patients (HCV-HFM). The HCV-specific effector $CD8^+$ T cells were readily detected by ELIspot in freshly isolated PBMCs of HCV-HFM. Furthermore, combination of cell depletion ELIspot analyses showed that the effector cells were of the $CD8^+$ $CD45RO^+$ $CD28^-$ phenotype. The persistence of effector $CD8^+$ T cells specific for both these epitopes in uninfected HCV-HFM suggested that: (1) an immunological memory is associated with a subclinical infection without any evidence of hepatitis in a large cohort of HCV-exposed individuals; and (2) these cells should be capable of prompt HCV-specific effector function in vivo, possibly providing antiviral protection.

Finally, a series of studies also addressed the identification of HLA class II restricted epitopes because HLA class II-restricted T-cell response to HCV antigens is believed to influence the final outcome of hepatitis C. In a study by Lamonaca et al. [125], 22 subjects with acute HCV infection were studied and followed for an average time of 29 months. Several highly immunogenic T-cell epitopes were identified within core, NS3, and NS4. All of the epitopes are immunodominant, highly conserved among the known HCV isolates, and promiscuous.

B. Identification of T-Cell Epitopes in Human Immunodeficiency Virus

A number of research groups have applied the strategies and tools described above to the identification of HIV-derived epitopes [119,127,141–150]. A first study [126] tested the antigenicity and immunogenicity of peptides capable of binding to multiple HLA class I molecules of the A3-like supertype. Primary in vitro cultures of lymphocytes from healthy donors, as well as in vitro restimulation of lymphocytes from HIV-infected individuals, were utilized. Several of the peptides that were capable of binding more than one HLA-A3 supertype molecule were also found to be immunogenic in the context of this same group of HLA molecules (degenerate CTL recognition). Some of the CTL lines thus generated demonstrated even promiscuous recognition of the cognate epitope in the context of more than one A3 supertype molecule. Thus, similar peptide binding was demonstrated to be reflected in a remarkable similarity in the peptide-MHC complex structures engaged by the TCR and responsible for T-cell activation.

To gain additional insights into a potential correlation between recognition of supertype epitopes and clinical outcome, responses of long-term nonprogressors (LTNPs) [128] were analyzed. The LTNPs represent a minority of HIV-infected individuals characterized by stable or even increasing CD4$^+$ T-cell count and by stronger immune responses against HIV than progressors. A panel of A2 and A3 supertype epitopes was tested. ELIspot and specific major histocompatibility complex (MHC)-peptide tetramers detected HIV-specific effector and memory CD8$^+$ T cells. Both effector and memory resting cells were contained within a CD8$^+$ population with memory CD45RO$^+$ phenotype, with the former being CD28$^-$ and the latter CD28$^+$. Remarkably, all A2 and A3 supertype peptides tested were recognized by the PBMCs of infected individuals.

An independent study [127] described the immunological characterization of a number of novel HIV-1-specific, HLA-A2-restricted CTL epitopes that share a high degree of conservation within HIV-1 and a strong binding to different alleles of the HLA-A2 superfamily. Among the novel epitopes identified by the approaches described above were the first reported CTL epitope in the Vpr protein and two epitopes immunodominant among the HLA-A2-restricted CTL responses of individuals with acute and chronic HIV-1 infection. These may be valuable for vaccine design and testing and for assessing the natural immune response to infection.

Finally, because HIV-specific helper T lymphocytes (HTLs) play a key role in the immune control of HIV-1 infection and, as such, are an important target of potential HIV-1 vaccines, Wilson et al. [119] also embarked in a systematic study to identify HIV-derived HTL epitopes. Accordingly, conserved HIV-1-derived peptides bearing an HLA-DR binding supermotif were tested for binding to a panel of the most representative HLA-DR molecules. Eleven highly cross-reactive peptides were identified as binders, and all peptides elicited proliferative responses with PBMCs derived from multiple HIV-infected donors for each peptide. Several HIV-infected subjects recognized multiple peptides, and a strong association existed between the recognition of the parental recombinant HIV-1 protein and the corresponding HTL peptides, suggesting that these peptides represent epitopes that are processed and presented during the course of natural HIV-1 infection.

The aim of the HIV project in the TB/HIV Research Laboratory has been to use bioinformatics tools to design a "World Clade" HIV vaccine that will induce T-cell responses against the broadest possible range of HIV isolates. The HIV sequences database was downloaded from the LANL website (http://www.lanl.gov). Peptides were selected for their conservation across HIV-1 isolates using Conservatrix and screened for potential MHC class I binding using EpiMatrix. From the pool of peptides screened by EpiMatrix and Conservatrix, a total of 100 peptides were selected based on their restriction by the following MHC-I alleles: A2, A11, A3, and B7—25 peptides being restricted by each allele. Each set of 25 peptides contained one published positive control for the corresponding HLA allele. Assays using PBMCs from non-HIV-infected subjects were also performed. No responses to the selected HIV-1 peptides were observed in these negative control assays.

All the positive control peptides and 72% of the predicted peptides tested in the binding assays bound to the corresponding HLA allele. ELIspot results obtained from PBMCs derived from HIV-infected patients indicated that 44% of the B7 peptides, 40% of the A11 peptides, 24% of the A2 peptides, and 64% of the A3 peptides elicited IFN-γ secretion. These novel T epitopes were conserved in as many as 1238 HIV-1 strains, including strains from Africa, Asia, and the Americas. These data showed that candidate T-cell epitopes predicted using the previously described bioinformatics tools were able to bind to the corresponding HLA molecules and were recognized by T cells from healthy HIV-infected patients. The novel epitopes identified here would therefore have to have been selected from naturally processed T-cell epitopes generated during HIV infection. Because these epitopes are highly conserved among HIV isolates, they can be presented by prevalent MHC class I alleles and can induce cross-clade T-cell activation.

In theory, inclusion of these epitopes in an HIV vaccine will induce a pool of anti-HIV T-cell memory clones able to recognize immunogenic and highly conserved HIV epitopes in the vaccine recipients. The recruitment of these memory T cells during the acute phase of infection would lead to a faster and more effective elimination of the infected cells, limiting the scope of the infection.

Transgenic mouse models are currently being utilized to test the ability of string-of-epitopes constructs such as these to generate an immune response against the corresponding epitopes. Another system that may prove useful in testing the efficacy of a multiepitope vaccine is the in vitro generation of de novo CTL responses using dendritic cells as APCs [151]. However, unlike in vivo systems, "in vitro immunization" may only approximate the strength and duration of the induced immune response.

C. Identifying T-Cell Epitopes in the Tuberculosis Genome

Various models of Mtb infection have indicated a central role for MHC class I-restricted CD8$^+$ T cells in protective immunity. Accordingly, one study performed by Cho et al. [152] investigated which antigens and epitopes of Mtb proteins were presented by infected cells to CD8$^+$ T cells. In that study, 40 Mtb proteins were searched for HLA class I A*0201 binding motifs. Predicted high-affinity binding peptides were assayed for recognition by CTL. Three epitopes, derived from three different antigens thymidylate synthase [ThyA(30-38)], RNA polymerase β-subunit [RpoB(127-135)], and a putative phosphate transport system permease protein A-1 [PstA1(75-83)], were identified when they were recognized by CD8$^+$ T cells of patients recovering from Mtb infection. Furthermore, CD8$^+$ T-cell lines specific for these antigens specifically recognized Mtb-infected macrophages, as demonstrated by production of IFN-γ or lysis of the infected target cells, and reduced the viability of the intracellular Mtb, providing evidence that CD8$^+$ T-cell recognition of MHC class I-restricted epitopes of these Mtb antigens might contribute to effective immunity.

Several Mtb genomes have been sequenced and made available to researchers. Accordingly, the group at the TB/HIV Research Laboratory has analyzed the TIGR Mtb CDC-1551 genome, the H37Rv genome, and the available sequenced fragments (contigs) of the BCG genome for T-cell epitope content. In collaboration with EpiVax, the TB/HIV Research Laboratory has performed two genome scans. The initial focus of these scans has been on secreted antigens, because they have been shown to induce a strong TH1 immune response in the early phase of infection in patients [153,154], as well as upregulated proteins, because they are expressed during bacterial growth and may therefore play an important role in latent Mtb infection. Seventeen peptides were selected for synthesis from each genome scan based on the following criteria: a high EpiMatrix (EBP) score for MHC class II binding and potential MHC promiscuity. The first-pass analysis resulted in a 95% reduction in the number of peptides to be tested (Fig. 2). These peptides were tested in thymidine incorporation T-cell proliferation assays and IFN-γ ELIspot assays. Immunogenic epitopes were assayed for recognition by T cells in healthy Mtb-infected individuals. In the genome scan for secreted antigens, 11 of 17 tested peptides were recognized in T-cell proliferation and ELIspot assays. From this set of 11 immunogenic peptides, one novel immunodominant T-cell epitope that induced IFN-γ secretion in 15 of 27 Mtb-infected patients was identified. In the genome scan for upregulated proteins, 13 of 17 peptides induced IFN-γ release. This pilot study represents the first step in a genome-derived TB vaccine project funded by the Sequella Global TB foundation.

VII. THE ROLE OF BREADTH AND MULTISPECIFICITY IN SUCCESSFUL IMMUNE RESPONSES AND VACCINE DESIGN

T-cell responses against certain T-cell specificities may go undetected during the course of natural immunity because of the fact that the corresponding epitopes are poorly generated by natural processing—the breakdown of the pathogen-derived proteins within the cells of the host [16,76,84,92, 155–163]. The issue of whether a given epitope is generated (or not) by natural antigen processing in sufficient amounts to allow for T-cell recognition is a crucial one. This is because the ultimate targets of T-cell responses are cells producing the naturally processed antigen, such as infected cells or cancer cells. Hence, a T-cell response that does not recognize the cancer cells or the infected cell would be useless ultimately in terms of prevention, control, or eradication of the disease.

However, the particular assay system utilized can influence whether a given peptide is scored as being generated by natural processing or not. For example, a given HCV-derived epitope elicited T cells that did not recognize natu-

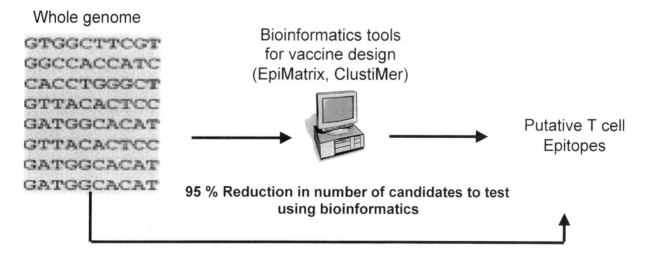

Figure 2 T-cell epitope mapping from the genome.

rally processed HCV antigens expressed by transfected cells, as determined by chromium release killing assays. However, the same CTL line was fully capable of recognizing the same transfected cells, if the production of IFN-γ was utilized as a readout [164]. In a different study [165], it was similarly shown that HBV peptide-specific CTL lines apparently incapable of killing endogenous targets or even producing significant amounts of IFN-γ in vitro were nonetheless capable of controlling viral replication in vivo in HBV transgenic mice.

Collectively, these examples illustrate that it is not safe to conclude that the failure to detect a response against a given epitope means that a particular epitope is nonimmunogenic or that it is not generated by natural processing. As long as the peptide binds to MHC molecules with the required affinity, failure to detect CTL response or recognition of naturally processed antigen under a given condition does not preclude the possibility of detecting immunogenicity under different conditions.

As noted above, in certain cases, the recognition of a particular epitope results in the suppression of other epitope-specific responses. This ability of an epitope to dominate a response is relative. The hierarchy of epitope recognition can be altered by the prior experience of the immune system as in memory T cells [166]. Likewise, the deletion of the immunodominant epitope from a protein antigen can also dramatically change the pattern of epitope recognition, resulting in the activation of T cells against previously subdominant peptides [74].

Finally, a complex interplay between T cells, APCs, and antigen production during natural infection also influences immunodominance. T cells specific for a given epitope might be present in higher numbers than those for other epitopes, or they may be stimulated earlier or more vigorously because their corresponding peptides are produced in greater abundance or bind with higher affinity to MHC. Their dominant expansion can limit the expansion of other T-cell specificities by competition for space or nutrients, competition for cell–cell interactions, and simply because a vigorous dominant response might rapidly eliminate or decrease the pathogen concentration before other specificities are effectively stimulated [167,168]. In these cases, immunization with epitope-based vaccines and immunogens offers an opportunity to alter immunodominance patterns and obtain responses directed against subdominant as well as dominant epitopes.

Immunodominance can be very profound, resulting in only one or few specificities dominating the response to a given pathogen and a large fraction of activated T cells specific for a single epitope/MHC combination. This rather absolute type of immunodominance is actually frequently observed in the mouse but more rarely in humans. Indeed, it has been shown in a number of different cases that human responses are often multispecific, directed against multiple proteins derived from a given pathogen, and broad, directed against multiple epitopes within a given protein [169,170]. For example, simple perusal of the Los Alamos HIV database (hivweb.lanl.gov/immunology/index.html) reveals that several hundred different HIV-derived T-cell epitopes have already been defined. These facts are hard to reconcile with certain dogmatic and simplistic views of immunodominance.

Indeed, it would appear that, depending on the particular type of situation and perhaps animal species considered, either a narrow response or broad multispecific response can be obtained.

The issues raised above have broad implications for the design and evaluation of vaccines directed against infectious diseases and cancer. According to one point of view, effective vaccines should focus on and optimize responses for one or a few immunodominant epitopes. The rationale for this argument is that this strategy would most closely mimic natural immune responses. However, in our view, the opposite is true, and vaccine constructs eliciting broad and multispecific immune responses offer several advantages, discussed in more detail in the present and following sections.

What are the characteristics of successful versus unsuccessful immune responses? In the case of HBV infection, individuals that recover from acute hepatitis and clear the virus are characterized as having a very broad and often multispecific T-cell response. In contrast, chronically infected individuals have weak and less diverse responses [132]. In chimpanzees experimentally infected with HCV, spontaneous clearance of the virus is accompanied by a vigorous and multispecific T-cell response, whereas chimpanzees with restricted responses remained chronically infected [171]. In the case of malaria, immunity from P. falciparum challenge is achieved by vaccination with parasites inactivated by irradiation. In the case of these individuals, recall memory responses directed against multiple epitopes, restricted by multiple HLA alleles and derived from each of four different antigens, were demonstrated [118,122].

In the case of chronic HIV infection, long-term nonprogressors are characterized by the presence of low viral loads and potent, broadly reactive HIV-1-specific CTL responses [104,105,172–174]. Thus, the breadth of CTL responses appears to be critical to the control of the virus in these persons as responses focused on limited numbers of viral gene products are more often associated with viral persistence and more rapid disease progression [175,176].

The observations described above raise the question of why a multispecific response may be more effective. A number of different factors should be considered. First, a multispecific response might offer a key advantage in terms of accessing a higher number of precursors. The overall disease-relevant immune response is the total number of immune T cells, which is the sum of the T cells specific for each epitope. By accessing more epitopes, and therefore a higher number of precursors, a more vigorous response can be obtained. A higher number of precursors can also offer another distinct temporal advantage. Because following encounter with the pathogen-derived epitopes, T-cell precursors divide exponentially, accessing more precursors leads to achieving a set level of active T cells sooner. This temporal advantage can play a key role in allowing the immune system to outpace the pathogens, which also is dividing exponentially.

Second, another important advantage of multispecific and broad responses is that they counteract escape from immune surveillance resulting from pathogen's heterogeneity, either already existing at the time of infection, or originating by mutation or loss of expression of the targeted antigen. It is well appreciated that mutation rates play a key role in the persistence of pathogens such as HIV, HCV, and *P. falciparum*. Any given sequence, placed under immune pressure, will have a certain mutation rate, which then defines the probability of selecting for a mutated pathogen, now potentially invisible to the T-cell response. However, if responses against two epitopes are present, the probability of a pathogen simultaneously mutating both epitopes is the product of the probabilities of each epitope mutating separately. It is a well-established paradigm that responses directed against multiple pathogen targets, such as T-cell epitopes, greatly decrease the probability of pathogen escape.

Likewise, monospecific responses could also select a tumor variant that had lost expression of the targeted antigen. However, it is logical to assume that targeting multiple tumor antigens would significantly decrease the probability of tumor escape because that would require loss of antigen expression to occur twice.

VIII. OPTIMIZING EPITOPE-BASED VACCINES

Enhancing the immunogenicity of multiepitope vaccines has been approached in several ways. One approach has focused on how best to package multiple epitopes in a vaccine construct. One option is to present the epitopes as a "string of beads," without any spacer sequences separating the individual epitopes. Indeed, some studies have indicated that flanking sequences have minimal effects on epitope presentation [177]. The actual role of flanking spacer sequences is currently under investigation, partly because our understanding of how multiepitope constructs are processed remains incomplete. In a "string of beads" construct, the individual epitopes are usually very closely apposed, without their natural flanking sequences; this has raised concern that their proteolytic processing may be compromised and that peptides other than the specific peptides of interest may be generated as a result of the processing [178,179]. There is some evidence that the introduction of spacer sequences to separate the individual epitopes may therefore help focus the immune response on the specific epitopes [180]. A study by Velders et al. [181] compared the immunogenicity of two similar HPV epitope string DNA constructs that differed only in the presence or absence of spacers between the epitopes, and found that the addition of AAY spacers between the epitopes was crucial for the epitope-induced tumor protection.

A recent study by Livingston et al. illustrated how a comprehensive strategy can be derived to optimize a multiepitope vaccine construct. These authors derived empirical rules to maximize proteosomal cleavage and epitope immunogenicity. A bioinformatic tool (EpiSort) was next derived to generate optimal spacer sequences tailored to each epitope pair, simultaneously optimizing for proteosomal cleavage and minimizing the occurrence of undesired junctional epitopes. The effectiveness of this strategy has been verified in several different disease models, by the use of transfected target cells and HLA transgenic mice [96].

Costimulatory molecules play a central role in the initiation of T-cell immune responses [182]. CD28 and CTLA4 represent the costimulatory receptors on T cells, and B7 molecules represent their corresponding ligands on APCs. Several studies carried out in murine models suggest that the APC signal mediated via CD28 is required for TCR-mediated T-cell activation [183]. CTLA4, on the other hand, appears to play an antagonistic role in T-cell activation. Two members of the B7 family have been identified: B7-1 (CD80) and B7-2 (CD86). These two molecules show comparable affinity to CD28 molecules and may differentially activate Th1 or Th2 immune responses [182]. Lack of costimulation can lead to T-cell tolerance. Peptide epitopes presented by nonprofessional APCs may fail to activate T cells if signal 1 is delivered in the absence of signal 2, and instead may lead to T-cell anergy. Because of the role played by costimulatory molecules in the initiation of T-cell responses, they can be manipulated to either stimulate the immune system, to potentially prevent infection, or to inhibit the immune system, for immunotherapy against allergies and autoimmune diseases. The addition of costimulatory molecules or cytokines to vaccine constructs has been used successfully to amplify responses to vaccines [141,184–190].

One additional strategy to enhance CTL responses is to target the T-cell epitopes of interest to the proteasome of the host cell [191]. It is known that the ubiquitination of proteins acts as a tag to target proteins to the proteasome and to enhance the proteolytic degradation of the introduced epitopes within the cell. Similarly, targeting the epitopes for either secretion or cell membrane expression can enhance Th responses. Past studies have exploited lysosome-associated membrane proteins (LAMPs), which, when fused to foreign antigens, can target antigens for lysosomal entry and destruction and enhanced class II presentation [192].

Another major strategy that takes advantage of bioinformatics methods described here for predicting peptide binding to MHC molecules is epitope enhancement—the modification of the epitope sequence to enhance immunogenicity [79,141,189]. The sequence modifications may be designed to increase the affinity for the MHC molecule or to increase the affinity of the peptide-MHC complex for the TCR. In the former approach, one can modify anchor residues that are suboptimal or alter secondary anchors [46,193].

The matrix algorithms for predicting binding to MHC molecules lend themselves well to this approach, although empirical methods and screening of combinatorial libraries can also be used [194]. Epitope enhancement has been used successfully to improve CTL epitopes for HIV [195], a hepatitis C viral antigen [196], and melanoma tumor antigens [197–199], as well as an HIV helper T-cell epitope [200,201], to name a few examples.

In the latter case, it was found that the enhanced helper epitope, attached to an unmodified CTL epitope, not only induced more CTL and better protection against a viral challenge, but also qualitatively changed the helper response, skewing it toward Th1 phenotype. This was shown to be due to increased induction by the higher-affinity peptide of CD40L on the helper T-cell, which greatly increased IL-12 production by dendritic cells, making them more polarizing and in turn skewing the Th cells toward Th1, as well as making the dendritic cells more effective at stimulating a CTL response [200]. The alternative approach, of increasing the affinity of the peptide-MHC complex for the TCR, has also been used successfully for improving the immunogenicity of tumor antigens [202–204].

Until recently, there was no simple way to predict alterations that would improve binding to the TCR, except in the rare cases when a crystal structure of the TCR-peptide-MHC complex was available. However, recently, Tangri et al. examined a large number of cases and found a pattern of conserved substitutions at positions 3, 5, and 7 in the CTL epitope sequence that were likely to result in increased affinity for the TCR. This discovery allows a more streamlined systematic approach to identifying good candidates for this type of epitope enhancement [205]. As the bioinformatics approaches to predicting epitopes improve further, these will likely be applicable to the prediction of sequence modifications for epitope enhancement as well. Such improved epitopes are likely to be critical in the cases of chronic viral infections, in which the natural response to the native pathogen is not sufficient to eradicate the infection.

Finally, it is widely appreciated that dose, schedule, and route of immunization can significantly influence the nature of the generated immune response. The role of vaccine dose and route of immunization varies with vaccine design (synthetic peptide, genetic recombinant vector, and so on). In general, low doses and slow release of antigen appear to facilitate optimal T-cell activation. In contrast, high doses of antigen are more prone to induce T-cell tolerance. A delicate balance exists between the induction and the anergization of protective T-cell responses. Therefore, an immunization program should be carefully designed to target the desired immune response—stimulation in the case of an infection, and tolerance in the case of allergies or autoimmune diseases.

IX. PRECLINICAL ASSESSMENT OF THE IMMUNOGENICITY OF EPITOPE-BASED VACCINES

After using in vitro T-cell assays to select for naturally processed T-cell epitopes, it is important to evaluate the ability of vaccines derived from these epitopes to induce an immune response in vivo. Transgenic mice expressing human MHC class I or class II molecules represent a suitable preclinical model for this purpose. The advantage of using HLA transgenic animals is that they can develop physiologically relevant HLA-restricted T-cell responses. Transgenic mouse strains that express either the entire most common HLA-A, HLA-B, and HLA-DR molecules [78,81,206,207] have been developed. HLA-A2 transgenic mice have been used to assess the immunogenicity of peptides that bind to HLA-A2. An excellent correlation has been found between CTL responses in infected individuals and CTL responses induced in immunized HLA transgenic mice [78,80,208–213]. The use of HLA transgenic mice to assay and to optimize multiepitope-based vaccines has been described in detail by the studies described above. An alternative assay, which allows the direct evaluation of the amount of each epitope generated by a given vaccine construct, has also been reported. This "antigenicity assay" takes advantage of human cells transfected with a given vaccine candidate, assayed in parallel to untransfected cells and a dose titration of synthetic epitope [96,214].

Induction of the desired immune response with defined T-cell epitopes facilitates the monitoring of the specificity of the immune response using new epitope-specific reagents such as MHC dimers and tetramers. The MHC tetramers were first developed just a few years ago by Altman and Safrit [215] and Altman et al. [216], who have written several excellent reviews on the topic. These specialized constructs bear four MHC molecules complexed with β_2 microglobulin and a specific pathogen-derived peptide ligand. Tetramers can bind directly to T cells that recognize the MHC-peptide complex. They can be used for direct ex vivo analysis of the frequency and phenotypes of epitope-specific T cells by flow cytometric technique. Tetramers permit the following types of experimental confirmations of epitope-specific T-cell responses in vivo: (1) direct quantitation of the number of epitope-specific T cells prior to and following vaccination; (2) phenotyping of responding T cells (examination for cell surface markers such as CD8, CD4, CD38, and additional activation markers); (3) monitoring of the immune response to specific epitopes following vaccination; and (4) direct evaluation of the effect of combinations of epitopes, epitope spacers or linkers, and signal sequences on T-cell responses. These reagents will prove to be useful as epitope-driven vaccines move into Phase I trials, as they provide a means of directly measuring and timing immune response to the vaccine. Likewise, intracellular cytokine staining flow cytometry assays and ELIspot assays can be used to enumerate cells responding to a given antigen or epitope.

X. ADVANTAGES OF EPITOPE-BASED VACCINES AS COMPARED TO WHOLE PROTEIN VACCINES

The use of whole protein as a vaccine allows not only the induction of cellular immune responses, but also the induction of humoral immune responses. However, immunization with whole organisms or proteins does not always induce the desired immune response. Immunization with the whole protein typically induces an immune response against the immunodominant epitopes, which may apply selective pressure on the pathogen to evolve to mutate its immunodominant epitopes [217–219]. Examples of such a selection pressure, characterized in several pathogens, including HCV [220], HIV [221], and *Plasmodium* [217,218], result in immune escape by the pathogens. Thus, the induction of immunity against epitopes that are subdominant, highly conserved, and critical to the life cycle of the pathogen may be useful for the design of therapeutic vaccines. A number of recent studies of vaccines against viral diseases have demonstrated that CTL responses to subdominant epitopes can compensate for the loss of a dominant epitope and can provide efficient protection [166,222]. Another potential disadvantage of using whole proteins as vaccines is that immunization with pathogenic functional antigens can lead to toxicity and potential complications in the host [223]. These adverse effects can be minimized by using a T-cell epitope vaccine that contains immunogenic epitopes for the induction of protective immunity, and that excludes epitopes that can induce harmful immune responses.

Another disadvantage of whole protein-based vaccines in the setting of cancer therapeutics was addressed in a study by Disis et al. These investigators found that peptide-based, (but not whole protein), vaccines elicited immunity against an oncogenic self-protein [224]. It has been proposed that tolerance to self-proteins is directed only to dominant epitopes of proteins and not to subdominant epitopes [100,225]. Tolerance can therefore be circumvented by immunization with subdominant epitopes, not whole protein.

Perhaps the most important advantage of epitope-driven vaccines is their superior potency [214]. Because of the knowledge of the exact epitope recognized and targeted for immunization, each epitope can actually be optimized in terms of MHC binding, proteolytic processing, and TCR recognition, as detailed in the preceding paragraphs.

XI. CONCLUSION

Bioinformatics and high-throughput MHC-peptide binding assays are ushering in a new era of vaccine design. The ability to induce an immune response to a broad repertoire of epitopes that are universally recognized across continents and across genetic backgrounds is considered to be a critical characteristic of an effective vaccine. Opportunities for epitope discovery are expanding as the number of pathogens that are entirely sequenced approaches 100 and as access to these data improves. Epitope-driven vaccines that are designed and optimized, based on our current knowledge and understanding of the mechanics of immunogenicity and immunodominance, are now approaching testing in clinical trials in humans.

ACKNOWLEDGMENT

Epimmune's algorithms are available to the academic and industrial community on a collaborative basis (asettte@epimmune.com). EpiMatrix and associated algorithm Conservatrix were licensed from Brown University in 1998 and have been further developed by EpiVax (annied@epivax.com). EpiMatrix is also available on-line for use with HIV sequences at http://tbhiv.biomed.brown.edu/. Additional resources available on-line include the predictive matrix algorithm independently developed by Parker et al. http://bimas.dcrt.nih.gov/molbio/hla_bind/ and one by Rammensee et al. http://syfpeithi.bmi-heidelberg.com/Scripts/MHC-Server.dll/Info.htm.

REFERENCES

1. Elliott T, et al. Peptide-induced conformational change of the class I heavy chain. Nature 1991; 351(6325):402–406.

2. Falk K, et al. Allele-specific motifs revealed by sequencing of self-peptides eluted from MHC molecules. Nature 1991; 351(6324):290–296.

3. Brown JH, et al. Three-dimensional structure of the human class II histocompatibility antigen HLA-DR1. Nature 1993; 364(6432):33–39.

4. Chicz RM, et al. Specificity and promiscuity among naturally processed peptides bound to HLA-DR alleles. J Exp Med 1993; 178(1):27–47.

5. Unanue ER. Cellular studies on antigen presentation by class II MHC molecules. Curr Opin Immunol 1992; 4(1):63–69.

6. O'Sullivan W, et al. On the interaction of promiscuous antigenic peptides with different DR alleles. Identification of common structural motifs. J Immunol 1991; 147(8):2663–2669.

7. Sette A, et al. Invariant chain peptides in most HLA-DR molecules of an antigen-processing mutant. Science 1992; 258(5089):1801–1804.

8. Hunt DF, et al. Peptides presented to the immune system by the murine class II major histocompatibility complex molecule I-Ad. Science 1992; 256(5065):1817–1820.

9. Campbell DJ, et al. Bacterial proteins can be processed by macrophages in a transporter associated with antigen processing-independent, cysteine protease-dependent manner for presentation by MHC class I molecules. J Immunol 2000; 164(1):168–175.

10. Paz P, et al. Discrete proteolytic intermediates in the MHC class I antigen processing pathway and MHC I-dependent peptide trimming in the ER. Immunity 1999; 11(2):241–251.

11. Serwold T, Shastri N. Specific proteolytic cleavages limit the diversity of the pool of peptides available to MHC class I molecules in living cells. J Immunol 1999; 162(8):4712–4719.

12. Shastri N, et al. Presentation of endogenous peptide/MHC class I complexes is profoundly influenced by specific C-terminal flanking residues. J Immunol 1995; 155(9):4339–4346.

13. Rock KL, et al. Inhibitors of the proteasome block the degradation of most cell proteins and the generation of peptides presented on MHC class I molecules. Cell 1994; 78(5):761–771.

14. Van Kaer L, et al. Altered peptidase and viral-specific T cell response in LMP2 mutant mice. Immunity 1994; 1:533–541.

15. Cascio P, et al. 26S proteasomes and immunoproteasomes produce mainly N-extended versions of an antigenic peptide. EMBO J 2001; 20(10):2357–2366.

16. Yewdell JW, Bennink JR. Cut and trim: generating MHC class I peptide ligands. Curr Opin Immunol 2001; 13(1):13–18.

17. Chen W, et al. Immunoproteasomes shape immunodominance hierarchies of antiviral CD8(+) T cells at the levels of T cell repertoire and presentation of viral antigens. J Exp Med 2001; 193(11):1319–1326.

18. Vinitsky A, et al. Inhibition of the proteolytic activity of the multicatalytic proteinase complex (proteasome) by substrate-related peptidyl aldehydes. J Biol Chem 1994; 269(47):29860–29866.

19. Vinitsky A, et al. The generation of MHC class I-associated peptides is only partially inhibited by proteasome inhibitors: involvement of nonproteasomal cytosolic proteases in antigen processing? J Immunol 1997; 159(2):554–564.

20. Toes RE, et al. Discrete cleavage motifs of constitutive and immunoproteasomes revealed by quantitative analysis of cleavage products. J Exp Med 2001; 194:1–12.

21. Trowsdale J, et al. Sequences encoded in the class II region of the MHC related to the "ABC" superfamily of transporters. Nature 1990; 348(6303):741–744.

22. Van Endert PM, et al. The peptide-binding motif for the

human transporter associated with antigen processing. J Exp Med 1995; 182(6):1883–1895.

23. van Endert PM. Genes regulating MHC class I processing of antigen. Curr Opin Immunol 1999; 11(1):82–88.

24. Androlewicz MJ, Cresswell P. Human transporters associated with antigen processing possess a promiscuous peptide-binding site. Immunity 1994; 1:7–14.

25. Germain RN, Margulies DH. The biochemistry and cell biology of antigen processing and presentation. Annu Rev Immunol 1993; 11:403–450.

26. Appella E, et al. Synthetic antigenic peptides as a new strategy for immunotherapy of cancer. Biomed Pept Proteins Nucleic Acids 1995; 1(3):177–184.

27. Demotz S, et al. Characterization of a naturally processed MHC class II-restricted T-cell determinant of hen egg lysozyme. Nature 1989; 342(6250):682–684.

28. German RN, et al. Processing and presentation of endocytically acquired protein antigens by MHC class II and class I molecules. Immunol Rev 1996; 151:5–30.

29. Morris P, et al. E An essential role for HLA-DM in antigen presentation by class II major histocompatibility molecules. Nature 1994; 368(6471):551–554.

30. Sloan VS, et al. Mediation by HLA-DM of dissociation of peptides from HLA-DR. Nature 1995; 375(6534):802–806.

31. Sherman MA, et al. DM enhances peptide binding to class II MHC by release of invariant chain-derived peptide. Immunity 1995; 3(2):197–205.

32. DeLisi C, Berzofsky JA. T-cell antigenic sites tend to be amphipathic structures. Proc Natl Acad Sci USA 1985; 82(20):7048–7052.

33. Rothbard JB, Taylor WR. A sequence pattern common to T cell epitopes. EMBO J 1988; 7(1):93–100.

34. Meister GE, et al. Two novel T cell epitope prediction algorithms based on MHC-binding motifs; comparison of predicted and published epitopes from *Mycobacterium tuberculosis* and HIV protein sequences. Vaccine 1995; 13:581.

35. Sette A, et al. Structural characteristics of an antigen required for its interaction with Ia and recognition by T cells. Nature 1987; 328(6129):395–399.

36. Sette A, et al. I-Ad-binding peptides derived from unrelated protein antigens share a common structural motif. J Immunol 1988; 141:45–48.

37. Sette AA, et al. Structural requirements for the interaction between peptide antigens and I-Ed molecules. J Immunol 1989; 143:3289–3294.

38. Carbone FR. Conformational constraints involved in MHC class I restricted antigen presentation. Int Rev Immunol 1991; 7(2):129–138.

39. Romero P, et al. H-2Kd-restricted antigenic peptides share a simple binding motif. J Exp Med 1991; 174(3):603–612.

40. Jardetzky TS. Identification of self peptides bound to purified HLA-B27. Nature 1991; 353(6342):326–329.

41. Leighton J, et al. Comparison of structural requirements for interaction of the same peptide with I-Ek and I-Ed molecules in the activation of MHC class II-restricted T cells. J Immunol 1991; 147(1):198–204.

42. Geluk A, et al. HLA-DR3 molecules can bind peptides carrying two alternative specific submotifs. J Immunol 1994; 152(12):5742–5748.

43. Wall KA, et al. A disease-related epitope of Torpedo acetylcholine receptor. Residues involved in I-Ab binding, self-nonself discrimination, and TCR antagonism. J Immunol 1994; 152(9):4526–4536.

44. Sidney J, et al. Definition of a DQ3.1-specific binding motif. J Immunol 1994; 152(9):4516–4525.

45. Sette A, et al. HLA DR4w4-binding motifs illustrate the biochemical basis of degeneracy and specificity in peptide–DR interactions. J Immunol 1993; 151(6):3163–3170.

46. Ruppert J, et al. Prominent role of secondary anchor residues in peptide binding to HLA-A2.1 molecules. Cell 1993; 74:929–937.

47. Sidney J, et al. DRB1*0301 molecules recognize a structural motif distinct from the one recognized by most DR beta 1 alleles. J Immunol 1992; 149(8):2634–2640.

48. O'Sullivan D, et al. Truncation analysis of several DR binding epitopes. J Immunol 1991; 146(4):1240–1246.

49. Kondo A, et al. Two distinct HLA-A*0101-specific submotifs illustrate alternative peptide binding modes. Immunogenetics 1997; 45(4):249–258.

50. Lipford GB, et al. Primary in vivo responses to ovalbumin. Probing the predictive value of the Kb binding motif. J Immunol 1993; 150:1212.

51. Parker KC, et al. Scheme for ranking potential HLA-A2 binding peptides based on independent binding of individual peptide side chains. J Immunol 1994; 152:163.

52. Hammer J, et al. Precise prediction of major histocompatibility complex class II–peptide interaction based on peptide side chain scanning. J Exp Med 1994; 180:2353–2358.

53. Sette A, et al. Prediction of major histocompatibility complex binding regions of protein antigens by sequence pattern analysis. Proc Natl Acad Sci USA 1989; 86(9):3296–3300.

54. Parker KC, et al. Peptide binding to MHC class I molecules: implications for antigenic peptide prediction. Immunol Res 1995; 14(1):34–57.

55. Davenport MP, et al. An empirical method for the prediction of T-cell epitopes. Immunogenetics 1995; 42(5).

56. Jesdale BM, et al. Matrix-based prediction of MHC binding peptides: the EpiMatrix algorithm, reagent for HIV research. Vaccines '97. Cold Spring Harbor, NY: Cold Spring Harbor Press, 1997:127–134.

57. De Groot AS, et al. An interactive web site providing MHC ligand predictions: application to HIV research. AIDS Res Hum Retrovir 1997; 13(7):539–541.

58. Leggatt GR, et al. The importance of pairwise interactions between peptide residues in the delineation of T cell receptor specificity. J Immunol 1998; 161:4728–4735.

59. Ruppert J, et al. Class I MHC–peptide interaction: structural and functional aspects. Behring-Inst-Mitt 1994; 94:48–60.

60. Schafer JA, et al. Prediction of well-conserved HIV-1 ligands using a matrix-based algorithm, EpiMatrix. Vaccine 1998; 16:1880–1884.

61. Altuvia Y, et al. Sequence features that correlate with MHC restriction. Mol Immunol 1994; 31:1–19.

62. Altuvia Y, et al. Ranking potential binding peptides to MHC molecules by a computational threading approach. J Mol Biol 1995; 249:244–250.

63. Gulukota K, DeLisi C. HLA allele selection for designing peptide vaccines. Genet Anal 1996; 13:81–86.

64. Altuvia Y, et al. A structure-based algorithm to predict potential binding peptides to MHC molecules with hydrophobic binding pockets. Hum Immunol 1997; 58(1):1–11.

65. Schueler-Furman O, et al. Structure-based prediction of binding peptides to MHC class I molecules: application to a broad range of MHC alleles. Protein Sci 2000; 9(9):1838–1846.

66. Logean A, et al. Customized versus universal scoring functions: application to class I MHC-peptide binding free energy predictions. Bioorg Med Chem Lett 2001; 11(5):675–679.

67. Sette A, et al. The relationship between class I binding affinity and immunogenicity of potential cytotoxic T cell epitopes. J Immunol 1994; 153(12):5586–5592.

68. Brusic V, et al. MHCPEP, a database of MHC-binding peptides: update 1997. Nucleic Acids Res 1998; 26(1):368–371.

69. Sturniolo T, et al. Generation of tissue-specific and promiscuous HLA ligand databases using DNA microarrays and virtual HLA class II matrices. Nat Biotechnol 1999; 17(6):555–561.

70. Zhang C, et al. Structural principles that govern the peptide-binding motifs of class I MHC molecules. J Mol Biol 1998; 281(5):929–947.

71. Sette A, Sidney J. Nine major HLA class I supertypes account for the vast preponderance of HLA-A and -B polymorphism. Immunogenetics 1999; 50(3-4):201–212.

72. Sette A, Sidney J. HLA supertypes and supermotifs: a functional perspective on HLA polymorphism. Curr Opin Immunol 1998; 10(4):478–482.

73. Kast WM, et al. Role of HLA-A motifs in identification of potential CTL epitopes in human papillomavirus type 16 E6 and E7 proteins. J Immunol 1994; 152(8):3904–3912.

74. Van der Most RG, et al. Uncovering subdominant cytotoxic T-lymphocyte responses in lymphocytic choriomeningitis virus-infected BALB/c mice. J Virol 1997; 71(7):5110–5114.

75. Van der Most RG, et al. Analysis of cytotoxic T cell responses to dominant and subdominant epitopes during acute and chronic lymphocytic choriomeningitis virus infection. J Immunol 1996; 157(12):5543–5554.

76. Van der Most RG, et al. Identification of Db- and Kb-restricted subdominant cytotoxic T-cell responses in lymphocytic choriomeningitis virus-infected mice. Virology 1998; 240(1):158–167.

77. Vitiello A, et al. Immunodominance analysis of CTL responses to influenza PR8 virus reveals two new dominant and subdominant Kb-restricted epitopes. J Immunol 1996; 157(12):5555–5562.

78. Wentworth PA, et al. Differences and similarities in the A2.1-restricted cytotoxic T cell repertoire in humans and human leukocyte antigen-transgenic mice. Eur J Immunol 1996; 26(1):97–101.

79. Berzofsky JA. Epitope selection and design of synthetic vaccines: molecular approaches to enhancing immunogenicity and crossreactivity of engineered vaccines. Ann NY Acad Sci 1993; 690:256–264.

80. Shirai M, et al. CTL responses of HLA-A2.1-transgenic mice specific for hepatitis C viral peptides predict epitopes for CTL of humans carrying HLA-A2.1. J Immunol 1995; 154:2733–2742.

81. Alexander J, et al. Derivation of HLA-A11/Kb transgenic mice: functional CTL repertoire and recognition of human A11-restricted CTL epitopes. J Immunol 1997; 159(10):4753–4761.

82. Kubo RT, et al. Definition of specific peptide motifs for four major HLA-A alleles. J Immunol 1994; 152(8):3913–3924.

83. DiBrino M, et al. Identification of the peptide binding motif for HLA-B44, one of the most common HLA-B alleles in the Caucasian population. Biochemistry 1995; 34(32):10130–10138.

84. York IA, et al. Proteolysis and class I major histocompatibility complex antigen presentation. Immunol Rev 1999; 172:49–66.

85. Mo XY, et al. Distinct proteolytic processes generate the C and N termini of MHC class I-binding peptides. J Immunol 1999; 163:5851–5859.

86. Daniel S, et al. Relationship between peptide selectivities of human transporters associated with antigen processing and HLA class I molecules. J Immunol 1998; 161:617–624.

87. Lauvau G, et al. Human transporters associated with antigen processing (TAPs) select epitope precursor peptides for processing in the endoplasmic reticulum and presentation to T cells. J Exp Med 1999; 190:1227–1240.

88. Neefjes J, et al. Analysis of the fine specificity of rat, mouse and human TAP peptide transporters. Eur J Immunol 1995; 25:1133–1136.

89. Berzofsky JA, Berkower IJ. Immunogenicity and antigen structure. In: WE Paul, ed. Fundamental Immunology. Philadelphia: Lippincott-Raven, 1999:651–699.

90. Wherry EJ, et al. The induction of virus-specific CTL as a function of increasing epitope expression: responses rise steadily until excessively high levels of epitope are attained. J Immunol 1999; 163(7):3735–3745.

91. Bergmann CC, et al. Differential effects of flanking residues on presentation of epitopes from chimeric peptides. J Virol 1994; 68(8):5306–5310.

92. Yewdell JW. Not such a dismal science: the economics of protein synthesis, folding, degradation and antigen processing. Trends Cell Biol 2001; 11(7):294–297.

93. Mo AX, et al. Sequences that flank subdominant and cryptic epitopes influence the proteolytic generation of MHC class I-presented peptides. J Immunol 2000; 164(8):4003–4010.

94. Fahmy TM, et al. Increased TCR avidity after T cell activation: a mechanism for sensing low-density antigen. Immunity 2001; 14(2):135–143.

95. Alexander MA, et al. Correlation between CD8 dependency and determinant density using peptide-induced. Ld-restricted cytotoxic T lymphocytes. J Exp Med 1991; 173(4):849–858.

96. Livingston BD, et al. Optimization of epitope processing enhances immunogenicity of multiepitope DNA vaccines. Vaccine 2001; 19(32):4652–4660.

97. Deng H, et al. The involvement of antigen processing in determinant selection by class II MHC and its relationship to immunodominance. APMIS Acta Pathol Microbiol Immunol Scand 1993; 101(9):655–662.

98. Yewdell JW, Bennink JR. Immunodominance in major histocompatibility complex class I-restricted T lymphocyte responses. Annu Rev Immunol 1999; 17:51–88.

99. Berzofsky JA. Immunodominance in T lymphocyte recognition. Immunol Lett 1988; 18(2):83–92.

100. Sercarz EE, Lehmann PV, Ametani A, Benichou G, Miller A, Moudgil K. Dominance and crypticity of T cell antigenic determinants. Annu Rev Immunol 1993; 11:729–766.

101. Schaeffer EB, et al. Relative contribution of "determinant selection" and "holes in the T-cell repertoire" to T-cell responses. Proc Natl Acad Sci USA 1989; 86(12):4649–4653.

102. Rosenthal AS. Determinant selection and macrophage function in genetic control of the immune response. Immunol Rev 1978; 40:136–152.

103. Klein J. Immunology. New York: John Wiley and Sons, 1982:299–302.

104. Cao Y, et al. Virologic and immunologic characterization of long-term survivors of human immunodeficiency virus type 1 infection. N Engl J Med 1995; 332(4):201–208.

105. Ferbas J, et al. Virus burden in long-term survivors of human immunodeficiency virus (HIV) infection is a determinant of anti-HIV CD8+ lymphocyte activity. J Infect Dis 1995; 172(2):329–339.

106. Sidney J, et al. Majority of peptides binding HLA-A*0201 with high affinity crossreact with other A2-supertype molecules. Hum Immunol 2001; 62(11):1200–1216.

107. Livingston BD, et al. Immunization with the HBV core 18-27 epitope elicits CTL responses in humans expressing different HLA-A2 supertype molecules. Hum Immunol 1999; 60(11):1013–1017.

108. Sidney J, et al. The HLA-A*0207 peptide binding repertoire is limited to a subset of the A*0201 repertoire. Hum Immunol 1997; 58(1):12–20.

109. Sidney J, et al. Specificity and degeneracy in peptide binding to HLA-B7-like class I molecules. J Immunol 1996; 157(8):3480–3490.

110. Sidney J, et al. Definition of an HLA-A3-like supermotif demonstrates the overlapping peptide-binding repertoires of common HLA molecules. Hum Immunol 1996; 45(2):79–93.

111. del Guercio MF, et al. Binding of a peptide antigen to multiple HLA alleles allows definition of an A2-like supertype. J Immunol 1995; 154(2):685–693.

112. Bertoni R, et al. Human class I supertypes and CTL repertoires extend to chimpanzees. J Immunol 1998; 161(8):4447–4455.

113. McKinney DM, et al. Identification of five different Patr class I molecules that bind HLA supertype peptides and definition of their peptide binding motifs. J Immunol 2000; 165(8):4414–4422.

114. Urvater JA, et al. Gorillas with spondyloarthropathies express an MHC class I molecule with only limited sequence similarity to HLA-B27 that binds peptides with arginine at P2. J Immunol 2001; 166(5):3334–3344.

115. Dzuris JL, et al. Conserved MHC class I peptide binding motif between humans and rhesus macaques. J Immunol 2000; 164(1):283–291.

116. Dzuris JL, et al. Molecular determinants of peptide binding to two common rhesus macaque major histocompatibility complex class ii molecules. J Virol 2001; 75(22):10958–10968.

117. Allen TM, et al. Characterization of the peptide binding motif of a rhesus MHC class I molecule (Mamu-A*01) that binds an immunodominant CTL epitope from simian immunodeficiency virus. J Immunol 1998; 160(12):6062–6071.

118. Doolan DL, et al. HLA-DR-promiscuous T cell epitopes from *Plasmodium falciparum* pre-erythrocytic-stage antigens restricted by multiple HLA class II alleles. J Immunol 2000; 165(2):1123–1137.

119. Wilson CC, et al. Identification and antigenicity of broadly cross-reactive and conserved human immunodeficiency virus type 1-derived helper T-lymphocyte epitopes. J Virol 2001; 75(9):4195–4207.

120. Southwood S, et al. Several common HLA-DR types share largely overlapping peptide binding repertoires. J Immunol 1998; 160(7):3363–3373.

121. Bertoni R, et al. Human histocompatibility leukocyte antigen-binding supermotifs predict broadly cross-reactive cytotoxic T lymphocyte responses in patients with acute hepatitis. J Clin Invest 1997; 100(3):503–513.

122. Doolan DL, et al. Degenerate cytotoxic T cell epitopes from *P. falciparum* restricted by multiple HLA-A and HLA-B supertype alleles. Immunity 1997; 7(1):97–112.

123. Chang KM, et al. Identification of HLA-A3- and -B7-restricted CTL response to hepatitis C virus in patients with acute and chronic hepatitis C. J Immunol 1999; 162(2):1156–1164.

124. Scognamiglio P, et al. Presence of effector CD8$^+$ T cells in hepatitis C virus-exposed healthy seronegative donors. J Immunol 1999; 162(11):6681–6689.

125. Lamonaca V, et al. Conserved hepatitis C virus sequences are highly immunogenic for CD4(+) T cells: implications for vaccine development. Hepatology 1999; 30(4):1088–1098.

126. Threlkeld SC, et al. Degenerate and promiscuous recognition by CTL of peptides presented by the MHC class I A3-like superfamily: implications for vaccine development. J Immunol 1997; 159(4):1648–1657.

127. Altfeld MA, et al. Identification of novel HLA-A2-restricted human immunodeficiency virus type 1-specific cytotoxic T-lymphocyte epitopes predicted by the HLA-A2 supertype peptide-binding motif. J Virol 2001; 75(3):1301–1311.

128. Propato A, et al. Spreading of HIV-specific CD8$^+$ T-cell repertoire in long-term nonprogressors and its role in the control of viral load and disease activity. Hum Immunol 2001; 62(6):561–576.

129. Cerny A, et al. The class I restricted cytotoxic T lymphocyte response to predetermined epitopes in the hepatitis B and C viruses. In: Oldstone MBA, ed. Current Topics in Microbiology and Immunology. Vol. 189. Heidelberg: Springer-Verlag, 1994:169–186.

130. Wentworth PA, et al. Identification of A2-restricted hepatitis C virus-specific cytotoxic T lymphocyte epitopes from conserved regions of the viral genome. Int Immunol 1996; 8(5):651–659.

131. De Groot AS, et al. Designing HIV-1 vaccines to reflect viral diversity and the global context of HIV/AIDS. AIDScience 2001; 1:2.

132. Chisari FV, Ferrari C. Hepatitis B virus immunopathogenesis. Annu Rev Immunol 1995; 13, 29–60.

133. Missale G, et al. HLA-A31- and HLA-Aw68-restricted cytotoxic T cell responses to a single hepatitis B virus nucleocapsid epitope during acute viral hepatitis. J Exp Med 1993; 177(3):751–762.

134. Rehermann B, et al. The cytotoxic T lymphocyte response to multiple hepatitis B virus polymerase epitopes during and after acute viral hepatitis. J Exp Med 1995; 181:1047–1058.

135. Battegay M, et al. Patients with chronic hepatitis C have circulating cytotoxic T cells which recognize hepatitis C virus-encoded peptides binding to HLA-A2.1 molecules. J Virol 1995; 69:2462–2470.

136. Kurokohchi K, et al. Use of recombinant protein to identify a motif-negative human CTL epitope presented by HLA-A2 in the hepatitis C virus NS3 region. J Virol 1996; 70:232–240.

137. Shirai M, et al. An epitope in hepatitis C virus core region recognized by cytotoxic T cells in mice and humans. J Virol 1994; 68:3334–3342.

138. Koziel MJ, et al. Hepatitis C virus (HCV)-specific cytotoxic T lymphocytes recognize epitopes in the core and envelope proteins of HCV. J Virol 1993; 67:7522–7532.

139. Koziel MJ, et al. HLA class I-restricted cytotoxic T lymphocytes specific for hepatitis C virus. Identification of multiple epitopes and characterization of patterns of cytokine release. J Clin Invest 1995; 96:2311–2321.

140. He XS, et al. Quantitative analysis of hepatitis C virus-specific CD8(+) T cells in peripheral blood and liver using peptide-MHC tetramers. Proc Natl Acad Sci USA 1999; 96(10):5692–5697.

141. Berzofsky JA, et al. Approaches to improve engineered vaccines for human immunodeficiency virus (HIV) and other viruses that cause chronic infections. Immunol Rev 1999; 170:151–172.

142. Berzofsky JA, et al. Construction of peptides encompassing multideterminant clusters of HIV envelope to induce in vitro T-cell responses in mice and humans of multiple MHC types. J Clin Invest 1991; 88:876–884.

143. Cease KB, et al. Helper T cell antigenic site identification in the AIDS virus gp120 envelope protein and induction of immunity in mice to the native protein using a 16-residue synthetic peptide. Proc Natl Acad Sci USA 1987; 84:4249–4253.

144. Clerici M, et al. Detection of cytotoxic T lymphocytes specific for synthetic peptides of gp160 in HIV-seropositive individuals. J Immunol 1991; 146:2214–2219.

145. Clerici M, et al. Interleukin-2 production used to detect antigenic peptide recognition by T-helper lymphocytes from asymptomatic HIV seropositive individuals. Nature 1989; 339:383–385.

146. Hosmalin A, et al. An epitope in HIV-1 reverse transcriptase recognized by both mouse and human CTL. Proc Natl Acad Sci USA 1990; 87:2344–2348.

147. Takahashi H, et al. An immunodominant epitope of the

HIV gp160 envelope glycoprotein recognized by class I MHC molecule-restricted murine cytotoxic T lymphocytes. Proc Natl Acad Sci USA 1988; 85:3105–3109.

148. McMichael AJ, Walker BD. Cytotoxic T lymphocyte epitopes: implications for HIV vaccines. AIDS 1994; 8(Suppl 1):S155–S173.

149. Nixon DF, et al. HIV-1 gag-specific cytotoxic T lymphocytes defined with recombinant vaccinia virus and synthetic peptides. Nature 1988; 336:484–487.

150. Walker BD, et al. Long-term culture and fine specificity of human cytotoxic T lymphocyte clones reactive with human immunodeficiency virus type 1. Proc Natl Acad Sci USA 1989; 86:9514–9518.

151. Wilson CC, et al. HIV-1-specific CTL responses primed in vitro by blood-derived dendritic cells and Th1-biasing cytokines. J Immunol 1999; 162(5):3070–3078.

152. Cho S, et al. Antimicrobial activity of MHC class I-restricted CD8$^+$ T cells in human tuberculosis. Proc Natl Acad Sci USA 2000; 97(22):12210–12215.

153. Ulrichs T, et al. Differential T cell responses to *Mycobacterium tuberculosis* ESAT6 in tuberculosis patients and healthy donors. Eur J Immunol 1998; 29(2):725725.

154. Ravn P, et al. Human T cell responses to the ESAT-6 antigen from *Mycobacterium tuberculosis*. J Infect Dis 1999; 179(3):637–645.

155. Mellman I, Steinman RM. Dendritic cells: specialized and regulated antigen processing machines. Cell 2001; 106(3):255–258.

156. Watts C, Powis S. Pathways of antigen processing and presentation. Rev Immunogenet 1999; 1(1):60–74.

157. Stoltze L, et al. The function of the proteasome system in MHC class I antigen processing. Immunol Today 2000; 21(7):317–319.

158. Nakagawa TY, Rudensky AY. The role of lysosomal proteinases in MHC class II-mediated antigen processing and presentation. Immunol Rev 1999; 172:121–129.

159. Niedermann G, et al. The specificity of proteasomes: impact on MHC class I processing and presentation of antigens. Immunol Rev 1999; 172:29–48.

160. Lankat-Buttgereit B, Tampe R. The transporter associated with antigen processing TAP: structure and function. FEBS Lett 1999; 464(3):108–112.

161. Gallimore A, et al. Hierarchies of antigen-specific cytotoxic T-cell responses. Immunol Rev 1998; 164:29–36.

162. Mellman IT, Steinman RM. Antigen processing for amateurs and professionals. Trends Cell Biol 1998; 8(6):231–237.

163. Pamer E, Cresswell P. Mechanisms of MHC class I-restricted antigen processing. Annu Rev Immunol 1998; 16:323–358.

164. Alexander J, et al. Recognition of a novel naturally processed, A2 restricted, HCV-NS4 epitope triggers IFN-gamma release in absence of detectable cytopathicity. Hum Immunol 1998; 59(12):776–782.

165. Sette AD, et al. Overcoming T cell tolerance to the hepatitis B virus surface antigen in hepatitis B virus-transgenic mice. J Immunol 2001; 166(2):1389–1397.

166. Cole GA, et al. Efficient priming of CD8$^+$ memory T cells specific for a subdominant epitope following Sendai virus infection. J Immunol 1997; 158(9):4301–4309.

167. Grufman P, et al. T cell competition for the antigen-presenting cell as a model for immunodominance in the cytotoxic T lymphocyte response against minor histocompatibility antigens. Eur J Immunol 1999; 29(7):2197–2204.

168. Chen W, et al. Dissecting the multifactorial causes of immunodominance in class I-restricted T cell responses to viruses. Immunity 2000; 12(1):83–93.

169. Gianfrani C, et al. Human memory CTL response specific for influenza A virus is broad and multispecific. Hum Immunol 2000; 61(5):438–452.

170. Jameson J, et al. Human cytotoxic T-lymphocyte repertoire to influenza A viruses. J Virol 1998; 72(11):8682–8689.

171. Cooper S, et al. Analysis of a successful immune response against hepatitis C virus. Immunity 1999; 10(4):439–449.

172. Pantaleo G, et al. Studies in subjects with long-term nonprogressive human immunodeficiency virus infection. N Engl J Med 1995; 332(4):209–216.

173. Rinaldo C, et al. High levels of anti-human immunodeficiency virus type 1 (HIV-1) memory cytotoxic T-lymphocyte activity and low viral load are associated with lack of disease in HIV-1-infected long-term nonprogressors. J Virol 1995; 69(9):5838–5842.

174. Rowland-Jones S. Long-term non-progression in HIV infection: clinico pathological issues. J Infect 1999; 38(2):67–70.

175. Harrer T, et al. Cytotoxic T lymphocytes in asymptomatic long-term nonprogressing HIV-1 infection. Breadth and specificity of the response and relation to in vivo viral quasispecies in a person with prolonged infection and low viral load. J Immunol 1996; 156(7):2616–2623.

176. Gillespie GM, et al. Functional heterogeneity and high frequencies of cytomegalovirus-specific CD8(+) T lymphocytes in healthy seropositive donors. J Virol 2000; 74(17):8140–8150.

177. An LL, Whitton JL. A multivalent minigene vaccine, containing B-cell, cytotoxic T-lymphocyte, and Th epitopes from several microbes, induces appropriate responses in vivo and confers protection against more than one pathogen. J Virol 1997; 71(3):2292–2302.

178. An LL, Whitton JL. Multivalent minigene vaccines against infectious disease. Curr Opin Mol Ther 1999; 1(1):16–21.

179. Moudgil KD, et al. Modulation of the immunogenicity of antigenic determinants by their flanking residues. Immunol Today 1998; 19(5):217–220.

180. Livingston BD, et al. Development of HTL epitope-based vaccine for prophylaxis and immunotherapy of HIV Second International Conference on Vaccine Development and Immunotherapy in HIV, San Juan, Puerto Rico, 2001.

181. Velders MP, et al. Defined flanking spacers and enhanced proteolysis is essential for eradication of established tumors by an epitope string DNA vaccine. J Immunol 2001; 166(9):5366–5373.

182. Kuchroo VK, et al. B7-1 and B7-2 costimulatory molecules activate differentially the Th1/Th2 developmental pathways: application to autoimmune disease therapy. Cell 1995; 80(5):707–718.

183. Shahinian A, et al. Differential T cell costimulatory requirements in CD28-deficient mice. Science 1993; 261(5121):609–612.

184. Sin JI, et al. Modulation of cellular responses by plasmid CD40L: CD40L plasmid vectors enhance antigen-specific helper T cell type 1 CD4$^+$ T cell-mediated protective immunity against herpes simplex virus type 2 in vivo. Hum Gene Ther 2001; 12:1091–1102.

185. Hodge JW, et al. A triad of costimulatory molecules synergize to amplify T-cell activation. Cancer Res 1999; 59:5800–5807.

186. Zhu M, et al. Enhanced activation of human T cells via avipox vector-mediated hyperexpression of a triad of costimulatory molecules in human dendritic cells. Cancer Res 2001; 61:3725–3734.

187. Ahlers JD, et al. Cytokine-in-adjuvant steering of the immune response phenotype to HIV-1 vaccine constructs: GM-CSF and TNFa synergize with IL-12 to enhance induction of CTL. J Immunol 1997; 158:3947–3958.

188. Belyakov IM, et al. Interplay of cytokines and adjuvants in the regulation of mucosal and systemic HIV-specific cytotoxic T lymphocytes. J Immunol 2000; 165:6454–6462.

189. Berzofsky JA, et al. Strategies for designing and optimizing

new generation vaccines. Nat Rev Immunol 2001; 1:209–219.

190. Iwasaki A, et al. Enhanced CTL responses mediated by plasmid DNA immunogens encoding costimulatory molecules and cytokines. J Immunol 1997; 158:4591–4601.

191. Tobery TW, Siliciano RF. Targeting of HIV-1 antigens for rapid intracellular degradation enhances cytotoxic T lymphocyte (CTL) recognition and the induction of de novo CTL responses in vivo after immunization. J Exp Med 1997; 185(5):909–920.

192. Rodriguez F, Whitton JL. Enhancing DNA immunization. Virology 2000; 268(2):233–238.

193. Boehncke W-H, et al. The importance of dominant negative effects of amino acids side chain substitution in peptide–MHC molecule interactions and T cell recognition. J Immunol 1993; 150:331–341.

194. La Rosa C, et al. Enhanced immune activity of cytotoxic T-lymphocyte epitope analogs derived from positional scanning synthetic combinatorial libraries. Blood 2001; 97:1776–1786.

195. Pogue RR, et al. Amino-terminal alteration of the HLA-A* 0201-restricted human immunodeficiency virus pol peptide increases complex stability and in vitro immunogenicity. Proc Natl Acad Sci USA 1995; 92:8166–8170.

196. Sarobe P, et al. Enhanced in vitro potency and in vivo immunogenicity of a CTL epitope from hepatitis C virus core protein following amino acid replacement at secondary HLA-A2.1 binding positions. J Clin Invest 1998; 102:1239–1248.

197. Rosenberg SA, et al. Immunologic and therapeutic evaluation of a synthetic peptide vaccine for the treatment of patients with metastatic melanoma. Nat Med 1998; 4:321–327.

198. Parkhurst MR, et al. Improved induction of melanoma-reactive CTL with peptides from the melanoma antigen gp100 modified at HLA-A*0201-binding residues. J Immunol 1996; 157(6):2539–2548.

199. Topalian SL, et al. Melanoma-specific CD4+ T cells recognize nonmutated HLA-DR-restricted tyrosinase epitopes. J Exp Med 1996; 183(5):1965–1971.

200. Ahlers JD, et al. High affinity T-helper epitope induces complementary helper and APC polarization, increased CTL and protection against viral infection. J Clin Invest 2001; 108:1677–1685.

201. Ahlers JD, et al. Enhanced immunogenicity of HIV-1 vaccine construct by modification of the native peptide sequence. Proc Natl Acad Sci USA 1997; 94(20):10856–10861.

202. Fong L, et al. Altered peptide ligand vaccination with Flt3 ligand expanded dendritic cells for tumor immunotherapy. Proc Natl Acad Sci USA 2001; 98:8809–8814.

203. Slansky JE, et al. Enhanced antigen-specific antitumor immunity with altered peptide ligands that stabilize the MHC-peptide-TCR complex. Immunity 2000; 13:529–538.

204. Zaremba S, et al. Identification of an enhancer agonist cytotoxic T lymphocyte peptide from human carcinoembryonic antigen. Cancer Res 1997; 57:4570–4577.

205. Tangri S, et al. Structural features of peptide analogs of human histocompatibility leukocyte antigen class I epitopes that are more potent and immunogenic than wild-type peptide. J Exp Med 2001; 194:833–846.

206. Das P, et al. HLA transgenic mice as models of human autoimmune diseases. Rev Immunogenet 2000; 2(1):105–114.

207. Taneja V, David CS. HLA class II transgenic mice as models of human diseases. Immunol Rev 1999; 169:67–79.

208. Diamond DJ, et al. Development of a candidate HLA A*0201 restricted peptide-based vaccine against human cytomegalovirus infection. Blood 1997; 90(5):1751–1767.

209. Firat H, et al. H-2 class I knockout, HLA-A2.1-transgenic mice: a versatile animal model for preclinical evaluation of antitumor immunotherapeutic strategies. Eur J Immunol 1999; 29(10):3112–3121.

210. Ressing ME, et al. Human CTL epitopes encoded by human papillomavirus type 16 E6 and E7 identified through in vivo and in vitro immunogenicity studies of HLA-A*0201-binding peptides. J Immunol 1995; 154:5934–5943.

211. Le A-XT, et al. Cytotoxic T cell responses in HLA-A2.1 transgenic mice: recognition of HLA alloantigens and utilization of HLA-A2.1 as a restriction element. J Immunol 1989; 142:1366–1371.

212. Man S, et al. Definition of a human T cell epitope from influenza A non-structural protein 1 using HLA-A2.1 transgenic mice. Int Immunol 1995; 7:597–605.

213. Vitiello A, et al. Analysis of the HLA-restricted influenza-specific cytotoxic T lymphocyte response in transgenic mice carrying a chimeric human-mouse class I major histocompatibility complex. J Exp Med 1991; 173(4):1007–1015.

214. Ishioka GY, et al. Utilization of MHC class I transgenic mice for development of minigene DNA vaccines encoding multiple HLA-restricted CTL epitopes. J Immunol 1999; 162(7):3915–3925.

215. Altman JD, Safrit JT. MHC tetramer analyses of CD8+ T cell responses to HIV and SIV. Int Virol, 1998:36–42.

216. Altman JD, et al. Phenotypic analysis of antigen, specific T lymphocytes. Science 1996; 274(5284):94–96.

217. Udhayakumar V, et al. Antigenic diversity in the circumsporozoite protein of Plasmodium falciparum abrogates cytotoxic-T-cell recognition. Infect Immun 1994; 62(4):1410–1413.

218. Roberts DJ, et al. Rapid switching to multiple antigenic and adhesive phenotypes in malaria. Nature 1992; 357(6380): 689–692.

219. Rowland-Jones SL, et al. Human immunodeficiency virus variants that escape cytotoxic T-cell recognition. AIDS Res Hum Retrovir 1992; 8(8):1353–1354.

220. Wang H, Eckels DD. Mutations in immunodominant T cell epitopes derived from the nonstructural 3 protein of hepatitis C virus have the potential for generating escape variants that may have important consequences for T cell recognition. J Immunol 1999; 162(7):4177–4183.

221. Phillips RE, et al. Human immunodeficiency virus genetic variation that can escape cytotoxic T cell recognition. Nature 1991; 354:453–459.

222. Gegin C, Lehmann-Grube F. Control of acute infection with lymphocytic choriomeningitis virus in mice that cannot present an immunodominant viral cytotoxic T lymphocyte epitope. J Immunol Methods 1992; 149(10):3331–3338.

223. Levy JA. Pathogenesis of human immunodeficiency virus infection. Microbiol Rev 1993; 57(1):183–289.

224. Disis ML, et al. Peptide-based, but not whole protein, vaccines elicit immunity to HER-2/neu, oncogenic self-protein. J Immunol 1996; 156(9):3151–3158.

225. Cibotti R, et al. Tolerance to a self-protein involves its immunodominant but does not involve its subdominant determinants. Proc Natl Acad Sci USA 1992; 89(1):416–420.

16

The Challenge of Inducing Protection in Very Young Infants

Claire-Anne Siegrist
University of Geneva, Geneva, Switzerland

I. INTRODUCTION

Currently used infant vaccines and schedules mostly induce protection after several vaccine doses, i.e., only at several months of age. As result of this delayed induction of protection, whooping cough still annually results in 360,000 infant deaths despite administration of three doses of diphtheria–tetanus–pertussis vaccine to 80% of children before their first birthday [1], and infants too young to have yet completed their three-dose vaccination schedule remain at a significant risk of pertussis [2]. At a global level, more than 2.5 million infant deaths annually result from acute respiratory and diarrheal infections, which could be prevented by immunization against a relatively limited number of viral and bacterial pathogens [3]. However, to prevent these infant deaths, vaccines and immunization strategies would have to safely induce protective responses more rapidly after birth, prior to pathogen exposure, which frequently occurs very early in life. The challenge, which will also have to be met by novel vaccines against major later killers, such as tuberculosis, malaria, and HIV, is thus to induce early protection despite the immaturity of the neonatal immune system and the presence of antibodies of maternal origin. The objective of this chapter is to review the current understanding of the determinants that may either limit or support the induction of vaccine responses in neonates and very young infants, and to highlight areas in which further research is needed.

II. CHALLENGES FOR THE INDUCTION OF ANTIBODY RESPONSES IN EARLY LIFE

A. Limitations of Early Life Antibody Responses

1. Limited Infant Responses to Polysaccharide Antigens

Infant and toddler responses to most bacterial capsular polysaccharides (PS) are markedly limited, which contributes to their high susceptibility to infections with encapsulated bacteria such as *Haemophilus influenzae* (HIB), *Streptococcus pneumoniae*, and *Neisseria meningitidis*. The same limitations affect most polysaccharide vaccines, which remain poorly immunogenic before the age of 2 years and exhibit an age-dependent increase in vaccine efficacy between 2 and 10 years of age [4]. Factors that limit infant responses to PS include (1) low complement activity, which limits the deposition of C3d on bacterial PS; (2) weak expression of surface C3d-receptors (CD21) on infant B lymphocytes, limiting synergy between B cell receptor and complement receptor-mediated activation; and (3) structural immaturity of the splenic marginal zone [5] to which C3d-bound PS preferentially localizes in adults. Altogether, these factors limit the capacity of marginal zone B cells and B1 cells to rapidly respond to particulate bacterial antigens [6]. The recognition of this limitation, intrinsic to infant and toddlers, led to the development of glycoconjugate vaccines that attach bacterial PS to a carrier protein. Processing and presentation of carrier peptide fragments at the surface of antigen-presenting-cells (APC) recruits CD4$^+$ T cells, which provide costimulation to infant B cells and thus induce immunogenic and protective responses in young infants. Despite the strong immunogenicity of glycoconjugate vaccines, the magnitude of IgG antibody responses they elicit does depend on age at administration: As an example, a single dose of HIB-conjugate vaccine elicits progressively higher serum anticapsular antibody concentrations when administered at 2–3, 4–6, or 8–17 months [7].

2. Limited Early Life Antibody Responses to Protein Antigens

The magnitude of IgG antibody responses that may be elicited by protein antigens, whether in subunit or live attenuated vaccines, is also directly related to age at immunization (Table 1). The influence of immune immaturity on currently available protein-based vaccines (such as combined diphtheria–tetanus–pertussis or hepatitis B vaccines) may not be directly assessed, as these vaccines do not induce significant antibody responses to a single vaccine dose even

Table 1 Characteristics of Early Life Compared to Adult Responses to Conventional Vaccines[a]

Characteristics	Duration
Magnitude of antibody responses	
age-dependent limited induction of IgG responses to protein Ag	≤12–24 months
limited persistence of IgG Ab responses	≤12 months (?)
age-dependent limited induction of IgG responses to most polysaccharides	≤18–24 months
efficient induction of memory B cells	At birth (?)
Quality of antibody responses	
age-dependent limited IgG2 responses	≤12–18 months
age-dependent limitation of IgG repertoire	≥8–12 months (?)
limited avidity of IgG antibodies compared to adult	(?)
Antigen-specific T cell responses	
efficient T cell priming	At or before birth
age-dependent limited primary IFN-γ responses	≥12 months (?)
age-dependent limited CTL responses	≥9–12 months (?)
adultlike IL-12 production by dendritic cells	≥12 months (?)

[a] Schematic comparison of main characteristics, although notable exceptions may exist.
(?) Limited data available; notable influence of antigen/vaccine type.

in adults. Although early rapid vaccination schedules (i.e., immunization at 2–3–4 months of age) elicit lower antibody titers and lower seroconversion rates than immunization at 2–4–6 or 3–5–12 months of age [8], this not only reflects immune immaturity but also the shorter time period available for affinity maturation of vaccine-induced B cells. In contrast, the stepwise increase of antibody concentrations following measles [9–11] or mumps [12] immunization when immunization is delayed from 6 to 9, 12, or 15 months of age directly reflects the influence of age at immunization.

The mechanisms that limit early life antibody responses to protein antigens, whether included in protein, subunit, inactivated, or live attenuated vaccines, are not yet fully understood. Recent studies assessing the influence of age on antibody responses to human vaccines in neonatal, infant, and adult mice yielded observations very similar to those of human infants, providing that immunization was initiated ≥7 days of age (rather than in the immediate neonatal period) to compensate for the greater immaturity of newborn mice (reviewed in Ref. 13). Studies assessing the various stages of antigen-specific B cell differentiation in these preclinical models of early life immunization demonstrated that the weaker antibody responses to alum-adjuvanted protein vaccines (tetanus, pertussis) reflect a delayed and weaker induction of primary antibody-secreting-cells (ASC) in infant mice [14]. This could reflect immaturity of neonatal B cells, CD4[+] T cells, or APC, as well as that of additional determinants such as the postnatal development of the microarchitecture of lymphoid organs. The definition of the relative contribution of each of these factors to the limited capacity of inducing early life B cells to differentiate into ASC, and the identification of strategies likely to circumvent such immaturity-associated limitations, require additional studies.

3. Limited Duration of Early Life Antibody Responses

Another challenge for early life immunization is that the strong antibody responses that are eventually elicited after several doses of immunogenic vaccines (such as tetanus or acellular pertussis vaccines) are of a shorter duration than those elicited >12 months of age. This rapid decline of IgG antibodies within 6–12 months requires repeat vaccine administration already in the second year of life, a strategy that is difficult to implement in many countries of the world. A similar finding is that early (<12 months) immunization could similarly be associated with waning immunity against measles, which is not observed following immunization at an older age [15]. The shorter persistence of IgG antibodies elicited in infancy is likely to reflect a limited in vivo half-life of plasma cells generated in early life, which is believed to depend on their developmental history, their homing capacity, as well as the supporting capacity of their environment. In mice, long-lived plasma cells are essentially located in the bone marrow. Our recent observation of a limited establishment of the bone marrow pool of long-lived plasmocytes in early life is thus of significant interest [14]. Should a similar limited homing of plasmocytes toward the bone marrow occur in infants, it would explain the shorter kinetics of their early life antibody responses. This can hardly be studied directly in humans, and studies in preclinical models will be required to eventually identify the contributing factors/molecules.

4. Does Early Life Immunization Limit the Quality of Antibody Responses?

Whether early life immunization results in antibodies of a different quality is an important question. Infant vaccines preferentially elicit IgG antibodies regardless of age at administration [16]. However, infant immunization mainly elicits IgG1 and IgG3 isotypes, and IgG2 antibodies remain weak during the first 18 months of life [17] even for vaccines that induce preferential IgG2 responses in adults (Table 1).

The relative capacity to induce high-avidity antibodies in early life is of significant concern, as avidity is a direct marker of functional efficacy. Infants indeed produce Ab of a significantly lower avidity (with absent bactericidal activity) following *N. meningitidis* infection as compared to older children and somatic hypermutation of Ig genes in infant B cells slowly increases between 2 and 10 months of age, with evidence for selection only from 6 months onward [18,19]. In infant mice, studies with hapten-conjugated antigens had demonstrated years ago that the capacity to enter into an efficient antibody maturation process was age-related. All together, this generated the concern that early life immunization may be associated with induction of antibodies of a weaker functional efficacy. However, we recently observed that in contrast to hapten-based vaccines, two human infant protein vaccines (tetanus and pertussis toxoids) induce an adult-like neonatal murine Ab avidity maturation process [20]. In accordance, several studies have now demonstrated that the affinity maturation machinery is already functional in the first year of life [21]. As studies in infant mice have shown that vaccines may differ in their capacity of inducing—or not inducing—an adultlike avidity maturation process, clinical studies comparing avidity maturation following immunization of infants and unprimed children/ adults are required to define the relative capacity of inducing high-avidity antibodies in early life and identify its determinants.

B. Does Early Immunization Induce Neonatal Tolerance or Priming of Memory Cells?

Inducing tolerance by neonatal immunization is a concern that has originated from many murine studies. However, in contrast to newborn mice and their profoundly immature immune system, human neonatal immunization induced either enhanced or conserved subsequent infant responses. There are only few reports of hyporesponsiveness to subsequent vaccine doses following neonatal immunization with whole-cell pertussis vaccines, PRP-OMPc, or *N. meningitidis* group C polysaccharides (MenC PS). In contrast, neonatal immunization generally induces early priming of memory cells. This is best illustrated by neonatal immunization with oral polio and hepatitis B vaccines: Despite limited antibody responses to the priming dose (<10% seroconversion), secondary response patterns are clearly observed following boosting at 1 month of age (reviewed in Ref. 13). Thus as observed in murine models, certain vaccine antigens/delivery systems/adjuvants are clearly able to activate neonatal human B cells and trigger their differentiation into memory B cells, despite their limited capacity to drive B cell differentiation toward IgG-secreting plasmocytes. Surprisingly, neonatal administration of certain strongly immunogenic infant vaccines (such as tetanus toxoid vaccine) did not result into enhanced responses to subsequent vaccine doses. Thus whether priming of memory cells may or may not be achieved by neonatal immunization currently cannot be predicted. As this is likely to prove essential for vaccine-mediated prevention in early life, through early prime–later boost immunization strategies, further studies are required so as to identify the determinants of neonatal priming.

C. Influence of Maternal Antibodies on Early Life Antibody Responses

It has long been recognized that residual maternal IgG antibodies (MatAb) passively transferred during gestation may inhibit infant vaccine responses to measles and oral poliomyelitis vaccines, and more recently that they may also affect responses to nonlive vaccines (reviewed in Ref. 13). The main determinant of MatAb-mediated inhibition of antibody responses was identified as the titer of MatAb present at the time of immunization or rather as the ratio between vaccine antigen and MatAb [22–24]. Indeed, reducing MatAb titer at time of immunization or enhancing the dose of vaccine antigen may both circumvent the inhibition of infant antibody responses, in human and murine infants. This is best explained by the fact that following introduction of a vaccine antigen into a host with preexisting passive antibodies, MatAb readily bind to specific B cell vaccine epitopes, preventing access of infant B cells to the same determinants. If the vaccine antigen/MatAb ratio is low, this prevents access of infant B cells to B cell epitopes and therefore inhibits their differentiation into antibody-secreting cells. At a higher ratio, some B cell epitopes may remain unmasked by MatAb and thus available for binding by infant B cells and priming of B cell responses. Thus strategies to circumvent MatAb inhibition of vaccine antibody responses currently mainly include delayed vaccine administration, awaiting decline of MatAb or use of higher vaccine doses. Whether slow-release vaccines or certain delivery systems could better shield B cell epitopes from MatAb is an interesting possibility that awaits confirmation. In theory, mucosal vaccines should prove better able at escaping from MatAb inhibition, as concentrations of MatAb reaching infant mucosae are significantly lower than those reaching their serum. However, this may only be the case for immune responses directly elicited at the mucosal surface and not into the draining lymph nodes where MatAb concentration is higher.

D. Perspectives for Enhancing Early Life Antibody Responses

In neonatal and infant murine models of immunization, certain adjuvant formulations are able to significantly enhance early life vaccine responses, whereas others fail to do so despite their strong adjuvanticity in adult animals (reviewed in Ref. 13). However, none of the adjuvant formulations tested so far proved capable of correcting the limitation of early antibody responses elicited following neonatal compared to adult immunization. This might unfortunately also be the case in human infants. Recently, coadministration of bacillus Calmette–Guerin (BCG) at time of neonatal hepatitis B immunization was shown to strongly enhance (50-fold) HBsAg antibody titers after the third vaccine dose compared to control infants [25], an influence likely to reflect the known maturation influence exerted by BCG on dendritic cells (DC). This observation thus suggests that enhancing DC/T cells/B cells interaction may have a positive influence on the magnitude of antibody responses elicited in neonates. Unfortunately, antibody responses to the first neonatal dose of HbsAg were only marginally enhanced by BCG coadministration. Although it cannot be excluded that this reflects in part the relatively weak immunogenicity of a single dose of hepatitis B vaccine even in adult hosts with mature DC, several months and/or vaccine doses were required for BCG to mediate its enhancing influence on neonatal antibody responses. This is similar to observations gathered with a large panel of adjuvants in murine models (review in Ref. 26) and may indicate that some limiting factors are not corrected by enhanced DC/T cells/B cells activation.

Novel antigen delivery systems, such as DNA vaccines, have not yet been tested in human neonates but were extensively studied in neonatal animal models. DNA vaccines induced similar antibody responses in newborn and adult mice (reviewed in Ref. 26) but failed to induce stronger early life antibody responses than those elicited by conventional protein/subunit/live attenuated vaccines. Accordingly, DNA immunization of newborn/infant nonhuman primates against hepatitis B, HIV, or influenza also resulted in weak antibody responses [27], and sequential bleeding indicated lack of antibody responses prior to 4 or 8 weeks of age, after 2 or 3 vaccine doses [28]. Thus vaccine formulations/delivery systems capable of rapidly inducing strong antibody responses in early life have not yet been identified. This calls for a better understanding of the limiting factors that they should be able to circumvent. Indeed, although early priming–later boosting strategies are currently the most promising strategies for enhancing early life antibody responses, time required for completion of such strategies is likely to be a limiting factor against pathogens for which exposure occurs very early in life.

III. CHALLENGES TO THE INDUCTION OF STRONG T CELL RESPONSES IN EARLY LIFE

A. Characteristics of Early Life CD4$^+$ and CD8$^+$ T Cell Responses

In contrast to the slow maturation of antibody responses, acquisition of antigen-specific T cell responses is an early event, as shown by in utero priming of fetal T cell responses to allergens. However, the age-dependent maturation and differentiation of Th1 (IFN-γ secreting) and Th2 (IL-4, IL-5, IL-13 secreting) T cell responses is yet poorly characterized (Table 1). T cell proliferative responses following BCG were stronger when administration was delayed from birth until 2–6 months of age in some studies, whereas adultlike IFN-γ responses to neonatal BCG were reported in *The Gambia*

[29]. In contrast, Gambian infants showed defective IFN-γ responses during the primary phase of the response to oral polio vaccine (29a) as compared to adults. Analyses of T cell responses to measles and mumps vaccines indicated similar antigen-specific T cell proliferative and IFN-γ responses in infants immunized at 6, 9, or 12 months of age, but lower infant responses than those of adult controls [12,30]. Infant T cells also showed a limited capacity to increase their IFN-γ release in response to IL-12 supplementation [30]. A limitation of these MMR/OPV/BCG studies is that they could not include previously unprimed naive adult controls. Thus to precisely define the influence of immune immaturity on T cell differentiation awaits additional clinical evidence.

Little is yet known on the maturation of human infant CD8$^+$ cytotoxic responses (CTLs) responses. Although infection-induced CTLs may be detected within the first weeks of life, CTL responses could also be age- and vaccine-dependent [31–33]. As an example, CTLs were recovered in infants following influenza infection, but not following immunization with a live influenza vaccine, suggesting that a certain immunogenicity threshold had only been reached in infected infants [32]. Thus it seems likely that the maturation of CD8$^+$ cytotoxic responses will prove age and vaccine type dependent in human as in mice, although far more studies are required to clarify this important issue.

B. Which Are the Factors Limiting Early Life T Cell Responses?

Studies assessing the determinants of early life T cell responses are currently limited to murine models of early life immunization. They indicate that antigen-specific T cell responses may be readily elicited at an early stage, but that early immunization is associated with lower IFN-γ responses (and higher IL-5, IL-4, and IL-13 responses) to most conventional vaccines (reviewed in Ref. 13). Early life murine immunization results in limited induction of Th1-driven IgG2a antibodies and of CTL responses. Altogether, these observations suggest a preferential differentiation of early life murine T cell responses to viral/protein vaccines toward the Th2 pathway, as a "default" developmental pathway (reviewed in Ref. 34). This is considered as reflecting suboptimal APC–T cell interactions. Evidence that neonatal APC function (assessed by IL-12 production) may be immature has indeed been provided in mice, and recently also in human cord blood monocyte-derived cells [35]. Available data suggests that a limited IL-12/IFN-γ release capacity may persist during the first year of life [36]. Suboptimal APC–T cell interactions could also result from deficient T cell costimulation, and transient differences in CD40L/CD154 expression between neonatal and adult T cells have indeed been reported both in mice and humans. Studies should now better define the relative influence of the immaturity of neonatal APC, neonatal T cells, and/or of the microenvironment in which APC–T cell interactions take place, so as to indicate potentially effective immunomodulation strategies.

C. Influence of Maternal Antibodies on Neonatal CD4+ and CD8+ Vaccine Responses

In contrast to the inhibiting influence of maternal antibodies (MatAb) on infant antibody responses, it was recently demonstrated that MatAb leave CD4+ and CD8+ T cell responses largely unaffected. This was first observed in mice, under experimental conditions in which high titers of MatAb completely abrogated antibody responses but did not affect either CD4+ T cell proliferative and cytokine responses [23,24] nor CTL responses [24,37,38]. In human infants, measles and mumps immunization also leaves infant CD4+ T cell proliferative and INF-γ responses unaffected despite inhibition of antibody responses by MatAb that present at immunization [10,12,30]. Accordingly, measles-specific T cell responses were measured in 86.8% of 6-month-old infants immunized in the presence of MatAb, whereas antibody responses were only observed in 36.7% [39]. This inhibition of B cell but not of T cell responses is best explained by the efficient uptake of antigen–antibody immune complexes by APC. Following processing, vaccine-derived antigenic peptides are thus presented at the APC cell surface, allowing priming of CD4+ and CD8+ T cells to independently occur of the inhibition of B cell responses. This early T cell priming is likely to explain the reduced measles morbidity and mortality observed in vaccinated infants who failed to seroconvert because of the presence of maternal antibodies. It could also significantly facilitate early prime–later boost strategies in early human life, as shown in mice [24].

D. Perspectives for Enhancement of Early Life CD4+ and CD8+ Vaccine Responses

Studies in mice have clearly demonstrated that adultlike T cell responses may be induced already in the neonatal period by novel delivery systems and/or adjuvants. This has been repeatedly achieved by DNA immunization against a panel of vaccine antigens (reviewed in Ref. 26) and the induction of adultlike CD4+ and CD8+ T cell responses appears as a generic property of most DNA vaccines. This could result in part from prolonged antigenic exposure, allowing both prolonged immune stimulation and ongoing immune maturation to occur. However, induction of adultlike neonatal Th1 and CTL responses was also achieved by certain adjuvants, including by oligonucleotides containing immunostimulating CpG motifs [40,41], which are present in DNA plasmids, as well as by certain nonpersistent novel delivery systems.

The current understanding is that neonatal T cells may have greater requirements than adult T cells for costimulatory signals, such that the induction of Th1 and CTL neonatal responses essentially reflects the relative capacity of vaccines to activate neonatal APCs to thresholds sufficient—or not sufficient—for optimal T cell activation to occur. In mice, mimicking (IL-12 supplementation) or triggering (CD40) optimal APC activation is sufficient to induce adultlike IFN-γ and CTL neonatal responses. Recently, the novel MF-59 adjuvant was reported as increasing human lymphoproliferative responses to recombinant HIV gp120 following immunization at birth, 2 weeks, 2 months, and 5 months of age [42]. Although cytokine responses were not measured, it seems reasonable to expect that certain adjuvant formulations or delivery systems may prove capable of enhancing early life Th1 responses, representing a major progress in the control of early infections with intracellular pathogens. However, the recent observation that neonatal BCG enhanced both Th1 and Th2 responses to coadministered HbsAg antigens despite its strong Th1-driving capacity [25] calls for much more detailed investigations of the capacity of modulating neonatal T cell responses.

IV. CONCLUSION AND PERSPECTIVES

The rapid induction of strong antibody responses in very early life is yet an unmet challenge both in preclinical and clinical studies, calling for a better understanding of the determinants of this important limitation. However, immune immaturity may not prevent early induction of memory B cells that may be recalled by subsequent boosting. The limited capacity for early life INF-γ and CTL responses appear to essentially result from suboptimal APC–T cell interactions, and thus might be overcome by use of specific adjuvants or delivery systems enhancing such interactions. As the optimal immunogenicity/reactogenicity balance of these new vaccine formulations will have to be defined in very young populations, specific ethical and regulatory considerations should be rapidly addressed.

ACKNOWLEDGMENTS

The author is most grateful to the support provided by the Fondation Mérieux and to all who participated in or supported the studies performed in the WHO Collaborating Center for Neonatal Vaccinology.

REFERENCES

1. Ivanoff B, Robertson SE. Pertussis: a worldwide problem. Dev Biol Stand 1997; 89:3–13.
2. Halperin SA, et al. Epidemiological features of pertussis in hospitalized patients in Canada, 1991–1997: report of the Immunization Monitoring Program-Active (IMPACT). Clin Infect Dis 1999; 28:1238–1243.
3. World Health Organization. Maternal Health and Safe Motherhood Programme. MSM96.7 1996.
4. De Wals P, et al. Impact of a mass immunization campaign against serogroup C meningococcus in the Province of Quebec, Canada. Bull WHO 1996; 74:407–411.
5. Timens W, et al. Immaturity of the human splenic marginal zone in infancy. Possible contribution to the deficient infant immune response. J Immunol 1989; 143:3200–3206.
6. Martin F, et al. Marginal zone and B1 B cells unite in the early response against T-independent blood-borne particulate antigens. Immunity 2001; 14:617–629.
7. Einhorn MS, et al. Immunogenicity in infants of *Haemophilus influenzae* type b polysaccharide in a conjugate

vaccine with *Neisseria meningitidis* outer-membrane protein. Lancet 1986; 2:299–302.

8. Booy R, et al. Immunogenicity of combined diphtheria, tetanus, and pertussis vaccine given at 2, 3, and 4 months versus 3, 5, and 9 months of age. Lancet 1992; 339:507–510.

9. Johnson CE, et al. Measles vaccine immunogenicity in 6-versus 15-month-old infants born to mothers in the measles vaccine era. Pediatrics 1994; 93:939–944.

10. Gans HA, et al. Deficiency of the humoral immune response to measles vaccine in infants immunized at age 6 months. JAMA 1998; 280:527–532.

11. Klinge J, et al. Comparison of immunogenicity and reactogenicity of a measles, mumps and rubella (MMR) vaccine in German children vaccinated at 9–11, 12–14 or 15–17 months of age. Vaccine 2000; 18:3134–3140.

12. Gans H, Lugauer S, Korn K, Heininger U, Stehr K. Immune responses to measles and mumps vaccination of infants at 6, 9, and 12 months. J Infect Dis 2001; 184:817–826.

13. Siegrist C. Neonatal and early life vaccinology. Vaccine 2001; 19:3331–3346.

14. Pihlgren M, et al. Delayed and deficient establishment of the long-term bone marrow plasma cell pool during early life. Eur J Immunol 2001; 31:939–946.

15. Whittle HC, et al. Effect of subclinical infection on maintaining immunity against measles in vaccinated children in West Africa. Lancet 1999; 353:98–102.

16. Ambrosino DM, et al. IgG1, IgG2 and IgM responses to two *Haemophilus influenzae* type b conjugate vaccines in young infants. Pediatr Infect Dis J 1992; 11:855–859.

17. Plebani A, et al. Serum IgG subclass concentrations in healthy subjects at different age: age normal percentile charts. Eur J Pediatr 1989; 149:164–167.

18. Cai J, et al. Extensive and selective mutation of a rearranged VH5 gene in human B cell chronic lymphocytic leukemia. J Exp Med 1992; 176:1073–1081.

19. Ridings J, et al. Somatic hypermutation of immunoglobulin genes in human neonates. Clin Exp Immunol 1997; 108:366–374.

20. Schallert N, et al. Generation of adult-like antibody avidity profiles after early-life immunization with protein vaccines. Eur J Immunol 2002; 32:752–760.

21. Goldblatt D, et al. Antibody avidity as a surrogate marker of successful priming by *Haemophilus influenzae* type b conjugate vaccines following infant immunization. J Infect Dis 1998; 177:1112–1115.

22. Markowitz LE, et al. Changing levels of measles antibody titers in women and children in the United States: impact on response to vaccination. Kaiser Permanent Measles Vaccine Trial Team. Pediatrics 1996; 97:53–58.

23. Siegrist CA, et al. Determinants of infant responses to vaccines in presence of maternal antibodies. Vaccine 1998; 16:1409–1414.

24. Siegrist CA, et al. Influence of maternal antibodies on vaccine responses: inhibition of antibody but not T cell responses allows successful early prime-boost strategies in mice. Eur J Immunol 1998; 28:4138–4148.

25. Ota MO, et al. Influence of *Mycobacterium bovis* bacillus Calmette–Guerin on antibody and cytokine responses to human neonatal vaccination. J Immunol 2002; 168:919–925.

26. Bot A. DNA vaccination and the immune responsiveness of neonates. Int Rev Immunol 2000; 19:221–245.

27. Prince AM, et al. Successful nucleic acid based immunization of newborn chimpanzees against hepatitis B virus. Vaccine 1997; 15:916–919.

28. Bot A, et al. Induction of antibody response by DNA immunization of newborn baboons against influenza virus. Viral Immunol 1999; 12:91–96.

29. Vekemans J, et al. Neonatal bacillus Calmette–Guerin vaccination induces adult-like IFN-gamma production by CD4+ T lymphocytes. Eur J Immunol 2001; 31:1531–1535.

29a. Vekemans J, et al. T cell responses to vaccines in infants: defective IFN-gamma production after polio vaccination. Clin Exp Immunol 2002; 127: 495–498.

30. Gans HA, et al. IL-12, IFN-gamma, and T cell proliferation to measles in immunized infants. J Immunol 1999; 162: 5569–5575.

31. Chiba Y, et al. Development of cell-mediated cytotoxic immunity to respiratory syncytial virus in human infants following naturally acquired infection. J Med Virol 1989; 28:133–139.

32. Mbawuike IN, et al. Cytotoxic T lymphocyte responses of infants after natural infection or immunization with live cold-recombinant or inactivated influenza A virus vaccine. J Med Virol 1996; 50:105–111.

33. Jaye A, et al. Ex vivo analysis of cytotoxic T lymphocytes to measles antigens during infection and after vaccination in Gambian children. J Clin Invest 1998; 102:1969–1977.

34. Adkins B. Development of neonatal Th1/Th2 function. Int Rev Immunol 2000; 19:157–171.

35. Goriely S, et al. Deficient IL-12(p35) gene expression by dendritic cells derived from neonatal monocytes. J Immunol 2001; 166:2141–2146.

36. Chougnet C, et al. Influence of human immunodeficiency virus-infected maternal environment on development of infant interleukin-12 production. J Infect Dis 2000; 181: 1590–1597.

37. Martinez X, et al. Combining DNA and protein vaccines for early life immunization against respiratory syncytial virus in mice. Eur J Immunol 1999; 29:3390–3400.

38. Bangham CR. Passively acquired antibodies to respiratory syncytial virus impair the secondary cytotoxic T-cell response in the neonatal mouse. Immunology 1986; 59:37–41.

39. Pabst HF, et al. Cell-mediated and antibody immune responses to AIK-C and Connaught monovalent measles vaccine given to 6 month old infants. Vaccine 1999; 17:1910–1918.

40. Kovarik J, et al. CpG oligodeoxynucleotides can circumvent the Th2 polarization of neonatal responses to vaccines but may fail to fully redirect Th2 responses established by neonatal priming. J Immunol 1999; 162:1611–1617.

41. Brazolot Millan CL, et al. CpG DNA can induce strong Th1 humoral and cell-mediated immune responses against hepatitis B surface antigen in young mice. Proc Natl Acad Sci U S A 1998; 95:15553–15558.

42. Borkowsky W, et al. Lymphoproliferative responses to recombinant HIV-1 envelope antigens in neonates and infants receiving gp120 vaccines. AIDS Clinical Trial Group 230 Collaborators. J Infect Dis 2000; 181:890–896.

17

Vaccination and Autoimmunity

Paul-Henri Lambert
University of Geneva, Geneva, Switzerland

Michel Goldman
Hôpital Erasme, Brussels, Belgium

I. INTRODUCTION

Diseases encompassing manifestations caused by an auto-immune process are not infrequent and are known to appear in age groups that are often selected as targets for vaccination programs. Therefore, in the context of a rapidly increasing number of vaccination events, it is not surprising that the question of a potential interaction between vaccines and autoimmune diseases is being raised with increasing insistence.

It is estimated that as much as 5% of the population in Western countries suffer from autoimmune diseases [1]. These disorders represent a growing burden for health budgets as their incidence has significantly increased over the last few years, as documented for type I diabetes [2] and multiple sclerosis [3]. It is generally assumed that autoimmune disorders result from complex interactions between genetic traits and environmental factors. Indeed, although there is a frequent concordance of autoimmune diseases among monozygotic twins [4], the concordance rate is lower than expected. Similarly, changes in the incidence of type I diabetes and multiple sclerosis when children from a given population migrate from one region to another [5,6] strongly suggest a critical role for environmental causes in addition to genetic predisposition. In most autoimmune diseases the trigger has not been formally identified, leaving room for hypotheses and allegations not always substantiated by facts. Mechanisms leading to autoimmune responses and to their occasional translation into autoimmune diseases are now better understood. Autoimmune responses result from the combined effects of antigen-specific stimulations of the immune system and of an antigen-nonspecific activation of antigen-presenting cells in the context of a genetically determined predisposition. Most often such responses are not followed by any clinical manifestations unless additional events favor disease expression, e.g., a localized inflammatory process at tissue level.

The role of infections has been occasionally demonstrated either as an etiologic factor or as a triggering event in autoimmune diseases. Well-known examples are the post-streptococcal heart disease or the Guillain–Barré syndrome that follows *Campylobacter jejuni* infections. Such observations have emphasized the multifactorial immunological pathogenesis of secondary autoimmune pathology. First, there is a potential role of antigenic similarities between some microbial molecules and host antigens (antigenic mimicry). Second, infection-related signals that trigger innate immunity appear to play an essential role in enhancing the immunogenicity of host antigens or of host-mimicking epitopes, and in possibly overcoming regulatory mechanisms that limit autoimmune responses. It should be stressed that post-infectious autoimmune responses are not infrequent, whereas associated autoimmune diseases remain rare events and often require additional infection-related inflammatory processes.

It is on the basis of such observations that questions are raised regarding the potential risk of autoimmune responses and of autoimmune diseases following vaccination. Is there a significant risk that some vaccines may induce autoimmune responses through the introduction of microbial epitopes that cross-react with host antigens? Can adjuvant-containing vaccines trigger the clinical expression of an underlying autoimmune process through a "nonspecific" activation of antigen-presenting cells and the release of inflammatory cytokines? Until now, answers to these questions have been largely based on epidemiological studies, with limitations due to the difficulty in assessing the frequency of relatively rare events during clinical trials or post-marketing surveillance. When considered as a whole, autoimmune diseases affect up to 5% of the general population in industrialized countries, but many specific autoimmune diseases have a relatively low natural incidence. Whereas diseases such as rheumatoid arthritis may reach 1% prevalence, others such as multiple sclerosis or SLE are less frequent (around 0.1%) and many others are relatively rare diseases. Therefore, for most of these clinical entities, only very large epidemiological studies or huge clinical trials would allow for a consistent assessment of the relative risk of vaccine-related effects.

Understanding the mechanisms by which autoimmune responses are generated and how they may or may not lead to autoimmune diseases is of paramount importance in defining the real risk of vaccine-associated autoimmune reaction. During the course of vaccine development, it is now becoming conceivable that a comprehensive and multidisciplinary approach would help to reduce to a minimum the risk that a new vaccine would induce autoimmune manifestations. Later, once the new vaccine is largely used in public health programs, systems should be in place to readily assess observations or allegations of unexpected autoimmune adverse effects. Although in the last few years, there has been a dramatic increase in the number of such allegations, it is somewhat reassuring to see that autoimmune adverse effects were only demonstrated in very few instances.

II. INFECTIOUS AGENTS AS TRIGGER OF AUTOIMMUNE DISEASES

The prototype of autoimmune disease of infectious origin is rheumatic fever. It is caused by an anti-streptococcal immune response that cross-reacts with cardiac myosin [7]. Another well-documented example is the Guillain–Barré syndrome occurring in the course of C. jejuni infection, which is mediated by anti-bacterial lipopolysaccharide antibodies that cross-react with human gangliosides [8]. Similarly, antibodies directed against the Tax protein of the human T-lymphotropic virus type 1 (HTLV-1) and cross-reacting with the heterogeneous nuclear ribonucleoprotein-A1 (hnRNP-A1) self-antigen were demonstrated in HTLV-1-associated myelopathy/tropical spastic paraparesis [9]. Although cross-reactivity between viral peptides and self-antigens was documented in type I diabetes and multiple sclerosis and despite circumstantial observations linking the overexpression of these diseases to previous viral infections, a clear-cut relation between the onset of organ-specific autoimmunity and viral infection has not been firmly established, except for type 1 diabetes in the context of congenital rubella [10–12]. In systemic autoimmune diseases, the role of viruses is also suspected, especially in systemic lupus erythematosus. However, such a role has only been clearly demonstrated in mixed cryoglobulinemia, a disease associated with hepatitis C [13].

It has also been suggested that some long-term complications of infections might be of autoimmune origin. This is the case for reactive arthritis consecutive to infection with intracellular bacteria, including Chlamydia, Salmonella, Shigella, Borrelia, and Yersinia species. In these diseases there is evidence of a persistent pathogenic immune response involving T lymphocytes, but whether such T-cell responses are directed against cross-reactive self-antigens or maintained by persistent bacterial antigens is still an open question [14,15]. In Lyme arthritis, the identification of an immuno-dominant epitope of the outer surface protein A of Borrelia burgdorfi (Osp A) displaying significant homology with human LFA-1, an adhesion molecule of the β2 integrin family, provided convincing evidence for an autoimmune mechanism [16]. Indeed, cross-reactive T-cell responses to OspA and LFA-1 were observed in blood and synovial fluid of patients with antibiotic-resistant chronic Lyme arthritis [16].

The role of infections as etiological agents of human autoimmune disease has been demonstrated in only a few instances. However, their involvement in the exacerbation of a pre-existing autoimmune disorder is rather well established. For example, in multiple sclerosis, epidemiological data strongly suggest that relapses of the disease can be triggered by both bacterial and viral infections [17,18]. Several vaccine-preventable infections are well known to negatively influence the course of defined autoimmune diseases. Vaccination in such cases is highly recommended (e.g., influenza vaccination in patients with multiple sclerosis) [19] because no exacerbation has been recorded following the use of any of the current vaccines.

III. MECHANISMS OF AUTOIMMUNITY INDUCED BY INFECTIOUS AGENTS

It is generally assumed that activation and clonal expansion of autoreactive T lymphocytes represent critical steps in the pathogenesis of autoimmune diseases. Infections might be responsible for these key events through several non-mutually exclusive mechanisms including molecular mimicry, enhanced presentation of self-antigens, bystander activation, and impaired T-cell regulation [15].

A. Molecular Mimicry

The molecular mimicry hypothesis is based on sequence homologies between microbial peptides and self-antigen epitopes. At the T-cell level, this concept was initially established in an experimental model in which immunization with a hepatitis B virus polymerase peptide containing a six amino-acid sequence of rabbit myelin basic protein (MBP) elicited an anti-MBP T-cell response leading to autoimmune encephalomyelitis [20]. The demonstration that a viral infection in itself can lead to autoimmune pathology caused by molecular mimicry was established in a murine model of herpes simplex keratitis, in which pathogenic autoreactive T-cell clones were shown to cross-react with a peptide from the UL6 protein of the herpes simplex virus [21]. Indeed, a single amino acid mutation in the UL6 T-cell epitope was sufficient to limit the capacity of the mutant virus to induce autoimmune corneal lesions [22]. Conclusive evidence that a viral infection can induce pathogenic autoreactive T cells was also provided in a model of Theiler's murine encephalomyelitis virus encoding a mimicking peptide [23]. Molecular mimicry at the level of epitopes recognized by CD8[+] T lymphocytes may also be involved in autoimmunity. This was shown in a model of inflammatory bowel disease induced in immuno-deficient mice by CD8[+] T-cell clones directed against mycobacterial heat shock protein hsp60, which cross-react with hsp60 self antigen [24].

B cell epitope mimicry also occurs. Functional mimicry of host proteins is quite widespread, as it allows pathogens not only to evade an immune response but also to use cellular receptors as port of entry. Such functional mimicry of human glycosphingolipids by lipopolysaccharides (LPS) from several Neisseria species and from Haemophilus influenzae may have evolved to serve this function [25]. Structural homology with autoimmune implications has been identified. A tetrasaccharide of the LPS core of the gastrointestinal pathogen C. jejuni can induce antibodies to human gangliosides and may be causally implicated in the autoimmune Guillain–Barré syndrome [26]. In contrast, it is well known that Lewis-like polysaccharide antigens from certain Helicobacter pylori strains induce antibodies that cross-react with gastric mucosa antigens and appear to contribute to atrophic gastritis in man [27].

B. Enhanced Presentation of Self-Antigens

Infection can promote processing and presentation of self-antigens by several mechanisms. First, cellular damage locally induced by viral or bacterial infection can result in the release of sequestered self-antigens that stimulate autoreactive T cells. This was clearly demonstrated in autoimmune diabetes induced by coxsackievirus B4 infection in mice [28]. Second, the local inflammatory reaction elicited in tissues by microbial products can trigger dendritic cell maturation, which represents a key step in the induction phase of immune responses. Microbial products that engage Toll-like receptors on dendritic cells can induce the up-regulation of membrane expression of MHC and costimulatory molecules and the secretion of cytokines, particularly interleukin (IL)-12, which promote T-cell activation [29]. Third, a T-cell response directed toward a single self-peptide can "spread" to other self-epitopes during an inflammatory reaction. This process of "epitope spreading" has been well-documented in murine models of encephalomyelitis [15].

C. Bystander Activation

The release of cytokines such as IL-12 can promote bystander activation of memory T cells and occasionally trigger autoimmune reactions when such autoreactive cells do pre-exist. Using murine models of encephalomyelitis, Shevach et al. demonstrated that quiescent autoreactive T cells could differentiate into pathogenic Th1 effectors in the presence of microbial products that induce IL-12 synthesis [30,31]. Likewise, Fujinami demonstrated that IL-12-inducing viral infections could elicit relapses of autoimmune encephalomyelitis, in a nonantigen-specific manner, in myelin-primed animals [32]. A salient feature of bystander activation is its limited duration. In order to observe an exacerbation of EAE one should provide the triggering signal within a relatively restricted window of time after the aetiological stimuli that "primed" the animal for disease. In addition, disease exacerbation occurs within weeks after bystander activation and is not usually seen after longer delays [32].

D. Regulatory T Cells

There is growing evidence that regulatory T cells are instrumental in controlling autoreactive T cells both in neonates and adults [33,34]. Indeed, depletion of regulatory CD25+ T cells promotes autoimmunity although in adult animals this maneuver is not sufficient by itself and requires administration of self-antigen [34]. It is likely that infectious agents could have profound influences, either positive or negative, on regulatory T cells. This represents an increasingly important area of investigation that will probably deserve attention during the course of vaccine development.

IV. THE RISK OF VACCINE-ASSOCIATED AUTOIMMUNITY

There exist no general criteria for diagnosing vaccine-related autoimmune disease and this question has to be analyzed on a case-by-case basis. In general, appropriate epidemiological studies are essential before seriously considering that a particular autoimmune clinical condition might be associated with a given vaccination. This can then be followed by the determination of known biological markers of the identified autoimmune disease in other vaccinees. However, it is always relevant to compare the level of vaccine-related risk to that associated with the corresponding natural infection, for the population at large or for specific subgroups to be identified

Criteria underpinning vaccine adverse event causality assessment have been established by WHO [35]. Some of these criteria particularly apply to autoimmune diseases and may be summarized as follows:

(1) Consistency. The association of a purported autoimmune event with the administration of a vaccine should be consistent, i.e., the findings should be replicable in different localities, by different investigators not unduly influencing one another, and by different methods of investigation, all leading to the same conclusion(s).

(2) Strength of the association. The association should be strong in the magnitude of the association (in an epidemiological sense).

(3) Specificity. The association should be distinctive and the adverse event should be linked uniquely or specifically with the vaccine concerned, rather than its occurring frequently, spontaneously, or commonly in association with other external stimuli or conditions. An adverse event may be caused by a vaccine adjuvant or additive, rather than by the active component of the vaccine. In this case, it might spuriously influence the specificity of the association between vaccine and adverse event.

(4) Temporal relation. There should be a clear temporal relationship between the vaccine and the adverse event, in that receipt of the vaccine should precede the earliest manifestation of the event or a clear exacerbation of an ongoing condition. The timing is important: long delays (over 2 months)

are not the rule. Indeed, the induction or the acceleration of autoimmune tissue lesions that have been observed following some acute infections (e.g., *C. jejuni* or influenza) has always occurred within weeks of the infectious event.

Therefore an association between vaccine administration and an autoimmune adverse event is most likely to be considered strong when the evidence is based on:

1. Well-conducted human studies that demonstrate a clear association in a study design that is determined a priori for testing the hypothesis of such association. Such studies will normally be one of the following, in descending order of probability of achieving the objective of the study: randomized controlled clinical trials, cohort studies, case control studies, and controlled case-series analyses. Case reports, however numerous and complete, do not fulfil the requirements for testing hypotheses. When autoimmune events appear attributable to a vaccine, it is important to determine whether there is a predisposed set of subjects (by age, population, genetic, immunological, environmental, ethnic, sociological, or underlying disease conditions). Such predisposition is most likely to be identified in case-controlled studies.
2. An association that is demonstrated in more than one human study and consistent among the studies. The studies would need to have been well conducted, by different investigators, in different populations, with results that are consistent, despite different study designs.
3. Pathology similarities: In the case of future vaccines against infections known to be associated with autoimmune complications (e.g., post-group A streptococcal rheumatic heart disease), vaccine-associated autoimmune adverse events should closely resemble these infection-associated complications.
4. A nonrandom temporal relationship between administration and the adverse incident.

There should be a strict definition of the autoimmune adverse event in clinical, pathological, and biochemical terms, as far as that is achievable. The frequency in the nonimmunized population of the adverse event should be substantially different from that in the immunized population.

A. Vaccine-Attributable Autoimmune Diseases

It is only in a few rare cases that autoimmune pathology has been firmly considered as attributable to the use of modern vaccines. For example, a form of Guillain–Barré Syndrome (GBS, polyradiculoneuritis) was found associated with the 1976–1977 vaccination campaign against swine influenza using the A/New Jersey/8/76 swine-flu vaccine [36]. The estimated attributable risk of vaccine-related GBS in the adult population was just under one case per 100,000 vaccinations and the period of increased risk in swine-flu vaccinated versus nonvaccinated individuals was concentrated

primarily within the 5-week period after vaccination (relative risk: 7.60). Although this original Centers for Disease Control study demonstrated a statistical association and suggested a causal relation between the two events, controversy has persisted for several years. The causal relation was reassessed and confirmed in a later study focusing on cases observed in Michigan and Minnesota [37]. The relative risk of developing Guillain–Barre syndrome in the vaccinated population of these two states, as compared to swine-flu nonvaccinated individuals, during the 6 weeks following vaccination was 7.10, whereas the excess cases of Guillain–Barre syndrome during the first 6 weeks attributed to the vaccine was 8.6 per million vaccinees in Michigan and 9.7 per million vaccinees in Minnesota. The pathogenic mechanisms involved are still unknown. With subsequent influenza vaccines, no significant increase in the development of Guillain–Barré syndrome was noted [38] and it is currently assumed that the risk of developing the Guillain–Barré syndrome following vaccination (one additional case per million persons vaccinated) is substantially less than the risk for severe influenza and influenza-related complications [39].

Another example of confirmed autoimmune adverse effect of vaccination is idiopathic thrombocytopenia (ITP) that may occur after measles-mumps-rubella (MMR) vaccination [40–44]. The reported frequency of clinically apparent ITP after this vaccine is around 1 in 30,000 vaccinated children. In one study [40], the relative incidence in the 6-week post-immunization risk period has been estimated at 3.27 (95% CI: 1.49 to 7.16) when compared to the control period. In about two thirds of the patients, platelet counts under 20,000 have been recorded. The clinical course of MMR-related ITP is usually transient but it is not infrequently associated with bleeding and, as shown in a study conducted in Finland, it can occasionally be severe [45]. In this latter study, there was an increase in platelet-associated immunoglobulin in 10 out of 15 patients whereas circulating antiplatelet autoantibodies, specific for platelet glycoprotein IIb/IIIa, were detected in 5 out of 15 patients. These findings are compatible with an autoimmune mechanism triggered by immune response to MMR vaccination. However, it should be noted that the risk for thrombocytopenia following natural rubella (1/3000) or measles (1/6000) infections is much greater than after vaccination [39]. Patients with a history of previous immune thrombocytopenic purpura are prone to develop this complication and in these individuals the risk of vaccination should be weighed against that of being exposed to the corresponding viral diseases [46].

B. Vaccine-Related Allegations of Autoimmune Adverse Effects

The advent of new vaccines and the increasing number of highly publicized reports that claim a link between certain immunizations and autoimmune disease have led to public concern over the risk of inducing autoimmune disease by immunization. For example, in France there has been concern over the potential association of multiple sclerosis with hepatitis B vaccination. Similarly, the influence of childhood vaccination on type 1 diabetes has been questioned in the United States. Such allegations, even if they are not confirmed, may have detrimental effects on vaccination programs at a global level and therefore require a very particular attention.

C. Hepatitis B and Multiple Sclerosis

The possible association of hepatitis B (HB) vaccination with the development of multiple sclerosis (MS) was primarily questioned in France, following the report of 35 cases of primary demyelinating events occurring at one Paris hospital between 1991 and 1997, within 8 weeks of recombinant HB vaccine injection [47–49].

The neurological manifestations were similar to those observed in MS. There were inflammatory changes in the cerebrospinal fluid and high signal intensity lesions were observed in the cerebral white matter on T2-weighted MR images. After a mean follow-up of 3 years, half of them became clinically definite MS. These neurological manifestations occurred in individuals considered at higher risk for MS: a preponderance of women, mean age near 30 years, overrepresentation of the DR2 HLA antigen, and a positive family history of MS. These observations rapidly called the attention of the French pharmaco-vigilance system and from 1993 through 1999, several hundred cases with similar demographic and clinical characteristics were identified. It is essential to note that this episode occurred in a very special context. In France, close to 25 million people received the HB vaccine during this period, of which 18 million were adults, and this represented about 40% of the population of the country. No cases were reported in children under 3 years

of age. Since these initial reports, at least 10 studies aiming at defining the significance of such observations have now been completed. They are summarized in Table 1. There was no significant association between hepatitis B vaccination and the occurrence of demyelinating events or MS in any of these studies. However, a common feature was an insufficient statistical power to definitely exclude such an association. Two studies are particularly illustrative of the difficulty in interpreting these data. First, a retrospective, hospital-based case-control study was carried out on patients experiencing the first episode of CNS demyelination during the 2-year period from January 1994–December 1995 [50] (121 cases and 121 matched controls). Adjusted odds ratios (OR) obtained from conditional logistic regression between a CNS demyelination and HB vaccine exposure during the previous 60 days were 1.7 (CI 95%, 0.5–6.3) and, during the previous 61–180 days, 1.5 (CI 95%, 0.5–5.3). Second, a population-based case-control study using the general practice database in the United Kingdom analyzed 360 cases with incident MS and 140 cases of central demyelination. Each case was matched with up to six controls [51]. The OR for exposure to HB vaccine in the 0–12-month period was 1.6 (CI 95%, 0.6–4.0).

However, two recent studies bear particular weight in confirming the lack of a significant association between hepatitis B vaccination and the occurrence of MS. Confavreux et al. [52] conducted a case-crossover study in patients included in the European Database for Multiple Sclerosis who had a relapse between 1993 and 1997. The index relapse was the first relapse confirmed by a visit to a neurologist and

Table 1 Clinical Studies of the Association Between Multiple Sclerosis or Demyelinating Diseases with Hepatitis B Vaccination

Analysis	Study site	RR/OR (time interval)	CI 95%	Ref.
MS, first episode	USA	0.7 (24 months)	0.3–1.8	[53]
		0.9 (any time)	0.5–1.6	
MS, relapses	Europe	0.71 (2 months)	0.4–1.3	[52]
Acute demyelination	France	1.7 (2 months)	0.5–6.3	[50]
		1.5 (2–6 months)	0.5–5.3	
MS, first episode	Canada	*5/288657 (pre-vaccination period, 1986–1992)*		[54]
		9/289651 (post-vaccination period, 1992–1998)		
MS, first episode	USA	1.3 (6 months)	0.4–4.8	[55]
		1.0 (12 months)	0.3–3.0	
		2.0, 0.9 (36 months)	0.4–2.1	
Acute demyelination	United States	1.09	0.7–1.7	[56]
MS, relapses	France	*0.6/year (incidence before vaccination)*		[57]
		0.5/year (incidence after vaccination)		
Acute demyelination	France	1.05 (2 months, expected 102.7 vs. observed 108/7.18 million vaccinees)		[58]
MS, first episode and acute demyelination	UK	1.6 (12 months)	0.6–4.0	[59]
Acute demyelination	US	0.6 (2 months)	01–4.6	[60]

RR = Relative risk, OR = odds risk.

preceded by a relapse-free period of at least 12 months. Exposure to vaccination in the 2-month risk period immediately preceding the relapse was compared with that in the four previous 2-month control periods for the calculation of relative risks. Of 643 patients with relapses of multiple sclerosis, 2.3% had been vaccinated during the preceding 2-month risk period as compared with 2.8% to 4.0% who were vaccinated during one or more of the four control periods. The relative risk of relapse associated with exposure to any vaccination during the previous 2 months was 0.71 (95% CI, 0.40 to 1.26). There was no increase in the specific short-term risk of relapse associated with hepatitis B.

Another recent study [53] also excluded a possible link between hepatitis B (HB) vaccine and multiple sclerosis. These authors conducted a nested case-control study in two large cohorts of nurses in the United States: those in the Nurses' Health Study (which has followed 121,700 women since 1976) and those in the Nurses' Health Study II (which has followed 116,671 women since 1989). For each woman with multiple sclerosis, five healthy women and one woman with breast cancer were selected as controls. The analyses included 192 women with multiple sclerosis and 645 matched controls. The multivariate relative risk of multiple sclerosis associated with exposure to the hepatitis B vaccine at any time before the onset of the disease was 0.9 (95% CI, 0.5 to 1.6). The relative risk associated with hepatitis B vaccination within 2 years before the onset of the disease was 0.7 (95% CI, 0.3 to 1.8). The results were similar in analyses restricted to women with multiple sclerosis that began after the introduction of the recombinant hepatitis B vaccine.

These reassuring data are consistent with the fact that, since the integration of hepatitis B vaccine into national childhood immunization schedules in over 125 countries, it has been used in more than 500 million persons and has proved to be among the safest vaccines yet developed.

D. Vaccination and Diabetes

Type 1 diabetes [formerly known as insulin-dependent diabetes mellitus (IDDM) or juvenile diabetes] results from autoimmune destruction of pancreatic β-cells in genetically susceptible individuals exposed to environmental risk factors. The incidence is particularly high in some geographic areas, e.g., Finland and Sardinia, where it can reach 40 cases per 100,000. During the last decades, there has been a regular increase of the incidence of type 1 diabetes in most countries of the world. In a recent European multicenter study covering the period 1989–1994, the annual rate of increase in incidence was found to be 3–4%, with a particularly rapid rate of increase in children under 4 years of age (6.3%) [61].

In this context, it is not surprising that the potential role of childhood vaccines as triggering event for this disease has been questioned. This possibility has been evaluated in a few epidemiologic studies. A case-control study conducted in Sweden in the mid-1980s did not observe any significant effect of vaccination against tuberculosis, smallpox, tetanus, Pertussis, rubella on odd-risk for diabetes [62]. However, some authors [63,64] have hypothesized that the timing of vaccination may be of importance and that certain vaccines

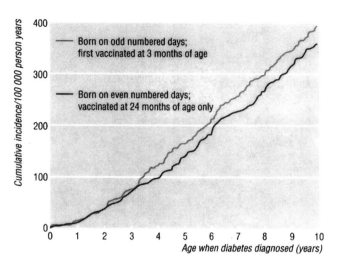

Figure 1 Cumulative incidence of type 1 diabetes per 100,000 person years in Finnish children aged 10 years or under. Comparison of children vaccinated first at the age of 3 months with children vaccinated at the age of 24 months only [65]. There was no statistically significant differences between these two groups (relative risk: 1.01).

(e.g., *Haemophilus influenzae* type b, Hib), if given at 2 months of life or later, may increase the risk of type 1 diabetes. This was not confirmed by a 10-year follow-up study of over 100,000 Finnish children involved in a clinical trial of Hib vaccine (Fig. 1). There was no increased risk of diabetes when comparing children who had received four doses of vaccine at 3, 4, 6, and 14 to 18 months of age with children who received only one dose at 24 months of age [65].

A recent study conducted in four large health maintenance organizations (HMOs) in the USA did not observe any association between administration of routine childhood vaccines and the risk of type 1 diabetes. There was no influence of the timing of hepatitis B or Hib vaccination on the diabetes risk [66].

Therefore, at this stage, there are no serious indications of any significant influence of current childhood vaccines on the occurrence of type 1 diabetes.

V. NEW GENERATION VACCINES AND AUTOIMMUNITY: APPROACHES TOWARD EARLY RISK ASSESSMENT

During the course of vaccine development, only a comprehensive and multidisciplinary strategy may help to reduce the theoretical risk that a new vaccine would induce autoimmune manifestations. First, one should question whether clinical manifestations of an autoimmune nature are known to be associated with the infectious disease that will be the target of the new vaccine. If such events have been reported, e.g., for group A streptococcal diseases, attention should be given to avoid reproducing the natural disease pathogenic process. This may include the identification and the exclusion of naturally pathogenic epitopes. Second, potential molecular and immunological mimicry between vaccine antigens and host components should be extensively and critically analyzed through an intelligent combination of bio-informatics and immunological studies. One should keep in mind that, by itself, an identified mimicry is of little pathogenic significance. Information should be gathered on the relative ability of such epitopes to bind to human MHC molecules, to be processed by human antigen-presenting cells, and to be recognized by autoreactive T cells. Molecular mimicry in itself is not sufficient to trigger autoimmune pathology and other factors intrinsic to infections such as tissue damage and long-lasting inflammatory reaction might be required as well. For example, a recently developed Lyme disease vaccine was shown to contain an immunodominant epitope of the outer surface protein A of *Borrelia burgdorfi* (Osp A) displaying significant homology with human LFA-1, an adhesion molecule of the β2 integrin family. Although this raised concern about the safety of this vaccine, there was no evidence for an increased incidence of arthritis in individuals having received the Lyme vaccine [39]. Third, indicative information can be obtained through the use of ad hoc experimental models of autoimmune diseases. Different vaccine formulations and adjuvants can be compared regarding their potential capacity to induce or enhance the expression of pathology in relevant models. For example, there are models of experimental allergic encephalitis which are sensitive to the administration of IL-12 inducing microbial products and can help to compare the nonspecific effects of different adjuvants or vaccine formulations [32]. Fourth, appropriate immunological investigations (e.g., autoimmune serology) may be systematically included in phase I–III clinical trials. On an ad hoc basis, clinical surveillance of potential autoimmune adverse effects may have to be included in the monitoring protocol. Such surveillance will have to be extended through the postmarketing stage if specific rare events have to be ruled out.

VI. CONCLUSION

Isolated case reports and increased attention in the media to possible side effects of vaccines have dramatically modified the perception by the medical community and the public of the risk of autoimmunity elicited by vaccination, despite the lack of epidemiological support for such a concern. Although available data are reassuring, we must remain vigilant as the risk of autoimmunity associated with some of the new generation vaccines might be increased as compared to current vaccines. A number of new adjuvants that are being developed aim at inducing strong Th1-type immune responses against viruses or other intracellular pathogens. Such effects may occasionally favor the expression of underlying autoimmune diseases or induce autoimmune responses in exceptional cases when the vaccine antigens contain immuno-dominant epitopes that cross-react with self-antigens. Special attention should be given to adjuvants acting as strong inducers of IL-12 synthesis [27,28]. Cancer vaccines based on dendritic cells pulsed with tumor antigens might also carry a significant risk of autoimmunity induction [39,40].

Finally, it is of paramount importance to keep in mind that the mere occurrence of autoimmune markers (autoreactive antibodies or T cells) is a frequent phenomenon in a normal population and that pathological expression, i.e., the development of an autoimmune disease, is by far much less frequent.

REFERENCES

1. Jacobson DL, Gange SJ, Rose NR, Graham NM. Epidemiology and estimated population burden of selected autoimmune diseases in the United States. Clin Immunol Immunopathol 1997; 84:223–243.
2. Onkamo P, Vaananen S, Karvonen M, Tuomilehto J. Worldwide increase in incidence of Type I diabetes—the analysis of the data on published incidence trends. Diabetologia 1999; 42:1395–1403.
3. Wynn DR, Rodriguez M, O'Fallon WM, Kurland LT. A reappraisal of the epidemiology of multiple sclerosis in Olmsted County, Minnesota. Neurology 1990; 40:780–786.
4. Salvetti M, Ristori G, Bomprezzi R, Pozzilli P, Leslie RD. Twins: mirrors of the immune system. Immunol Today 2000; 21:342–347.
5. Noseworthy JH, Lucchinetti C, Rodriguez M, Weinshenke BG. Multiple sclerosis. N Engl J Med 2000; 343:938–952.
6. Dahlquist G. The aetiology of type 1 diabetes: an epidemiological perspective. Acta Paediatr Suppl 1998; 425:5–10.
7. Cunningham MW, Antone SM, Smart M, Liu R, Kosanke S. Molecular analysis of human cardiac myosin-cross-reactive B- and T-cell epitopes of the group A streptococcal M5 protein. Infect Immun 1997; 65:3913–3923.
8. Rees JH, Soudain SE, Gregson NA, Hughes RA. *Campylobacter jejuni* infection and Guillain–Barre syndrome. N Engl J Med 1995; 333:1374–1379.
9. Levin MC, Lee SM, Kalume F, Morcos Y, Dohan FC Jr, Hasty KA, Callaway JC, Zunt J, Desiderio D, Stuart JM. Autoimmunity due to molecular mimicry as a cause of neurological disease. Nat Med 2002; 8:509–513.
10. Davidson A, Diamond B. Autoimmune diseases. N Engl J Med 2001; 345:340–350.
11. Robles DT, Eisenbarth GS. Type 1A diabetes induced by infection and immunization. J Autoimmun 2001; 16:355–362.
12. Clarke WL, Shaver KA, Bright GM, Rogol AD, Nance WE. Autoimmunity in congenital rubella syndrome. J Pediatr 1984; 104:370–373.
13. Ferri C, Zignego AL. Relation between infection and autoimmunity in mixed cryoglobulinemia. Curr Opin Rheumatol 2000; 12:53–60.
14. Benoist C, Mathis D. Autoimmunity provoked by infection: how good is the case for T cell epitope mimicry? Nat Immunol 2001; 2:797–801.
15. Wucherpfennig KW. Mechanisms for the induction of autoimmunity by infectious agents. J Clin Invest 2001; 108:1097–1104.
16. Gross DM, Forsthuber T, Tary-Lehmann M, Etling C, Ito K, Nagy ZA, Field JA, Steere AC, Huber BT. Identification of LFA-1 as a candidate autoantigen in treatment-resistant Lyme arthritis. Science 1998; 281:703–706.
17. Rapp NS, Gilroy J, Lerner AM. Role of bacterial infection in exacerbation of multiple sclerosis. Am J Phys Med Rehabil 1995; 74:415–418.
18. Andersen O, Lygner PE, Bergstrom T, Andersson M, Vahlne A. Viral infections trigger multiple sclerosis relapses: a prospective seroepidemiological study. J Neurol 1993; 240:417–422.
19. De Keyser J, Zwanikken C, Boon M. Effects of influenza

vaccination and influenza illness on exacerbations in multiple sclerosis. J Neurol Sci 1998; 159:51–53.

20. Fujinami RS, Oldstone MB. Amino acid homology between the encephalitogenic site of myelin basic protein and virus: mechanism for autoimmunity. Science 1985; 230:1043–1045.

21. Zhao ZS, Granucci F, Yeh L, Schaffer PA, Cantor H. Molecular mimicry by herpes simplex virus-type 1: autoimmune disease after viral infection. Science 1998; 279:1344–1347.

22. Panoutsakopoulou V, Sanchirico ME, Huster KM, Jansson M, Granucci F, Shim DJ, Wucherpfennig KW, Cantor H. Analysis of the relationship between viral infection and autoimmune disease. Immunity 2001; 15:137–147.

23. Olson JK, Croxford JL, Calenoff MA, Dal. Canto MC, Miller SD. A virus-induced molecular mimicry model of multiple sclerosis. J Clin Invest 2001; 108:311–318.

24. Steinhoff U, Brinkmann V, Klemm U, Aichele P, Seiler P, Brandt U, Bland PW, Prinz I, Zugel U, Kaufmann SH. Autoimmune intestinal pathology induced by hsp60-specific CD8 T cells. Immunity 1999; 11:349–358.

25. Harvey HA, Swords WE, Apicella MA. The mimicry of human glycolipids and glycosphingolipids by the lipooligosaccharides of pathogenic neisseria and haemophilus. J Autoimmun 2001; 16:257–262.

26. Moran AP, Prendergast MM, Hogan EL. Sialosyl-galactose: a common denominator of Guillain–Barre and related disorders? J Neurol Sci 2002; 196:1–7.

27. Moran AP, Prendergast MM. Molecular mimicry in *Campylobacter jejuni* and *Helicobacter pylori* lipopolysaccharides: contribution of gastrointestinal infections to autoimmunity. J Autoimmun 2001; 16:241–256.

28. Horwitz MS, Ilic A, Fine C, Rodriguez E, Sarvetnick N. Presented antigen from damaged pancreatic beta cells activates autoreactive T cells in virus-mediated autoimmune diabetes. J Clin Invest 2002; 109:79–87.

29. Medzhitov R, Janeway CA Jr. Decoding the patterns of self and nonself by the innate immune system. Science 2002; 296:298–300.

30. Segal BM, Klinman DM, Shevach EM. Microbial products induce autoimmune disease by an IL-12-dependent pathway. J Immunol 1997; 158:5087–5090.

31. Segal BM, Chang JT, Shevach EM. CpG oligonucleotides are potent adjuvants for the activation of autoreactive encephalitogenic T cells in vivo. J Immunol 2000; 164:5683–5688.

32. Theil DJ, Tsunoda I, Rodriguez F, Whitton JL, Fujinami RS. Viruses can silently prime for and trigger central nervous system autoimmune disease. J Neurovirol 2001; 7:220–227.

33. Shevach EM. Regulatory T cells in autoimmunity*. Annu Rev Immunol 2000; 18:423–449.

34. McHugh RS, Shevach EM. Cutting edge: depletion of CD4 (+)CD25(+) regulatory T cells is necessary, but not sufficient, for induction of organ-specific autoimmune disease. J Immunol 2002; 168:5979–5983.

35. WHO Global Advisory Committee for Vaccine Safety. Causality assessment of adverse events following immunization. WER 2001: 85–92.

36. Schonberger LB, Bregman DJ, Sullivan-Bolyai JZ, Keenly-side RA, Ziegler DW, Retailliau HF, Eddins DL, Bryan JA. Guillain–Barre syndrome following vaccination in the National Influenza Immunization Program, United States, 1976–1977. Am J Epidemiol 1979; 110:105–123.

37. Safranek TJ, Lawrence DN, Kurland LT, Culver DH, Wiederholt WC, Hayner NS, Osterholm MT, O'Brien P, Hughes JM. Reassessment of the association between Guillain–Barre syndrome and receipt of swine influenza vaccine in 1976–1977: results of a two-state study. Expert Neurology Group. Am J Epidemiol 1991; 133:940–951.

38. Lasky T, Terracciano GJ, Magder L, Koski CL, Ballesteros M, Nash D, Clark S, Haber P, Stolley PD, Schonberger LB,

39. Chen RT. The Guillain–Barre syndrome and the 1992–1993 and 1993–1994 influenza vaccines. N Engl J Med 1998; 339:1797–1802.

40. Chen RT, Pless R, Destefano F. Epidemiology of autoimmune reactions induced by vaccination. J Autoimmun 2001; 16:309–318.

41. Miller E, Waight P, Farrington CP, Andrews N, Stowe J, Taylor B. Idiopathic thrombocytopenic purpura and MMR vaccine. Arch Dis Child 2001; 84:227–229.

42. Vlacha V, Forman EN, Miron D, Peter G. Recurrent thrombocytopenic purpura after repeated measles–mumps–rubella vaccination. Pediatrics 1996; 97:738–739.

43. Oski FA, Naiman JL. Effect of live measles vaccine on the platelet count. N Engl J Med 1966; 275:352–356.

44. Jonville-Bera AP, Autret E, Galy-Eyraud C, Hessel L. Thrombocytopenic purpura after measles, mumps and rubella vaccination: a retrospective survey by the French regional pharmacovigilance centres and pasteur-merieux serums et vaccins. Pediatr Infect Dis J 1996; 15:44–48.

45. Beeler J, Varricchio F, Wise R. Thrombocytopenia after immunization with measles vaccines: review of the vaccine adverse events reporting system (1990 to 1994). Pediatr Infect Dis J 1996; 15:88–90.

46. Nieminen U, Peltola H, Syrjala MT, Makipernaa A, Kekomaki R. Acute thrombocytopenic purpura following measles, mumps and rubella vaccination. A report on 23 patients. Acta Paediatr 1993; 82:267–270.

47. Pool V, Chen R, Rhodes P. Indications for measles–mumps–rubella vaccination in a child with prior thrombocytopenia purpura. Pediatr Infect Dis J 1997; 16:423–424.

48. Gout O, Théodorou I, Liblau R., et al. Central nervous system demyelination after recombinant hepatitis B vaccination report of 25 cases. Neurology, 1997:48.

49. Gout O, Lyon-Caen O. Sclerotic plaques and vaccination against hepatitis B. Rev Neurol (Paris) 1998; 154:205–207.

50. Tourbah A, Gout O, Liblau R, Lyon-Caen O, Bougniot C, Iba-Zizen MT, Cabanis EA. Encephalitis after hepatitis B vaccination: recurrent disseminated encephalitis or MS? Neurology 1999; 53:396–401.

51. Touze E, Gout O, Verdier-Taillefer MH, Lyon-Caen O, Alperovitch A. The first episode of central nervous system demyelinization and hepatitis B virus vaccination. Rev Neurol (Paris) 2000; 156:242–246.

52. Sturkenboom MC, Wolfson C, Roullet E, Heinzlef O, Abenhaim L. Demyelination, multiple sclerosis, and hepatitis B vaccination: a population-based study in the U.K. Neurology, 2000:54.

53. Confavreux C, Suissa S, Saddier P, Bourdes V, Vukusic S. Vaccinations and the risk of relapse in multiple sclerosis. Vaccines in multiple sclerosis study group. N Engl J Med 2001; 344:319–326.

54. Ascherio A, Zhang SM, Hernan MA, Olek MJ, Coplan PM, Brodovicz K, Walker AM. Hepatitis B vaccination and the risk of multiple sclerosis. N Engl J Med 2001; 344:327–332.

55. Sadovnick AD, Scheifele DW. School-based hepatitis B vaccination programme and adolescent multiple sclerosis. Lancet 2000; 355:549–550.

56. Zipp F, Weil JG, Einhaupl KM. No increase in demyelinating diseases after hepatitis B vaccination. Nat Med 1999; 5: 964–965.

57. Verstraeten TM. Risk of demyelinating disease after hepatitis B vaccination. European Society for Paediatric Infectious Diseases, 2001.

58. Coustans M, Brunet P, De Marco O. Demyelinating disease and hepatitis B vaccination: survey of 735 patients seen at MS clinic. Neurology 2000:54.

59. Fourrier A, Begaud B, Alperovitch A, Verdier-Taillefer MH, Touze E, Decker N, Imbs JL. Hepatitis B vaccine and first

episodes of central nervous system demyelinating disorders: a comparison between reported and expected number of cases. Br J Clin Pharmacol 2001; 51:489–490.

59. Sturkenboom M, Abenhaim L, Wolfson C, Roulet E, Heinzelf O, Gout O. Vaccination, demyelination and multiple sclerosis study (VDAMS): a population-based study in the UK. Pharmacoepidemiol Drug Safety 1999:88.

60. Weil J. The incidence of central nervous system demyelinating disease following hepatitis B vaccination. In International Conference on Pharmacoepidemiology, 1998.

61. Variation and trends in incidence of childhood diabetes in Europe. EURODIAB ACE Study Group. Lancet 2000; 355: 873–876.

62. Blom L, Nystrom L, Dahlquist G. The Swedish childhood diabetes study. Vaccinations and infections as risk determinants for diabetes in childhood. Diabetologia 1991; 34:176–181.

63. Classen JB, Classen DC. Immunization in the first month of life may explain decline in incidence of IDDM in The Netherlands. Autoimmunity 1999; 31:43–45.

64. Classen JB, Classen DC. Association between type 1 diabetes and hib vaccine. Causal relation is likely. BMJ 1999; 319: 1133.

65. Karvonen M, Cepaitis Z, Tuomilehto J. Association between type 1 diabetes and Haemophilus influenzae type b vaccination: birth cohort study. BMJ 1999; 318:1169–1172.

66. DeStefano F, Mullooly JP, Okoro CA, Chen RT, Marcy SM, Ward JI, Vadheim CM, Black SB, Shinefield HR, Davis RL, Bohlke K. Childhood vaccinations, vaccination timing, and risk of type 1 diabetes mellitus. Pediatrics 2001; 108: E112.

18
Adjuvants for the Future

Richard T. Kenney
Iomai Corporation, Gaithersburg, Maryland, U.S.A.

Robert Edelman
University of Maryland School of Medicine, Baltimore, Maryland, U.S.A.

In 1925, Ramon demonstrated that it was possible to artificially increase antigen-specific levels of diphtheria or tetanus antitoxin by the addition of bread crumbs, agar, tapioca, starch oil, lecithin, or saponin to the vaccines [1]. Since then, aluminum hydroxide has become the dominant reagent used and is the only adjuvant currently used in licensed vaccines in the United States. The field has become much more sophisticated in the past decade with the introduction of numerous new adjuvants and new concepts regarding the mechanisms of action. In this brief chapter, we review the modern adjuvants administered to enhance a variety of experimental vaccines in human. After a more general discussion of adjuvants, including their definition, mechanisms of action, and safety, we will discuss clinical trials of investigational adjuvants. For additional study of this complex subject, including a historical perspective, the reader is referred to recent published reviews of vaccine adjuvants (Refs. [2–5] and references therein).

Interest in vaccine adjuvants is growing rapidly for several reasons. First, dozens of new vaccine candidates have emerged over the past decade against infectious agents, cancer, fertility, and allergic and autoimmune diseases; many of these candidates require adjuvants. Second, the Children's Vaccine Initiative (CVI), initiated in 1990 [6], and the Global Alliance for Vaccines (GAVI), initiated in 1999 [7], have helped to energize political and public health interest in vaccine adjuvants by establishing ambitious goals for enhancing present vaccines and for developing new ones. Finally, refinements in the fields of analytical biochemistry, macromolecular purification, recombinant technology, and improved understanding of immunological mechanisms and disease pathogenesis have helped to improve the technical basis for adjuvant development and application.

I. DEFINITIONS

The term "adjuvant" (from the Latin *adjuvare*, meaning *to help*) was coined in 1926 by Ramon for a substance used in combination with a specific antigen that produces more immunity than the antigen used alone [8]. The enormous diversity of compounds that increase specific immune responses to an antigen and thus function as vaccine adjuvants makes any classification system somewhat arbitrary. Adjuvants can be loosely categorized in terms of their physical nature as 1) mineral salts; 2) mycobacterial, bacterial, and plant derivatives; 3) surface-active agents and microparticles; 4) polymers, cytokines, vitamins, and hormones; and 5) synthetic constructs. Those listed in Table 1 are examples of immunopotentiators used during the past 25 years. They are grouped according to origin rather than mechanism of action because the mechanisms for most adjuvants are incompletely understood. Agents in Table 1 are reported to augment specific antigens; nonspecific enhancers of the immune response that principally stimulate innate immunity are largely excluded. A comprehensive list of adjuvants, beyond the scope of this chapter, is available and updated by the NIAID [9].

A "carrier" is an immunogenic protein to which a hapten or a weakly immunogenic antigen is bound [10]. A carrier may also be a living organism (or vector) bearing genes for expression of the foreign hapten or antigen on its surface. A naked DNA vaccine is a carrier in the sense that it entails injection into the host of a plasmid-based DNA vector that encodes the production of the protein antigen [11]. Carriers increase the immune response by providing T-cell help to the hapten or antigen.

A "vehicle" provides the substrate for the adjuvant, the antigen, or the antigen–carrier complex. Unlike the carriers

Table 1 Classes of Modern Vaccine Adjuvants, Carriers, and Vehicles

Adjuvants			
Mineral salts	Mycobacterial, bacterial, and plant derivatives	Surface-active agents and microparticles	Polymers
Aluminum hydroxide (Alhydrogel; Rehydragel®), aluminum, and calcium phosphate gel	Complete Freund's adjuvant (killed *M. tuberculosis*), DETOX™ (MPL plus cell wall skeleton of *Mycobacterium phlei*), Bacillus Calmette Guérin (BCG), muramyl dipeptides and tripeptides, dipalmitoyl phosphatidylethanolamine-MTP (MTP-PE), monophosphoryl lipid A (MPL®), gamma inulin/alum (Algammulin), *Klebsiella pneumoniae* glycoprotein, *Bordetella pertussis*, *Corynebacterium parvum*, cholera toxin, cholera B subunit, *E. coli* heat-labile toxin (LT)	Saponin (Stimulon™ QS-21, Quil-A), immune-stimulating complexes (ISCOMS™), Avridine®, nonionic block copolymers (CRL1005, Pluronic® L121), virosomes, dimethyl dioctadecyl-ammonium bromide (DDA)	Dextran, double-stranded polynucleotides (Poly rA:Poly rU), acetylated polymannose (Acemannan), sulfolipopolysaccharide, polymethyl methacrylate (PMMA), acrylic acid-allyl sucrose (Carbopol), polyphosphazene (Admumer™), β-glucan (Pleuran, Algal Glucan)

Cytokines, vitamins, and hormones	Synthetic constructs	Carriers	Vehicles
GM-CSF, IFN-α, IFN-γ, IL-1β, IL-2, IL-6, IL-7, IL-12, cytokine-containing liposomes, vitamin A, D₃ (Calcitriol), E, human growth hormone, dehydroepiandrosterone (DHEA)	Imidazo-quinolines (Imiquimod, S-28463), glycolipid bay R1005, stearyl tyrosine, DTP-GDP (ImmTher™), DTP-DPP (Theramide™), threonyl-MDP 7-allyl-8-oxoguanosine (Loxoribine), multiantigen peptide (MAP) system, linear polymerization of haptenic peptides, peptide linkage to T-cell or B-cell epitopes	Bacterial toxoids (tetanus, diphtheria, pseudomonas A, pertussis), meningococcal outer membrane proteins (proteosomes), fatty acids, Ty viruslike particles, nucleic acid vaccines, living vectors (vaccinia virus, adenovirus, canary pox, polio virus, BCG, attenuated *Salmonella*, *Vibrio cholerae*, and *Shigella*), protein cochleates	Mineral oil (IFA, Montanide®, Specol) and vegetable oil (peanut, olive, sesame) emulsions, squalene and squalane emulsions (MF59, SAF, SPT), lipid-containing vesicles (liposomes [DMPC, DMPG], Sendai proteoliposomes, virosomes [IRIV]), biodegradable polymer microspheres (lactide and glycolide polymers (PLGA, PGA, PLA), proteinoid microspheres (PODDS™), polyphosphazene, protein cochleates, edible plants

listed in Table 1, vehicles are not themselves immunogenic. Like carriers, most vehicles can enhance antigens alone and so sometimes are considered to be another class of adjuvants, although their immunostimulatory effects are often augmented by the addition of conventional adjuvants to constitute "adjuvant formulations." Thus, an "adjuvant formulation" is composed of an adjuvant in a suitable vehicle. Many examples of such adjuvant formulations have been tested in humans [12–15] (cf. Table 2).

II. MECHANISMS OF ACTION

Adjuvants can select for or modulate humoral or cell-mediated immunity and they can do this in several ways. First, antigen processing can be modulated, leading to vaccines that can elicit both helper T cells and cytotoxic lymphocytes (CTLs) (reviewed in Refs. [16–18]). Second, depending upon the adjuvant, the immune response can be modulated in favor of type 1 or type 2 immune responses [16,17,19]. For example, complete Freund's adjuvant and the QS-21 adjuvant can elicit DTH and MHC class I CTL responses when mixed with protein antigens, peptides, or inactivated viruses [20]. Many other adjuvants, such as aluminum salts [19] and nonionic block polymers [3] elicit principally antibody responses when combined with protein antigens or inactivated organisms, perhaps by activating APCs by an IL-4-dependent mechanism [21]. Third, adjuvants can modulate the immune response by preferentially stimulating Th1 or Th2 CD4$^+$ T-helper cells [22]. The Th1 response is accompanied by secretion of interleukin-2 (IL-2), interferon-gamma (IFN-γ), and TNF-β leading to a CMI response, including activation of macrophages and CTLs and high levels of IgG2a antibodies in mice. The Th2 response is modulated by secretion of IL-4, IL-5, IL-6, and IL-10, which provide better help for B-cell responses, including those of IgG1, IgE, and IgA isotypes in mice. Aluminum salts principally stimulate the Th2 response [23], whereas the Th1 response is stimulated by many adjuvants, such as muramyl dipeptide, monophosphoryl lipid A, and QS-21 [16,24,25].

Vaccine adjuvants can modulate antibody avidity, specificity, quantity, isotype, and subclass against epitopes on complex immunogens [26–29]. For example, only certain adjuvants, vehicles, and adjuvant formulations can induce the development of the protective IgG2a antibody isotype against *Plasmodium yoelii* [28]. The ability of adjuvants to influence so many parameters of the immune response greatly complicates the process of finding an effective adjuvant, because our knowledge of how any one adjuvant operates on a cellular level is insufficient to support a completely rational approach for matching the vaccine antigen with the proper adjuvant. Consequently, many investigators advocate an empirical approach for antigen selection based on the balance between toxicity and adjuvanticity in animals. Unfortunately, no validated animal models exist that can substitute for comparing adjuvants directly in humans [30,31]. Decades of experimental studies in laboratory mammals have shown that successful predictions about the safety, potency, or efficacy in humans of a

particular adjuvant cannot be reliably made in these models. The effect of adjuvants are modulated strongly by 1) the nature and dose of the immunogen; 2) the nature and dose of the adjuvant, carrier, or vehicle in the formulation; 3) the stability of the formulation; 4) the immunization schedule; 5) the route of administration; 6) the species of animal; and 7) the genetic and other biological variations within species, including their immune status.

III. SAFETY

During the past 75 years many adjuvants have been developed, but they were never accepted for routine vaccination because of their immediate toxicity and fear of delayed side effects. The current attitude regarding risk benefits of vaccination favors safety over efficacy when a vaccine is given to a healthy population of children and adults. In high-risk groups, including patients with cancer and AIDS, and for therapeutic vaccines an additional level of toxicity may be acceptable if the benefit of the vaccine was substantial. Unfortunately, the absolute safety of adjuvanted vaccines, or any vaccine, cannot be guaranteed, so the risks must be minimized. Undesirable reactions can be grouped as either local or systemic.

The most frequent local adverse effects are tenderness and swelling, with the most severe ones involving the formation of painful abscesses and nodules at the inoculum site. The mechanisms for such severe local reactions include the following: 1) contamination of the vaccine at the time of formulation with reactogenic chemicals and microbial products; 2) instability of the vaccine on storage with breakdown into reactogenic side products; 3) formation of inflammatory immune complexes at the inoculation site by combination of the adjuvanted vaccine with preexisting antibodies resulting in an Arthus-type reaction; and 4) poor biodegradability of the adjuvanted vaccine resulting in prolonged persistence in the tissues and reactive granuloma formation. Such local reactions are of special concern for depot-type adjuvants, such as aluminum salts, oil emulsions, liposomes, biodegradable polymer microspheres, and living vectors such as BCG.

Severe local reactions in humans followed subcutaneous injections of incomplete Freund's adjuvant (IFA), a mineral oil emulsion, using early formulations made with a mannide monooleate stabilizer that contained free fatty acid impurities. However, these lesions did not occur with IFA injected intramuscularly and that contained the stabilizer without impurities (reviewed in Refs. [30,32]). IFA has been administered to more than a million people worldwide [32–35]. Despite the apparent long-term safety of this adjuvant [36], the risk/benefit ratio is felt to be too high for commercial use.

To date, vaccine adjuvants have caused few severe acute systemic adverse effects. More theoretical risks include the induction of autoimmunity or cancer. Fortunately, in 10-, 18-, and 35-year follow-up studies, the incidence of cancer and autoimmune and collagen disorders in 18,000 persons who received oil-emulsion influenza vaccine in the early 1950s was not different from that in persons given aqueous vaccines [33,36–38]. It requires decades of expensive and time-consuming follow-up for such low-incidence reactions to be identified, and, at present, a mechanism for the systematic, active follow-up of vaccinees given experimental adjuvants is not available [39]. Anterior chamber uveitis has been reported with *N*-acetylmuramyl-L-alanyl-D-isogluta-mine (MDP) and several MDP analogues in rabbits [40] and monkeys [41], and has been systematically sought in at least one adjuvant vaccine study involving 110 volunteers, but it was not found there [42]. Adjuvant-associated arthritis [43,44] has not been reported in humans, even after long-term follow-up [34,36,45]. Anaphylactic reactions, angioedema, urticaria, and vasculitis have been described following the administration of the majority of vaccines, although severe events are rare [31]. Finally, a syndrome known as macrophagic myofasciitis (MMF), characterized by diffuse arthromyalgias and fatigue in connection with muscle infiltration by macrophages and lymphocytes, was recently linked to alum-containing vaccinations in France [46], although a causal association has not been established.

IV. REGULATORY ISSUES

In concert with the progress of the International Conference on Harmonization of Technical Requirements for Registration of Pharmaceuticals for Human Use (ICH), worldwide regulatory guidance on the development and testing of vaccines has expanded significantly in the last few years. Documents covering nearly every aspect of drug and biological development are being created and revised in an effort to enhance and standardize the quality, safety, and efficacy of pharmaceutical products (http://www.ich.org, http://www.fda.gov/cber/guidelines.htm, http://www.emea.eu.int). However, advice directed specifically at the development of adjuvants is lacking. It is important to note that as a rule adjuvants are not licensed on their own. Because each combination of one or more antigens with an adjuvant has its own unique safety and efficacy profile, they are licensed and regulated as individual products in combination.

V. EXPERIMENTAL ADJUVANTS IN HUMANS

The number of commercially feasible adjuvants tested in animals and humans (Table 1) is too large to review in this short chapter. Instead, a smaller number of modern adjuvants or adjuvant formulations used to enhance a variety of experimental vaccines in humans (Table 2) will be considered. The development of experimental adjuvants has been driven principally by the failure of aluminum compounds to 1) enhance many vaccines in man [32], 2) enhance subunit vaccine antigens in animals [30,47,48], and 3) to stimulate cytotoxic T-cell responses [19]. In many instances, several adjuvants have been combined in one adjuvant formulation hoping to obtain a synergistic or additive effect.

A. Emulsion-Based Formulations

Two basic concepts have emerged in the manufacture of aqueous and oil combinations that describe the dispersion of one liquid as particles within a second liquid that is continuous [49]. Surfactants, which are compounds that contain both polar and nonpolar groups, are added to stabilize the emulsions. Their hydrophilic/lipophilic balance determines the state of the emulsion that forms. Water-in-oil (W/O) emulsions that Freund used were initially very unstable and viscous and caused strong local reactions, yet they are very efficient at inducing an immune response to weak antigens. Newer oils and surfactants are now used that allow the development of stable fluid emulsions that are safer [49].

Mineral oils in W/O emulsions, such as IFA, stay at the injection site and are slowly eliminated by macrophages or metabolized to fatty acids, triglycerides, phospholipids, or sterols [50]. Protein antigens are released very slowly from this matrix. Proprietary, highly refined emulsifiers from the mannide monooleate family in a natural metabolizable oil solution were developed by SEPPIC (Paris, France), named Montanide ISA 51 and ISA 720. Both Montanide adjuvants induce a strong immune response, but severe local reactions may limit their use.

Oil-in-water (O/W) preparations containing small particles of oil dispersed in an aqueous continuous phase are more easily cleared from the injection site. The droplets with antigen can be endocytosed by APCs or readily pass from the injection site to lymphatics [51]. A major part of the effort to develop immunostimulators as vaccine adjuvants has been devoted to the characterization of mycobacterial cell wall components and their analogues as additions to these preparations [32,52,53]. The most studied component of the cell wall has been the muramyl dipeptide, MDP. Three promising derivatives of MDP were developed because of MDP's residual toxicity and pyrogenicity; they include a butyl-ester derivative (Murabutide™) [54,55], threonyl-MDP [56,57], and muramyl tripeptide dipalmitoyl phosphatidylethanolamine (MTP-PE) [48,57]. Because MDP in water provides only a modest adjuvant effect in mice [58,59] and in humans [54], threonyl-MDP and MTP-PE have been administered in oil emulsion vehicles in attempts to improve potency.

The Syntex adjuvant formulation (SAF) preparation (Syntex Research, Palo Alto, CA) is an oil-in-water emulsion vehicle. The vehicle contains 5% squalane, 2.5% Pluronic® L121, and 0.2% polysorbate 80 (Tween® 80) in phosphate-buffered saline, pH 7.4 [14,51]. Squalane, used in several modern adjuvant emulsions, is a metabolizable oil used in many over-the-counter drugs and cosmetics. Pluronic® 121 is a nonionic block copolymer discussed below. SAF elicits both cell-mediated (lymphocyte blastogenic) and humoral responses. MTP-PE, which is often added to SAF, probably acts by inducing immunoregulatory cytokines, whereas the emulsion vehicle and Pluronic® L121 facilitate presentation of antigens to responding lymphocytes. In humans, SAF and SAF + threonyl-MDP have been compared to other adjuvanted HIV gp120 vaccines; the results showed SAF preparations to be immunogenic but highly reactogenic.

In addition to the inclusion of MF-59 in various experimental and licensed vaccines in Europe [57,60–62], several other oil-in-water emulsions are under development by SmithKline Beecham in Rixensart, Belgium. AS02 (formerly known as SBAS2) is a proprietary O/W emulsion containing

Table 2 Selected Clinical Trials of Experimental Adjuvanted Vaccines

Vaccine	Vehicle, adjuvant, or formulation	Vaccine	Vehicle, adjuvant, or formulation
Viral		**Parasitic**	
HIV-1 *env2–3*	MTP-PE/squalene emulsion [15]	Leishmania peptides	MDP (Murabutide®) [150]
	MTP-PE/MF59 [124]	Inactivated *L. major*	BCG bacteria [151,152]
HIV-1 gp120/gp160	Alum [125]	Malaria CS, RTS,S	Interferon-alpha [117,153]
	MF59 + MDP-PE, MTP-PE [126,127]		Interferon-gamma [117]
	MF59 ± Alum [60]		DETOX™ [12,84]
	SAF + threonyl-MDP, QS-21, MPL®,		MPL®/liposomes + alum [13,154]
	Liposome/MPL ± alum [42]		MPL® + alum [87]
HIV p17/p24	Ty-VLP [128]		QS-21 + alum [155]
HIV-1 inact.	IFA (Montanide®) [129–131]		AS02 [63,64]
HIV TAB9	Montanide ISA 720 [132,133]		
Influenza	IFA [34,36]	Malaria blood stage	Montanide ISA 720 [156,157]
	MTP-PE/squalene emulsion [134]	**Cancer**	
	MF59 [57]	*Solid tumors*	
	ISCOMS [107]	ras peptides	DETOX™ [158]
	Liposome [135]	EGF-TT, EGF-P64k	Alum [159]
	QS-21 + MPL [136]	HCG-DT	Nonionic block copolymer [160]
	Virosomes or MF59 [137,138]	*Colon*	
Inactivated polio	IFA [45]	hCG peptide	Nor-MDP/squalene emulsion [161]
Hepatitis B	IFN-γ [139,140], IFN-α [141]	*Breast*	
	Interleukin-2 [142,143]	Synthetic glycoconjugate	DETOX™ [83]
	MPL® [85,86]	*Cervix*	
	MPL® + alum [66,144]	HPV16 L1 VLP	Alum or MF59 [62,162]
	GM-CSF [113]	*Ovary*	
	DNA vaccination [145]	Glycoconjugate	DETOX™ [82]
Herpes simplex gp's	MPL® + aluminum [74,88,89]	*Melanoma*	
	MF59 [57,61]	Cell lysates	DETOX™ [79–81]
Bacterial		Melanoma liposomes	Interleukin-2 [163]
Tetanus toxoid	MDP (Murabutide®) [54]	**Antifertility**	
Clostridium difficile	Alum [146]	hCG peptide	Nor-MDP/squalene [164,165]
ETEC	LT [98,99]		
S. pyogenes M prot.	MDP (Murabutide®) [147]		
Borrelia OspA	Alum [148]		
	rBCG [149]		
S. pneumoniae	MPL ± alum [78]		

monophosphoryl lipid A (MPL®) and QS-21 that causes strong antibody responses as well as Th1 and CTL cellular responses. Phase 1/2 studies have been conducted in malaria, most recently with RTS,S, a circumsporozoite (CS) subunit antigen fused to the hepatitis S antigen [63]. RTS,S with AS02 demonstrated efficacy in a Phase 2b field trial in the Gambia [64]. Similar emulsions have been studied with human papilloma virus (HPV)-induced genital warts in a therapeutic setting [65], with hepatitis BsAg [66], and with multiple HIV vaccine formulations [67].

B. Monophosphoryl Lipid A (MPL®)

The adjuvant effect of lipopolysaccharide (LPS) was described in 1956 [68]. Most of the adjuvanticity and toxicity of LPS are associated with the lipid A region of the molecule [69]. The LPS of *Salmonella minnesota* R595 has been detoxified without destroying its adjuvant activity by exposing the LPS to mild hydrolytic treatment [70]. The resultant monophosphoryl derivative of lipid A, called MPL® by

Corixa Corporation (Hamilton, MT), is a highly adaptable molecule that can be used effectively in many adjuvant formulations [24,71]. Such formulations include antigen in saline [72], oil-in-water emulsions [72,73], aluminum salts (a combination also called AS04) [66,74], and in liposomes [13]. The immunopotentiating nature of MPL® may be associated with its capacity to induce cytokines, such as IL-12 [24], IFN-γ, IL-1, and IL-2 in mouse and human macrophages [75,76]. MPL® promotes antigen-specific DTH and a predominant murine IgG2a immunoglobulin response characteristic of TH1 help [77]. Numerous animal and human studies testify to the utility of MPL® as an adjuvant, used alone or combined effectively with other adjuvants and vehicles for capsular polysaccharide, protein, and peptide antigens [24,71,78]. In the past decade, many clinical studies have utilized MPL® or DETOX™ (MPL® plus cell wall skeleton of *Mycobacterium phlei* in a squalane-in-water emulsion vehicle) as vaccine adjuvants in volunteers [12,13,66,67,74,79–92] (Table 2). The DETOX™ adjuvant formulation has been used as therapeutic vaccines for melanoma [80,81], ovarian cancer [82], and breast cancer [83] with modest clinical success.

C. Exotoxins

The bacterial ADP-ribosylating exotoxins (bAREs) represent a potent group of proteins that have been studied as enteric, nasal, and topical adjuvants for decades, and this category includes both licensed and experimental vaccines. Cholera toxin B subunit is used to enhance the mucosal immune response in a licensed whole-cell cholera vaccine (Dukoral, PowderJect Pharmaceuticals, PLC, Oxford, UK) that contains 10^{11} killed *V. cholerae* O1 organisms including classical and El Tor Inaba and Ogawa strains [93]. The vaccine afforded a high level of protection (85%) against both classical and El Tor strains in the first 6 months [94]. However, the efficacy against El Tor waned by 36 months, particularly in young children [95]. The addition of the cholera toxin B subunit also provides short-lived efficacy (67% at 3 months) against traveler's diarrhea associated with heat-labile toxin (LT) producing enterotoxigenic *E. coli* (ETEC) [93,96].

In addition to its use in a licensed intranasal virosomal influenza vaccine (see earlier), recombinant LT, which is one of the most potent mucosal adjuvants [97], was recently shown to be safe and immunogenic by transcutaneous immunization (TCI) in humans [98]. LT-specific IgG and IgA antibodies were present in both stool and urine, implying the induction of a strong mucosal immune response. The potent activation of epidermal Langerhans cells allows LT to adjuvant the response to a coadministered antigen as well [99]. Serological and antibody-secreting cell (ASC) responses to the LT and the *E. coli* surface antigen CS6 were comparable to those seen following a protective oral challenge, suggesting that TCI can potentially elicit effective immunity similar to natural infection with ETEC [99]. Other groups are using detoxified mutants of LT to explore the potential for oral or nasal vaccination [100–102].

D. Saponins

Saponins are triterpene glycosides that can be isolated from the bark of the *Quillaja saponaria* Molina tree, a species native to South America [25]. A partially purified saponin, Quil A, has been used widely as an adjuvant in veterinary vaccines [103]. Quil A is a heterogeneous mixture of glycosides. Analysis by HPLC reveals at least 24 peaks that vary in their adjuvanticity and toxicity in mice [104]. Quil A has also been tested extensively as part of immune-stimulating complexes (ISCOMs), which are cagelike, 40-nm particles consisting of antigen, cholesterol, phospholipids, and Quil A [105]. Despite their potent adjuvanticity, ISCOM vaccines have only recently been administered to humans because of the local and systemic toxicity of Quil A in mice [105,106]. An influenza ISCOM vaccine for humans containing a less toxic saponin fraction is under development that shows a strong cellular immune response [107].

QS-21 (Stimulon™) is one of at least 24 structurally distinct triterpene glycosides isolated from Quil A. QS-21 was chosen for development by the Antigenics, Inc. (Fra-

mingham, MA), because it demonstrated the proper balance of low mouse toxicity and maximum adjuvanticity, and it eliminated the problem of lot-to-lot variation characteristic of Quil A. QS-21 is novel in that it can improve the immunogenicity of protein, and polysaccharide antigens [108] in a variety of small animals, dogs, or primates. It also uniquely stimulates both humoral and cell-mediated immunity, including potent class I-restricted cytotoxic T-lymphocyte responses to subunit antigens [109].

E. Nonionic Block Copolymers

The copolymer adjuvants are simple linear chains or blocks of polymers of hydrophobic polyoxypropylene, flanked by two chains of hydrophilic polyoxyethylene. A large number of copolymer adjuvants have been synthesized by varying the constituent chains [110]. Nonionic block copolymers are currently used commercially in over-the-counter products, including shampoos, mouthwashes, and cosmetics. Copolymers are adhesive molecules that bind antigens to hydrophobic surfaces, such as oil drops or cells [111]. Evidence suggests that proteins bound to copolymer are held firmly in a condensed fashion and retain much of their native B-cell epitope confirmation when presented to macrophages and dendritic cells for immune processing [111]. The activation of complement by contact with the copolymer surface augments the adjuvant effect. A block polymer of ethylene oxide and propylene oxide (Pluronic® L121) has been used in humans as a component of the Syntex adjuvant formulation. Several preparations of block polymers developed by Vaxcel, Inc. (Norcross, GA) are awaiting clinical trial [110,112].

F. Cytokines

The use of cytokines as vaccine adjuvants has been encouraged by better understanding of cytokine mechanisms and by the commercial availability of recombinant (IFN-γ) and granulocyte-macrophage stimulating factor (GM-CSF). Many cytokines (e.g., IL-3, IL-6, IL-11, GM-CSF) are capable of enhancing various immune responses when administered repeatedly. The cytokines with the greatest potential are those administered in a single dose at or near the time of antigen injection; cytokines administered in this practical way include IFN-α, IFN-γ, IL-1, IL-2, IL-12, and GM-CSF. The adjuvant effects of these cytokines in animals or humans have been reviewed in detail [113–115]. Trial results to date have failed to document a strong adjuvant effect for cytokines in humans [116]. It appears that cytokines have not reached their potential, because the in vivo functions of cytokine networks are complex and incompletely understood. A cytokine can enhance, inhibit, or have no effect, depending on the dose, timing, and animal species, and which of these effects predominates is not always predictable [117,118].

G. Immunostimulatory Oligonucleotides: CpGs

Just as bacterial DNA can activate immune cells, synthetic oligodeoxynucleotides (ODNs) containing unmethylated CpG dinucleotides in particular base contexts (CpG motifs) stimulate the innate immune system to induce protection in mice and primates [119,120]. Either alone or in combination with a vaccine, they can activate human B cells, DC, and NK cells [121] and trigger an immune cascade that includes the production of cytokines, chemokines, and IgM to protect against infection. CpG ODN are extremely efficient inducers of Th1 immunity and CTLs, and can allow a 10- to 100-fold reduction in the dose of antigen, presumably because of the increased efficiency of antigen presentation by DC [122]. Preliminary reports from human studies indicate safety should be expected in allergenic, cancer, and infectious vaccine applications, even at high doses [123].

VI. SUMMARY AND CONCLUSION

Every adjuvant has a complex and often multifactorial immunological mechanism, usually poorly understood in vivo. Adjuvant safety, including the real and theoretical risks of administering vaccine adjuvants to humans, is a critical component that can enhance or retard vaccine development. In addition to the problem of safety, at least four other issues impede the orderly development of adjuvanted vaccines. These include inconsistent immunopotentiation by candidate adjuvants, the unreliability of reference aluminum adjuvants, marked variation in response to the same adjuvant by different animal models, and the inability to consistently predict protective efficacy by immunoassays.

The most studied experimental adjuvants in man include aluminum compounds, oil-based emulsions with or without muramyl dipeptide, monophosphoryl (detoxified) lipid A, the triterpene glycoside QS-21, nonionic block copolymers, and several cytokines. In preclinical studies of adjuvants and vaccines, the same adjuvant can enhance, inhibit, or have no effect at all. The more important determinants of immunogenicity include the nature and dose of the immunogen, the stability of the adjuvant formulation, the schedule and route of immunization, and the animal species and strain studied. In addition to immunological enhancement without toxicity and successful protection against challenge, choice of adjuvant for a clinical trial may depend upon cost and commercial availability. Future vaccine development will focus increasingly on unique synthetic antigen constructs, DNA, and live-vector vaccines to avoid administration of extraneous chemical or biological adjuvants to humans. Until those are broadly available, the rational development of classical and novel adjuvants will continue to be one of the most important challenges for the vaccinologist.

REFERENCES

1. Ramon G. Sur l'augmentation anormale de l'antitoxine chez les chevaux producteurs de serum antidiphthérique. Bull Soc Cent Med Vet 1925; 101:227–234.
2. O'Hagan DT. Vaccine Adjuvants. Preparation Methods and Research Protocols. Totowa, NJ: Humana Press, 2000.
3. Hunter RL. Overview of vaccine adjuvants: present and future. Vaccine 2002; 20:S7–S12.
4. Kenney RT, et al. Second meeting on novel adjuvants currently in/close to human clinical testing. Vaccine 2002; 20: 2155–2163.
5. Edelman R. The development and use of vaccine adjuvants. Mol Biotechnol 2002; 21:129–148.
6. Douglas RG. The children's vaccine initiative—will it work? J Infect Dis 1993; 168:269–274.
7. Wittet S. Introducing GAVI and the Global Fund for Children's Vaccines. Vaccine 2000; 19:385–386.
8. Ramon G. Procédés pour accroitre la production des antitoxines. Ann Inst Pasteur 1926; 40:1–10.
9. Vogel FR, et al. A Compendium of Vaccine Adjuvants and Excipients. 2d ed. NIH/NIAID/DMID, http://www.niaid. nih.gov/aidsvaccine/pdf/compendium.pdf, 2001.
10. Edelman R, Tacket CO. Adjuvants. Int Rev Immunol 1990; 7:51–66.
11. Fynan EF, et al. DNA vaccines: protective immunizations by parenteral, mucosal, and gene-gun inoculations. Proc Natl Acad Sci U S A 1993; 90:11478–11482.
12. Hoffman SL, et al. Safety, immunogenicity, and efficacy of a malaria sporozoite vaccine administered with monophosphoryl lipid A, cell wall skeleton of mycobacteria, and squalane as adjuvant. Am J Trop Med Hyg 1994; 51:603–612.
13. Fries LF, et al. Liposomal malaria vaccine in humans: a safe and potent adjuvant strategy. Proc Natl Acad Sci U S A 1992; 89:358–362.
14. Lidgate DM, Byars NE. Development of an emulsion-based muramyl dipeptide adjuvant formulation for vaccines. In: Powell MF, Newman MJ, eds. Vaccine Design: The Subunit and Adjuvant Approach. New York: Plenum Press, 1995:313–324.
15. Wintsch J, et al. Safety and immunogenicity of a genetically engineered human immunodeficiency virus vaccine. J Infect Dis 1991; 163:219–225.
16. Cooper PD. The selective induction of different immune responses by vaccine adjuvants. In: Ada GL, ed. Strategies in Vaccine Design. Austin, TX: Landes, 1994:125–158.
17. Newman MJ, Powell MF. Immunological and formulation design considerations for subunit vaccines. In: Powell MF, Newman MJ, eds. Vaccine Design: The Subunit and Adjuvant Approach. New York: Plenum Press, 1995:1–42.
18. Schijns VE. Activation and of adaptive immune responses by vaccine adjuvants. Veterinary Sciences Tomorrow 2001; 3. http://www.vetscite.org (accessed August 2001).
19. HogenEsch H. Mechanisms of stimulation of the immune response by aluminum adjuvants. Vaccine 2002; 20:S34–S39.
20. Newman MJ, et al. Induction of cross-reactive cytotoxic T-lymphocyte responses specific for HIV-1 gp120 using saponin adjuvant (QS-21) supplemented subunit vaccine formulations. Vaccine 1997; 15:1001–1007.
21. Ulanova M, et al. The common vaccine adjuvant aluminum hydroxide up-regulates accessory properties of human monocytes via an interleukin-4-dependent mechanism. Infect Immun 2001; 69:1151–1159.
22. Yip HC, et al. Adjuvant-guided type-1 and type-2 immunity: infectious/noninfectious dichotomy defines the class of response. J Immunol 1999; 162:3942–3949.
23. Gupta RK, Siber GR. Comparison of adjuvant activities of aluminium phosphate, calcium phosphate and stearyl tyrosine for tetanus toxoid. Biologicals 1994; 22:53–63.
24. Ulrich JT, Myers KR. Monophosphoryl lipid A as an adjuvant: past experiences and new directions. In: Powell MF, Newman MJ, eds. The Subunit and Adjuvant Approach. New York: Plenum Press, 1995:495–524.
25. Kensil C, et al. Structural and immunological characterization of the vaccine adjuvant QS-21. In: Powell MF, Newman MJ, eds. Vaccine Design: The Subunit and Adjuvant Approach. New York: Plenum Press, 1995:525–542.
26. Hui GS, et al. Influence of adjuvants on the antibody specificity to the *Plasmodium falciparum* major merozoite surface protein, gp195. J Immunol 1991; 147:3935–3941.
27. Kenney JS, et al. Influence of adjuvants on the quantity,

affinity, isotype and epitope specificity of murine antibodies. J Immunol Methods 1989; 121:157–166.

28. Hunter RL, Lal AA. Copolymer adjuvants in malaria vaccine development. Am J Trop Med Hyg 1994; 50:52–58.

29. Siegrist CA, et al. Addition of CpG-containing oligonucleotides to a hepatitis B vaccine markedly enhances the antibody avidity maturation process in healthy adults. In: 5th Annual Conference on Vaccine Research. Washington, DC: National Foundation for Infectious Diseases, 2002 (Abstract No. S37).

30. Alving CR. Design and selection of vaccine adjuvants: animal models and human trials. Vaccine 2002; 20(suppl 3): S56–64.

31. Descotes J, et al. Vaccines: predicting the risk of allergy and autoimmunity. Toxicology 2002; 174:45–51.

32. Edelman R. Vaccine adjuvants. Rev Infect Dis 1980; 2:370–383.

33. Davenport FM. Seventeen years' experience with mineral oil adjuvant influenza virus vaccines. Ann Allergy 1968; 26:288–292.

34. Stuart-Harris CH. Adjuvant influenza vaccines. Bull World Health Organ 1969; 41:617–621.

35. Chang JC, et al. Adjuvant activity of incomplete Freund's adjuvant. Adv Drug Deliv Rev 1998; 32:173–186.

36. Beebe GW, et al. Long-term mortality follow-up of Army recruits who received adjuvant influenza virus vaccine in 1951–1953. Am J Epidemiol 1972; 95:337–346.

37. Beebe GW, et al. Follow-up study on army personnel who received adjuvant influenza virus vaccine 1951–53. Am J Med Sci 1964; 247:385–406.

38. Page WF, et al. Long-term follow-up of Army recruits immunized with Freund's incomplete adjuvanted vaccine. Vaccine Res 1993; 2:141–149.

39. Jacobson RM, et al. Adverse events and vaccination—the lack of power and predictability of infrequent events in prelicensure study. Vaccine 2001; 19:2428–2433.

40. Waters RV, et al. Uveitis induction in the rabbit by muramyl dipeptides. Infect Immun 1986; 51:816–825.

41. Allison AC, Byars NE. Immunological adjuvants: desirable properties and side-effects. Mol Immunol 1991; 28:279–284.

42. McElrath MJ. Adjuvant effects on human immune responses in recipients of candidate HIV vaccines. In: IBC Conference: Novel Vaccine Strategies for Mucosal Immunisation, Genetic Approaches, and Adjuvants, Rockville, MD, 1994.

43. Kleinau S, et al. Adjuvant oils induce arthritis in the DA rat. I. Characterization of the disease and evidence for an immunological involvement. J Autoimmun 1991; 4:871–880.

44. Murray R, et al. Mineral oil adjuvants: biological and chemical studies. Ann Allergy 1972; 30:146–151.

45. Salk J, Salk D. Control of influenza and poliomyelitis with killed virus vaccines. Science 1977; 195:834–847.

46. Gherardi RK, et al. Macrophagic myofasciitis lesions assess long-term persistence of vaccine-derived aluminium hydroxide in muscle. Brain 2001; 124:1821–1831.

47. Haigwood NL, et al. Native but not denatured recombinant human immunodeficiency virus type 1 gp120 generates broad-spectrum neutralizing antibodies in baboons. J Virol 1992; 66:172–182.

48. Sanchez-Pescador L, et al. The effect of adjuvants on the efficacy of a recombinant herpes simplex virus glycoprotein vaccine. J Immunol 1988; 141:1720–1727.

49. Aucouturier J, et al. Adjuvants designed for veterinary and human vaccines. Vaccine 2001; 19:2666–2672.

50. Bollinger JN, et al. Metabolic fate of mineral oil adjuvants using 14C-labeled tracers I: mineral oil. J Pharm Sci 1970; 59:1084–1088.

51. Allison AC. Squalene and squalane emulsions as adjuvants. Methods 1999; 19:87–93.

52. Gupta RK, Siber GR. Adjuvants for human vaccines—current status, problems and future prospects. Vaccine 1995; 13:1263–1276.

53. White RG, et al. Correlation of adjuvant activity and chemical structure of wax D fractions of mycobacteria. Immunology 1964; 7:158–163.

54. Telzak E, et al. Clinical evaluation of the immunoadjuvant murabutide, a derivative of MDP, administered with a tetanus toxoid vaccine. J Infect Dis 1986; 153:628–633.

55. Chedid LA, et al. Biological activity of a new synthetic muramyl peptide adjuvant devoid of pyrogenicity. Infect Immun 1982; 35:417–424.

56. Byars NE, et al. Enhancement of antibody responses to influenza B virus haemagglutinin by use of a new adjuvant formulation. Vaccine 1990; 8:49–56.

57. Ott G, et al. MF59. Design and evaluation of a safe and potent adjuvant for human vaccines. Pharm Biotechnol 1995; 6:277–296.

58. Audibert F, et al. Dissociation of immunostimulant activities of muramyl dipeptide (MDP) by linking amino-acids or peptides to the glutaminyl residue. Biochem Biophys Res Commun 1980; 96:915–923.

59. Tamura M, et al. Effects of muramyl dipeptide derivatives as adjuvants on the induction of antibody response to recombinant hepatitis B surface antigen. Vaccine 1995; 13:77–82.

60. McElrath MJ, et al. A phase II study of two HIV type 1 envelope vaccines, comparing their immunogenicity in populations at risk for acquiring HIV type 1 infection. AIDS Vaccine Evaluation Group. AIDS Res Hum Retroviruses 2000; 16:907–919.

61. Straus SE, et al. Immunotherapy of recurrent genital herpes with recombinant herpes simplex virus type 2 glycoproteins D and B: results of a placebo-controlled vaccine trial. J Infect Dis 1997; 176:1129–1134.

62. Koutsky LA, et al. A controlled trial of a human papillomavirus type 16 vaccine. N Engl J Med 2002; 347:1645–1651.

63. Stoute JA, et al. A preliminary evaluation of a recombinant circumsporozoite protein vaccine against Plasmodium falciparum malaria. RTS,S Malaria Vaccine Evaluation Group. N Engl J Med 1997; 336:86–91.

64. Bojang KA, et al. Efficacy of RTS,S/AS02 malaria vaccine against Plasmodium falciparum infection in semi-immune adult men in The Gambia: a randomised trial. Lancet 2001; 358:1927–1934.

65. Gerard CM, et al. Therapeutic potential of protein and adjuvant vaccinations on tumour growth. Vaccine 2001; 19:2583–2589.

66. Desombere I, et al. Immune response of HLA DQ2 positive subjects, vaccinated with HBsAg/AS04, a hepatitis B vaccine with a novel adjuvant. Vaccine 2002; 20:2597–2602.

67. McCormack S, et al. A phase I trial in HIV negative healthy volunteers evaluating the effect of potent adjuvants on immunogenicity of a recombinant gp120W61D derived from dual tropic R5X4 HIV-1ACH320. Vaccine 2000; 18:1166–1177.

68. Johnson AG, et al. Studies on the O antigen of Salmonella typhosa V. Enhancement of antibody response to protein antigens by the purified lipopolysaccharide. J Exp Med 1956; 103:225–246.

69. Luderitz O, et al. Endotoxins of gram-negative bacteria. Pharmacol Ther 1981; 15:383–402.

70. Myers KR, et al. A critical determinant of lipid A endotoxic activity. In: Nowotny A, Spitzer JJ, Ziegler EJ, eds. Cellular and Molecular Aspects of Endotoxin Reactions. Amsterdam: Elsevier, 1996:145–156.

71. Baldridge JR, Crane RT. Monophosphoryl lipid A (MPL)

formulations for the next generation of vaccines. Methods 1999; 19:103–107.

72. Schneerson R, et al. Evaluation of monophosphoryl lipid A (MPL) as an adjuvant. Enhancement of the serum antibody response in mice to polysaccharide–protein conjugates by concurrent injection with MPL. J Immunol 1991; 147:2136–2140.

73. Garg M, Subbarao B. Immune responses of systemic and mucosal lymphoid organs to Pnu-Imune vaccine as a function of age and the efficacy of monophosphoryl lipid A as an adjuvant. Infect Immun 1992; 60:2329–2336.

74. Leroux-Roels G, et al. Immunogenicity and reactogenicity of a recombinant HSV-2 glycoprotein D vaccine with or without monophosphoryl lipid A in HSV seronegative and seropositive subjects. In: 33rd Interscience Conference on Antimicrobial Agents and Chemotherapy. Washington, DC: American Society for Microbiology, 1993.

75. Dijkstra J, et al. Modulation of the biological activity of bacterial endotoxin by incorporation into liposomes. J Immunol 1987; 138:2663–2670.

76. Carozzi S, et al. Effect of monophosphoryl lipid A on the in vitro function of peritoneal leukocytes from uremic patients on continuous ambulatory peritoneal dialysis. J Clin Microbiol 1989; 27:1748–1753.

77. Gustafson GL, Rhodes MJ. Bacterial cell wall products as adjuvants: early interferon gamma as a marker for adjuvants that enhance protective immunity. Res Immunol 1992; 143:483–488.

78. Vernacchio L, et al. Effect of monophosphoryl lipid A (MPL®) on T-helper cells when administered as an adjuvant with pneumocococcal–CRM(197) conjugate vaccine in healthy toddlers. Vaccine 2002; 20:3658–3667.

79. Schultz N, et al. Effect of DETOX as an adjuvant for melanoma vaccine. Vaccine 1995; 13:503–508.

80. Mitchell MS, et al. Active-specific immunotherapy for melanoma. J Clin Oncol 1990; 8:856–869.

81. Elliott GT, et al. Interim results of a phase II multicenter clinical trial evaluating the activity of a therapeutic allogeneic melanoma vaccine (theraccine) in the treatment of disseminated malignant melanoma. Semin Surg Oncol 1993; 9:264–272.

82. MacLean GD, et al. Active immunization of human ovarian cancer patients against a common carcinoma (Thomsen-Friedenreich) determinant using a synthetic carbohydrate antigen. J Immunother 1992; 11:292–305.

83. MacLean GD, et al. Immunization of breast cancer patients using a synthetic sialyl-Tn glycoconjugate plus Detox adjuvant. Cancer Immunol Immunother 1993; 36:215–222.

84. Rickman LS, et al. Use of adjuvant containing mycobacterial cell-wall skeleton, monophosphoryl lipid A, and squalane in malaria circumsporozoite protein vaccine. Lancet 1991; 337:998–1001.

85. Van Damme P, et al. Safety, humoral, and cellular immunity of a recombinant hepatitis B vaccine with monophosphoryl lipid A in healthy volunteers. In: 33rd Interscience Conference on Antimicrobial Agents and Chemotherapy. Washington, DC: American Society for Microbiology, 1993.

86. Thoelen S, et al. Immunogenicity of a recombinant hepatitis B vaccine with monophosphoryl lipid A administered following various two-dose schedules. In: 33rd Interscience Conference on Antimicrobial Agents and Chemotherapy. Washington, DC: American Society for Microbiology, 1993.

87. Gordon DM, et al. Safety, immunogenicity, and efficacy of a recombinantly produced *Plasmodium falciparum* circumsporozoite protein–hepatitis B surface antigen subunit vaccine. J Infect Dis 1995; 171:1576–1585.

88. Leroux-Roels G, et al. Persistence of humoral and cellular immune response and booster effect following vaccination with Herpes Simplex (gD2t) candidate vaccine with MPL.

In: 34th Interscience Conference on Antimicrobial Agents and Chemotherapy. Washington, DC: American Society for Microbiology, 1994.

89. Koutsoukos M, et al. Induction of cell mediated immune responses in man with vaccines against Herpes Simplex Virus based on glycoprotein D. In: 34th Interscience Conference on Antimicrobial Agents and Chemotherapy. Washington, DC: American Society for Microbiology, 1994.

90. Thoelen S, et al. Safety and immunogenicity of a hepatitis B vaccine formulated with a novel adjuvant system. Vaccine 1998; 16:708–714.

91. Drachenberg KJ, et al. A well-tolerated grass pollen-specific allergy vaccine containing a novel adjuvant, monophosphoryl lipid A, reduces allergic symptoms after only four preseasonal injections. Allergy 2001; 56:498–505.

92. Le TP, et al. Immunogenicity of *Plasmodium falciparum* circumsporozoite protein multiple antigen peptide vaccine formulated with different adjuvants. Vaccine 1998; 16:305–312.

93. Ryan ET, Calderwood SB. Cholera vaccines. Clin Infect Dis 2000; 31:561–565.

94. Clemens JD, et al. Field trial of oral cholera vaccines in Bangladesh. Lancet 1986; 2:124–127.

95. van Loon FP, et al. Field trial of inactivated oral cholera vaccines in Bangladesh: results from 5 years of follow-up. Vaccine 1996; 14:162–166.

96. Clemens JD, et al. Cross-protection by B subunit-whole cell cholera vaccine against diarrhea associated with heat-labile toxin-producing enterotoxigenic *Escherichia coli*: results of a large-scale field trial. J Infect Dis 1988; 158:372–377.

97. Singh M, O'Hagan D. Advances in vaccine adjuvants. Nat Biotechnol 1999; 17:1075–1081.

98. Glenn GM, et al. Transcutaneous immunization: a human vaccine delivery strategy using a patch. Nat Med 2000; 6:1403–1406.

99. Güereña-Burgueño F, et al. Safety and immunogenicity of a prototype enterotoxigenic *Escherichia coli* vaccine administered transcutaneously. Infect Immun 2002; 70:1874–1880.

100. Barackman JD, et al. Oral administration of influenza vaccine in combination with the adjuvants LT-K63 and LT-R72 induces potent immune responses comparable to or stronger than traditional intramuscular immunization. Clin Diagn Lab Immunol 2001; 8:652–657.

101. Ryan EJ, et al. Mutants of *Escherichia coli* heat-labile toxin act as effective mucosal adjuvants for nasal delivery of an acellular pertussis vaccine: differential effects of the nontoxic AB complex and enzyme activity on Th1 and Th2 cells. Infect Immun 1999; 67:6270–6280.

102. Kotloff KL, et al. Safety and immunogenicity of oral inactivated whole-cell *Helicobacter pylori* vaccine with adjuvant among volunteers with or without subclinical infection. Infect Immun 2001; 69:3581–3590.

103. Campbell JB, Peerbaye YA. Saponin. Res Immunol 1992; 143:526–530. Discussion, 577–578.

104. Kensil CR, et al. Separation and characterization of saponins with adjuvant activity from *Quillaja saponaria* Molina cortex. J Immunol 1991; 146:431–437.

105. Rimmelzwaan GF, Osterhaus A. A novel generation of viral vaccines based on the ISCOM matrix. In: Powell MF, Newman MJ, eds. Vaccine Design: The Subunit and Adjuvant Approach. New York: Plenum Press, 1995:543–558.

106. Rönnberg B, et al. Adjuvant activity of non-toxic *Quillaja saponaria* Molina components for use in ISCOM matrix. Vaccine 1995; 13:1375–1382.

107. Ennis FA, et al. Augmentation of human influenza A virus-specific cytotoxic T lymphocyte memory by influenza vaccine and adjuvanted carriers (ISCOMS). Virology 1999; 259:256–261.

108. Coughlin RT, et al. Adjuvant activity of QS-21 for experimental *E. coli* 018 polysaccharide vaccines. Vaccine 1995; 13:17–21.

109. Shirai M, et al. Helper-cytotoxic T lymphocyte (CTL) determinant linkage required for priming of anti-HIV CD8+ CTL in vivo with peptide vaccine constructs. J Immunol 1994; 152:543–556.

110. Brey RN. Development of vaccines based on formulations containing nonionic block polymers. In: Powell MF, Newman MJ, eds. Vaccine Design: The Subunit and Adjuvant Approach. New York: Plenum Press, 1995:297–312.

111. Hunter RL, Bennett B. The adjuvant activity of nonionic block polymer surfactants. II. Antibody formation and inflammation related to the structure of triblock and octablock copolymers. J Immunol 1984; 133:3167–3175.

112. Newman MJ, et al. Use of nonionic block copolymers in vaccines and therapeutics. Crit Rev Ther Drug Carrier Syst 1998; 15:89–142.

113. Lin R, et al. Present status of the use of cytokines as adjuvants with vaccines to protect against infectious diseases. Clin Infect Dis 1995; 21:1439–1449.

114. O'Hagan DT, et al. Recent developments in adjuvants for vaccines against infectious diseases. Biomol Eng 2001; 18:69–85.

115. Schijns VE. Induction and direction of immune responses by vaccine adjuvants. Crit Rev Immunol 2001; 21:75–85.

116. Evans TG, et al. The safety and efficacy of GM-CSF as an adjuvant in hepatitis B vaccination of chronic hemodialysis patients who have failed primary vaccination. Clin Nephrol 2000; 54:138–142.

117. Sturchler D, et al. Effects of interferons on immune response to a synthetic peptide malaria sporozoite vaccine in non-immune adults. Vaccine 1989; 7:457–461.

118. Heath AW, Playfair JH. Cytokines as immunological adjuvants. Vaccine 1992; 10:427–434.

119. Krieg AM, et al. CpG motifs in bacterial DNA trigger direct B-cell activation. Nature 1995; 374:546–549.

120. Verthelyi D, et al. CpG oligodeoxynucleotides as vaccine adjuvants in primates. J Immunol 2002; 168:1659–1663.

121. Verthelyi D, et al. Human peripheral blood cells differentially recognize and respond to two distinct CPG motifs. J Immunol 2001; 166:2372–2377.

122. Krieg AM. From bugs to drugs: therapeutic immunomodulation with oligodeoxynucleotides containing CpG sequences from bacterial DNA. Antisense Nucleic Acid Drug Dev 2001; 11:181–188.

123. Agrawal S, Kandimalla ER. Medicinal chemistry and therapeutic potential of CpG DNA. Trends Mol Med 2002; 8:114–121.

124. Keefer MC, et al. Safety and immunogenicity of Env 2–3, a human immunodeficiency virus type 1 candidate vaccine, in combination with a novel adjuvant, MTP-PE/MF59. NIAID AIDS Vaccine Evaluation Group. AIDS Res Hum Retroviruses 1996; 12:683–693.

125. Gorse GJ, et al. HIV-1MN recombinant glycoprotein 160 vaccine-induced cellular and humoral immunity boosted by HIV-1MN recombinant glycoprotein 120 vaccine. National Institute of Allergy and Infectious Diseases AIDS Vaccine Evaluation Group. AIDS Res Hum Retroviruses 1999; 15:115–132.

126. Kahn JO, et al. Clinical and immunologic responses to human immunodeficiency virus (HIV) type 1SF2 gp120 subunit vaccine combined with MF59 adjuvant with or without muramyl tripeptide dipalmitoyl phosphatidylethanolamine in non-HIV-infected human volunteers. J Infect Dis 1994; 170:1288–1291.

127. Graham BS, et al. Safety and immunogenicity of a candidate HIV-1 vaccine in healthy adults: recombinant glycoprotein (rgp) 120. A randomized, double-blind trial. NIAID AIDS Vaccine Evaluation Group. Ann Intern Med 1996; 125:270–279.

128. Klein MR, et al. Gag-specific immune responses after immunization with p17/p24:Ty virus-like particles in HIV type 1-seropositive individuals. AIDS Res Hum Retroviruses 1997; 13:393–399.

129. Trauger RJ, et al. Effect of immunization with inactivated gp120-depleted human immunodeficiency virus type 1 (HIV-1) immunogen on HIV-1 immunity, viral DNA, and percentage of CD4 cells. J Infect Dis 1994; 169:1256–1264.

130. Turner JL, et al. Double-blind placebo-controlled dose ranging study of Salk immunogen in asymptomatic patients with early human immunodeficiency virus infection (PoB3043) [B94 Abstract]. Program and Abstracts VIII International Conference on AIDS/III STD World Congress, Amsterdam, 1992.

131. Churdboonchart V, et al. A double-blind, adjuvant-controlled trial of human immunodeficiency virus type 1 (HIV-1) immunogen (Remune) monotherapy in asymptomatic, HIV-1-infected Thai subjects with CD4-cell counts of >300. Clin Diagn Lab Immunol 2000; 7:728–733.

132. Toledo H, et al. A phase I clinical trial of a multi-epitope polypeptide TAB9 combined with Montanide ISA 720 adjuvant in non-HIV-1 infected human volunteers. Vaccine 2001; 19:4328–4336.

133. Cano CA. The multi-epitope polypeptide approach in HIV-1 vaccine development. Genet Anal 1999; 15:149–153.

134. Keitel W, et al. Pilot evaluation of influenza virus vaccine (IVV) combined with adjuvant. Vaccine 1993; 11:909–913.

135. Powers DC, et al. In previously immunized elderly adults inactivated influenza A (H1N1) virus vaccines induce poor antibody responses that are not enhanced by liposome adjuvant. Vaccine 1995; 13:1330–1335.

136. Van Hoecke C, et al. Humoral and cellular immune responses to three formulations of inactivated split influenza vaccine (ISIV) adjuvanted with QS-21. In: 35th Interscience Conference on Antimicrobial Agents and Chemotherapy. Washington, DC: American Society for Microbiology, 1995.

137. Baldo V, et al. Comparison of three different influenza vaccines in institutionalised elderly. Vaccine 2001; 19:3472–3475.

138. Pregliasco F, et al. Immunogenicity and safety of three commercial influenza vaccines in institutionalized elderly. Aging (Milano) 2001; 13:38–43.

139. Quiroga JA, et al. Recombinant gamma-interferon as adjuvant to hepatitis B vaccine in hemodialysis patients. Hepatology 1990; 12:661–663.

140. Patou G, et al. Gamma interferon as an adjuvant to hepatitis B vaccine [abstract]. J Interferon Res 1989; 9:S261.

141. Grob PJ, et al. Interferon as an adjuvant for hepatitis B vaccination in non-and low-responder populations. Eur J Clin Microbiol 1984; 3:195–198.

142. Meuer SC, et al. Low-dose interleukin-2 induces systemic immune responses against HBsAg in immunodeficient non-responders to hepatitis B vaccination. Lancet 1989; 1:15–18.

143. Jungers P, et al. Randomised placebo-controlled trial of recombinant interleukin-2 in chronic uraemic patients who are non-responders to hepatitis B vaccine. Lancet 1994; 344:856–857.

144. Jacques P, et al. The immunogenicity and reactogenicity profile of a candidate hepatitis B vaccine in an adult vaccine non-responder population. Vaccine 2002; 20:3644–3649.

145. Tacket CO, et al. Phase 1 safety and immune response studies of a DNA vaccine encoding hepatitis B surface antigen delivered by a gene delivery device. Vaccine 1999; 17:2826–2829.

146. Kotloff KL, et al. Safety and immunogenicity of increasing doses of a *Clostridium difficile* toxoid vaccine administered to healthy adults. Infect Immun 2001; 69:988–995.

147. Olberling F, et al. Enhancement of antibody response to a natural fragment of streptococcal M protein by Murabitide administered to healthy volunteers. Int J Immunol 1983; 1983:398.

148. Feder HM Jr, et al. Immunogenicity of a recombinant *Borrelia burgdorferi* outer surface protein A vaccine against Lyme disease in children. J Pediatr 1999; 135:575–579.

149. Edelman R, et al. Safety and immunogenicity of recombinant Bacille Calmette–Guerin (rBCG) expressing *Borrelia burgdorferi* outer surface protein A (OspA) lipoprotein in adult volunteers: a candidate Lyme disease vaccine. Vaccine 1999; 17:904–914.

150. Monjour L, et al. Protective immunity against cutaneous leishmaniasis achieved by partly purified vaccine in a volunteer. Lancet 1986; 1:1490.

151. Khalil EA, et al. Autoclaved *Leishmania major* vaccine for prevention of visceral leishmaniasis: a randomised, double-blind, BCG-controlled trial in Sudan. Lancet 2000; 356: 1565–1569.

152. Satti IN, et al. Immunogenicity and safety of autoclaved *Leishmania major* plus BCG vaccine in healthy Sudanese volunteers. Vaccine 2001; 19:2100–2106.

153. Sturchler D, et al. Interferon-alpha and synthetic peptide malaria sporozoite vaccine in non-immune adults: antibody response after 40 weeks. Bull World Health Organ 1990; 68(suppl):38–41.

154. Heppner DG, et al. Safety, immunogenicity, and efficacy of *Plasmodium falciparum* repeatless circumsporozoite protein vaccine encapsulated in liposomes. J Infect Dis 1996; 174: 361–366.

155. Nardin EH, et al. Synthetic malaria peptide vaccine elicits high levels of antibodies in vaccinees of defined HLA genotypes. J Infect Dis 2000; 182:1486–1496.

156. Genton B, et al. Safety and immunogenicity of a three-component blood-stage malaria vaccine in adults living in an endemic area of Papua New Guinea. Vaccine 2000; 18:2504–2511.

157. Saul A, et al. Human phase I vaccine trials of 3 recombinant asexual stage malaria antigens with Montanide ISA720 adjuvant. Vaccine 1999; 17:3145–3159.

158. Khleif SN, et al. A phase I vaccine trial with peptides reflecting ras oncogene mutations of solid tumors. J Immunother 1999; 22:155–165.

159. Gonzalez G, et al. A novel cancer vaccine composed of human-recombinant epidermal growth factor linked to a carrier protein: report of a pilot clinical trial. Ann Oncol 1998; 9:431–435.

160. Triozzi PL, et al. Effects of a beta-human chorionic gonadotropin subunit immunogen administered in aqueous solution with a novel nonionic block copolymer adjuvant in patients with advanced cancer. Clin Cancer Res 1997; 3: 2355–2362.

161. Triozzi PL, et al. Phase Ib trial of a synthetic beta human chorionic gonadotropin vaccine in patients with metastatic cancer. Ann N Y Acad Sci 1993; 690:358–359.

162. Harro CD, et al. Safety and immunogenicity trial in adult volunteers of a human papillomavirus 16 L1 virus-like particle vaccine. J Natl Cancer Inst 2001; 93:284–292.

163. Adler A, et al. Allogeneic human liposomal melanoma vaccine with or without IL-2 in metastatic melanoma patients: clinical and immunobiological effects. Cancer Biother 1995; 10:293–306.

164. Jones WR, et al. Phase I clinical trial of a World Health Organisation birth control vaccine. Lancet 1988; 1:1295–1298.

165. Snyder LL, et al. Synthetic hormone/growth factor subunit vaccine with application to antifertility and cancer. In: Powell MF, Newman MJ, eds. Vaccine Design: The Subunit and Adjuvant Approach. New York: Plenum Press, 1995:907–930.

19

MF59 Adjuvant Emulsion

Audino Podda and Giuseppe Del Giudice
Chiron S.r.l., Siena, Italy

I. INTRODUCTION

Most of the existing vaccines share two general characteristics; with very few exceptions, they are parenterally administered. In addition, they are formulated together with adjuvants with the aim of enhancing their immunogenicity. The need for the use of adjuvants is particularly evident for highly purified recombinant or subunit antigens, which are generally very poorly immunogenic when delivered as such. Adjuvants can significantly influence the outcome of the immune response to vaccine molecules, both quantitatively and qualitatively. As a consequence, the use of inappropriate adjuvants may adversely affect the development of new vaccines either by the conventional approach to antigen selection or by the emerging genomic approach [1].

Major efforts have been made in the past decades to develop new vaccine adjuvants; a very long list of adjuvants has been proposed and several of them have even been tested in humans in association with a variety of vaccines or vaccine candidates [2]. Despite all these efforts, aluminum salts, the first vaccine adjuvants introduced during the 1920s, remain the standard adjuvants admitted worldwide for human use. Several reasons have determined this negative outcome in adjuvant research. For sure, safety has represented one of the major limiting factors in the introduction of new adjuvants. On the other hand, not all adjuvants are equally effective for all vaccine constructs. For example, it is well known that aluminum salts fail to exert appropriate adjuvanticity for influenza vaccines, for some Hib conjugate vaccines, and for some recombinant antigens and synthetic peptides [2].

In 1997, the MF59 adjuvant emulsion was the first new adjuvant to be licensed for human use 70 years after the introduction of aluminum salts and remains the only adjuvant licensed for human use in addition to alum. MF59 was licensed after the successful outcome of a long-lasting preclinical experience and an extensive clinical testing that yielded a database of more than 20,000 subjects, 12,000 of which were immunized with one or more doses of the influenza adjuvanted vaccine. Today MF59 is licensed in most European countries and its safety has been supported

by more than ten million doses of vaccine distributed so far. In this chapter, we will briefly summarize the characteristics of the MF59 adjuvant; we will go through the animal testing with various vaccines and comment on the immune response induced; finally, we will give some details on the extensive clinical experience not only with the licensed influenza vaccine, but also with other investigational vaccines, safely and efficiently tested in different age groups.

II. THE MF59 ADJUVANT

MF59 is an oil-in-water emulsion consisting of small (< 250 nm in diameter), uniform, and stable microparticles made by a drop of oil surrounded by a coat of water droplets held onto the oil by surface detergents. The oil is the natural and fully metabolizable squalene. This oil is obtained from shark liver and is also found in humans as a natural metabolite of cholesterol and is a normal component of cell membranes. Squalene droplets are stabilized by addition of two emulsifiers, a water-soluble surfactant, the polyoxyethylene sorbitan monoleate (Tween 80), and an oil-soluble surfactant, sorbitan trioleate (Span 85) [3].

For manufacturing of stable and uniform emulsions, a key point is to keep the number of large particles down to a minimum because large particles act as nucleation sites for further aggregation during storage, potentially leading to phase separation. Indeed, emulsions tend to be thermodynamically unstable systems, subject to flocculation and coalescence during storage. For MF59, the reduction in the number of large particles is achieved by microfluidization and filtration of the emulsion through a 0.22-μm membrane. This procedure removes 99.5% of particles larger than 1.2 μm, so that particles of this size are < 0.1% in the final bulk. The mean particle size, the squalene concentration, and the pH remain unchanged from initial values for at least 3 years at 4°C, providing an excellent stability to vaccine formulations adjuvanted with MF59. Importantly, the number of large particle per milliliter of MF59 also remained stably very low during the same period of time.

A wide variety of vaccine antigens have been formulated with MF59, either premixed in a single container or in separate vials to be mixed just before use. It is interesting to note that antigens successfully formulated in a single container with MF59 can have quite diverse physical–chemical characteristics. Some are fully soluble antigens, such as the HSV-2 gD protein; others are hydrophobic, representing proteins with an intrinsic ability to self-associate or to associate with lipid bilayers or emulsions, such as the influenza HA. Finally, other proteins are particulate antigens, such as HBsAg containing the preS region. All this shows the large versatility of the MF59 as a stable vaccine adjuvant.

III. MECHANISM OF ADJUVANTICITY OF MF59 AND QUALITY OF IMMUNE RESPONSE INDUCED

Although vaccine adjuvants have been used for more than 70 years, very little is known on the exact mechanisms behind their biological effect. The depot effect postulated for aluminum salts and other adjuvants cannot explain, by itself, all the immunological phenomena that are triggered by vaccine adjuvants, and that bring the activation and recruitment of professional antigen-presenting cells (APC), which, in turn, induce the activation and expansion of antigen-specific T cell and then B cell populations.

During the past few years, a big explosion of research has been experienced in the field of innate immunity [4]. This has brought the recognition of several molecules and their relevant ligands important in the first line of defense against invading microorganisms. These findings are turning out to be instrumental in the understanding of the mechanisms of adjuvanticity of several substances, mainly those derived from bacterial components. The family of the Toll-like receptors (TLR), first described in *Drosophila*, is emerging as a key player in the delivery of initial signals not only by invading pathogens, but also by some of their ingredients, which can be used as vaccine adjuvants. Activation of cells by lipopolysaccharides (LPS) requires the presence on APC of an intact TLR4: This will induce the expression of inflammatory cytokines and of costimulatory molecules [5]. In addition to LPS, TLR4 is also implicated in the recognition of the heat shock protein of 60 kDa (hsp60) [6] and of lipoteichoic acid [7], which have been known for a while for their adjuvant activity [2]. By forming heterodimers with TLR1 and TLR6, TLR2 recognizes several microbial components, such as peptidoglycan, bacterial lipoproteins, and zymosan [8,9]. It is likely that the strong adjuvant activity of complete Freund's adjuvant, which contains mycobacteria, and of monophosphoryl lipid A (MPL), derived from the bacterial cell wall, may be at least partly explained by the interaction with TLR2. Finally, the strong immunostimulatory effect of unmethylated CpG DNA oligonucleotides, which leads to the strong induction of Th1-type response, has been shown to be mediated by a specific recognition of TLR9 by these motifs [10]. This leads to the activation of macrophages and dendritic cells (DC), upregulation of major histocompatibility complex (MHC) class I molecules and of costimulatory molecules, and to the production of pro-inflammatory (Th1-type) cytokines.

The MF59 does not contain any microbial component. Thus there is no indication that its mechanism(s) of action may be mediated by iterations with Toll-like receptors. The fine mechanisms of MF59 adjuvanticity are still unknown. Studies conducted with fluorescent-labeled MF59 have shown that 4 hr after intramuscular (i.m.) administration, 36% of the injected adjuvant was in the muscle and that the peak of localization in the draining lymph nodes was maximal 2 days after injection. It is noteworthy that the presence of the adjuvant did not influence the distribution of the coadministered antigen (HSV-2 gD), which was cleared from the site of injection independently of MF59. Using the same technology, it was shown that 2 days after i.m. injection, MF59 localized inside cells that had all the characteristics of APC, mainly of mature macrophages. Administration of MF59 clearly induced a significant influx of macrophages at the site of injection, which was significantly suppressed in mice deficient for the chemokine receptor 2 (CCR2) [11,12].

Irrespective of its mechanism(s) of action, the available data strongly support the notion that MF59 predominantly induces Th2-type immune responses, as evidenced by the immunoglobulin isotypes and by the cytokines induced after immunization in mice. Indeed, mice immunized with MF59-adjuvanted influenza vaccine exhibited significant increase in the levels of IL-5 and IL-6 (but not of IFN-γ) [13,14], which peaked already 3–12 hr after immunization [13]. A more pronounced IL-4 and IL-5 induction was also observed in mice immunized with the HSV-2 gD2 antigen given together with MF59 [15]. In agreement with the cytokine data, mouse receiving MF59-adjuvanted flu vaccine [14], HSV-2 gD2 antigen [15], or *Neisseria meningitidis* outer membrane proteins [16] produced higher titers of antigen-specific IgG1 than IgG2a. An in-depth knowledge of the mechanism(s) behind the adjuvanticity of MF59 will shed light on the propensity of this adjuvant to preferentially induce Th2-type immune responses.

IV. THE PRECLINICAL EXPERIENCE WITH MF59-ADJUVANTED VACCINES

MF59 has been utilized by several groups, both inside and outside Chiron Corporation, to evaluate the enhancement of the immunogenicity and of the efficacy of several vaccine constructs in various animal models. In several cases, as with influenza vaccine, HSV-2 antigens, human immunodeficiency virus (HIV) antigens, hepatitis C virus (HCV) antigens, etc., these studies have been instrumental to move to clinical studies in humans. The clinical experience with MF59 is now so wide, also in consideration of the existence of licensed MF59-adjuvanted vaccines, that we will only give an overview of the preclinical experience with this adjuvant limited to a few model vaccines to give more emphasis to the clinical studies at all ages, from elderly people to newborns, which have confirmed in humans some of the findings obtained in animals. Those readers interested in a detailed description of the animal studies performed with MF59-adjuvanted vaccines and appeared in literature up to now (Spring 2002) are referred to in Table 1, which provides an almost comprehensive list of the published papers.

Table 1 Summary of the Major Studies Carried Out in Animals with Immunogens Adjuvanted with MF59

Microorganism	Antigen(s)	Animal species	Comments	Ref.
HSV-2	gD2	Hartley guinea pigs	Therapeutic efficacy of the vaccine against recurrent genital disease.	[23]
	gB2, gD2	NZW rabbits	Periocular (subconjunctival) therapeutic immunization in HSV-1-infected rabbits induces an 8–60-fold increase in antibody titers and reduction of viral shedding.	[25]
	gD1, gD2	NZW rabbits	Therapeutic efficacy with reduced recurrence of herpetic keratitis after periocular immunization. With gD1 reduced viral shedding.	[28]
	gB2, gD2	NZW rabbits	Prophylactic efficacy against HSV-1 infection (conjunctivitis, iritis) after periocular, but not after systemic immunization.	[27]
	gB2, gD2	NZW rabbits	Therapeutic efficacy after periocular, but not after systemic immunization: less viral shedding and specific IgA in the tears.	[26]
	gD2	BALB/c mice	More pronounced Th2-type immune response than PLG	[15]
	gD2	BALB/c mice	High serum IgG titers and high neutralizing antibody titers	[57]
	gD2	Hartley guinea pigs	Protection against intravaginal challenge	[24]
Influenza virus	Subunit vaccine	BALB/c mice	Pronounced Th2-type profile of serum cytokines	[13]
	Split vaccine	BALB/c mice, Syrian hamsters, Hartley guinea pigs, NZW rabbits, Beagle dogs, goats	Very strong enhancement of the antibody response. Tested with and without MTP, which gives little increase in antibody response.	[17]
	Subunit vaccine	BALB/c mice	Significant enhancement of the antibody response in old mice, and in old mice previously infected with influenza virus. Pronounced Th2-type immune response.	[14]
	Subunit vaccine	BALB/c mice	Protection against intranasal challenge, long-lasting	[18]
	Subunit vaccine	BALB/c mice	Intranasal administration for priming and boosting	[58]
HIV-1	gp120	Chimpanzees	One animal fully protected against homologous challenge. The other animal with transient infection.	[29]
	gp120	Chimpanzees	After priming with adenovirus and boost with MF59, three out of four animals had neutralizing antibodies and were protected. Antibodies and protection persisted.	[30]
	gp120	Rhesus monkeys	Heterologous boosting does not protect.	[59]
	gp120	Rhesus monkeys	Three out of four with full protection against challenge with SHIV. In the fourth monkey, transient infection.	[31]
	gp120, p24	BALB/c mice, baboons	Together with PLG, enhancement of antibody and cellular responses.	[60]
HBV	HbsAg + preS2	Baboons	Stronger and faster induction of protective antibody titers (>10 mIU/mL) that alum adjuvanted vaccine and than commercially available vaccines	[19]
HCV	E1–E2	Chimpanzees	Full protection against homologous challenge with the highest antibody titers, or milder disease	[20]
HPV-16b	E7	DBA/2, BALB/c mice	Induction of specific CD8+ CTL similar to that achieved with vaccinia virus	[61]
HPV-6b	VLPs	BALB/c mice	Strong serum IgG response.	[62]
H. influenzae b, N. meningitidis C	Conjugate vaccine (oligosaccharide + CRM197)	Baboons	In 1–4 months old animals, 7-fold enhancement of the antibody response and 5–10-fold increase of bactericidal antibody titers. Induction of strong B cell memory	[32]
N. meningitidis	Outer membrane complexes	BALB/c mice	Enhancement of IgG antibody and of bactericidal antibody titers.	[16]
E. coli	FimH adhesin	Cynomolgus monkeys	After bladder challenge, three out of four protected against bacteriuria and pyuria.	[34]
Plasmodium falciparum	MSP1	Aotus monkeys	Lower antibody responses than with Freund's; no protection against challenge.	[63]

A. Influenza Virus

It is commonly accepted that influenza vaccine is mainly recommended for elderly people who are at higher risk of contracting serious and life-threatening complications following influenza infection. Unadjuvanted, split, and subunit vaccines are commonly available. However, there is a general agreement on the need to enhance the immunogenicity and the efficacy of these vaccines, especially at the elderly age when the ability of the immune system to mount strong and efficacious responses generally decreases. It is known that aluminum salts do not work as adjuvants for these vaccines.

A very large experience has been acquired in the past 10 years on the use of MF59 as a strong adjuvant to enhance the immunogenicity of the influenza vaccine in several animal species, including old mice. Indeed, MF59 was proved to strongly enhance the immunogenicity of flu vaccines in mice, hamsters, guinea pigs, dogs, and goats inducing antibody titers 5 to > 100 times higher than those obtained in the absence of adjuvants [17]. It is noteworthy that old mice responded very poorly to immunization with a conventional (nonadjuvanted) subunit vaccine, as compared to young, fully immune competent mice. However, when old mice were immunized with the same vaccine admixed together with MF59, antigen-specific antibody titers increased at levels normally encountered in young animals [14]. Importantly, this enhancement of the immune response to the vaccine was not affected by a preexisting immunity to the virus, because post-immunization antibody titers remained high in mice that had been previously infected with a homologous viral strain [14]. These data are of particular importance because vaccination against influenza is routinely carried out every year, and a preexisting immunity can negatively affect the efficacy of subsequent vaccinations. Additional studies very clearly showed that the use of the adjuvant MF59 permitted to decrease the amount of vaccine to be used per dose to induce a strong immune response, to significantly decrease the viral load in the lungs of mice, and to significantly protect against an infectious challenge, even 126 and 200 days post immunization [18].

B. Hepatitis B Virus and Hepatitis C Virus

A dramatically strong adjuvanticity was exerted by MF59 in baboons for a CHO-derived hepatitis B virus (HBV) vaccine containing the preS2 component [19]. As compared to a similar vaccine adjuvanted with aluminum hydroxide, or with two commercially available vaccines, the MF59-adjuvanted vaccine generated protective levels of antibodies (i.e., > 10 mIU/mL) in a larger number of animals, with antibody titers higher than up to 127-fold than those obtained with conventional vaccines. These very high protective antibody titers were still persisting several months after the third immunization. These results have been, then, successfully confirmed in humans vaccinated with the MF59-adjuvanted HBV vaccine (see below).

If vaccines against HBV exist, although their effectiveness can be ameliorated, vaccines against HCV are not available. Using the E1–E2 envelope glycoproteins derived from an eukaryotic expression system, it was shown that immunization together with MF59 (plus MTP) induced a strong antigen-specific antibody response. The animals with the highest antibody titers were fully protected against an infectious challenge with the homologous virus, whereas the two vaccinated monkeys that became infected exhibited an infection and a disease milder than those observed in control monkeys [20]. It was subsequently shown that such protection could have been mediated by antibodies able to specifically inhibit the binding of the E1 glycoprotein to its cell receptor [21]. This finding was instrumental in the discovery of CD81 as the receptor for HCV [22].

C. Herpes Simplex Virus and Human Immunodeficiency Virus

The efficacy of MF59-adjuvanted vaccines was also demonstrated in experimental models of infection with herpes simplex virus (HSV) and HIV. Immunization with the gD2 recombinant proteins along with MF59 efficiently protected guinea pigs against recurrent genital disease both therapeutically [23] and prophylactically [24]. In addition, periocular (subconjunctival) immunization of rabbits with gB and gD proteins efficiently prevented HSV-1 infection in the eye (conjunctivitis, iritis) [25–28]. The same procedure exhibited therapeutic efficacy against herpetic keratitis [25–28].

Most of the chimpanzees immunized with recombinant gp120 given with MF59, either as such [29] or as a boost to a primary immunization provided with adenoviruses expressing the gp120 [30], were protected against a challenge with homologous HIV. Similar good levels of protection were achieved in immunized rhesus monkeys subsequently challenged with SHIV [31].

D. Bacterial Vaccines

An important objective for future vaccines or vaccination strategies will be to anticipate the timing of immunization to confer protection right after birth, mainly for those diseases, such as meningitis, which have a particularly high morbidity during the very first months of life. Using infant baboons as an experimental model, it was shown that MF59 significantly enhanced the protective (bactericidal) antibody response to bacterial capsular polysaccharides of *Haemophilus influenzae* type b and of group C *N. meningitidis*, when they were given as conjugate vaccines [32]. As compared to the conventional alum-adjuvanted vaccines, the vaccine containing MF59 induced five to seven times higher titers of bactericidal antibodies, which still persisted at these high levels 31 weeks after the third immunization.

Uropathogenic *Escherichia coli* is the major cause of urinary tract infections. FimH is an adhesin crucial in the colonization of the urinary bladder mucosa [33]. Immunization of cynomolgus monkeys immunized three times with recombinant FimH plus MF59 induced a strong and sustained antigen-specific antibody response. Very importantly, three out of four monkeys were protected against bacteriuria and pyuria from a challenge with an infectious uropathogenic *E. coli* isolate [34].

V. CLINICAL EXPERIENCE

Extensive clinical research programs have been carried out for the development of several MF59-adjuvanted vaccines, mostly against viral diseases. The clinical experience spaced across all age groups; depending on the type of vaccine, clinical trials with MF59-adjuvanted vaccines have been performed in elderly subjects, younger adults, adolescents, children, and even newborns in some cases.

A. Adult Immunization

1. Influenza Virus Vaccine

Conventional influenza vaccines are highly effective (70–90%) in young adults, particularly when the vaccine composition closely matches the epidemic influenza strain [35–37]. However, their efficacy considerably drops in elderly subjects. More specifically, conventional vaccines have a limited efficacy to protect the elderly from an influenza infection, as shown in a review of influenza vaccine effectiveness in elderly subjects, which reports a reduction in mortality of 74% and 47% (institutionalized and noninstitutionalized subjects, respectively), but a prevention of clinical illness in only 33% and 5% of the subjects [38]. The reduced immunogenicity of influenza vaccines in elderly subjects [39,40] is one of the factors that might explain the decreased efficacy of conventional influenza vaccines in this age group [38,41,42]. As shown in the preclinical studies, MF59 significantly increases the response to influenza vaccination in aged mice with depressed antibody and cellular immune response, as well as altered cytokine response [3,14]. Therefore the preclinical data and the medical need to develop more immunogenic vaccines for the elderly have targeted the clinical development of this adjuvanted vaccine for the elderly age group. This is the reason why the great majority of the over 20,000 subjects evaluated in the clinical development program of the MF59-adjuvanted influenza vaccine were elderly subjects [43].

Most of these clinical trials were aimed to compare the safety and immunogenicity of the new vaccine with that of nonadjuvanted conventional vaccines. Influenza vaccines, because of the frequent change in their antigenic composition, are normally administered every year; therefore it is extremely important to evaluate the profile of any new influenza vaccine also after repeated administrations. This approach was followed in the clinical development of the MF59-adjuvanted vaccine whose safety and immunogenicity profiles were evaluated after repeated immunization during three consecutive influenza seasons [44,45].

Safety. In elderly subjects, MF59-adjuvanted influenza vaccine is safe and very well tolerated. Because of the presence of the adjuvant, the rates of local adverse reactions, particularly local pain, were increased in the recipients of the MF59 vaccine; however, most of the reactions were mild in nature, of short duration, and qualitatively similar to those induced by control vaccines [43–47]. Additionally, the repeated immunization of elderly subjects with the adjuvanted vaccine across subsequent influenza seasons did not exhibit any increased reactogenicity [44,45]. More clinically relevant adverse events, also monitored during the clinical trials, were rare and quantitatively similar to those induced or temporally associated with control vaccines [43].

Immunogenicity. The immune response to immunization was assessed by standard and validated procedures

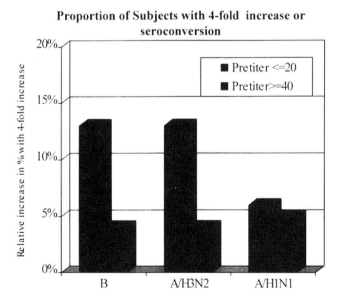

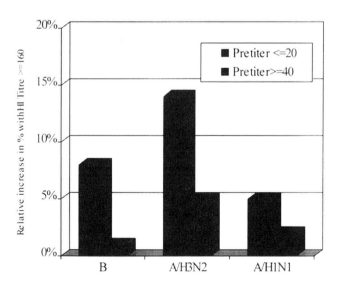

Figure 1 Increased adjuvant effect in elderly subjects susceptible to influenza. The MF59 adjuvant effect on the immunogenicity of subunit influenza antigens is enhanced in elderly subjects with low preimmunization titer. Both the proportion of subjects with fourfold increase or seroconversion and that of subjects with highly protective postimmunization titers (i.e., ≥160) are significantly higher in subjects with low preimmunization titers (i.e., ≤20). (From Ref. 43.)

(haemagglutination inhibition assay), which are known to correlate with clinical protection [48–52]. The statistical analyses were based on several immunogenicity measures, including geometric mean titers and ratios, proportions of subjects with seroconversion and proportions of subjects achieving accepted thresholds of protection [i.e., 40 (PL50) and 160 (PL90)] after immunization [53].

The adjuvant effect of MF59, resulting in an increased immunogenicity compared to conventional vaccines, particularly for the A/H3N2 and B strains, was a consistent finding of clinical trials in elderly [43–47]. This enhanced immunogenicity of MF59-adjuvanted flu vaccines was also observed after repeated immunization [44,45]. Additional analyses were performed and helped to better characterize the immunogenicity profile of the new vaccine. More specifically, the adjuvant effect of MF59 was greater in the subsets of the elderly population, which are more likely to develop influenza and the most serious complications of the disease. As a matter of fact, an increased adjuvant effect was shown in elderly subjects with a low titer of specific antibodies before

immunization (Figure 1) and in subjects affected by chronic underlying conditions, such as respiratory and cardiovascular diseases and/or diabetes mellitus [43]. Another important finding from immunogenicity analyses was the increased immunogenicity against heterovariant strains of influenza viruses. This phenomenon might be important in case of flu outbreaks caused by strains that do not entirely match those included in the vaccine available for immunization [44,45] (Figure 2).

Influenza Pandemic Vaccines. The prepandemic alert consequent to the A/H5N1 outbreak in Hong Kong in 1997, prompted public health authorities to focus on pandemic preparedness plans. In these plans, the availability of effective pandemic vaccines is always considered as one of the key tools to be made available to face these potentially catastrophic events. In this context, the role of MF59 as a primary ingredient of a pandemic influenza vaccine was considered and clinically explored. A study performed in young adults, immunized with increasing concentrations of A/H5N3 antigen with and without MF59, clearly showed

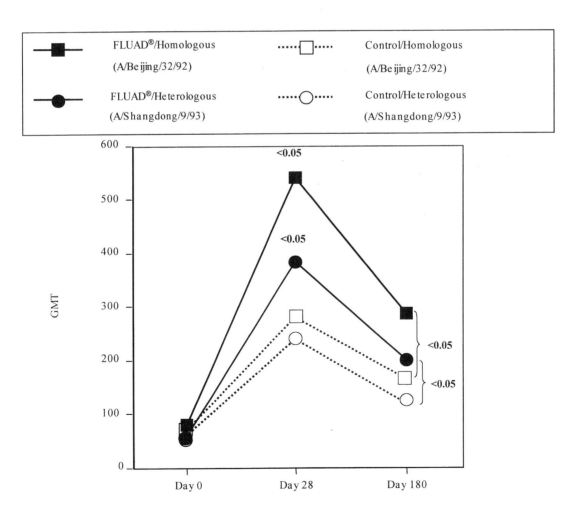

Figure 2 Increased immunogenicity against heterologous influenza strains. The addition of MF59 increases the immune response of subunit influenza antigens not only against the vaccine homologous H3N2 strain (i.e., A/Beijing/32/92), but also against an heterologous H3N2 strain (i.e., A/Shangdong/9/93). The difference between the two vaccines is still significant 6 months after immunization. (From Ref. 45.)

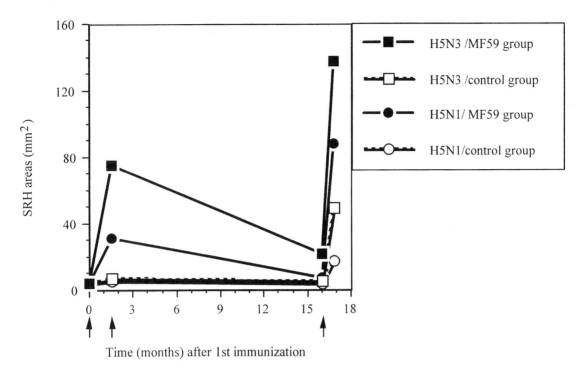

Figure 3 Increased immunogenicity against potentially pandemic influenza strains. The addition of MF59 dramatically increases the immunogenicity against potentially pandemic influenza strains in naive young volunteers and determines a more potent booster response in subjects previously primed with the same vaccine. (From Ref. 55.)

that conventional nonadjuvanted subunit vaccines are very poorly immunogenic against the homologous vaccine strain A/H5N3 and even less against the heterologous wild A/H5N1 Hong Kong strain [54]. By contrast, the addition of MF59 elicited high titers of protective antibodies, even with a reduced antigen concentration (7.5 μg/dose in a two-dose schedule) [54]. A second trial demonstrated that a primary immunization with a MF59 vaccine not only allows a better priming, but also determines a longer persistence of protective antibody titers and a better booster response up to 16 months after the primary immunization [55] (Figure 3). In light of the expected severe consequences of an influenza pandemic, these data are very relevant and underline the major role that an innovative adjuvant like MF59 can play in a public health emergency in terms of both increased clinical protection and greater availability of vaccine doses.

2. Hepatitis B Virus Vaccine

Safe and immunogenic vaccines for the prevention of hepatitis B are already available. However, also in this case, there is the need for improvement, particularly with regard to the schedule of immunization, currently requiring three doses at 0, 1, and 6 months, and to the immunogenicity of the vaccine in some high-risk populations, who should be offered an earlier and more complete protection. Because of the very promising preclinical data obtained in baboons [19] with a PreS2 + S hepatitis virus vaccine, produced in CHO cells and adjuvanted with MF59, this vaccine has also been evaluated in seronegative human healthy volunteers.

Vaccines received either the adjuvanted vaccine or a licensed, alum-based vaccine according to three different immunization schedules (i.e., 0 and 2 months; 0 and 6 months; and 0, 1, and 6 months). Despite a higher rate of local reactions, the adjuvanted vaccine was overall well tolerated. After the first immunization, 89% of recipients of the adjuvanted vaccine had protective (10 mIU/mL) anti HBs antibodies compared to 12% of subjects immunized with the licensed vaccine; additionally, more than 50% had a post-immunization titer 10-fold higher than the protective threshold [56] (Table 2). The geometric mean titer after the first dose was more than 100-fold greater than that of the licensed vaccine. The difference between the two vaccines was still statistically significant 6 months after a single dose

Table 2 The Addition of MF59 Enhances the Response to HBV Vaccine. A Protective Titer of Anti-HbsAg Antibody (i.e., > 10 mIU/mL) Is Obtained in 89% of the Recipients of MF59 Adjuvanted HBV Vaccine Already After the First Dose Compared to 12% in the Control Group Immunized with an Unadjuvanted HBV Vaccine

Anti-HBs antibody titers (mlU/mL)	HB vaccine + MF59	Comparator
> 10	89%	12%
> 100	52%	6%
> 1000	10%	2%

Source: Ref. 56.

in terms of both seroprotection rate (94% versus 69%) and GMT (161 mIU/mL versus 11 mIU/mL) [56]. Antibody responses following the second and third immunizations were still significantly higher in the MF59 group compared to the licensed vaccine (Figure 4). In particular, it was clinically important that all subjects in the MF59 group, after the second dose, regardless of its timing (1, 2, or 6 months after the first dose), had titers 10-fold greater than the protective threshold of 10 mIU/mL. Additionally, two doses of the MF59 vaccine (given at 0 and 1 month) elicited the same level of antibody titers as three doses of the licensed vaccine given at 0, 1, and 6 months [56] (Figure 4). In summary, the clinical experience with the PreS2 + S hepatitis B virus vaccine adjuvanted with MF59 highlights the adjuvant effect of MF59, which, with a very reasonable safety profile, increases the immunogenicity of the vaccine, allows the use of a two-dose schedule over a short period of time, and might be considered for a better prophylaxis of hypo- or nonresponders to the current vaccine.

3. Herpes Simplex Virus Vaccine

A very large clinical experience has been acquired with an experimental recombinant HSV vaccine formulated with MF59 adjuvant and given to adult volunteers. The vaccine consists of the two recombinant glycoproteins gD2 and gB2, which represent the target of specific antibodies with neutralizing activity. Three immunizations with these proteins together with MF59 was shown to be very well tolerated. In HSV-seronegative subjects, this vaccine induced specific neutralizing antibody titers and T cells at frequencies equal or higher than those obtained in naturally infected individuals. Also in HSV-seropositive subjects, the antibody response induced by vaccination was higher than that acquired with natural infection [64], suggesting a boosting effect of the vaccine on the immune response primed by the natural infection [65]. Interestingly, intramuscular vaccination also induced high titers of gD2- and gB2-specific IgA and IgG antibodies in the cervical secretions of vaccinated women [66].

Tested in phase III trials in more than 2000 HSV-2-seronegative individuals, this vaccine was shown to reduce

the acquisition rate of HSV-2 by 50% during the first 5 months of the trial, as compared to placebo, but not on the overall follow up of the study. In addition, the vaccine did not influence the duration of the first nor of the subsequent HSV-2 genital episodes [67]. In HSV-2-seropositive individuals, immunization with this vaccine did not affect the frequency of the recurrence of the genital lesions, but significantly reduced the duration and the severity of the first clinically confirmed herpes lesion [65].

B. Pediatric Immunization

Vaccination early in life can have different advantages over conventional pediatric immunization, including those of reducing morbidity and disease transmission in the first months of life. However, the peculiarities of the neonatal immune system [68] impose the need for particular vaccination strategies acceptably safe and sufficiently strong to induce protective immunity. The MF59 adjuvant has been tested in toddlers and infants using candidate vaccines against cytomegalovirus (CMV) and HIV.

1. Cytomegalovirus Vaccine

The safety and immunogenicity of a recombinant CMV gB protein from CHO cells was extensively tested in adult volunteers. Following three immunizations over a period of 6 months, seronegative subjects mounted a strong and sustained antibody responses, which was higher than that induced by the same protein formulated with aluminum hydroxide and that commonly found in naturally CMV infected patients [69,70]. Interestingly, lower doses of the vaccine (5–30 μg) induced better responses than higher doses. Furthermore, immunization with this vaccine induced gB-specific mucosal IgG and IgA antibodies [71] and good and sustained production of IFN-γ upon in vitro restimulation of peripheral blood mononuclear cells with the gB protein [72].

Child-to-child transmission of CMV is very common and children may represent the source of infection for their parents. Thus early vaccination against CMV may contribute to prevent congenital infection. The safety and immunogenicity of the gB recombinant vaccine adjuvanted with MF59 was tested in seronegative toddlers aged between 12 and 35 months [73]. After three doses (20 μg each), the MF59-adjuvanted gB-based vaccine exhibited a very high immunogenicity. Vaccine-specific antibody titers were > 100 times higher than those observed after the first dose, at least six times higher than those normally found in the adults immunized with the same vaccine, and higher than those found in adults naturally infected with CMV. Thus such a vaccine may represent a tool to reduce CMV transmission among infants and to reduce congenital CMV by providing maternal immunity against primary maternal infection.

2. Human Immunodeficiency Virus

A recombinant HIV vaccine construct consisting of the gp120 from HIV-SF2 adjuvanted with MF59 has been investigated for its safety and immunogenicity in adults before being tested in infants at birth. Indeed, at doses

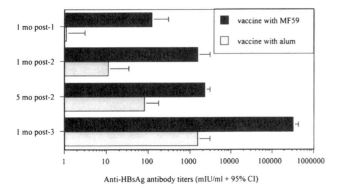

Figure 4 Increased immunogenicity against HbsAg. The immunogenicity of the MF59-adjuvanted vaccine is significantly higher after each of three doses administered at 0, 1, and 6 months. (From Ref. 56.)

ranging between 25 and 100 μg and after three doses given over a period of 6 months, followed by one or two booster doses, the MF59-adjuvanted vaccine was very well tolerated, both in adult American and Thai volunteers [74–77]. Moderate to severe side effects were observed only when the formulation contained MTP-PE [75,76]. Interestingly, after three immunizations, all the vaccinated individuals developed strain-specific neutralizing antibodies, and about two-third of them exhibited antibodies that cross-neutralized other HIV strain (e.g., HIV-MN) [74,75,77]. Also, a very strong antigen-specific proliferative response was consistently observed in these trials in adults.

Vaccination against HIV at birth of infants born from HIV-infected mothers may offer the advantage of preventing the infection. However, the presence of maternal antibodies may indeed limit the efficacy of a vaccine given so early. The recombinant gp120–SF2 protein formulated with MF59 was shown to be totally safe when given at doses of 5, 15, or 50 μg at birth (within the first 72 hr of life) and then 4, 12, and 20 weeks later [78]. This vaccination schedule (or even shorter) induced specific antibody responses in 87% of the infants [79]. Interestingly, the MF59-adjuvanted gp120-SF2 vaccine was much stronger than an alum-adjuvanted gp120-MN vaccine in inducing cell proliferative responses when administered at birth [80]. Indeed, very low doses (e.g., 5 μg) of the MF59-adjuvanted vaccine induced strong proliferative responses to the homologous gp120 protein in about 80% of the infants, and in 50% of the infants even to an heterologous protein, thus largely exceeding the results obtained with the alum-adjuvanted vaccine containing the recombinant protein at doses ranging from 30 to 300 μg per dose (Figure 5). These results are in full agreement with those obtained in adults with the pandemic influenza vaccine showing that the use of MF59 as an adjuvant can induce stronger responses with lower doses of the vaccine.

VI. CONCLUSIONS

After extensive studies in different preclinical models, MF59, as part of an influenza vaccine, is now one of the few vaccine adjuvants already licensed for human use. Additionally, MF59 is under clinical investigation as adjuvant of several other vaccines, both bacterial and viral. Although currently licensed for use in elderly, the results in toddlers and infant studies with candidate vaccines against CMV and HIV have shown that this adjuvant can be safely used for vaccination also in the youngest age groups. This may pave the way to the neonatal use of vaccines for prevention of infections that peculiarly affect this age (e.g., pertussis) or for prevention of neonatal transmission of pathogens such as CMV and HIV. In addition, the results obtained with the pandemic flu vaccines and with the HIV candidate vaccine clearly show that the use of MF59 can allow a significant reduction of the amount of antigens required to induce strong and protective immune responses; the same data have also shown that a better response is achieved not only against homologous, but also heterologous, strains of the targeted infectious agent. In conclusion, the experience with MF59 suggests that this adjuvant can play an important role to strengthen and broaden the immune response against several pathogens and can be used, with a very good safety profile, in all age groups, from elderly to children and even newborns.

ACKNOWLEDGMENTS

The authors are grateful to Anne-Marie Duliège for insights on pediatric immunization with MF59-adjuvanted vaccines and to Maria Bernadotte for assistance in manuscript preparation

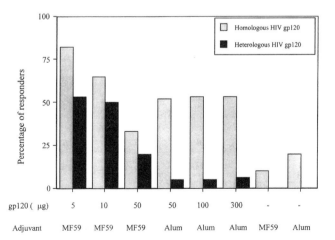

Figure 5 Increased responses against homologous and heterologous HIV gP120. Percentages of vaccine recipients with positive cell proliferative responses to homologous and heterologous HIV antigens are significantly greater compared to an alum adjuvanted vaccine. (From Ref. 80.)

REFERENCES

1. Rappuoli R. Reverse vaccinology. Curr Opin Microbiol 2000; 3:445–450.
2. Edelman R. An overview of adjuvant use. In: O'Hagan D, ed. Vaccine Adjuvants: Preparation Methods and Research Protocols. Totowa, NJ: Humana Press, 2000:1–27.
3. Ott G, et al. The adjuvant MF59: a 10-year perspective. In: O'Hagan D, ed. Vaccine Adjuvants: Preparation Methods and Research Protocols. Totowa, NJ: Humana Press, 2000: 211–228.
4. Janeway CA Jr., Medzhitov R. Innate immune recognition. Annu Rev Immunol 2002; 20:197–216.
5. Medzhitov R, et al. A human homologue of the *Drosophila* Toll protein signals activation of adaptive immunity. Nature 1997; 388:394–397.
6. Ohashi K, et al. Heat shock protein 60 is a putative endogenous ligand of the toll-like receptor-4 complex. J Immunol 2000; 164:558–561.
7. Takeuchi O, et al. Differential roles of TLR2 and TLR4 in recognition of gram-negative and gram-positive bacterial cell wall components. Immunity 1999; 11:443–451.
8. Aliprantis AO, et al. Cell activation and apoptosis by bacterial lipoproteins through toll-like receptor-2. Science 1999; 285:736–739.
9. Brightbill HD, et al. Host defense mechanisms triggered by microbial lipoproteins through toll-like receptors. Science 1999; 285:732–736.

10. Hemmi H, et al. A Toll-like receptor recognizes bacterial DNA. Nature 2000; 408:740–745.

11. Dupuis M, et al. Dendritic cells internalize vaccine adjuvant after intramuscular injection. Cell Immunol 1998; 186:18–27.

12. Dupuis M, et al. Distribution of adjuvant MF59 and antigen gD2 after intramuscular injection in mice. Vaccine 2000; 18:434–439.

13. Valensi JPM, et al. Systemic cytokine profiles in BALB/c mice immunized with trivalent influenza vaccine containing MF59 oil emulsion and other advanced adjuvants. J Immunol 1994; 153:4029–4039.

14. Higgins DA, et al. MF59 enhances the immunogenicity of influenza vaccine in both young and old mice. Vaccine 1996; 14:478–484.

15. Singh M, et al. A comparison of biodegradable microparticles and MF59 as systemic adjuvants for recombinant gD from HSV-2. Vaccine 1998; 16:1822–1827.

16. Steeghs L, et al. Immunogenicity of outer membrane proteins in a lipopolysaccharide-deficient mutant of Neisseria meningitidis: influence of adjuvants on the immune response. Infect Immun 1999; 67:4988–4993.

17. Ott G, et al. Enhancement of humoral response against human influenza vaccine with the simple submicron oil/water emulsion adjuvant MF59. Vaccine 1995; 13:1557–1562.

18. Cataldo DM, van Nest G. The adjuvant MF59 increases the immunogenicity and protective efficacy of subunit influenza vaccine in mice. Vaccine 1997; 15:1710–1715.

19. Traquina P, et al. MF59 adjuvant enhances the antibody response to recombinant hepatitis B surface antigen vaccine in primates. J Infect Dis 1996; 174:1168–1175.

20. Choo QL, et al. Vaccination of chimpanzees against infection by the hepatitis C virus. Proc Natl Acad Sci U S A 1994; 91:1294–1298.

21. Rosa D, et al. A quantitative test to estimate neutralizing antibodies to the hepatitis C virus: cytofluorimetric assessment of envelope glycoprotein 2 binding to target cells. Proc Natl Acad Sci U S A 1996; 93:1759–1763.

22. Pileri P, et al. Binding of hepatitis C virus to CD81. Science 1998; 282:938–941.

23. Burke RL, et al. The influence of adjuvant on the therapeutic efficacy of a recombinant genital herpes vaccine. J Infect Dis 1994; 170:1110–1119.

24. O'Hagan D, et al. Intranasal immunization with recombinant gD2 reduces disease severity and mortality following genital challenge with herpes simplex virus type 2 in guinea pigs. Vaccine 1999; 17:2229–2236.

25. Nesburn AB, et al. Vaccine therapy of ocular herpes simplex virus (HSV) infection: periocular vaccination reduces spontaneous ocular HSV type 1 shedding in latently infected rabbits. J Virol 1994; 68:4092–5084.

26. Nesburn AB, et al. Therapeutic periocular vaccination with a subunit vaccine induces higher levels of herpes simplex virus-specific tear secretory immunoglobulin A than systemic vaccination and provides protection against recurrent spontaneous ocular shedding of virus in latently infected rabbits. Virology 1998; 252:200–209.

27. Nesburn AB, et al. Local periocular vaccination protects against eye disease more effectively than systemic vaccination following primary ocular herpes simplex virus infection in rabbits. J Virol 1998; 72:7715–7721.

28. Nesburn AB, et al. A therapeutic vaccine reduces recurrent herpes simplex virus type 1 corneal disease. Investig Ophthalmol Vis Sci 1998; 39:1163–1170.

29. El-Amad Z, et al. Resistance of chimpanzees immunized with recombinant gp120SF2 to challenge with HIV-1SF2. AIDS 1995; 9:1313–1322.

30. Zolla-Pazner S, et al. Induction of neutralizing antibodies to T-cell line-adapted and primary human immunodeficiency virus type 1 isolates with a prime-boost vaccine regimen in chimpanzees. J Virol 1998; 72:1052–1059.

31. Verschoor EJ, et al. Comparison of immunity generated by nucleic acid-, MF59-, and ISCOM-formulated human immunodeficiency virus type 1 vaccines in rhesus macaques: evidence for viral clearance. J Virol 1999; 73:3292–3300.

32. Granoff DM, et al. MF59 adjuvant enhances antibody responses to infant baboons immunized with Haemophilus influenzae type b and Neisseria meningitidis group C oligosaccharide-CRM197 conjugate vaccine. Infect Immun 1997; 65:1710–1715.

33. Langermann S, et al. Prevention of mucosal Escherichia coli infection by FimH-adhesin-based systemic vaccination. Science 1997; 276:607–611.

34. Langermann S, et al. Vaccination with FimH adhesin protects cynomolgus monkeys from colonization and infection by uropathogenic Escherichia coli. J Infect Dis 2000; 181:774–778.

35. ACIP. Prevention and Control of Influenza. MMWR 2001; 50(RR-04):1–46.

36. Fiebach N, Beckett W. Prevention of respiratory infections in adults—influenza and pneumococcal vaccines. Arch Intern Med November 1994; 54(22):2545–2557.

37. Monto AS. The clinical efficacy of influenza vaccination. PharmacoEconomics 1996; 9(Suppl. 3):16–22.

38. Strassburg MA, et al. Influenza in the elderly: report of an outbreak and review of vaccine effectiveness reports. Vaccine 1986 March; 4(1):38–44.

39. Keren G, et al. Failure of influenza vaccination in the aged. J Med Virol 1988 May; 25(1):85–89.

40. Phair J, et al. Failure to respond to influenza vaccine in the aged: correlation with B-cell number and function. J Lab Clin Med 1978 November; 92(5):822–828.

41. Arden NH, et al. Safety and immunogenicity of a 45-microgram supplemental dose of inactivated split-virus influenza B vaccine in the elderly. J Infect Dis 1986 April; 153(4):805–806.

42. Barker WH, Mullooly JP. Effectiveness of inactivated influenza vaccine among non-institutionalised elderly persons. In: Kendal AP, Patriarca PA, eds. Options for the Control of Influenza. New York, NY: Alan R. Liss, Inc, 1986:169–182.

43. Podda A. The adjuvanted influenza vaccines with novel adjuvants: experience with the MF59-adjuvanted vaccine. Vaccine 2001 March 21; 19(17–19):2673–2680.

44. Minutello M, et al. Safety and immunogenicity of an inactivated subunit influenza virus vaccine combined with MF59 adjuvant emulsion in elderly subjects, immunized for three consecutive influenza seasons. Vaccine 1999 January; 17(2):99–104.

45. De Donato S, et al. Safety and immunogenicity of MF59-adjuvanted influenza vaccine in the elderly. Vaccine 1999 August 6; 17(23–24):3094–3101.

46. Gasparini R, et al. Increased immunogenicity of the MF59-adjuvanted influenza vaccine compared to a conventional subunit vaccine in elderly subjects. Eur J Epidemiol 2001; 17(2):135–140.

47. Baldo V, et al. Comparison of three different influenza vaccines in institutionalised elderly. Vaccine 2001 May 14; 19(25–26):3472–3475.

48. Potter CW, Oxford JS. Determinants of immunity to influenza infection in man. Br Med Bull 1979 Jan; 35(1):69–75 (Review).

49. Davies JR, Grilli A. Natural or vaccine induced antibody as predictor of immunity in the face of natural challenge with influenza viruses. Epidemiol Infect 1989; 102:325–333 (Published erratum appears in Epidemiol Infect August 1989; 103 (1): 217).

50. Hobson D, et al. The role of serum haemagglutination-inhibiting antibody in protection against challenge infection

with influenza A2 and B viruses. J Hyg (Lond) 1972; 70(4): 767–777.

51. Masurel N, Laufer J. A one year study of trivalent influenza vaccines in primed and unprimed volunteers: immunogenicity, clinical reactions and protection. J Hyg (Camb) 1984; 92:263–276.

52. Wesselius-De Casparis A, et al. Field trial with human and equine influenza vaccines in children: protection and antibody titers. Bull WHO 1972; 46(2):151–157.

53. Palache AM. Influenza vaccination: the effect of dose and age on the antibody response: a methodological evaluation of serological vaccination studies. [Ph.D. thesis]. Rotterdam: Erasmus Univ., 1991; (4):82–119.

54. Nicholson KG, et al. Safety and antigenicity of non-adjuvanted and MF59-adjuvanted influenza A/Duck/Singapore/97 (H5N3) vaccine: a randomised trial of two potential vaccines against H5N1 influenza. Lancet 2001 June 16; 357 (9272):1937–1943.

55. Stephenson I, et al. Planning for the next influenza pandemic: Boosting immunity to influenza H5N1 with MF59-adjuvanted H5N3 A/Duck/Singapore/97 vaccine in a primed human population. Submitted. 2002.

56. Heineman TC, et al. A randomized, controlled study in adults of the immunogenicity of a novel hepatitis B vaccine containing MF59 adjuvant. Vaccine 1999 July 16; 17(22): 2769–2778.

57. Ugozzoli M, et al. Intranasal immunization of mice with herpes simplex type 2 recombinant gD2: the effect of adjuvants on mucosal and serum antibody responses. Immunology 1998; 93:563–571.

58. Barchfeld GL, et al. The adjuvants MF59 and LT-K63 enhance the mucosal and systemic immunogenicity of subunit influenza vaccine administered intranasally in mice. Vaccine 1999 February 26; 17(7–8):695–704.

59. Verschoor EJ, et al. Efforts to broaden HIV-1-specific immunity by boosting with heterologous peptides or envelope protein and the influence of prior exposure to virus. J Med Primatol 1999; 28:224–232.

60. O'Hagan DT, et al. Microparticles in MF59, a potent adjuvant combination for a recombinant protein vaccine against HIV-1. Vaccine 2000 March 6; 18(17):1793–1801.

61. Zhu X, et al. Both immunization with protein and recombinant vaccinia virus can stimulate CTL specific for the E7 protein of human papilloma virus 16 in H-2d mice. Scand J Immunol 1995 November; 42(5):557–563.

62. Greer CE, et al. The comparison of the effect of LTR72 and MF59 adjuvants on mouse humoral response to intranasal immunisation with human papillomavirus type 6b (HPV-6b) virus-like particles. Vaccine 2000 December 8; 19(9–10):1008–1012.

63. Stowers AW, et al. Efficacy of two alternate vaccines based on *Plasmodium falciparum* merozoite surface protein 1 in an Aotus challenge trial. Infect Immun 2001 March; 69(3):1536–1546.

64. Langenberg AGM, et al. A recombinant glycoprotein vaccine for herpes simplex type 2: safety and immunogenicity. Ann Intern Med 1995; 122:889–898.

65. Straus SE, et al. Immunotherapy of recurrent genital herpes with recombinant herpes simplex virus type 2 glycoproteins D and B: results of a placebo-controlled vaccine trial. J Infect Dis 1997; 176:1129–1134.

66. Ashley RL, et al. Cervical antibody responses to a herpes simplex type 2 glycoprotein subunit vaccine. J Infect Dis 1998; 178:1–7.

67. Corey L, et al. Recombinant glycoprotein vaccine for the prevention of genital HSV-2 infection. Two randomized controlled trials. JAMA 1999; 282:331–340.

68. Siegrist CA. Neonatal and early life vaccinology. Vaccine 2001, May 14; 19(25–26):3331–3346 (Review).

69. Pass RP, et al. A subunit cytomegalovirus vaccine based on recombinant envelope glycoprotein B and a new adjuvant. J Infect Dis 1999; 180:970–975.

70. Frey SE, et al. Effects of antigen dose and immunization regimens on antibody responses to a cytomegalovirus glycoprotein B subunit vaccine. J Infect Dis 1999; 180:1700–1703.

71. Wang JB, et al. Mucosal antibodies to human cytomegalovirus glycoprotein B occur following both natural infection and immunization with human cytomegalovirus vaccines. J Infect Dis 1996; 174:387–392.

72. Bernstein DI, et al. Effect of previous or simultaneous immunization with canarypox expressing cytomegalovirus (CMV) glycoprotein B (gB) on response to subunit gB vaccine plus MF59 in healthy CMV-seronegative adults. J Infect Dis 2002; 185:686–690.

73. Mitchell DK, et al. Immunogenicity of a recombinant human cytomegalovirus gB vaccine in seronegative toddlers. Pediatr Infect Dis J 2002; 21:133–138.

74. Kahn JO, et al. Clinical and immunological responses to human immunodeficiency virus (HIV) type 1-SF2 gp120 subunit vaccine combined with MF59 adjuvant with or without mutamyl tripeptide dipalmitoyl phosphatidylethanolamine in non-HIV-infected human volunteers. J Infect Dis 1994; 170: 1288–1291.

75. Graham BS, et al. NIAID AIDS Vaccine Evaluation Group. Safety and immunogenicity of a candidate HIV-1 vaccine in healthy adults: recombinant glycoprotein (rgp) 120. A randomized, double-blind trial. Ann Intern Med 1996; 125:270–279.

76. Keefer MC, et al. Safety and immunogenicity of Env 2–3, a human immunodeficiency virus type 1 candidate vaccine, in combination with a novel adjuvant, MTP–PE/MF59. NIAID AIDS Vaccine Evaluation Group. AIDS Res Hum Retrovir 1996; 12:683–693.

77. Nitayaphan S, et al. AFRIMS–RIHES Vaccine Evaluation Group. A phase I/II trial of HIV SF2 gp120/MF59 vaccine in seronegative Thais. Vaccine 2000; 18:1448–1455.

78. Cunningham CK, et al. Pediatric AIDS Clinical Trials Group 230 Collaborators. Safety of 2 recombinant human immunodeficiency virus type 1 (HIV-1) envelope vaccines in neonates born to HIV-1-infected women. Clin Infect Dis 2001; 32:801–807.

79. McFarland EJ, et al. Pediatric AIDS Clinical Trials Group 230 Collaborators. Human immunodeficiency virus type 1 (HIV-1) gp120-specific antibodies in neonates receiving an HIV-1 recombinant gp120 vaccine. J Infect Dis 2001; 184: 1331–1335.

80. Borkowsky W, et al. Pediatric AIDS Clinical Trials Group 230 Collaborators. Lymphoproliferative responses to recombinant HIV-1 envelope antigens in neonates and infants receiving gp120 vaccines. J Infect Dis 2000; 181:890–896.

20

Immune-Enhancing Sequences (CpG Motifs), Cytokines, and Other Immunomodulatory Moieties

Sanjay Gurunathan
Aventis Pasteur, Swiftwater, Pennsylvania, U.S.A.

Dennis M. Klinman
Food and Drug Administration, Bethesda, Maryland, U.S.A.

Robert A. Seder
National Institutes of Health, Bethesda, Maryland, U.S.A.

I. INTRODUCTION

The goal of vaccination is to provide protection against a particular infection. Vaccines induce protection through a variety of immune mechanisms. Understanding the immune mechanisms, often referred to as "immune correlates of protection," can facilitate the rational design of vaccines. The humoral immune response through the production of antibodies appears to be the immune correlate by which a majority of current vaccines induce protection, most notably against viral or bacterial infections. For many other infectious diseases, however, the cellular immune response through $CD4^+$ and $CD8^+$ T cells is also important for immune protection. Indeed, a major impediment to the development of successful vaccines against HIV, malaria, and *Mycobacterium tuberculosis* infection has been the failure to induce and sustain long-term cellular immune responses sufficient to mediate protection. Thus, in considering vaccine design, especially for the aforementioned infections in which cellular immune responses might be critical in mediating protection, attention should be given not only to maximizing the magnitude of the immune response but also to the qualitative aspects of the immune response.

The immune response can be segregated into two major compartments designated the innate and adaptive immune systems. The innate response relies on immediate recognition of antigenic structures common to many microorganisms by a selected set of immune cells [1–3]. The adaptive immune response is made up of B and T lymphocytes that have unique receptors specific to various microbial antigens.

The goal of vaccination is to enhance the number of antigen-specific B and T cells against a given pathogen sufficient to provide protection following an infectious challenge. Recently, there have been several exciting discoveries showing that the innate immune response has an additional important role in regulating the adaptive immune response, especially the cellular immune response. Innate immune recognition of infectious pathogens is mediated by pattern recognition receptors, called Toll-like receptors [4–6], which are expressed on various cells of the innate immune response including the major antigen-presenting cells (APCs) (macrophages, dendritic cells [DCs], and B cells) responsible for T-cell activation. This innate recognition pathway leads to an increase in APC function that can strongly influence the initial adaptive immune response generated by immunization. These observations of how innate immune responses can affect adaptive immunity have tremendous importance for vaccine design, especially when cellular immune responses are required as discussed below.

T cells comprise a major part of the adaptive immune response. $CD4^+$ T cells recognize antigens that have been processed through the exogenous pathway by APC expressing MHC class II histocompatibility molecules. $CD4^+$ T cells become activated, and differentiation can occur into functional subsets termed T helper 1 (Th1)-and T helper 2 (Th2)-type cells. Th1 cells produce the cytokine IFN-γ, whereas Th2 cells produce the cytokine IL-4 [7,8]. Th1 cells, through their production of IFN-γ, mediate killing for a variety of intracellular infections and will be critical in generating a vaccine against *M. tuberculosis* as well as other intracellular infections. $CD8^+$ T cells recognize antigens processed and presented by cells expressing MHC class I molecules and have a critical role in mediating protection in many infections including HIV and malaria. While all currently licensed vaccines (killed/inactivated, whole-cell, recombinant protein, or live attenuated) generate humoral immune responses, a potential shortcoming of nonlive vaccines is their relative inefficiency in generating cellular immune (Th1 or CD8$^+$ T cell) responses. Although live attenuated vaccines allow for efficient MHC class I presentation of antigen that can stimulate CD8$^+$ T-cell responses, the use of live attenuated vaccines may be precluded for several intracellular infections due to safety and/or manufacturing concerns.

Together, these findings have prompted investigation into how cellular immune responses can be generated using nonlive antigens. In this regard, there has been a focus on using specific immune adjuvants to induce such responses. At present, aluminum adjuvants (alum) are the only approved adjuvants for use in humans in the United States. Although alum enhances antibody production, it has little effect on influencing cellular immune responses and in fact may facilitate a type of cellular immune response (Th2) that would provide no protective efficacy against intracellular infections [9]. As the cellular and molecular mechanisms of immune activation for both humoral and cellular responses are more clearly understood, it is now possible to use immunomodulators as vaccine adjuvants with a cellular and molecular basis for how they work. The focus of this chapter will be to review how cytokines, costimulatory molecules, and cytosine phosphate guanosine (CpG) oligodeoxynucleotides (ODNs) can be used as vaccine adjuvants to induce long-term humoral and cellular immune responses sufficient to mediate protection against infectious and neoplastic disease.

II. CYTOKINES AS IMMUNE ADJUVANTS

Much of the early work using cytokines as vaccine adjuvants or treatments in neoplastic disease was done with recombinant proteins delivered systemically. As most cytokines are small proteins with very short half-life in vivo, recent work has focused on using plasmid DNA encoding specific cytokine genes given with DNA encoding an antigen as a potential method to deliver the cytokine to the same site as the antigen. This would potentially mitigate side effects associated with giving high doses of cytokine proteins systemically. In addition, cytokine DNA might allow for more sustained persistence in vivo, albeit at lower levels than what would be achieved by giving cytokine protein. The majority of studies have used plasmid DNA vaccines encoding cytokines codelivered with the DNA encoding the antigen in the same inoculation. This is clearly the most practical regimen for use. One notable exception is the use of a plasmid DNA encoding a fusion protein for IL-2 [10,11]. In this instance, optimal induction of immune responses occurred when the cytokine DNA was given 2 days following DNA encoding the antigen. This might be explained by the kinetics of T-cell activation. The optimal effect of IL-2 would occur once T cells were activated and expressed the IL-2 receptor α chain.

This might indeed take 1 or 2 days and would explain the importance of the kinetics for this particular cytokine. These data raise an important point: the timing and even the ratio of cytokine to DNA encoding the antigen should be carefully studied in experimental models to determine the best way to administer the vaccine for optimizing an immune response. This information can then be used as the basis to develop a usable and practical regimen in humans.

Cytokines have been shown to be effective immune modulators at several key points within the generation and maintenance of the immune response. First, depending on the type of immune response required, a potentially important issue would be to target the vaccine toward a specific APC. In this regard, cytokines such as granulocyte–macrophage colony-stimulating factor (GM-CSF) (see Table 1) or FLT-3 ligand [76] have been shown to be potent stimulators of DC and have been used as proteins and/or plasmid DNA as vaccine adjuvants with varying efficacy in mice, primates, and humans. It is important to note that there is substantial heterogeneity in the type and function of DCs that can markedly effect the immune response generated [77]. Thus, while the targeting of DC for vaccination is a burgeoning area of vaccine research for a variety of diseases (infectious, autoimmune, neoplastic), the maturation and specific type of DC is an additional and important consideration when using such a targeted approach. Second, cytokines can act directly on T cells to facilitate T-cell proliferation. IL-2 is the most intensively studied cytokine for clinical use in humans for both infectious and neoplastic diseases and is a potent inducer of both CD4$^+$ and CD8$^+$ T-cell proliferation. Recently, IL-15 has been shown to be a critical factor in sustaining CD8$^+$ memory T cells [78] and is currently being studied as a vaccine adjuvant to enhance the maintenance of CD8$^+$ T-cell responses. Finally, cytokines can influence the qualitative aspects of the immune response. For CD4$^+$ Th responses, IL-12 is the most potent inducer of Th1 responses, while IL-4 induces Th2 responses [79,80]. Thus, in instances where the immune correlates of protection are known, it is possible to choose a cytokine regimen to specifically induce the immune response to achieve the desired effect.

A summary of studies using such an approach is shown in Table 1. For CD4$^+$ T helper responses, coinjection of IFN-γ-, IL-12-, or IL-18-encoding plasmids has been shown to enhance induction of Th1 responses, while cytokines IL-4, IL-5, IL-10, and IL-13 have generated a predominantly Th2 response. Other cytokines encoding plasmids, such as TGF-β and IL-10, have been shown to decrease T-cell proliferative responses and have been used to downregulate the immune response [40,70]. In this regard, IL-10 and TGF-β might be useful in vaccines against specific autoimmune diseases in which the goal is to inhibit proinflammatory immune responses or generate T regulatory cells. The use of cytokines to both augment and inhibit immune responses for infections and autoimmune diseases, respectively, raises an important issue. Thus, induction of long-term cellular immune responses required for protection against infection is balanced by the risk of autoimmune disease due to the presence of a persistent cellular immune response. For CD8$^+$ T-cell

Table 1 Effects of Cytokine DNA on Humoral and Cellular Immune Response

Cytokine adjuvant	Antibody	Cellular response	CTL	References
IL-1	↑ IgG ↑ IgG2a	↑ CTL ↑ IFN-γ	↑ Proliferation	12–14
IL-2	↑ IgG ↑ IgG2a ↑ IgG1[a]	↑ Proliferation ↑ IFN-γ	↑ CTL	14–27
IL-4	↑ IgG1 ↑ IgG	↑ Proliferation ↓ DTH ↑ IL-4	No enhancement	13, 15, 18, 20, 21, 23, 28–31
IL-5	↑ IgG	± Proliferation	No enhancement	15, 30
IL-6			Improves survival post viral challenge	32–34
IL-7	↑ IgG2a, ↑ IgG1	↑ IFN-γ		19, 35
IL-8		↑ Neutrophils		14, 36, 37
IL-10	↑ IgG ↓ IgG2a ↓ IgG1[a]	↓ DTH ↓ Proliferation ↓ IFN-γ ↓ TNF-α ↓ Neutrophil activity		15, 21, 26, 38–42
IL-12	↑ Ig2a ↑ or ↓ IgG1[a] ↑ or ↓ IgG[a]	↑ DTH ↑ Proliferation ↑ IFN-γ	↑ CTL	13, 15, 19–21, 28, 43–54
IL-13				23
IL-15	↑ IgG[a]	± ↑ Proliferation	↑ CTL	14, 15, 26, 30, 55
IL-18	↑ IgG	↑ Proliferation	↑ CTL	15, 50, 52, 56–59
TNF-α and –β	↑ IgG	↑ Proliferation	↑ CTL	15, 60
GM-CSF	↑ IgG ↑ IgG2a and IgG1[a]	↑ Proliferation	↑ CTL ↑ IFN-γ ↑ ? IL-4	13, 18, 20, 21, 27, 28, 30, 44, 60–68
TGF-β	No change in IgG or IgG2a ↑ IgG1	↓ DTH ↓ Proliferation ↓ IL-4 ↓ IL5 ↓ IFN-γ ↑ IL-10 ↓ TNF-α ↓ WBC		14, 69, 70
IFN-γ	↑ IgG2a ↑ or ↓ IgG[a]	↑ or ↓ Proliferation ↑ IFN-γ ↓ IL-5 ↓ Eosinophils	↑ CTL	13, 14, 24, 30, 50, 60, 64, 71, 72
IFN-α and –β		Reduced viral replication Reduced tumor burden		73–75

[a] Studies not in agreement.

responses, a broad array of cytokines (e.g., IL-2, IL-12, IL-15, IL-18, and GM-CSF) have been shown to increase such responses.

III. COSTIMULATORY MOLECULES AS IMMUNE ADJUVANTS

Initiation of an immune response involves recognition of antigen in the context of MHC class II and class I for activation of CD4$^+$ and CD8$^+$ T cells, respectively. In addition, several accessory or costimulatory molecules that exist on T cells and APC allow for enhanced activation and expansion of T-cell responses and can further increase the functional capacity of APCs. Several of these adhesive and costimulatory ligand/receptor molecules have been exploited as potential vaccine adjuvants for both T and APC activation.

The most widely studied costimulatory molecules for plasmid DNA vaccines have been CD80, CD86, and CD40 ligand (Table 2). In the course of initial T-cell activation, CD80 and CD86, through interaction with CD28 on the T cell, augment T-cell activation. Plasmid DNA encoding either CD80 or CD86 has been used with varying efficacy to augment cellular immune responses, notably CD8 responses. Another costimulatory molecule, CD40 ligand, is induced upon T-cell activation and interacts with B cells, DC, and macrophages expressing its cognate ligand CD40. This interaction is critical for both B-cell activation and immunoglobulin (Ig) class switching and enhances DC activation, resulting in upregulation of CD80 and CD86 production of cytokines such as IL-12. Studies using CD40 ligand DNA have demonstrated striking increases in antibody production as well as induction of Th1 responses and enhancement in CTL responses. This immune enhancement fits well with a profile for a vaccine adjuvant to induce a broad immune response that can be used in a variety of infectious diseases and cancer models. A final approach is to direct antigen directly to APCs to improve immunogenicity. To this end, plasmid encoding a fusion protein of CTLA-4, a ligand for CD80 and CD86 antigen would target the antigen to APCs by binding to CD80 or CD86 on the APC. A brief summary of these studies is provided in Table 2.

IV. CHEMOKINES

In addition to the exciting developments in understanding the role of cytokines and costimulatory molecules in the immune response and their role in vaccines, a very active area of recent research is the role and function of chemokines and chemokine receptors. Chemokines were initially shown to be important in mediating leukocyte extravasation and navigation (with selectins and integrins). In addition, flexible regulation of chemokine receptors is seen during activation and differentiation of lymphocytes. Thus, chemokines can selectively induce, modulate, and prevent cellular immune interactions and conceivably will find therapeutic application. Several studies using molecules from the chemokine superfamily have shown that codelivery of these chemokines not only modulates immune responses but also impacts protection from disease. Of particular interest is a study using plasmid DNA encoding CCR7 ligands SLC and ELC as immunoregulators [95]. CCR7 is a homing receptor for DC into secondary lymphoid organs. Consequently, provision of SLC and ELC can influence migration of DC into lymphoid tissue and increase the efficiency of immune induction. Data from this study suggest that coimmunization with CCR7 ligands increased antibody production, T-cell-mediated immunity (antigen-specific CD4 T-cell proliferation and CD8 cytolytic activity), and the number of DCs in secondary lymphoid tissues. Table 3 is a brief summary of the immune responses seen in studying the effects of chemokine DNA in vivo.

Table 2 Effects of Costimulatory and Adhesion Molecule DNA on Humoral and Cellular Immunity

Adjuvant	Antibody	Cellular response	CTL	References
B7-1 (CD80)			↑ CTL[a]	44, 81–85
B7-2 (CD86)		↑ DTH ↑ Proliferation	↑ CTL[a]	44, 81–83, 86–88
CD40L	↑ IgG2a ↑ IgG, ↑ IgG1[a]	↑ IFN-γ	↑ CTL	46, 89, 90
ICAM-1 (CD54)		↑ Proliferation ↑ IFN-γ ↑ Chemokines	↑ CTL	91, 92
LFA-3		↑ Proliferation ↑ IFN-γ ↑ Chemokines	↑ CTL	91, 92
L-selectin	↑ IgG ↑ IgG2a > IgG1	↑ Proliferation		93, 94
CTLA-4	↑ IgG ↑ IgG1 > IgG2a	↑ Proliferation		93, 94

[a] Studies not in agreement.

Table 3 Effects of Chemokine DNA on Humoral and Cellular Immunity

Adjuvant	Antibody	Cellular response	CTL	References
Chemokines (CXC)				
IL-8	↑ IgG, ↑ IgG2a	↑ Proliferation ↑ IL-2 ↑ IFN-γ		14, 96, 97
IP-10	↑ IgG1	↓ IFN-γ	↑ CTL with IL-12 coinjection	54, 96, 97
	↓ IgG2a			
MIP-2	↑ IgG ↑ IgG2a	↑ Proliferation ↑ IL-2 and IFN-γ	No ↑	98
Chemokines (CC)				
RANTES	↑ IgG[a] ↑ IgG2a	↑ Proliferation ↑ IL-2 ↑ IFN-γ	↑ CTL	96, 97, 99–101
MCP-1	↑ IgG ↑ IgG1[a]	↑ Proliferation ↑ IL-2 and IL-4	No ↑	96, 98, 100–102
MIP-1α	↑ IgG ↑ IgG2a[a] ↑ IgG1[a]	↑ Proliferation ↑ IL-2 and IL-4	↑ CTL	97, 98, 100–103
MIP-1β	↑ IgG	↑ Proliferation ↑ IL-2 and IFN-γ	No ↑	98, 100, 101
SLC	↑ IgG ↑ IgG2a	↑ Proliferation ↑ IL-2 and IFN-γ	↑ CTL	95
ELC	↑ IgG ↑ IgG2a	↑ Proliferation ↑ IL-2, IFN-γ, IL-4	CTL ↑	95

[a] Studies not in agreement.

V.   IMMUNE ENHANCING CpG SEQUENCES

A.   Mechanisms of CpG Sequences and Their Effects on Immune Response

Yamamoto and his colleagues made the seminal observation that synthetic ODNs with sequences patterned after those found in bacterial DNA were immunostimulatory. They reported that purified bacterial DNA and synthetic ODNs expressing palindromic sequences could activate natural killer cells to secrete IFN-γ [104,105]. Subsequently, studies by Krieg et al. and Klinman et al. showed that the critical immunostimulatory motif consisted of an unmethylated CpG dinucleotide with appropriate flanking regions. In mice, this CpG should be flanked by two 5′ purines and two 3′ pyrimidines [106,107]. Such motifs are 20-fold more common in microbial than mammalian DNA, due to differences in the frequency of use and the methylation pattern of CpG dinucleotides in prokaryotes vs. eukaryotes [108,109].

CpG motifs have been shown to directly activate B cells to proliferate and secrete antibody [106]. CpG ODNs also directly trigger professional APCs (DCs, macrophages) to differentiate, mature, and/or secrete cytokines [107,110,111]. Most recently, Hemmi and his colleagues established that Toll-like receptor 9 is involved in recognition of CpG motifs in mice [112], a finding confirmed for the human response to CpG DNA [113]. As noted above, Toll-like receptors are pattern-recognition receptors that are expressed on various cells including the major APCs (macrophages, DCs). Acti-

vation of APCs via Toll-like receptor 9 has been shown to improve APC function both by enhancing expression of activation and costimulatory molecules on APCs and by induction of proinflammatory cytokines and chemokines such as IL-6, IL-12, tumor necrosis factor alpha (TNF-α), IFN-α, MIP1-β, and MIP-1α [107,114–116]. In turn, these activated APCs can enhance the activity of natural killer cells and induce both Th1 and CTL responses. The enhancement of natural killer and T cells provides a striking example of how CpG ODNs, through their effect on APCs, influence the innate and adaptive immune response, respectively (Figure 1). Together, this broad-based immune enhancement profile has generated considerable interest in harnessing the immunostimulatory properties of CpG motifs for use as vaccine adjuvants for vaccines in which humoral and cellular immune responses are required.

B.   The Role of CpG Motifs in Mediating Immune Responses by DNA Vaccines

Over the past 10 years, a growing body of literature has demonstrated that plasmid DNA vaccination can induce broad cellular immune responses in rodents and nonhuman primates. Early work has shown that some of the potency of DNA vaccines is due to the presence of CpG motifs within the backbone of the plasmid itself. First, these plasmids mimic the ability of bacterial DNA and CpG ODN to stimulate the host immune response [117]. For example, in

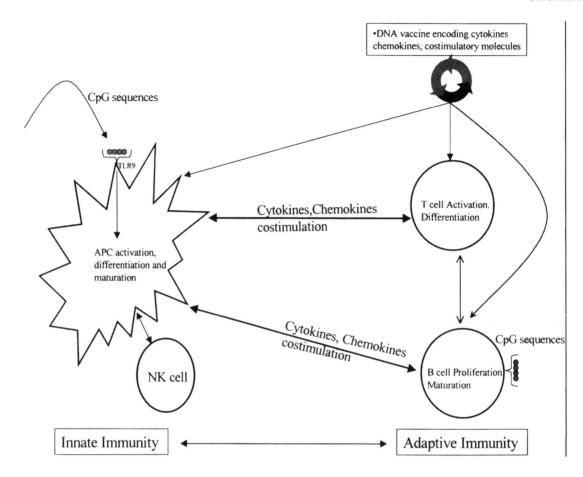

Figure 1   Role of CpG ODN and/or plasmid DNA in linking innate and adaptive immune responses. Innate immune recognition of bacterial DNA or CpG motifs is mediated by Toll-like receptor 9 (TLR9) expressed on APCs (DCs, macrophages, and B cells). Activation through TLR-9 can lead to enhancement in APC function, through secretion of cytokines and chemokines and an increase in costimulatory molecules leading to activation of both natural killer cells and T cells. CpG motifs can also directly stimulate B cells via TLR9 to enhance B-cell activation and antibody production. Plasmid DNA encoding specific cytokines, chemokines, or costimulatory molecule genes can be codelivered with plasmid DNA encoding specific antigens. These immunostimulatory DNA enhance APC function (e.g., GM-CSF, CD40L), T-cell activation (e.g., IL-2, CD80, and CD86), CD4$^+$ T-cell differentiation (e.g., IL-12, IL-4), B-cell activation (e.g., IL-2, CD40L), and immune cell trafficking (e.g., chemokines).

vitro studies involving murine spleen cells show that bacterial DNA plasmids (with or without protein-encoding inserts) trigger a five-to eightfold increase in the number of lymphocytes secreting IgM, IL-6, IL-12, and IFN-γ. This is similar to the level of immune stimulation elicited by bacterial DNA or CpG ODN. Second, when these CpG motifs in the plasmid backbone are methylated using Sss-I CpG methylase, the plasmid's ability to trigger this cytokine and IgM production is concomitantly reduced [115,117]. Third, the nature of the immune response elicited by coadministration of CpG ODNs and protein antigens is similar to the response elicited by DNA vaccine encoding the same antigen (in vivo mimics the pattern induced by a CpG-dominated response) [118–120]. Specifically, DNA vaccines preferentially stimulate the production of antigen-specific IFN-γ and IgG2a antibodies. Compared with the response elicited against the same protein in Freund's adjuvant, the levels of IFN-γ and IgG2a production induced by a DNA vaccine is

greater than threefold higher, whereas production of IL-4 and IgG1 antibodies may actually be reduced [121].

Based on these findings, researchers examined whether the activity of a DNA vaccine could be improved by increasing the number of CpG motifs present in the plasmid backbone. In this regard, substituting a CpG-containing ampR gene for a kanR-selectable marker in a β-gal-encoding plasmid elicited a higher IgG antibody response, more CTL, and greater IFN-γ production than did the original vector [115]. The same effect was observed when CpG motifs were added elsewhere in plasmid backbone by other groups [117,121–126]. In general, adding CpG motifs to a DNA vaccine either increases the magnitude of the resultant in vivo response or decreases the amount of vaccine required to induce a significant response [117,121–126]. Further evidence of the contribution of CpG motifs to the immunogenicity of a DNA vaccine derives from studies in which synthetic CpG ODNs were coadministered with DNA plasmids. Mice primed and boosted with DNA vaccine plus CpG ODNs developed antigen-specific IgG and IFN-γ responses up to an order of magnitude greater than those in animals receiving DNA vaccine alone [117,127]. The magnitude of this CpG effect was greatest when mice were immunized with low doses of DNA vaccine, presumably because CpG motifs in the vector served the same function at high plasmid concentrations. It should also be noted that sequences present in mammalian DNA can block immune activation by bacterial CpG sequences [126]. This may account for the inability of mammalian DNA, which contains some unmethylated CpG motifs (albeit at a lower frequency than bacterial DNA), to persistently stimulate the host immune system; however, an excess of control ODNs can inhibit uptake of CpG ODNs [128]. This inhibition abrogated the ability of CpG DNA to induce immune stimulation, interfering with cytokine production and stress kinase activation [128,129]. Recent work by Krieg et al. [126] confirmed that the immunostimulatory activity of CpG ODNs could be blocked by certain non-CpG motifs. They found that eliminating such suppressive motifs (tandem repeats of GpC) from the plasmid backbone of a DNA vaccine improved vaccine immunogenicity by up to threefold [122]. Alternatively, while eliminating suppressive motifs might enhance the immunogenicity of a plasmid, these observations suggest that adding stimulatory CpG motifs to a plasmid could significantly improve the resultant DNA vaccine's ability to induce a protective immune response; however, in using this approach, CpG motifs appear to be limited in their ability to augment antibody and cytokine production in vivo. In one study, introducing 16 additional CpG motifs into the plasmid backbone improved the humoral immune response of a DNA vaccine, whereas introducing 50 such motifs was detrimental [122]. Not only the number but the placement and sequence of CpG motifs may be important. Efforts are under way to determine whether different motifs can preferentially induce specific types of immune response and to identify regions in the plasmid where addition of CpG motifs provides the greatest benefit. These efforts are likely to yield vectors with significantly improved immunostimulatory capacity for clinical use.

C. The Role of Synthetic CpG ODNs as Vaccine Adjuvant

Several studies have examined the ability of CpG ODNs to boost the immune response elicited by a variety of protein antigens. Ovalbumin (OVA) was the model antigen widely used in early studies. Normal mice immunized with soluble OVA generated a modest serum IgG anti-OVA response; addition of CpG ODNs to the OVA increased the resultant antibody response by approximately fourfold [121]. It was quickly recognized that the immunogenicity of the ODN–antigen combination might be improved if these components were prevented from diffusing away from the injection site. Thus, methods for linking ODN to the antigen were investigated, including coemulsifying them in incomplete Freund's adjuvant, coencapsulating them in liposomes, or coupling them together ionically or covalently [132]. In each case, the immune response elicited by the antigen–ODN

complex triggered an antigen-specific IgG response at least 10-fold greater than free antigen plus CpG ODN and > 50-fold higher than antigen alone [119,121,125,132]. Throughout these studies, control ODN (lacking the critical CpG dinucleotide) had no significant effect on immunogenicity, demonstrating that the adjuvant effect was CpG dependent. Consistent with results from studies of DNA vaccines, combining CpG ODN with antigen significantly altered the isotype profile of the subsequent immune response. For example, OVA alone primarily elicits an IgG1 response (IgG1:IgG2a ratio ranging from 6 to 9), whereas inclusion of CpG ODN increases production of IgG2a antibodies [119,121,125,132]. The enhanced ratio of IgG2a:IgG1 in mice is correlative with a Th1 response and is consistent with studies showing that protein plus CpG ODN indeed induces potent Th1 responses [130,133]. In addition to enhancing antibody and Th1 responses, CpG ODNs have also been shown to activate DCs, leading to presentation of soluble proteins to class I-restricted T cells, and to induce CTL responses [134–136].

Moreover, physically conjugated antigen and CpG ODN has been shown to enhance uptake by DC in mice [137] and to induce substantially higher CTL responses than protein and CpG given together but not conjugated [136,138]. These observations in mouse models have potential importance in human studies in allowing a protein-based vaccine to induce both Th1 and CD8/CTL responses, which in the case of CD8 responses are normally limited to live attenuated vaccines. Subsequent studies have established that CpG ODNs could boost the response to other protein- or peptide-based vaccines [119,121,125,130,131]. This includes evidence that the antibody, T cell, and protective responses of normal mice to agents—including the gp33 glycoprotein-derived peptide from lymphocytic choriomeningitis virus [139], tetanus and diphtheria toxoids [140], and proteins from HIV, influenza, herpes, brucella, and hepatitis-were all increased by coadministration of CpG ODNs [141–144].

As above, optimal adjuvanticity required that the ODN be given in the same immunization with the antigen. Under such conditions, improved immune responses were induced when the CpG ODN–antigen mixtures were administered by a variety of routes including intramuscular, intranasal, oral, and subcutaneous [141].

D. CpG ODNs Have Different Immune-Stimulating Properties Based on Sequence

Because of evolutionary divergence in CpG recognition between species, CpG ODNs that are highly active in rodents are poorly immunostimulatory in primates and vice versa [121,145–148]. Several groups succeeded in identifying CpG ODNs capable of stimulating human B cells [147–150], natural killer cells [151], and/or macrophages/monocytes to proliferate, mature and/or secrete [147,151,152]. These were subsequently used in preclinical and clinical studies evaluating the activity and safety of these agents in vivo. Recent studies show that human peripheral blood mononuclear cells recognize and respond to two distinct types of

CpG ODNs [147,153]. K-type ODNs have phosphorothioate backbones, encode multiple TCGTT and/or TCGTA motifs, and primarily stimulate B cells and macrophages to proliferate and produce IgM and/or IL-6 [147]. D-type ODNs have phosphodiester backbones and contain a single hexameric purine/pyrimidine/CG/purine/pyrimidine motif flanked by self-complementary bases that form a stem-loop structure capped at the 3′ end by a poly G tail [147]. D-type ODNs trigger maturation of APCs and preferentially induce secretion of IFN-α and IFN-γ. These findings raise the intriguing possibility that CpG ODNs may be tailored to activate specific cell types and thus support precisely the type of immune response required to provide maximal protection against a specific target pathogen [147,150].

Because rodents respond poorly to the motifs that strongly activate human peripheral blood mononuclear cells, preclinical studies evaluated the response of nonhuman primates to these ODNs. Results from several laboratories show that peripheral blood mononuclear cells from rhesus macaques, Aotus monkeys, and chimpanzees recognize and respond to the same D-and K-type ODNs that are active in humans [147,148,150,153–155]. Based on previous studies in mice, the adjuvant activity of CpG ODNs was tested in primates using the model antigen OVA. Rhesus macaques were immunized and boosted with OVA plus D-type, K-type, or control ODN. Alum was used to cross-link ODNs to the antigen. Monkeys immunized with D ODN plus OVA increased their IgG anti-OVA response by nearly 500-fold after primary and secondary immunization [156]. By comparison, K ODN boosted the IgG antibody response by sevenfold after primary and 35-fold after secondary immunization. Further studies established that CpG ODN could boost the in vivo response of primates to protein-or peptide-based vaccines. For example, the antigen-specific serum IgG response of Aotus monkeys immunized with a synthetic malaria peptide vaccine was significantly increased by inclusion of an ODN expressing multiple CpG motifs [154,155]. Control ODN had no effect on peptide immunogenicity. Similarly, nonhuman primates vaccinated with the hepatitis B antigen plus CpG ODN developed 15-fold higher antihepatitis antibody titers than did animals immunized with the vaccine alone [157]. One study established that the protective efficacy of a leishmanial protein was improved by coadministration of CpG ODN. Rhesus macaques were immunized and boosted with alum-adsorbed heat-killed leishmania vaccine (HKLV) plus K or D ODN. In this model system, generation of antigen-specific IFN-γ production is strongly associated with parasitic control. When these animals were challenged with *L. major* metacyclic promastigotes, animals vaccinated with HKLV-alum plus D ODN developed smaller lesions than those of controls [156].

VI. SAFETY

The use of DNA vaccines, plasmid-encoded immunomodulators, and CpG motifs as vaccine adjuvants raises several safety concerns, particularly because newborns, children, and healthy adults are common vaccine recipients. Concerns include the possibility that potent immunostimulatory activity may 1) enhance the immunogenicity of self-proteins, thereby triggering development of autoimmune disease or 2) stimulate production of cytokines that alter the subsequent host response to pathogens or other vaccines [158].

These concerns are supported by evidence that bacterial DNA can induce production of anti-double-stranded-DNA autoantibodies in normal mice and accelerate development of autoimmune disease in lupus-prone animals [159–161]. Furthermore, CpG motifs present in bacterial DNA and CpG ODN have been shown to stimulate production of IL-6 and block the apoptotic death of activated lymphocytes, both functions that predispose to the development of systemic lupus erythematosus by facilitating persistent B-cell activation [162–167]. These findings led several groups to investigate whether systemic autoimmune disease was induced or accelerated by the CpG motifs [168]. Results show that shortly after CpG DNA treatment, the number of IgG anti-DNA-secreting B cells rises by two-to threefold [169]. This is accompanied by a 35% to 60% increase in serum IgG anti-DNA antibody titer. This modest rise in autoantibody level did not, however, cause disease in normal mice or accelerate disease in lupus-prone animals [168–171]. The situation is somewhat more complex for organ-specific autoimmune disease, whose induction is promoted by the type of Th1 response preferentially triggered by CpG motifs. In an IL-12-dependent model of experimental allergic encephalomyelitis, animals treated with CpG DNA and then challenged with myelin basic protein developed autoreactive Th1 effector cells that caused experimental allergic encephalomyelitis [172]. In a molecular mimicry model, CpG motifs acted as potent immunoactivators, inducing autoimmune myocarditis when coinjected with *Chlamydia*-derived antigen [173]. These findings indicate that CpG motifs may trigger deleterious autoimmune reactions under certain circumstances.

In addition to concerns with regard to autoimmunity, potential safety concerns also arise from vaccines/adjuvants that can elicit potent or persistent stimulation of the host immune system. An important component of immune homeostasis is balance in the production of Th1 cytokines (which promote cell-mediated immunity) and Th2 cytokines (which facilitate humoral immune responses or counter-regulate Th1 responses). Overproduction of one type of cytokine can disrupt immune homeostasis, altering the host response to other vaccines, susceptibility to infection, and predisposition to develop autoimmune disease. In this regard, mice treated repeatedly with CpG ODN develop a statistically significant twofold increase in serum IgM levels and in the number of spleen and lymph node cells secreting IL-6 and IFN-γ in vivo. They also showed a modest decrease in the number of cells actively secreting IL-4 [174]. These effects persist for the duration of ODN therapy but return to baseline by 1 month after cessation of treatment. Several reports indicate that CpG ODN can be toxic if administered with lipopolysaccharide or D-galactosamine [175]. Finally, while the use of cytokine-encoding plasmids is growing in popularity, relatively little information is available on their long-term safety. Although no serious side effects have been reported following the administration of cytokine-encoding plasmids in animals [176], it is unclear whether systematic efforts to detect such events were undertaken.

Despite concern that DNA vaccines/CpG ODN might have adverse effect on the host, there is no evidence that even multiple doses of CpG ODN are directly toxic under normal conditions. Moreover, major toxicity has not been reported among the hundreds of normal human volunteers exposed to CpG motifs in plasmid DNA vaccines.

VII. CONCLUSIONS

Identifying agents that boost antigen-specific immune responses is an important goal of vaccine research. Our increased understanding of the role of cellular immunity in mediating protection against a variety of infections, combined with a molecular basis for inducing long-term memory cellular immune responses, should provide a strong foundation for developing successful vaccines for a variety of diseases. The use of CpG ODNs and immunomodulators described above has generated much enthusiasm in moving toward this goal.

REFERENCES

1. Hoffmann JA, et al. Phylogenetic perspectives in innate immunity. Science 1999; 284:1313–1318.
2. Medzhitov R, Janeway CA Jr. Innate immunity: the virtues of a monoclonal system of recognition. Cell 1997; 91:295–298.
3. Medzhitov R, Janeway CA Jr. Innate immunity. N Engl J Med 2000; 343:338–344.
4. Medzhitov R, et al. A human homologue of the Drosophila Toll protein signals activation of adaptive immunity. Nature 1997; 388:394–397.
5. Poltorak A, et al. Defective LPS signaling in C3H/HeJ and C57BL/10ScCr mice: mutations in Tlr4 gene. Science 1998; 282:2085–2088.
6. Aderem A, Ulevitch RJ. Toll-like receptors in the induction of the innate immune response. Nature 2000; 406:782–787.
7. Seder RA, Paul WE. Acquisition of lymphokine-producing phenotype by CD4$^+$ T cells. Annu Rev Immunol 1994; 12:635–673.
8. O'Garra A. Cytokines induce the development of functionally heterogeneous T helper cell subsets. Immunity 1998; 8:275–283.
9. Lindblad EB, et al. Adjuvant modulation of immune responses to tuberculosis subunit vaccines. Infect Immun 1997; 65:623–629.
10. Barouch DH, et al. Augmentation and suppression of immune responses to an HIV-1 DNA vaccine by plasmid cytokine/Ig administration. J Immunol 1998; 161:1875–1882.
11. Barouch DH, et al. Augmentation of immune responses to HIV-1 and simian immunodeficiency virus DNA vaccines by IL-2/Ig plasmid administration in rhesus monkeys. Proc Natl Acad Sci U S A 2000; 97:4192–4197.
12. Hakim I, et al. A nine-amino acid peptide from IL-1β augments antitumor immune responses induced by protein and DNA vaccines. J Immunol 1996; 157:5503–5511.
13. Maecker HT, et al. DNA vaccination with cytokine fusion constructs biases the immune response to ovalbumin. Vaccine 1997; 15:1687–1696.
14. Min W, et al. Adjuvant effects of IL-1β, IL-2, IL-8, IL-15,

15. IFN-α, IFN-γ TGF-β4 and lymphotactin on DNA vaccination against Eimeria acervulina. Vaccine 2001; 20:267–274.
15. Kim JJ, et al. Modulation of amplitude and direction of in vivo immune responses by co-administration of cytokine gene expression cassettes with DNA immunogens. Eur J Immunol 1998; 28:1089–1103.
16. Raz E, et al. Systemic immunological effects of cytokine genes injected into skeletal muscle. Proc Natl Acad Sci U S A 1993; 90:4523–4527.
17. Chow YH, et al. Improvement of hepatitis B virus DNA vaccines by plasmids coexpressing hepatitis B surface antigen and interleukin-2. J Virol 1997; 71:169–178.
18. Geissler M, et al. Enhancement of cellular and humoral immune responses to hepatitis C virus core protein using DNA-based vaccines augmented with cytokine-expressing plasmids. J Immunol 1997; 158:1231–1237.
19. Prayaga SK, et al. Manipulation of HIV-1 gp120-specific immune responses elicited via gene gun-based DNA immunization. Vaccine 1997; 15:1349–1352.
20. Chow YH, et al. Development of Th1 and Th2 populations and the nature of immune responses to hepatitis B virus DNA vaccines can be modulated by codelivery of various cytokine genes. J Immunol 1998; 160:1320–1329.
21. Kim JJ, et al. Cytokine molecular adjuvants modulate immune responses induced by DNA vaccine constructs for HIV-1 and SIV. J Interferon Cytokine Res 1999; 19:77–84.
22. Kim JJ, et al. Modulation of antigen-specific cellular immune responses to DNA vaccination in rhesus macaques through the use of IL-2, IFN-γ, or IL-4 gene adjuvants. Vaccine 2001; 19:2496–2505.
23. Kim JJ, et al. Coimmunization with IFN-γ or IL-2, but not IL-13 or IL-4 cDNA can enhance Th1-type DNA vaccine-induced immune responses in vivo. J Interferon Cytokine Res 2000; 20:311–319.
24. Kim JJ, et al. Modulation of antigen-specific humoral responses in rhesus macaques by using cytokine cDNAs as DNA vaccine adjuvants. J Virol 2000; 74:3427–3429.
25. Xin KQ, et al. Intranasal administration of human immunodeficiency virus type-1 (HIV-1) DNA vaccine with interleukin-2 expression plasmid enhances cell-mediated immunity against HIV-1. Immunology 1998; 94:438–444.
26. Sin JI, et al. In vivo modulation of vaccine-induced immune responses toward a Th1 phenotype increases potency and vaccine effectiveness in a herpes simplex virus type 2 mouse model. J Virol 1999; 73:501–509.
27. Nobiron I, et al. Cytokine adjuvancy of BVDV DNA vaccine enhances both humoral and cellular immune responses in mice. Vaccine 2001; 9:4226–4235.
28. Okada E, et al. Intranasal immunization of a DNA vaccine with IL-12-and granulocyte macrophage colony-stimulating factor (GM-CSF)-expressing plasmids in liposomes induces strong mucosal and cell-mediated immune responses against HIV-1 antigens. J Immunol 1997; 159:3638–3647.
29. Lim YS, et al. Vaccination with an ovalbumin/interleukin-4 fusion DNA efficiently induces Th2 cell-mediated immune responses in an ovalbumin-specific manner. Arch Pharm Res 1998; 21:537–542.
30. Scheerlinck JP, et al. The immune response to a DNA vaccine can be modulated by co-delivery of cytokine genes using a DNA prime-protein boost strategy. Vaccine 2001; 9:4053–4060.
31. Garren H, et al. Combination of gene delivery and DNA vaccination to protect from and reverse Th1 autoimmune disease via deviation to the Th2 pathway. Immunity 2001; 15:15–22.
32. Larsen DL, et al. Coadministration of DNA encoding interleukin-6 and hemagglutinin confers protection from influenza virus challenge in mice. J Virol 1998; 72:1704–1708.
33. Lee SW, et al. IL-6 induces long-term protective immunity

against a lethal challenge of influenza virus. Vaccine 1999; 17:490–496.

34. Olsen CW. DNA vaccination against influenza viruses: a review with emphasis on equine and swine influenza. Vet Microbiol 2000; 74:149–164.

35. Sin JI, et al. Interleukin 7 can enhance antigen-specific cytotoxic T-lymphocyte and/or Th2-type immune responses in vivo. Clin Diagn Lab Immunol 2000; 7:751–758.

36. Kim JJ, et al. Chemokine gene adjuvants can modulate immune responses induced by DNA vaccines. J Interferon Cytokine Res 2000; 20:487–498.

37. Sin J, et al. DNA vaccines encoding interleukin-8 and RANTES enhance antigen-specific Th1-type CD4$^+$ T-cell-mediated protective immunity against herpes simplex virus type 2 in vivo. J Virol 2000; 74:11173–11180.

38. Rogy MA, et al. Human tumor necrosis factor receptor (p55) and interleukin 10 gene transfer in the mouse reduces mortality to lethal endotoxemia and also attenuates local inflammatory responses. J Exp Med 1995; 181:2289–2293.

39. Daheshia M, et al. Suppression of ongoing ocular inflammatory disease by topical administration of plasmid DNA encoding IL-10. J Immunol 1997; 159:1945–1952.

40. Manickan E, et al. Modulation of virus-induced delayed-type hypersensitivity by plasmid DNA encoding the cytokine interleukin-10. Immunology 1998; 94:129–134.

41. Chun S, et al. Immune modulation by IL-10 gene transfer via viral vector and plasmid DNA: implication for gene therapy. Cell Immunol 1999; 194:194–204.

42. Chun S, et al. Distribution fate and mechanism of immune modulation following mucosal delivery of plasmid DNA encoding IL-10. J Immunol 1999; 163:2393–2402.

43. Gurunathan S, et al. Vaccine requirements for sustained cellular immunity to an intracellular parasitic infection. Nat Med 1998; 4:1409–1415.

44. Iwasaki A, et al. Enhanced CTL responses mediated by plasmid DNA immunogens encoding costimulatory molecules and cytokines. J Immunol 1997; 158:4591–4601.

45. Kim JJ, et al. In vivo engineering of a cellular immune response by coadministration of IL-12 expression vector with a DNA immunogen. J Immunol 1997; 158:816–826.

46. Gurunathan S, et al. CD40 ligand/trimer DNA enhances both humoral and cellular immune responses and induces protective immunity to infectious and tumor challenge. J Immunol 1998; 161:4563–4571.

47. Tsuji T, et al. Enhancement of cell-mediated immunity against HIV-1 induced by coinoculation of plasmid-encoded HIV-1 antigen with plasmid expressing IL-12. J Immunol 1997; 158:4008–4013.

48. Rakhmilevich AL, et al. Gene gun-mediated skin transfection with interleukin 12 gene results in regression of established primary and metastatic murine tumors. Proc Natl Acad Sci U S A 1996; 93:6291–6296.

49. Kim JJ, et al. Development of a multicomponent candidate vaccine for HIV-1. Vaccine 1997; 15:879–883.

50. Kim JJ, et al. Antigen-specific humoral and cellular immune responses can be modulated in rhesus macaques through the use of IFN-γ, IL-12, or IL-18 gene adjuvants. J Med Primatol 1999; 28:214–223.

51. Gherardi MM, et al. Interleukin-12 (IL-12) enhancement of the cellular immune response against human immunodeficiency virus Type 1 env antigen in a DNA prime/vaccinia virus boost vaccine regimen is time and dose dependent: suppressive effects of IL-12 boost are mediated by nitric oxide. J Virol 2000; 74:6278–6286.

52. Hanlon L, et al. Feline leukemia virus DNA vaccine efficacy is enhanced by coadministration with interleukin-12 (IL-12) and IL-18 expression vectors. J Virol 2001; 75:8424–8433.

53. Dunham SP, et al. Protection against feline immunodeficiency virus using replication defective proviral DNA vaccines with feline interleukin-12 and -18. Vaccine 2002; 20:1483–1496.

54. Narvaiza I, et al. Intratumoral coinjection of two adenoviruses, one encoding the chemokine IFN-γ-inducible protein-10 and another encoding IL-12, results in marked antitumoral synergy. J Immunol 2000; 164:3112–3122.

55. Xin KQ, et al. IL-15 expression plasmid enhances cell-mediated immunity induced by an HIV-1 DNA vaccine. Vaccine 1999; 17:858–866.

56. Maecker HT, et al. Vaccination with allergen-IL-18 fusion DNA protects against, and reverses established, airway hyperreactivity in a murine asthma model. J Immunol 2001; 166:959–965.

57. Billaut-Mulot O, et al. Modulation of cellular and humoral immune responses to a multiepitopic HIV-1 DNA vaccine by interleukin-18 DNA immunization/viral protein boost. Vaccine 2001; 9:2803–2811.

58. Kim SH, et al. Efficient induction of antigen-specific, T helper type 1-mediated immune responses by intramuscular injection with ovalbumin/interleukin-18 fusion DNA. Vaccine 2001; 19:4107–4114.

59. Dupre L, et al. Immunostimulatory effect of IL-18-encoding plasmid in DNA vaccination against murine Schistosoma mansoni infection. Vaccine 2001; 19:1373–1380.

60. Lewis PJ, et al. Polynucleotide vaccines in animals: enhancing and modulating responses. Vaccine 1997; 15:861–864.

61. Svanholm C, et al. Amplification of T-cell and antibody responses in DNA-based immunization with HIV-1 Nef by co-injection with a GM-CSF expression vector. Scand J Immunol 1997; 46:298–303.

62. Weiss WR, et al. A plasmid encoding murine granulocyte-macrophage colony-stimulating factor increases protection conferred by a malaria DNA vaccine. J Immunol 1998; 161: 2325–2332.

63. Lee AH, et al. DNA inoculations with HIV-1 recombinant genomes that express cytokine genes enhance HIV-1 specific immune responses. Vaccine 1999; 17:473–479.

64. Xiang Z, Ertl HC. Manipulation of the immune response to a plasmid-encoded viral antigen by coinoculation with plasmids expressing cytokines. Immunity 1995; 2:129–135.

65. Sin JI, et al. Protective immunity against heterologous challenge with encephalomyocarditis virus by VP1 DNA vaccination: effect of coinjection with a granulocyte-macrophage colony stimulating factor gene. Vaccine 1997; 15:1827–1833.

66. Sin JI, et al. Enhancement of protective humoral (Th2) and cell-mediated (Th1) immune responses against herpes simplex virus-2 through co-delivery of granulocyte-macrophage colony-stimulating factor expression cassettes. Eur J Immunol 1998; 28:3530–3540.

67. Kusakabe K, et al. The timing of GM-CSF expression plasmid administration influences the Th1/Th2 response induced by an HIV-1-specific DNA vaccine. J Immunol 2000; 164: 3102–3111.

68. Sedegah M, et al. Improving protective immunity induced by DNA-based immunization: priming with antigen and GM-CSF-encoding plasmid DNA and boosting with antigen-expressing recombinant poxvirus. J Immunol 2000; 164: 5905–5912.

69. Song XY, et al. Plasmid DNA encoding transforming growth factor-β1 suppresses chronic disease in a streptococcal cell wall-induced arthritis model. J Clin Invest 1998; 101: 2615–2621.

70. Kuklin NA, et al. Immunomodulation by mucosal gene transfer using TGF-β DNA. J Clin Invest 1998; 102:438–444.

71. Lim YS, et al. Potentiation of antigen specific, Th1 immune responses by multiple DNA vaccination with ovalbumin/interferon-γ hybrid construct. Immunology 1998; 94:135–141.

72. Xiang ZQ, et al. The effect of interferon-γ on genetic immunization. Vaccine 1997; 15:896–898.

73. Yeow WS, et al. Antiviral activities of individual murine IFN-α subtypes in vivo: intramuscular injection of IFN expression constructs reduces cytomegalovirus replication. J Immunol 1998; 160:2932–2939.

74. Horton HM, et al. A gene therapy for cancer using intramuscular injection of plasmid DNA encoding interferon α. Proc Natl Acad Sci U S A 1999; 96:1553–1558.

75. Cui B, Carr DJ. A plasmid construct encoding murine interferon β antagonizes the replication of herpes simplex virus type I in vitro and in vivo. J Neuroimmunol 2000; 108:92–102.

76. Pulendran B, et al. Prevention of peripheral tolerance by a dendritic cell growth factor: Flt3 ligand as an adjuvant. J Exp Med 1998; 188:2075–2082.

77. Reis e Sousa C. Dendritic cells as sensors of infection. Immunity 2001; 14:495–498.

78. Zhang X, et al. Potent and selective stimulation of memory-phenotype CD8⁺ T cells in vivo by IL-15. Immunity 1998; 8:591–599.

79. Seder RA, and Paul WE. Acquisition of lymphokine-producing phenotype by CD4+ T cells. Annual Review of Immunology 1994; 12:635–673.

80. O'Garra A. Cytokines induce the development of functionally heterogeneous T helper cell subsets. Immunity 1998; 8: 275–283.

81. Corr M, et al. Costimulation provided by DNA immunization enhances antitumor immunity. J Immunol 1997; 159: 4999–5004.

82. Horspool JH, et al. Nucleic acid vaccine-induced immune responses require CD28 costimulation and are regulated by CTLA4. J Immunol 1998; 160:2706–2714.

83. Flo J, et al. Modulation of the immune response to DNA vaccine by co-delivery of costimulatry molecules. Immunology 2000; 100:259–267.

84. Tsuji T, et al. Immunomodulatory effects of a plasmid expressing B7−2 on human immunodeficiency virus-1-specific cell-mediated immunity induced by a plasmid encoding the viral antigen. Eur J Immunol 1997; 27:782–787.

85. Kim JJ, et al. Engineering of in vivo immune responses to DNA immunization via codelivery of costimulatory molecule genes. Nat Biotechnol 1997; 15:641–646.

86. Agadjanyan MG, et al. CD86 (B7-2) can function to drive MHC-restricted antigen-specific CTL responses in vivo. J Immunol 1999; 162:3417–3427.

87. Kim JJ, et al. Engineering DNA vaccines via co-delivery of co-stimulatory molecule genes. Vaccine 1998; 16:1828–1835.

88. Flo J, et al. Codelivery of DNA coding for the soluble form of CD86 results in the down-regulation of the immune response to DNA vaccines. Cell Immunol 2001; 209:120–131.

89. Mendoza RB, et al. Immunostimulatory effects of a plasmid expressing CD40 ligand (CD154) on gene immunization. J Immunol 1997; 159:5777–5781.

90. Sin JI, et al. Modulation of cellular responses by plasmid CD40L: CD40L plasmid vectors enhance antigen-specific helper T cell type 1 CD4⁺ T cell-mediated protective immunity against herpes simplex virus type 2 in vivo. Hum Gene Ther 2001; 12:1091–1102.

91. Kim JJ, et al. Intracellular adhesion molecule-1 modulates beta-chemokines and directly costimulates T cells in vivo. J Clin Invest 1999; 103:869–877.

92. Sin JI, et al. LFA-3 plasmid DNA enhances antigen-specific humoral-and cellular-mediated protective immunity against herpes simplex virus-2 in vivo: involvement of CD4⁺ T cells in protection. Cell Immunol 2000; 203:19–28.

93. Boyle JS, et al. Enhanced responses to a DNA vaccine encoding a fusion antigen that is directed to sites of immune induction. Nature 1998; 392:408–411.

94. Drew DR, et al. The comparative efficacy of CTLA-4 and L-selectin targeted DNA vaccines in mice and sheep. Vaccine 2001; 19:4417–4428.

95. Eo SK, et al. Immunopotentiation of DNA vaccine against herpes simplex virus via co-delivery of plasmid DNA expressing CCR7 ligands. Vaccine 2001; 19:4685–4693.

96. Sin J, et al. DNA vaccines encoding interleukin-8 and RANTES enhance antigen-specific Th1-type CD4⁺ T-cell-mediated protective immunity against herpes simplex virus type 2 in vivo. J Virol 2000; 74:11173–11180.

97. Kim JJ, et al. Chemokine gene adjuvants can modulate immune responses induced by DNA vaccines. J Interferon Cytokine Res 2000; 20:487–498.

98. Eo SK, et al. Modulation of immunity against herpes simplex virus infection via mucosal genetic transfer of plasmid DNA encoding chemokines. J Virol 2001; 75:569–578.

99. Xin KQ, et al. Immunization of RANTES expression plasmid with a DNA vaccine enhances HIV-1-specific immunity. Clin Immunol 1999; 92:90–96.

100. Youssef S, et al. C–C chemokine-encoding DNA vaccines enhance breakdown of tolerance to their gene products and treat ongoing adjuvant arthritis. J Clin Invest 2000; 106:361–671.

101. Youssef S, et al. Long-lasting protective immunity to experimental autoimmune encephalomyelitis following vaccination with naked DNA encoding C–C chemokines. J Immunol 1998; 161:3870–3879.

102. Youssef S, et al. Prevention of experimental autoimmune encephalomyelitis by MIP-1α and MCP-1 naked DNA vaccines. J Autoimmun 1999; 13:21–29.

103. Lu Y, et al. Macrophage inflammatory protein-1α (MIP-1α) expression plasmid enhances DNA vaccine-induced immune response against HIV-1. Clin Exp Immunol 1999; 115:335–341.

104. Yamamoto S, et al. Unique palindromic sequences in synthetic oligonucleotides are required to induce IFN and augment IFN-mediated natural killer activity. J Immunol 1992; 148:4072–4076.

105. Yamamoto S, et al. DNA from bacteria, but not vertebrates, induces interferons, activate NK cells and inhibits tumor growth. Microbiol Immunol 1992; 36:983–997.

106. Krieg AM, et al. CpG motifs in bacterial DNA trigger direct B-cell activation. Nature 1995; 374:546–549.

107. Klinman DM, et al. CpG motifs present in bacteria DNA rapidly induce lymphocytes to secrete interleukin 6, interleukin 12, and interferon γ. Proc Natl Acad Sci U S A 1996; 93:2879–2883.

108. Cardon LR, et al. Pervasive CpG suppression in animal mitochondrial genomes. Proc Natl Acad Sci U S A 1994; 91:3799–3803.

109. Razin A, Friedman J. DNA methylation and its possible biological roles. Prog Nucleic Acid Res Mol Biol 1981; 25: 33–52.

110. Stacey KJ, et al. Macrophages ingest and are activated by bacterial DNA. J Immunol 1996; 157:2116–2122.

111. Jakob T, et al. Activation of cutaneous dendritic cells by CpG-containing oligodeoxynucleotides: a role for dendritic cells in the augmentation of Th1 responses by immunostimulatory DNA. J Immunol 1998; 161:3042–3049.

112. Hemmi H, et al. A Toll-like receptor recognizes bacterial DNA. Nature 2000; 408:740–745.

113. Bauer S, et al. Human TLR9 confers responsiveness to bacterial DNA via species-specific CpG-motif recognition. Proc Natl Acad Sci U S A 2001; 98:9237–9242.

114. Halpern MD, et al. Bacterial DNA induces murine interferon-γ production by stimulation of interleukin-12 and tumor necrosis factor-α. Cell Immunol 1996; 167:72–78.

115. Sato Y, et al. Immunostimulatory DNA sequences necessary for effective intradermal gene immunization. Science 1996; 273:352–354.

116. Takeshita S, et al. CpG oligodeoxynucleotides induce murine macrophages to up-regulate chemokine mRNA expression. Cell Immunol 2000; 206:101–106.

117. Klinman DM, et al. Contribution of CpG motifs to the immunogenicity of DNA vaccines. J Immunol 1997; 158: 3635–3639.

118. Brazolot Millan CL, et al. CpG DNA can induce strong Th1 humoral and cell-mediated immune responses against hepatitis B surface antigen in young mice. Proc Natl Acad Sci U S A 1998; 95:15553–15558.

119. Davis HL, et al. CpG DNA is a potent enhancer of specific immunity in mice immunized with recombinant hepatitis B surface antigen. J Immunol 1998; 160:870–876.

120. Klinman DM. Therapeutic applications of CpG-containing oligodeoxynucleotides. Antisense Nucleic Acid Drug Dev 1998; 8:181–184.

121. Klinman DM, et al. CpG motifs as immune adjuvants. Vaccine 1999; 17:19–25.

122. Krieg AM, Davis HL. Enhancing vaccines with immune stimulatory CpG DNA. Curr Opin Mol Ther 2001; 3:15–24.

123. Davis HL. Use of CpG DNA for enhancing specific immune responses. Curr Top Microbiol Immunol 2000; 247:171–183.

124. McCluskie MJ, et al. The role of CpG in DNA vaccines. Springer Semin Immunopathol 2000; 22:125–132.

125. Roman M, et al. Immunostimulatory DNA sequences function as T helper-1-promoting adjuvants. Nat Med 1997; 3: 849–854.

126. Krieg AM, et al. Sequence motifs in adenoviral DNA block immune activation by stimulatory CpG motifs. Proc Natl Acad Sci U S A 1998; 95:12631–12636.

127. Klinman DM, et al. CpG DNA augments the immunogenicity of plasmid DNA vaccines. Curr Top Microbiol Immunol 2000; 247:131–142.

128. Weeratna R, et al. Reduction of antigen expression from DNA vaccines by coadministered oligodeoxynucleotides. Antisense Nucleic Acid Drug Dev 1998; 8:351–356.

129. Hacker H, et al. CpG-DNA-specific activation of antigen-presenting cells requires stress kinase activity and is preceded by non-specific endocytosis and endosomal maturation. EMBO J 1998; 17:6230–6240.

130. Chu RS, et al. CpG oligodeoxynucleotides act as adjuvants that switch on T helper (Th1) immunity. J Exp Med 1997; 186:1623–1631.

131. Tighe H, et al. Conjugation of immunostimulatory DNA to the short ragweed allergen amb a 1 enhances its immunogenicity and reduces its allergenicity. J Allergy Clin Immunol 2000; 106:124–134.

132. Gursel I, et al. Sterically stabilized cationic liposomes improve the uptake and immunostimulatory activity of CpG oligonucleotides. J Immunol 2001; 167:3324–3328.

133. Chu RS, et al. CpG DNA switches on Th1 immunity and modulates antigen-presenting cell function. Curr Top Microbiol Immunol 2000; 247:199–210.

134. Sparwasser T, et al. Bacterial CpG-DNA activates dendritic cells in vivo: T helper cell-independent cytotoxic T cell responses to soluble proteins. Eur J Immunol 2000; 30:3591–3597.

135. Davila E, Celis E. Repeated administration of cytosine-phosphorothiolated guanine-containing oligonucleotides together with peptide/protein immunization results in enhanced CTL responses with anti-tumor activity. J Immunol 2000; 165:539–547.

136. Cho HJ, et al. Immunostimulatory DNA-based vaccines induce cytotoxic lymphocyte activity by a T-helper cell-independent mechanism. Nat Biotechnol 2000; 18:509–514.

137. Shirota H, et al. Novel roles of CpG oligodeoxynucleotides

138. Tighe H, et al. Conjugation of protein to immunostimulatory DNA results in a rapid, long-lasting and potent induction of cell-mediated and humoral immunity. Eur J Immunol 2000; 30:1939–1947.

139. Oxenius A, et al. CpG-containing oligonucleotides are efficient adjuvants for induction of protective antiviral immune responses with T-cell peptide vaccines. J Virol 1999; 73: 4120–4126.

140. Eastcott JW, et al. Oligonucleotide containing CpG motifs enhances immune response to mucosally or systemically administered tetanus toxoid. Vaccine 2001; 19:1636–1642.

141. McCluskie MJ, Davis HL. CpG DNA is a potent enhancer of systemic and mucosal immune responses against hepatitis B surface antigen with intranasal administration to mice. J Immunol 1998; 161:4463–4466.

142. Gallichan WS, et al. Intranasal immunization with CpG oligodeoxynucleotides as an adjuvant dramatically increases IgA and protection against herpes simplex virus-2 in the genital tract. J Immunol 2001; 166:3451–3457.

143. AlMariri A, et al. Protection of BALB/c mice against Brucella abortus 544 challenge by vaccination with bacterioferritin or P39 recombinant proteins with CpG oligodeoxynucleotides as adjuvant. Infect Immun 2001; 69:4816–4822.

144. von Hunolstein C, et al. The adjuvant effect of synthetic oligodeoxynucleotide containing CpG motif converts the anti-Haemophilus influenzae type b glycoconjugates into efficient anti-polysaccharide and anti-carrier polyvalent vaccines. Vaccine 2001; 9:3058–3066.

145. Bauer M, et al. DNA activates human immune cells through a CpG sequence-dependent manner. Immunology 1999; 97: 699–705.

146. Hartmann G, Krieg AM. Mechanism and function of a newly identified CpG DNA motif in human primary B cells. J Immunol 2000; 164:944–952.

147. Verthelyi D, et al. Human peripheral blood cells differentially recognize and respond to two distinct CpG motifs. J Immunol 2001; 166:2372–2377.

148. Hartmann G, et al. Delineation of a CpG phosphorothioate oligodeoxinucleotide for activating primate immune responses in vitro and in vivo. J Immunol 2000; 164:1617–1624.

149. Liang H, et al. Activation of human B cells by phosphorothioate oligodeoxynucleotides. J Clin Invest 1996; 98:1119–1129.

150. Ballas ZK, et al. Divergent therapeutic and immunological effects of oligonucleotides with distinct CpG motifs. J Immunol 2001; 167:4878–4886.

151. Ballas ZK, et al. Induction of NK activity in murine and human cells by CpG motifs in oligodeoxynucleotides and bacterial DNA. J Immunol 1996; 157:1840–1845.

152. Hartmann G, et al. CpG DNA: A potential signal for growth, activation and maturation of human dendritic cells. Proc Natl Acad Sci U S A 1999; 96:9305–9310.

153. Gursel M, et al. Differential and competitive activation of human immune cells by distinct classes of CpG oligodeoxynucleotides. J Leukocyte Biol 2002; 71:813–820.

154. Davis HL, et al. CpG DNA overcomes hyporesponsiveness to hepatitis B vaccine in orangutans. Vaccine 2000; 19, 1920–1924.

155. Jones TR, et al. Synthetic oligodeoxynucleotides containing CpG motifs enhance immunogenic vaccine in Aotus monkeys. Vaccine 1999; 17:3065–3071.

156. Verthelyi D, et al. CpG oligodeoxynucleotides as vaccine adjuvants in primates. J Immunol 2001; 168:1659–1663.

157. Hartmann G, et al. Delineation of a CpG phosphorothioate

oligodeoxynucleotide for activating primate immune responses in vitro and in vivo. J Immunol. 2000 Feb 1; 164(3): 1617–1624.

158. Klinman DM, et al. DNA vaccines: safety and efficacy issues. Springer Semin Immunopathol 1997; 19:245–256.

159. Gilkeson GS, et al. Induction of immune-mediated glomerulonephritis in normal mice immunized with bacterial DNA. Clin Immunol Immunopathol 1993; 68:283–292.

160. Gilkeson GS, et al. Induction of cross-reactive anti-dsDNA antibodies in preautoimmune NZB/NZW mice by immunization with bacterial DNA. J Clin Invest 1995; 95:1398–1402.

161. Steinberg AD, et al. Theoretical and experimental approaches to generalized autoimmunity. Immunol Rev 1990; 118:129–163.

162. Klinman DM, et al. Polyclonal B cell activation in lupus-prone mice precedes and predicts the development of autoimmune disease. J Clin Invest 1990; 86:1249–1254.

163. Klinman DM, Steinberg AD. Systemic autoimmune disease arises from polyclonal B cell activation. J Exp Med 1987; 165:1755–1760.

164. Linker-Israeli M, et al. Elevated levels of endogenous IL-6 in systemic lupus erythematosus. A putative role in pathogenesis. J Immunol 1991; 147:117–123.

165. Watanabe-Fukunaga R, et al. Lymphoproliferation disorder in mice explained by defects in Fas antigen that mediates apoptosis. Nature 1992; 356:314–317.

166. Krieg AM. CpG DNA: a pathogenic factor in systemic lupus erythematosus? J Clin Immunol 1995; 15:284–292.

167. Yi AK, et al. CpG DNA rescue of murine B lymphoma cells from anti-IgM-induced growth arrest and programmed cell death is associated with increased expression of c-myc and bcl-xL. J Immunol 1996; 157:4918–4925.

168. Katsumi A, et al. Humoral and cellular immunity to an encoded protein induced by direct DNA injection. Hum Gene Ther 1994; 5:1335–1339.

169. Mor G, et al. Do DNA vaccines induce autoimmune disease? Hum Gene Ther 1997; 8:293–300.

170. Xiang ZQ, et al. Immune responses to nucleic acid vaccines to rabies virus. Virology 1995; 209:569–579.

171. Gilkeson GS, et al. Effects of bacterial DNA on cytokine production by (NZB/NZW)F1 mice. J Immunol 1998; 161: 3890–3895.

172. Segal BM, et al. Microbial products induce autoimmune disease by an IL-12-dependent pathway. J Immunol 1997; 158:5087–5090.

173. Bachmaier K, et al. Chlamydia infections and heart disease linked through antigenic mimicry. Science 1999; 283:1335–1339.

174. Klinman DM, et al. Repeated administration of synthetic oligodeoxynucleotides expressing CpG motifs provides long-term protection against bacterial infection. Infect Immun 1999; 67:5658–5663.

175. Sparwasser T, et al. Macrophages sense pathogens via DNA motifs: induction of tumor necrosis factor-α-mediated shock. Eur J Immunol 1997; 27:1671–1679.

176. Parker SE, et al. Safety of a GM-CSF adjuvant-plasmid DNA malaria vaccine. Gene Ther 2001; 8:1011–1023.

21

Use of Genetically Detoxified Mutants of Cholera and *Escherichia coli* Heat-Labile Enterotoxins as Mucosal Adjuvants

Gordon Dougan
Imperial College of Science, Technology and Medicine, London, England

Gill Douce
University of Glasgow, Glasgow, Scotland

I. INTRODUCTION

Vaccination remains one of the most cost-effective methods of medical intervention in the battle to reduce human morbidity and mortality from infectious disease in the 21st century. However, its use remains limited due to the existence of many challenging scientific and ethical issues including the high cost of development and licensing, public acceptance of new technologies used in the generation of such vaccines, and high cost of litigation that may result from vaccine failure or damage. Yet the potential for worldwide protection and, in some cases such as smallpox, complete eradication of disease has driven scientists to consider the generation and development of new, effective, cheap, and easy to administer vaccines. To this end, vaccines that induce high levels of protection following a single immunization would be of great benefit, especially if they could be administered without the use of needles. In addition, it is thought that the stimulation of protective immune responses at the natural site of infection is necessary to achieve high levels of efficacy against some infectious agents. This may result in not only the protection of the individual, but also the reduction of the circulation of pathogens in the community and enhancement of herd immunity. For these and other related reasons, there has been a consistent and continuing interest in the development of vaccines that can be delivered via mucosal surfaces (particularly oral and nasal vaccines) [1]. However, the fact that so few mucosal vaccines are in current use indicates that there are significant barriers to their development. These include the fact that most soluble antigens are poorly immunogenic when delivered directly to the host via mucosal surfaces. Even antigens such as tetanus toxoid that are potent immunogens when administered parenterally are weak mucosal immunogens [2]. Stimulation of such responses is limited, as although these surfaces have evolved to deal with the threat of microorganisms and their toxic products, protective immunity has to be induced without simultaneously mounting inappropriate immune responses to food and harmless environmental antigens. Hence there is a sophisticated network of immune regulation operating at the surfaces of the body that control immune responses in an antigen-specific manner [3–5]. Unfortunately, despite intensive investigation, these regulatory mechanisms are currently poorly understood. However, we have known for many years that live pathogens can act as mucosal immunogens, stimulating local and, in some cases, systemic immune responses during infection [6]. Using this information, attenuated derivatives of pathogens and their close relations have been created that can stimulate protective immunity without causing disease. Such live mucosal vaccines are considered elsewhere in this volume.

Immune responses to such pathogens are dependent on the production of a number of pathogen-associated antigens that target host cells, often in a tissue-specific way. Some of these products, including some adhesions and toxins, have been shown to have the ability to act as mucosal immunogens in their native (cell binding) form [7–9]. Hence the mucosal immune system may have some capacity to recognize potentially dangerous antigens produced by pathogens and mount appropriate immune responses against them. Many immune cells express receptors that recognize degenerate pathogen products such as DNA, lipopolysaccharide, and other features distinct to microbes. These include the Toll receptors that lead to signal pathways associated with the activation of innate immune responses [10]. Many adjuvants have the capacity to activate innate immunity via Toll receptors, although it is likely that many other mechanisms remain to be discovered.

Perhaps the most powerful mucosal immunogens identified to date are members of the bacterial enterotoxin family that includes cholera toxin (CT) and the different heat-labile toxins (LT) produced by *Escherichia coli*. Cholera toxin and labile toxin can stimulate potent local and systemic responses to themselves when delivered to the mucosal surfaces of a number of different animals [11]. In addition to being potent mucosal immunogens, LT and CT can activate local and systemic immune responses to uncoupled or (chemically or genetically) coupled antigens that are co-administered to the same mucosal surface in some animals (e.g., mice). Thus LT and CT act as potent mucosal adjuvants [11,12]. Cholera toxin and LT have relatively low toxicity in mice and can be readily used in microgram quantities to adjuvant immune responses to both nasally and orally co-administered proteins, polysaccharides, protein/polysaccharide conjugates, and even whole microorganisms [13,14]. However, in other species, including man, they are toxic and in their native form are not ideal for use as vaccine components [15].

II. STRUCTURAL AND FUNCTIONAL RELATIONSHIPS BETWEEN LABILE TOXIN AND CHOLERA TOXIN

Cholera toxin and labile toxin belong to the AB class of bacterial toxins and share a high degree of homology in both their primary [16] (80% identity) and tertiary structures [17]. The toxins are hetero-oligomeric complexes each composed of an enzymatic A subunit (CT-A or LT-A) and five identical B subunits (CT-B or LT-B) [17,18]. The A subunit is responsible for toxicity, while the pentameric B oligomer binds to receptor(s) on the surface of eukaryotic cells. The A subunit contains an ADP-ribosyltransferase activity which is able to transfer an ADP-ribose group from NAD to host proteins, including the α subunit of the GTP-binding protein Gs that activates adenylate cyclase in mammalian cells. The A subunit is associated with the B subunit via the A2 domain that forms an extended α helix which enters the central cavity of the B subunit oligomer. This A2 domain differs between CT and LT, being nicked in CT but initially unnicked in LT [19]. The A subunit is also able to associate with other eukaryotic proteins, and although cAMP accumulation is thought to lead to toxicity, other factors may provide some contribution to this effect. The B oligomer of these toxins is a pentameric protein of ~ 55 kDa, which contain five identical polypeptide monomers of ~ 11 kDa. These monomers form a compact, protease, and pH-resistant structure, which forms spontaneously even in the absence of the A subunit. The receptor-binding activity of both CT-B and LT-B is specific for polysaccharide groups. Cholera toxin-B binds predominantly to ganglioside GM1, which is almost certainly the major toxin receptor [20]. Labile toxin-B is more promiscuous in that in addition to GM1, it also binds to other molecules including glycosphingolipids and glycoproteins [21–23]. When LT or CT binds to host cells via the B subunit,

they are rapidly internalized into vesicles that undergo retrograde trafficking to the Golgi rather than via the conventional endocytic pathway to lysosomes. During this transport, the A and B subunits remain associated; however, they eventually dissociate and the A subunit is transported via the Golgi to the endoplasmic reticulum and thence to the cytosol. In the cytosol, the A subunits interact with a number of proteins referred to as ADP-ribosylation factors or ARFs. ADP-ribosylation factors normally play a key role in vesicular membrane trafficking, but here, they contribute to the activation of the A subunits [24]. The NAD and ARF binding domains are believed to be distinct on both LT-A and CT-A [25]. When associated together, the A and B subunits form a tightly compact holotoxin structure, which is significantly resistant to denaturation, dissociation, and protease degradation. These characteristics may contribute to the longevity of the toxins at the mucosal surfaces of the body and may play a key contribution to the unique immunogenicity and potentially adjuvanticity of the molecules.

Labile toxin and cholera toxin can induce mucosal IgA and systemic Ig responses after mucosal administration both to themselves and to certain co-administered bystander molecules [26]. Thus they apparently activate immunocompetent cells at mucosal surfaces that are normally regulated to be nonresponders to mucosally delivered antigen. The mucosal immune system is highly organized, and many immune cells are located in specific lymphoid tissues such as those associated with the Peyer's patches of the intestine (the gut-associated lymphoid tissues or GALT). Despite the high degree of homology that exists between CT and LTs, most immunological studies indicate subtle differences in the adjuvant activity of these proteins, with CT-mediated adjuvanticity apparently accompanied by a preferential activation of T helper 2 (Th2) type CD4+ cell populations. In contrast, polarization of the response is less pronounced when LT is used as an adjuvant, with both Th1 and Th2 cells being activated [27]. These differences may reflect subtle differences that exist in the binding of the proteins to their receptors, inherent stability of the holotoxin molecule, trafficking and activation of secondary messengers within the cell, and the level of enzymatic activation once inside the cell. It is also important to recognize that there is considerable variation in the type of T cell immunity (Th1 vs. Th2) reported from different laboratories using LT and CT as mucosal adjuvants. Thus many factors such as toxin purity, animal health, and variations in local experimental practice may influence the type of immunity induced. Nevertheless, both CT and LT have been consistently shown to be potent mucosal adjuvants of both humoral and cellular immune responses in the mouse and other animals [28,29].

The potent mucosal adjuvant activity of LT and CT has attracted considerable interest from immunologists keen to investigate the mechanisms of mucosal adjuvanticity associated with defined molecules. However, despite much intensive investigation, we still do not understand how these enterotoxins act as mucosal adjuvants. One problem is the fact that the mechanism is likely to involve multiple steps in which different cell types operating in a strictly regulated environment are required to interact. Thus work in vitro using purified cellular components and these toxins may provide potentially misleading clues about these mechanisms. Labile toxin and cholera toxin can induce both CD4- and CD8-associated immune responses to bystander antigens [30]. Cholera toxin can induce CD4 T cells secreting interleukin (IL)-4, IL-5, IL-6, and IL-10 which may provide help for antibody class switching to IgG and IgA [27]. Cholera toxin and labile toxin can induce the production of CD8 cytotoxic lymphocytes that can contribute to the protection against disease [31,32]. One area that could be of vital importance is antigen presentation. Treatment of both B cells and macrophages with CT and LT is known to influence the levels of expression of the B7-1 and B7-2 signal molecules, implicating B7/CD28 signaling in adjuvant activity [33]. CD40 may also play a role in adjuvanticity as LT and CT lose some adjuvant activity in CD40 gene knockout mice, although this defect has not been linked directly to CD40–CD40 ligand interactions [27]. Interestingly, CT, rather than LT, has been shown in vitro to reduce expression of CD40 on CD4 cells [34], which may help to explain the greater polarization of Th2 responses observed when CT rather than LT is used as an adjuvant. Cholera toxin and labile toxin can also influence antigen presentation by dendritic cells. Cholera toxin-treated dendritic cells upregulate HLA-DR molecule expression on their surface, increase B7-1 and B7-2 expression, and are able to prime naive T cells, driving the polarization toward Th2 [35]. Cholera toxin treatment also influences chemokine receptor expression [35]. Clearly, more work will be needed in this area if we are to define the immunological mechanisms underpinning this adjuvant activity.

III. THE ADJUVANTICITY OF NONTOXIC MUTANT DERIVATIVES OF LABILE TOXIN AND CHOLERA TOXIN

A key question concerning the mechanism of mucosal antigenicity associated with CT and LT is whether toxicity is linked to adjuvanticity. Early studies using CT-B or LT-B purified by biochemical means from wild-type, fully toxic enterotoxins proved difficult to interpret because of the potential contamination of the nontoxic B subunits with small amounts of the fully toxic parent toxins. Controlled experiments showed that even very small levels of LT or CT toxin contamination could enhance significantly any adjuvant activity associated with the B subunits [36]. Hence investigators turned to the use of highly purified preparations of recombinant proteins produced by heterologous expression hosts that did not produce the wild-type toxins. Production and testing of these recombinant proteins have allowed us to clarify the contribution of the different characteristics and domains of LT and CT to the adjuvant activity of these proteins. Overall studies with the recombinant B subunits in different systems indicate that both LT-B and CT-B retain some ability to act as mucosal adjuvants. Most data indicate that both B subunits are weaker adjuvants than the holotoxins, although there is no universal agreement about this between different laboratories. Labile toxin-B appears to retain

a more potent adjuvant capacity than CT-B, possibly because LT-B is a more stable pentamer than CT-B [37]. Labile toxin-B may also have a more substantial effect on trafficking (vasculation and protein retention in vesicles) than CT-B, potentially influencing the length of time antigens are presented to the immune system [38].

A number of groups have generated mutations in the B subunit that obliterate or reduce the ability of this subunit to bind to its receptor. From these studies, it appears that receptor-binding activity contributes significantly to adjuvant activity [39,40], although this is not a consistent finding as some nonbinding mutants may retain some adjuvant activity particularly following nasal delivery [41] which is a more sensitive route than oral immunization. Recently, a novel B subunit mutant has been described which is able to bind GM1 and traffic to the Golgi but is unable to influence immunomodulation (by either the B subunit alone or the holotoxin if genetically created in this molecule). This mutant LTH57A [42], in which the histidine at position 57 of the B subunit has been changed for an arginine, is believed to result in a more rigid protein structure. It has been postulated that this reduction in flexibility prevents interaction with membrane proteins that are important in the activation of secondary signal pathways within the host cell, which are important for adjuvanticity.

In addition to work with the B subunits, many different site-directed mutants of LT and CT have been created, and these have been used to monitor the relationship between structure and function with respect to adjuvant activity [26]. Many mutations in the toxins generate mutant derivatives that are either unstable, unable to form AB complexes, or have properties indistinguishable from wild-type toxins [26]. However, some site-directed mutants are able to form stable AB complexes but exhibit either severely reduced or undetectable levels of toxicity or ADP-ribosyltransferase activity [43]. Of these mutants, LTK63, CTK63 (harboring inactivating lysine substitutions at position 63 of the respective A subunits), and CTE112K (harboring a lysine substitution at position 112 of the CT-A subunit) [44,45] have been studied in most detail. These molecules form stable holotoxoid complexes but do not detectably direct the accumulation of cAMP in target cells. They do not appear to ADP-ribosylate host proteins and are nontoxic when incubated with cultured cells or evaluated in ligated intestinal loop assays [46]. LTK63 also retains the ability to interact with ARFs. The crystal structure of LTK63 has been solved and compared directly to the wild-type LT parental toxin. The two molecules show indistinguishable identity except for a bulge in the active site associated with the lysine at position 63 [47]. LTK63 has been consistently shown to retain significant adjuvant activity, capable of adjuvanting both CD4- and CD8-associated immune responses [30,31]. However, CTK63 is a poor mucosal adjuvant [48]. The adjuvant activity of LTK63 also appears to be consistently greater than LT-B in direct comparisons using identical bystander molecules [49]. CTE112K appears to exhibit similar properties to LTK63 in terms of the level of adjuvant activity [50]. Thus these experiments conclusively show that mutants of LT and CT with undetectable activity can retain adjuvant activity.

Several mutant derivatives have been created that have significantly reduced toxicity and enzymatic activity but retained some adjuvant activity. These include LTR72 [51] and CTS106 [48]. Both these molecules are excellent mucosal adjuvants with levels of activity approaching those of the wild-type toxins. Other mutant derivatives with reduced activity have been created by introducing mutations into the protease-sensitive loop of LT. LTG192 is perhaps best characterized by this class and has an arginine replaced by a glycine at position 192 of the A subunit [52] which reduces the efficiency of protease nicking associated with the A2 domain of the toxin. In vitro, the mutant is completely trypsin-resistant, however, in vivo, proteases other than trypsin can cleave the loop and activate the toxin, resulting in detectable toxicity [46]. LTG192 retains significant adjuvanticity [53], and ongoing human trials are expected to establish the safety profile of this adjuvant.

From the above studies, it appears that several characteristics of the LT/CT classes of enterotoxins contribute to adjuvant activity. Binding to receptors has been shown to be relevant for this activity, as has stability of the holotoxin structure. However, the fact that nontoxic mutants of both LT and CT retain greater adjuvant activity than the B subunit alone suggests that the formation of the holotoxoid may contribute towards the increased activity of these proteins at immune-inductive sites in vivo. Generation of these mutants has allowed us to see that although enzymatic activity and toxicity are not essential for adjuvant activity, they contribute to it. A dose–response curve measuring the adjuvant activity of different LT derivatives at different immunization doses has shown that a few nanograms of LT-B or LTK63 have no obvious adjuvant activity when administered intranasally to mice with bystander antigens [51]. However, increasing the amount of LTK63 reveals adjuvant activity at concentrations lower than that required for showing similar levels of activity with LT-B. In contrast, wild-type LT exhibits adjuvant activity at much lower doses than either LTK63 or LT-B. However, the activity of LT increases in a dose-dependent manner, following the curve of LTK63, suggesting that the influence of enzymatic activity can become saturated. Interestingly, the mutant LTR72, which has reduced toxic activity, behaved in a manner intermediate to LTK63 and LT in these assays. Thus enzymatic activity acts in a dose-independent manner, whereas the nontoxic AB complex acts in a manner dependent on dose. The inactivated A subunit may enhance LT-B-associated activity by increasing the resistance of the complex to denaturing factors. Also, the LT-A subunit of LTK63 is still delivered via the Golgi to the cell cytosol, and the interaction of this subunit with host factors such as ARF may play important roles in adjuvanticity. Clearly, the mechanism of adjuvanticity is complex and is likely to be multifactorial.

Some investigations have been made comparing the immunological properties of LT and CT mutant derivatives to wild-type toxins. CTE112K retains a Th2-type activation profile associated with the upregulation of B7 on antigen-presenting cells [45]. LTK63 enhances a mixed Th1/Th2-type response, whereas LTK72 promotes a more Th2-type response [54]. LTK63 and LT-B apparently enhance IL-12 and

interferon γ production as well as NFk-B activation levels comparable to both LT and LTR72 [55].

IV. CLINICAL EVALUATION OF LABILE TOXIN AND MUTANT DERIVATIVES AS MUCOSAL ADJUVANTS

Although many studies have now been performed in animal models using these adjuvants, very few have been conducted in human volunteers. In fact, most clinical studies to date have actually used the wild-type LT to evaluate the potential of this molecule as a mucosal adjuvant. Early studies with wild-type cholera-like enterotoxins in volunteers showed that microgram quantities could induce diarrhea when ingested orally [15]. Despite this observation, wild-type enterotoxins have been fed to volunteers as potential adjuvants. In one study, wild-type LT was used to immunize volunteers along with a recombinant urease from *Helicobacter pylori* [56]. Volunteers received several doses of vaccine and were divided into groups who received different amounts of urease together with LT. A number of the volunteers who received LT developed diarrhea, and although immune responses to *H. pylori* urease were detected, the adjuvant activity of LT was not clearly demonstrated. Human LT has also been formulated into a virosome preparation containing the hemagglutinin of influenza virus, and this vaccine has been administered intranasally to many people in Switzerland [57]. In preregistration volunteer studies, vaccine formulations containing hemagglutinin were prepared with or without LT and administered as two independent intranasal sprays. This immunization regime induced a humoral immune response to hemagglutinin that was equivalent to a single parenteral immunization and was associated with an anti-hemagglutinin IgA response in the nasal secretions of the volunteers. Incorporation of LT apparently enhanced the immune response to the virus antigen, demonstrating some adjuvant activity with LT in humans.

A study using the protease-sensitive mutant LTG192 as an adjuvant has recently been reported in human volunteers. In these studies, the protein was admixed with a formalin-inactivated whole cell *H. pylori* antigen with or without LTG192 [58]. The oral immunization was performed using both *H. pylori*-free and infected volunteers. Following vaccination, some of the volunteers developed diarrhea and other adverse events were reported. However, significant increases were detected in the production of anti-*H. pylori* IgA at appropriate mucosal sites (fecal and salivary) in the group receiving high doses of *H. pylori* cells, and lympho-proliferative responses associated with the generation of IFN-γ were detected in some volunteers.

Progress towards further volunteer studies using mutant LT molecules has recently been inhibited by concerns that these holotoxoid molecules may traffic to the brain through olfactory nerves particularly following intranasal immunization [59]. Wild-type toxin has been used in combination with commercial influenza vaccine [57], although safety follow-ups on the patients should have revealed some side effects. Other studies have found no olfactory involvement following intranasal immunization [60]. It is reasonable to hypothesize that in this case, the use of a nontoxic mutant of these adjuvants would additionally minimize the risk of serious adverse events.

V. CONCLUSION

Over the last 5 years, much progress has been made in the generation, development, and testing of bacterial enterotoxins as mucosal adjuvants. Using molecular techniques, a collection of mutants was generated which have allowed us to assign a role for binding, holotoxin structure, and enzymatic activity in the adjuvant activity of these proteins. Much work still remains especially regarding the specific immune mechanisms activated by such toxins, and further clinical trials are urgently needed in this area if LT- or CT-based mucosal adjuvants are ever to find use in human vaccines. Another exciting approach that could offer potential practical benefits in the future is the design of novel artificial mucosal adjuvants based on LT/CT components or mimetic equivalents [61].

ACKNOWLEDGMENTS

This work was supported by grants from The Wellcome Trust and EU (MUCIMM and NEOVAC).

REFERENCES

1. Levine MM, Dougan G. Optimism over vaccines administered through mucosal surfaces. Lancet 1998; 351:1375–1376.
2. Douce G, Turcotte C, Cropley I, Roberts M, Pizza M, Domenghini M, Rappuoli R, Dougan G. Mutants of *Escherichia coli* heat labile toxin that lack ADP-ribosyltransferase activity act as nontoxic mucosal adjuvants. Proc Natl Acad Sci U S A 1995; 92:16644–16648.
3. Czerkinsky C, Anjuere F, McGhee JR, George-Chandy A, Holmgren J, Kieny MP, Fujiyashi K, Mestecky JF, Pierrefite-Carle V, Rask C, Sun JB. Mucosal immunity and tolerance: relevance to vaccine development. Immunol Rev 1999; 170:197–222.
4. Nagler-Anderson C. Man the barrier! Strategic defences in the intestinal mucosa. Nat Rev Immunol 2001; 1:59–67.
5. Hayday A, Viney JL. The ins and outs of body surface immunology. Science 2000; 290:97–100.
6. Tacket CO, Sztein MB, Losonsky GA, Wasserman SS, Nataro JP, Edelman R, Pickard D, Dougan G, Chatfield SN, Levine MM. Safety of live oral *Salmonella typhi* vaccine strains with deletions in *htrA* and *aroC aroD* and immune response in humans. Infect Immun 1997; 65:452–456.
7. Jespersgaard C, Hajishengallis G, Huang Y, Russell MW, Smith DJ, Michalek SM. Protective immunity against *Streptococcus mutans* infection in mice after intranasal immunization with the glucan-binding region of *S. mutans* glucosyltransferase. Infect Immun 1999; 67:6543–6549.
8. Van den Broeck W, Cox E, Goddeeris BM. Induction of immune responses in pigs following oral administration of purified F4 fimbriae. Vaccine 1999; 17:2020–2029.
9. Cropley I, Douce G, Roberts M, Chatfield S, Pizza M, Marsili I, Rappuoli R, Dougan GD. Mucosal and systemic immunogenicity of a recombinant, non-ADP-ribosylating pertussis toxin: effects of formaldehyde treatment. Vaccine 1995; 13:16448–16648.
10. Medzhitov R. Toll-like receptors and innate immunity. Nat Rev Immunol 2001; 1:135–145.
11. Lycke N, Holmgren J. Strong adjuvant effects of cholera toxin on gut mucosal immune responses to orally presented antigens. Immunology 1986; 39:301–308.
12. Holmgren J, Lycke N, Czerkinsky C. Cholera toxin and cholera B subunit as oral-mucosal adjuvant and antigen vector systems. Vaccine 1993; 11:1179–1181.
13. Jakobsen H, Schulz D, Pizza M, Rappuoli R, Jonsdottir I. Intranasal immunisation with pneumococcal polysaccharide conjugate vaccines with nontoxic mutants of *Escherichia coli* heat-labile enterotoxins as adjuvants protects mice against invasive pneumococcal infections. Infect Immun 1999; 67:5892–5897.
14. Rollwagen, FM, Pacheco, ND, Clements, JD, Pavlovaskis, O, Rollins, DM, Walker, RI. Killed *Campylobacter* elicits immune responses and protection when administered with an oral adjuvant. Infect Immun 1993; 11:1316–1320.
15. Levine MM, Kaper JB, Black RE, Clements ML. New knowledge on pathogenesis of bacterial enteric infections as applied to vaccine development. Microbiol Rev 1983; 47: 510–550.
16. Spicer EK, Kavanaugh WM, Dallas WS, Falkow S, Konigsberg WH, Schafer DE. Sequence homologies between A subunits of *Escherichia coli* and *Vibrio cholerae* enterotoxins. Proc Natl Acad Sci U S A 1981; 78:50–54.
17. Sixma TK, Kalk KH, Van Zanten BA, Dauter Z, Kingma J, Witholt B, Hol WGJ. Refined structure of *Escherichia coli* heat-labile enterotoxin, a close relative of cholera toxin. J Mol Biol 1993; 230:890–918.
18. Sixma TK, Pronk SE, Kalk KH, Wartna ES, Van Zanten BA, Witholt B, Hol WGJ. Crystal structure of cholera related heat labile toxin from *Escherichia coli*. Nature 1991; 351:371–377.
19. Grant CCR, Messer RJ, Cieplak W. Role of trypsin-like cleavage at arginine 192 in the enzymatic and cytotoxic activities of *Escherichia coli* heat-labile enterotoxin. Infect Immun 1994; 62:4270–4278.
20. Holmgren J, Lonnroth I, Svennerholm L. Fixation and inactivation of cholera toxin by GM1 ganglioside. Scand J Infect Dis 1973; 5:77–78.
21. Holmgren J, Lindblad M, Fredman P, Svennerholm L, Myrvold H. Comparison of receptors for cholera and *Escherichia coli* enterotoxins in human intestine. Gastroenterology 1985; 89:27–35.
22. Holmgren J, Fredman P, Lindblad M, Svennerholm AM, Svennerholm L. Rabbit intestinal glycoprotein receptor for *Escherichia coli* heat-labile enterotoxin lacking affinity for cholera toxin. Infect Immun 1982; 38:424–433.
23. Teneberg S, Hirst TR, Angstrom J, Karlsson KA. Comparison of the glycolipid-binding specificities of cholera toxin and porcine *Escherichia coli* heat-labile enterotoxin: identification of a receptor-active non-ganglioside glycolipid for the heat-labile toxin in infant rabbit small intestine. Glycoconj J 1994; 11:533–540.
24. Zhu X, Kahn RA. The *Escherichia coli* heat labile toxin (LTA1) binds to Golgi membranes and alters Golgi and cell morphologies using ARF-dependent processes. J Biol Chem 2001; 276:25014–25021.
25. Stevens LA, Moss J, Vaughan M, Pizza M, Rappuoli R. Effects of site-directed mutagenesis of *Escherichia coli* heat labile enterotoxin on ADP-ribosyltransferase activity and interaction with ADP-ribosylation factors. Infect Immun 1999; 67:259–265.
26. Rappuoli R, Pizza M, Douce G, Dougan G. Structure and mucosal adjuvanticity of cholera and *Escherichia coli* heat labile enterotoxins. Immunol Today 1999; 20:493–500.
27. Yamamoto M, Kiyono H, Kweon M-N, Yamamoto S, Fujihashi K, Kurazono H, Imaoka K, Bluethemann H, Takahashi I, Takeda Y, Azuma M, McGhee JR. Enterotoxin

adjuvants have direct effects on T cells and antigen presenting cells that result in either interleukin-4 dependent or -independent immune responses. J Infect Dis 2000; 182:180–190.

28. Lee CK. Vaccination against *Helicobacter pylori* in non-human primate models and humans. Scand J Immunol 2001; 53:437–442.

29. Yuan L, Iosef C, Azevedo MS, Kim Y, Qian Y, Geyer A, Nguyen TV, Chang KO, Saif LJ. Protective immunity and antibody-secreting cell responses elicited by combined oral attenuated Wa human rotavirus and intranasal Wa 2/6-VLPs with mutant *Escherichia coli* heat-labile toxin in gnotobiotic pigs. J Virol 2001; 75:9229–9238.

30. Simmons CP, Mastroeni P, Fowler R, Ghaem-Maghami M, Lycke N, Pizza M, Rappuoli R, Dougan G. MHC class I restricted cytotoxic lymphocyte responses induced by enterotoxin based mucosal adjuvants. J Immunol 1999; 163:6502–6510.

31. Partidos CD, Salani BF, Pizza M, Rappuoli R. Heat-labile enterotoxin of *Escherichia coli* and its site-directed mutant LTK63 enhance the proliferative and cytotoxic T-cell responses to intranasally co-immunized synthetic peptides. Immunol Lett 1999; 67:209–216.

32. Jones HP, Hodge LM, Fujihashi K, Kiyono H, McGhee JR, Simecka JW. The pulmonary environment promotes Th2 cell responses after nasal-pulmonary immunisation with antigen alone, but Th1 responses are induced during instances of intense immune stimulation. J Immunol 2001; 167:4518–4526.

33. Cong C, Weaver CT, Elson CO. The mucosal adjuvanticity of cholera toxin involves enhancement of costimulatory activity by selective up-regulation of B7.2 expression. J Immunol 1997; 159:5301–5308.

34. Martin M, Metzinger DJ, Michalek SM, Connell TD, Russell MW. Distinct cytokine regulation by cholera toxin and type II heat-labile toxins involves differential regulation of CD 40 ligand on CD4+ T cells. Infect Immun 2001; 69:4486–4492.

35. Gagliardi MC, Sallusto F, Marinaro M, Langenkamp A, Lanzavecchia A, De Magistris M-T. Cholera toxin induces maturation of human dendritic cells and licences them for Th2 priming. Eur J Immunol 2000; 30:2394–2403.

36. Tamura S, Asanuma H, Tomita T, Komase K, Kawahara K, Danbara H, Hattori N, Watanabe K, Suzuki Y, Nagamine T. *Escherichia coli* heat-labile enterotoxin B subunits supplemented with a trace amount of the holotoxin as an adjuvant for nasal influenza vaccine. Vaccine 1994; 12:1083–1089.

37. Millar DG, Hirst TR, Snider DP. *Escherichia coli* heat-labile enterotoxin B subunit is a more potent mucosal adjuvant than its closely related homologue, the B subunit of cholera toxin. Infect Immun 2001; 69:3476–3482.

38. Millar DG, Hirst TR. Cholera toxin and *Escherichia coli* enterotoxin B subunits inhibit macrophage-mediated antigen processing and presentation: evidence for antigen persistence in non-acidic recycling endosomal compartments. Cell Microbiol 2001; 3:311–329.

39. Nasher TO, Williams NA, Hirst TR. Importance of receptor binding in the immunogenicity, adjuvanticity and therapeutic properties of cholera toxin and *Escherichia coli* heat-labile toxin. Med Microbiol Immunol 1998; 187:3–10.

40. Nasher TO, Webb HM, Eaglestone S, Williams NA, Hirst TR. Potent immunogenicity of the B subunits of *Escherichia coli* heat-labile enterotoxin: receptor binding is essential and induces modulation of lymphocyte subsets. Proc Natl Acad Sci U S A 1996; 93:226–230.

41. Guidry JJ, Cardenas L, Cheng E, Clements JD. Role of receptor binding in toxicity, immunogenicity, and adjuvanticity of *Escherichia coli* heat-labile toxin. Infect Immun 1997; 65:4943–4950.

42. Aman AT, Fraser S, Merritt EA, Rodigherio C, Kenny M,

Ahn M, Hol WGJ, Williams NA, Lencer WI, Hirst TR. A mutant cholera toxin B subunit that binds GM1-ganglioside but lacks immunomodulatory or toxic activity. Proc Natl Acad Sci U S A 2001; 98:8536–8541.

43. Tsuji T, Inoue T, Miyama A, Okamoto K, Honda T, Miwanti T. A single amino acid substitution in the A subunit of *Escherichia coli* enterotoxin results in a loss of its toxic activity. J Biol Chem 1990; 265:22520–22525.

44. Yamamoto S, Takeda Y, Yamamoto M, Kurazono H, Imaoka K, Yamamoto M, Fujihashi K, Noda M, Kiyono H, McGhee JR. Mutants in the ADP-ribosyltransferase cleft of cholera toxin lack diarrheagenicity but retain adjuvanticity. J Exp Med 1997; 185:1203–1210.

45. Yamamoto S, Kiyono H, Yamamoto M, Imaoka K, Yamamoto M, Fujihashi K, Van Ginkel FW, Noda M, Takeda Y, McGhee JR. A nontoxic mutant of cholera toxin elicits Th2-type responses for enhanced mucosal immunity. Proc Natl Acad Sci U S A 1997; 94:5267–5272.

46. Giannelli V, Fontana MR, Giuliani MM, Guangcai D, Rappuoli R, Pizza M. Protease susceptibility and toxicity of heat-labile enterotoxins with a mutation in the active site or in the protease-sensitive loop. Infect Immun 1997; 65:331–334.

47. van den Akker F, Pizza M, Rappuoli R, Hol WG. Crystal structure of a non-toxic mutant of heat-labile enterotoxin, which is a potent mucosal adjuvant. Protein Sci 1997; 6:2650–2654.

48. Douce G, Fontana M, Pizza M, Rappuoli R, Dougan G. Intranasal immunogenicity and adjuvanticity of site-directed mutant derivatives of cholera toxin. Infect Immun 1997; 65:2821–2828.

49. Douce G, Giuliani MM, Giannelli V, Pizza MG, Rappuoli R, Dougan G. Mucosal immunogenicity of genetically detoxified derivatives of heat labile toxin from *Escherichia coli*. Vaccine 1998; 16:1065–1073.

50. Yamamoto M, McGhee JR, Hagiwara Y, Otake S, Kiyono H. Genetically manipulated bacterial toxin as a new generation mucosal adjuvant. Scand J Immunol 2001; 53:211–217.

51. Giuliani MM, Del Giudice G, Giannelli V, Dougan G, Douce G, Rappuoli R, Pizza M. Mucosal adjuvanticity and immunogenicity of LTR72, a novel mutant of *Escherichia coli* heat-labile enterotoxin with partial knockout of ADP-ribosyltransferase activity. J Exp Med 1998; 187:1123–1132.

52. Dickinson BL, Clements JD. Dissociation of *Escherichia coli* heat-labile enterotoxin adjuvanticity from ADP–ribosyltransferase activity. Infect Immun 1995; 63:1617–1623.

53. Cheng E, Cardenas-Freytag L, Clements JD. The role of cAMP in mucosal adjuvanticity of *Escherichia coli* heat-labile enterotoxin (LT). Vaccine 2000; 18:38–49.

54. Ryan EJ, McNeela E, Murphy GA, Stewart H, O'Hagan D, Pizza M, Rappuoli R, Mills KHG. Mutants of *Escherichia coli* heat-labile toxin act as effective mucosal adjuvants for nasal delivery of acellular pertussis vaccine:differential effects of nontoxic AB complex and enzyme activity on Th1 and Th2 cells. Infect Immun 1999; 67:6270–6280.

55. Ryan EJ, McNeela E, Pizza M, Rappuoli R, O'Neill L, Mills KHG. Modulation of innate and acquired immune responses by *Escherichia coli* heat-labile toxin: distinct pro- and anti-inflammatory effects of the nontoxic AB complex and the enzyme activity. J Immunol 2000; 165:5750–5759.

56. Michetti P, Kreiss C, Kotloff KL, Porta N, Blanco JL, Bachmann D, Herranz M, Saldinger PF, Corthesy-Theulaz I, Losonsky G, Nichols R, Simon J, Stolte M, Ackerman S, Monath TP, Blum AL, adults. OiwuaEch-leisaiiHp-i. Oral immunization with urease and *Escherichia coli* heat-labile enterotoxin is safe and immunogenic in *Helicobacter pylori*-infected adults. Gastroenterology 1999; 116:804–812.

57. Gluck R, Mischler R, Durrer P, Fruer E, Lang AB, Herzog

C, Cryz SJ. Safety and immunogenicity of intranasally administered inactivated trivalent virosome-formulated influenza vaccine containing *Escherichia coli* heat-labile toxin as a mucosal adjuvant. J Infect Dis 2000; 181:1129–1132.

58. Kotloff KI, Sztein MB, Wasserman SS, Losonsky GA, DiLorenzo SC, Walker RI. Safety and immunogenicity of oral inactivated whole-cell *Helicobacter pylori* vaccine with adjuvant among volunteers with or without subclinical infection. Infect Immun 2001; 69:3581–3590.

59. Van Ginkel FW, Jackson RJ, Yuki Y, McGhee JR. Cutting edge: the mucosal adjuvant cholera toxin redirects vaccine proteins into olfactory tissues. J Immunol 2000; 165:4778–4782.

60. Hagiwara Y, Iwasaki T, Asanuma H, Sato Y, Sata T, Aizawa C, Kurata T, Tamura S-I. Effects of intranasal administration of cholera toxin (or *Escherichia coli* heat-labile enterotoxin) B subunits supplemented with a trace amount of the holotoxin on the brain. Vaccine 2001; 19: 1652–1660.

61. Agren LC, Ekman L, Lowenalder B, Lycke NY. Genetically engineered nontoxic vaccine adjuvant that combines B cell targeting with immunomodulation by cholera toxin A1 subunit. J Immunol 1997; 158:3936–3946.

22
Recent Developments in Vaccine Delivery Systems

Derek T. O'Hagan
Chiron Corporation, Emeryville, California, U.S.A.

I. INTRODUCTION

This chapter reviews recent developments in the use of vaccine adjuvants, which function primarily as "vaccine delivery systems." Hence I will focus on emulsion, liposome, iscom, and microparticle-based adjuvants, whose principal mode of action is the delivery of antigens into the key cells and/or sites that are responsible for the induction of immune responses. Immunological adjuvants were originally described by Ramon [1] as "substances used in combination with a specific antigen that produced a more robust immune response than the antigen alone." This broad definition encompasses a very wide range of materials [2], including a range of particulate delivery systems. Generally, immunological adjuvants have proven notoriously difficult to classify in any rational way, primarily because their mechanisms of action are often ill defined. Although this chapter will focus primarily on particulate adjuvants, in many situations these have been combined with additional adjuvants. Primarily, adjuvants are components of bacteria and viruses, or synthetic agents that mimic these, and are recognized as "danger signals" by receptors on innate immune cells, including the toll-like receptors (TLRs), which trigger the release of a cascade of proinflammatory cytokines [3]. Hence, many adjuvants have been referred to as representing pathogen-associated molecular patterns (PAMPs), although synthetic molecules can also be used as mimics. A full discussion of both adjuvants and delivery systems is beyond the scope of this chapter, but has been reviewed recently [4]. For an optimal adjuvant effect, it is becoming increasingly common to use delivery systems to target both antigen and adjuvants into the same immunocompetent cells. In these situations, it becomes even more difficult to determine the mechanism of action for the combined adjuvant formulation. In many studies that will be discussed in this chapter, it is clear that synergies between adjuvants and delivery systems are possible and optimal vaccine formulations using a variety of components.

Although many approaches have been extensively evaluated over the years, the only adjuvants currently approved by the U.S. Food and Drug Administration are aluminum-based mineral salts (generically called alum). Alum has been used as an adjuvant for many years, but its mechanism of action still remains poorly defined. It was originally thought to provide a "depot" effect, resulting in persistence of antigen at the injection site following immunization. However, studies involving radiolabeled antigens have brought this assumption into question [5]. Recent work has indicated that alum upregulates costimulatory signals on human monocytes and promotes the release of IL-4 [6]. It has also been suggested that alum adsorption may make an important contribution to a reduction in toxicity for some vaccines because of the adsorption of contaminating endotoxin [7]. Nevertheless, although alum has a good safety record, comparative studies show that it is a weak adjuvant for antibody induction to protein subunit antigens, a poor adjuvant for cell-mediated immunity (CMI) in general, and ineffective for the induction of cytotoxic T lymphocytes (CTLs) [8]. Moreover, alum adjuvants can induce IgE antibody responses and have been associated with allergic reactions in some subjects [8,9]. Therefore, there is an urgent need for the development of new-generation adjuvants, which can induce potent CMI, including CTL responses, work with a broad range of antigens, to include recombinant proteins and DNA vaccines, and be appropriate for different routes of delivery, to include mucosal immunization.

A key issue in adjuvant development is toxicity, since safety concerns have restricted the development of adjuvants since alum was first introduced more than 50 years ago [10]. Many experimental adjuvants and delivery systems have advanced to clinical trials and some have demonstrated high potency, but most have proven too toxic for routine clinical use. For prophylactic immunization in healthy individuals, only adjuvants that induce minimal adverse effects will prove acceptable. In contrast, for adjuvants that are designed to be used in life-threatening situations, e.g., as a component of cancer vaccines, the acceptable level of adverse events would likely be increased. This might also be true for adjuvants to be used in vaccines as therapeutic agents in people already infected with pathogens with life-threatening consequences, e.g., HIV and HCV. This review will focus primarily on antigen delivery systems to be used in prophylactic or therapeutic vaccines against infectious diseases. Developments in cancer vaccines have recently been reviewed elsewhere [11,12].

Following the discovery of some very potent adjuvant molecules in recent years, including synthetic oligonucleotides based on unmethylated bacterial DNA (CpG DNA), there has been some concern that these potent adjuvants might activate immunity to such an extent that autoimmune conditions might be triggered. This is a reasonable concern for adjuvant actives that mimic components of pathogenic microorganisms and provide potent proinflammatory signals. However, the timing and localization of the proinflammatory stimuli may prove to be important. In this context, limiting the systemic distribution of the adjuvants and focusing their effects specifically onto the key immune cells is likely to be beneficial. Hence, an important contribution of particulate delivery systems may be to limit the toxicity of adjuvants by limiting their systemic distribution following injection. Additional practical issues important for the development of adjuvants and delivery systems include biodegradability, stability, ease of manufacture, cost, and applicability to a wide range of vaccines. Ideally, for ease of administration and enhanced patient compliance, the adjuvant should allow the vaccine to be administered by a mucosal route, preferably orally.

II. THE ROLE OF ADJUVANTS IN VACCINE DEVELOPMENT

The precise mechanisms of action of most adjuvants still remain only partially understood, and this has impeded the rational development of new adjuvants. Immunization activates a complex cascade of innate and adaptive responses, and the primary effect of the adjuvant is often difficult to discern. However, if the geographical concept of immune reactivity is accepted, in which antigens that do not reach the local lymph nodes do not induce responses [13], it becomes easier to propose mechanistic interpretations for the important effects of some adjuvants, particularly those that function mainly as delivery systems. If antigens that do not reach lymph nodes do not induce responses, then any adjuvant that enhances delivery of the antigen to the node may be expected to induce an enhanced response. Antigen delivery to lymph nodes may be enhanced in a number of ways; the adjuvant may increase cellular infiltration into the injection site, so that more cells are present to take up antigen, it may directly promote the uptake of antigen into antigen-presenting cells (APCs) through activating phagocytosis, or it may directly deliver the antigen to the local lymph node by exiting from the injection site and moving into the lymphatics. The most important APCs involved in antigen capture are thought to be dendritic cells (DCs), which have the unique ability to present antigen to naive T cells in lymph nodes. However, macrophages are also known to be important APCs and their role may be underappreciated.

III. PARTICULATE ANTIGEN DELIVERY SYSTEMS

The use of particulate antigen delivery systems as alternative approaches or in combination with adjuvant molecules has been evaluated extensively. Particulate adjuvants (e.g., emulsions, microparticles, immunostimulatory complexes [iscoms], liposomes, virosomes, and viruslike particles) have comparable dimensions to the pathogens that the immune system evolved to combat. Therefore, these particulates are normally taken up efficiently by phagocytic cells of the innate immune system and function mainly to deliver associated antigen into these key cells. Adjuvant molecules, often PAMPs, may also be included in particulate delivery systems to further enhance the level of response or to focus the response through a desired pathway, e.g., Th1 or Th2. In addition, formulating potent adjuvants into delivery systems may limit adverse events through restricting the systemic distribution of the adjuvant.

A. Emulsions

A potent oil-in-water (o/w) emulsion adjuvant, the syntex adjuvant formulation (SAF) [14], was developed using a biodegradable oil (squalane) in the 1980s, as a replacement for Freund's adjuvants. Freund's complete adjuvant (FCA) is a potent but toxic water in mineral-oil-in-water (w/o) adjuvant, which includes Arlacel A as a detergent and contains killed mycobacteria [15]. Incomplete Freund's adjuvant, which does not contain mycobacteria, is still in use for cancer vaccines and as an immunotherapeutic vaccine in HIV-infected individuals [16]. However, mineral oil adjuvants are generally considered too toxic for routine use in prophylactic vaccines. SAF also contained a bacterial cell-wall-based synthetic adjuvant, threonyl muramyl dipeptide (t-MDP), and a nonionic surfactant, poloxamer L121, but proved too toxic for widespread use in humans [10]. Therefore, a squalene o/w emulsion was developed (MF59), without the presence of additional adjuvants, which proved to be potent, but with an acceptable safety profile [17]. Squalene, which is commercially derived from shark liver oil, is an intermediate in human steroid hormone biosynthesis and is a direct synthetic precursor to cholesterol. MF59 enhanced the immunogenicity of influenza vaccine in small animal models [18–20] and was shown to be a more potent adjuvant than alum for hepatitis B vaccine (HBV) in baboons [21]. Subsequently, the safety and immunogenicity of MF59-adjuvanted influenza vaccine (FLUAD™) was confirmed in elderly subjects in clinical trials [22,23], and these data allowed the approval of this product for licensure in Italy in 1997 and for several additional countries through mutual recognition in 2000. Recent clinical data have shown that the potency of MF59 as an adjuvant for influenza vaccine may be particularly advantageous in the face of a potential pandemic strain [24]. The potency of MF59 for HBV has also been confirmed in a human clinical trial [25], in which MF59 was shown to be 100-fold more potent than the commercial alum-adjuvanted vaccine (Figure 1). In addition, MF59 has also been shown to be an effective adjuvant for a protein/polysaccharide conjugate vaccine in infant

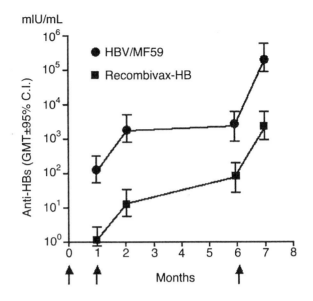

Figure 1 MF59 in combination with a novel recombinant hepatitis B vaccine (HBV) induced significantly higher antibody responses in humans (n = 230 subjects in total, receiving either vaccine) than the commercially available alum-adsorbed vaccine (Recombivax).

baboons [26]. Studies with labeled MF59 have shown that it is taken up by macrophages and DCs, both at the site of injection and in local lymph nodes [27]. Hence, it is thought that the principal mode of action of MF59 is to induce macrophage recruitment into the injection site and uptake and migration of the adjuvant and antigen to local lymph nodes. Apoptosis of MF59-carrying macrophages may then occur in lymph nodes, with transfer of apoptopic bodies to DCs [28]. Experience in the clinic (>18,000 subjects immunized in Chiron-sponsored clinical trials) with HIV, HSV, CMV, HBV, and influenza has shown that MF59 is safe and well tolerated in adults and children [29–32]. In addition, MF59 was shown to be safe and well tolerated in newborn infants in an HIV vaccine trial [33]. Moreover, MF59 can be used with recombinant proteins as an effective booster vaccine in individuals primed with a live virus vaccine [34] or with DNA [35]. In summary, MF59 is a safe and well-tolerated adjuvant in humans and is effective for the induction of potent antibody responses and CD4$^+$ T-cell responses. However, in most studies, MF59 has been ineffective for CTL induction. Nevertheless, a modified MF59 emulsion was recently described as a delivery system for DNA vaccines, which might be expected to induce CTL responses [36].

In many studies, emulsions have also been used as delivery systems for additional adjuvants, including monophosphoryl lipid A (MPL) derived from gram-negative bacteria and QS21, a purified fraction of Quil A from *Quillaja saponaria*. This approach allows adjuvant molecules to be targeted for enhanced uptake by APC. For example, an o/w emulsion containing MPL and QS21 induced protection in a mouse model of malaria that was

comparable or better than the levels of protection induced with the vaccine in FCA [37]. The o/w adjuvant formulation (called SBAS-2) subsequently showed protective efficacy against an experimental challenge in human volunteers exposed to infected mosquitoes, although protection was of short duration [38]. In a subsequent trial with recombinant HIV-1 env protein, SBAS-2 induced high titers and proliferative T-cell responses, but did not induce CTL or primary isolate neutralizing antibodies [39]. In addition, the formulation was associated with a significant number of adverse events and the reactogenicity profile appeared to preclude its use for most if not all prophylactic vaccines. The high reactogenicity appears to be caused by the presence of QS21, but may be reduced by modifications to the formulation and the addition of excipients [40]. In addition, there have been suggestions that the potency of Quil-based adjuvants may be adversely affected by degradation of this component [41]. Emulsion formulations of MPL and QS21 may have potential as adjuvants for cancer vaccines [42] and other therapeutic vaccines. An alternative emulsion-based approach involves the use of the Montanide series of adjuvants, which are based on the surfactant, mannide oleate [43,44]. The w/o mineral oil (Drakeol) adjuvant (ISA-51) has been evaluated as a therapeutic vaccine in HIV-infected individuals [45]. However, as discussed earlier, because of significant adverse effects, mineral oil adjuvants are unlikely to be considered as acceptable for prophylactic vaccines. An alternative approach, comprising a w/o non-mineral-oil emulsion (ISA-720), has also been evaluated in a malaria vaccine trial [43]. However, although potent, the adjuvant (ISA-720) induced severe local reactions in some volunteers and may prove too toxic for routine use in prophylactic vaccines [46,47].

B. Liposomes

Liposomes are phospholipid vesicles that are used as drug delivery systems in several commercially available products. At least five liposomal products are on the market and at least another 10 are currently in clinical trials. Most of the formulations on the market use the naturally occurring phosphatidyl choline as neutral lipid, with fatty acyl chains of varying lengths and degrees of saturation to build membranes. Cholesterol is often included to modulate membrane rigidity and to reduce instability. A variety of liposomal formulations have been evaluated both as adjuvants and as delivery systems [48,49]. However, liposomes have often been used in complex adjuvant formulations, with many including MPL, which makes it difficult to determine the contribution of the liposome to the overall adjuvant effect. Recently, liposomes were described as effective delivery systems for T-independent antigens, when they were used in combination with CpG DNA [50]. In addition, Gursel et al. [51] reported that cationic liposomes were effective delivery systems for CpG adjuvants.

Liposomal vaccines based on viral membrane proteins (virosomes) without additional immunostimulators have been extensively evaluated in the clinic and are approved as products in Europe for hepatitis A and influenza [52]. Immunopotentiating reconstituted influenza virosomes

(IRIV) are unilamellar liposomes comprising mainly phosphatidyl choline, with influenza hemagglutinin intercalated into the membrane. The use of viral membrane proteins in the formation of virosomes offers the opportunity to exploit the targeting and fusogenic properties of the native viral membrane proteins, perhaps resulting in effective delivery of entrapped antigens into the cytosol for CTL induction [53]. An alternative approach to vaccine delivery that may have some advantages over traditional liposomes has been described using "archaeosomes," which are vesicles prepared from the polar lipids of *Archaeobacteria* [54]. Archaeosomes have been shown to induce more potent responses than traditional liposomes [55,56]. Cationic lipid vesicles have also been described recently, which comprise cationic cholesterol derivatives with or without neutral phospholipids [57]. The best results were obtained with cationic vesicles to which antigen was bound to the surface, which greatly outperformed neutral liposomes that did not bind antigen [57]. In addition, oil-in-water liposomal formulations were recently described in which mineral oil was emulsified in the presence of liposomes, which donated phospholipids as stabilizers [58]. Clearly, this is a very complex formulation, which would need to show a dramatic improvement over alternatives before it can be accepted as a significant advance in the field. Modified liposomal structures termed "cochleates" are also being evaluated as systemic and mucosal adjuvants in small animal models [59].

C. Immunostimulatory Complexes

The immunostimulatory fractions from *Q. saponaria* (Quil A) have been incorporated into lipid particles comprising cholesterol, phospholipids, and cell membrane antigens, which are called iscoms [60]. The principal advantage of the preparation of iscoms is to allow a reduction in the dose of the hemolytic Quil A adjuvant and to target the formulation directly to APCs. In addition, within the iscoms structure, the Quil A is bound to cholesterol and is not free to interact with cell membranes. Therefore, the hemolytic activity of the saponins is significantly reduced [60,61]. It is well established that iscoms induce cytokine production in a range of mouse strains, and a recent study has indicated that the induction of IL-12 is key to the adjuvant effect [62]. However, strong IFN-γ responses have also been described [63]. In a study in macaques, influenza iscoms were shown to be more immunogenic than a classical subunit vaccine and induced enhanced protective efficacy [64]. A similar formulation has been evaluated in human clinical trials and successfully induced a CTL response [65]. In a comparative study in rhesus macaques, although iscoms induced a potent Th1 response against a recombinant HIV-1 env antigen, while MF59 induced a Th2 response, both vaccines offered a similar degree of protection against challenge [66]. Iscoms are generally accepted as the most potent adjuvant approach for the induction of CTL responses with recombinant proteins in preclinical models [67]. For example, in a recent study, we demonstrated the induction of potent long-lasting CTL responses in rhesus macaques immunized with recombinant core antigen from hepatitis C virus adsorbed to novel iscoms [68]. In addition, potent T-cell proliferative responses

have been induced in primates with iscoms containing CMV, flu, HIV, and EBV antigens [60–69]. However, the efficacy for CTL induction and the safety profile of iscoms need to be further established in human subjects, although initial studies are encouraging [70]. In addition, a potential problem with iscoms is that inclusion of antigens into the adjuvant is often difficult, and may require extensive antigen modification [71]. Nevertheless, recent work has identified novel ways by which some antigens can be effectively associated with iscoms without significant formulation difficulties [68–72]. In addition, simplified approaches to the preparation of iscoms have also been described [73], as well as approaches to isolate Quil-based saponins, with less heterogeneity [74].

D. Alternative Lipid Vehicles for Vaccine Delivery

An alternative approach involving lipid vesicles has also been described involving nonionic surfactant vesicle, or "niosomes," which have induced potent responses in small animal models [75]. In addition, it has been suggested that an important component of the adjuvant effect of synthetic lipopeptide antigens is their ability to aggregate into particulate structures [76]. Although binding of lipopeptides to TLR2 is also important to their adjuvant effect [77]. Nevertheless, the potency of lipopeptides has been shown to be enhanced by their formulation into particulate delivery systems [78].

E. Microparticles

Antigen uptake by APC is enhanced by association of antigens with polymeric microparticles, or by the use of polymers or proteins that self-assemble into particles. The biodegradable and biocompatible polyesters, the polylactide-co-glycolides (PLGs) are the primary candidates for the development of microparticles as adjuvants, because they have been used in humans for many years as suture material and as controlled-release drug delivery systems [79,80]. The adjuvant effect achieved through the encapsulation of antigens into PLG microparticles was first demonstrated more than 10 years ago [81–84]. Microparticles appear to function mainly as delivery systems, targeting associated antigens into APCs. In contrast to alum adjuvants, PLG microparticles are effective for the induction of CTL responses in small animal models [78,85–87]. Microparticles also have significant potential as delivery systems for DNA vaccines [4,88–90]. We recently described a novel approach in which cationic microparticles with adsorbed plasmids were used to dramatically enhance the potency of DNA vaccines [89–91] (Figure 2). Importantly, the cationic microparticles enhanced both antibody and T-cell responses in a range of animal models, including nonhuman primates; they efficiently adsorbed DNA and can be designed to deliver several plasmids simultaneously on the same formulation at a range of different loading levels [90,91]. The microparticles appear to be effective mainly as a consequence of efficient delivery of the adsorbed plasmids into DC [92]. Similar anionic microparticles can also be used for effective delivery of adsorbed proteins and have been shown to be effective for

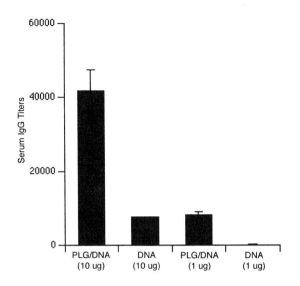

Figure 2 Serum IgG antibody titers in groups of mice (n = 10) immunized intramuscularly with 1 or 10 µg DNA encoding HIV-1 p55 gag adsorbed to cationic microparticles or as naked DNA.

CTL induction in mice [93]. In addition, cationic microparticles can be used as delivery systems for adsorbed adjuvants, including CpG DNA [94]. Surprisingly, the potency of microparticles as an adjuvant can be significantly enhanced by their combination with MF59 emulsion [95]. A particularly attractive feature of microparticles is their ability to control the rate of release of entrapped antigens [96,97]. Controlled release of antigen may allow the development of *single-dose vaccines*, which would result in improved vaccine compliance, particularly in the developing world. However, although microparticles have significant potential for the development of single-dose vaccines, work is needed to ensure the stability of antigens entrapped in microparticles, and progress has been slow [98]. On several occasions, it has been shown that controlled-release microparticles work optimally for bacterial toxoids when they are combined with alum [97], and this approach may be evaluated in the clinic in the near future [99].

F. Alternative Particulate Adjuvants

Polymers that self-assemble into particulates (poloxamers) [100], or soluble polymers (polyphosphazenes) [101], may also be used as adjuvants, but the safety and tolerability of these approaches need to be further evaluated. A recent study suggested an adjuvant effect for CRL1005, a nonionic block copolymer (poloxamer) for a DNA vaccine in rhesus macaques [102]. However, in this same study, a combination adjuvant involving alum and MPL did not appear to provide any benefit for the DNA vaccine [102]. Recombinant proteins that naturally self-assemble into particles can also be used to enhance delivery of antigens to APC. The first recombinant protein vaccine that was developed, based on hepatitis B surface antigen (HBsAg), was expressed in yeast as a particulate protein [103]. Recombinant HBsAg is po-

tently immunogenic and can be used to prime CTL responses [104]. HBsAg and other viruslike particles (VLPs) can also be used as delivery systems for coexpressed antigens [105]. Recombinant Ty VLPs from *Saccharomyces cerevisiae* carrying a string of up to 15 CTL epitopes from *Plasmodium* species have been shown to prime protective CTL responses in mice following a single immunization [106]. In addition, Ty VLPs have also been shown to induce CTL activity in macaques against coexpressed SIV p27 [107]. Clinical trials of Ty VLPs have shown them to be safe and immunogenic in humans [108].

IV. ALTERNATIVE ROUTES OF IMMUNIZATION

Although most vaccines have traditionally been administered by intramuscular or subcutaneous immunization, mucosal delivery of vaccines offers a number of important advantages, including easier administration, reduced adverse effects, and the potential for frequent boosting. In addition, local immunization induces mucosal immunity at the sites where many pathogens initially establish infection of hosts. Oral immunization would be particularly advantageous in isolated communities, where access to health care professionals is difficult. Moreover, mucosal immunization would avoid the potential problem of infection caused by the reuse of needles. Several orally administered vaccines are commercially available, which are based on live-attenuated organisms, including polio, *Vibrio cholerae*, and *Salmonella enterica* serovar Typhi. In addition, a wide range of approaches is currently being evaluated for mucosal delivery of vaccines [109], including many approaches involving nonliving adjuvants and delivery systems.

The most attractive route for mucosal immunization is oral, because of the ease and acceptability of administration through this route. However, because of the presence of low acidity in the stomach, an extensive range of digestive enzymes in the intestine and a protective coating of mucus that limits access to the mucosal epithelium, oral immunization has proven extremely difficult with nonliving antigens. However, novel delivery systems and adjuvants may be used to significantly enhance responses following oral immunization.

A. Mucosal Immunization with Antigen Delivery Systems

In mice, oral immunization with PLG microparticles of 1–10 µm has been shown to induce potent mucosal and systemic immunity to entrapped antigens [110–113]. In addition, mucosal immunization with microparticles has been shown to induce protection against challenge with *Bordetella pertussis* [114–117], *Chlamydia trachomatis* [118], *Yersinia pestis* [119], *Brucella ovis* [120], *Salmonella typhimurium* [121], and *Streptococcus pneumoniae* [122]. In primates, initial studies involving mucosal immunization with microparticles were encouraging, although oral immunization was not as effective as delivery to the respiratory tract. Mucosal immunization with inactivated SIV in microparticles induced protective immunity against intravaginal challenge [123].

Also in primates, mucosal immunization with microparticles induced protection against aerosol challenge with staphylococcal enterotoxin B [124]. Nevertheless, studies undertaken so far involving oral immunization with PLG microparticles in larger animal models and human clinical trials have been largely disappointing [125–127]. However, difficulty in translating observations from smaller to larger animals and humans is not unique to microparticle formulations. Generally speaking, although small animal models are necessary screening tools to be used for mucosal immunization studies, they are unlikely to prove predictive of potency in larger animal models and humans. This applies particularly to approaches for oral immunization, since the gastrointestinal tract and mucosal immune tissues of both small and large animal models are very different from humans. The potential of microparticles and other polymeric delivery systems for mucosal delivery of vaccines was recently reviewed in detail [128], as too was the use of a broader range of antigen delivery systems [129]. Although much of the literature has focused on PLG microparticles, several alternative approaches involving microencapsulation in different polymers have also been described [128]. While many have used similar sized microparticles (1–10 μm), some groups have described the use of larger microparticles that are designed to protect antigens against degradation in the stomach and to release it in the intestine [128]. Nevertheless, given the significant challenges associated with oral immunization using nonliving delivery systems, simple protection against stomach degradation is unlikely to prove successful without the inclusion of additional formulation components, including adjuvants. Moreover, although advantages are often claimed for alternative polymers to PLG, comparisons are rarely made and it is often difficult to understand what the likely advantages are, particularly when the microparticles are of similar dimensions. The ability of 1 to 10μm microparticles of any composition to perform effectively following mucosal administration is largely a consequence of their uptake into the specialized mucosal associated lymphoid tissue (MALT) [130]. However, the majority of literature in this area has concluded that the extent of uptake of microparticles into lymphoid tissue following oral delivery is very low [130], imposing a strict limitation on the likely success of microparticles for oral delivery. Nevertheless, although most of the studies undertaken so far have described microparticle uptake following oral delivery, uptake of microparticles following intranasal delivery was recently described in mice [119]. In addition, comparative studies have indicated that microparticles are one of the most potent adjuvants available for nasal delivery of recombinant protein vaccines in small animal models [131] (Figure 3A and B). In addition, microparticles also have potential for intranasal delivery of DNA vaccines [132] (Figure 4). While microparticles retain significant potential for mucosal delivery of vaccines, particularly for the intranasal route, their potency may be improved by use in combination with additional adjuvants. In a recent study in a large animal model, the potency of mutants of heat labile enterotoxin from *Escherichia coli* as mucosal adjuvants for an influenza vaccine was improved by formulation into a novel microsphere delivery system [133] (Figure 4A and B). The combination of optimal delivery

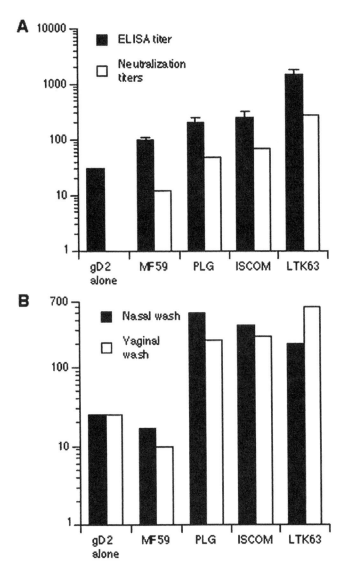

Figure 3 Serum IgG antibody and neutralization titers (A) and mucosal IgA titers in nasal and vaginal wash samples (B) following intranasal immunization in mice with a recombinant glycoprotein (gD2) from herpes simplex virus type 2 in combination with MF59 emulsion, PLG microparticles, ISCOMs, or LTK63 adjuvants. Titers were determined 2 weeks after three monthly immunizations with 10μg HSV gD2 in combination with adjuvants.

system and adjuvant is likely to be a prerequisite for the development of effective oral vaccines, since the challenges faced should not be underestimated. Accumulated experimental evidence suggests that simple encapsulation of vaccines into microparticles is unlikely to result in the successful development of oral vaccines and improvements in the current technology are needed [134]. Nevertheless, microparticles continue to show significant promise as delivery systems for intranasal immunization [135]. However, most of these data have been generated in small animal models and the performance of microparticles for intranasal immuniza-

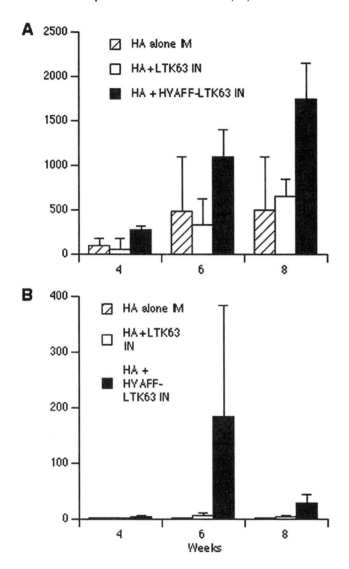

Figure 4   Serum IgG (A) and nasal wash IgA (Ab) antibody (B) responses following immunization in pigs ($n = 4$) with influenza vaccine (HA) alone IM, IN with mucosal adjuvant LTK63, or IN with bioadhesive hyaluronic acid (HYAFF) microspheres in combination with LTK63. Pigs were immunized at 0 and 4 weeks with 25 µg HA alone IM or 25 µg HA in combination with 100 µg LTK63 IN.

tion in larger animals and humans remains to be evaluated. Although the stability of antigens following microencapsulation into PLG microparticles can present significant problems, recent work has suggested that microparticles with adsorbed antigens may also be used for mucosal immunization [136,137]. These approaches are similar to the approach described earlier involving the preparation of PLG microparticles with adsorbent surfaces for antigen delivery [93]. In addition, particulate polymeric lamellae with adsorbed antigens may also be used for mucosal immunization [138]. Alternatively, significant success has been achieved recently by using soluble polymers or microparticles of chitosan for mucosal immunization [139,140]. In recent studies, micro-

particles have also shown some promise for mucosal delivery of DNA [141–143]. Nevertheless, optimal responses are likely to be achieved with microparticle formulations that have been modified to maintain the integrity of entrapped DNA [143,144].

A wide range of alternative delivery systems, including liposomes and iscoms, has also been evaluated for mucosal delivery of vaccines [129]. The development of polymerized liposomes, which show enhanced stability in the gut, offers potential for the development of oral vaccines [145], particularly if the delivery system can be targeted for optimal uptake into the M cells [146]. Nevertheless, this approach represents a very complex delivery system that might prove difficult and expensive to manufacture at large scale. However, work continues to identify the optimal targeting agents for use in the gastrointestinal tract [147]. Significant success has been achieved in the clinic using IRIV as an influenza vaccine for intranasal immunization and the approach appears to be safe and immunogenic [148–150]. Nevertheless, although the safety data were sufficient to allow this product to be introduced into the market in Switzerland in 2000, the inclusion of wild type, heat-labile enterotoxin from *E. coli* as an adjuvant in the vaccine will ensure that there will be close monitoring of this approach postlicensure. Unfortunately, the clinical data indicated that potent immune responses were not induced by IRIV in the absence of the enterotoxin adjuvant [148]. Iscoms can also be used for intranasal delivery of vaccines [151], including influenza [152].

Another alternative delivery system for mucosal immunization is represented by proteosomes, which are formed from the outer membrane proteins from *Neisseria meningitidis* [153]. Proteosomes were recently used for intranasal delivery of influenza vaccine in mice [154] and of *Shigella sonnei* LPS antigen in man [155].

V.   FUTURE DEVELOPMENTS IN VACCINE ADJUVANTS AND DELIVERY SYSTEMS

Several recent issues have served to highlight the urgent need for the development of new and improved vaccines. These have included the following: 1) the inability of traditional approaches to enable the successful development of vaccines against "difficult" organisms, including those that establish chronic infections, e.g., HIV and HCV; 2) the emergence of new diseases, e.g., Ebola, West Nile, and nvCJD; 3) the reemergence of "old" infections, e.g., TB; and 4) the continuing spread of antibiotic-resistant bacteria. A likely component of new and improved vaccines will be more potent adjuvants and delivery systems. The adjuvant formulations to be used in these vaccines may have to closely mimic an infection to elicit protective immunity. This may be achieved through the use of particulate antigen delivery systems that have similar dimensions to pathogens and are able to target antigens to macrophages and DCs. In addition, it may also be necessary to deliver one or more adjuvant active molecules, which will more fully activate the innate response and may result in the desired type of adaptive response. If this hypothesis is correct, it suggests that a delicate balance must be maintained between the desired initiation of immune responses and avoidance of the problems potentially associated with an overly robust response, e.g., local tissue damage and systemic cytokine release. Many new-generation vaccines will require the induction of potent CMI, including CTL responses, to be effective. Accumulated research shows that induction of CTL is difficult with proteins and may require much stronger stimulation of the immune system than is normally required for a humoral response. Therefore, DNA remains an attractive approach for many pathogens, but needs to be delivered more effectively to improve its potency in humans. Microparticle-based delivery systems are showing considerable promise in this area.

Targeted delivery of adjuvants and antigens to specific cell types or tissues may reduce potential toxic effects and help to achieve a specific desired response. Targeting may be achieved at several different levels to include tissue specific delivery to local lymph nodes, cell-specific targeting to APC, or targeting to subcellular compartments, e.g., the proteasome to promote class I presentation or the nucleus for DNA vaccines. Most antigen delivery systems are effective, largely as a consequence of their "passive" uptake into macrophages and DCs following injection. However, "active" targeting may also be achieved through the use of ligands designed to specifically interact with preferred cell types. For example, the literature shows that lectins have been successfully used to target antigens [156], liposomes [157], and microparticles [158] to the M cells of MALT following mucosal delivery. An alternative targeting ligand is the mannose receptor, which has been used to target liposomes to APCs [159]. Further developments in the delivery of adjuvants may be achieved through the identification of the recognition mechanisms of specific receptors on APC, which might be extra or intracellular. If the receptors are intracellular, such as TLR 4 [160], then a means to promote uptake of the adjuvant by the relevant cells may be required for optimal efficacy. We have shown recently how synergy may be achieved through the combination of an adjuvant, an antigen, and a delivery system to induce potent immune responses [94]. Moreover, a similar synergy may also be achieved for mucosally administered vaccines [133].

Future developments in adjuvants are likely to include the development of more site-specific delivery systems for both mucosal and systemic administration. In addition, the identification of specific receptors on APCs is likely to allow targeting of adjuvants for the optimal induction of potent and specific immune responses. However, further developments in novel adjuvants will likely be driven by a better understanding of the mechanism of action of currently available adjuvants and this is an area of research that requires additional work.

ACKNOWLEDGMENTS

I would like to acknowledge the contributions of my colleagues in the Vaccine Delivery Group at Chiron Corporation, including Manmohan Singh, Mildred Ugozzoli, Michael Vajdy, Jina Kazzaz, Elawati Soenawan, and Maylene Briones, who were responsible for generating the data included in this chapter. I would also like to thank Nelle Cronen for help in the chapter preparation.

REFERENCES

1. Ramon G. Sur la toxine et surranatoxine diphtheriques. Ann Inst Pasteur 1924; 38:1.
2. Vogel FR, Powell MF. A compendium of vaccine adjuvants and excipients. In: Powell MF, Newman MJ, eds. Vaccine Design: The Subunit and Adjuvant Approach. New York: Plenum Press, 1995:141–228.
3. Bendelac A, Medzhitov R. Adjuvants of immunity: harnessing innate immunity to promote adaptive immunity. J Exp Med 2002; 195:F19–F23.
4. O'Hagan DT, et al. Recent developments in adjuvants for vaccines against infectious diseases. Biomol Eng 2001; 18: 69–85.
5. Gupta RK, et al. In vivo distribution of radioactivity in mice after injection of biodegradable polymer microspheres containing 14C-labeled tetanus toxoid. Vaccine 1996; 14: 1412–1416.
6. Ulanova M, et al. The common vaccine adjuvant aluminum hydroxide up-regulates accessory properties of human monocytes via an interleukin-4-dependent mechanism. Infect Immun 2001; 69:1151–1159.
7. Shi Y, et al. Detoxification of endotoxin by aluminum hydroxide adjuvant. Vaccine 2001; 19:1747–1752.
8. Gupta RK. Aluminum compounds as vaccine adjuvants. Adv Drug Deliv Rev 1998; 32:155–172.
9. Relyveld EH, et al. Rational approaches to reduce adverse reactions in man to vaccines containing tetanus and diphtheria toxoids. Vaccine 1998; 16:1016–1023.
10. Edelman R. Adjuvants for the future. In: Levine MM, Woodrow GC, Kaper JB, Cobon GS, eds. New Generation Vaccines. New York: Marcel Dekker, 1997:173–192.
11. Moingeon P. Cancer vaccines. Vaccine 2001; 19:1305–1326.
12. Rosenberg SA. Progress in human tumour immunology and immunotherapy. Nature 2001; 411:380–384.
13. Zinkernagel RM, et al. Antigen localisation regulates immune responses in a dose- and time-dependent fashion: a geographical view of immune reactivity. Immunol Rev 1997; 156:199–209.
14. Allison AC, Byars NE. An adjuvant formulation that selectively elicits the formation of antibodies of protective isotypes and of cell-mediated immunity. J Immunol Methods 1986; 95:157–168.
15. Lindblad EB. Freund's adjuvants. In: O'Hagan D, ed. Vaccine Adjuvants: preparation methods and research protocols. Totowa, NJ: Humana Press, 2000:49–64.
16. Trauger RJ, et al. Safety and immunogenicity of a gp120-depleted, inactivated HIV-1 immunogen: results of a double-blind, adjuvant controlled trial. J Acquir Immune Defic Syndr Hum Retrovirol 1995; 10:S74–S82.
17. Ott G, et al. MF59: design and evaluation of a safe and potent adjuvant for human vaccines. In: Powell MF, Newman MJ, eds. Vaccine Design: The Subunit and Adjuvant Approach. New York: Plenum Press, 1995:277–296.
18. Cataldo DM, Van Nest G. The adjuvant MF59 increases the immunogenicity and protective efficacy of subunit influenza vaccine in mice. Vaccine 1997; 15:1710–1715.
19. Higgins DA, et al. MF59 adjuvant enhances the immunogenicity of influenza vaccine in both young and old mice. Vaccine 1996; 14:478–484.
20. O'Hagan DT, et al. Recent advances in vaccine adjuvants: the development of MF59 emulsion and polymeric microparticles. Mol Med Today 1997; 3:69–75.
21. Traquina P, et al. MF59 adjuvant enhances the antibody

response to recombinant hepatitis B surface antigen vaccine in primates. J Infect Dis 1996; 174:1168–1175.

22. Menegon T, et al. Influenza vaccines: antibody responses to split virus and MF59-adjuvanted subunit virus in an adult population. Eur J Epidemiol 1999; 15:573–576.

23. DeDonato S, et al. Safety and immunogenicity of MF59-adjuvanted influenza vaccine in the elderly. Vaccine 1999; 17:3094–3101.

24. Nicholson K, et al. Confronting a potential H5N1 pandemic: a randomised controlled trial of conventional and MF59 adjuvanted influenza A/Duck/Singapore/97 (H5N3) surface antigen vaccine. Lancet 2001; 9272:357.

25. Heineman TC, et al. A randomized, controlled study in adults of the immunogenicity of a novel hepatitis B vaccine containing MF59 adjuvant. Vaccine 1999; 17:2769–2778.

26. Granoff DM, et al. MF59 adjuvant enhances antibody responses of infant baboons immunized with *Haemophilus influenzae* type b and *Neisseria meningitidis* group C oligo-saccharide-CRM197 conjugate vaccine. Infect Immun 1997; 65:1710–1715.

27. Dupuis M, et al. Dendritic cells internalize vaccine adjuvant after intramuscular injection. Cell Immunol 1998; 186:18–27.

28. Dupuis M, et al. Immunization with the adjuvant MF59 induces macrophage trafficking and apoptosis. Eur J Immunol 2001; 31:2910–2918.

29. Pass RF, et al. A subunit cytomegalovirus vaccine based on recombinant envelope glycoprotein B and a new adjuvant. J Infect Dis 1999; 180:970–975.

30. Nitayaphan S, et al. A phase I/II trial of HIV SF2 gp120/MF59 vaccine in seronegative Thais. Vaccine 2000; 18:1448–1455.

31. Kahn JO, et al. Clinical and immunologic responses to human immunodeficiency virus (HIV) type 1SF2 gp120 subunit vaccine combined with MF59 adjuvant with or without muramyl tripeptide dipalmitoyl phosphatidyletha-nolamine in non-HIV-infected human volunteers. J Infect Dis 1994; 170:1288–1291.

32. Langenberg AG, et al. A recombinant glycoprotein vaccine for herpes simplex virus type 2: safety and immunogenicity [published erratum appears in Ann Intern Med 1995 Sep 1;123(5):395]. Ann Intern Med 1995; 122:889–898.

33. Cunningham CK, et al. Safety of 2 recombinant human immunodeficiency virus type 1 (hiv-1) envelope vaccines in neonates born to hiv-1-infected women. Clin Infect Dis 2001; 32:801–807.

34. Team AVEGP. Cellular and humoral immune responses to a canarypox vaccine containing human immunodeficiency virus type 1 Env, Gag, and Pro in combination with rgp120. J Infect Dis 2001; 183:563–570.

35. Fuller DH, et al. Enhancement of immunodeficiency virus-specific immune responses in DNA-immunized rhesus macaques. Vaccine 1997; 15:924–926.

36. Ott G, et al. A cationic sub-micron emulsion (MF59/DOTAP) is an effective delivery system for DNA vaccines. J Control Release 2002; 79:1–5.

37. Ling IT, et al. Immunization against the murine malaria parasite *Haemophilus influenzae* using a recombinant protein with adjuvants developed for clinical use. Vaccine 1997; 15:1562–1567.

38. Stoute JA, et al. A preliminary evaluation of a recombinant circumsporozoite protein vaccine against *Plasmodium falciparum* malaria. RTS,S Malaria Vaccine Evaluation Group. N Engl J Med 1997; 336:86–91.

39. McCormack S, et al. A phase I trial in HIV negative healthy volunteers evaluating the effect of potent adjuvants on immunogenicity of a recombinant gp120W61D derived from dual tropic R5X4 HIV-1ACH320. Vaccine 2000; 18:1166–1177.

40. Waite DC, et al. Three double-blind, randomized trials evaluating the safety and tolerance of different formulations of the saponin adjuvant QS-21. Vaccine 2001; 19: 3957–3967.

41. Marciani DJ, et al. Altered immunomodulating and toxicological properties of degraded *Quillaja saponaria* Molina saponins. Int Immunopharmacol 2001; 1:813–818.

42. Gerard CM, et al. Therapeutic potential of protein and adjuvant vaccinations on tumour growth. Vaccine 2001; 19: 2583–2589.

43. Lawrence GW, et al. Phase I trial in humans of an oil-based adjuvant SEPPIC MONTANIDE ISA 720. Vaccine 1997; 15:176–178.

44. Aucouturier J, et al. Efficacy and safety of new adjuvants. Ann N Y Acad Sci 2000; 916:600–604.

45. Gringeri A, et al. Safety and immunogenicity of HIV-1 Tat toxoid in immunocompromised HIV-1-infected patients. J Hum Virol 1998; 1:293–298.

46. Toledo H, et al. A phase I clinical trial of a multi-epitope polypeptide TAB9 combined with Montanide ISA 720 adjuvant in non-HIV-1 infected human volunteers. Vaccine 2001; 19:4328–4336.

47. Genton B, et al. Safety and immunogenicity of a three-component blood-stage malaria vaccine in adults living in an endemic area of Papua New Guinea. Vaccine 2000; 18: 2504–2511.

48. Alving CR. Immunologic aspects of liposomes: presentation and processing of liposomal protein and phospholipid antigens. Biochim Biophys Acta 1992; 1113:307–322.

49. Gregoriadis G. Immunological adjuvants: a role for liposomes. Immunol Today 1990; 11:89–97.

50. Li WM, et al. Enhanced immune response to T-independent antigen by using CpG oligodeoxynucleotides encapsulated in liposomes. Vaccine 2001; 20:148–157.

51. Gursel I, et al. Sterically stabilized cationic liposomes improve the uptake and immunostimulatory activity of CpG oligonucleotides. J Immunol 2001; 167:3324–3328.

52. Ambrosch F, et al. Immunogenicity and protectivity of a new liposomal hepatitis A vaccine. Vaccine 1997; 15:1209–1213.

53. Bungener DT, et al. Virosomes as an antigen delivery system. J Liposome Res 2000; 10:329–338.

54. Krishnan L, et al. Archaeosome vaccine adjuvants induce strong humoral, cell-mediated, and memory responses: comparison to conventional liposomes and alum. Infect Immun 2000; 68:54–63.

55. Krishnan L, et al. Archaeosomes induce long-term CD8+ cytotoxic T cell response to entrapped soluble protein by the exogenous cytosolic pathway, in the absence of CD4+ T cell help. J Immunol 2000; 165:5177–5185.

56. Conlan JW, et al. Immunization of mice with lipopeptide antigens encapsulated in novel liposomes prepared from the polar lipids of various *Archaeobacteria* elicits rapid and prolonged specific protective immunity against infection with the facultative intracellular pathogen, *Listeria monocytogenes*. Vaccine 2001; 19:3509–3517.

57. Guy B, et al. Design, characterization and preclinical efficacy of a cationic lipid adjuvant for influenza split vaccine. Vaccine 2001; 19:1794–1805.

58. Muderhwa JM, et al. Oil-in-water liposomal emulsions: characterization and potential use in vaccine delivery. J Pharm Sci 1999; 88:1332–1339.

59. Gould-Fogerite S, et al. Targeting immune response induction with cochleate and liposome-based vaccines. Adv Drug Deliv Rev 1998; 32:273–287.

60. Barr IG, et al. ISCOMs and other saponin based adjuvants. Adv Drug Deliv Rev 1998; 32:247–271.

61. Soltysik S, et al. Structure/function studies of QS-21 adjuvant: assessment of triterpene aldehyde and glucuronic

acid roles in adjuvant function. Vaccine 1995; 13:1403–1410.

62. Smith RE, et al. Immune-stimulating complexes induce an IL-12-dependent cascade of innate immune responses. J Immunol 1999; 162:5536–5546.

63. Emery DL, et al. Influence of antigens and adjuvants on the production of gamma-interferon and antibody by ovine lymphocytes. Immunol Cell Biol 1990; 68(Pt 2):127–136.

64. Rimmelzwaan GF, et al. Induction of protective immunity against influenza virus in a macaque model: comparison of conventional and iscom vaccines. J Gen Virol 1997; 78:757–765.

65. Ennis FA, et al. Augmentation of human influenza A virus-specific cytotoxic T lymphocyte memory by influenza vaccine and adjuvanted carriers (ISCOMS). Virology 1999; 259:256–261.

66. Verschoor EJ, et al. Comparison of immunity generated by nucleic acid-, MF59-, and ISCOM-formulated human immunodeficiency virus type 1 vaccines in Rhesus macaques: evidence for viral clearance. J Virol 1999; 73:3292–3300.

67. Le TT, et al. Cytotoxic T cell polyepitope vaccines delivered by ISCOMs. Vaccine 2001; 19:4669–4675.

68. Polakos NK, et al. Characterization of hepatitis C virus core-specific immune responses primed in rhesus macaques by a nonclassical ISCOM vaccine. J Immunol 2001; 166:3589–3598.

69. Sjolander A, et al. Immune responses to ISCOM((R)) formulations in animal and primate models. Vaccine 2001; 19:2661–2665.

70. Bates J, et al. IscomT adjuvant—a promising adjuvant for influenza virus vaccines. In: Brown LE, Hampson AW, Webster RG, eds. Options for the Control of Influenza III. Amsterdam: Elsevier Science, 1996:661–667.

71. Lovgren-Bengtsson K, Morein B. The ISCOM™ technology. In: O'Hagan D, ed. Vaccine Adjuvants: Preparation Methods and Research Protocols. Totowa, NJ: Humana Press, 2000:239–258.

72. Andersson C, et al. Protection against respiratory syncytial virus (RSV) elicited in mice by plasmid DNA immunisation encoding a secreted RSV G protein-derived antigen. FEMS Immunol Med Microbiol 2000; 29:247–253.

73. Copland MJ, et al. Hydration of lipid films with an aqueous solution of Quil A: a simple method for the preparation of immune-stimulating complexes. Int J Pharm 2000; 196:135–139.

74. Kamstrup S, et al. Preparation and characterisation of quillaja saponin with less heterogeneity than Quil-A. Vaccine 2000; 18:2244–2249.

75. Brewer JM, et al. Lipid vesicle size determines the Th1 or Th2 response to entrapped antigen. J Immunol 1998; 161:4000–4007.

76. Tsunoda I, et al. Lipopeptide particles as the immunologically active component of CTL inducing vaccines. Vaccine 1999; 17:675–685.

77. Aliprantis AO, et al. Cell activation and apoptosis by bacterial lipoproteins through toll-like receptor-2. Science 1999; 285:736–739.

78. Nixon DF, et al. Synthetic peptides entrapped in microparticles can elicit cytotoxic T cell activity. Vaccine 1996; 14:1523–1530.

79. Okada H, Toguchi H. Biodegradable microspheres in drug delivery. Crit Rev Ther Drug Carr Sys 1995; 12:1–99.

80. Putney SD, Burke PA. Improving protein therapeutics with sustained-release formulations [published erratum appears in Nat Biotechnol 1998 May; 16(5):478]. Nat Biotechnol 1998; 16:153–157.

81. Eldridge JH, et al. Biodegradable and biocompatible poly (DL-lactide-co-glycolide) microspheres as an adjuvant for

82. O'Hagan DT, et al. Biodegradable microparticles as controlled release antigen delivery systems. Immunology 1991; 73:239–242.

83. O'Hagan DT, et al. Controlled release microparticles for vaccine development. Vaccine 1991; 9:768–771.

84. O'Hagan DT, et al. Long-term antibody responses in mice following subcutaneous immunization with ovalbumin entrapped in biodegradable microparticles. Vaccine 1993; 11:965–969.

85. Maloy KJ, et al. Induction of mucosal and systemic immune responses by immunization with ovalbumin entrapped in poly(lactide-co-glycolide) microparticles. Immunology 1994; 81:661–667.

86. Moore A, et al. Immunization with a soluble recombinant HIV protein entrapped in biodegradable microparticles induces HIV-specific CD8+ cytotoxic T lymphocytes and CD4+ Th1 cells. Vaccine 1995; 13:1741–1749.

87. Peter K, et al. Induction of a cytotoxic T-cell response to HIV-1 proteins with short synthetic peptides and human compatible adjuvants. Vaccine 2001; 19:4121–4129.

88. Hedley ML, Curley J, Urban R. Microspheres containing plasmid-encoded antigens elicit cytotoxic T-cell responses. Nat Med 1998; 4:365–368.

89. Singh M, et al. Cationic microparticles: a potent delivery system for DNA vaccines. Proc Natl Acad Sci USA 2000; 97:811–816.

90. Briones M. The preparation, characterization, and evaluation of cationic microparticles for DNA vaccine delivery. Pharm Res 2001; 18:709–711.

91. O'Hagan D, et al. Induction of potent immune responses by cationic microparticles with adsorbed HIV DNA vaccines. J Virol 2001; 75:9037–9043.

92. Denis-Mize KS, et al. Plasmid DNA adsorbed onto PLG-CTAB microparticles mediates target gene expression and antigen presentation by dendritic cells. Gene Ther 2000; 7:2105–2112.

93. Kazzaz J, et al. Novel anionic microparticles are a potent adjuvant for the induction of cytotoxic T lymphocytes against recombinant p55 gag from HIV-1. J Control Release 2000; 67:347–356.

94. Singh M, et al. Cationic microparticles are an effective delivery system for immune stimulatory CpG DNA. Pharm Res 2001; 18:1476–1479.

95. O'Hagan DT, et al. Microparticles in MF59, a potent adjuvant combination for a recombinant protein vaccine against HIV-1. Vaccine 2000; 18:1793–1801.

96. O'Hagan DT. Prospects for the development of new and improved vaccines through the use of microencapsulation technology. In: Levine MM, Woodrow GC, Kaper JB, Cobon GS, eds. New Generation Vaccines. New York: Marcel Dekker, 1997:215–228.

97. O'Hagan DT, et al. Poly(lactide-co-glycolide) microparticles for the development of single-dose controlled-release vaccines. Adv Drug Deliv Rev 1998; 32:225–246.

98. Jiang W, Schwendeman SP. Stabilization of a model formalinized protein antigen encapsulated in poly(lactide-co-glycolide)-based microspheres. J Pharm Sci 2001; 90:1558–1569.

99. Johansen P, et al. Revisiting PLA/PLGA microspheres: an analysis of their potential in parenteral vaccination. Eur J Pharm Biopharm 2000; 50:129–146.

100. Newman MJ, et al. Development of adjuvant-active nonionic block copolymers. Adv Drug Deliv Rev 1998; 32:199–223.

101. Payne LG, et al. Poly[di(carboxylatophenoxy)phosphazene] (PCPP) is a potent immunoadjuvant for an influenza vaccine. Vaccine 1998; 16:92–98.

staphylococcal enterotoxin B toxoid which enhances the level of toxin-neutralizing antibodies. Infect Immun 1991; 59:2978–2986.

102. Shiver JW, et al. Replication-incompetent adenoviral vaccine vector elicits effective anti-immunodeficiency-virus immunity. Nature 2002; 415:331–335.

103. Valenzuela P, et al. Synthesis and assembly of hepatitis B virus surface antigen particles in yeast. Nature 1982; 298: 347–350.

104. Schirmbeck R, et al. Nucleic-acid vaccination primes hepatitis-b virus surface antigen-specific cytotoxic T-lymphocytes in nonresponder mice. J Virol 1995; 69:5929–5934.

105. Gilbert SC. Virus-like particles as vaccine adjuvants. In: O'Hagan D, ed. Vaccine Adjuvants: Preparation Methods and Research Protocols. Totowa, NJ: Humana Press, 2000:197–210.

106. Gilbert SC, et al. A protein particle vaccine containing multiple malaria epitopes. Nat Biotechnol 1997; 15:1280–1284.

107. Klavinskis LS, et al. Mucosal or targeted lymph node immunization of macaques with a particulate SIVp27 protein elicits virus-specific CTL in the genito-rectal mucosa and draining lymph nodes. J Immunol 1996; 157:2521–2527.

108. Martin SJ, et al. Immunization of human HIV-seronegative volunteers with recombinant p17/p24:Ty virus-like particles elicits HIV-1 p24-specific cellular and humoral immune responses. AIDS 1993; 7:1315–1323.

109. Levine MM, Dougan G. Optimism over vaccines administered via mucosal surfaces. Lancet 1998; 351:1375–1376.

110. Challacombe SJ, et al. Enhanced secretory IgA and systemic IgG antibody responses after oral immunization with biodegradable microparticles containing antigen. Immunology 1992; 76:164–168.

111. Challacombe SJ, et al. Salivary, gut, vaginal and nasal antibody responses after oral immunization with biodegradable microparticles. Vaccine 1997; 15:169–175.

112. Eldridge JH, et al. Controlled vaccine release in the gut-associated lymphoid tissues. I. Orally administered biodegradable microspheres target the Peyer's patches. J Control Release 1990; 11:205–214.

113. O'Hagan DT. Microparticles as oral vaccines. In: O'Hagan DT, ed. Novel Delivery Systems for Oral Vaccines. Boca Raton: CRC Press, 1994:175–205.

114. Cahill ES, et al. Immune responses and protection against *Bordetella pertussis* infection after intranasal immunization of mice with filamentous haemagglutinin in solution or incorporated in biodegradable microparticles. Vaccine 1995; 13:455–462.

115. Jones DH, et al. Orally administered microencapsulated *Bordetella pertussis* fimbriae protect mice from *B. pertussis* respiratory infection. Infect Immun 1996; 64:489–494.

116. Shahin R, et al. Adjuvanticity and protective immunity elicited by *Bordetella pertussis* antigens encapsulated in poly(DL-lactide-co-glycolide) microspheres. Infect Immun 1995; 63:1195–1200.

117. Conway MA, et al. Protection against *Bordetella pertussis* infection following parenteral or oral immunization with antigens entrapped in biodegradable particles: effect of formulation and route of immunization on induction of Th1 and Th2 cells. Vaccine 2001; 19:1940–1950.

118. Whittum-Hudson JA, et al. Oral immunization with an anti-idiotypic antibody to the exoglycolipid antigen protects against experimental *Chlamydia trachomatis* infection. Nat Med 1996; 2:1116–1121.

119. Eyles JE, et al. Tissue distribution of radioactivity following intranasal administration of radioactive microspheres. J Pharm Pharmacol 2001; 53:601–607.

120. Murillo M, et al. A *Brucella ovis* antigenic complex bearing poly-varepsilon-caprolactone microparticles confer protection against experimental brucellosis in mice. Vaccine 2001; 19:4099–4106.

121. Allaoui-Attarki K, et al. Protective immunity against *Salmonella typhimurium* elicited in mice by oral vaccination with phosphorylcholine encapsulated in poly(DL-lactide-co-glycolide) microspheres. Infect Immun 1997; 65:853–857.

122. Seo JY, et al. Cross-protective immunity of mice induced by oral immunization with pneumococcal surface adhesin a encapsulated in microspheres. Infect Immun 2002; 70: 1143–1149.

123. Marx PA, et al. Protection against vaginal SIV transmission with microencapsulated vaccine. Science 1993; 260: 1323–1327.

124. Tseng J, et al. Humoral immunity to aerosolized staphylococcal enterotoxin B (SEB), a superantigen, in monkeys vaccinated with SEB toxoid-containing microspheres. Infect Immun 1995; 63:2880–2885.

125. Tacket CO, et al. Enteral immunization and challenge of volunteers given enterotoxigenic *E. coli* CFA/II encapsulated in biodegradable microspheres. Vaccine 1994; 12: 1270–1274.

126. Lambert JS, et al. A Phase I safety and immunogenicity trial of UBI microparticulate monovalent HIV-1 MN oral peptide immunogen with parenteral boost in HIV-1 seronegative human subjects. Vaccine 2001; 19:3033–3042.

127. Felder CB, et al. Microencapsulated enterotoxigenic *Escherichia coli* and detached fimbriae for peroral vaccination of pigs. Vaccine 2000; 19:706–715.

128. O'Hagan D, et al. Microparticles and polymers for the mucosal delivery of vaccines. Adv Drug Deliv Rev 1998; 34:305–320.

129. Michalek SM, et al. Antigen delivery systems: nonliving microparticles, liposomes, cochleates, and ISCOMS. In: Ogra PL, Mestecky J, Lamm ME, Strober W, Bienenstrock J, McGhee JR, eds. Mucosal Immunology. 2d ed. San Diego: Academic Press, 1999:759–778.

130. O'Hagan DT. The intestinal uptake of particles and the implications for drug and antigen delivery. J Anat 1996; 189(Pt 3):477–482.

131. Ugozzoli M, et al. Intranasal immunization of mice with herpes simplex virus type 2 recombinant gD2: the effect of adjuvants on mucosal and serum antibody responses. Immunology 1998; 93:563–571.

132. Singh M, et al. Mucosal immunization with HIV-1 gag DNA on cationic microparticles prolongs gene expression and enhances local and systemic immunity. Vaccine 2001; 20:594–602.

133. Singh M, et al. Hyaluronic acid biopolymers for mucosal delivery of vaccines. In: Abatangelo G, Weigel PH, eds. New Frontiers in Medical Sciences: Redefining Hyaluronan. Amsterdam: Elsevier Science, 2000:163–170.

134. Brayden DJ. Oral vaccination in man using antigens in particles: current status. Eur J Pharm Sci 2001; 14:183–189.

135. Vajdy M, O'Hagan DT. Microparticles for intranasal immunization. Adv Drug Deliv Rev 2001; 51:127–141.

136. Jung T, et al. Tetanus toxoid loaded nanoparticles from sulfobutylated poly(vinyl alcohol)-graft-poly(lactide-co-glycolide): evaluation of antibody response after oral and nasal application in mice. Pharm Res 2001; 18:352–360.

137. Flick-Smith HC, et al. Mucosal or parenteral administration of microsphere-associated *Bacillus anthracis* protective antigen protects against anthrax infection in mice. Infect Immun 2002; 70:2022–2028.

138. Jabbal-Gill I, et al. Polymeric lamellar substrate particles for intranasal vaccination. Adv Drug Deliv Rev 2001; 51: 97–111.

139. Illum L, et al. Chitosan as a novel nasal delivery system for vaccines. Adv Drug Deliv Rev 2001; 51:81–96.

140. van der Lubben IM, et al. Chitosan for mucosal vaccination. Adv Drug Deliv Rev 2001; 52:139–144.

141. Jones DH, et al. Poly(DL-lactide-co-glycolide)-encapsulated plasmid DNA elicits systemic and mucosal antibody

responses to encoded protein after oral administration. Vaccine 1997; 15:814–817.

142. Mathiowitz E. Biologically erodable microspheres as potential oral drug delivery systems. Nature 1997; 386: 410–414.

143. Singh M, et al. A novel bioadhesive intranasal delivery system for inactivated influenza vaccine. J Control Release 2001: 267–276.

144. Ando S, et al. PLGA microspheres containing plasmid DNA: preservation of supercoiled DNA via cryopreparation and carbohydrate stabilization. J Pharm Sci 1999; 88:126–130.

145. Chen H, et al. Polymerized liposomes as potential oral vaccine carriers: stability and bioavailability. J Control Release 1996; 42:263–272.

146. Clark MA, et al. Targeting polymerised liposome vaccine carriers to intestinal M cells. Vaccine 2001; 20:208–217.

147. Pinilla C, Lambkin I. Targeting approaches to oral drug delivery. Expert Opin Biol Ther 2002; 2:67–73.

148. Gluck U, et al. Phase 1 evaluation of intranasal virosomal influenza vaccine with and without *Escherichia coli* heat-labile toxin in adult volunteers. J Virol 1999; 73:7780–7786.

149. Gluck R, et al. Safety and immunogenicity of intranasally administered inactivated trivalent virosome-formulated influenza vaccine containing *Escherichia coli* heat-labile toxin as a mucosal adjuvant. J Infect Dis 2000; 181: 1129–1132.

150. di Valserra MDB, et al. An open-label comparison of the immunogenicity and tolerability of intranasal and intramuscular formulations of virosomal influenza vaccine in healthy adults. Clin Ther 2002; 24:100–111.

151. Hu J, et al. Simian immunodeficiency virus rapidly penetrates the cervicovaginal mucosa after intravaginal inoculation and infects intraepithelial dendritic cells. J Virol 2000; 74:6087–6095.

152. Sjolander S, et al. Intranasal immunisation with influenza-ISCOM induces strong mucosal as well as systemic antibody and cytotoxic T-lymphocyte responses. Vaccine 2001; 19:4072–4080.

153. Lowell GH. Proteosomes for improved nasal, oral or injectable vaccines. In: Levine MM, Woodrow GC, Kaper JB, Cobon GS, eds. New Generation Vaccines. 2d ed. New York: Marcel Dekker, 1997:193–206.

154. Plante M, et al. Nasal immunization with subunit proteosome influenza vaccines induces serum HAI, mucosal IgA and protection against influenza challenge. Vaccine 2001; 20:218–225.

155. Fries LF, et al. Safety and immunogenicity of a proteosome-*Shigella flexneri* 2a lipopolysaccharide vaccine administered intranasally to healthy adults. Infect Immun 2001; 69:4545–4553.

156. Giannasca PJ, et al. Targeted delivery of antigen to hamster nasal lymphoid tissue with M-cell-directed lectins. Infect Immun 1997; 65:4288–4298.

157. Chen H, et al. Lectin-bearing polymerized liposomes as potential oral vaccine carriers. Pharm Res 1996; 13:1378–1383.

158. Foster N, et al. *Ulex europaeus* 1 lectin targets microspheres to mouse Peyer's patch M-cells in vivo. Vaccine 1998; 16:536–541.

159. Toda S, et al. HIV-1-specific cell-mediated immune responses induced by DNA vaccination were enhanced by mannan-coated liposomes and inhibited by anti-interferon-gamma antibody. Immunology 1997; 92:111–117.

160. Hornef MW, et al. Toll-like receptor 4 resides in the golgi apparatus and colocalizes with internalized lipopolysaccharide in intestinal epithelial cells. J Exp Med 2002; 195: 559–570.

23
Proteosome™ Technology for Vaccines and Adjuvants

George H. Lowell, David Burt, and Greg White
ID Biomedical Corporation of Quebec, Montreal, Quebec, Canada

Louis Fries
ID Biomedical Corporation of Maryland, Baltimore, Maryland, U.S.A.

I. BACKGROUND AND CHARACTERIZATION

A. Background

Successful subunit vaccines are comprised of two essential components. The first component is the antigen to which protective immune responses are to be generated. Such antigens may be proteins, polysaccharides, or lipopolysaccharides (LPS) purified from target organisms, or recombinant somatic proteins, genetically or chemically detoxified toxins, or synthetic peptides. Using defined products has the advantage of including only those moieties required for protective immune responses while excluding extraneous or toxic cellular or nuclear components commonly present in whole microorganisms or crude extracts. The second component is comprised of the adjuvant and/or vaccine delivery vehicle, which provides structure and/or immunostimulation. This component promotes antigen recognition, presentation, and processing in a manner that generates optimal immune responses of the types and at the sites required to provide protective immunity.

A great challenge of vaccine delivery and adjuvant research is to develop safe subunit mucosal vaccines that elicit protective mucosal immunity. Antigens adequately immunogenic when injected with adjuvant are frequently wholly ineffective when administered mucosally. Ideally, a mucosal vaccine would also provide systemic immunity when needed. Another much sought goal has been the development of vaccines that direct immune responses toward enhanced Type 1 T-cell immunity, which can be critical to eliciting protective responses for certain prophylactic or therapeutic vaccines. This chapter focuses on the development of Proteosome™-based delivery platforms and adjuvants to provide improved prophylactic and therapeutic vaccines against a variety of diseases. The ability of Proteosome technology to effectively and simultaneously confer both nasal immunogenicity as well as Type 1 immunity will

be highlighted. The advantages of Proteosome nasal vaccine delivery, demonstrated in both preclinical studies as well as in multiple human clinical trials, will be presented.

B. Design

The Proteosome nomenclature was selected to emphasize the distinctive physical and biological properties of preparations of outer membrane proteins (OMPs), particularly from meningococci [1–3] and other *Neisseria* [4,5]. Proteosome proteins are highly hydrophobic, reflecting their role as transmembrane proteins and porins [4,6,7]. When isolated by detergent extraction, their hydrophobic protein–protein interactions cause them to naturally self-assemble into multimolecular, membranous nanoparticles with morphological characteristics of vesicles, up to several hundred nanometers in diameter. Such Proteosome particles may be readily disassociated into vesicle membrane or multimolecular fragments to a variable extent, depending on the type and the strength of detergent chosen for their isolation, storage, or Proteosome vaccine formulation [1–8]. Indeed, the ability of Proteosome vaccine particles to be reconstituted upon substantial detergent removal is a key advantage of the simplicity of Proteosome vaccine design.

1. Proteosome™ Noncovalent Complex Vaccines

The primary mode of creating Proteosome-based vaccines is to process a mixture of detergent-solubilized Proteosome particles and amphiphilic antigens in a manner that facilitates noncovalent complexing or association of the antigens with Proteosome particles while effecting marked diminution of the solubilizing detergent. This process can result in soluble Proteosome vaccine particles when antigen hydrophobic "anchor" moieties sufficiently satisfy Proteosome hydrophobic sites while antigen hydrophilic moieties remain exposed, creating a hydrophilic microenvironment around the Proteosome vaccines [1–5,7,8]. Resultant Proteosome vaccines are thereby comprised of noncovalent complexes or associations in which reconstituted Proteosome multimolecular nanoparticles are studded with intercalating amphiphilic antigen. The current lead example of this Proteosome vaccine system is FluINsure™, a nasal Proteosome influenza vaccine currently in Phase 2 clinical trials under development [9] at ID Biomedical Corporation (IDB).

2.   Proteosome™ IVX-908 Vaccine Adjuvant

A second approach to developing Proteosome-based vaccines is to formulate a mixture of vaccine antigen with a soluble preformed Proteosome adjuvant preparation comprised of Proteosome particles complexed with LPS. This system, tentatively called IVX-908 [10], differs from the first Proteosome system described in that vaccine antigens adjuvanted by IVX-908 (a) may be either amphiphilic or entirely hydrophilic and devoid of recognizable hydrophobic "anchor" moieties, and (b) are formulated by mixing antigens with the preformed LPS-solubilized Proteosome particles. IVX-908 is referred to as an adjuvant because the immunostimulatory properties of Proteosome particles (see below) are complemented by the well-described adjuvant properties of native LPS it contains and because it is effective when simply mixed with the antigen (although antigen interaction with IVX-908 particles has not been ruled out). Given the substantial amount of LPS in IVX-908, it is germane that a favorable safety profile of an IVX-908 prototype given nasally alone (as a Proteosome *Shigella* LPS vaccine) has already been demonstrated in both preclinical toxicity studies as well as in Phase 1 and Phase 2 clinical trials [11,12].

C.   Mechanisms of Action

1.   Proteosome™ Vaccine Delivery Vehicle Characteristics—Particulate and Hydrophobic Structure

Proteosome particles are considered to serve as vaccine delivery vehicles for antigens associated with them by virtue of their nanoparticulate, multimolecular, vesicle-like nature. Proteosome vaccine particles and particle clusters are generally comparable to the size of certain viruses, ranging in size from 20 to 800 nm in diameter, depending on the type and the amount of antigen formulated. This biophysical characteristic, mandating that vaccine antigens associated with Proteosome particles are treated as particles rather than as soluble proteins, is deemed to benefit from immunogenicity because components of the immune system characteristically recognize and respond to particles differently and frequently more efficiently than they do soluble antigens. In addition, the hydrophobicity of both Proteosome porin proteins and the hydrophobic anchor of amphiphilic antigens associated with Proteosome particles may contribute to vaccine delivery capabilities by inhibiting antigen degradation, facilitating antigen uptake, and/or directing antigen processing to intracellular pathways that promote Type 1 T-cell responses. In this regard, the major OMPs in *Neisseria meningitides* Proteosome particles, PorA (class 1) and PorB (class 2 or 3), are protein porins that naturally form trimers that constitute pores allowing anion exchange through the

bacterial membrane [5,6]. That these neisserial porins can, in vitro, translocate and insert into host cell membranes [6] suggests that Proteosome vaccine delivery function may be related to these unique porin properties. Although from the particulate or hydrophobic perspective, Proteosome particles may be viewed as having some commonality with certain microsphere [13], liposome [14], or other lipid-based vaccine delivery vehicles [15,16]; the intrinsic porin protein properties of Proteosome particles as well as the immunostimulatory capacity (described below) clearly distinguish them from the "inert" systems that rely only on their particulate nature to promote immune responsiveness.

2.   Proteosome™ Adjuvant Characteristics—Immunostimulation

Proteosome adjuvant potential was first suggested by the ability of Proteosome OMPs to initiate B-cell activation as measured by B-cell proliferation and polyclonal antibody secretion in both human [17] and murine [18–20] cells. The murine mitogenicity experiments showed that OMP activation was not LPS-mediated [18,20–22]. This is significant because LPS is a well-known adjuvant and B-cell mitogen [23] and a minor component of Proteosome preparations (<2% in typical IDB Proteosome preparations). In these experiments, Proteosome proteins induced B-cell activation in C3H/HeJ mice that are resistant to LPS stimulation [18–22] due to a natural point mutation in the gene encoding the Toll-like receptor (TLR) 4 [24] necessary for LPS-mediated signal transduction [25]. Over the last several years, Wetzler et al. have provided considerable evidence to support the mechanism of Proteosome adjuvanticity. First, they demonstrated that *Neisseria* OMP recognize and upregulate B7.2 (CD86) costimulatory ligand on B-cell antigen-presenting cells, which results in augmented costimulation of T cells by interacting with its counterreceptor, CD28 [20]. They then showed, using TLR2 knockout mice, that this OMP-mediated activation is due to induction of NfkB nuclear translocation dependent upon B-cell expression of MyD88 and TLR2, but not TLR4 [26]. Porin OMP activation was therefore clearly differentiated from LPS activation, which depends on TLR4 and not TLR2 [25,27]. Most recently, they reported that Proteosome PorB (class 2 or 3) protein also induces maturation of professional APCs as shown by upregulation of B7.2, class I, and class II MHC molecules on C3H/HeJ dendritic cell (DC) surfaces with concomitant enhanced DC allostimulatory activity [28]. This increased expression of B7.2 costimulatory molecules on B cells and DC provides the "second signal" that increases their capacity to costimulate T cells by lowering the threshold number of T-cell receptors required to trigger T-cell responses at a given antigen dose [29]. The result is increased T-cell sensitivity to antigenic stimulation and enhanced immune responses.

These data support the theory of the involvement of TLRs with innate immunity and bacterial adjuvant functions [26,30] now including, in addition to Proteosome porins with TLR2, peptidoglycan and lipoprotein with TLR2 [30], LPS with TLR4, and CpG DNA motifs with TLR9 [31]. Promotion of expression of TLRs on B cell and DC APCs with subsequent upregulation of the efficiency of APC processing and presentation of antigens to T cells appears to be the key to understanding the mechanism of Proteosome-mediated adjuvanticity and may also explain Proteosome vaccine promotion of Type 1 T-cell responses. Furthermore, the report [32] that alveolar macrophages present antigen inefficiently to CD4$^+$ T cells due to defective expression of B7 costimulatory cell surface molecules supports the concept that the nasal Proteosome vaccine advantage is to provide APC TLR activation to effect enhanced respiratory immunogenicity. And last, in addition to vaccine delivery and adjuvant activity, complexing antigen to Proteosome particles may provide broader or exclusive T-cell help for antigens that alone lack the ability to effectively stimulate helper T cells.

The role of TLRs in the adjuvanticity of Proteosome-based vaccines is also particularly relevant to the mechanism of action of the LPS-bearing Proteosome adjuvant, IVX-908, because both Type 2 and Type 4 TLR stimulation can be expected to contribute to adjuvanticity due to the presence of LPS, a known TLR4 stimulant, in IVX-908. Moreover, IVX-908 can be effective without formulating the antigen with Proteosome particles to facilitate complexing; hence, the "vaccine delivery" role is not applicable and the "adjuvant" role is paramount.

D. Safety for Human Use

Safety is the first prerequisite in choosing a system to improve vaccines and is a prime consideration in developing Proteosome platform technology. Meningococcal (Mgc) OMPs comparable to those present in Proteosome vaccines have been safely given parenterally to hundreds of millions of children in a *Haemophilus influenzae* Type b (Hib) conjugate vaccine licensed for infants and adults since 1990 [33]. In this Hib vaccine, Mgc OMPs are covalently linked via bigeneric spacers to Hib polyribosyl ribitol phosphate (PRP) polysaccharide to serve as carrier proteins for PRP so that the vaccine can provide bactericidal anti-PRP IgG antibodies [33]. Similar Mgc OMP preparations have also been hydrophobically complexed to Mgc capsular polysaccharide and given by injection to millions of children and adults in clinical trials designed to protect against meningococcal disease [7]. Most significantly, nasal Proteosome vaccines (including FluINsure and IVX-908) have demonstrated a good safety profile in ~500 persons in Phase 1 and Phase 2 clinical trials of influenza and *Shigella* vaccines. Indeed, in GLP-compliant toxicity studies performed prior to these trials, nasal Proteosome vaccines were successfully evaluated in over 1500 animals using dose levels up to 30-fold greater than projected human doses on a weight-adjusted basis.

E. Versatility for a Variety of Antigen Types for Immunoprophylactic and Immunotherapeutic Vaccines

Any antigen with a hydrophobic moiety available for interacting with Proteosome particles is suitable without modification for use in Proteosome vaccines. Such antigens include natural or recombinant transmembrane or envelope proteins with native hydrophobic amino acid anchor sequences and lipopolysaccharides, polysaccharides, or gangliosides with natural covalently bound lipid components. For LPS (and

hence, IVX-908), noncovalent complexing, verified by size exclusion HPLC [34] or standard chromatography [35], occurs via OMP interaction with LPS lipid A, whereas the *O*-polysaccharide, oriented outside the Proteosome particles, effectively solubilizes the hydrophobic OMPs such that the complex can be terminally sterilized by passage through a 0.22-μm membrane filter. Recombinant proteins can also be made suitable by inserting synthetic nucleotides coding for a hydrophobic anchor sequence into the recombinant genetical sequence toward either the carboxyl or amino terminus. Hydrophobic anchors can also be covalently coupled to antigens after purification. Synthetic peptides are particularly applicable for Proteosome vaccines because a hydrophobic anchor can be readily added toward either terminus of the peptide during synthesis. For any such antigens, either fatty acyl groups (e.g., lauroyl) or a series of 5–21 hydrophobic amino acids can serve as the hydrophobic anchor. A cysteine situated between the epitope and the anchor can be important to peptide immunogenicity perhaps due to cysteic dimerization of both the anchor and the peptide with resultant increases in stability of Proteosome interactions with antigen. The hydrophobic region of antigens responsible for Proteosome interaction may be subtle, as suggested by use of formalinized toxoids whose cross-linked free amino groups may serve this purpose.

Antigens should be oriented so that important epitopes are neither buried nor altered during formulation or complexing with vaccine adjuvants or delivery vehicles. This can be problematical for covalent complexing. Noncovalent complexing to Proteosome particles avoids this problem because antigens complex via hydrophobic moieties distal from important epitopes (which are usually highly hydrophilic [36]). This unidirectional binding of antigens to Proteosome particles allows antigen epitopes to remain unaltered and exposed for recognition by antigen processing cells. Optimal peptide or recombinant protein orientation can be determined by selecting the appropriate position for the hydrophobic anchor. For native transmembrane proteins, such as influenza hemagglutinin (HA), the antigen is posited to insert into the Proteosome particles much as it does in the native viral membrane, thereby promoting maintenance of its native antigenic three-dimensional structure.

The versatility of Proteosome-based vaccines has been further broadened by the IVX-908 adjuvant system because IVX-908 can be mixed with either amphiphilic or nonamphiphilic antigens, and the latter may be more readily available for certain vaccines. Versatility is further emphasized because, in addition to prophylactic vaccines against infectious diseases, IVX-908 is especially suited for nasal immunotherapeutic allergy vaccines, which benefit Type 1 immunity and the shift of immune response patterns away from the allergic responses associated with Type 2 immunity.

F. Simplicity of Scale-Up and Guanylic Acid Production

There has been much progress over the past several years in the scale-up and guanylic acid (GMP) manufacture of Proteosome particles and vaccines. To date, >30 Proteosome lots (>10 GMP and >20 development lots) purified from more than eight bacterial cell paste lots have been produced with demonstrated consistency under a high level of quality systems oversight. The robustness and scalability of the Proteosome production process have allowed successful technology transfer/production at four sites including an FDA-inspected and FDA-licensed facility. Proteosome particles have maintained protein stability and integrity after more than 3 years at $-20°C$ in bulk storage and for 1 month at $40°C$ in accelerated stability studies. A Proteosome protein consistency profile with low level of residuals has been verified by LC-MS, SDS-PAGE/Western blots, RP-HPLC, N-terminal sequencing, and amino acid analysis. Proteosome vaccines and IVX-908 have inherently favorable stability profiles at clinical storage ($4°C$) demonstrated by retention of vaccine complex and protein integrity, particle size stability, and vaccine potency. IVX-908 and Proteosome vaccines can also retain potency after lyophilization and reconstitution (when the antigen tolerates lyophilization). Proteosome vaccines and IVX-908 are produced by a simple, scaleable 1-day process designed to promote optimal noncovalent complexing or association of Proteosome particles with antigen (or, for IVX-908, with LPS) while the solubilizing detergent is removed. This process allows production technology used in preclinical research to be consistent with that performed in scale-up GMP production suites for human clinical trials and for commercial production. Moreover, the simple and efficient design of the key manufacturing method (diafiltration/ultrafiltration) attests to the demonstrated ease of Proteosome vaccine formulation with a variety of antigens and allows for cost-effective production and inexpensive cost of goods favorable for commercial development.

II. NASAL VACCINES FOR RESPIRATORY DISEASES

A. Influenza

1. Background

The Proteosome vaccine application that has made the greatest advance toward commercialization is FluINsure, the nasal Proteosome-based vaccine for influenza under development by ID Biomedical Corporation. Each year in North America and Western Europe, an estimated 57 million cases of influenza occur, leading to at least 210,000 hospitalizations and as many as 70,000 deaths [37]. Most deaths occur in the elderly [38], but there is a significant disease burden in infants [39] and preschool children, who also serve as major disseminators of the virus [20]. Although licensed injectable influenza vaccines reduce morbidity and mortality, vaccination compliance, especially in high-risk groups such as infants and the elderly, is often low [37]. In addition, despite being at least 70% effective in preventing influenza illness in healthy adults [41], the virus-specific serum antibodies elicited by current injectable influenza vaccines limit the spread of the virus, but are relatively ineffective at preventing infection or shortening viral shedding [37]. Moreover, current injectable vaccines are significantly less immunogenic (40–60%) in the elderly [42] and require two injected doses yearly in children [40]—two situations that further limit vaccine acceptance. Reduced compliance and immunogenicity ensure that large sectors of the population remain at high risk of infection and complications caused by influenza.

2. Rationale

FluINsure is efficiently manufactured using the diafiltration technology designed to remove solubilizing detergents and to facilitate Proteosome association with antigen. The antigens in trivalent FluINsure are three conventional "split-flu" influenza antigens comparable to those used yearly in all currently licensed inactivated injectable influenza vaccines. Like conventional intramuscular vaccines, FluINsure dosing is based on hemagglutininin (HA) content. FluINsure is a nasal spray vaccine with fewer safety issues because it is a nonliving, subunit vaccine that, unlike live influenza nasal vaccines, is noninfectious and cannot be transmitted from person to person or have unwanted interactions with wild-type viruses. FluINsure also has potential to provide decreased morbidity against influenza compared to intramuscular vaccines because, in addition to producing serum HAI antibodies, FluINsure elicits antiviral secretory IgA antibodies in nasal passages where influenza invades. Indeed, such nasal antibodies have been shown to be a strong correlate of reduced infection and illness [37,49,50]. Each of these factors (user-friendly needle-free vaccination, good safety profile, decreased safety concerns, and potential for more complete immunity) is expected to increase vaccination compliance in all age groups.

3. Preclinical Immunogenicity Studies

Murine studies of nasal Proteosome influenza vaccines showed induction of virus-specific serum IgG, HAI, and virus-neutralizing antibodies in titers equivalent to those induced by HA vaccine antigens given in the same dose as classical inactivated intramuscular vaccines, or as a sublethal infection with homologous virus [43,44]. Induction of statistically significant virus-specific serum IgA responses, as well as nasal and pulmonary IgA responses including neutralizing antibodies in lung washes, was found in mice immunized nasally with Proteosome influenza vaccine, but not those of mice given the intramuscular vaccine or given the flu antigen without Proteosome particles. In addition, the nasal Proteosome vaccine generated virus-reactive T cells that produced the Type 1 cytokine interferon gamma (IFN-γ) without activating Type 2 cytokine (IL-5) responses. These data were in marked contrast to immunization either intramuscularly or nasally with influenza antigen alone, which resulted in strong IL-5 responses and less IFN-γ, indicating a mixed Type 2/Type 1 response [44]. The pattern of strong Type 1 T-cell responses shown by the Proteosome influenza vaccine is consistent with the pattern typically associated with cytotoxic T-cell induction that prevents the spread of influenza virus. Furthermore, nasal Proteosome influenza vaccine induced solid protection against a lethal respiratory challenge of homologous mouse-adapted virus [44].

Subsequent murine studies were designed to verify the applicability of trivalent formulations of FluINsure for human use showing that (a) H1, H3, and B influenza proteins in FluINsure were immunogenic, and that (b) FluINsure can be given periodically to provide immunity to new or recurrent circulating strains. This is important because influenza vaccines are routinely given every year to match newly emerging circulating strains of influenza virus. In experiments designed to mimic the human experience, mice were reimmunized with a nasal Proteosome influenza vaccine 9 months after (1) receiving the identical Proteosome vaccine, or (2) exposure to antigens of an older strain of influenza given in the form of either (a) a nasal Proteosome influenza vaccine, (b) a standard intramuscular split-flu vaccine, or (c) live influenza virus. In each of these experimental situations, high levels of serum and mucosal antibodies that recognized the strain of influenza present in the Proteosome vaccine used for reimmunization were induced. These data indicate that yearly administration of nasal Proteosome influenza vaccine can be immunogenic for the most recent strain administered, whether the subject was previously exposed to influenza antigens as either a nasal Proteosome vaccine, a standard intramuscular vaccine, or influenza infection [45].

4. Preclinical Toxicity Studies

Nasal Proteosome influenza vaccines were studied in 400 mice, a relevant animal model in which both influenza disease and influenza vaccine-induced protective immunity can be studied. All studies used a three-dose series, with the last dose given in the presence of a documented preexisting immune response. These studies evaluated dose levels up to 20-fold greater than projected human doses on a weight-adjusted basis. No vaccine-attributable weight loss or clinical findings, no changes in blood hematological or chemical parameters, and no vaccine-attributable pathology in any organ (including the nose, sinuses, upper respiratory tract, or adjacent central nervous system tissues such as the olfactory bulb) were found in any animal. The observed absence of pathology in neural tissue was especially important to nasal Proteosome vaccine development because advanced development of other powerful nasal adjuvants [notably those of the cholera toxin (CT) and *Escherichia coli* heat-labile toxin (LT) family] has been significantly impeded due to the finding of olfactory bulb toxicity in mice [46] and the inability to rule out an association with facial nerve palsy in humans (AP news report).

5. Clinical Studies of FluINsure™ Nasal Proteosome™ Influenza Vaccines

As of this writing, seven Phase 1 or Phase 2 dose-escalating clinical trials of FluINsure using single-dose (15, 30, or 45 µg HA) and two-dose (7.5, 15, or 30 µg of HA per dose) regimens with placebo or vaccine comparator controls have enrolled 500 healthy adults in the United States and Canada. These trials to date include two Phase 1 trials of a monovalent (A/Beijing/H1N1) prototype [47], and a Phase 1 [48] and four Phase 2 trials of trivalent FluINsure. Safety data from this clinical experience indicate that FluINsure is well tolerated. Systemic reactions did not exceed those of the standard intramuscular influenza vaccine in one study, and could not be distinguished from those following placebo doses in another trial. No vaccine recipient has had fever. The only local reactions significantly associated with active nasal vaccine in both parallel and crossover study designs, mild and short-lived nasal stuffiness, and/or rhinorrhea occur in

30–60% of vaccinees (exceeding placebo recipients by 10–20%) and only rarely are reported to interfere with normal daily activities in any way. Immunogenicity data in humans have been similarly very encouraging. Significant increases in serum hemagglutination-inhibiting (HAI) antibodies are induced to all strains and at all dose regimens tested, and the observed dose response is shallow, suggesting that the clinically useful nasal dose of influenza antigen when given in FluINsure may be similar to, or only modestly higher than, the dose now used for intramuscular immunization. In addition, statistically significant rises in secreted IgA antibodies in nasal fluid are found in all treatment groups, and are especially high and persistent in recipients of two-dose regimens. This suggests that an important immune response is produced on the respiratory mucosa, where it can meet the invading virus before infection is established. Indeed, specific sIgA in the nose is documented to be a strong correlate of reduced infection rate, limited viral replication, and reduced illness in influenza challenge studies in adults [37,49,50]. Preliminary data in subjects from the first trivalent study indicate that potentially protective immune responses, consisting of one or more of a serum reciprocal HAI titer of ≥ 40, a ≥ 4-fold rise in HAI titer, and/or a significant rise in virus-specific nasal wash secretory IgA, are found, for H1, H3, and B strains, respectively, in 74%, 90%, and 95% of one-dose vaccinees and 83%, 94%, and 100%, respectively, of two-dose vaccinees. It is particularly encouraging that subjects nonimmune before immunization (serum reciprocal HAI titers <40) show comparable values. These serum HAI and nasal sIgA responses appear at least equal, and often superior, to those elicited by nasal immunization with live cold-adapted influenza virus vaccines in similar adult populations [51]. These data were so encouraging, that two of the placebo-controlled double-blind Phase 2 immunogenicity trials were followed by an experimental challenge of subjects with live influenza to demonstrate FluINsure-induced protection against influenza illness. While all the data from both challenge studies are not available as of the writing of this chapter, ID Biomedical has announced that the safety and immunogenicity results from the first challenge trial are consistent with the previous results cited above and furthermore, that the optimal regimen of FluINsure elicited 100% protection against laboratory confirmed influenza illness. With the success of these studies, a large field trial is scheduled for late 2003 to show efficacy during the winter 2003–2004 influenza season.

6. Preclinical Influenza Pandemic Preparedness Studies

FluINsure is eminently suitable for pandemic influenza vaccine preparedness because its manufacture is just as readily accomplished with split-flu conventional antigens as it is with recombinant HA (rHA) produced in tissue culture [52]. Nasal immunization of mice with baculovirus-derived rHA formulated into Proteosome vaccines using dialysis technology resulted in higher levels of HAI antibodies and antiviral IgG in serum than mice immunized intramuscularly with the same doses of rHA alone. In addition, only the Proteosome rHA vaccine induced antiviral IgA in lung and nasal respiratory fluids. Furthermore, as shown by analysis of IgG isotype ratios and cytokine (γ-IFN, IL-5, and IL-2) secretion from restimulated spleen cells, the nasal Proteosome rHA vaccine clearly elicited responses that were more strongly of the Type 1 phenotype than rHA alone. Live virus challenge studies showed that immunization with either the Proteosome rHA vaccine nasally or rHA alone intramuscular totally protected against death by lethal challenge; nevertheless, protection against morbidity, as measured by significant weight loss, was higher in mice immunized nasally with Proteosome rHA vaccine compared to mice given rHA alone by either the nasal or intramuscular route. This study expands the type of influenza antigen that can be used in FluINsure to include recombinant proteins and is a significant asset to pandemic preparedness because availability of conventional egg-derived influenza antigens from pandemic influenza strains may be problematical.

7. Preclinical Influenza Studies with the Lipopolysaccharides-Bearing Proteosome Adjuvant, IVX-908

In mouse studies, nasal immunization with IVX-908, mixed with either conventional split-flu antigen preparations or baculovirus rHA, resulted in strong stimulation of serum HAI, serum IgG, and lung IgA titers [10]. These responses were of the Type 1 phenotype as measured by high IFN-γ and absent IL-5 secretion, and were strongly protective against mortality and morbidity due to live virus challenge. Because IVX-908 can adjuvant immune responses either with amphiphilic or soluble antigens (see "Allergies" below), this technology is a promising candidate as a nasal vaccine adjuvant for a variety of viral or bacterial antigens.

8. Preclinical Studies with Influenza Viral Peptides

A study of nasal Proteosome vaccines using influenza peptides showed that Proteosome vaccines containing influenza peptides representing T-cell and B-cell influenza-specific epitopes can protect a murine model of viral influenza infection [53]. Mice were immunized nasally with Proteosome peptide vaccines containing one to three influenza peptides: a conserved HA B-cell peptide for protective antibodies and two nucleoprotein peptides with either a T-helper cell or cytotoxic T-cell (CTL) epitope. The Proteosome vaccines containing the B-cell epitope elicited antivirus IgA in the lung and Proteosome vaccines containing T-cell epitopes induced proliferative responses and histological evidence of cellular immunity in mouse lungs and spleen. The latter correlated with protective immunity shown by reduction in lung viral titers in mice challenged 2 months after immunization with Proteosome vaccines containing both B-cell and T-cell epitopes [53]. These results support the concept that Proteosome technology is a versatile intranasal delivery platform for multivalent peptide vaccines that enhance humoral and cellular immunity against microbial pathogens.

B. Biothreat Agents

1. Plague

Plague is caused by *Yersinia pestis* bacteria responsible for over 150 recorded epidemics and pandemics and is recog-

nized as a major potential bioterrorism threat agent. Plague pneumonia is highly contagious because large numbers of bacteria can rapidly spread through coughing and initial symptoms are similar to the flu. For effective biodefense against plague, it is of paramount importance that a vaccine prevent the pneumonic form of infection and there is no such licensed vaccine. In collaborative studies between the U.S. Army Medical Research Institute for Infectious Diseases and IDB, nasal immunization of mice with a Proteosome-based Plague vaccine consisting of IVX-908 plus the recombinant fusion protein F1-V induced high levels of antiplague IgG antibodies in serum as well as IgA antibodies in respiratory lavage fluids. Most importantly, this vaccine with 1 μg or 2.5 μg IVX-908 elicited 100% protection against death in mice challenged either 35 or 55 days post-immunization by exposure to an aerosol containing 169 LD50s (inhaled dose) of lethal plague bacteria.

2. Staphylococcal Enterotoxin B and Ricin

Staphylococcal enterotoxin B belongs to a family of *Staphylococcus aureus* superantigen [54] exotoxins that causes human food poisoning and nonmenstrual toxic shock syndrome (TSS) [55,56]. In nonhuman primates, SEB results in lethal shock after aerosol exposure and is therefore a potential biological weapon [57,58]. Nasal immunization of mice with formalinized SEB toxoid formulated with Proteosome particles elicited high levels of anti-SEB serum IgG as well as IgA in lung and intestinal secretions, and afforded significant protection against lethal intramuscular or respiratory SEB challenge in murine models of intoxication [59]. In contrast, intranasal or intramuscular immunization with toxoid in saline without Proteosome particles was not significantly protective against challenge by either route. Immunogenicity and efficacy were confirmed in the nonhuman primate aerosol challenge model of SEB intoxication [60]. Monkeys primed intramuscular (with alum) and boosted twice either intramuscular or intratracheally with the Proteosome SEB toxoid vaccine showed anamnestic anti-SEB serum IgG rises in all monkeys. Strong IgA responses in sera and in bronchial secretions were elicited both pre-SEB and post-SEB challenge only in monkeys boosted intratracheally [60]. The Proteosome SEB toxoid vaccine was efficacious by both routes, protecting 100% of monkeys against severe symptomatology and death from exposure to a 15 LD$_{50}$ dose of aerosolized SEB [60]. Nasal immunization of mice with Proteosome vaccines containing SEB or ricin peptides also elicited antitoxin IgA in lung and intestinal lavage fluids as well as serum IgG [61,62].

3. Brucella

To develop a vaccine against respiratory exposure to *Brucella*, a potential biological threat agent, mice and guinea pigs were intranasally immunized with meningococcal OMPs hydrophobically complexed to *Brucella melitensis* LPS [63] using techniques comparable to those described for Proteosome *Shigella* LPS vaccines [35]. High and persistent levels of anti-*Brucella* LPS serum IgG and high IgG and IgA lung lavage fluid antibodies and antibody-secreting cells in lungs, cervical lymph nodes, and spleen were found

[63,64]. Mice were protected against respiratory challenge with virulent *B. melitensis* as shown by reduced bacterial dissemination to spleen and liver, although the course of the lung infection was unaltered [64].

C. Allergies

Allergic individuals respond to allergen proteins by producing Type 2 T-cell cytokines (e.g., IL-4 and IL-5), which direct or reflect IgE production that leads to allergic symptoms. Allergy immunotherapy "desensitization" vaccine strategies reverse allergic disease in allergic individuals by switching antiallergen immune responses from the Type 2 to the Type 1 phenotype with production of Type 1 cytokines such as interferon gamma. For conventional immunotherapy to show benefits, however, weekly and monthly injections with allergen extracts are required for up to 3 years. Proteosome-based allergy immunotherapy is designed to achieve the same switch in phenotype via nasal administration and is designed to be beneficial more quickly. The major allergen of birch tree pollen, BetV1, induces Type 2 allergic responses (high IL-5, low IFN-γ, and high IgE) when given nasally in a mouse model of allergic disease. In marked contrast, when recombinant protein BetV1 or an allergen extract containing BetV1 are given nasally with Proteosome particles or, especially, with IVX-908, to naïve or sensitized mice, the immune response switches to a Type 1 phenotype against the allergen with production of high IFN-γ levels and low levels of IL-5 and serum IgE [10,65]. Furthermore, sensitized animals treated with allergen extract plus IVX-908 and subsequently exposed to the allergen kept their Type 1 phenotype, whereas mice untreated or given allergen alone maintained their Type 2 phenotype with higher levels of Type 2 cytokines and serum IgE.

III. NASAL VACCINES FOR GASTROINTESTINAL AND SEXUALLY TRANSMITTED DISEASES

A. Shigella

1. Preclinical Immunogenicity and Protection Studies in Small Animals and Nonhuman Primates

Shigella sonnei and *Shigella flexneri* are major causes of dysentery and diarrhea in residents of developing countries and in travelers to such locations from developed countries [66,67]. The *O*-specific polysaccharides of LPS of shigellae are the protective antigens for shigellosis, and local intestinal type-specific antibodies are considered a prime protective mechanism against enteric *Shigella* infections [68]. Either nasal or intragastric immunization of mice with Proteosome *Shigella* LPS vaccines for *S. flexneri* 2a and *S. sonnei* induced homologous anti-*Shigella* LPS IgG and IgA in sera and in bronchial and intestinal mucosal lavage secretions, although nasal immunization required 10- to 100-fold lower doses and resulted in serum antibody levels that persisted and was strongly elevated for > 1 year [34,35,69]. Also, guinea pigs nasally immunized with a Proteosome *S. sonnei* vaccine acquired high levels of anti-LPS IgA and IgG antibody-secreting cells (ASCs) in cervical lymph nodes [34,70]. Same day administration of Proteosome *S. sonnei* and *S. flexneri*

2a vaccines was as immunogenic as either given alone, indicating that multivalent Proteosome *Shigella* vaccines strains are practical [34,71]. Nasal immunization in small (5 µL) volumes to deliver vaccine only to the nasaopharynx elicited comparable IgG and IgA antibody levels in sera and in intestinal mucosa [72], confirming that respiratory immunization can induce the common mucosal immune system to secrete antibodies at nonrespiratory sites [34,35,71–73].

Two models of *Shigella* infections demonstrated efficacy of Proteosome *Shigella* LPS vaccines. Either intranasal or intragastric immunization conferred significant homologous protection against keratoconjunctivitis (*Shigella* eye infection) in the Sereny Test [35], data that further supported the common mucosal immune system. Efficacy of nasal or intragastric Proteosome *Shigella* LPS vaccines was also demonstrated in protection studies against fatal suppurative pneumonia in a murine challenge model of *Shigella* infection [34,69,72]. The ability of Proteosome vaccines to safely present LPS in a nontoxic form is underscored by the lack of observed toxicity of Proteosome LPS vaccines, whereas the same amount of LPS given alone was toxic to mice [69].

Safety and immunogenicity were also shown in two nonhuman primate studies in which 30 rhesus monkeys were immunized with Proteosome vaccines for *S. sonnei* [34,74]. The Proteosome LPS vaccines were well tolerated without noticeable adverse reactions. In the first study, three doses of Proteosome *S. sonnei* LPS given as intranasal nose drops [74] elicited 4- to 2048-fold serum IgG rises in 14 of 15 monkeys. In the second study, all monkeys immunized intratracheally or by intranasal spray responded with high serum IgG titer rises 128- to 4096-fold and 8- to 10,240-fold, respectively, whereas orogastric immunization elicited 4- to 32-fold rises in only three of five monkeys. In addition, all monkeys immunized intratracheally showed at least fourfold IgA rises in sera and bronchial lavage fluids, and twofold to fourfold serum IgA rises were elicited in all intranasal immunized monkeys [34].

Toxicity studies were performed prior to clinical trials of Proteosome LPS vaccines for *S. sonnei* and *S. flexneri* 2a vaccines, utilizing a total of 760 rodents, each immunized three times. Doses up to 30 times the human exposure on a weight-adjusted basis were given nasally in small volumes to conscious animals (to avoid vaccine aspiration). These exposures were both clinically and histologically benign, with no tissue damage or pathology of the upper or lower respiratory tract or other adjacent tissues including the olfactory bulb. Only minor increased nasal-associated lymphoid tissue cellularity was noted and, consistent with a normal response to vaccine antigen exposure and processing, resolved in animals sacrificed after a recovery period.

2. Clinical Studies of *Shigella* Vaccines

Three dose-escalating Phase 1 or Phase 2 safety and immunogenicity trials of Proteosome vaccines for *S. sonnei* or *S. flexneri* 2a have been performed, enrolling 135 subjects, of which 111 received Proteosome vaccines nasally [11,12,75]. Doses, given in a two-dose regimen 14 days apart, ranged from 100 to 1500 µg of Proteosome protein and contained comparable amounts of *Shigella* LPS. In summary, clinical safety analysis showed that the vaccines were well tolerated even at the highest doses. There were no fevers, no sustained illness, and no serious or unexpected adverse events attributable to the vaccine. Repeated ENT exam 2 and 7 days after each dose showed no inflammation, mucosal lesions, otitis, or sinusitis. Transient nasal congestion, clear rhinorrhea, or mild nasal irritation that occurred in approximately one-half to two-thirds of vaccinees was generally mild and short-lived (2–3 days) and greater than 95% of vaccine doses caused no complaint that interfered with daily activities; all complaints were less after the second dose. Immunogenicity analyses showed that O-polysaccharide-specific immune responses were consistently evoked in multiple compartments: 90–100% responded with ASCs (IgA was strongest); 60–90% responded with serum antibodies (fourfold GMT increases in IgG and IgA were typical at 1-mg doses); IgA and IgG responses (3.5- to 6-fold at 1-mg doses) were found in stool; and IgA responses were detected in urine [11,12,75].

An experimental challenge trial was performed in which 14 vaccinees and 13 placebo recipients, at intervals ranging from 27 to 62 days after their last dose of test article, ingested 500 CFU of freshly prepared *S. flexneri* 2a in sodium bicarbonate buffer [76]. Although protective efficacy (PE) against any disease (diarrhea, dysentery, or fever) was 36% ($P = 0.04$), volunteers challenged <48 days postimmunization showed 78% PE ($P = 0.003$) against fever and 56% PE ($P = 0.03$) against severe symptoms. Increased levels of *S. flexneri* 2a-specific serum IgA after immunization (but not prior to immunization) were associated with a lower frequency of diarrhea ($P = 0.02$) and a lower frequency of any disease ($P = 0.01$), whereas serum IgG and blood ASC levels were not found to be predictive. These data are the first demonstration of human protection against any enteric disease by a subunit nasal vaccine and delivery system [76]. The increased protection against severe disease <48 days after immunization suggests that improved efficacy might be achieved by monthly booster doses. This strategy may be practical for high-risk individuals such as short-term military or civilian travelers to endemic areas.

B. Human Immunodeficiency Virus

Mucosal vaccines that induce immunity at intestinal and vaginal sites are designed to contribute to protection against HIV by reducing the likelihood of viral acquisition and dissemination at these entry portals [77]. Mucosal vaccination may also generate systemic immune responses to help reduce the systemic HIV burden. Mice were immunized nasally with the recombinant envelope protein rgp160, complexed to Proteosome particles [78], and delivered either in saline, with a nanoemulsion (Emulsomes™; Pharmos Corp., Iselin, NJ) containing a mucoadhesive biopolymer, or with cholera toxin B subunit (CTB). (Emulsomes are a novel lipoidal particulate vehicle with features intermediate between liposomes and oil-in-water emulsions [79].) Nasal immunization with the Proteosome rgp160 vaccine elicited improved anti-HIV IgG and IgA titers in serum and in vaginal, intestinal, and lung fluids and in fecal pellets and broadened the number of gp160 epitopes recognized compared to immunizing with rgp160 alone, and combining the Proteosome vaccine with either Emulsomes or CTB often

increased effectiveness [78]. The ability of nasal Proteosome vaccines to enhance anti-HIV IgG and IgA immune responses 2–3 logs in sera, in vaginal, intestinal, and lung secretions, and in fecal extracts [78] was confirmed [80] with a native HIV-1 oligomeric gp160 (oligo-gp160) [81] protein that has greater potential to elicit neutralizing antibodies. The demonstration of neutralizing antibodies in vaginal and lung secretions as well as in sera was unique to nasal Proteosome oligo-gp160 immunization in this study [80] and is particularly encouraging for human trials of this mucosal AIDS vaccine.

IV. PARENTERAL VACCINES

A. Proteins

1. Parasitic and Viral Diseases: Schistosomiasis, Malaria, and Human Immunodeficiency Virus

For schistosomiasis, an intramuscular Proteosome vaccine containing an extracted 38- to 40-kDa *Schistosoma mansoni* antigen induced high levels of antibodies that mediated complement-dependant antischistosomal activity as well as in vivo protection, with >70% decrease in worm burden while immunization without Proteosome technology was not protective [82]. In another study, immunizing with a recombinant 62-kDa *S. mansoni* antigen formulated with Proteosomes elicited the most consistent and highest levels (83%) of protection [83]. In malaria studies in mice and rabbits, intramuscular immunization with any of three proteosome vaccines made with recombinant *Plasmodium falciparum* circumsporozoite proteins containing carboxyl terminus hydrophobic amino acids (that were either native to the molecule, or were recombinantly added) enhanced specific serum IgG responses up to 50-fold [84]. These data confirm the applicability of recombinant proteins with native or synthetic anchors for antiparasite intramuscular Proteosome vaccines. Similarly, Proteosome vaccines made with HIV rgp160 given intramuscularly in saline, with alum or with a submicron emulsion (SME), improved the magnitude and the breadth of antibody responses compared to rgp160 alone [87]. Strong CTL responses were also elicited by proteosome vaccines, especially when delivered in SME.

2. Toxin Diseases: Enterohemorrhagic *E. coli* Shiga-Like Toxin-1 and Staphylococcal Enterotoxin B

Enterohemorrhagic *E. coli* that produce shiga-like toxins are important enteric pathogens that induce both hemorrhagic colitis and hemolytic uremic syndrome (HUS) [85]. Subcutaneous immunization with SLT-1B (the B subunit of SLT-1) formulated with Proteosomes plus alum induced anti-SLT-1B IgG that neutralized SLT-1 cytotoxicity in vitro and conferred significant protection against weight loss, gross and microscopical intestinal vascular lesions, and edema associated with RDEC-H19A challenge [86] in a rabbit model of human EHEC colitis. In addition, in models of SEB intoxication, intramuscular immunization with formalinized SEB toxoid plus proteosomes with or without alum enhanced antitoxin serum IgG levels compared to SEB toxoid alone and significantly protected mice against lethal systemic or respiratory SEB intoxication [59] and monkeys challenged by aerosol with 15 LD_{50} of SEB [60].

B. Peptides

Complexing Proteosome particles to dozens of peptides derived from malaria, trypanosome, streptococci, SEB, and ricin antigens via lipid or hydrophobic anchors synthetically linked to the peptides resulted in highly improved intramuscular immunogenicity [1–3,62,88] and, using computer modeling, led to identification of a protective ricin peptide vaccine [89]. Another elegant use of a Proteosome peptide vaccine utilized the creation of a peptide mimicking a polysaccharide antigenic determinant. Computer analysis of the variable regions of an anti-idiotypic monoclonal antibody (MAb) mimicking meningococcal group C polysaccharide (MCP) elucidated the immunogenic site on the anti-id MAb responsible for inducing anti-MCP responses. Mice immunized with a Proteosome vaccine containing a peptide representing the MAb protective domain developed high-serum anti-MCP IgG and IgM that protected sensitized mice against virulent meningococci as measured by both survival (100%) and bacteremia clearing [90].

C. Polysaccharides and Detoxified Lipopolysaccharides

The safety and immunogenicity of injectable Proteosome vaccines were emphasized by large clinical trials testing OMPs complexed to polysaccharides for vaccines against meningitis [7]. In other studies, immunization with a detoxified J5 LPS complexed to Proteosome OMPs [91] was used to produce rabbit IgG that passively protected neutropenic rats against lethal challenge with *Pseudomonas aeruginosa*. Because J5 antibodies elicited by this vaccine bound several types of gram-negative bacteria, the authors suggested that such vaccines have potential as a vaccine against gram-negative septicemia caused by a wide variety of bacteria.

D. Cancer Cell Surface Gangliosides

A Proteosome vaccine containing GD3 ganglioside complexed via its hydrophobic ceramide component induced high anti-GD3 IgM antibody levels that mediated complement-dependant lysis of melanoma tumor cells, whereas numerous other formulations did not [92]. In other studies, a GM3 ganglioside complexed to Proteosome particles induced antimelanoma cell IgG responses that mediated complement-mediated cytotoxicity, suppressed tumor growth, and prolonged survival in mice challenged with live melanoma cells [93]. These data suggest that Proteosome technology is a promising candidate to augment antiganglioside responses for cancer immunotherapy vaccines.

V. CONCLUSIONS AND FUTURE DIRECTIONS

This chapter has highlighted several advances in the understanding and application of Proteosome delivery vehicles and adjuvants, particularly for nasal vaccines. The finding that B-cell activation by Proteosome porin proteins depends on TLR2 activation with concomitant upregulation of expression of B7.2, MHC-1, and MHC-2 costimulatory molecules on APCs, including both B cells and dendritic cells, allows classification of Proteosome stimulatory adjuvant activity with that of other known adjuvants that stimulate APCs. This, combined with the nanoparticulate structure of Proteosome vaccines, has provided conceptual grounds for understanding the basis of Proteosome enhancement of vaccine-induced immunity. Further work on the mechanism of action of Proteosome-based vaccines on the mucosal level would also be informative because the potential contribution of mucosal uptake and/or processing and presentation by Proteosome particles and adjuvants at mucosal sites is not currently completely clear. As shown by animal and/or human studies for vaccines against intestinal or sexually transmitted diseases such as shigellosis and AIDS, nasal Proteosome vaccines do stimulate the common mucosal immune system to provide mucosal antibodies at sites distal to the respiratory tract. The results of the nasal Proteosome *Shigella* vaccine in a human challenge study demonstrating significant protection against severe disease and fever is a significant advance for nasal subunit vaccines even though the level and duration of protection found needed improvement. Indeed, such improvement might be accomplished by more frequent nasal spray booster immunizations—a prospect not unreasonable for high-risk individuals exposed to infection by *Shigella* or HIV.

The most rapid advances in nasal vaccines will likely occur against respiratory targets. The progress of the nasal Proteosome influenza vaccine, FluINsure, from murine studies to Phase 1 and Phase 2 clinical trials, and to experimental challenge studies demonstrating protection in people over the last few years along with the upcoming field trial attests to the rapidity with which these vaccines can be developed for human use. The preclinical safety, immunogenicity, and toxicity package available for nasal Proteosome vaccines is now quite extensive. The success of FluINsure using split product viral protein preparations in human studies suggests that similar vaccines could be developed for other respiratory viral infections such as RSV, measles, and PIV, all of which display protective transmembrane proteins on their surface. Another important respiratory target for nasal Proteosome vaccines is against biothreat agents and preliminary data using IVX-908 vaccine showing protection of mice against a high lethal aerosol challenge with *Y. pestis* (plague) have significance for nasal vaccination against other biothreat agents such as anthrax, ricin, and SEB.

The ability of Proteosome vaccines and adjuvants, even when delivered nasally, to switch immune responses of antigens from Type 2 to Type 1 phenotype (with IFN-γ production) has several important implications. First, generation of Type 1 immunity indicates that cell-mediated mechanisms including CTL responses would be expected. This would be beneficial to influenza vaccines by providing cellular immunity that is considered to be important in reducing clinical morbidity from viral infection and eliminating the last traces of virus inside cells that may be otherwise unavailable to antibodies. This would complement the demonstrated ability of mucosal IgA, also induced by nasal vaccines such as FluINsure, to neutralize viruses in cells. Second, it is now accepted that certain vaccines, notably against RSV, must provide Type 1 immunity in order to avoid the vaccine-associated pathology and adverse reactions found in the 1960s using formalin-inactivated viral vaccines with alum. Third, stimulation of Type 1 immunity opens the avenue of Proteosome therapeutic vaccines for allergy, currently under active investigation, where generating Type 1 responses is the fundamental basis for allergy immunotherapy as well as for cancer vaccines. The addition of IVX-908 as a Proteosome-based nasal adjuvant that is effective even when mixed with antigen devoid of hydrophobic anchors also expands the applicability of Proteosome technology.

The upgrade in the characterization, scale-up, and stability package for Proteosome vaccines has allowed rapid advancement of Proteosome-based products toward use in commercial vaccine products. Continued progress over the next several years in research, development, and advanced clinical trials leading to commercialization of Proteosome nasal vaccines and adjuvants is eagerly anticipated.

ACKNOWLEDGMENT

We thank Dr. Philip R. Glade, M.D., whose advice, recommendation, encouragement, and inspiration at a critical time made this work possible.

REFERENCES

1. Lowell GH, et al. Peptides bound to proteosomes via hydrophobic feet become highly immunogenic without adjuvants. J Exp Med 1988; 167:658–663.
2. Lowell GH, et al. Proteosome–lipopeptide vaccines: enhancement of immunogenicity for malaria CS peptides. Science 1988; 240:800–802.
3. Lowell GH, et al. Designing highly immunogenic vaccines by complexing synthetic malaria, trypanosome or streptococcal peptides to proteosomes via hydrophobic amino acid or lauric acid feet. In: Lasky L, ed. Technical Advances in Vaccine Development. New York: Alan R. Liss, 1988:423–443.
4. Wetzler LM, et al. Gonococcal porin vaccine evaluation: comparison of por proteosomes, liposomes, and blebs isolated from rmp deletion mutants. J Infect Dis 1992; 166:551–555.
5. Wetzler LM. Immunopotentiating ability of neisserial major outer membrane proteins. Use as an adjuvant for poorly immunogenic substances and potential use in vaccines. Ann NY Acad Sci 1994; 730:367–370.
6. Lynch EC, et al. Studies of porins spontaneously transferred from whole cells and reconstituted from purified proteins of *Neisseria gonorrhea* and *Neisseria meningitides*. Biophys J 1984; 45:104–107.
7. Rappuoli R, et al. Meningococcal conjugate and protein-based vaccines. In: Levine MM, et al., eds. New Generation Vaccines. 3rd ed. New York: Marcel Dekker, 2003:421–426.
8. Frasch CE, Peppler MS. Protection against group B *Neisseria meningitides* disease: preparation of soluble protein and protein–polysaccharide immunogens. Infect Immun 1982; 37:271–280.

9. Halperin S, et al. Phase I safety and immunogenicity of FluINsure, proteosome–trivalent influenza vaccine, given nasally to adults. The 42nd Interscience Conference on Antimicrobial Agents and Chemotherapy (ICAAC), San Diego, September 27–30, 2002.
10. Jones T, et al. IVX-908—a novel mucosal adjuvant for induction of enhanced serum IgG, mucosal IgA and Type 1 cytokine responses. 11th International Congress of Mucosal Immunology, Orlando, FL, June 16–20, 2002.
11. Fries LF, et al. Safety and immunogenicity of a proteosome–*Shigella flexneri* 2a lipopolysaccharide vaccine administered intranasally to healthy adults. Infect Immun 2001; 69:4545–4553.
12. Mckenzie R, et al. Safety and immunogenicity of an intranasal vaccine for *Shigella flexneri*. 39th Annual Meeting of the Infectious Diseases Society of America, San Francisco, October 25–28, 2001.
13. O'Hagan DT. Recent developments in vaccine delivery systems. In: Levine MM, et al., eds. New Generation Vaccines. 3rd ed. New York: Marcel Dekker, 2003:259–270.
14. Alving CL. Vaccines against atherosclerosis. In: Levine MM, et al., eds. New Generation Vaccines. 3rd ed. New York: Marcel Dekker, 2003:1003–1010.
15. Mannino RJ, Gould-Fogerite S. Antigen cochleate preparations for oral and systemic vaccination. In: Levine MM, Woodrow GC, eds. New Generation Vaccines. New York: Marcel Dekker, 2002:229–237.
16. Kenney RT, Edelman R. Adjuvants for the future. In: Levine MM, et al., eds. New Generation Vaccines. 3rd ed. New York: Marcel Dekker, 2003:213–223.
17. Lowell GH, et al. Mitogenesis and polyclonal activation of human B lymphocytes by meningococcal outer membrane proteins. Intersci Conf Antimicrob Agents Chemother 1981; 21:691.
18. Solow RS, et al. Studies of mitogenicity and adjuvanticity of meningococcal outer membrane proteins in mice. Fed Proc 1982; 41:830.
19. Liu MA, et al. A vaccine carrier derived from *Neisseria meningitidis* with mitogenic activity for lymphocytes. Proc Natl Acad Sci USA 1992; 89:4633–4637.
20. Wetzler LM, et al. Neisserial porins induce B lymphocytes to express co-stimulatory B7-2 molecules and to proliferate. J Exp Med 1996; 183:1151–1159.
21. Mackinnon FG, et al. The role of B/T costimulatory signals in the immunopotentiating activity of neisserial porin. J Infect Dis 1999; 180:755–761.
22. Bhasin N, et al. *Neisseria meningitidis* lipopolysaccharide modulates the specific humoral immune response to neisserial porins but has no effect on porin-induced upregulation of costimulatory ligand B7-2. Infect Immun 2001; 69:5031–5036.
23. Skidmore BJ, et al. Immunologic properties of bacterial lipopolysaccharide (LPS): III. Genetic linkage between the in vitro mitogenic and in vivo adjuvant properties of LPS. J Exp Med 1976; 143:143–150.
24. Poltorak A, et al. Defective LPS signaling in C3H/HeJ and C57BL/10ScCr mice: mutations in Tlr4 gene. Science 1998; 282:2085–2088.
25. Chow JC, et al. Toll-like receptor-4 mediates lipopolysaccharide-induced signal transduction. J Biol Chem 1999; 274:10689–10692.
26. Massari P, et al. Cutting edge: immune stimulation by neisserial porins is Toll-like receptor 2 and MyD88 dependent. J Immunol 2002; 168:1533–1537.
27. Heine H, et al. Cutting edge: cells that carry A null allele for Toll-like receptor 2 are capable of responding to endotoxin. J Immunol 1999; 162:6971–6975.
28. Singleton TE, et al. *Neisseira meningitides* PorB induces dendritic cell maturation. ASM General Meeting, Washington, DC, May 19–23.

29. Viola A, Lanzavecchia A. T cell activation determined by T cell receptor number and tunable thresholds. Science 1996; 273:104–106.

30. Takeuchi O, Akira S. Toll-like receptors; their physiological role and signal transduction system. Int Immunopharmacol 2001; 1:625–635.

31. Takeshita F, et al. Cutting edge: role of Toll-like receptor 9 in CpG DNA-induced activation of human cells. J Immunol 2001; 167:3555–3558.

32. Chelen CJ, et al. Human alveolar macrophages present antigen ineffectively due to defective expression of B7 costimulatory cell surface molecules. J Clin Invest 1995; 95:1415–1421.

33. Ward JE, Zangwill KM. Haemophilus influenzae vaccines. In: Plotkin SA, Orenstein WA, eds. Vaccines. 3rd ed. Philadelphia: WB Saunders Co., 1999:183–221.

34. Lowell GH, et al. Status of pre-clinical and Phase 1 studies of proteosome *Shigella* vaccines. Proceedings of the Seventh USA/IDF Conference on Infectious Diseases and Vaccines of Military Importance, Gaithersburg, MD, 1995.

35. Orr N, et al. Immunogenicity and efficacy of oral or intranasal *Shigella flexneri* 2a and *Shigella sonnei* proteosome–lipopolysaccharide vaccines in animal models. Infect Immun 1993; 61:2390–2395.

36. Hopp TP, Woods KR. Prediction of protein antigenic determinants from amino acid sequences. Proc Natl Acad Sci USA 1981; 78:3824–3828.

37. Betts RF, Treanor JJ. Approaches to improved influenza vaccination. Vaccine 2000; 18:1690–1695.

38. Webster RG. Immunity to influenza in the elderly. Vaccine 2000; 18:1686–1689.

39. Glezen WP, et al. Influenza virus infection in infants. Pediatr Infect Dis J 1997; 16:1065–1068.

40. Monto AS, et al. Effect of vaccination of a school-age population upon the course of an A2-Hong Kong influenza epidemic. Bull World Health Organ 1969; 41:537–542.

41. Demicheli V, et al. Prevention and early treatment of influenza in healthy adults. Vaccine 2000; 18:957–1030.

42. Gross PA, et al. The efficacy of influenza vaccine in elderly persons. Ann Intern Med 1995; 123:518–527.

43. Plante M, et al. Nasal proteosome subunit flu vaccines elicit enhanced mucosal IgA, and serum HAI and protection comparable to conventional injectable flu vaccine. Conference on Options for the Control of I.V. Influenza, Crete, September 23–28, 2000.

44. Plante M, et al. Nasal immunization with subunit proteosome influenza vaccines induces serum HAI, mucosal IgA and protection against influenza challenge. Vaccine 2001; 20: 218–225.

45. Burt D, et al. Nasal proteosome–flu vaccines induce enhanced serum and mucosal antibodies in previously infected or immunized hosts. Fifth Annual Conference on Vaccine Research (NFID), Baltimore, MD, May 6–8, 2002.

46. Bourguignon P, et al. Reactogenicity and passage into the brain of enterotoxins and CPG-oligonucleotides administered intranasally to mice. Fourth Annual Conference on Vaccine Research, Arlington, VA, April 23–25, 2001:53.

47. Treanor J, et al. Phase I evaluation of an intranasal proteosome–influenza vaccine in healthy adults. 4th Annual National Foundation for Infectious Diseases (NFID) Conference on Vaccine Research, V.A. Arlington, 2001.

48. Halperin S, et al. Phase I safety and immunogenicity of FluINsure, proteosome–trivalent influenza vaccine, given nasally to adults. The 42nd Interscience Conference on Antimicrobial Agents and Chemotherapy (ICAAC), San Diego, 2002.

49. Clements ML, et al. Serum and nasal wash antibodies associated with resistance to experimental challenge with influenza A wild-type virus. J Clin Microbiol 1986; 24:157–160.

50. Beyer WEP, et al. Cold-adapted live influenza vaccine versus inactivated vaccine: systemic vaccine reactions, local and systemic antibody response, and vaccine efficacy. A meta-analysis. Vaccine 2002; 20:1340–1353.

51. Treanor JJ, et al. Evaluation of trivalent, live, cold-adapted (CAIV-T) and inactivated (TIV) influenza vaccines in prevention of virus infection and illness following challenge of adults with wild-type influenza A (H1N1). A (H3N2) and B viruses. Vaccine 2000; 18:899–906.

52. Jones DH, et al. Nasal proteosome influenza vaccine using a baculovirus hemagglutinin induces improved mucosal and systemic immunity. 4th Annual Conference on Vaccine Research, Arlington, VA, April 23–25, 2001.

53. Levi R, et al. Intranasal immunization of mice against influenza with synthetic peptides anchored to proteosomes. Vaccine 1995; 13:1353–1359.

54. Marrak P, Kappler J. The staphylococcal enterotoxins and their relatives. Science 1990; 248:705–711.

55. Schlievert PM. Role of superantigens in human disease. J Infect Dis 1993; 167:997–1002.

56. Spero L, et al. Enterotoxins of staphylococci. In: Hardegree MC, Tu AT, eds. Handbook of Natural Toxins. New York: Marcel Dekker, 1988:131–163.

57. Mattix ME, et al. Aerosolized staphylococcal enterotoxin B-induced pulmonary lesions in rhesus monkeys (*Macaca mulatta*). Toxicol Pathol 1995; 23:262–268.

58. Hunt RE, et al. Host respiratory protection for lethal staphylococcal enterotoxin B. In: Kamely D, Bannister KA, Sasmore RM, eds. Army Sciences: The New Frontiers: Military and Civilian Applications. Wyoming: Borg Biomedical Books, 1993:71–78.

59. Lowell GH, et al. Intranasal and intramuscular proteosome–staphylococcal enterotoxin B (SEB) toxoid vaccines: immunogenicity and efficacy against lethal SEB intoxication in mice. Infect Immun 1995; 64:1706–1713.

60. Lowell GH, et al. Immunogenicity and efficacy against lethal aerosolized staphylococcal enterotoxin B challenge in monkeys by intramuscular and respiratory delivery of proteosome–toxoid vaccines. Infect Immun 1996; 64:4686–4693.

61. Aboud-Pirak E, et al. Parenteral or intranasal proteosome–lipopeptide vaccines using staphylococcal enterotoxin B or ricin peptides to induce anti-protein toxin serum IgG or respiratory IgA in mice. American Society for Microbiology, Annual Meeting, Atlanta, GA, 1993:152.

62. Kaminski R, et al. Comparison of induction of respiratory IgA and serum IgG by intranasal and parenteral proteosome vaccines formulated with staphylococcal enterotoxin B toxoids or ricin peptides. Med Def Biosci Rev 1993; 3: 1443.

63. Van de Verg LL, et al. Outer membrane protein of *Neisseria meningitidis* as a mucosal adjuvant for lipopolysaccharide of *Brucella melitensis* in mouse and guinea pig intranasal immunization models. Infect Immun 1996; 64:5263–5268.

64. Bhattacharjee AK, et al. Protection of mice against brucellosis by intranasal immunization with *Brucella melitensis* lipopolysaccharide as a noncovalent complex with *Neisseria meningitidis* group B outer membrane protein. Infect Immun 2002; 70:3324–3329.

65. Rioux CR, et al. Induction of Type 1 immune responses against Bet v 1a allergens in mice by proteosome based mucosal adjuvants. American Academy of Allergy Asthma and Immunology Conference, New York City, March 1–6, 2002.

66. Lee LA, et al. Hyperendemic shigellosis in the United States: a review of surveillance data for 1967–1988. J Infect Dis 1991; 164:894–900.

67. Stoll BJ, et al. Epidemiologic and clinical features of patients infected with *Shigella* who attended a diarrheal disease hospital in Bangladesh. J Infect Dis 1982; 146:177–183.

68. Kotloff K, et al. Overview of live vaccines against *Shigella*.

In: Levine MM, et al., eds. New Generation Vaccines. 3rd ed. New York: Marcel Dekker, 2003:723–735.

69. Mallett CP, et al. Intranasal or intragastric immunization with proteosome–Shigella lipopolysaccharide vaccines protect against lethal pneumonia in a murine model of Shigella infection. Infect Immun 1995; 63:2382–2386.

70. Van De Verg LL, et al. Intranasal immunization with LPS of Brucella or Shigella complexed with Neisseria meningitidis OMP in murine and guinea pig models. 95th General Meeting of the American Society for Microbiology (Abstract), Washington, DC, 1995.

71. Orr N, et al. Development of a bivalent Shigella flexneri 2a/Shigella sonnei vaccine composed of LPS–proteosome hydophobic complex. Proceedings of the 35th Interscience Conference. Antimicrob Agents Chemother, 1995:159.

72. Mallett CP, et al. Efficacy and immunogenicity studies of mucosal proteosome–Shigella LPS vaccines in a murine intranasal challenge model of Shigella infection. 9th International Congress of Immunology, San Francisco, CA, 1995.

73. Orr N, et al. Enhancement of anti-Shigella LPS responses by addition of cholera toxin B subunit (CTB) to oral or intranasal proteosome–Shigella flexneri 2a LPS vaccines. Infect Immun 1994; 62:5198–5200.

74. Lowell GH, et al. Mucosal immunogenicity in non-human primates of proteosome–Shigella sonnei lipopolysaccharide vaccines. 95th General Meeting of the American Society for Microbiology, Washington, DC, 1995.

75. Mallett CP, et al. Immunogenicity of a proteosome–Plesiomonas shigelloides LPS vaccine for Shigella sonnei in human volunteers. American Society for Microbiology, 97th General Meeting, Miami Beach, FL, 1997.

76. Durbin A, et al. Intranasal immunization with proteosome–Shigella flexneri 2a LPS vaccine: factors associated with protection in a volunteer challenge model. 39th Annual Meeting of the Infectious Diseases Society of America, San Francisco, October 25–28, 2001.

77. Forrest BD. Women, HIV and mucosal immunity. Lancet 1991; 337:679–835.

78. Lowell GH, et al. Proteosomes, Emulsomes and cholera toxin B improve nasal immunogenicity of human immunodeficiency virus gp160: induction of serum, intestinal, vaginal and lung IgA and IgG in mice. J Infect Dis 1997; 175:292–301.

79. Amselem S, et al. Emulsomes, a novel drug delivery technology. Int Symp Control Release Bioact Mater 1994; 21:668–669.

80. VanCott T, et al. HIV-1 neutralizing antibodies in the genital and respiratory tracts of mice intransally immunized with oligomeric gp160. J Immunol 1998; 160:2000–2012.

81. VanCott TC, et al. Characterization of a soluble oligomeric HIV-1 gp160 protein as a potential immunogen. J Immunol Methods 1995; 183:103–117.

82. Tarrab-Hazdai R, et al. Proteosome delivery of a protective 9B-antigen against Schistosoma mansoni vaccine. Int J Immunopharmacol 1999; 21:205–218.

83. Soisson LMA, et al. Induction of protective immunity in mice using a 62-kDa recombinant fragment of a Schistosoma mansoni surface antigen. J Immunol 1992; 149:36123612.

84. Lowell GH, et al. A recombinant P. falciparum circumsporozoite (CS) protein (R32Ft) designed with a hydrophobic decapeptide anchor: purification and immunogenicity in CS-repeat responder and non-responder mice either without adjuvants or hydrophobically complexed to proteosomes. Proceedings of the Pre-Erythrocytic Stage Malaria Vaccine Development: Current Status and Future Prospects Conference, Bethesda, MD, April 12–15, 1989. Am Soc Trop Med Hyg (Abstr 61), 1989.

85. Pickering LK, et al. Hemolytic–uremic syndrome and enterohemorrhagic Escherichia coli. Pediatr Infect Dis J 1994; 13:459–476.

86. Noel J, et al. Parenteral immunization with shiga like toxin B subunit in proteosomes protects in a model of enterohemorrhagic E. coli (EHEC) colitis. Annual Meeting of the North American Society for Pediatric Gastroenterology.

87. Kaminski R, et al. Immunization with gp160 plus proteosomes, sub-micron emulsions and/or alum to enhance HIV peptide and protein antibody responses. Vaccine Res 1996; 4:189–206.

88. Ruegg CL, et al. Preparation of proteosome-based vaccines: correlation of immunogenicity with physical characteristics. J Immunol Methods 1990; 135:101–108.

89. Aboud-Pirak E, et al. Identification of a neutralizing epitope on ricin A chain and application of its 3D structure to design peptide vaccines that protect against ricin intoxication. Med Def Biosci Rev 1993; 3:1431.

90. Westerink MAJ, et al. Peptide mimicry of the meningococcal group C capsular polysaccharide. Proc Soc Natl Acad Sci USA 1995; 92:4021–4025.

91. Bhattarcharjee AK, et al. A noncovalent complex vaccine prepared with detoxified Escherichia coli J5 (Rc chemotype) LPS and Neisseria meningitidis group B outer membrane protein produces protective antibodies against gram-negative bacteremia. J Infect Dis 1996; 173:1156–1163.

92. Livingston PO, et al. GD3/proteosome vaccines induce consistent IgM antibodies against the ganglioside GD3. Vaccine 1993; 11:1199.

93. Alonso DF, et al. A novel hydrophobized GM3 ganglioside/Neisseria meningitides outer-membrane–protein complex vaccine induces tumor protection in B16 murine melanoma. Int J Oncol 1999; 15:59–66.

24
Viruslike Particle (VLP) Vaccines

Margaret E. Conner
Baylor College of Medicine and Veterans Affairs Medical Center, Houston, Texas, U.S.A.

Mary K. Estes
Baylor College of Medicine, Houston, Texas, U.S.A.

I. INTRODUCTION

Viruslike particles (VLPs) are nonreplicating, virus capsids made using recombinant DNA technology that mimic the structure of native virions [1,2]. They generally are formed when viral structural protein(s) are synthesized in eukaryotic or prokaryotic expression systems and the proteins self-assemble to form particles. VLPs are not infectious because they lack the viral genome. VLPs can be simple and formed by expression of one viral capsid protein (papillomavirus, parvovirus, calicivirus, hepatitis B core protein) or by coexpression of multiple proteins that form more complex capsid structures (orbivirus, Ebola virus, herpesvirus, and rotavirus). VLPs can be produced for both nonenveloped and enveloped RNA and DNA viruses. VLPs mimic the immunogenicity of native virions because they display authentic or near-authentic conformational epitopes. VLPs are being investigated in many viral systems as subunit vaccines and as vectors to carry other proteins, peptides, or nucleic acids for gene transfer, gene therapy, or DNA vaccines (Table 1). VLPs provide vaccine approaches in systems where native virions cannot be readily isolated or produced (e.g., papillomavirus, Ebola virus, or Norwalk virus) and traditional vaccine approaches are not possible [3–5]. VLPs are also useful reagents in these same systems to produce diagnostic reagents or to evaluate immune responses in vaccine trials [5–9].

VLPs are advantageous as vaccines because they can induce both arms of the immune system, they display a large repertoire of antigenic sites, and they display discontinuous epitopes that structurally mimic virus particles. In many cases, VLP vaccines are in preclinical testing in animal models, but some have progressed to Phase I or II clinical trials [4,6,10–13,33]. An important advantage of VLPs as vaccines is their apparent high safety compared to live or inactivated vaccine approaches. VLPs are safe both to produce and to

handle, and safe to administer as vaccines or carriers because when produced in baculovirus or yeast they lack mammalian cell proteins or mammalian-derived pathogens [14]. In addition, they are a safe alternative for vaccines for viruses for which a more traditional attenuated or inactivated vaccine approach is not feasible because of the serious consequences of a reversion to virulence or failure in inactivation (e.g., HIV or papillomavirus) [1,2]. Because VLPs are noninfectious and do not contain nucleic acid, there is no possibility of reversion to virulence, integration into the host genome, and spread to nonvaccinated individuals. These are important safety advantages, especially because of their potential safety in multiple populations including children and the increasing numbers of immunocompromised hosts throughout the world.

VLPs can be produced or expressed in many expression systems, including mammalian cells (HIV, Ebola, influenza, HTLV-I, rotavirus), baculovirus (orbivirus, rotavirus, Norwalk virus, papillomavirus, HIV), yeast (HBV, HPV, HIV), recombinant vaccinia (HIV), *Salmonella* (HPV L1), *Escherichia coli* (HPV, polyomavirus, HCV), alphavirus replicons (Norwalk virus), and plants (HBV, Norwalk virus, HPV, rotavirus) [1,13,15–24]. Baculovirus expression systems have been commonly used for expression of VLPs used in preclinical testing; these and other systems such as yeast and bacterial expression systems may be adapted for vaccine production. The system of choice depends on the particular VLP being produced. Assembly of some VLPs requires authentic posttranslation modifications of viral proteins possible only in eukaryotic cells, and some viral gene sequences are toxic in bacteria or yeast [16,25]. In these cases, modifications of the expression system or changes in codon usage may overcome initial potential disadvantages. Yields of VLPs have not been reported for all VLPs in the different expression systems, but reported yields range from ~3 to 65 mg/L [5,19,26–29]. Yields for VLPs composed of single

Table 1 Examples of VLPs for Different Vaccines for Different Diseases

| VLP | Vaccine to prevent | Immunogenic or protective in: | | References |
		Animals	Humans	
Reoviridae				
Rotavirus	Diarrheal disease	Yes	NT	28, 90, 105, 107, 108, 114, 121, 122
Orbivirus	Bluetongue	Yes	NA	14, 29
Calicivirus				
Norwalk virus	Diarrheal disease	Yes	Yes	5, 6, 20, 40, 64, 67, 69
Rabbit hemorrhagic disease virus	Hepatitis in rabbits	Yes	NA	123, 124
Human immunodeficiency virus	AIDS	Yes	Yes	18, 26, 42, 125, 126
Influenza virus	Respiratory disease	Yes	NT	127–129
Hepatitis E virus	Hepatitis	Yes	NT	38, 130
Hepatitis C virus	Hepatitis	Yes	NT	21, 131
Ebola virus	Hemorrhagic disease	NT	NT	3, 132
Papillomavirus	Cervical and anogenital cancer	Yes	Yes	11–13, 33, 34, 133
Papillomavirus	Autoimmunity-carrier	Yes	NT	118
Papillomavirus	Carrier	Yes		43, 44, 134
Porcine parvovirus	Carrier	Yes	NT	41, 45, 46, 135–137
Polyomavirus	Carrier	Yes	NT	23, 138–140
Hepatitis B virus core	Carrier	Yes	NT	47, 141–145
Hepatitis B virus (surface antigen)	Carrier	Yes	NT	141, 146
Hepatitis E virus	Carrier	Yes	NT	39
HIV	Carrier	NT	NT	147
Calicivirus	Carrier	Yes	NT	148
Ty-VLPs	Carrier or adjuvant	Yes	Yes	18, 149, 150

NT, not tested.
NA, not applicable.

proteins generally exceed yields for multiple protein VLPs because of a limitation of total protein production in cells. Vectors that contain and express multiple gene sequences can increase yields for more complex VLPs [28,29].

II. VLPs AS VACCINES

VLPs provide a vaccine immunogen with an ordered structure and intact conformational epitopes. VLP immunogenicity is dependent on ordered structure because disrupted VLPs or mutant proteins that are able to aggregate, but not self-assemble to form VLPs, are much less or nonimmunogenic [4,13,30,31]. VLPs are typically highly immunogenic and often do not need the coadministration of adjuvants to induce antibody responses but adjuvants may improve immunogenicity and protection [4,11,32–34]. VLPs are immunogenic or protective at doses ranging from 0.1 to 250 µg. Immunogenic or protective doses of VLPs are reported for parenteral or intranasal immunizations with doses from 0.3 to 50 µg [29,32–37] and for oral immunizations 10–200 µg [32,33,37–40].

VLPs are typically effective inducers of neutralizing antibodies. For most pathogens, vaccine-induced protection

against disease is dependent on the presence of neutralizing antibodies at the time of subsequent exposure to the pathogen. However, an advantage of VLPs is that they can also induce T-cell responses, as measured by bulk culture proliferation assays and cytotoxic T-lymphocyte assays, and VLPs can be presented by both class I and II MHC pathways. VLPs induce both cytotoxic and helper T cells, frequently without the addition of adjuvant, and can confer protection from virus challenge. However, more potent induction of cytotoxic T-cell responses may occur when adjuvants or other moieties that activate antigen-presenting cells are included in the vaccine [31,41–48]. While VLPs are strong inducers of immune responses, they may induce different or more limited immune effector responses compared to responses to native virus infection [49,50]. Different VLPs may be processed by antigen presenting cells differently or induce different immune mediators, even if the VLPs are similar in size and structure (papillomavirus versus polyomavirus) [31,51]. The route of VLP administration and adjuvant can also affect the immune response. Papillomavirus VLPs administered parenterally induce vaginal IgG but not IgA, whereas orally administered VLPs induce vaginal IgA [37]. Taken together, these data suggest that although presentation of structure is an important parameter of VLP-induced

Table 2 Summary of Characteristics of Rotavirus and Norwalk virus VLPs as Vaccines

| Experimental system | Immunogenic | | Induce | | Adjuvant | | Protective administered | | | Human trials | Proteins included in VLPs |
	Systemic	Mucosal	Neutralizing antibodies	T cells	Required	Act as	Mucosal	Parenteral	Carrier		
Rotavirus	Yes	Yes	Yes	NT	No	NT	Yes	Yes	NT	No	VP2, VP4, VP6, VP7
Calicivirus (NV)	Yes	Yes	?	Yes	No	No	?	?	NT	Yes	ORF2, ORF3

NT, not tested.
?, currently not able to test.

immune responses, other factors also affect the immune response induced by VLPs.

The remainder of this chapter will focus on use of viruslike particles as vaccines for mucosal diseases, specifically enteric infections caused by Norwalk virus and rotavirus. These systems are being emphasized because these VLPs have undergone extensive preclinical testing and Norwalk virus VLPs are in Phase I clinical trials (Table 2).

III. NORWALK VIRUS AND ROTAVIRUS VLPs

Candidate VLP vaccines are being pursued for two enteric viral pathogens, rotavirus and Norwalk virus (Figure 1).

Both viruses cause acute, local gastrointestinal infections of humans and both are also important pathogens in many animal species. Rotavirus is the leading cause of severe dehydrating and diarrhea-associated deaths (400–600,000) in young children worldwide. Norwalk and related human caliciviruses are the leading viral cause of epidemic food- and water-borne diarrheal and vomiting illness in all age groups. The human caliciviruses are considered "emerging pathogens" because of the rapidly expanding disease burden attributed to infections with these viruses as new tests for diagnosis have become available. The caliciviruses are also considered Class B biodefense pathogens because of their apparent low infectious dose and potential to cause large outbreaks of waterborne, and possibly airborne, disease.

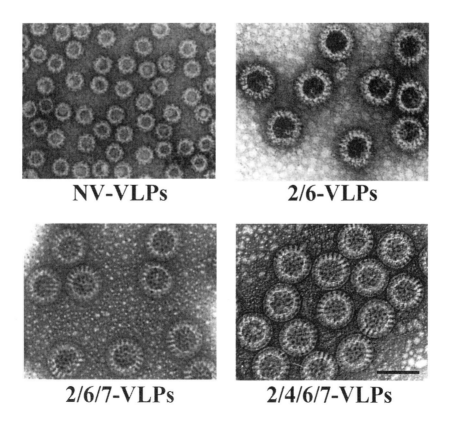

NV-VLPs   **2/6-VLPs**

2/6/7-VLPs   **2/4/6/7-VLPs**

Figure 1 Norwalk virus and rotavirus VLPs produced in Sf9 cells and used for vaccine studies in humans and animals.

Challenges for development of effective vaccines for both rotavirus and Norwalk virus include the need to induce mucosal immune responses to protect from diarrheal disease and the need to target the vaccine to young children, particularly for rotavirus. We review below the progress toward development of Norwalk virus and rotavirus VLP vaccines for use in humans and animals.

A. Norwalk Virus and Norwalk-Like Viruses

Norwalk virus is the prototype virus of the *Norovirus* (NoVs) genus of the genetically diverse, single-stranded RNA viruses belonging to the family *Caliciviridae* [52–54]. In the United States, NoVos cause an estimated 23 million episodes of illness, 50,000 hospitalizations, and 300 deaths each year [55]. NLVs can be transmitted by fecally contaminated food and water and by direct person-to-person contact or through droplets from infected persons [56,57]. Outbreaks are a particular concern in elderly residents of nursing homes [58], military personnel [59], and travelers [60]. The use of new diagnostic assays to detect these genetically diverse pathogens has rapidly determined that these viruses cause significantly more infections than previously recognized and they infect all age groups [61]. The clinical manifestations of NLV infections include sudden onset of vomiting and/or diarrhea after a 24- to 48-hr incubation period that typically lasts 12–24 hr [56,62]. The increasing disease burden and significance of infections in selected settings, combined with the discovery that the expressed capsid protein of Norwalk virus folds spontaneously into VLPs that lack nucleic acid [63] and have desirable properties for use as a subunit vaccine, have stimulated vaccine development [64,67]. Norwalk virus VLPs have been made using baculovirus vectors [63] and a Venezuelan equine encephalitis replicon system [20].

Studies with NV VLPs also serve as an excellent model to dissect and understand effective strategies for mucosal immunization with nonreplicating antigens because of the following useful properties. First, the VLPs are stable at low pH so they can be administered orally. Second, they can be lyophilized and stored at 4 °C in water or phosphate-buffered saline (PBS) for at least 3 years without degradation. Third, the VLPs are easily made by using the baculovirus expression system; yields of more than 22 mg per 9×10^8 cells are obtained in sufficient purity for vaccine evaluation and successful crystallization [65]. Fourth, the unique structure of the single protein that folds to make a VLP, and mutational studies, suggest these particles can be modified to be an antigen-delivery system [65,66]. Finally, rNV VLPs are immunogenic when tested in inbred and outbred mice, and in volunteers following oral administration, even in the absence of a mucosal adjuvant [5,6].

Norwalk virus is a noncultivatable human pathogen, and there are no small animal models available to study pathogenesis or protection from disease. Therefore, the immunogenicity of VLPs has been tested in mice and confirmed in volunteers. Efficacy studies will require reestablishing a human challenge model [6,68]. Preclinical studies in mice administered rNV VLPs have shown that these nonreplicat-

ing vaccines are immunogenic when administered by systemic and mucosal (intranasal and oral) routes [5,40,69]. Immunizations have been given in the presence or absence of a mucosal adjuvant, either cholera toxin or mutant *E. coli* heat-labile toxin LT(R192G), and rNV specific IgG and fecal IgA were evaluated by ELISA. Intranasal delivery of rNV VLPs is more effective than the oral route at inducing serum IgG and intestinal IgA responses to low doses of rNV particles. Vaginal responses of female mice given VLPs by the intranasal and oral routes are also induced. All mice that receive two immunizations with low intranasal doses (10 or 25 μg) of rNV VLPs and the majority of mice that received two high doses orally (200 μg) in the absence of adjuvant produce rNV-specific serum IgG responses, fecal responses, and vaginal responses. These experiments show that low doses of nonreplicating rNV VLPs are immunogenic when administered by the intranasal route, high doses are immunogenic by the oral route in the absence of adjuvant, and these VLPs represent a candidate mucosal vaccine for Norwalk virus infections in humans.

Based on the preclinical responses in mice, Phase I studies have evaluated oral administration of two doses (100 μg and 250 μg) of rNV VLPs without adjuvant to healthy, adult volunteers [6]. The VLPs were safe and immunogenic. Serum IgG responses to the VLPs were dose-dependent, and all vaccinees given 250 μg responded with serum IgG titers. Most of the volunteers responded after the first dose and showed no increase in serum IgG titer after the second dose. However, the maximal titers of serum antibody induced by VLP immunization were lower than titers seen following infection with Norwalk virus. A follow-up Phase I study evaluating escalating doses (250, 500, and 2000 μg) of VLPs administered to volunteers that measured systemic and mucosal (stool, saliva, vaginal, and semen) humoral and cellular immune responses confirmed the vaccines are safe [10]. All vaccinees developed significant rises in IgA antibody secreting cells after vaccination. Ninety percent of vaccinees who received 250 μg developed rises in serum IgG anti-VLP antibody, and neither the rates of seroconversion nor titers increased at the higher doses. About 30–40% of volunteers developed salivary, fecal, or genital fluid IgA antibody and lymphoproliferative responses and interferon-γ production were observed transiently in vaccinees who received the 250 and 500 μg, but not 2000 μg of VLPs [10]. Other studies have shown that mice and volunteers fed potatoes that express NV capsid protein also respond and produce antibodies [70,71]; these studies show proof of concept for edible vaccines for viruses whose capsid proteins can form VLPs (see Chapter 28).

Because rNV VLPs are immunogenic in the absence of adjuvant, experiments have evaluated if rNV VLPs can function as a mucosal adjuvant by evaluating the immune responses to two soluble proteins, keyhole limpet hemocyanin (KLH) and chicken egg albumin (OVA). Under the conditions tested, rNV VLPs did not enhance the serum IgG or fecal IgA response to these soluble proteins when coadministered by the intranasal or oral route [40]. However, because the two test antigens used in these studies have the capability to induce tolerance, further studies should reevaluate adjuvant activity using other antigens.

Overall, studies with rNV VLPs have shown that adult antibody-positive volunteers respond to rNV VLPs in a manner similar to naïve mice. Studies to increase the immunogenicity of VLPs in volunteers using a mucosal adjuvant and to test the efficacy of VLPs against Norwalk virus challenge are planned. If successful, further studies to determine if heterotypic protection against other types of NLVs can be induced with immunization with a single VLP. Mice immunized with a single type of NLV VLP can produce cross-reactive antibodies to other types of NLVs so the potential exists for inducing cross-protection [72].

B. Rotavirus

Rotaviruses cause nearly 50% of diarrheal disease in infants and young children worldwide; 30% of all children develop a rotavirus infection before 9 months of age and 80% within the first 3 years of life [73]. The peak age of disease of children in developing countries is younger than in developed countries and is frequently between 3 and 6 months of age [74–76]. Rotavirus infections cause disease ranging from asymptomatic infections to severe, dehydrating, fatal diarrhea. Rotaviral-related diarrheal deaths are rare in developed countries but in developing countries cause an estimated annual 352,000–592,000 deaths [77,78]. In the United States, rotavirus is a major health concern, causing 55,000 hospitalizations, 500,000 physician visits, and 20–40 deaths, which is estimated to cost more than one billion dollars annually [73,79]. Most children in the world are infected with rotavirus multiple times but, typically, it is the first rotavirus infection that is most severe. For these reasons, the development of a rotavirus vaccine to prevent severe dehydrating diarrhea in young children is a major global health priority.

There are many serotypes of rotavirus that infect children, and multiple serotypes of rotavirus circulate concurrently. Rotaviruses have a dual serotype classification system of P and G types, based on two neutralization antigens, VP4 and VP7, respectively [80]. Rotavirus disease worldwide has been most frequently associated with G1–G4 types [81,82] and targeted in vaccine development. However, unusual serotypes may be rising in prevalence or may be more important than G1–G4 serotypes in specific locales [74–76,83]. There is conflicting information from animal models, natural outbreaks in children, and vaccine studies as to whether protection from rotavirus disease is entirely homotypic or whether heterotypic protection is achievable [84]. Immune correlates of protection for rotavirus have not been clearly defined in children or animals, but intestinal antibodies are thought to be of primary importance in protection [84,85]. Protection from rotavirus infection or disease correlates in some, but not all, studies with neutralizing antibodies or IgA. In the absence of IgA, other factors, possibly local IgG can protect from rotavirus infection [86,87].

1. Rotavirus Animal Models for Vaccine Testing

There are multiple animal models for rotavirus. The advantages and disadvantages of each animal model system have been reviewed and reported elsewhere and will only be briefly summarized here [85,88–90]. Young calves and gnotobiotic piglets are susceptible to rotavirus infection and develop diarrhea up to at least 6 weeks of age. There are three rotavirus small animal models, adult rabbits, mice, and rats [91–94]. Diarrheal disease is severely age-restricted in rabbits, mice, and rats to animals <14 days of age. Therefore, protection from diarrhea is studied in neonatal animals and protection from infection is studied in adult rabbits, mice, and rats [95]. Following primary rotavirus infection, rabbits and mice, but not rats, develop sterilizing immunity and cannot be reinfected with rotavirus [91–93]. Different vaccine formulations and immunization regimens have been tested in mice, rabbits, and piglets; the results from these studies do not always concur, and it is not yet clear which model will accurately predict responses in children.

Traditional vaccine approaches for rotavirus are being actively pursued and have been reviewed elsewhere [85,96]. Live rotavirus vaccines have been licensed for use in children or are in field trials. Live attenuated human and human and animal rotavirus reassortant rotavirus vaccines can protect children from severe rotavirus disease. The safety of live attenuated rotavirus vaccines has been questioned in light of the adverse event (intussusception) associated with RotaShield® vaccine and its subsequent removal from the market [97]. Inactivated rotaviruses, DNA vaccines, and recombinant protein vaccines have also been tested in animal models and exhibit variable efficacy dependent on the immunogen and animal model in which it was tested [85,90,98–101]. Safety concerns about live attenuated vaccines and the availability of the technology to make subunit vaccines have led to the pursuit of subunit vaccination strategies. VLPs have been studied most extensively of any rotavirus subunit approach.

2. Rotavirus VLP Vaccines to Induce Active Immunity

Rotavirus VLPs are made by coinfecting insect cells with baculovirus recombinants that express rotavirus structural proteins; these proteins self-assemble into VLPs that are morphologically and antigenically similar to rotavirus [27,28,32,36,102]. Rotaviruses are composed of three concentric capsid layers but intermediate noninfectious subviral particles are also formed. Expressing VP2 alone produces single-layered VLPs [103]. Coexpression of the rotavirus proteins VP2 and VP6 that form the innermost and middle capsid layers of rotavirus particles, respectively, produces double-layered 2/6-VLPs. Coexpression of VP4 with VP2 and VP6 form double-layered VLPs with VP4 spikes (2/4/6-VLPs) [27]. Coexpression of VP2, VP6, and VP7 produces triple-layered 2/6/7-VLPs. Coexpression of VP2, VP4, VP6, and VP7 results in 2/4/6/7-VLPs that are complete triple-layered VLPs with the VP4 spike protein. Double-layered 6/7-VLPs comprised of the middle and outer capsid proteins can form but are not as homogeneous or stable as 2/6/7-VLPs [35]. Chimeric rotavirus VLPs are readily formed with individual rotavirus proteins from different rotavirus strains or with one protein from two different rotavirus strains on one particle [27]. One advantage of VLP vaccines is the potential ability to easily interchange genes encoding proteins from different P and G serotypes that may allow development of geographic-specific vaccine formulations. Complete and subviral VLPs induce active immunity in adult rabbits, adult mice, and gnotobiotic piglets, and induce passive protection in neonatal mice and calves.

The availability of different formulations of VLPs allowed the pursuit of which proteins provide protection from rotavirus and whether neutralizing antibodies are necessary to induce protection in the various models. Vaccination studies have focused on 2/6-, 2/6/7-, and 2/4/6/7-VLPs, which have been administered parenterally (intramuscularly) or mucosally (orally or intranasally). The following section briefly reviews current data and discusses what has been learned with each formulation of VLPs given by the different routes and in different animal models for both active and passive vaccination strategies. Each vaccine formulation is discussed separately and the results with different formulations and routes of administration are compared.

2/6-VLPs. Double-layered 2/6-VLPs do not contain the rotavirus neutralization antigens (VP4, VP7) and fail to induce neutralizing antibodies in mice or rabbits [32,36]. Therefore, if rotavirus-specific neutralizing antibodies were an absolute requirement for protection, 2/6-VLPs would not provide any protection. However, if efficacious, 2/6-VLPs would be a relatively simple two-component vaccine to make that can be produced in high yields [28] and might induce more cross-protective antibodies to VP6 than VLP formulations with VP4 and VP7. Such 2/6-VLPs have been administered to rabbits, mice, and pigs intranasally, orally, or intramuscularly and protection against infection (rabbits, mice) or diarrheal disease (pigs) assessed. The results with 2/6-VLPs vary depending on the animal model in which they were tested and the route of administration.

2/6-VLPs are immunogenic in mice [28,32,104,105], rabbits [36], and piglets [106–108] by all routes tested, with the exception of intranasal administration in rabbits [28]. The immunogenicity and protection of 2/6-VLPs are enhanced for all routes of administration tested by inclusion of adjuvants. Protective efficacy of 2/6-VLPs varies by animal model. In mice, 2/6-VLP immunization provides at least partial protection from infection by all routes and intranasal immunization provides high levels of protection. In rabbits, 2/6-VLPs administered intramuscularly or intranasally are not protective or are generally less efficacious than other VLP formulations (see below). In piglets, 2/6-VLPs are not protective alone either intranasally or orally even with multiple doses, but they provide moderate protective efficacy against diarrhea and virus shedding as part of prime-boost immunization protocol with live attenuated rotavirus. Immunization of mice and rabbits with 2/6-VLPs results in widely variable protection in individual animals within groups. For example, the mean levels of protection induced by 2/6-VLPs administered intramuscularly in rabbits are low (5–41%) but individual rabbits are highly protected (up to 94%). Overall, immunization with 2/6-VLPs appears to be a promising vaccine candidate for use in a prime-boost strategy with other vaccine formulations or for strategies to induce passive immunity (see below). However, the utility

of 2/6 VLPs alone as an immunogen for active immunity remains unresolved.

2/6/7-VLPs. Triple-layered 2/6/7-VLPs that contain VP7, one of the rotavirus neutralization antigens, have been tested to determine if the presence of VP7 increases the protective efficacy of VLPs. If protection is dependent on neutralizing antibody independently induced by VP4 and VP7, then the inclusion of VP7 would be protective. Compared to 2/6-VLPs, 2/6/7-VLPs would be the next least complex VLP formulation to produce commercially. 2/6/7-VLPs have been tested in mice by all three routes and in rabbits by intramuscular administration.

In mice, intranasal administration of 2/6/7-VLPs induces 100% protection from a low-challenge dose in mice and is superior to orally administered 2/6/7-VLPs [32]. 2/6/7-VLPs provide low (5%) to partial (53%) protection when administered orally at 25- or 100-μg doses, respectively [32]. Parenteral administration of 2/6/7-VLPs induces high levels of both homotypic and heterotypic protection when administered with QS-21, but not aluminum phosphate [109]. Double-layered 6/7-VLPs are similarly immunogenic to triple-layered 2/6/7-VLPs when administered intramuscularly to mice but 6/7-VLPs are less stable than 2/6/7-VLPs [35]. In rabbits, two 50-μg doses of 2/6/7-VLPs administered intramuscularly provide low (28%) to moderate (58%) mean protection but individual rabbits were highly protected [36]. 2/6/7-VLPs can induce higher levels of protection. However, the protective efficacy of 2/6/7-VLPs is not significantly different than 2/6-VLPs administered either intranasally or orally in mice, or intramuscularly in rabbits, indicating that in mice and rabbits with the regimens tested, inclusion of VP7 in VLPs does not increase protective efficacy against infection. Whether inclusion of VP7 in VLPs is important in protection against disease (diarrhea) remains to be determined.

2/4/6/7-VLPs. Native rotavirus virions are composed of triple capsid layers with the spike protein. Triple-layered 2/4/6/7-VLPs that contain both the neutralization antigens VP7 and VP4 have been tested to determine if VLPs, similar to complete rotavirus virions would increase the protective efficacy of VLPs. 2/4/6/7-VLPs contain both neutralization antigens (VP4 and VP7) and are capable of binding to cells via VP4, the viral attachment protein [27]. 2/4/6/7-VLPs have been tested in mice by all three routes and in rabbits by intramuscular administration.

Parenteral administration of 2/4/6/7-VLPs or inactivated SA11 rotavirus to rabbits with QS-21 induces higher levels (84–100%) of protection than either 2/6- or 2/6/7-VLPs (5–58% protection) [36]. In addition, serotype G1 and G3 2/4/6/7-VLPs induce both heterotypic and homotypic protection from rotavirus infection. Protection of rabbits by VLPs correlates moderately with the inclusion of VP4, indicating that VP4 enhances, but is not absolutely required to induce protection. Mice parenterally administered G1 2/4/6/7-VLPs develop both homotypic and heterotypic (G3) immunity but the protective efficacy in mice has not been evaluated [102]. Mice immunized orally or intranasally with 2/4/6/7-VLPs develop moderate levels of protection against a high challenge dose (Warfield, Estes, and Conner, unpublished data). 2/4/6/7-VLPs can be highly protective against infection in both mice and rabbits, supporting the need to test whether the VLPs will stimulate high levels of protection against rotavirus diarrhea.

3. Rotavirus VLP Vaccines to Induce Passive Immunity

VLPs have been investigated to induce passive immunity for veterinary use. Induction of passive immunity by vaccination of dams is an important strategy to protect young farm animals during the first few weeks of life when they are most vulnerable to mortality from rotavirus disease. This model has also been used in mice to test what antibodies are essential to protect pups against rotavirus-induced diarrhea in the neonatal period. A similar strategy may also prove efficacious to protect young infants in developing countries where rotavirus infection and disease occur early in life.

VLP vaccination of dams serves to boost preexisting rotavirus-specific antibody titers in the dams shortly before parturition to increase the titers of rotavirus-specific antibody in the colostrum and milk ingested by the young animal. This vaccination strategy has proven effective with live or inactivated rotavirus vaccines in cows [110,111]. Intramuscular immunization, followed by booster intramammary injections of 2/4/6/7-VLPs or 2/6-VLPs with adjuvant to pregnant cows, significantly increases rotavirus-specific antibody titers in milk and colostrum compared to control cows [112]. Calves fed this colostrum and challenged with rotavirus are protected from diarrhea and virus shedding [113]. 2/4/6/7-VLPs are somewhat superior to 2/6-VLP vaccines.

Passive immunization studies performed in the mouse model have shown that intranasal immunization of mice with 2/6- or 2/6/7-VLPs (VP7 G6), with or without adjuvant, induces serum and lactogenic antibodies in the mouse dams [114]. Protection from rotavirus diarrhea was observed in a high percentage of pups whose mothers were immunized with 2/6/7-VLPs (73%) but not 2/6-VLPs (29%). Unexpectedly, heterotypic protection from challenge by a rotavirus serotype different from the VLP serotype was not observed. The protection against diarrhea induced by 2/6-VLP immunization of cows, but not mice, is likely because naïve seronegative mice were vaccinated with 2/6-VLPs, whereas cows vaccinated with 2/6-VLPs had preexisting antibodies to rotavirus acquired from natural infections. Thus, although both 2/4/6/7- and 2/6-VLPs could readily induce antibodies in either situation, only 2/6/7-VLPs would induce neutralizing antibodies in the naïve animal. These results suggest that neutralizing antibodies are required to provide protection from diarrhea.

A maternal vaccination approach for humans either alone or in combination with an active vaccination program in children may be useful and highly effective in developing countries where primary rotavirus infections occur earlier and breast-feeding is practiced widely. Maternal vaccination of pregnant women might provide longer-lasting protection from severe diarrhea and reduce mortality in young children. Vaccination of pregnant women would require safe non-replicating vaccines. VLPs seem to be an ideal candidate for such an approach. VLPs boost preexisting antibody responses in pigs and induce protective levels of lactogenic immunity in cows and mice [90,112–114], so it is expected they will boost responses in antibody-positive women as well.

4. Rotavirus VLP Summary

All the preclinical data with rotavirus VLPs support the testing of rotavirus VLPs in humans. Rotavirus VLPs alone are immunogenic and at least partially protective by all routes tested. Coadministration of adjuvants increases immunogenicity, lowers the protective dose of VLPs and may enhance the longevity of the protective immune response. Mucosal administration of rotavirus VLPs to humans provides many advantages, including ease of delivery, elimination of the need for needles, and cost especially in the developing world where vaccines are most urgently needed but where health-care funding is limited. Intranasal delivery of VLPs is a very effective route of administration to induce rotavirus-specific antibody in the intestine in two of the three animal models in which it has been tested. Comparisons of doses between oral and intranasal routes of immunization indicate that intranasal delivery of VLPs induces higher levels of protection and requires up to 10-fold lower doses of VLPs than needed to achieve low to moderate protection when VLPs are administered orally. Intranasal administration of VLPs may be superior to oral administration because of limited degradation in respiratory compared to intestinal tract, increased retention of and interaction of VLPs with M cells or lymphocytes, and differences in antigen uptake or processing. However, it is not clear whether intranasal administration of vaccines and adjuvants will be approved soon for use in humans because of possible introduction of any potential pathogen or toxin into the brain via the olfactory bulb [115–117]. Further work is needed to determine if this highly promising vaccination route will be safe for use in humans. Studies are under way to understand the differences in immunogenicity and protective efficacy induced by the two mucosal routes and to determine if modifications to the vaccine protocol or VLPs themselves can reduce the variability in protection and enhance the immunogenicity and protective efficacy of orally administered VLPs. Additional studies of parenteral administration of VLPs to induce mucosal protection are also warranted. Studies in human subjects, which are long overdue, may help to delineate some of these factors and define which animal model(s) are most predictive of responses in children or pregnant women, the target populations for rotavirus VLP vaccines.

IV. CONCLUSIONS

VLPs are a promising candidate for parenterally and mucosally administered subunit vaccines to prevent diarrheal diseases. Rotavirus VLPs have been extensively tested in animal models and await testing in humans. Norwalk VLPs are immunogenic in both animals and humans but protective efficacy needs to be tested in humans when a human challenge model can be reestablished. VLP vaccines for sexually transmitted infections caused by papillomavirus are also being actively pursued and are currently in preclinical through Phase II clinical trials (see Chapter 85) [33]. When studies with VLPs or other subunit vaccines were first envisioned, one of the theoretical problems raised was the expectation that ingested nonreplicating immunogens would result in tolerance to the immunogen, not protective immune responses. In fact, oral administration of VLPs or other immunogens may ultimately prove useful to specifically downregulate autoimmune responses [118]. However, data with VLPs applied orally or ingested in plant material as edible vaccines (see Chapter 28) indicate that particulate VLP vaccines administered orally are immunogenic and they can induce protection. Oral administration is a promising vaccination route, if we can overcome some limitations, including relatively high doses required and for rotavirus the need for nontoxic mucosal adjuvants. It has been proposed that live virus vaccines work more effectively than subunit vaccines because live virus stimulates more components of the immune system than subunit vaccines [49,50,119,120]. Further work is needed to understand the differences in immunity and protection induced by VLPs and live virus infections and to determine if VLP-induced protection can be enhanced to levels obtained by live virus vaccines. These challenges should be met by inclusion of efficacious and safe adjuvants, or directed engineering or targeting of VLPs without induction of potential safety concerns associated with the same live virus vaccines.

ACKNOWLEDGMENTS

The authors are grateful to our students, postdoctoral fellows, and colleagues who have worked with us to demonstrate the effectiveness of VLPs as immunogens and to understand their mechanisms of inducing immunity.

Supported by Applied Technology program grants 04949-033 and 004949-055 from the Texas Higher Education Coordinating Board, National Institutes of Health training grants T32-DK07664, General Clinical Research Center grants M01 RR00188, N01 A165229, DK56338, and R01 A124998, and Office of Medical Research Service Department of Veterans Affairs.

REFERENCES

1. Ulrich R, et al. Chimaera and its modern virus-like descendants. Intervirology 1996; 39(1–2):126–132.
2. Kruger DH, et al. Chimeric virus-like particles as vaccines. Biol Chem 1999; 380(3):275–276.
3. Bavari S, et al. Lipid raft microdomains: a gateway for compartmentalized trafficking of Ebola and Marburg viruses. J Exp Med 2002; 195(5):593–602.
4. Schiller J, Lowy D. Papillomavirus-like particle vaccines. J Natl Cancer Inst Monogr 2001; 28:50–54.
5. Ball JM, et al. Oral immunization with recombinant Norwalk virus-like particles induces a systemic and mucosal immune response in mice. J Virol 1998; 72:1345–1353.
6. Ball JM, et al. Recombinant Norwalk virus-like particles given orally to volunteers: phase I study. Gastroenterology 1999; 117(1):40–48.
7. Studentsov YY, et al. Enhanced enzyme-linked immunosorbent assay for detection of antibodies to virus-like particles of human papillomavirus. J Clin Microbiol 2002; 40(5):1755–1760.
8. Bousarghin L, et al. Detection of neutralizing antibodies against human papillomaviruses (HPV) by inhibition of gene transfer mediated by HPV pseudovirions. J Clin Microbiol 2002; 40(3):926–932.
9. Li TC, et al. Empty virus-like particle-based enzyme-linked immunosorbent assay for antibodies to hepatitis E virus. J Med Virol 2000; 62(3):327–333.
10. Tacket CO, et al. Humoral, mucosal, and cellular immune responses to oral Norwalk virus-like particles (VLPs) in volunteers. Clin Immunol 2003. In press.
11. Zhang LF, et al. HPV6b virus like particles are potent immunogens without adjuvant in man. Vaccine 2000; 18(11–12):1051–1058.
12. Evans TG, et al. A Phase 1 study of a recombinant viruslike particle vaccine against human papillomavirus type 11 in healthy adult volunteers. J Infect Dis 2001; 183(10):1485–1493.
13. Schiller JT, Hidesheim A. Developing HPV virus-like particle vaccines to prevent cervical cancer: a progress report. J Clin Virol 2000; 19(1–2):67–74.
14. Roy P. Genetically engineered particulate virus-like structures and their use as vaccine delivery systems. Intervirology 1996; 39(1–2):62–71.
15. O'Brien GJ, et al. Rotavirus VP6 expressed by PVX vectors in Nicotiana benthamiana coats PVX rods and also assembles into viruslike particles. Virology 2000; 270(2):444–453.
16. Bouamr F, et al. Differential budding efficiencies of human T-cell leukemia virus type I (HTLV-I) Gag and Gag-Pro polyproteins from insect and mammalian cells. Virology 2000; 278(2):597–609.
17. Buonaguro L, et al. High efficient production of Pr55(gag) virus-like particles expressing multiple HIV-1 epitopes, including a gp120 protein derived from an Ugandan HIV-1 isolate of A subtype. Antiviral Res 2001; 49(1):35–47.
18. Weber J, et al. Immunogenicity of the yeast recombinant p17/p24:Ty virus-like particles (p24-VLP) in healthy volunteers. Vaccine 1995; 13(9):831–834.
19. Chen XS, et al. Papillomavirus capsid protein expression in Escherichia coli: purification and assembly of HPV11 and HPV16 L1. J Mol Biol 2001; 307(1):173–182.
20. Harrington PR, et al. Systemic, mucosal, and heterotypic immune induction in mice inoculated with Venezuelan equine encephalitis replicons expressing Norwalk virus-like particles. J Virol 2002; 76(2):730–742.
21. Lorenzo LJ, et al. Assembly of truncated HCV core antigen into virus-like particles in Escherichia coli. Biochem Biophys Res Commun 2001; 281(4):962–965.
22. Sasnauskas K, et al. Yeast cells allow high-level expression and formation of polyomavirus-like particles. Biol Chem 1999; 380(3):381–386.
23. Gleiter S, Lilie H. Coupling of antibodies via protein Z on modified polyoma virus-like particles. Protein Sci 2001; 10(2):434–444.
24. Tacket CO, et al. Human immune responses to a novel Norwalk virus vaccine delivered in transgenic potatoes. J Infect Dis 2000; 182:302–305.
25. Sutton DW, et al. Synthetic cryIIIA gene from Bacillus thuringiensis improved for high expression in plants. Transgenic Res 1992; 1(5):228–236.
26. Wagner R, et al. Safety and immunogenicity of recombinant human immunodeficiency virus-like particles in rodents and rhesus macaques. Intervirology 1996; 39(1–2):93–103.

27. Crawford SE, et al. Characterization of virus-like particles produced by the expression of rotavirus capsid proteins in insect cells. J Virol 1994; 68(9):5945–5952.

28. Bertolotti-Ciarlet A, et al. Comparison of immunogenicity and protective efficacy of rotavirus 2/6-virus-like particles (VLPs) produced in a dual expression baculovirus vector, administered intramuscularly, intranasally or orally to mice. Vaccine 2003; 21:3885–3900.

29. Pearson LD, Roy P. Genetically engineered multi-component virus-like particles as veterinary vaccines. Immunol Cell Biol 1993; 71(Pt 5):381–389.

30. Slupetzky K, et al. Chimeric papillomavirus-like particles expressing a foreign epitope on capsid surface loops. J Gen Virol 2001; 82(Pt 11):2799–2804.

31. Lenz P, et al. Papillomavirus-like particles induce acute activation of dendritic cells. J Immunol 2001; 166(9):5346–5355.

32. O'Neal CM, et al. Rotavirus virus-particles administered mucosally induce protective immunity. J Virol 1997; 71(11):8707–8717.

33. Koutsky LA, et al. A controlled trial of a human papillomavirus Type 16 vaccine. NEJM 2002; 347:1645–1651.

34. Breitburd F, Coursaget P. Human papillomavirus vaccines. Semin Cancer Biol 1999; 9(6):431–444.

35. Madore HP, et al. Biochemical and immunologic comparison of virus-like particles for a rotavirus subunit vaccine. Vaccine 1999; 17:2461–2471.

36. Ciarlet M, et al. Subunit rotavirus vaccine administered parenterally to rabbits induces protective immunity. J Virol 1998; 72:9233–9246.

37. Gerber S, et al. Human papillomavirus virus-like particles are efficient oral immunogens when coadministered with Escherichia coli heat-labile enterotoxin mutant R192G or CpG DNA. J Virol 2001; 75(10):4752–4760.

38. Li T, et al. Oral administration of hepatitis E virus-like particles induces a systemic and mucosal immune response in mice. Vaccine 2001; 19(25–26):3476–3484.

39. Niikura M, et al. Chimeric recombinant hepatitis E virus-like particles as an oral vaccine vehicle presenting foreign epitopes. Virology 2002; 293(2):273–280.

40. Guerrero RA, et al. Recombinant Norwalk virus-like particles administered intranasally to mice induce systemic and mucosal (fecal and vaginal) immune responses. J Virol 2001; 75(20):9713–9722.

41. Lo-Man R, et al. A recombinant virus-like particle system derived from parvovirus as an efficient antigen carrier to elicit a polarized Th1 immune response without adjuvant. Eur J Immunol 1998; 28(4):1401–1407.

42. Paliard X, et al. Priming of strong, broad, and long-lived HIV type 1 p55gag-specific CD8+ cytotoxic T cells after administration of a virus-like particle vaccine in rhesus macaques. AIDS Res Hum Retroviruses 2000; 16(3):273–282.

43. Liu WJ, et al. Papillomavirus virus-like particles for the delivery of multiple cytotoxic T cell epitopes. Virology 2000; 273(2):374–382.

44. Peng S, et al. Papillomavirus virus-like particles can deliver defined CTL epitopes to the MHC class I pathway. Virology 1998; 240(1):147–157.

45. Sedlik C, et al. Recombinant parvovirus-like particles as an antigen carrier: a novel nonreplicative exogenous antigen to elicit protective antiviral cytotoxic T cells. Proc Natl Acad Sci U S A 1997; 94(14):7503–7508.

46. Sedlik C, et al. In vivo induction of a high-avidity, high-frequency cytotoxic T-lymphocyte response is associated with antiviral protective immunity. J Virol 2000; 74(13):5769–5775.

47. Storni T, et al. Critical role for activation of antigen-presenting cells in priming of cytotoxic T cell responses after

vaccination with virus-like particles. J Immunol 2002; 168(6):2880–2886.

48. Moron G, et al. CD8alpha− CD11b+ dendritic cells present exogenous virus-like particles to CD8+ T cells and subsequently express CD8alpha and CD205 molecules. J Exp Med 2002; 195(10):1233–1245.

49. Szomolanyi-Tsuda E, et al. T-cell-independent immunoglobulin G responses in vivo are elicited by live-virus infection but not by immunization with viral proteins or virus-like particles. J Virol 1998; 72(8):6665–6670.

50. Szomolanyi-Tsuda E, Welsh RM. T-cell-independent antiviral antibody responses. Curr Opin Immunol 1998; 10(4):431–435.

51. Charpilienne A, et al. Individual rotavirus-like particles containing 120 molecules of fluorescent protein are visible in living cells. J Biol Chem 2001; 276(31):29361–29367.

52. Jiang X, et al. Norwalk virus genome: cloning and characterization. Science 1990; 250:1580–1583.

53. Green KY, et al. Caliciviridae. In: van Regenmortel M, Fauquet CM, Bishop DHL, Carsten E, Estes MK, Lemon SM, et al., eds. Virus Taxonomy: 7th Report of the International Committee on Taxonomy of Viruses. Orlando, FL: Academic Press, 2000:725–735.

54. Lopman BA, et al. Human caliciviruses in Europe. J Clin Virol 2002; 24:137–160.

55. Mead PS, et al. Food-related illness and death in the United States. Emerg Infect Dis 1999; 5(5):607–625.

56. Green KY, et al. Human caliciviruses. In: Knipe DM, Howley PM, eds. Fields Virology. Philadephia: Lippincott Williams & Wilkins, 2001:841–874.

57. Harrington PR, et al. Binding of Norwalk virus-like particles to ABH histo-blood group antigens is blocked by antisera from infected human volunteers or experimentally vaccinated mice. J Virol 2002; 76:12335–12343.

58. Green KY, et al. A predominant role for Norwalk-like viruses as agents of epidemic gastroenteritis in Maryland nursing homes for the elderly. J Infect Dis 2002; 185(2):133–146.

59. McCarthy M, et al. Norwalk-like virus infection in military forces: epidemic potential, sporadic disease, and the future direction of prevention and control efforts. J Infect Dis 2000; 181(suppl 2):S387–S391.

60. Brown CM, et al. Outbreak of Norwalk virus in a Caribbean island resort: application of molecular diagnostics to ascertain the vehicle of infection. Epidemiol Infect 2001; 126(3):425–432.

61. Atmar RL, Estes MK. Diagnosis of noncultivatable gastroenteritis viruses, the human caliciviruses. Clin Microbiol Rev 2001; 14:15–37.

62. Graham DY, et al. Norwalk virus infection of volunteers: new insights based on improved assays. J Infect Dis 1994; 170: 14:34–43.

63. Jiang X, et al. Expression, self-assembly, and antigenicity of the Norwalk virus capsid protein. J Virol 1992; 66:6527–6532.

64. Estes MK, et al. Norwalk virus vaccines: challenges and progress. J Infect Dis 2000; 181(S2):S367–S373.

65. Prasad BVV, et al. X-ray crystallographic structure of the Norwalk virus capsid. Science 1999; 286(5438):287–290.

66. Bertolotti-Ciarlet A, et al. Structural requirements for the assembly of Norwalk virus-like particles. J Virol 2002; 76(8):4044–4055.

67. Periwal SB, et al. A modified cholera holotoxin CT-E29H enhances systemic and mucosal immune responses to recombinant Norwalk virus–virus-like particle vaccine. Vaccine 2003; 21:376–385.

68. Graham DY, et al. Norwalk virus infection of volunteers: new insights based on improved assays. J Infect Dis 1994; 170(1):34–43.

69. Harrington PR, et al. Systemic, mucosal, and heterotypic immune induction in mice inoculated with Venezuelan equine encephalitis replicons expressing Norwalk virus-like particles. J Virol 2002; 76(2):730–742.

70. Mason HS, et al. Expression of Norwalk virus capsid protein in transgenic tobacco and potato and its oral immunogenicity in mice. Proc Natl Acad Sci U S A 1996; 93(11):5335–5340.

71. Tacket CO, et al. Human immune responses to a novel Norwalk virus vaccine delivered in transgenic potatoes. J Infect Dis 2000; 182(1):302–305.

72. Kitamoto N, et al. Cross-reactivity among several recombinant calicivirus virus-like particles (VLPs) with monoclonal antibodies obtained from mice immunized orally with one type of VLP. J Clin Microbiol 2002; 40(7):2459–2465.

73. Tucker AW, et al. Cost-effectiveness analysis of a rotavirus immunization program for the United States. JAMA 1998; 279(17):1371–1376.

74. Kilgore PE, et al. Neonatal rotavirus infection in Bangladesh: strain characterization and risk factors for nosocomial infection. Pediatr Infect Dis J 1996; 15(8):672–677.

75. Cunliffe NA, et al. Epidemiology of rotavirus diarrhoea in Africa: a review to assess the need for rotavirus immunization. Bull World Health Organ 1998; 76(5):525–537.

76. Jain V, et al. Epidemiology of rotavirus in India. Indian J Pediatr 2001; 68(9):855–862.

77. Parashar UD, et al. Global illness and deaths caused by rotavirus disease in children. Emerg Infect Dis 2003; 95:565–572.

78. Institute of Medicine. The prospectives for immunizing against rotavirus. New Vaccine Development: Establishing Priorities, Diseases of Importance in Developing Countries. Vol. II. Washington, DC: National Academy Press, 1986: 308–318.

79. Glass RI, et al. The epidemiology of rotavirus diarrhea in the United States: surveillance and estimates of disease burden. J Infect Dis 1996; 174(suppl 1):S5–S11.

80. Estes MK. Rotaviruses and their replication. In: Fields BN, Knipe DM, Howley PM, eds. Field's Virology. Philadelphia: Lippincott-Raven Publishers, 1997:1625–1655.

81. Kapikian AZ, et al. Jennerian and modified Jennerian approach to vaccination against rotavirus diarrhea using a quadrivalent rhesus rotavirus (RRV) and human-RRV reassortant vaccine. Arch Virol 1996; 6(suppl 12):163–175.

82. Midthun K, Kapikian AZ. Rotavirus vaccines: an overview. Clin Microbiol Rev 1996; 9(3):423–434.

83. Cunliffe NA, et al. The expanding diversity of rotaviruses. Lancet 2002; 359(9307):640–642.

84. Jiang B, et al. The role of serum antibodies in the protection against rotavirus disease: an overview. Clin Infect Dis 2002; 34(10):1351–1361.

85. Conner ME, et al. Development of a mucosal rotavirus vaccine. In: Kiyono H, Ogra PL, McGhee JR, eds. Mucosal Vaccines. San Diego, CA: Academic Press, 1996:325–344.

86. Conner ME, et al. Rotavirus vaccine administered parenterally induces protective immunity. J Virol 1993; 67(11): 6633–6641.

87. O'Neal CM, et al. Protection of the villus epithelial cells of the small intestine from rotavirus infection does not require immunoglobulin A. J Virol 2000; 74:4102–4109.

88. Ciarlet M, Conner ME. Evaluation of rotavirus vaccines in small animal models. In: Gray J, Desselberger U, eds. Rotaviruses: Methods and Protocols. Totowa, NJ: Humana Press, 2000:147–187.

89. Greenberg HB, et al. Rotavirus pathology and pathophysiology. Curr Top Microbiol Immunol 1994; 185:255–283.

90. Yuan L, Saif LJ. Induction of mucosal immune responses and protection against enteric viruses: rotavirus infection of gnotobiotic pigs as a model. Vet Immunol Immunopathol 2002; 87(3–4):147–160.

91. Conner ME, et al. Rabbit model of rotavirus infection. J Virol 1988; 62:1625–1633.

92. Ward RL, et al. Development of an adult mouse model for studies on protection against rotavirus. J Virol 1990; 64: 5070–5075.

93. Ciarlet M, et al. Group A rotavirus infection and age-dependent diarrheal disease in rats: a new animal model to study the pathophysiology of rotavirus infection. J Virol 2002; 76(1):41–57.

94. Guerin-Danan C, et al. Development of a heterologous model in germfree suckling rats for studies of rotavirus diarrhea. J Virol 1998; 72(11):9298–9302.

95. Conner ME, Ramig RF. Viral enteric diseases. In: Nathanson N, Ahmed R, Gonzalez-Scarano F, Griffin DE, Holmes KV, Murphy FA, eds. Viral Pathogenesis. Philadelphia: Lippincott-Raven Publishers, 1997:713–743.

96. Offit PA. The rotavirus vaccine. J Clin Virol 1998; 11(3): 155–159.

97. Withdrawal of rotavirus vaccine recommendation. MMWR Morb Mortal Wkly Rep 1999; 48(43):1007.

98. Coffin SE, et al. Immunologic correlates of protection against rotavirus challenge after intramuscular immunization of mice. J Virol 1997; 71(10):7851–7856.

99. McNeal MM, et al. Stimulation of local immunity and protection in mice by intramuscular immunization with triple- or double-layered rotavirus particles and QS-21. Virology 1998; 243:158–166.

100. Herrmann JE, et al. Immune responses and protection obtained by oral immunization with rotavirus VP4 and VP7 DNA vaccines encapsulated in microparticles. Virology 1999; 259(1):148–153.

101. Choi AH, et al. Antibody-independent protection against rotavirus infection of mice stimulated by intranasal immunization with chimeric VP4 or VP6 protein. J Virol 1999; 73(9):7574–7581.

102. Crawford SE, et al. Heterotypic protection and induction of a broad heterotypic neutralization response by rotavirus-like particles. J Virol 1999; 73(6):4813–4822.

103. Labbe M, et al. Expression of rotavirus VP2 produces empty corelike particles. J Virol 1991; 65:2946–2952.

104. O'Neal CM, et al. Rotavirus 2/6 viruslike particles administered intranasally with cholera toxin, Escherichia coli heat-labile toxin (LT), and LT-R192G induce protection from rotavirus challenge. J Virol 1998; 72(4):3390–3393.

105. Siadat-Pajouh M, Cai L. Protective efficacy of rotavirus 2/6-virus-like particles combined with CT-E29H, a detoxified cholera toxin adjuvant. Viral Immunol 2001; 14(1):31–47.

106. Yuan L, et al. Intranasal administration of 2/6-rotavirus-like particles with mutant Escherichia coli heat-labile toxin (LT-R192G) induces antibody-secreting cell responses but not protective immunity in gnotobiotic pigs. J Virol 2000; 74(19):8843–8853.

107. Yuan L, et al. Protective immunity and antibody-secreting cell responses elicited by combined oral attenuated Wa human rotavirus and intranasal Wa 2/6-VLPs with mutant Escherichia coli heat-labile toxin in gnotobiotic pigs. J Virol 2001; 75(19):9229–9238.

108. Iosef C, et al. Systemic and intestinal antibody secreting cell responses and protection in gnotobiotic pigs immunized orally with attenuated Wa human rotavirus and Wa 2/6-rotavirus-like-particles associated with immunostimulating complexes. Vaccine 2002; 20(13–14):1741–1753.

109. Jiang B, et al. Heterotypic protection against rotavirus infection in mice vaccinated with virus-like particles. Vaccine 1999; 17:1005–1013.

110. Saif LJ, et al. Passive immunity to bovine rotavirus in newborn calves fed colostrum supplements from immunized or nonimmunized cows. Infect Immun 1983; 41:1118–1131.

111. Saif LJ, et al. Immune response of pregnant cows to bovine rotavirus immunization. Am J Vet Res 1984; 45:49–58.

112. Fernandez FM, et al. Isotype-specific antibody responses to rotavirus and virus proteins in cows inoculated with subunit vaccines composed of recombinant SA11 rotavirus core-like particles (CLP) or virus-like particles (VLP). Vaccine 1996; 14(14):1303–1312.

113. Fernández FM, et al. Passive immunity to bovine rotavirus in newborn calves fed colostrum supplements from cows immunized with recombinant SA11 rotavirus core-like particle (CLP) or virus-like particle (VLP) vaccines. Vaccine 1998; 16(5):507–516.

114. Coste A, et al. Nasal immunization of mice with virus-like particles protects offspring against rotavirus diarrhea. J Virol 2000; 74(19):8966–8971.

115. Fujihashi K, et al. A dilemma for mucosal vaccination: efficacy versus toxicity using enterotoxin-based adjuvants. Vaccine 2002; 20(19–20):2431–2438.

116. van Ginkel FW, et al. Cutting edge: the mucosal adjuvant cholera toxin redirects vaccine proteins into olfactory tissues. J Immunol 2000; 165(9):4778–4782.

117. Safety evaluation of toxin adjuvants delivered intranasally. http://www.niaid.nih.gov/dmid/enteric/intranasal.htm. Accessed July 9, 2001.

118. Chackerian B, et al. Conjugation of a self-antigen to papillomavirus-like particles allows for efficient induction of protective autoantibodies. J Clin Invest 2001; 108(3):415–423.

119. Zinkernagel RM, et al. Antigen localisation regulates immune responses in a dose- and time-dependent fashion: a geographical view of immune reactivity. Immunol Rev 1997; 156:199–209.

120. Zinkernagel RM, et al. On immunological memory. Annu Rev Immunol 1996; 14:333–367.

121. Kim Y, et al. Lactogenic antibody responses in cows vaccinated with recombinant bovine rotavirus-like particles (VLPs) of two serotypes or inactivated bovine rotavirus vaccines. Vaccine 2002; 20(7–8):1248–1258.

122. Fromantin C, et al. Rotavirus 2/6 virus-like particles administered intranasally in mice, with or without the mucosal adjuvants cholera toxin and *Escherichia coli* heat-labile toxin, induce a Th1/Th2-like immune response. J Virol 2001; 75(22):11010–11016.

123. Plana-Duran J, et al. Oral immunization of rabbits with VP60 particles confers protection against rabbit hemorrhagic disease. Arch Virol 1996; 141(8):1423–1436.

124. Nagesha HS, et al. Neutralizing monoclonal antibodies against three serotypes of porcine rotavirus. J Virol 1989; 63:3545–3549.

125. Montefiori DC, et al. Induction of neutralizing antibodies and gag-specific cellular immune responses to an R5 primary isolate of human immunodeficiency virus type 1 in rhesus macaques. J Virol 2001; 75(13):5879–5890.

126. Luo L, et al. Induction of V3-specific cytotoxic T lymphocyte responses by HIV *gag* particles carrying multiple immunodominant V3 epitopes of gp120. Virology 1998; 240:316–325.

127. Watanabe T, et al. Immunogenicity and protective efficacy of replication-incompetent influenza virus-like particles. J Virol 2002; 76(2):767–773.

128. Latham T, Galarza JM. Formation of wild-type and chimeric influenza virus-like particles following simultaneous expression of only four structural proteins. J Virol 2001; 75(13):6154–6165.

129. Gomez-Puertas P, et al. Efficient formation of influenza virus-like particles: dependence on the expression levels of viral proteins. J Gen Virol 1999; 80(Pt 7):1635–1645.

130. Li TC, et al. Expression and self-assembly of empty virus-like particles of hepatitis E virus. J Virol 1997; 71(10):7207–7213.

131. Acosta-Rivero N, et al. Characterization of the HCV core virus-like particles produced in the methylotrophic yeast *Pichia pastoris*. Biochem Biophys Res Commun 2001; 287(1):122–125.

132. Noda T, Sagara H, Suzuki E, Takada A, Kida H, Kawaoka Y. Ebola virus VP40 drives the formation of virus-like filamentous particles along with GP. J Virol 2002; 76(10): 4855–4865.

133. Balmelli C, et al. Nasal immunization of mice with human papillomavirus type 16 virus-like particles elicits neutralizing antibodies in mucosal secretions. J Virol 1998; 72(10): 8220–8229.

134. Liu XS, et al. Route of administration of chimeric BPV1 VLP determines the character of the induced immune responses. Immunol Cell Biol 2002; 80(1):21–29.

135. Sedlik C, et al. Intranasal delivery of recombinant parvovirus-like particles elicits cytotoxic T-cell and neutralizing antibody responses. J Virol 1999; 73(4):2739–2744.

136. Maranga L, et al. Large scale production and downstream processing of a recombinant porcine parvovirus vaccine. Appl Microbiol Biotechnol 2002; 59(1):45–50.

137. Rueda P, et al. Minor replacements in the insertion site provoke major differences in the induction of antibody responses by chimeric parvovirus-like particles. Virology 1999; 263(1):89–99.

138. Touze A, et al. Gene transfer using human polyomavirus BK virus-like particles expressed in insect cells. J Gen Virol 2001; 82(Pt 12):3005–3009.

139. Clark B, et al. Immunity against both polyomavirus VP1 and a transgene product induced following intranasal delivery of VP1 pseudocapsid–DNA complexes. J Gen Virol 2001; 82(Pt 11):2791–2797.

140. Goldmann C, et al. Molecular cloning and expression of major structural protein VP1 of the human polyomavirus JC virus: formation of virus-like particles useful for immunological and therapeutic studies. J Virol 1999; 73(5): 4465–4469.

141. Pumpens P, et al. Evaluation of HBs, HBc, and frCP virus-like particles for expression of human papillomavirus 16 E7 oncoprotein epitopes. Intervirology 2002; 45(1):24–32.

142. Pumpens P, Grens E. HBV core particles as a carrier for B cell/T cell epitopes. Intervirology 2001; 44(2–3):98–114.

143. Koletzki D, et al. Puumala (PUU) hantavirus strain differences and insertion positions in the hepatitis B virus core antigen influence B-cell immunogenicity and protective potential of core-derived particles. Virology 2000; 276(2): 364–375.

144. Ulrich R, et al. New chimaeric hepatitis B virus core particles carrying hantavirus (serotype Puumala) epitopes: immunogenicity and protection against virus challenge. J Biotechnol 1999; 73(2–3):141–153.

145. Koletzki D, et al. HBV core particles allow the insertion and surface exposure of the entire potentially protective region of Puumala hantavirus nucleocapsid protein. Biol Chem 1999; 380(3):325–333.

146. Netter HJ, et al. Antigenicity and immunogenicity of novel chimeric hepatitis B surface antigen particles with exposed hepatitis C virus epitopes. J Virol 2001; 75(5):2130–2141.

147. Garnier L, et al. Incorporation of pseudorabies virus gD into human immunodeficiency virus type 1 Gag particles produced in baculovirus-infected cells. J Virol 1995; 69(7): 4060–4068.

148. Nagesha HS, et al. Virus-like particles of calicivirus as epitope carriers. Arch Virol 1999; 144(12):2429–2439.

149. Gilbert SC, et al. Ty virus-like particles, DNA vaccines and Modified Vaccinia Virus Ankara; comparisons and combinations. Biol Chem 1999; 380(3):299–303.

150. Kingsman SM, Kingsman AJ. Polyvalent recombinant antigens: a new vaccine strategy. Vaccine 1988; 6(4):304–306.

25

Immunostimulating Reconstituted Influenza Virosomes

Reinhard Glueck

Berna Biotech Ltd., Bern, Switzerland

I. INTRODUCTION

New vaccine formulations have been under study over the last years, which are directed not only against infectious agents, but also against antigen structures related to certain types of cancer, allergies, and autoimmune disorders [1–4]. Subunit vaccine research investigated the use of small antigens or portions of them known to be protective, for example, synthetic peptides, recombinant antigens, bacterial toxoids, polysaccharides, lipopolysaccharides, and protein structures. However, the successful development of the majority of these vaccines, due to their generally low immunogenicity, has been dependent on adjuvants; even antigens that are sufficiently immunogenic when injected with an adjuvant are often less effective when administered by mucosal route.

Sometimes, classic alum-salts, which have been for years the only adjuvant licensed for human use, are not optimal immune enhancers. In fact, their activity, based on a local inflammatory response, may produce undesirable side effects. In addition, when used as an adjuvant for small proteins [5], alum-salts have proven to be less effective (Table 1).

Pathogens with complete intact proteins are effective immunogens. Their surface glycoproteins contain B cell epitopes in certain regions which recognize the B cell lymphocytes, which then manufacture and secrete antibodies inhibiting pathogenic infection [6]. As a survival mechanism, some pathogens have mutated to sabotage the immune system by adapting their surface glycoproteins to contain regions termed dominant B cell epitopes, as in the case of the human immunodeficiency virus (HIV) and malaria. Moreover, the antibodies reacting against these regions do not interfere with the infectivity of the pathogen and, in some cases, even serve to enhance pathogenic infectivity. These dominant B cell epitopes can suppress the immune response to weakly immunogenic neutralizing B cell epitopes while stimulating the host immune response to themselves, hence sabotaging the immune system and guaranteeing continued survival.

The search for better adjuvants and more efficient carrier systems received impetus from the successful studies on liposomes carried out during the past 26 years since Allison and Gregoriadis [7] first demonstrated that liposomes enhanced the antibody response to the diphtheria toxoid. Liposomes, vesicles comprised of phospholipids, have been used as tool to investigate areas bridging from biophysics to cell biology and medicine [8–12]. In particular, they have been shown to be effective adjuvants for a large number of protein antigens [7,13,14]. When used in subunit vaccines against viral disease, they were demonstrated to efficiently present the surface glycoproteins of many enveloped viruses by anchoring the viral glycoprotein into the liposomal bilayer via a transmembrane segment and assuming a conformation analogous to their native structure in the viral envelope, culminating in stimulation of a protective immune response.

Synthetic peptides are only weakly or nonimmunogenic when used alone as a vaccine [15]. This necessitated the use of a large highly immunogenic protein as a carrier system, covalently coupling the peptide. However, because there was no relationship to the pathogen which the vaccine was designed against, these carrier systems, although helpful in producing an initial antibody response, did not evoke pathogen-specific T cell help. This meant that when one was vaccinated with a peptide–carrier complex subsequently challenged with the pathogen, a primary rather than a secondary response resulted. Booster immunizations unfortunately led to a stronger antibody response to the carrier and a lesser one to the peptide.

To test the hypothesis that anchorage of a peptide in the liposomal bilayer might mimic the normal presentation of antigen on an infectious agent thereby potentiating the immune response to the peptide, peptides were covalently linked to a phospholipid, providing a hydrophobic anchorage into the phospholipid bilayer. When viral envelope proteins or peptides representing defined Th cell epitopes are combined into the same phospholipid matrix as a B cell epitope, it stimulates the T helper cells, and a highly efficient immunogen is produced. Sequences, which are not recognized by T helper cells, do not elicit antibody responses even

Table 1 IRIV Combination Vaccine vs. Single Alum Vaccines

Immunogen	Day 0			Day 28		
	Adjuvant	GMT[a] (IU/mL)	p		GMT[a]	p
α-diph. toxoid	Alum	0.4	0.4		0.7 IU/ml	0.00007
	IRIV	0.8			3.2 IU/ml	
α-tet. toxoid	Alum	4.3	0.07		13.1 IU/ml	0.00002
	IRIV	6.6			45.2 IU/ml	
HBs	Alum	292	0.4		6373 IU/ml	0.002
	IRIV	343			13'204 IU/ml	
HAV	Alum	8.0	0.6		252 mIU/mL	0.08
	IRIV	7.0			361 mIU/mL	

[a] Geometric mean titers (alum $n = 26$, IRIV $n = 27$) for diphtheria, tetanus, hepatitis B, and hepatitis A.
Source: Ref. 34.

when formulated into peptide–phospholipid complexes [16–18].

A crucial aspect of the mechanism in which peptide epitopes are presented to CD8+, MHC Class I-restricted cytotoxic T lymphocytes, is the capacity to introduce antigen into the cytoplasm but not the endosomes of antigen-presenting cells. To mimic this mechanism, the integration of lipid-linked membrane proteins into the lipid bilayer of large, mainly unilamellar liposomes was attempted by Gould-Fogerite and Mannino in 1985 [19]. The glycoproteins of influenza viruses maintain their activities of receptor binding and receptor-induced endocytosis when reconstituted into protein lipid vesicles, which have been named virosomes [20]. An effective delivery vehicle for antigens, drugs, proteins, and DNA water-soluble materials can also be encapsulated within the virosomes.

II. IMMUNOPOTENTIATING RECONSTITUTED INFLUENZA VIROSOMES

Virosomes also proved to be effective as an immunogen in mice, rabbits, and monkeys and were able to stimulate strong CD8+ cytotoxic T cell responses (CTL) to lipid bilayer-integrated glycoproteins or lipid-linked peptides, as well as to encapsulated peptides, proteins, and formalin-fixed whole viruses [21–27]. Immunostimulating reconstituted influenza virosomes are unilamellar, spherical vesicles with an approximate mean diameter of 120 to 170 nm. They have short spiked surface projections of 10–15 nm (Figure 1). They are initially prepared by detergent removal of influenza surface glycoproteins and a mixture of natural and synthetic phospholipids containing 70% egg yolk phosphatidylcholine (EYPC), 20% phosphatidylethanolamine (PE), and 10% envelope phospholipids originating from H1N1 influenza virus (A/Singapore/6/86) [28] (Figure 2). Egg yolk phosphatidylcholine is well tolerated in man and has been an important constituent in commercial solutions for i.v. applications in undernourished persons. Egg yolk phosphatidylcholine has been used in nearly all liposomal preparations which were produced for the enhancement of immune responses. Phosphatidylethanolamine was chosen for two

reasons. First, in the case of the hepatitis A virus, attachment to the host cell occurs via binding into PE regions of the cell membrane. Furthermore, it has been shown that liposomes containing PE are able to directly stimulate B cells to produce antibodies without any T cell determinant being present [38]. There were several reasons for including influenza virus envelope glycoproteins. The hemagglutinin (HA) plays a key role in the mode of action of the immunostimulating reconstituted influenza virosomes (IRIVs). Hemagglutinin is the major antigen of influenza virus, containing epitopes on both HA-1 and HA-2 polypeptides, and is responsible for the fusion of the virus with the endosomal membrane [39,40]. The HA-1 globular head groups contain the sialic acid site for HA, and it is therefore expected that the IRIVs bind to such receptors of antigen-presenting cells, e.g., macrophages and lymphocytes initiating a successful immune response. The entry of influenza viruses into cells occurs through HA receptor-mediated endocytosis [41]. It is likely that this mechanism also functions with the IRIV particles. The HA-2 subunit of HA mediates the fusion of viral and endosomal membranes, which is required in order to initiate infection of cells. At the low pH of the host cell endosome (~pH 5), a conformational change occurs in the HA that is a prerequisite for fusion to occur. Fusion activity tests have shown that there was no difference of activity between influenza virus and IRIV. It is suspected that this mediates the rapid release of the transported antigen into the membranes of the target cells [42].

Studies providing evidence for further immunopotentiating effects of influenza virus hemagglutinin were described describing the stimulation of peritoneal B lymphocytes by HA, a so-called B cell "superstimulatory" antigen [43,44]. This study implied that the superstimulatory glycoprotein adapted itself to activate not only conventional B2 cells, but a B cell subset as well, representing a major defense against invading microorganisms. The predilection of B1 cells to build up an immediate immune response against microbial antigen is paralleled by its increased susceptibility to cross-react with "third-party" antigen. This phenomenon has been further investigated by showing that this new example of B cell stimulation by multivalent type-2 antigen (e.g., HA) seems to be mediated by a phosphatidylinositol and Ca^{2+}-independent signaling pathway [43,44]. It was also reported that B cell superstimulatory influenza virus (H2-subtype) induced B cell proliferation by a protein kinase C (PKC)-activating, Ca2 + -independent mechanism.

The enzyme neuraminidase (NA) is a tetramer composed of four equal, spherical subunits hydrophobically embedded in the membrane by a central stalk and is the second glycoprotein exposed on the IRIV surface. Neuraminidase catalyzes the cleavage of N-acetylneuraminic acid (sialic acid) from bound sugar residues [45]. This process leads to decreased viscosity in mucus and allows the influenza virus to have easier access to epithelial cells (which could be useful in the development of a nasal virosomal vaccine). In the cell membrane, the same process leads to the destruction of the HA receptor. Consequently, newly formed virus particles do not adhere to the host cell membrane after budding, and aggregation of the viruses is prevented. Therefore NA allows the influenza virus to retain its mobility. With IRIVs, these characteristics are useful, so that after coupling with HA, IRIVs not taken up by phagocytosis could be cleaved off again and would therefore not be lost. As a side benefit, it would come to bear that the reduction in

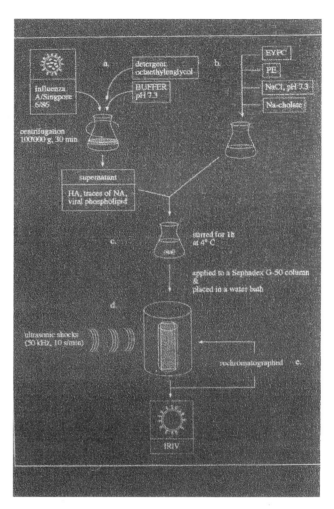

Figure 2 Production scheme for IRIVs egg yolk phosphatidylcholine (EYPC), phosphatidylethanolamine (PE), hemagglutinin (HA), and neuraminidase (NA).

viscosity of the mucus would be found to be useful when developing an intranasal vaccine.

III. PROPOSED MECHANISM OF ACTION—VIROSOMES IN GENERAL

One feature of a virosomal vaccine is that along with the vaccine antigen, the virosomes contain hemagglutinin (and the subchains HA-1 and HA-2) which enables the antigen to be conveyed into immunocompetent cells. All humans, at some time or another, have been exposed to influenza, thus priming their immune systems to HA, which is the major antigen of the influenza virus [34,62,63]. It is thought that the HA enables the virosomes to bind to macrophages and other immunocompetent cells, which have been primed to influenza virus [42], and then enters the cells by endocytosis, mediated by HA-1 receptors [41]. After exposure to the low pH (~5) of cell endosomes, the HA-2 undergoes conformational changes and induces fusion of the virosome and endosome membranes [64].

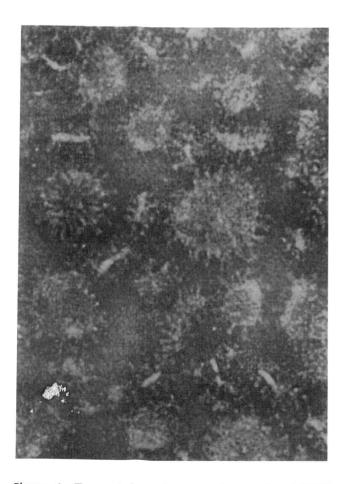

Figure 1 Transmission electron micrograph of IRIV (×100,000). The electron micrograph of the IRIVs shows spherical unilamellar vesicles with a mean diameter of ~150 nm. The vesicles show spike projections of ~15 nm, which originate from influenza glycoproteins (E.M. by T. Wyler, Bern).

The endoplasmic reticulum manufactures major histocompatibility class II (MHC II) molecules which are then transported through the Golgi apparatus and the trans-Golgi reticulum [65]. The MHC class II molecules join with endosomes containing antigens which were proteolyzed to antigenic peptides [66]. The invariant chain is then removed from the MHC class II molecules by cathepsins B and D, enabling binding to the processed antigenic peptides. The MHC class II molecule/antigenic peptide complex is then transported to the cell surface, initiating a specific humoral and/or cellular immune response [42,65,67].

As stated above, it is thought that the influenza glycoprotein neuraminidase, which is included when isolating the HA when formulating the virosomes, works as an enzyme to catalyze the cleavage of sialic acid (N-acetylneuraminic acid) from membrane-bound sugar residues [45], and it is theorized that it might destroy the virosomal HA when bound to cell membranes. This might contribute to the increase of the availability of the vaccine, as the neuraminidase may release the virosomes which are fruitlessly bound to cells [42].

Cephalin has also been shown to stimulate B cells without the presence of T cell determinants [38]. Cephalin also appears to facilitate binding of hepatitis A virions to virosomes [42].

IV. OVERVIEW OF THE EVOLUTION OF VIROSOMAL VACCINES

The natural biocharacteristics of IRIVs as adjuvants were demonstrated in several different prototypical systems. Virosomes were first utilized in the commercial development of a hepatitis A vaccine which contained formalin-inactivated and highly purified hepatitis A viruses (HAV) of strain RG-SB, cultured on human diploid cells, electrostatically coupled to the IRIV vesicle [28]. The surface spikes of hemagglutinin and neuraminidase of three influenza strains were attached to the virosomal membrane, with successful clinical results. The antigen is believed to be attached to the liposomal vesicles by interacting with phospholipids probably corresponding to its natural receptor on hepatocytes.

Then, a combined hepatitis A and hepatitis B vaccine based on virosomes was produced. The highly purified, inactivated hepatitis A virions and the hepatitis B surface antigens (HBsAg) genetically engineered in yeast were covalently coupled to the surface of the virosome [51].

Combination vaccines were then developed in a combined diphtheria–tetanus–hepatitis A vaccine. The diphtheria toxoid, the alpha-tetanus toxoid, the beta-tetanus toxoid, and the inactivated hepatitis A virion were covalently bound via cross-linker molecules to the IRIV surface. A "supercombined" vaccine based on virosomes was also developed, containing covalently bound HAV, HBs, diphtheria, alpha- and-beta tetanus, as well as HA and NA from three different influenza strains [33,35]. Today, several different virosomal vaccines are registered in European, Asian, and American countries.

V. A CLOSER LOOK AT A SUCCESSFUL VIROSOMAL HEPATITIS A VACCINE (STRAIN RG-SB)

As mentioned earlier, the first vaccine was developed from the hepatitis A strain RG-SB, cultured on MRC-5 human diploid cells and inactivated by formalin, and the vaccine antigen was adsorbed onto virosomes. In clinical trials, a dosage of 0.5-mL suspension of 500 radioimmunoassay units of inactivated hepatitis A antigen was injected into the deltoid muscle. Relative to the World Health Organization reference sera information, a protective level of antibodies is generally considered to be $\geq$20 IU/L, as determined by enzyme-linked immunosorbent assay (ELISA) [68].

The first hepatitis A vaccine was extensively tested and went through several chemical analyses, in vitro tests, preclinical trials, and, ultimately, large clinical trials consisting of several thousands of volunteers [28,32,46,47]. Initial studies compared three different formulations. In two of the formulations, the inactivated hepatitis A virus was adsorbed onto virosomes or aluminum hydroxide. The third formulation contained only soluble hepatitis A with no adjuvant [31,32]. Local reactions occurred at a significantly reduced rate in the virosomal vaccine [30–32], and the IRIV vaccine induced a more rapid immune response, with statistically higher rate of seroconversion at day 14 accompanied by a higher geometric mean titer (GMT) (Table 2).

In the larger phase 3 clinical studies, in adults and children, seroconversion [$\geq$20 ELISA units per liter of anti-hepatitis A virus (anti-HAV) antibodies] was induced in almost all volunteers within 4 weeks (usually 2 weeks) of vaccination with the virosomal hepatitis A vaccine (500 ra-

Table 2 Kinetics of the Immune Response Following Immunization with Different Hepatitis A Vaccines

Vaccine formulation[a]	Geometric mean titer (% $\geq$20 IU/mL)				
	Day 0	Day 14	Day 28	Day 180	Day 352[b]
Fluid	<20	16 (30)	388 (100)	211 (80)	39 (50)
AL (OH)$_3$	<20	21 (44)	871 (100)	535 (95)	57 (60)
IRIV	<20	140 (100)	831 (100)	1499 (100)	655 (100)

[a] One dose of each vaccine formulation contained 1000 radioimmunoassay units of HAV antigen and was administered to 40 healthy adults.
[b] Data from 14, 10, and 22 subjects immunized with fluid, AL (OH)$_3$, or IRIV vaccines, respectively.
Source: Ref. 59.

dioimmunoassay units), as demonstrated in noncomparative studies [28–30].

By 4 weeks postimmunization, seroconversion rates were still around 98–100%. Antibody titers were still rising during the 4th and 26th week after vaccination and were lasting mainly over one year with GMT of the IRIV vaccine recipients >10-fold higher than for the other two vaccine groups [28,47,48].

Booster injections of the virosomal vaccine 12 months after the initial dose increased antihepatitis A virus (anti-HAV) antibody titers by 11–40-fold. Following the administration of the booster injection, 100% of the volunteers seroconverted [48].

Studies were carried out for 3 years (with a booster vaccination after 1 year) and showed high anti-HAV antibody titers; protection against hepatitis A infection has been estimated to last for over ten years.

A schedule of a single-dose immunization was tested and found effective, reaching protective antibody titers in ≥95% of vaccinated subjects [30–32,49,50] and protecting from hepatitis A outbreaks and endemic disease [49,50].

Data collected from immunogenicity studies and results from multiple field trials have proven that virosomal hepatitis A vaccination (strain RG-SB) is effective in protecting against hepatitis A infection.

VI. IRIV-BASED INFLUENZA VACCINE

With the exciting results achieved with the virosomal hepatitis A vaccine, attention was turned toward a vaccine against influenza.

The safety and immunogenicity of a trivalent virosomal influenza vaccine was compared with the effects of a commercial whole-virus vaccine and with a subunit vaccine in the elderly [59,70,83]. Elderly as well as immunocompromised patients are at increased risk of complications associated with influenza because of an increasingly poorly functioning immune system [3,70–74]. At that time, the available vaccines were efficacious only in particular settings and suffered from several limitations. Infants and young children require two doses of vaccine spaced 1–2 months apart, and the available vaccines at that time did not result in high, long-lasting protective immune responses. Long-lasting protective immune responses were also lacking in the elderly, but only a single dose of vaccine could be administered per year. This variable immunogenicity was one of the most important reasons for low vaccine uptake among these two groups. Although the existing vaccines were well tolerated, occasionally moderate to severe reactions precluded giving further doses [75,76]. Given the wide variation in immune responses to influenza vaccines, new vaccines which combine an improved immunogenicity with a low rate of side effects were clearly needed.

The search for vaccines with improved immunogenicity [77,78] stimulated the development of formulations with whole virus and subunit vaccines containing new adjuvants and antigen-free delivery systems [81–84]. The new strategies pointed to preparations able to target both local and systemic antibody responses since mucosal immunity constitutes the first line of defense for the host against influenza pathogens and is a major component of the immunological cell-mediated response in the upper and lower respiratory tract passages.

We then became interested in studying the virosomal vaccine concept for other routes of vaccination, in particular, for the intranasal vaccination.

VII. VIROSOME-FORMULATED INFLUENZA VACCINE FOR PARENTERAL ADMINISTRATION

Virosomes were confirmed to posses significant adjuvantal properties and increased immunoprotective activity when administered as a trivalent influenza vaccine formulation. The results from an early comparative clinical investigation [69] against commercial whole virion and subunit vaccines demonstrated a higher seroconversion rate (a fourfold or greater rise in anti-HA titer) and a significantly greater protection rate (individuals with antibody titers ≥1:40) in subjects vaccinated with the virosome formulation when compared with the existing commercial formula [69].

Further studies confirmed similar results of immunogenicity and safety with the virosome-formulated influenza vaccine [85,87,106]. The virosomes bind to antigen-presenting cells by the influenza virus surface glycoproteins HA and are internalized by receptor-mediated endocytosis, then the virosomes fuse with the membranes of the endosomal cell. This process provides optimal processing and presentation of the antigens to immunocompetent cells.

However, presently used injectable influenza vaccines stimulate serum HA-specific immunoglobulin G (IgG) of HA inhibition antibody in the majority of healthy individuals, but they give a significant rise in HA-specific nasal IgA antibodies in only a minority of subjects.

VIII. POTENTIAL FOR AN INTRANASALLY ADMINISTERED INFLUENZA VACCINE

The reduced ability of parenteral vaccines to elicit an immunological response at the mucosa, the site of influenza virus entry and propagation, as confirmed by animal experiments [86], is an important determinant of the suboptimal protective capacity of current vaccines. It may also be particularly relevant when considering that mucosal immunity represents the first line of defense for the host and is a major component of the immunological cell-mediated response in the upper and lower respiratory tract. The need to improve vaccine efficacy has led to the development of an intranasal virosome-based influenza vaccine. An efficient vaccine applied to the site of virus entry, i.e., intranasal, may be expected to stimulate humoral and cellular immune responses at both mucosal and systemic levels [87,88]. A further advantage of an intranasal influenza vaccine is the needle-free administration that may improve vaccine coverage due to greater patient acceptance particularly in risk groups. Thus the high tolerability of virosome-based influenza vaccines, namely, Inflexal V, combined with intranasal administration should provide a safe and effective vaccine that is easy to use.

IX. OTHER VIROSOMAL-BASED VACCINES

A. Combined Vaccines

Surface antigens of many viruses when covalently coupled to IRIVs were shown to be immunogenic. Clinical trials with combined IRIV vaccines are still in phase I and II clinical trials; however, some preliminary results have already been published [33–35].

Combined hepatitis A–hepatitis B (HBs) vaccine on a virosomal basis has also been formulated by mixing inactivated HAV virions with hepatitis B surface antigen genetically grown on yeast, and it showed a better effect than that of the commercial monovalent alum products available [35].

Other combinations such as diphtheria–tetanus (DT)–hepatitis A vaccine, where diphtheria toxoid, α-tetanus toxoid, β-tetanus toxoid, and inactivated virions are covalently bound to the surface of virosomal particles by using cross-linker molecules, are being evaluated because alternatives are needed to current alum-adsorbed DT vaccines, which require two or three doses to be effective and are often accompanied by pain at the injection site.

The IRIV-based formulations appeared to be superior to the alum-based vaccines not only in terms of immunogenicity, but also protectively as reported in mice experiments, where an IRIV-based toxoid vaccine (diphtheria and tetanus) was compared to a standard alum-adsorbed toxoid vaccine in mice. In vitro tests and challenge experiments showed that influenza-primed mice had a threefold higher neutralizing and protective antibody titers after receiving the new vaccine, compared to the group receiving the classical alum formulation [60].

Another "supercombined" vaccine was constructed by binding HAV, HBs, diphtheria toxoid, α- and β-tetanus toxoids, and, respectively, Ha and NA of three different influenza strains type A and B with very interesting results in a series of clinical trials on human volunteers [51].

After exclusion of epitope-specific suppression by single components, particularly diphtheria and tetanus antigens showed "antigenic competition" on the HAV and possibly on the HBs antigens.

By reducing the diphtheria and tetanus toxoid subunits, the immune response to these antigens could be increased and antigenic suppression on other antigens was completely removed [34].

First results on the immunogenicity and tolerability of the combined vaccine, compared with that of the corresponding single vaccines, are shown in Table 3.

B. Nucleic Acid and Peptide-Based Vaccines

The generation of an effective cell-mediated immune response (CMI) is an important factor in the overcoming of certain viral infections. Therefore the ability to generate CMI in addition to antibodies production is a wished feature of a vaccine against virus infection. In the last years, several experiments of DNA vaccination by using plasmid vectors have been showing promising results [52–54] in the induction of humoral and CMI responses.

Because of the need of high quantities of DNA and many vaccination doses, several new delivery systems to target cells have been tested to optimize immunogenicity, including viral and lipid-based methods [55,56].

Virosomes are also being studied as a carrier system for nucleic acid vaccines, particularly to potentiate the poor uptake in target cells of antisense oligonucleotides (ODNs), considered as promising therapeutic agents against viral diseases, in cancer therapy, or as immunomodulators.

Recent data showed evidence that ODNs encapsulated into fusogenic, reconstituted cationic influenza virosomes (better interactions between positively charged lipids on virosomes and negatively charged oligonucleotides) are rapidly and efficiently internalized into cancer cells due to mediation of the fusion activity of the hemagglutinin of the influenza virus [57]. In these experiments, the addition of cationic virosomes containing antisense L-*myc* ODNs in the picomolar range to small-cell-lung-cancer cultures overexpressing the L-myc oncogene induced inhibitory effect on thymidine uptake by those cells.

During this process, the content of oligonucleotides is released into the cytoplasm where they stay protected from

Table 3 Combined Commercial Di, Te, Hepatitis A and Hepatitis B Vaccines vs. an IRIV Supercombined with the same Antigens

Adverse events	Commercial vaccine	IRIV Supercombined
Pain grade 2 or 3	82%	24%
Induration	41%	23%
Redness	37%	9%
Redness average:		
Area	left: 3800 mm^2	2 mm^2
	right:1034 mm^2	
Swelling	48%	27%
General symptoms:		
Headache, nausea, etc.	78%	28%

Source: Ref. 34.

enzymatic degradation; this protection could be efficacious also in the blood, an important feature for a future in vivo application of this type of vaccine.

Investigations carried out on influenza virosomes used as a tumor-associated antigen-gene delivery system also showed very promising results [58].

For these experiments, engineered plasmid (GC90) expressing the parathyroid hormone-related peptide (PTH-rP) associated with prostate and lung tumor cells was inserted on influenza virosomes (GC90V). The ability of such virosomes including PTH-rP plasmids to elicit a multiepitopic CTL-mediated immune response in vitro and in a mouse model has been described, providing a rationale for investigating this system in clinical trials of active specific anticancer immunotherapy.

Further studies will include clinical trials with GC90V to elucidate the possible in vivo ability to migrate in tumor tissue where they could have an antitumor effect.

The efficacy of mumps DNA vaccine delivered by virosomes administered intranasally in mice was recently described [61]. In this study, a plasmid vector expressing viral hemagglutinin or the fusion protein associated with virosomes was tested for humoral, mucosal, and cell-mediated response. Results showed production of specific s-IgA in respiratory tract and circulating IgG antibody in the blood. PCR techniques revealed the presence of the plasmid 1 month after immunization. DNA–influenza virosome composition was shown to be safe and nontoxic in mice at doses also producing a good immune response. Doses as small as 5 μg DNA were sufficient to induce an immune barrier to prevent infection at the mucosal entry site [61].

Virosomes were used as a delivery system for the development of a synthetic peptide-based malaria vaccine SPf66 [36]. Mice were immunized twice intramuscularly with peptide-loaded virosomes, and the amount of elicited anti-SPf66 IgG was determined by ELISA. Titers were higher and immunization doses were lower for the SPf66-IRIV vaccine than with alum-adsorbed, when mice were preimmunized with a commercial whole virus vaccine because of the priming effect. Monoclonal antibodies produced by four B cell hybridoma clones derived from a mouse vaccinated with IRIV formulation cross-reacted with *Plasmodium falciparum* blood stage parasites in immunofluorescence tests, and all were specific for the merozoite protein-1-derived 83.1 portion of SPf66. In this study, biomolecular interaction analyses and sequencing data provided evidence that a synthetic peptide vaccine delivered virosomally has great potential as a combined vaccine targeted against several antigens as well as against multiple pathogens.

An HIV vaccine, based on genetically modified glycoprotein and nonstructural peptides, and a vaccine against hepatitis C and respiratory synctial virus (RSV) by using the virosomal carrier system are all under study [37].

X. CONCLUSION

Immunostimulating reconstituted influenza virosomal vaccines comprised of viral glycoproteins, bacterial toxoid, inactivated virus, recombinant proteins, synthetic peptides, and DNA plasmids or polynucleotides were formulated and tested. The safety profile of IRIV vaccines has been excellent, and the immunopotentiating effect was superior to comparable alum-based vaccines.

Compared to alum-adsorbed vaccines, they elicit far fewer local reactions. Both local and systemic reactions are predominantly mild and transient. Additionally, immunization with IRIVs does not induce a serum antiphospholipid antibody response even after repeated doses of vaccine have been administered. IRIV-based vaccines are currently manufactured on a large scale and are available under the brand names Epaxal® for hepatitis A and Inflexal V® for influenza. New formulations of antigens incorporated into IRIVs are undergoing testing and clinical evaluation.

REFERENCES

1. Millgrom H, Fick RB Jr, Su JQ, et al. Treatment of allergic asthma with monoclonal anti-IgE antibody. rhuMAb-E25 Study Group. N Engl J Med 1999; 341:1966–1973.
2. Hellström KE, Chen L. Antitumor vaccines. In: Levine MM, Woodrow GC, Kaper JB, Cobon GS, eds. New Generation Vaccines. 2d ed. 1997:1095–1115.
3. Couch RB, Kasel JA, Glezen WP, Cate TR, Six HR, Taber LH, Frank AL, Greenberg SB, Zahradnik JM, Keital WA. Influenza: its control in persons and populations. J Infect Dis 1986; 153:431–440.
4. Cox NJ, Subbarao K. Influenza. Lancet 1999; October 9; 354(9186):1277–1282.
5. Gupta RK, Relyveld EH, Lindblad EB, Bizzini B, Ben-Efraim S, Gupta CK. Adjuvants—a balance between their toxicity and adjuvanticity. Vaccine 1993; 11:293–305.
6. Zanetti M, Sercarz E, Sal J. The immunology of a new generation of vaccines. Immunol Today 1987; 8:18–23.
7. Allison AC, Gregoriadis G. Liposomes as immunological adjuvants. Nature 1974; 252:252–255.
8. Duzzqunes N, Papahadiopoulos D. Ionotropic effects on phospholipid membranes: calcium/magnesium specificity in binding, fluidity and fusion. In: Aloja RC, ed. Membrane Fluidity in Biology. New York: Academic Press, 1983:187–197.
9. Lüscher-Mattli M, Glueck R, Kempf R, Zanoni-Grassi M. A comparative study of the effect of dextran sulfate on the fusion and the in vitro replication of influenza A and B, Semliki Forest, vesicular stomatitis, rabies Sendai and mumps virus. Arch Virol 1993; 130:317–326.
10. Gregoriadis G, Leathwood PD. Enzyme entrapment in liposomes. FEBS Lett 1971; 14:95–99.
11. Hafeman DG, Lewis TJ, McConnel HM. Triggering of the macrophage and neutrophil respiratory burst by antibody bound to a spin-label phospholipid hapten in model lipid bilayer membranes. Biochemistry 1980; 19:5387–5394.
12. Papahadiopoulos D. Cholesterol and cell-membrane functions: a hypothesis concerning the etiology of arteriosclerosis. J Theor Biol 1974; 43:329–337.
13. Morein B, Simons K. Subunit vaccines against enveloped viruses: virosomes, micelles and other protein complexes. Vaccine 1985; 3:83–93.
14. Boudreault A, Thibodeau L. Mouse response to influenza immunosomes. Vaccine 1985; 3:231–234.
15. Muller GM, Shapira M, Arnon R. Anti-influenza response achieved by immunization with a synthetic conjugate. Proc Natl Acad Sci USA 1982; 79:569–573.
16. Goodman-Snitkoff G, Good MR, Berzofsky JA, Mannino RJ. Role of intrastructural/intermolecular help in immuni-

zation with peptide–phospholipid complexes. J Immunol 1991; 147:410–415.

17. Goodman-Snitkoff G, Eisele LE, Heimer EP, Felix AM, Andersen TT, Fuerst TR, Mannino RJ. Defining minimal requirements for antibody production to peptide antigens. Vaccine 1990; 8:257–262.

18. Mannino RJ, Gould-Fogerite S. Lipid matrix-based vaccines for mucosal and systemic immunization. In: Powell MF, Newman MJ, eds. Vaccine Design: The Subunit and Adjuvant Approach. New York: Plenum Press, 1995:363.

19. Gould-Fogerite S, Mannino RJ. Rotary dialysis: 1st application to the production of large liposomes and large proteoliposomes (protein–lipid vesicles) with high encapsulation efficiency and efficient reconstitution of membrane proteins. Anal Biochem 1985; 148:15.

20. Bron R, Ortiz A, Dijkstra J, Stegmann T, Wilschut J. Preparation, properties, and applications of reconstituted influenza virus envelopes (virosomes). Methods Enzymol 1993; 220:313–331.

21. Miller MD, Gould-Fogerite S, Shen L, Woods RM, Koenig S, Mannino RJ, Letvin NL. Vaccination of rhesus monkeys with synthetic peptide in a fusogenic proteoliposome elicits simian immunodeficiency virus specific CD8+ cytotoxic T lymphocytes. J Exp Med 1992; 176:1739–1744.

22. Gould-Fogerite S, Edghill-Smith Y, Kheiri M, Wang Z, Das K, Feketeova E, Canki M, Mannino RJ. Lipid matrix-based subunit vaccines: a structure–function approach to oral and parenteral immunizations. AIDS Res Hum Retrovir 1994; 10:99.

23. Mannino RJ, Gould-Fogerite S. Lipid matrix-based vaccines for mucosal and systemic immunization. In: Powell MF, Newman MJ, eds. Vaccine Design: The Subunit and Adjuvant Approach. New York: Plenum Press, 1995:363.

24. Gregoriadis G. Immunological adjuvants: a role for liposomes. Immunol Today 1990; 11:89–97.

25. Pregliasco F, Mensi C, Serpilli W, Speccher L, Masella P, Belloni A. Immunogenicity and safety of three commercial influenza vaccines in institutionalized elderly. Ageing (Milano) Feb 2001; 13(1):38–43.

26. Glueck R, Mischler R, Durrer P, Furer E, Lang AB, Herzog C, Cryz SJ Jr. Safety and immunogenicity of intranasally administered inactivated trivalent virosome-formulated influenza vaccine containing Escherichia coli heat-labile toxin as a mucosal adjuvant. J Infect Dis Mar 2000; 181(3):1129–1132.

27. Nerome K, Yoshioka Y, Ishida M, Okuma K, Oka T, Kataoka T, Inoue Oya A. Development of a new type of influenza subunit vaccine made by muramyldipeptide-liposome: enhancement of humoral and cellular immune responses. Vaccine Oct 1990; 8(5):503–509.

28. Glueck R, Mischler R, Brantschen S, Just M, Althaus B, Cryz SJ Jr. Immunopotentiating reconstituted influenza virosomes (IRIV) vaccine delivery system for immunization against hepatitis A. J Clin Invest 1992; 90:2491–2495.

29. Argentini C, D'Ugo E, Bruni R, Glueck R, Giuseppetti R, Rapicetta M. Sequence and phylogenetic analysis of the VP1 gene in two cell culture-adapted HAV strain from a unique pathogenic isolate. Virus Gene 1995; 10:37–43.

30. Lea AP, Balfour JA. Virosomal hepatitis A vaccine (strain RG-SB): a preliminary review of its immunogenicity protective efficacy and tolerability in at-risk populations. BioDrugs 1997; 7:232–248.

31. Bovier P, Loutan L, Farinelly T, et al. Cross-immunogenicity of a booster dose of a virosomal hepatitis A vaccine in healthy travellers after basic immunization with an alum-based hepatitis A vaccine [abstr]. European Conference on Tropical Medicine, Hamburg, Germany, 1995:22–26.

32. Holzer BR, Hatz C, Schmidt-Sissolak D, et al. Immunogenicity and adverse effects of inactivated virosome versus

alum-adsorbed hepatitis A vaccine: a randomized controlled trial. Vaccine 1996; 14:982–986.

33. Just M. Experience with IRIV as carrier for hepatitis A and other antigens. Abstract No. 277. Third Conference on International Travel Medicine, Paris, 1993:25–29.

34. Glueck R. Liposomal hepatitis A vaccine and liposomal multi-antigen combination vaccines. J Liposome Res 1995; 5:456–479.

35. Glueck R. Towards a universal IRIV, vaccine. Abstract No. 259. Third Conference on International Travel Medicine, Paris, France, 1993:25–29.

36. Poeltl-Frank F, Zurbriggen R, Helg A, Stuart F, Robinson J, Glueck R, Pluschke G. Use of reconstituted influenza virosomes as an immunopotentiating delivery system for a peptide-based vaccine. Clin Exp Immunol 1999; 117:496–503.

37. Hunziker IP, Zurbriggen R, Glueck R, Cerny A, Pichler WJ. Loaded with viral hepatitis C (HCV) peptides deliver them into the MHC class I pathway. Keystone Symposium in Snowbird, April 12–17.

38. Garcon NM, Six HR. Universal vaccine carrier. Liposomes that provide T-dependent help to weak antigens. J Immunol Jun 1, 1991; 146(11):3697–3702.

39. Tsurudome M, Glück R, Graf R, Falchetto R, Schaller U, Brunner J. Lipid interactions of the hemagglutinin HA2NH2-terminal segment during influenza virus-induced membrane fusion. J Biol Chem 1992; 267/28:20225–20232.

40. Durrer P, Galli C, Hoenke S, Corti C, Glück R, Vorherr T, Brunner J. H+-induced membrane insertion of influenza virus hemagglutinin involves the HA2 amino-terminal fusion peptide but not the coiled coil region. J Biol Chem 1996; 271/23:13417–13421.

41. Matlin KS, Reggio H, Helenius A, Simmons K. Infections entry pathway of influenza virus in a canine kidney cell line. J Cell Biol 1981; 91:601–613.

42. Glück R. Liposomal presentation of antigens for human vaccines. In: Powell MR, Newman MJ, eds. Vaccine Design. New York: Plenum Press, 1995a:325–345.

43. Rott O, Charreire J, Mignon-Godefroy K, Cash E. B Cell superstimulatory influenza virus activates peritoneal B cells. J Immunol 1995a; 155:134–142.

44. Rott O, Charreire J, Semichon M, Bismuth G, Cash E. B Cell superstimulatory influenza virus (H2 subtype) induces B cell proliferation by a PKC-activating, Ca2+-independent mechanism. J Immunol 1995b; 154:2092–2103.

45. Air GM, Laver WG. The neuraminidase of influenza virus. Proteins 1989; 6:341–356.

46. Wegmann A, Zellmayer M, Glueck R, Finkel B, Flückiger A, Berger R, Just M. Immunogenität und Stabilität eines aluminiumfreien liposomalen Hepatitis A-Impfstoff (Epaxal Berna). Schweiz Med Wochenschr 1994; 124:2053–2056.

47. Just M, Berger R, Drechsler H, Brantschen S, Glueck R. A single vaccination with an inactivated hepatitis A vaccine induces protective antibodies after only two weeks. Vaccine 1992; 10(11):737–739.

48. Loutan L, Bovier P, Althaus B, Glueck R. Inactivated virosome hepatitis A vaccine. Lancet 1994; (343):322–324.

49. Poovorawan Y, Theamboonlers A, Chumdermpadetsuk S, et al. Safety, immunogenicity, and kinetics of the immune response to a single dose of virosome-formulated hepatitis A vaccine in Thais. Vaccine 1995; 13:891–893.

50. Poovorawan Y, Theamboonlers A, Chumdermpadetsuk S, et al. Control of a hepatitis A outbreak by active immunization of high-risk susceptible subjects. J Infect Dis 1994; 169:228–229.

51. Mengiardi B, Berger R, Just M, Glück R. Virosomes as carriers for combined vaccines. Vaccine Oct. 1995; 13(14):1306–1315.

52. Wolff JA, Malone RW, Williams P, Chong W, Acsadi G,

Jani A, Felgner PL. Direct gene transfer into mouse muscle in vivo. Science 1990; 247:1465–1468.

53. Tang DC, Devit M, Johnston SA. Genetic immunisation is a simple method for eliciting an immune response. Nature 1992; 356:152–154.

54. Rimmelzwann GF, Osterhaus ADME. Cytotoxic T-lymphocyte memory: role in cross-protective immunity against influenza? Vaccine 1995; 13/8:703–705.

55. Trapnell BC, Gorziglia M. Gene therapy using adenoviral vectors. Curr Opin Biotechnol 1994; 5:617–625.

56. Ruysschaert JM, El Ouahabi A, Willeaume V, Huez G, Fuks R, Vandenbranden M, Di Stefano P. A novel cationic amphiphile transfection of mammalian cells. Biochem Biophys Res Commun 1994; 203:1622–1628.

57. Waelti ER, Glueck R. Delivery to cancer cells of antisense L-*myc* oligonucleotides incorporated in fusogenic, cationic-lipid reconstituted influenza-virus envelopes (cationic virosomes). Int J Cancer 1998; 77:728–733.

58. Correale P, Cusi MG, Sabatino M, Micheli L, Pozzessere D, Nencini C, Valensin PE, Petrioli R, Giorgi G, Zurbriggen R, Gluck R, Francini G. Tumour-associated antigen (TAA)-specific cytotoxic T cell (CTL) response in vitro and in a mouse model, induced by TAA-plasmids delivered by influenza virosomes. Eur J Cancer Nov 2001; 37(16):2097–2103.

59. Cryz SJ, Glueck R. Immunopotentiating reconstituted influenza virosomes as a novel antigen delivery system. In: Brown F, Haaheim LR, eds. Modulation of the Immune Response to Vaccine Antigens. Vol. 92. Dev Biol Stand. Basel: Karger, 1998:219–223.

60. Zurbriggen R, Glueck R. Immunogenicity of IRIV-versus alum-adjuvanted diphtheria and tetanus toxoid vaccines in influenza primed mice. Vaccine 1999; 17:1301–1305.

61. Cusi MG, Zurbriggen R, Valassina M, Bianchi S, Durrer P, Valensin PE, Donati M, Glueck R. Intranasal immunisation with mumps virus DNA vaccine delivered by influenza virosomes elicits mucosal and systemic immunity. Virology 2000; 277:111–118.

62. Jackson DC, Crabb BS, Poumbourious P, et al. Three antibody molecules can bind simultaneously to each monomer of the tetramer of influenza virus neuraminidase and the trimer of influenza virus hemagglutinin. Arch Virol 1991; 116:45–56.

63. Taylor AH, Haberman AM, Gerhard W, et al. Structure–function relationships among highly diverse T cells that recognise a determinant from influenza virus hemagglutinin. J Exp Med 1990; 162:1643–1651.

64. Wiley DC, Skehel JJ. The structure and function of the hemagglutinin membrane glycoprotein of influenza virus. Ann Rev Biochem 1987; 56:365–394.

65. Roitt I. Essential Immunology. 8th ed. Oxford, UK: Blackwell, 1994.

66. Neefjes JJ, Stoolorz V, Peters PJ, et al. The biosynthetic pathway of MHC class II molecules but not class I molecules intersected the endocatotic route. Cell 1990; 61:171–183.

67. Alving CR. Liposomal vaccines: clinical status and immunological presentation for humoral and cellular immunity. Ann N Y Acad Sci May 31, 1995; 754:143–152.

68. Ambrosch F, Wiedermann G, Jonas S, et al. Immunogenicity and protectivity of a new liposomal hepatitis A vaccine. Vaccine Aug 1997; 15(11):1209–1213.

69. Glück R, Mischler R, Finkel B, Que JU, Scarpa B, Cryz SJ. Immunogenicity of new virosome influenza vaccine in the elderly people. Lancet 1994; 344:160–163.

70. Kohn RP. Cause of death in very old people. JAMA 1982; 246:2793–2797.

71. Perrotta DM, Decker M, Glezen WP. Acute respiratory disease. Hospitalization as a measure of impact of epidemic influenza. Am J Epidemiol 1985; 122:468–476.

72. Oliveira EC, Marik PE, Colice G. Influenza pneumonia: a descriptive study. Chest June 2001; 119(6):1717–1723.

73. Castle SC. Clinical relevance of age-related immune dysfunction. Clin Infect Dis Aug. 2000; 31(2):578–585.

74. Chien, JW, Johnson, JL. Viral pneumonias. Epidemic respiratory virus. Postgrad Med Mar. 2000; 107(3):41–42, 45–47, 51–52.

75. Zei T, Neri M, Iorio AM. Immunogenicity of trivalent subunit and split influenza vaccines (1989–1990 winter season) in volunteers of different age groups. Vaccine 1991; 9:613–617.

76. Wright PF, Cherry JD, Foy HM, et al. Antigenicity and reactogenicity of influenza A/USSR/77 virus vaccine in children—a multicenter evaluation of dosage and safety. Rev Infect Dis Jul–Aug 1983; 5(4):758–764.

77. Gauthey L, Toscani L, Schira J-C. Vaccination contre la grippe en Suisse. Soz Präventivmed 1997; 42(suppl 2):107–111.

78. Fedson DS, Hirota Y, Shin HK, et al. Influenza vaccination in 22 developed countries: an update to 1995. Vaccine 1997; 15:1506–1511.

79. Gruber WC, Campbell PW, Thompson JM, et al. Comparison of live and inactivated vaccines in cystic fibrosis patients and their families: results of a 3-year study. J Infect Dis 1994; 169:241–247.

80. Anon. Prevention and control of influenza: recommendations of the Advisory Committee on Immunization practices (ACIP), Centers for Disease Control and Prevention. MMWR Morb Mort Wkly Rep 1998; 47:1–26.

81. Dunn C, Goa KL. Zanamivir—a review of its use in influenza. Drugs 1999; 58:761–784.

82. Glueck R, Mischler R, Finkel B, Que JU, Scarpa B, Cryz SJ Jr. Immunogenicity of new virosome influenza vaccine in elderly people. Lancet 1994; 344:160–163.

83. Conne P, Gauthey L, Vernet P, Althaus B, Que J, Finkel B, Glueck R, Cryz SJ Jr. Immunogenicity of trivalent subunits versus virosome-formulated influenza vaccines in geriatric patients. Vaccine 1997; 15:1675–1679.

84. Holm KJ, Goa KL. Liposomal influenza vaccine. BioDrugs 1999; 11:137–144.

85. Glück R, Wegmann A. Influenza vaccination in the elderly. Dev Comp Immunol 1997; 21(6):501–507.

86. Hu KF, Lovgren-Bengtsson K, Morein B. Immunostimulating complexes (ISCOMs) for nasal vaccination. Adv Drug Deliv Rev Sep 23, 2001; 51(1–3):149–159.

87. McGhee JR, Kiyono H. New perspectives in vaccine development: mucosal immunity to infections. Infect Agents Dis 1993; 2:55–73.

88. Holmgren J. Mucosal immunity and vaccination. FEMS Microbiol Immunol 1991; 89:1–10.

26

Plants as a Production and Delivery Vehicle for Orally Delivered Subunit Vaccines

Tsafrir S. Mor, Hugh S. Mason, Charles J. Arntzen, and Guy A. Cardineau
Arizona State University, Tempe, Arizona, U.S.A.

Dwayne D. Kirk
Arizona State University, Tempe, Arizona, and Boyce Thompson Institute, Ithaca, New York, U.S.A.

I. INTRODUCTION

A major focus of biotechnology is the improvement of human health around the globe. It is anticipated that the genomic revolution will greatly expand our knowledge of the molecular basis of many diseases and pathological states. Combining this knowledge with powerful screening techniques will be used in the development of safe and efficacious drugs for the prevention, diagnosis, and treatment of disease, including new vaccines and vaccine technologies. Unfortunately, the availability of these new treatments for use by all those who need them greatly depends on economic considerations such as the cost of their development, production, and delivery. Therefore, a major challenge of biotechnology is to reduce clinical innovations to economically viable practice, and the production and oral delivery of plant-derived vaccines is a step in that direction.

II. WHY PRODUCTION AND DELIVERY OF VACCINES IN PLANTS MAKE SENSE

Despite the public health success of current vaccines in controlling various infectious diseases, there are limitations in the technology as we are faced with many emerging infectious diseases, some of which are the result of pathogens that have the ability to mutate rapidly to circumvent vaccination, as well as the unprecedented reality of bioterrorism. Production and delivery can be an issue in vaccine development, and manufacturing may be hampered by high costs for vaccines against many of the pathogens for which vaccines are needed. Furthermore, for certain live vaccines, attenuation may impact immunogenic properties, making such vaccines ineffective or unsafe.

Mucosal immune responses, characterized by production of secretory antibodies such as secretory immunoglobulin A (sIgA) and the transport of these antibodies across the epithelium, represent a first line of defense against pathogens that colonize and infect mucosal surfaces. As a result, stimulation of the mucosal immune system may be a particularly advantageous route of vaccination. Furthermore, mucosal vaccines that can be delivered by oral or nasal route have the advantage of not requiring the use of needles, and are perhaps safer and may result in improved patient compliance. Consequently, vaccine development focuses on finding alternatives to traditional vaccines in terms of both immunogen source and route of administration.

Subunit vaccines, especially those that target the mucosal immune system, can potentially fill this gap in vaccine development. To create these vaccines, a gene encoding an antigenic determinant from an infectious agent is cloned, put under the control of an appropriate expression system, and transferred into a host organism. The transgenic host will then produce a "subunit" of the pathogen, a protein that cannot cause disease but can elicit a protective immune response against the pathogen. In most studies of the last 15 years, subunit vaccines have been purified from transgenic "production hosts" (e.g., cultured yeast cells) and have been delivered via injection to immunize against a specific disease. To date, the only recombinant subunit vaccines licensed for use in humans are a yeast-derived hepatitis B vaccine and an *Escherichia coli* recombinant Lyme disease vaccine, which are delivered by intramuscular injection.

While still in experimental stages of development, plant-produced, orally delivered subunit vaccines provide a strategy to efficiently improve modes of production, distribution, and administration. Such plant-based vaccines merge innovations in medical science and plant biology. Since the emergence of the original idea about 13 years ago [1], it has been embraced by a growing number of laboratories in the academia and industry. Work in this field was reported in the previous edition of this volume [2], and due to the subject's interdisciplinary nature, importance, and appeal, it continues to be periodically reviewed [3–10]. In this chapter, we present an update on advances in the technology and, in particular, on recent Phase I clinical trials run in the United States. We also address areas of research that require further attention if plant-based vaccines are to become a viable reality and contributor to world health.

III. EXPRESSION OF ANTIGENIC PROTEINS IN PLANTS

Plants can cost-effectively produce large amounts of functional proteins, free of animal pathogens, and production can be increased to agricultural scale. As a result, transgenic plants have emerged as a promising alternative to available fermentation-based production systems for valuable pharmaceuticals. The ability of a plant to produce, correctly process, and assemble complex foreign proteins from a variety of organisms is well documented and is based on extensive research during the past two decades in the realms of plant molecular biology, plant transformation, and regeneration. This work has not been confined to the developed world, as many scientists and public health authorities in developing counties have embraced the new technology for the possible future benefit of their people. Regardless of the many reported successes, expressing a particular recombinant protein to significant levels in plants remains an empirical exercise, which often requires custom tailoring and optimization. Unfortunately, except for a few rules of thumb, insights gained while studying one protein are not always readily transferable when approaching a different expression project. However, when focused on the endproduct, such as a plant-expressed antigen as a vaccine candidate, the expenditure of time, effort, and resources directed at gene optimization can significantly contribute to success. A few studies (e.g., Richter et al. [11]) have attempted to address the issues surrounding the low levels of expression of recombinant proteins that may sometimes occur in transgenic plants. Questions regarding the "how, where, and when" to express a transgene to allow maximal accumulation of its product while retaining its functional properties have been addressed by many workers in the field of agricultural biotechnology. It is especially important in the case of plant-based vaccines, where the goal is sufficient dosage and minimal processing of antigenic proteins in edible plant tissue, to ensure that sufficient quantities survive passage through the stomach to elicit a clinically relevant immune response.

IV. PLANT-DERIVED VACCINES IN CLINICAL TRIALS

The genesis of the concept of plant-based vaccines occurred in 1986 [12] and was first documented in a patent application entitled "Oral Immunization by Transgenic Plants" known in the field as the "Curtiss–Cardineau Patent" after its inventors [1]. Although this publication is the first description

of the plant expression of an antigen of an important mucosal pathogen (*Streptococcus mutans*) and the subsequent feeding of transgenic plant tissue to elicit a secretory immune response, the results of the work were never reported in the scientific literature. Shortly afterward, in 1992, a paper describing the expression of hepatitis B surface antigen (HBsAg) in tobacco plants was published by Mason et al. [13], who proposed that this recombinant protein produced in plants could serve as a vaccine candidate. Following the publication of their pioneering paper, Arntzen and Mason continued to develop the concept of plant-based vaccines and reported on their work in a succession of papers. The initial report focused on the expression and structural consideration of the plant-produced HBsAg, which assembled into 22-nm virus-like particles (VLPs) similarly to the yeast-derived commercial vaccine antigen. Partially purified and concentrated tobacco-derived HBsAg was used in parenteral immunization experiments in mice, demonstrating its ability to invoke the expected B and T lymphocytic responses [14]. In order to further prove that plant-derived HBsAg could stimulate mucosal immune responses via an oral route, the group refocused their attention to expression in potato tubers [11]. Surprisingly, the plant-derived material proved superior to the yeast-derived antigen in both priming and boosting immune responses in mice [11,15]. Success in these preclinical trials led to Phase I clinical trials with HBsAg potatoes (Thanavala, Mason, and Arntzen, submitted for publication). To complement the efforts with HBV vaccine, Arntzen and Mason explored plant expression of other vaccine candidates following essentially the same experimental approach. Progress on two of these antigens, the labile toxin B subunit (LT-B) of enterotoxigenic *E. coli* (ETEC) and the capsid protein of Norwalk virus (NVCP), actually occurred more rapidly than did their work on HBsAg [16–20]. These antigens of two important enteric pathogens may represent examples of the ideal oral subunit vaccine candidate. Both are oligomers: LT-B is a pentamer, which has a high affinity to GM_1 gangliosides present on mucosal cells [16], whereas NVCP can form VLPs [19]. Furthermore, both have evolved to survive the extreme conditions of the stomach and infect (in the case of NV) or colonize (in the case of *E. coli*) the gut epithelium.

Another apparent advantage associated with plant expression of these proteins was accumulation to higher levels in potato tuber than that seen with HBsAg. Significantly, both assembled correctly into functional oligomers that could elicit oral immune responses in animals [17,19] and humans [18,20]. The Phase I clinical trial with potato tubers expressing LT-B not only provided the proof of concept that orally delivered, plant-based vaccines could result in an immune response in humans, but also shared the distinction of being one of the first experiments with a pharmaceutical product derived from a transgenic plant that were conducted in humans. Results of a clinical experiment with plant-derived monoclonal antibodies against *S. mutans* were published in the same issue of *Nature Medicine* [21].

The clinical trials were intended to test both the safety and immunogenicity of plant-produced LT-B, NVCP, and HBsAg (Phase I/II) [18,20] (Thanavala et al., unpublished manuscript). In all three trials, individuals who consumed raw potato tubers containing 0.3–1.0 mg of the antigens developed antibody responses. It is important to note that three very different pathogens are represented by the three antigens and represent viral (NV and HBV), bacterial (*E. coli*), enteric (NV and *E. coli*), as well as nonenteric (HBV) organisms. The titers of mucosal and systemic antibodies in some of the test subjects suggest that they would be protected from infection [18,20] and provide the basis for anticipated wider-scale clinical trials with these antigens.

V. PLANT-DERIVED VACCINES CAN PROVIDE PROTECTION AGAINST A PATHOGEN CHALLENGE

The initial successes of early clinical trials encouraged other groups to explore the ability of plants to produce, fold, and assemble other vaccine candidates for the prevention of human and animal diseases. Various laboratories reported on efforts to produce transgenic plant-based vaccines for oral delivery to protect against human viruses such as rabies [22], respiratory syncytial virus (RSV) [23], measles [24], rotavirus [25–27], hepatitis B [28], and human cytomegalovirus [29,30]. Advances toward plant-based vaccines targeting cholera [27,31–33] and ETEC [27,34] were also reported.

Plant-derived oral vaccines for veterinary use are aimed at foot and mouth disease virus (FMDV) [35–38], swine-transmissible gastroenteritis virus (TGEV) [10,39–41], rabbit hemorrhagic disease virus [42], and *Mannheimia haemolytica*, the bacterial agent that causes shipping fever [43].

Although high titers of secretory and circulating antibodies following oral vaccination with plant-derived vaccines is an important immune correlate, proof of efficacy requires that vaccination results in immune system memory to provide long-lasting protection against a pathogen challenge. In a few cases [17], surrogate protection assays have been performed. By contrast, veterinary vaccines provide an opportunity to assess the degree of immune protection more directly. The series of papers published by Carrillo et al. [35,36] and Wigdorovitz et al. [37] serves as an excellent example of this methodological approach in a veterinary context. Their first report described the use of a model plant system (*Arabidopsis thaliana*) for the expression of the VP1 protein of FMDV [35]. Plant extracts containing VP1 provided full protection in mice after parenteral delivery and constituted the first demonstration of protection by a recombinant vaccine candidate produced in transgenic plants. Further studies using a larger number of mice immunized with extracts from transgenic potatoes [36] corroborated the initial work. They next expressed VP1 in alfalfa and delivered the transgenic plant material orally to mice. Despite low antigen expression, they achieved 70% protection against a virulent challenge after repeated oral boosting [37].

VI. FORMING MULTIVALENT AND MULTICOMPONENT VACCINES

The design of vaccines to stimulate several facets of the immune system, such as induction of strong humoral and mucosal responses as well as effective cellular immune responses, is highly desirable. Similarly, combination vaccines targeting multiple pathogens in one formulation are preferred. Therefore, developing both multivalent and multicomponent plant-based vaccines provides both efficacious and cost-effective immunization strategies. Plants harboring transgenes encoding the antigens of several pathogens—either by direct transformation or sexual crosses of individually transformed lines, or the blending of separately transformed plant tissues—can easily fulfill this need.

An alternative approach to achieve the same goal was taken by Yu and Langridge [27]. In their paper, they describe a recombinant multicomponent vaccine based on cholera toxin (CT). They fused peptides containing important protective epitopes derived from two other enteric pathogens—ETEC, which causes bacterial traveler's diarrhea, and rotavirus, which causes acute viral gastroenteritis—to the CT-A2 and CT-B subunits of CT, respectively. The two recombinant CT subunit fusions were expressed from a single bidirectional promoter, ensuring a coordinated expression pattern for the two gene fusions and potentially facilitating the assembly of the chimeric holotoxin. In this approach, CT provides a scaffold for presentation of the protective epitopes, acts as a mucosal targeting molecule without toxic effect due to use of the nontoxic CT-A2 and B subunits, and is itself a vaccine candidate. The recombinant protein represents a trivalent vaccine that can elicit significant mucosal and humoral responses against *Vibrio cholerae*, ETEC, and rotavirus. Mice, orally immunized with potatoes expressing these recombinant antigens, developed immune memory B cells as well as helper T cell type 1 (Th1) responses, which are indicators of successful immunization. Further, pups of immunized dams were protected from challenge with rotavirus, with a significantly lower morbidity rate as compared to controls. These results provide robust evidence for a vaccine strategy employing chimeric microbiological proteins expressed in plants.

VII. PLANT–VIRAL VECTORS AS ALTERNATIVE EXPRESSION SYSTEMS

Low-level antigen expression in transgenic plants (0.01–2% of total soluble protein) remains a critical issue. Up to three doses of 100 g of raw potato tubers expressing LT-B were needed in the clinical trials described above to elicit a significant immune response [18,20]. It is likely that antigens with less immunogenic potential would require substantially larger doses to be effective. Even with more palatable alternatives to potatoes, such as tomatoes, low levels of antigen expression could severely limit the utility of any vaccine product.

Recently, plant viral expression vectors have been constructed to allow efficient expression of recombinant proteins in plants [44–46]. These vectors are transgenic viruses incorporating a foreign gene that expresses a recombinant product as the virus spreads throughout the plant. Although plant virus-based vectors have been useful in directing the expression of medically important transgenes, such as single-chain antibodies [47] and a hepatitis C virus hypervariable region 1/CT-B fusion [48], there may be certain insert size limitations. Alternatively, some plant virus vectors make use of coat–protein peptide fusions [49–51]. Viral vectors based on tobamoviruses, such as tobacco mosaic virus, have received the most attention [48,51–53]. Other plant virus vectors that have been described are based on potyviruses (e.g., plum poxvirus) [54], comoviruses (e.g., cowpea mosaic virus) [53,55,56], and bromoviruses (e.g., alfalfa mosaic virus) [57].

The selection of antigens expressed by viral vectors is also impressive, including bacterial pathogens such as *V. cholerae* [27,48], *Staphylococcus aureus* [58], and *Pseudomonas aeruginosa* [53,59,60]. An even larger selection of viral antigens has been expressed via plant viral vectors such as hepatitis C virus [48], RSV [57], rotavirus [61], human immunodeficiency virus [49,62,63], rabies [49,51], mink enteritis virus [56], canine parvovirus [56,64,65], FMDV [38], and rabbit hemorrhagic disease virus [54].

In most cases, viral vectors result in increased accumulation of the expressed recombinant antigens. Accumulation levels of the FMDV VP1 protein were low when the gene was expressed in stably transformed plants on the order of 0.005–0.01% total soluble protein [35,36,38], but were substantially higher when the antigen was expressed using a tobamovirus vector, approaching up to 150 µg/g fresh weight, or approximately 15% total protein [38]. Interestingly, it is not uncommon to see similarly high levels of expression of stably integrated recombinant gene products in transgenic seeds without the use of viral vectors [10]. The success of viral expression vectors relies primarily on the fact that plant viruses are very efficient pathogens, employing very small genomes to infect their hosts. However, disadvantages include genetic instability due to recombination among viruses to remove inserted sequences, a requirement for individual plant inoculation and environmental concerns regarding the release of agronomically important plant pathogens. All of these issues will need to be addressed with further research if viral vectors are to become a successful alternative to current plant transformation systems.

VIII. PLASTID TRANSFORMATION

Over the past several years, data have been published on the transformation and expression of transgenes in plant chloroplasts, thereby taking advantage of the semiautonomous genetic machinery of these organelles [8,66–68]. Potential advantages of this system are high ploidy state, high transcription and translation rates, and the lack of gene silencing, all of which can contribute to high levels of foreign protein accumulation. Although site-directed integration through homologous recombination appears to be a requirement, it might also provide more control of genetic engineering and increased uniformity of transgene expression [8,67, 69,70]. Additionally, one can make use of polycistronic operons, much like a bacterial system, to permit coordinated expression of multiple genes [70,71]. Lastly, and of great importance particularly for biopharmaceutical crops, environmental transgene containment is ensured through the strictly maternal inheritance of plastids in most species [72].

Direct transformation of chloroplasts results in high levels of protein accumulation, up to several percent of total soluble protein, which is considerably more than those reported for other systems. In one case involving an operon from *Bacillus thuringiensis*, more than 40% was reported [70]. Pharmaceutically important proteins expressed in plastids include human somatotropin [67], a biodegradable synthetic polymer [73], and also CT-B as a vaccine candidate [33].

Plastid transformation has recently been extended to the experimental model plant *A. thaliana* [74] and two important solanaceous crop species, potato [75] and tomato [68]. In relation to the latter two crops, transgene expression and recombinant protein accumulation were observed to occur in plastids that are specific for these two plants: potato tuber amyloplasts and tomato fruit chromoplasts. This is of particular importance because it provides expression in the edible tissues of these plants.

Unique advantages and disadvantages of plastid expression depend on the prokaryotic nature of the organelle, but so do its shortcomings. For example, *N*-glycosylation strictly depends on the endomembrane system, which might preclude utility for viral antigens. However, in the case of prokaryotic antigens, or proteins and antigens that do not need to be glycosylated, plastids may offer some distinct advantages.

IX. OTHER TARGETS OF PLANT-EXPRESSED ANTIGENS

Transgenic plants have been proposed for the production of autoantigens. One concept is the expression of human autoantigens to treat autoimmune diseases by tolerizing the immune system rather than stimulating it. An autoantigen implicated in diabetes, glutamic acid dehydrogenase (GAD), was produced in plants and fed to nude obese diabetic (NOD) mice, which have a particular susceptibility to the development of diabetes. This resulted in a reduction in pancreatic islet inflammation, an indication that immunotolerance had occurred [76]. Arakawa et al. [77] used a similar approach by feeding plant tissues expressing either proinsulin or a CT-B/proinsulin fusion to NOD mice, and they also observed a reduction in pancreatitis. This result suggested that they had immunotolerized the mice against this type of cytotoxic T cell-mediated autoimmune disease. In this case, reduction of pancreatic inflammation coincided with increase in anti-insulin antibodies, mostly of the IgG1 isotype, leading to the conclusion that the cytotoxic T-cell response is suppressed. They were able to enhance this effect with the addition of a second antigen fusion, CT-B/GAD. It is interesting to note that the reduction in pancreatitis was considerably greater with the fusions than with the autoantigens alone, supporting targeting or adjuvant activity due to the CT-B component. We should also mention the differences in feeding protocols used in these two experiments. Ma et al. [76] fed very large amounts of recombinant GAD (1–1.5 mg/mouse/day) daily for 4 weeks, a more frequently used toleration protocol. Arakawa et al. [77], on the other hand, fed potato containing 20 µg of the CT-B–proinsulin fusion protein in five doses over a 4-week period, which is almost identical to the feeding regimen they had reported to be effective in eliciting protective immune responses against foreign antigens [27]. As Arakawa et al. suggested in their paper and as mentioned above, perhaps the fusion to CT-B may facilitate the presentation of the antigen to the gut-associated lymphoid tissue to enhance the response. The control of mammalian wild species experiencing overpopulation in a humane and effective manner through the use of edible immunocontraceptive vaccines provides another option for the technology [78,79]. The approach is used to express in plants a protein or a carrier protein harboring an antigenic epitope of an essential component of the mammalian reproductive system with the intention of inducing a humoral response, upon feeding by the animal, that results in sterility. The animal would remain sterile coincident with immune memory, or until the next boosting vaccination. Antigenic targets reportedly under investigation include the gonadotropin-releasing hormone and ZP3 from the zona pellucida of the mammalian ovulated egg [79,80]. Although effectiveness is still under study, this application is bound to meet considerable objections, the principal one of which is the danger these broadly cross-reacting vaccines potentially present to other mammalian species that will have access to them. This is a legitimate environmental concern that must be addressed.

X. ISSUES AND CHALLENGES

The remarkable growth of the field of plant-produced, orally delivered vaccines, from its germination well over a decade ago in a couple of laboratories to a research area involving many laboratories around the world, has occurred despite initial skepticism by many in the scientific, and particularly the immunology, community. The idea was initially advocated principally by plant biologists, yet has advanced to date through three successful Phase I human clinical trials. Successful development of the technology comes in spite of deficiencies in our understanding of mucosal immunity. In fact, many of the original criticisms are still valid and we have been able to identify other areas that will require investigation in order to bring this technology out of the laboratory to become a functional reality. These issues should be seen as challenges rather than impenetrable roadblocks.

In no particular order, we see issues associated with addressing concerns about oral tolerance; the identification and use of oral adjuvants; the potential impact of glycosylation of antigen proteins in plants, dosing concentration and timing, selection of the optimal plant production system, and control of antigen expression within the plant to enhance expression level; and location and the determination of processing protocols for optimal delivery to both facilitate patient compliance and enhance the immune response.

The concept of an edible vaccine presents itself to some immunologists as a contradiction in terms. They argue that the most common response to food antigens is an induced state of specific unresponsiveness, which is called oral tolerance [83–85]. From a tolerance perspective, we must be cognitive of the fact that tolerance plays an important role in the response of the host to environmental antigens and to resident microflora. At the very least, it certainly would be counterproductive should a vaccine candidate induce long-term tolerance rather than a protective immune response.

The issue is further complicated by reports in the literature of the use of comparable experimental approaches with similar constructs and feeding regimens to induce either immune responses or tolerance [27,77]. The issue of oral tolerance is quite controversial within the immunology community, reflecting the complexity of the phenomenon. Clearly, avoidance of tolerance to antigenic determinants of pathogens delivered via plant-based vaccines is critical. Dosing regimens must be employed to prevent such an outcome. Additionally, optimal concentration of antigen provided in both primary inoculum and subsequent boosting, as well as the timing of the boosting, will need to be determined empirically. Due to the high levels of antigen anticipated to be necessary for oral delivery and appropriate stimulation of the mucosa-associated lymphoid tissue, it is likely that some sort of adjuvant will be required for optimal response. Identification of appropriate adjuvants is another focus of research in this area. The inclusion of nontoxic mutant forms of CT or LT as part of a formulation may be one approach [86], whereas the identification of additional potential oral adjuvants should also be pursued. For example, plant products such as lectins and saponins are being explored for their oral adjuvanticity [62,81,82].

We know that plants glycosylate proteins and this can be used to our advantage. However, we also know that carbohydrate side chains, while added at the same sites in plants and animals, have slightly different structures. What we do not know is if that is, or will be, important in the immune response. In some instances, it has been reported that the expression levels of the antigens are so low and that an unrealistic quantity of plant material would have to be consumed to achieve meaningful immune responses. As a result, concerns regarding the unpredictable and highly variable levels of expression are relevant. These are recurrent problematic themes that can be solved by improving the expression systems. Careful identification and selection of the host plant married to optimization of expression vectors and/or novel expression systems may provide a solution to low expression level. Furthermore, compartmentalization of expression in discrete tissues may provide additional benefits with regard to controlled expression, level of protein antigen produced, and stability, and may also impact processing concerns. In fact, minimal processing and creation of edible vaccine "batches" may contribute to a solution of the variability problem. Currently available food processing technologies may be employed to generate formulations that are not only more concentrated but have delivery advantages as well (Kirk, in preparation). It is important to note that even with the limitations of variable and/or modest antigen levels, edible vaccines were able to establish clinically relevant immune responses in adult human volunteers. Further research can only lead to improvements in the system.

REFERENCES

1. Curtiss R III, Cardineau GA. Oral Immunization by Transgenic Plants. World Intellectual Property Organization, 1990; PCT/US89/03799.
2. Arntzen CJ, Mason HS. Oral vaccine production in the edible tissues of transgenic plants. In: Levine MM, Woodrow

GC, Kaper JB, Cobon GS, eds. New Generation Vaccines. 2d ed. New York: Marcel Dekker, 1997:263–277.

3. Mason HS, Arntzen CJ. Transgenic plants as vaccine production systems. Trends Biotechnol 1995; 13:388–392.

4. Mor TS, et al. Edible vaccines: a concept comes of age. Trends Microbiol 1998; 6:449–453.

5. Fischer R, et al. Towards molecular farming in the future: moving from diagnostic protein and antibody production in microbes to plants. Biotechnol Appl Biochem 1999; 30:101–108.

6. Tacket CO, Mason HS. A review of oral vaccination with transgenic vegetables. Microbes Infect 1999; 1:777–783.

7. Walmsley AM, Arntzen CJ. Plants for delivery of edible vaccines. Curr Opin Biotechnol 2000; 11:126–129.

8. Daniell H, et al. Medical molecular farming: production of antibodies, biopharmaceuticals and edible vaccines in plants. Trends Plant Sci 2001; 6:9–226.

9. Koprowski H, Yusibov V. The green revolution: plants as heterologous expression vectors. Vaccine 2000 19:2735–2741.

10. Streatfield SJ, et al. Plant-based vaccines: unique advantages. Vaccine 2001; 19:2742–2748.

11. Richter LJ, et al. Production of hepatitis B surface antigen in transgenic plants for oral immunization. Nat Biotechnol 2000; 18:1167–1171.

12. Curtiss R III. Genetically modified plants for use as oral immunogens. Mucosal Immunol Update 1999; 7:9–11.

13. Mason HS, et al. Expression of hepatitis B surface antigen in transgenic plants. Proc Natl Acad Sci USA 1992; 89:11745–11749.

14. Thanavala Y, et al. Immunogenicity of transgenic plant-derived hepatitis B surface antigen. Proc Natl Acad Sci USA 1995; 92:3358–3361.

15. Kong Q, et al. Oral immunization with hepatitis B surface antigen expressed in transgenic plants. Proc Natl Acad Sci USA 2001; 98:11539–11544.

16. Haq TA, et al. Oral Immunization with a recombinant bacterial antigen produced in transgenic plants. Science 1995; 268:714–716.

17. Mason HS, et al. Edible vaccine protects mice against E. coli heat-labile enterotoxin (LT): potatoes expressing a synthetic LT-B gene. Vaccine 1998; 16:1336–1343.

18. Tacket CO, et al. Immunogenicity in humans of a recombinant bacterial-antigen delivered in transgenic potato. Nat Med 1998; 4:607–609.

19. Mason HS, et al. Expression of Norwalk virus capsid protein in transgenic tobacco and protein and its oral immunogenicity in mice. Proc Natl Acad Sci USA 1996; 93: 5335–5340.

20. Tacket CO, et al. Human immune responses to a novel Norwalk virus vaccine delivered in transgenic potatoes. J Infect Dis 2000; 182:302–305.

21. Ma JK, et al. Characterization of a recombinant plant monoclonal secretory antibody and preventive immunotherapy in humans. Nat Med 1998; 4:601–606.

22. McGarvey PB, et al. Expression of the rabies virus glycoprotein in transgenic tomatoes. Bio/technology 1995; 13: 1484–1487.

23. Sandhu JS, et al. Oral immunization of mice with transgenic tomato fruit expressing respiratory syncytial virus-F protein induces a systemic immune response. Transgenic Res 2000; 9:127–135.

24. Huang Z, et al. Plant-derived measles virus hemagglutinin protein induces neutralizing antibodies in mice. Vaccine 2001; 19:2163–2171.

25. Mor TS, et al. Expression of rotavirus proteins in transgenic plants. In: Altman A, Ziv M, Izhar S, eds. Plant Biotechnology and In Vitro Biology in the 21st Century. Dordrecht: Kluwer, 1998:521–524.

26. Chung IS, et al. Production of recombinant rotavirus VP6 from a suspension culture of transgenic tomato (Lycopersicon esculentum Mill.) cells. Biotechnol Lett 2000; 22:251–255.

27. Yu J, Langridge WH. A plant-based multicomponent vaccine protects mice from enteric diseases. Nat Biotechnol 2001; 19:548–552.

28. Kapusta J, et al. A plant-derived edible vaccine against hepatitis B virus. FASEB J 1999; 13:1796–1799. [published erratum appears in FASEB J 1999; 13 (15):2339].

29. Tackaberry ES, et al. Development of biopharmaceuticals in plant expression systems: cloning, expression and immunological reactivity of human cytomegalovirus glycoprotein B (UL55) in seeds of transgenic tobacco. Vaccine 1999; 17: 3020–3029.

30. Wright KE, et al. Sorting of glycoprotein B from human cytomegalovirus to protein storage vesicles in seeds of transgenic tobacco. Transgenic Res 2001; 10:177–181.

31. Arakawa T, et al. Expression of cholera toxin B subunit oligomers in transgenic potato plants. Transgenic Res 1997; 6:403–413.

32. Arakawa T, et al. Efficacy of a food plant based oral cholera toxin B subunit vaccine. Nat Biotechnol 1998; 16:292–297.

33. Daniell H, et al. Expression of the native cholera toxin b subunit gene and assembly as functional oligomers in transgenic tobacco chloroplasts. J Mol Biol 2001; 311:1001–1009.

34. Lauterslager TG, et al. Oral immunization of naive and primed animals with transgenic potato tubers expressing LT-B. Vaccine 2001; 19:2749–2755.

35. Carrillo C, et al. Protective immune response to foot-and-mouth disease virus with VP1 expressed in transgenic plants. J Virol 1998; 72:1688–1690.

36. Carrillo C, et al. Induction of a virus-specific antibody response to foot and mouth disease virus using the structural protein VP1 expressed in transgenic potato plants. Viral Immunol 2001; 14:49–57.

37. Wigdorovitz A, et al. Induction of a protective antibody response to foot and mouth disease virus in mice following oral or parenteral immunization with alfalfa transgenic plants expressing the viral structural protein VP1. Virology 1999; 255:347–353.

38. Wigdorovitz A, et al. Protection of mice against challenge with foot and mouth disease virus (FMDV) by immunization with foliar extracts from plants infected with recombinant tobacco mosaic virus expressing the FMDV structural protein VP1. Virology 1999; 264:85–91.

39. Gomez N, et al. Expression of immunogenic glycoprotein S polypeptides from transmissible gastroenteritis coronavirus in transgenic plants. Virology 1998; 249:352–358.

40. Gomez N, et al. Oral immunogenicity of the plant derived spike protein from swine-transmissible gastroenteritis coronavirus. Arch Virol 2000; 145:1725–1732.

41. Tuboly T, et al. Immunogenicity of porcine transmissible gastroenteritis virus spike protein expressed in plants. Vaccine 2000; 18:2023–2028.

42. Castanon S, et al. Immunization with potato plants expressing VP60 protein protects against rabbit hemorrhagic disease virus. J Virol 1999; 73:4452–4455.

43. Lee RW, et al. Towards development of an edible vaccine against bovine pneumonic pasteurellosis using transgenic white clover expressing a Mannheimia haemolytica A1 leukotoxin 50 fusion protein. Infect Immun 2001; 69:5786–5793.

44. Timmermans MCP, et al. Geminiviruses and their uses as extrachromosomal replicons. Annu Rev Plant Physiol Plant Mol Biol 1994; 45:79–112.

45. Scholthof HB, et al. Plant virus gene vectors for transient expression of foreign proteins in plants. Annu Rev Phytopathol, 1996; 34:299–323.

46. Palmer KE, Rybicki EP. The use of geminiviruses in biotechnology and plant biology, with particular focus on Mastreviruses. Plant Sci 1997; 129:115–130.

47. McCormick AA, et al. Rapid production of specific vaccines for lymphoma by expression of the tumor-derived single-chain Fv epitopes in tobacco plants. Proc Natl Acad Sci USA 1999; 96:703–708.

48. Nemchinov LG, et al. Development of a plant-derived sub-unit vaccine candidate against hepatitis C virus. Arch Virol 2000; 145:2557–2573.

49. Yusibov V, et al. Antigens produced in plants by infection with chimeric plant viruses immunize against rabies virus and HIV-1. Proc Natl Acad Sci USA 1997; 94:5784–5788.

50. Johnson J, et al. Presentation of heterologous peptides on plant viruses: genetics, structure and function. Annu Rev Phytopathol 1997; 35:67–86.

51. Modelska A, et al. Immunization against rabies with plant-derived antigen. Proc Natl Acad Sci USA 1998; 95:2481–2485.

52. Turpen TH. Tobacco mosaic virus and the virescence of biotechnology. Philos Trans R Soc Lond B Biol Sci 1999; 354:665–673.

53. Gilleland HE, et al. Chimeric animal and plant viruses expressing epitopes of outer membrane protein F as a combined vaccine against *Pseudomonas aeruginosa* lung infection. FEMS Immunol Med Microbiol 2000; 27:291–29.

54. Fernandez-Fernandez MR, et al. Protection of rabbits against rabbit hemorrhagic disease virus by immunization with the VP60 protein expressed in plants with a potyvirus-based vector. Virology 2001; 280:283–291.

55. Brennan FR, et al. Cowpea mosaic virus as a vaccine carrier of heterologous antigens. Mol Biotechnol 2001; 17:15–26.

56. Dalsgaard K, et al. Plant-derived vaccine protects target animals against a viral disease. Nat Biotechnol 1997; 15:248–252.

57. Belanger H, et al. Human respiratory syncytial virus vaccine antigen produced in plants. FASEB J 2000; 14:2323–2328.

58. Brennan FR, et al. Immunogenicity of peptides derived from a fibronectin-binding protein of *S. aureus* expressed on two different plant viruses. Vaccine 1999; 17:1846–1857.

59. Brennan FR, et al. *Pseudomonas aeruginosa* outer-membrane protein F epitopes are highly immunogenic in mice when expressed on a plant virus. Microbiology 1999; 145: 211–220.

60. Staczek J, et al. Immunization with a chimeric tobacco mosaic virus containing an epitope of outer membrane protein F of *Pseudomonas aeruginosa* provides protection against challenge with *P. aeruginosa*. Vaccine 2000; 18: 2266–2274.

61. O'Brien GJ, et al. Rotavirus VP6 expressed by PVX vectors in *Nicotiana benthamiana* coats PVX rods and also assembles into virus-like particles. Virology 2000; 270:444–453.

62. McInerney TL, et al. Analysis of the ability of five adjuvants to enhance immune responses to a chimeric plant virus displaying an HIV-1 peptide. Vaccine 1999; 17:1359–1368.

63. Marusic C, et al. Chimeric plant virus particles as immunogens for inducing murine and human immune responses against human immunodeficiency virus type 1. J Virol 2001; 75:8434–8439.

64. Gil F, et al. High-yield expression of a viral peptide vaccine in transgenic plants. FEBS Lett 2001; 488:13–17.

65. Langeveld JP, et al. Inactivated recombinant plant virus protects dogs from a lethal challenge with canine parvovirus. Vaccine 2001; 19:3661–3670.

66. Heifetz PB. Genetic engineering of the chloroplast. Biochimie 2000; 82:655–666.

67. Staub JM, et al. High-yield production of a human therapeutic protein in tobacco chloroplasts. Nat Biotechnol 2000; 18:333–338.

68. Ruf S, et al. Stable genetic transformation of tomato plastids and expression of a foreign protein in fruit. Nat Biotechnol 2001; 19:870–875.

69. McBride KE, et al. Amplification of a chimeric *Bacillus* gene in chloroplasts leads to an extraordinary level of an insecticidal protein in tobacco. Bio/technology 1995; 13:362–365.

70. De Cosa B, et al. Overexpression of the Bt cry2Aa2 operon in chloroplasts leads to formation of insecticidal crystals. Nat Biotechnol 2001; 19:71–74.

71. Staub JM, Maliga P. Expression of a chimeric *uidA* gene indicates that polycistronic mRNAs are efficiently translated in tobacco plastids. Plant J 1995; 7:845–848.

72. Daniell H, et al. Containment of herbicide resistance through genetic engineering of the chloroplast genome. Nat Biotechnol 1998; 16:345–348.

73. Guda C, et al. Stable expression of a biodegradable protein-based polymer in tobacco protoplasts. Plant Cell Rep 2000; 19:257–262.

74. Sikdar SR, et al. Plastid transformation in *Arabidopsis thaliana*. Plant Cell Rep 1998; 18:20–24.

75. Sidorov VA, et al. Technical Advance: stable chloroplast transformation in potato: use of green fluorescent protein as a plastid marker. Plant J 1999; 19:209–216.

76. Ma SW, et al. Transgenic plants expressing autoantigens fed to mice to induce oral immune tolerance. Nat Med 1997; 3:793–796.

77. Arakawa T, et al. A plant-based cholera toxin B subunit–insulin fusion protein protects against the development of autoimmune diabetes. Nat Biotechnol 1998; 16:934–938.

78. Smith G, et al. Plant-derived immunocontraceptive vaccines. Reprod Fertil Dev 1997; 9:85–89.

79. Walmsley AM, et al. Transgenic plants as vectors for delivery of animal immunocontraceptive vaccines. FASEB J 1999; 13:A290.

80. Fitchen J, et al. Plant virus expressing hybrid coat protein with added murine epitope elicits autoantibody response. Vaccine 1995; 13, 1051–1057.

81. Singh M, O'Hagan D. Advances in vaccine adjuvants. Nat Biotechnol 1999; 17:1075–1081.

82. Lavelle EC, et al. The identification of plant lectins with mucosal adjuvant activity. Immunology 2001; 102:77–86.

83. Simecka JW. Mucosal immunity of the gastrointestinal tract and oral tolerance. Adv Drug Deliv Rev 1998; 34:235–259.

84. Mayer L, et al. Oral tolerance to protein antigens. Allergy 2001; 56:12–15.

85. Garside P, Mowat AM. Oral tolerance. Semin Immunol 2001; 13:177–185.

86. Dickinson BL, Clements JD. Use of *Escherichia coli* heat-labile enterotoxin as an oral adjuvant. In: Kiyono H, Ogra PL, McGhee JR, eds. Mucosal Vaccines. San Diego: Academic Press, Inc., 1996:73–87.

27

Vaccinia Virus and Other Poxviruses as Live Vectors

Bernard Moss

National Institute of Allergy and Infectious Diseases, National Institutes of Health, Bethesda, Maryland, U.S.A.

I. VACCINIA VIRUS AS A HUMAN VACCINE FOR SMALLPOX

On May 14, 1796, Edward Jenner inoculated 8-year-old James Phipps with cowpox virus obtained from an infection on the hand of Sarah Nelmes, a milkmaid. Subsequent events established that this simple procedure provided complete protection against smallpox and formed the basis for its ultimate eradication: The last case of endemic smallpox was in 1977 [1]. The prophylactic effect of vaccination was due to the close genetic and antigenic relationships between variola virus, the causative agent of smallpox, and its more benign relatives cowpox virus and vaccinia virus. The latter virus may have been isolated from an infected horse and, presumably because of its milder reactivity, was substituted for cowpox virus [2]. Vaccinia virus was economical to produce, active in low amounts, heat stable, resistant to freeze drying, simple to administer, relatively safe, and provided long-lasting immunity. Of equal importance for smallpox eradication, however, were the ease of diagnosis of the disease, variola's lack of antigenic variation, and the absence of latently infected human or animal reservoirs. Although the vaccine was immediately successful, eradication of smallpox proved difficult for logistical reasons. In 1967, the World Health Organization implemented a new intensified global ring vaccination strategy that ultimately contained and eliminated variola virus from nature. Nevertheless, registered stocks of variola virus are preserved in both the United States and Russia. With the eradication of smallpox, the general need for vaccination was eliminated and the practice largely stopped. As a result, most people are now susceptible to variola virus, as well as other orthopoxviruses such as monkeypox virus. As a precaution against the possible reintroduction by terrorists of variola virus from an unregistered stock, a new tissue-culture-derived vaccinia virus vaccine will soon be available. In addition, attenuated strains of vaccinia virus are being evaluated as safer alternatives to the conventional vaccine.

Soon after the eradication of smallpox and the cessation of general vaccination, the ability to produce recombinant vaccinia viruses that express genes of other microorganisms was developed [3,4]. Such genetically engineered viruses have been used extensively as research tools to establish the targets of humoral and cell-mediated immunity and are being evaluated as live recombinant vaccines. Similar approaches have been used to generate immunogenic avipoxvirus recombinants [5,6] and could be applied to other poxviruses.

II. CONSTRUCTION OF POXVIRUS EXPRESSION VECTORS

A. Insertion of Foreign DNA into the Poxvirus Genome

The development of expression vectors depended on an understanding of the molecular biology of poxviruses, a subject that is reviewed in detail elsewhere [7]. The distinctive characteristics of vaccinia virus (and other poxviruses) include the following: a large, complex, enveloped virion containing enzymes for mRNA synthesis; a genome composed of a linear, double-stranded DNA molecule of about 200,000 base pairs; and the ability to replicate within the cytoplasm of infected cells. Detailed protocols for preparing and characterizing recombinant vaccinia viruses are available [8–11] and only general concepts are dealt with here.

The large size of the vaccinia virus genome posed an initial hurdle to the incorporation of foreign genetic material. In addition, the viral DNA is not infectious because enzymes contained within the virion are essential for gene expression. However, it was known that recombination occurs between homologous DNA sequences of poxviruses [12]. Furthermore, recombination was shown to occur between virus-derived genomic DNA and either subgenomic DNA fragments [13,14] or recombinant plasmids [15] that had been transfected into the cell. The latter finding provided a way of inserting foreign DNA into the vaccinia virus genome: A plasmid containing a foreign gene flanked with vaccinia DNA is transfected into an infected cell, allowing homologous recombination to occur during DNA replication.

Of course, for the recombinant vaccinia virus to remain infectious, the foreign DNA must not interrupt any vital viral function. This was not an obstacle, however, because there are many nonessential vaccinia virus genes and it is possible to insert DNA between genes. In this manner, foreign DNA segments as large as 25,000 base pairs were recombined into the vaccinia virus genome [16]. Several methods are available to select recombinant viruses or distinguish the plaques from the parental virus. Similar methods have been used to generate recombinant avian poxviruses.

Two additional methods have been used to form recombinant vaccinia viruses. Both depend on the in vitro cleavage of the vaccinia virus genome at a unique restriction endonuclease site. In one procedure, a DNA fragment containing the foreign DNA is ligated to the cleaved genome, which is then transfected into cells infected with a helper virus—either a temperature-sensitive vaccinia virus or an avian poxvirus [17,18]. The procedure is especially useful for very large DNA inserts or to avoid intermediate cloning in bacteria. Alternatively, three-way recombination can be achieved by transfecting the cleaved genome and a foreign DNA segment with flanking vaccinia virus sequences into cells infected with a helper virus [19,20].

B. Expression of Foreign Genes

Poxviruses encode their own transcription system, which includes a multisubunit RNA polymerase, stage-specific transcription factors, poly(A) polymerase, and capping and methylating enzymes [7]. Because the DNA sequences that are recognized by the viral transcription system are unique, the use of poxvirus promoters for foreign gene expression is obligatory. Vaccinia virus gene expression is temporally regulated: Early-stage genes are transcribed before DNA replication and intermediate and late-stage genes are transcribed after DNA replication. Some genes are expressed throughout infection because they have two promoters. A foreign gene inserted into the vaccinia virus genome will be regulated in a predictable manner, depending on the vaccinia virus promoter placed adjacent to it. In general, high expression is obtained by using late promoters derived from vaccinia virus genes encoding major structural proteins, but early or early/late promoters are best for expression in antigen-presenting cells and inducing cytotoxic T-cell responses [21,22]. Therefore, synthetic early/late promoters have been designed [23,24]. Because vaccinia virus can accommodate large amounts of additional DNA, multiple genes can be expressed using vaccinia virus vectors.

Care needs to be taken in choosing the form of the foreign gene to be expressed. Most importantly, only continuous open reading frames may be used, as splicing does not occur in the cytoplasm. This problem is avoided by using cDNA copies of mRNAs. In addition, any cryptic poxvirus early transcription termination signals, TTTTTNT in which N is any nucleotide, should be eliminated [25].

C. General Methods of Isolating Recombinant Poxviruses

Vaccinia virus is cytopathic and produces large plaques on monolayers of appropriate cell lines; most virus isolation procedures depend on the discrimination of plaques formed by parental and recombinant viruses. Recombinant viruses can be recognized by the presence of foreign DNA sequences or expression of the gene products. Thus, plaques can be screened by hybridization to specific DNA [26] or by binding to antibody [8]. However, because recombinants usually comprise less than 0.1% of the progeny, additional selection or screening methods have been devised.

To facilitate the process of recombinant virus formation, plasmid transfer vectors have been constructed in which a vaccinia virus promoter followed by unique restriction endonuclease sites has been inserted into the vaccinia virus DNA needed for homologous recombination. The first of these general transfer vectors used the vaccinia virus thymidine kinase (TK) gene as the site for promoter insertion to provide a method for the selection of recombinant viruses [27]. The selection depends on the disruption of the TK gene upon recombination of the foreign DNA into the vaccinia virus genome. The basis for the selection is the lethal effect of the incorporation of certain nucleoside analogs into viral DNA and the need for a functional TK for this to occur. Other selection approaches depend on the cotransfer of a dominant selectable marker along with the foreign gene. Genes encoding the neomycin-resistance [28], guanine phosphoribosyltransferase [29,30], hygromycin-resistance [31], puromycin-resistance [32], and herpes simplex virus TK [33] genes have been used for this purpose.

Several screening methods, some of which may be used in conjunction with selection procedures, have been developed. These include the cotransfer of the β-galactosidase [34], β-glucuronidase [35], or enhanced green fluorescent protein [36] genes, which allow the color staining or fluorescence of recombinant plaques. Still other screening methods depend on the plaque phenotype of the recombinant virus [37] or host range [38].

D. Hybrid Expression Vectors

A high-expression system with great utility for protein synthesis in cultured cells, rather than for live virus immunization, has been developed. This innovation took advantage of the bacteriophage T7 (or related SP6) RNA polymerase, which is a single-subunit enzyme with high catalytic activity and strict promoter specificity. By attaching a vaccinia virus promoter to the T7 or SP6 RNA polymerase gene, recombinant vaccinia viruses that express bacteriophage RNA polymerase have been constructed [39,40]. Cells are infected with the latter and then either transfected with a plasmid that has a foreign gene regulated by the bacteriophage promoter or coinfected with a second vaccinia virus that has the bacteriophage promoter regulated foreign gene [39,41]. Inducible systems have been developed in which both the T7 RNA polymerase gene and the T7 promoter regulated foreign gene are in the same virus [42]. Expression can be enhanced by inserting the untranslated leader sequence of encephalomyocarditis virus before the initiation codon [43].

E. Fidelity of Expression

Excellent results have been obtained using vaccinia virus vectors to express foreign genes from viral, prokaryotic, or eukaryotic sources. Factors that contribute to the high success rate include the cytoplasmic site of expression and concomitant use of vaccinia transcription factors. The cytoplasmic site avoids potential problems related to cryptic splice sites, processing, and nuclear-cytoplasmic transport. For example, the structural proteins of HIV-1 were expressed without the need for regulatory factors *rev* and *tat* [44,45].

The proteins made by recombinant vaccinia viruses are usually processed and transported in a manner similar to that occurring in uninfected cells. For example, N- and O-glycosylation [46], proteolytic cleavage [44,47], polarized membrane insertion [48], and nuclear transport [49] all occur. Biologically active enzymes, such as reverse transcriptase [45] and bacteriophage T7 RNA polymerase [45] and ion channel proteins [50] are made. Perhaps most striking is the expression of multiple genes by recombinant vaccinia virus leading to the assembly of infectious RNA virus particles [51–53].

III. RECOMBINANT VACCINIA VIRUS VACCINES

A. Experimental Vaccines

Vaccinia virus can infect most mammalian as well as avian species, making it a useful vector for studying the immune response to proteins of both human and veterinary pathogens. Recombinant vaccinia viruses are standard laboratory tools for defining protective antigens and fine-mapping immunogenic epitopes from infectious agents. Prophylactic, live recombinant vaccinia viruses have protected animals from challenge with numerous viruses, bacteria, and parasites [54]. In addition, poxvirus vectors expressing tumor antigens have been investigated for the immunoprophylaxis and immunotherapy of tumors in animal models [55–58].

B. Immunogenicity

A particular advantage of vaccinia virus as a recombinant vaccine vector is its ability to mimic the immune responses elicited by viral antigens during the course of a natural infection. Consequently, cell-mediated as well as humoral immunity is evoked [59]. Antibody responses induced by recombinant vaccinia virus can be as high as those induced by natural infection [60]. Mice vaccinated with a recombinant expressing herpes simplex virus (HSV) glycoprotein D were still protected from a lethal challenge with HSV one year after vaccination [61], and macaques vaccinated with a simian type D retrovirus (SRV-2) envelope glycoprotein recombinant were still protected against SRV-2 two years after vaccination [62].

Route and dose of vaccinia virus are important in eliciting efficient immune responses. Dermal inoculation is considered to be the most immunogenic route in man, apparently reflecting a preferred site of replication of orthopoxviruses as well as the presence of a large number of antigen-presenting cells. Percutaneous vaccination with vaccinia virus produced significantly higher antibody titers and a longer duration of immunity than subcutaneous vaccination [63,64]. Intramuscular vaccination of mice with a rabies virus nucleoprotein recombinant was substantially less im-

munogenic than intradermal inoculation [65]. In primate species, there was a linear relationship between the size of skin lesions formed by vaccinia/RSV recombinants and titers of RSV neutralizing antibody [66]. Intradermal vaccination of mice and hamsters with a vaccinia/influenza HA recombinant elicited mainly IgG, which prevented lower respiratory infection; intranasal inoculation induced secretory IgA production and prevented both upper and lower respiratory tract infections [67]. Limited testing of oral smallpox vaccine in humans indicated that vaccinia is immunogenic when administered by this route. Successful oral vaccinations of domestic and wild animals with vaccinia/rabies glycoprotein recombinants [68,69] may be mediated by replication in tonsillar or buccal tissue [70]. Furthermore, intrajejunal vaccination of mice with vaccinia-influenza recombinants leads to generalized mucosal immunity against influenza [71]. Oral or intranasal routes of inoculation could potentially be exploited with other vaccinia-based veterinary or human vaccines.

Although disease protection correlates with vaccine-induced antibody titers in some cases, other vaccinia recombinants appear to protect by priming for immunoglobulin and/or inducing effector lymphocyte responses. In some cases, it is difficult to discriminate between these two possibilities. A vaccinia/hepatitis B surface antigen (HBsAg) recombinant failed to stimulate protective titers of anti-HBsAg antibody in chimpanzees, but did protect against disease. Apparently, vaccinated animals were primed for accelerated antibody production and possibly cell-mediated immunity [72]. Similarly, a recombinant expressing the bovine leukemia virus envelope glycoprotein failed to elicit neutralizing antibodies, but partially protected vaccinated animals presumably through induction of cell-mediated immunity [73]. When a recombinant virus expresses only internal structural or regulatory proteins, which cannot induce neutralizing antibody, protection is attributed to cytotoxic T-cell responses. For example, mice vaccinated with vaccinia/influenza nucleoprotein recombinants developed lower respiratory tract infections after challenge with influenza A virus, but had reduced symptoms, and some were protected from death [74]. The protection from influenza in mice vaccinated with vaccinia/influenza NP appeared to be CTL mediated, because vaccination was effective only in murine strains capable of generating a strong anti-NP CTL response. Similarly, recombinants expressing the rabies virus nucleoprotein did not prevent illness, but prevented fatal rabies in dogs [75]. A vaccinia recombinant expressing the murine cytomegalovirus immediate early protein pp89, an internal protein that regulates gene expression, afforded partial protection against a lethal challenge [76]. Depletion of vaccinated mice with anti-CD8 antiserum abrogated protection, and adoptive transfer of $CD8^+$ lymphocytes from vaccinia/pp89-primed animals into unvaccinated animals limited murine cytomegalovirus replication [76,77]. In addition, $CD4^+$ effector T cells may mediate the protective immunity induced by certain vaccinia/measles recombinants [78]. Recombinant vaccinia viruses that express simian immunodeficiency virus gag-pol proteins have provided protection in a monkey challenge model [79,80].

Effector T cells may also play a central role in the antitumor response elicited by vaccinia recombinants. Although antibodies to tumor antigens are often present postvaccination, CTLs were likely mediators of tumor regression in a murine mastocytoma model [81].

Several techniques have been developed to improve the immunogenicity of live recombinant vaccinia vaccines. Because the magnitude of the response may be dependent on the amount of foreign protein expressed, a high level of protein production is desirable. This can be achieved by using strong natural or synthetic vaccinia promoters [23,24, 82,83]. Elimination of cryptic vaccinia transcription termination sequences from an HIV envelope gene boosted the level of HIV env production in infected cells [25]. Moreover, the corresponding recombinant virus was more immunogenic than the vector containing the termination sequence, as determined by anti-gp160 antibody titers in vaccinated mice, and by enhanced lysis of infected human CTL target cells.

Immunogenicity may also be enhanced by altering protein presentation on the surface of infected cells. Fusion of a secreted malarial blood stage antigen to the murine immunoglobulin G transmembrane anchor sequence resulted in surface expression of the protein and a greatly enhanced antibody response [84]. A related strategy has been used in which repeating epitopes of the malarial circumsporozoite protein (CSP) were fused to the ectodomains of the RSV glycoprotein G, thereby enhancing anti-CSP antibody titers in vaccinated animals [85]. Elimination of proteolytic cleavage sites from the HIV env gene prevented release of gp120 from the env precursor gp160, and the resulting recombinant produced a stronger anti-gp120 antibody response in vaccinated animals, presumably by increasing the amount of surface-associated gp120 [86].

The incorporation of additional helper T-cell epitopes in expressed antigens may also increase immunogenicity through enhanced recruitment and proliferation of B cells. A short peptide derived from the sequence of the neutralizing epitope of the viral capsid protein VP1 of foot-and-mouth disease virus produced a weak antibody response in cattle and pigs. However, fusion of the VP1 epitope to hepatitis B core protein (HBcAg) led to a dramatic increase in antibody titers in animals vaccinated with the purified protein expressed by recombinant vaccinia virus and greatly enhanced virus neutralization [87]. Inclusion of murine helper T-cell epitopes led to increased titers of antimalarial antibodies in mice vaccinated with a CSP fusion construct [88].

Protein targeting may also enhance immunogenicity. Fusion of antigen genes to endoplasmic reticulum or lysosomal targeting sequences may direct expressed proteins into intracellular compartments where processing for antigenic recognition is facilitated, boosting the immune response to viral and tumor-associated antigens. In one case, endoplasmic reticulum targeting was reported to increase CD8$^+$ T-cell recognition of tumor cells [81]. Fusion of HIV gp160 sequences to the lysosomal targeting sequence LAMP-1 boosted the CD4$^+$, class II-restricted effector T-cell response to the expressed peptide, through enhanced transport of peptide into processing compartments [89]. In addition, boosted antibody titers, lymphoproliferative, and CD4$^+$ CTL responses followed immunization with a vaccinia LAMP-1/human papillomavirus E7 construct, as compared to the standard construct [90].

Recombinant poxviruses that coexpress certain cytokines or other mediators exhibit increased immune responses. Expression of interleukin-2 enhanced the serum IgG response to influenza nucleoprotein [91] and expression of interleukin-5 or -6 increased the secretory IgA response to influenza HA following intranasal vaccination [92]. Interleukin-2 coexpression with β-galactosidase enhanced activity against β-galactosidase-expressing tumors in mice [93]. Similarly, expression of granulocyte/macrophage colony-stimulating factor produced by recombinant avian poxviruses enriched the regional lymph nodes with antigen-presenting cells and acted as an immunoadjuvant [94]. Expression of the CD28 ligand B7 by recombinant vaccinia viruses enhanced antitumor activity in mice by mediating a Th1-type T-cell response [95]. Synergistic effects were reported for a triad of costimulatory molecules, namely, B7-1, ICAM-1, and LFA-3 [96].

Heterologous priming and recombinant poxvirus boosting greatly enhanced T-cell responses. This was first noted using a recombinant influenza virus as the prime followed by a recombinant vaccinia virus [97]. This approach works particularly well using a DNA prime followed by a vaccinia virus or avipoxvirus boost [98–100]. The generally accepted explanation is that immune competition between the many poxvirus proteins and the recombinant protein limits the extent of the immune response to the latter. However, if the animal has already made a primary immune response to the recombinant protein, then the recombinant vaccinia virus can specifically boost this.

The presence of maternal antibodies is a major obstacle to vaccination of infants with some attenuated viruses such as measles and also diminishes the immune response to recombinant vaccines. Passive administration of antiserum to influenza A [101] or respiratory syncytial virus (RSV) [102,103] abrogated both the desired antibody response and disease protection mediated by vaccinia-based influenza or RSV vaccines. Replication of the recombinant viruses and stimulation of antibodies to vaccinia proteins was unaffected, indicating that antibodies to the influenza or RSV proteins produced specific immune interference. Normal immune responses were restored after waiting for clearance of passively administered antibodies to measles virus in mice repeatedly vaccinated with vaccinia/measles recombinants [104]. The inhibitory effect depends on the level of passive antibody, however, and a recombinant vaccinia virus provided significant protection of monkeys against measles infection [105]. Changing the site of inoculation may partially overcome passive blockade of antigen, because intranasal administration of vaccinia/RSV vectors was significantly more immunogenic than dermal administration in cotton rats given anti-RSV antiserum parenterally [106].

Existing immunity to the vector is a potential problem with any live recombinant virus, and holds true for vaccinia virus [61,107]. Because of the cessation of smallpox vaccination in the early 1970s, individuals under 30 are generally vaccinia naive. Systemic immunity to vaccinia virus can be circumvented to some extent by administering the recombinant vaccine by a mucosal route [108]. Repeated vaccination or priming with a DNA vaccine may also be useful. Because of their large genetic differences, immunity to vaccinia does not appreciably affect vaccination with avipox vectors.

C. Safety

During the extensive use of vaccinia virus as a smallpox vaccine, adverse reactions in addition to the routine swelling and soreness at the site of administration and low-grade fever were frequently observed. The most serious of these were progressive or disseminated infection in immunocompromised individuals, eczema vaccinatum, and postvaccinal encephalitis or encephalopathy in infants. The incidence of the latter was reported to vary with different vaccine strains, ranging from 1 in 2,000, for the Copenhagen strain, to 1 in 200,000 or more for the New York City Board of Health (Wyeth) and Lister strains [1,109]. There is a fear that adverse reactions would be even more prevalent now because of the high incidence of HIV, use of immunosuppressive drugs in transplant patients, and increased atopic dermatitis.

Before to the eradication of smallpox, highly attenuated strains of vaccinia virus were made by serial passage in tissue culture [1]. The strain most extensively tested in humans, called modified vaccinia virus Ankara (MVA), was passed 570 times in cultured chick embryo cells and induces only a slight reddening at the site of inoculation [110,111]. MVA has multiple gene deletions [112,113] resulting in an inability to replicate efficiently in human and most other mammalian cells [114–117]. Further studies indicated that replication is blocked at a step in virus assembly and that early and late viral or recombinant protein synthesis occurs normally [118]. Remarkably, recombinant MVA strains seem to induce as good an immune response in mouse and monkey models as replicating strains [119,120]. Avian poxviruses, which are naturally host restricted in mammalian cells, also provide a safe vector system [121].

With knowledge of the vaccinia virus genome sequence and functions of many genes [7], it has become possible to attenuate vaccinia virus by making specific deletions [122,123]. NYVAC, a genetically engineered vaccinia virus with many of the same deletions as MVA, appears safe and immunogenic although it has not been as extensively tested in humans [124,125].

Coexpression of genes encoding certain immunomodulators attenuates live recombinant vaccinia viruses. Human interleukin-2 expression prevented generalized lethal vaccinia infection in immunodeficient athymic nude mice [91,126]. This appeared to be mediated by elevation of natural killer cells and interferon-γ activity in mice vaccinated with the recombinants [127–129]. Interleukin-2 expression also attenuated recombinant vaccinia viruses in normal, immunocompetent rodents [91,130] and primate species [131,132] without significantly reducing vector immunogenicity. Similar results have been achieved with recombinant vaccinia viruses expressing interferon-γ [133] and tumor necrosis factor-α [134].

Increased safety of vaccinia virus might be achieved by altering the route of inoculation, although this could diminish immunogenicity [63,64]. Subcutaneous, intramuscular, and oral routes may reduce the risk of person-to-person

spread of virus but still leave the risk of progressive infection in the immunocompromised host.

Given recent successes in the development of antiviral drugs, it should be possible to identify effective chemotherapeutic interventions for vaccinia virus [135]. This could provide a "safety net" for the rare but serious adverse effects of vaccination. Certain DNA replication inhibitors such as Cidofovir and derivatives appear particularly promising [136–139].

D. Veterinary Applications

Both vaccinia virus and avian poxviruses are being used as veterinary vaccines. Successful oral vaccination of animals with a vaccinia virus rabies glycoprotein vaccine [140,141] led to its extensive field testing as a wildlife vaccine. Live recombinant vaccinia-vaccine-impregnated bait, scattered in areas where rabies is endemic, produced a protective immune response in most animals. Raccoons [69] and foxes [68] were targeted in the United States and Europe, respectively. The vaccinia virus rabies glycoprotein vaccine contributed to the elimination of rabies in a red fox population in Belgium [142]. A raccoon poxvirus recombinant expressing rabies virus glycoprotein has also been shown to be effective as an oral vaccine [143]. A bait strategy has been proposed to control the fertility of wild or feral animal populations by using live recombinant vaccines expressing antifertility immunogens such as β-chorionic gonadotropin [144].

Recombinant vaccinia viruses that express vesicular stomatitis virus [145] or rinderpest [146] glycoprotein genes were shown to protect cattle against the respective pathogens. The rinderpest vaccine provides long-lasting protection and because of its economical production and ease of administration would be attractive for remote areas of the developing world [147]. A recombinant capripoxvirus expressing the hemagglutinin protein gene has also been proposed as a rinderpest vaccine [148]. Live recombinant vaccinia viruses have been shown to protect chickens against avian influenza [149] and Newcastle disease [150]. Many other recombinant vaccinia viruses have been shown to be effective against pathogens in small animal models.

Avian poxvirus recombinants are immunogenic in chickens and have been shown to protect against avian influenza virus [151–153], Newcastle disease virus [154], infectious bursal disease virus [155–157], and infectious bronchitis virus [158]. Fowlpox virus vaccines against Newcastle disease virus and avian influenza virus have been licensed. Avian poxviruses are also immunogenic in nonavian species [6], and the demonstration that recombinant canarypox vectors protect canine distemper virus [159], feline leukemia virus [160], and rabies virus [161] have led to veterinary vaccines.

E. Clinical Applications

Many recombinant poxviruses that express genes of human pathogens have been tested for immunogenicity in small animal models and no attempt will be made to summarize them all here. Instead, this review will be limited to selected candidate vaccines that have been used clinically or in nonhuman primates. Also largely omitted from this review are the attempts to develop therapeutic cancer vaccines using poxvirus vectors [162]. The demonstration that a recombinant vaccinia virus could protect chimpanzees against hepatitis B virus gave credibility to poxvirus vectors [72,163], although the existence of licensed vaccines against this disease hindered its further development. Recombinant vaccinia viruses expressing Epstein–Barr virus glycoprotein provided protection in marmosets [164,165] and in a small clinical trial [166]. Phase I and II clinical trials have been performed with a recombinant vaccinia virus Hantaan vaccine [167]. After two doses by the subcutaneous route, Hantaan virus neutralizing antibodies were detected in 72% of vaccinia virus naïve but in only 26% of vaccinia virus immune volunteers. An MVA expressing a truncated dengue type 2 E protein protected monkeys against a challenge [168].

Phase I trials of canarypox vectors expressing human cytomegalovirus glycoprotein B or phosphoprotein 65 were reported. The glycoprotein vaccine induced only a weak antibody response even after multiple inoculations but primed for a subsequent boost with an attenuated human cytomegalovirus [169]; the phosphoprotein vaccine induced a cytotoxic T-cell response in all subjects [170]. In another study, priming with a canarypox glycoprotein B vaccine and boosting with the subunit protein was not more immunogenic than priming and boosting with the subunit protein [171]. A canarypox rabies glycoprotein vaccine elicited dose-dependent antibody responses that were in the protective range, although lower than that of the standard human diploid rabies vaccine [172].

A recombinant NYVAC expressing seven genes from all stages of the *Plasmodium falciparum* life cycle was tested in a Phase I/II efficacy trial [173]. Antibody responses were low, but cell-mediated immunity was detected in most volunteers. After challenge with five infected mosquitoes, only 1 of 35 was uninfected, but there was a small but significant delay to parasite development in the experimental group compared to the control. A prime-boost immunization regimen using DNA followed by recombinant MVA induced strong cellular immune responses against the *P. falciparum* TRAP antigen in chimpanzees [174]. A multistage, multiantigen DNA prime and canarypox boost malaria vaccine provided partial protection against *Plasmodium knowlesi* in rhesus macaques [175].

Live attenuated measles vaccines are ineffective in the presence of maternal antibody, indicating a need for a vaccine that can be used during the first 6 months of life. Passive antibody studies in primates gave some hope that recombinant MVA expressing the measles F and HA genes may provide some protection under these conditions [105,176].

The most extensive preclinical and clinical investigations of recombinant poxviruses have involved those expressing HIV or related SIV genes. Recombinant vaccinia viruses were used to demonstrate CTL in HIV-infected humans [177,178]. The first clinical studies, performed with a recombinant vaccinia virus that expresses the HIV envelope gene gp160, provided evidence for safety but were not highly immunogenic [179,180]. A history of prior smallpox vaccination did not prevent an antibody response to gp160,

although vaccinia naive subjects in general developed a more vigorous antibody response. Priming followed by boosting with recombinant purified protein, however, produced a strong anamnestic response, with the production of type-specific neutralizing antibody [181,182]. Similar results were obtained using a recombinant canarypox expressing gp160 alone or with a gp160 boost [183]. Other canarypox virus vectors expressed HIV gag, protease, pol, and nef as well as envelope and induced CTL memory in 61% of volunteers at some time during the clinical trial [184]. Preclinical studies of MVA-based SIV and simian human immunodeficiency virus (SHIV) vaccines have shown great promise. MVA alone or preceded by a DNA boost induced high gag and env CTL levels in macaques [100,185,186]. When given prophylactically, such vaccines significantly lower the viral loads and protect macaques against CD4 depletion and clinical illness caused by to SIV or SHIV challenge [100,120,187,188]. In one DNA prime and MVA boost study, expression of env plus gag and pol provided more uniform protection than expression of gag and pol alone [189]. Phase 1 studies with recombinant MVA HIV vaccines have just started.

Because vaccinia virus vectors have the capacity to incorporate at least 25,000 bp of extra DNA [16], the concept of polyvalent vaccines is extremely attractive. Recombinant vaccinia viruses that simultaneously express three or more foreign proteins have been constructed [190,191]. Besides enhancing risk/benefit ratios, polyvalency would circumvent the reduction in immunogenicity of live vectors accompanying revaccination. The logistics of developing such a polyvalent vaccine, however, may prove daunting.

REFERENCES

1. Fenne F, et al. Smallpox and its eradication. Geneva: World Health Organization, 1988:1460.
2. Baxby D. The origins of vaccinia virus. J Infect Dis 1977; 136:453–455.
3. Mackett M, et al. Vaccinia virus: a selectable eukaryotic cloning and expression vector. Proc Natl Acad Sci USA 1982; 79:7415–7419.
4. Panicali D, Paoletti E. Construction of poxviruses as cloning vectors: insertion of the thymidine kinase gene from herpes simplex virus into the DNA of infectious vaccinia virus. Proc Natl Acad Sci USA 1982; 79:4927–4931.
5. Boyle DB, Coupar BEH. Construction of recombinant fowlpox viruses as vectors for poultry vaccines. Virus Res 1988; 10:343–356.
6. Taylor J, et al. Recombinant fowlpox virus inducing protective immunity in non-avian species. Vaccine 1988; 6:497–503.
7. Moss B. Poxviridae: the viruses and their replication. In: Knipe DM, Howley PM, eds. Fields Virology. Vol. 2. Philadelphia: Lippincott Williams and Wilkins, 2001:2849–2883.
8. Earl PL. Generation of recombinant vaccinia viruses. In: Ausubel FM, Brent R, Kingston RE, et al., eds. Current Protocols in Molecular Biology. Vol. 2. New York: Greene Publishing Associates and Wiley Interscience, 1998:16.17.1–16.17.19.
9. Earl PL, et al. Preparation of cell cultures and vaccinia virus stocks. In: Ausubel FM, Brent R, Kingston RE, et al., eds. Current Protocols in Molecular Biology. Vol. 2. New York: John Wiley and Sons, 1998:16.16.1–16.16.3.

10. Moss B, Earl P. Expression of proteins in mammalian cells using vaccinia viral vectors. Overview of the vaccinia virus expression system. In: Ausubel FM, Brent R, Kingston RE, et al., eds. Current Protocols in Molecular Biology Vol. 2. New York: Greene Publishing Associates and Wiley Interscience, 1998:16.15.1–16.15.5.

11. Earl PL, Moss B. Characterization of recombinant vaccinia viruses and their products. In: Ausubel FM, Brent R, Kingston RE, et al., eds. Current Protocols in Molecular Biology. Vol. 2. New York: Greene Publishing Associates and Wiley Interscience, 1998:16.18.1–16.18.11.

12. Fenner F, Comben BM. Genetic studies with mammalian poxviruses. I. Demonstration of recombination between two strains of poxviruses. Virology 1958; 5:530–548.

13. Sam CK, Dumbell KR. Expression of poxvirus DNA in coinfected cells and marker rescue of thermosensitive mutants by subgenomic fragments of DNA. Ann Virol 1981; 132E:135–150.

14. Nakano E, et al. Molecular genetics of vaccinia virus: demonstration of marker rescue. Proc Natl Acad Sci USA 1982; 79:1593–1596.

15. Weir JP, et al. Mapping of the vaccinia virus thymidine kinase gene by marker rescue and by cell-free translation of selected mRNA. Proc Natl Acad Sci USA 1982; 79:1210–1214.

16. Smith GL, Moss B. Infectious poxvirus vectors have capacity for at least 25,000 base pairs of foreign DNA. Gene 1983; 25:21–28.

17. Pfleiderer M, et al. A novel vaccinia virus expression system allowing construction of recombinants without the need for selection markers, plasmids and bacterial hosts. J Gen Virol 1995; 76:2957–2962.

18. Merchlinsky M, et al. Construction and characterization of vaccinia direct ligation vectors. Virology 1997; 238:444–451.

19. Smith ES, et al. Lethality-based selection of recombinant genes in mammalian cells: application to identifying tumor antigens. Nat Med 2001; 7:967–972.

20. Timiryasova TM, et al. Construction of recombinant vaccinia viruses using PUV-inactivated virus as a helper. Biotechniques 2001; 31:534–540.

21. Townsend A, et al. Defective presentation to class I-restricted cytotoxic T lymphocytes in vaccinia-infected cells is overcome by enhanced degradation of antigen. J Exp Med 1988; 168:1211–1224.

22. Bronte V, et al. Antigen expression by dendritic cells correlates with the therapeutic effectiveness of a model recombinant poxvirus tumor vaccine. Proc Natl Acad Sci USA 1997; 93:3183–3188.

23. Chakrabarti S, et al. Compact, synthetic, vaccinia virus early/late promoter for protein expression. Biotechniques 1997; 21:1904–1907.

24. Wyatt LS, et al. Development of a replication-deficient recombinant vaccinia virus vaccine effective against parainfluenza virus 3 infection in an animal model. Vaccine 1996; 14:1451–1458.

25. Earl PL, et al. Removal of cryptic poxvirus transcription termination signals from the human immunodeficiency virus type 1 envelope gene enhances expression and immunogenicity of a recombinant vaccinia virus. J Virol 1990; 64:2448–2451.

26. Paoletti E. Construction of live vaccines using genetically engineered poxviruses: biological activity of vaccinia virus recombinants expressing the hepatitis B virus surface antigen and the herpes simplex virus glycoprotein D. Proc Natl Acad Sci USA 1984; 81:193–197.

27. Mackett M, et al. General method for production and selection of infectious vaccinia virus recombinants expressing foreign genes. J Virol 1984; 49:857–864.

28. Franke CA, et al. Neomycin resistance as a dominant selectable marker for selection and isolation of vaccinia virus recombinants. Mol Cell Biol 1985; 5:1918–1924.

29. Falkner FG, Moss B. *Escherichia coli gpt* gene provides dominant selection for vaccinia virus open reading frame expression vectors. J Virol 1988; 62:1849–1854.

30. Boyle DB, Coupar BEH. A dominant selectable marker for the construction of recombinant poxviruses. Gene 1988; 65:123–128.

31. Zhou J, et al. The hygromycin-resistance-encoding gene as a selection marker for vaccinia virus recombinants. Gene 1991; 107:307–312.

32. Sanchez-Puig JM, et al. Puromycin resistance (pac) gene as a selectable marker in vaccinia virus. Gene 2000; 257:57–65.

33. Coupar BEH, et al. A general method for the construction of recombinant vaccinia viruses expressing multiple foreign genes. Gene 1988; 68:1–10.

34. Chakrabarti S, et al. Vaccinia virus expression vector: coexpression of β-galactosidase provides visual screening of recombinant virus plaques. Mol Cell Biol 1985; 5:3403–3409.

35. Carroll MW, Moss B. *E. coli* β-glucuronidase (GUS) as a marker for recombinant vaccinia viruses. Biotechniques 1995; 19:352–355.

36. Ward BM, Moss B. Visualization of intracellular movement of vaccinia virus virions containing a green fluorescent protein-B5R membrane protein chimera. J Virol 2001; 75:4802–4813.

37. Blasco R, Moss B. Selection of recombinant vaccinia viruses on the basis of plaque formation. Gene 1995; 158:157–162.

38. Perkus ME, et al. Cloning and expression of foreign genes in vaccinia virus, using a host range selection system. J Virol 1989; 63:3829–3836.

39. Fuerst TR, et al. Eukaryotic transient-expression system based on recombinant vaccinia virus that synthesizes bacteriophage T7 RNA polymerase. Proc Natl Acad Sci USA 1986; 83:8122–8126.

40. Usdin TB, et al. SP6 RNA polymerase containing vaccinia virus for rapid expression of cloned genes in tissue culture. Biotechniques 1993; 14:222–224.

41. Fuerst TR, et al. Use of a hybrid vaccinia virus T7 RNA polymerase system for expression of target genes. Mol Cell Biol 1987; 7:2538–2544.

42. Ward GA, et al. Stringent chemical and thermal regulation of recombinant gene expression by vaccinia virus vectors in mammalian cells. Proc Natl Acad Sci USA 1995; 92:6773–6777.

43. Elroy-Stein O, et al. Cap-independent translation of mRNA conferred by encephalomyocarditis virus 5' sequence improves the performance of the vaccinia virus/bacteriophage T7 hybrid expression system. Proc Natl Acad Sci USA 1989; 86:6126–6130.

44. Chakrabarti S, et al. Expression of the HTLV-III envelope gene by a recombinant vaccinia virus. Nature 1986; 320:535–537.

45. Flexner C, et al. Characterization of human immunodeficiency virus gag/pol gene products expressed by recombinant vaccinia viruses. Virology 1988; 166:339–349.

46. Elango N, et al. Resistance to human respiratory syncytial virus (RSV) infection induced by immunization of cotton rats with a recombinant vaccinia virus expressing the RSV G glycoprotein. Proc Natl Acad Sci USA 1986; 83:1906–1911.

47. Rice CM, et al. Expression of Sindbis virus structural proteins via recombinant vaccinia virus: synthesis, processing, and incorporation into mature Sindbis virions. J Virol 1985; 56:227–239.

48. Stephens EB, et al. Surface expression of viral glycoproteins is polarized in epithelial cells infected with recombinant vaccinia virus vectors. EMBO J 1986; 5:237–245.

49. Stomatos N, et al. Expression of polyomavirus virion

proteins by a vaccinia virus vector: association of VP1 and VP2 with the nuclear framework. J Virol 1987; 61:516–525.

50. Leonard RJ, et al. Expression of *Drosophila* Shaker potassium channels in mammalian cells infected with recombinant vaccinia virus. Proc Natl Acad Sci USA 1989; 86:7629–7633.

51. Schnell MJ, et al. Infectious rabies viruses from cloned cDNA. EMBO J 1994; 13:4195–4204.

52. Whelan SPJ, et al. Efficient recovery of infectious vesicular stomatitis virus entirely from cDNA clones. Proc Natl Acad Sci USA 1995; 92:8388–8392.

53. Collins PL, et al. Production of infectious human respiratory syncytial virus from cloned cDNA confirms an essential role for the transcription elongation factor from the 5′ proximal open reading frame of the M2 mRNA in gene expression and provides a capability for vaccine development. Virology 1995; 92:11563–11567.

54. Moss B. Genetically engineered poxviruses for recombinant gene expression, vaccination, and safety. Proc Natl Acad Sci USA 1996; 93:11341–11348.

55. Lathe R, et al. Tumor prevention and rejection with recombinant vaccinia virus. Nature 1987; 326:878–880.

56. Carroll MW, et al. Highly attenuated modified vaccinia virus Ankara (MVA) as an effective recombinant vector: a murine tumor model. Vaccine 1997; 15:387–394.

57. Wang M, et al. Active immunotherapy of cancer with a non-replicating recombinant fowlpox virus encoding a model tumor-associated antigen. J Immunol 1995; 154:4685–4692.

58. Kantor J, et al. Antitumor activity and immune responses induced by a recombinant carcinoembryonic antigen-vaccinia virus vaccine. J Natl Cancer Inst 1992; 84:1084–1091.

59. Bennink JR. Recombinant vaccinia virus primes and stimulates influenza virus HA-specific CTL. Nature 1984; 311:578–579.

60. Durbin A, et al. The immunogenicity and efficacy of intranasally or parenterally administered replication-deficient vaccinia-parainfluenza virus type 3 recombinants in rhesus monkeys. Vaccine 1998; 16:1324–1330.

61. Rooney JF, et al. Immunization with a vaccinia virus recombinant expressing herpes simplex virus type 1 glycoprotein D: long-term protection and effect of revaccination. J Virol 1988; 161:269–275.

62. Benveniste RE, et al. Long-term protection of macaques against high-dose type D retrovirus challenge after immunization with recombinant vaccinia virus expressing envelope glycoproteins. J Med Primatol 1993; 22:74–79.

63. Galasso GJ, et al. Clinical and serological study of four smallpox vaccines comparing variations of dose and route of administration. J Infect Dis 1977; 135:131–186.

64. McClain DJ, et al. Immunologic responses to vaccinia vaccines administered by different routes. J Infect Dis 1997; 175:756–763.

65. Sumner JW, et al. Protection of mice with vaccinia virus recombinants that express the rabies nucleoprotein. Virology 1991; 183:703–710.

66. Olmsted RA, et al. Evaluation in non-human primates of the safety, immunogenicity and efficacy of recombinant vaccinia viruses expressing the F or G glycoprotein of respiratory syncytial virus. Vaccine 1988; 6:519–524.

67. Bender BS, et al. Oral immunization with a replication-deficient recombinant vaccinia virus protects mice against influenza. J Virol 1996; 70:6418–6424.

68. Blancou J, et al. Oral vaccination of the fox against rabies using a live recombinant vaccinia virus. Nature 1986; 322:373–375.

69. Rupprecht CE, et al. Oral immunization and protection of raccoons (*Procyon lotor*) with a vaccinia-rabies glycoprotein recombinant virus vaccine. Proc Natl Acad Sci USA 1986; 83:7947–7950.

70. Thomas I, et al. Primary multiplication site of the vaccinia-rabies glycoprotein recombinant virus administered to foxes by the oral route. J Gen Virol 1990; 71:37–42.

71. Meitin C, et al. Enteric immunization of mice against influenza with recombinant vaccinia. Proc Natl Acad Sci USA 1994; 91:11187–11191.

72. Moss B, et al. Live recombinant vaccinia virus protects chimpanzees against hepatitis B. Nature 1984; 311:67–69.

73. Ohishi K, et al. Protective immunity against bovine leukaemia virus (BLV) induced in carrier sheep by inoculation with a vaccinia virus-BLV env recombinant—association with cell-mediated immunity. J Gen Virol 1991; 72:1887–1892.

74. Andrew ME, et al. Cell-mediated immune response to influenza virus antigens expressed by vaccinia virus recombinants. Microb Path 1986; 1:443–452.

75. Fekadu M, et al. Sickness and recovery of dogs challenged with a street rabies virus after vaccination with a vaccinia virus recombinant expressing rabies virus N-protein. J Virol 1992; 66:2601–2604.

76. Jonjic S, et al. A nonstructural viral protein expressed by a recombinant vaccinia virus protects against lethal cytomegalovirus infection. J Virol 1988; 62:1653–1658.

77. Del Val M, et al. Molecular basis for cytolytic T-lymphocyte recognition of the murine cytomegalovirus immediate-early protein pp89. J Virol 1988; 62:3965–3972.

78. Bankamp B, et al. Measles virus nucleocapsid protein protects rats from encephalitis. J Virol 1991; 65:1695–1700.

79. Ourmanov I, et al. Comparative efficacy of recombinant modified vaccinia virus ankara expressing simian immunodeficiency virus (SIV) gag-Pol and/or env in macaques challenged with pathogenic SIV. J Virol 2000; 74:2740–2751.

80. Seth A, et al. Immunization with a modified vaccinia virus expressing simian immunodeficiency virus (SIV) gag-Pol primes for an anamnestic gag-specific cytotoxic T-lymphocyte response and is associated with reduction of viremia after SIV challenge. J Virol 2000; 74:2502–2509.

81. Irvine KR, et al. Synthetic oligonucleotide expressed by a recombinant vaccinia virus elicits therapeutic CTL. J Immunol 1995; 154:4651–4657.

82. Davison AJ, Moss B. The structure of vaccinia virus early promoters. J Mol Biol 1989; 210:749–769.

83. Davison AJ, Moss B. The structure of vaccinia virus late promoters. J Mol Biol 1989; 210:771–784.

84. Langford DJ, et al. Anchoring a secreted plasmodium antigen on the surface of recombinant vaccinia virus infected cells increases its immunogenicity. Mol Cell Biol 1986; 6:3191–3199.

85. Vijaya S, et al. Transport to the cell surface of a peptide sequence attached to the truncated C terminus of an N-terminally anchored integral membrane protein. Mol Cell Biol 1988; 1988:1709–1714.

86. Kieny MP, et al. Improved antigenicity of the HIV env protein by cleavage site removal. Protein Eng 1988; 2:219–225.

87. Clarke BE, et al. Improved immunogenicity of a peptide epitope after fusion to hepatitis B core protein. Nature 1987; 330:381–384.

88. Good MF, et al. Construction of synthetic immunogen: use of new T-helper epitope on malaria circumsporozoite protein. Science 1987; 235:1059–1062.

89. Rowell JF, et al. Lysosome-associated membrane protein-1-mediated targeting of the HIV-1 envelope protein to an endosomal/lysosomal compartment enhances its presentation to MHC class II-restricted T cells. J Immunol 1995; 155:1818–1828.

90. Wu TC, et al. Engineering an intracellular pathway for major histocompatibility complex class II presentation of antigens. Proc Natl Acad Sci USA 1995; 92:11671–11675.

91. Flexner C, et al. Prevention of vaccinia virus infection in immunodeficient nude mice by vector-directed IL-2 expression. Nature 1987; 330:259–262.

92. Ramsay AJ, et al. The role of interleukin-6 in mucosal IgA antibody responses in vivo. Science 1994; 264:561–563.

93. Bronte V, et al. IL-2 enhances the function of recombinant poxvirus-based vaccines in the treatment of established pulmonary metastases. J Immunol 1995; 154:5282–5292.

94. Kass E, et al. Granulocyte/macrophage-colony stimulating factor produced by recombinant avian poxviruses enriches the regional lymph nodes with antigen-presenting cells and acts as an immunoadjuvant. Cancer Res 2001; 61:206–214.

95. Rao JB, et al. IL-12 is an effective adjuvant to recombinant vaccinia virus-based tumor vaccines. Enhancement by simultaneous B7-1 expression. J Immunol 1996; 156:3357–3365.

96. Hodge JW, et al. A triad of costimulatory molecules synergize to amplify T-cell activation. Cancer Res 1999; 59:5800–5807.

97. Li S, et al. Priming with recombinant influenza virus followed by administration of recombinant vaccinia virus induces CD8$^+$ T-cell-mediated protective immunity against malaria. Proc Natl Acad Sci USA 1993; 90:5214–5218.

98. Kent SJ, et al. Enhanced T-cell immunogenicity and protective efficacy of a human immunodeficiency virus type 1 vaccine regimen consisting of consecutive priming with DNA and boosting with recombinant fowlpox virus. J Virol 1998; 72:10180–10188.

99. Schneider J, et al. Enhanced immunogenicity for CD8+ T cell induction and complete protective efficacy of malaria DNA vaccination by boosting with modified vaccinia virus Ankara. Nat Med 1998; 4:397–402.

100. Amara RR, et al. Control of a mucosal challenge and prevention of AIDS by a multiprotein DNA/MVA vaccine. Science 2001; 292:69–74.

101. Johnson MP, et al. Passive immune serum inhibits antibody response to recombinant vaccinia virus. In: Ginsberg H, Brown FD, Lerner RA, Chanock RM, eds. New Chemical and Genetic Approaches to Vaccination. Cold Spring Harbor: Cold Spring Harbor Laboratory Press, 1988:189–192.

102. Murphy BR, et al. Passive transfer of respiratory syncytial virus (RSV) antiserum suppresses the immune response to the RSV fusion (F) and large (G) glycoprotein expressed by recombinant vaccinia viruses. J Virol 1988; 62:3907–3910.

103. Durbin AP, et al. Comparison of the immunogenicity and efficacy of a replication-defective vaccinia virus expressing antigens of human parainfluenza virus Type 3 (HPIV3) with those of a live attenuated HPIV3 vaccine candidate in rhesus monkeys passively immunized with PIV3 antibodies. J Infect Dis 1999; 179:1345–1351.

104. Galletti R, et al. Passively administered antibody suppresses the induction of measles virus antibodies by vaccinia–measles recombinant viruses. Vaccine 1995; 13:197–201.

105. Stittelaar KJ, et al. Protective immunity in macaques vaccinated with a modified vaccinia virus Ankara-based measles virus vaccine in the presence of passively acquired antibodies. J Virol 2000; 74:4236–4243.

106. Murphy BR, et al. Immunosuppression of the antibody response to respiratory syncytial virus (RSV) by pre-existing serum antibodies: partial prevention by topical infection of the respiratory tract with vaccinia virus-RSV recombinants. J Gen Virol 1989; 70:2185–2190.

107. Kündig TM, et al. Vaccination with two different vaccinia recombinant viruses: long term inhibition of secondary vaccination. Vaccine 1993; 11:1154–1158.

108. Belyakov IM, et al. Mucosal vaccination overcomes the barrier to recombinant vaccinia immunization caused by preexisting poxvirus immunity. Proc Natl Acad Sci USA 1999; 96:4512–4517.

109. Lane JM, et al. Complications of smallpox vaccination, 1968.

110. Mayr A, et al. Der pockenimpfstamm MVA: marker, genetische struktur, erfahrungen mit der parenteralen schutzimpfung und verhalten im abwehrgeschwächten organismus. Zentralbl Bakteriol Hyg 1978; 167:375–390.

111. Stickl H, et al. MVA-Stufenimpfung gegen Pocken. Klinische Erprobung des attenuierten Pocken-Lebendimpfstoffes Stamm MVA. Dtsch Med Wochenschr 1974; 99: 2386–2392.

112. Meyer H, et al. Mapping of deletions in the genome of the highly attenuated vaccinia virus MVA and their influence on virulence. J Gen Virol 1991; 72:1031–1038.

113. Antoine G, et al. The complete genomic sequence of the modified vaccinia Ankara strain: comparison with other orthopoxviruses. Virology 1998; 244:365–396.

114. Drexler I, et al. Highly attenuated modified vaccinia virus Ankara replicates in baby hamster kidney cells, a potential host for virus propagation, but not in various human transformed and primary cells. J Gen Virol 1998; 79:347–352.

115. Carroll M, Moss B. Host range and cytopathogenicity of the highly attenuated MVA strain of vaccinia virus: propagation and generation of recombinant viruses in a nonhuman mammalian cell line. Virology 1997; 238:198–211.

116. Blanchard TJ, et al. Modified vaccinia virus Ankara undergoes limited replication in human cells and lacks several immunomodulatory proteins: implications for use as a human vaccine. J Gen Virol 1998; 79:1159–1167.

117. Wyatt LS, et al. Marker rescue of the host range restricted defects of modified vaccinia virus Ankara. Virology 1998; 251:334–342.

118. Sutter G, Moss B. Nonreplicating vaccinia vector efficiently expresses recombinant genes. Proc Natl Acad Sci USA 1992; 89:10847–10851.

119. Sutter G, et al. A recombinant vector derived from the host range-restricted and highly attenuated MVA strain of vaccinia virus stimulates protective immunity in mice to influenza virus. Vaccine 1994; 12:1032–1040.

120. Hirsch VM, et al. Patterns of viral replication correlate with outcome in simian immunodeficiency virus (SIV)-infected macaques: effect of prior immunization with a trivalent SIV vaccine in modified vaccinia virus Ankara. J Virol 1996; 70:3741–3752.

121. Taylor J, et al. Biological and immunogenic properties of a canarypox–rabies recombinant, ALVAC-RG (vCP65) in non-avian species. Vaccine 1995; 13:539–549.

122. Buller RML, et al. Decreased virulence of recombinant vaccinia virus expression vectors is associated with a thymidine kinase-negative phenotype. Nature 1985; 317:813–815.

123. Buller RML, et al. Deletion of the vaccinia virus growth factor gene reduces virus virulence. J Virol 1988; 62:866–874.

124. Tartaglia J, et al. NYVAC—a highly attenuated strain of vaccinia virus. Virology 1992; 188:217–232.

125. Paoletti E. Applications of poxvirus vectors to vaccination: an update. Proc Natl Acad Sci USA 1996; 93:11349–11353.

126. Ramshaw A, et al. Recovery of immunodeficient mice from a vaccinia virus/IL-2 recombinant infection. Nature 1987; 329:545–546.

127. Hugin AW, et al. Clearance of recombinant vaccinia virus expressing IL-2: role of local host immune responses. Cell Immunol 1993; 152:499–509.

128. Karupiah G, et al. Interferon γ is involved in the recovery of athymic nude mice from recombinant vaccinia virus interleukin-2 infection. J Exp Med 1990; 172:1495–1503.

129. Karupiah G, et al. Elevated natural killer cell responses in mice infected with recombinant vaccinia virus encoding murine IL-2. J Immunol 1990; 144:290–298.

130. Karupiah G, et al. Immunobiology of infection with recombinant vaccinia virus encoding murine IL-2—mecha-

National surveillance in the United States. N Engl J Med 1969; 281:1201–1208.

nisms of rapid viral clearance in immunocompetent mice. J Immunol 1991; 147:4327–4332.

131. Flexner C, et al. Attenuation and immunogenicity in primates of vaccinia virus recombinants expressing human interleukin-2. Vaccine 1990; 8:17–22.

132. Ruby J, et al. Response of monkeys to vaccination with recombinant vaccinia virus which coexpress HIV gp160 and human interleukin-2. Immunol Cell Biol 1990; 68:113–117.

133. Kohonen-Corish MRJ, et al. Immunodeficient mice recover from infection with vaccinia virus expressing interferon-γ. Eur J Immunol 1990; 20:157–161.

134. Sambhi SK, et al. Local production of tumor necrosis factor encoded by recombinant vaccinia virus Is effective in controlling viral replication In vivo. Proc Natl Acad Sci USA 1991; 88:4025–4029.

135. De Clercq E. Vaccinia virus inhibitors as a paradigm for the chemotherapy of poxvirus infections. Clin Microbiol Rev 2001; 14:382–397.

136. Bray M, et al. Cidofovir protects mice against lethal aerosol or intranasal cowpox virus challenge. J Infect Dis 2000; 181:10–19.

137. Smee DF, et al. Treatment of lethal vaccinia virus respiratory infections in mice with Cidofovir. Antivir Chem Chemother 2001; 12:71–76.

138. Smee DF. Treatment of lethal cowpox virus respiratory infections in mice with 2-amino-7-(1,3-dihydroxy-2-propoxy)methyl purine and its orally active diacetate ester prodrug. Antiviral Res 2002; 54:113–120.

139. Kern ER, et al. Enhanced inhibition of orthopoxvirus replication in vitro by alkoxyalkyl esters of Cidofovir and cyclic Cidofovir. Antimicrob Agents Chemother 2002; 46:991–995.

140. Wiktor TJ, et al. Protection from rabies by a vaccinia virus recombinant containing the rabies virus glycoprotein gene. Proc Natl Acad Sci USA 1984; 81:7194–7198.

141. Kieny MP, et al. Expression of rabies virus glycoprotein from a recombinant vaccinia virus. Nature, 1984, 312.

142. Brochier B, et al. Elimination of sylvatic rabies in Belgium by oral vaccination of the red fox (*Vulpes vulpes*). Ann Med Vet 2001; 145:293–305.

143. Esposito JJ, et al. Successful oral rabies vaccination of raccoons with raccoon poxvirus recombinants expressing rabies virus glycoprotein. Virology 1988; 167:313–316.

144. Boyle DB. Disease and fertility control in wildlife and feral animal populations: options for vaccine delivery using vectors. Reprod Fertil Dev 1994; 6:393–400.

145. Mackett M, et al. Vaccinia virus recombinants: expression of VSV genes and protective immunization of mice and cattle. Science 1985; 227:433–435.

146. Yilma T, et al. Protection of cattle against rinderpest with vaccinia virus recombinants expressing the HA or F gene. Science 1988; 242:1058–1061.

147. Verardi PH, et al. Long-term sterilizing immunity to rinderpest in cattle vaccinated with a recombinant vaccinia virus expressing high levels of the fusion and hemagglutinin glycoproteins. J Virol 2002; 76:484–491.

148. Romero CH, et al. Recombinant capripoxvirus expressing the hemagglutinin protein gene of rinderpest virus: protection of cattle against rinderpest and lumpy skin disease. Virology 1994; 204:425–429.

149. Chambers TM, et al. Protection of chickens from lethal influenza infection by vaccinia-expressed hemagglutinin. Virology 1988; 167:414–421.

150. Nishino Y, et al. Analysis of the protective effect of the haemagglutinin-neuraminidase protein in Newcastle disease virus infection. J Gen Virol 1991; 72:1187–1190.

151. Taylor J, et al. Protective immunity against avian influenza induced by a fowlpox virus recombinant. Vaccine 1988; 6: 504–508.

152. Webster RG, et al. Efficacy of nucleoprotein and haemagglutinin antigens expressed in fowlpox virus as vaccine for influenza in chickens. Vaccine 1991; 9:303–308.

153. Boyle DB, et al. Vaccinating chickens against avian influenza with fowlpox recombinants expressing the H7 haemagglutinin. Aust Vet J 2000; 78:44–48.

154. Boursnell ME, et al. A recombinant fowlpox virus expressing the hemagglutinin-neuraminidase gene of Newcastle disease virus (NDV) protects chickens against challenge by NDV. Virology 1990; 178:297–300.

155. Bayliss CD, et al. A recombinant fowlpox virus that expresses the VP2 antigen of infectious bursal disease virus induces protection against mortality caused by the virus. Arch Virol 1991; 120:193–205.

156. Shaw I, Davison TF. Protection from IBDV-induced bursal damage by a recombinant fowlpox vaccine, fpIBD1, is dependent on the titre of challenge virus and chicken genotype. Vaccine 2000; 18:3230–3241.

157. Tsukamoto K, et al. Dual-viral vector approach induced strong and long-lasting protective immunity against very virulent infectious bursal disease virus. Virology 2000; 269:257–267.

158. Yu L, Liu W, et al. Study of protection by recombinant fowl poxvirus expressing C-terminal nucleocapsid protein of infectious bronchitis virus against challenge. Avian Dis 2001; 45:340–348.

159. Welter J, et al. Vaccination against canine distemper virus infection in infant ferrets with and without maternal antibody protection, using recombinant attenuated poxvirus vaccines. J Virol 2000; 74:6358–6367.

160. Tartaglia J, et al. Protection of cats against feline leukemia virus by vaccination with a canarypox virus recombinant, ALVAC-FL. J Virol 1993; 67:2370–2375.

161. Taylor J, et al. Efficacy studies on a canarypox–rabies recombinant virus. Vaccine 1991; 9:190–193.

162. Mastrangelo MJ, et al. Poxvirus vectors: orphaned and underappreciated. J Clin Invest 2000; 105:1031–1034.

163. Smith GL, et al. Infectious vaccinia virus recombinants that express hepatitis B antigen. Nature 1983; 302:490–495.

164. Morgan MW, et al. Recombinant vaccinia virus expressing Epstein–Barr virus glycoprotein gp340 protects cottontop tamarins against EB virus-induced malignant lymphomas. J Med Virol 1988; 25:189–195.

165. Mackett M. Immunisation of common marmosets with vaccinia virus expressing Epstein–Barr virus (EBV) gp340 and challenge with EBV. J Med Virol 1996; 50:263–271.

166. Gu SY, et al. First EBV vaccine trial in humans using recombinant vaccinia virus expressing the major membrane antigen. Dev Biol Stand 1995; 84:171–177.

167. McClain DJ, et al. Clinical evaluation of a vaccinia-vectored Hantaan virus vaccine. J Med Virol 2000; 60:77–85.

168. Men R, et al. Immunization of rhesus monkeys with a recombinant of modified vaccinia virus Ankara expressing a truncated envelope glycoprotein of dengue type 2 virus induced resistance to dengue type 2 virus challenge. Vaccine 2000; 18:3113–3122.

169. Adler SP, et al. A canarypox vector expressing cytomegalovirus (CMV) glycoprotein B primes for antibody responses to a live attenuated CMV vaccine (Towne). J Infect Dis 1999; 180:843–846.

170. Berencsi K, et al. A canarypox vector-expressing cytomegalovirus (CMV) phosphoprotein 65 induces long-lasting cytotoxic T cell responses in human CMV-seronegative subjects. J Infect Dis 2001; 183:1171–1179.

171. Bernstein DI, et al. Effect of previous or simultaneous immunization with canarypox expressing cytomegalovirus (CMV) glycoprotein B (gB) on response to subunit gB vaccine plus MF59 in healthy CMV-seronegative adults. J Infect Dis 2002; 185:686–690.

172. Fries LF, et al. Human safety and immunogenicity of a canarypox–rabies glycoprotein recombinant vaccine: an alternative poxvirus vector system. Vaccine 1996; 14:428–434.

173. Ockenhouse CF, et al. Phase I/IIa safety, immunogenicity, and efficacy trial of NYVAC-Pf7, a pox-vectored, multiantigen, multistage vaccine candidate for *Plasmodium falciparum* malaria. J Infect Dis 1998; 177:1664–1673.

174. Schneider J. A prime-boost immunisation regimen using DNA followed by recombinant modified vaccinia virus Ankara induces strong cellular immune responses against the *Plasmodium falciparum* TRAP antigen in chimpanzees. Vaccine 2001; 19:4595–4602.

175. Rogers WO, et al. Multistage multiantigen heterologous prime boost vaccine for *Plasmodium knowlesi* malaria provides partial protection in rhesus macaques. Infect Immun 2001; 69:5565–5572.

176. Zhu YD, et al. Evaluation of recombinant vaccinia virus—measles vaccines in infant rhesus macaques with preexisting measles antibody. Virology 2000; 276:202–213.

177. Walker BD, et al. HIV-1 reverse transcriptase is a target for cytotoxic T lymphocytes in infected individuals. Science 1988; 240:64–66.

178. Walker BD, et al. HIV-specific cytotoxic T lymphocytes in seropositive individuals. Nature 1987; 328:345–348.

179. Graham BS, et al. Vaccination of vaccinia-naive adults with human immunodeficiency virus type-1 gp160 recombinant vaccinia virus in a blinded, controlled, randomized clinical trial. J Infect Dis 1992; 166:244–252.

180. Cooney EL, et al. Safety of and immunological response to a recombinant vaccinia virus vaccine expressing HIV envelope glycoprotein. Lancet 1991; 337:567–572.

181. Graham BS, et al. Augmentation of human immunodeficiency virus type-1 neutralizing antibody by priming with gp160 recombinant vaccinia and boosting with rgp160 in vaccinia-naive adults. J Infect Dis 1993; 167:533–537.

182. Cooney EL, et al. Enhanced immunity to human immunodeficiency virus (HIV) envelope elicited by a combined vaccine regimen consisting of priming with a vaccinia recombinant expressing HIV envelope and boosting with gp160-protein. Proc Natl Acad Sci USA 1993; 90:1882–1886.

183. Clements-Mann ML, et al. Immune responses to human immunodeficiency virus (HIV) type 1 induced by canarypox expressing HIV-1(MN) gp120, HIV-1(SF2) recombinant gp120, or both vaccines in seronegative adults. J Infect Dis 1998; 177:1230–1246.

184. Evans TG, et al. A canarypox vaccine expressing multiple human immunodeficiency virus type 1 genes given alone or with rgp120 elicits broad and durable CD8(+) cytotoxic T lymphocyte responses in seronegative volunteers. J Infect Dis 1999; 180:290–298.

185. Seth A, et al. Recombinant MVA-SIV *gag pol* elicits cytotoxic T lymphocytes in rhesus monkeys detected by an MHC class I/peptide tetramer. Proc Natl Acad Sci USA 1998; 95:10112–10116.

186. Hanke T, et al. Effective induction of simian immunodeficiency virus-specific cytotoxic T lymphocytes in macaques by using a multiepitope gene and DNA prime-modified vaccinia virus Ankara boost vaccination regimen. J Virol 1999; 73:7524–7532.

187. Barouch DH, et al. Reduction of simian–human immunodeficiency virus 89.6P viremia in rhesus monkeys by recombinant modified vaccinia virus Ankara vaccination. J Virol 2001; 75:5151–5158.

188. Earl PL, et al. Comparison of vaccine strategies using recombinant env-gag-pol MVA with or without an oligomeric env protein boost in the SHIV rhesus macaque model. Virology 2002; 294:270–281.

189. Amara RR, et al. Critical role for Env as well as Gag-Pol in control of a simian–human immunodeficiency virus 89.6P challenge by a DNA prime/recombinant modified vaccinia virus Ankara vaccine. J Virol 2002; 76:6138–6146.

190. Flexner C, et al. Successful vaccination with a polyvalent live vector despite existing immunity to an expressed antigen. Nature 1988; 335:259–262.

191. Perkus ME, et al. Recombinant vaccinia virus: immunization against multiple pathogens. Science 1985; 229:981–984.

28

Live Adenovirus Recombinants as Vaccine Vectors

L. Jean Patterson, Bo Peng, Xinli Nan, and Marjorie Robert-Guroff
National Cancer Institute, National Institutes of Health, Bethesda, Maryland, U.S.A.

I. INTRODUCTION

Live virus vaccines characteristically induce cellular and humoral immunity and produce long-lasting protection. Early live vaccines were attenuated usually by repeated in vitro passaging. Advances in biochemical and molecular biological techniques have allowed the engineering of mutant and recombinant live viral vectors, which avoids the dangers inherent in spontaneously attenuated viruses by lessening the possibility of reversion to virulence, yet confers some of the advantages of live vaccines.

II. ADVANTAGES OF ADENOVIRUS-VECTORED VACCINES

Engineered adenovirus (Ad) vectors offer a number of attractive features for vaccine design (for reviews, see Refs. 1–4). Adenoviruses are independent of host cell division for virus replication. They infect a variety of postmitotic cells and have a broad tissue tropism, including the respiratory tract, eye, intestine, liver, skeletal muscle, brain, and heart. They can be easily administered intranasally or orally, and their replication in the epithelium of the upper respiratory track and gut elicits mucosal immunity essential for the prevention of mucosally and sexually transmitted infections. During infection, up to 10^4 progeny virions are produced per cell, and are easily purified to titers of 10^{12} particles per milliliter. As naked viruses, Ads are more stable than enveloped viruses, an important feature for vaccines to be used worldwide in underdeveloped areas. They also exhibit genetic stability. They do not integrate into the host genome, but persist extrachromosomally [5], minimizing risks of insertional mutagenesis and cellular gene activation. Because Ad has been studied extensively as a model of RNA processing and gene expression in mammalian cells, its molecular biology and host interactions are well understood.

III. ADENOVIRUS BIOLOGY AND MOLECULAR BIOLOGY

Adenoviruses were initially isolated from human pediatric adenoid tissues and respiratory secretions [6,7], and subsequently from tissues of monkeys, birds, pigs, horses, and cows [8]. Human Ads are the etiological agents for diseases ranging from pharyngitis to pneumonia, conjunctivitis, hepatitis, and acute hemorrhagic cystitis [9,10]. However, only one third of all Ad serotypes causes disease, and most Ad infections are subclinical. Only 3–7% of febrile illnesses in the civilian adult population are attributable to Ads, and a slightly higher 5–10% in children [9].

The Ad virion forms a characteristic 70- to 100-nm icosahedral particle, which lacks a lipid envelope (Figure 1A). The outer capsid is made up of the hexon, penton, and fiber proteins, in addition to a number of minor cement proteins. The core contains Ad DNA, closely associated with proteins of varied function [1,8]. The Ad enters cells via a receptor-mediated pathway, binding to the coxsackie/adenovirus receptor (CAR) via the protruding fiber protein [1, 11,12]. Subsequently, internalization is mediated by specific binding of the penton base to cellular integrins [13], which help define Ad tropism. Integrin $\alpha v\beta 5$ is expressed at the major sites of primary Ad infection in vivo, including bronchial and intestinal epithelium [14]. All human Ads bind to CAR except subgroup B Ads, which recognize a different receptor [15].

Other than chimpanzees, few animal models exist for the study of human Ad infection, as most Ads are species-specific. Group C Ads replicate in the lungs of cotton rats, allowing the study of Ad-induced pneumonia [16]. Although Ads do not replicate in mice, high-dose infection of mice results in virus entry and early gene expression [17], providing a model for assessment of gene transduction, expression, and immunogenicity. An Ad5 host range mutant, with a point mutation in the DNA-binding protein, replicates in

A. Adenovirus virion structure.

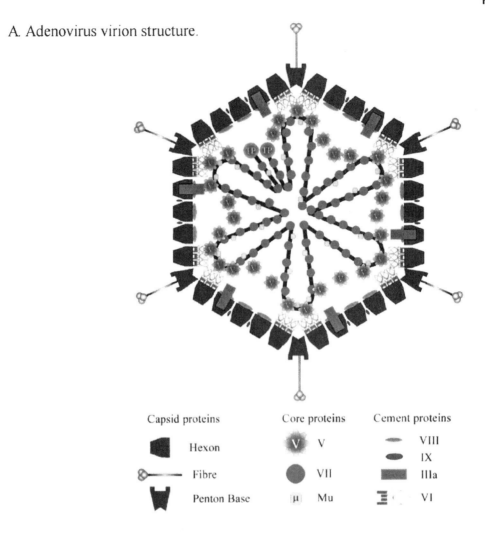

B. Adenovirus genome.

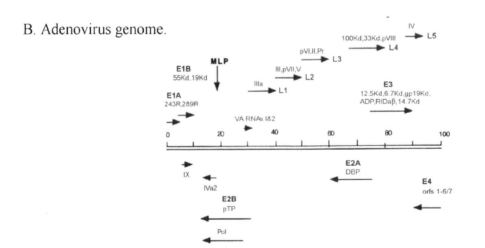

Figure 1 Schematic of the Ad virion and the Ad genome. In (B), the arrows indicate directional transcription of Ad genes. "E" designates early mRNA products (E1–E4), whereas late mRNAs are denoted as L1–L5. MLP = major late promoter. VA RNAs (1 and 2) are not translated and play a role in regulating host defense mechanisms. IVa2- and IX-expressed proteins are transcriptional activators of the MLP. (From Ref. 1.)

simian cells [18], allowing preclinical study of Ad recombinant vaccines in nonhuman primates.

The association of Ad12 with tumor production in rodents [19] suggested that Ads might be oncogenic for humans. Although human Ads are able to transform cultured rodent cells, only a few subtypes cause tumor formation in rats and hamsters [8]. A recent report, as yet unconfirmed, suggested that Ad oncogenicity in rodents was due to a "hit-and-run" mechanism, with Ad being required for initiation but not for maintenance of the transformed state [20]. Importantly with regard to vaccine safety, despite their long use as wild-type vaccines, Ads have never been associated with human cancer [21].

The Ad genome is a linear, double-stranded DNA of around 36 kb with an inverted terminal repeat (ITR) at each extremity. The left ITR contains an origin of replication, and a required cis-acting packaging sequence is located in its immediate vicinity. The replication cycle of Ad (reviewed in Ref. 8) consists of early and late phases, before and after the onset of viral DNA replication, respectively. In the early phase, viral regulatory genes are expressed noncontiguously from five early transcription units: E1A, E1B, E2, E3, and E4 (Figure 1B). E1 genes, essential for replication, encode the predominant regulatory proteins and are required for the activation of all other early expressed genes. Two E1A polypeptides are expressed first and modulate the transcription of early Ad genes and some cellular genes, rendering the cell susceptible to viral infection [1,3]. Interactions with the tumor suppressor protein, pRB, lead to disruption of normal cellular control processes and quiescent cells begin synthesizing DNA. E1B encodes the E1B-55 kDa protein that binds the tumor suppressor p53, blocks its normal function, and thus contributes to cell cycle progression. Together with the E1B-55 kDa protein, the E1B-19 kDa protein blocks E1A-induced apoptosis, thereby contributing to cell growth.

A DNA-binding protein, preterminal protein, and polymerase, all required for DNA replication, are encoded by the E2 region. The E3 region, in contrast, is nonessential for virus growth, but its gene products are important for regulation of host antiviral immunity. The best characterized 19K protein binds MHC class I molecules with high affinity and retains them in the endoplasmic reticulum, thereby blocking transport to the surface and antigen presentation to T cells [22,23]. The 14.7K protein inhibits tumor necrosis factor (TNF)-mediated lysis of Ad-infected cells [24].

The E4 region (reviewed in Ref. 25) orchestrates the transition from early to late gene expression and downregulates host cell gene expression in preparation for virion assembly [3]. E4 gene products have complex functions impacting transcriptional regulation, mRNA transport, and DNA replication. Of six identified E4-encoded polypeptides, E4 Orf3 and Orf6 proteins are of special interest. Both increase viral late protein production, facilitating accumulation of cytoplasmic mRNA posttranscriptionally. In addition, Orf6 complexes with the E1B-55K protein to increase nuclear export of mRNAs while inhibiting cellular mRNA export. Both Orf3 and Orf6 stabilize unprocessed nuclear late RNA, thus increasing RNA available for maturation and transport. Both proteins are important for splicing events, and both participate in Ad DNA replication. Impor-

tantly, the E4 Orf6 protein binds p53 [26] (thus blocking p53-induced apoptosis) and, together with E1A, transforms rodent cells [27]. The Ad9 E4 Orf1 protein also appears to have transforming properties and has been correlated with mammary tumorigenesis in rodents [28].

Overall, E4-deleted Ad vectors might be safer. In addition to loss of transforming potential, they induce significantly less vector toxicity and inflammation in vivo [29]. But E4-deleted Ads also poorly express transgenes from exogenous promoters [29,30]. E4 gene complexity must be carefully considered in vector design. Provision of selected E4 Orf genes in packaging cells, rather than vectors, may supply important functions for transgene expression while avoiding safety concerns.

The late phase of Ad infection is initiated by activation of the major late promoter (MLP) following DNA replication. This transcription unit is processed to generate five families of late mRNAs (L1–L5) and then is translated into viral structural proteins, leading to assembly and maturation of infectious virus. In permissive cells, the early phase of infection may take about 6–8 hr, whereas virus production occurs after another 4–6 hr in the late phase. Cell lysis begins to occur 24–72 hr after infection [9].

IV. EVOLUTION OF ADENOVIRUS RECOMBINANT VECTORS

Gene therapy research has yielded much of what is known about Ad vectors and complementing cell lines. Thousands of Ad vectors have been generated, most of them derived from either Ad2 or Ad5, the genomes of which are well characterized. Because its icosahedral capsid is rigid, Ad can package DNA only up to 105% of its genome size [31]. Adenovirus late proteins provide the structural framework of the virion particle and are essential. Therefore, deletion of Ad early region genes has been generally exploited to create a variety of Ad vectors with increased cloning capacity.

Most recombinant Ads are generated by insertion of foreign genes into deleted E1 or E3 regions, resulting in Ad vectors with different natures (Table 1): replication competent E3-deleted vectors and replication-defective E1-deleted vectors. To express transgenes from replication-defective Ad vectors, an expression cassette is introduced with the transgene under the control of an exogenous promoter.

E3-deleted replication-competent Ad vectors can accommodate a transgene of 3–4 kb, large enough for most foreign gene inserts. Replication-defective vectors lacking both E1 and E3 regions can accommodate larger inserts up to 7–8 kb. Deletion of additional early genes can further increase cloning capacity and may also lessen host immunity to the Ad vector, thus leading to greater persistence of transgene expression. Replication-defective Ad vectors with additional deletions in the E2a, E2b, or E4 region allow inserts up to 10 kb [32–35]. They exhibit reduced expression of early and late virus proteins and, in some cases, extended persistence of transduced liver cells [35–37]. Conflicting results, however, have shown that mice, which received vectors defective in E1, E3, and E4 or E1, E3, and E2A and lacking a transgene, exhibited similar vector persistence and anti-

Table 1 Characteristics of Replication-Competent and Replication-Defective Ad Vectors

Characteristic	Replication competent	Replication defective		
		First generation	Second generation	"Gutless"
Deletion	E3	E1, E3	E1, E2, E3; E1, E3, E4; E1, E2a, E3, partial E4	All but ITRs and ψ
Clone capacity (kb)	3–4	7–8	~10	~35
Effective dose	10^5–10^7	10^9–10^{11}	10^9–10^{11}	10^9–10^{11}
Helper virus	Not required	Not required	Not required	Required
Packaging cells	Not required	*293* (HEK + Ad5 bases 1-4344) [71,72] *911* (HEK + Ad5 bases 79-5789) [74] *PER.C6* (HER + Ad5 bases 459-3510) [75] *GH329* (HeLa + Ad5 bases 511-3924) [76]	*E2T* (293 + E2a; tetracycline regulated) [103] *IGRP2* (293 + E4 Orf6 and Orf7; dexamethasone-inducible MMTV-LTR) [104] *293 Orf6* (293 + E4 Orf6; Zn^{2+}-inducible metallothionein promoter) [77] *C7* (293 + Ad polymerase + pTP) [105] *A70.S54* (A549 + Ad5-E1, Ad5-E2a, Ad5-E4; dexamethasone-inducible) [106]	*293-Cre* [41], *293FLP* [107,108]

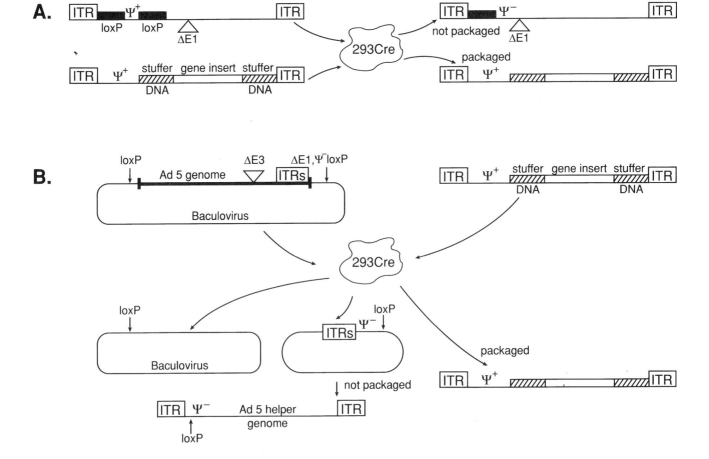

Figure 2 Strategies for production of HD-Ad. (A) Reprinted in slightly modified form. (From Ref. 41.) (B) Reprinted in slightly modified form. (From Ref. 42.)

viral immune response compared to a simple E1- and E3-deleted vector [38]. Furthermore, in the absence of transgene expression, mouse cellular immunity played a minor role in eliminating the Ad vector [38].

Persistence of transgene expression is influenced by host immunity to both the transgene and the vector. A completely "gutless" Ad vector has been proposed to combat the latter. In addition to reducing immunity to vector components, a gutless vector would provide the greatest possible cloning capacity and would theoretically be safer, as all viral genes except the ITRs and packaging signal would be eliminated. This strategy is not without problems, however. To maintain the optimal packaging size of approximately 75% of the wild-type genome length [39], "stuffer" DNA, which can significantly influence persistence of transgene expression [40], is required. Furthermore, gutless Ad vectors depend on helper virus to supply structural components of the virion. Production of helper-dependent Ad vectors (HD-Ads) has been complicated by difficulties in separating HD-Ad recombinant virus from the helper. Among several strategies, the best known uses Cre recombinase to remove the helper virus packaging signal between engineered loxP recognition sites (Figure 2A) [41], producing HD-Ad recombinants containing approximately 0.1% helper virus. A modification of this strategy, using baculovirus, lacks a packaging signal in the helper component (Figure 2B) and is reported to completely eliminate helper contamination [42]. This approach, however, requires further development of alternate packaging cells lacking overlap in the E1 region, in order to avoid eventual emergence of replication-competent adenovirus (RCA).

V. ISSUES IN APPLICATION OF ADENOVIRUS VECTORS FOR VACCINE DEVELOPMENT

Desirable features of Ad vaccine vectors differ from optimal gene therapy vectors. A critical decision in vaccine design is use of a replication-competent or replication-defective Ad vector. Comparative studies with regard to vaccine efficacy and immunogenicity have yet to be carried out. Further characteristics of these vectors are summarized in Table 1. Vector choice is influenced by the expression and persistence of the transgene, safety, and potential to propagate the vector at levels necessary for manufacture and use. Other elements of Ad vector design concern the choice of serotype, and whether vector targeting is desired.

Replication-competent Ad vectors have been used for immunization where viral replication is desired to increase the amount of immunogen [9]. They provide higher levels of gene expression than replication-incompetent vectors because the Ad MLP, which controls transgene expression, is greatly enhanced by a cis-acting function linked to Ad replication itself, resulting in a potent promoter. Importantly, these vectors continue to generate large amounts of viral mRNA with each infection cycle. In contrast, transgene expression of replication-defective vectors with a dormant MLP is limited, as its expression is solely dependent on a heterologous promoter.

Strong immune responses result from highly expressed transgenes. Cytotoxic T lymphocytes (CTLs) develop against both transgenes and Ad antigens, and eventually clear Ad-infected cells. Replication-competent Ad recombinants, because they spread from cell to cell, may persist longer, thereby inducing a more potent and long-lasting CTL response. Although replication-defective Ad vectors have demonstrated high levels of transgene expression in vitro, expression is short-lived in vivo. This may relate to their inability to initiate new infections in vivo, resulting in rapid elimination by CTL.

Avoidance of toxicity and immunopathological responses is critical for vaccines that will be administered to healthy people. Oral wild-type Ad4 and Ad7 vaccines were used for over 25 years to protect against acute upper respiratory disease in military personnel. Over 100 million people were vaccinated safely and effectively [43]. With this extensive safety profile, replication-competent Ad vectors with simple E3 deletions would seem to be vectors of choice. They can be easily constructed and manufactured. Moreover, they may elicit better CTL activity compared to wild-type virus, as their ability to down-modulate MHC class I is impaired. However, intranasal administration of Ad5-E3-deleted vector to cotton rats has elicited greater lung pathology compared to wild-type Ad5 [44], raising safety concerns. Effects of E3 region gene products are not always predictable, however. Cloned expression of the E3-19 kDa protein failed to suppress either CTL or natural killer (NK) cell responses to vaccinia virus in infected mice [45]. In addition, E3-deleted bovine adenovirus vaccines showed no enhanced pathogenic effect when administered to cattle [46]. We examined lung pathology in cotton rats following intranasal administration of candidate Ad4-HIVenv and HIVgag vaccines [47]. Although Ad4 did not replicate in the rats, only Ad early gene expression is sufficient to induce immunopathology due to host inflammatory cytokine and virus-specific CTL responses [17,48]. The increased lung pathology elicited by the Ad4-E3-deleted vector compared to wild-type Ad4 was abrogated when HIVenv or HIVgag was inserted into the E3 region. The responsible mechanism remains to be elucidated, but could be related to immune-suppressive properties of the inserted HIV genes [47].

These results bode well for the use of replication-competent Ad recombinant vaccines. Oral and intranasal administration of Ad-E3-deleted recombinant vaccines to nonhuman primates and people has not caused any significant clinical sequelae [49–58]. This, in part, reflects the low doses sufficient to elicit desired immune responses. Ad4 and Ad7 wild-type vaccines typically were administered orally at doses of 10^7 TCID$_{50}$ [59]. The Ad4 vaccine has been given intranasally to Ad-seropositive and Ad-seronegative people at doses of 2×10^5 and 4×10^4 TCID$_{50}$, respectively [60], with no serious side effects.

In contrast to the benign sequelae observed following low-dose administration of replication-competent Ad vaccines, clinically significant inflammatory responses in humans have resulted following treatment with replication-defective Ad recombinants at high dose to achieve desired levels of transgene expression [61]. In animals, doses of 5×10^{10} plaque-forming units (pfu) or more replication-defective Ad recombinants are necessary for transgene expression [62]. Dose-dependent toxicity includes an acute-phase response with rapid release of inflammatory cytokines and recruitment of host cell defenses [63–65]. The CTL- and NK-mediated responses subsequently elicit late-phase toxicity [63]. High doses of Ad can also elicit toxicity via induction of multiple signaling cascades upon interaction of numerous virions with Ad receptors on many cells types. In addition, at high multiplicity of infection, replication-defective Ad vectors may self-replicate, leading to greater tissue inflammation [1]. Many cells have E1-like proteins able to activate Ad-E2 genes, facilitating Ad replication and late protein synthesis [66–68].

Vector toxicity is also dependent on route of administration. High-dose immunization via the upper respiratory tract, desirable in a vaccine to induce mucosal immunity, is problematical. Repeated intranasal doses of 10^9 pfu of replication-defective Ad recombinant have been safely tolerated [69,70]. An intranasal dose of 10^{10} pfu, however, produced local mucosal inflammation. Overall, a delicate balance between immunogen expression and Ad-associated toxicity must be achieved.

The availability of permissive cell lines for vector propagation is another important consideration in the design of Ad-vectored vaccines. Replication-competent Ad vectors can grow in many cell lines of epithelial origin, including HeLa (human cervical carcinoma), A549 (human lung carcinoma) cells, and primary cells. However, E1 gene functions must be provided in trans for growth of replication-defective Ad vectors. Historically, transformed human embryonic kidney 293 cells containing the first 4344 bp of the Ad5 genome [71,72], which express the E1 gene products, have been used. The 293 cells have good growth characteristics, produce extremely high yields of E1-deleted Ad recombinant viruses, and are easily transfected by DNA plasmids. However, the extensive homology between the Ad5 genomic sequence in 293 cells and standard E1-deleted Ad vectors provides a substantial risk of generating RCAs that have recovered E1 genes by recombination during viral production [73]. Recently, human embryonic retinoblasts (HERs) were transformed by Ad [74], and cell lines containing smaller portions of the Ad5-E1 region that prevent RCA were developed [75,76]. However, appropriately matched Ad vectors are also required to prevent RCA development during Ad recombinant production.

With design of second-generation and gutless Ad vectors, additional packaging lines became necessary to complement functions of deleted early region genes (Table 1), or to provide a helper virus function. In some cases, expression of early region gene products was toxic for cells, and these were introduced under the control of inducible promoters. The extent to which replication-defective Ad vectors based on different serotypes will require packaging lines with serotype-matched inserts is not known. The 293 Orf6 cells, for example, containing the Ad5-E1 and Ad5-E4 Orf6 genes, support the growth of Ad7 replication-defective vectors [77]. The choice of producer cells is critical for vaccine development. Weighing the risk–benefit of live vaccines for healthy people elicits greater caution than gene therapies for patients, where potential treatment success may outweigh associated cell line risks. These include potential oncogenicity and undetected exogenous or endogenous viruses or viral

sequences. To avoid such risks, vaccines must be produced in well-characterized cells and shown free of contaminating cellular DNA.

A further consideration in Ad vector design is the Ad vector subtype. At issue is whether preexisting immunity in the population to the vector will preclude effective immunization. Repeated administration of Ad recombinants in gene therapy trials led to loss of transgene expression, due to rapid elimination of the Ad recombinant by host immune responses. For vaccination, repeated frequent immunizations may not be optimal for induction of strong, persistent immune responses, including memory cells [78]. Moreover, preexisting immunity to Ad does not necessarily limit the response to the transgene. Two sequential immunizations of rhesus macaques with an Ad5 host range mutant expressing SIV gene products were able to boost cellular immune responses to the expressed proteins [56] (J Zhao, Y Lou, LJ Patterson, N Malkevitch, M Robert-Guroff, unpublished observations). Immunization of cattle with preexisting high antibody titers to Ad with a bovine Ad3 bovine herpes virus recombinant successfully elicited strong immune responses and protected the animals from a subsequent bovine herpes virus challenge [46].

There are currently 49 recognized Ad serotypes and two additional subtype candidates, Ad50 and Ad51 [79]. However, little is known concerning current Ad seroprevalence worldwide. Most serological studies in healthy individuals were carried out in the 1960s on Ad subtypes 1–7 (Figure 3). Later studies focused on the enteric Ads, subtypes 40 and 41. Virus isolations from patients in the 1960s and 1970s showed that Ad2 and Ad1 were most prevalent [80]. Whether these patterns hold today is unknown. However, the great variety of Ad serotypes provides a means for sequential immunization with Ad vectors of different subtype, should preexisting immunity be a problem. Our HIV vaccine studies have used sequential immunizations with Ad5, Ad7, and Ad4-HIV recombinants in chimpanzees [52–54]. Gene therapy experiments have also established the feasibility of this approach [81,82]. After cessation of the Ad4 and Ad7 US military vaccination program, 88% of new recruits lack protective antibodies to both Ad4 and Ad7 [83]. Thus, these subtypes are reasonable choices for Ad vector development. Animal Ad vectors may also circumvent preexisting immunity to human Ads. A replication-defective chimpanzee Ad68 vector with little homology to human Ads is under development [84].

A final consideration in the design of Ad vaccine vectors concerns targeting desired cell types. Delivery of Ad to potent antigen-presenting dendritic cells has been achieved by targeting cell surface CD40 with a bispecific antibody [85]. A chimeric virus made by switching the less permissive subgroup C Ad5 fiber with one from subgroup B (Ad35) gave 100-fold better transgene expression [86]. Similarly, substitution with fibers from Ad40 or Ad41 that infect primarily gut tissue may help target Ad vaccines to mucosal inductive sites. Ad recombinants with knobless fibers, replaced with a moiety to provide the fiber trimerization function and a targeting ligand, can also alter viral tropism and retarget vectors to specific cell types [87]. Generation of Ad recombinants independent of CAR for

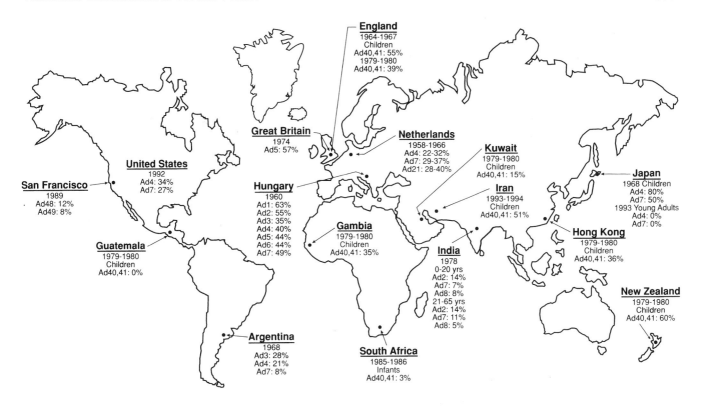

Figure 3 Worldwide seroprevalence of adenovirus subtypes. Seroprevalence in healthy individuals without symptoms of upper respiratory tract or gastrointestinal infection is reported. Dates provided are from the cited references or date of publication. (From Refs. 83,109–118.)

cell entry, including retargeting complexes composed of the CAR ectodomain fused to targeting ligands, were recently reviewed [88].

VI. ADENOVIRUS VACCINE APPLICATIONS

It is beyond the scope of this chapter to summarize the innumerable vaccine strategies to which Ad recombinants have been applied, including those designed for veterinary use. Studies with Ad recombinants that targeted a broad array of viruses causing human disease and resulting in protection were recently reviewed [2]. Nonviral diseases, such as malaria, have also been targeted effectively by Ad recombinant vaccines [78]. We will conclude, rather, with brief comments on two areas under intensive efforts of vaccine development: HIV/AIDS and cancer immunotherapy.

For HIV/AIDS vaccines, significant progress has been made using replication-competent Ad recombinants. The rationale is based on chimpanzee studies, which suggested that better replication of Ad-HIV recombinants in vivo leads to enhanced immune responses and greater protection [52–54]. Overall, a combination approach of Ad-HIV or Ad-SIV recombinant priming followed by boosting with envelope protein has elicited humoral, cellular, and mucosal immunity [49–57]. The vaccinated chimpanzees, in particular, showed persistent potent immune responses with significant protec-

tion against homologous and heterologus HIV challenges and provided the basis for moving forward into Phase I human trials. Other groups are utilizing replication-defective Ad recombinants deleted in E1 and E3 [89–92]. Recently, application of the chimpanzee Ad68 vector has been described [93]. In lieu of second-generation vectors, improved expression of HIV/SIV-inserted genes has been achieved by removing instability elements from targeted genes [94], or by altering codons to those preferentially utilized in mammalian cells [92]. Combination DNA priming, followed by Ad recombinant boosting, has led to enhanced immune responses, recently demonstrated with Ad-SIV vaccines in monkeys [92]. The potential of this approach is further exemplified by the synergistic immune responses seen in monkeys primed with an Ebola virus DNA vaccine and boosted with an Ad-Ebola recombinant. The animals were completely protected against a lethal Ebola virus challenge [95].

Adenovirus recombinant vectors are also being applied in the rapidly growing area of cancer vaccine development. Adenovirus recombinants can effectively deliver various therapeutic immune modulators, but recently have been used to immunize against tumor components themselves. Among the earliest strategies, mice immunized with Ad recombinants expressing the melanoma antigens MART-1 or gp100 were protected from a murine B16 melanoma challenge [96]. The safety of this approach was later confirmed in Phase I human trials [97]. Enhancement of immunity to melanoma antigens has been demonstrated by immunization of mice with Ad-gp100-transduced dendritic cells [98]. In other approaches, protection against B-cell and T-cell lymphomas has been described using Ad-B-cell lymphoma idiotypes [99] and an Ad-chimeric T-cell antigen receptor [100], respectively. An Ad-prostate-specific membrane antigen recombinant induced an immune response in people, thereby breaking tolerance to a self-antigen [101]. Ad-HPV16 vaccines have suppressed the growth of tumors in mice [102]. The use of vaccine strategies shown to enhance immune responses against infectious agents will undoubtedly have benefit in the cancer vaccine field.

VII. CONCLUDING REMARKS

Overall, live Ad recombinants have a broad potential for vaccine strategies against both infectious diseases and cancer. The long history of safety and efficacy of wild-type vaccines, the flexibility afforded by the numerous subtypes, the vast body of knowledge accumulated through gene therapy studies, and the already extensive accumulation of appropriate vectors and associated cell lines should stimulate and facilitate their further development for vaccine use.

REFERENCES

1. Russell WC. Update on adenovirus and its vectors. J Gen Virol 2000; 81:2573–2604.
2. Peng B, Robert-Guroff M. Adenovirus recombinants as vehicles for AIDS vaccine development. Curr Top Virol 1999; 1: 45–60.
3. Imler JL. Adenovirus vectors as recombinant viral vaccines. Vaccine 1995; 13:1143–1151.
4. Wilkinson GW, Borysiewicz LK. Gene therapy and viral vaccination: the interface. Br Med Bull 1995; 51:205–1216.
5. Harui A, et al. Frequency and stability of chromosomal integration of adenovirus vectors. J Virol 1999; 73:6141–6146.
6. Rowe WP, et al. Isolation of a cytopathogenic agent from human adenoids undergoing spontaneous degeneration in tissue culture. Proc Soc Exp Biol Med 1953; 84:570–573.
7. Hilleman MR, Werner JH. Recovery of new agents from patients with acute respiratory illness. Proc Soc Exp Biol Med 1954; 85:183–188.
8. Shenk T. Adenoviridae: the viruses and their replication. In: Fields BN, Knipe DM, Howley PM, Chanock RM, Melnick JL, Monath TP, Roizman B, Straus SE, eds. Fields Virology. Vol. 2. Philadelphia: Lippincott-Raven, 1996:2111–2148.
9. Horwitz MS. Adenoviruses. In: Fields BN, Knipe DM, Howley PM, Chanock RM, Melnick JL, Monath TP, Roizman B, Straus SE, eds. Fields Virology Vol 2. Philadelphia: Lippincott-Raven, 1996:2149–2169.
10. Ginsberg HS, Prince GA. The molecular basis of adenovirus pathogenesis. Infect Agents Dis 1994; 3:1–8.
11. Bergelson JM, et al. Isolation of a common receptor for coxsackie B viruses and adenoviruses 2 and 5. Science 1997; 275:1320–1323.
12. Tomko RP, et al. HCAR and MCAR: the human and mouse cellular receptors for subgroup C adenoviruses and group B coxsackieviruses. Proc Natl Acad Sci USA 1997; 94:3352–3356.

13. Wickham TJ, et al. Integrins αvβ3 and αvβ5 promote adenovirus internalization but not virus attachment. Cell 1993; 73:309–319.
14. Mette SA, et al. Distribution of integrin cell adhesion receptors on normal bronchial epithelial cells and lung cancer cells in vitro and in vivo. Am J Res Respir Cell Mol Biol 1993; 8:562–572.
15. Roelvink PW, et al. The coxsackievirus–adenovirus receptor protein can function as a cellular attachment protein for adenovirus serotypes from subgroups A, C, D, E, and F. J Virol 1998; 72:7909–7915.
16. Prince GA, et al. Pathogenesis of adenovirus type 5 pneumonia in cotton rats. J Virol 1993; 67:101–111.
17. Ginsberg HS, et al. A mouse model for investigating the molecular pathogenesis of adenovirus pneumonia. Proc Natl Acad Sci USA 1991; 88:1651–1655.
18. Cheng S-M, et al. Coexpression of the simian immunodeficiency virus env and rev proteins by a recombinant human adenovirus host range mutant. J Virol 1992; 66:6721–6727.
19. Graham FL. Transformation by and oncogenicity of human adenoviruses and their DNA. In: Ginsberg HS, ed. The Adenoviruses. New York: Plenum, 1984:339–398.
20. Nevels M, et al. "Hit-and-run" transformation by adenovirus oncogenes. J Virol 2001; 75:3089–3094.
21. Green M, et al. Analysis of human tonsil and cancer DNAs and RNAs for sequences of group C (serotypes 1, 2, 5, and 6) human adenoviruses. Proc Natl Acad Sci USA 1979; 76: 6606–6610.
22. Paabo S, et al. Structural and functional dissection of an MHC class I antigen-binding adenovirus glycoprotein. EMBO J 1986; 5:1921–1927.
23. Wold WS, Gooding LR. Region E3 of adenovirus: a cassette of genes involved in host immunosurveillance and virus–cell interactions. Virology 1991; 184:1–8.
24. Gooding LR, et al. A 14,700 MW protein from the E3 region of adenovirus inhibits cytolysis by tumor necrosis factor. Cell 1988; 53:341–346.
25. Leppard KN. E4 gene function in adenovirus, adenovirus vector and adeno-associated virus infections. J Gen Virol 1997; 78:2131–2138.
26. Dobner T, et al. Blockage by adenovirus E4orf6 of transcriptional activation by the p53 tumor suppressor. Science 1996; 272:1470–1473.
27. Moore MA, et al. Oncogenic potential of the adenovirus E4orf6 protein. Proc Natl Acad Sci USA 1996; 93:11295–11301.
28. Javier RT. Adenovirus type 9 E4 open reading frame 1 encodes a transforming protein required for the production of mammary tumors in rats. J Virol 1994; 68:3917–3924.
29. Christ M, et al. Modulation of the inflammatory properties and hepatotoxicity of recombinant adenovirus vectors by the viral E4 gene products. Hum Gene Ther 2000; 11:415–427.
30. Grave L, et al. Differential influence of the E4 adenoviral genes on viral and cellular promoters. J Gene Med 2000; 2: 433–443.
31. Bett A, et al. Packaging capacity and stability of human adenovirus type 5 vectors. J Virol 1993; 67:5911–5921.
32. Fang B, et al. Lack of persistence of E1-recombinant adenoviral vectors containing a temperature-sensitive E2A mutation in immunocompetent mice and hemophilia B dogs. Gene Ther 1996; 3:217–222.
33. Gorziglia MI, et al. Elimination of both E1 and E2 from adenovirus vectors further improves prospects for in vivo human gene therapy. J Virol 1996; 70:4173–4178.
34. Zhou H, et al. Development of a complementing cell line and a system for construction of adenovirus vectors with E1 and E2a deleted. J Virol 1996; 70:7030–7038.
35. Gao GP, et al. Biology of adenovirus vectors with E1 and

E4 deletions for liver-directed gene therapy. J Virol 1996; 70:8934–8943.

36. Engelhardt JF, et al. Ablation of E2A in recombinant adenoviruses improves transgene persistence and decreases inflammatory response in mouse liver. Proc Natl Acad Sci USA 1996; 91:6196–6200.

37. Dedieu JF, et al. Long-term gene delivery into the livers of immunocompetent mice with E1/E4-defective adenoviruses. J Virol 1997; 71:4626–4637.

38. Lusky M, et al. In vitro and in vivo biology of recombinant adenovirus vectors with E1, E1/E2A, or E1/E4 deleted. J Virol 1998; 72:2022–2032.

39. Parks RJ, Graham FL. A helper-dependent system for adenovirus vector production helps define a lower limit for efficient DNA packaging. J Virol 1997; 71:3293–3298.

40. Parks RJ, et al. Effects of stuffer DNA on transgene expression from helper-dependent adenovirus vectors. J Virol 1999; 73:8027–8034.

41. Parks RJ, et al. A helper-dependent adenovirus vector system: removal of helper virus by Cre-mediated excision of the viral packaging signal. Proc Natl Acad Sci USA 1996; 93:13565–13570.

42. Cheshenko N, et al. A novel system for the production of fully deleted adenovirus vectors that does not require helper adenovirus. Gene Ther 2001; 8:846–854.

43. Rubin BA, Rorke LB. In: Plotkin SA, Mortimer EA, eds. Vaccines. Philadelphia: W.B. Saunders Company, 1988:492–515.

44. Ginsberg HS, et al. Role of early region 3 (E3) in pathogenesis of adenovirus disease. Proc Natl Acad Sci USA 1989; 86:3823–3827.

45. Cox JH, et al. Expression of adenovirus E3/19K protein does not alter mouse MHC class I-restricted responses to vaccinia virus. Virology 1994; 204:558–562.

46. Babiuk LA, Tikoo SK. Adenoviruses as vectors for delivering vaccines to mucosal surfaces. J Biotechnol 2000; 83:105–113.

47. Patterson LJ. et al. Insertion of HIV-1 genes into Ad4ΔE3 vector abrogates increased pathogenesis in cotton rats due to E3 deletion. Virology 2002; 292:107–113.

48. Ginsberg HS, et al. Role of early genes in pathogenesis of adenovirus pneumonia. Proc Natl Acad Sci USA 1990; 87:6191–6195.

49. Lubeck MD, et al. Immunogenicity and efficacy testing in chimpanzees of a oral hepatitis B vaccine based on live recombinant adenovirus. Proc Natl Acad Sci USA 1989; 86:6763–6767.

50. Natuk RJ, et al. Immunogenicity of recombinant human adenovirus–human immunodeficiency virus vaccines in chimpanzees. AIDS Res Hum Retrovir 1993; 9:395–404.

51. Lubeck MD, et al. Immunogenicity of recombinant adenovirus–human immunodeficiency virus vaccines in chimpanzees following intranasal administration. AIDS Res Hum Retrovir 1994; 10:1443–1449.

52. Lubeck MD, et al. Long-term protection of chimpanzees against high-dose HIV-1 challenge induced by immunization. Nat Med 1997; 3:651–658.

53. Zolla-Pazner S, et al. Induction of neutralizing antibodies in chimpanzees to T-cell line-adapted and primary human immunodeficiency virus type 1 isolates with a prime/boost vaccine regimen in chimpanzees. J Virol 1998; 72:1052–1059.

54. Robert-Guroff M, et al. Vaccine protection against a heterologous, non-syncytium-inducing, primary human immunodeficiency virus. J Virol 1998; 72:10275–10280.

55. Buge SL, et al. An adenovirus–simian immunodeficiency virus env vaccine elicits humoral, cellular, and mucosal immune responses in rhesus macaques and decreases viral burden following vaginal challenge. J Virol 1997; 71:8531–8541.

56. Buge SL, et al. Factors associated with slow disease progression in macaques immunized with an adenovirus–simian immunodeficiency virus (SIV) envelope priming–gp120 boosting regimen and challenged vaginally with SIVmac251. J Virol 1999; 73:7430–7440. (Erratum in J Virol 1999;73:9692).

57. Patterson LJ, et al. A conformational C4 peptide polymer vaccine coupled with live recombinant vector priming is immunogenic but does not protect against rectal SIV challenge. AIDS Res Hum Retrovir 2001; 17:837–849.

58. Tacket CO, et al. Initial safety and immunogenicity studies of an oral recombinant adenohepatitis B vaccine. Vaccine 1992; 10:673.

59. Takafuji ET, et al. Simultaneous administration of live, enteric-coated adenovirus types 4, 7, and 21 vaccines: safety and immunogenicity. J Infect Dis 1979; 140:48–53.

60. Smith TJ, et al. Experimental respiratory infection with type 4 adenovirus vaccine in volunteers: clinical and immunological responses. J Infect Dis 1970; 122:239–248.

61. Knorr D. Serious adverse event on NIH human gene transfer protocol no. 9512-139. A Phase I study of adenovector mediated gene transfer to liver in adults with partial ornithine transcarbamylase deficiency. Memorandum of September 21, 1999. Office of Recombinant DNA Activities at NIH, 1999.

62. Lozier JN, et al. Adenovirus-mediated expression of human coagulation factor IX in the rhesus macaque is associated with dose-limiting toxicity. Blood 1999; 94:3968–3975.

63. Brenner M. Gene transfer by adenovectors. Blood 1999; 94:3965–3967.

64. Lee B, et al. Hepatocyte gene therapy in a large animal: a neonatal bovine model of citrullinemia. Proc Natl Acad Sci USA 1999; 96:3981–3986.

65. O'Neal WK, et al. Toxicological comparison of E2a-deleted and first-generation adenoviral vectors expressing alpha1-antitrypsin after systemic delivery. Hum Gene Ther 1998; 9:1587–1598.

66. Imperiale MJ, et al. Common control of the heat shock gene and early adenovirus genes: evidence of a cellular E1a-like activity. Mol Cell Biol 1984; 4:867–874.

67. Spergel JM, Chen-Kiang S. Interleukin 5 enhances a cellular activity that functionally substitutes for E1a protein in transactivation. Proc Natl Acad Sci USA 1991; 88:6472–6476.

68. Spergel JM, et al. NF-IL6, a member of the C/EBP family, regulates E1a-responsive promoters in absence of E1a. J Virol 1992; 66:1021–1030.

69. Knowles MR, et al. A controlled study of adenovirus-vector-mediated gene transfer in the nasal epithelium of patients with cystic fibrosis. N Engl J Med 1995; 333:823–831.

70. Zabner J, et al. Repeat administration of an adenovirus vector encoding cystic fibrosis transmembrane conductance regulator to the nasal epithelium of patients with cystic fibrosis. J Clin Invest 1996; 97:1504–1511.

71. Graham FL, et al. Characteristics of a human cell line transformed by DNA from human adenovirus type 5. J Gen Virol 1977; 36:59–74.

72. Louis N, et al. Cloning and sequencing of the cellular–viral junctions from the human adenovirus type 5 transformed 293 cell line. Virology 1997; 233:423–429.

73. Mehtali M. Complementation cell lines for viral vectors to be used in gene therapy. Cytotechnology 1996; 19:43–54.

74. Fallaux FJ, et al. Characterization of 911: a new helper cell line for the titration and propagation of early region 1-deleted adenoviral vectors. Hum Gene Ther 1996; 7:215–222.

75. Fallaux FJ, et al. New helper cells and matched early region 1-deleted adenovirus vectors prevent generation of replication-competent adenoviruses. Hum Gene Ther 1998; 9:1909–1917.

76. Gao G-P, et al. A cell line for high-yield production of E1-deleted adenovirus vectors without the emergence of replication-competent virus. Hum Gene Ther 2000; 11:213–219.

77. Brough DE, et al. A gene transfer vector–cell line system for complete functional complementation of adenovirus early regions E1 and E4. J Virol 1996; 70:6497–6501.

78. Bruna-Romero O, et al. Complete, long-lasting protection against malaria of mice primed and boosted with two distinct viral vectors expressing the same plasmodial antigen. Proc Natl Acad Sci USA 2001; 98:11491–11496.

79. De Jong JC, et al. Adenovirus from human immunodeficiency virus-infected individuals, including two strains that represent new candidate serotype Ad50 and Ad51 of species B1 and D, respectively. J Clin Microbiol 1999; 37:3940–3945.

80. Schmitz H, et al. Worldwide epidemiology of human adenovirus infections. Am J Epidemiol 1983; 117:455–466.

81. Mastrangeli A, et al. "Sero-switch" adenovirus-mediated in vivo gene transfer: circumvention of anti-adenovirus humoral immune defenses against repeat adenovirus vector administration by changing the adenovirus serotype. Hum Gene Ther 1996; 7:79–89.

82. Morral N, et al. Administration of helper-dependent adenoviral vectors and sequential delivery of different vector serotype for long-term liver-directed gene transfer in baboons. Proc Natl Acad Sci USA 1999; 96:12816–12821.

83. Ludwig SL, et al. Prevalence of antibodies to adenovirus serotypes 4 and 7 among unimmunized US army trainees: results of a retrospective nationwide seroprevalence survey. J Infect Dis 1998; 178:1776–1778.

84. Farina SF, et al. Replication-defective vector based on a chimpanzee adenovirus. J Virol 2001; 75:11603–11613.

85. Tillman BW, et al. Adenoviral vectors targeted to CD40 enhance the efficacy of dendritic cell-based vaccination against human papillomavirus 16-induced tumor cells in a murine model. Cancer Res 2000; 60:5456–5463.

86. Rea D, et al. Highly efficient transduction of human monocyte-derived dendritic cells with subgroup B fiber-modified adenovirus vectors enhance transgene-encoded antigen presentation to cytotoxic T cells. J Immunol 2001; 166:5236–5244.

87. van Beusechem VW, et al. Recombinant adenovirus vectors with knobless fibers for targeted gene transfer. Gene Ther 2000; 7:1940–1946.

88. Krasnykh V, et al. Advanced generation adenoviral vectors possess augmented gene transfer efficiency based upon coxsackie adenovirus receptor-independent cellular entry capacity. Cancer Res 2000; 60:6784–6787.

89. Bruce CB, et al. Replication-deficient recombinant adenoviruses expressing the human immunodeficiency virus env antigen can induce both humoral and CTL immune responses in mice. J Gen Virol 1999; 80:2621–2628.

90. Chenciner N, et al. Enhancement of humoral immunity to SIVenv following simultaneous inoculation of mice by three recombinant adenoviruses encoding SIVenv/poliovirus chimeras, Tat and Rev. AIDS Res Hum Retrovir 1997; 13:801–806.

91. Flanagan B, et al. A recombinant human adenovirus expressing the simian immunodeficiency virus Gag antigen can induce long-lived immune responses in mice. J Gen Virol 1997; 78:991–997.

92. Shiver J. Merck's HIV vaccine program: research approaches and critical issues. Presented at the AIDS Vaccine 2001 Meeting, Philadelphia, PA, September 5–8, 2001.

93. Fitzgerald J, et al. A novel vaccine to HIV-1 gag based on a replication-defective adenovirus recombinant of the chimpanzee serotype 68. Presented at the AIDS Vaccine 2001 Meeting, Philadelphia, PA, September 5–8, 2001.

94. Schwartz S, et al. Mutational inactivation of an inhibitory sequence in human immunodeficiency virus type 1 results in Rev-independent gag expression. J Virol 1992; 7:176–182.

95. Sullivan N, et al. Development of a preventive vaccine for Ebola virus infection in primates. Nature 2000; 408:605–609.

96. Zhai Y, et al. Antigen-specific tumor vaccines. Development and characterization of recombinant adenoviruses encoding MART1 or gp100 for cancer therapy. J Immunol 1996; 156:700–710.

97. Rosenberg SA, et al. Immunizing patients with metastatic melanoma using recombinant adenoviruses encoding MART-1 or gp100 melanoma antigens. J Natl Cancer Inst 1998; 90:1894–1900.

98. Wan Y, et al. Enhanced immune response to the melanoma antigen gp100 using recombinant adenovirus-transduced dendritic cells. Cell Immunol 1999; 198:131–138.

99. Timmerman JM, et al. Idiotype-encoding recombinant adenoviruses provide protective immunity against murine B-cell lymphomas. Blood 2001; 97:1370–1377.

100. Wong CP, Levy R. Recombinant adenovirus vaccine encoding a chimeric T-cell antigen receptor induces protective immunity against a T-cell lymphoma. Cancer Res 2000; 60:2689–2695.

101. Mincheff M, et al. Naked DNA and adenovirus immunizations for immunotherapy of prostate cancer: a phase I/II clinical trial. Eur Urol 2000; 38:208–217.

102. Liu DW, et al. Induction of CD8 T cells by vaccination with recombinant adenovirus expressing human papillomavirus type 16 E5 gene reduces tumor growth. J Virol 2000; 74:9083–9089.

103. Zhou H, Beaudet AL. A new vector system with inducible E2a cell line for production of higher titer and safer adenoviral vectors. Virology 2000; 275:348–357.

104. Yeh P, et al. Efficient dual transcomplementation of adenovirus E1 and E4 regions from a 293-derived cell line expressing a minimal E4 functional unit. J Virol 1996; 70:559–565.

105. Amalfitano A, Chamberlain JS. Isolation and characterization of packaging cell lines that coexpress the adenovirus E1, DNA polymerase, and preterminal proteins: implications for gene therapy. Gene Ther 1997; 4:258–263.

106. Gorzigia MI, et al. Generation of an adenovirus vector lacking E1, E2a, E3, and all of E4 except open reading frame 3. J Virol 1999; 73:6048–6055.

107. Ng P, et al. Development of a FLP/frt system for generating helper-dependent adenoviral vectors. Mol Ther 2001; 3:809–815.

108. Umana P, et al. Efficient FLPe recombinase enables scalable production of helper-dependent adenoviral vectors with negligible helper-virus contamination. Nat Biotechnol 2001; 19:582–585.

109. Evans AS. Serologic studies of acute respiratory infections in military personnel. Yale J Biol Med 1975; 48:201–209.

110. Mathur A, et al. Prevalence of neutralizing antibodies against adenoviruses at Lucknow. Indian J Med Res 1978; 67:19–26.

111. Van Der Veen J, et al. Patterns of infections with adenovirus types 4, 7, and 21 in military recruits during a 9-year survey. J Hyg Camb 1969; 67:255–268.

112. Alwen J, Emmerson AM. Antibodies against adeno-, cytomegalo- and rubella viruses in Australia-antigen-negative sera from patients with infectious hepatitis. J Hyg Camb 1974; 72:433–439.

113. Sakamoto M, et al. Longitudinal investigation of epidemiologic feature of adenovirus infections in acute respiratory illnesses among children in Yamagata, Japan (1986–1991). Tohoku J Exp Med 1995; 175:185–193.

114. Tiemessen CT, et al. Infection by enteric adenoviruses, rotaviruses, and other agents in a rural African environment. J Med Virol 1989; 28:176–182.

115. Kidd AH, et al. Antibodies to fastidious faecal adenoviruses (species 40 and 41) in sera from children. J Med Virol 1983; 11:333–341.

116. Crawford-Miksza L, Schnurr DP. Seroepidemiology of new AIDS-associated adenoviruses among the San Francisco Men's Health Study. J Med Virol 1996; 50:230–236.

117. Saderi H, et al. Antibodies to enteric adenoviruses (Ad40 and Ad41) in sera from Iranian children. J Clin Virol 2000; 16:145–147.

118. Nasz I, Toth M. Antibodies against adenoviruses. Lancet 1960; I:285.

29

RNA Virus Replicon Vaccines

Nancy L. Davis and Robert E. Johnston
University of North Carolina, Chapel Hill, North Carolina, U.S.A.

I. INTRODUCTION

Expression systems based on single-stranded RNA viruses offer exciting prospects for their application as vaccines. The relatively recent development of cDNA-based genetic systems for a substantial number of these viruses has made possible the directed manipulation of RNA virus genomes, the discovery of substantial genomic plasticity in these virus systems, and their reconfiguration as vaccine vectors. While not directly germane to a discussion of vaccines, pioneering work with infectious clones of poliovirus [1], positive-strand RNA plant viruses [2,3], and rabies virus [4] was key in guiding the subsequent development of analogous reverse genetic systems for other RNA viruses and vaccine vectors derived from them.

Single-stranded RNA virus vectors can be conveniently divided into those based on positive- or negative-stranded genomes. Positive-stranded genomes have the same sequence as mRNA. The first step in genome replication, the translation of the replicase enzymes from the parental RNA genome, directly occurs upon introduction of the genomic RNA into cells. Therefore when the RNA genome alone is introduced into a cell by any one of a number of transfection methods, it is infectious without the need of any exogenous viral proteins. For genetic manipulation of a positive-strand RNA genome, cDNA clones may be constructed with the viral sequences downstream of a phage RNA polymerase promoter. Linearization of the plasmid downstream of the viral sequences and in vitro transcription with the cognate phage RNA polymerase result in the production of positive-strand RNA replicas of the viral genome which are infectious after transfection into cells.

Negative-stranded RNA genomes carry their genetic information in the complementary sense relative to mRNA. Therefore successful virus propagation requires that the viral replicase/transcriptase enzymes active in the earliest stages of intracellular replication be introduced into the cell along with the genome. In systems designed for reverse genetics of negative-stranded viruses, in vitro transcripts from cDNA clones (usually transcripts which are the positive sense complement of the genome) are introduced into cells where the replicase proteins are being expressed from a second expression system (often the vaccinia T7 system).

With either positive or negative sense RNA genomes, the systems used to regenerate infectious viruses from cDNA clones have also been employed to add immunizing genes from target pathogens to the viral genomes. This results in a fully infectious and propagation competent virus vector which expresses an exogenous immunogen in addition to a full complement of viral proteins in the successive cells it infects. A second iteration on this theme is the substitution of an immunogen gene for one or more of the structural protein genes of the vector virus. The resulting RNA genome is self-replicating inside an appropriate cell, thus the term "replicon." The replicon expresses the immunizing gene and can be packaged into "replicon particles" when the structural proteins are produced *in trans* within the same cell. When inoculated into an animal or human, the replicon particles target to those cells normally infected first by the complete virus, the replicon genome expresses the immunizing gene, but the infection cannot be propagated to additional cells because of the absence of the structural protein genes from the replicon genome. Thus replicon particles can provide safe and effective immunization against a variety of pathogens.

II. REPLICON VACCINE VECTORS DERIVED FROM POSITIVE-STRAND RNA VIRUSES

A. Propagation Competent Vectors

1. Alphaviruses

Propagation competent vectors express an immunizing gene in the context of a complete virus genome. For instance, the alphavirus promoter for transcription of the subgenomic mRNA has been defined by deletion and point mutation analysis [5], and a second copy of this promoter can be inserted into the genome either immediately upstream of the original subgenomic promoter or between the end of the structural protein genes and the beginning of the 3' untranslated region [6,7]. As alphaviruses contain an icosahedral nucleocapsid, which presumably limits the total genome size, the size of exogenous RNA that can be added is also limited. Genes of up to 2.3 kb have been inserted and successfully used in murine immunization experiments [8], although genes in the 1-kb range are more stable upon passage of the virus [9]. Increased stability also may be associated with insertion at the upstream site [9].

2. Coronaviruses

Coronaviruses express their genes from a 3' coterminal nested set of mRNAs in which sequences at the 5' end of the genome are fused with the beginning of each mRNA immediately upstream of the coding sequence for each of the coronavirus genes. Although the precise mechanism whereby this occurs remains a matter of some controversy, the necessary *cis*-acting signals at the beginning of each gene have been well defined. An exogenous immunizing gene may be inserted between native coronavirus genes, and the gene will be expressed if the *cis*-acting intergenic region signals are included at its 5' end [10].

3. Picornaviruses

In picornavirus propagation competent vectors, short, foreign epitope sequences have been substituted for external loops on the poliovirus capsid structure, resulting in an immune response to those epitopes following infection with the chimeric poliovirus [11]. In a second iteration, the immunizing gene is placed either upstream of the major capsid genes or at the P1/P2 junction, maintaining the genomic open reading frame (ORF). As picornavirus genes are expressed as a single ORF, an additional internal ribosome entry site is utilized [12], or additional viral protease cleavage sites are placed as appropriate to excise the expressed protein from the polyprotein precursor [13]. Immunization with such vectors protected mice against a model tumor challenge [14]. Crotty et al. [15,16] overcame the inherently limited insertion size in such vectors by expressing a population of relatively short overlapping coding sequences from genes many times larger than the insertion maximum. Immunization of macaques with the population of vector viruses resulted in significant immunity to simian immunodeficiency virus (SIV), and significant protection upon challenge.

4. Flaviviruses

Flaviviruses have also been modified in a manner analogous to picornaviruses. A malaria epitope has been inserted into the E protein of the yellow fever vaccine strain, 17D [17], and 17D has been utilized to express a model tumor antigen and protect against tumor challenge [18]. The 17D virus, as well as attenuated dengue fever virus subtypes, has been utilized for the production of flavivirus chimeras in which the prM and E genes of a flavivirus to be vaccinated against are exchanged for the same genes in one of the vaccine virus backbones [19,20]. The goal is to take advantage of the attenuating mutations embedded in the vaccine backbone to create alternative live virus vaccines for the agents supplying the exogenous prM and E genes. Early stage clinical trials of this concept are underway [21].

5. Advantages and Disadvantages of Propagation Competent Vectors

Propagation competent vectors are essentially live virus vaccines and share some of their advantages and disadvantages. Because they are propagation-competent, they should be inexpensive to produce, and amplification in the vaccinee should allow immunization at a relatively low dose. The biological characteristics of the parent virus backbone also contribute to the characteristics of the vector. For example, in the case of poliovirus vectors, oral vaccination and induction of mucosal immunity are potentially significant advantages of this approach. However, the ability of propagation competent vectors to amplify in the host also imposes several challenges. The first of these is the necessity of maintaining an attenuated phenotype. In most of these systems, the insertion of the exogenous gene is itself a strongly attenuating mutation, and this can be supplemented with other defined attenuating mutations to make reversion a rare event. Second, the stability of the inserted gene is critical to the ability to immunize with the vectored gene. Third, inclusion of all the viral genes in addition to the vectored gene limits the size of the heterologous sequence that may be accommodated within the viral capsid, especially icosahedral capsids. Finally, the inclusion of all the viral genes in these vectors means that immunization will induce strong vector-specific immunity, perhaps limiting the ability of such vectors to be used for boosting or to be subsequently used in the same individuals for immunization against additional pathogens. In those instances where an existing human vaccine is utilized as the vector, the ability to vaccinate with the exogenous gene may be limited by preexisting immunity to the vector itself.

B. Replicon Vectors

Replicon vectors derived from positive-strand RNA viruses are essentially self-replicating machines designed to amplify the mRNA for the exogenous genes that they carry. By substituting an immunizing gene for one or more viral structural protein genes, the immunizing gene can be expressed to high level. The replicon genome can be packaged into virions by supplying the structural proteins in trans, thus producing a replicon particle capable of delivering the replicon genome to the same target cells as those normally infected by the wild-type virus. Because replicon genomes typically do not carry the genes for structural proteins, they are suicide vectors incapable of propagation beyond the initially infected cell.

RNA replicons based on poliovirus, the alphaviruses [Semliki Forest (SFV), Sindbis (SIN), Venezuelan equine encephalitis (VEE), and South African Arbovirus 86 (S.A.AR86)], the flavivirus Kunjin and the coronavirus transmissible gastroenteritis virus have been produced and tested for their ability to induce protective immune responses in experimental animals, including nonhuman primates in some cases. A human Phase I clinical trial with a VEE replicon expressing the human immunodeficiency virus (HIV) clade C gag gene has been initiated.

1. Alphaviruses

The antecedents of alphavirus replicon systems are found in the work of the Rice, Schlesinger, and Strauss laboratories, which constructed the first cDNA clones of alphaviruses, mapped the *cis*-acting signals required for alphavirus RNA replication and encapsidation, and showed that alphavirus RNAs could be modified to express exogenous genes [5–7,22–27]. Replicon expression systems have now been derived from several alphaviruses including SFV [28,29], SIN [30], VEE [31,32], and S.A.AR86 [33]. A replicon system based on a related Togavirus, rubella, also was recently described [34].

The structural protein genes, normally expressed to high level from a subgenomic mRNA, are deleted from alphavirus replicon systems and replaced by the immunizing gene. Thus, the gene of interest is expressed in replicon infected cells to levels approaching 20% of the total cell protein. In the SFV and SIN systems, high-level expression depends on the presence of a translational enhancer sequence extending from the subgenomic mRNA start site through approximately 200 nucleotides into the capsid gene [35,36]. Although the cells are eventually killed as a result of replicon infection, the absence of the structural protein genes prolongs the period of maximal expression [37]. Moreover, mutant alphavirus replicons have been selected which are capable of persistent infection and expression [38–41].

Packaging of alphavirus replicon genomes into replicon particles has been accomplished either by coelectroporation of in vitro replicon and helper structural protein transcripts [29,30,32], or by the establishment of stable cell lines constitutively expressing transcripts for the structural proteins [42]. In either case, the helper transcripts contain the *cis*-acting 5′ and 3′ ends of the cognate alphavirus, a deletion in the nonstructural gene region (deleting replicase function and the *cis*-acting packaging signal), and the native subgenomic promoter followed by the structural protein genes. Therefore in the presence of the cognate alphavirus replicon transcript, the structural protein helper RNAs are replicated, and the structural protein genes are expressed from the native 26S promoter. In the packaging cell lines, the helper transcripts are constitutively expressed but are not translated until introduction of the replicon RNA, either by electroporation or by infection with previously packaged replicon particles. Complementation occurs between the replicase functions inherent in the replicon RNA and the structural proteins supplied by the helper RNAs in these transfected cells, and replicon particles are assembled. These contain only the replicon RNA as a result of the absence of a packaging signal on the helper RNAs.

Alphavirus RNAs are capable of low-level recombination [43], and alphavirus particles can copackage multiple RNAs [30]. In the context of alphavirus packaging systems, either can result in the production of propagation competent genomes. Expressing the capsid and glycoprotein genes from separate helper RNAs significantly reduces the generation of propagation competent virions contaminating replicon particle preparations [32,42,44].

Replicon particles provide an efficient system for delivery of the replicon genome into cells in vivo. The effectiveness of the VEE replicon system may be attributable in part to the ability of VEE replicon particles to target and replicate within dendritic cells in lymph nodes of mice [45] and primates (West et al., personal communication). The SIN variants, selected from laboratory adapted strains for increased ability to target dendritic cells, may improve the ability of SIN replicon particles to induce immune responses [46]. However, other studies suggest that wild-type SIN itself targets efficiently to dendritic cells in vivo [47]. The SFV replicon particles also appear to target lymphoid tissue [48].

Replicon RNAs derived from alphaviruses have also been directly delivered into animals [49–53], although degradation of the RNA prior to entry into cells may limit this approach. Alternatively, cDNAs driven by eukaryotic promoters have been used to express self-replicating replicon RNAs [54–57]. In the case of cDNA delivery, the efficiency of transcription in and exit from the nucleus may limit effectiveness in a vaccine context [58].

Alphavirus replicon particle vaccines have been tested in a variety of animal models of disease. Humoral, cellular, and mucosal immunity have been demonstrated in mice, and in primates there is clear induction of both antibodies and cytotoxic T cells. Pushko et al. [32] described the protection of mice from intranasal (IN) influenza challenge by using VEE replicon particles expressing the hemagglutinin (HA) protein of influenza strain A/PR/8/34. Challenge virus replication was reduced by greater than 4 logs in the nose and could not be detected by in situ hybridization (Davis et al., personal communication). VEE replicon particle immunization against the A/HK/156/97 HA protected mice and chickens against challenge with the human pathogenic Hong Kong origin H5N1 virus [59]. Protection with VEE replicon particles has also been reported for equine arteritis virus in horses [60,61] and for rodent models of Lassa fever, Ebola, and botulinum toxin [62–64]. In primates, partial protection against simian immunodeficiency virus challenge has been demonstrated [65], and complete protection of primates against a high-dose challenge of Marburg virus was achieved [66]. Immunization with VEE replicon particles expressing the E7 protein from human papilloma virus 16 completely protected mice against tumor establishment in a murine model and led to eradication of established tumors in 67% of the animals [67].

The SIN- and SFV-based replicon vectors, either as naked RNA, as DNA-launched replicon genomes, or as replicon particles, have also induced varying degrees of immune response and protection in animal challenge models. These include influenza in mice [53,68–71], infectious bronchitis and infectious bursal disease viruses in chickens [72,73], flaviviruses in mice and sheep [53,74,75], herpes simplex in mice [57], tumor immunotherapy [76–83], immunodeficiency virus models in rodents and macaques [84–90], hepatitis C in conventional and HLA-A2.1 transgenic mice [91–93], *Plas-*

modium falciparum in mice [52,70], and respiratory syncytial virus in mice [53,94].

2. Picornaviruses

Kaplan and Racaniello [95] identified the sequences not essential for replication of poliovirus RNA, setting the stage for Ansardi et al. [96], who devised a poliovirus replicon system in which immunizing genes replace the P1 segment of the polio genome. Transfection of the replicon RNA and coinfection with vaccinia expressing the substituted poliovirus structural protein genes results in the production of poliovirus replicon particles, as well as the vaccinia helper. The polio replicon particles may be amplified by continued passage of the mixed population followed by separation of the much larger vaccinia virions from the polio replicon particles. This system has been utilized for immunization against a variety of bacterial and viral pathogens (e.g., *Helicobacter pylori* [97]; HIV/SIV [98–101]; tetanus toxin C-fragment [102]), and for tumor immunotherapy and viral induced lysis of tumors [103,104]. Following the poliovirus example, other picornaviruses, such as rhinoviruses, also are being developed as vaccine vectors [105].

3. Flaviviruses

Flavivirus genomes are organized as a single long ORF encoding the structural proteins at the 5′ end and the replicative nonstructural proteins in the 3′ portion of the genomic RNA. Replicons of Kunjin virus have been constructed in which the structural proteins are replaced with the gene of interest in a cDNA clone of the virus genome [106]. Much like the poliovirus replicons, electroporation of in vitro transcripts from the modified cDNA results in synthesis of the heterologous gene. Packaging of the Kunjin replicon genome into flavivirus-like particles is accomplished by supplying the structural proteins in trans from an SFV replicon [107]. Whether delivered into an animal as a naked RNA, as a cDNA placed behind a eukaryotic promoter, or as a Kunjin replicon particle, this system induces humoral and cellular immune responses to heterologous antigens [108]. A noncytopathic version of the Kunjin replicon has also been developed and may improve the capacity for immunization and/or enable gene therapy applications [109].

4. Coronaviruses

Coronavirus replicons are in the early stages of development but they hold promise as vaccine vectors because of their potential for expression of large gene cassettes. Heterologous genes have been inserted into the genome of transmissible gastroenteritis virus after deletion of genes required for either virus replication or assembly. The required genes are supplied in trans by a helper virus [110], or by an alphavirus replicon expressing the helper genes [111].

5. Advantages and Disadvantages of Replicon Vectors

Replicon vectors combine some of the features of live virus and subunit vaccines. They initiate a partial replication cycle in vivo, which allows the production of immunizing genes in the context of viral replication, much as what would occur with a live virus. The major product of that replication, however, is one or more protein subunits derived from the target pathogen. In a sense, replicon vectors represent the implantation of a subunit vaccine factory into the vaccinee, using the vaccinee's own cells for in situ production of the subunit vaccine. The absence of viral structural protein genes in the replicon RNA allows immunization with the vectored immunogen without raising high levels of immunity to the replicon particles themselves, facilitating booster inoculations as well as the sequential immunization of the same individual with the same vector expressing genes from other pathogens. Positive-strand RNA replicon vaccines can be delivered as self-replicating naked RNAs or as cDNAs from which self-replicating RNA replicons can be transcribed by cellular polymerases. This feature may facilitate the rapid development of new vaccines, as Good Manufacturing Practice (GMP) production of DNAs is straightforward and DNA vaccines will have been well characterized. The deletion of the vector's structural protein genes has two implications. First, it leaves room for larger inserted sequences than the related propagation competent vectors, and second, it makes replicon vectors inherently safe. Additional safety features can be built into the system, e.g., by using helper systems which reduce or eliminate the possibility of regenerating a propagation competent virus, including known attenuating mutations in the replicon genome and/or the structural protein genes used for packaging into replicon particles, and developing sensitive assays for the detection of propagation competent viruses in replicon particle preparations. However, a number of practical questions remain. No results of human trials are yet available for any of these systems, and for some, primate experiments have yet to be initiated. The GMP production of replicon particles may be problematic, with low relative yields in approved cell substrates and no packaging cell lines yet established in cell substrates likely to be approved for GMP production. These difficulties will be magnified in adapting these processes to commercial scale. Notwithstanding these issues, replicon vaccines derived from positive-strand RNA viruses have shown tremendous promise in experimental systems and certainly merit continued effort to resolve these potential limitations.

A number of review articles have been published on expression systems derived from positive-strand RNA viruses [112–124].

III. REPLICON VACCINE VECTORS DERIVED FROM NEGATIVE-STRAND RNA VIRUSES

Negative-strand viruses share advantages with positive-strand viruses when configured as vaccine vectors. Both have evolved mechanisms for high-level protein expression, and neither directs the integration of foreign genetic material into the genome of the host. However, now that systems have been established for the efficient recovery of recombinants of several negative-strand RNA viruses, and specific signals for gene expression have been defined, members of this group of viruses offer these additional advantages. First, viruses with segmented genomes and/or filamentous nucleocapsids are able to accommodate additional whole gene segments, or large gene insertions. Second, many are infectious by the intranasal (IN) route and deliver heterologous immunogens to the respiratory mucosa. Third, multiple serotypes exist in many cases, which facilitates effective booster strategies. Finally, in several cases, safe and effective vaccine strains have been reproduced as full-length cDNA clones and are available as the starting point for development of vaccine vectors.

A. Influenza Virus

Influenza virus is a member of the orthomyxovirus family, with a genome of eight segments of negative-sense RNA. These encode 10 viral proteins, the three polymerase proteins, PB2, PB1, and PA, the nucleoproteins, NP and NEP (NS2), the nonstructural protein, NS1, the membrane associated proteins, M1 and M2, and the transmembrane spike glycoproteins, neurominidase (NA) and hemagglutinin (HA). Fifteen distinct hemagglutinin subtypes and nine different NA subtypes have been identified, which could be alternated in sequential immunizations for improved boosting (see Section 3.2 below). Influenza virus differs from other RNA viruses in that genome replication and transcription occur in the nucleus of infected cells, although the life cycle does not involve a DNA intermediate. M1 and M2 are both expressed from the same genome segment by way of an unspliced (M1) or a spliced (M2) mRNA, as are NS1 and NS2. NS1 protein, which regulates mRNA export from the nucleus [125] and its translation in the cytoplasm [126], and inhibits the host interferon response [127], is the only nonstructural protein, and the only protein not required for viability. It has been possible, by using techniques described below, to generate viable viruses that contain more than eight segments.

Strategies for genetic engineering of influenza virus have been recently reviewed by Neumann and Kawaoka [128], and will be only briefly summarized here. Recombinant DNA technology has been a part of the study of influenza virus since the first system was described in 1989 by Luytjes et al. [129]. This initial technique was helper-virus-dependent. It combined the in vitro transcription and reconstitution of an influenza viral ribonucleoprotein (RNP) segment with RNP transfection. This was followed by helper virus superinfection and counterselection of helper virus to produce a pure stock of viable recombinant virus. The first published demonstration included the modification of influenza virus to drive the expression of chloramphenicol acetyltransferase (CAT), and influenza virus-based expression vectors were born [129]. The construction of RNA polymerase I-driven expression plasmids to produce all eight influenza vRNA segments, followed by cotransfection with influenza protein expression plasmids allowed generation of recombinant influenza virus entirely from cDNA, eliminated the need for helper virus, and opened up all 10 genes to genetic analysis [130–132].

Several approaches have been used to express foreign genes from influenza virus (reviewed in Refs. [133,134]). In an approach called epitope grafting, peptides were inserted to produce chimeric HA or NA proteins. Influenza vectors in which foreign peptides replaced the antigen B site of HA were used to immunize mice, and elicited serum antibodies, mucosal immune responses and/or CD8+ T cell responses against several disease agents, such as HIV [135–138], malaria [139,140], and *Pseudomonas aeruginosa* [141].

The stalk region of NA can also accommodate foreign sequence, and although this site may not efficiently present B cell epitopes [133,142], it has been used to induce specific CD8+ T cell responses against lymphocytic choriomeningitis virus [143], model tumor antigens [144], and malaria [145]. The strategy of epitope grafting is limited with respect to the amount and character of the foreign sequence that can be inserted without detrimental effects on the viability of the recombinant vector.

Efficient incorporation of a third, heterologous transmembrane glycoprotein into both the plasma membrane of infected cells and the envelope of recombinant virus has been demonstrated by Zhou et al. [146]. This was accomplished by helper virus rescue of a ninth genome segment expressed from an RNA polymerase I-driven plasmid that encoded a chimeric protein (the HA cytoplasmic region fused to the transmembrane anchor and ectodomain of classical swine fever virus (CSFV) E2 protein). The initial proportion of recombinant virus was maintained on passage because of the inclusion of an upregulated viral promoter on the engineered ninth genome segment. The performance of this vector as a vaccine for CSFV has not yet been reported.

The NS1 gene presents an attractive site for the insertion of foreign sequences. It is a true nonstructural protein which varies in size among different isolates, and thus may have fewer size constraints than a structural protein. It is abundant in influenza-infected cells. In infected animals, both NS1-specific antibody [147] and cytotoxic T lymphocytes (CTLs) [148] have been reported. Finally, the abrogation of its function as an interferon antagonist has been shown to significantly attenuate influenza virus virulence [127,149,150]. A recombinant NS genome segment was engineered to express a truncated NS1 protein fused to a self-cleaving foot-and-mouth disease virus (FMDV) protease domain followed by an HIV-1 Nef-derived polypeptide. This segment was rescued into viable virus by using a high-efficiency helper system for NS mutants [151]. The engineered NS-Nef virus replicated as well as the parent virus in most in vitro culture conditions, and was stable through five serial passages. In mice, IN inoculation of the NS-Nef virus produced no clinical signs and no virus replication in the nose or lung, which represented a significant reduction in virulence compared to the parent virus. However, the attenuated virus vector did replicate sufficiently to induce Nef-specific serum antibody and CD8+ T cells in the spleen and in lymph nodes of the respiratory tract and urogenital tract. A successful booster immunization was achieved by using a second analogous vaccine vector with a distinct HA subtype.

It has been possible to engineer influenza genome segments for expression of bicistronic mRNAs in which two open reading frames are separated by a mammalian internal ribosomal entry site or IRES. Garcia-Sastre et al. [152] constructed two such altered NA segments that contained (5′ to 3′) the HA signal sequence, a part of the HIV-1 gp41 ectodomain, a transmembrane region and cytoplasmic tail derived from either gp41 or HA, a BiP IRES, and the intact NA gene. The recombinant viruses, whose viability was dependent on the translation of the NA gene downstream of the IRES, grew to 0.5–1.5 log lower titers than the wild-type virus. Cells infected with both viruses contained the predicted gp41-related polypeptide, and the presence of the HA transmembrane region and cytoplasmic tail resulted in efficient transport of the foreign protein to the plasma membrane for incorporation into the virion envelope. Tests of the immune response to this vector have not been reported. A similar vector was constructed for *P. falciparum* and shown to induce specific CD8 + CTLs [140]. Improvements in this type of vector might include the use of a different, more efficiently replicated genome segment, such as HA, or the identification of a more active IRES.

Vaccinia-T7-based [153] and plasmid-based [154] systems have been established for the production of nonpropagating influenza virus-like particles (VLPs). An RNA polymerase I-driven plasmid was engineered to express a vRNA with an antisense copy of green fluorescent protein. The VLPs containing the synthetic vRNA were packaged by cotransfection of plasmids expressing the influenza structural proteins. By analogy to replicon particles of positive-strand viruses, single-cycle vector particles that contain a vRNA expressing a gene of interest as well as vRNA segments for PA, PB1, PB2, and NP (required for transcription and replication of the foreign sequence) would deliver the foreign gene to influenza virus susceptible cells for in vivo expression, but be unable to spread in the host. Also, a nonpropagating influenza virus vaccine vector could be based on the work of Watanabe et al. [155], who engineered an NS2-knockout virus that is replication-defective and highly immunogenic in mice.

B. Rhabdoviruses

The best known members of the Rhabdovirus family are vesicular stomatitis virus (VSV) and rabies virus, both of which have been exploited as vaccine vectors. Rhabdoviruses contain nonsegmented, negative-sense RNA genomes and are classified with Paramyxoviruses and Filoviruses in the order Mononegavirales. Genomic RNA is approximately 11 kb in length, and encodes the nucleocapsid protein (N), phosphoprotein (P, previously NS, a cofactor in viral RNA synthesis), matrix protein (M), spike glycoprotein (G), and RNA-dependent RNA polymerase (L). All five viral proteins are found in the virus particle. Sequential transcription of these five genes by the viral transcriptase complex occurs on the nucleoprotein-encapsidated genome and is regulated by *cis*-acting signal sequences, including the 3′ polymerase entry site and gene-start, polyadenylation, and gene-stop sequences flanking each gene. The level of gene expression is directly related to gene position relative to the 3′ end of the RNP template, such that rearrangement of the viral genes leads to slower growth in cultured cells and attenuation of virus virulence in the animal host [156]. These rearranged genomes are stable on passage, as homologous recombination does not occur. There are three known serotypes of VSV, but only a single serotype of rabies virus. Specific mu-

tations in both the VSV and rabies virus glycoproteins have been shown to attenuate virulence, and there is a live attenuated vaccine for rabies that is safe in many animal species. Although VSV is cytopathic in cell culture, rabies virus does not shut off host protein synthesis in cultured cells. VSV has a wide host range, from insects to man, and causes a mild, flu-like illness in humans. Laboratory animals can be infected by subcutaneous, intracranial or IN routes.

Vesicular stomatitis virus RNA transcription has been characterized in depth by elegant in vitro reconstitution studies. Further insights into the virus life cycle were gained by using cells infected with defective deletion mutants and transfected with virus protein expression plasmids, or by using cells cotransfected with cDNAs expressing either deletion mutant genomes or synthetic minigenomes and virus proteins. Schnell et al. [4], working with rabies virus, first demonstrated cDNA-based replication of a full-length recombinant rhabdovirus genome, by using the transfection of T7-driven RNA expression plasmids for transcription of both the complete genome complement (or antigenome) and the mRNAs for the N, P, and L proteins, followed by infection with vaccinia virus expressing T7 bacteriophage RNA polymerase. In the 8 years since this signal success, this strategy has been successfully used to produce recombinant VSV and several paramyxoviruses (see below). More recently, vaccinia virus-free systems for both rabies virus and VSV have been developed [157,158].

Functional gene-stop and gene-start signal sequences were inserted into the rabies virus genome sequence and recovered in viable virus as part of the demonstration that a recombinant rabies virus could be produced from cDNA [4]. Shortly thereafter, stable expression of a reporter protein from a sixth VSV gene flanked by minimal start and stop signals and inserted between the G and L genes was obtained [159]. This basic strategy has been used in the construction of several expression and vaccine vectors (some of which are described in Schnell et al. [160]), which have allowed the characterization of this system.

It was expected, based on the well-known ability of VSV to incorporate heterologous glycoproteins into its virions, that heterologous glycoproteins expressed from VSV vectors would become part of analogous mosaic virions or psuedotypes. Viable viruses carrying genes for CD4, measles virus hemagglutinin (MH) or measles virus fusion protein (MF) were produced from cDNAs and were shown to contain varying amounts of the foreign protein inserted into their virion envelopes. The additional gene increased the length of the bullet-shaped particles, presumably because of the increased length of the filamentous ribonucleocapsid, and reduced, to varying degrees, the level of virus replication in cultured cells. In many but not in all cases, no VSV-specific sequence was needed to drive incorporation of the additional glycoprotein into the virion envelope. The efficiency of VSV G incorporation into virions was not affected, suggesting that the new membrane protein occupied extra space in the envelope. By electron microscopy, each virus particle contained both proteins. This type of replication-competent VSV vaccine vector has been tested in animal models against measles virus [161], influenza virus [162,163], respiratory syncytial virus [164,165], HIV-1 (see below), and bovine viral diarrhea virus [166]. The VSV vector expressing measles virus H protein was used to vaccinate cotton rats intranasally in a measles virus challenge experiment [161]. In contrast to the attenuated live virus measles vaccine, the VSV vaccine vector was able to induce protective levels of serum neutralizing antibody even in the presence of maternal antibody. In vitro, virions carrying both VSV G and measles H protein on their surface (at 30% the level of G) were easily neutralized by VSV-specific antiserum, but required very high titers of measles-specific serum for neutralization. Thus the additional envelope glycoprotein is highly immunogenic, but is nonfunctional in the vector replication cycle, and when bound to moderate amounts of cognate antibody, does not interfere with G-driven VSV infection. This vaccine vector approach is promising in cases such as measles, where vaccination in the presence of maternal antibody is needed to prevent dangerous early childhood infections.

Haglund et al. [167] demonstrated that viable VSV vectors could express two foreign proteins from two additional mRNAs with only a threefold reduction in titer. The HIV-1 *gag* gene was positioned between M and G, and the *env* gene between G and L in the same recombinant VSV genome. HIV virus-like particles (VLPs) as well as VSV vector particles were produced. HIV gp160 was incorporated only into VLPs, while VSV G was found in both.

A cocktail approach, mixing vaccine vectors expressing either SIV Gag or an HIV Env/VSV G chimeric protein, was used in a SHIV89.6P challenge experiment in macaques [168]. HIV-specific neutralizing antibody was induced, and cellular immune responses were detected against both proteins in most vaccinated monkeys. All the vaccinated animals were infected upon SIV 89.6P challenge, but were able to control their virus loads and remain disease-free for several months.

Two concerns surround the use of propagation competent VSV vectors: (1) the febrile, flu-like illness associated with human infection [169], as well as residual reactogenicity in mice of IN-administered vaccine vectors; and (2) induction of levels of antivector antibody that prevent effective booster immunizations [163,170]. Some improvements of propagation competent vectors have been explored. Recombinant VSV mutants carrying deletions in the cytoplasmic tail of G that were significantly attenuated relative to the parent virus have been described, and vaccine vectors carrying these mutations and expressing influenza HA showed comparable immunogenicity in mice to the parent vector [163,171]. In addition, effective boosting in the presence of anti-VSV antibody has been achieved by constructing vaccine vectors with G proteins of three alternate serotypes [170].

In an alternate approach, both vector virulence and antivector immunity are addressed by the use of nonpropagating G-deleted vectors. It is possible to engineer a recombinant virus whose G gene is replaced with that for a heterologous glycoprotein. This virus can be maintained on cells that provide G in trans. However, following a single passage through normal cells, nonpropagating virions carry primarily the heterologous envelope protein. When such vectors were constructed with influenza HA, RSV G, or RSV F, each of the three proteins was incorporated into virions that did not spread in cell culture. However, RSV F did function to produce syncytia in vector-infected cells. In mice, the vectors inoculated IN produced no clinical signs, and gave complete protection against disease [171,165]. In contrast, the analogous vector lacking the VSV G gene and expressing an HIV-1 gp160 chimeric protein with the VSV G transmembrane and cytoplasmic domains was infectious. Gp160 substituted for G in the virus envelope to produce a "surrogate virus," which was able to grow efficiently in HIV-susceptible cells [172]. This was also true, in reverse, for vectors expressing cellular CD4 and CXCR4, which mediated entry of vector particles into HIV-infected cells with gp160 on their surface [173]. The utility of this approach may depend, therefore, on the ability of the heterologous glycoprotein to produce a propagation-competent recombinant virus, and its resulting biological properties.

Vaccine vectors have also been based on rabies virus. Advantages of this vector system include the availability of a vaccine strain shown to be safe in many animal species, the less cytopathic nature of infection in cultured cells, and the possibility of oral immunization [174]. A vector in which HIV-1 gp160 was inserted between the G and L genes was inoculated intraperitoneally (IP) into mice and primed a neutralizing antibody response to HIV [174] and a cross-reactive anti-HIV CTL response [175]. The IP immunization of mice with an analogous vector expressing HIV-1 Gag induced HIV gag-specific CD8+ CTLs. G-deficient rabies virus vectors expressing a chimeric HIV-1 gp160-G protein (with the rabies virus G protein cytoplasmic domain) contained gp160 in their envelope, showed reduced replication in vitro compared to G-containing vectors and displayed the cell tropism of HIV-1 [176].

C. Paramyxoviruses

The Paramyxovirus family includes two subfamilies, the Paramyxovirinae subfamily, with the respiroviruses (e.g., Sendai virus, human parainfluenza, and bovine parainfluenza), the rubulaviruses [New Castle disease virus (NDV) and simian virus 5 (SV5)], and the morbilliviruses (measles and rinderpest viruses), and the Pneumovirinae subfamily, with the pneumoviruses (human and bovine respiratory syncytial viruses) and the metapneumoviruses. Paramyxoviruses contain nonsegmented negative-sense RNA genomes in filamentous ribonucleocapsids enclosed in polymorphic envelopes. They share patterns of gene expression and regulation with the simpler rhabdoviruses, but carry additional genes. For example, all paramyxoviruses have two distinct glycoprotein spikes, one for attachment and the other for fusion with the host cell membrane. Several recombinant paramyxoviruses have been recovered from genomic cDNA clones by using techniques analogous to those described for rhabdoviruses. Reverse genetics systems have been reported for measles virus, respiratory syncytial virus, Sendai virus, Rinderpest virus, human parainfluenza type 3 (hPIV-3), and simian virus 5 (SV5) (reviewed by Roberts and Rose [177]). More recently, recombinant bovine PIV-3 [178] and New Castle disease virus (NDV) [179] have been recovered. Work with these systems has made significant contributions to the understanding of the replication cycles of these viruses and, in some cases, has allowed determinants of attenuation to be mapped and candidate vaccine vectors to be constructed.

A large body of work with genomic cDNA clones of RSV and PIV3 has been previously summarized [180]. The ability to rescue recombinant human and bovine RSV spurred the development of candidate live attenuated RSV vaccines (reviewed in Collins et al. [181]). These were constructed by introducing single and multiple mutations originally identified in cold-passaged and/or chemically mutated strains [182–188], by deleting genes not required for growth in cultured cells [181,189,190,191,192,193] or by replacing the G and F genes of recombinant bovine RSV with human RSV G and F [194].

The RSV genome was engineered to express the CAT reporter gene by linking its coding sequence to flanking RSV gene-start and gene-stop signals and inserting them between the G and F genes of the cDNA encoding the RSV antigenome. Expression was maintained on passage in spite of the fact that the additional small gene reduced virus yield in vitro by 20-fold [195]. A dual-specificity, propagation-competent RSV vaccine candidate was produced by inserting the RSV subgroup B G protein between the F and M2 genes of recombinant subgroup A RSV [196]. This virus vector showed a 1 $\log_{10}$ reduction in peak titer in vitro and both glycoproteins were expressed in infected cells. However, insertion into virion envelopes was not assayed.

In 1997, two groups reported the recovery of human PIV3 from full-length cDNA [197,198]. By analogy to RSV, recombinant hPIV3 has been used to test attenuating mutations for inclusion in a live, attenuated vaccine [199–202]. Bovine PIV3 shows restricted replication in human cells and in the primate respiratory tract, and is attenuated in humans [203,204]. Three recombinant human and bovine PIV3 chimeras have been constructed and tested for attenuation. Two were based on hPIV3 cDNA with its N gene [205], or F and HN genes [206] replaced by those from bovine PIV3. The third was based on a bovine PIV3 cDNA with its F and HN genes replaced by those from hPIV3 [178,206]. The reverse genetics system for human PIV3 also has been used as a starting point for development of vaccine candidates against the closely related human pathogens, hPIV1 [207–210], and hPIV2 [211].

Dual-specificity paramyxovirus vaccine candidates have been produced by adding genes to a full-length cDNA as described for RSV subgroups A and B above. In this strategy, the original recombinant virus becomes a vaccine vector, and an attenuated bivalent or trivalent vaccine strain is produced. In initial experiments with recombinant hPIV3, the insertion of an additional transcribed but noncoding sequence between the HN and L genes was shown to contribute in and of itself to attenuation in hamsters [212]. The insertion of the coding sequence for measles virus HA protein at any one of several intergenic sites in the hPIV-3 cDNA was similarly attenuating [213]. When administered intranasally, this bivalent vaccine candidate induced a protective immune response against hPIV challenge in hamsters, and a level of measles virus neutralizing antibody in excess of that known to protect humans. The IN administration may allow the successful immunization of infants against these two respiratory pathogens even in the presence of maternal

antimeasles neutralizing antibodies in the serum. A similar approach was taken by using the attenuated bovine–human PIV3 chimera (F and HN genes of hPIV3 in the bovine PIV3 backbone). The insertion of either the RSV G or F protein as the first gene transcribed, upstream of the PIV3 N gene, produced a bivalent vaccine that protected hamsters against challenge with both hPIV3 and RSV [214]. This result was the basis for construction of two recombinant PIV3 chimeras containing G and F genes from either RSV subgroup A or B, and a test in monkeys [215]. The levels of neutralizing antibody against both PIV3 and RSV were comparable to those induced by RSV infection or by infection with the bovine–human PIV3 vector. These studies describe an attractive strategy for mucosal vaccination against two of the most important respiratory pathogens of infants.

Reverse genetics for measles virus has led to the rescue of recombinant measles virus expressing several heterologous reporter proteins and immunogens [216,217]. This work is based on a full-length cDNA of the Edmonston B vaccine strain, which has a long history of safe and effective human use. In addition, the targeting of measles virus to macrophages and dendritic cells may be important in induction of immune responses to a vectored immunogen. Recombinant measles virus expressing the surface antigen of hepatitis B virus induced antihepatitis B virus antibody in a mouse model for measles virus infection [218], and measles virus vectors stably expressed immunogens of simian immunodeficiency virus with only a minor effect on growth kinetics [219]. A vaccination strategy based on recombinant measles virus has been proposed that would replace the current early-life measles vaccine with a cocktail of vectors expressing heterologous immunogens.

Simian virus 5, although it can infect and replicate in most cultured cells lines, induces very little cell death in most cell lines tested, and can persistently infect cultured cells. This property was exploited by Parks et al. [220] to produce a recombinant SV5 vector for controlled cell killing. SV5 was engineered to express the herpes simplex thymidine kinase gene inserted between its HN and L genes, and shown to replicate in several cell lines without extensive cytopathic effect. However, infection coupled with treatment with acyclovir or gancyclovir, drugs that become toxic when phosphorylated by TK, led to extensive cell death. The use of this virus vector for targeted killing of cancer cells depends on the ability to engineer the SV5 HN protein for specific cell targeting in vivo. More recently, induction of a strong cellular immune response by recombinant SV5 has been demonstrated [221].

There are many reminders that the vaccine vector approach is an empirical one. For example, expression of mumps glycoproteins by a measles virus vector was unexpectedly very deleterious to virus growth [219]. Also, expression of foot-and-mouth disease genes by an attenuated recombinant rinderpest virus did not induce any detectable immune response to FMDV, nor did it protect cattle against FMDV infection [222], in spite of the fact that vaccination with an analogous rinderpest virus vaccine vector for influenza HA was highly immunogenic in cattle [223].

A vaccine vector based on a full-length cDNA of the Newcastle disease virus (NDV) veterinary vaccine strain,

Hitchner B1, was described by Nakaya et al. [179], who tested for the expression of either CAT or influenza HA from genes inserted between the P and M genes. The expressed HA protein was incorporated into the infected cell plasma membrane and virion envelope, and viral titers were reduced 20-fold. The addition of the HA gene attenuated even further the virulence of the NDV vaccine strain for embryonated eggs. The intraperitoneal or intravenous immunization of mice induced HA-specific serum antibody and protected against a lethal influenza virus challenge. NDV vaccine vectors present the possibility of bivalent poultry vaccines, as well as human use vaccines.

A vaccine vector for SIV was based on recombinant Sendai virus. Macaques were immunized intranasally with SIV Gag-expressing Sendai virus, either alone or following an initial immunization with a DNA vector, and then challenged with pathogenic SHIV. The Sendai vector contributed to induction of a protective immune response when used as a booster [224]. A nonpropagating Sendai virus-based vector also has been reported. This defective recombinant virus does not carry a functional gene for F, the fusion protein, and can be propagated only in cells that provide F protein in trans, but is able to enter susceptible cells, replicate its RNA genome and express the heterologous gene to high levels [225]. It cannot spread either by production of infectious virus progeny or by cell-to-cell fusion.

IV. CONCLUSION

RNA virus genomes, reconfigured to express heterologous antigen genes, have great potential as vaccine vectors. Levels of expression are generally high, the plasticity of RNA genomes will allow innovative use of their coding capacity, knowledge of virulence determinants will insure safety, and the variety of potential vaccine vectors will obviate problems of antivector immunity. However, this field is relatively young, and significant hurdles must be surmounted as RNA virus vectors progress from the laboratory to human use vaccine products. Few of these concepts have moved from tests in mice to experiments in nonhuman primates, and fewer still have progressed to human trials. In addition, some of these laboratory-derived systems are not particularly well suited for GMP production at commercial scale. Nevertheless, the potential of RNA virus-based replicon strategies for improvement of existing vaccines and for derivation of new ones places these rapidly developing vaccine concepts at the leading edge among new vaccine technologies.

REFERENCES

1. Racaniello VR, Baltimore D. Cloned poliovirus complementary DNA is infectious in mammalian cells. Science 1981; 214:916–919.
2. Ahlquist P, et al. Multicomponent RNA plant virus infection derived from cloned viral cDNA. Proc Natl Acad Sci USA 1984; 81:7066–7070.
3. French R, et al. Bacterial gene inserted in an engineered RNA virus: efficient expression in monocotyledonous plant cells. Science 1986; 231:1294–1297.
4. Schnell M, et al. Infectious rabies viruses from cloned cDNA. EMBO J 1994; 13:4195–4203.
5. Levis R, et al. The promoter for Sindbis virus RNA-dependent subgenomic RNA transcription. J Virol 1990; 64: 1726–1733.
6. Levis R, et al. Engineered defective interfering RNAs of Sindbis virus express bacterial chloramphenicol acetyltransferase in avian cells. Proc Natl Acad Sci USA 1987; 84: 4811–4815.
7. Hahn CS, et al. Infectious Sindbis virus transient expression vectors for studying antigen processing and presentation. Proc Natl Acad Sci USA 1992; 89:2679–2683.
8. Caley IJ, et al. Humoral, mucosal and cellular immunity in response to a human immunodeficiency virus type 1 immunogen expressed by a Venezuelan equine encephalitis virus vaccine vector. J Virol 1997; 71:3031–3038.
9. Caley IJ, et al. Venezuelan equine encephalitis virus vectors expressing HIV-1 proteins: vector design strategies for improved vaccine efficacy. Vaccine 1999; 17:3124–3135.
10. Masters PS. Reverse genetics of the largest RNA viruses. Adv Virus Res 1999; 53:245–264.
11. Evans DJ, et al. An engineered poliovirus chimera elicits broadly reactive HIV-1 neutralizing antibodies. Nature 1989; 339:385–388.
12. Alexander L, et al. Poliovirus containing picornavirus type 1 and/or type 2 internal ribosomal entry site elements: genetic hybrids and the expression of a foreign gene. Proc Natl Acad Sci USA 1994; 91:1406–1410.
13. Andino R, et al. Engineering poliovirus as a vaccine vector for the expression of diverse antigens. Science 1994; 265: 1448–1451.
14. Mandl S, et al. Poliovirus vaccine vectors elicit antigen-specific cytotoxic T cells and protect mice against lethal challenge with malignant melanoma cells expressing a model antigen. Proc Natl Acad Sci USA 1998; 95:8216–8221.
15. Crotty S, et al. Mucosal immunization of cynomolgus macaques with two serotypes of live poliovirus vectors expressing simian immunodeficiency virus antigens: stimulation of humoral, mucosal and cellular immunity. J Virol 1999; 73:9485–9495.
16. Crotty S, et al. Protection against simian immunodeficiency virus vaginal challenge by using Sabin poliovirus vectors. J Virol 2001; 75:7435–7452.
17. Bonaldo MC, et al. Surface expression of an immunodominant malaria protein B cell epitope by yellow fever virus. J Mol Biol 2002; 315:873–885.
18. McAllister A, et al. Recombinant yellow fever viruses are effective therapeutic vaccines for treatment of murine experimental solid tumors and pulmonary metastases. J Virol 2000; 74:9197–9205.
19. Bray M, Lai CJ. Construction of intertypic chimeric dengue viruses by substitution of structural protein genes. Proc Natl Acad Sci USA 1991; 88:10342–10346.
20. Chambers TJ, et al. Yellow fever/Japanese encephalitis chimeric viruses: construction and biological properties. J Virol 1999; 73:3095–3101.
21. Monath TP, et al. Clinical proof of principle for ChimeriVax: recombinant live, attenuated vaccines against flavivirus infections. Vaccine 2002; 20:1004–1018.
22. Strauss EG, et al. Complete nucleotide sequence of the genomic RNA of Sindbis virus. Virology 1984; 133:92–110.
23. Rice CM, et al. Production of infectious RNA transcripts from Sindbis virus cDNA clones: mapping of lethal mutations, rescue of a temperature-sensitive marker, and in vitro mutagenesis to generate defined mutants. J Virol 1987; 61:3809–3819.
24. Weiss B, et al. Evidence for specificity in the encapsidation of Sindbis RNAs. J Virol 1989; 63:5310–5318.
25. Xiong C, et al. Sindbis virus: an efficient, broad host range

vector for gene expression in animal cells. Science 1989; 243: 1188–1191.

26. Geigenmuller-Gnirke U, et al. Complementation between Sindbis viral RNAs produces infectious particles with a bipartite genome. Proc Natl Acad Sci USA 1991; 88:3253–3257.

27. Strauss JH, Strauss EG. The alphaviruses: gene expression, replication, and evolution. Microbiol Rev 1994; 58:491–562.

28. Liljeström P, et al. In vitro mutagenesis of a full-length cDNA clone of Semliki Forest virus: the small 6,000-molecular-weight membrane protein modulates virus release. J Virol 1991; 65:4107–4113.

29. Liljeström P, Garoff H. A new generation of animal cell expression vectors based on the Semliki Forest virus replicon. Bio/Technology 1991; 9:1356–1361.

30. Bredenbeek PJ, et al. Sindbis virus expression vectors: packaging of RNA replicons by using defective helper RNAs. J Virol 1993; 67:6439–6446.

31. Davis NL, et al. In vitro synthesis of infectious Venezuelan equine encephalitis virus RNA from a cDNA clone: analysis of a viable deletion mutant. Virology 1989; 171:189–204.

32. Pushko P, et al. Replicon–helper systems from attenuated Venezuelan equine encephalitis virus: expression of heterologous genes in vitro and immunization against heterologous pathogens in vivo. Virology 1997; 239:389–401.

33. Heise MT, et al. Sindbis-group alphavirus replication in periosteum and endosteum of long bones in adult mice. J Virol 2000; 74:9294–9299.

34. Tzeng WP, et al. Rubella virus DI RNAs and replicons: requirement for nonstructural proteins acting in cis for amplification by helper virus. Virology 2001; 289:63–73.

35. Frolov I, Schlesinger S. Translation of Sindbis virus mRNA: effects of sequences downstream of the initiating codon. J Virol 1994; 68:8111–8117.

36. Frolov I, Schlesinger S. Translation of Sindbis virus mRNA: analysis of sequences downstream of the initiating AUG codon that enhance translation. J Virol 1996; 70:1182–1190.

37. Frolov I, Schlesinger S. Comparison of the effects of Sindbis virus and Sindbis virus replicons on host cell protein synthesis and cytopathogenicity in BHK cells. J Virol 1994; 68:1721–1727.

38. Dryga SA, et al. Identification of mutations in a Sindbis virus variant able to establish persistent infection in BHK cells; the importance of a mutation in the nsP2 gene. Virol 1997; 228:74–83.

39. Agapov EV, et al. Noncytopathic Sindbis virus RNA vectors for heterologous gene expression. Proc Natl Acad Sci USA 1998; 95:12989–12994.

40. Frolov I, et al. Selection of RNA replicons capable of persistent noncytopathic replication in mammalian cells. J Virol 1999; 73:3854–3865.

41. Perri S, et al. Replicon vectors derived from Sindbis virus and Semliki forest virus that establish persistent replication in host cells. J Virol 2000; 74:9802–9807.

42. Polo JM, et al. Stable alphavirus packaging cell lines for Sindbis virus-and Semliki Forest virus-derived vectors. Proc Natl Acad Sci USA 1999; 96:4598–4603.

43. Raju R, et al. Genesis of Sindbis virus by in vivo recombination of nonreplicative RNA precursors. J Virol 1995; 69:7391–7401.

44. Smerdou C, Liljeström P. Two-helper RNA system for production of recombinant Semliki forest virus particles. J Virol 1999b; 73:1092–1098.

45. MacDonald GH, Johnston RE. The role of dendritic cell targeting in Venezuelan equine encephalitis virus pathogenesis. J Virol 2000; 74:914–922.

46. Gardner JP, et al. Infection of human dendritic cells by a Sindbis virus replicon vector is determined by a single amino acid substitution in the E2 glycoprotein. J Virol 2000 Dec; 74(24):11849–11857.

47. Ryman KD, et al. Type 1 interferon protects adult mice from fatal Sindbis virus infection and is an important determinant of cell and tissue tropism. J Virol 2000; 74:3366–3378.

48. Morris-Downes MM, et al. Semliki forest virus-based vaccines: persistence, distribution and pathological analysis in two animal systems. Vaccine 2001; 19:1978–1988.

49. Brand D, et al. Comparative analysis of humoral immune responses to HIV type 1 envelope glycoproteins in mice immunized with a DNA vaccine, recombinant Semliki forest virus RNA, or recombinant Semliki forest virus particles. AIDS Res Hum Retrovir 1998; 14:1369–1377.

50. Giraud A, et al. Generation of monoclonal antibodies to native human immunodeficiency virus type 1 envelope glycoprotein by immunization of mice with naked RNA. J Virol Methods 1999; 79:75–84.

51. Vignuzzi M, et al. Naked RNA immunization with replicons derived from poliovirus and Semliki forest virus genomes for the generation of a cytotoxic T cell response against the influenza A virus nucleoprotein. J Gen Virol 2001; 82:1737–1747.

52. Andersson C, et al. Comparative immunization study using RNA and DNA constructs encoding a part of the Plasmodium falciparum antigen Pf332. Scand J Immunol 2001; 54:117–124.

53. Fleeton MN, et al. Self-replicative RNA vaccines elicit protection against influenza A virus, respiratory syncytial virus, and a tickborne encephalitis virus. J Infect Dis 2001; 183:1395–1398.

54. Driver DA, et al. Layered amplification of gene expression with a DNA gene delivery system. Ann NY Acad Sci 1995; 772:261–264.

55. Dubensky TW Jr, et al. Sindbis virus DNA-based expression vectors: utility for in vitro and in vivo gene transfer. J Virol 1996; 70:508–519.

56. Berglund P, et al. Enhancing immune responses using suicidal DNA vaccines. Nat Biotechnol 1998; 16:562–565.

57. Hariharan MJ, et al. DNA immunization against herpes simplex virus: enhanced efficacy using a Sindbis virus-based vector. J Virol 1998; 72:950–958.

58. Kamrud KI, et al. Comparison of the protective efficacy of naked DNA, DNA-based Sindbis replicon, and packaged Sindbis replicon vectors expressing Hantavirus structural genes in hamsters. Virology 1999; 263:209–219.

59. Schultz-Cherry S, et al. Influenza virus (A/HK/156/97) hemagglutinin expressed by an alphavirus replicon system protects chickens against lethal infection with Hong Kong-origin H5N1 viruses. Virology 2000; 278:55–59.

60. Balasuriya UBR, et al. Expression of the two major envelope proteins of equine arteritis virus as a heterodimer is necessary for induction of neutralizing antibodies in mice immunized with recombinant Venezuelan equine encephalitis virus replicon particles. J Virol 2000; 74:10623–10630.

61. Balasuriya UBR, et al. Alphavirus replicon particles expressing the two major envelope proteins of equine arteritis virus induce high level protection against challenge with virulent virus in vaccinated horses. Vaccine 2002; 20:1609–1617.

62. Pushko P, et al. Recombinant RNA replicons derived from attenuated Venezuelan equine encephalitis virus protect guinea pigs and mice from Ebola hemorrhagic fever virus. Vaccine 2000 Aug 15; 19(1):142–153.

63. Pushko P, et al. Individual and bivalent vaccines based on alphavirus replicons protect guinea pigs against infection with Lassa and Ebola viruses. J Virol 2001 Dec; 75(23): 11677–11685.

64. Lee JS, et al. Candidate vaccine against botulinum neurotoxin serotype A derived from a Venezuelan equine encephalitis virus vector system. Infect Immun 2001 Sep; 69(9): 5709–5715.

65. Davis NL, et al. Vaccination of macaques against pathogenic simian immunodeficiency virus with Venezuelan equine encephalitis virus replicon particles. J Virol 2000; 74:371–378.

66. Hevey M, et al. Marburg virus vaccines based upon alphavirus replicons protect guinea pigs and nonhuman primates. Virology 1998 Nov 10; 251(1):28–37.

67. Velders MP, et al. Eradication of established tumors by vaccination with Venezuelan equine encephalitis virus replicon particles delivering human papillomavirus 16 E7 RNA. Cancer Res 2001; 61:7861–7867.

68. Zhou X, et al. Self-replicating Semliki forest virus RNA as recombinant vaccine. Vaccine 1994; 12:1510–1514.

69. Zhou X, et al. Generation of cytotoxic and humoral immune responses by nonreplicative recombinant Semliki forest virus. Proc Natl Acad Sci USA 1995; 92:3009–3013.

70. Tsuji M, et al. Recombinant Sindbis viruses expressing a cytotoxic T-lymphocyte epitope of a malaria parasite or of influenza virus elicit protection against the corresponding pathogen in mice. J Virol 1998; 72:6907–6910.

71. Berglund P, et al. Immunization with recombinant Semliki forest virus induces protection against influenza challenge in mice. Vaccine 1999; 17:497–507.

72. Seo SH, et al. The carboxyl-terminal 120-residue polypeptide of infectious bronchitis virus nucleocapsid induces cytotoxic T lymphocytes and protects chickens from acute infection. J Virol 1997; 71:7889–7894.

73. Phenix KV, et al. Recombinant Semliki forest virus vector exhibits potential for avian virus vaccine development. Vaccine 2001; 19:3116–3123.

74. Colombage G, et al. DNA-based and alphavirus-vectored immunization with prM and E proteins elicits long-lived and protective immunity against the flavivirus, Murray Valley encephalitis virus. Virology 1998; 250:151–163.

75. Morris-Downes MM, et al. A recombinant Semliki forest virus particle vaccine encoding the prME and NS1 proteins of louping ill virus is effective in a sheep challenge model. Vaccine 2001; 19:3877–3884.

76. Colmenero P, et al. Induction of P815 tumor immunity by recombinant Semliki forest virus expressing the P1A gene. Gene Ther 1999; 6:1728–1733.

77. Daemen T, et al. Genetic immunization against cervical carcinoma: induction of cytotoxic T lymphocyte activity with a recombinant alphavirus vector expressing human papillomavirus type 16 E6 and E7. Gene Ther 2000; 7:1859–1866.

78. Leitner WW, et al. Enhancement of tumor-specific immune response with plasmid DNA replicon vectors. Cancer Res 2000; 60:51–55.

79. Lachman LB, et al. DNA vaccination against neu reduces breast cancer incidence and metastasis in mice. Cancer Gene Ther 2001; 8:259–268.

80. Yamanaka R, et al. Enhancement of antitumor immune response in glioma models in mice by genetically modified dendritic cells pulsed with Semliki forest virus-mediated complementary DNA. J Neurosurg 2001; 94:474–481.

81. Cheng WF, et al. Enhancement of Sindbis virus self-replicating RNA vaccine potency by linkage of Mycobacterium tuberculosis heat shock protein 70 gene to an antigen gene. J Immunol 2001; 166:6218–6226.

82. Cheng WF, et al. Cancer immunotherapy using Sindbis virus replicon particles encoding a VP22-antigen fusion. Hum Gene Ther 2002; 13:553–568.

83. Daemen T, et al. Immunization strategy against cervical cancer involving an alphavirus vector expressing high levels of a stable fusion protein of human papillomavirus 16 E6 and E7. Gene Ther 2002; 9:85–94.

84. Mossman SP, et al. Protection against lethal simian immunodeficiency virus SIVsmmPBj14 disease by a recombinant Semliki forest virus gp160 vaccine and by a gp120 vaccine. J Virol 1996; 70:1953–1960.

85. Berglund P, et al. Outcome of immunization of cynomolgus monkeys with recombinant Semliki forest virus encoding human immunodeficiency virus type 1 envelope protein and challenge with a high dose of SHIV-4 virus. AIDS Res Hum Retrovir 1997; 13:1487–1495.

86. Rosenwirth B, et al. An anti-HIV strategy combining chemotherapy and therapeutic vaccination. J Med Primatol 1999; 28:195–205.

87. Notka F, et al. Construction and characterization of recombinant VLPs and Semliki forest virus live vectors for comparative evaluation in the SHIV monkey model. Biol Chem 1999a; 380:341–352.

88. Notka F, et al. Accelerated clearance of SHIV in rhesus monkeys by virus-like particle vaccines is dependent on induction of neutralizing antibodies. Vaccine 1999b; 18:291–301.

89. Vajdy M, et al. Human immunodeficiency virus type 1 Gag-specific vaginal immunity and protection after local immunizations with Sindbis virus-based replicon particles. J Infect Dis 2001; 184:1613–1616.

90. Nilsson C, et al. Enhanced simian immunodeficiency virus-specific immune responses in macaques induced by priming with recombinant Semliki forest virus and boosting with modified vaccinia virus Ankara. Vaccine 2001; 19:3526–3536.

91. Vidalin O, et al. Use of conventional or replicating nucleic acid-based vaccines and recombinant Semliki forest virus-derived particles for the induction of immune responses against hepatitis C virus core and E2 antigens. Virology 2000; 276:259–270.

92. Brinster C, et al. Different hepatitis C virus nonstructural protein 3 (Ns3)-DNA-expressing vaccines induce in HLA-A2.1 transgenic mice stable cytotoxic T lymphocytes that target one major epitope. Hepatology 2001; 34:1206–1217.

93. Brinster C, et al. Hepatitis C virus non-structural protein 3-specific cellular immune responses following single or combined immunization with DNA or recombinant Semliki forest virus particles. J Gen Virol 2002; 83:369–381.

94. Andersson C, et al. Protection against respiratory syncytial virus (RSV) elicited in mice by plasmid DNA immunization encoding a secreted RSV G protein-derived antigen. FEMS Immunol Med Microbial 2000; 29:247–253.

95. Kaplan G, Racaniello VR. Construction and characterization of poliovirus subgenomic replicons. J Virol 1988; 62:1687–1696.

96. Ansardi DC, et al. Complementation of a poliovirus defective genome by a recombinant vaccinia virus which provides poliovirus P1 capsid precursor in trans. J Virol 1993; 67:3684–3690.

97. Novak MJ, et al. Poliovirus replicons encoding the B subunit of Helicobacter pylori urease elicit a Th1 associated immune response. Vaccine 1999; 17:2384–2391.

98. Morrow CD, et al. New approaches for mucosal vaccines for AIDS: encapsidation and serial passage of poliovirus replicons that express HIV-1 proteins on infection. AIDS Res Hum Retrovir 1994; 10(suppl 2):S61–S68.

99. Moldoveanu Z, et al. Immune responses induced by administration of encapsidated poliovirus replicons which express HIV-1 gag and envelope proteins. Vaccine 1995; 13:1013–1022.

100. Porter DC, et al. Release of virus-like particles from cells infected with poliovirus replicons which express human immunodeficiency virus type 1 gag. J Virol 1996; 70:2643–2649.

101. Anderson MJ, et al. Characterization of the expression and immunogenicity of poliovirus replicons that encode simian

immunodeficiency virus SIVmac239 Gag or envelope SU proteins. AIDS Res Hum Retrovir 1997; 13:53–62.

102. Porter DC, et al. Immunization of mice with poliovirus replicons expressing the C-fragment of tetanus toxin protects against lethal challenge with tetanus toxin. Vaccine 1997; 15:257–264.

103. Ansardi DC, et al. Characterization of poliovirus replicons encoding carcinoembryonic antigen. Cancer Res 1994; 54: 6359–6364.

104. Ansardi DC, et al. RNA replicons derived form poliovirus are directly oncolytic for human tumor cells of diverse origins. Cancer Res 2001; 61:8470–8479.

105. Dollenmaier G, et al. Membrane-associated respiratory syncytial virus F protein expressed from a human rhinovirus type 14 vector is immunogenic. Virol 2001; 281:216–230.

106. Khromykh AA, Westaway EG. Subgenomic replicons of the flavivirus Kunjin: construction and applications. J Virol 1997; 71:1497–1505.

107. Khromykh AA, et al. Encapsidation of the flavivirus Kunjin replicon RNA by using a complementation system providing Kunjin virus structural proteins in trans. J Virol 1998; 72:5967–5977.

108. Anraku I, et al. Kunjin virus replicon vaccine vectors induce protective CD8(+) T-cell immunity. J Virol 2002; 76:3791–3799.

109. Varnavski AN, Khromykh AA. Noncytopathic flavivirus replicon RNA-based system for expression and delivery of heterologous genes. Virology 1999; 255:366–375.

110. Alonso S, et al. In vitro and in vivo expression of foreign genes by transmissible gastroenteritis coronavirus-derived minigenomes. J Gen Virol Mar 2002; 83(Pt 3):567–579.

111. Curtis KM, et al. Heterologous gene expression from transmissible gastroenteritis virus replicon particles. J Virol Feb 2002; 76(3):1422–1434.

112. Huang HV, et al. RNA viruses as gene expression vectors. Virus Genes 1989; 3:85–91.

113. Girard M, et al. The use of picornaviruses as vectors for the engineering of live recombinant vaccines. Biologicals 1995; 23:165–169.

114. Atkins GJ, et al. Manipulation of the Semliki forest virus genome and its potential for vaccine construction. Mol Biotechnol 1996; 5:33–38.

115. Frolov I, et al. Alphavirus-based expression vectors: strategies and applications. Proc Natl Acad Sci USA 1996; 93: 11371–11377.

116. Morrow CD, et al. Recombinant viruses as vectors for mucosal immunity. Curr Top Microbiol Immunol 1999; 236:255–273.

117. Palese P. RNA virus vectors: where are we and where do we need to go? Proc Natl Acad Sci USA 1998; 95:12750–12752.

118. Smerdou C, Liljeström P. Non-viral amplification systems for gene transfer: vectors based on alphaviruses. Curr Opin Mol Ther 1999; 1:244–251.

119. Schlesinger S, Dubensky TW Jr. Alphavirus vectors for gene expression and vaccines. Curr Opin Biotechnol 1999; 10:434–439.

120. Hewson R. RNA viruses: emerging vectors for vaccination and gene therapy. Mol Med Today 2000; 6:28–35.

121. Khromykh AA, et al. Replicon-based vectors of positive strand RNA viruses. Curr Opin Mol Ther 2000; 2:555–569.

122. Polo JM, et al. Alphavirus DNA and particle replicons for vaccines and gene therapy. Dev Biol 2000; 104:181–185.

123. Schlesinger S. Alphavirus vectors: development and potential therapeutic applications. Expert Opin Biol Ther 2001; 1:177–191.

124. Enjuanes L, et al. Coronavirus derived expression systems. Progress and problems. Adv Exp Med Biol 2001; 494:309–321.

125. Alonso-Caplen FV, et al. Nucleocytoplasmic transport: the influenza virus NS1 protein regulates the transport of spliced NS2 mRNA and its precursor NS1 mRNA. Genes Dev 1992; 6:255–267.

126. Enami K, et al. Influenza virus NS1 protein stimulates translation of the M1 protein. J Virol 1994; 68:1432–1437.

127. Garcia-Sastre A, et al. Influenza A virus lacking the NS1 gene replicates in interferon-deficient systems. Virology 1998; 252:324–330.

128. Neumann G, Kawaoka Y. Reverse genetics of influenza virus. Virology 2001; 287:243–250.

129. Luytjes W, et al. Amplification, expression and packaging of a foreign gene by influenza virus. Cell 1989; 58:1107–1113.

130. Fodor E, et al. Rescue of influenza A virus from recombinant DNA. J Virol 1999; 73:9679–9682.

131. Neumann G, et al. Generation of influenza A viruses entirely from cloned cDNAs. Proc Natl Acad Sci 1999; 96: 9345–9350.

132. Pekosz A, et al. Reverse genetics of negative strand RNA viruses: closing the circle. Proc Natl Acad Sci 1999; 96: 8804–8806.

133. Garcia-Sastre A, Palese P. Influenza virus vectors. Biologicals 1995; 23:171–178.

134. Palese P, et al. Negative-strand RNA viruses: genetic engineering and applications. Proc Natl Acad Sci 1996; 93: 11354–11358.

135. Li S, et al. Chimeric influenza virus induces neutralizing antibodies and cytotoxic T cells against human immunodeficiency virus type 1. J Virol 1993; 67:6659–6666.

136. Muster T, et al. Mucosal model of immunization against human immunodeficiency virus type 1 with a chimeric influenza virus. J Virol 1995; 69:6678–6686.

137. Ferko B, et al. Chimeric influenza virus replicating predominantly in the murine upper respiratory tract induces local immune responses against human immunodeficiency virus type 1 in the genital tract. J Infect Dis 1998; 178:1359–1368.

138. Gonzalo RM, et al. Enhanced CD8 + T cell response to HIV-1 env by combined immunization with influenza and vaccinia virus recombinants. Vaccine 1999; 17:887–892.

139. Li S, et al. Priming with recombinant influenza virus followed by administration of recombinant vaccinia virus induces CD8 + T-cell-mediated protective immunity against malaria. Proc Natl Acad Sci 1993; 90:5214–5218.

140. Miyahira Y, et al. Recombinant viruses expressing a human malaria antigen can elicit potentially protective immune CD8 + responses in mice. Proc Natl Acad Sci 1998; 95: 3954–3959.

141. Gilleland HE, et al. Chimeric animal and plant viruses expressing epitopes of outer membrane protein F as a combined vaccine against *Pseudomonas aeruginosa* lung infection. FEMS Immunol Med Microbiol 2000; 27:291–297.

142. Luo G, et al. Alterations of the stalk of the influenza virus neuraminidase: deletions and insertions. Vir Res 1993; 29: 141–153.

143. Castrucci MR, et al. Protection against lethal lymphocytic choriomeningitis virus (LCMV) infection by immunization of mice with an influenza virus containing an LCMV epitope recognized by cytotoxic T lymphocytes. J Virol 1994; 68:3486–3490.

144. Restifo NP, et al. Transfectant influenza viruses are effective recombinant immunogens in the treatment of experimental cancer. Virology 1998; 249:89–97.

145. Rodrigues M, et al. Influenza and vaccinia viruses expressing malaria CD8 + T and B cell epitopes. J Immunol 1994; 153:4636–4648.

146. Zhou Y, et al. Membrane-anchored incorporation of a foreign protein in recombinant influenza virions. Virology 1998; 246:83–94.

147. Birch-Machin I, et al. Expression of the nonstructural protein NS1 of equine influenza A virus: detection of anti-NS1 antibody in post infection equine sera. J Virol Methods 1997; 65:255–263.

148. Man S, et al. Definition of a human T cell epitope from influenza A non-structural protein 1 using HLA-A2.1 transgenic mice. Int Immunol 1995; 7:597–605.

149. Talon J, et al. Influenza A and B viruses expressing altered NS1 proteins: a vaccine approach. Proc Natl Acad Sci 2000; 97:4309–4314.

150. Garcia-Sastre A. Inhibition of interferon-mediated antiviral responses by influenza A viruses and other negative-strand RNA viruses. Virology 2001; 279:375–384.

151. Ferko B, et al. Hyperattenuated recombinant influenza A virus nonstructural-protein-encoding vectors induce human immunodeficiency virus type 1 Nef-specific systemic and mucosal immune responses in mice. J Virol 2001; 75:8899–8908.

152. Garcia-Sastre A, et al. Use of a mammalian internal ribosomal entry site element for expression of a foreign protein by a transfectant influenza virus. J Virol 1994; 68:6254–6261.

153. Gomez-Puertas P, et al. Efficient formation of influenza virus-like particles: dependence on the expression levels of viral proteins. J Gen Virol 1999; 80:1635–1645.

154. Neumann G, et al. Plasmid-driven formation of influenza virus-like particles. J Virol 2000; 74:547–551.

155. Watanabe T, et al. Immunogenicity and protective efficacy of replication-incompetent influenza virus-like particles. J Virol 2002; 76:767–773.

156. Wertz GW, et al. Gene rearrangement attenuates expression and lethality of a nonsegmented negative strand RNA virus. Proc Natl Acad Sci 1998; 95:3501–3506.

157. Harty RN, et al. Vaccinia virus-free recovery of vesicular stomatitis virus. J Mol Microbiol Biotechnol 2001; 3:513–517.

158. Finke S, Conzelmann KK. Virus promoters determine interference by defective RNAs: selective amplification of mini-RNA vectors and rescue from cDNA by a 3′ copy-back ambisense rabies virus. J Virol 1999; 73:3818–3825.

159. Schnell MJ, et al. The minimal conserved transcription stop–start signal promotes stable expression of a foreign gene in vesicular stomatitis virus. J Virol 1996; 70:2318–2323.

160. Schnell MJ, et al. Foreign glycoproteins expressed from recombinant vesicular stomatitis viruses are incorporated efficiently into virus particles. Proc Natl Acad Sci 1996; 93:11359–11365.

161. Schlereth B, et al. Successful vaccine-induced serconversion by single-dose immunization in the presence of measles virus-specific maternal antibodies. J Virol 2000; 74:4652–4657.

162. Kretzschmar E, et al. High-efficiency incorporation of functional influenza virus glycoproteins into recombinant vesicular stomatitis viruses. J Virol 1997; 71:5982–5989.

163. Roberts A, et al. Vaccination with a recombinant vesicular stomatitis virus expressing an influenza virus hemagglutinin provides complete protection from influenza virus challenge. J Virol 1998; 72:4704–4711.

164. Kahn JS, et al. Recombinant vesicular stomatitis virus expressing respiratory syncytial virus (RSV) glycoproteins: RSV fusion protein can mediate infection and cell fusion. Virology 1999; 254:81–91.

165. Kahn JS, et al. Replication-competent or attenuated, non-propagating vesicular stomatitis viruses expressing respiratory syncytial virus (RSV) antigens protect mice against RSV challenge. J Virol 2001; 75:11079–11087.

166. Grigera PR, et al. Presence of bovine viral diarrhea virus (BVDV) E2 glycoprotein in VSV recombinant particles and induction of neutralizing BVDV antibodies in mice. Virus Res 2000; 69:3–15.

167. Haglund K, et al. Expression of human immunodeficiency virus type 1 Gag protein precursor and envelope proteins from a vesicular stomatitis virus recombinant: high-level production of virus-like particles containing HIV envelope. Virology 2000; 268:112–121.

168. Rose NF, et al. An effective AIDS vaccine based on live attenuated vesicular stomatitis virus recombinants. Cell 2001; 106:539–549.

169. Johnson KM, et al. Clinical and serological response to laboratory-acquired human infection by Indiana type vesicular stomatitis virus (VSV). Am J Trop Med Hyg 1966; 15:244–246.

170. Rose NF, et al. Glycoprotein exchange vectors based on vesicular stomatitis virus allow effective boosting and generation of neutralizing antibodies to a primary isolate of human immunodeficiency virus type 1. J Virol 2000; 74:10903–10910.

171. Roberts A, et al. Attenuated vesicular stomatitis viruses as vaccine vectors. J Virol 1999; 73:3723–3732.

172. Boritz E, et al. Replication-competent rhabdoviruses with human immunodeficiency virus type 1 coats and green fluorescent protein; entry by a pH-independent pathway. J Virol 1999; 73:6937–6945.

173. Schnell MJ, et al. Construction of a novel virus that targets HIV-1-infected cells and controls HIV-1 infection. Cell 1997; 90:849–857.

174. Schnell MJ, et al. Recombinant rabies virus as potential live-viral vaccines for HIV-1. Proc Natl Acad Sci 2000; 97:3544–3549.

175. McGettigan JP, et al. Rabies virus-based vectors expressing human immunodeficiency virus type 1 (HIV-1) envelope protein induce a strong, cross-reactive cytotoxic t-lymphocyte response against envelope proteins from different HIV-1 isolates. J Virol 2001; 75:4430–4434.

176. Foley HD, et al. Rhabdovirus-based vectors with human immunodeficiency virus type 1 (HIV-1) envelopes display HIV-1-like tropism and target human dendritic cells. J Virol 2002; 76:19–31.

177. Roberts A, Rose JK. Recovery of negative-strand RNA viruses from plasmid DNAs: a positive approach revitalizes a negative field. Virology 1998; 247:1–6.

178. Haller AA, et al. Expression of the surface glycoproteins of human parainfluenza virus type 3 by bovine parainfluenza virus type 3, a novel attenuated virus vaccine vector. J Virol 2000; 74:11626–11635.

179. Nakaya T, et al. Recombinant Newcastle disease virus as a vaccine vector. J Virol 2001; 75:11868–11873.

180. Murphy BR, Collins PL. Current status of respiratory syncytial virus (RSV) and parainfluenza virus type 3 (PIV3) vaccine development; memorandum from a joint WHO/NIAID meeting. Bull WHO 1997; 75:307–313.

181. Collins PL, et al. Rational design of live-attenuated recombinant vaccine virus for human respiratory syncytial virus by reverse genetics. Adv Vir Res 1999; 54:423–451.

182. Juhasz K, et al. The temperature-sensitive (ts) phenotype of a cold-passaged (cp) live attenuated respiratory syncytial virus vaccine candidate, designated cpts530, results from a single amino acid substitution in the L protein. J Virol 1997; 71:5814–5819.

183. Whitehead SS, et al. Recombinant respiratory syncytial virus (RSV) bearing a set of mutations from cold-passaged RSV is attenuated in chimpanzees. J Virol 1998; 72:4467–4471.

184. Whitehead SS, et al. A single nucleotide substitution in the transcription start signal of the M2 gene of respiratory syncytial virus vaccine candidate cpts248/404 is the major determinant of the temperature-sensitive and attenuation phenotypes. Virology 1998; 247:232–239.

185. Whitehead SS, et al. Recombinant respiratory syncytial

virus bearing a deletion of either the NS2 or SH gene is attenuated in chimpanzees. J Virol 1999; 73:871–877.

186. Juhasz K, et al. The two amino acid substitutions in the L protein of cpts530/1009, a live-attenuated respiratory syncytial virus candidate vaccine, are independent temperature-sensitive and attenuation mutations. Vaccine 1999; 17:1416–1424.

187. Juhasz K, et al. The major attenuating mutations of the respiratory syncytial virus vaccine candidate cpts530/1009 specify temperature-sensitive defects in transcription and replication and a non-temperature-sensitive alteration in mRNA termination. J Virol 1999; 73:5176–5180.

188. Crowe JE Jr, et al. Acquisition of the ts phenotype by a chemically mutagenized cold-passaged human respiratory syncytial virus vaccine candidate results from the acquisition of a single mutation in the polymerase (L) gene. Virus Genes 1996; 13:269–273.

189. Bukreyev A, et al. Recombinant respiratory syncytial virus from which the entire SH gene has been deleted grows efficiently in cell culture and exhibits site-specific attenuation in the respiratory tract of the mouse. J Virol 1997; 71:8973–8982.

190. Whitehead SS, et al. Addition of a missense mutations present in the L gene of respiratory syncytial virus (RSV) cpts530/1030 to RSV vaccine candidate cpts248/404 increases its attenuation and temperature sensitivity. J Virol 1999; 73:3438–3442.

191. Teng MN, et al. Recombinant respiratory syncytial virus that does not express the NS1 or M2-2 protein is highly attenuated and immunogenic in chimpanzees. J Virol 2000; 74:9317–9321.

192. Jin H, et al. Respiratory syncytial virus that lacks open reading frame 2 of the M2 gene (M2-2) has altered growth characteristics and is attenuated in rodents. J Virol 2000; 74:74–82.

193. Jin H, et al. Recombinant respiratory syncytial viruses with deletions in the NS1, NS2, SH and M2-2 genes are attenuated in vitro and in vivo. Virology 2000; 273:210–218.

194. Buchholz UJ, et al. Chimeric bovine respiratory syncytial virus with glycoprotein gene substitutions from human respiratory syncytial virus (HRSV): effects on host range and evaluation as a live-attenuated HRSV vaccine. J Virol 2000; 74:1187–1199.

195. Bukreyev A, et al. Recovery of infectious respiratory syncytial virus expressing an additional, foreign gene. J Virol 1996; 70:6634–6641.

196. Jin H, et al. Recombinant human respiratory syncytial virus (RSV) from cDNA and construction of subgroup A and B chimeric RSV. Virology 1998; 251:206–214.

197. Hoffman MA, Banerjee AK. An infectious clone of human parainfluenza virus type 3. J Virol 1997; 71:4272–4277.

198. Durbin AP, et al. Recovery of infectious human parainfluenza virus type 3 from cDNA. Virology 1997; 235:323–332.

199. Skiadopoulos MH, et al. Three amino acid substitutions in the L protein of the human parainfluenza virus type 3 cp45 live attenuated vaccine candidate contribute to its temperature-sensitive and attenuation phenotypes. J Virol 1998; 72:1762–1768.

200. Skiadopoulos MH, et al. Identification of mutations contributing to the temperature-sensitive, cold-adapted, and attenuation phenotypes of the live-attenuated cold-passage 45 (cp45) human parainfluenza virus 3 candidate vaccine. J Virol 1999; 73:1374–1381.

201. Skiadopoulos MH, et al. Attenuation of the recombinant human parainfluenza virus type 3 cp45 candidate vaccine virus is augmented by importation of the respiratory syncytial virus cpts530 L polymerase mutation. Virology 1999; 260:125–135.

202. Durbin AP, et al. Mutations in the C, D, and V open reading frames of human parainfluenza virus type 3 attenuate replication in rodents and primates. Virology 1999; 261:319–330.

203. Coelingh K, et al. Attenuation of bovine parainfluenza virus type 3 in nonhuman primates and its ability to confer immunity to human parainfluenza virus type 3 challenge. J Infect Dis 1996; 157:655–662.

204. Karron RA, et al. Evaluation of a live attenuated bovine parainfluenza type 3 vaccine in two-to six-month old infants. Pediatr Infect Dis J 1996; 15:650–654.

205. Bailly JE, et al. A recombinant human parainfluenza virus type 3 (PIV3) in which the nucleocapsid N protein has been replaced by that of bovine PIV3 is attenuated in primates. J Virol 2000; 74:3188–3195.

206. Schmidt AC, et al. Bovine parainfluenza virus type 3 (BIV3) fusion and hemagglutinin-neuraminidase glycoproteins make an important contribution to the restricted replication of BPIV3 in primates. J Virol 2000; 74:8922–8929.

207. Tao T, et al. Recovery of a fully viable chimeric human parainfluenza virus (PIV) type 3 in which the hemagglutinin-neuraminidase and fusion glycoproteins have been replaced by those of PIV type 1. J Virol 1998; 72:2955–2961.

208. Tao T, et al. A live attenuated chimeric recombinant parainfluenza virus (PIV) encoding the internal proteins of PIV type 3 and the surface glycoproteins of PIV type 1 induces complete resistance to PIV1 challenge and partial resistance to PIV3 challenge. Vaccine 1999; 17:1100–1108.

209. Tao T. A live attenuated recombinant chimeric parainfluenza virus (PIV) candidate vaccine containing the hemagglutinin-neuraminidase and fusion glycoproteins of PIV1 and the remaining proteins from PIV3 induces resistance to PIV1 even in animals immune to PIV3. Vaccine 2000; 18:1359–1366.

210. Skiadopoulos MH, et al. Generation of a parainfluenza virus type 1 vaccine candidate by replacing the HN and F glycoproteins of the live-attenuated PIV3 cp45 vaccine virus with their PIV1 counterparts. Vaccine 1999; 18:503–510.

211. Tao T, et al. Replacement of the ectodomains of the hemagglutinin-neuraminidase and fusion glycoproteins of recombinant parainfluenza virus type 3 (PIV3) with their counterparts from PIV2 yields attenuated PIV2 vaccine candidates. J Virol 2000; 74:6448–6458.

212. Skiadopoulos MH, et al. Long nucleotide insertions between the HN and L protein coding regions of human parainfluenza virus type 3 yield viruses with temperature-sensitive and attenuation phenotypes. Virology 2000; 272:225–234.

213. Durbin AP, et al. Human parainfluenza virus type 3 (PIV3) expressing the hemagglutinin protein of measles virus provides a potential method for immunization against measles virus and PIV3 in early infancy. J Virol 2000; 74:6821–6831.

214. Schmidt AC, et al. Recombinant bovine/human parainfluenza virus type 3 (B/HPIV3) expressing the respiratory syncytial virus (RSV) G and F proteins can be used to achieve simultaneous mucosal immunization against RSV and HPIV3). J Virol 2001; 75:4594–4603.

215. Schmidt AC, et al. Mucosal immunization of Rhesus monkeys against respiratory syncytial virus subgroups A and B and human parainfluenza virus type 3 by using a live cDNA-derived vaccine based on a host range-attenuated bovine parainfluenza virus type 3 vector backbone. J Virol 2002; 76:1089–1099.

216. Spielhofer P, et al. Chimeric measles viruses with a foreign envelope. J Virol 1998; 72:2150–2159.

217. Singh M, Billeter MA. A recombinant measles virus expressing biologically active human interleukin-12. J Gen Virol 1999; 80:101–106.

218. Singh M, et al. A recombinant measles virus expressing

hepatitis B virus surface antigen induces humoral immune responses in genetically modified mice. J Virol 1999; 73: 4823–4828.

219. Wang Z, et al. Recombinant measles viruses expressing heterologous antigens of mumps and simian immunodeficiency viruses. Vaccine 2001; 19:2329–2336.

220. Parks GD, et al. Controlled cell killing by a recombinant nonsegmented negative-strand RNA virus. Virology 2002; 293:192–203.

221. Parks GD, Alexander-Miller MA. High avidity cytotoxic T lymphocytes to a foreign antigen are efficiently activated following immunization with a recombinant paramyxovirus, simian virus 5. J Gen Virol 2002; 83:1167–1172.

222. Baron MD, et al. Expression in cattle of epitopes of a heterologous virus using a recombinant rinderpest virus. J Gen Virol 1999; 80:2031–2039.

223. Walsh EP, et al. Recombinant rinderpest vaccines expressing membrane-anchored proteins as genetic markers: evidence of exclusion of marker protein from the virus envelope. J Virol 2000; 74:10165–10175.

224. Matano T, et al. Rapid appearance of secondary immune responses and protection from acute CD4 depletion after a highly pathogenic immunodeficiency virus challenge in macaques vaccinated with a DNA prime/Sendai virus vector boost regimen. J Virol 2001; 75:11891–11896.

225. Li HO, et al. A cytoplasmic RNA vector derived from nontransmissible Sendai virus with efficient gene transfer and expression. J Virol 2000; 74:6564–6569.

30

Attenuated *Salmonella* and *Shigella* as Live Vectors Carrying Either Prokaryotic or Eukaryotic Expression Systems

James E. Galen, Marcela F. Pasetti, Marcelo B. Sztein, Eileen M. Barry, and Myron M. Levine
University of Maryland School of Medicine, Baltimore, Maryland, U.S.A.

I. INTRODUCTION

A vaccinology strategy that has generated much optimism in recent years is the use of attenuated strains of bacteria to carry protective antigens of foreign, unrelated pathogens and to deliver those heterologous antigens to the immune system, thereby resulting in protective immune responses [1,2]. Initially, the strategy focused on engineering the attenuated strains to express foreign proteins and polysaccharide antigens directly [3–7]. Subsequently, bacterial live vectors were modified to carry DNA vaccine plasmids (i.e., foreign genes on plasmids controlled by eukaryotic regulation elements) [5,6,8–13]. In this approach, the bacteria deliver the DNA vaccine plasmids to the host cells, particularly antigen-presenting cells [e.g., dendritic cells (DCs), macrophages, and B lymphocytes] where the foreign antigen is subsequently expressed.

An array of bacteria has been utilized as live vectors [4]. These include attenuated strains derived from wild-type pathogens such as *Salmonella enterica* serovar *Typhi* (*S. typhi*) [14–18] and *S. enterica* serovar *Typhimurium* (*S. typhimurium*) [19–21], *Shigella* [22–25], *Vibrio cholerae* [26–28], *Listeria monocytogenes* [29], *Mycobacterium bovis* (Bacille Calmette Guerin, BCG) [30], and *Yersinia enterocolitica* [31]. Other investigators have chosen to utilize as bacterial live vectors nonpathogenic strains derived from normal flora such as *Streptococcus gordonii* [32] or other sources such as *Lactobacillus casei* [33] and *Lactococcus lactis* [34].

Attenuated strains of *Salmonella* and *Shigella* are particularly versatile because they can deliver to the mammalian immune system foreign antigens produced either by the vectors themselves (by means of prokaryotic expression systems), or by eukaryotic cells (by means of eukaryotic expression plasmids). In addition, such strains are administered by mucosal rather than parenteral routes, an approach that can increase vaccination compliance and can avoid problems of injection safety that are associated with the use of parenteral immunization in developing countries

[35,36]. Moreover, *S. Typhi* and *Shigella* live vector vaccines are amenable to relatively economical manufacture compared to tissue culture-based, conjugate, or purified subunit vaccines. This review will focus on the use of *Salmonella* and *Shigella* as live vectors. We will first briefly describe common themes of virulence and regulation in *Salmonella* and *Shigella* to provide a context for emerging strategies in the engineering of prokaryotic expression systems. We will also summarize recent progress in live vector delivery of DNA vaccines and will review the immunology of *Salmonella*-based and *Shigella*-based live vectors carrying either prokaryotic or eukaryotic expression systems.

II. VIRULENCE AND REGULATION IN *SALMONELLA* AND *SHIGELLA*

To be fully pathogenic, both *Salmonella* and *Shigella* require a variety of virulence genes, which are scattered throughout the chromosome as well as residing on large virulence plasmids in the case *S. Typhimurium* and *Shigella*. Because the genomic sequences of *S. Typhi* [37] and *S. Typhimurium* [38] have recently been described, we will focus on the organization of virulence determinants within these genomes and draw parallels to *Shigella* where possible.

Controlled expression of genomic virulence factors is accomplished at several different levels, the most basic of which involves the clustering of virulence functions into large pathogenicity islands which can be up to 134 kb in size. Analysis of the genomes of *S. Typhi* and *S. Typhimurium* has revealed the presence of at least nine [37,38] and perhaps 12 [39] *Salmonella* pathogenicity islands (SPIs) common to both serovars. If one considers the pathogenesis of *Salmonella* in terms of biochemical events occurring prior to eukaryotic cell invasion and those following invasion, the functions encoded by the SPI-1 and SPI-2 islands are immediately seen to play key roles. The SPI-1 locus encodes a contact-dependent type III secretion system, which specifically targets effector molecules to eukaryotic target cells, thereby allowing invasion to proceed [40]. Once inside a eukaryotic cell, a number of factors are required for intracellular survival and colonization of deeper tissues. Synthesis of these factors involves coordinated expression from several SPIs [41], including the SPI-2 locus, which encodes a second contact-dependent type III secretion system that delivers many of these molecules [42,43]; a detailed study of the mechanisms of such effector molecules is currently underway.

A type III secretion system also resides within the virulence plasmid of *Shigella*. The complete sequence of the 214-kb virulence plasmid from *S. flexneri* serotype 5 [44] reveals a 31-kb *virB–spa40* island encoding the type III secretion apparatus and IpaA–D effector proteins, as well as additional pathogenicity factors distributed around the plasmid. Analysis by Parsot and Sansonetti [45] reveals significant homology between the IpaA–D effector proteins and SPI-1-encoded effector proteins; in addition, extensive homologies between both secretion apparatuses were noted.

III. ATTENUATED *SALMONELLA* AND *SHIGELLA* AS LIVE VECTORS DELIVERING HETEROLOGOUS ANTIGENS

With increasingly detailed knowledge of *Salmonella* and *Shigella* genomics and mechanisms of pathogenicity, precise mutations were introduced, resulting in the development of attenuated vaccine strains with minimal reactogenicity and yet highly protective against disease (see Levine et al., Chapter 43 and Kotloff et al., Chapter 61 of this volume). It was also attractive to use such attenuated strains as live vectors to present foreign (heterologous) antigens from unrelated human pathogens, creating a multivalent vaccine that could elicit both homologous and heterologous protective immune responses.

Heterologous antigen expression within live vector strains may involve either chromosomal or plasmid loci, and a wide variety of plasmid-based expression technology are now available for achieving the appropriate expression levels required to elicit the appropriate and relevant immune response(s). However, often overlooked in live vector engineering is the effect that expression plasmids (and the heterologous antigens they typically encode) can exert on the fitness of a live vector. The notable burden placed upon live vectors carrying multicopy plasmids is the cumulative result of a metabolic cascade triggered by two processes: (1) the replication and maintenance of expression plasmids [46–48], and (2) the transcription and translation of the various plasmid-encoded functions including the heterologous antigen(s). It is therefore not surprising that plasmid-bearing bacteria grow more slowly than plasmidless bacteria [49–53], and this explains why growth rate decreases as copy number increases [46,47]. Reduced growth rate is the inevitable consequence of metabolic burden, which in turn is the cumulative result of a number of physiological perturbations. Because this creates a selective pressure for loss of resident plasmids in the absence of selection, significant loss of expression plasmids from live vectors may occur after

immunization, accompanied by reduced immunogenicity and reduced protective efficacy. Clearly, spontaneous plasmid loss would remove any metabolic burden and allow plasmidless bacteria to quickly outgrow the population of plasmid-bearing bacteria. Such a shift in antigen expression within a population of live vector bacteria would be expected to reduce the efficiency of stimulating immune responses specific to the foreign antigen.

A. Chromosomal Expression Systems

Several approaches have been applied to reduce metabolic burden while ensuring consistent immunogenic levels of expression for a given heterologous antigen. Chromosomal integration of expression cassettes into nonessential loci has been successful for the expression of otherwise toxic eukaryotic antigens from *Plasmodium falciparum* and *Leishmania mexicana* within *S. Typhi* live vectors, but expression levels resulted in modest immune responses [54,55]. In a clever attempt to increase heterologous antigen expression levels while still minimizing toxicity, Santiago-Machuca et al. [56] introduced expression cassettes onto multicopy plasmids in which transcription of the heterologous gene is controlled by the extremely powerful bacteriophage T7 promoter; expression of the cognate T7 polymerase was encoded within a *S. Typhi* chromosomally integrated expression cassette, controlled in turn by a promoter responding to an environmental cue (anaerobiosis), likely to be encountered within immunized hosts. Expression levels in vitro were tightly regulated with high induction ratios, but the immunogenicity of such constructs has not yet been tested.

One further variation on the theme of chromosomally integrated transcriptional control elements driving expression of plasmid-based antigen cassettes was recently reported in *S. Typhi* by Qian and Pan [57]. They described the construction of a chromosomally encoded tetracycline repressor (*tetR*) used to control the expression of a plasmid-encoded 42-kDa merozoite surface protein 1 fragment (MSP-1$_{42}$) from *P. falciparum*, under the control of a tightly regulated tetracycline response promoter; in the absence of the anhydrotetracycline inducer, antigen expression is quantitatively shut down. Although antibodies against MSP-1$_{42}$ were not observed in mice immunized intraperitoneally (i.p.) (possibly due to improperly folded cytoplasmic antigen expression), a greater concern for this approach is the need to coadminister an antibiotic with the inoculum to achieve regulated antigen expression. However, *tetR* mutants, which activate transcription in the *absence* of tetracycline inducer while maintaining tight regulation of the target antigen cassette in the presence of inducer, are now available [58].

B. Plasmid-Based Expression Systems

Nonchromosomally regulated expression of multicopy heterologous antigen cassettes can be achieved either at the level of transcription, translation, or both. Work done by Chatfield et al. [19] clearly demonstrated that constitutive expression in *S. Typhimurium*, using the powerful *tac* promoter (P_{tac}) to express fragment C of tetanus toxin (fragC) from a multicopy plasmid, resulted in no detectable anti-fragC antibodies. Isogenic expression using the reengineered *nirB* promoter P_{nir15}, which responds to the environmental signal of low oxygen, elicited protective anti-fragC responses after challenge with 50 LD_{50} of tetanus toxin [19]. It was further demonstrated that plasmids carrying the constitutive P_{tac}–fragC cassette were rapidly lost in vivo from bacteria colonizing deep tissues [19].

This concept of using "in vivo-induced" expression cassettes to enhance the stability of multicopy plasmids, thereby improving relevant immune response(s), was soon expanded to include eukaryotic antigens from parasites such as *Schistosoma* [59] and *Leishmania* [60]. Elegant work by Bumann [61] clearly demonstrates that regulated expression of foreign antigens strongly influences the immunogenicity of live vectors by affecting colonization levels of the live vector. When comparing constitutive expression of green fluorescent protein (GFP) fusions from P_{tac} vs. regulated expression from the PhoQ/PhoP-controlled P_{pagC}, Bumann showed that although both constructs induced comparable cellular immune responses, doses almost 1000-fold lower were sufficient for live vectors expressing antigen from P_{pagC}. Using two-color flow cytometry, Bumann [62] has gone on to quantitate the in vivo induction ratios of various promoters controlling *Salmonella* virulence, including P_{phoP}, P_{pagC} (positively controlled by PhoP and induced within macrophages [63,64]), P_{sicA} (from SPI-1), P_{ssaH} (from SPI-2), and P_{sifA} (controlled by SPI-2 [65]). Such work raises the possibility of influencing the host's immune response by using well-characterized promoters of differing strengths to deliver antigen to different compartments of an immunized host and to influence the immune response.

Further refinements to expression plasmid stability have addressed the inheritance of these plasmids within a population of dividing live vectors. To prevent plasmidless daughter cells from overtaking a growing population, conditionally lethal systems were engineered such that plasmid loss quickly led to cell death. In one variation, mutations were engineered into chromosomal loci encoding critical metabolic enzymes such as aspartate β-semialdehyde dehydrogenase (Asd), which were complemented by plasmid-encoded genes [66]. Therefore, plasmid loss removed the capacity to synthesize necessary metabolites resulting in cell lysis. Another variation involves expression plasmids, which encode a toxin–antitoxin system in which the protective antitoxin is unstable and requires constant synthesis from resident expression plasmids; plasmid loss activates the toxin, again leading to cell lysis [50,67,68]. To remove the random partitioning of multicopy plasmids during cell division, plasmid segregation functions were also introduced to ensure nonrandom inheritance of plasmids into all daughter cells [68].

However, it is not enough to optimize in vivo expression levels and plasmid stability to secure an appropriate immune response [69]. Problems with inherent antigen toxicity may diminish the colonizing ability of live vectors and lower the levels of antigen delivered to immunological induction sites. In addition, proper folding may be required for conformationally specific epitopes to trigger protective serum antibody responses. For example, neutralizing serum antibodies

against the critical 19-kDa carboxyl terminal domain of MSP-1 are only observed when the six disulfide bridges of the terminal domain are properly folded [70,71]; this is unlikely to efficiently occur for antigens made within the reducing environment of the live vector cytoplasm.

In attempts to address potential toxicity and folding problems, various antigen export technologies have been developed for surface or extracellular secretion of foreign proteins. Impressive success has been achieved using a novel surface display technology based on engineering of expression cassettes derived from the *Pseudomonas syringe* ice nucleation protein (Inp); the versatility and the promise of this approach are illustrated by recent reports of the display of properly folded eukaryotic antigens such as the human immunodeficiency virus type 1 glycoprotein gp120 on the surface of *Escherichia coli* [72], and the construction of an immunogenic multivalent hepatitis B surface antigen/hepatitis C core protein displayed on the surface of the licensed *S. Typhi* vaccine strain Ty21a [73].

In addition to surface display, secretion of heterologous antigens out of *Salmonella* live vectors has been reported by several groups to enhance the immune response to a foreign protein. Hess et al. [74] reported that cytoplasmic expression of the protective T-cell antigen listeriolysin O (LLO) within recombinant *Salmonella* vaccine strains did not confer protection in mice against lethal challenge with virulent *L. monocytogenes*. However, in-frame insertion of LLO within a truncated form of the *E. coli* hemolysin A (HlyA) allowed extracellular secretion of this fusion in the presence of the coexpressed *E. coli* HlyB/HlyD/TolC export apparatus, and resulted in protection against lethal challenge with *L. monocytogenes*.

Similar results were reported by Russmann et al. [75] wherein secretion via the SPI-1-encoded type III secretion system of an eight-amino-acid immunodominant epitope from the murine lymphocytic choriomeningitis virus (LCMV) conferred a protective class I-restricted cytotoxic T lymphocyte (CTL) response against an intracerebral lethal challenge with virulent LCMV, not observed for the cytoplasmically expressed epitope. This type III secretion-mediated approach was recently used to improve upon the protective immune response in mice against lethal challenge with *L. monocytogenes*, using the heterologous *Yersinia* outer membrane protein E (YopE) as a carrier for carboxyl-terminal fusions of LLO and p60 domains consisting of >300 residues [76]. As of this writing, the use of SPI-2 mediated secretion to enhance the immunogenicity of heterologous antigens delivered within target cells such as macrophages has not yet been reported.

C. *Shigella* Live Vectors

Use of attenuated *Shigella* as live vectors is rapidly advancing. Initial attempts at using *Shigella* as a live vector employed the ΔaroD *S. flexneri* vaccine strain SFL124. Heterologous antigens from the related *S. dysenteriae* were successfully expressed from chromosomal cassettes, including surface-expressed O-antigenic determinants, as well as a Shiga toxin B subunit ($Stx1_B$) fusion secreted from SFL124 through a chromosomally encoded *E. coli* HlyA type I secretion operon [77,78]. Multicopy expression plasmids have also been used in *Shigella* for the expression of foreign antigens in various subcellular locations. Colonization factors from enterotoxigenic *E. coli* (ETEC) [79], as well as fragC of tetanus toxin [24], have been cytoplasmically synthesized, whereas rotavirus VP4 was expressed as a fusion with *E. coli* maltose-binding protein and localized either to the cytoplasm or periplasmic space [80]. Outright secretion through the *Shigella* type III secretion system of a poliovirus VP1-neutralizing epitope was accomplished using IpaC–C3 hybrid protein fusions [81]. In addition, stabilized expression plasmids developed for *Salmonella* live vectors have recently been used in Δ*guaBA S. flexneri* 2a live vectors to express several ETEC fimbrial colonization factors plus LT antigens from a single expression plasmid [23,25].

IV. IMMUNE RESPONSES INDUCED BY *SALMONELLA* AND *SHIGELLA* EXPRESSING HETEROLOGOUS ANTIGENS

Attenuated *Salmonella* and *Shigella* strains have remarkable potential as mucosal live vectors expressing heterologous antigens, as they can stimulate a wide array of humoral and cellular immune responses. Serum IgG antibodies, secretory IgA (sIgA), T-cell proliferation, cytokine production, and MHC class I-restricted CTL responses have been demonstrated in animal models [16,24,25,82,83] and humans [84–86]. It is likely that the tropism of these bacteria for dendritic cells and macrophages allows "direct delivery" of antigens into professional antigen-presenting cells (APCs) at inductive sites of the immune system.

Mucosal and systemic responses against bacterial and foreign antigens have been demonstrated with *S. Typhimurium* -expressing fragC [19,87–89], *Y. pestis* F1 capsular antigens [90], influenza A nucleoprotein [75], ETEC fimbria [91], *M. tuberculosis*- and *M. bovis*-secreted T-cell antigen ESAT-6 [92], *L. major* gp63 [60,93], *Plasmodium* spp. sporozoite and merozoite surface proteins [94], *Helicobacter pylori* urease [95], *Streptococcus* spp. antigens [96], hepatitis B antigen [97], and herpes simplex [98] and measles virus B and T epitopes [99]. *Salmonella* infection induces activation of macrophages and DCs by increasing surface expression of MHC class I, MHC class II, and costimulatory molecules as well as cytokine production. These immunoregulatory activities are believed to enhance the ability of APC to activate specific T cells during the initial stages of the immune response, including antigen processing and presentation, as well as the subsequent lymphocyte expansion and generation of memory T cells. [100]. Antigens expressed by recombinant *Salmonella* strains can be presented by DCs in the context of MHC class II and MHC class I molecules, thus inducing both Th1-type and Th2-type cell-mediated responses. For example, it has been shown that bacterial live vectors expressing foreign antigens can induce CTL responses [101], which proved critical to confer prolonged protection [101]. Antigen-specific long-term memory mucosal responses have also been described [102].

As mentioned above, *S. Typhi* strains have been engineered to express a variety of heterologous antigens. *S. Typhi*

strains CVD 908, CVD 908-*htrA*, and CVD 915 expressing fragC elicited high levels of serum IgG antitetanus toxin and fragC antibodies when delivered to mice intranasally (i.n.) [16,103–105]. In addition to humoral responses, CVD 915 expressing fragC induced antigen-specific T-cell proliferation and Th1 cytokines [103]. Mice immunized intranasally with CVD 908 expressing pertussis toxin subunit S1 fused to fragC developed serum pertussis-neutralizing antibodies [15]. Lee et al. [73] adapted *S. Typhi* strain Ty21a to express HBsAg and HCV antigens on the cell surface and demonstrated induction of high levels of serum antibodies against both antigens in intranasally immunized mice. *S. Typhi* strain CVD 908 expressing *L. mexicana* gp63 given to mice orally elicited a broad antigen-specific T-cell-mediated immunity, including T-cell proliferation, IL-2 secretion, and CTL responses, which conferred significant protection against wild-type strain of *L. mexicana mexicana* challenge [55].

Immunization using *Shigella* as a mucosal live vector has also been successful. Mice immunized intranasally or intravenously (i.v.) with *S. flexneri* 2a SC602-expressing IpaC–C3 neutralizing epitope of the poliovirus VP1 as hybrid protein elicited serum IgG and local IgA and IgG anti-C3 and Ipa [81]. *S. flexneri* 2a CVD 1203 expressing *E. coli* (ETEC) colonization factor CS3 fimbriae (CFA) induced sIgA and serum IgG anti-CS3 in mice and guinea pigs immunized orally and intranasally. Of note, the nasal route was shown to be more efficient in inducing significantly higher immune responses in both animal models [79]. Using a similar approach, Altboum et al. [23] coexpressed ETEC CS2 and CS3 fimbriae in *S. flexneri* 2a CVD 1204 and showed the presence of sIgA and serum IgG against *Shigella* LPS, CS2, and CS3 antigens in guinea pigs immunized intranasally. In both reports, the animals were protected following conjunctival challenge with virulent *S. flexneri* 2a [23,79]. *S. flexneri* 2a CVD 1204 carrying fragC was able to induce potent serum IgG responses to fragC (neutralizing tetanus toxin in vivo) as well as serum IgG and sIgA against bacteria LPS that protected them from ocular *S. flexneri* challenge [24]. Koprowski et al. [25] adapted *S. flexneri* CVD 1204 to coexpress ETEC CFA/1 and genetically detoxified ETEC heat-labile toxin derivatives LThK63 or LThR72, showing the production of IgG and sIgA anti-CFA/I and LTh antibodies in guinea pigs immunized intranasally, which also produced sIgA and serum IgG anti-*S. flexneri* 2a LPS.

This impressive array of immune responses induced by bacterial live vectors carrying foreign antigens provides a strong rationale for the continuing evaluation of this approach in the development of vaccines for human use against a wide variety of pathogenic organisms.

V. ATTENUATED *SALMONELLA* AND *SHIGELLA* AS LIVE VECTORS DELIVERING DEOXYRIBONUCLEIC ACID VACCINES

DNA vaccines, in general, consist of plasmid vectors that encode foreign antigens under control of a eukaryotic promoter. In animal studies and in the few clinical trials, DNA vaccines have been traditionally given intramuscularly (i.m.) or adsorbed to gold particles and inoculated intradermally (i.d.) with a gene gun; either route has produced strong cellular as well as humoral responses, particularly in animal models. A major disadvantage of this approach is that large amounts of DNA are required as the efficiency of the DNA uptake is low and dose-dependent. In addition, parenteral DNA delivery does not induce strong mucosal responses, and the manufacturing of highly purified DNA vaccines can be extremely expensive [106].

Bacterial live vectors represent an attractive alternative to limitations encountered with purified DNA vaccines [8, 13,107]. In this approach, DNA vaccine plasmids are delivered by the live vector to host APCs after cell invasion, where encoded heterologous antigens are expressed using the cellular machinery. Thus, this strategy combines the advantages of mucosal delivery of a live carrier with efficiently targeted DNA vaccination. This can be particularly relevant to elicit cell-mediated immunity against intracellular organisms that gain access through the mucosal surfaces. Moreover, bacterial components such as unmethylated CpG motifs in the bacterial DNA [108] and lipopolysaccharide can serve as adjuvants, thus potentiating the immunogenicity of the foreign antigen. The possibility of selecting sophisticated gene expression systems [109], or the coadministration of immunomodulators such as cytokines and costimulatory molecules [108], makes live vector-mediated DNA vaccination an appealing approach to tailor immune responses [6]. As with prokaryotic systems, antigen expression cassettes could be manipulated to specify transport to a particular eukaryotic cellular compartment, or to influence their processing, thus enhancing immunogenicity [110].

Shigella appears to be particularly efficient in the delivery of DNA vaccines, as many strains retain a functional IpaB that allows the bacteria to break out of the phagolysosome and enter the cytosol. Upon death and disruption of the attenuated bacteria, the DNA vaccine plasmid is released and can enter the nucleus of the eukaryotic target cell. In the first report of live vectors used to deliver a DNA vaccine, Sizemore et al. [111,112] showed that *S. flexneri* 2a can successfully deliver a DNA vaccine encoding β-galactosidase and can induce specific serum antibodies and T-cell proliferation. Subsequently, Fennelly et al. [113] used a similar strategy to deliver a DNA vaccine encoding measles virus antigens and demonstrated induction of specific antibodies and T-cell proliferation. Anderson et al. [24] used *S. flexneri* 2a CVD 1204 to deliver a DNA vaccine encoding tetanus toxin fragC and observed potent serum responses to fragC in guinea pigs immunized intranasally. Devico et al. [114], Shata and Hone [115], and Shata et al. [116] reported the induction of CD8$^+$ T-cell responses and protective antiviral immunity using *S. flexneri* 2a CVD 1203 delivering DNA plasmids encoding HIV gp120 and gp140. Examples of in vivo studies using *Salmonella* and *Shigella* as gene delivery systems are summarized in Table 1.

Despite the fact that *Salmonella* remains in the phagosomal compartment and does not escape into the cytoplasm as do *Listeria* or *Shigella*, several groups have demonstrated the delivery of DNA vaccines and immunogenicity of DNA-encoded antigens. In fact, *Salmonella* delivering these eu-

karyotic expression vectors have been shown to induce cellular and humoral immune responses against bacterial pathogens [117,118] and their toxins [103], viruses [113,119,120], as well as tumor antigens [121]. Interestingly, *Salmonella*-mediated delivery of DNA vaccines appears to be more effective at inducing mucosal cell-mediated immune responses than intramuscular immunization with purified DNA [119]. *Salmonella* DNA delivery can even be more efficient at induction of both cellular and humoral systemic immune responses when compared with prokaryotic antigen expressions [103,118].

Although it is unclear how the plasmid DNA is transported from the phagosomal compartment into the nucleus, it has been suggested that plasmids released from lysed bacteria may reach the cytoplasm of the host cell by leakiness from the atypical vacuolar compartment in which the live vector resided [6]. This has been supported by the observations that bacterial invasion is necessary but not sufficient for efficient gene transfer and, in fact, escape of bacteria or plasmid DNA from the primary vacuole is required for gene transfer to occur [107]. In this context, different strategies have been devised to facilitate DNA delivery to the cytosol to improve immunogenicity of DNA live vector vaccines [122]. Gentschev et al. [123] constructed a *Salmonella* strain equipped with the Hly secretion system, which disrupts the phagosomal membrane and releases the *Salmonella* into the cytosol; this construct exhibited an enhanced ability to transfect mammalian cells. DNA delivery via recombinant *Salmonella* strains in the presence of phagosomal escape properties was successfully used to direct macrophage presentation of DNA-encoded antigen within MHC class I and to stimulate specific CD8$^+$ T cells in vitro [124].

It has also been observed that efficient DNA delivery can be achieved by inducing programmed bacterial lysis, which would enhance the release of DNA constructs into the eukaryotic cytosol [125]. Thus, Sizemore et al. [111] and Vecino et al. [126] used an attenuated *Shigella* strain that cannot synthesize diaminopimelic (DAP) acid, an essential cell wall component. In vivo starvation for DAP eventually causes bacterial cell lysis and DNA release. Recently, Jain and Mekalanos [127] showed that the incorporation of lambda phage S and R in an inducible lysis system for *S. Typhimurium* can be useful to finely regulate bacterial lysis within mucosal tissue or APC and more efficiently release DNA vaccines. It is puzzling, however, that wild-type intracellular bacteria (without mechanisms to favor cell lysis or DNA release) can still deliver DNA into mammalian cells [107]. It is possible that a yet unidentified specific phagosome-to-cytosol transport process could exist for the translocation of the plasmids molecules across the phagosomal membrane; such a pathway was recently reported for protein antigens in DC [128]. Another hypothesis raises the possibility that *Salmonella*-induced apoptotic macrophages containing antigenic material might be engulfed by bystander APCs, mainly DCs, facilitating antigen presentation by crosspriming [129].

In a recent publication, Vecino et al. [126] investigated the ability of *S. flexneri* 15D, *S. Typhi* Ty21a, and *S. Typhimurium* SL7207 given intranasally to deliver DNA plasmids encoding HIV gp120 and SIV Nef and to induce

Table 1 Selected Studies Evaluating Preclinical *Salmonella* and *Shigella* as Delivery Vehicles for DNA Vaccine Plasmids

Strain (mutation)	DNA-encoding antigen[a]	Animal model[b]	Dose, route[c]	*Salmonella* and *Shigella* live vectors delivering DNA plasmids — Immune response to foreign antigens			Immune response to the live vector[d]	Reference
				Ab[e]	CMI[f]	Protection[g]		
S. Typhimurium SL7207 (*aroA*)	*E. coli* β-gal *L. monocytogenes* Act A, LLO	BALB/c mice	1–4; o.g.	High IgG; IgG1 IgG2a	T-cell proliferation, IFN-γ, IL-4, CTL	*L. monocytogenes* challenge + LLO; Act	NA	[118]
S. Typhimurium SL7207	*E. coli* β-gal-TAA	BALB/c mice	1–4; o.g.	IgG, IgG2a, IgM; IgA	IFN-γ CD8+ CTL	+ β-gal tumor challenge	NA	[121,140]
S. Typhimurium 22-11 Δpur	*C. trachomatis* MOMP	BALB/c mice	4; o.g.	IgG2a; IgA	DTH, T-cell proliferation; IFN-γ (naked DNA)	+/– *C. trachomatis* (MoPn) pulmonary challenge	NA	[117]
S. Typhimurium SL7207	Murine melanoma gp100 and TRP2 human gp100	C57BL-6J mice	3; o.g.	NA	MHC class I CD8+ CTL, IFN-γ	+ Melanoma challenge; tumor rejection; growth suppression	NA	[141,142]
S. Typhimurium SL7207	IFN-γ gene	C57BL-6 GKO mice	o.g.	NR	Restores IFN-γ in GKO mice	NR	+ Resistance to bacteria in GKO mice	[143]
S. Typhimurium SL7207	Self-antigen murine TH	A/J mice	1, o.g.	NA	TIL CD4+, CD8+	+ Neuroblastoma challenge; tumor reduction	NA	[144]
S. Typhimurium SL5000 (*aroA*)	hCD40L	BALB/c mice	1, o.g.	NA	TIL CD4+, CD8+ FasL+	+ B-cell lymphoma challenge; longer survival	NA	[145]
S. Typhimurium SL7237 (*aroA*)	*E. coli* β-gal *L. monocytogenes* Act A, LLO	BALB/c DBA/2 C57BL/6 NIH-Swiss	1–4; o.g., i.n.	Serum and mucosal Abs	T-cell proliferation, CTL	*L. monocytogenes* challenge + LLO	NA	[110]
S. Typhimurium SL7207	*E. coli* β-gal	BALB/c and SCID mice	3; o.g.	IgM+ cells in LN and TIL, low IgG	CD8+ memory; CTL in TIL; LN and spleen; IL-12; IFN-γ, LAK, IL-10, IL-14	+ Renal carcinoma LacZ challenge, tumor growth retardation	NA	[146]
S. Typhimurium 7207	HBsAg	BALB/c mice	1, o.g.	Low IgM and IgG	CTL, high IFN-γ, low IL-4	NA	NA	[147]
S. Typhimurium 7207	HSV gD	BALB/c mice	3; o.g.	Serum IgG, IgG1, IgG2a, low IgA	CD4+ activation, DTH, IFN-γ SC in PP, spleen and ILN; IFN-γ in vaginal tissue	+ Intravaginal HSV challenge, control infection and viral shedding	NA	[119]

Vector	Antigen	Animal model	No.; route	Antibody	CMI	Protection/challenge	Other	Ref.
S. Typhimurium SL7207	HIV Env epitopes	BALB/c mice	1–3; o.g.	NA	CD8⁺ IFN-γ in spleen, PP	NA	NA	[120]
S. Typhimurium SL7207	hCEA	C57BL/6J CEA tg mice	3; o.g.	IgM, IgG	MHC class I CD8⁺ CTL, IFN-γ, IL-12, GM-CSF	+Tumor rejection; +lethal challenge with murine colon carcinoma	NA	[148]
S. Typhi Ty21a (*rpoS, galE, Vi⁻*)	Measles virus NP	BALB/c mice	1; i.p.	NA	CTL	NA	NA	[113]
S. Typhi CVD 915 (Δ*guaBA*)	Tetanus toxin frag C	BALB/c mice	2; i.n.	High serum IgG1, IgG2a, IgG2b	T-cell proliferation in CLN and spleen; IFN-γ in spleen	NA	IgG anti-LPS and H, T-cell proliferation in LN and spleen; IFN-γ; IL-2, IL-12	[103]
S. Typhi Ty21a (*rpoS, galE, Vi⁻*)	HBsAg	BALB/c mice	1; o.g.	Total Io and IgM	NA	NA	IgM anti-LPS	[149]
S. flexneri 2a 15D (Δ*asd*)	β-gal	BALB/c mice	2; i.n.	IgG	T-cell proliferation in spleen	NA	NA	[111,112]
S. flexneri 2a 15D (Δ*asd*)	Measles virus F, H and NP	BALB/cJ mice	1–3; i.n.	IgG; IgA low IgG2a, IgG1	CD8⁺ CTL IFN-γ in spleen	NA	NA	[113]
S. flexneri 2a CVD1204 (Δ*guaBA, virG*)	Tetanus toxin fragC	Guinea pigs	2; i.n.	High IgG; IgG2 > IgG1	NA	+*S. flexneri* wild-type challenge	Serum IgG and sIgA to LPS	[24]
S. flexneri 2a CVD1203 (Δ*aroA, virG*)	HIV gp120	BALB/c mice	1; i.n.	NA	CD8⁺ IFN-γ SC	+Vaccinia-*env* challenge	NA	[114,115]
S. flexneri 2a 15D (Δ*asd*), *S. Typhi* Ty21a (*rpoS, galE, Vi⁻*), *S. Typhimurium* SL7207 (*aroA*)	HIV gp120 SIV *nef*	BALB/c mice	3; i.n.	Serum IgG, vaginal IgA to gp120	*nef* and gp120-specific CD8⁺ IFN-γ SC in spleen	NA	NA	[126]

a Antigens: β-gal = *E. coli* β-galactosidase; Act A = *L. monocytogenes* protein membrane protein; LLO = *L. monocytogenes* listeriolisin; TAA = tumor-associated antigen; MOMP = major outer membrane protein of *Chlamydia trachomatis* mouse pneumonitis strain; gp = glycoprotein; TRP2 = melanoma-associated antigen tyrosinase-related protein 2; TH = tyrosine hydroxylase; HBSAg = hepatitis B surface antigen; HSV gD = herpes simplex virus glycoprotein D; hCEA = human carcinoembryonic self-antigen; measles virus fusion (F), hemagglutinin (h), and nucleoprotein (NP).

b Tg = transgenic; GKO = IFN-γ knock out mice.

c Routes of immunization: o.g. = orogastric; i.n. = intranasally; i.p. = intraperitoneal.

d H = *S. Typhi* flagella antigen; sIgA = secretory (mucosal) IgA.

e NA = not available (not tested in the study or data not provided); NR = not relevant for the model.

f CMI = cell-mediated immunity; CTL = cytotoxic lymphocyte; DHR = delayed hypersensitivity reaction; TIL = tumor-infiltrating lymphocytes; SC = secreting cells; LAK = lymphocyte-activated killer.

g MoPn = *C. trachomatis* mouse pneumonitis.

Table 2 Selected Phase I and Phase II Human Clinical Trials Evaluating the Safety, Immunogenicity, and Efficacy of Attenuated *S. enterica* serovar *Typhi* and *S. enterica* serovar *Typhimurium* Constructs Expressing Foreign Antigens Using Prokaryotic Expression Systems

	Foreign antigen expressed	Expression system	Site of expression	Clinical response	Number of doses, route	Immune response to vector antigens	Immune response to foreign antigen	Protection	Reference
S. Typhi									
Ty21a[a], *rpoS, galE, Vi*[-]	*V. cholerae* O1 Inaba LPS	Plasmid	Surface	Well tolerated	3, oral	Moderate	5/14[b]	25% Efficacy against El Tor Inaba cholera challenge	[132]
Ty21a[a], *rpoS, galE, Vi*[-]	*H. pylori* urease A and B	Plasmid	Cytoplasm	Well tolerated	3, oral	Modest	3/9[c]	NA	[137]
CVD 908, *aroC, aroD*	*P. falciparum* CSP	Chromosome	Cytoplasm	Well tolerated	2, oral	Strong	3/10[d]	NA	[54]
CVD 908-*htrA, aroC, aroD, htrA*	fragC of tetanus toxin	Plasmid	Cytoplasm	Well tolerated	1 oral	Strong	Low dose, 0/3[e]; high dose, 1/1[f]	NA	[133]
c4073, *cya, crp, cdt, asd*	HBV core pre-S	Stabilized plasmid	Cytoplasm	Well tolerated	1 oral, (n = 7), 1 rectal (n = 6)	Strong after oral; weak after rectal	0/7 oral; 1/6 rectal[f]	NA	[138]
Ty800, *phoP, phoQ, purB*	*H. pylori* urease A and B	Stabilized plasmid	Cytoplasm	Well tolerated	1 oral	Strong	0/8	NA	[134]
CVD 908-*htrA, aroC, aroD, htrA*	*H. pylori* urease A and B	Plasmid	Cytoplasm	Well tolerated	2, oral	Strong	Low dose, 0/4; high dose, 2/8 IgA[g] and 7/8 IgG[h]	NA	[136]
S. Typhimurium									
ATCC 14028 *phoP, phoQ, purB*	*H. pylori* urease A and B	Stabilized plasmid	Cytoplasm	Moderately reactogenic	1, oral	Strong	3/6[h]	NA	[135]

[a] Ty21a was developed using chemical mutagenesis and therefore has many other mutations besides the three listed.
[b] Serum vibriocidal antibody.
[c] Cell-mediated immune responses.
[d] Two subjects manifested serum antibody responses (ELISA against purified protein or indirect immunofluorescent assay against whole sporozoites). One subject mounted a specific MHC class I-restricted, CD8[+] cytotoxic lymphocyte response.
[e] Results in subjects lacking tetanus antitoxin at baseline.
[f] Serum antibody.
[g] IgA antibody secreting cell response.
[h] IgG antibody secreting cell response.

immune responses, in comparison with the traditional intramuscular DNA vaccination. Among the three strains evaluated, *S. flexneri* induced the highest responses, measured by CD8$^+$ IFN-γ-secreting T cells, in spleen after three doses. These responses were comparable to those induced by intramuscular immunization. Of note, mucosal IgA responses were higher in the *S. flexneri* group than following intramuscular immunization.

Despite the evidence that *Salmonella* and *Shigella* can successfully deliver DNA vaccines in animal models, it is unclear whether this approach will be effective in humans. A more precise understanding of the mechanisms involved, further evaluation of ways to optimize the DNA delivery, and safety issues (including the possibility of DNA integration into the host cell genome or induction of autoimmunity) need to be carefully addressed before this vaccine strategy can be evaluated in volunteers.

VI. HUMAN CLINICAL TRIALS WITH ATTENUATED *SALMONELLA* AND *SHIGELLA* EXPRESSING FOREIGN ANTIGENS

Although studies in murine, guinea pig, and other animal models with attenuated *Salmonella* live vectors expressing foreign antigens have clearly demonstrated the feasibility of this vaccine strategy, heretofore, only a few Phase I and Phase II clinical trials have been carried out in humans. Clinical trials with *Shigella* live vectors have not yet been initiated but are imminent. Salient results of these trials are summarized in Table 2.

Early studies with Ty21a expressing *S. sonnei* O-polysaccharide or *V. cholerae* O1 Inaba lipopolysaccharide established that *S. Typhi* live vectors bearing foreign surface antigens could stimulate relevant immune responses (*S. sonnei* O-antibody and Inaba vibriocidal antibody) and could confer protection against experimental shigellosis and cholera, respectively. However, the efficacy of the Ty21a construct expressing *S. sonnei* was inconsistent [130,131] and the level of protection (25% efficacy) of the Ty21a construct expressing Inaba LPS was low [132], impeding further development of those vaccines.

Oral immunization of young adults with two doses of *S. Typhi* live vector CVD 908 expressing the circumsporozoite protein of *P. falciparum* set two milestones [54]. First, this construct documented that *S. Typhi* live vectors could elicit antibody responses to a protein antigen in humans. Second, this *S. Typhi* live vector stimulated CD8$^+$ MHC class I-restricted cytotoxic lymphocytes that recognized targets bearing CSP, demonstrating that *Typhi* live vectors could elicit relevant cell-mediated effector responses in humans [54].

Immunization of adults with a single oral dose of CVD 908-*htrA* carrying a plasmid-encoding fragC of tetanus toxin elicited enhanced proliferative responses and stimulated protective levels of tetanus antitoxin in a seronegative subject [133]. The importance of the latter observation is to demonstrate that a single oral dose of a *S. Typhi* live vector can elicit a type of protective immune response that is generally thought to require parenteral immunization. Re-cent clinical trials have illuminated the influence of the specific live vector on the immune response to a given heterologous antigen. In a Phase I clinical trial of an attenuated *S. Typhi* Ty800 live vector expressing *H. pylori* urease A and B from stabilized expression plasmids, no immune response was observed against the heterologous antigen despite a strong response against live vector antigens [134]. When this urease antigen was expressed from the identical expression plasmid introduced into an attenuated *S. Typhimurium* live vector, vaccination stimulated strong responses to the live vector as well as antiurease antibodies in three of six subjects, but this live vector was not well tolerated clinically [135]. However, a recent preliminary report by McKenzie et al. [136] using CVD 908-*htrA* to express *H. pylori* urease resulted in impressive and encouraging dose-dependent responses to both live vector and heterologous antigen; when immunizing with 5×10^9 colony-forming units (cfu), urease-specific IgG ASC responses were detected in seven of eight subjects, and urease-specific fecal IgA responses were detected in 50% of vaccinees.

Clinical trials with other live vector constructs have given generally modest results [17,134,137–139]. In some of these clinical trials, the *S. Typhi* live vectors failed to elicit a detectable immune response to the foreign antigen, despite immunogenicity of the identical (or homologous *S. Typhimurium*) constructs when tested in preclinical animal models. Regrettably, none of the human clinical trials with *Salmonella* live vectors, heretofore, has utilized constructs that would be considered optimal.

REFERENCES

1. Dougan G, et al. Live oral *Salmonella* vaccines: potential use of attenuated strains as carriers of heterologous antigens to the immune system. Parasite Immunol 1987; 9:151–160.
2. Levine MM, et al. Attenuated *Salmonella* as carriers for the expression of foreign antigens. Microecol Ther 1990; 19:23–32.
3. Levine MM, et al. Attenuated *Salmonella* as live oral vaccines against typhoid fever and as live vectors. J Biotechnol 1996; 44:193–196.
4. Medina E, Guzman CA. Use of live bacterial vaccine vectors for antigen delivery: potential and limitations. Vaccine 2001; 19:1573–1580.
5. Mollenkopf H, et al. Intracellular bacteria as targets and carriers for vaccination. Biol Chem 2001; 382:521–532.
6. Drabner B, Guzman CA. Elicitation of predictable immune responses by using live bacterial vectors. Biomol Eng 2001; 17:75–82.
7. Stocker BA. Aromatic-dependent *Salmonella* as anti-bacterial vaccines and as presenters of heterologous antigens or of DNA encoding them. J Biotechnol 2000; 83:45–50.
8. Dietrich G, et al. Bacterial systems for the delivery of eukaryotic antigen expression vectors. Antisense Nucleic Acid Drug Dev 2000; 10:391–399.
9. Dietrich G, et al. Gram-positive and gram-negative bacteria as carrier systems for DNA vaccines. Vaccine 2001; 19:2506–2512.
10. Dietrich G, et al. Delivery of DNA vaccines by attenuated intracellular bacteria. Immunol Today 1999; 20:251–253.
11. Dietrich G, Goebel W. DNA vaccine delivery by attenuated intracellular bacteria. Subcell Biochem 2000; 33:541–557.
12. Weiss S, Krusch S. Bacteria-mediated transfer of eukaryotic

expression plasmids into mammalian host cells. Biol Chem 2001; 382:533–541.

13. Weiss S, Chakraborty T. Transfer of eukaryotic expression plasmids to mammalian host cells by bacterial carriers. Curr Opin Biotechnol 2001; 12:467–472.

14. Chatfield SN, et al. Construction of a genetically defined *Salmonella typhi* Ty2 *aroA*, *aroC* mutant for the engineering of a candidate oral typhoid-tetanus vaccine. Vaccine 1992; 10:53–60.

15. Barry EM, et al. Expression and immunogenicity of pertussis toxin S1 subunit–tetanus toxin fragment C fusions in *Salmonella typhi* vaccine strain CVD 908. Infect Immun 1996; 64:4172–4181.

16. Galen JE, et al. A murine model of intranasal immunization to assess the immunogenicity of attenuated *Salmonella typhi* live vector vaccines in stimulating serum antibody responses to expressed foreign antigens. Vaccine 1997; 15:700–708.

17. Tacket CO, et al. Safety and immunogenicity in humans of an attenuated *Salmonella typhi* vaccine vector strain expressing plasmid-encoded hepatitis B antigens stabilized by the Asd-balanced lethal vector system. Infect Immun 1997; 65:3381–3385.

18. Wang JY, et al. Construction, genotypic and phenotypic characterization, and immunogenicity of attenuated ΔguaguaBA *Salmonella enterica* serovar Typhi strain CVD 915. Infect Immun 2001; 69:4734–4741.

19. Chatfield SN, et al. Use of the *nirB* promoter to direct the stable expression of heterologous antigens in *Salmonella* oral vaccine strains: development of a single-dose oral tetanus vaccine. Biotechnology (NY) 1992; 10:888–892.

20. Schodel F, et al. Hybrid hepatitis B virus core antigen as a vaccine carrier moiety: II. Expression in avirulent *Salmonella* spp. for mucosal immunization. Adv Exp Med Biol 1996; 397:15–21.

21. Nayak AR, et al. A live recombinant avirulent oral *Salmonella* vaccine expressing pneumococcal surface protein A induces protective responses against *Streptococcus pneumoniae*. Infect Immun 1998; 66:3744–3751.

22. Noriega F, et al. Engineered ΔguaB-A, *virG Shigella flexneri* 2a strain CVD 1205: construction, safety, immunogenicity, and potential efficacy as a mucosal vaccine. Infect Immun 1996; 64:3055–3061.

23. Altboum Z, et al. Attenuated *Shigella flexneri* 2a Delta guaBA strain CVD 1204 expressing enterotoxigenic *Escherichia coli* (ETEC) CS2 and CS3 fimbriae as a live mucosal vaccine against *Shigella* and ETEC infection. Infect Immun 2001; 69:3150–3158.

24. Anderson RJ, et al. DeltaguaBA attenuated *Shigella flexneri* 2a strain CVD 1204 as a *Shigella* vaccine and as a live mucosal delivery system for fragment C of tetanus toxin. Vaccine 2000; 18:2193–2202.

25. Koprowski H, et al. Attenuated *Shigella flexneri* 2a vaccine strain CVD 1204 expressing colonization factor antigen I and mutant heat-labile enterotoxin of enterotoxigenic *Escherichia coli*. Infect Immun 2000; 68:4884–4892.

26. Butterton JR, et al. Coexpression of the B subunit of Shiga toxin 1 and EaeA from enterohemorrhagic *Escherichia coli* in *Vibrio cholerae* vaccine strains. Infect Immun 1997; 65:2127–2135.

27. Ryan ET, et al. Protective immunity against *Clostridium difficile* toxin A induced by oral immunization with a live, attenuated *Vibrio cholerae* vector strain. Infect Immun 1997; 65:2941–2949.

28. Ryan ET, et al. Oral immunization with attenuated vaccine strains of *Vibrio cholerae* expressing a dodecapeptide repeat of the serine-rich *Entamoeba histolytica* protein fused to the cholera toxin B subunit induces systemic and mucosal antiamebic and anti-*V. cholerae* antibody responses in mice. Infect Immun 1997; 65:3118–3125.

29. Frankel FR, et al. Induction of cell-mediated immune responses to human immunodeficiency virus type 1 Gag protein by using *Listeria monocytogenes* as a live vaccine vector. J Immunol 1995; 155:4775–4782.

30. Edelman R, et al. Safety and immunogenicity of recombinant Bacille Calmette–Guerin (rBCG) expressing *Borrelia burgdorferi* outer surface protein A (OspA) lipoprotein in adult volunteers: a candidate Lyme disease vaccine. Vaccine 1999; 17:904–914.

31. Igwe EI, et al. Rational live oral carrier vaccine design by mutating virulence-associated genes of *Yersinia enterocolitica*. Infect Immun 1999; 67:5500–5507.

32. Medaglini D, et al. Mucosal and systemic immune responses to a recombinant protein expressed on the surface of the oral commensal bacterium *Streptococcus gordonii* after oral colonization. Proc Natl Acad Sci 1995; 92:6868–6872.

33. Zegers ND, et al. Expression of the protective antigen of *Bacillus anthracis* by *Lactobacillus casei*: towards the development of an oral vaccine against anthrax. J Appl Microbiol 1999; 87:309–314.

34. Steidler L, et al. Mucosal delivery of murine interleukin-2 (IL-2) and IL-6 by recombinant strains of *Lactococcus lactis* coexpressing antigen and cytokine. Infect Immun 1998; 66:3183–3189.

35. Sirard JC, et al. Live attenuated *Salmonella*: a paradigm of mucosal vaccines. Immunol Rev 1999; 171:5–26.

36. Phalipon A, Sansonetti P. Live attenuated *Shigella flexneri* mutants as vaccine candidates against shigellosis and vectors for antigen delivery. Biologicals 1995; 23:125–134.

37. Parkhill J, et al. Complete genome sequence of a multiple drug resistant *Salmonella enterica* serovar Typhi CT18. Nature 2001; 413:848–852.

38. McClelland M, et al. Complete genome sequence of *Salmonella enterica* serovar Typhimurium LT2. Nature 2001; 413:852–856.

39. Hansen-Wester I, Hensel M. Genome-based identification of chromosomal regions specific for *Salmonella* spp. Infect Immun 2002; 70:2351–2360.

40. Lostroh CP, Lee CA. The *Salmonella* pathogenicity island-1 type III secretion system. Microbes Infect 2001; 3:1281–1291.

41. Marcus SL, et al. *Salmonella* pathogenicity islands: big virulence in small packages. Microbes Infect 2000; 2:145–156.

42. Hansen-Wester I, Hensel M. *Salmonella* pathogenicity islands encoding type III secretion systems. Microbes Infect 2001; 3:549–559.

43. Hensel M. *Salmonella* pathogenicity island 2. Mol Microbiol 2000; 36:1015–1023.

44. Buchrieser C, et al. The virulence plasmid pWR100 and the repertoire of proteins secreted by the type III secretion apparatus of *Shigella flexneri*. Mol Microbiol 2000; 38:760–771.

45. Parsot C, Sansonetti P. The virulence plasmid of shigellae: an archipelago of pathogenicity islands? In: Kaper JB, Hacker J, eds. Pathogenicity Islands and Other Mobile Virulence Elements. Washington, DC: ASM Press, 1999:151–165.

46. Bailey JE. Host–vector interactions in *Escherichia coli*. In: Fiechter, A ed. Advances in Biochemical Engineering. Biotechnology, 1993. Berlin: Springer-Verlag, 1993:29–77.

47. Glick BR. Metabolic load and heterologous gene expression. Biotechnol Adv 1995; 13:247–261.

48. Smith MA, Bidochka MJ. Bacterial fitness and plasmid loss: the importance of culture conditions and plasmid size. Can J Microbiol 1998; 44:351–355.

49. Pecota DC, et al. Combining the *hok/sok*, *parDE*, and *pnd* postsegregational killer loci to enhance plasmid stability. Appl Environ Microbiol 1997; 63:1917–1924.

50. Boe L, et al. Effects of genes exerting growth inhibition and

plasmid stability on plasmid maintenance. J Bacteriol 1987; 169:4646–4650.

51. McDermott PJ, et al. Adaptation of *Escherichia coli* growth rates to the presence of pBR322. Lett Appl Microbiol 1993; 17:139–143.

52. Wu K, Wood TK. Evaluation of the *hok/sok* killer locus for enhanced plasmid stability. Biotechnol Bioeng 1994; 44:912–921.

53. Summers DK. Timing, self-control and sense of direction are the secrets of multicopy plasmid stability. Mol Microbiol 1998; 29:1137–1145.

54. Gonzalez C, et al. *Salmonella typhi* vaccine strain CVD 908 expressing the circumsporozoite protein of *Plasmodium falciparum*: strain construction and safety and immunogenicity in humans. J Infect Dis 1994; 169:927–931.

55. Gonzalez CR, et al. Immunogenicity of a *Salmonella typhi* CVD 908 candidate vaccine strain expressing the major surface protein gp63 of *Leishmania mexicana mexicana*. Vaccine 1998; 16:1043–1052.

56. Santiago-Machuca AE, et al. Attenuated *Salmonella enterica* serovar *Typhi* live vector with inducible chromosomal expression of the T7 RNA polymerase and its evaluation with reporter genes. Plasmid 2002; 47:108–119.

57. Qian F, Pan W. Construction of a *tetR*-integrated *Salmonella enterica* serovar Typhi CVD908 strain that tightly controls expression of the major merozoite surface protein of *Plasmodium falciparum* for applications in human vaccine production. Infect Immun 2002; 70:2029–2038.

58. Gossen M, Bujard H. Tight control of gene expression in mammalian cells by tetracycline-responsive promoters. Proc Natl Acad Sci USA 1992; 89:5547–5551.

59. Khan CM, et al. Construction, expression, and immunogenicity of multiple tandem copies of the *Schistosoma mansoni* peptide 115–131 of the P28 glutathione *S*-transferase expressed as C-terminal fusions to tetanus toxin fragment C in a live aro-attenuated vaccine strain of *Salmonella*. J Immunol 1994; 153:5634–5642.

60. McSorley SJ, et al. Vaccine efficacy of *Salmonella* strains expressing glycoprotein 63 with different promoters. Infect Immun 1997; 65:171–178.

61. Bumann D. Regulated antigen expression in live recombinant *Salmonella enterica* serovar Typhimurium strongly affects colonization capabilities and specific $CD4^+$-T-cell responses. Infect Immun 2001; 69:7493–7500.

62. Bumann D. Examination of *Salmonella* gene expression in an infected mammalian host using the green fluorescent protein and two-colour flow cytometry. Mol Microbiol 2002; 43:1269–1283.

63. Hohmann EL, et al. Macrophage-inducible expression of a model antigen in *Salmonella typhimurium* enhances immunogenicity. Proc Natl Acad Sci USA 1995; 92:2904–2908.

64. Dunstan SJ, et al. Use of in vivo-regulated promoters to deliver antigens from attenuated *Salmonella enterica* var Typhimurium. Infect Immun 1999; 67:5133–5141.

65. Hansen-Wester I, et al. Type III secretion of *Salmonella enterica* serovar Typhimurium translocated effectors and SseFG. Infect Immun 2002; 70:1403–1409.

66. Galan JE, et al. Cloning and characterization of the *asd* gene of *Salmonella typhimurium*: use in stable maintenance of recombinant plasmids in *Salmonella* vaccine strains. Gene 1990; 94:29–35.

67. Gerdes K, et al. Stable inheritance of plasmid R1 requires two different loci. J Bacteriol 1985; 161:292–298.

68. Galen JE, et al. Optimization of plasmid maintenance in the attenuated live vector vaccine strain *Salmonella typhi* CVD 908-*htrA*. Infect Immun 1999; 67:6424–6433.

69. Galen JE, Levine MM. Can a "flawless" live vector vaccine strain be engineered? Trends Microbiol 2001; 9:372–376.

70. Chang SP, et al. A carboxyl-terminal fragment of *Plasmodium falciparum* gp195 expressed by a recombinant baculovirus induces antibodies that completely inhibit parasite growth. J Immunol 1992; 149:548–555.

71. Uthaipibull C, et al. Inhibitory and blocking monoclonal antibody epitopes on merozoite surface protein 1 of the malaria parasite *Plasmodium falciparum*. J Mol Biol 2001; 307:1381–1394.

72. Kwak Y-D, et al. Cell surface display of human immunodeficiency virus type 1 gp120 on *Escherichia coli* by using ice nucleation protein. Clin Diagn Lab Immunol 1999; 6:499–503.

73. Lee J-S, et al. Surface-displayed viral antigens on *Salmonella* carrier vaccine. Nat Biotechnol 2000; 18:645–648.

74. Hess J, et al. Superior efficacy of secreted over somatic antigen display in recombinant *Salmonella* vaccine induced protection against listeriosis. Proc Natl Acad Sci 1996; 93:1458–1463.

75. Russmann H, et al. Delivery of epitopes by the *Salmonella* type III secretion system for vaccine development. Science 1998; 281:565–568.

76. Russmann H, et al. Protection against murine listeriosis by oral vaccination with recombinant *Salmonella* expressing hybrid *Yersinia* type III proteins. J Immunol 2001; 167:357–365.

77. Klee SR, et al. Construction and characterization of a live attenuated vaccine candidate against *Shigella dysenteriae* type 1. Infect Immun 1997; 65:2112–2118.

78. Tzschaschel BD, et al. Towards a vaccine candidate against *Shigella dysenteriae* 1: expression of the Shiga toxin B-subunit in an attenuated *Shigella flexneri aroD* carrier strain. Microb Pathog 1996; 21:277–288.

79. Noriega F, et al. Further characterization of $\Delta aroA$, $\Delta virG$ *Shigella flexneri* 2a strain CVD 1203 as a mucosal *Shigella* vaccine and as a live vector vaccine for delivering antigens of enterotoxigenic *Escherichia coli*. Infect Immun 1996; 64:23–27.

80. Loy AL, et al. Immune response to rotavirus VP4 expressed in an attenuated strain of *Shigella flexneri*. FEMS Immunol Med Microbiol 1999; 25:283–288.

81. Barzu S, et al. Immunogenicity of IpaC-hybrid proteins expressed in the *Shigella flexneri* 2a vaccine candidate SC602. Infect Immun 1998; 66:77–82.

82. Mittrucker HW, Kaufmann SH. Immune response to infection with *Salmonella typhimurium* in mice. J Leukoc Biol 2000; 67:457–463.

83. Pasetti MF, et al. *Salmonella enterica* serovar Typhi live vector vaccines delivered intranasally elicit regional and systemic specific $CD8^+$ major histocompatibility class I-restricted cytotoxic T lymphocytes. Infect Immun 2002; 70:4009–4018.

84. Kotloff KL, et al. *Shigella flexneri* 2a strain CVD 1207, with specific deletions in virG, sen, set, and guaBA, is highly attenuated in humans. Infect Immun 2000; 68:1034–1039.

85. Tacket CO, et al. Safety of live oral *Salmonella Typhi* vaccine strains with deletions in *htrA* and *aroC aroD* and immune responses in humans. Infect Immun 1997; 65:452–456.

86. Tacket CO, et al. Phase 2 clinical trial of attenuated *Salmonella enterica* serovar Typhi oral live vector vaccine CVD 908-*htrA* in US volunteers. Infect Immun 2000; 68:1196–1201.

87. Allen JS, et al. Kinetics of the mucosal antibody secreting cell response and evidence of specific lymphocyte migration to the lung after oral immunisation with attenuated *S. enterica* var. *typhimurium*. FEMS Immunol Med Microbiol 2000; 27:275–281.

88. Fairweather NF, et al. Oral vaccination of mice against tetanus by use of a live attenuated *Salmonella* carrier. Infect Immun 1990; 58:1323–1326.

89. VanCott JL, et al. Regulation of mucosal and systemic antibody responses by T helper cell subsets, macrophages, and derived cytokines following oral immunization with live recombinant *Salmonella*. J Immunol 1996; 156:1504–1514.

90. Titball RW, Williamson ED. Vaccination against bubonic and pneumonic plague. Vaccine 2001; 19:4175–4184.

91. Ascon MA, et al. Oral immunization with a *Salmonella typhimurium* vaccine vector expressing recombinant enterotoxigenic *Escherichia coli* K99 fimbriae elicits elevated antibody titers for protective immunity. Infect Immun 1998; 66:5470–5476.

92. Mollenkopf HJ, et al. Protective efficacy against tuberculosis of ESAT-6 secreted by a live *Salmonella typhimurium* vaccine carrier strain and expressed by naked DNA. Vaccine 2001; 19:4028–4035.

93. Xu D, et al. Protective effect on *Leishmania major* infection of migration inhibitory factor, TNF-alpha, and IFN-gamma administered orally via attenuated *Salmonella typhimurium*. J Immunol 1998; 160:1285–1289.

94. Gomez-Duarte OG, et al. Expression, extracellular secretion, and immunogenicity of the *Plasmodium falciparum* sporozoite surface protein 2 in *Salmonella* vaccine strains. Infect Immun 2001; 69:1192–1198.

95. Gomez-Duarte OG, et al. Protection of mice against gastric colonization by *Helicobacter pylori* by single oral dose immunization with attenuated *Salmonella typhimurium* producing urease subunits A and B. Vaccine 1998; 16:460–471.

96. Jespersgaard C, et al. Effect of attenuated *Salmonella enterica* serovar Typhimurium expressing a *Streptococcus mutans* antigen on secondary responses to the cloned protein. Infect Immun 2001; 69:6604–6611.

97. Nardelli-Haefliger D, et al. Nasal vaccination with attenuated *Salmonella typhimurium* strains expressing the Hepatitis B nucleocapsid: dose response analysis. Vaccine 2001; 19:2854–2861.

98. Karem KL, et al. Protective immunity against herpes simplex virus (HSV) type 1 following oral administration of recombinant *Salmonella typhimurium* vaccine strains expressing HSV antigens. J Gen Virol 1997; 78:427–434.

99. Spreng S, et al. *Salmonella* vaccines secreting measles virus epitopes induce protective immune responses against measles virus encephalitis. Microbes Infect 2000; 2:1687–1692.

100. Yrlid U, et al. *Salmonella* infection of bone marrow-derived macrophages and dendritic cells: influence on antigen presentation and initiating an immune response. FEMS Immunol Med Microbiol 2000; 27:313–320.

101. Shams H, et al. Induction of specific CD8$^+$ memory T cells and long lasting protection following immunization with *Salmonella typhimurium* expressing a lymphocytic choriomeningitis MHC class I-restricted epitope. Vaccine 2001; 20:577–585.

102. Kohler JJ, et al. Long-term immunological memory induced by recombinant oral *Salmonella* vaccine vectors. Infect Immun 2000; 68:4370–4373.

103. Pasetti MF, et al. Attenuated delta*guaBA Salmonella typhi* vaccine strain CVD 915 as a live vector utilizing prokaryotic or eukaryotic expression systems to deliver foreign antigens and elicit immune responses. Clin Immunol 1999; 92:76–89.

104. Pasetti MF, et al. A comparison of immunogenicity and in vivo distribution of *Salmonella enterica* serovar Typhi and Typhimurium live vector vaccines delivered by mucosal routes in the murine model. Vaccine 2000; 18:3208–3213.

105. Pickett TE, et al. In vivo characterization of the murine intranasal model for assessing the immunogenicity of attenuated *Salmonella enterica* serovar Typhi strains as live mucosal vaccines and as live vectors. Infect Immun 2000; 68:205–213.

106. Gurunathan S, et al. DNA vaccines: immunology, application, and optimization. Annu Rev Immunol 2000; 18:927–974.

107. Grillot-Courvalin C, et al. Wild-type intracellular bacteria deliver DNA into mammalian cells. Cell Microbiol 2002; 4:177–186.

108. McKenzie BS, et al. Nucleic acid vaccines: tasks and tactics. Immunol Res 2001; 24:225–244.

109. Polo JM, et al. Alphavirus DNA and particle replicons for vaccines and gene therapy. Dev Biol (Basel) 2000; 104:181–185.

110. Darji A, et al. Oral delivery of DNA vaccines using attenuated *Salmonella typhimurium* as carrier. FEMS Immunol Med Microbiol 2000; 27:341–349.

111. Sizemore DR, et al. Attenuated *Shigella* as a DNA delivery vehicle for DNA-mediated immunization. Science 1995; 270:299–302.

112. Sizemore DR, et al. Attenuated bacteria as a DNA delivery vehicle for DNA-mediated immunization. Vaccine 1997; 15:804–807.

113. Fennelly GJ, et al. Mucosal DNA vaccine immunization against measles with a highly attenuated *Shigella flexneri* vector. J Immunol 1999; 162:1603–1610.

114. Devico AL, et al. Development of an oral prime-boost strategy to elicit broadly neutralizing antibodies against HIV-1. Vaccine 2002; 20:1968–1974.

115. Shata MT, Hone DM. Vaccination with a *Shigella* DNA vaccine vector induces antigen-specific CD8(+) T cells and antiviral protective immunity. J Virol 2001; 75:9665–9670.

116. Shata MT, et al. Recent advances with recombinant bacterial vaccine vectors. Mol Med Today 2000; 6:66–71.

117. Brunham RC, Zhang D. Transgene as vaccine for *Chlamydia*. Am Heart J 1999; 138:S519–S522.

118. Darji A, et al. Oral somatic transgene vaccination using attenuated *S. typhimurium*. Cell 1997; 91:765–775.

119. Flo J, et al. Oral transgene vaccination mediated by attenuated salmonellae is an effective method to prevent Herpes simplex virus-2 induced disease in mice. Vaccine 2001; 19:1772–1782.

120. Shata MT, et al. Mucosal and systemic HIV-1 Env-specific CD8(+) T-cells develop after intragastric vaccination with a *Salmonella* Env DNA vaccine vector. Vaccine 2001; 20:623–629.

121. Paglia P, et al. Gene transfer in dendritic cells, induced by oral DNA vaccination with *Salmonella typhimurium*, results in protective immunity against a murine fibrosarcoma. Blood 1998; 92:3172–3176.

122. Dietrich G. Current status and future perspectives of DNA vaccine delivery by attenuated intracellular bacteria. Arch Immunol Ther Exp (Warszawa) 2000; 48:177–182.

123. Gentschev I, et al. Recombinant attenuated bacteria for the delivery of subunit vaccines. Vaccine 2001; 19:2621–2628.

124. Catic A, et al. Introduction of protein or DNA delivered via recombinant *Salmonella typhimurium* into the major histocompatibility complex class I presentation pathway of macrophages. Microbes Infect 1999; 1:113–121.

125. Courvalin P, et al. Gene transfer from bacteria to mammalian cells. C R Acad Sci Ser 3 1995; 318:1207–1212.

126. Vecino WH, et al. Mucosal DNA vaccination with highly attenuated *Shigella* is superior to attenuated *Salmonella* and comparable to intramuscular DNA vaccination for T cells against HIV. Immunol Lett 2002; 82:197–204.

127. Jain V, Mekalanos JJ. Use of lambda phage S and R gene products in an inducible lysis system for *Vibrio cholerae*- and *Salmonella enterica* serovar *Typhimurium*-based DNA vaccine delivery systems. Infect Immun 2000; 68:986–989.

128. Rodriguez A, et al. Selective transport of internalized antigens to the cytosol for MHC class I presentation in dendritic cells. Nat Cell Biol 1999; 1:362–368.

129. Yrlid U, Wick MJ. *Salmonella*-induced apoptosis of infected macrophages results in presentation of a bacteria-encoded antigen after uptake by bystander dendritic cells. J Exp Med 2000; 191:613–624.

130. Black RE, et al. Prevention of shigellosis by a *Salmonella typhi–Shigella sonnei* bivalent vaccine. J Infect Dis 1987; 155: 1260–1265.

131. Herrington DA, et al. Studies in volunteers to evaluate candidate *Shigella* vaccines: further experience with a bivalent *Salmonella typhi–Shigella sonnei* vaccine and protection conferred by previous *Shigella sonnei* disease. Vaccine 1990; 8: 353–357.

132. Tacket CO, et al. Safety, immunogenicity, and efficacy against cholera challenge in humans of a typhoid–cholera hybrid vaccine derived from *Salmonella typhi* Ty21a. Infect Immun 1990; 58:1620–1627.

133. Tacket CO, et al. Safety and immune responses to attenuated *Salmonella enterica* serovar typhi oral live vector vaccines expressing tetanus toxin fragment C. Clin Immunol 2000; 97:146–153.

134. DiPetrillo MD, et al. Safety and immunogenicity of phoP/phoQ-deleted *Salmonella typhi* expressing *Helicobacter pylori* urease in adult volunteers. Vaccine 1999; 18:449–459.

135. Angelakopoulos H, Hohmann EL. Pilot study of phoP/phoQ-deleted *Salmonella enterica* serovar *Typhimurium* expressing *Helicobacter pylori* urease in adult volunteers. Infect Immun 2000; 68:2135–2141.

136. McKenzie R, et al. A phase I study of the safety and immunogenicity of two attenuated *Salmonella typhi* vectors expressing the urease vaccine antigen of *H. pylori*. ASM 102nd General Meeting Abstract, 2002, E-45-E-45E-45-E-45.

137. Bumann D, et al. Safety and immunogenicity of live recombinant *Salmonella enterica* serovar Typhi Ty21a expressing urease A and B from *Helicobacter pylori* in human volunteers. Vaccine 2001; 20:845–852.

138. Nardelli-Haefliger D, et al. Oral and rectal immunization of adult female volunteers with a recombinant attenuated *Salmonella typhi* vaccine strain. Infect Immun 1996; 64: 5219–5224.

139. Tramont EC, et al. Safety and antigenicity of typhoid–*Shigella sonnei* vaccine (strain 5076-1C). J Infect Dis 1984; 149: 133–136.

140. Medina E, et al. *Salmonella* vaccine carrier strains: effective delivery system to trigger anti-tumor immunity by oral route. Eur J Immunol 1999; 29:693–699.

141. Xiang R, et al. An autologous oral DNA vaccine protects against murine melanoma. Proc Natl Acad Sci USA 2000; 97:5492–5497.

142. Cochlovius B, et al. Oral DNA vaccination: antigen uptake and presentation by dendritic cells elicits protective immunity. Immunol Lett 2002; 80:89–96.

143. Paglia P, et al. In vivo correction of genetic defects of monocyte/macrophages using attenuated *Salmonella* as oral vectors for targeted gene delivery. Gene Ther 2000; 7:1725–1730.

144. Lode HN, et al. Tyrosine hydroxylase-based DNA-vaccination is effective against murine neuroblastoma. Med Pediatr Oncol 2000; 35:641–646.

145. Urashima M, et al. An oral CD40 ligand gene therapy against lymphoma using attenuated *Salmonella typhimurium*. Blood 2000; 95:1258–1263.

146. Zoller M, Christ O. Prophylactic tumor vaccination: comparison of effector mechanisms initiated by protein versus DNA vaccination. J Immunol 2001; 166:3440–3450.

147. Woo PC, et al. Unique immunogenicity of hepatitis B virus DNA vaccine presented by live-attenuated *Salmonella typhimurium*. Vaccine 2001; 19:2945–2954.

148. Xiang R, et al. A dual-function DNA vaccine encoding carcinoembryonic antigen and CD40 ligand trimer induces T cell-mediated protective immunity against colon cancer in carcinoembryonic antigen-transgenic mice. J Immunol 2001; 167:4560–4565.

149. Woo PC, et al. Enhancement by ampicillin of antibody responses induced by a protein antigen and a DNA vaccine carried by live-attenuated *Salmonella enterica* serovar Typhi. Clin Diagn Lab Immunol 2000; 7:596–599.

31
DNA Vaccines

Indresh K. Srivastava and Jeffrey B. Ulmer
Chiron Corporation, Emeryville, California, U.S.A.

Margaret A. Liu
Transgene Inc., Strasbourg, France

I. INTRODUCTION

Compared to other conventional vaccine technologies, such as adjuvanted protein, recombinant vector, and attenuated pathogens, the concept of DNA vaccination is relatively simple. A specific gene of interest from a particular pathogen is cloned into a plasmid containing a powerful promoter active in eukaryotic cells and, upon injection into vaccinees, the antigen is produced in situ. The expressed protein is then processed and presented to the immune system by the MHC class-1 restricted pathway for CTL induction, the MHC class-II restricted pathway for the induction of helper T (Th) cell responses and to B cells for the induction of antibodies. It has been known for quite some time that direct inoculation of linear or plasmid DNA could result in gene expression in vivo [1,2]. The power of this technology for inducing potent immune responses and its potential for vaccine application was demonstrated by Tang et al. [3], Ulmer et al. [4], Fynan et al. [5], Wang et al. [6], and many others in different animal models. Using the gene gun to deliver plasmid DNA into the skin of mice, Tang et al. [3] demonstrated the induction of antibody responses. Ulmer et al. [4] first demonstrated the induction of CTL responses and proof of principle for protective efficacy of a DNA vaccine encoding influenza nucleoprotein (NP). Specifically, these animals were protected from both morbidity and mortality upon lethal challenge with a heterosubtypic strain of influenza A virus. While substantial antibody responses were also generated against NP, protection was demonstrated to be cell mediated [4]. Later that same year, DNA vaccine studies were extended to other diseases such as HIV [6], rabies virus [7], and hepatitis B [8]. These early studies established several important features of DNA vaccines: 1) both antibody and cellular immune responses can be induced; 2) immune responses can be induced by different routes of immunization (intramuscular and epidermal); and 3) it is possible to express foreign genes in vivo with proper structure and conforma-

tion, as judged by the induction of neutralizing antibodies. Since then, DNA immunization has been used successfully to induce immune responses in animal species from mice to humans with DNA encoding antigens from various sources such as HIV [9–14], herpes simplex virus-1 (HSV-1) [15–18], HSV-2 [19–21], rabies [7,22–24], hepatitis C [25,26], tuberculosis [27–30], malaria [31–34], mycoplasma [35], toxoplasma [36–40], rotavirus [41–43], Ebola virus [44–46], and many others. In addition to infectious diseases, the DNA vaccine strategy has been shown to be potentially a very powerful tool in animal models of allergy, asthma, and cancer.

This review will focus on the ability of DNA vaccines to induce humoral and cellular responses against a wide variety of infectious agents, and the current approaches being developed to enhance the efficacy of DNA vaccines.

II. HUMORAL IMMUNE RESPONSES

Antibodies against viral proteins induced by DNA vaccines were first demonstrated by intramuscular injection of DNA encoding influenza NP and hemagglutinin (HA) [4]. The ability of DNA vaccines to induce appreciable antiviral antibodies was subsequently confirmed by several other investigators with other genes from influenza [47–52], HIV [53–58], rabies virus [7,23,59–61], and hepatitis B virus [62]. Since then, the DNA vaccine approach has been used extensively to induce antibody responses against various viral, bacterial, parasitic, fungal, tumor, and eukaryotic proteins.

In general, the antibodies induced by DNA vaccination are predominantly of the IgG subtype with lower levels of serum IgA and IgM [52,63]. The quantity and quality of the antibody responses induced by DNA vaccination appear to be influenced by the nature and type of immunogen, animal species, and also by the method and site of DNA delivery. First, as with protein-based vaccines, the inherent antigenicity of the protein expressed by DNA vaccines in part determines the potency of the immune responses induced. However, increased antibody responses can be achieved by expressing antigens as secreted proteins, or as fusion proteins with other antigens or helper T-cell epitopes [64–66]. Second, antibodies induced by DNA vaccines in small animals such as mice are durable and long lasting as shown with influenza [67,68], hepatitis B [69], hepatitis C [25], plasmodia [70–72], leishmania [73–75], and other animal models. In general, though, antibodies induced in nonhuman primates by DNA vaccination are of lower titer and rather short-lived [76,77]. However, this is partly due to a species-related phenomenon, because even potent protein subunit vaccines induce short-lived antibodies in primates [76]. Finally, it has been shown that DNA vaccines can successfully be delivered via different routes, such as intramuscular, intravenous, intranasal, oral, intraepidermal, intrarectal and intravaginal [57,68,78–83], and more recently intrasplenic [84] and intrahepatic [85]. However, the most common routes are intramuscular needle injections and gene gun-mediated epidermal delivery. The nature of how DNA vaccines are delivered with these two modes of vaccination is fundamentally different. After i.m. injection, myocytes are the primary cells transfected, and uptake of DNA is passive and very inefficient [86]. Whereas the gene gun propels DNA-coated gold beads directly into cells of the dermis and epidermis, including antigen presenting cells (APCs). As a consequence, less DNA is required for induction of immune responses by the gene-gun route [5,87,88]. But there is currently a limitation on the mass of DNA that can be delivered by the gene gun and the difference in immune priming can be overcome simply by injecting more DNA. Interestingly, the type of helper T-cell response induced by the gene gun is sometimes qualitatively different. For example, in almost all cases, i.m. injection of DNA induces dominant Th1-type responses, as shown by the induction of IgG2a antibody responses in mice, increased levels of IFN-γ production, and little IL-4 production [88–90]. In contrast, gene gun-mediated epidermal delivery of DNA has been shown in some instances to induce more of a balanced Th1/Th2-type response, as shown by the induction of IgG1 antibodies, increased levels of IL-4 production, and lower levels of IFN-γ production [88,89,91]. The reason for these differences is not yet known, but it may involve the site of antigen production (i.e., myocytes versus skin cells) or differential stimulation of the innate immune system (e.g., via immunostimulatory CpG sequences).

For many infectious diseases caused by pathogens that enter the host through mucosal surfaces, such as HIV, induction of mucosal immunity may be desirable for effective prophylaxis. So far, intramuscular injection, gene gun-mediated delivery, or mucosal delivery of naked plasmid DNA have been rather limited in their ability to induce secretory mucosal IgA responses. However, mucosal delivery of formulated plasmid DNA, such as with cationic lipids [92], monophosphoryl lipid A [93], QS-21 [94], encapsulation in ploy(lactide-coglycolide) (PLG) microparticles [95–98], macroaggregated polyethyleneimine-albumin conjugates [99], and biodegradable alginate microspheres [100], is effective at inducing secretory IgA responses at mucosal sites. This increased effectiveness was likely due to protection of DNA from digestion and more efficient delivery of DNA

into cells of the mucosal immune system. Using a different approach, Wang et al. reported the induction of strong mucosal immunity against simian immunodeficiency virus in primates using DNA expressing intact noninfectious virions [101]. The levels of secretory IgA observed in the rectal secretions of the immunized primates were even higher than the levels achieved through the natural infection. Thus development of DNA vaccine technologies capable of enhancing local IgA responses will be important for the prevention of infectious diseases.

III. CYTOTOXIC T-CELL RESPONSES

One of the potential advantages of DNA vaccines, compared to certain other types of vaccines, is their ability to induce cellular responses. DNA vaccines induce potent long-lasting cellular responses mediated by MHC class-1 restricted CD8+ cytotoxic T lymphocytes (CTL). Effector CTL recognizing appropriate MHC-restricted peptides have been demonstrated in mice immunized with DNA encoding NP from influenza A virus [4,49,66,102–104], hepatitis B surface [105] and core antigen [106], and HIV Env [107–109] and gag antigens [109–111], and many others. DNA vaccine-induced CTL were also capable of killing virus-infected targets, thereby demonstrating recognition of endogenously processed epitopes. It has been shown that CTL induced in mice by DNA vaccination can persist for more than 2 years after immunization [67,112,113], demonstrating the longevity of CTL responses. In addition, the ability of DNA vaccines to prime CTL in nonhuman primates has been demonstrated, where long-lived and broad responses can be achieved [76,114–118]. In several independent experiments, one or two intramuscular injections of plasmid DNA encoding HIV env or gag genes induced MHC-class 1-restricted CTL in primates [114]. For example, anti-Env CTL was detected for at least 11 months after the last immunization [114] and gag DNA induced CTL against multiple discrete epitopes [110], demonstrating the longevity and breadth of these responses. Also, gene gun-mediated immunization of rhesus macaques with plasmid DNA encoding simian immunodeficiency virus (SIV) Env and Gag induced Env-specific CTL [110]. Intramuscular and intravenous administration of the same plasmids combined with gene gun-mediated immunization induced Env- and Gag-specific CTL responses. The efficiency of DNA vaccines for the induction of potent CTL responses, like antibodies, is also influenced by the route and site of immunization, as well as on the immunization regimen. In general, multiple immunizations are necessary to induce strong responses; however, the number and frequency appear to be important. Fuller and Haynes [91] have shown that gene gun-mediated delivery of HIV-1 env DNA vaccine induced strong CTL and weak antibody responses after one, two, or three immunizations. However, a fourth immunization caused a significant drop in CTL levels with a significant increase in antibody titers. A corresponding decrease in IFN-γ and increase in IL-4 was also observed along with this change in the nature and profile of immune response. However, other investigators demonstrated that repeated immunization boosted the CTL levels against influenza NP [119] and HIV Env [109,114], and in both these instances the nature of response remained of Th1 type [89]. Thus the optimum dose and regimen may be different for different DNA vaccines. In addition, differences with the quality and quantity of T-cell responses observed with different routes of DNA administration may be due to fundamental differences in how antigens are processed and presented to the immune system. After i.m. injection, CTL are primed mainly via cross-presentation [120], where expression of antigens directly by APCs is important for CTL priming by the gene gun [121].

DNA vaccines have been tested in human clinical trials for initial safety and immunogenicity. Clinical trials using DNA vaccines either alone or in combination with a live vector boost have been conducted for herpes, influenza, hepatitis B, HIV, malaria, and several cancers. For example, Phase I clinical trials were initiated to evaluate the safety and immunogenicity of HIV-1 *env/rev* DNA constructs in infected and uninfected human subjects [122–126]. The uninfected human subjects that received the highest dose of DNA vaccine induced antigen-specific lymphoproliferative responses and antigen-specific production of interferon-γ and β-chemokines [124]. In the infected individuals, HIV-1 *env/rev* DNA vaccine construct modestly boosted the env-specific antibodies; however, no consistent effect was observed on cellular responses to HIV. In a separate study, HIV regulatory genes such as rev, nef, and tat were also evaluated in a Phase I clinical trial. Immunization of infected individuals with these genes resulted in enhanced cellular responses without any consistent changes in lymphocyte subsets or viral load [122,123,125,126]. The DNA vaccines were well tolerated in a broad dose range from 20 μg up to 2500 μg, as no significant local or systemic reactions were observed in human subjects [123,127].

In a Phase I clinical trial for a malaria DNA vaccine, it has been shown that three intramuscular immunizations of a *Plasmodium falciparum* circumsporozoitem (PfCSP) construct induced antigen-specific, genetically restricted CD8 + T-cell-dependent CTL. The cellular responses were directed against multiple epitopes and were restricted by six HLA class I alleles [32]. In the same study, despite induction of significant CTL responses, DNA vaccination failed to induce detectable antigen specific antibodies in any of the volunteers [127]. Phase I trials have also been conducted with the gene gun, where DNA encoding hepatitis B surface antigen induced both humoral and cellular immune responses (CD4 + and CD8 + T cells) [128]. A Phase I trial of an experimental HIV vaccine was recently initiated in Kenya, which involved a DNA vaccine encoding an HIV subtype A *gag* gene as a fusion with several discrete CTL epitopes from other HIV genes [129]. The DNA vaccine was administered by the gene gun and was the first component of a prime-boost vaccination strategy, which will be followed by a recombinant vaccinia virus vector [130]. In addition, Phase I clinical trials have been initiated in healthy and HIV-infected human volunteers to perform a head-to-head comparison of HIV DNA vaccines delivered as naked DNA and/or by a recombinant adenovirus [131]. Phase I/II trials are also ongoing using DNA immunogens as potential immunotherapies for cancer, including carcinoembryonic antigen

(CEA) for colon cancer, human follicular lymphoma, and a T-cell receptor Vβ for cutaneous T-cell lymphoma. The next year or two should reveal in detail the potency of new DNA vaccine technologies for inducing immune responses in humans.

IV. PROTECTION BY DNA VACCINES IN PRECLINICAL DISEASE MODELS

The influenza virus model was used to demonstrate that immune responses induced by DNA vaccination could protect mice against a lethal viral challenge [4]. The protection observed was due to NP-specific cellular responses, as passive transfer of immune serum from the immunized mice did not protect naïve mice against the challenge infection, although the serum contained high levels of specific antibodies to NP. In addition, adoptive transfer of splenocytes from the immunized mice protected naïve mice against lethal challenge infection [132]. Furthermore, both CD4 + and CD8 + T cells played a role in protection [102]. In addition to influenza, the protective efficacy of DNA vaccines has been demonstrated against many other diseases such as herpes simplex virus [16,18,133], rabies virus [22–24], cottontail rabbit papilloma virus [113], hepatitis B virus [128,134], Plasmodia [31,70,135,136], SIV/SHIV [58,137–140], rotavirus [97], LCMV [141], and others.

Strong CTL responses were induced by DNA vaccines encoding HIV-1 Env and SIV Gag in primates and these animals were successfully protected from challenge with chimeric SHIV virus [117,118,142,143]. However, strong antibody responses are not induced by DNA vaccines alone. Thus considerable attention has been focused on prime/boost strategies involving recombinant proteins or vectors to induce protective immune responses in primates. Along these lines, Amara et al. have demonstrated that priming of rhesus macaques with plasmid DNA encoding multiple proteins of SIV (Gag, Pol, Vif, Vpr) and HIV (Env, Tat and Rev) and boosting with recombinant modified vaccinia Ankara expressing SIV Gag and Pol and HIV Env induced potent CTL but weak antibody responses [117]. These animals were protected from AIDS upon mucosal challenge with highly pathogenic SHIV. In a separate study, protection from SHIV challenge has been induced in primates primed with an HIV-1 *env* DNA and boosted with recombinant oligomeric gp140 protein [142]. Barouch et al. have demonstrated the enhanced efficacy of DNA vaccine in inducing CTL and humoral responses by coadministration of HIV-1 Env- and SIVmac239 Gag-encoding plasmids with a plasmid encoding IL-2/Ig in rhesus macaques [118]. Upon challenge with pathogenic SHIV-89.6, these animals were able to control their viremia and were also protected against clinical AIDS. Finally, recombinant adenovirus vectors have successfully been used to boost CTL responses and protection in primate models of SIV [143] and ebola virus [46].

The efficacy of DNA vaccines for inducing protective responses in diseases where protection is mediated by antibodies has been shown against influenza [5,47,52,76], rabies [23], HSV [15,144], human papilloma virus [113], Ebola virus [46], and others. The effectiveness of DNA vaccines at inducing protective levels of antibodies is perhaps surprising, given the very low level of antigen produced by cells of the vaccinated host. This is particularly true for proteins that are poorly expressed (e.g., major capsid protein of papilloma virus) [113]. Possible explanations could include the duration of protein expression and the potential for preservation of conformation-specific epitopes by production of antigen in situ. In a DNA prime-protein boost study, Barnett et al. demonstrated the induction of strong neutralizing antibody responses in rabbits and rhesus macaques by intramuscular and intradermal injection of plasmid DNA encoding an oligomeric form of HIV-1 Env (o-gp140) followed by boosting with Env protein (o-gp140ΔV2 SF162) [53]. These antibodies neutralized both homologous and heterologous primary isolates, and initially protected rhesus macaques from challenge with pathogenic SHIV SF162P4 [142]. In this study, the primary control of the viremia was likely exerted by antibodies as the animals were depleted of CD8+ T cells prior to challenge.

The requirements for the expression, folding, and intracellular transport of bacterial and parasite proteins compared to viral proteins are different. Nevertheless, the DNA vaccine approach is quite effective at inducing protective responses in preclinical models of bacterial and parasitic diseases. In some of these models, protection is thought to be mediated by T cells, such as tuberculosis [27,145], *Mycoplasma pulmonis* infection [35], malaria [70,135,136,146], and leishmaniasis [147]. In these cases, processing and presentation of DNA-encoded antigens to T cells are unlikely to be affected by the source of the antigen (i.e., virus versus bacteria). In contrast, expression of bacterial antigens in cells of the eukaryotic host, where posttranslational modification and folding of the protein may be different than in the organism, may have an effect on the quality of antibody responses. Nevertheless, it is possible to induce protective immunity based on antibody responses with DNA encoding bacterial antigens, such as tetanus toxin C fragment [148] and *Salmonella typhi* OmpC porin [149].

In general, DNA vaccines are effective at inducing CTL, but less so at inducing T-helper responses and humoral responses, as compared to other means of immunization (e.g., adjuvanted recombinant protein, inactivated virus). To overcome these limitations, several approaches have been used to increase the potency of DNA vaccines, such as 1) optimization of vectors and genes of interest, in order to achieve higher levels of expression of antigen; 2) coadministration of plasmid DNA encoding immunologically active proteins such as chemokines, cytokines, costimulatory molecules, in order to enhance immune responses against encoded antigens; and 3) targeted DNA delivery into cells by either formulated DNA, physical delivery technology or vector systems, in order to overcome some of the barriers to effective transfection of cells in situ.

V. VECTOR AND GENE OPTIMIZATION

Expression studies using reporter genes indicate that only picogram to nanogram quantities of protein are expressed in vivo after administration of plasmid DNA [2,150]. While only small amounts of antigen may be sufficient for presentation to MHC class-1 molecules for induction of potent CTL responses, this may be a limiting factor in inducing potent humoral responses. To compound this problem, certain antigens from pathogens are not efficiently expressed by mammalian cells. For example, codon usage, mRNA instability, and dependence on coexpression of other genes (e.g., *rev*-dependence in HIV) can lead to suboptimal levels of expression of prokaryotic genes in eukaryotic cells. Therefore increasing gene expression by DNA vaccines is a reasonable strategy for increasing the potency of immune responses, and several approaches have been successful. First, the choice of promoter, enhancer, intron, polyadenylation, and transcriptional termination vector sequences can affect gene expression. The promoter/enhancer element of cytomegalovirus (CMV) is most commonly used in DNA vaccines and offers a high level of gene expression in a variety of cells. However, one potential disadvantage of the CMV promoter is that its activity may be downregulated by high levels of IFN-γ and TNF-α [151], which may be produced locally in response to DNA vaccines. Second, Haas et al. demonstrated that optimizing the nucleotide sequence of HIV genes to reflect the preferential codon usage in the mammalian cells can result in higher levels of gene expression [152]. Using codon optimization and also by removing certain inhibitory sequences, zur Megede et al. increased HIV *gag* expression by 1000-fold in vitro, with a corresponding substantial increase in immunogenicity in mice and primates [111]. Third, fusion of poorly expressed sequences with highly expressed heterologous proteins can increase the production of the target gene. For example, Wu and Barry showed that HIV *env* gene fused to the "C" termini of GFP or human protein alpha1-antitrypsin resulted in better anti-Env immune responses [153]. In addition to expression levels, localization of the encoded protein can affect the quantity and quality of DNA vaccine-induced immune responses. In general, secreted forms of the antigens compared to those targeted to the cytosol or plasma membrane are more effective at inducing antibody and helper T-cell responses, whereas cytosolic targeting may be preferred for CTL induction. However, this is not always the case, as membrane-bound antigens can induce high levels of antibodies [144] and secreted antigens can be effective for CTL [154]. The effectiveness of DNA vaccines for inducing CTL responses also may be enhanced by inducing rapid degradation of antigen by proteasomes, which can sometimes be achieved by expression as a fusion protein with ubiquitin [155,156]. In addition to intracellular targeting of antigen, extracellular targeting also can be effective. For example, expression of the gene of interest as a fusion protein with ligands such as CTLA4 [65,157], L-selectin [157,158], IgG-Fc [159], and chemokines [160], which target the cell surface receptors of APCs, have been shown to enhance both cellular and humoral immunity of DNA vaccines. In a related approach, expression as a fusion protein with a heat-shock protein increased potency [161], possibly by facilitating cross-priming via delivery of antigen to and activation of APCs. These previous examples have focused on the production of most or all of the antigens. This allows for determinant selection of T-cell epitopes by the vaccinated host.

In order to focus the immune response on specific T-cell epitopes, DNA vaccines encoding minimal epitopes [49, 162,163], strings of epitopes [49,104,129,164], and epitopes in the context of other proteins [49,165] have all shown to be effective at priming MHC class I- and class II-restricted responses. Therefore for efficient induction of cellular and humoral immunity by a given DNA vaccine the form of antigen should be evaluated on a case-by-case basis.

VI. ADJUVANTS FOR DNA VACCINES

To modulate or enhance immune responses induced by DNA vaccines, coadministration of biologically active molecules such as cytokines, chemokines and costimulatory molecules have been used extensively. The role of these biological or genetic adjuvants for DNA vaccines has been reviewed in detail [166]. Following are a few examples to demonstrate the potential of this approach. In general, coadministration of IL-2, a potent stimulator of cellular immunity that induces the proliferation and differentiation of T cells, B cells, and NK cells, enhances both cellular and humoral immune responses against DNA vaccine antigens [26,167]. For example, Barouch et al. have shown that coadministration of IL-2 as a fusion protein with the Fc portion of immunoglobulin G significantly enhanced the DNA vaccine-induced protective immune responses against HIV and SIV antigens in mice and rhesus macaques [12,168]. Intramuscular and intranasal coadministration of DNA encoding another cytokine, IL-12, has enhanced cellular and T-helper responses and downregulated humoral responses induced by DNA vaccines against various antigens [169–173]. In addition, Iwasaki et al. have shown that coadministration of IL-12 can overcome unresponsiveness of certain antigens [174]. DNA encoding other Th-1 inducing cytokines, such as IL-15 and IL-18, were also evaluated for their capability to modulate immune responses induced by DNA vaccines [169]. Interestingly, in contrast to IL-2 and IL-12, coadministration of IL-15 and IL-18 with DNA vaccines significantly enhanced antibody and proliferative responses but had little effect upon cellular responses [169,170,175]. In general, coadministration of DNA encoding Th-2-type cytokines, such as IL-4, IL-5, and IL-10, as might be expected significantly enhanced the magnitude of antibody responses induced by DNA vaccines [68,175]. In addition, IL-4 DNA inhibited cellular responses [68], which may limit the application of this cytokine as an adjuvant for antiviral vaccines. Coadministration of DNA encoding GM-CSF, a pro-inflammatory cytokine, has been shown to enhance antigen-specific cellular, humoral, and T-helper responses [176,177], as has been observed with antigens from HIV [92,178,179], influenza [174], HCV [26], encephalomyocarditis virus [180], rabies [90], and plasmodia [181,182]. Furthermore, coinjection of GM-CSF DNA has also improved the protective efficacy in models of rabies [90] and malaria [181,182]. The effect of GM-CSF DNA appears to be dependent upon the mode and route of DNA delivery, as no enhancement was seen with gene gun-mediated epidermal delivery [183]. Other pro-inflammatory cytokines, such as TNF-α and TNF-β, also were effective at enhancing the

antibody and proliferative responses in rodents [175]; however, only TNF-α DNA was effective for CTL [175].

Another strategy to enhance the potency of DNA vaccine is coadministration of DNA encoding costimulatory molecules such as B7.1 (CD80), B7.2 (CD86), and CD40. For example, coinjection of CD86 DNA resulted in a substantial increase in CTL responses against influenza NP [174] and HIV-1 antigens [184,185]. Whether these effects are a consequence of rendering non-APCs capable of priming CTL or of further activation of professional APCs already expressing these costimulatory molecules remains to be determined.

In summary, DNA encoding many cytokines or costimulatory molecules have increased the potency of DNA vaccines. Further development of these genetic adjuvants will require careful evaluation of the safety of potential long-term intracellular expression of these biologically active molecules. So far, GM-CSF DNA has been evaluated in nonhuman primates and human clinical studies with a malaria DNA vaccine.

VII. IMMUNOSTIMULATORY ACTIVITY OF DNA VACCINES

The inherent immunostimulatory activity of bacterial DNA has received widespread attention, particularly in the context of DNA-based adjuvants for proteins. It has been shown that oligonucleotides containing particular sequences surrounding CpG dinucleotides can stimulate B cells to proliferate and secrete immunoglobulins, activate APCs, and stimulate the production of cytokines [186,187]. These CpG sequences signal the innate immune system through Toll-like receptor 9 [188–191], and their role in the potency of DNA vaccines is illustrated as follows. First, plasmid DNA vaccines containing extra CpG motifs can induce stronger antibody and CTL responses [192]. However, this does not always result in more potent DNA vaccines, suggesting that context may be important. Second, methylation abrogates DNA vaccine potency [193]. This likely reflects a means by which the innate immune system recognizes pathogen-derived DNA as distinct from host DNA. Finally, the potency of plasmid DNA can also be enhanced by coadministration of noncoding plasmid DNA [194], presumably by providing additional CpG motifs. Efforts to codeliver plasmid DNA with CpG oliognucleotides, however, resulted in reduced DNA vaccine expression and immunogenicity [195], suggesting competition between the plasmid and the oligonucleotide. Thus appropriate DNA delivery or formulation will be required to take full advantage of CpG oliognucleotides for enhancing the potency of DNA vaccines.

VIII. DNA VACCINE DELIVERY SYSTEMS

Conventional methods of DNA vaccine delivery include direct intramuscular injection of plasmid DNA into muscle and gene gun delivery into skin, neither of which provides optimal immune responses. Intramuscular injection is suboptimal because only a small fraction of muscle cells are transfected due to inefficient uptake of DNA by cells. Antigen presenting cells can also be transfected but the efficiency is very low. Using fluorescently tagged plasmid DNA, Dupuis et al. demonstrated that after intramuscular injection 1) distribution of DNA within the injected tissue was rather limited; 2) uptake of DNA by myocytes and APCs was low; and 3) the majority of labeled DNA was phagocytosed and degraded by macrophages [86]. Therefore approaches to facilitate distribution of DNA throughout the tissue, increase transfection of muscle cells or APCs, prevent DNA degradation, or enhance the release of DNA out of endosomes may all be of help in the enhancing potency of DNA vaccines. With regard to DNA delivery, three promising general approaches have been shown to enhance the potency of DNA vaccines: 1) physical methods of delivery of the plasmid DNA into cells; 2) particle-mediated delivery of plasmid DNA to APCs; and 3) viral or bacterial vectors.

IX. PHYSICAL METHODS

Physical or mechanical methods have been used effectively to facilitate DNA delivery in vivo. The main technologies include the gene gun (previously discussed), needle-free devices, electroporation, and hydrostatic pressure. Needle-free devices (such as the Biojector) are commonly used for administration of various drugs and vaccines, and offer the advantages of less invasiveness (i.e., no needle) and better distribution of inoculum. For DNA vaccines, the Biojector has shown some effectiveness in enhancing immune responses in animal models [34,196] and is being evaluated in a clinical trial involving a malaria DNA vaccine. Recently, it has been shown that electroporation treatment of tissue in vivo after DNA vaccination results in higher gene expression [197] and markedly enhanced cellular and humoral responses in small and large animal models [198–200]. Electroporation has long been used to transfect cells in vitro due to a transient disruption of the plasma membrane, thereby facilitating uptake of DNA. The precise mechanism by which electroporation facilitates DNA delivery in vivo and the factors influencing the enhancement of the immune response are not clear but may involve an increased DNA distribution within the tissue (i.e., iontophoresis) and delivery directly through membranes (i.e., electroporation). It is also possible that an inflammatory response at the site of treatment may contribute to the enhanced immunogenicity of DNA vaccines. Because of the physical nature of the enhanced delivery of DNA by electroporation and the effectiveness in large animals, this technology holds much promise for use in humans. However, issues related to tolerability, safety, and feasibility will need to be examined and may limit its use, in the first instances, to therapeutic applications. Finally, increased DNA delivery can be achieved through brute force using hydrostatic pressure [201]. This is accomplished by i.v. injection of large volumes of DNA solution, followed by restriction of blood flow to the injected limb, and results in substantially higher levels of gene expression in endothelial and muscle cells. As such, this approach would seem to be best suited to gene therapy but could conceivably be considered for therapeutic vaccination.

X. PARTICLE-MEDIATED DELIVERY OF DNA VACCINES

Ideally, one would prefer to have a simple formulation of DNA that could be administered by conventional means, without the need for a device. In theory, DNA formulations could provide the following: 1) increased DNA stability (i.e., protection from nuclease digestion in tissues); 2) a depot for slow-release of DNA over a period of days or weeks; 3) facilitated uptake of DNA by cells; 4) targeting of DNA to specialized cells (e.g., APCs); and 5) inclusion of adjuvants to stimulate immune responses. To this end, several polymers that condense or interact with DNA have been tried, with varying degrees of success. Some examples include poly(-ethylenimine) [202], polyvinyl pyrrolidone [203], dendrimers [204,205], chitosan [206], and poly(DL-lactide-co-glcolide) (PLG) [95,207,208]. The best studied of these in the context of DNA vaccines is PLG, and the rationale is twofold. First, methods for encapsulation of compounds into PLG microparticles are well established and these formulations have been used for slow-release delivery of various entities. Encapsulation of plasmid DNA in PLG microparticles has been shown to be effective for oral delivery of DNA vaccines, presumably by protection from degradation in the gut [95,96,209]. Second, PLG can be made into particles of uniform size and lends itself to formulation with DNA into or onto particles of ˜1 μm in diameter, which should be readily internalized by APCs. Indeed, it has been shown that DNA vaccines adsorbed onto the surface of PLG microparticles substantially increased humoral and cellular immune responses [207,210], and the mechanism appears to involve targeting DNA to APCs [211]. Potential advantages of surface adsorption are that it avoids the harsh conditions of encapsulation of DNA and allows for the rapid release of DNA from the surface once inside the cell, thereby acting as an efficient delivery system.

XI. USE OF LIVE VIRAL AND BACTERIAL VECTORS FOR VACCINE DELIVERY

Use of live attenuated organisms is very effective at inducing potent immune responses. However, because of safety issues, this technology may be problematic for enhancing the immune responses against chronic deadly diseases such as HIV [212]. For example, it has been shown that an attenuated SIV can cause an AIDS-like disease in monkeys [213]. A potential alternative is to deliver genes encoding antigens using heterologous live viral or bacterial vectors. Some of the viral vectors that have been tested for DNA or RNA vaccine applications include vaccinia [116,117,129,214], canarypox [215–218], yellow fever-Japanese encephalitis [219], rabies [220], canine herpes virus [221], adenovirus [143,222,223], varicella-zoster [224], poliovirus [225,226], and alphaviruses [227–229]. However, because the antigens are encoded by the viral genomes, these vectors are not plasmid DNA delivery systems per se. Whereas various bacterial vectors have been used for such purposes. The ability of bacteria to readily enter cells of the respiratory and gastrointestinal mucosa provides an efficient delivery of DNA to immunologically relevant cells. For example, *Shigella* spp. are Gram-negative bacteria that enter cells via phagocytosis. To facilitate delivery of plasmid DNA vaccines out of the bacteria and into the cytosol, Sizemore et al. engineered a strain of *Shigella* with an unstable cell wall, which was shown to be effective at inducing humoral and cellular immune responses [230,231]. *Listeria monocytogenes* is another Gram-positive bacteria that enters the cytosol of infected cells and has been successfully used to deliver plasmid DNA [232–234]. Yet another bacterial vector that has been shown to be effective for DNA delivery is *Salmonella* [235–238]. In this case, though, the bacteria remains in the phagosomal compartment of the host cell and it is not clear how the plasmid DNA is delivered to the cytosol. The use of certain bacterial vectors offers potential advantages, such as a substantial safety profile in humans (e.g., BCG, *S. typhi* TY21a), the possibility of inducing systemic and local responses, and they may provide synergy with DNA vaccines in a prime/boost regimen. However, as with viral vectors, preexisting immunity may limit the effectiveness of DNA delivery.

XII. SUMMARY

In conclusion, a substantial amount of work has been done on DNA vaccines since 1990, only a fraction of which has been cited here. During this time, work in animal models has shed light on the limitations of DNA vaccines, how they work, and how one may be able to increase their potency. First-generation DNA vaccines (i.e., naked DNA) have so far demonstrated limited effectiveness in larger animals, including humans. However, substantial advancements have been made over the past several years on improved DNA vectors and delivery, and on the use of adjuvants (biologic and genetic). The potency of these second-generation DNA vaccines in humans remains to be fully determined, but they represent significant advancements toward the development of protective DNA vaccines for humans.

REFERENCES

1. Benvenisty N, Reshef L. Direct introduction of genes into rats and expression of the genes. Proc Natl Acad Sci USA 1986; 83:9551–9555.
2. Wolff JA, et al. Direct gene transfer into mouse muscle in vivo. Science 1990; 247:1465–1468.
3. Tang DC, et al. Genetic immunization is a simple method for eliciting an immune response. Nature 1992; 356:152–154.
4. Ulmer JB, et al. Heterologous protection against influenza by injection of DNA encoding a viral protein. Science 1993; 259:1745–1749.
5. Fynan EF, et al. DNA vaccines: protective immunizations by parenteral, mucosal, and gene-gun inoculations. Proc Natl Acad Sci USA 1993; 90:11478–11482.
6. Wang B, et al. Gene inoculation generates immune responses against human immunodeficiency virus type 1. Proc Natl Acad Sci USA 1993; 90:4156–4160.
7. Xiang ZQ, et al. Vaccination with a plasmid vector carrying the rabies virus glycoprotein gene induces protective immunity against rabies virus. Virology 1994; 199:132–140.
8. Davis HL, et al. DNA-based immunization induces con-

9. tinuous secretion of hepatitis B surface antigen and high levels of circulating antibody. Hum Mol Genet 1993; 2: 1847–1851.
9. Lu S, et al. Use of DNAs expressing HIV-1 Env and non-infectious HIV-1 particles to raise antibody responses in mice. Virology 1995; 209:147–154.
10. Shiver JW, et al. Anti-HIV env immunities elicited by nucleic acid vaccines. Vaccine 1997; 15:884–887.
11. Ishii N, et al. Cationic liposomes are a strong adjuvant for a DNA vaccine of human immunodeficiency virus type 1. AIDS Res Hum Retrovir 1997; 13:1421–1428.
12. Barouch DH, et al. Augmentation and suppression of immune responses to an HIV-1 DNA vaccine by plasmid cytokine/Ig administration. J Immunol 1998; 161:1875–1882.
13. Barouch DH, et al. Elicitation of high-frequency cytotoxic T-lymphocyte responses against both dominant and subdominant simian–human immunodeficiency virus epitopes by DNA vaccination of rhesus monkeys. J Virol 2001; 75: 2462–2467.
14. Asakura Y, et al. DNA-plasmids of HIV-1 induce systemic and mucosal immune responses. Biol Chem 1999; 380:375–379.
15. Bourne N, et al. DNA immunization confers protective immunity on mice challenged intravaginally with herpes simplex virus type 2. Vaccine 1996; 14:1230–1234.
16. Nass PH, et al. Protective immunity against herpes simplex virus generated by DNA vaccination compared to natural infection. Vaccine 2001; 19:1538–1546.
17. Caselli E, et al. Local and systemic inoculation of DNA or protein gB1s-based vaccines induce a protective immunity against rabbit ocular HSV-1 infection. Vaccine 2000; 19: 1225–1231.
18. Caselli E, et al. Mice genetic immunization with plasmid DNA encoding a secreted form of HSV-1 gB induces a protective immune response against herpes simplex virus type 1 infection. Intervirology 2001; 44:1–7.
19. McClements WL, et al. The prophylactic effect of immunization with DNA encoding herpes simplex virus glycoproteins on HSV-induced disease in guinea pigs. Vaccine 1997; 15:857–860.
20. Mester JC, et al. Immunity induced by DNA immunization with herpes simplex virus type 2 glycoproteins B and C. Vaccine 1999; 18:875–883.
21. Strasser JE, et al. Herpes simplex virus DNA vaccine efficacy: effect of glycoprotein D plasmid constructs. J Infect Dis 2000; 182:1304–1310.
22. Ray NB, et al. Nanogram quantities of plasmid DNA encoding the rabies virus glycoprotein protect mice against lethal rabies virus infection. Vaccine 1997; 15:892–895.
23. Lodmell DL, et al. DNA immunization protects nonhuman primates against rabies virus. Nat Med 1998; 4:949–952.
24. Lodmell DL, et al. Gene gun particle-mediated vaccination with plasmid DNA confers protective immunity against rabies virus infection. Vaccine 1998; 16:115–118.
25. Lagging LM, et al. Immune-responses to plasmid DNA encoding the hepatitis-C virus core protein. J Virol 1995; 69: 5859–5863.
26. Geissler M, et al. Enhancement of cellular and humoral immune responses to hepatitis C virus core protein using DNA-based vaccines augmented with cytokine-expressing plasmids. J Immunol 1997; 158:1231–1237.
27. Huygen K, et al. Immunogenicity and protective efficacy of a tuberculosis DNA vaccine. Nat Med 1996; 2:893–898.
28. Montgomery DL, et al. Induction of humoral and cellular immune responses by vaccination with *M. tuberculosis* antigen 85 DNA. Cell Mol Biol 1997; 43:285–292.
29. Ulmer JB, et al. Expression and immunogenicity of *Mycobacterium tuberculosis* antigen 85 by DNA vaccination. Vaccine 1997; 15:792–794.

30. Lozes E, et al. Immunogenicity and efficacy of a tuberculosis DNA vaccine encoding the components of the secreted antigen 85 complex. Vaccine 1997; 15:830–833.

31. Hoffman SL, et al. Protection against malaria by immunization with a *Plasmodium yoelii* circumsporozoite protein nucleic acid vaccine. Vaccine 1994; 12:1529–1533.

32. Wang R, et al. Induction of antigen-specific cytotoxic T lymphocytes in humans by a malaria DNA vaccine. Science 1998; 282:476–480.

33. Gurunathan S, et al. DNA vaccines: immunology, application, and optimization. Annu Rev Immunol 2000; 18:927–974.

34. Aguiar JC, et al. Enhancement of the immune response in rabbits to a malaria DNA vaccine by immunization with a needle-free jet device. Vaccine 2001; 20:275–280.

35. Barry MA, et al. Protection against mycoplasma-infection using expression-library immunization. Nature 1995; 377:632–635.

36. Angus CW, et al. Nucleic acid vaccination against *Toxoplasma gondii* in mice. J Eukaryot Microbiol 1996; 43:117S.

37. Angus CW, et al. Immunization with a DNA plasmid encoding the SAG1 (P30) protein of *Toxoplasma gondii* is immunogenic and protective in rodents. J Infect Dis 2000; 181:317–324.

38. Vercammen M, et al. DNA vaccination with genes encoding *Toxoplasma gondii* antigens GRA1, GRA7, and ROP2 induces partially protective immunity against lethal challenge in mice. Infect Immun 2000; 68:38–45.

39. Desolme B, et al. Induction of protective immunity against toxoplasmosis in mice by DNA immunization with a plasmid encoding *Toxoplasma gondii* GRA4 gene. Vaccine 2000; 18:2512–2521.

40. Leyva R, et al. Genetic immunization with plasmid DNA coding for the ROP2 protein of *Toxoplasma gondii*. Parasitol Res 2001; 87:70–79.

41. Herrmann J, et al. DNA vaccines against rotavirus infections. Arch Virol Suppl 1996; 12:207–215.

42. Chen SC, et al. Protective immunity induced by rotavirus DNA vaccines. Vaccine 1997; 15:899–902.

43. Yang K, et al. Immune responses and protection obtained with rotavirus VP6 DNA vaccines given by intramuscular injection. Vaccine 2001; 19:3285–3291.

44. Vanderzanden L, et al. DNA vaccines expressing either the GP or NP genes of Ebola virus protect mice from lethal challenge. Virology 1998; 246:134–144.

45. Xu L, et al. Immunization for Ebola virus infection. Nat Med 1998; 4:37–42.

46. Sullivan NJ, Sanchez A, Rollin PE, Yang ZY, Nabel GJ. Development of a preventive vaccine for Ebola virus infection in primates. Nature 2000; 408:605–609.

47. Webster RG, et al. Protection of ferrets against influenza challenge with a DNA vaccine to the hemagglutinin. Vaccine 1994; 12:1495–1498.

48. Chen Z, et al. Protection and antibody responses in different strains of mouse immunized with plasmid DNAs encoding influenza virus haemagglutinin, neuraminidase and nucleoprotein. J Gen Virol 1999; 80:2559–2564.

49. Fomsgaard A, et al. Induction of cytotoxic T-cell responses by gene gun DNA vaccination with minigenes encoding influenza A virus HA and NP CTL-epitopes. Vaccine 1999; 18:681–691.

50. Bot A, et al. Induction of humoral and cellular immunity against influenza virus by immunization of newborn mice with a plasmid bearing a hemagglutinin gene. Int Immunol 1997; 9:1641–1650.

51. Robinson HL, et al. DNA immunization for influenza virus: studies using hemagglutinin- and nucleoprotein-expressing DNAs. J Infect Dis 1997; 176(Suppl 1):S50–S55.

52. Deck RR, et al. Characterization of humoral immune responses induced by an influenza hemagglutinin DNA vaccine. Vaccine 1997; 15:71–78.

53. Barnett SW, et al. The ability of an oligomeric human immunodeficiency virus type 1 (HIV-1) envelope antigen to elicit neutralizing antibodies against primary HIV-1 isolates is improved following partial deletion of the second hypervariable region. J Virol 2001; 75:5526–5540.

54. Vinner L, et al. Gene gun DNA vaccination with Rev-independent synthetic HIV-1 gp160 envelope gene using mammalian codons. Vaccine 1999; 17:2166–2175.

55. Richmond JF, et al. Studies of the neutralizing activity and avidity of anti-human immunodeficiency virus type 1 Env antibody elicited by DNA priming and protein boosting. J Virol 1998; 72:9092–9100.

56. Agadjanyan MG, et al. An HIV type 2 DNA vaccine induces cross-reactive immune responses against HIV type 2 and SIV. AIDS Res Hum Retrovir 1997; 13:1561–1572.

57. Prayaga SK, et al. Manipulation of HIV 1 gp120 specific immune responses elicited via gene gun based DNA immunization. Vaccine Aug–Sep 1997; 15:1349–1352.

58. Fuller DH, et al. Enhancement of immunodeficiency virus-specific immune responses in DNA-immunized rhesus macaques. Vaccine 1997; 15:924–926.

59. Xiang ZQ, et al. Immune-responses to nucleic-acid vaccines to rabies virus. Virology 1995; 209:569–579.

60. Lodmell DL, et al. DNA vaccination of mice against rabies virus: effects of the route of vaccination and the adjuvant monophosphoryl lipid A (MPL). Vaccine 2000; 18:1059–1066.

61. Osorio JE, et al. Immunization of dogs and cats with a DNA vaccine against rabies virus. Vaccine 1999; 17:1109–1116.

62. Davis HL, et al. DNA vaccine for hepatitis B: evidence for immunogenicity in chimpanzees and comparison with other vaccines. Proc Natl Acad Sci USA 1996; 93:7213–7218.

63. Justewicz DM, et al. Antibody-forming cell response to virus challenge in mice immunized with DNA encoding the influenza virus hemagglutinin. J Virol 1995; 69:7712–7717.

64. Ross TM, et al. C3d enhancement of antibodies to hemagglutinin accelerates protection against influenza virus challenge. Nat Immunol 2000; 1:127–131.

65. Deliyannis G, et al. A fusion DNA vaccine that targets antigen-presenting cells increases protection from viral challenge. Proc Natl Acad Sci USA 2000; 97:6676–6680.

66. Fu TM, et al. Induction of MHC class I-restricted CTL response by DNA immunization with ubiquitin-influenza virus nucleoprotein fusion antigens. Vaccine 1998; 16:1711–1717.

67. Yankauckas MA, et al. Long-term anti-nucleoprotein cellular and humoral immunity is induced by intramuscular injection of plasmid DNA containing NP gene. DNA Cell Biol 1993; 12:771–776.

68. Raz E, et al. Intradermal gene immunization: the possible role of DNA uptake in the induction of cellular immunity to viruses. Proc Natl Acad Sci USA 1994; 91:9519–9523.

69. Michel ML, et al. DNA-mediated immunization to the hepatitis B surface antigen in mice: aspects of the humoral response mimic hepatitis B viral infection in humans. Proc Natl Acad Sci USA 1995; 92:5307–5311.

70. Gardner M, et al. DNA vaccines against malaria: immunogenicity and protection in a rodent model. J Pharm Sci 1996; 85:124–130.

71. Kang Y, et al. Comparison of humoral immune responses elicited by DNA and protein vaccines based on merozoite surface protein-1 from *Plasmodium yoelii*, a rodent malaria parasite. J Immunol 1998; 161, 4211–4219.

72. Sanchez GI, et al. Immunogenicity and protective efficacy of a *Plasmodium yoelii* Hsp60 DNA vaccine in BALB/c mice. Infect Immun 2001; 69:3897–3905.

73. Gurunathan S, et al. Vaccination with DNA encoding the immunodominant lack parasite antigen confers protective immunity to mice infected with leishmania major. J Exp Med 1997; 186:1137–1147.

74. Walker PS, et al. Genetic immunization with glycoprotein 63 cDNA results in a helper T cell type 1 immune response and protection in a murine model of leishmaniasis. Hum Gene Ther 1998; 9:1899–1907.

75. Mendez S, et al. The potency and durability of DNA- and protein-based vaccines against *Leishmania major* evaluated using low-dose, intradermal challenge. J Immunol 2001; 166:5122–5128.

76. Donnelly JJ, et al. Preclinical efficacy of a prototype DNA vaccine: enhanced protection against antigenic drift in influenza virus. Nat Med 1995; 1:583–587.

77. Lu S, Arthos J, Montefiori DC, et al. Simian immunodeficiency virus DNA vaccine trial in macaques. J Virol 1996; 70:3978–3991.

78. Davis HL, et al. Direct gene transfer in skeletal muscle: plasmid DNA-based immunization against the hepatitis B virus surface antigen. Vaccine 1994; 12:1503–1509.

79. Sasaki S, et al. Comparison of intranasal and intramuscular immunization against human immunodeficiency virus type 1 with a DNA-monophosphoryl lipid A adjuvant vaccine. Infect Immun 1998; 66:823–826.

80. Hamajima K, et al. Intranasal administration of HIV-DNA vaccine formulated with a polymer, carboxymethylcellulose, augments mucosal antibody production and cell-mediated immune response. Clin Immunol Immunopathol 1998; 88: 205–210.

81. Hamajima K, et al. Systemic and mucosal immune responses in mice after rectal and vaginal immunization with HIV-DNA vaccine. Clin Immunol 2002; 102:12–18.

82. Wang L, et al. Differences in epitope recognition, isotype and titer of antisera to *Plasmodium falciparum* merozoite surface protein 4 raised by different modes of DNA or protein immunization. Vaccine 2000; 19:816–824.

83. Weiss R, et al. Genetic vaccination against malaria infection by intradermal and epidermal injections of a plasmid containing the gene encoding the *Plasmodium berghei* circumsporozoite protein. Infect Immun 2000; 68:5914–5919.

84. Gerloni M, et al. Somatic transgene immunization with DNA encoding an immunoglobulin heavy chain. DNA Cell Biol 1997; 16:611–625.

85. Kamei A, et al. Induction of hepatitis C virus-specific cytotoxic T lymphocytes in mice by an intrahepatic inoculation with an expression plasmid. Virology 2000; 273:120–126.

86. Dupuis M, et al. Distribution of DNA vaccines determines their immunogenicity after intramuscular injection in mice. J Immunol 2000; 165:2850–2858.

87. Pertmer TM, et al. Gene gun-based nucleic-acid immunization—elicitation of humoral and cytotoxic T-lymphocyte responses following epidermal delivery of nanogram quantities of DNA. Vaccine 1995; 13:1427–1430.

88. Feltquate DM, et al. Different T helper cell types and antibody isotypes generated by saline and gene gun DNA immunization. J Immunol 1997; 158:2278–2284.

89. Pertmer TM, et al. Influenza virus nucleoprotein-specific immunoglobulin G subclass and cytokine responses elicited by DNA vaccination are dependent on the route of vector DNA delivery. J Virol 1996; 70:6119–6125.

90. Xiang Z, Ertl HC. Manipulation of the immune response to a plasmid-encoded viral antigen by coinoculation with plasmids expressing cytokines. Immunity 1995; 2:129–135.

91. Fuller DH, Haynes JR. A qualitative progression in HIV type-1 glycoprotein-120-specific cytotoxic cellular and humoral immune-responses in mice receiving a DNA-based glycoprotein-120 vaccine. AIDS Res Human Retrovir 1994; 10:1433–1441.

92. Okada E, et al. Intranasal immunization of a DNA vaccine with IL-12- and granulocyte-macrophage colony-stimulating factor (GM-CSF)-expressing plasmids in liposomes induces strong mucosal and cell-mediated immune responses against HIV-1 antigens. J Immunol 1997; 159:3638–3647.

93. Sasaki S, et al. Monophosphoryl lipid a enhances both humoral and cell mediated immune responses to DNA vaccination against human immunodeficiency virus type 1. Infect Immun 1997; 65:3520–3528.

94. Sasaki S, et al. Induction of systemic and mucosal immune responses to human immunodeficiency virus type 1 by a DNA vaccine formulated with QS-21 saponin adjuvant via intramuscular and intranasal routes. J Virol 1998; 72:4931–4939.

95. Jones DH, et al. Poly(DL-lactide-co-glycolide)-encapsulated plasmid DNA elicits systemic and mucosal antibody responses to encoded protein after oral administration. Vaccine 1997; 15:814–817.

96. Chen SC, et al. Protective immunity induced by oral immunization with a rotavirus DNA vaccine encapsulated in microparticles. J Virol 1998; 72:5757–5761.

97. Herrmann JE, et al. Immune responses and protection obtained by oral immunization with rotavirus VP4 and VP7 DNA vaccines encapsulated in microparticles. Virology 1999; 259:148–153.

98. Vajdy M, O'Hagan DT. Microparticles for intranasal immunization. Adv Drug Deliv Rev 2001; 51:127–141.

99. Orson FM, et al. Genetic immunization with lung-targeting macroaggregated polyethyleneimine-albumin conjugates elicits combined systemic and mucosal immune responses. J Immunol 2000; 164:6313–6321.

100. Mittal SK, et al. Immunization with DNA, adenovirus or both in biodegradable alginate microspheres: effect of route of inoculation on immune response. Vaccine 2000; 19:253–263.

101. Wang SW, et al. Effective induction of simian immunodeficiency virus-specific systemic and mucosal immune responses in primates by vaccination with proviral DNA producing intact but noninfectious virions. J Virol 2000; 74: 10514–10522.

102. Ulmer JB, et al. Protective CD4+ and CD8+ T cells against influenza virus induced by vaccination with nucleoprotein DNA. J Virol 1998; 72:5648–5653.

103. Fu TM, et al. Protective cellular immunity: cytotoxic T-lymphocyte responses against dominant and recessive epitopes of influenza virus nucleoprotein induced by DNA immunization. J Virol 1997; 71:2715–2721.

104. Thomson SA, et al. Delivery of multiple CD8 cytotoxic T cell epitopes by DNA vaccination. J Immunol 1998; 160: 1717–1723.

105. Schirmbeck R, et al. Nucleic-acid vaccination primes hepatitis-B virus surface antigen-specific cytotoxic T-lymphocytes in nonresponder mice. J Virol 1995; 69:5929–5934.

106. Kuhober A, et al. DNA immunization induces antibody and cytotoxic T cell responses to hepatitis B core antigen in H-2b mice. J Immunol 1996; 156:3687–3695.

107. Liu J, et al. Regulated expression of a dominant negative form of Rev improves resistance to HIV replication in T cells. Gene Ther 1994; 1:32–37.

108. Okuda K, et al. Induction of potent humoral and cell-mediated immune responses following direct injection of DNA encoding the HIV type 1 env and rev gene products. AIDS Res Hum Retrovir 1995; 11:933–943.

109. Shiver JW, et al. Cytotoxic T lymphocyte and helper T cell responses following HIV polynucleotide vaccination. Ann N Y Acad Sci 1995; 772:198–208.

110. Yasutomi Y, et al. Simian immunodeficiency virus-specific cytotoxic T-lymphocyte induction through DNA vaccination of rhesus monkeys. J Virol 1996; 70:678–681.

111. zur Megede J. Increased expression and immunogenicity of sequence-modified human immunodeficiency virus type 1 gag gene. J Virol 2000; 74:2628–2635.

112. Ulmer JB, et al. Immunization against viral proteins with naked DNA. Ann N Y Acad Sci 1995; 772:117–125.

113. Donnelly JJ, et al. Protection against papillomavirus with a polynucleotide vaccine. J Infect Dis 1996; 173:314–320.

114. Liu MA, et al. Vaccination of mice and nonhuman primates using HIV-gene-containing DNA. Antibiot Chemother 1996; 48:100–104.

115. Buge SL, et al. Factors associated with slow disease progression in macaques immunized with an adenovirus-simian immunodeficiency virus (SIV) envelope priming-gp120 boosting regimen and challenged vaginally with SIVmac251. J Virol 1999; 73:7430–7440.

116. Allen TM, et al. Induction of AIDS virus-specific CTL activity in fresh, unstimulated peripheral blood lymphocytes from rhesus macaques vaccinated with a DNA prime/ modified vaccinia virus Ankara boost regimen. J Immunol 2000; 164:4968–4978.

117. Amara RR, et al. Control of a mucosal challenge and prevention of AIDS by a multiprotein DNA/MVA vaccine. Science 2001; 292:69–74.

118. Barouch DH, et al. Control of viremia and prevention of clinical AIDS in rhesus monkeys by cytokine-augmented DNA vaccination. Science 2000; 290:486–492.

119. Donnelly JJ, et al. Protective efficacy of intramuscular immunization with naked DNA. Ann N Y Acad Sci 1995; 772:40–46.

120. Corr M, et al. In vivo priming by DNA injection occurs predominantly by antigen transfer. J Immunol 1999; 163: 4721–4727.

121. Porgador A, et al. Predominant role for directly transfected dendritic cells in antigen presentation to CD8+ T cells after gene gun immunization. J Exp Med 1998; 188:p1075–p1082.

122. MacGregor RR, et al. First human trial of a DNA-based vaccine for treatment of human immunodeficiency virus type 1 infection: safety and host response. J Infect Dis 1998; 178:92–100.

123. MacGregor RR, et al. Safety and immune responses to a DNA-based human immunodeficiency virus (HIV) type I Env/Rev vaccine in HIV-infected recipients: follow-up data. J Infect Dis 2000; 181:406.

124. Boyer JD, et al. Vaccination of seronegative volunteers with a human immunodeficiency virus type 1 env/rev DNA vaccine induces antigen-specific proliferation and lymphocyte production of beta-chemokines. J Infect Dis 2000; 181: 476–483.

125. Calarota S, et al. Cellular cytotoxic response induced by DNA vaccination in HIV-1-infected patients. Lancet 1998; 351:1320–1325.

126. Calarota SA, et al. Immune responses in asymptomatic HIV-1-infected patients after HIV-DNA immunization followed by highly active antiretroviral treatment. J Immunol 1999; 163:2330–2338.

127. Le TP, et al. Safety, tolerability and humoral immune responses after intramuscular administration of a malaria DNA vaccine to healthy adult volunteers. Vaccine 2000; 18: 1893–9019.

128. Roy MJ, et al. Induction of antigen-specific CD8+ T cells, T helper cells, and protective levels of antibody in humans by particle-mediated administration of a hepatitis B virus DNA vaccine. Vaccine 2000; 19:764–778.

129. Hanke T, McMichael A. Pre-clinical development of a multi-CTL epitope-based DNA prime MVA boost vaccine for AIDS. Immunol Lett 1999; 66:177–181.

130. Stephenson J. Vaccine aimed at African HIV to begin trials. JAMA 2000; 284:683.

131. Cohen J. AIDS research. Merck reemerges with a bold AIDS vaccine effort. Science 2001; 292:24–25.

132. Fu TM, et al. Dose dependence of CTL precursor frequency induced by a DNA vaccine and correlation with protective immunity against influenza virus challenge. J Immunol 1999; 162:4163–4170.

133. Talaat AM, et al. A combination vaccine confers full protection against co-infections with influenza, herpes simplex and respiratory syncytial viruses. Vaccine 2001; 20: 538–544.

134. Prince AM, et al. Successful nucleic acid based immunization of newborn chimpanzees against hepatitis B virus. Vaccine 1997; 15:916–919.

135. Becker SI, et al. Protection of mice against *Plasmodium yoelii* sporozoite challenge with *P. yoelii* merozoite surface protein 1 DNA vaccines. Infect Immun 1998; 66:3457–3461.

136. Smooker PM, et al. Expression library immunization protects mice against a challenge with virulent rodent malaria. Vaccine 2000; 18:2533–2540.

137. Haigwood NL, et al. Protection from pathogenic SIV challenge using multigenic DNA vaccines. Immunol Lett 1999; 66:183–188.

138. Habel A, et al. DNA vaccine protection against challenge with simian/human immunodeficiency virus 89.6 in rhesus macaques. Dev Biol (Basel) 2000; 104:101–105.

139. Kim JJ, et al. Modulation of antigen-specific cellular immune responses to DNA vaccination in rhesus macaques through the use of IL-2, IFN-gamma, or IL-4 gene adjuvants. Vaccine 2001; 19:2496–2505.

140. McKay PF, et al. Vaccine protection against functional CTL abnormalities in simian human immunodeficiency virus-infected rhesus monkeys. J Immunol 2002; 168:332–337.

141. Yokoyama M, et al. DNA immunization confers protection against lethal lymphocytic choriomeningitis virus-infection. J Virol 1995; 69:2684–2688.

142. Cherpelis S, et al. DNA vaccination with the human immunodeficiency virus type 1 SF162DeltaV2 envelope elicits immune responses that offer partial protection from simian/ human immunodeficiency virus infection to CD8(+) T-cell-depleted rhesus macaques. J Virol 2001; 75:1547–1550.

143. Shiver JW, et al. Replication-incompetent adenoviral vaccine vector elicits effective anti-immunodeficiency-virus immunity. Nature 2002; 415:331–335.

144. McClements WL, et al. Immunization with DNA vaccines encoding glycoprotein D or glycoprotein B, alone or in combination, induces protective immunity in animal models of herpes simplex virus-2 disease. Proc Natl Acad Sci USA 1996; 93:11414–11420.

145. Tascon RE, et al. Vaccination against tuberculosis by DNA injection. Nat Med 1996; 2:888–892.

146. Daubersies P, et al. Protection against *Plasmodium falciparum* malaria in chimpanzees by immunization with the conserved pre-erythrocytic liver-stage antigen 3. Nat Med 2000; 6:1258–1263.

147. Xu D, Liew FY. Protection against leishmaniasis by injection of DNA encoding a major surface glycoprotein, gp63, of l-major. Immunol 1995; 84:173–176.

148. Anderson R, et al. Immune response in mice following immunization with DNA encoding fragment C of tetanus toxin. Infect Immun 1996; 64:3168–3173.

149. Lopez-Macias C, et al. Induction of antibodies against Salmonella *typhi* OmpC porin by naked DNA immunization. Ann N Y Acad Sci 1995; 772:285–288.

150. Manthorpe M, et al. Gene-therapy by intramuscular injection of plasmid DNA-studies on firefly luciferase gene-expression in mice. Hum Gene Ther 1993; 4:419–431.

151. Qin L, et al. Promoter attenuation in gene therapy: interferon-gamma and tumor necrosis factor-alpha inhibit transgene expression. Hum Gene Ther 1997; 8:2019–2029.

152. Haas J, et al. Codon usage limitation in the expression of HIV-1 envelope glycoprotein. Curr Biol 1996; 6:315–324.

153. Wu L, Barry MA. Fusion protein vectors to increase protein production and evaluate the immunogenicity of genetic vaccines. Mol Ther 2000; 2:288–297.

154. Baldwin SL, et al. Immunogenicity and protective efficacy of DNA vaccines encoding secreted and non-secreted forms of *Mycobacterium tuberculosis* Ag85A. Tuber Lung Dis 1999; 79:251–259.

155. Tobery TW, Siliciano RF. Targeting of HIV-1 antigens for rapid intracellular degradation enhances cytotoxic T lymphocyte (CTL) recognition and the induction of de novo CTL responses in vivo after immunization. J Exp Med 1997; 185:909–920.

156. Rodriguez F, et al. DNA immunization: ubiquitination of a viral protein enhances cytotoxic T-lymphocyte induction and antiviral protection but abrogates antibody induction. J Virol 1997; 71:8497–8503.

157. Lew AM, et al. Site-directed immune responses in DNA vaccines encoding ligand–antigen fusions. Vaccine 2000; 18: 1681–1685.

158. Drew DR, et al. The comparative efficacy of CTLA-4 and L-selectin targeted DNA vaccines in mice and sheep. Vaccine 2001; 19:4417–4428.

159. You Z, et al. Targeting dendritic cells to enhance DNA vaccine potency. Cancer Res 2001; 61:3704–3711.

160. Biragyn A, Kwak LW. B-cell malignancies as a model for cancer vaccines: from prototype protein to next generation genetic chemokine fusions. Immunol Rev 1999; 170:115–126.

161. Planelles L, et al. DNA immunization with *Trypanosoma cruzi* HSP70 fused to the KMP11 protein elicits a cytotoxic and humoral immune response against the antigen and leads to protection. Infect Immun 2001; 69:6558–6563.

162. Iwasaki A, Barber BH. Induction by DNA immunization of a protective antitumor cytotoxic T lymphocyte response against a minimal-epitope-expressing tumor. Cancer Immunol Immunother 1998; 45:273–279.

163. Iwasaki A, et al. Epitope-specific cytotoxic T lymphocyte induction by minigene DNA immunization. Vaccine 1999; 17:2081–2088.

164. Livingston BD, et al. Optimization of epitope processing enhances immunogenicity of multiepitope DNA vaccines. Vaccine 2001; 19:4652–4660.

165. Leifert JA, et al. Enhancing T cell activation and antiviral protection by introducing the HIV-1 protein transduction domain into a DNA vaccine. Hum Gene Ther 2001; 12: 1881–1892.

166. Sasaki S, et al. The search for a potent DNA vaccine against AIDS: the enhancement of immunogenicity by chemical and genetic adjuvants. Anticancer Res 1998; 18:3907–3916.

167. Chow YH, et al. Improvement of hepatitis B virus DNA vaccines by plasmids coexpressing hepatitis B surface antigen and interleukin-2. J Virol 1997; 71:169–178.

168. Barouch DH, Letvin NL. DNA vaccination for HIV-1 and SIV. Intervirology 2000; 43:282–287.

169. Kim JJ, et al. In vivo engineering of a cellular immune response by coadministration of IL-12 expression vector with a DNA immunogen. J Immunol 1997; 158:816–826.

170. Tsuji T, et al. Enhancement of cell-mediated immunity against HIV-1 induced by coinoculation of plasmid-encoded HIV-1 antigen with plasmid expressing IL-12. J Immunol 1997; 158:4008–4013.

171. Maecker HT, et al. DNA vaccination with cytokine fusion constructs biases the immune response to ovalbumin. Vaccine Oct 1997; 15:1687–1696.

172. Chow YH, et al. Development of Th1 and Th2 populations and the nature of immune responses to hepatitis B virus DNA vaccines can be modulated by co-delivery of various cytokine genes. J Immunol 1998; 160:1320–1329.

173. Tuting T, et al. Autologous human monocyte-derived dendritic cells genetically modified to express melanoma antigens elicit primary cytotoxic T cell responses in vitro: enhancement by cotransfection of genes encoding the Th1-biasing cytokines IL-12 and IFN-alpha. J Immunol 1998; 160:1139–1147.

174. Iwasaki A, et al. Enhanced CTL responses mediated by plasmid DNA immunogens encoding costimulatory molecules and cytokines. J Immunol 1997; 158:4591–4601.

175. Kim JJ, et al. Modulation of amplitude and direction of in vivo immune responses by co-administration of cytokine gene expression cassettes with DNA immunogens. Eur J Immunol 1998; 28:1089–1103.

176. Morrissey PJ, et al. Granulocyte-macrophage colony-stimulating factor augments the primary antibody response by enhancing the function of antigen-presenting cells. J Immunol 1987; 139:1113–1119.

177. Heufler C, et al. Granulocyte/macrophage colony-stimulating factor and interleukin 1 mediate the maturation of murine epidermal Langerhans cells into potent immunostimulatory dendritic cells. J Exp Med 1988; 167:700–705.

178. Kusakabe K, et al. The timing of GM-CSF expression plasmid administration influences the Th1/Th2 response induced by an HIV-1-specific DNA vaccine. J Immunol 2000; 164:3102–3111.

179. Kim JJ, et al. Chemokine gene adjuvants can modulate immune responses induced by DNA vaccines. J Interferon Cytokine Res 2000; 20:487–498.

180. Sin JI, et al. Protective immunity against heterologous challenge with encephalomyocarditis virus by VP1 DNA vaccination: effect of coinjection with a granulocyte-macrophage colony stimulating factor gene. Vaccine 1997; 15: 1827–1833.

181. Sedegah M, et al. Improving protective immunity induced by DNA-based immunization: priming with antigen and GM-CSF-encoding plasmid DNA and boosting with antigen-expressing recombinant poxvirus. J Immunol 2000; 164:5905–5912.

182. Weiss WR, et al. A plasmid encoding murine granulocyte-macrophage colony-stimulating factor increases protection conferred by a malaria DNA vaccine. J Immunol 1998; 161: 2325–2332.

183. Conry RM, et al. Selected strategies to augment polynucleotide immunization. Gene Ther 1996; 3:67–74.

184. Kim JJ, et al. Engineering of in vivo immune responses to DNA immunization via codelivery of costimulatory molecule genes. Nat Biotechnol 1997; 15:641–646.

185. Santra S, et al. B7 co-stimulatory requirements differ for induction of immune responses by DNA, protein and recombinant pox virus vaccination. Eur J Immunol 2000; 30:2650–2659.

186. Krieg AM, et al. CpG motifs in bacterial DNA trigger direct B-cell activation. Nature 1995; 374:546–549.

187. Iho S, et al. Oligodeoxynucleotides containing palindrome sequences with internal 5′-CpG-3′ act directly on human NK and activated T cells to induce IFN-gamma production in vitro. J Immunol 1999; 163:3642–3652.

188. Chuang TH, et al. Toll-like receptor 9 mediates CpG-DNA signaling. J Leukoc Biol 2002; 71:538–544.

189. Krug A, et al. Toll-like receptor expression reveals CpG DNA as a unique microbial stimulus for plasmacytoid dendritic cells which synergizes with CD40 ligand to induce high amounts of IL-12. Eur J Immunol 2001; 31:3026–3037.

190. Takeshita F, et al. Cutting edge: role of Toll-like receptor 9 in CpG DNA-induced activation of human cells. J Immunol 2001; 167:3555–3558.

191. Hemmi H, et al. A Toll-like receptor recognizes bacterial DNA. Nature 2000; 408:740–745.

192. Sato Y, et al. Immunostimulatory DNA sequences neces-

sary for effective intradermal gene immunization. Science 1996; 273:352–354.

193. Elkins KL, et al. Bacterial DNA containing CpG motifs stimulates lymphocyte-dependent protection of mice against lethal infection with intracellular bacteria. J Immunol 1999; 162:2291–2298.

194. Donnelly JJ, et al. DNA vaccines. Ann Rev Immunol 1997; 15:617–648.

195. Weeratna R, et al. Reduction of antigen expression from DNA vaccines by coadministered oligodeoxynucleotides. Antisense Nucleic Acid Drug Dev 1998; 8:351–356.

196. Manam S, et al. Plasmid DNA vaccines: tissue distribution and effects of DNA sequence, adjuvants and delivery method on integration into host DNA. Intervirology 2000; 43:273–281.

197. Mathiesen I. Electropermeabilization of skeletal muscle enhances gene transfer in vivo. Gene Ther 1999; 6:508–514.

198. Zucchelli S, et al. Enhancing B- and T-cell immune response to a hepatitis C virus E2 DNA vaccine by intramuscular electrical gene transfer. J Virol 2000; 74:11598–11607.

199. Selby M, et al. Enhancement of DNA vaccine potency by electroporation in vivo. J Biotechnol 2000; 83:147–152.

200. Widera G, et al. Increased DNA vaccine delivery and immunogenicity by electroporation in vivo. J Immunol 2000; 164:4635–4640.

201. Budker V, et al. The efficient expression of intravascularly delivered DNA in rat muscle. Gene Ther 1998; 5:272–276.

202. Kircheis R, Wightman L, Wagner E. Design and gene delivery activity of modified polyethylenimines. Adv Drug Deliv Rev 2001; 53:341–358.

203. Perez C, et al. Poly(lactic acid)-poly(ethylene glycol) nanoparticles as new carriers for the delivery of plasmid DNA. J Control Release 2001; 75:211–224.

204. Sato N, et al. Tumor targeting and imaging of intraperitoneal tumors by use of antisense oligo-DNA complexed with dendrimers and/or avidin in mice. Clin Cancer Res 2001; 7:3606–3612.

205. Rudolph C, et al. In vivo gene delivery to the lung using polyethylenimine and fractured polyamidoamine dendrimers. J Gene Med 2000; 2:269–278.

206. Illum L, et al. Chitosan as a novel nasal delivery system for vaccines. Adv Drug Deliv Rev 2001; 51:81–96.

207. Singh M, et al. Cationic microparticles: a potent delivery system for DNA vaccines. Proc Natl Acad Sci USA 2000; 97:811–816.

208. O'Hagan D, et al. Recent developments in adjuvants for vaccines against infectious diseases. Biomol Eng 2001; 18:69–85.

209. Jones DH, et al. Oral delivery of micro-encapsulated DNA vaccines. Dev Biol Stand 1998; 92:149–155.

210. O'Hagan D, et al. Induction of potent immune responses by cationic microparticles with adsorbed HIV DNA vaccines. J Virol 2001; 75:9037–9043.

211. Denis-Mize KS, et al. Plasmid DNA adsorbed onto cationic microparticles mediates target gene expression and antigen presentation by dendritic cells. Gene Ther 2000; 7:2105–2112.

212. Johnson RP. Live attenuated AIDS vaccines: hazards and hopes. Nat Med 1999; 5:154–155.

213. Baba TW, et al. Live attenuated, multiply deleted simian immunodeficiency virus causes AIDS in infant and adult macaques. Nat Med 1999; 5:194–203.

214. Holzer GW, et al. Highly efficient induction of protective immunity by a vaccinia virus vector defective in late gene expression. J Virol 1999; 73:4536–4542.

215. Belshe RB, et al. Induction of immune responses to HIV-1 by canarypox virus (ALVAC) HIV-1 and gp120 SF-2 recombinant vaccines in uninfected volunteers. NIAID AIDS Vaccine Evaluation Group. AIDS 1998; 12:2407–2415.

216. Adler SP, et al. A canarypox vector expressing cytomegalovirus (CMV) glycoprotein B primes for antibody responses to a live attenuated CMV vaccine (Towne). J Infect Dis 1999; 180:843–846.

217. Evans TG, et al. A canarypox vaccine expressing multiple human immunodeficiency virus type 1 genes given alone or with rgp120 elicits broad and durable CD8+ cytotoxic T lymphocyte responses in seronegative volunteers. J Infect Dis 1999; 180:290–298.

218. Salmon-Ceron D, et al. Safety and immunogenicity of a live recombinant canarypox virus expressing HIV type 1 gp120 MN MN tm/gag/protease LAI (ALVAC-HIV, vCP205) followed by a p24E-V3 MN synthetic peptide (CLTB-36) administered in healthy volunteers at low risk for HIV infection. AGIS Group and L'Agence Nationale de Recherches sur Le Sida. AIDS Res Hum Retrovir 1999; 15:633–645.

219. Guirakhoo F, et al. Immunogenicity, genetic stability, and protective efficacy of a recombinant, chimeric yellow fever-Japanese encephalitis virus (ChimeriVax-JE) as a live, attenuated vaccine candidate against Japanese encephalitis. Virology 1999; 257:363–372.

220. Schnell MJ, et al. Recombinant rabies virus as potential live-viral vaccines for HIV-1. Proc Natl Acad Sci USA 2000; 97:3544–3549.

221. Xuan X, et al. Biological and immunogenic properties of rabies virus glycoprotein expressed by canine herpesvirus vector. Vaccine 1998; 16:969–976.

222. Callebaut P, et al. An adenovirus recombinant expressing the spike glycoprotein of porcine respiratory coronavirus is immunogenic in swine. J Gen Virol 1996; 77:309–313.

223. Xiang ZQ, et al. Induction of genital immunity by DNA priming and intranasal booster immunization with a replication-defective adenoviral recombinant. J Immunol 1999; 162:6716–6723.

224. Heineman TC, et al. Immunization with recombinant varicella-zoster virus expressing herpes simplex virus type 2 glycoprotein D reduces the severity of genital herpes in guinea pigs. J Virol 1995; 69:8109–8113.

225. Mattion NM, et al. Attenuated poliovirus strain as a live vector: expression of regions of rotavirus outer capsid protein VP7 by using recombinant Sabin 3 viruses. J Virol 1994; 68:3925–3933.

226. Crotty S, et al. Mucosal immunization of cynomolgus macaques with two serotypes of live poliovirus vectors expressing simian immunodeficiency virus antigens: stimulation of humoral, mucosal, and cellular immunity. J Virol 1999; 73:9485–9495.

227. Davis NL, et al. Vaccination of macaques against pathogenic simian immunodeficiency virus with Venezuelan equine encephalitis virus replicon particles. J Virol 2000; 74:371–378.

228. Perri S, et al. Replicon vectors derived from Sindbis virus and Semliki forest virus that establish persistent replication in host cells. J Virol 2000; 74:9802–9807.

229. Berglund P, et al. Immunization with recombinant Semliki Forest virus induces protection against influenza challenge in mice. Vaccine 1999; 17:497–507.

230. Sizemore DR, et al. Attenuated Shigella zas a DNA delivery vehicle for DNA-mediated immunization. Science 1995; 270:299–302.

231. Sizemore DR, et al. Attenuated bacteria as a DNA delivery vehicle for DNA-mediated immunization. Vaccine 1997; 15:804–807.

232. Dietrich G, et al. Delivery of antigen-encoding plasmid DNA into the cytosol of macrophages by attenuated suicide Listeria monocytogenes. Nat Biotechnol 1998; 16:181–185.

233. Frankel FR, et al. Induction of cell-mediated immune responses to human immunodeficiency virus type 1 Gag pro-

tein by using *Listeria monocytogenes* as a live vaccine vector. J Immunol 1995; 155:4775–4782.

234. Soussi N, et al. Listeria monocytogenes as a short-lived delivery system for the induction of type 1 cell-mediated immunity against the p36/LACK antigen of *Leishmania major*. Infect Immun 2000; 68:1498–1506.

235. Darji A, et al. Oral somatic transgene vaccination using attenuated *S. typhimurium*. Cell 1997; 91:765–775.

236. Jain V, Mekalanos JJ. Use of lambda phage S and R gene products in an inducible lysis system for *Vibrio cholerae-* and *Salmonella enterica* serovar Typhimurium-based DNA vaccine delivery systems. Infect Immun 2000; 68:986–989.

237. Tacket CO, et al. Phase 2 clinical trial of attenuated *Salmonella enterica* serovar Typhi oral live vector vaccine CVD 908-*htrA* in U.S. volunteers. Infect Immun 2000; 68: 1196–1201.

238. Flo J, et al. Oral transgene vaccination mediated by attenuated Salmonellae is an effective method to prevent Herpes simplex virus-2 induced disease in mice. Vaccine 2001; 19: 1772–1782.

32

DNA-Modified Virus Ankara and Other Heterologous Prime-Boost Immunization Strategies for Effector T Cell Induction

Adrian V. S. Hill
University of Oxford, John Radcliffe Hospital, Oxford, England

Joerg Schneider
Oxxon Pharmaccines Ltd., Oxford, England

Andrew J. McMichael
Oxford University, Oxford, England

I. INTRODUCTION

In recent years, there has been increasing interest in immunization approaches that seek to generate protective immunity through effector T cell induction. An improved capacity to induce such T cells would facilitate the development of vaccines against a variety of intracellular pathogens including malaria, HIV/AIDS, and tuberculosis, three of the most important infectious diseases of the developing world. Also, a capacity to induce high-level persistent T cell responses could revolutionize the field of therapeutic vaccines and allow the development of immunotherapeutics for persistent viral infections such as hepatitis C virus and HIV and malignancies such as melanoma and breast cancer. Although vaccination studies aimed at inducing cellular immunity have often focused on CD8 + cytotoxic T cells as the main effector cells, it is becoming clear that CD4 + effector T cells may be of value in several diseases.

Numerous studies of subunit vaccines with the widely used alum adjuvant have shown that nonparticulate antigens with alum generally induce few or no CD8 + T cells, leading to the assessment of a wide variety of alternative vaccine delivery systems for CTL induction. These have included peptides with a variety of adjuvants, lipopeptides, particulate vaccines such as recombinant Ty-virus-like particles, DNA vaccines, and viral and bacterial vectors. Although all of these approaches have succeeded in inducing CD8 T cell re-

sponses, often, the magnitude of the induced responses and their durability has been insufficient to induce useful levels of protection.

In this chapter, we shall review an increasingly widely used approach to inducing high-level effector T cell responses that requires the sequential use of two different vaccines both encoding the same epitopes or antigen. Such heterologous prime–boost immunization [1–3] can be employed with a variety of the so-called priming vaccines and a more limited variety of boosting vaccines. However, because there is now the most extensive preclinical and clinical experience with DNA as a priming agent and the recombinant viral vector, modified virus Ankara, as a boosting agent, this particular prime–boost combination will be the focus of this chapter.

We shall initially review the background to the discovery of the immunogenicity and efficacy of this heterologous prime–boost immunization approach. Then we shall give some examples and characteristics of this immunization approach in small animal models and discuss the likely underlying mechanisms. Next, available data from nonhuman primate studies will be reviewed before summarizing recent clinical data suggesting that marked synergy is also observed with the use of this prime–boost approach in humans. Recent clinical data showing good safety of this approach and unprecedented levels of effector T cell induction suggest that further development of such strategies should contribute to the development of new therapeutic as well as prophylactic vaccines.

II. BACKGROUND STUDIES

The development of improved means of inducing strong T cell responses has advanced in parallel with, and been facilitated by, new immunoassays allowing more sensitive measures of specific T cell numbers and function. The original assay for CD8 T cells was the chromium release assay which, although providing an assay of effector function, has limited sensitivity and requires radiolabeling of target cells and usually many days of expansion of T cells in in vitro culture to allow their detection. Although precursor frequencies were measurable using chromium release assays along with limiting dilution methods, these often underestimate the overall effector frequency [4]. Newer assays such as the ex vivo ELISPOT assays of cytokines [5,6] allow quantification of lower numbers of T cells and have a much greater measurement range, so that 10–1000-fold changes in immunogenicity can be measured. The γ-interferon ELISPOT assay in particular has become widely used to enumerate induced CD4 and CD8 T cell in both preclinical and clinical studies [7,8]. Flowcytometric methods of enumerating specific cells in the presence and the absence of antigens allow the characterization of the induced response using intracellular staining of cytokines and other mediators [9]. Finally, the introduction of fluorescently labeled MHC-peptide tetramer reagents has provided an elegant and sensitive method of both staining and sorting specific vaccine-induced T cells [10].

The discovery and widespread adoption of DNA vaccination in the 1990s are described elsewhere in this volume. The ease of generation of plasmids and their ability to induce both humoral and cellular immune responses in small animals led to numerous studies of DNA vaccines and, subsequently, to attempts to improve their immunogenicity and protective efficacy. Heterologous prime–boost immunization may thus be seen as one of the many means that have been employed in attempts to improve the performance of DNA vaccines.

However, heterologous prime–boost immunization approaches also build on 15–20 years of experience with using recombinant viral vectors, particularly recombinant poxviruses as candidate vaccines. Recombinant vaccinia viruses were generated in the early 1980s and shown to be capable of inducing protective T cell responses in small animals [11,12]. In 1988, Taylor et al. [13] showed that a recombinant avipoxvirus, fowlpox, was able to induce humoral and cellular immune responses in mammals, although the avipoxviruses cannot replicate in mammalian cells. Subsequently, large numbers of recombinant canarypox vectors have been evaluated in phase I/II clinical trials for several diseases including HIV, but, generally, these failed to generate strong effector T cell responses in most vaccines [14]. Recombinant nonreplicating orthopoxviruses such as modified vaccinia virus Ankara (MVA) [15] and NYVAC [16] may be more immunogenic. MVA was generated from the virulent replicating CVA strain of vaccinia virus by Mayr [17] by over 500 passages in chick embryo fibroblasts and

used briefly as a smallpox vaccine. NYVAC is a molecularly attenuated virus made from the Copenhagen strain of vaccinia virus.

Attempts to improve the efficacy of poxvirus or DNA vaccines by adding another type of subunit vaccine initially employed protein-adjuvant boosting. Several studies showed enhanced immunogenicity particularly for antibody responses, but this appears to represent an additive effect without synergy between the components [18,19]. In particular, effector T cell responses are not substantially enhanced by this approach. In retrospect, the first heterologous prime–boost immunization experiment that probably induced markedly enhanced CD8 T cell responses was reported by Li et al. [20] in a murine malaria model with the *Plasmodium yoelii* parasite. Greater protective efficacy was observed when a priming immunization with a recombinant influenza virus was followed by a boosting immunization with a recombinant replicating vaccinia virus encoding the same antigen than homologous immunization or the opposite order of immunization. T cell assays were not reported prechallenge, and the authors speculated that administering the vaccinia virus second might have enhanced homing of protective T cells to the liver, the target organ for protective T cell in preerythrocytic malaria models. Later analyses showed that this viral vector prime–boost approach did enhance T cell immunogenicity [21]. At about this time, DNA priming and fowlpox vector boosting was reported to enhance protection and antibody levels in an influenza model [22], but CD8 T cells were not measured after the fowlpox boost.

In 1995, what was apparently the first study of DNA followed by MVA immunization was initiated as part of studies of malaria vaccination in a chimpanzee model [23]. Boosting of animals primed with DNA by recombinant MVAs enhanced CD4 and CD8 T cell responses measured in ELISPOT assays, and murine studies employing both plasmid DNA and Ty-virus-like particles soon revealed markedly enhanced T cell immunogenicity and protective efficacy mediated by effector CD8 T cells [1,3,24,25]. Several of the principles of prime–boost immunization using nonreplicating viruses as boosting agents were elucidated in this series of studies that will be reviewed in more detail.

III. MURINE STUDIES

Schneider et al. [1] described some key features of heterologous prime–boost immunization with DNA and MVA vectors using the *Plasmodium berghei* malaria model. Immunization with DNA followed at a 2-week interval by recombinant MVA induced a 5–10-fold greater level of CD8 T cells compared to immunization with either vector used in a homologous prime–boost regime (Figure 1). This enhanced immunogenicity was associated with a transformation in the level of observed efficacy against sporozoite challenge from 0–20% to 80–100% (Table 1). This was the first time that high-level protective efficacy had been achieved in this murine malaria model. The order of immunization was critical with MVA priming and DNA boosting neither more immunogenic nor protective than MVA used alone. Also, coadministration of DNA and MVA was

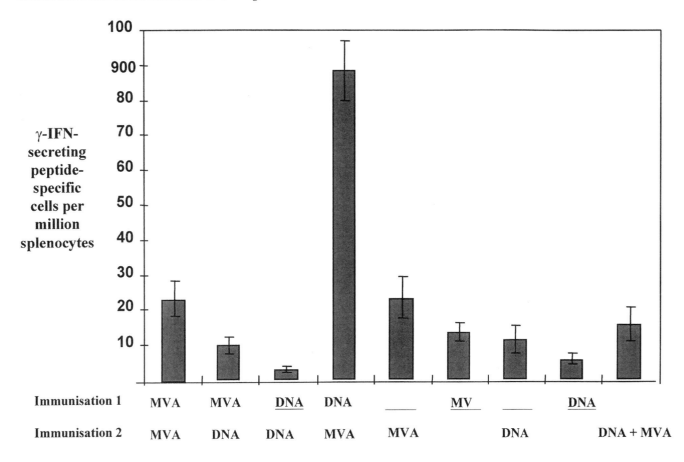

Figure 1 Immunogenicity of various prime–boost immunization regimes. The CD8 T cell response to a nonamer Kd-restricted epitope in the CS protein of *P. berghei* was measured by gamma-interferon ELISPOT assay of Balb/c mouse splenocytes after various immunization regimes, shown on the *X*-axis legend. The interval between immunizations was 14 days [1].

ineffective and a minimum 9-day interval between priming and boosting was required for high-level immunogenicity [2]. In these studies, CD8 T cells were measured to an immunodominant H2-Kd-restricted class I T cell epitope, termed pb9, in the *P. berghei* circumsporozoite (CS) protein using γ-interferon ELISPOT assays and chromium release assays. However, the marked increment in T cell immunogenicity was more evident in the ELISPOT assay than the less quantitative chromium release assay. Subsequent studies with a pb9-specific tetramer reagent confirmed these findings and, interestingly, revealed substantially greater numbers of induced pb9-specific T cells than the ELISPOT assay (Sheu et al., unpublished data).

In studies of the route of MVA immunization, intradermal administration of MVA was more immunogenic and protective than intramuscular or subcutaneous MVA and almost as immunogenic as intravenous MVA [1]. DNA was an efficient priming agent when delivered either intramuscularly or intradermally using a gene gun [26]. A striking and then surprising finding was made in comparisons of the

Table 1 Prime–Boost Immunization Studies with Viral Boosting

Species	Target organism	Reference
Mice	*P. berghei*	[1]
	P. yoelii	[27]
	P. falciparum	[20]
	Influenza	[26]
	HBV	(Schneider et al., unpublished)
	HCV	[64]
	HIV	[3]
	HSV	[65]
	HPV	[66]
	M. tuberculosis	[37,38]
	Tumors	[30,31]
Primates	*P. falciparum*	[23]
	P. knowlesi	[52]
	HBV	[39]
	SIV/HIV	[40–42]

boosting ability of replicating and nonreplicating strains of vaccinia virus. The nonreplicating MVA strain was more immunogenic than the replicating Western Reserve (WR) strain of vaccinia virus both as a priming and a boosting agent [1]. The mechanistic basis of this counterintuitive observation remains unclear, but this adds to the potential clinical utility of the MVA strain. In more limited studies, the nonreplicating NYVAC strain also appeared more immunogenic and protective than the WR strain.

The view that protective efficacy was mediated directly by CD8 T cells was supported by the use of constructs encoding only the nine amino acids of pb9 from the *P. berghei* genome, as these proved as immunogenic and protective as constructs encoding the entire CS antigen [1,25]. In the C57/BL6 mouse strain that is very sensitive to malaria infection, complete protective efficacy could also be induced using a mixture of constructs encoding the *P. berghei* CS and thrombospondin-related adhesion protein (TRAP) sporozoite antigens [1]. Data on prime–boost immunization in the *P. yoelii* malaria model with the NYVAC vector as a boosting agent showed comparable enhanced immunogenicity and protective efficacy [27]. Parallel studies of immunogenicity of an HIV epitope in mice indicated that this prime–boost principle was not limited to malaria antigens [3], and this has been extensively confirmed with examples of the capacity of poxvirus vectors to boost CD8 T cells now provided for epitopes from numerous viruses, bacteria, and parasites in a variety of species (Table 2). Epitopes have been encoded singly, as parts of whole antigens, as polyepitope strings, as parts of polyproteins, and in initial clinical trials as parts of polyepitope-protein constructs (see below).

In parallel with these DNA–MVA studies of malaria in mice, studies of Ty-virus-like particles followed by MVA boosting demonstrated enhanced immunogenicity and protective efficacy [24,25]. This suggested that the principle of prime–boost immunization owed little if anything to particular properties of DNA as a priming agent, and this has been extensively illustrated. A large variety of vaccine types have now been shown to prime CD8 T cells efficiently for a subsequent poxvirus boost. These include recombinant influenza virus [20], lipopeptides [28], protein with adjuvant, bacterial vectors, and several other viral vectors (e.g., adenovirus [29], see below).

The potential utility of heterologous prime–boost immunization for cancer immunotherapy has also been dem-

onstrated in small animal models. DNA and MVA vaccines encoding an epitope string that included the P1A tumor epitope were protective against mastocytoma tumor development in a prophylactic vaccination model in mice (Schneider et al., unpublished). Constructs designed for human use have also been immunogenic in mice [30]. Using beta-galactosidase as a model antigen, Irvine et al. [31] showed enhanced immunogenicity of heterologous prime–boost regimes using either fowlpox or replicating vaccinia as boosting vectors. Heterologous prime–boost regimes were more protective than homologous regimes against challenge with a murine colon carcinoma cell line transfected with the beta-galactosidase gene. In studies of vaccinia and fowlpox vectors expressing carcinoembryonic antigen as well as co-stimulatory molecules, enhanced immunogenicity was again observed with heterologous prime–boost immunization [32]. Anderson et al. (submitted for publication) studied an attenuated strain of fowlpox termed FP9 [33] and showed it to be particularly effective at induction of CD8 T cell responses compared to the widely used Webster's strain of fowlpox virus. In heterologous prime–boost studies with the *P. berghei* CS protein, FP9–MVA and MVA–FP9 immunization was considerably more immunogenic than DNA–MVA immunization with a concomitant increase in protective efficacy against sporozoite challenge. This study showed directly that T cell cross-reactivity postimmunization was minimal between the avipoxvirus and orthopoxvirus vectors.

There has recently been increasing interest in recombinant nonreplicating adenovirus vectors as alternatives to either DNA or MVA in prime–boost immunization regimes. In the *P. berghei* malaria model, recombinant adenovirus was shown to be capable of priming and boosting CD8 T cell responses, and adenovirus priming followed by MVA boosting was more protective using the intradermal route of immunization than intramuscular DNA followed by intradermal MVA [29]. In studies in the *P. yoelii* malaria model replication-defective adenovirus was a particularly immunogenic priming agent and could be boosted by replicating vaccinia [34,35].

An important feature of prime–boost immunization is that priming of T cell responses may occur by natural infection. Both *Plasmodium falciparum* and *P. berghei* malaria sporozoites were found to induce very weak T cell responses that could be substantially boosted by replicating vaccinia virus and MVA, respectively [28] (Schneider et al., unpublished). This observation may have important impli-

Table 2 Heterologous Prime–Boost Immunization and Protection Against *Plasmodium Berghei* Sporozoite Challenge [1]

Immunization 1	Immunization 2	No. of infected	% Protection
DNA-CS+-TRAP	DNA-CS+-TRAP	5/5	0
MVA-CS+-TRAP	MVA-CS+-TRAP	4/5	20
DNA-CS	MVA-CS	0/10	100
DNA-TRAP	MVA-TRAP	2/16	88
DNA-CS+-TRAP	MVA-CS+-TRAP	0/10	100
MVA-CS+-TRAP	DNA-CS+-TRAP	5/5	0
DNA-epitope	MVA-epitope	0/10	100
None	None	9/10	10

cations for the use of these vectors as therapeutic vaccines, suggesting that in a therapeutic setting, the use of the boosting vector alone might induce strong T cell responses.

The duration of induced T cell responses has been assessed in some limited studies after DNA–MVA immunization in small animals. In the *P. berghei* model, protective efficacy had dropped from 100% at 14 days following the MVA immunization to 60% at day 150 (Schneider et al., unpublished). In the *P. yoelii* model in mice, protection of 70–100% persisted for 20 weeks and dropped to 30–40% by 28 weeks [36]. At this latter time point, effector CD8 T cells had declined from 12–20% of splenic CD8 T cells at 2 weeks to 6%. Complete protection at 3 1/2 months after priming was reported with an adenovirus–vaccinia immunization regime in the *P. yoelii* model. In this regime, better immunogenicity and protection were observed after increasing the interval between priming and boosting from 2 to 8 weeks [35]. More detailed comparative studies of the durability of induced T responses with different prime–boost regimes would be valuable.

Although DNA–MVA immunization was originally used to induce strong CD8 T cell responses, it has turned out to be a surprisingly effective means of inducing γ-interferon secreting CD4+ T cells. This was clearly illustrated in a tuberculosis model where Th1-type CD4 T cells are of particular protective importance [37]. Using antigens and a mouse strain where no CD8 T cell response was detectable, the strongest CD4 T cell responses were induced by three DNA immunizations followed by an MVA boost. However, in contrast to findings with CD8 T cell responses, CD4 T cell responses were as strong following single dose MVA–DNA prime–boost immunization as with DNA–MVA immunization. Using the gene for a major secreted antigen of *Mycobacterium tuberculosis*, Ag85A, as an insert, both CD4 and CD8 T cell responses were induced by DNA–MVA immunization with protective efficacy equivalent to the BCG vaccine [38] (Figure 2).

One of the potential concerns with viral vector boosting is that the vector might not be reusable for subsequent immunization against the same or another pathogen because of antivector immunity. However, Sheu et al. (submitted for publication) showed that DNA-recombinant MVA immunization retained good immunogenicity in MVA immune mice, although the immunogenicity of homologous recombinant MVA immunization was substantially compromised. Thus mice immunized with DNA and MVA encoding malaria antigens could generate strong T cell responses when subsequently immunized with DNA and MVA vectors encoding an influenza antigen.

The capacity of nonreplicating poxviruses and adenoviruses to boost CD8 T cell responses naturally led to studies of triple vector immunization in which the capacity of a third vector heterologous to both the first and second is assessed. Disappointingly, in murine studies with the *P. berghei* CS antigen, no improvement in immunogenicity was observed over prime–boost immunization alone assessing various combinations of DNA, adenovirus, MVA, and fowlpox vectors in triple immunization regimes [29] (Anderson et al., unpublished).

Several vaccine delivery systems have now been assessed for their capacity to boost preexisting CD8 T cell responses. MVA and other nonreplicating poxviruses appear to boost most effectively and better than replicating orthopoxviruses. Avipoxviruses, which do not replicate in mammalian cells, can also boost efficiently perhaps less so than the orthopoxviruses. Nonreplicating adenoviruses also boost effectively in mice and are also very immunogenic priming agents. However, in general plasmid DNA, peptides, lipopeptides, and proteins either as particles or with adjuvants are relatively ineffective as boosting agents [1,25,28].

IV. NONHUMAN PRIMATE STUDIES

Studies in nonhuman primates have made an important contribution to the development of heterologous prime–boost immunization strategies. This has been facilitated by the application of new ELISPOT and tetramer assays to studies in nonhuman primates and by the availability of relevant challenge models in several species. In an early study of chimpanzees ELISPOT responses to a malaria pre-erythrocytic antigen, TRAP were not detected after DNA immunizations but were evident after boosting with recombinant MVA [23]. A chimpanzee infected with hepatitis B virus was immunized with DNA and remained viremic, but a booster immunization with a recombinant canarypox vector also expressing the hepatitis B surface antigen led to the clearance of HBV DNA [39]. However, the most substantial data on primate immunization come from HIV and SIV studies.

Prime–boost immunizations have been tested in macaques to generate CD8 T cell responses specific for simian immunodeficiency virus (SIV) or hybrid HIV–SIV viruses, SHIV. Pig-tailed macaques, immunized by DNA and then recombinant fowlpox expressing HIV proteins, were protected against HIV challenge [40]. Protection was associated with good CD8 T cell responses; however, HIV only weakly

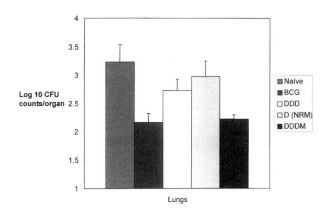

Figure 2 Protective efficacy against tuberculosis of DNA–MVA immunization with constructs expressing a major secreted antigen of *M. tuberculosis*, antigen 85A. Colony forming units were measured in lung tissue after various immunization regimes and compared with no vaccination and BCG vaccination. NRM = nonrecombinant MVA. (From Ref. 38.)

infects this macaque species, and this may not be a very robust model of HIV vaccine protection. In rhesus macaques, immunization with DNA encoding HIV and SIV protein epitopes, followed by MVA recombinant for the same DNA, could generate strong CD8 T cell responses, measured by tetramer staining, to the immunodominant epitope presented by the Mamu A01 class I MHC type [41]. Prior DNA priming was essential for the strong response after the MVA boost. Amara et al. [42,43] took this a stage further and showed that monkeys primed with DNA and boosted with MVA were able to survive challenge with the highly aggressive SHIV 89.6P virus. The immunity was not sterilizing, but virus loads were reduced by a thousand-fold and CD4 T cell counts remained stable. It was of interest that the challenge was 7 months after the last MVA immunization so protection was long-lived. Similar results have been obtained in macaques immunized by DNA that encodes the SIV gag protein, followed by recombinant adenovirus expressing the same protein [44]. Again, animals were not completely protected from SHIV 89.6 challenge but survived and did not lose CD4 T cells. However, a warning note for this type of study comes from a study where similar levels of protection against this virus were achieved in rhesus macaques using DNA and interleukin-2, but one animal became sick when the virus mutated a critical amino acid residue in the epitope and was no longer controlled by the T cell response [45]. Another note of caution comes from a study where DNA- and MVA-immunized macaques were challenged with the slightly less aggressive virus SIV 239 and showed only marginal transient reduction of virus level compared to controls [46]. It is not clear why this is so, but the route of DNA immunization, intramuscular in the former study compared to intradermal by gene gun in the latter study, could contribute if the intradermal route favors Th2 responses [47]. In both studies, the level of SIV-specific CD8 T cells was high and very similar. It is also possible that protection might actually be better at late time points after vaccine immunization.

There have been studies of challenge with each vaccine component alone. DNA immunization followed by recombinant adenovirus gave better protection in macaques than either alone or DNA followed by recombinant MVA [44]. However, two studies have shown that quite good protection against SHIV 89.6P challenge could be obtained by recombinant MVA alone [48,49]. These studies are focused on monkeys with the Mamu A*01 MHC type, and the epitope usually monitored seems to be very immunodominant, whether delivered by SIV, DNA, recombinant adenovirus, or recombinant MVA. This may not be true of other epitopes in which case the DNA priming step may be needed so that the MVA generates a T cell response to the inserted gene product.

There has been one study that used the DNA prime, recombinant adenovirus boost approach to protect macaques from Ebola virus [50]. Both humoral and cellular immune responses were generated. The level of protection was impressive.

These results in macaques, which have been immunized by DNA followed by MVA, therefore confirm the results in rodents showing that DNA prime and MVA or adenovirus boost gives better T cell responses and better protection than either component alone.

Macaques also provide a valuable model for preclinical testing of malaria vaccines. Rogers et al. [51] have evaluated DNA priming and both canarypox and NYVAC vectors as boosting agents in the *Plasmodium knowlesi* simian malaria model. Using a mixture of two pre-erythrocytic antigens and two blood stage antigens, detectable protection was induced with the DNA–canarypox regime and higher levels of protection with the DNA–NYVAC prime–boost regime [52].

Macaques are not naturally infected by the major human malarias, but they are very susceptible to the human tuberculosis bacillus, *M. tuberculosis*. The long time scale of vaccine efficacy studies for tuberculosis has led to increasing interest in macaques as both an immunogenicity and efficacy model [53] for new tuberculosis vaccines. Goonetilleke et al. (unpublished) have evaluated prime–boost immunization strategies in macaques using a major secreted antigen of *M. tuberculosis*, Ag85A, as an insert in both MVA and FP9 vectors, with or without priming with the BCG vaccine. Strong CD8 T cell responses could be induced by a triple immunization regime employing a BCG prime and MVA and FP9 booster immunizations.

V. CLINICAL TRIALS

A. Malaria

In 1999, a series of heterologous prime–boost immunization trials were initiated in Oxford to ask whether heterologous prime–boost immunization with DNA and MVA vectors showed enhanced immunogenicity over the individual vaccines and to determine whether any efficacy could be achieved against sporozoite challenge [54]. Clinical trials are in progress of DNA–MVA immunization for malaria using as an insert a polyepitope string used to an entire pre-erythrocytic protein antigen, thrombospondin-related adhesion protein (TRAP) (Figure 3). The epitope string includes 14 CD8 T cell epitopes from six different pre-erythrocytic *P. falciparum* antigens and six other B cell or CD4 T cell epitopes. Doses of DNA from 0.5 to 2.0 mg have been delivered intramuscularly with a needle or a much lower dose of 4 μm delivered intradermally with the Powderject Vaccines ballistic device or "gene gun." MVA has been delivered intradermally with doses of 3×10^7 to 1.5×10^8 pfu. Overall, in over 150 vaccinees receiving either DNA or MVA or both, the safety profile of both of these vaccines has been good without any severe or serious adverse events [54a,54b].

T cell immunogenicity has been assessed in these studies principally with ex vivo ELISPOT assays to peptides spanning the entire insert sequence. Both CD4 and CD8 T cell responses have been observed, and these are focused more on the TRAP antigen than the string of largely CD8 T cell epitopes. A summary of the T cell immunogenicity observed in a series of small-scale studies is presented in Figure 4 [54b]. The time point shown is 7 days after the last immunization, at about the time of peak immunogenicity. The use of DNA and MVA at various doses induced detectable but modest immunogenicity with arithmetic mean responses measured

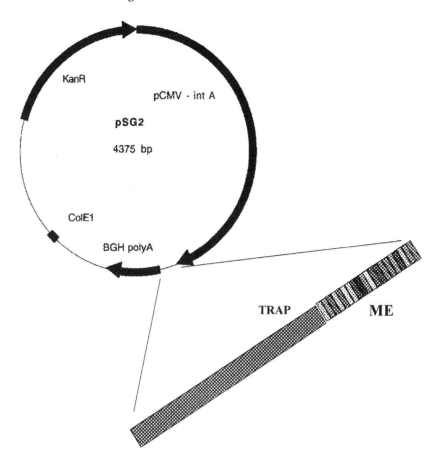

Figure 3 Plasmid DNA construct used for DNA–MVA malaria clinical trials. The insert is an entire pre-erythrocytic antigen, thrombospondin-related adhesion protein fused in-frame to the C-terminus of a polyepitope string of 20 peptides, including 14 CD8 T cell epitopes from six different *P. falciparum* pre-erythrocytic antigens [24].

as under 100 per million peripheral blood mononuclear cells (PBMCs) by summing responses across the different peptide pools used in the assays. Importantly, substantially higher immunogenicity was observed with DNA–MVA heterologous prime–boost immunization, particularly using the higher dose regimes. In the regime with three priming DNA immunizations, a mean response of over 1000/million was observed 7 days after the first MVA boost (Figure 5). Responses were higher with a 3-week interval between the third DNA immunization and the MVA than with an 8-week interval. In this high responder group, the responses measured were predominantly CD4 rather than CD8 peptide-specific cells.

Polymorphism in major antigens is a significant difficulty in malaria vaccine development, and the TRAP antigen used in these vaccine constructs shows such variation. The strain used in the DNA and MVA vaccine constructs is from the T9/96 *P. falciparum* parasite that differs by about 6% in sequence from the 3D7 parasite strain generally used in human malaria sporozoite challenge studies [55]. Analysis in ELISPOT assays of T cell responses to both strains of TRAP showed substantial but incomplete T cell cross-reactivity. Sporozoite challenge studies in volunteers immu-

nized with various regimes showed a significant delay in time to patent parasitemia in volunteers immunized with DNA–MVA heterologous prime–boost immunization regimes but not with homologous immunization regimes (McConkey et al., submitted for publication). The efficacy observed with DNA–MVA in this sporozoite challenge study is encouraging in that this is the first time protection has been achieved with a subunit vaccine against heterologous strain challenge, and the estimated reduction in parasite numbers in the liver is of the order of 75%. Given that the dose of parasites used in the challenge model may be an order of magnitude larger than a natural field infection, greater efficacy may be observed in field studies.

Phase I trials of DNA–MVA immunization in Gambians naturally exposed to malaria have been undertaken with a view to larger-scale efficacy trials in this population [54a]. T cell responses evoked by natural infection against the ME-TRAP insert are low and of the order of 25 SFUs/million PBMCs, much lower than what can be achieved by DNA–MVA vaccination. In Gambians, safety data have been satisfactory and T cell immunogenicity is equal to or greater than that observed in nonimmune European volunteers [54a]. Furthermore, the cross-reactivity of the induced

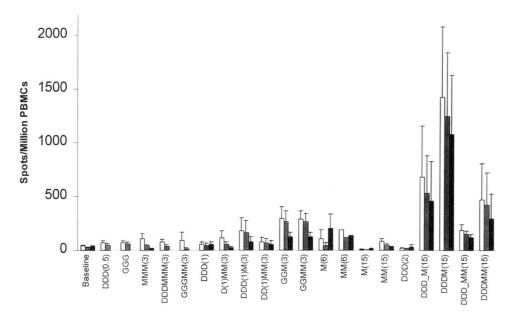

Figure 4 γ-Interferon ELISPOT responses to pools of peptides from the ME-TRAP malaria insert 7 days after various DNA and/ or MVA vaccination regimes showing summed net responses to pools of peptides from all of the vaccine insert, from the T9/96 strain of TRAP encoded in the vaccine, and from TRAP from another *P. falciparum* strain, 3D7. The bracketed numerals included in the regimen names correspond to the dosage of vaccine, in milligram for DNA and pfu×10⁷ for MVA. The arithmetic mean of the responses for the subjects in that group are presented with an error bar to indicate the standard error of the mean. (From Ref 54b.)

T cell responses between strains was greater than in nonimmune vaccines. Phase IIb studies in larger numbers of adults of the efficacy of DNA–MVA against malaria infection are planned for the near future.

The greater immunogenicity of FP9–MVA than DNA–MVA prime–boost immunization observed in studies of murine malaria (Anderson et al., submitted for publication) led to the clinical assessment of an FP9 construct encoding the same insert as the DNA and MVA vaccines. Again, much higher T cell responses were observed with FP9–MVA

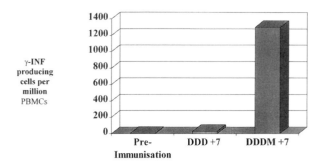

Figure 5 Immunogenicity of DNA immunization compared to DNA–MVA immunization. T cell responses to the ME-TRAP insert (Figure 3) were measured in eight volunteers prevaccination, 7 days following three DNA immunizations with 2 mg per dose and 7 days following a booster immunization with MVA encoding the same insert. (From Ref 54b.)

immunization than with homologous prime–boost immunization, and significant efficacy was observed against sporozoite challenge (Webster et al., unpublished). Although some volunteers immunized thus have been fully protected against sporozoite challenge, further analysis is required to determine whether DNA–MVA or FP9–MVA immunization regimes will be more immunogenic or protective.

In both the DNA–MVA and FP9–MVA studies, antibody responses induced to the malaria insert have been low or absent, indicating that in their current formulations, these approaches, like DNA vaccines used alone, induce low level or no antibody responses. Conversely, this finding implies that the protection observed in the malaria challenge studies is almost certainly cell-mediated rather than antibody-mediated.

In summary, these malaria studies have demonstrated that the DNA–MVA immunization in humans can be used safely and can generate effector T cell responses apparently higher than previously reported for any other subunit vaccination approach. Initial evidence of protection in malaria challenge studies is encouraging, and field studies are planned to assess the utility of this approach in a natural field setting.

B. HIV

Attempts are in progress to make a vaccine that stimulates CD8 and CD4 T cells specific for HIV in humans. Early studies showed that relatively low doses of DNA immunization (<1 mg) elicit transient T cell responses in HIV-uninfected volunteers [56]. Similarly, recombinant canarypox vaccines have stimulated relatively weak T cell responses, particularly CD8 T cells [14,57,58].

A series of trials of DNA, MVA, and DNA plus MVA have recently been completed in Oxford and Nairobi, Kenya (Mwau et al., submitted for publication; Anzala et al., in preparation). The vaccine is a synthetic DNA construct which comprises HIV clade A consensus gag p24 and p17. DNA, encoding a string of 25 epitopes from other HIV proteins, was added to the 3′ end [59]. The latter include the gag epitope presented by Mamu A*01 and a gp120 V3 loop peptide presented by H2-Kd. Thus the vaccine could be tested in mice and macaques [60]. The MVA is recombinant for the same DNA construct. In humans, the DNA stimulated weak responses at early time points, but, surprisingly, strong CD4 and CD8 responses appeared 6 and 12 months after vaccination, possibly reflecting persistence of the DNA at the site of injection. MVA gave a more classical CD8 T cell response to a nonpersisting virus, but not all volunteers responded to the inserted sequence. Boosting of DNA-primed volunteers with MVA elicited good CD4 and CD8 responses. All volunteers who were given the DNA and MVA responded, and the quality of the response differed from that induced by MVA alone. Both vaccines appeared safe.

Further larger-scale trials are in progress, testing different doses of the vaccines, different routes, and schedules. If the vaccines prove to be safe and stimulate strong and broad T cell responses, it is planned to test them in efficacy trials in East Africa, countries where the A clade virus is predominant.

In a parallel series of clinical trials in humans, Emini et al. (http://www.retroconference.org/2002) have shown that DNA encoding HIV B clade gag, given by intramuscular injection, elicited definite T cell responses in some volunteers. The same construct presented by recombinant adenovirus gave stronger T cell responses, especially in recipients with lower levels of preexisting neutralizing antibody. Prime–boost studies are in progress.

These early studies in humans are reasonably encouraging. Some response is elicited by the main vaccine components, and optimization of the prime–boost approaches should result in enhanced T cell responses. Most of the current studies are focused on T cell responses, but it will be informative to monitor antibody responses as well.

Besides the prophylactic studies, there are some therapeutic studies that are aimed at stimulating T cell immunity in HIV-infected patients who are on antiretroviral drug treatment. If the T cell responses can be enhanced, it may be possible to withdraw drug treatment and maintain immunological control of the virus.

C. Hepatitis B Virus Therapeutic Vaccination

One of the main objectives of strategies aimed at improving effector T cell responses is to allow therapeutic vaccination. Many such attempts have targeted the hepatitis B virus because most individuals manage to mount a sufficient immune response postinfection to effect viral clearance. However, others who fail to do so comprise 15% of adults in some developing countries and about 350 million individuals worldwide. These carriers are at substantially increased risk of hepatocellular carcinoma. Current treatments for hepatitis B virus infection offer only transient suppression of virus load with antivirals or low responder rates using alpha interferon. The rationale for developing a therapeutic CD8+ T cell inducing vaccine derives from preclinical and clinical observations. In a murine HBV model, Guidotti and Chisari [61] demonstrated that INF-γ secreting CD8+ T cells suppress transcription of viral genes. In murine studies, DNA–MVA immunization showed substantially enhanced CD8 T cell responses compared to vaccination with either DNA or MVA alone. A phase I trial of DNA and MVA vaccines encoding the hepatitis B surface antigen has been undertaken in the United Kingdom, and preliminary data show good safety and induced cellular immune responses. In The Gambia, a phase II trial with viral clearance as an outcome measure has commenced. In this trial, a potential synergistic effect of DNA–MVA prime–boost vaccination and the use of the antiviral drug lamivudine are being assessed.

D. Melanoma and Other Cancers

The identification of tumor-associated antigens (TAA) recognized by CD8+ T cells offers targets for recombinant antigen delivery systems. There are now many CD8+ T cell epitopes available to target the cellular immune response to the tumor. Melanoma is the best-studied human malignancy in which numerous TAA have been identified. Currently, there are several products being tested using recombinant gene-based antigen delivery systems with the aim of inducing a tumor-specific CD8+ T cell response. The use of multiple antigens or CD8+ T cell epitope strings may induce a multispecific CD8+ T cell response minimizing the occurrence of antigen-loss variants and may increase the safety of these gene-based vaccines, particularly for newly identified TAAs whose biological roles are poorly understood. Epitope string-based DNA and MVA melanoma vaccines [30] have been tested in stages II and IV melanoma patients. A CD8+ T cell epitope string containing seven different epitopes presented by HLA-A2 and HLA-A1 derived from five different melanoma TAA was safe. An expansion of melanoma-specific CD8+ T cells was detected in the majority of the vaccinees, particularly following heterologous priming and boosting.

In a phase I trial of patients with tumors expressing the carcinoembryonic antigen, fowlpox and replicating vaccinia viral vectors were assessed in heterologous prime–boost immunization regimes. Stronger T cell responses were observed by boosting vaccine-primed patients with the fowlpox vaccine than the opposite order of immunization [62]. The use of heterologous boost–boost cycles (for example, recombinant MVA followed by recombinant adenovirus followed by recombinant fowlpox virus) is particularly attractive for chronic conditions such as cancer.

VI. CONCLUSIONS AND PROSPECTS

Attempts to induce the high-level effector T cell responses with subunit vaccines are at an early stage of development.

Prime–boost strategies grew out of attempts to optimize protective CD8 T cell responses in mice and have entered clinical trials relatively rapidly. Safety data with both the DNA vaccines and the attenuated viral vectors tested to date in these trials look reassuring. As hoped for, some very high effector T cell levels have been achieved, at least as compared to previous subunit vaccination approaches. However, a major unknown is the level of response that will be required to provide protection in various diseases. Extrapolation from animal models is of limited value in making such estimates, and challenge studies, where feasible and ethical, may be of greater value in the short term. The characteristics of the induced responses with DNA-based vaccines appear different to protein-adjuvant strategies, with the former inducing higher effector T cell numbers but lower T cell proliferative responses as well as lower level antibody induction. Another key issue, particularly for prophylactic vaccination, remains the durability of induced T cell responses. In the malaria clinical trials discussed above, responses are maximal 1–2 weeks after the booster vaccination and decline to a plateau at about 28 days. How well sustained these responses are over subsequent years requires characterization.

It is likely that improvements to both the priming and boosting compositions of the DNA–MVA approach will be forthcoming. Improvements by adding cytokines or other types of adjuvant to DNA vaccines are discussed elsewhere in this volume. MVA may be improved, in principle, by addition of adjuvants or by modifications to the vector. The latter includes further deletion of genes that may dampen immune responses and also addition of extraneous genes such as cytokines and chemokines that may improve immunogenicity. Such modifications may either increase immunogenicity and efficacy at current doses or reduce the dose of the vector that is required for a defined response. This could be particularly important for DNA vaccines where current milligram doses may prove expensive for prophylactic vaccination in developing countries. It remains unclear whether optimization of the doses and regime of boosting will allow lower doses of DNA to be used in a prime in humans, but studies in mice suggest that this may be possible [63].

One of the attractions of DNA vaccines is the generic nature of the manufacturing process and the limited modification of this process required with a different plasmid. Furthermore, it is likely that DNA vaccines may be distributable without a cold chain, of great importance in some developing countries. Similar considerations apply to the use of recombinant poxvirus vaccines. Cost of manufacture is likely to be lower for these, the approach is generic, readily transferable to developing country manufacturers, and poxviruses may be freeze-dried. The WHO has previously used a poxvirus vaccine worldwide to eliminate smallpox.

Despite the efforts being made to assess DNA–MVA vaccines for malaria and HIV prophylaxis in Africa, the route to market for other diseases may be shorter. Demonstration of convincing efficacy against persistent viral infections or even malignancies might require smaller trials and less time. The capacity to induce readily measurable effector T cell responses to pathogen and tumor antigens with these vectors should allow rapid assessment of the potential of induced T cells to reduce viral load or effect viral clearance in diseases such as persistent HBV and HCV infection as well as against HIV. The greater challenge of therapeutic vaccination against malignancies could be pursued with greater confidence if measurable T cell responses against tumor antigens prove to be inducible in the majority of patients by prime–boost vaccination strategies.

REFERENCES

1. Schneider J, et al. Enhanced immunogenicity for CD8+ T cell induction and complete protective efficacy of malaria DNA vaccination by boosting with modified vaccinia virus Ankara. Nat Med 1998; 4:397–402.
2. Schneider J, et al. Induction of CD8+ T cells using heterologous prime–boost immunisation strategies. Immunol Rev 1999; 170:29–38.
3. Hanke T, et al. Enhancement of MHC class I-restricted peptide-specific T cell induction by a DNA prime/MVA boost vaccination regime. Vaccine 1998; 16:439–445.
4. Goulder PJ, et al. Functionally inert HIV-specific cytotoxic T lymphocytes do not play a major role in chronically infected adults and children. J Exp Med 2000; 192:1819–1832.
5. Hutchings PR, et al. The detection and enumeration of cytokine-secreting cells in mice and man and the clinical application of these assays. J Immunol Methods 1989; 120:1–8.
6. Kabilan L, et al. Number of cells from *Plasmodium falciparum*-immune donors that produce gamma interferon in vitro in response to Pf155/RESA, a malaria vaccine candidate antigen. Infect Immun 1990; 58:2989–2994.
7. Miyahira Y, et al. Quantification of antigen specific CD8+ T cells using an ELISPOT assay. J Immunol Methods 1995; 181: 45–54.
8. Lalvani A, et al. Rapid effector function in CD8+ memory T cells. J Exp Med 1997; 186:859–865.
9. Jin X, et al. Safety and immunogenicity of ALVAC vCP1452 and recombinant gp160 in newly human immunodeficiency virus type 1-infected patients treated with prolonged highly active antiretroviral therapy. J Virol 2002; 76:2206–2216.
10. Altman JD, et al. Phenotypic analysis of antigen-specific T lymphocytes. Science 1996; 274:94–96.
11. Panicali D, Paoletti E. Construction of poxviruses as cloning vectors: insertion of the thymidine kinase gene from herpes simplex virus into the DNA of infectious vaccinia virus. Proc Natl Acad Sci USA 1982; 79:4927–4931.
12. Smith GL, et al. Infectious vaccinia virus recombinants that express hepatitis B virus surface antigen. Nature 1983; 302: 490–495.
13. Taylor J, et al. Recombinant fowlpox virus inducing protective immunity in non-avian species. Vaccine 1988; 6:497–503.
14. Belshe RB, et al. Safety and immunogenicity of a canarypox-vectored human immunodeficiency virus Type 1 vaccine with or without gp120: a phase 2 study in higher- and lower-risk volunteers. J Infect Dis 2001; 183:1343–1352.
15. Sutter G, Moss B. Nonreplicating vaccinia vector efficiently expresses recombinant genes. Proc Natl Acad Sci USA 1992; 89:10847–10851.
16. Tartaglia J, et al. NYVAC: a highly attenuated strain of vaccinia virus. Virology 1992; 188:217–232.
17. Mayr A. Historical review of smallpox, the eradication of smallpox and the attenuated smallpox MVA vaccine. Berl Munch Tierarztl Wochenschr 1999; 112:322–328.
18. Gorse GJ, et al. Vaccine-induced antibodies to native and recombinant human immunodeficiency virus type 1 envelope glycoproteins. NIAID AIDS Vaccine Clinical Trials Network. Vaccine 1994; 12:912–918.

19. Letvin NL, et al. Potent, protective anti-HIV immune responses generated by bimodal HIV envelope DNA plus protein vaccination. Proc Natl Acad Sci USA 1997; 94:9378–9383.

20. Li S, et al. Priming with recombinant influenza virus followed by administration of recombinant vaccinia virus induces CD8+ T-cell-mediated protective immunity against malaria. Proc Natl Acad Sci USA 1993; 90:5214–5218.

21. Murata K, et al. Characterization of in vivo primary and secondary CD8+ T cell responses induced by recombinant influenza and vaccinia viruses. Cell Immunol 1996; 173:96–107.

22. Ramsay AJ, et al. DNA vaccination against virus infection and enhancement of antiviral immunity following consecutive immunization with DNA and viral vectors. Immunol Cell Biol 1997; 75:382–388.

23. Schneider J, et al. A prime–boost immunisation regimen using DNA followed by recombinant modified vaccinia virus Ankara induces strong cellular immune responses against the *Plasmodium falciparum* TRAP antigen in chimpanzees. Vaccine 2001; 19:4595–4602.

24. Gilbert SC, et al. A protein particle vaccine containing multiple malaria epitopes. Nat Biotechnol 1997; 15:1280–1284.

25. Plebanski M, et al. Protection from *Plasmodium berghei* infection by priming and boosting T cells to a single class I-restricted epitope with recombinant carriers suitable for human use. Eur J Immunol 1998; 28:4345–4355.

26. Degano P, et al. Gene gun intradermal DNA immunization followed by boosting with modified vaccinia virus Ankara: enhanced CD8+ T cell immunogenicity and protective efficacy in the influenza and malaria models. Vaccine 1999; 18:623–632.

27. Sedegah M, et al. Boosting with recombinant vaccinia increases immunogenicity and protective efficacy of malaria DNA vaccine. Proc Natl Acad Sci USA 1998; 95:7648–7653.

28. Miyahira Y, et al. Recombinant viruses expressing a human malaria antigen can elicit potentially protective immune CD8(+) responses in mice. Proc Natl Acad Sci USA 1998; 95:3954–3959. [In Process Citation].

29. Gilbert SC, et al. Enhanced CD8 T cell immunogenicity and protective efficacy in a mouse malaria model using a recombinant adenoviral vaccine in heterologous prime–boost immunisation regimes. Vaccine 2002; 20:1039–1045.

30. Palmowski MJ, et al. Competition between CTL narrows the immune response induced by prime–boost vaccination protocols. J Immunol 2002; 168:4391–4398.

31. Irvine KR, et al. Enhancing efficacy of recombinant anticancer vaccines with prime/boost regimens that use two different vectors. J Natl Cancer Inst 1997; 89:1595–1601.

32. Grosenbach DW, et al. Synergy of vaccine strategies to amplify antigen-specific immune responses and antitumor effects. Cancer Res 2001; 61:4497–4505.

33. Mockett B, et al. Comparison of the locations of homologous fowlpox and vaccinia virus genes reveals major genome reorganization. J Gen Virol 1992; 73(Pt 10):2661–2668.

34. Rodrigues EG, et al. Single immunizing dose of recombinant adenovirus efficiently induces CD8+ T cell-mediated protective immunity against malaria. J Immunol 1997; 158:1268–1274.

35. Bruna-Romero O, et al. Complete, long-lasting protection against malaria of mice primed and boosted with two distinct viral vectors expressing the same plasmodial antigen. Proc Natl Acad Sci USA 2001; 98:11491–11496.

36. Sedegah M, et al. Persistence of protective immunity to malaria induced by DNA priming and poxvirus boosting: characterization of effector and memory CD8(+)-T-cell populations. Infect Immun 2002; 70:3493–3499.

37. McShane H, et al. Enhanced immunogenicity of CD4(+) t-cell responses and protective efficacy of a DNA-modified vaccinia virus Ankara prime–boost vaccination regimen for murine tuberculosis. Infect Immun 2001; 69:681–686.

38. McShane H, et al. Protective immunity against Mycobacterium tuberculosis induced by dendritic cells pulsed with both CD8(+)- and CD4(+)-T-cell epitopes from antigen 85A. Infect Immun 2002; 70:1623–1626.

39. Pancholi P, et al. DNA prime/canarypox boost-based immunotherapy of chronic hepatitis B virus infection in a chimpanzee. Hepatology 2001; 33:448–454.

40. Kent SJ, et al. Enhanced T-cell immunogenicity and protective efficacy of a human immunodeficiency virus type 1 vaccine regimen consisting of consecutive priming with DNA and boosting with recombinant fowlpox virus. J Virol 1998; 72:10180–10188.

41. Hanke T, et al. Effective induction of simian immunodeficiency virus-specific cytotoxic T lymphocytes in macaques by using a multiepitope gene and DNA prime-modified vaccinia virus Ankara boost vaccination regimen. J Virol 1999; 73:7524–7532.

42. Amara RR, et al. Control of a mucosal challenge and prevention of AIDS by a multiprotein DNA/MVA vaccine. Science 2001; 292:69–74.

43. Amara RR, et al. Critical role for Env as well as Gag-Pol in control of a simian-human immunodeficiency virus 89.6P challenge by a DNA prime/recombinant modified vaccinia virus Ankara vaccine. J Virol 2002; 76:6138–6146.

44. Shiver JW, et al. Replication-incompetent adenoviral vaccine vector elicits effective anti-immunodeficiency-virus immunity. Nature 2002; 415:331–335.

45. Barouch DH, et al. Eventual AIDS vaccine failure in a rhesus monkey by viral escape from cytotoxic T lymphocytes. Nature 2002; 415:335–339.

46. Horton H, et al. Immunization of rhesus macaques with a DNA prime/modified vaccinia virus Ankara boost regimen induces broad simian immunodeficiency virus (SIV)-specific T-cell responses and reduces initial viral replication but does not prevent disease progression following challenge with pathogenic SIVmac239. J Virol 2002; 76:7187–7202.

47. McCluskie MJ, et al. Route and method of delivery of DNA vaccine influence immune responses in mice and non-human primates. Mol Med 1999; 5:287–300.

48. Amara RR, et al. Different patterns of immune responses but similar control of a simian-human immunodeficiency virus 89.6P mucosal challenge by modified vaccinia virus Ankara (MVA) and DNA/MVA vaccines. J Virol 2002; 76:7625–7631.

49. Barouch DH, et al. Reduction of simian-human immunodeficiency virus 89.6P viremia in rhesus monkeys by recombinant modified vaccinia virus Ankara vaccination. J Virol 2001; 75:5151–5158.

50. Sullivan NJ, et al. Development of a preventive vaccine for Ebola virus infection in primates. Nature 2000; 408:605–609.

51. Rogers WO, et al. Multistage multiantigen heterologous prime boost vaccine for *Plasmodium knowlesi* malaria provides partial protection in rhesus macaques. Infect Immun 2001; 69:5565–5572.

52. Rogers WO, et al. Protection of rhesus macaques against lethal *Plasmodium knowlesi* malaria by a heterologous DNA priming and poxvirus boosting immunization regimen. Infect Immun 2002; 70:4329–4335.

53. Langermans JA, et al. Divergent effect of bacillus Calmette–Guerin (BCG) vaccination on Mycobacterium tuberculosis infection in highly related macaque species: implications for primate models in tuberculosis vaccine research. Proc Natl Acad Sci USA 2001; 98:11497–11502.

54. Hill AV, et al. DNA-based vaccines for malaria: a heterologous prime–boost immunisation strategy. Dev Biol (Basel) 2000; 104:171–179.

54a. Moorthy VS, et al. Safety of DNA and modified vaccinia virus Ankara vaccines against liver-stage P. falciparum malaria in non-immune volunteers. Vaccine 2003; 21:2004–2011.

54b. McConkey SJ, et al. Enhanced T-cell immunogenicity of plasmid DNA vaccines boosted by recombinant modified vaccinia virus Ankara in humans. Nat Med 2003; 9:729–735.

55. Robson KJ, et al. Polymorphism of the TRAP gene of *Plasmodium falciparum*. Proc R Soc Lond B Biol Sci 1990; 242:205–216.

56. Boyer JD, et al. Vaccination of seronegative volunteers with a human immunodeficiency virus type 1 env/rev DNA vaccine induces antigen-specific proliferation and lymphocyte production of beta-chemokines. J Infect Dis 2000; 181:476–483.

57. Gupta K, et al. Safety and immunogenicity of a high-titered canarypox vaccine in combination with rgp120 in a diverse population of HIV-1-uninfected adults: AIDS Vaccine Evaluation Group Protocol 022A. J Acquir Immune Defic Syndr 2002; 29:254–261.

58. Evans TG, et al. Evaluation of canarypox-induced CD8(+) responses following immunization by measuring the effector population IFNgamma production. Immunol Lett 2001; 77:7–15.

59. Hanke T, McMichael AJ. Design and construction of an experimental HIV-1 vaccine for a year-2000 clinical trial in Kenya. Nat Med 2000; 6:951–955.

60. Wee EG, et al. A DNA/MVA-based candidate human immunodeficiency virus vaccine for Kenya induces multi-specific T cell responses in rhesus macaques. J Gen Virol 2002; 83:75–80.

61. Guidotti LG, Chisari FV. Noncytolytic control of viral infections by the innate and adaptive immune response. Annu Rev Immunol 2001; 19:65–91.

62. Marshall JL, et al. Phase I study in advanced cancer patients of a diversified prime-and-boost vaccination protocol using recombinant vaccinia virus and recombinant nonreplicating avipox virus to elicit anti-carcinoembryonic antigen immune responses. J Clin Oncol 2000; 18:3964–3973.

63. Sedegah M, et al. Improving protective immunity induced by DNA-based immunization: priming with antigen and GM-CSF-encoding plasmid DNA and boosting with antigen-expressing recombinant poxvirus. J Immunol 2000; 164:5905–5912.

64. Pancholi P, et al. DNA prime-canarypox boost with polycistronic hepatitis C virus (HCV) genes generates potent immune responses to HCV structural and nonstructural proteins. J Infect Dis 2000; 182:18–27.

65. Eo SK, et al. Prime–boost immunization with DNA vaccine: mucosal route of administration changes the rules. J Immunol 2001; 166:5473–5479.

66. van der Burg SH, et al. Pre-clinical safety and efficacy of TA-CIN, a recombinant HPV16 L2E6E7 fusion protein vaccine, in homologous and heterologous prime–boost regimens. Vaccine 2001; 19:3652–3660.

33

Mucosal Immunization and Needle-Free Injection Devices

Myron M. Levine and James D. Campbell
University of Maryland School of Medicine, Baltimore, Maryland, U.S.A.

I. INTRODUCTION

Currently, most vaccines are administered parenterally by needle and syringe. However, in industrialized countries, a proportion of children and adults have an aversion to injections. Therefore, administering vaccines without needles would be expected to increase compliance. Indeed, concern among parents about the number of injections that must be given to infants and toddlers in order to deliver the recommended vaccines has been a strong impetus for the development of infant combination vaccines. Moreover, the administration of vaccines by needle and syringe poses occupational safety risks for health care providers. This could emerge as a more substantive issue in the future should it become necessary to immunize large populations expeditiously in response to a bioterror or emerging infection emergency.

The role of needles and syringes in immunization practice is even more problematic in developing countries, where there are efforts to increase immunization coverage and to introduce new vaccines. Except for the oral polio vaccine, all the other vaccines recommended by the Expanded Program on Immunization (EPI) are given parenterally, using needles and syringes. However, in developing countries, injection safety is a notorious problem [1,2], as improper practices involving nonsterile needles and syringes (often used from one subject to another) cause abscesses and transmit bloodborne pathogens (e.g., hepatitis B and C and HIV) [2]. Although parenteral vaccination accounts for only a fraction of the injections given by health workers, nevertheless, immunization must be held to a higher standard because it involves healthy individuals. The Global Alliance for Vaccines and Immunization (GAVI) and its associated Vaccine Fund are addressing the difficulties faced by immunization services in developing countries. As part of its concept, GAVI supports the vision that immunization in the future would be more efficient, economical, and effective if all vaccines could be administered without the need for injection by needles.

Three broad strategies are being advocated for needle-free administration of vaccines, each with its own advan-tages [3]. The first strategy involves mucosal immunization; the second is based on injection using needle-free devices; the third involves transcutaneous immunization. Because transcutaneous immunization is covered in the chapter authored by Glenn, this chapter will limit itself to reviewing mucosal immunization and needle-free injection devices.

II. VACCINES DELIVERED VIA MUCOSAL SURFACES

A. Potential and Practical Mucosal Sites for Administering Vaccines

Whereas the human oral, nasal, rectal, conjunctival, and vaginal mucosa are all amenable to the application of vaccines for immunization, not all options are equally practical. For example, the rectal route, which is highly efficient at eliciting immune responses [4–6], would be unpopular in a number of cultures globally. Although antigens can be immunogenic after instillation into the conjunctival sac [7,8], some antigens might elicit conjunctival inflammation which, on occasion, might secondarily lead to purulent conjunctivitis. The vaginal mucosa, despite having relatively sparse inductive sites, can serve as a route for immunization against certain infections in females [9]. Thus, in practical terms, oral and nasal administration are the most suitable options for all ages and both genders [10].

B. Inductive Sites for Immune Responses

Aggregates of mucosa-associated lymphoid tissue are found along the mucosa of the gastrointestinal, respiratory, and genitourinary tracts. These include the gut-associated lymphoid tissue (GALT), bronchus-associated lymphoid tissue (BALT), and the nasal associated lymphoid tissues (NALT). Specialized microfold (M) cells overlying the mucosa-associated lymphoid tissues in the intestine and the nose constitute competent portals by which antigens (including vaccines) can reach the underlying inductive sites for initiation of immune responses [11]. These inductive sites are rich in antigen-presenting cells (macrophages, dendritic cells, etc.), in addition to the B and T lymphocytes that are present. Several reviews contain detailed descriptions of the anatomic architecture and cell types observed in the mucosa-associated lymphoid tissue [11–13].

The gastrointestinal and upper respiratory mucosa are constantly exposed to antigens from resident normal bacterial flora of the gut and nasopharynx, food, and inhaled materials. As a consequence, the mucosa of these anatomical sites can develop tolerance to an antigen, such that either a local immune response is not elicited or it is muted. This is more likely to occur if the antigen is delivered in a soluble form and given repetitively. Repetitive oral administration of a soluble antigen can also lead to systemic tolerance manifested by a diminished ability to mount an immune response upon parenteral administration of the same antigen [14]. Notably, as discussed later in this chapter, by administering the antigen of interest in a specialized delivery system or by coadministering strong adjuvants, potent immune mucosal and systemic responses can be elicited.

C. Immune Effector Responses

Mucosally administered vaccines work well in preventing infections limited to the mucosal surfaces (e.g., cholera) [15,16], or those caused by pathogens that invade via the mucosa (e.g., poliomyelitis, *Salmonella* Typhi) [17–19]. Dimeric secretory immunoglobulin A (SlgA) is, by far, the predominant immunoglobulin found in gastrointestinal and respiratory tract mucosal secretions, saliva, and breast milk. Mucosal SlgA can mediate protection by neutralizing toxins, preventing virus entry into cells, or by inhibiting the fimbriae and other virulence adhesins that bacteria utilize to attach to epithelial cell receptors.

Because of the preponderance of SlgA in mucosal secretions, steps involved in the generation of this effector response have been the most extensively studied. Initial exposure of naive B lymphocytes to antigen in inductive sites in the mucosa-associated lymphoid sites (e.g., Peyer's patches, NALT) and draining regional lymph nodes, is followed by clonal expansion, isotype switching, affinity maturation, and migration [20,21]. At approximately 7–10 days following the administration of the mucosal vaccine, the migrating cells can be detected as antibody secreting cells (ASCs) found among peripheral blood mononuclear cells [22–29]. Mucosal immunization predominantly elicits lgA ASCs that carry on their surface the $\alpha_4\beta_7$ homing receptor that directs them back to the lamina propria in mucosal sites [30,31]; they mainly return (but not exclusively) to the anatomic area from which they originated. The distribution of ASCs (mainly lgA) and memory B cells, upon their return to the mucosa, accounts for both the compartmentalization of the mucosal immune system (SlgA responses are usually strongest at the site of induction) and the phenomenon of the "common mucosal immune system" (whereby SlgA responses can often be detected in mucosal sites remote from the inductive site).

There is reason to believe that if the relevant immune responses can be generated, systemic infections (including those that do not involve initial invasion from a mucosal surface, e.g., malaria) and toxicoses (e.g., tetanus) can also be prevented by administering the appropriate vaccines via mucosal surfaces [32]. Indeed, properly formulated, mucosally administered vaccines can stimulate virtually any relevant type of immune response: serum lgG neutralizing antibodies against toxins [32–34] and viruses [35–37], and the full array of cell-mediated immune responses including lymphocyte proliferation [38,39], cytokine production [38], and $CD8^+$ cytotoxic lymphocyte activity [38,40–42], in addition to stimulating mucosal secretory lgA antibodies [25,43–48].

D. Duration of Protection Conferred by Mucosally Administered Vaccines

It was previously taught that vaccines administered via mucosal surfaces can only elicit relatively short-term protection. However, there are multiple examples of mucosal vaccines that have conferred long-term protection and have elicited long-lived immune responses that correlate with protection. For example, an enteric-coated capsule formulation of Ty21a live oral typhoid vaccine conferred 62% protection over 7 years of follow-up, and a more effective liquid formulation conferred 78% protection over 5 years of follow-up [49]. A prototype nonliving oral cholera vaccine consisting of B subunit and inactivated whole vibrios conferred 56% protection over 3 years of follow-up [50]. Titers of serum neutralizing antibody remain elevated for years following oral immunization with Sabin live oral polio vaccine [51].

E. Oral Vaccines

Both live and nonliving antigens can be delivered orally with good results. The trivalent attenuated Sabin poliovirus vaccine, the keystone of the global poliomyelitis eradication program, constitutes a paradigm that has encouraged the development and use of other live attenuated vaccines administered orally that have been licensed or are near licensure. The Sabin oral polio vaccine sets the standard for ease of administration to subjects of any age. Other licensed oral vaccines include the following: Ty21a [49,52], live oral cholera vaccine strain CVD 103-HgR [53], and nonliving cholera vaccines [16,54]. Overall, the experience with oral vaccines has been highly satisfactory. Nevertheless, problems have emerged. Postlicensure surveillance in the United States detected a rare association between tetravalent reassortant rhesus rotavirus vaccine and intestinal intussusception [55] that ultimately led to withdrawal of the vaccine from the market. As a consequence of this experience, new generation rotavirus vaccines that are under development are addressing the risk of possible intussusception through large prelicensure clinical trials.

Another problem that is being investigated is why some, particularly live, oral vaccines appear to be less immunogenic among individuals in developing countries, compared to their counterparts in industrialized countries [56,56–61]. Factors that can play a role include the presence of small bowel bacterial overgrowth [62], competing enteric viruses, or intestinal helminths [63].

Various platform technologies are creating promising oral vaccine candidates. These include bacterial and viral live vectors expressing foreign antigens [32,64–67], DNA vaccines administered directly [68–70] or via bacterial vectors [71–74], transgenic plant "edible vaccines" [75,76], and various nonliving antigen delivery systems (liposomes, proteosomes, polylactide/polyglycolide microspheres, etc.), among others. Clinical trials with these technologies have generated mixed results [32,75,77], some of which have been promising [32,75].

F. Nasal Vaccines

Nonliving and live antigens delivered nasally can also be highly immunogenic and protective. Indeed, in recent years considerable experience has been gained with an array of intranasal vaccines, recognizing that NALT is a particularly competent site for inducing immune responses. Based on its safety, immunogenicity and efficacy [78,79], live cold-adapted trivalent influenza vaccine, administered by a convenient single-use spray device that painlessly delivers vaccine to the nasal mucosa, has been licensed by the Food and Drug Administration (FDA) (albeit initially restricted to use in certain age groups).

Various soluble and particulate nonliving antigens have been administered intranasally with varying success. Research is seeking well-tolerated adjuvants and antigen delivery systems to enhance immunologic responses to nonliving vaccines administered via the nasal mucosal surface. Cholera toxin (CT) and heat-labile enterotoxin (LT) of enterotoxigenic *Escherichia coli* are powerful adjuvants that enhance local SIgA and serum antibody responses to coadministered soluble or particulate antigens. While these toxin adjuvants are unacceptable as human oral adjuvants (because as little as 5.0 μg can cause severe diarrhea) [80], they have been investigated for nasal administration. Wild-type LT adjuvant was incorporated into a nasal nonliving influenza vaccine used in Europe [81]. The vaccine was well tolerated and immunogenic in prelicensure clinical trials. However, postlicensure surveillance identified a likely association with cases of Bell's palsy, resulting in the withdrawal of that nasal influenza vaccine from the market. It is hypothesized that the promiscuous ganglioside binding mediated by the LT B subunits allowed toxin molecules to adsorb to facial nerve fibers and to translocate proximally, possibly resulting in neuronal damage [82].

Efforts have been made to develop adjuvants that retain the potency and versatility of LT and CT for enhancing immune responses to coadministered antigens, but with greatly improved safety profiles. One strategy has been to engineer mutant LT and CT molecules that exhibit reduced toxicity but retain adjuvanticity [83,84]. Theoretical safety concerns remain to be resolved with these proteins because, in some species, the unaltered ganglioside binding properties of the mutant LT and CT molecules allow uptake by nasal olfactory nerve fibers and retrograde transport to the olfactory lobes of the brain [82]. It is not known whether such neuronal transport of mutant LT and CT occurs in humans as well and, if so, what consequences might ensue. Accordingly, clinical trials using mutant toxins administered intranasally are carefully surveying for possible adverse effects.

Safer intranasal adjuvants must be developed to realize more fully the potential of intranasal immunization with nonliving antigens. Several encouraging breakthroughs have been reported. One attractive adjuvant, referred to as CTA1-DD, links enzymatically active subunit A of CT to an Ig receptor binding peptide [85], thereby targeting the immune system's B cells [85]. One may envision that adjuvants like CTA1-DD could be coadministered intranasally with existing diphtheria, tetanus, pertussis (DTP), hepatitis B virus (HBV), and Hib conjugate vaccines, as well as other relevant vaccines (e.g., pneumococcal and meningococcal conjugates, or common protein vaccines), resulting in the stimulation of potent mucosal and systemic immune responses.

Another promising approach involves the use of the mucoadhesive polycationic polysaccharide "chitosan" as an antigen delivery system. Chitosan increases the transport of antigen across the nasal epithelium by means altering intercellular tight junctions and decreases the mucociliary clearance of antigen [86,87]. In a Phase I human clinical trial, diphtheria toxin CRM_{197}, given intranasally in a chitosan delivery system, elicited significantly higher serum neutralizing antitoxin titers and SIgA antibodies than CRM_{197} administered without chitosan [34].

These encouraging intranasal vaccine delivery strategies still have major hurdles to overcome. One of the most important challenges will be to assess their effectiveness in immunizing infants in developing countries, recognizing that in such infants, upper respiratory infections and nasal discharge are highly prevalent.

G. Aerosol Measles Vaccine

Mass immunization campaigns in Latin America and pilot campaigns in Southern Africa with parenteral measles vaccine administered by needle and syringe have decreased measles incidence and mortality. Nevertheless, field experiences make it clear that such campaigns would be logistically simpler and safer if measles vaccine could be administered without needles. Measles vaccine administered by aerosol (creating small particles that reach the lung) is highly immunogenic and efficacious [35,88]. The early aerosol measles vaccine devices that generated the highly encouraging clinical results had limitations in rapidity, portability, or robustness. Much improved, more compact, simpler, and robust new devices are currently under evaluation in monkey studies and human clinical trials.

III. NEEDLE-FREE INJECTION DEVICES

A. Jet Injectors

Jet injectors are needle-free devices that propel liquid (nonliving or live) vaccine under high pressure through a minute orifice so that it pierces the integument to reach the dermis, subcutaneous tissue, or muscle, as desired. Needle-free jet injectors stimulate immune responses that are similar in magnitude and character to vaccine injected by needle and syringe. Vaccination with some jet injectors elicits higher rates of local reactions than needle and syringe. From the 1950s to the 1980s, high-workload, multiple-use-nozzle jet injectors were widely utilized in mass immunization campaigns in less-developed countries to deliver smallpox, measles, yellow fever, and other vaccines [89]. Multidose vials (containing up to 50 doses) permitted these devices to vaccinate 600–1000 subjects each hour using the same dose chamber, fluid path, and nozzle on consecutive subjects. The dosing chamber was automatically replenished from the multidose vial following each injection. In the mid-1980s, it came to be recognized that multiple-use-nozzle jet injectors could inadvertently transmit blood-borne infections (e.g., hepatitis B), albeit rarely [90]. Safety concerns stemming from the emerging global pandemic of HIV led health authorities to discontinue the utilization of the high-workload, multiple-use-nozzle jet injectors.

The anthrax emergency in the USA in late 2001 has prompted public health authorities to contemplate how they might conduct mass immunization campaigns if their jurisdiction is confronted by a bioterror event. Concern over how to administer, en masse and rapidly, vaccines against bioterror agents has reawakened interest in new high workload devices. One device of interest is a multiple-use-nozzle jet injector that incorporates a disposable cap to reduce the risk of splash back of blood or serum onto the nozzle after injection. Other injectors of interest employ disposable cartridges that disable after use. If large clinical trials convincingly document the safety of these devices, they could be utilized in mass campaigns in developing countries

(e.g., against measles and meningitis) as well as for use in campaigns in industrialized countries.

Single-dose jet injector devices also exist for administering vaccines under lower workload situations. These devices utilize disposable cartridges and nozzles for individual patients to avoid cross contamination [91]. Currently, in physician's offices and clinics in industrialized countries, some needle-free injection devices (e.g., Biojector 2000®) (Figure 1) are employed to administer vaccines to subjects who have extreme aversion to needles, and to avoid needle-stick injuries among health care workers [91,92]. These devices are not yet affordable for routine use in developing countries. A perceived drawback of the current devices in some venues is that vaccine must be transferred from its vial into the cartridge by means of a needle or special adaptor; this could pose safety problems in developing country settings [93]. On the other hand, this intermediate step is advantageous for reconstituting lyophilized vaccines. The need for the intermediate step could be entirely eliminated if manufacturers prefilled vaccines directly into universal standard single-dose cartridges that could fit a variety of injectors. One such experimental system, the Imule® cartridge [94], when inserted into a hand-wound spring-powered injector (Mini-Imojet®) [94], gave promising results in pediatric and adult clinical vaccine trials in both industrialized and developing countries [94].

A yet-to-be licensed needle-free jet injector that is highly promising, particularly from the purview of logistical practicality and ergonomics, is LectraJet HS® (Figure 2). This high-speed jet injection system has been designed as a "kit,"

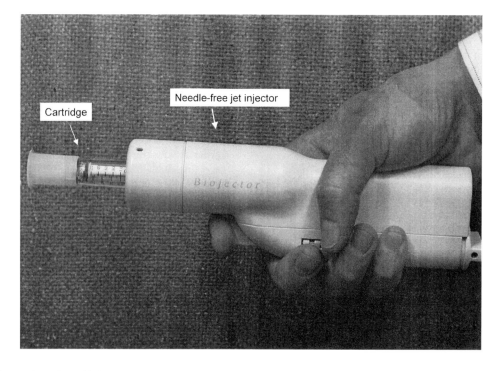

Figure 1 Biojector 2000®, a high-pressure, gas-driven, needle-free jet injector licensed by the FDA for the intramuscular or subcutaneous administration of vaccines. By attaching this device to a large tank of CO_2, it can be adapted for use in high-workload situations.

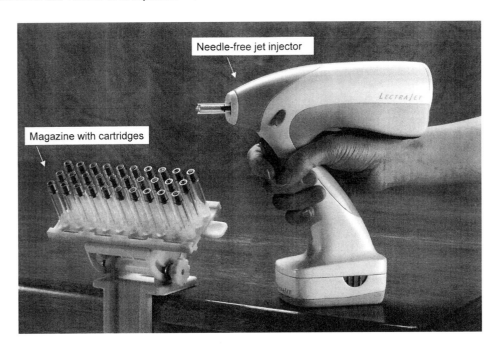

Figure 2 LectraJet HS®, a promising (but as yet unlicensed) high-workload, ergonomic jet injection system with disposable, single-use vaccine cartridges (shown in a multiple-cartridge magazine). (Published with permission of the manufacturer, DCI, Inc.)

containing everything needed for a large-scale, high-workload scenario. The system uses an individual auto-disable cartridge for each patient that is filled on-site. To maximize speed during high workload situations, the prefilled cartridge is extracted from a "magazine," the injection is administered, the used cartridge is discarded into a trash receptacle with the push of a button, and the injector is then ready to rearm with another cartridge from the magazine. The LectraJet HS® is electrically powered via rechargeable batteries or via an electrical outlet. For use in developing countries, where electrical power may not be reliable, manual power is also available. Notably, in addition to their usefulness in delivering a variety of protein and polysaccharides subunit vaccines, polysaccharide–protein conjugates, combination vaccines, and live attenuated viral vaccines, needle-free devices have also successfully delivered DNA vaccines in clinical trials [95].

IV. SUMMARY COMMENT

Advances in mucosal immunization, improved needle-free injection devices, and the rapidly developing field of transcutaneous immunization all engender optimism that vaccines will be increasingly administered without the need for needles. Because each of these strategies has its own particular advantages, it is likely that all three will be needed to realize the ultimate vision when all immunizations in all age groups will be administered without needles.

REFERENCES

1. Aylward B, et al. Reducing the risk of unsafe injections in immunization programmes: financial and operational implications of various injection technologies. Bull WHO 1995; 73:531–540.
2. Simonsen L, et al. Unsafe injections in the developing world and transmission of bloodborne pathogens: a review. Bull WHO 1999; 77:789–800.
3. Levine MM. Can needle-free administration of vaccines become the norm in global immunization? Nat Med 2003; 9: 99–103.
4. Forrest BD, et al. Specific immune response in humans following rectal delivery of live typhoid vaccine. Vaccine 1990; 8:209–211.
5. Kantele A, et al. Differences in immune responses induced by oral and rectal immunizations with *Salmonella typhi* Ty21a: evidence for compartmentalization within the common mucosal immune system in humans. Infect Immun 1998; 66: 5630–5635.
6. Jertborn M, et al. Local and systemic immune responses to rectal administration of recombinant cholera toxin B subunit in humans. Infect Immun 2001; 69:4125–4128.
7. Black FL, Sheridan SR. Studies on an attenuated measles-virus vaccine: IV. Administration of vaccine by several routes. N Engl J Med 1960; 263:165–169.
8. McCrumb FR Jr., et al. Studies with live attenuated measles-virus vaccine: I. Clinical and immunologic responses in institutionalized children. Am J Dis Child 1961; 101:689–700.
9. Kozlowski PA, et al. Mucosal vaccination strategies for women. J Infect Dis 1999; 179(suppl 3):S493–S498.
10. Levine MM, Dougan G. Optimism over vaccines administered via mucosal surfaces. Lancet 1998; 351:1375–1376.
11. Neutra MR, et al. Epithelial M cells: gateways for mucosal infection and immunization. Cell 1996; 86:345–348.
12. Brandtzaeg P, et al. Mucosal immunity—a major adaptive defence mechanism. Behring Inst Mitt 1997; 98:1–23.
13. Farstad IN, et al. Immunoglobulin A cell distribution in the human small intestine: phenotypic and functional characteristics. Immunology 2000; 101:354–363.
14. Czerkinsky C, et al. Mucosal immunity and tolerance: relevance to vaccine development. Immunol Rev 1999; 170:197–222.

15. Tacket CO, et al. Randomized, double-blind, placebo-controlled, multicentered trial of the efficacy of a single dose of live oral cholera vaccine CVD 103-HgR in preventing cholera following challenge with *Vibrio cholerae* O1 El Tor Inaba three months after vaccination. Infect Immun 1999; 67:6341–6345.

16. Sanchez JL, et al. Protective efficacy of oral whole-cell/recombinant-B-subunit cholera vaccine in Peruvian military recruits. Lancet 1994; 344:1273–1276.

17. Sabin AB. Oral poliovirus vaccine. History of its development and prospects for eradication of poliomyelitis. J Am Med Assoc 1965; 194:130–134.

18. Levine MM, et al. Large-scale field trial of Ty21a live oral typhoid vaccine in enteric-coated capsule formulation. Lancet 1987; 1:1049–1052.

19. Levine MM, et al. Comparison of enteric-coated capsules and liquid formulation of Ty21a typhoid vaccine in randomised controlled field trial. Lancet 1990; 336:891–894.

20. McHeyzer-Williams MG, Ahmed R. B cell memory and the long-lived plasma cell. Curr Opin Immunol 1999; 11:172–179.

21. Manz RA, et al. Humoral immunity and long-lived plasma cells. Curr Opin Immunol 2002; 14:517–521.

22. Kantele A. Antibody-secreting cells in the evaluation of the immunogenicity of an oral vaccine. Vaccine 1990; 8:321–326.

23. Tacket CO, et al. Clinical acceptability and immunogenicity of CVD 908 *Salmonella typhi* vaccine strain. Vaccine 1992; 10:443–446.

24. Jertborn M, et al. Dose-dependent circulating immunoglobulin. A antibody-secreting cell and serum antibody responses in Swedish volunteers to an oral inactivated enterotoxigenic *Escherichia coli* vaccine. Clin Diagn Lab Immunol 2001; 8:424–428.

25. Jertborn M, et al. Intestinal and systemic immune responses in humans after oral immunization with a bivalent B subunit-O1/O139 whole cell cholera vaccine. Vaccine 1996; 14:1459–1465.

26. Losonsky GA, et al. Secondary *Vibrio cholerae*-specific cellular antibody responses following wild-type homologous challenge in people vaccinated with CVD 103-HgR live oral cholera vaccine: changes with time and lack of correlation with protection. Infect Immun 1993; 61:729–733.

27. Kotloff KL, et al. Safety, immunogenicity, and transmissibility in humans of CVD 1203, a live oral *Shigella flexneri* 2a vaccine candidate attenuated by deletions in aroA and virG. Infect Immun 1996; 64:4542–4548.

28. Kotloff KL, et al. *Shigella flexneri* 2a Strain CVD 1207, with specific deletions in virG, sen, set, and guaBA, is highly attenuated in humans. Infect Immun 2000; 68:1034–1039.

29. Van de Verg L, et al. Specific immunoglobulin A-secreting cells in peripheral blood of humans following oral immunization with a bivalent *Salmonella typhi–Shigella sonnei* vaccine or infection by pathogenic *S. sonnei*. Infect Immun 1990; 58:2002–2004.

30. Kantele A, et al. Homing potentials of circulating lymphocytes in humans depend on the site of activation: oral, but not parenteral, typhoid vaccination induces circulating antibody-secreting cells that all bear homing receptors directing them to the gut. J Immunol 1997; 158:574–579.

31. Quiding-Jarbrink M, et al. Induction of compartmentalized B-cell responses in human tonsils. Infect Immun 1995; 63:853–857.

32. Tacket CO, et al. Safety and immune responses to attenuated *Salmonella enterica* serovar typhi oral live vector vaccines expressing tetanus toxin fragment C. Clin Immunol 2000; 97:146–153.

33. Aggerbeck H, et al. Intranasal booster vaccination against diphtheria and tetanus in man. Vaccine 1997; 15:307–316.

34. Mills KH, et al. Protective levels of diphtheria-neutralizing antibody induced in healthy volunteers by unilateral priming–boosting intranasal immunization associated with restricted ipsilateral mucosal secretory immunoglobulin a. Infect Immun 2003; 71:726–732.

35. Dilraj A, et al. Response to different measles vaccine strains given by aerosol and subcutaneous routes to schoolchildren: a randomised trial. Lancet 2000; 355:798–803.

36. Dilraj A, et al. Persistence of measles antibody two years after revaccination by aerosol or subcutaneous routes. Pediatr Infect Dis J 2000; 19:1211–1213.

37. Faden H, et al. Comparative evaluation of immunization with live attenuated and enhanced-potency inactivated trivalent poliovirus vaccines in childhood: systemic and local immune responses. J Infect Dis 1990; 162:1291–1297.

38. Sztein MB, et al. Cytokine production patterns and lymphoproliferative responses in volunteers orally immunized with attenuated vaccine strains of *Salmonella typhi*. J Infect Dis 1994; 170:1508–1517.

39. Murphy JR, et al. Characteristics of humoral and cellular immunity to *Salmonella typhi* in residents of typhoid-endemic and typhoid-free regions. J Infect Dis 1987; 156:1005–1009.

40. Sztein MB, et al. Cytotoxic T lymphocytes after oral immunization with attenuated vaccine strains of *Salmonella typhi* in humans. J Immunol 1995; 155:3987–3993.

41. Salerno-Goncalves R, et al. Characterization of CD8(+) effector T cell responses in volunteers immunized with *Salmonella enterica* serovar Typhi strain Ty21a typhoid vaccine. J Immunol 2002; 169:2196–2203.

42. Salerno-Goncalves R, et al. Concomitant Induction of CD4(+) and CD8(+) T cell responses in volunteers immunized with *Salmonella enterica* serovar typhi strain CVD 908-htrA. J Immunol 2003; 170:2734–2741.

43. Losonsky GA, et al. Systemic and mucosal immune responses to rhesus rotavirus vaccine MMU 18006. Pediatr Infect Dis J 1988; 7:388–393.

44. Forrest BD. Impairment of immunogenicity of *Salmonella typhi* Ty21a due to preexisting cross-reacting intestinal antibodies. J Infect Dis 1992; 166:210–212.

45. Sarasombath S, et al. Systemic and intestinal immunities after different typhoid vaccinations. Asian Pacific J Allergy Immunol 1987; 5:53–61.

46. Clements ML, et al. Advantage of live attenuated cold-adapted influenza A virus over inactivated vaccine for A/Washington/80 (H_3N_2) wild-type virus infection. Lancet 1984; 1:705–708.

47. Ogra PL, Karzon DT. Distribution of poliovirus antibody in serum, nasopharynx and alimentary tract following segmental immunization of lower alimentary tract with poliovaccine. J Immunol 1969; 102:1423–1430.

48. Ogra PL, Karzon DT. Poliovirus antibody response in serum and nasal secretions following intranasal inoculation with inactivated poliovaccine. J Immunol 1969; 102:15–23.

49. Levine MM, et al. Duration of efficacy of ty21a, attenuated salmonella typhi live oral vaccine. Vaccine 1999; 17(suppl 2):S22–S27.

50. Clemens JD, et al. Field trial of cholera vaccines in Bangladesh: results from three year follow-up. Lancet 1990; 335:270–273.

51. Rousseau WE, et al. Persistence of poliovirus neutralizing antibodies eight years after immunization with live, attenuated-virus vaccine. N Engl J Med 1973; 289:1357–1359.

52. Levine MM, et al. Typhoid vaccines come of age. Pediatr Infect Dis J 1989; 8:374–381.

53. Levine MM, Kaper JB. Live oral cholera vaccine: from principle to product. Bull Inst Pasteur 1995; 93:243–253.

54. Trach DD, et al. Field trial of a locally produced, killed, oral cholera vaccine in Vietnam. Lancet 1997; 349:231–235.

55. Murphy TV, et al. Intussusception among infants given an oral rotavirus vaccine. N Engl J Med 2001; 344:564–572.

56. John TJ, Jayabal P. Oral polio vaccination of children in the

tropics: I. The poor seroconversion rates and the absence of viral interference. Am J Epidemiol 1972; 96:263–269.

57. Gotuzzo E, et al. Safety, immonogenicity, and excretion pattern of single-dose live oral cholera vaccine CVD 103-HgR in Peruvian adults of high and low socioeconomic levels. Infect Immun 1993; 61:3994–3997.

58. Hanlon P, et al. Trial of an attenuated bovine rotavirus vaccine (RIT 4237) in Gambian infants. Lancet 1987; 1: 1342–1345.

59. Suharyono, et al. Safety and immunogenicity of single-dose live oral cholera vaccine CVD 103-HgR in 5–9-year-old Indonesian children. Lancet 1992; 340:689–694.

60. John TJ. Problems with oral poliovaccine in India. Indian Pediatr 1972; 9:252–256.

61. Patriarca PA, et al. Factors affecting the immunogenicity of oral poliovirus vaccine in developing countries: review. Rev Infect Dis 1991; 13:926–929.

62. Lagos R, et al. Effect of small bowel bacterial overgrowth on the immunogenicity of single-dose live oral cholera vaccine CVD 103-HgR. J Infect Dis 1999; 180:1709–1712.

63. Cooper PJ, et al. Albendazole treatment of children with ascariasis enhances the vibriocidal antibody response to the live attenuated oral cholera vaccine CVD 103-HgR. J Infect Dis 2000; 182:1199–1206.

64. Gonzalez C, et al. *Salmonella typhi* vaccine strain CVD 908 expressing the circumsporozoite protein of *Plasmodium falciparum*: strain construction and safety and immunogenicity in humans. J Infect Dis 1994; 169:927–931.

65. Monath TP, et al. Clinical proof of principle for ChimeriVax: recombinant live, attenuated vaccines against flavivirus infections. Vaccine 2002; 20:1004–1018.

66. Belshe RB, et al. Safety and immunogencity of a canarypox-vectored human immunodeficiency virus Type 1 vaccine with or without gp120: a phase 2 study in higher- and lower-risk volunteers. J Infect Dis 2001; 183:1343–1352.

67. Bland J, Clements J. Protecting the world's children: the story of WHO's immunization programme. World Health Forum 1998; 19:162–173.

68. Bartholomeusz RCA, et al. Gut immunity to typhoid—the immune response to a live oral typhoid vaccine, Ty21a. J Gastroenterol Hepatol 1986; 1:61–67.

69. Wu Y, et al. M cell-targeted DNA vaccination. Proc Natl Acad Sci U S A 2001; 98:9318–9323.

70. Link H, et al. Vaccination with autologous dendritic cells: from experimental autoimmune encephalomyelitis to multiple sclerosis. J Neuroimmunol 2001; 114:1–7.

71. Pasetti MF, et al. Attenuated ΔguaBA *Salmonella typhi* vaccine strain CVD 915 as a live vector utilizing prokaryotic or eukaryotic expression systems to deliver foreign antigens and elicit immune responses. Clin Immunol 1999; 92:76–89.

72. Anderson R, et al. ΔguaBA attenuated *Shigella flexneri* 2a strain CVD 1204 as a *Shigella* vaccine and as a live mucosal system for fragment C of tetanus toxin. Vaccine 2000; 18:2193–2202.

73. Fennelly GJ, et al. Mucosal DNA vaccine immunization against measles with a highly attenuated *Shigella flexneri* vector. J Immunol 1999; 162:1603–1610.

74. Shata MT, Hone DM. Vaccination with a *Shigella* DNA vaccine vector induces antigen-specific CD8(+) T cells and antiviral protective immunity. J Virol 2001; 75:9665–9670.

75. Tacket CO, et al. Immunogenicity in humans of a recombinant bacterial antigen delivered in a transgenic potato. Nat Med 1998; 4:607–609.

76. Tacket CO, et al. Human immune responses to a novel norwalk virus vaccine delivered in transgenic potatoes. J Infect Dis 2000; 182:302–305.

77. Tacket CO, et al. Enteral immunization and challenge of volunteers given enterotoxigenic *E. coli* CFA/II encapsulated in biodegradable microspheres. Vaccine 1994; 12:1270–1274.

78. Belshe RB, et al. The efficacy of live attenuated, cold-adapted, trivalent, intranasal influenza virus vaccine in children. N Engl J Med 1998; 338:1405–1412.

79. King JC Jr., et al. Safety and immunogenicity of low and high doses of trivalent live cold-adapted influenza vaccine administered intranasally as drops or spray to healthy children. J Infect Dis 1998; 177:1394–1397.

80. Levine M, et al. New knowledge on pathogenesis of bacterial enteric infections as applied to vaccine development. Microbiol Rev 1983; 47:510–550.

81. Gluck R, et al. Safety and immunogenicity of intranasally administered inactivated trivalent virosome-formulated influenza vaccine containing *Escherichia coli* heat-labile toxin as a mucosal adjuvant. J Infect Dis 2000; 181:1129–1132.

82. Van Ginkel FW, et al. Cutting edge: the mucosal adjuvant cholera toxin redirects vaccine proteins into olfactory tissues. J Immunol 2000; 165:4778–4782.

83. Douce G, et al. Mutants of *Escherichia coli* heat-labile toxin lacking ADP-ribosyltransferase activity act as nontoxic, mucosal adjuvants. Proc Natl Acad Sci U S A 1995; 92: 1644–1648.

84. Yamamoto S, et al. Mutants in the ADP-ribosyltransferase cleft of cholera toxin lack diarrhea genicity but retain adjuvanticity. J Exp Med 1997; 185:1203–1210.

85. Agren LC, et al. Adjuvanticity of the cholera toxin A1-based gene fusion protein, CTA1-DD, is critically dependent on the ADP-ribosyltransferase and Ig-binding activity. J Immunol 1999; 162:2432–2440.

86. Aspden TJ, et al. Chitosan as a nasal delivery system: the effect of chitosan solutions on in vitro and in vivo mucociliary transport rates in human turbinates and volunteers. J Pharm Sci 1997; 86:509–513.

87. Bacon A, et al. Carbohydrate biopolymers enhance antibody response to mucosally delivered vaccine antigens. Infect Immun 2000; 68:5764–5770.

88. Fernandez-de Castro J, et al. La vacunacion antisarampionosa en Mexico por el metodo de aerosol. Salud Publ Mex 1997; 39:53–60.

89. Hingson RA, et al. The historical development of jet injection and envisioned uses in mass immunization and mass therapy based upon two decades experience. Milit Med 1963; 128:516–524.

90. Canter J, et al. An outbreak of hepatitis B associate with jet injections in a weight reduction clinic. Arch Intern Med 1990; 150:1923–1927.

91. Cohen Reis E, et al. Taking the sting out of shots: control of vaccination-associated pain and adverse reactions. Pediatr Ann 1998; 27:375–386.

92. Jackson LA, et al. Safety and immunogenicity of varying dosages of trivalent inactivated influenza vaccine administered by needle-free jet injectors. Vaccine 2001; 19:4703–4709.

93. Jodar L, et al. Ensuring vaccine safety in immunization programmes—a WHO perspective. Vaccine 2001; 19:1594–1605.

94. Parent dC I, et al. Clinical immunogenicity and tolerance studies of liquid vaccines delivered by jet-injector and a new single-use cartridge (Imule): comparison with standard syringe injection. Imule Investigators Group. Vaccine 1997; 15:449–458.

95. Roy MJ, et al. Induction of antigen-specific CD8+ T cells, T helper cells, and protective levels of antibody in humans by particle-mediated administration of a hepatitis B virus DNA vaccine. Vaccine 2000; 19:764–778.

34

Transcutaneous Immunization

Gregory M. Glenn and Richard T. Kenney
IOMAI Corporation, Gaithersburg, Maryland, U.S.A.

I. INTRODUCTION

Transcutaneous immunization (TCI) and skin immune system targeting techniques are new vaccine delivery methods poised to have a major impact on approaches to immunization. Previously, the skin was seen as an impervious barrier for large molecules such as antigens and as an obstacle for vaccine delivery. Recently, our work and those of others have shown that the skin, most especially the epidermis, is an accessible and competent immune environment that is suitable for vaccine delivery. This led to a host of recent work that has focused on antigen delivery into the skin using a patch or similar means, and the establishment of a new vaccine delivery paradigm.

There are several compelling reasons to consider the skin as an important site for vaccine delivery. First, the skin contains a readily accessible and dense population of highly efficient antigen-presenting cells (APCs), which are an attractive target for vaccine delivery. Second, the newest and most promising vaccine developments encompass a variety of strategies for immunostimulation that enhance and focus the immune response to specific antigens. However, the advantages of immunostimulation are inevitably accompanied by acute safety risks associated with systemic adverse reactions to the immunostimulating compounds. Delivery of very potent immunostimulating compounds to the skin holds great promise for avoiding this complication. Thus, we suggest that the primary reason for considering the skin as a target for vaccine delivery is the potential for safe and potent immunostimulation. However, there are also practical aspects to patch-based skin delivery strategies that make this approach attractive. The Centers for Disease Control and Prevention, the World Health Organization, and the Global Alliance for Vaccines and Immunization have rated needle-free delivery as a priority for new development in vaccine delivery due to the risk of needle-born transmission of disease and hopes for increased compliance [1,2]. The simplicity of skin delivery strategies would improve access to and compliance with vaccination globally. In the developing world, needle-free administration of vaccines across the skin would diminish the inadvertent transmission of infection (hepatitis B, hepatitis C, and human immunodeficiency virus) by reused, improperly sterilized needles and syringes.

In this chapter, we describe the scientific rationale for TCI as a strategy that counters some long-held notions regarding skin penetration and immune responses in the skin. We also briefly review the interactions between Langerhans cell (LC) biology and both adjuvants and microbes delivered into the skin. We then focus on the growing body of data showing that transcutaneous immunization results in relevant and robust immune responses. Finally, we discuss the near-term goals and development hurdles faced by skin immune system targeting strategies.

II. BARRIERS AND TARGETS FOR TRANSCUTANEOUS IMMUNIZATION

Transcutaneous immunization is a vaccine delivery technique that focuses on delivery of vaccine components through the stratum corneum (SC) into the skin. The stratum corneum, the outer protective layer of the epidermis, is composed principally of quiescent, keratin-filled epidermal cells encased in a mortar of surrounding lipids that are secreted by maturing keratinocytes (Figure 1). The stratum corneum is widely accepted as the principal barrier to penetration [3]. The living epidermis that underlies the SC is composed primarily (95%) of epidermal keratinocytes, but also includes a significant population (3–5%) of immune surveillance cells [4] called Langerhans cells (Figure 1). In fact, 25% of the total skin surface area in humans is undergirded by Langerhans cells, which are evenly distributed among the viable keratinocytes [5]. Langerhans cells thus form an extensive, highly superficial network barrier of immune cells at the very surface of the skin. The considerable dedication of biological resources committed to immune surveillance in the superficial layers of the skin indicates that the SC is often penetrated by microbes, and suggests that it could be penetrated for purposes of immunization. The fact that TCI has been used in mice, rabbits, guinea pigs, cats,

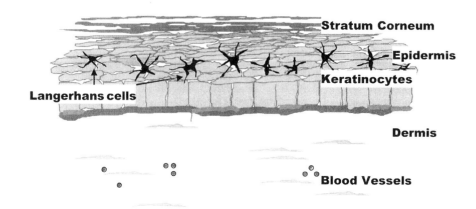

Figure 1 Langerhans cells are found in the epidermis among epidermal keratinocytes and represent highly superficial immune surveillance cells.

dogs, cattle, sheep, and humans has validated this premise [6–8].

Several strategies have emerged for the penetration of the SC. Occlusion, wetting of the skin, and other techniques lead to hydration of the SC. Hydration of the SC results in swelling of the keratinocytes, pooling of fluid in the intercellular spaces, and dramatic microscopic changes in the SC structure [9]; yet, remarkably, these changes have no lasting effect once the skin is allowed to dry. Hydrated SC clearly allows antigens to pass through the skin, although the transit pathways utilized by antigens to traverse the stratum corneum are unknown at this time. Transdermal drug delivery of polar drugs is thought to occur through aqueous intercellular channels formed between the keratinocytes, and it is reasonable to presume similar pathways for antigen delivery [9]. It has been important to conceptually differentiate TCI—the delivery of antigens (which are relatively large molecules) through the SC to the epidermal immune cells—from transdermal drug delivery. The latter generally delivers relatively small molecules through the epidermis and basement membrane, then into the dermis to blood vessels where the drug is adsorbed and carried to distant sites. The importance of this distinction in terminology is illustrated by the widely held maxim that only molecules < 500–1000 Da could penetrate the skin [3,10, 11]. Although this may be true for transdermal delivery of drugs, which have a tortuous and long pathway through the skin, we have definitively shown that very large antigens can be delivered into the skin using TCI [7,12,13]. Because the SC is the limiting barrier for penetration by both transcutaneous and transdermal techniques, the techniques and materials utilized (patches, formulations, and packaging) have provided a wealth of practical strategies for vaccine delivery to the skin.

The SC is breached by hair follicles and sweat ducts. These appendages are thought to play only a minor role in transdermal drug delivery [3]. Despite some evidence in mice that TCI using DNA may utilize hair follicles as a pathway for skin penetration [14], hair follicles and sweat glands are unlikely to be a significant pathway for vaccine and adjuvant delivery to skin dendritic cells [15–17]. This is supported by

the observation that outbred CD1 mice with normal hair follicle development and hairless SKH mice with sparse vestigial follicles respond equally well to topical immunization with tetanus toxoid (TTx) adjuvanted with heat-labile enterotoxin from *Escherichia coli* (LT). CD1 mice develop high-titer (ELISA units, EU = 652,000) serum IgG to tetanus that is not significantly different from the immune response elicited by hairless SKH mice (EU = 941,000) [17a].

A more likely pathway for vaccine delivery is by passive diffusion of vaccine and adjuvant from the skin surface into the most superficial cell layers in the epidermis. Simultaneous loading of antigen and GM1 receptor-mediated binding of LT by LCs is a more direct and efficient way to deliver vaccines and antigens into the skin. Although the most significant barrier to topical immunization is the SC, it is a fragile barrier that can be easily disrupted, allowing antigens to more readily diffuse to the target cell population. This concept is demonstrated when split virus influenza vaccine (A/Panama) adjuvanted with LT is applied to intact skin that has been pretreated to disrupt the SC. As illustrated in Figure 2, shaved intact mouse skin was hydrated with saline, or the skin was pretreated with emery paper (10 strokes) to disrupt the SC, or the SC was disrupted with D-Squame tape (10×) or 3M™ tape (10×). Immediately following the pretreatment, a solution containing 25 μg of A/Panama and 10 μg of LT was applied to the pretreated skin for 1 hr and rinsed to remove excess vaccine. After three immunizations every other week, serum was collected and evaluated for antibody titers to A/Panama. As illustrated in Figure 2, the serum antibody response to topical immunization was increased 10-fold to 300-fold by disrupting the SC immediately prior to topical application of the influenza vaccine with the LT adjuvant. The magnitude of the immune response is highly dependent upon codelivery of LT with the antigen, which provides the essential second signal necessary for the activation and mobilization of antigen-loaded LCs. Disruption of the SC as described is not normally accompanied by clinically apparent local reactions. The combination of hydration and SC disruption, using a swab or similar simple step, may improve the efficiency and therefore enhance the immune responses to

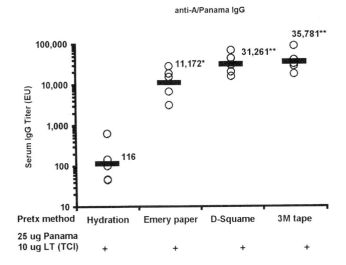

Figure 2 Improved topical delivery of influenza split virus vaccine by disruption of the stratum corneum. C57BL/6 mice were shaved on the dorsal caudal surface 2 days prior to topical immunization. Exposed skin was hydrated by gently rubbing (20 strokes) with a saline-saturated gauze sponge. The SC was disrupted by mild abrasion with emery paper (10 soft strokes) or tape stripping with D-Squame (10×) or 3M tape (10×). A solution consisting of 25 µg of A/Panama and 10 µg of LT was applied to the pretreated skin for 1 hr and then washed off with warm water. Groups were immunized three times (days 0, 14, and 28) and serum was collected 2 weeks after the third immunization on day 42. Serum antibody titers to A/Panama were determined by enzyme-linked immunosorbent assay (ELISA), and titers were reported as ELISA units, the serum dilution equal to 1 OD unit at 405 nm. The geometrical mean titer for each group is indicated. Serum elicited by hydration pretreatment was compared to antibody titers elicited by skin pretreatment with emery paper or tape stripping. *$P = 0.012$; **$P \leq 0.006$.

antigens delivered by this method, while continuing to be well tolerated and practical.

III. ADJUVANTS AND TRANSCUTANEOUS IMMUNIZATION

Adjuvants are used to augment the immune response to vaccine antigens as well as to direct the qualitative response, and are amply discussed elsewhere [18]. The induction of robust immune responses following TCI is dependent on the presence of an adjuvant in the formulation [6,12,19,20]. The use of adjuvants targeting potent APCs opens a host of possibilities for manipulation of the immune response and for enhancement of efficacy through augmentation of the immune response.

The greatest experience using adjuvants for TCI has been with the bacterial ADP-ribosylating exotoxins (bAREs), which include cholera toxin (CT), LT [21–25], and their mutants [18,20,26]. Bacterial ADP-ribosylating exotoxins have had extensive use as adjuvants via intranasal and oral routes and have generated data that can be applied

to their use on the skin. Transcutaneous immunization is similar to intranasal or oral immunization, as the simple admixture of CT or LT with a coadministered antigen such as TTx or influenza hemagglutinin results in markedly higher antibody levels compared to the administration of antigens alone, which can themselves elicit immune responses [6,12,20]. Similarly, bAREs administered either intranasally or by TCI can induce cellular immune responses to coadministered antigens mediated by CD4$^+$ or CD8$^+$ T-cells [16,27–29].

Among the bAREs, there are several adjuvant choices for TCI. Native CT and LT cause diarrhea when mixed in buffer solution and ingested by fasting subjects [23,30]. Accordingly, mutant toxins that have adjuvant activity similar to the native toxins but are much less prone to induce gastrointestinal side effects have been engineered should a skin patch containing the adjuvant be inadvertently ingested [26,29]. However, these side effects are of little relevance to TCI. Purified cholera toxin B-subunit (pCTB), which harbors trace amounts of holotoxin, is also a potent adjuvant on the skin in contrast to recombinant CTB (rCTB), which is far less potent but readily induces anti-CTB antibodies [20]. Other adjuvants, including bacterial DNA, cytokines, and LPS, have been shown to act as adjuvants, but their comparative potency on the skin needs to be evaluated [20]. However, the data suggest that a wide variety of adjuvants function in the context of the skin.

IV. LANGERHANS CELLS AND TRANSCUTANEOUS IMMUNIZATION

Langerhans cells are thought to be the principal target in TCI. They are bone marrow-derived APCs that migrate to and reside in the epidermis, where they sample antigens and migrate out of the skin in low numbers to the draining lymph nodes. Langerhans cells are known to increase their rate of migration out of the skin in response to activating stimuli such as infectious agents, adjuvants, contact sensitizers, and cytokines, and to travel to the lymph node where antigen presentation to T cells occurs [4]. In immune pathologies, such as topically induced delayed-type hypersensitivity (DTH), sensitized T cells generated from previous antigen exposure migrate back to a site where antigen is present in the skin and produce local inflammation [31], but this afferent arm of DTH is not a necessary or typical component of TCI. This is best illustrated in human immunization studies using multiple applications of LT that can induce robust boostable immune responses in the absence of clinical or histological evidence of DTH [7], and have been confirmed in other laboratories [32,33].

The role of LCs in TCI is not fully characterized at this time, but there are accumulating data that clearly implicate the LC as the principal target. Intradermal administration of adjuvants, including bacterial DNA (CPGs as well as *E. coli* DNA), LPS, or TNFα as LC activators [4,34,35], induces classical markers of LC activation by FACS analysis of LCs in epidermal digests, including upregulation of MHC class II and the costimulatory molecule CD86, and downregulation of E-cadherin (mediates LC adhesion to keratinocytes). Morphological changes and depletion of LCs from the epidermis in response to topical application of contact sensitizers, intradermally delivered LPS and cytokines [36], or viruses [37,38] are readily observed in stained epidermal sheets. After topical application of CT, LCs from epidermal sheet digests analyzed by flow cytometry similarly demonstrate upregulation of MHC class II and CD86, and downregulation of E-cadherin, in conjunction with morphological changes in LCs in epidermal sheets fluorescently stained for MHC class II [39]. When LT is placed on the skin, increased numbers of activated CD11c$^+$ cells are found in the draining lymph node, and both labeled adjuvant and antigen are seen in association with these cells after TCI, suggesting that these dendritic cells are loaded with adjuvant and antigen by TCI techniques [40]. Investigators using live inactivated herpes virus with CT delivered by TCI-stimulated potent T-cell response protected mice against challenge [32], and this was accompanied by increased numbers of LCs migrating out of the skin into the draining lymph nodes. In a cutaneous viral infection model using West Nile or Semliki Forest virus delivered intradermally by injection [41], increases in the number of activated murine LCs in the draining lymph node (MHC class II$^+$/NLDC145$^+$/E-cadherin$^+$) and concomitant depletion of epidermal LCs in the skin were noted. When these viruses were inactivated by exposure to ultraviolet irradiation, the LC migration and depletion were abrogated, suggesting that the viral replication had LC-activating effects. Similarly,

increased numbers of fluorescein isothiocyanate (FITC)-loaded dendritic cells have been detected in the draining lymph node after topical application of adjuvant (Figure 3). These cells also show upregulation of CD86 in response to LT (Panel C), suggesting that their maturation has been prompted by the addition of adjuvants. In total, these data suggest that LCs are the primary target cells for TCI.

V. IMMUNE RESPONSES TO TRANSCUTANEOUS IMMUNIZATION

Transcutaneous immunization represents a fundamental insight for vaccine delivery. Beginning with the observation that CT could be used as an adjuvant for topical immunization with toxoid antigens [6], we have shown that a wide variety of adjuvants and antigens can be used to induce robust systemic and mucosal immunity via this topical immunization technique [8,20,42]. Although the mechanisms by which adjuvants exert their effects are under investigation [21,43–45], their enhancing effects are well described [24], and the wealth of data in this field has been directly applicable to TCI. We have primarily focused on CT, LT, and their derivatives, given their potency and the breadth of available information on these adjuvants [21,44,46].

Because TCI represents a departure from other routes of immunization, it was important to test whether TCI could

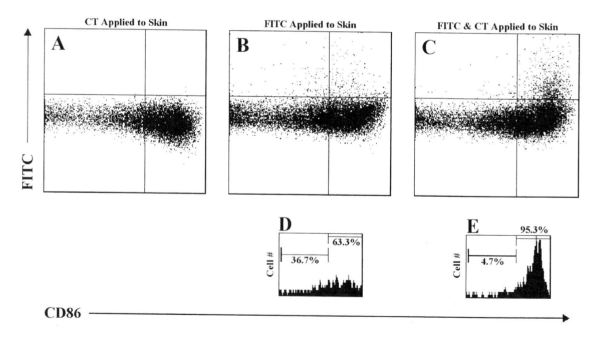

Figure 3 Upregulation of CD86 on dendritic cells isolated from draining lymph nodes after topical application of cholera toxin and fluorecein isothiocyanate. C57BL/6 mice ($n = 5$) were transcutaneously immunized on the lower back with CT (A), FITC (B and D), or FITC coadministered with CT for 1 hr (C and E). Twenty hours after immunization, the draining (inguinal) lymph nodes were excised, and single cell suspensions of the lymph nodes were produced, stained for CD86 and I-A^b, or CD86 and CD11c, and analyzed by flow cytometry. Dot plots in panels (A)–(C) were gated on large, MHC class II^{High} cells. Similar results were obtained by gating on large CD11c$^+$ cells. Histograms in panels (D) and (E) were gated on FITC$^+$ cells in panels (B) and (C), respectively, and display the percentages of CD86^{High} and CD86^{Low} populations. Similar CD86 populations were observed by gating on large CD11c^{High} FITC$^+$ cells. (From Crit Rev Ther Drug Carrier Syst 2001;18(5):503–525.)

result in classical immune responses such as those induced by other routes of immunization. The use of adjuvant on the skin results in both primary and secondary serum antibody responses to coadministered antigens when boosting is conducted using CT or LT as adjuvants [42] (Figure 4). Mice immunized with CT or LT alone and subsequently boosted demonstrate a typical secondary antibody response to the toxins. Serial repeated immunization with the same adjuvant and different antigens may readily be achieved despite the presence of high-titer antibodies to the adjuvant (Figure 4)

[42]. Additionally, TCI appears to induce boostable, long-lasting immune responses. As shown in Figure 5, mice immunized with diphtheria toxoid (DT) and CT had little decline in their immune responses over 9 months.

The memory responses seen after boosting immunizations using TCI suggest that T-cell responses are induced [27]. This is evident using a variety of adjuvants. Mice were immunized with TTx and one of the following adjuvants: CT, rCTB, pCTB (which contains trace holotoxin activity), LT, and a mutant of LT known as LTR192G, which has

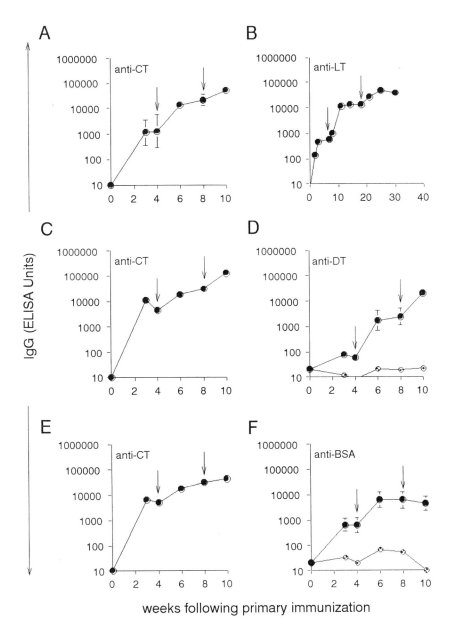

Figure 4 Kinetics of the IgG (H + L) antibody response to CT (A, C, E), LT (B), DT (D), or BSA (F) in animals immunized and boosted (arrows) by the transcutaneous route. BALB/c mice (*n* = 5) were immunized with (A) CT alone (100 μg), (B) LT alone (100 μg), (C and D) CT + DT (100 μg of CT, 100 μg of DT), and (D) DT alone (100 μg of DT). Gray circles in (D) indicate antibody levels to DT in mice vaccinated without using CT as adjuvant. Antibodies were measured by ELISA at multiple time points. The results are reported as the mean±SEM. Similar results were obtained in two independent experiments. (From Crit Rev Ther Drug Carrier Syst 2001;18(5):503–525.)

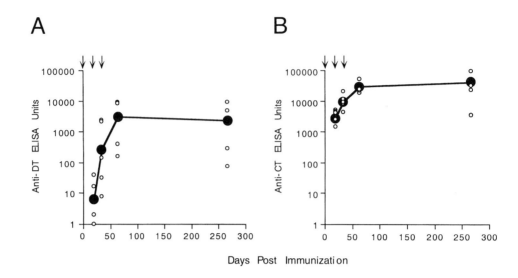

Figure 5 Serum IgG antibody responses to DT and CT. C57BL/6 ($n = 5$) mice were immunized three times with DT and CT at 0, 3, and 6 weeks (arrows). Individual (open circles) and geometrical mean (closed circles). Anti-DT (A) or anti-CT (B) IgG antibodies are shown over 9 months and reported as ELISA units.

equivalent adjuvant capabilities as native LT but has decreased potential for causing diarrhea on ingestion [47]. The antibody responses to TTx were similar for all adjuvants except rCTB, which lacks the ribosyl transferase activity associated with the A subunit [20]. T-cell proliferative responses in spleen and lymph node preparations from mice revealed the induction of tetanus-specific immunity, as well as mixed but predominantly Th2 cytokine profiles, as

assessed by matching the relatively higher serum anti-TTx IgG1 compared to IgG2a [27]. In a separate experiment, we also examined whether priming by the intramuscular route with TTx and alum, which was known to induce T-cell memory, could be followed by a booster immunization on the skin to induce secondary responses [27]. As shown in Table 1, intramuscularly primed animals respond vigorously to topical boosting, producing high levels of anti-TTx anti-

Table 1 Serum Anti-TTx IgG in Mice Primed Intramuscularly with TTx and Boosted Transcutaneously with CT and TTx[a]

First immunization		Second immunization		Third immunization	
TTx, IM[b]	EU (range)[c]	10 µg of CT + TTx, TCI[d]	EU (range)	10 µg of CT + TTx, TCI	EU (range)
2.0 Lf[e]	4467 (912–28,010)	50 Lf	44,360 (9,320–264,000)	ND[f]	ND
0.5 Lf	953 (60–6,640)	12.5 Lf	122,100 (20,030–346,300)	12.5 Lf	163,190 (110,180–391,230)
0.05 Lf	81 (49–212)	12.5 Lf	27,320 (10,560–52,500)	12.5 Lf	154,280 (12,800–268,000)
0.005 Lf	65 (41–100)	12.5 Lf	9,560 (2,080–32,990)	12.5 Lf	90,080 (45,800–276,500)
ND	ND	50 Lf	11 (3–67)	50 Lf	11,630 (4,420–31,290)

[a] Sera samples analyzed before immunization were all <36 ELISA units.
[b] The amount of TTx in Lf administered with alum in an intramuscular (i.m.) injection.
[c] EU = ELISA unit; range is the low and high limits of TTx-specific EU measured for each group of mice ($n = 5$).
[d] The amount of TTx in Lf coadministered with 10 µg of CT by transcutaneous immunization (TCI).
[e] 1 Lf is equivalent to 2 µg of protein.
[f] ND, not done.
Source: From Hamond et al. Transcutaneous immunization: T cell responses and boosting of existing immunity. Vaccine 2001;19:2705–2707, with permission from Elsevier Science.

bodies. Taken together, these studies demonstrated that TCI and classical routes of immunization such as injection induce T-cell responses, which underlie the robust immune responses that follow boosting and are necessary for immunoprotection.

The role of the adjuvant appears to be critical to the induction of high levels of antibodies to a coadministered antigen. Transcutaneous immunization, with increasing doses of LT as adjuvant and different doses of TTx as antigen, produced robust levels of anti-TTx antibodies that are clearly dependent on the presence of adjuvant [20] (Figure 6). The same animals were fully protected against systemic tetanus toxin challenge, and only animals receiving adjuvant with the antigen were fully protected [20]. Others have shown that anti-diphtheria toxin antibodies generated by TCI in the presence of adjuvant neutralize the highly potent diphtheria toxin [15]. Thus, the use of adjuvants greatly amplifies the immune response to antigen on the skin, and the use of adjuvant patches and clinically accepted skin preparation techniques has allowed the effective immu-

nization of mice with adjuvant/antigen doses at 0.5/5 μg, respectively. These and other studies have shown that the antibodies induced by TCI in the presence of adjuvant are robust [20], functional [13], and can lead to protection in disease settings [17,20,32].

VI. MUCOSAL RESPONSES TO TRANSCUTANEOUS IMMUNIZATION

Topical immunization with LT and CT as adjuvants clearly induces both IgG and IgA antibodies in mucosal secretions of mice [48,49]. We have postulated that the skin immune system may be an extension of the mucosal immune system. The mucosa and skin share similar elements, including LCs and secretory organs, and the presence of IgA such as that found in the sweat glands [50,51]. Furthermore, microorganisms found on the skin demonstrate coating with immunoglobulins, including IgA and the secretory component of IgA [52,53]. Thus, the skin immune system has immunological

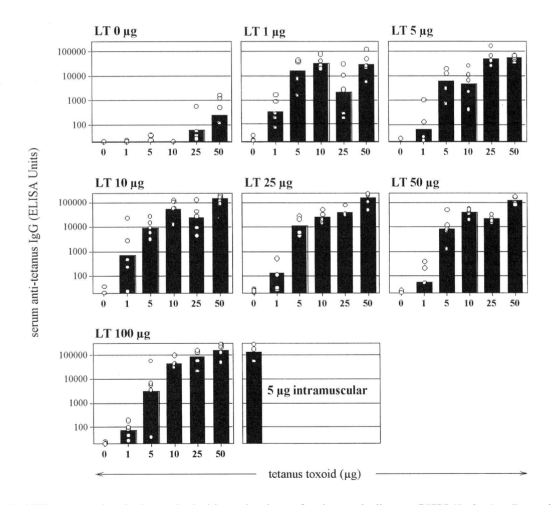

Figure 6   Anti-TTx response in mice immunized with varying doses of antigen and adjuvant. C57BL/6 mice ($n = 5$) were immunized on the skin with LT (doses indicated above each panel) and TTx (doses indicated on the x-axis) at 0, 4 and 7 weeks. The intramuscular group was immunized with alum and TTx (5 μg) doses at 0, 4, and 8 weeks. Serum collected 2 weeks after final immunization was assayed for TTx-specific IgG by ELISA. The geometrical mean (bar) and individual values (open circles) are shown for each group. (From Infect Immun 2000; 68(9):5306–5313.)

responses to microbes that are mucosal-like, suggesting that the skin and the mucosal immune system may be related.

The topical application of bAREs, such as LT, CT, and coadministered antigens, induces antibodies that can be detected at the mucosa [20,32,48], as well as mucosal cellular responses [33]. Mice immunized transcutaneously with CT produce anti-CT IgG and IgA antibodies in the stool and pulmonary secretions (Figure 7) that are toxin-neutralizing [48]. IgG antibodies to the coadministered antigen have been detected in the mucosa in several settings [20,32,42], and IgA antibodies to tetanus and herpes antigens have been detected in mice immunized topically with CT and TTx or inactivated herpes virus [32,33]. The detection of antibodies in the stool and lung wash of immunized mice suggests that antibody-secreting cells have homed to the mucosa; it has been shown that anti-TTx antibody secreting cell (ASCs) can be detected in the vaginal mucosa of mice immunized topically using CT and TTx [33], but migration of LCs to the gut may also

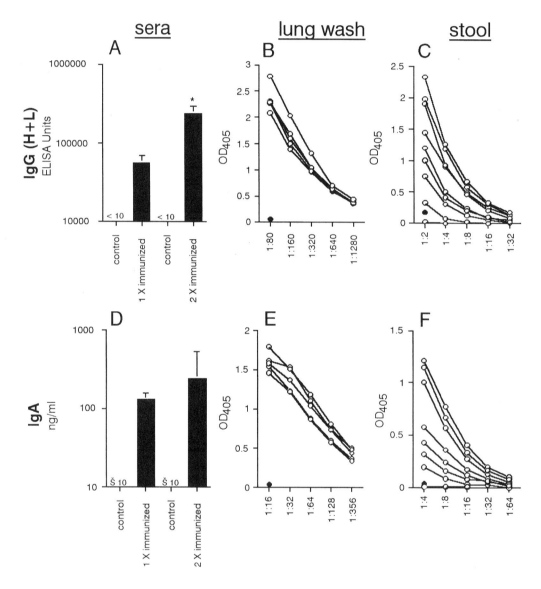

Figure 7   Sera (A and D), mucosal lung (B and E), and stool (C and F) antibody responses to CT after TCI. In panels (A) and (D), C57BL/6 mice were immunized transcutaneously at 0, or at 0 and 3 weeks with 100 µg of CT. Data shown are the geometrical mean ± SEM for ELISA measurements from five individual animals. *A statistically significant ($p < 0.05$) difference between the titers measured in the 1× and 2× immunization groups. In panels (B) and (E), C57BL/6 mice were immunized transcutaneously at 0 week; lung washes were collected at 3 weeks. IgG and IgA levels were assessed by ELISA; the titers (OD = 405 nm) from individual animals are shown. In panels (C) and (F), C57BL/6 mice were immunized transcutaneously at 0 week, and single stool pellets were collected immediately after defecation at 6 weeks. IgG and IgA levels were assessed in fecal homogenates by ELISA; the dilution curves from eight (F) or nine (C) individual animals are shown. (●) Indicates the maximal level of anti-CT IgG or anti-CT IgA Ab detected in control lung washes from mice immunized with an irrelevant protein (B and E) or in 1/2 dilutions of stool from unimmunized mice (C and F). (From Crit Rev Ther Drug Carrier Syst 2001;18(5):503–525.)

explain these findings [49]. Alternatively, antibodies may represent transudates into the mucosal secretions, although recent data have shown that anti-LT antibodies detected in the stool and lung wash contain the secretory component of IgA, indicating that local antibody production occurs [13]. Plasmid DNA immunization delivered by TCI similarly induced both serum IgG and fecal IgA against the M protein encoded in the plasmid, and elicited a protective immune response on influenza virus challenges [17]. Anti-LT IgG and IgA antibodies were found in humans immunized topically with LT, which is consistent with the repeated observations in mice [7]. The presence of antibodies in the secretions of animals immunized by TCI raises many mechanistic questions, but the data suggest that induction of mucosal and systemic responses by TCI may be used to enhance vaccine efficacy.

VII. HUMAN STUDIES

There are a number of potential targets for the creation of new vaccines delivered via the skin. The goals at this early stage of human studies have been to demonstrate the safety and clinical utility of TCI with various antigens, to begin to optimize their delivery by studying skin preparations and patch types, and to assess the immune responses induced.

The initial clinical study used LT alone, capitalizing on its ability to act both as an antigen and an adjuvant, in a dose-escalation format to assess the safety and immune response to simple liquid application of LT to unprepared skin [7]. Eighteen healthy volunteers received 25, 50, 250, or 500 µg of an LT solution that was added to a simple gauze pad under an adhesive patch and applied to the upper arm, without skin pretreatment, for 6 hr, with a boost at 12 weeks. Six in the 500-µg LT group returned for a third immunization 35 weeks after the first immunization. No serious vaccine-related adverse reactions were observed, either systemically or locally (at the site of immunization). Histological sections of biopsies taken at the dosing sites were normal, consistent with the absence of DTH clinically. Langerhans cells visualized in the same biopsy using anti-CD1a staining consistently demonstrated enlarged or rounded LC cell bodies at the site of immunization at 24 and 48 hr compared to the control biopsies from the opposite arm, similar to the chronically activated LCs seen in sections of the tonsilar crypts in the mouth [54] and in sections from mice topically exposed to CT [39].

Both systemic and mucosal immune responses to LT were achieved using TCI. All subjects in the high-dose group produced a greater than fourfold rise in serum antibodies against LT, with clear boosting responses (Figure 8), along with IgG or IgA antibodies against LT in either the urine or stool. This group had a 14.6- and 7.2-mean fold rise in serum anti-LT IgG and IgA, respectively, at 44 weeks. Antibodies against LT were durable and persisted long after the second immunization, with a clear booster response after the second and third doses. There were minimal responses in other dosing groups.

The importance of the role of the adjuvant in the induction of immune responses to a coadministered antigen

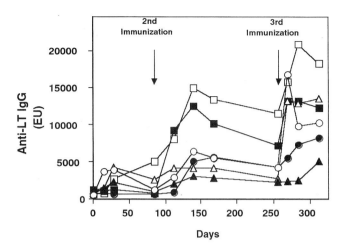

Figure 8 Individual human serum IgG antibody responses to LT. Six volunteers were immunized using a patch containing 500 µg of LT placed on the upper arm for 6 hr at 0, 12, and 35 weeks. Individual anti-LT IgG antibodies are shown over the time course of the trial and reported as ELISA units, the inverse dilution at which the sera yield an optical density of 1.0. (From Crit Rev Ther Drug Carrier Syst 2001;18(5):503–525.)

was initially tested in the context of *E. coli*-related traveler's diarrhea using the colonization factor CS6, a multisubunit intestinal epithelial cell-binding protein [55]. Normal adult volunteers were enrolled in a dose-escalating study of 250, 500, 1000, or 2000 µg of CS6 alone or with 500 µg of LT dosed at 0, 1, and 3 months [12]. Fourteen of 19 volunteers (74%) in the combined groups had mild DTH skin reactions with the second or third dose. No other adverse events correlated with vaccine administration. As shown in Figure 8, volunteers receiving LT as adjuvant produced serum anti-CS6 IgG and IgA. The response to LT was very robust in comparison to the previous trial (above), and may be explained by the use of simple skin preparation steps before application of the patch. Overall, when CS6 was given with LT, 68% and 53% had anti-CS6 IgG and IgA, respectively, and 100% and 90% had anti-LT IgG and IgA, respectively. This anti-CS6 response compares favorably to that observed when volunteers were experimentally challenged with CS6-expressing ETEC strain B7A, whereupon 35% and 31% of the subjects developed anti-CS6 IgG and IgA, respectively [56,57]. The anti-LT response that occurs when LT serves as the adjuvant in TCI would likely contribute further to protection against LT toxin-induced diarrheal disease [58]. Antibody-secreting cells were also measured in the peripheral blood. In the combined-dose TCI groups, 37% and 42% developed anti-CS6 IgG and IgA ASCs, respectively, compared to 50% that developed anti-CS6 IgA ASCs following challenge, historically [57]. There were no immune responses seen in the CS6 alone groups.

The vaccination provided prolonged immunity, and a booster effect to both LT and CS6 was seen once again (Figure 9). The two highest-dose groups had the strongest anti-CS6 IgG response. There was a marked IgG response to

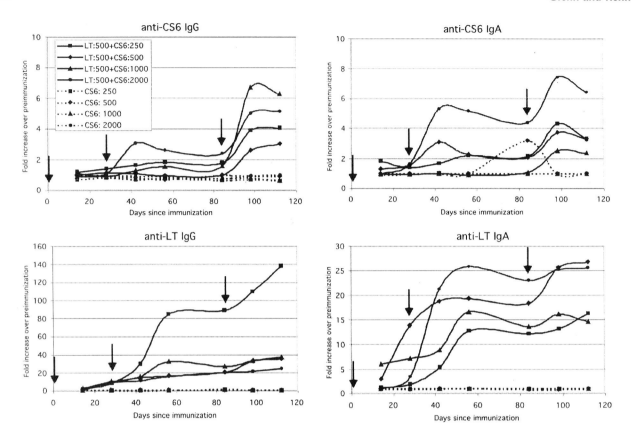

Figure 9 Human serum IgG and IgA responses to coadministered CS6 and LT. Normal adult volunteers were enrolled in a dose-escalating study of 250, 500, 1000, or 2000 μg of CS6 alone or with 500 μg of LT dosed at 0, 1, and 3 months (arrows). The mean serological response for each group is shown over the time course of the trial and reported as fold increase of ELISA units over baseline.

LT, particularly in the lowest-dose CS6 group. This may indicate some degree of competition for antigen presentation, such that more APCs were available for the LT to act as an antigen when the ratio of CS6/ to LT was lower. The lack of response to CS6 without LT and clear responses in the presence of LT confirmed the universal finding in animal studies that the adjuvant plays a critical role in TCI. Favorable induction of an immune response in comparison with the one seen after a live challenge suggests that the vaccination may provide a similar degree of protection.

Finally, optimization of TCI requires evaluation of new strategies in the human setting. Preclinical studies suggested that the dose of LT could be dramatically reduced with retention of immunogenicity by altering the SC. The effect of mild disruption of the SC on the delivery of LT was explored with commercially available medical products, including abrasive pads used to enhance EKG signal conductivity, or adhesive tapes used to evaluate skin hydration [17a]. We compared the immunogenicity of LT on human skin pretreated with hydration alone in a high-dose (400 μg of LT) group, compared with hydration, mild abrasion, or tape stripping in lower-dose (50 μg of LT) groups of normal volunteers.

SC disruption achieved about a four-times-greater immune response compared to hydration alone. Three weeks after the second dose, there was a significant increase in the

GMT fold rise of LT-specific IgG and IgA in the pretreatment group compared with hydration alone, as well as in the tape-stripping group with IgA. SC disruption and tape stripping consistently achieved a greater than twofold rise in geometrical mean titer for each patient in those groups (100% response rate). The titers were persistent, with no significant decrease in any group at 6 months. These results suggest that this is a safe method of delivering LT, although a self-limited, mild, irritant dermatitis was occasionally observed. Overall, this study demonstrated that with effective skin pretreatment to disrupt the SC, the dose of LT can be decreased by at least a log with no decrease in immunogenicity. Further refinements of the pretreatment methodology should allow a simple approach for use in final commercialization in conjunction with a patch.

VIII. CONCLUSION

Over the past few decades, clinicians have witnessed the tremendous positive impact of new vaccine products such as the Hib and, more recently, meningococcal C vaccines [59,60], which sprang from a basic observation [61]. Development of the original observation into a deliverable product required a great deal of formulation studies, preclinical testing, and clinical testing. Without underestimating the effort required to create a vaccine formulation delivered by a patch, certain strategies may compress the development time frame for a TCI-based product. Transdermal patch materials and manufacturing strategies, established vaccine antigens such as tetanus and influenza that are currently licensed, and adjuvants that are commercially manufactured are being utilized to accelerate development. In cooperation with the Food and Drug administration (FDA), we have conducted several Phase I trials, which have demonstrated the safety and immunogenicity of this approach, and product development trials are underway. Additionally, preclinical development has clearly shown that low doses of adjuvant may be optimal, and doses of antigen in the range of doses given parenterally can be effective. Translation of these findings into the clinic will be an important goal. More widespread use of TCI in other laboratories, publication and dissemination of related data and techniques, and adoption of this approach by industry suggest that transcutaneous immunization will move from an investigational observation to a product in the future.

REFERENCES

1. Fletcher MA, Saliou P. Vaccines and infectious disease. EXS 2000; 89:69–88.
2. WHO. Reducing the Risk of Unsafe Injections in Immunization Programmes: The Role of Injection Equipment. Geneva, Switzerland: World Health Organization, 1996.
3. Barry BW. Dermatologic formulations. In: Bronaugh RL, Maibach HI, eds. Percutaneous Absorption: Methods, Methodology, Drug Delivery. New York: Marcel Dekker, 1985:33.
4. Jakob T, Udey MC. Epidermal Langerhans cells: from neurons to nature's adjuvants. Adv Dermatol 1999; 14:209–258.
5. Yu RC, et al. Morphological and quantitative analyses of normal epidermal Langerhans cells using confocal scanning laser microscopy. Br J Dermatol 1994; 131:843–848.
6. Glenn GM, et al. Skin immunization made possible by cholera toxin. Nature 1998; 391:851.
7. Glenn GM, et al. Transcutaneous immunization: a human vaccine delivery strategy using a patch. Nat Med 2000; 6:1403–1406.
8. Hammond SA, et al. Transcutaneous immunization of domestic animals: opportunities and challenges. Adv Drug Deliv Rev 2000; 43:45–55.
9. Roberts MS, Walker M. Water, the most natural penetration enhancer. In: Walters KA, Hadgraft J, eds. Pharmaceutical Skin Penetration Enhancement 1993; Vol. 59. New York: Marcel Dekker, 1993.
10. Rietschel RI, Fowler JF. Fisher's Contact Dermatitis. 4th ed. Baltimore, MD: Williams and Wilkins, 1995.
11. Wester RC, Maibach HI. Percutaneous absorption of drugs. Clin Pharmacokinet 1992; 23: 253–266.
12. Güereña-Burgueño F, et al. Safety and immunogenicity of a prototype enterotoxigenic Escherichia coli vaccine administered transcutaneously. Infect Immun 2002; 70:1874–1880.
13. Yu J, et al. Transcutaneous immunization using colonization factor and heat labile enterotoxin induces correlates of protective immunity for enterotoxigenic Escherichia coli. Infect Immun 2002; 70:1056–1068.
14. Fan H, et al. Immunization via hair follicles by topical application of naked DNA to normal skin. Nat Biotechnol 1999; 17:870–872.
15. Hammond SA, et al. Transcutaneous immunization: an emerging route of immunization and potent immunostimu-

16. Seo N, et al. Percutaneous peptide immunization via corneum barrier-disrupted murine skin for experimental tumor immunoprophylaxis. Proc Natl Acad Sci USA 2000; 97:371–376.
17. Watabe S, et al. Protection against influenza virus challenge by topical application of influenza DNA vaccine. Vaccine 2001; 19:4434–4444.
17a. Glenn GM, et al. Transcutaneous immunization and immunostimulant strategies: capitalizing on the immunocompetence of the skin. Expert Rev Vaccines 2003; 2:253–267.
18. O'Hagan DT, ed. Methods in Molecular Medicine 2000; Vol. 42. Totowa, NJ: Humana Press, Inc., 2000.
19. Baca-Estrada ME, et al. Effects of IL-12 on immune responses induced by transcutaneous immunization with antigens formulated in a novel lipid-based biphasic delivery system. Vaccine 2000; 18: 1847–1854.
20. Scharton-Kersten T, et al. Transcutaneous immunization with bacterial ADP-ribosylating exotoxins, subunits, and unrelated adjuvants. Infect Immun 2000; 68:5306–5313.
21. Freytag LC, Clements JD. Bacterial toxins as mucosal adjuvants. Curr Top Microbiol Immunol 1999; 236:215–236.
22. Gluck R, et al. Safety and immunogenicity of intranasally administered inactivated trivalent virosome-formulated influenza vaccine containing Escherichia coli heat-labile toxin as a mucosal adjuvant. J Infect Dis 2000; 181:1129–1132.
23. Michetti P, et al. Oral immunization with urease and Escherichia coli heat-labile enterotoxin is safe and immunogenic in Helicobacter pylori-infected adults. Gastroenterology 1999; 116:804–812.
24. Snider DP. The mucosal adjuvant activities of ADP-ribosylating bacterial enterotoxins. Crit Rev Immunol 1995; 15:317–348.
25. Weltzin R, et al. Parenteral adjuvant activities of Escherichia coli heat-labile toxin and its B subunit for immunization of mice against gastric Helicobacter pylori infection. Infect Immun 2000; 68:2775–2782.
26. Dickinson BL, Clements JD. Dissociation of Escherichia coli heat-labile enterotoxin adjuvanticity from ADP-ribosyltransferase activity. Infect Immun 1995; 63:1617–1623.
27. Hammond SA, et al. Transcutaneous immunization: T-cell responses and boosting of existing immunity. Vaccine 2001; 19:2701–2707.
28. Porgador A, et al. Intranasal immunization with CTL epitope peptides from HIV-1 or ovalbumin and the mucosal adjuvant cholera toxin induces peptide-specific CTLs and protection against tumor development in vivo. J Immunol 1997; 158:834–841.
29. Neidleman JA, et al. Mutant heat-labile enterotoxins as adjuvants for CTL induction. In: O'Hagan D ed. Vaccine Adjuvants: Preparation Methods and Research Protocols 2000; Vol. 42, Totowa, NJ: Humana Press, 2000:327–336.
30. Levine MM, et al. New knowledge on pathogenesis of bacterial enteric infections as applied to vaccine development. Microbiol Rev 1983; 47:510–550.
31. Murphy GF, et al. Phenotypic transformation of macrophages to Langerhans cells in the skin. Am J Pathol 1986; 123:401–406.
32. El-Ghorr AA, et al. Transcutaneous immunisation with herpes simplex virus stimulates immunity in mice. FEMS Immunol Med Microbiol 2000; 29:255–261.
33. Gockel CM, et al. Transcutaneous immunization induces mucosal and systemic immunity: a potent method for targeting immunity to the female reproductive tract. Mol Immunol 2000; 37:537–544.
34. Jakob T, et al. Bacterial DNA and CpG-containing

lation strategy. Crit Rev Ther Drug Carrier Syst 2001; 18:503–526.

oligodeoxynucleotides activate cutaneous dendritic cells and induce IL-12 production: implications for the augmentation of Th1 responses. Int Arch Allergy Immunol 1999; 118:457–461.

35. Kremer IB, et al. Intradermal granulocyte–macrophage colony-stimulating factor alters cutaneous antigen-presenting cells and differentially affects local versus distant immunization in humans. Clin Immunol 2000; 96:29–37.

36. Aiba S, Katz SI. Phenotypic and functional characteristics of in vivo-activated Langerhans cells. J Immunol 1990; 145: 2791–2796.

37. Hernando RA, et al. Changes in epidermal Langerhans cells, gamma delta T cells and CD4 T cells after intradermal infection with recombinant vaccinia virus expressing cytokine genes. Immunol Cell Biol 1994; 72:383–389.

38. Nagao S, et al. Langerhans cells at the sites of vaccinia virus inoculation. Arch Dermatol Res 1976; 256:23–31.

39. Vassell R, et al. Activation of Langerhans cells following transcutaneous immunization. 5th National Symposium, Basic Aspects of Vaccines, Bethesda, MD, 1999.

40. Guebre-Xabier M, et al. Immunostimulant patch containing heat labile enterotoxin from *E. coli* enhances immune responses to injected influenza vaccine through activation of skin dendritic cells. J Virol 2003; 77:5218–5225.

41. Johnston LJ, et al. Phenotypic changes in Langerhans cells after infection with arboviruses: a role in the immune response to epidermally acquired viral infection. J Virol 1996; 70:4761–4766.

42. Glenn GM, et al. Transcutaneous immunization with bacterial ADP-ribosylating exotoxins as antigens and adjuvants. Infect Immun 1999; 67:1100–1106.

43. Akira S, et al. Toll-like receptors: critical proteins linking innate and acquired immunity. Nat Immunol 2001; 2:675–680.

44. Lycke N. The mechanism of cholera toxin adjuvanticity. Res Immunol 1997; 148:504–520.

45. Williams NA, et al. Immune modulation by the cholera-like enterotoxins: from adjuvant to therapeutic. Immunol Today 1999; 20:95–101.

46. Singh M, O'Hagan D. Advances in vaccine adjuvants. Nat Biotechnol 1999; 17:1075–1081.

47. Kotloff KL, et al. Safety and immunogenicity of oral inactivated whole-cell *Helicobacter pylori* vaccine with adjuvant among volunteers with or without subclinical infection. Infect Immun 2001; 69:3581–3590.

48. Glenn GM, et al. Transcutaneous immunization with cholera toxin protects mice against lethal mucosal toxin challenge. J Immunol 1998; 161:3211–3214.

49. Enioutina EY, et al. The induction of systemic and mucosal immune responses to antigen–adjuvant compositions administered into the skin: alterations in the migratory properties of dendritic cells appears to be important for stimulating mucosal immunity. Vaccine 2000; 18:2753–2767.

50. Gebhart W, et al. IgA in human skin appendages. In: Caputo R, ed. Immunodermatology. Rome: CIC Edizioni Internationali, 1987:185.

51. Okada T, et al. Identification of secretory immunoglobulin A in human sweat and sweat glands. J Invest Dermatol 1988; 90:648–651.

52. Hard GC. Electron microscopic examination of *Corynebacterium ovis*. J Bacteriol 1969; 97:1480–1485.

53. Metze D, et al. Immunoglobulins coat microorganisms of skin surface: a comparative immunohistochemical and ultrastructural study of cutaneous and oral microbial symbionts. J Invest Dermatol 1991; 96:439–445.

54. Noble B, et al. Microanatomical distribution of dendritic cells in normal tonsils. Acta Otolaryngol Suppl 1996; 523:94–97.

55. Wolf MK, et al. The CS6 colonization factor of human enterotoxigenic *Escherichia coli* contains two heterologous major subunits. FEMS Microbiol Lett 1997; 148:35–42.

56. Levine MM, et al. Immunity to enterotoxigenic *Escherichia coli*. Infect Immun 1979; 23:729–736.

57. Wolf M, et al. Use of the human challenge model to characterize the immune response to the colonization factors of enterotoxigenic *Escherichia coli* (ETEC). The 35th Joint Conference of the U.S.–Japan Cooperative Medical Science Program, Baltimore, MD, 1999.

58. Clemens JD, et al. Cross-protection by B subunit-whole cell cholera vaccine against diarrhea associated with heat-labile toxin-producing enterotoxigenic *Escherichia coli*: results of a large-scale field trial. J Infect Dis 1988; 158:372–377.

59. Miller E, et al. Planning, registration, and implementation of an immunisation campaign against meningococcal serogroup C disease in the UK: a success story. Vaccine 2001; 20(suppl 1):S58–S67.

60. Robbins JB, et al. The 1996 Albert Lasker Medical Research Awards. Prevention of systemic infections, especially meningitis, caused by *Haemophilus influenzae* type b. Impact on public health and implications for other polysaccharide-based vaccines. JAMA 1996; 276:1181–1185.

61. Schneerson R, et al. Preparation, characterization, and immunogenicity of *Haemophilus influenzae* type b polysaccharide–protein conjugates. J Exp Med 1980; 152:361–376.

35

Combination Vaccines for Routine Infant Immunization

Margaret B. Rennels
University of Maryland School of Medicine, Baltimore, Maryland, U.S.A.

Rosanna M. Lagos
Centro para Vacunas en Desarrollo-Chile, Santiago, Chile

Kathryn M. Edwards
Vanderbilt University School of Medicine, Nashville, Tennessee, U.S.A.

I. INTRODUCTION

A combination vaccine consists of two or more immunogens which are physically combined and administered at the same time in the same anatomic site. In this chapter, a sign (+) will be used to indicate the vaccines administered simultaneously but at separate anatomic sites, and a virgule (/) will indicate combined vaccines. The administration of multiple antigens in the same syringe eliminates the need for separate injections, which is painful for the child, time-consuming for medical personnel, and economically costly. Although many combination vaccines have been routinely used for decades, more are needed. Pediatric combination vaccines presently licensed or under development are listed in Table 1 [1]. This chapter will consider the negative consequences of multiple injections, potential problems from combining vaccines, regulatory perspectives, existing combination vaccines, and combinations under evaluation.

The following five new parenteral vaccines have been introduced into many routine infant vaccination schedules in the last 15 years: conjugate *Haemophilus influenzae* type b (Hib), conjugate multivalent pneumococcal vaccine, trivalent inactivated poliovirus (IPV), varicella (V), and hepatitis B (HB). Hepatitis A (HA) vaccine is also administered to young children in some areas with high hepatitis A endemicity. A consequence of this successful development and deployment of new pediatric vaccines is that the number of injections a child in the United States, for example, receives in the first 18 months of life has increased from 4 to 20. Consequently, 25% of U.S. parents surveyed felt that their children's immune systems were weakened by too many vaccines [2]. This has led some parents to choose to forego some vaccines or to request extra visits to complete the

immunization series. These developments threaten to diminish the high immunization levels many have worked so hard to achieve.

Combining vaccines into one syringe may result in a combination product with enhanced reactogenicity, or diminished immunogenicity, or efficacy, compared to the separately administered vaccines. There are several mechanisms proposed to explain how one vaccine might interfere with the immunogenicity of another when mixed together. Physical or chemical interaction between components of the vaccines might alter the conformation of the necessary epitope. As an example, studies of the combined inactivated polio vaccine (IPV) and diphtheria toxoid–tetanus toxoid–whole cell pertussis (DTwP) vaccine demonstrated that the preservative thimerosal can destroy the potency of IPV [3]. The pertussis component also lost potency over time, possibly as a result of the destruction of antigen or formulation without merthiolate stabilizer [4,5]. Mixing an adjuvanted vaccine with one that does not contain an adjuvant may result in the displacement of the one vaccine from its adjuvant, resulting in diminished immune response to that component. Interference between components of live viral vaccines has also occurred. One such instance was the reduced seroconversion to the mumps component of the bivalent Urabe Am9/Schwartz mumps–measles vaccine [6]. Viral strain interference is thought to be a consequence of competition for mucosal receptors or lymphocyte binding sites. It is also possible that the immune responses, such as interferon production, stimulated by one vaccine viral strain may interfere with the replication of another virus strain. Therefore, new combinations of vaccine products must be evaluated with the same methods and rigor as if it were a new vaccine.

Table 1 Pediatric Combination Vaccines Presently Licensed or Under Development[a]

| Combination vaccine[b] | Producers or vendors of licensed vaccines | | Under development[c] |
	Licensed in the United States	Licensed outside the United States	
Td–IPV		AvP-Fr, AvP-Ca, AP MSD	
DT–IPV		AvP-Ca, AP MSD	
DT–HB		AP MSD	
DTP–IPV		AvP-Ca, AvP-Fr, AP MSD	
DTP–Hib	AvP-US, WL	AvP-Ca, AvP-Fr, AP MSD, GSK, WL	
DTP–Hib–IPV		AvP-Ca, AvP-Fr, AP MSD	
DTP–HB		GSK	
DTP–Hib–HB		GSK	
DTaP–IPV		AvP-Ca, AP MSD, NAVA, GSK	
DTaP–Hib	AvP-US[d]	AvP-Fr, GSK	
DTaP–IPV–Hib		AvP-Ca, AP MSD, GSK	
DTaP–HB		GSK	
DTaP–IPV–HB	GSK	GSK	
DTaP–Hib–HB			Yes
DTaP–Hib–IPV–HB		AP MSD, GSK	
DTaP–Hib–IPV–HB–HA			Yes
HB–Hib	Merck	AP MSD	
HB-HA	GSK	GSK	
MMR–V			Yes
PnC–MnC			Yes
PnC–MnC–Hib			Yes

Abbreviations: aP, acellular pertussis vaccine; AvP, Aventis Pasteur (formerly Pasteur Mérieux Connaught; Ca, Fr, US, and AP MSD designate, respectively, vaccines sourced from the Canadian, French, and US subsidiaries or the AvP–Merck European joint venture); D, diphtheria toxoid vaccine; HA, hepatitis A vaccine; HB, hepatitis B vaccine; Hib, conjugate *H. influenzae* type b vaccine; IPV, enhanced inactivated trivalent poliovirus vaccine; MMR–V, measles, mumps, rubella, and varicella vaccine; MnC, meningococcal conjugate vaccine; NAVA, North American Vaccine; P, whole-cell pertussis vaccine; PnC, pneumococcal conjugate vaccine; GSK, GlaxoSmithKline; T, tetanus toxoid vaccine; WL, Wyeth Lederle Vaccines and Pediatrics.

[a] Products combining only multiple serotypes of a single pathogen are excluded, as are DT, DTP, DTaP, OPV, IPV, and MMR themselves. Only those manufacturers who distribute their products globally are listed; other manufacturers may produce some products (e.g., DTP–IPV) for local or regional use. Some products represent components derived from, or joint efforts of, more than one manufacturer, in such cases, their principal distributor is shown.

[b] No discrimination is made between products distributed in combined form and those distributed in separate containers, for combination at the time of use.

[c] Indicated vaccines may be under development by more than one company.

[d] Licensed for the fourth (booster) dose only.

Source: Ref. 1.

II. REGULATORY ASPECTS

Each country or region has separate regulatory agencies responsible for licensure or registration of new combination vaccines. The Food and Drug Administration (FDA) of the United States must follow the Code of Federal Regulation (CFR). Two codes directly apply to the approval of combination products. One of these, 21 CFR 300.50, states that a fixed combination prescription drug must demonstrate that each component makes a contribution to the claimed treatment effects, and that the dosage is such that it is safe and effective. It is further stipulated in 21 CFR 601.25(d)(4) that safe and effective active components may be combined if each component makes a contribution to the claimed effects, combining does not decrease purity, potency, safety, or effectiveness of the individual component, and when used correctly, provides preventive therapy or treatment. The

FDA issued in 1997 a "Guidance for industry for the evaluation of combination vaccines for preventable diseases: Product, testing and clinical studies" to assist the industry in the manufacture and testing of combination vaccines.

III. DESIGN OF COMBINATION VACCINE TRIALS

The safety, immunogenicity ($\pm$efficacy) of combination vaccines must be compared to that of the individual components in prospective, randomized, blinded trials. Two general approaches may be used. The fully combined final product (A/B/C/D) may be compared to each of its components (A + B + C + D). A disadvantage of this method is that it requires multiple arms (2^n), and the sample sizes are large. It also carries the danger that if there is enhanced reactogenicity or diminished immunogenicity with the combination, it cannot be determined which component(s) was (were) responsible. Therefore the evaluation method most commonly used is to proceed in a stepwise manner. If the ultimate goal is to combine four vaccines (A/B/C/D), the initial study compares bivalent A/B to A + B. If no interference is observed with the bivalent vaccine, the next evaluation will be of A/B/C vs. A/B + C. If that is successful, then a final study comparing A/B/C + D vs. A/B/C/D would be performed.

The optimal study compares the protective efficacy of the components of a combination vaccine to its separately administered components. This may not be possible if the routine use of the single component has dramatically reduced or eliminated the disease under study. A trial that demonstrates efficacy in one country may be used to support licensure in a different country if a bridging study is performed, showing that the immunogenicity of the vaccine component in the second population is similar to that in the original efficacy study. The use of serologic markers of protection is another approach. For example, the presence of neutralizing antibody to polioviruses may be considered proof of immunity to infection. Therefore, if a poliovirus vaccine is combined with another product, one simply must demonstrate that the combination product stimulates neutralizing antibodies to the three poliovirus strains contained in the vaccine. This method is only feasible with diseases for which serologic correlates of protection have been established, such as diphtheria, tetanus, hepatitis B, and, arguably, *H. influenzae* type b (Hib). Unfortunately, immunologic correlates of protection are not recognized (or are not widely accepted) for many pathogens, including *Bordetella pertussis* and *Streptococcus pneumoniae*.

The statistical approach to the evaluation of combination vaccines is to demonstrate the noninferiority (one-sided equivalence) of the components in the combination compared to the components administered separately [7]. Immune response end-points in noninferiority trials are the geometric mean concentration (GMC) and/or the proportion of children achieving a defined level of antibodies. The trial is designed to reject the null hypothesis that the combination is inferior by a predetermined amount. In comparisons of GMCs, the null hypotheses (H_0) for each component is $H_0: \theta = \mu_{combined}/\mu_{separate} \leq \theta_0$. The choice of H_0 is based on what is thought to be a clinically meaningful difference and, by necessity, may sometimes be arbitrary. For evaluation of differences in the proportion of responding vaccinees, the null hypotheses for each component is $H_0: \delta = P_{combination} - P_{separate} \leq -\delta_0$. Here, again, the value of δ is determined by what is judged to be clinically meaningful.

Successfully combined vaccines in widespread use for many years include DTwP, IPV, measles–mumps–rubella (MMR) vaccine, DTwP/*H. influenzae* type b (Hib), Hib/hepatitis B (HB), 23-valent polysaccharide pneumococcal vaccine, quadrivalent polysaccharide meningococcal vaccine, and the trivalent inactivated influenza vaccines. These combination products will not be discussed further in this chapter. Attention will be focused on vaccines that have not been universally accepted by regulatory bodies.

A. Diphtheria Toxoid–Tetanus Toxoid–Acellular Pertussis (DTaP) Combined with Inactivated Poliovirus Vaccine, with or Without Hepatitis B

Combining IPV with either DTwP or a DTaP containing two pertussis antigens (aP$_2$) has been reported to result in decreased geometric mean titers (GMTs) of antibody to pertussis antigens [8,9]. Precise serological correlates of protection have not been determined for protection against pertussis, thus the biological significance of diminished pertussis antibody levels is unknown. Also, 100% of children administered three doses of the DTaP$_2$/IPV vaccine had fourfold increase of antibody to pertussis toxin (PT) and filamentous hemagglutinin (FHA), and the GMC of neutralizing antibody to all three poliovirus serotypes were actually higher among children administered the DTaP$_2$/IPV combination compared to those receiving the vaccines simultaneously at separate anatomic locations [8].

The combination of DTaP$_3$/HepB/IPV (Infanrix$_{DTPa-HepB-IPV}$) has been extensively evaluated in German and U.S. children, who received vaccine at a 3-, 4-, 5-month or a 2-, 4-, 6-month schedule. Immune responses following combination vaccine that were noninferior compared to separately administered vaccines included: (1) the rates of seroprotection against diphtheria, tetanus, all three types of poliovirus, and hepatitis B; and (2) the GMCs of antibodies to pertussis toxin, and pertactin. The GMCs of antibody to FHA were lower in those children given the combination vaccine [10]. However, efficacy studies of pertussis vaccines suggest that the role of FHA in protection against disease is minimal [11]. Children given the combination vaccine experienced higher rates of low-grade fever but no differences in the rates of high fever were observed [10]. Children who received a birth dose of hepatitis B vaccine and were subsequently given the combined DTaP$_3$/HepB/IPV experienced no more reactions than those who had not been given a birth dose. (Presented at the Vaccines and Related Biologics Products Advisory Committee, FDA, Bethesda, MD, 3/7/01. www.fda.gov/ohrms/dockets/ac/cber01.htm.)

B. DTaP/Hib (±IPV and/or -HB) Combinations

The successful combination of DTwP and Hib vaccines was, in retrospect, deceptively simple. The reconstitution of conjugate Hib vaccines with DTwP vaccines was accomplished with generally no significant increase in reactogenicity or decrease in immunogenicity of the antibody response to the polyribosyl-ribitol-phosphate (PRP) component [12–14]. Unfortunately, this same experience was not generally repeated when lyophilized conjugate Hib vaccines were reconstituted with liquid DTaP vaccines. Statistically significant diminution in the immune response to the Hib component (PRP) has occurred with three of four DTaP/Hib products evaluated after the primary series of vaccinations in infancy, Table 2 [9,15–24]. The mechanism(s) responsible for this diminution is unclear. Hypotheses include: (1) loss of the adjuvant effect of whole cell pertussis vaccine, (2) carrier-induced epitopic suppression [18,25,26], (3) effects on anti-

Table 2 Comparison of Anti-PRP Seroresponses to Combined and Separately Administered Hib Containing Vaccine After the Primary Infants Series

Vaccine	Reference (Location)	Schedule	% >0.15 µg/mL	% >1.0 µg/mL	GMC
DTaP$_2$[a]/IPV/PRP-T	[9] (Chile)	2, 4, 6 mo.	99.3	97.1	7.5
DTaP$_2$/IPV + PRP-T			99.3	96.3	14.0
DTaP$_2$/PRP-T	[15] (United States)	2, 4, 6 mo.	94.7	85.3	4.3
DTaP$_2$ + PRP-T			100	100	7.0
DTaP$_2$/PRP-T	[22] (United States)	2, 4, 6 mo.	94	79	3.2
DTaP$_2$ + PRP-T			98	80	4.4
DTaP$_3$/HB/PRP-T	[16] (U.S.A.)	2, 4, 6 mo.	81.3	58.2	1.2
DTaP$_3$ + HB + PRP-T			93.8	87.5	5.5
DTaP$_3$/IPV/PRP-T	[20] (Canada)	2, 4, 6 mo.	96.4	66.3	1.6
DTaP$_3$/IPV + PRP-T			95.1	76.5	3.2
DTaP$_3$/HB/IPV/PRP-T	[24] (Germany)	2, 3, 4 mo.	99.3	77.2	2.6
DTaP$_3$ + HB + IPV + PRP-T			100	88.2	4.5
DTaP$_3$/HB/PRP-T	[23] (United States)	2, 4, 6 mo.	87.8	71.3	1.6
DTaP$_3$ + HB + PRP-T			98.3	90.4	6.15
DTaP$_5$/IPV/PRP-T	[19] (Canada)	2, 4, 6 mo.	98.5	84.7	3.8
DTaP$_5$/IPV + PRP-T					5.0
DTaP$_5$/PRP-T	[21] (Taiwan)	2, 4, 6 mo.	100	98.5	13.0
DTaP$_5$ + PRP-T			100	95.3	11.8

[a] Subscript indicates number of pertussis antigens.

gen capture, processing or presentation [18], or (4) interference with lymphocyte recognition and responses. An alternative explanation offered is that Hib conjugate vaccine may be incompatible with the aluminum adjuvant in DTaP vaccines [25]. Interestingly, suppression of the immune response to PRP has not been observed following the infant primary series of the combination vaccine consisting of the five-component DTaP$_5$, manufactured by Aventis Pasteur, with IPV and PRP-T (Table 2). It is unclear why this product has been an exception. Hepatitis B has also been added to the DTaP$_5$/IPV/PRP-T mixture. Following this hexavalent combination, the postdose GMC of antibody against PRP and hepatitis B surface antigen (HBsAg) was lower in the DTaP$_5$/IPV/PRP-T/HB group than the DTaP$_5$/IPV/PRP-T + HB group. However, the seroprotection rates, defined as anti-PRP antibody level ≥0.15 µg/mL and anti-HBsAg ≥10 IU/mL, were noninferior in the fully combined vaccine group [27].

The GMC of antibody to tetanus toxoid has also been observed to be lower, following vaccination with DTaP/PRP-T combinations [8,14,21]. However, all children achieved the putative protective level of 0.1 IU/mL of antitoxin. Reduction in antibody responses to the tetanus toxoid contained in DTaP/Hib combinations has not been a problem.

The biological significance of diminished anti-PRP responses following primary immunization with DTaP/Hib combinations is actively debated. The obvious concern is that lower levels of antibody may translate into an increase in carriage of *H. influenzae* type b organisms in the population, leading to loss of herd immunity and to increase in disease rates, as what has occurred in Alaska [28]. However, the postprimary series GMT, achieved after immunization in many of the studies with DTaP/Hib combinations, have

often been higher than seen historically following the licensed Hib vaccines. It also has been shown that children with low or even undetectable antibodies to PRP after intake of a DTaP/PRP-T combination are primed for an anamnestic response. Evidence for this includes demonstration of rapid development of high levels of anti-PRP after a fourth dose of either conjugated or unconjugated PRP given to toddlers [16,20,29–31] and the observation that the antibodies produced by these children to the fourth dose are primarily IgG1 [29] and are of high affinity [32,33]—primarily indicating a T-cell-dependent response. There is disagreement about whether the anamnestic response will occur with sufficient rapidity to consistently protect children against invasive disease. Some older children presenting with *H. influenzae* type b meningitis have high levels of anti-PRP antibodies shortly after hospitalization for disease, which suggests that they may have been primed but not protected from invasive infection [34]. Both priming and existing serum antibody are probably important in protection against invasive disease [35].

There are reassuring surveillance data indicating the reliable effectiveness of DTaP/Hib combination vaccines against *H. influenzae* type b invasive disease in German children. Two surveillance systems, one-hospital based and one laboratory-based, were utilized for detection of invasive Hib disease in 1998 and 1999. Although only 70% of children had received three doses of the DTaP/Hib-containing vaccines in the first year of life, the overall vaccine effectiveness among children given at least one dose was 97.5% (95% CI, 96.3–98.4). Vaccine effectiveness was 98.8% (98.2–99.3) following three doses of combination vaccine [36]. The demonstration of population-based field effectiveness is compelling evidence that these DTaP/Hib combinations have been successfully utilized in German children. It is unclear whether these results can be safely extrapolated to other populations of children living in different circumstances.

C. Hepatitis A/Hepatitis B Combination

The inactivated hepatitis A vaccine and recombinant hepatitis B vaccines manufactured by GlaxoSmithKline Biologicals have been combined, and, in the United States, are approved as a three-dose series (0, 1, and 6 months) in individuals 18 years and older. Safety of the vaccine has been evaluated in 2165 adults. Systemic and local reactions experienced were similar to those seen following monovalent hepatitis B immunization [37]. After two doses of vaccine, 98.8% of recipients achieved a putative protective titer of antibody to hepatitis A, but only 78.2% had an anti-HBsAg titer of ≥ 10 mIU/mL, subsequently necessitating a third dose [38]. This combination vaccine is indicated for individuals at risk of exposure to both hepatitis A and hepatitis B.

IV. INVESTIGATIONAL COMBINATION VACCINES

A. Measles–Mumps–Rubella–Varicella Vaccine (MMRV)

Soon after the completion of development of the Oka strain vaccine against varicella, efforts began to combine it with the combined measles–mumps–rubella vaccine. With the initial vaccine compositions, the measles component interfered with the immune response to the varicella component [39–41], necessitating the adjustment of the quantity of varicella in the vaccine. A new formulation of MMRV has been reported to elicit equivalent or better GMT and seroconversion rates to all component of the vaccine compared to separately administered MMR + V [42]. Licensure of this product will save children one injection at 12–15 months of age. It is not yet known whether the quadrivalent MMRV or the MMR will be recommended for the second preschool dose. Cost of the vaccine will be an important determining factor.

B. Conjugate Combination Vaccines

The currently available seven-valent pneumococcal vaccine conjugated to CRM_{197} (7vPnC) contains serotypes—4, 6B, 9V, 14, 18C, 19F, and 23F. These seven serotypes are responsible for approximately 85% of cases of invasive disease in the industrialized world [43]. Serotypes 1 and 5 also are important causes of pneumococcal infection in certain pediatric groups in the United States, such as southwest Native American, older children, and children in the developing world. The addition of serotypes 1 and 5 to the current heptavalent vaccine would extend protection to these groups of children.

It has been estimated that *Neisseria meningitidis* serogroup C causes more sepsis and meningitis in children less than 2 years of age than any of the individual pneumococcal serotypes in the heptavalent pneumococcal vaccine [43,44].

Conjugate meningococcal serogroup C (MnC) vaccine has been licensed and widely used in Great Britain and parts of Canada. Introduction of a separate, injectable MnC vaccine may not be readily accepted in the United States. Therefore safety and immunogenicity studies of a nine-valent pneumococcal vaccine conjugated to CRM_{197}/meningococcal group C conjugated to CRM_{197} (9vPnC–MnCC)$\pm H.$ influenzae type b conjugate to CRM_{197} (HbOC) are underway. The preliminary results of a study of a three-dose schedule at 2, 4, and 6 months of age indicate that the combination vaccines are no more reactogenic than separately injected 7vPnC and HbOC vaccines. The humoral immune responses to the seven pneumococcal vaccine serotypes by both the 9vPnC/MnCC and 9vPnc/MnCC/HbOC were noninferior to those stimulated by 7vPnC. Anti-PRP responses in the 9vPnc/MnCC/HbOC were diminished compared to those of recipients of separately administered HbOC and 7vPnC, but the anti-PRP responses in the 9v-MnCC+HbOC group satisfied the criteria for noninferiority. Primary IgG responses to MnC and pneumococcal types 1 and 5 were observed. These preliminary results suggest that 9vPnC/MnCC is acceptably reactogenic and immunogenic, and should be further developed [45].

Introduction of new parenteral vaccines into the routine childhood immunization schedule will require the licensure and availability of further combinations of vaccines. If surveillance data from additional countries employing DTaP/Hib combination vaccines indicate the control of Hib disease, perhaps the criteria for establishment of immunologic noninferiority may be reexamined. Ongoing communication and cooperation among investigators, industry, and regulatory bodies will be necessary to advance this important field.

REFERENCES

1. Decker MD. Principles of pediatric combination vaccines and practical issues related to use in clinical practice. Pediatr Infect Dis J 2001; 20:S14.
2. Gellin BG, et al. Do parents understand immunizations? A national telephone survey. Pediatrics 2000; 106:1097–1102.
3. Corkill JM. The stability of the components in DTP–poliomyelitis and DPT–poliomyelitis–measles vaccines. Symposia Series in Immunological Standardization 7. Basel: Karger, 1967:165–178.
4. Pittman M. Instability of pertussis vaccine component in quadruple antigen vaccine, diphtheria, and tetanus toxoids and pertussis and poliomyelitis vaccines. J Am Med Assoc 1962; 181:25–30.
5. Edsall G, et al. Significance of the loss of potency in the pertussis component of certain lots of "quadruple antigen". N Engl J Med 1962; 267:687–689.
6. André FE, Peetermans J. Effect of simultaneous administration of live mumps vaccines on the "take rate" of live mumps vaccines. In: IABS Congress on Use and Standardization of Combined Vaccines. Amsterdam, The Netherlands, 1985. Dev Biol Stand 1986; Vol. 65:101–107.
7. Blackwelder WC. Similarity/equivalence trials for combination vaccines. Ann NY Acad Sci 1995; 754:321–328.
8. Halperin SA, et al. Effect of inactivated poliovirus vaccine on the antibody response to *Bordetella pertussis* antigens when combined with diphtheria pertussis–tetanus vaccine. Clin Infect Dis 1996; 22:59–62.

9. Lagos R, et al. Clinical acceptability and immunogenicity of a pentavalent parenteral combination vaccine containing diphtheria, tetanus, acellular pertussis, inactivated poliomyelitis and *Haemophilus influenzae* type b conjugate antigens in two-, four-, and six-month-old Chilean infants. Pediatr Infect Dis J 1998; 17:294–304.

10. Yeh SH, et al. Safety and immunogenicity of a pentavalent diphtheria, tetanus, pertussis, hepatitis B and polio combination vaccine in infants. Pediatr Infect Dis J 2001; 20:973–980.

11. Storsaeter J, et al. Levels of anti-pertussis antibodies related to protection after household exposure to *Bordetella pertussis*. Vaccine 1998; 16:1907–1916.

12. Watemberg N, et al. Safety and immunogenicity of *Haemophilus* type b-tetanus protein conjugate vaccine, mixed in the same syringe with diphtheria–tetanus–pertussis vaccine in young infants. Pediatr Infect Dis J 1991; 10:758–761.

13. Paradiso PR, et al. Safety and immunogenicity of a combined diphtheria, tetanus, pertussis and influenzae type b vaccine in young infants. Pediatrics 1993; 92:827–832.

14. Kaplan S, et al. Immunogenicity and safety of *Haemophilus influenzae* type b-tetanus protein conjugate vaccine alone or mixed with diphtheria–tetanus–pertussis vaccine in infants. J Pediatr 1994; 124:323–327.

15. Pichichero ME, et al. Vaccine antigen interactions after a combination diphtheria–tetanus toxoid–acellular pertussis/purified capsular polysaccharide of *Haemophilus influenzae* type b-tetanus toxoid vaccine in two-, four-, and six-month-old infants. Pediatr Infect Dis J 1997; 16:863–870.

16. Pichichero ME, Passador S. Administration of combined diphtheria and tetanus toxoids and pertussis vaccine, hepatitis b vaccine, and *Haemophilus influenzae* type b (Hib) vaccine to infants. Clin Infect Dis 1997; 25:1378–1384.

17. Shinefield H, Black S, Ray P, Lewis N, Adelman T, Ensor K, Hohenboken CA, Hohenboken M, Hackell J. Immunogenicity of combined DTaP–HbOC vaccine (Wyeth–Lederle) in infants and toddler follow-up: evidence of immunologic interference. Presented at the European Society for Pediatric Infectious Disease. Paris, France, 1997.

18. Dagan R, et al. Reduced responses to multiple vaccines sharing common protein epitopes that are administered simultaneously to infants. Infect Immun 1998; 66:2093–2098.

19. Mills E, et al. Safety and immunogenicity of a combined five-component pertussis diphtheria—tetanus-inactivated poliomyelitis–*Haemophilus* b conjugate vaccine administered to infants at two, four and six months of age. Vaccine 1998; 16:576–585.

20. Halperin SA, et al. Safety and immunogenicity of *Haemophilus influenzae*–tetanus toxoid conjugate vaccine given separately or in combination with a three-component acellular pertussis vaccine combined with diphtheria and tetanus toxoids and inactivated poliovirus vaccine for the first four doses. Clin Infect Dis 1999; 28:995–1001.

21. Lee C-Y, et al. An evaluation of the safety and immunogenicity of a five component acellular pertussis, diphtheria, and tetanus toxoid vaccine (DTaP) when combined with a *Haemophilus influenzae* type b-tetanus toxoid conjugate vaccine (PRP-T) in Taiwanese infants. Pediatrics 1999; 103:25–30.

22. Rennels MB, et al. Diminution of the anti-polyribosylribitol phosphate response to a combined diphtheria–tetanus–acellular pertussis/*Haemophilus influenzae* type b vaccine by concurrent inactivated poliovirus vaccination. Pediatr Infect Dis J 2000; 19:417–423.

23. Greenberg DP, et al. Immunogenicity of a *Haemophilus influenzae* type b –tetanus toxoid conjugate vaccine when mixed with a diphtheria –tetanus acellular pertussis–hepatitis B combination vaccine. Pediatr Infect Dis J 2000; 19:1135–1140.

24. Schmitt HJ, et al. Primary vaccination of infants with diphtheria–tetanus–acellular pertussis–hepatitis B virus-inactivated polio virus and *Haemophilus influenzae* type b vaccines given as either separate or mixed injections. J Pediatr 2000; 137:304–312.

25. Insel RA. Potential alterations in immunogenicity by combining or simultaneously administering vaccine components. Ann NY Acad Sci 1995; 754:35–47.

26. Eskola J, et al. Randomized trial of the effect of co-administration with acellular pertussis DTP vaccine on immunogenicity of *Haemophilus influenzae* type b conjugate vaccine. Lancet 1996; 348:1688–1692.

27. Mallet E, et al. Immunogenicity and safety of a new liquid hexavalent combined vaccine compared with separate administration of reference licensed vaccines in infants. Pediatr Infect Dis J 2000; 19:1119–1127.

28. Galil K, et al. Reemergence of invasive *Haemophilus influenzae* type b disease in a well-vaccinated population in remote Alaska. J Infect Dis 1999; 179:101–106.

29. Zepp F, et al. Evidence for induction of polysaccharide-specific B-cell memory in the 1st year of life: plain *Haemophilus influenzae* type b-PRP (Hib) boosters children primed with a tetanus-conjugate Hib–DTaP–HBV combined vaccine. Eur J Pediatr 1997; 156:18–24.

30. Bell F, et al. Effect of combination with an acellular pertussis, diphtheria, tetanus vaccine on antibody response to Hib vaccine (PRP-T). Vaccine, 1998, 16637–16642.

31. Goldblatt D, et al. The induction of immunologic memory after vaccination with *Haemophilus influenzae* type b conjugate and acellular pertussis containing diphtheria, tetanus, and pertussis vaccine combination. J Infect Dis 1999; 180:538–541.

32. Pichichero ME, et al. Kinetics of booster responses to *Haemophilus influenzae* type b conjugate after combined diphtheria–tetanus–acellular pertussis *Haemophilus influenzae* type b vaccination in infants. Pediatr Infect Dis J 1999; 18:1106–1108.

33. Poolman J, et al. Clinical relevance of lower Hib response in DTaP-based combination vaccines. Vaccine 2001; 19:2280–2285.

34. Anderson P, et al. A high degree of natural immunologic priming to the capsular polysaccharide may not prevent *Haemophilus influenzae* type b meningitis. Pediatr Infect Dis J 2000; 19:589–591.

35. Lucas AH, Granoff DM. Imperfect memory and the development of *Haemophilus influenzae* type b disease. Pediatr Infect Dis J 2000; 19:235–239.

36. Schmitt H-J, et al. *Haemophilus influenzae* type b disease: impact and effectiveness of diphtheria–tetanus toxoids–acellular pertussis (-inactivated poliovirus)/*Haemophilus influenzae* type b combination vaccines. Pediatr Infect Dis J 2001; 20:767–774.

37. Czeschinski PA, et al. Hepatitis A and hepatitis B vaccinations: immunogenicity of combined vaccine and of simultaneously or separately applied single vaccines. Vaccine 2000; 18:1074–1080.

38. MMWR. Notice to Readers: FDA approval for a combined hepatitis A and B vaccine. MMWR 2001; 50:806–807.

39. Brunell PA, et al. Combined vaccine against measles, mumps, rubella and varicella. Pediatrics 1988; 81:779–784.

40. Berger R, Just M. Interference between strains in live virus vaccines. II. Combined vaccination with varicella and measles–mumps–rubella vaccine. J Biol Standard 1988; 16:275–279.

41. White CJ, et al. Measles, mumps, rubella, and varicella combination vaccine: safety and immunogenicity alone and in combination with other vaccines given to children. Clin Infect Dis 1997; 25:925–931.

42. Shinefield HR, et al. Evaluation of a new formulation of a

quadrivalent measles, mumps, rubella, and varicella (MMRV) vaccine in healthy infants. Soc Pediatr Res 2000; 47:276A.

43. Butler JC, et al. Serotype distribution of *Streptococcus pneumoniae* infections among preschool children in the United States, 1978–1994: implications for development of a conjugate vaccine. J Infect Dis 1995; 171:885–889.

44. Rosenstein NE, et al. The changing epidemiology of menin-gococcal disease in the United States, 1992–1996. J Infect Dis 1999; 180:1894–1901.

45. Rennels M, et al. Safety and immunogenicity of combined conjugate 9-valent *S. pneumoniae*-meningococcal group C and *Haemophilus influenzae* b–9vPnC–MnCC (HbOC–9vPnC–MnCC) vaccine. 41st Interscience Conference on Antimicrobial Agents and Chemotherapy. Chicago, IL, 2001: A2039.

36

Meningococcal Conjugate and Protein-Based Vaccines

Rino Rappuoli
Chiron S.r.l., Siena, Italy

Andrew J. Pollard and E. Richard Moxon
University of Oxford, John Radcliffe Hospital, Oxford, England

Neisseria meningitidis remains as one of the leading infectious causes of death in childhood in many industrialized countries and a cause of devastating epidemics in nonindustrialized nations. About 500,000 cases of endemic meningococcal infection are thought to occur annually worldwide [1], with the greatest burden of disease in Africa and Asia. Of great public health importance, meningococci are the cause of cyclic epidemic meningitis in Africa [2] and Asia [3], and occasional outbreaks have been associated with population movements and overcrowding in other regions over the past half century [4].

Currently, five serogroups of meningococci, A, B, C, Y, and W135, defined by the biochemistry of their polysaccharide capsule, are responsible for almost all meningococcal disease, although the overall proportions of cases caused by each serogroup vary widely around the globe. In industrialized nations, serogroup B meningococci cause 30–70% of cases of sporadic meningococcal disease [5–7], and have been responsible for pockets of persistently increased rates of disease [8–10]. Serogroup C meningococci are particularly associated with small outbreaks of disease among teenagers and young adults and sporadic disease in individuals of other ages [6]. Serogroup Y disease is uncommon in the United Kingdom but accounts for up to 30% of cases in the United States [6], and rates of Y-disease may also be on the rise in some parts of Canada [7]. Occasional sporadic disease caused by W135 meningococci had been largely ignored until a recent large outbreak among pilgrims to the Hajj in 2000 [11]. Although the epidemiological characteristics of disease caused by each serogroup are intriguingly different, the clinical features of invasive disease are mostly indistinguishable. The shifting epidemiological patterns of meningococcal carriage and disease are poorly understood, and the lack of predictability concerning the future spatial and temporal distribution of this pathogen must be taken into account as vaccines are developed. Nonetheless, several new vaccine initiatives provide the possibility of a major reduction in the global burden of this disease during the coming decade. The contribution of vaccines in the control of meningococcal disease is particularly important because of the rapidity of its onset, and the short window of time that may exist between health, acquisition of meningococci, fulminant disease, and death. Antibiotics and specialist intensive care have significantly reduced the mortality rate from meningococcal septicaemia [12] in specialized centers in industrialized countries. However, the timely and universal availability of such treatment cannot be provided for most of the world, particularly in countries where access to antibiotics and primary health care, let alone sophisticated intensive management, is virtually unavailable on a day-to-day basis. Widespread control of meningococcal disease is an important public health goal, and immunization is the only realistic means to achieve this aim.

The bedrock of progress rests on the crucial role of capsular polysaccharides (PS) of meningococci in virulence and the protective role of serum antibodies to these surface-exposed carbohydrate antigens.

The protective role of antibodies able to promote complement-mediated killing of bacteria [bactericidal activity (BCA)] was demonstrated in the 1960s [13]. This information was used to develop and license vaccines composed of purified capsular polysaccharides, which are currently available as bivalent vaccines against serogroups A and C, or as tetravalent vaccines against serogroups A, C, Y, and W135. Although there is proven efficacy for MenA and C plain polysaccharides (PS), polysaccharide vaccines are still used only in people at increased risk (for instance, military recruits), or in response to outbreaks. They have never been considered for universal vaccination because of several shortcomings that compromise their utility. Specifically, immunization with MenA PS does not confer long-term protection (it is effective for about 6 years), and MenC PS is unsatisfactory as a vaccine in children aged less than 2 years. Most importantly, polysaccharide vaccines do not induce immunological memory. Improved immunogenicity and immunological memory-mediated longer-term protection, especially in infants and young children, can be realized through conjugation of the capsular PS to carrier proteins. Described for the first time in 1992 [14], conjugate/protein–polysaccharide vaccines (CV) were introduced into the U.K. primary infant schedule in November 1999 against MenC, after many years of careful assessment of their safety and immunogenicity. They had a major impact on disease caused by Serogroup C meningococci in childhood in the United Kingdom [15, see Chapter 45)]. MenC CVs have also been licensed in other countries around Europe [16] and in Canada [7]. Furthermore, combination A/C conjugate vaccines have already been proven immunogenic in clinical trials performed in infants and children [17], while combinations of A, C, Y, and W135 protein–polysaccharide CVs are underway, and there is a reasonable expectation that these combination meningococcal vaccines will be available within a few years, and will provide effective protection from infancy onward. This optimism has been boosted by the announcement of significant funding from *The Bill and Melinda Gates Foundation* in July 2001. This initiative and, in addition, further development of a serogroup A/C conjugate vaccine under the direction of the Global Alliance for Vaccines and Immunization (GAVI) could halt the cycle of epidemic disease in Africa [18].

Progress toward the global control of disease caused by A, C, Y, and W135 must be tempered in view of the current failure to find a solution to the problem of MenB disease. The highest attack rate of meningococcal disease is in children under 5 years of age and, at this age, 50% of disease is caused by MenB in the USA (1992–1996) [6], 39% in Canada (1985–2000) [7], and more than 65% in the UK (1999–2000) [5].

The major stumbling block concerning a MenB vaccine is that the polysaccharide capsule is a homopolymer of sialic acid, chemically identical to polysaccharides found in human tissues, especially fetal brain during development [19]. Hence the Group B capsule is seen by the immune system as a self-antigen; this may partly account for its poor immunogenicity, even after its conjugation to a protein carrier [20]. Although the lack of immunogenicity of the sialic acid capsule is a major problem in the development of a MenB vaccine, research efforts in this area continue because of the attractiveness of a vaccine antigen that is, by definition, shared across this group of meningococci. There are obvious attractions to employing an approach using principles that have successfully worked for other capsular polysaccharides. Jennings and workers have pioneered an innovation in which chemical modification of the polysaccharide (*N*-propionylation) retains immunogenic epitopes. This approach has resulted in the development of a protein–polysaccharide conjugate vaccine that elicits functional (bactericidal) antibody in both mice and nonhuman primates [21,22]. Some of the antibodies elicited have activity against polysialic acid and therefore have the potential to be auto-reactive in humans, although no deleterious effects have been noted in early human trials (P. Fusco and Baxter, personal commu-

nication, 2001). Nonetheless, there is a strong sense that the strategy of polysaccharide–protein conjugation is not attractive to vaccine developers who anticipate ethical and regulatory difficulties that may be difficult, if not impossible, to resolve in taking forward these vaccines as commercially viable propositions. However, other antibodies that arise after immunization with a conjugate *N*-propionylated serogroup B polysaccharide vaccine do not cross-react with human tissues. A derivative approach that might avoid the cross-reactivity issue is to use molecular mimetics of non-autoreactive epitopes as potentially safe serogroup B vaccine antigens [23].

The problems encountered in the development of MenB polysaccharide-based vaccines has resulted in the consideration of a variety of alternative candidates, some of which have already shown encouraging efficacy in clinical trials; others are being rigorously evaluated in early-phase clinical trials and preclinical development programs.

Evaluation of the potential utility of these alternative MenB vaccine candidates is difficult because of the lack of an accepted laboratory surrogate of protection. Other than to capsular polysaccharides, no defined level of circulating antibody to serogroup B meningococci relates to protection against invasive disease. However, indirect evidence suggests that a certain titer of bactericidal antibody (dilutions of serum that can kill meningococci in the laboratory in the presence of complement) might be correlated with protection at the population level [13].

Because of these difficulties in realizing an effective MenB polysaccharide vaccine, investigators have turned their attention to other bacterial surface structures as vaccines. Potentially, surface-exposed components of the cell envelope of meningococci include a large number of outer membrane proteins (OMPs), lipoproteins, and lipopolysaccharide (LPS).

The OMPs of MenB have been extensively studied as potential vaccine constituents since the 1970s. A drawback to their candidacy as vaccines is that these proteins tend to be highly variable not only among different MenB isolates, but also within clonal populations of the same strain. As a consequence, any outer membrane protein from a single strain is unlikely to provide cross-protection to all other MenB strains. Furthermore, the antigenic regions of many of these protein structures evolve rapidly within bacterial populations because of the natural selection on carriage strains, especially through the acquired host immune clearance mechanisms mediated by local and systemic B cells. Despite these problems, outer membrane-based vaccine candidates have reached trials and one is currently in routine use in Central and South America [24]. However, to date, there is little convincing evidence that these vaccines are effective in young children in whom the attack rates for invasive MenB disease are highest.

The earliest OMP vaccines comprised of insoluble aggregates of outer membrane proteins that were poorly immunogenic in humans [25]. Purified OMPs noncovalently complexed to meningococcal C-polysaccharide were tested in a trial in Chile and resulted in substantial protection in older children and young adults (70%), but were poorly protective in children less than 5 years of age [26]. To im-

Table 1 Summary of the Efficacy Trials Against Meningococcus B Performed with Outer Membrane Vesicle Vaccines

Trial (year)	Vaccine (strain)	Doses	Efficacy, adults (age)	Efficacy, children (age)	Efficacy, infants (age)	Efficacy, total	Ref.
Norway 1988–1991	NIPH 15:P1.7,16	2 doses	87% (10 mo) 57% (29 mo) (13–16 yr)	/	/		[26]
Cuba 1987–1989	Finlay 4:P1.19,15	2 doses	83% (10–14 yr)	/	/		[23]
Brazil 1990–1991	Finlay 4:P1.19,15	2 doses	74% (>48 mo)	47% (24–47 mo)	−37% (<24 mo)	54%	[27]
Chile (Iquique) 1987–1989	Cuban type 15:P1.7b,3	2 doses	70% (30 mo) (5–21 yr)	/	−23% (30 mo) (1–4 yr)	51%	[25]

prove immunogenicity, OMP vaccines were produced in spheres of bacterial outer membrane, known as outer membrane vesicles (OMVs) [26]. These OMV vaccines have now been evaluated in large-scale trials (Table 1) and, using two doses, have resulted in substantial protection in older children [24,26,27], but not in children under 4 years of age [24,26,28,29]. Furthermore, bactericidal antibody tends to be directed to the serogroup B meningococcal "type strain" included in the vaccine (Table 2, [30,31]).

The major target of protective immunity in these OMV vaccines is PorA, a porin that is the basis of the subserotyping system of meningococci, and therefore known to be antigenically variable. The role of PorA as a target for protective antibodies, the problem of its variability, and the lack of cross-strain protection have stimulated research culminating in second-generation OMV vaccines. This approach used genetic techniques so that six different PorA proteins, expressed in two engineered strains, were included. Phase II trials in various age groups have demonstrated variable and, overall, disappointing immunogenicity to each PorA type [32]. Furthermore, mutations in the genes encoding this protein are common and result in evasion of complement-mediated killing of the organism, further complicating the success of this approach [33].

Nonetheless, the observation that some protection and induction of bactericidal antibody directed against the vaccine strain is induced with monovalent OMV vaccines suggests that these vaccines may be of use in outbreaks of serogroup B disease caused by a single "type strain" of

bacteria. For example, over the past decade, the rates of MenB disease in New Zealand are 4–20 times higher than other industrialized countries [8]. In July 2001, the Ministry of Health in New Zealand announced plans for further development of a monovalent OMV vaccine with Chiron Corporation in conjunction with the National Institute for Public Health (NIPH), Norway, in the hope of halting serogroup B disease [34]. Considering the antigenic variability of PorA and the disappointing efficacy of OMV vaccines in children, preclinical research into other surface-exposed membrane proteins as vaccine candidates has been undertaken. Antigenic variability or inconsistent accessibility to antibodies across genetically different strains has proved to be problematical and none has been taken forward into clinical trials except for the transferrin binding protein (TbpB), for which the immunogenicity was disappointing [35].

In addition to surface expressed proteins, another major component of the cell envelope of all gram-negative bacteria, including meningococci, is lipopolysaccharide (LPS). The potential use of LPS as a vaccine has been impeded by concerns about toxicity, especially through lipid A (endotoxin) and the molecular mimicry of *N. meningitidis* glycoforms, especially lacto-*N*-tetraose, expressed on human cells. However, there is now compelling evidence to support the potential of meningococcal LPS as a vaccine, or as a component of one. Evidence of protection by antibodies to the LPS has been documented in animals [36,37] and humans [38,39], although antibodies induced by outer membrane vesicle vaccines retaining LPS lacked bactericidal activity

Table 2 Strain Specificity of the Immuno-Response in Infants and Children After Immunization with OMV Vaccines

Test strain	Bactericidal activity, Norwegian vaccine			Bactericidal activity, Cuban vaccine		
	Infants	Children	Adults	Infants	Children	Adults
Chile	12	35	60	10	31	37
Cuban	2	24	46	**90**	**78**	**67**
Norwegian	**98**	**98**	**96**	31	41	56

Comparison of bactericidal responses against homologous and heterologous strains induced in infants, children, and adults in a clinical trial in Iquique (Chile) using the Cuban and Norwegian OMV vaccines. As shown, three doses of OMV vaccines induce good bactericidal titers against the homologous strain at all ages. No or low titers found against heterologous strain in infants and children, respectively.

Table 3 Bactericidal Activity Against a Panel of Different Strains Induced by Three Prototype Antigens Against Meningococcus B

	B	B	B	B	B	B	A	C	C
Strain	2996	BZ232	1000	MC58	NGH38	394/98	F612	C11	BZ133
OMP	16,000	2048	–	–	–	–	–	–	–
OMV	65,000	8000	–	2048	–	–	32,000	–	–
Non-OMP	65,000	512	4000	8000	32,000	4000	8000	1024	16,000

OMP is a purified outer membrane protein with a predicted typical beta-barrel structure spanning the outer membrane. OMV is a typical OMV vaccine produced from strains 2996. Non-OMP is a new surface-exposed protein discovered with the genomic approach.

[40,41]. A Phase 1 study of detoxified LPS (immunotypes L3, 7, and 9) was immunogenic, but most of the functional antibody was directed against OMPs [42]. Nontoxic LPS vaccines have been also produced by conjugating the core saccharide to protein carriers, but this strategy failed to induce antibodies with bactericidal activity [43–45]. A different approach, one also addressing the unproven but theoretical concern of an autoimmune response induced by lacto-*N*-tetraose, has resulted in vaccines based on the inner core region of LPS. This component is relatively conserved across the species, and there is strong evidence to indicate the accessibility of inner core epitopes to antibodies based on studies of in vitro grown and ex vivo organisms [46,47]. Monoclonal antibodies (Mabs) specific for inner core epitopes indicate that that these structures can be targets for bactericidal activity and protective immune responses in animals (infant rats) challenged with some, but not all, strains of meningococci [48].

I. GENOME-BASED DISCOVERY OF NEW ANTIGENS

The recent availability of two meningococcal genomes [49, 50] allowed to pursue vaccine development in a new way that was named "reverse vaccinology" [51]. Novel potential vaccine candidates were identified in silico using computer programs and subsequently expressed as recombinant fusion-proteins in *Escherichia coli*. The recombinant antigens were then purified and used to immunize mice. Finally, the sera obtained were tested in vitro for their ability to kill bacteria in the presence of exogenous complement. The work was performed while the sequence was in progress and by the time the sequence was published, the first screening for new antigens was also completed. Computer analysis identified approximately 600 potential antigens predicted to be surface-exposed. A total of 370 of these were successfully expressed in *E. coli*, purified, and then used to immunize mice. Of the 370 sera tested, 29 showed bactericidal activity. As soon as the 29 novel antigens had been identified, a lot of work was put into their characterization in order to select those that induced the best bactericidal activity against all strains. In a first approach, the genes of the novel antigens were sequenced in a panel of strains representative of the genetic variability of the worldwide population of meningococcus B. Surprisingly, many of the novel genes were found to be quite conserved among genetically diverse strains, suggesting that some of the novel proteins could be used to develop a vaccine against all serogroup B meningocci. Finally, the bactericidal activity induced by all of them was tested against a panel of genetically diverse strains. Some of the novel antigens were indeed found to induce a bactericidal activity against most of the strains tested; however, many induced bactericidal activity only against a subgroup of them. Table 3 compares the immune response against a recombinant OMP, an OMV-based vaccine, and a recombinant protein found by the genomic approach. As shown, while the recombinant OMP and the OMV vaccine induce bactericidal antibodies against a subset of strains, the genome-derived antigen is able to induce immunity against all strains tested. The proteins inducing the most cross-reacting bactericidal response are now being studied alone or in combination in order to find a vaccine formulation that, hopefully, is going to be effective against all strains. The combination of several antigens in the vaccine formulation should be able to avoid the generation of escape mutants, which are to be expected for single antigens. One of the antigens identified by genome screening (GNA 33), although conserved in sequence, was found to induce immunity against only a subgroup of strains having P1.2 porin. It was found that this antigen contains a QTP (Q = glutamine; T = threonine; P = proline) peptide, which induces strong antibodies against the loop 4 of porin A, where the QTP sequence is also present. This example shows that the genome-based approach not only finds genuine antigens, but can also pick up mimetic antigens which induce protective immunity against other targets present in the bacterium [52].

Protein antigens have been found not only by using the genomic approach, but also by using more conventional techniques. The best known of these is NspA, a protein of the outer membrane which is well conserved among strains and induces bactericidal antibodies against many but not all of them [53,54].

II. CONCLUSIONS

Polysaccharide vaccines against serogroups A, C, Y, and W135 of meningococcus have been available for decades and have been useful for immunization of at-risk groups and control of outbreaks. They have never been used for general immunization because they provide a short-term immunity with no memory and, in most of the cases, they do not work in infants and children. A conjugate vaccine against meningococcus C, licensed in the United Kingdom in 1999, has been extremely effective in eliminating the disease in all ages, showing that conjugate vaccines are an excellent solution for the prevention of meningococcus. In fact, they induce immunological memory and are efficacious at all ages. Conjugates against serogroups A, Y, and W135 are also in development, and are expected to be licensed within 3–6 years. The conjugation approach cannot be applied as such to serogroup B because the capsular polysaccharide is a polysialic acid identical to a self-antigen. To avoid this problem, a number of alternative approaches have been tested. These include the chemical modification of the polysaccharide, the use of OMVs, the use of the core structure of the LPS, and the search for conserved proteins inducing a bactericidal response. The use of the whole genomic sequence to identify novel protein targets has provided many novel antigens. It is reasonable to hope that within the next decade, we may have vaccines for the universal prevention of all meningococcal diseases.

REFERENCES

1. Tikhomirov E, et al. Meningococcal disease: public health burden and control. World Health Stat Q 1997; 50:170–177.
2. Lapeyssonnie L. La meningite cerebro-spinale en Afrique. Bull WHO 1963; 28:3–114.
3. Wang JF, et al. Clonal and antigenic analysis of serogroup A *Neisseria meningitidis* with particular reference to epidemiological features of epidemic meningitis in the People's Republic of China. Infect Immun 1992; 60:5267–5282.
4. Achtman M. Global Epidemiology of Meningococcal Disease. In: Cartwright K, ed. Meningococcal Disease. Chichester: John Wiley and Sons, 1995:159–175.
5. Communicable Disease Surveillance Centre and the Meningococcal Reference Unit. Invasive Meningococcal Infections, England and Wales, by age and serogroup. 2001; http://www.phls.co.uk/facts/Mening/N%20Mening/meni-Quarters.htm.
6. Rosenstein NE, et al. The changing epidemiology of meningococcal disease in the United States, 1992–1996. J Infect Dis 1999; 180:1894–1901.
7. Pollard AJ, National Committee on Immunization (NACI). Statement on recommended use of pneumococcal conjugate vaccine. An Advisory Committee Statement (ACS). National Advisory Committee on Immunization (NACI). Can Commun Dis Rev 2002; 28(Pt2):1–32.
8. Baker M, et al. Household crowding a major risk factor for epidemic meningococcal disease in Auckland children. Pediatr Infect Dis J 2000; 19:983–990.
9. Diermayer M, et al. Epidemic serogroup B meningococcal disease in Oregon: the evolving epidemiology of the ET-5 strain. J Am Med Assoc 1999; 281:1493–1497.
10. Stuart JM, et al. An outbreak of meningococcal disease in Stonehouse: planning and execution of a large-scale survey. Epidemiol Infect 1987; 99:579–589.
11. Centers for Disease Control and Prevention. Update: assessment of risk for meningococcal disease associated with the Hajj 2001. Morb Mort Wkly Rep 2001; 50:221–222.
12. Levin M, et al. Improved survival in children admitted to intensive care with meningococcal disease. In: 2nd Annual Spring Meeting of the Royal College of Paediatrics and Child Health. University of York: Royal College of Paediatric and Child Health, 1998.
13. Goldschneider I, et al. Human immunity to the meningococcus. I. The role of humoral antibodies. J Exp Med 1969; 129:1307–1326.
14. Costantino P, et al. Development and phase I clinical testing of a conjugate vaccine against meningococcus A and C. Vaccine 1992; 10:691–698.
15. Ramsay ME, et al. Efficacy of meningococcal serogroup C conjugate vaccine in teenagers and toddlers in England. Lancet 2001; 357:195–196.
16. Cartwright K, et al. Meningococcal disease in Europe: epidemiology, mortality and prevention with conjugate vaccines. Vaccine 2001; 19:4347–4356.
17. Fairley CK, et al. Conjugate meningococcal serogroup A and C vaccine: reactogenicity and immunogenicity in United Kingdom infants. Infect Dis 1996; 174:1360–1363.
18. World Health Organisation. The Meningitis Vaccine Project. 2001; http://www.who.int/vaccines/intermediate/meningococcus.htm.
19. Finne J, et al. An IgG monoclonal antibody to group B meningococci cross-reacts with developmentally regulated polysialic acid units of glycoproteins in neural and extraneural tissues. J Immunol 1987; 138:4402–4407.
20. Bartoloni A, et al. Immunogenicity of meningococcal B polysaccharide conjugated to tetanus toxoid or CRM197 via adipic acid dihydrazide. Vaccine 1995; 13:463–470.
21. Fusco PC, et al. Preclinical evaluation of a novel group B meningococcal conjugate vaccine that elicits bactericidal activity in both mice and nonhuman primates. J Infect Dis 1997; 175:364–372.
22. Jennings H, et al. *N*-PropionylatedGroup b meningococcal polysaccharide mimics a unique epitope on Group B *Neisseria meningitidis*. J Exp Med 1987; 165:1207–1211.
23. Granoff DM, et al. Bactericidal monoclonal antibodies that define unique meningococcal B polysaccharide epitopes that do not cross-react with human polysialic acid. J Immunol 1998; 160:5028–5036.
24. Sierra GV, et al. Vaccine against group B *Neisseria meningitidis*: protection trial and mass vaccination results in Cuba. NIPH Ann 1991; 14:195–207. Discussion 208–210.
25. Zollinger WD, et al. Safety and immunogenicity of a *Neisseria meningitidis* type 2 protein vaccine in animals and humans. J Infect Dis 1978; 137:728–739.
26. Boslego J, et al. Efficacy, safety, and immunogenicity of a meningococcal group B (15:P1.3) outer membrane protein vaccine in Iquique, Chile. Chilean National Committee for Meningococcal Disease. Vaccine 1995; 13:821–829.
27. Bjune G, et al. Effect of outer membrane vesicle vaccine against group B meningococcal disease in Norway. Lancet 1991; 338:1093–1096.
28. de Moraes JC, et al. Protective efficacy of a serogroup B meningococcal vaccine in Sao Paulo, Brazil. Lancet 1992; 340:1074–1078.
29. Noronha CP, Struchiner CJ, Halloran ME. Assessment of the direct effectiveness of BC meningococcal vaccine in Rio de Janeiro, Brazil: a case-control study. Int J Epidemiol 1995; 24:1050–1057.
30. Perkins BA, et al. Immunogenicity of two efficacious outer membrane protein-based serogroup B meningococcal vaccines among young adults in Iceland. J Infect Dis 1998; 177:683–691.
31. Tappero JW, et al. Immunogenicity of 2 serogroup B outer-membrane protein meningococcal vaccines: a randomized controlled trial in Chile. J Am Med Assoc 1999; 281:1520–1527.
32. Cartwright K, et al. Immunogenicity and reactogenicity in UK infants of a novel meningococcal vesicle vaccine containing multiple class 1 (PorA) outer membrane proteins. Vaccine 1999; 17:2612–2619.
33. de Kleijn ED, et al. Immunogenicity and safety of a hexavalent meningococcal outer-membrane- vesicle vaccine in children of 2–3 and 7–8 years of age. Vaccine 2000; 18:1456–1466.
34. New Zealand Ministry of Health. Development of meningococcal vaccine to begin. 2001; http://www.moh.gov.nz/moh.nsf/wpg_Index/News + and + Issues-Index.

35. Danve B, et al. Safety and immunogenicity of a *Neisseria meningitidis* group B transferrin binding protein vaccine in adults. In: Eleventh International Pathogenic Neisseria Conference. EDK, Paris: Nice, 1998.

36. Saukkonen K, et al. Comparative evaluation of potential components for group B meningococcal vaccine by passive protection in the infant rat and in vitro bactericidal assay. Vaccine 1989; 7:325–328.

37. Zollinger WD, et al. Bactericidal antibody responses of juvenile rhesus monkeys to Neisseria meningitidis conjugate B polysaccharide vaccines. Neisseria 94: Proceedings of the Ninth International Pathogenic Neisseria Conference. Winchester, England, Sept 26–30, 1994:441–442.

38. Griffiss JM, et al. Immune response of infants and children to disseminated infections with *Neisseria meningitidis*. J Infect Dis 1984; 150:71–79.

39. Plested JS, et al. Functional opsonic activity of human serum antibodies to inner core lipopolysaccharide (galE) of serogroup B meningococci measured by flow cytometry. Infect Immun May 2001; 69:3203–3213.

40. Rosenqvist E, et al. The 5C protein of *Neisseria meningitidis* is highly immunogenic in humans and induces bactericidal antibodies. J Infect Dis 1993; 167:1065–1073.

41. Rosenqvist E, et al. Human antibody responses to meningococcal outer membrane antigens after three doses of the Norwegian group B meningococcal vaccine. Infect Immun 1995; 63:4642–4652.

42. Zollinger WD, et al. Phase I safety and immunogenicity study of a meningococcal outer membrane protein, detoxified LPS vaccine. Frontiers in Vaccine Research. Hanasaari, Finland, Sept 9–11 1991.

43. Jennings HJ, et al. Conjugation of meningococcal lipopolysaccharide R type oligosaccharides to tetanus toxoid as route to a potential vaccine against group B Neisseria meningococcal lipopolysaccharide R type oligosaccharides to tetanus toxoid as route to a potential vaccine against group B *Neisseria meningitidis*. Infect Immun 1984; 43:407–412.

44. Verheul AF, et al. Preparation, characterisation, and immunogenicity of meningococcal immunotype L2 and L3,7,9 phosphoethanolamine group-containing oligosaccharide–protein conjugates. Infect Immun 1991; 59:843–851.

45. Verheul AF, et al. Meningococcal lipopolysaccharide (LPS)-derived oligosaccharide–protein conjugates evoke outer membrane protein- but not LPS-specific bactericidal antibodies in mice: influence of adjuvants. Infect Immun 1993; 61:187–196.

46. Andersen SR, et al. Cross-reactive polyclonal antibodies to the inner core of lipopolysaccharide from *Neisseria meningitidis*. Infect Immun 2002; 70:1293–1300.

47. Plested JS, et al. Conservation and accessibility of an inner core lipopolysaccharide epitope of *Neisseria meningitidis*. Infect Immun 1999; 67:5417–5426.

48. Plested JS, et al. Functional opsonic activity of human serum antibodies to inner core lipopolysaccharide (gale) of serogroup b meningococci measured by flow cytometry. Infect Immun 2001; 69:3203–3213.

49. Tettelin H, et al. Complete genome sequence of *Neisseria meningitidis* serogroup B strain MC58. Science 2000; 287: 1809–1815.

50. Parkhill J, et al. Complete DNA sequence of a serogroup A strain of *Neisseria meningitidis* Z2491. Nature 2000; 404:451–452.

51. Pizza M, et al. Whole genome sequencing to identify vaccine candidates against serogroup B meningococcus. Science 2000; 287:1816–1820.

52. Granoff DM, et al. A novel mimetic antigen eliciting protective antibody to *Neisseria meningitidis*. J Immunol 2001; 167:6487–6496.

53. Martin D, et al. Highly conserved *Neisseria meningitidis* surface protein confers protection against experimental infection. J Exp Med 1997; 185(7):1173–1183.

54. Moe GR, et al. Functional activity of anti-Neisserial surface protein A monoclonal antibodies against strains of *Neisseria meningitidis* serogroup B. Infect Immun 2001; 69:3762–3771.

37

The Postlicensure Impact of *Haemophilus influenzae* Type b and Serogroup C *Neisseria meningitidis* Conjugate Vaccines

Jay Wenger
World Health Organization, Geneva, Switzerland

Helen Campbell and Elizabeth Miller
Communicable Disease Surveillance Center, London, England

David Salisbury
Department of Health, London, England

I. BACKGROUND

Polysaccharide–protein conjugate vaccines are new tools for the prevention of serious disease caused by encapsulated bacteria. Conjugate vaccines to prevent disease caused by *Haemophilus influenzae* type b (Hib) and serogroup C meningococcus (SCM) have already been introduced into routine national immunization programs. In this chapter, we review development and implementation of these vaccines, and present data from countries demonstrating their striking impact.

A. The Bacteria

H. influenzae and *Neisseria meningitidis* are unrelated bacteria which share a number of characteristics, the most obvious being their tendency to cause bacterial meningitis and septicemia in humans.

H. influenzae is a gram-negative cocco-bacillus which colonizes the human oropharynx. A minority of these organisms have polysaccharide capsules. The encapsulated strains are characterized based on the antigenic properties of the capsule. Of the six serologically identified types (designated a–f), organisms with the type b capsule (Hib) are the most virulent.

As humans are the only biologically relevant reservoir of *H. influenzae*, transmission of the organism occurs by person-to-person spread, usually through direct or indirect exchange of oropharyngeal secretions. After introduction into the oropharynx, *H. influenzae* may establish relatively long-term colonization (often lasting several months or

more), or primarily in the case of Hib, may invade through the mucosa and enter the bloodstream. Once in the blood, the organism multiplies and may seed other sites, such as the meninges, joint spaces, or soft tissue. If Hib remains unchecked, clinical sepsis may follow, with or without manifestations of localized disease. *H. influenzae* may also cause lower respiratory tract infection, presumably by aspiration or direct extension from the oropharynx, but only a minority of these respiratory tract infections result in bacteremia.

N. meningitidis is a gram-negative coccus with a polysaccharide capsule. The capsular polysaccharides of meningococcus define the serogroup. Five serogroups are associated with human disease, of which A, B, and C are the most important in terms of morbidity and mortality worldwide, accounting for 90% or more of disease. All three serogroups may cause endemic disease. Serogroup A strains have caused most of the major outbreaks, especially in the African meningitis belt. Recently, outbreaks in Africa caused by serogroup W135 have been reported. Serogroups B and C have been associated with outbreaks in the developed world, usually with substantially lower incidence rates than those in the meningitis belt. Humans are the only recognized host for *N. meningitidis* and there is no known animal or environmental reservoir.

N. meningitidis, similar to Hib, also colonizes the human oropharynx. Meningococcus is highly adapted to this commensal existence in humans, with a range of strategies for evasion of the immune response. The carrier state may last for a few days to months; it provides a reservoir for infection and enhances the immunity of the host. Similar to Hib, invasive disease—primarily meningitis and/or sepsis—may follow carriage, but meningococcus is a less common cause of pneumonia than Hib.

B. Epidemiology of Disease: Hib

Although Hib disease incidence, age distribution, and presentation vary with socioeconomic and geographic factors, the bulk of disease occurs in children less than 5 years of age. Table 1 shows the incidence of invasive Hib disease and meningitis in children less than 5 years of age in selected areas [1–8]. In the United States, overall rates of invasive disease from various studies in the prevaccine era ranged from 50 to 100 cases per 100,000 children below 5 years of age, with rates of meningitis between 30 and 60 per 100,000. Rates of disease in Europe tended to be somewhat lower, with rates of all invasive disease usually between 30 and 60 cases per 100,000 children below 5 years of age. Rates of disease in Latin America and the Middle East tend to be similar to those in Europe, while those in Africa are somewhat higher. Although additional studies are ongoing in Asia, current data suggests that the incidence of Hib disease in many Asian countries (e.g., China, Japan, South Korea, Singapore) is substantially lower than in Europe or the United States. Some population groups have much higher rates of meningitis and invasive disease, for example, 200–300 cases per 100,000 children below 5 years of age among Aboriginal Australians and Native Americans.

Table 1 also demonstrates that, in addition to variation in disease incidence, substantial variation exists in the age distribution of disease. In the United States, prior to immunization, somewhat over one-half of *H. influenzae* meningitis in children less than 5 years of age occurred in children under 1 year of age, with peak incidence in children 6–8 months of age. In contrast, in many developing countries, a substantially larger proportion of cases occur in children less than 1 year old. In western Europe, the age distribution is shifted in the other direction, so that less than 50% of all cases occur in children less than 1 year of age and nearly half occur in those between ages 1 and 3 years.

Hib may cause meningitis, epiglottitis, bacteremia without focus, facial cellulitis, pneumonia, arthritis, and other infections. Disease manifestation and outcome also vary by socioeconomic status and geography. In much of the developed world, meningitis is the most common form of invasive disease. Meningitis represented 60–70% of all invasive *H. influenzae* disease in children in the United States before widespread immunization. The case fatality rate for meningitis in the United States has ranged from between 3% and 6% since 1985. Morbidity from meningitis includes sensorineural deafness in up to 15% of survivors and other neurological deficits less commonly. In comparison with Western countries, meningitis occurs at a younger age and has a higher mortality in many developing countries. For example, the case fatality rate in rural Africa is often between 30% and 45%. Although epiglottitis was the next most common manifestation of Hib disease in developed countries in North America and Europe, in many developing countries epiglottitis is a rare entity. The primary manifestation of *H. influenzae* disease in developing countries may be lower respiratory tract infection. Hib accounted for about 20% of chest x-ray documented clinical bacterial pneumonia in field trials of Hib conjugate vaccines in the Gambia and Chile [9,10].

C. Epidemiology of Disease: Serogroup C Meningococcus

In contrast to Hib, which causes a relatively stable burden of childhood meningitis in a given country, meningococci not only contribute a continuing burden of endemic disease, but also cause epidemics with widely varying rates, occurring at unpredictable intervals. Worldwide, there are around 1.2 million cases of endemic and epidemic meningococcal disease each year, with an estimated 135,000 deaths [11]. The disease can occur anywhere, but the largest and most frequent epidemics arise in the African meningitis belt, where epidemic waves of meningococcal disease occur every 5–12 years, usually attributable to serogroup A organisms with serogroup C and W135 strains playing a smaller role. Emergency mass immunization using meningococcal serogroup A and C polysaccharide vaccine is initiated within this area, when the incidence rate reaches a predefined epidemic threshold level [12]. Rates of disease are highest during hot and dry weather and subside with the onset of the

Table 1 Epidemiology of Hib Disease in Selected Areas

Country	Incidence, children <5 yrs (cases/10^5)		% of Meningitis	
	All	Meningitis	In <1-yr-olds	In <2-yr-olds
Sweden (1)	60	27	32	55
Iceland (1)	63	43		71
United Kingdom (2)	36	25	48	76
United States (3)	59	37	55	84
Chile (4)	22	15	64	89
Gambia (5)	–	60	83	94
Niger (6)	–	51	84	93
Kuwait (7)	–	14	69	90
China (Hong Kong) (8)	3	2	35	70

rains. During epidemics in Africa meningococcal disease is generally more prevalent in older age groups, although this is not always the case [13].

Certain factors are thought to increase susceptibility to meningococcal infection including climate, crowded living conditions, upper respiratory tract infection, and waning population immunity. Disease onset is often sudden and even with correct treatment, individuals may be left with severe disabling sequelae, in particular, brain damage and loss of limbs. The case fatality rate is high—10–20% of all cases of meningococcal disease die—but varies with serogroup, clinical presentation (meningitis, sepsis), and the availability of prompt antibiotic treatment.

In developed countries (as well as developing countries outside the meningitis belt), serogroups B and C predominate as a cause of invasive disease. Through the period 1993–1996, the overall incidence of meningococcal disease within countries in Europe was 1.1 per 100,000 [14]. The incidence rate of meningococcal disease increased within Europe to 1.5 per 100,000 in 1997/1998 and to 1.7 per 100,000 in1998/1999. Within Europe, there is variation in both the overall incidence of meningococcal infection, probably reflecting real differences in epidemiology but also in national ascertainment, and the proportion of cases that occur as a result of serogroup C infection (Table 2). During the 1990s, increased incidence of group C disease was observed in England and Wales (Figure 1), Finland, Greece [15], Spain [16], and the Republic of Ireland [17]) among others. Between 1993 and 1996, serogroup C cases rose from 26% to 32% of cases in Europe, with the number of cases increasing by 35% [14].

During the 1980s, the annual incidence of invasive meningococcal disease in Canada increased slowly from a low of 0.8 per 100,000, and serogroup C began to account for

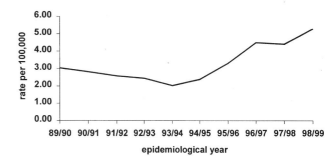

Figure 1 Incidence of confirmed cases of all meningococcal disease by epidemiological year (1 July–30 June), England and Wales, 1989/1990 to 1998/1999. (Health Protection Agency, Meningococcal Reference Unit, England.)

a larger proportion of cases [18]. The proportion of serogroup C cases increased significantly from 24% in 1985 to 65% in 1992, against a background of increasing incidence of all meningococcal infection. The 14.5% case fatality rate for serogroup C disease was higher than that for other serogroups. Much of the increase was accounted for by the emergence of a particular strain of serotype C:2a that was associated with a high case fatality and sequelae rate. There was considerable geographical variation across the regions, and Quebec introduced a mass immunization campaign in which polysaccharide vaccine was offered free to all those aged 6 months to 20 years from December 1992 to March 1993 [19]. At the time that the campaign started in 1993, the incidence of serogroup C disease was 1.4 per 100,000 and this decreased to 0.3 per 100,000 by 1998. There was no evidence of protection in those under 2 years of age and protection began to decrease within 2 years of immunization in other age groups.

The United States has a relatively low incidence of meningococcal disease, with an annual incidence ranging from approximately 0.8–1.3 per 100,000 population [20]. In 1998/1999, cases with a confirmed serogroup in the United States were equally distributed among serogroups B (30.5%), C (29.4%), and Y (31.5%). Outbreaks of serogroup C meningococcal disease began to occur more frequently in the United Sates from the early 1990s [21]. These outbreaks were dispersed geographically throughout the United States and disproportionately affected adults and school aged children, in comparison to sporadic cases.

Throughout the developed world, the peak incidence of meningococcal C disease is in children aged under 2 years of age with a secondary peak in individuals aged between 15 and 18 years. Unlike disease due to meningococcal B or Hib infection, the death rates are highest in those aged between 15 and 18 years, as illustrated in Figure 2 for England and Wales. In 1998/1999, about 25.6% of cases in reporting European countries occurred in those aged 1–4 years old and 20.4% in those aged 15–19 years old [22]. About a third (37%) of serogroup C cases were aged less than 5 years in that epidemiological year, compared to about half (48%) of group B. The age distribution changes during epidemics, with an increase in the proportion of cases observed in

Table 2 Rates and Distribution of Culture-Confirmed Cases of Meningococcal Disease in Selected Countries: Europe 1999

Country and incidence	Proportion of cases serogroup C
< 1 case/100,000	
France	22
Germany	22
Italy	23
1–3 cases/100,000	
Denmark	14
Norway	14
Spain[a]	38
> 3 cases/100,000	
England and Wales	38
Iceland	48
Ireland	32
Netherlands	14
Average Europe (17 contributing countries)	
1.3 cases/100,000	30

[a] Reference Laboratory, Spain
Source: Ref. 23.

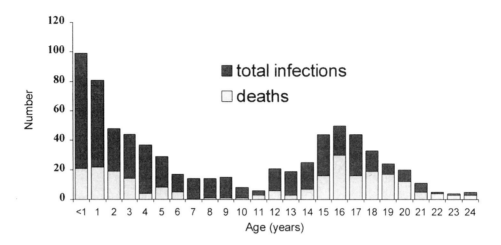

Figure 2 Meningococcal serogroup C disease and deaths by age. Isolates referred to the Public Health Laboratory Service in1998/ 1999. (Health Protection Agency, Meningococcal Reference Unit, England.)

teenagers and young adults. There is clear seasonal variation with the highest incidence of disease, endemic and outbreaks, in the winter months. Case fatality rates tend to be relatively high, but there is significant variation in the rates reported, for example, the rates in Australia, Canada, and European countries are approximately 10–15% [14,18,23]; whereas in the United States, the case fatality rate appears to be very low at 3.4% [20].

II. HIB VACCINE DEVELOPMENT AND IMPACT

A. Immunology and Development

In spite of differences in age-specific rates and disease manifestations and regardless of socioeconomic status or geographic area, the major burden of Hib disease was in children less than 2 years of age, and it was in that group that effective immunization was crucial. A major advance in understanding immunity to this disease resulted when Fothergill and Wright [24] demonstrated an inverse correlation between disease rates and whole-blood killing activity by comparing age-specific incidence data with laboratory data in persons of different ages. Hib disease incidence was lowest in newborns (who had maternally derived immunity) and older children (who apparently acquired immunity through carriage of Hib or cross-reactive bacteria) and highest at the nadir of whole-blood bactericidal activity between ages 5 and 11 months. Subsequent studies demonstrated that antibody to the type b capsular polysaccharide, polyribosyl-ribitol-phosphate (PRP), was the primary component of immunity.

Initial attempts to make Hib vaccines were focused on development of vaccines with PRP alone. Immunogenicity studies of the polysaccharide vaccine showed measurable antibody levels in children 2 years of age and older, but absent or poor immunogenicity in younger children. A large-scale double-blind study of PRP vaccine in Finland in children 3 months to 5 years of age [25] showed >90% efficacy for children who received vaccine at age 18 months or in

older, but no protection in younger children. The vaccine was licensed in the United States in 1985, but a series of postmarketing efficacy studies in different U.S. populations showed, at best, moderate efficacy (point estimates of efficacy between 47% and 80% in children 2 years and older), and one study showed no statistically significant protective effect [26].

Although the PRP vaccines were ultimately disappointing as a public health measure, evaluation of these vaccines contributed to development of the newer conjugates. Robbins and coworkers [27] had suggested that the protective level of anti-PRP antibody was between 0.06 and 0.1 μg/mL, based on studies of healthy adults (who are not at risk for Hib disease) and persons with immunoglobulin deficiency who were routinely receiving intravenous immune globuline. Kayhty et al. [28] reviewed data from the Finnish PRP efficacy trial and estimated, based on rates of disease, vaccine efficacy, and postvaccination antibody, that 0.15 μg/mL of anti-PRP antibody was adequate for protection at the time of "challenge," and that a postimmunization peak level of 1.0 μg/mL indicated long-term protection of up to 1 year. Although the actual "protective level" of antibody required is still debated, the levels of 0.15 and 1.0 μg/mL are generally used by researchers reporting immunogenicity data for Hib vaccines.

The poor immunogenicity and efficacy of PRP vaccines in those at greatest risk for disease was due to the T-cell-independent nature of PRP as an immunogen. Failure to stimulate T-cell interaction led to little or no primary immunological response in infant immune systems, and a failure to prime cells for subsequent booster responses to additional doses. In contrast, T-cell-dependent antigens, such as diphtheria and tetanus toxoid, did accomplish these tasks, although several doses were required. Earlier work by Avery and Gobel [29] showed that coupling strong antigens (such as proteins) to otherwise poor immunogens could result in a credible response to the formerly inactive component. Several investigators developed protein poly- or oligosaccharide conjugates. Each of these vaccines differed not only in the conjugated protein but also in the size of the saccharide chain used and the presence or absence of a "spacer" between the protein and the saccharide unit, among other things (Table 3).

Not surprisingly, most studies showed that immunogenicity of these vaccines differs. Table 4 shows results of one comparative study [30]. PRP-D, HbOC, and PRP-T behaved similarly, each requiring two or three doses to reach substantial antibody levels. However, in most studies, PRP-D shows the poorest immunogenicity, often with less than 60% of vaccines achieving 1.0 µg/mL after three doses [31,32]. In contrast, most HbOC and PRP-T recipients routinely achieve higher levels after three doses. Recipients of PRP-OMP demonstrate a markedly different pattern. After one dose of this vaccine, a majority of recipients achieve antibody levels of 1.0 µg/mL. In part, because of these immunogenicity differences, PRP-D, HbOC and PRP-T have generally been evaluated in three-dose primary regimens, while PRP-OMP has been evaluated as a two-dose primary series. Regardless of which vaccine was used for the primary series, antibody levels decline after the third dose, so that one year after the third dose, the circulating level of anti-PRP antibody is relatively low. In the United States, a booster dose has been recommended after a primary series of each of these vaccines at 12–15 months of age. In booster studies, each of these vaccines demonstrated the ability to prime T cells for response to subsequent booster doses. These studies also highlight the issue of whether circulating antibody levels are essential for protection induced by the conjugate vaccines as they were for protection by polysaccharide vaccines [33]. Because the conjugates induce immunological memory, which may rapidly respond to challenge by Hib, they may obviate the need for preexisting circulating antibody at time of challenge.

Widespread use of Hib conjugate vaccines did not occur until large, prospective efficacy studies were completed. The first conjugate vaccine to be formally evaluated in a prospective efficacy study was PRP-D [34]. In 1986, a total of 114,000 infants (98% of all eligible Finnish infants) were involved in a prospective randomized field trial with PRP-D. Overall protective efficacy was 94% (95% CI, 83–98%) with 90% after three doses and 100% efficacy after the fourth (booster) dose. However, Ward et al. subsequently evaluated this vaccine in a randomized, controlled trial among Native Alaskans and did not find evidence of significant efficacy in that population (point estimate 35%; 95% CI, 57–73%) [35]. Extensive review of the Alaska study did not reveal any methodological problems that may have led to an inaccurate

Table 4 Immunogenicity of *Haemophilus influenzae* Type b Vaccine Among Infants [30]

Vaccine	Baseline	Postdose 1	Postdose 2	Postdose 3
PRP-D	0.07[a]	–	0.08	0.28
PRP-OMP	0.11	0.83	0.84	1.14
HbOC	0.07	0.09	0.13	3.08
PRP-T	0.10	0.05	0.30	3.64

[a] µg/mL of serum.

estimate of efficacy. The immunogenicity of the vaccine at both sites was similar and relatively poor. One explanation for the disparate results has centered on the difference in the epidemiology of disease in the two sites—with relatively low disease incidence and high socioeconomic status in Finland and very high incidence of disease and markedly different lifestyles in Alaska. Nevertheless, the failure of the vaccine in Alaska, even in the face of the somewhat vague notion of higher disease "pressure," found a serious problem with the vaccine.

HbOC was evaluated in a large Northern California health maintenance organization by Black et al. [36]. The study demonstrated significant efficacy for children who completed a series of three doses at 2, 4, and 6 months of age (100%; 95% CI, 68–100%). No efficacy was demonstrated for fewer doses, but the study was too small to estimate efficacy in those not receiving the recommended schedule. A subsequent case-control efficacy study by Vadheim et al. [37] did demonstrate the efficacy of one (71%; 95% CI, 38–87%) and two doses (89%; 95% CI, 60–97%) and confirmed the efficacy of three doses (94%; 95% CI, 68–99%). Santosham et al. [38] demonstrated the efficacy of 97% in persons who received a single dose of PRP-OMP. Prospective evaluations of PRP-T were halted in the United States after licensure of HbOC and PRP-OMP for infants, but prior to the implementation of nationwide Hib vaccination in the United Kingdom, a prospective controlled community intervention study was conducted in the Oxford health region (population about 2,500,000) to assess the efficacy of PRP-T vaccine [39]. Doses of PRP-T were given at 2, 3, and 4 months of age. A booster dose was not offered in the second year of life. The uptake of PRP-T was in excess of 90%, with nearly 28,000 infants being vaccinated. By January 1, 1993, the estimated efficacy of vaccination with PRP-T was 95% with only one vaccine failure.

Table 3 Hib Conjugate Vaccines: Selected Characteristics

Vaccine	Polysaccharide	Linkage	Protein carrier
PRP-D	medium	6-carbon	diphtheria toxoid
HbOC	small	none	CRM_{197} mutant C diphtheria toxin
PRP-OMP	medium	thioether	*N. meningitidis* group B outer membrane protein
PRP-T	large	6-carbon	tetanus toxoid

Hib conjugate vaccines demonstrated another unexpected but important benefit over PRP vaccines—reduction of nasopharyngeal carriage of Hib among immunized children. In a carriage study in Finland, 725 healthy children attending clinic for a routine examination were enrolled between April 1987 and October 1990. Up to October 1988, Hib carriage was found to be 3.5% in 3-year-old children (who had not received PRP-D vaccine) [40]. None of the 327 vaccinated children sampled thereafter were carriers. Subsequent studies in the United States in populations receiving primarily PRP-D, HbOC, and PRP-OMP confirmed the following results: (1) decreased carriage among immunized children compared to unimmunized children [41] and (2) drastically reduced carriage rates (< 1%) in children 2–5 years old compared to historical levels [42]. A carriage study in Oxford, England, has also demonstrated the impact of PRP-T on Hib carriage rates. In the 6 months after completion of the accelerated vaccination schedule, only 1.5% of PRP-T recipients carried the Hib organism, compared with a 6.3% carriage rate in control infants (relative risk, 4.3) [43].

B. Impact of Hib Immunization Regimens

1. The United States

Hib immunization was introduced in the U.S. population in three distinct stages, based on the availability of efficacy and immunogenicity data. The PRP vaccines were licensed for children 24–60 months of age (and those 18–24 months if in day care) in April 1985. Uptake of these vaccines was slow, however, and estimates of vaccine coverage of the eligible age group were rarely more than 35–40%. The PRP vaccines were the only Hib vaccines in use in the United States from mid-1985 through December 1987, when PRP-D was licensed for use in children between 18 and 60 months of age, based on the Finnish PRP-D efficacy trial. Although HbOC and PRP-OMP were subsequently licensed for use in this older age group, between December 1987 and late 1990, PRP-D was used for the vast majority of children who received Hib conjugate vaccines. In October 1990, following the Northern California efficacy study, HbOC was licensed for use in infants beginning at 2 months of age in a three-dose primary series. Between 1990 and 1993, at least 90% of all vaccine distributed in the United States for infant immunization was HbOC. Thus for all practical purposes, children were immunized with PRP vaccines at 18–24 months between 1985 and 1987, with PRP-D at 18 months between 1987 and 1990, and with HbOC beginning at 2 months between 1990 and 1993.

A variety of surveillance systems were used to evaluate the impact of these programs. The Centers for Disease Control and Prevention (CDC) coordinated a passive national system for reporting bacterial meningitis beginning in 1977. Although many states did not participate, between 1980 and 1991, a total of 20 states reported consistently. Adams et al. published data from this system comparing reported rates of meningitis caused by *H. influenzae*, *N. meningitidis*, and *S. pneumoniae* in children less than 5 years of age [44]. Although rates of disease caused by the meningococcus and pneumococcus changed very little, between 1988 and 1991, the rate of *H. influenzae* meningitis dropped by over 80%. The incidence of *H. influenzae* meningitis declined only marginally during the PRP years, consistent with the moderate efficacy of the vaccine and low coverage. The major decline in incidence occurred during the time when PRP-D was being used in older children (1988–1990) and continued after introducing HbOC and PRP-OMP for infants (Figure 3).

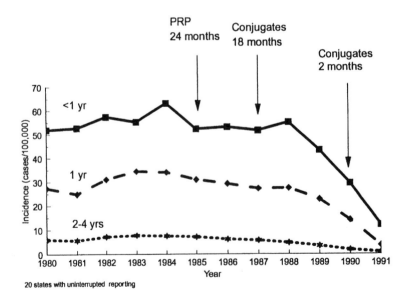

Figure 3   Age-specific incidence of *H. influenzae* meningitis in the United States between 1980 and 1991 (National Bacterial Meningitis Reporting System, Ref. 1). Rates in children less than 1 year old shown with solid line, rates in children 12–23 months old shown by hatched line, and rates for children 2–4 years old shown by dotted line. Licensure dates for polysaccharide vaccine (PRP) and conjugate vaccines are shown by arrows.

The rapidity of the decline between 1988 and 1990 came as a surprise, given the fact that most disease occurred in age groups younger than those for which the vaccine was licensed. Evaluation of age-specific decline in disease incidence (Figure 3) confirmed a significant decline in disease even in children less than 1 year of age. Adams et al. [44] and Murphy et al. [45] found similar results from prospective, population-based laboratory surveillance studies.

Data from other sources confirmed the decline in *H. influenzae* disease. Several groups used multistate or national hospital discharge data to identify decreased hospital admissions for *H. influenzae* disease. Schoendorf and colleagues used national mortality data to confirm that although deaths attributed to *H. influenzae* meningitis had been declining slowly since 1980, a significant change in the rate of decline occurred in both children less than 1 year of age and those between 1 and 4 years of age beginning in 1989, shortly after introduction of Hib conjugate vaccines in older children [46].

The remarkable success of Hib conjugate vaccines, with the unexpected benefit of herd immunity attributed to reduction in oropharyngeal carriage, led to hope for rapid elimination of Hib disease among children less than 5 years old in the United States. The early reduction in disease incidence was accomplished in spite of less than optimal vaccination coverage. Although accurate national coverage data for Hib vaccines are not available for most of the time between 1985 and 1991, estimates from case-control and focused immunization coverage studies suggest overall immunization rates in the late 1980s through 1990 probably were not above 60% and were probably much lower.

Recent data from the CDC showed that by the year 2000, 93% of children in the United States received at least three doses of the Hib conjugate vaccines. The overall rates of invasive Hib disease fell from about 100 out of 100,000 children less than 5 years of age in the prevaccine era to 0.23 out of 100,000 by the year 2000 [47]. This suggests less than 100 cases of Hib disease are identified each year in the United States. Notably, nontype b disease remained at low levels throughout the 10-year period (Figure 4).

As Hib disease has declined in incidence, some investigators raised the possibility of other organisms filling the disease "niche" left by Hib. Several early studies found no evidence for such "replacement disease" caused by other *H. influenzae* types or other organisms. Neither the National Bacterial Meningitis Surveillance System nor national mortality data showed increase disease due to meningococcus or pneumococcus through 1991, when major declines in Hib disease occurred. Similarly, laboratory-based studies of disease caused by nontype b *H. influenzae* did not show increased rates, Figure 4 [47–49]. Continued surveillance for increased rates of disease by any of these agents in appropriate. However, the role of Hib in human disease was largely a function of the characteristics of the organism, including virulence of the Hib capsule, transmission modalities, and other organism-specific factors; it is unlikely that having another organism filling the ecological niche in the human oropharynx that Hib once filled is sufficient to cause substantial amounts of human disease.

2. The United Kingdom

The United Kingdom began routine vaccination against Hib in October 1992. A catch-up program of vaccination against Hib was mounted in the first year after vaccine introduction. It aimed to cover infants and young children up to 4 years of age by offering those below 1 year of age three doses of PRP-T at monthly intervals, while children aged 13 months to 4 years of age were given HbOC as a single dose. Just over a year after the launch, the average national uptake figure for PRP-T in the accelerated schedule was 92% (varying within a tight range of 89–96% for the United Kingdom's 15 health regions) [50], and the uptake for children aged 1–4 years was around 75% [51].

Coincident with the introduction of Hib conjugate vaccines into the routine immunization schedule in the United Kingdom in 1992, a national prospective surveillance study to detect cases of invasive *H. influenzae* disease in vaccine recipients was undertaken [52]. It sought to determine the incidence of vaccine failure in a large population and to estimate the effectiveness of PRP-T in the field, particularly in the longer term in the absence of a booster dose.

The Hib vaccination program was highly effective, resulting in over 97% reduction in disease incidence in children under 5 years of age in the postvaccination compared with the prevaccine era, from 31 per 100,000 to 0.67 per 100,000 in 1998 in England and Wales (Figure 5). The percentage reduction in disease in infants who would have completed routine primary immunization with three doses of vaccine remained remarkably steady over a period of 3 years, such that in children aged 5–11 months, percentage reduction was 99.4% (95% CI, 98.9–99.6%), in those 12–23 months of age 98.0% (95% CI, 97.0–98.6%), and in those 60–71 months of age, 97.3% (95% CI, 79.2–99.7%) [52]. This high level of population protection was maintained in spite of a gradual and progressive loss in antibody in children, such that by age 72 months, 32% of children had less than 0.15 µg/mL of anti-PRP antibody, a level previously associated with protection. However, from 1999 a small increase in Hib disease in all age groups, in particular

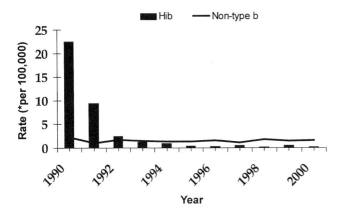

Figure 4 Race-adjusted incidence rate of *H. influenzae* type b and nontype b invasive disease detected among children aged < 5 years—United States, 1990–2000. (From Ref. 47.)

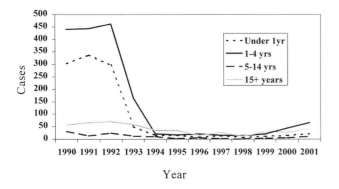

Figure 5 Invasive Hib infections by age group, 1990–2001, England and Wales. (HRU/CDSC, London, UK.)

those under 5 years who had received 3 doses of Hib vaccine in infancy, was observed (Fig. 5) [52a].

Although overall program effectiveness remains high, the direct protection afforded by the vaccine in the United Kingdom, as measured by the screening method [53,54] was estimated at only 56.7% (95% CI, 42.5–67.4%) between October 1993 and December 2001, incorporating the period of observed increase in disease [52b]. Taking underestimate of vaccine coverage into account, true efficacy may lie nearer 71.8%. Both of these figures are lower than previously published but those earlier figures were based on comparison of attack rates before and the reduction in rates after the introduction of Hib vaccine in vaccinated children [52]. The difference between vaccine efficacy and percentage reduction in disease incidence in vaccinated children confirms the generation of a herd immunity effect. Efficacy was significantly lower in children vaccinated in infancy rather than as part of the UK catch-up cohort; it declined with time since immunization and was significantly lower in a period when DTaP-Hib vaccine was used where previously wholecell DTP-Hib was used exclusively. These findings following the observed increase in cases in all age groups in recent years aided the decision by the Department of Health to

implement a second Hib catch-up campaign in the United Kingdom in 2003 for children between 6 months and 4 years of age [52c]. The need for a routine booster dose in the U.K. program is being kept under review.

3. The Gambia

The Gambia was the first country in Africa in which the efficacy of Hib conjugate vaccine was evaluated, and which introduced the vaccine into its routine infant immunization program. Critical impact data were provided from each experience. During a randomized, controlled efficacy trial performed from 1993 through 1995, the vaccine was 94% effective against Hib meningitis [9]. More importantly, vaccinated children had 21% fewer episodes of chest x-ray documented bacterial pneumonia than unvaccinated children. In this study population, for every case of invasive Hib disease prevented, at least three cases of chest x-ray documented pneumonia were prevented.

Soon after the vaccine trial ended, the vaccine was introduced into the routine program. Figure 6 shows the impact of the various Hib vaccine interventions on rate of Hib meningitis in children less than 1 year of age in The Gambia [56]. Two baseline studies confirmed rates of over 200 per 100,000 before immunization began. As a result of the trial, during which an estimated 40% of the at-risk population was immunized, the overall rate of disease dropped by over 50%. After the trial, there was a gap in immunization, when no vaccine was given for approximately 16 months. The rate of Hib disease remained stable. Subsequently, Hib vaccine was introduced as a routine infant immunization (without a catch-up program) and although rates of disease did not change in the first year, the second full year after introduction saw a drop to 21 per 100,000 (95% CI, 7–48%). Several points can be made from these Gambian data. First, the initial impact of the Hib trial was greater than would be expected from vaccination of 40% of the at-risk population, again suggesting the influence of herd immunity. Second, during the interim period when no vaccine was available, Hib disease rates remained low. This phenomenon has been observed in other countries where Hib vaccine was started,

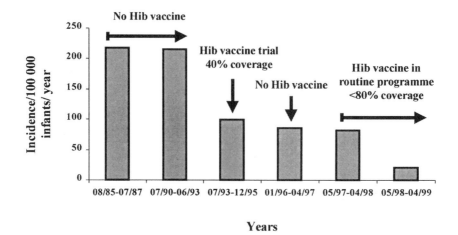

Figure 6 Incidence rate of *H. influenzae* disease in The Gambia. (From Ref. 56.)

then discontinued, and then restarted. This may be due in part to immunization of the (now) older cohort in the previous year, thus leaving siblings of the incoming birth cohort less likely to carry, and subsequently transmit, the organism. Finally, reinstitution of vaccination, even with less than 80% coverage, resulted in a reduction of over 90%, again, most likely because of the impact on carriage and herd immunity.

4. Uruguay

The government of Uruguay introduced Hib vaccine in 1994. Introduction included immunization of the incoming birth cohort, and catch-up immunization of children up to 5 years of age. Figure 7 shows the number of cases notified to the national government before, during, and after introduction [57]. The Uruguayan experience is a striking example of the rapidity with which Hib vaccine introduction can reduce disease burden, especially when introduced with a catch-up campaign. By vaccinating older children, from whom carriage is most likely transmitted to higher-risk infants, maximal impact on organism transmission can be realized. It must be recognized, of course, that conduct of catch-up campaigns require substantially greater resources and vaccine supply than introduction into the routine infant immunization program alone.

5. Saudi Arabia

Saudi Arabia introduced Hib vaccine nationally in 2002. However, before the national program was put in place, specific populations were offered vaccine, including the families and dependants of employees of the National Guard. Data from the Fahad National Guard Hospital was recently published showing effect of introduction of Hib vaccine into this population [58]. A constant decline in cases was seen over a 3-year period, such that by the last year, there was an 80% reduction in Hib meningitis in this population (Figure 8). The somewhat gradual decline in Hib disease is consistent with other countries, such as Chile and the United States, which did not conduct simultaneous introduction into the infant program and mass catch-up campaigns of all children up to 5 years of age. Another factor which may have contributed to the slower decline in incidence is that the entire country was not being immunized, so

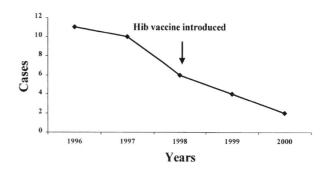

Figure 8 Number of cases of Hib AQ_1pr > meningitis in children less than 5 years of age at King Fahad Hospital, Saudi Arabia. (From Ref. 58.)

a full "herd" immunity effect could not occur because of the constant reintroduction of the bacteria from children outside the vaccinated group. The clear impact of Hib vaccination in spite of this epidemiological setting is very encouraging.

III. MENINGOCOCCAL C VACCINE DEVELOPMENT AND IMPACT

A. Immunology and Development

The pathophysiology and epidemiology of serogroup C meningococcal disease are similar in some respects to that of Hib, and present some of the same difficulties for vaccine development. The highest attack rate for serogroup C meningococcal disease in the developed world occurs in infancy with a secondary peak in teenagers and young adults. As for Hib, meningococcal capsular polysaccharides are poorly immunogenic in young children. The more immunogenic surface-protein antigens are highly variable and vaccines directed at these antigens would require multiple components. Thus the mechanisms that enable sustained colonization of human hosts have also made vaccine development problematic.

Capsular antigens have been crucial in the development of licensed vaccines against meningococcal C disease [59]. Promising results from early trials of a multivalent pneumococcal polysaccharide vaccine demonstrated that capsular polysaccharides could elicit protective immune responses. Initial trials of candidate meningococcal A and C polysaccharide preparations were disappointing but a new purification technique, developed in the 1960s, enabled the production of highly purified, high molecular weight meningococcal polysaccharides. These were shown to be safe and highly immunogenic in adults and older children and are the basis of the presently licensed bivalent A and C and tetravalent A, C, W135, and Y meningococcal polysaccharide vaccines. However, meningococcal polysaccharide capsules usually act as T-cell-independent antigens. This means that T-lymphocytes are usually not involved in the induction of immune responses against these antigens [60]. T-independent responses are age-dependent, not generally occurring before 18 months of age, and do not induce immunological memory. Consequently, currently licensed polysaccharide vaccines are

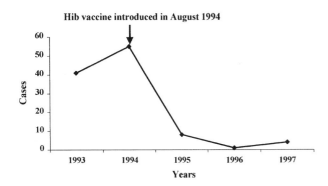

Figure 7 Number of cases of Hib meningitis in Uruguay. (From Ref. 57.)

ineffective in protecting young children against group C disease and do not provide long-term protection.

The relatively recent development of Hib conjugate vaccine was closely followed by the development of meningococcal conjugate vaccines. The vaccines are made from oligosaccharides derived from purified capsular polysaccharides that are chemically conjugated, using different methods, to tetanus toxoid or diphtheria CRM 197 carrier proteins to convert them into T-dependent antigens [61]. Clinical trials of meningococcal C conjugate (MCC) vaccines found them to be immunogenic in all age groups and their reactogenicity profiles were in line with other routinely recommended vaccines with no serious adverse events identified [62–66]. The vaccines also induced immunological memory, which lasted at least 5 years, and are expected to provide long-term immunity against meningococcal C disease [67]. More than 25,000 children received the vaccine in trials worldwide before the first MCC vaccine was licensed in the United Kingdom in September 1999. It was recognized that the low overall incidence of serogroup C disease made Phase III controlled efficacy trials impractical, and licensure was based on recognition that a correlate for protection already existed for serogroup C polysaccharide vaccines in the serum bactericidal assay [68].

B. Impact of Meningococcal C Conjugate Vaccines

As with many other developed countries, the incidence of laboratory-confirmed meningococcal infection of all types increased through the 1990s in England and Wales. The incidence rose from 2.8 per 100,000 in the 1990/1991 epidemiological year (running from July to June) to 5.3 per 100,000 in 1998/1999. The rise was partly a result of better ascertainment following the wide availability of more sensitive polymerase chain reaction (PCR) methods for the identification and serogrouping of meningococci [69,70].

Historically, approximately 60–70% of all confirmed meningococcal disease in England and Wales was caused by meningococcal B infection. Almost all of the remaining meningococcal infection (25–30%) was due to serotype C. The disease profile changed in the mid-1990s, when the incidence of meningococcal disease increased. Cases of serogroup C disease increased proportionately more than other serogroups, signifying a true rise in the level of endemic serogroup C infection rather than solely better ascertainment. Based on enhanced surveillance, it was estimated that annually there were 1500 cases of meningococcal C infection and that these caused 150 deaths in England and Wales [71]. Cases and deaths caused each year by serogroup C meningococci in those less than 18 years of age were separately estimated at 1137 and 72, respectively [72].

In November 1999, the United Kingdom became the first country in the world to introduce MCC immunization into the routine infant schedule. A national catch-up campaign began on November 1, 1999 and was planned to run over approximately 1 year. All children under 18 years of age (12 million in England and Wales) were offered MCC vaccine during the campaign. At the time that the campaign started, there was only one licensed MCC vaccine available and there were not enough MCC vaccine supplies for all children under

18 years [73]. Further supplies were phased in over the next 12 months as two other MCC vaccines were licensed. Therefore each age group was assigned a time to be immunized within the campaign schedule prioritized according to the profile of meningococcal C disease in the 0–18 years age range.

Vaccine was offered first to all children aged 15–17 years, the age group with the highest disease incidence (other than in those under 2 years of age), the highest risk of outbreaks, and the highest mortality rate. Very shortly after this, the vaccine was introduced into the routine infant schedule at 2, 3, and 4 months of age. The vaccine was offered to different age groups of children as supplies became available through the duration of the campaign, according to the priority assigned to each age group. Recorded MCC vaccine coverage for school children aged 5–17 years inclusive was 85%. Coverage for the catch-up groups of children aged 5 months to 4 years of age was recorded at 78%. Routine infant immunization by first birthday reached 89% coverage by the beginning of 2002 [74].

1. Impact on Disease

Cases of meningococcal B and C infection in all age groups are shown in Figure 9, for England and Wales, from January 1997 to March 2002 by quarter. This graph clearly demonstrates that, in the 2000/2001 epidemiological year (which runs from July 1 to June 30), Group B cases occurred at the levels previously recorded, while the level of Group C disease was markedly reduced. Group C cases decreased by 56% overall in 2000/2001, compared to 1998/1999.

With the exception of some university/college students offered meningococcal C polysaccharide vaccine only those aged 20 years and over were left completely unimmunized against meningococcal C disease up to the end of the 2000/ 2001 epidemiological year. The impact of the campaign in each age group targeted for immunization was rapid and marked and occurred in close temporal association to the introduction of the vaccine [75]. In the 2000/2001 epidemiological year, the numbers of confirmed cases of serogroup C disease were consistently 63–94% lower than 1998/1999 in every age group that was targeted for immunization with MCC vaccine in England. Table 5 summarizes the comparative number of group B and C cases in England in each age group for the 1998/1999 and 2000/2001 epidemiological years.

As summarized in Figure 10, in the 2000/2001 epidemiological year, the number of cases of meningococcal C disease in those aged 20 years and over in England was similar to the previous year (with a 6% decrease). The number of cases of group C disease in those under 20 years of age fell from 574 to 130, an overall decrease of 77%. In comparison, the number of cases of group B disease in those aged 20 years and over and under 20 years remained relatively stable with increases of 7% and 9%, respectively.

These data suggest that the changes in the epidemiology of meningococcal disease have been specific to serogroup C and to the age groups that were offered MCC vaccine. These general observations support the suggestion that any changes observed in serogroup C disease in immunized age groups were attributable to the MCC vaccine.

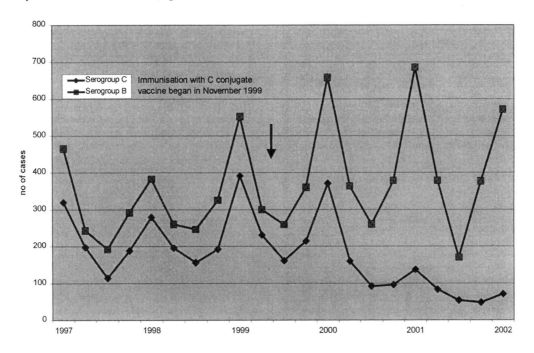

Figure 9 Laboratory confirmed cases of serogroup B and C meningococci in England and Wales. (Health Protection Agency, Meningococcal Reference Unit, England.)

The number of deaths following meningococcal C infection in England in individuals under 20 years of age fell in the epidemiological year 2000/2001 with 10 deaths compared to 73 deaths in 1998/1999 (source: Office of National Statistics). The number of deaths in those aged 20 years and over increased from 37 to 55 in the same time period: this was in line with the increase in the number of cases of meningococcal C infection seen in that age group over that period of time.

2. MCC Vaccine Efficacy

Up to the end of the 2000/2001 epidemiological year, immunization status had been determined in 98% of confirmed serogroup C cases in individuals eligible for immunization with MCC vaccine in England and Wales. The short-term efficacy of this MCC vaccine was 97% (95% CI, 77–99.9%) for teenagers and 92% (95% CI, 65–98%) for toddlers during the first 9 months following the introduction of the

vaccine [76]. After 18 months of follow-up in England, the estimated efficacy in 15- to 17-year-olds was 93% overall (95% CI, 79–96%) and 89% (95% CI, 72–96%) for toddlers [73]. The preliminary data on vaccination status of cases in each of the other vaccinated age group is consistent with a high vaccine efficacy in the short term. Surveillance is continuing in order to monitor long-term efficacy that will depend on the ability to mount a rapid booster response on exposure to the organism. This is particularly important in the light of recent changes in the epidemiology of Hib disease in the United Kingdom with associated changes in the effectiveness of the Hib vaccine program and as no meningococcal vaccine booster is currently given in the U.K. program.

3. Meningococcal Isolates

Concerns have been raised about the possibility of capsule switching arising from selection pressure by MCC vaccine on

Table 5 Impact of Serogroup C Meningococcal Conjugate Vaccine—Number of Cases of Confirmed Meningococcal B and C Disease in England in 1998/1999 and 2000/2001 Epidemiologic Years (July 1–June 30)

	Cases of serogroup C disease			Cases of serogroup B disease		
Age group	1998/1999	2000/2001	% Change	1998/1999	2000/2001	% Change
Under 1	98	18	−82%	311	337	8%
1–4 yr	194	42	−78%	376	509	35%
5–8 yr	71	26	−63%	93	119	28%
9–10 yr	18	1	−94%	29	26	−10%
11–14 yr	74	9	−88%	47	88	89%
15–19 yr[a]	190	34	−82%	139	182	31%
20 + yr	222	257	16%	283	347	23%

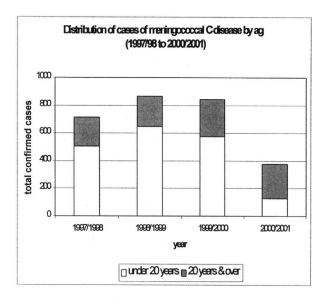

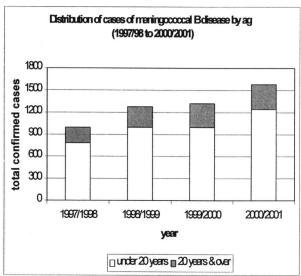

Figure 10 Distribution of cases of meningococcal C and B disease in England in age groups targeted and not targeted by meningococcal C conjugate vaccine (1997/1998 to 2000/2001). (Health Protection Agency, Meningococcal Reference Unit, England.)

serogroup C strains [77]. If capsule switching occurred more serogroup B strains would be expected to display P1.5/NT/NT or P1.5/P1.2/NT sero-subtype patterns (the common sero-subtypes of serogroup C). The analysis of sero-subtype for groups B and C for the years 2000 and 2001 showed no evidence of increases in group B organisms with sero-subtypes corresponding to the more common C strains (P1.5, P1.2) (personal correspondence Manchester Reference Unit). Therefore there is no evidence of capsule switching occurring to date.

4. Use of Meningococcal C Conjugate Vaccine in Other Countries

The meningococcal C conjugate vaccine was launched in the Republic of Ireland at the beginning of October 2000 against a background of high and increasing meningococcal C infection [17]. Ultimately, everyone under the age of 23 years will be offered the vaccine. Groups B and C are the predominant forms of invasive meningococcal disease seen in Ireland, accounting for approximately 60–65% and 30–35% of cases, respectively. The incidence of group C disease fell dramatically in 2000/2001 from 4.6 per 100,000 (167 cases, excluding 1 imported case) in 1999/2000 to 1.8 per 100,000 population (66 cases, excluding 1 imported case) in 2000/2001, a 61% reduction [78]. The incidence of group C had declined in all age groups other than the over 24 years age group during this period. The incidence of group B invasive meningococcal disease (IMD) also fell, but to a lesser extent, by 14% to 6.5 per 100,000 population in 2000/2001 from 7.6 per 100,000 population in 1999/2000.

There are currently recommendations for routine MCC vaccine use in the United Kingdom, Republic of Ireland, Luxembourg, and all regions in Spain (http://www.aepap.org/calvaces.htm). The vaccine has also been introduced into

Belgium and Greece, for administration on a voluntary basis by clinicians; use is said to be high in both countries [23]. The Netherlands and Madeira, an autonomous region of Portugal, propose to use the vaccine in 2002.

The vaccine has also been used in France and Hungary. In Canada, the Quebec government announced in the summer of 2001 that meningococcal C conjugate vaccine would be offered to all residents under the age of 20 years.

IV. CONCLUSIONS

The success of Hib conjugate vaccines in countries that have immunized the majority of children has been stunning, ranging from elimination of disease in nations with very high immunization coverage to declines of over 95% in countries with somewhat lower immunization rates. Similarly, early data on impact of the meningococcal C conjugate vaccine are impressive. Worldwide use of Hib and meningococcal C conjugate vaccines could lead to elimination of these infections. However, major obstacles stand in the way of achievement of this goal. Conjugate vaccines currently are expensive, and implementation of standard regimens into many national immunization programs schedules poses a daunting challenge for available health care resources, particularly in developing countries. Progress is needed in reducing production and distribution costs. Equally as important is interaction between ministries of health and immunization partners to enhance support for conjugate vaccine immunization programs. Accurate estimates of the burden of disease as well as clearly defined examples of impact are needed to contribute to the political will to use these vaccines. Continued surveillance for disease in countries that have introduced these vaccines is essential, both to identify poorly served populations, and to assess the impact of different strategies, for example, use of a booster dose of Hib vaccine. Finally, efforts to enhance routine immunization coverage, including improved logistics and decreasing dropout rates of children returning for multidose regimens are critical. Most of these challenges are common to all childhood immunization programs, however, and the existence of these new, effective tools for elimination of a much-feared disease of childhood can contribute to the will to overcome these obstacles for all vaccines.

REFERENCES

1. Claesson BA. Epidemiology of invasive *Haemophilus influenzae* type b disease in Scandinavia. Vaccine 1993; 11:530–533.
2. Booy R, Hodgson SA, Slack MPE, et al. Invasive *Haemophilus influenzae* type b disease in the Oxford region (1985–91). Arch Dis Child 1993; 69:225–228.
3. Wenger JD, Hightower AW, Facklam RR, et al. Bacterial meningitis in the United States, 1986: report of a multistate surveillance study. J Infect Dis 1990; 162:1316–1323.
4. Ferreccio C, Ortiz E, Astroza L, et al. A population-based retrospective assessment of the disease burden resulting from invasive *Haemophilus influenzae* in infants and young children in Santiago, Chile. Pediatr Infect Dis J 1990; 9:488–494.
5. Biljimer HA, van Alphen L, Greenwood BM, et al. The epidemiology of *Haemophilus influenzae* meningitis in children under five years of age in the Gambia, West Africa. J Infect Dis 1990; 161:1210–1215.
6. Campagne G, Schuchat A, Djibo S, et al. Epidemiology of bacterial meningitis in Niamey, Niger, 1981–96. Bull WHO 1999; 77:499–508.
7. Zaki M, Daoud AS, El Saleh Q, et al. Childhood bacterial meningitis in Kuwait. J Trop Med Hyg 1990; 93:7–11.
8. Lau YL, Yung R, Low L, et al. *Haemophilus influenzae* type b infections in Hong Kong. Pediatr Infect Dis J 1998; 17:S165–S169.
9. Mulholland K, Hilton S, Adegbola R, et al. Randomised trial of *Haemophilus influenae* type-b tetanus protein conjugate for prevention of pneumonia and meningitis in Gambian infants. Lancet 1997; 349:1191–1197.
10. Levine OS, Lagos R, Munoz A, et al. Defining the burden of pneumonia in children preventable by vaccination against *Haemophilus influenzae* type b. Pediatr Infect Dis J 1999; 18:1060–1064.
11. World Health Organisation. Epidemics of meningococcal disease, African meningitis belt, 2001. Weekly Epidemiological record 2001; 37:282–288.
12. Bovier PA, Wyss K, Au HJ. A cost-effectiveness analysis of vaccination strategies against *N. meningitidis* in sub-Saharan African countries. Soc Sci Med 1999; 48:1205–1220.
13. Hart CA, Cuevas LE. Meningococcal disease in Africa. Ann Trop Med Parasitol 1997; 91(7):777–785.
14. Connolly M, Noah N. Is group C meningococcal disease increasing in Europe? A report of surveillance of meningococcal infection in Europe 1993–6. Epidemiol Infect 1999; 122:41–49.
15. Kremastinou J, Tzanakaki G, Kansouzidou A, et al. Recent emergence of serogroup C disease in Greece. FEMS Immunol Med Microbiol 1999; 23:49–55.
16. Berron S, De La Fuente L, Martin E, et al. Increasing incidence of meningococcal disease in Spain associated with a new variant of serogroup C. Eur J Clin Microbiol Infect Dis 1998; 17:85–89.
17. Cafferkey M, Murphy K, Fitzgerald M, et al. Epidemiology of meningococcal disease in Ireland: a report on laboratory confirmed cases, July 1999 to June 2000. Epi-Insight 2000; 1(4):2–3.
18. Whalen CM, Hockin JC, Ryan A, et al. The changing epidemiology of invasive meningococcal disease in Canada, 1985 through 1992: emergence of a virulent clone of *Neisseria meningitidis*. J Am Med Assoc 1995; 273(5):390–394.
19. De Wals P, De Serres G, Niyonsenga T. Effectiveness of a mass immunisation campaign against serogroup C meningococcal disease in Quebec. J Am Med Assoc 2001; 285:177–181.
20. CDC. Prevention and control of meningococcal disease. Recommendations of the Advisory |Committee on Immunisation Practices. MMWR 2000; 49(RR07):1–10.
21. Jackson LA, Schuchat A, Reeves MW, et al. Serogroup C meningococcal outbreaks in the United States: an emerging threat. J Am Med Assoc 1995; 273(5):383–389.
22. Cartwright K, Noah N, Peltola H. Meningococcal Disease Advisory Board. Meningococcal disease in Europe: epidemiology, mortality, and prevention with conjugate vaccines. Report of a European advisory board meeting, Vienna, Austria, 6–8 October, 2000. Vaccine 2001; 31:4347–4356.
23. Commission of the European Communities. Surveillance network for invasive Neisseria meningitidis in Europe—1999 and 2000. Final Report. http://www.euibis.org/documents/meningo19992000.pdf.
24. Fothergill LD, Wright J. Influenzal meningitis: the relation of age incidence to the bactericidal power of blood against the causal organism. J Immunol 1993; 24:273–284.
25. Peltola H, Kaytty H, Sivonen A, et al. *Haemophilus influenzae* type b capsular polysaccharide vaccine in children: a double-blind field study of 100,000 vaccinees 3 months to 5 years of age in Finland. Pediatrics 1977; 60:730–737.
26. Ward JI, Broome CV, Harrison LH, et al. *Haemophilus influenzae* type b vaccines: lessons for the future. Pediatrics 1988; 81:886–892.
27. Robbins JB, Parke JC, Schneerson R, et al. Quantitative measurement of "natural" and immunization induced *Haemophilus influenzae* type b capsular polysaccharide antibodies. Pediatr Res 1973; 7:103–110.
28. Kayhty H, Peltola H, Karanko V, et al. The protective level of serum antibodies to the capsular polysaccharide of *Haemophilus influenzae* type b. J Infect Dis 1983; 147:1100.
29. Avery OT, Goebel WF. Chemo–immunological studies on conjugated carbohydrate–proteins: II. Immunological specificity of synthetic sugar–protein antigens. J Exp Med 1929; 50:522–550.
30. Decker MD, Edwards KM, Bradley R, et al. Comparative trial in infants of four conjugate *Haemophilus influenzae* type b vaccines. J Pediatr 1992; 120:184–189.
31. Kayhty H, Eskola J, Peltola H, et al. Antibody responses to four *Haemophilus influenzae* type b conjugate vaccines. Am J Dis Child 1991; 145:223–227.
32. Peltola H, Eskola J, Kayhty H, et al. Clinical comparison of the *Haemophilus influenzae* type b polysaccharide-diphtheria toxoid and the oligosaccharide-CRM[197] protein vaccines in infancy. Arch Pediatr Adolesc Med 1994; 148:620–625.
33. Eskola J, Ward J, Dagan R, et al. Combined vaccination of *Haemophilus influenzae* type b conjugate and diphtheria–tetanus–pertussis containing acellular pertussis. Lancet 1999 Dec 11; 354(9195):2063–2068.
34. Eskola J, Kayhty H, Takala AK, et al. A randomized, prospective field trial of a conjugate vaccine in the protection of infants and young children against invasive *Haemophilus influenzae* type b disease. N Engl J Med 1990; 323:1381–1387.
35. Ward J, Brenneman G, Letson GW, et al. the Alaska *H influenzae* Vaccine Study Group. Limited efficacy of a *Haemophilus influenzae* type b conjugate vaccine in Alaskan native infants. N Engl J Med 1990; 323:1393–1401.

36. Black SB, Shinefeld HR, Fireman B, et al. the Northern California Kaiser Permanente Vaccine Study Center Pediatrics Group. Efficacy in infancy of oligosaccharide conjugate *Haemophilus influenzae* type b (HbOC) vaccine in a United States population of 61,080 children. Pediatry Infect Dis J 1991; 10:97–104.

37. Vadheim C, Greenberg D, Ericksen E, et al. Protection provided by *Haemophilus influenzae* type b conjugate vaccines in Los Angeles: a case-control study. Pediatr Infect Dis J 1994; 13:274–280.

38. Santosham M, Wolff M, Reid R, et al. The efficacy in Navaho infants of a conjugate vaccine consisting of *Haemophilus influenzae* type b polysaccharide and Neisseria meningitidis outer membrane protein complex. N Engl J Med 1991; 324:1767–1772.

39. Booy R, Hodgson S, Carpenter L, et al. Efficacy of *Haemophilus influenzae* type b conjugate vaccine PRP-T. Lancet 1994; 344:362–366.

40. Takala AK, Eskola J, Leinonen M, et al. Reduction of oropharyngeal carriage of *Haemophilus influenzae* type b (Hib) in children immunized with a Hib conjugate vaccine. J Infect Dis 1991; 164:982–986.

41. Murphy TV, Pastor P, Medley F, et al. Decreased Haemophilus colonization in children vaccinated with *Haemophilus influenzae* type b conjugate vaccine. J Pediatr 1993; 122:517–523.

42. Mohle-Boetani JC, Ajello G, Breneman E, et al. Carriage of *Haemophilus influenzae* type b in children after widespread vaccination with conjugate *Haemophilus influenzae* type b vaccines. Pediatr Infect Dis J 1993; 12:589–593.

43. Barbour ML, Mayon-White RT, Coles C, et al. The impact of conjugate vaccine on carriage of *Haemophilus influenzae* type b. J Infect Dis 1995; 171:93–98.

44. Adams WG, Deaver KA, Cochi SL, et al. Decline of childhood *Haemophilus influenzae* type b (Hib) disease in the Hib vaccine era. J Am Med Assoc 1993; 269:221–226.

45. Murphy TV, White KE, Pastor P, et al. Declining incidence of *Haemophilus influenzae* type b disease since introduction of vaccination. J Am Med Assoc 1993; 269:246–248.

46. Schoendorf KC, Adams WG, Kiely JL, et al. National trends in *Haemophilus influenzae* meningitis mortality and hospitalization among children, 1980 through 1991. Pediatrics 1994; 93:663–668.

47. Centers for Disease Control. Progress toward elimination of *Haemophilus influenzae* type b disease among infants and children—United States, 1998–2000. MMWR 2002; 51:234–237.

48. Wenger JD, Pierce R, Deaver KA, et al. Invasive *Haemophilus influenzae* disease: a population based evaluation of the role of capsular polysaccharide serotype. J Infect Dis 1992; 165(suppl 1):S34–S35.

49. Takala AK, Peltola H, Eskola J. Disappearance of epiglottitis during large-scale vaccination with *Haemophilus influenzae* type b conjugate vaccine among children in Finland. Laryngoscope 1994; 104:731–735.

50. White JM, Leon S, Begg NT. "COVER" (cover of vaccination evaluated rapidly). Commun Dis Rep 1994; 4:R51–52.

51. O'Brien H. Hib immunisation catch up program in North East Thames. Commun Dis Rep 1994; 4:R17–R18.

52. Heath PT, Booy R, Azzopardi HJ, et al. Antibody concentration and clinical protection after Hib conjugate vaccination in the United Kingdom. J Am Med Assoc 2000; 284:2334–2340.

52a. Trotter CL, Ramsay ME, Slack MPE. Rising incidence of *Haemophilus influenzae* type b disease in England and Wales indicates a need for a second catch-up campaign. Commun Dis Public Health 2003; 6:55–58.

52b. Ramsay ME, McVernon J, Andrews NJ, et al. Estimating *Haemophilus influenzae* Type b vaccine effectiveness in England and Wales by use of the screening method. JID 2003; 188:481–485 .

52c. Chief Medical Officer, Chief Nursing Officer, Chief Pharmaceutical Officer. Planned Hib vaccination catch-up campaign. PL/CMO/L Z-17-2003. http://www.doh.gov.uk/cmo/letters/cmo0301.htm.

53. Orenstein W, Bernier R, Dondero TJ, et al. Field evaluation of vaccine efficacy. Bull WHO 1985; 63:1055–1068.

54. Farrington CP. Estimation of vaccine effectiveness using the screening method. Int J Epidemiol 1995; 22:742–746.

55. Ramsay M, Handford S, Andrews N et al. An evaluation of *Haemophilus influenzae* type b (Hib) vaccination and description of risk factors for Hib vaccine failure in Europe, 1996–1998. Final Report to Directorate General XII of the European Union.

56. Adegbola RA, Usen SO, Weber M, et al. *Haemophilus influenzae* type b meningitis in The Gambia after introduction of a conjugate vaccine. Lancet 1999; 354:1091–1092.

57. Landaverde M, Di Fabio JL, Ruocco G, et al. Introduction de la vacuna conjugada contra Hib en Chile y Uruguay. Pan Am J Public Health 1999; 5:200–206.

58. Almuneef M, Alshaalan M, Memish Z, et al. Bacterial meningitis in Saudi Arabia: the impact of *Haemophilus influenzae* type b vaccination. J Chemother 2001; 13(suppl 1):34–39.

59. Feavers IM. Meningococcal vaccines and vaccine developments. In: Pollard AJ, Maiden MCJ, eds. Meningococcal Vaccines: Methods and Protocols. Totowa, NJ: Humana Press, 2001:1–22.

60. Pollard AJ, Goldblatt D. Immune response and host–pathogen interactions. In: Pollard AJ, Maiden MCJ, eds. Meningococcal Vaccines: Methods and Protocols. Totowa, NJ: Humana Press, 2001:23–40.

61. Lockhart S. Meningococcal serogroup C conjugate vaccines. A clinical review. Vacunas 2000; 1(3):126–129.

62. Fairley CK, Begg N, Borrow R, et al. Reactogenicity and immunogenicity of conjugate meningococcal serogroup A and C vaccine in UK infants. J Infect Dis 1996; 174:1360–1363.

63. Richmond PC, Miller E, Borrow R, et al. Meningococcal serogroup C conjugate vaccine is immunogenic in infancy and primes for memory. J Infect Dis 1999; 179:1569–1572.

64. Richmond P, Borrow R, Goldblatt D, et al. Ability of 3 different meningococcal C conjugate vaccines to induce immunologic memory after a single dose in UK toddlers. J Infect Dis 2001; 183:160–163.

65. MacLennan JM, Shackley F, Heath PT, et al. Safety, immunogenicity and induction of immunologic memory by a serogroup C meningococcal conjugate vaccine in infants. J Am Med Assoc 2000; 283(21):2795–2801.

66. Borrow R, Fox AJ, Richmond PC, et al. Induction of immunological memory in UK infants by a meningococcal A/C conjugate vaccine. Epidemiol Infect 2000; 124:427–432.

67. Borrow R, Goldblatt D, Andrews N, et al. Antibody persistence and immunological memory at age 4 years after meningococcal group C conjugate vaccination in children in the United Kingdom. J Infect Dis 2002; 186:1353–1357.

68. Farrington P, Miller E. Meningococcal vaccine trials. In: Pollard AJ, Maiden MCJ, eds. Meningococcal Vaccines: Methods and Protocols. Totowa, NJ: Humana Press, 2001: 371–394.

69. Guiver M, et al. Evaluation of the Applied Biosystems Automated Taqman PCR system for the detection of meningococcal DNA. FEMS Immunol Med Microbiol 2000; 28:173–179.

70. Kaczmarski E, Cartwright K. Control of meningococcal disease: guidance for microbiologists. Commun Dis Rep CDR Rev 1995; 5:R196–R198.

71. Anon. Vaccination programme for group C meningococcal infection is launched. Commun Dis Rep CDR Wkly 1999; 9(30):261–264.

72. Trotter CL, Edmunds JW. Modelling cost effectiveness of meningococcal serogroup C conjugate vaccination campaign in England and Wales. Br Med J 2002; 324:809–812.

73. Miller E, Salisbury D, Ramsay M. Planning, registration, and implementation of an immunisation campaign against meningococcal serogroup C disease in the UK: a success story. Vaccine 2001; 20:S58–S67.

74. COVER programme: October to December 2001. Vaccination coverage statistics for children up to 5 years of age in the United Kingdom. CDR Wkly 28 March 2002; 12(4)

(Available online at http://www.hpa.org.uk/cdr/PDFfiles/2002/cdr0402.pdf).

75. Anon. Meningococcal disease falls in vaccine recipients. CDR Wkly 2000; 10(15):133–136.

76. Ramsay M, Andrews N, Kaczmarski EB, Miller E. Efficacy of meningococcal serogroup C conjugate vaccine in teenagers and toddlers in England. Lancet 2001; 357:195–196.

77. Maiden MCJ, Spratt BG. Meningococcal conjugate vaccines: new opportunities and new challenges (commentary). Lancet 1999; 354:615–616.

78. Fitzgerald M, O'Flanagan D, Cafferkey M, Murphy K. Invasive meningococcal disease in Ireland 2000/2001. Epi-Insight 2001; 2(11):2–3.

38

Pneumococcal Protein–Polysaccharide Conjugate Vaccines

Orin S. Levine
Johns Hopkins Bloomberg School of Public Health, Baltimore, Maryland, U.S.A.

David L. Klein
National Institute of Allergy and Infectious Diseases, National Institutes of Health, Bethesda, Maryland, U.S.A.

Jay C. Butler
National Center for Infectious Diseases, Centers for Disease Control and Prevention, Anchorage, Alaska, U.S.A.

I. EPIDEMIOLOGY AND IMPLICATIONS FOR VACCINE DEVELOPMENT

Few infectious pathogens match the global impact of *Streptococcus pneumoniae* infections. In industrialized countries, *S. pneumoniae* is the most common identified bacterial cause of hospitalization for pneumonia, meningitis, and acute otitis media [1–3]. Invasive pneumococcal infections are most common among the very young (generally, 100–200 cases per 100,000 persons aged <2 years per year) and the elderly (45–90 per 100,000 persons aged >65 years per year) (Figure 1) [4–9]. Attack rates for persons aged 85 years and older are similar to those in infants [6]. These numbers translate into 106,000–175,000 hospitalizations and 7000–12,500 deaths in the United States annually [10]. Certain racial and ethnic groups, such as American Indians and Alaska Natives, are at increased risk for serious pneumococcal infections, as are individuals with underlying illnesses such as human immunodeficiency virus (HIV) [4,5,7–9,12,13].

In developing countries, pneumococcal infections are a major cause of morbidity and mortality among infants and young children. The World Health Organization (WHO) estimates that >1 million young children die annually of pneumococcal infections [14]. Greater than 90% of these deaths occur in the developing world and most of these deaths are attributed to pneumococcal pneumonia. Pneumococcal meningitis is severe, with a high case fatality rate (up to 50%, even with antibiotic therapy) and a high risk (~20–25%) of long-term disability among survivors [15,16] The burden of pneumococcal disease among adults in the developing world may also be substantial because acute respiratory infections are the leading infectious causes of adult mortality, *S. pneumoniae* is the leading etiological agent identified in adults hospitalized with severe pneumonia [17–21], and the prevalence of risk factors known to increase the risk of pneumococcal disease (such as HIV infection and cigarette smoking) is common in many developing countries [11,22].

Estimates of the burden of pneumococcal disease vary, depending on case definition and case finding methodology. The most specific definition of pneumococcal disease is based on the isolation of pneumococci from normally sterile body sites (e.g., blood, cerebrospinal fluid, and pleural fluid). The sensitivity of this definition, though, is low. Therefore, incidence rates based only on isolates from sterile body sites underestimate the overall disease burden. Case finding based on disease syndromes commonly caused by the pneumococcus, such as community-acquired pneumonia or acute otitis media, captures a more complete picture of the burden of pneumococcal disease, but these data are quite nonspecific. The accuracy and the specificity of alternative diagnostics, such as sputum Gram stain and culture, pleural fluid and urine antigen testing, polymerase chain reaction (PCR), and serological assays, are limited and can be unacceptably low among patients who are merely colonized with *S. pneumoniae* [23–33]. The challenges to accurate measurement of the burden of pneumococcal disease are exacerbated in developing countries [34] where few, if any, laboratory resources are consistently available for diagnosis.

A. Serotype Distribution

For vaccines directed against the capsular polysaccharides, the distribution of serotypes causing illness is critically important. For practical and economic reasons, only a limited

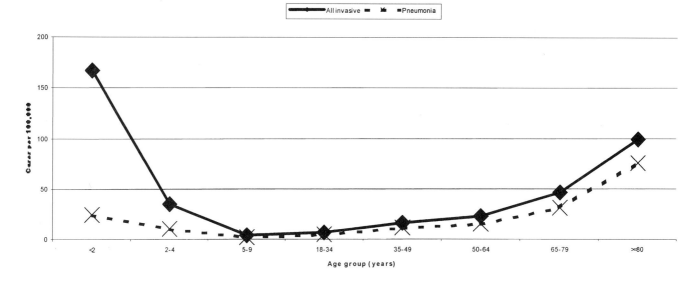

Figure 1 Age-specific incidence of pneumococcal disease in the United States, 1998.

number of serotypes are included in conjugate pneumococcal vaccine formulations [35]. The first licensed pneumococcal conjugate vaccine contains capsular polysaccharides of seven serotypes (4, 6B, 9V, 14, 18C, 19F, and 23F) (Table 1). Other vaccines under evaluation cover 9, 11, or 13 serotypes. To some degree, the relative importance of individual pneumococcal serotypes differs by age group, clinical syndrome, and geographical area, and over time. Optimal vaccine formulations need to target the serotypes that most commonly cause diseases among populations to be vaccinated.

The seven serotypes in the first licensed conjugate vaccine account for >80% of isolates from blood and cerebrospinal fluid of children aged <2 years in the United States compared with <60% of isolates from older children and adults [9]. Vaccine formulations that are based on the most prevalent serotypes among young children may not

provide optimal serotype coverage for the prevention of pneumococcal infections in adults. The addition of four serotypes to the seven-valent vaccine formulation (1, 3, 5, and 7A) would add coverage for <2% of isolates from children aged under 2 years, but would increase coverage by nearly 10% among older children and adults [9].

The distribution of serotypes causing otitis media differs from that of isolates causing bacteremia and meningitis. In national surveillance in the United States, the seven most common serotypes causing bacteremia and meningitis in children aged <6 years, plus serologically related serotypes (6A, 9A, 9L, 18B, and 18F), accounted for only 65% of 314 isolates from middle ear fluid during 1978–1994 [36]. Serotype 3 accounted for 9% of middle ear fluid isolates but <1% of blood or cerebrospinal fluid isolates. More recent data from the United States with a larger number of isolates

Table 1 The Seven Pneumococcal Serogroups Most Frequently Causing Invasive Disease Among Young Children, by Region

	Rank order of isolation frequency						
Region	First	Second	Third	Fourth	Fifth	Sixth	Seventh
United States and Canada	14 (27.8)	6 (17.0)	19 (14.3)	18 (8.6)	23 (7.4)	9 (6.3)	4 (6.3)
Asia	1 (11.7)	19 (10.8)	6 (9.9)	5 (9.1)	14 (8.0)	7 (6.4)	23 (5.3)
Africa	6 (23.8)	14 (18.9)	1 (12.7)	19 (11.7)	23 (4.2)	5 (4.0)	15 (3.8)
Europe	14 (18.7)	6 (15.4)	19 (12.7)	18 (9.6)	23 (8.1)	9 (6.3)	1 (6.1)
Latin America	14 (22)	6 (13.9)	5 (9.2)	1 (8.2)	19 (7.9)	23 (7.9)	18 (5.5)
Oceania	14 (24.0)	6 (15.9)	19 (14.2)	18 (6.6)	23 (6.4)	9 (6.3)	4 (4.2)

Serogroups included in seven-valent Pnc-CRM$_{197}$ are in bold. Numbers in parentheses are the proportion of all sterile site isolates for each serogroup. (From Ref. 45.)

show that the proportion of isolates that would be covered by the current heptavalent vaccine is much higher (>86%) during the first 3 years of life, but falls thereafter [37]. Preliminary data from a large international collaborative study that analyzed isolates obtained from over 3000 children with acute otitis media indicates that serotypes 6B, 14, 19F, and 23F were isolated most frequently among children aged 10–18 months, an age when the incidence of acute otitis media is highest (W. Hausdorff, personal communication). The prevalence of individual serotypes appears to shift slowly over a period of decades rather than years. At the Boston City Hospital, serotypes 1, 2, and 3 accounted for roughly one-half of isolates from all sites prior to 1950, but during 1979–1982, they accounted for <5%, whereas serogroups 4, 6, 14, 18, and 19 became increasingly common [38–41]. Of 3644 isolates from blood collected at 10 U.S. hospitals between 1967 and 1975, serotypes 1, 2, and 3 accounted for 8.5%, 0.3%, and 7.1%, respectively [42]. In contrast, among the >7000 blood isolates serotyped at Centers for Disease Control and Prevention (CDC) from 1978 to 1995, only one was serotype 2. In 1998, the proportion of serotype 1 and serotype 3 isolates from blood submitted to the CDC through population-based surveillance was down to 2.4% and 3.3%, respectively [9]. Factors contributing to the apparent decline in serotypes 1, 2, and 3 invasive diseases and the increases in disease caused by other serotypes are unknown.

Serotypes that most commonly cause invasive pneumococcal infection differ somewhat in various regions of the world. Serogroups 6, 14, and 19 are leading causes of invasive pediatric pneumococcal disease in all regions (Table 1) [43–45]. Serogroup 1 continues to be a common cause of invasive diseases in Asia, Africa, Latin America, and parts of Europe, but is uncommon in the United States, Canada, Oceania, and Scandinavia [45,46]. Differences in the prevalence of serotype 1 among ethnic groups also occur. In southern Israel, serotype 1 accounts for 10–14% of invasive infections among Jewish children compared with 32–38% of infections among Bedouins [47]. In Alaska, serotype 1 caused 7% of invasive infections among Alaska Native children aged <5 years during 1991–1998 but was recovered from only 1 of over 200 non-Native children [12].

Some investigators have suggested that the observed geographical variability in serotype distribution reflects variations in blood culture practices [48]. Prospective studies will be required to test this hypothesis.

The global acquired immune deficiency syndrome (AIDS) epidemic also influences serotype distributions [49,50]. In South Africa, a greater proportion of HIV-positive adults had invasive disease caused by serogroups usually associated with infection in children (6, 14, 19, and 23) compared with HIV-negative adults. Serotype 1 was less common among HIV-infected persons of all ages compared with those without HIV [51,52].

II. IMMUNOBIOLOGY AND VACCINE DESIGN

Immunization with a polysaccharide covalently coupled to an immunogenic protein elicits isotype switching primarily to IgG1, a strong memory response, and involvement of T-cell help [53,54]. These features, which are characteristic of T-dependent antigens, make good immunogens in young children and yield booster responses with repeated administration.

The development and production of conjugate vaccines is a complex process. The process must minimize structural, chemical, and stoichiometrical changes to the individual components (carrier protein and polysaccharide) and couple the polysaccharide directly to the protein carrier in a one-step reaction. This procedure also must be optimized for each polysaccharide in the vaccine.

The combination of vaccines into multivalent formulations can result in a decrease in immunogenicity of one or more components. In the case of conjugated vaccines, the underlying mechanism for this suppression is not well understood, but appears to be associated with increasing dosage of the carrier protein [55]—a phenomenon called "carrier-induced epitopic suppression." Some studies have shown that epitope suppression can occur when a subject is immunized with an antigen conjugated to a carrier molecule to which the subject is immunologically experienced [56–58].

Theoretically, protein carrier-induced epitope suppression could prevent the boosting effect for pneumococcal polysaccharide antigens in individuals already primed to the carrier. In humans, carrier-induced epitope suppression may be dependent on vaccine dose, which may be highly antigen-specific and, thus, quite unpredictable in individual volunteers [58]. Preexposure to the protein carrier has, in fact, led to immune enhancement for several protein antigens and for responses to Hib capsular polysaccharide. [54]. It will be necessary to determine whether different combinations of each conjugate, when part of multivalent formulations, result in a significant alteration in the immunogenicity of the combination vaccine components compared to the conjugates alone.

III. ISSUES IN MEASUREMENT OF THE IMMUNE RESPONSE TO CONJUGATE VACCINES

Licensure of new pneumococcal conjugate vaccines will need to be based on in vitro measures of immune response. This approach was successfully used to license a Hib conjugate vaccine in the United States in the 1990s. Approval was based upon the use of immune correlates of protection to show the comparability of the candidate with previously licensed Hib conjugates. A similar approach will be needed for approval of new pneumococcal conjugate vaccines.

Several issues complicate the establishment of immune correlates of protection. First, there are at least two measures of immune response that can be used to evaluate immunogenicity—serum IgG antibody concentration and opsonophagocytic activity. Second, the amount of antibody or opsonophagocytic antibody needed may vary by serotype, and hence require serotype-specific correlates. Third, the concentrations or titers that correlate with protection against invasive diseases may not be adequate for protection against mucosal infections such as pneumonia, otitis media, or carriage. Fourth, for the evaluation of vaccines that contain new serotypes not included in any existing licensed vaccine, comparison to licensed vaccines will not be possible.

Typically, pneumococcal conjugate vaccine immunogenicity has been measured as the concentration of specific serum IgG (expressed as μg/mL) antibody following vaccination. Measuring IgG antibody concentrations is useful because these antibodies enhance opsonization, complement-dependent phagocytosis, and killing of pneumococci by leukocytes and other phagocytic cells, and because the assay (an enzyme immunoassay) is relatively straightforward to standardize. Increases in serum IgG antibody concentration following primary vaccination are also generally accompanied by an increase in antibody avidity. Improved antibody avidity indicates immunological maturation and corresponds with the establishment of immunological memory. Immunological memory, not antibody concentration postimmunization, may be the effector mechanism ultimately responsible for protection against invasive disease.

Opsonophagocytic activity is a more rigorous measure of protection provided by antipolysaccharide antibodies. Antibody avidity correlates better with opsonophagocytic activity in vitro than with the concentration of serum IgG antibody [59], and protection against experimental challenge infection correlates better with opsonophagocytic activity than with total antibody concentration [60]. The role of subclass distribution of antibodies, alone or in combination with functional activity, remains to be determined. Attempts to standardize the opsonophagocytic assay among international laboratories are currently underway. An opsonophagocytic assay developed by scientists at the CDC uses the HL-60 tissue culture cell line, and has been validated against the traditionally used human peripheral blood polymophonuclear leukocytes. This assay is performed by flow cytometry using fluorescently labeled bacteria, and titers to multiple serotypes can be simultaneously estimated [61,62].

IV. CLINICAL EVALUATIONS IN INFANTS AND YOUNG CHILDREN

A. Safety

Pneumococcal conjugate vaccines are generally well tolerated among infants and toddlers. Currently, the pneumococcal conjugate vaccine with the most extensive safety evaluation is a seven-valent vaccine (Pnc-7 CRM$_{197}$, Prevnar™; Wyeth Vaccines, Pearl River, NY). Each dose of Pnc-7 CRM$_{197}$ contains 2 μg each of capsular polysaccharides from serotypes 4, 9V, 14, 19F, and 23F; 2 μg of oligosaccharide from serotype 18C; and 4 μg of polysaccharide from serotype 6B, conjugated to approximately 20 μg of a recombinant diphtheria toxoid, cross-reactive material (CRM) 197. Pnc-7 CRM$_{197}$ has been licensed and routinely used since 2000 in the United States. With this vaccine, local and systemic reactions such as swelling, redness, and fever are less frequently observed than with diphtheria–tetanus–whole cell pertussis (DTwP) vaccines, but more frequent than with

hepatitis B or diphtheria–tetanus–acellular pertussis (DTaP) vaccines [63,64] In a large randomized trial, vaccination with Pnc-7 CRM$_{197}$ was not associated with an increased risk of outpatient visits for allergic reactions, asthma, wheezing, shortness of breath, or breath holding within 3 days of any dose. Further evaluation of the long-term safety of pneumococcal conjugates is ongoing.

B. Immunogenicity

The antibody response varies by serotype and is potentially influenced by the type and dose of saccharide used, the protein carrier to which the saccharide is conjugated, the type of protein–saccharide linkage used, and the simultaneous coadministration of other vaccines. Immunogenicity studies in infants illustrate the effect of different types of saccharides. Daum et al. [65] examined the response of infants to three different antigen concentrations of multivalent polysaccharide and oligosaccharide vaccines containing up to five different serotypes. For nearly all serotypes included in the vaccine, the antibody concentrations following three doses of vaccine were greater in the infants who received the polysaccharide formulation compared to those who received the oligosaccharide formulation (Table 2) [65]. No significant differences were noted for any of the local reactions or measured adverse events associated with the two prototype vaccines. The polysaccharide formulation may be more immunogenic than a comparable oligosaccharide design because it displays more epitopes [66]. Further Phase II and Phase III studies have used the polysaccharide formulation.

The effect of the dose of protein–saccharide seems to vary by vaccine type. In the study by Daum et al. [65], the differences between doses (0.5, 2.0, and 5.0 μg) were minor in comparison to the differences between polysaccharide and oligosaccharide preparations (Table 2). With a four-valent PncT vaccine candidate, the antibody responses appeared to be inversely associated with the dose used [67]. The antibody concentrations were highest in the group that received 1 μg compared to groups that received 3- or 10-μg formulations.

The kinetics of the antibody response vary according to serotype. With a candidate five-valent Pnc-CRM$_{197}$ vaccine, increased antibody concentrations were seen after one dose for serotypes 18C and 19F and after two doses for serotypes 14 and 23F, but antibodies to 6B did not increase substantially until after three doses (Table 2) [65]. Similarly, an immunogenicity study of a quadrivalent vaccine manufactured by conjugating pneumococcal polysaccharides to outer membrane proteins of group B meningococcus (Pnc-OMP) infants showed good antibody responses to serotypes 14 and 19F following one or two doses of vaccine, but antibody increases were more gradual for serotypes 6B and 23F, with substantial concentrations not appearing until two or three doses [68].

The simultaneous administration of other vaccines also can impact the antibody response to some pneumococcal conjugate vaccines. Specifically, administration of acellular pertussis (aP) vaccine significantly reduces the immunogenicity of simultaneously administered pneumococcal saccha-

Table 2 Immunogenicity of Different Doses and Formulations of a Quinquevalent Pn-CRM$_{197}$ Vaccine in Infants

Serotypes	Time[a]	Control[b]	Geometrical mean titer (µg/mL IgG)					
			Ps[c] (5.0)	Os[d] (5.0)	Ps (2.0)	Os (2.0)	Ps (0.5)	Os (0.5)
6B	Pre	0.41	0.33	0.33	0.45	0.24	0.26	0.30
	Post 1	0.10	0.09	0.12	0.11	0.09	0.11	0.11
	Post 2	0.06	0.13	0.11	0.20	0.07	0.10	0.08
	Post 3	0.07	1.45	0.78	2.14	0.56	0.42	0.37
14	Pre	0.28	0.18	0.21	0.47	0.22	0.21	0.21
	Post 1	0.07	0.21	0.15	0.27	0.12	0.11	0.08
	Post 2	0.06	1.26	0.53	1.10	0.35	0.49	0.28
	Post 3	0.50	3.39	2.63	2.34	1.58	1.66	0.98
18C	Pre	0.30	0.23	0.24	0.30	0.21	0.20	0.27
	Post 1	0.10	0.42	0.41	0.71	0.41	0.45	0.30
	Post 2	0.05	1.95	1.48	1.91	1.32	1.15	1.02
	Post 3	0.05	3.09	2.63	2.82	2.34	1.95	2.14
19F	Pre	0.40	0.32	0.44	0.21	0.32	0.28	
	Post 1	0.13	0.43	0.11	0.41	0.10	0.32	0.12
	Post 2	0.06	1.74	0.12	1.74	0.09	1.07	0.11
	Post 3	0.05	2.29	0.56	2.19	0.43	1.62	0.44
23F	Pre	0.26	0.18	0.19	0.30	0.14	0.22	0.17
	Post 1	0.10	0.07	0.08	0.12	0.06	0.10	0.06
	Post 2	0.05	0.63	0.16	0.65	0.21	0.45	0.23
	Post 3	0.04	3.38	1.25	2.45	0.93	1.55	1.00

[a] Approximately 50 subjects were enrolled per group and immunized at 2, 4, and 6 months of age.
[b] Received combination diphtheria–tetanus–whole cell pertussis–Hib conjugate vaccine.
[c] Polysaccharide at 5.0, 2.0, or 0.5 µg per serotype.
[d] Oligosaccharide at 5.0, 2.0, or 0.5 µg per serotype.

rides conjugated to tetanus toxoid (T-conjugates), but not those conjugated to diphtheria toxoid (D-conjugates) [69]. The exact biological mechanism for this observation is unclear, but it is possible that wP vaccines provide a powerful adjuvant effect that is needed by the T-conjugates, but not the D-conjugates.

C. Efficacy

1. Seven-Valent Pnc-CRM$_{197}$

Three large-scale, randomized, controlled trials of this vaccine have been conducted in northern California, Finland, and the Apache and Navajo nations of the southwestern United States (Table 3).

Kaiser Permanente, Northern California. This individually randomized, controlled, double-blinded trial of efficacy served as the pivotal trial for the licensure of this vaccine [64]. The study was conducted among children enrolled in a large managed care plan, the Northern California Kaiser Permanente group. The trial was designed to assess the efficacy of a four-dose regimen for the prevention of culture-proven invasive pneumococcal disease in young children. A total of 37,868 infants were randomly assigned to receive either Pnc-7 CRM$_{197}$ or an investigational meningococcal serogroup C conjugate vaccine containing CRM$_{197}$ at the ages of 2, 4, 6, and 12–15 months.

Infants were followed in blinded fashion for a period of 3.5 years. In the intention-to-treat analysis, 49 cases of

culture-confirmed invasive pneumococcal diseases due to vaccine serotypes were observed among the control vaccine recipients versus three cases among the pneumococcal conjugate vaccine recipients for an efficacy of 93.9% (95% CI: 79.6, 98.5). The per-protocol analysis showed that only 1 of 40 cases occurred among recipients of the pneumococcal conjugate vaccine for an efficacy of 97.4% (95% CI: 82.7, 99.9). Subsequent analyses showed that partially vaccinated children (e.g., <3 doses of vaccine) were significantly protected against invasive disease.

Serotype specific efficacy was 100% for the serotypes 14, 18C, and 23F components, and 84.6% for serotype 19F. Data were not sufficient to determine efficacy for serotype 6B, 9V, or 4, or to determine whether there was significant cross-protection against other serotypes in the same serogroup (e.g., serotype 6B vaccination providing protection against serotype 6A disease).

The majority of invasive pneumococcal diseases detected during this trial were bacteremia without an obvious focus (30 of 52 cases detected). There were five cases of pneumococcal meningitis and six cases of sepsis in control vaccine recipients, with no cases of meningitis and one case of sepsis among the pneumococcal vaccine recipients. These results are encouraging, but effectiveness against the most severe manifestations of pneumococcal disease will most likely be documented through postlicensure surveillance studies.

In addition to the primary endpoint of invasive disease, Black et al. [64] were able to assess the vaccine's efficacy

Table 3 Results of Randomized, Controlled Trials of Pneumococcal Conjugate Vaccine Efficacy

| Trial site | Vaccines | | N | Efficacy (95% LL, UL) | | | |
	Pneumococcal	Control		Vaccine-type pneumococcal invasive disease	Vaccine-type otitis media	All pneumococcal otitis media	Radiographic pneumonia with consolidation
Northern California, USA	Seven-valent-CRM$_{197}$	MenC-CRM$_{197}$	37,868	97% (83, 100)			19% (6, 30)
Navajo and Apache Nations, USA	Seven-valent-CRM$_{197}$	MenC-CRM$_{197}$	8,292	77% (−9, 95); 83% (21, 96)[a]			−3% (−60, 33)
Finland	Seven-valent-CRM$_{197}$	Hepatitis B	1,662		57% (44, 67)	34% (21, 45)	
Finland	Seven-valent-OMP	Hepatitis B	1,666		56% (44, 66)		
South Africa	Nine-valent-CRM$_{197}$	Placebo	~40,000	HIV-negative: 85% (32, 98); HIV-positive: 58% (−1, 84)			HIV-negative: 22% (0, 40); HIV-positive: 6% (−21, 27)

[a] Intention-to-treat analysis

against clinically defined otitis media. In the intention-to-treat analysis, there were 17 cases of spontaneously ruptured tympanic membranes among controls and six cases among vaccinees for a point estimate of efficacy of 64.7% ($P = 0.035$). Of note, all the positive cultures among vaccinees were serotype 19F. The vaccine showed significant protection against endpoints that are more frequent but less specific than pneumococcal otitis media, including protection against clinically defined otitis media and ventilatory tube placement.

The efficacy against pneumonia with x-ray evidence of consolidation was also assessed in this study. The vaccine reduced the incidence of pneumonia with consolidation by 19% (95% CI: 6, 30).

Finland. An individually randomized, double-blinded, controlled trial of the efficacy of a four-dose regimen of the seven-valent Pnc-CRM$_{197}$ conjugate vaccine was conducted in three areas of Finland [63]. This trial's primary objective was to determine the efficacy of the vaccine for the prevention of acute otitis media due to pneumococcal serotypes included in the vaccine. Over a 3.5-year period, 1662 children were enrolled into the trial. Equal numbers of children received Pnc-CRM$_{197}$ vaccine or a control regimen of hepatitis B vaccine. This study was designed as a three-arm trial, with an equal number of children also receiving a candidate seven-valent vaccine using a different protein, the outer membrane protein of serogroup B *Neisseria meningitidis* (seven-valent Pnc-OMP). (For details of the results with the Pnc-OMP vaccine, see below.) Children were vaccinated at the ages of 2, 4, 6, and 12 months.

A standardized definition of acute otitis media was developed, which included signs, symptoms, and the appearance of the tympanic membrane. For the prevention of clinically defined episodes of acute otitis media, the protective efficacy estimate was 6% (95% CI: −4, 16). For the prevention of recurrent otitis media—defined as at least three episodes in 6 months, or four or more episodes in 12 months—the vaccine's efficacy was estimated at 16% (95% CI: −6, 35).

A unique feature of the Finnish trial was its ability to routinely carry out myringotomy to collect middle ear fluid for bacteriological culture from patients with acute otitis media. This allowed the study to assess the efficacy of the vaccine for the prevention of ear infections due to *S. pneumoniae*. The study showed significant protection against acute otitis media episodes due to pneumococci of serotypes included in the vaccine (VE = 57%; 95% CI: 44, 67), and also, significant protection against certain pneumococci of the same serogroup but of a different serotype—6A, 9N, 19A, 18B, and 23A (VE = 51%; 95% CI: 27, 67). Of note, there was a 33% increase in the risk of otitis media due to nonvaccine type pneumococci among vaccinees, which was of borderline statistical significance (VE = −33%; 95% CI: −80, 1). This finding of an increased risk of nonvaccine-type otitis media is not surprising given that other studies have shown that the vaccine reduces the prevalence of colonization with vaccine serotypes, but often is associated with an increase in colonization with nonvaccine serotypes (see below).

Navajo/Apache Nations. In this high-incidence population, a uniquely designed efficacy trial was conducted [70]. Unlike the other trials, where individual infants were randomized to a vaccine group, this study randomized on the basis of community units on an Indian reservation. This community-randomized trial of the efficacy of a four-dose regimen of the seven-valent Pnc-CRM$_{197}$ conjugate vaccine was unique among the trials with this vaccine because of its ability to measure the indirect (i.e., herd immunity) effects of vaccination. The control communities received the investigational meningococcal C conjugate vaccine; all participants and investigators were blinded to vaccine group allocations. The study's primary objective was to measure the effectiveness of community-wide vaccination for the prevention of invasive pneumococcal disease. Secondary objectives included an assessment of the impact of vaccination on pneumococcal carriage among vaccinees and the impact on transmission in households.

The trial enrolled 8292 infants from 8 randomization units. Enrollment and surveillance were truncated by the licensure of the vaccine in February 2000. In the per-protocol analysis, there were eight cases of vaccine-type invasive disease among control vaccinees and two cases among pneumococcal conjugate vaccinees (VE = 76.8%; 95% CI: −9, 95); the intention-to-treat analysis included three additional cases in the control group for a vaccine efficacy estimate of 82.6% (95% CI: 21, 96) [71].

2. Seven-Valent Pnc-OMP

Finland. This candidate vaccine's efficacy against serotype-specific otitis media was evaluated in the same randomized, controlled trial as the seven-valent Pnc-CRM$_{197}$ vaccine (see "Seven-Valent Pnc-CRM$_{197}$" for detailed information) [72]. In all, 835 children were enrolled in the Pnc-OMP group as compared to 831 in the hepatitis B vaccine group. Infants were vaccinated with Pnc-OMP at the ages of 2, 4, 6, and 12 months, except for the last 187 enrolled infants who received unconjugated pneumococcal polysaccharide vaccine at the age of 12 months.

The vaccine regimen was associated with a 56% reduction in acute otitis media due to vaccine serotypes (95% CI: 44, 66). Serotype-specific efficacy estimates ranged from a low of 37% (95% CI: 1, 59) for serotype 19F to a high of 82% (95% CI: 12, 96) for serotype 9V. Overall, the vaccine reduced the incidence of pneumococcal acute otitis media by 25% (95% CI: 11, 37). The overall frequency of acute otitis media, however, did not differ between the two groups.

3. Nine-Valent Pnc-CRM$_{197}$

South Africa. A randomized, placebo-controlled efficacy study was conducted in Soweto, an urban area near Johannesburg, South Africa. The trial was designed to assess the efficacy of a three-dose, accelerated regimen of vaccination (ages of 2, 3, and 4 months) for the prevention of invasive disease and x-ray-confirmed pneumonia in HIV-positive and HIV-negative infants and children. The preliminary results of the study were presented in May 2002 at the International Symposium on Pneumococci and Pneumococcal Diseases in Anchorage, AK.

In HIV-infected children, the vaccine provided 58% efficacy versus invasive pneumococcal diseases of vaccine serotypes (per-protocol analysis, 95% CI: −1, 84). The vaccine did not show a significant reduction in the incidence of pneumonia with consolidation (VE = 6%; 95% CI: −21, 27), but this finding is not surprising considering the substantial role of *Pneumocystis carinii* and other organisms as agents of pneumonia in HIV-infected children.

In HIV-uninfected children, the vaccine demonstrated highly significant efficacy against invasive pneumococcal diseases due to vaccine serotypes (VE = 85%; 95% CI: 32, 98). Against pneumonia with x-ray evidence of alveolar consolidation, the vaccine efficacy estimate was 22% (95% CI: 0.1, 40) ($P = 0.049$). Of relevance for public health purposes, in the per-protocol analysis, the vaccine prevented three times as many cases of x-ray pneumonia with consolidation (33 cases) as it did culture-confirmed invasive pneumococcal disease (11 cases), indicating that most of the cases of pneumococcal diseases prevented by this vaccine will be undetected by routine culture methods.

The Gambia. A randomized, placebo-controlled trial design is testing the efficacy of the nine-valent pneumococcal conjugate vaccine for the prevention of severe pneumococcal diseases including culture-confirmed invasive disease and x-ray-confirmed pneumonia [73]. The trial population includes infants born in two rural divisions of The Gambia. With a per-capita GNP of $300, a high infant mortality rate (~80/1000 live births), endemic malaria transmission, and limited health care access, the situation is typical of much of rural Africa. Results should be available by 2005.

4. Eleven-Valent Pnc-D/T

Bohol, Philippines. This trial is designed to evaluate the efficacy of Aventis' 11-valent pneumococcal conjugate vaccine for the prevention of radiographic pneumonia in an urban area of the Philippines on the island of Bohol. This vaccine is manufactured by linking pneumococcal polysaccharides with either diphtheria or tetanus toxoids. This randomized controlled trial aims to enroll ~ 12,000 infants. It is anticipated that the results of this trial will be available by 2005. Although Aventis does not plan to proceed with the licensure and commercialization of this pneumococcal vaccine, nevertheless, the trial will provide important information on the burden of pneumococcal pneumonia and the value of pneumococcal vaccination in an Asian setting.

5. Eleven-Valent Pnc-Protein D

Czech Republic. Glaxo SmithKline developed an 11-valent pneumococcal vaccine using, as a recombinant, a nonlipidated form of protein D (a highly conserved cell surface lipoprotein obtained from either capsulated or unencapsulated strains of *Haemophilus influenzae*) as the carrier protein [74].

This vaccine is being evaluated in a Phase III field trial in the Czech Republic that aims to enroll 5000 infants with vaccinations given at the ages of 3, 4, 5, and 12–15 months. The infants also receive diphtheria–tetanus–acellular pertussis vaccine at the same visit. The study is designed to determine efficacy against culture-proven otitis media due to vaccine serotypes. The results of the study are expected to be available by 2004.

V. CLINICAL EVALUATION IN THE ELDERLY

Persons over 65 years of age are at increased risk for contracting, or dying from, pneumococcal infection. Higher rates of pneumococcal disease in the elderly may be related to immunosenescence (age-related declines in immune function) resulting in losses of opsonizing antibody concentrations and functions in the elderly [75,76].

Two studies in adults examined the immunogenicity of a five-valent candidate pneumococcal CRM_{197} vaccine containing serotypes 6B, 14, 18C, 19F, and 23F [93,95]. The first study randomly assigned 46 "generally healthy" older adults age 50–85 years to either a conjugate vaccine (CRM_{197}) or a licensed polysaccharide vaccine [77]. Similar postvaccination geometrical mean antibody levels were reached for serotypes 6B, 14, and 18C for both vaccines. The conjugated vaccine tended to elicit lower levels of antibody to 19F and higher levels to 23F compared to the polysaccharide vaccine, but none of these differences was statistically significant [77]. The second study compared the same conjugate vaccine to a licensed polysaccharide vaccine in younger (age <45 years) and older (age >60 years) adults [78]. There were no statistically significant differences in antibody responses between the vaccines in either age group.

VI. CLINICAL EVALUATION IN PERSONS WITH UNDERLYING MEDICAL CONDITIONS

In 2000, the Advisory Committee on Immunization Practices (ACIP) of the U.S. Public Health Service issued guidelines on the use of conjugate and polysaccharide pneumococcal vaccines in persons with immunocompromising conditions. The ACIP did not recommend the use of pneumococcal conjugate vaccine in immunocompromised persons aged 5 years and older. There are currently no data from randomized trials assessing the efficacy of pneumococcal conjugate vaccine among persons immunocompromised by medical conditions or medications, but a number of studies have been conducted to determine the safety and immunogenicity of conjugate vaccines in these groups. These studies compare responses to conjugate pneumococcal vaccines among immunocompromised persons compared with healthy controls, assess responses to conjugate vaccines compared with responses to polysaccharide vaccines, and determine booster responses to conjugate or polysaccharide vaccines among immunocompromised persons previously vaccinated with a conjugate vaccine.

A. Sickle Cell Disease

Effective vaccines are needed for the prevention of life-threatening pneumococcal infections in infants and young children with sickle cell disease and related hemoglobinopathies [79,80]. The risk of pneumococcal infection increases dramatically within the first 6 months after birth, well before T-cell-independent immune responses to polysaccharide vaccines are developed. Infants with sickle cell disease who were vaccinated with Pnc-CRM$_{197}$ at the ages of 2, 4, and 6 months developed antibody responses comparable to those seen in infants without sickle cell disease [81]. Children aged 2 years and older with sickle cell disease who were primed with two doses of Pnc-7 CRM$_{197}$ 8 weeks apart responded with higher antibody concentrations to polysaccharide vaccine than did those who were previously unimmunized [82]. Antibodies induced by the booster dose of polysaccharide vaccine after priming with conjugate vaccine may have more functional activities than do antibodies that are present before vaccination [83]. Local reactions were not more common following the booster dose of polysaccharide vaccine compared to the priming doses of conjugate vaccine, even among patients with high prebooster antibody concentrations [81,82].

B. Human Immunodeficiency Virus-Infected Patients

In general, immune responses to pneumococcal conjugate vaccines are impaired in HIV-infected persons, particularly with more advanced HIV infection [84,85]. One exception is found in data from a study of 18 HIV-infected and 33 uninfected children aged 2–24 months where geometrical mean antibody concentrations were similar in the two groups 1 month after completing a three-dose primary series with a five-valent Pnc-CRM$_{197}$ vaccine [86].

No clear advantage of pneumococcal conjugate vaccine over polysaccharide vaccine has been identified for HIV-infected persons aged 2 years and older. The HIV-infected children aged 2–19 years responded to a five-valent Pnc-CRM$_{197}$ vaccine with greater antibody concentrations for some serotypes than did children receiving 23-valent polysaccharide vaccine [87]. Better responses to a single dose of conjugate vaccine compared with a single polysaccharide vaccine for selected serotypes have been found in some studies of HIV-infected adults with CD4$^+$ lymphocyte counts >200 [88] but not in others [85]. Among adults with more advanced AIDS (CD4 count <200), the response to 19F as part of a five-valent vaccine was inferior to that elicited by a 23-valent polysaccharide vaccine [85]. However, until immune correlates of protection disease are determined, it is unclear whether even statistically significant differences in an immune response are clinically relevant. Although more local reactions (primarily tenderness at the injection site) have been reported for HIV-infected adults

after vaccination with conjugate vaccines as compared with polysaccharide vaccine, serious untoward effects have not been reported in either group [85,88]. In addition, no changes in viral load during 24 weeks of follow-up were observed among 33 patients receiving one or two doses of the seven-valent Pnc-CRM$_{197}$ vaccine [89].

Incremental increases in antibody concentration and functional activity after a second dose of conjugate vaccine are limited in HIV-infected adults [84,88]. However, these data are considered inadequate at this time to justify the additional costs and efforts of the widespread use of pneumococcal conjugate vaccine.

C. Hodgkin's Disease

Patients treated for Hodgkin's disease are particularly susceptible to life-threatening pneumococcal infections. Although patients with Hodgkin's disease respond well to pneumococcal immunization before treatment, immune responses to polysaccharide vaccines are impaired for up to 2 years after treatment [90]. Responses to polysaccharide vaccine two or more years after a diagnosis of Hodgkin's disease do not differ from those of healthy controls [91]. Responses to a single dose of seven-valent Pnc-OMP vaccine in these patients were inferior to those elicited by polysaccharide vaccines [91]. However, the conjugate vaccine recipients responded better to a dose of 23-valent polysaccharide vaccine 1 year later than did patients who had not received conjugate vaccines, suggesting a possible role for conjugate vaccines for the immunological priming of patients with Hodgkin's disease [92].

D. Bone Marrow Transplant Patients

Opportunistic pneumococcal infection among persons undergoing allogeneic bone marrow transplantation occurs most commonly in the late recovery phase (>100 days after transplantation) [93]. Antibodies to pneumococcal capsular polysaccharides can be depressed for several years after transplantation [94]. IgG antibody responses to pneumococcal polysaccharide vaccine during the first 2 years after bone marrow transplantation are depressed and have low functional activity [95,96]. Prolonged depression of antipneumococcal antibodies and poor responses to pneumococcal polysaccharide vaccine are a particular problem for patients with graft-versus-host disease [97]. Antibody responses in a small number of patients vaccinated with a seven-valent OMP conjugate vaccine 1 year after bone marrow transplantation were similar to responses to pneumococcal polysaccharide vaccine [98].

Administering *H. influenzae* type b (Hib) conjugate vaccine to patients undergoing autologous bone marrow transplantation led to better anticapsular antibody responses to posttransplantation doses of Hib conjugate vaccine compared with patients who were not vaccinated before harvest [99]. Likewise, pretransplantation vaccination of stem cell donors with Hib conjugate vaccine produced higher total anti-polyribosylribitol phosphate (PRP) responses in allogeneic stem cell transplant recipients compared with recipients with unvaccinated donors [100]. Future work will assess similar strategies using pneumococcal conjugate vaccine for pretransplantation immunization.

VII. IMPACT OF ROUTINE IMMUNIZATION ON TRANSMISSION AND DISEASE

A. Effect of Conjugate Vaccination on Nasopharyngeal Colonization

Pneumococcal conjugate vaccines reduce colonization with vaccine serotypes. Klugman [101] reviewed four published and six unpublished studies of the effect of pneumococcal conjugate immunization on subsequent carriage of pneumococci in the nasopharynx (NP) [102–105]. These studies included seven different vaccine formulations, ranging from five-valent to 11-valent, given to infants or toddlers in five different schedules, and investigators collected NP specimens 1 month to 2 years after immunization. The effect on colonization by pneumococcal serotypes included in the vaccine was remarkably consistent. In all but one study, which measured colonization 2 years after primary immunization [101], pneumococcal conjugate vaccination was associated with significantly reduced colonization by vaccine serotypes.

Notably, in five of the studies reviewed by Klugman [101], pneumococcal conjugate vaccinees were significantly more likely to be colonized with nonvaccine pneumococcal serotypes [102–104]. In a large randomized trial of nine-valent Pnc-CRM$_{197}$ vaccine among toddlers in Israel, vaccination reduced colonization with several serotypes included in the vaccines (6B, 9V, 14, and 23F) but not 19F [106].

The increase in nonvaccine serotype pneumococcal colonization raises the question of whether the increase is due to "replacement" colonization by nonvaccine serotypes, or is the result of "unmasking" of existing nonvaccine type subpopulations [107]. Replacement occurs when vaccinated individuals, who are protected against colonization by vaccine serotypes, become relatively more susceptible to colonization by nonvaccine types, perhaps by allowing nonvaccine serotypes to compete more successfully for resources in the absence of competition from vaccine serotypes.

Unmasking implies that the observed increase in nonvaccine serotype carriage after vaccination is actually due to an increased likelihood of detection after the decline in the number of vaccine-type organisms. Most NP colonization studies are performed by directly plating specimens onto agar plates and then by selecting one or a few colonies for serotyping. This technique is sensitive for identifying the presence of any pneumococci, but insensitive for detecting colonization by multiple serotypes. Because individuals may be colonized with multiple serotype populations (e.g., one vaccine serotype and one nonvaccine serotype) and, in some cases, the minority serotype may account for only 10% or less of all pneumococci, the effect of vaccination may be to simply unmask the nonvaccine serotype populations by decreasing the density of vaccine serotypes on the agar plate [108]. Differentiating between serotype replace-

ment and unmasking can be difficult, but a recently developed statistical test by Lipsitch [109] helps to determine the likelihood of true replacement in the context of clinical trials.

Although pneumococcal conjugates were expected to be highly efficacious against systemic infections, it was largely a surprise to find that this parenterally administered vaccine protected against the acquisition of *S. pneumoniae* at mucosal surfaces. The mechanisms that mediate protection against mucosal infection are unclear. Typically, protection on mucosal surfaces is thought to be due to secretory IgA. However, the response to pneumococcal conjugates is overwhelmingly serum IgG antibody, with only low levels of salivary IgA demonstrable following primary immunization with pneumococcal conjugates [110,111]. Some authors have proposed that the effect on colonization is due to the production of high-serum IgG levels, which transude onto the mucosal surfaces, providing short-lived protection immediately following immunization [112] and, indeed, salivary IgG concentrations following immunization correlate with serum IgG concentrations [110]. It is likely that both IgA and IgG antibodies play a role in vivo [110].

Routine pneumococcal conjugate vaccination will likely have substantial indirect effects, which may be beneficial, detrimental, or both, at the individual and population levels. At the individual level, vaccination will likely reduce the risk of colonization by vaccine serotypes but also increase the risk of colonization, and perhaps disease, by nonvaccine serotypes. At the population level, widespread vaccination is likely to reduce the transmission of vaccine serotypes and hence induce herd immunity (i.e., reduce the risk of disease due to vaccine serotypes among vaccinated and unvaccinated persons). There is also the possibility that increases in colonization with nonvaccine serotypes will lead to increased transmission of the disease due to these types. Mathematical models by Lipsitch [107] indicate that replacement colonization and transmission are likely to occur, and that the extent to which they occur will be mediated by vaccination coverage, the efficacy of the vaccine against vaccine serotype colonization, and the degree of competition between vaccine and nonvaccine serotypes.

The overall impact of vaccination on pneumococcal disease rates will be a balance of these direct and indirect effects. In vaccinated children, an increased risk of acute otitis media caused by nonvaccine serotypes has been reported [63], but data from controlled trials do not indicate a greater risk of invasive disease from nonvaccine serotypes. Black et al. [113] reported that following the introduction of routine infant immunization with seven-valent Pnc-CRM$_{197}$ vaccine, the incidence of invasive disease due to vaccine serotypes decreased far greater than expected based on immunization coverage alone. For example, in the first year of routine vaccination, the incidence of disease among infants <1 year old decreased by 87% even though the proportion of infants fully vaccinated did not exceed 30% at any point and <67% of infants had received any pneumococcal conjugate vaccine dose. No increase in nonvaccine serotype invasive disease was reported. Postlicensure surveillance studies are needed to detect any clinically significant increased risk of invasive disease caused by nonvaccine serotypes.

B. Effect of Conjugate Vaccines on Nasopharyngeal Colonization with Antibiotic-Resistant Strains

Conjugate pneumococcal vaccines may reduce antibiotic-resistant infections by protecting infants from drug-resistant strains, by disrupting the transmission of drug-resistant organisms, and, perhaps, by lessening the selective pressure for antibiotic-resistant pneumococci by reducing antibiotic use in vaccinated children. During the 1990s, antimicrobial drug resistance was most common among the serotypes that are included in the seven-valent conjugate vaccine [114,115]. Although replacement by nonvaccine serotypes raises questions about the efficacy of conjugate vaccine in reducing overall transmission, drug resistance has been less common in the nonvaccine serotypes recovered from vaccinated children [101,103,105,116]. Thus, pneumococcal conjugate vaccines should reduce person-to-person transmission of drug-resistant strains. Ongoing surveillance and additional studies will be necessary to determine whether the emergence of antimicrobial resistance in nonvaccine serotypes will pose future challenges to the treatment of pneumococcal infections.

Results of a randomized, double-blinded trial in Israel show how pneumococcal conjugate vaccination may reduce the selective pressure of antibiotics that drives drug resistance [106]. Day care center attendees aged 12–35 months were randomized to vaccination with a nine-valent CRM_{197} pneumococcal conjugate vaccine or a control vaccine (*N. meningitidis* group C CRM_{197} conjugate) and followed monthly to bimonthly with nasopharyngeal swabs for 2 years. The history of illnesses and antibiotic use during the period since the previous visit were obtained during interviews with parents. Children receiving pneumococcal conjugate vaccine had fewer reported episodes of upper respiratory tract infections, lower respiratory problems, and otitis media than did control recipients. More importantly, the group receiving pneumococcal vaccine had 17% fewer days on antibiotics, including reductions of 10% for antibiotics taken for upper respiratory infections, 20% for otitis media, and 47% for lower respiratory tract problems.

C. Serotype Switching in Response to Immunological Pressure

The overwhelming majority of penicillin-resistant, multidrug-resistant *S. pneumoniae* isolates are associated with only a select few (e.g., types 6B, 14, 19F, and 23F) of the 90 different capsular types that may decorate the surface of the organism. These same four serotypes are the predominant players that cause invasive disease in infants. The restriction of these dangerous drug-resistant organisms to such a few key serotypes provided hope that the development of conjugate vaccines, which include these serotypes, would control some of the most dangerous strains of *S. pneumoniae* that cause widespread disease [117].

Recent work, however, has led to the discovery that multidrug-resistant strains could overcome the protective effects of a conjugate vaccine by acquiring DNA molecules from other pneumococci that allow expression of new capsular types [118]. In an outbreak among AIDS patients in New York, a multidrug-resistant pneumococcal clone, which represented a serotype 23F strain that had acquired the genes to express the capsule of serotype 3, was identified, thereby converting the strain to serotype 3 [119].

VIII. ISSUES FOR USE OF PNEUMOCOCCAL CONJUGATE VACCINES IN DEVELOPING COUNTRIES

With an estimated 1 million childhood deaths due to pneumococcal disease each year, the routine use of pneumococcal conjugate vaccines could substantially improve child health in developing countries. The successful introduction of these vaccines into developing countries will require efforts to overcome some major obstacles. The introduction process begins with researchers who generate an evidence base in developing countries, which shows the importance of pneumococcal disease, especially pneumococcal pneumonia, and the safety and effectiveness of the vaccines. This must in turn generate a local appreciation for the importance and value of vaccination. Experience with Hib conjugate vaccines has shown that the lack of local disease burden data was one of the major obstacles to the vaccine's uptake in developing countries [120].

Epidemiological differences and limitations in financial and programmatic resources limit the ability to extrapolate data from studies conducted in industrialized countries to developing countries. For example, efficacy studies conducted in industrialized countries have evaluated a four-dose regimen in which the second dose of vaccine was not given until at least the age of 4 months. In many developing countries, however, pneumococcal pneumonia among very young infants (i.e., less than 3 months old) is a major problem and most developing country programs give only three doses, not four, in the primary vaccination schedule. Studies of immunization regimens tailored to the epidemiology in developing countries are needed.

Pneumococcal conjugate vaccines will likely cost more than the vaccines that are currently part of the routine immunization program. The economic impact of pneumococcal disease and the cost-effectiveness of immunization must be assessed. Even with these efforts, substantial external assistance will be needed to make the vaccine available to the countries that need it the most—those countries with high infant and child mortality and few economic resources. The creation of the Vaccine Fund of the Global Alliance for Vaccines and Immunization (GAVI) represents a major step forward in this respect. The acceleration of pneumococcal vaccine use in these countries will be a major test for the alliance, and its success, or failure, will likely have major implications for vaccine development in the future.

REFERENCES

1. Marston BJ, et al. Incidence of community-acquired pneumonia requiring hospitalization. Results of a population-based active surveillance Study in Ohio. The Community-Based Pneumonia Incidence Study Group. Arch Intern Med 1997; 157:1709–1718.
2. Schuchat A, et al. Bacterial meningitis in the United States in 1995. N Engl J Med 1997; 337:970–976.
3. Del Beccaro MA, et al. Bacteriology of acute otitis media: a new perspective. J Pediatr 1992; 120:81–84.
4. Breiman RF, et al. Pneumococcal bacteremia in Charleston County, South Carolina. A decade later. Arch Intern Med 1990; 150:1401–1405.
5. Bennett NM, et al. Pneumococcal bacteremia in Monroe County, New York. Am J Public Health 1992; 82:1513–1516.
6. Plouffe JF, et al. Bacteremia with *Streptococcus pneumoniae*. Implications for therapy and prevention. Franklin County Pneumonia Study Group. JAMA 1996; 275:194–198.
7. Pastor P, et al. Invasive pneumococcal disease in Dallas County, Texas: results from population-based surveillance in 1995. Clin Infect Dis 1998; 26:590–595.
8. Harrison LH, et al. Invasive pneumococcal infection in Baltimore, MD: implications for immunization policy. Arch Intern Med 2000; 160:89–94.
9. Robinson KA, et al. Epidemiology of invasive *Streptococcus pneumoniae* infections in the United States, 1995–1998: opportunities for prevention in the conjugate vaccine era. JAMA 2001; 285:1729–1735.
10. Feikin DR, et al. Mortality from invasive pneumococcal pneumonia in the era of antibiotic resistance, 1995–1997. Am J Public Health 2000; 90:223–229.
11. Nuorti JP. Epidemiologic relation between HIV and invasive pneumococcal disease in San Francisco County, California. Ann Internal Med 2000; 132:182–190.
12. Rudolph KM, et al. Serotype distribution and antimicrobial resistance patterns of invasive isolates of *Streptococcus pneumoniae*: Alaska, 1991–1998. J Infect Dis 2000; 182:490–496.
13. Cortese MM, et al. High incidence rates of invasive pneumococcal disease in the White Mountain Apache population. Arch Intern Med 1992; 152:2277–2282.
14. WHO. Pneumococcal vaccines: WHO position paper. Wkly Epidemiol Rec 1999; 74:177–184.
15. Goetghebuer T, et al. Outcome of meningitis caused by *Streptococcus pneumoniae and Haemophilus influenzae* type b in children in The Gambia. Trop Med Int Health 2000; 5:207–213.
16. Campagne G, et al. Epidemiology of bacterial meningitis in Niamey, Niger, 1981–96. Bull World Health Organ 1999; 77:499–508.
17. Scott JA, et al. Aetiology, outcome, and risk factors for mortality among adults with acute pneumonia in Kenya. Lancet 2000; 355:1225–1230.
18. Barnes DJ, et al. The role of percutaneous lung aspiration in the bacteriological diagnosis of pneumonia in adults. Aust NZ J Med 1988; 187:754–757.
19. Macfarlane JT, et al. *Mycoplasma pneumoniae* and the aetiology of lobar pneumonia in northern Nigeria. Thorax 1979; 34:713–719.
20. Douglas RM, Devitt L. Pneumonia in New Guinea: I. Bacteriological findings in 632 adults with particular reference to *Haemophilus influenzae*. Med J Aust 1973; 1:42–49.
21. Bell M, et al. Seasonal variation in the etiology of bloodstream infections in a febrile inpatient population in a developing country. Int J Infect Dis 2002; 5:63–69.
22. Nuorti JP, et al. Cigarette smoking and invasive pneumo-

23. Roson B, et al. Prospective study of the usefulness of sputum Gram stain in the initial approach to community-acquired pneumonia requiring hospitalization. Clin Infect Dis 2000; 31:869–874.
24. Rusconi F, et al. Counterimmunoelectrophoresis and latex particle agglutination in the etiologic diagnosis of presumed bacterial pneumonia in pediatric patients. Pediatr Infect Dis J 1988; 7:781–785.
25. Scott JA, et al. Diagnosis of pneumococcal pneumonia in epidemiological studies: evaluation in Kenyan adults of a serotype-specific urine latex agglutination assay. Clin Infect Dis 1999; 28:764–769.
26. Ruiz-Gonzalez A, et al. Is *Streptococcus pneumoniae* the leading cause of pneumonia of unknown etiology? A microbiologic study of lung aspirates in consecutive patients with community-acquired pneumonia. Am J Med 1999; 106:385–390.
27. Murdoch DR, et al. Evaluation of a rapid immunochromatographic test for detection of *Streptococcus pneumoniae* antigen in urine samples from adults with community-acquired pneumonia. J Clin Microbiol 2001; 39:3495–3498.
28. Dominguez J, et al. Urinary antigen test for pneumococcal pneumonia. Chest 2001; 120:1748–1750.
29. Dowell SF, et al. Evaluation of Binax NOW, an assay for the detection of pneumococcal antigen in urine samples, performed among pediatric patients. Clin Infect Dis 2001; 32:824–825.
30. Gillespie SH, et al. Detection of *Streptococcus pneumoniae* in sputum samples by PCR. J Clin Microbiol 1994; 32:1308–1311.
31. Rudolph KM, et al. Evaluation of polymerase chain reaction for diagnosis of pneumococcal pneumonia. J Clin Microbiol 1993; 31:2661–2666.
32. Salo P, et al. Diagnosis of bacteremic pneumococcal pneumonia by amplification of pneumolysin gene fragment in serum. J Infect Dis 1995; 171:479–482.
33. Musher DM, et al. Nonspecificity of assaying for IgG antibody to pneumolysin in circulating immune complexes as a means to diagnose pneumococcal pneumonia. Clin Infect Dis 2001; 32:534–538.
34. Mulholland K. Magnitude of the problem of childhood pneumonia. Lancet 1999; 354:590–592.
35. Siber GR. Pneumococcal disease: prospects for a new generation of vaccines. Science 1994; 265:1385–1387.
36. Butler JC, et al. Serotype distribution of *Streptococcus pneumoniae* infections among preschool children in the United States, 1978–1994: implications for development of a conjugate vaccine. J Infect Dis 1995; 171:885–889.
37. Joloba ML, et al. Pneumococcal conjugate vaccine serotypes of *Streptococcus pneumoniae* isolates and the antimicrobial susceptibility of such isolates in children with otitis media. Clin Infect Dis 2001; 33:1489–1494.
38. Finland M, Barnes MW. Changes in occurrence of capsular serotypes of *Streptococcus pneumoniae* at Boston City Hospital during selected years between 1935 and 1974. J Clin Microbiol 1977; 5:154–166.
39. Barry MA, et al. Serotypes of *Streptococcus pneumoniae* isolated from blood cultures at Boston City Hospital between 1979 and 1982. J Infect Dis 1984; 149:449–452.
40. Tilghman FC, Finland M. Clinical significance of bacteremia in pneumococcal pneumonia. Arch Intern Med 1937; 59:602–619.
41. Babl FE, et al. Constancy of distribution of serogroups of invasive pneumococcal isolates among children: experience during 4 decades. Clin Infect Dis 2001; 32:1155–1161.
42. Austrian R, et al. Prevention of pneumococcal pneumonia

by vaccination. Trans Assoc Am Physicians 1976; 89:184–194.

43. Sniadack DH, et al. Potential interventions for the prevention of childhood pneumonia: geographic and temporal differences in serotype and serogroup distribution of sterile site pneumococcal isolates from children—implications for vaccine strategies. Pediatr Infect Dis J 1995; 14:503–510.

44. Scott JA, et al. Serogroup-specific epidemiology of *Streptococcus pneumoniae*: associations with age, sex, and geography in 7,000 episodes of invasive disease. Clin Infect Dis 1996; 22:973–981.

45. Hausdorff WP, et al. Which pneumococcal serogroups cause the most invasive disease: implications for conjugate vaccine formulation and use, Part I. Clin Infect Dis 2000; 30:100–121.

46. Eskola J, et al. Epidemiology of invasive pneumococcal infections in children in Finland. JAMA 1992; 268:3323–3327.

47. Dagan R, et al. Epidemiology of invasive childhood pneumococcal infections in Israel. The Israeli Pediatric Bacteremia and Meningitis Group. JAMA 1992; 268:3328–3332.

48. Hausdorff WP, et al. Geographical differences in invasive pneumococcal disease rates and serotype frequency in young children. Lancet 2001; 357:950–952.

49. Frankel RE, et al. Invasive pneumococcal disease: clinical features, serotypes, and antimicrobial resistance patterns in cases involving patients with and without human immunodeficiency virus infection. Clin Infect Dis 1996; 23:577–584.

50. Hibbs JR, et al. Prevalence of human immunodeficiency virus infection, mortality rate, and serogroup distribution among patients with pneumococcal bacteremia at Denver General Hospital, 1984–1994. Clin Infect Dis 1997; 25:195–199.

51. Jones N, et al. The impact of HIV on *Streptococcus pneumoniae* bacteraemia in a South African population. AIDS 1998; 12:2177–2184.

52. Crewe-Brown HH, et al. *Streptococcus pneumoniae* blood culture isolates from patients with and without human immunodeficiency virus infection: alterations in penicillin susceptibilities and in serogroups or serotypes. Clin Infect Dis 1997; 25:1165–1172.

53. Stein KE. Thymus-independent and thymus-dependent responses to polysaccharide antigens. J Infect Dis 1992; 165 (Suppl 1):S49–S52.

54. Granoff DM, et al. Induction of immunologic memory in infants primed with *Haemophilus influenzae* type b conjugate vaccines. J Infect Dis 1993; 168:663–671.

55. Dagan R, et al. Reduced response to multiple vaccines sharing common protein epitopes that are administered simultaneously to infants. Infect Immun 1998; 66:2093–2098.

56. Herzenberg LA, Tokuhisa T. Epitope-specific regulation: I. Carrier-specific induction of suppression for IgG anti-hapten antibody responses. J Exp Med 1982; 155:1730–1740.

57. Herzenberg LA, et al. Epitope-specific regulation: II. A bistable, IgH-restricted regulatory mechanism central to immunologic memory. J Exp Med 1982; 155:1741–1753.

58. DiJohn D, et al. Effect of priming with carrier on response to conjugate vaccine. Lancet 1989; 2:1415–1418.

59. Usinger WR, Lucas AH. Avidity as a determinant of the protective efficacy of human antibodies to pneumococcal capsular polysaccharides. Infect Immun 1999; 67:2366–2370.

60. Anttila M, et al. Avidity of IgG for *Streptococcus pneumoniae* type 6B and 23F polysaccharides in infants primed with pneumococcal conjugates and boosted with polysaccharide or conjugate vaccines. J Infect Dis 1998; 177:1614–1621.

61. Martinez JE, et al. A flow cytometric opsonophagocytic assay for measurement of functional antibodies elicited after vaccination with the 23-valent pneumococcal polysaccharide vaccine. Clin Diagn Lab Immunol 1999; 6:581–586.

62. Romero-Steiner S, et al. Standardization of an opsonophagocytic assay for the measurement of functional antibody activity against *Streptococcus pneumoniae* using differentiated HL-60 cells. Clin Diagn Lab Immunol 1997; 4:415–422.

63. Eskola J, et al. Efficacy of a pneumococcal conjugate vaccine against acute otitis media. N Engl J Med 2001; 344:403–409.

64. Black S, et al. Efficacy, safety and immunogenicity of heptavalent pneumococcal conjugate vaccine in children. Northern California Kaiser Permanente Vaccine Study Center Group. Pediatr Infect Dis J 2000; 19:187–195.

65. Daum RS, et al. Infant immunization with pneumococcal CRM$_{197}$ vaccines: effect of saccharide size on immunogenicity and interactions with simultaneously administered vaccines. J Infect Dis 1997; 176:445–455.

66. Steinhoff MC, et al. A randomized comparison of three bivalent *Streptococcus pneumoniae* glycoprotein conjugate vaccines in young children: effect of polysaccharide size and linkage characteristics. Pediatr Infect Dis J 1994; 13:368–372.

67. Ahman H, et al. Dose dependency of antibody response in infants and children to pneumococcal polysaccharides conjugated to tetanus toxoid. Vaccine 1999; 17:2726–2732.

68. Kayhty H, et al. Pneumococcal polysaccharide–meningococcal outer membrane protein complex conjugate vaccine is immunogenic in infants and children. J Infect Dis 1995; 172:1273–1278.

69. Dagan R, et al. Reduction in antibody responses to an 11-valent pneumococcal vaccine (PncT/D) when coadministered with a vaccine containing acellular pertussis (aP). Presented at the 42nd Interscience Conference on Antimicrobial Agents and Chemotherapy, San Diego, CA, September 27–30, 2002.

70. Moulton LH, et al. Design of a group-randomized *Streptococcus pneumoniae* vaccine trial. Control Clin Trials 2001; 22:438–452.

71. O'Brien KL, et al. Efficacy and safety of seven-valent conjugate pneumococcal vaccine in American Indian children: group randomised trial. Lancet 2003; 362:355–361.

72. Kilpi T, et al. Efficacy of a seven-valent pneumococcal conjugate vaccine (PncOMPC) against serotype-specific acute otitis media (AOM) caused by *Streptococcus pneumoniae* (Pnc). Presented at the 40th Interscience Conference on Antimicrobial Agents and Chemotherapy. Toronto, Ontario, Canada, September 2000.

73. Jaffar S, et al. Preparation for a pneumococcal vaccine trial in The Gambia: individual or community randomisation? Vaccine 1999; 18:633–640.

74. Bakaletz LO, et al. Protection against development of otitis media induced by nontypeable *Haemophilus influenzae* by both active and passive immunization in a chinchilla model of virus–bacterium superinfection. Infect Immun 1999; 67:2746–2762.

75. Musher DM, et al. Pneumococcal polysaccharide vaccine in young adults and older bronchitics: determination of IgG responses by ELISA and the effect of adsorption of serum with non-type-specific cell wall polysaccharide. J Infect Dis 1990; 161:728–735.

76. Ruben FL, Uhrin M. Specific immunoglobulin-class antibody responses in the elderly before and after 14-valent pneumococcal vaccine. J Infect Dis 1985; 151:845–849.

77. Powers DC, et al. Reactogenicity and immunogenicity of a protein-conjugated pneumococcal oligosaccharide vaccine in older adults. J Infect Dis 1996; 173:1014–1018.

78. Shelly MA, et al. Comparison of pneumococcal polysac-

charide and CRM$_{197}$-conjugated pneumococcal oligosaccharide vaccines in young and elderly adults. Infect Immun 1997; 65:242–247.

79. Daw NC, et al. Nasopharyngeal carriage of penicillin-resistant *Streptococcus pneumoniae* in children with sickle cell disease. Pediatrics 1997; 99:E7.

80. Steele RW, et al. Colonization with antibiotic-resistant *Streptococcus pneumoniae* in children with sickle-cell disease. J Pediatr 1996; 128:531–535.

81. O'Brien KL, et al. Safety and immunogenicity of heptavalent pneumococcal vaccine conjugated to CRM(197) among infants with sickle cell disease. Pneumococcal Conjugate Vaccine Study Group. Pediatrics 2000; 106: 965–972.

82. Vernacchio L, et al. Combined schedule of 7-valent pneumococcal conjugate vaccine followed by 23-valent pneumococcal vaccine in children and young adults with sickle cell disease. J Pediatr 1998; 133:275–278.

83. Vernacchio L, et al. Comparison of an opsonophagocytic assay and IgG ELISA to assess responses to pneumococcal polysaccharide and pneumococcal conjugate vaccines in children and young adults with sickle cell disease. J Infect Dis 2000; 181:1162–1166.

84. Kroon FP, et al. Enhanced antibody response to pneumococcal polysaccharide vaccine after prior immunization with conjugate pneumococcal vaccine in HIV-infected adults. Vaccine 2000; 19:886–894.

85. Ahmed F, et al. Effect of human immunodeficiency virus type 1 infection on the antibody response to a glycoprotein conjugate pneumococcal vaccine: results from a randomized trial. J Infect Dis 1996; 173:83–90.

86. King JCJ, et al. Safety and immunogenicity of three doses of a five-valent pneumococcal conjugate vaccine in children younger than two years with and without human immunodeficiency virus infection. Pediatrics 1997; 99:575–580.

87. King JCJ, et al. Comparison of the safety and immunogenicity of a pneumococcal conjugate with a licensed polysaccharide vaccine in human immunodeficiency virus and non-human immunodeficiency virus-infected children. Pediatr Infect Dis J 1996; 15:192–196.

88. Feikin DR, et al. Randomized trial of the quantitative and functional antibody responses to a 7-valent pneumococcal conjugate vaccine and/or 23-valent polysaccharide vaccine among HIV-infected adults. Vaccine 2001; 20:545–553.

89. Goetz MB, et al. Viral load response to a 7-valent pneumococcal conjugate vaccine, 23-valent polysaccharide vaccine or placebo among HIV-infected patients. AIDS, 2002; 16:1421–1423.

90. Siber GR, et al. Impaired antibody response to pneumococcal vaccine after treatment for Hodgkin's disease. N Engl J Med 1978; 299:442–448.

91. Molrine DC, et al. Antibody responses to polysaccharide and polysaccharide-conjugate vaccines after treatment of Hodgkin disease. Ann Internal Med 1995; 123:828–834.

92. Chan CY, et al. Pneumococcal conjugate vaccine primes for antibody responses to polysaccharide pneumococcal vaccine after treatment of Hodgkin's disease. J Infect Dis 1996; 173:256–258.

93. Winston DJ, et al. Pneumococcal infections after human bone-marrow transplantation. Ann Internal Med 1979; 91: 835–841.

94. Nordoy T, et al. Humoral immunity to viral and bacterial antigens in lymphoma patients 4–10 years after high-dose therapy with ABMT. Serological responses to revaccinations according to EBMT guidelines. Bone Marrow Transplant 2001; 28:681–687.

95. Spoulou V, et al. Kinetics of antibody concentration and avidity for the assessment of immune response to pneumococcal vaccine among children with bone marrow transplants. J Infect Dis 2000; 182:965–969.

96. Parkkali T, et al. Opsonophagocytic activity against *Streptococcus pneumoniae* type 19F in allogeneic BMT recipients before and after vaccination with pneumococcal polysaccharide vaccine. Bone Marrow Transplant 2001; 27:207–211.

97. Hammarstrom V, et al. Pneumococcal immunity and response to immunization with pneumococcal vaccine in bone marrow transplant patients: the influence of graft versus host reaction. Support Care Cancer 1993; 1:195–199.

98. Storek J, et al. IgG response to pneumococcal polysaccharide–protein conjugate appears similar to IgG response to polysaccharide in bone marrow transplant recipients and healthy adults. Clin Infect Dis 1997; 25:1253–1255.

99. Molrine DC, et al. *Haemophilus influenzae* type b (HIB)-conjugate immunization before bone marrow harvest in autologous bone marrow transplantation. Bone Marrow Transplant 1996; 17:1149–1155.

100. Molrine DC, et al. Donor immunization with *Haemophilus influenzae* type b (HIB)-conjugate vaccine in allogeneic bone marrow transplantation. Blood 1996; 87:3012–3018.

101. Klugman KP. Efficacy of pneumococcal conjugate vaccines and their effect on carriage and antimicrobial resistance. Lancet Infect Dis 2001; 1:85–91.

102. Obaro SK, et al. Carriage of pneumococci after pneumococcal vaccination. Lancet 1996; 348:271–272.

103. Mbelle N, et al. Immunogenicity and impact on nasopharyngeal carriage of a nonavalent pneumococcal conjugate vaccine. J Infect Dis 1999; 180:1171–1176.

104. Dagan R, et al. Reduction of pneumococcal nasopharyngeal carriage in early infancy after immunization with tetravalent pneumococcal vaccines conjugated to either tetanus toxoid or diphtheria toxoid. Pediatr Infect Dis J 1997; 16:1060–1064.

105. Dagan R, et al. Reduction of nasopharyngeal carriage of pneumococci during the second year of life by a heptavalent conjugate pneumococcal vaccine. J Infect Dis 1996; 174: 1271–1278.

106. Dagan R, et al. Effect of a conjugate pneumococcal vaccine on the occurrence of respiratory infections and antibiotic use in day-care center attendees. Pediatr Infect Dis J 2001; 20:951–958.

107. Lipsitch M. Vaccination against colonizing bacteria with multiple serotypes. Proc Natl Acad Sci USA 1997; 94:6571–6576.

108. Gratten M, et al. Multiple colonization of the upper respiratory tract of Papua New Guinea children with *Haemophilus influenzae* and *Streptococcus pneumoniae*. Southeast Asian J Trop Med Public Health 1989; 20:501–509.

109. Lipsitch M. Interpreting results from trials of pneumococcal conjugate vaccines: a statistical test for detecting vaccine-induced increases in carriage of nonvaccine serotypes. Am J Epidemiol 2001; 154:85–92.

110. Choo S, et al. Primary and booster salivary antibody responses to a 7-valent pneumococcal conjugate vaccine in infants. J Infect Dis 2000; 182:1260–1263.

111. Korkeila M, et al. Salivary anti-capsular antibodies in infants and children immunised with *Streptococcus pneumoniae* capsular polysaccharides conjugated to diphtheria or tetanus toxoid. Vaccine 2000; 18:1218–1226.

112. Robbins JB, et al. Hypothesis: how licensed vaccines confer protective immunity. Adv Exp Med Biol 1996; 397:169–182.

113. Black SB, et al. Postlicensure evaluation of the effectiveness of seven valent pneumococcal conjugate vaccine. Pediatr Infect Dis J 2001; 20:1105–1107.

114. Whitney CG, et al. Increasing prevalence of multidrug-resistant *Streptococcus pneumoniae* in the United States. N Engl J Med 2000; 343:1917–1924.

115. Dagan R, Fraser D. Conjugate pneumococcal vaccine and antibiotic-resistant *Streptococcus pneumoniae*: herd immun-

ity and reduction of otitis morbidity. Pediatr Infect Dis J 2000; 19:79–87.

116. Obaro S, Adegbola R. The pneumococcus: carriage, disease and conjugate vaccines. J Med Microbiol 2002; 51:98–104.

117. Peters TR, Edwards KM. The pneumococcal protein conjugate vaccines. J Pediatr 2000; 137:416–420.

118. Coffey TJ, et al. Recombinational exchanges at the capsular polysaccharide biosynthetic locus lead to frequent serotype changes among natural isolates of *Streptococcus pneumoniae*. Mol Microbiol 1998; 27:73–83.

119. Barnes DM, et al. Transmission of multidrug-resistant serotype 23F *Streptococcus pneumoniae* in group day care: evidence suggesting capsular transformation of the resistant strain in vivo. J Infect Dis 1995; 171:890–896.

120. Wenger JD, et al. Introduction of Hib conjugate vaccines in the non-industrialized world: experience in four 'newly adopting' countries. Vaccine 1999; 18:736–742.

39

Pneumococcal Common Proteins and Other Vaccine Strategies

David E. Briles and Susan K. Hollingshead
The University of Alabama at Birmingham, Birmingham, Alabama, U.S.A.

James C. Paton
University of Adelaide, Adelaide, Australia

I. DEVELOPMENT OF NOVEL VACCINES TO PNEUMOCOCCAL ANTIGENS

Streptococcus pneumoniae expresses a number of molecules, aside from capsular polysaccharide, that are able elicit protection. Figure 1 is a cartoon of the pneumococcal surface depicting many different pneumococcal surface structures. All of the labeled structures, except the cell membrane and cell wall, are able to elicit protective responses. Data for some of these molecules are stronger than those of others. Although the data demonstrating protection by antibody to IgA1 protease are limited, its high sequence diversity suggests that the antibody to this protein has a protective effect in man [1].

II. PHOSPHOCHOLINE/TEICHOIC ACIDS

Antibodies to the phosphocholine (PC) epitope of the teichoic and lipoteichoic acids of the pneumococcus are protective [2–6]. Although most of the work has been conducted with mouse antibodies, human antibody to PC protects in a mouse challenge model [3]. Phosphocholine is a common epitope on other respiratory bacterial pathogens [4,5]. Human C-reactive protein, which recognizes PC, protects mice against pneumococci [6] and *Haemophilus influenzae* [7]. Phosphocholine is considered an attractive vaccine candidate because it is invariant in structure and it is found on all pneumococci [8,9]. Shortcomings include the fact that it does not elicit memory responses, and antibodies to PC are less protective on a one-to-one basis than those to capsule [10]. Isolated phosphocholine-containing teichoic acid is not highly immunogenic in mice or humans. Purified lipoteichoic acid (F-antigen), however, is immunogenic [11,12] and can protect mice (Moon Nahm, manuscript in preparation). Immune responses to teichoic acids are readily elicited by immunization with killed intact pneumococci [13].

III. PNEUMOCOCCAL PROTEIN VACCINE ANTIGENS

One alternative to using polysaccharides or polysaccharide–protein conjugates is to develop a vaccine composed of protection-eliciting pneumococcal protein(s) [2]. Infants generally make good responses to protein antigens, and the immunogens of all successful nonliving pediatric vaccines are either proteins themselves, or make use of protein carriers. By including a few selected virulence proteins in a protein-based vaccine, it should be possible to target more than one virulence and invasion mechanism. Indeed, immunization with mixtures of pneumococcal proteins can be more protective in mice than individual proteins [14,15]. A protein vaccine would also have the advantage in that the recombinant proteins can be produced relatively inexpensively, a possibility that might make such vaccines more affordable worldwide.

Several pneumococcal proteins, PspA, PsaA, pneumolysin, neuraminidase, autolysin, and PspC, elicit protective immunity in mice against pneumococcal infection [16–23,15,24,25]. Each of these proteins is a virulence factor [2,24,25]. The capsule has long been believed to be required for virulence [26–28]. Studies with genetic exchange mutants have confirmed these expectations [29]. Based on the analysis of the pneumococcal genome and the use of in vivo gene selection systems, many additional protein vaccine candidates have been proposed [30–32].

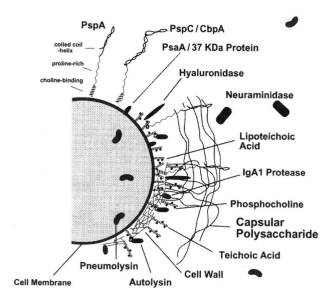

Figure 1 Cartoon showing the pneumococcal cell membrane, cell wall, and nine different components that are considered likely to be able to elicit protection against pneumococcal infection, invasion, or colonization. These molecules include the carbohydrates, capsular polysaccharide, teichoic acids, and lipoteichoic acid; as well as the protein PspA, PspC (CbpA), PsaA, pneumolysin, neuraminidase, hyaluronidase, and IgA1 protease.

A. PspA

Pneumococcal surface protein A (PspA) is expressed by all pneumococci [33] and, so far, is the only purified pneumococcal protein that has been used to immunize human volunteers [34]. Human antibodies elicited by immunization with rPspA protect mice from fatal sepsis with pneumococci [23]. As for size, PspA molecules from different strains range from about 65 to about 95 kDa [35]. The N-terminal half of the molecule is thought to have an α-helical antiparallel coiled coil structure [36,37].

The center of the molecule contains about 80 residues, which are about 40% proline, and in some molecules there is a 30-residue highly conserved, nonproline containing region in the center of the proline-rich region. The C-terminal end of the molecule is composed of 9–10 highly conserved, choline-binding repeats of 10 amino acids, each with a highly conserved 17 amino acid tail. The choline-binding domain attaches PspA noncovalently to the phosphocholine residues of the lipoteichoic acid (and possibly cell wall teichoic acid). Much of the α-helical domain of the molecule is highly immunogenic and exposed at the bacterial surface. Antibodies elicited by the α-helical domain protect against infection and the 100 amino acids near the C-terminal end of the α-helical domain is where major cross-protective epitopes of Rx1 (clade 2, family 1) PspA have been mapped [36,38–40,35].

Although PspA exhibits much structural variability [35], protective antibodies to it are quite cross-reactive

[38,23,24]. Much of the cross-protection appears to be elicited by epitopes encoded by the most C-terminal 100 amino acids of the α-helical region. Based on the amino-acid sequence of this region of PspA, we have divided all PspAs into six clades which comprise three families [35]. We have examined over 2000 strains of pneumococci collected from around the world and have found that at least 98% are in families 1 and 2, which are composed of clades 1 and 2, and 3 through 5, respectively (Hollingshead, manuscript in preparation). Although in strains of many capsular types the isolates are predominantly of members of a single PspA family, both major PspA families have been found in all major capsular types. Antibodies to PspA produced by five mammalian species were shown to be able to protect mice against intravenous infection with pneumococci expressing either family 1 or family 2 PspA [22–24]. Table 1 shows the results obtained when antibody PspA elicited in a monkey were used to passively protect mice (J. Monde and D. E. Briles, unpublished results). At least, some cross-protective immunity exists even between different PspA families, and makes it likely that a PspA vaccine need not contain more than one or few PspAs [22–24].

Although several biological properties of PspA are known, the relative importance of these properties in virulence is not known. It is important to resolve these questions if we are to have confidence that antibody to PspA will be as efficacious in man as it is in mice. Understanding PspA's mechanism of action should help us understand the pathogenesis of pneumococcal disease. Understanding the mechanism by which an antibody to PspA protects should aid in the development of a useful surrogate assay for evaluating human responses to PspA vaccines.

Pneumococcal surface protein A is probably not important for any metabolic or transport function. The net growth of pneumococci in media or in C3-deficient mice is not dependent on the expression of PspA [41]. Moreover, antibodies to PspA do not alter the growth or cause death of pneumococci in media [42], heparinized blood [3], or in C3-deficient mice (Briles and Szalai, unpublished results).

Table 1 Serum from a Rhesus Monkey Immunized with PspA Can Protect Mice from Fatal Infection with Capsular Type 3 *Streptococcus pneumoniae*

Immunogen	Dilution of serum	Numbers of mice		*P* vs. preimmune
		Alive	Dead	
No serum	No serum	0	3	
Preimmune	1/20	1	5	
	1/40	0	6	
	1/80	0	6	
Immune	1/20	6	0	
	1/40	6	0	< 0.0001
	1/80	4	2	

0.1 ml of passive serum given i.p. 1 hr before i.v. challenge with > 10 LD$_{50}$ of *S. pneumoniae*. *P*-value compares alive vs. dead mice via Fisher's Exact Test.

Pneumococcal surface protein A is required for full virulence of pneumococci [18,41,25]. Mice can be protected against pneumococcal sepsis and death with passive MAb and polyclonal anti-PspA [3,17,18,40] as well as by immunization with native and recombinant PspA [23,24,43,44], or with DNA vaccine encoding PspA [45,46].

Pneumococcal surface protein A is expressed on the surface of encapsulated pneumococci [47,37,42], but is measurably more exposed on nonencapsulated, as on encapsulated pneumococci (Hakansson and Briles, manuscript in preparation). Antibodies to PspA are not able to opsonize pneumococci for opsonophagocytosis and killing in vitro using standard techniques [3] (Briles, unpublished results; Moon Nahm, unpublished results), and they are not able to agglutinate pneumococci [42]. These observations are consistent with the expectation that the surface density and exposure of PspA epitopes is less than that of the repeating epitopes of capsular polysaccharides.

Serious pneumococcal infections are frequently associated with low levels of serum complement [48,49]. Pneumococcal capsular polysaccharides, teichoic acids, and lipoteichoic acids can all fix C' at least weakly through the alternative pathway [50–52]. This pathway of complement activation is required for most of the C' deposition on encapsulated pneumococci exposed to fresh human serum [53].

By use of the bystander C' activation assay, it was shown that one of our PspA$^-$ mutants activated more C' than PspA$^+$ pneumococci [54,55]. This has also been observed using Western blots to look at deposited C' fragments [41] and by using ELISA to detect C' deposited on the pneumococcal surface [56]. A most convincing in vitro demonstration that the presence of PspA affects the surface deposition of C' was obtained with a flow cytometry assay using live pneumococci (Ren et al., submitted). Evidence that PspA affects C' deposition in vivo has also come from our studies, where PspA$^+$ bearing and PspA$^-$ isogenic strains were injected into mice and the relative levels of C' in their sera were measured [41] (Figure 2). If the virulence function of PspA is to block C' fixation, then Ab–PspA might be able to block PspA's ability to inhibit C' fixation, and should thus increase the level of C' deposited on pneumococci [56].

PspA's ability to decrease C' deposition could explain PspA's effect on virulence, if the C' deposited on PspA$^-$ pneumococci enhanced opsonophagocytosis and killing in vivo. In mice lacking C3, neither the PspA nor the antibody to PspA affects virulence. These observations are consistent with the expectation that PspA's effect on C' activation may be important to its effect on virulence [57,57a,41]. The effect of PspA on opsonization by complement is further emphasized by the observation that Fc receptors do not appear to be required for the protective effects of antibodies to PspA. Even though the phagocytes of mice lacking Fc receptors FcγRI, FcγRIIB, and FcγRIII [58] fail to bind to IgG1, IgG2 and IgG2b, antibodies to PspA are almost as efficacious in these mice as in wild type-mice (Szalai et al., manuscript in preparation).

In light of the above results, it was a little surprising that the antibody to PspA efficiently mediates the binding of

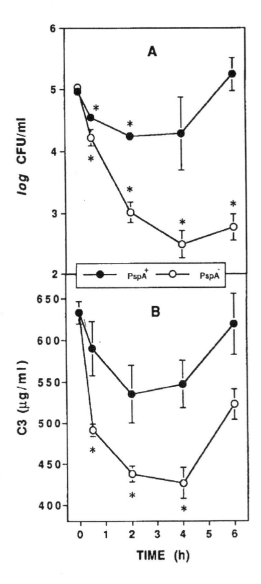

Figure 2 Expression of PspA by pneumococci inhibits complement activation and clearance of pneumococci during a bacteremic infection of CBA/N mice with 10^5 colony-forming units of PspA$^+$ or PspA-pneumococci. Blood was collected to quantitate bacteremia (A) and serum C3 (B). Data are presented as means ± standard errors of the means from a total of 15 mice per group. Asterisks indicate significant decreases ($P < 0.05$) in bacteremia or serum C3 concentrations compared to 0-hr (preinfection) values. (Adapted from Ref. 41.)

capsular type 3 pneumococci to phagocytes [55,59–61]. We refer to this binding as Ab-dependent adherence of bacteria to phagocytes (AABP). We have observed that AABP can be mediated by a normal human serum but that it is not observed using PspA$^-$ capsular type 3 pneumococci, suggesting that PspA might be a major mechanism by which this is mediated in nonimmune human sera (Briles and King, unpublished results). AABP with the pneumococcus occurs in both the presence or absence of C' [61] (Briles et al., unpublished results) and does not lead to killing of the opsonized pneumococci even when the C' levels of about 1/10 normal serum are used in the assay. Whether the attachment of pneumococci to phagocytes by anti-PspA may play a role in the killing, or clearance, of pneumococci in vivo is not known.

All PspA families and clades bind lactoferrin avidly and specifically [42,62] (Mirza, Hollingshead and Briles, unpublished results). The binding site for lactoferrin is within the clade-defining region of the α-helical domain [35,42]. This same region of PspA is also responsible for most of the cross-protective Ab elicited by PspA/Rx1 [38,22]. The ability of lactoferrin to bind to PspAs of different clades, despite the differences in sequences of different PspAs, suggests that lactoferrin's binding has functional significance. The extensive sequence differences within the region of PspA that binds lactoferrin suggest that the binding of PspA to lactoferrin may be dependent on protein conformation, rather than specific linear protein sequences. Our observation that Ab–PspA can inhibit the binding of lactoferrin to PspA (Mirza and Briles, unpublished results) indicates that whatever advantage pneumococci gain by binding lactoferrin, it can probably be blocked by the antibody to PspA.

Lactoferrin is present in all body secretions at concentrations ranging from 0.1 to 7 mg/mL [63]. It is produced by neutrophils during inflammation, and can reach blood levels of 0.2 mg/mL, with even higher local concentrations [63]. Lactoferrin effectively sequesters iron from most pathogens [64,65], including pneumococci [66]. Apolactoferrin (lacking iron) is bactericidal for many bacteria [67] including pneumococci. Killing by lactoferrin may be important within phagocytes [67] and possibly in secretions, but not in the blood, as its bactericidal effects are inhibited by serum (Mirza et al., manuscript in preparation). Lactoferrin has also been reported to enhance [68] or inhibit [69,70] C' activation, depending on the system studied. Thus it is possible that the binding of lactoferrin to PspA may enhance PspA's anticomplementary activity. It is also possible that the presence of PspA on pneumococci may interfere with lactoferrin-mediated killing.

At present, only indirect data support the contention that PspA antibodies protect against pneumococci in humans. If human antibody to PspA is protective, it should also select for variants in the antigenic structure of PspA. The bulk of the diversity of PspA is in the exposed portions of the molecule, not in the choline-binding domain. The extensive diversity of the exposed portions of the molecule suggests that in its primary host, man, immunity to PspA must reduce the chance that the pathogen is able to successfully colonize/infect and be transmitted to a new host.

Immunity to PspA could act at one or more steps in the infection process. Antibody to PspA is initially acquired transplacentally from the mother, and children subsequently develop their own titers of anti-PspA; this occurs rather slowly in children in response to pneumococcal carriage and infection [71–73]. However, the appearance of substantial levels of antibodies to PspA in children corresponds to the period of time in which young children begin to be relatively resistant to pneumococcal infection [74]. Some data indicate that invasive pneumococcal disease may be more frequent in children with low antibody levels to PspA than in those with

high levels of antibody to PspA [73]. In a human carriage challenge model, establishment of carriage leads to elevated PspA antibody levels. The same studies suggest that elevated antibody levels may protect against carriage in adults [75].

B. PspC

Another pneumococcal surface protein, variously called PspC, CbpA, SpSA, or Hic [76–81], plays a role in adherence and colonization [25,78], C3 binding [82], secretory IgA binding [77,80,81], factor H binding [83–85], and inhibition of alternative pathway C3 activation [85]. The multiple names for PspC has ensued partly because of the different activities of the protein, and partly because PspC is a variably mosaic protein which has allelic variants with significant differences in their domain structure [79,83,86]. The term "PspC" was the first name given to this family of allelic genes in gene bank, on September 26, 1996 [54,76,79]. The alleles of *pspC* that were originally described encoded a domain structure very similar to that of PspA. PspC consists of a choline-binding repeat and proline-rich domains that are indistinguishable from those of PspA. The size of the α-helical domain of PspC is within the range observed for the α-helical domain of PspA, and some PspC molecules have α-helical domains that are highly homologous to portions of the alpha helical domain of some PspA molecules [79].

While the PspC produced by about 75% of pneumococci have a choline-binding region indistinguishable from PspA [77,79] other pneumococci produce a PspC in which the choline-binding region is replaced by an LPXTG amino acid sequence motif, which is associated with attachment to the cell wall peptide cross-bridge by the enzyme sortase [83,86]. Eleven major groups of PspC proteins exist, and a nomenclature based on differences in the domain structures of the encoded proteins has been proposed [86].

Immunization with purified rPspC elicits protection against fatal sepsis, as well as nasopharyngeal carriage in mice [25,79]. Studies are needed to evaluate the breadth of protection afforded by this molecule and to compare the virulence roles and protection elicited by the different forms of PspC.

C. Pneumolysin

Pneumolysin is produced by virtually all strains of *S. pneumoniae*, and was one of the first pneumococcal proteins proposed as a vaccine antigen [87]. It is a member of a family of toxins referred to as the thiol-activated cytolysins (streptolysin-O and listeriolysin-O also belong to this group). These toxins initially interact with cholesterol in host cell membranes, after which they insert into the bilayer and oligomerize to form transmembrane pores, thereby bringing about cell lysis [88]. The ubiquity of cholesterol in animal cells accounts for the broad range of detrimental effects attributable to these toxins, many of which occur at sublytic concentrations. For pneumolysin, these effects include inhibition of the bactericidal activity of leukocytes, blockage of proliferative responses and Ig production by lymphocytes, reduction of ciliary beating of human respiratory epithelium, and direct cytotoxicity for respiratory endothelial and epithelial cells [89].

Pneumolysin is a bifunctional toxin that, in addition to its cytotoxic properties, binds the Fc region of human IgG and activates the classical complement pathway (with a concomitant reduction in serum opsonic activity) [90,91]. Thus pneumolysin may interfere with both phagocytic and ciliary clearance of pneumococci, by blocking humoral immune responses, and by aiding penetration of host tissues. Pneumolysin also directly induces inflammatory responses [92] and, under certain circumstances, can alter the inflammatory responses so that they are less protective than normal [93]. Injection of purified pneumolysin into rat lungs induces severe lobar pneumonia, histologically indistinguishable from that seen when virulent pneumococci are injected [94].

Defined pneumolysin-negative mutants of *S. pneumoniae* exhibit significantly reduced virulence in mouse models of sepsis and pneumonia [95]. When compared to the wild-type strain, intranasal challenge with pneumolysin-negative mutants results in a less severe inflammatory response, a reduced rate of multiplication within the lung, a reduced capacity to injure the alveolar–capillary barrier, and a delayed onset of bacteremia [96,97].

Although native pneumolysin is a protective immunogen in mice, it is not suitable as a human vaccine antigen, because of its toxicity. To overcome this, mutations have been introduced into the pneumolysin gene in regions essential for its cytotoxic and/or complement activation properties, resulting in the expression of nontoxic but immunogenic "pneumolysoids," which are easily purified from recombinant *Escherichia coli* expression systems [98]. Pneumolysin is a highly conserved protein, and extensive analysis of genes from a wide range of *S. pneumoniae* serotypes has detected negligible variation in deduced amino acid sequence, auguring well for broad coverage. Indeed, immunization of mice with a pneumolysoid carrying a Trp433–Phe mutation resulting in >99.5% reduction in cytotoxicity (designated as PdB) provided a significant degree of protection against all nine serotypes of *S. pneumoniae* that were tested [99].

Humans develop antibody to pneumolysin as a result of natural exposure to *S. pneumoniae*, and purified human antipneumolysin IgG passively protects mice from challenge with virulent pneumococci [100]. Thus it is anticipated that the various pneumolysoids will be immunogenic in humans. However, pneumolysoid may not provide a sufficient degree of protection to be an effective standalone human vaccine antigen. Pneumolysin is not displayed on the surface of the pneumococcus. Rather, it is located in the cytoplasm and released into the external milieu when pneumococci undergo spontaneous autolysis in some strains [21]. It also appears to be released by an as yet uncharacterized export mechanism in other pneumococci [101].

Antibodies to pneumolysin presumably impart protection by neutralization of the biological properties of the toxin, thereby impeding the kinetics of infection, rather than by stimulating opsonophagocytic clearance of the invading bacteria. Thus protein-based vaccines combining pneumolysoid with pneumococcal surface proteins capable of eliciting opsonic antibodies would be expected to be more effective (see Section 5).

D. Pneumococcal Surface Antigen A (PsaA)

Pneumococcal Surface Antigen A, a highly conserved 37-kDa surface protein produced by all pneumococci, was initially thought to be an adhesin based on sequence homology with putative lipoprotein adhesins of oral streptococci. It is actually metal-binding lipoprotein component of an ATP-binding cassette (ABC) transport system with specificity for Mn^{2+} [102]. Defined $PspA^-$ mutants of *S. pneumoniae* are virtually avirulent for mice and exhibit markedly reduced adherence in vitro to human type II pneumocytes [103]. This is presumed to be a consequence of a requirement for Mn as a cofactor, or for regulation of expression of other virulence factors (e.g., adhesins), and/or growth retardation due to an inability to scavenge this metal in vivo [104]. The avirulence of PspA-pneumococci might also be due, at least in part, to the fact that they are highly susceptible to oxidative stress [105].

Immunization of mice with purified PsaA confers partial protection against intraperitoneal challenge with *S. pneumoniae*, although it is less efficacious than either pneumolysoid or PspA [15]. The dimensions of PsaA (approximately 7 nm at its longest axis) [106] are such that if it is anchored to the outer face of the cell membrane via its N-terminal lipid moiety, it is unlikely to be exposed on the outer surface of the pneumococcus. Thus the observed protection is presumably attributable to in vivo blockade of ion transport, which necessitates the diffusion of antibody through the capsule and cell-wall layers. Penetration of antibody may well be influenced by the thickness of the capsule, which is believed to be upregulated during invasive infection. In contrast, pneumococci colonizing the nasopharynx are thought to downregulate capsule expression [107], thereby facilitating the interaction between surface adhesins and the host mucosa. Consistent with this hypothesis, the intranasal immunization of mice with PsaA significantly reduces the nasopharyngeal carriage of *S. pneumoniae* [14].

E. Autolysin

Autolysin, a *N*-acetylmuramoyl-L-alanine amidase [108], has been shown to be primarily responsible for pneumococcal autolysis, which follows pneumococcal death at the end of the growth phase in vitro. Isolated autolysin elicits protective immune responses [109] and is a virulence factor [110,111]. Observations that antibodies to autolysin and pneumolysin did not have synergistic protective effects led to the hypothesis that the virulence mechanism of autolysin was the autolytic release of pneumolysi, and that pneumolysin carried out the virulence functions [109]. This hypothesis was supported by the observation that, in capsular type 2 strain D39, mutations in either autolysin or pneumolysin reduced virulence in a lung inoculation model [111]; mutations in autolysin reduce virulence in this model more than mutations in pneumolysin.

F. Neuraminidase and Hyaluronidase

S. pneumoniae produces a large number of hydrolytic enzymes, some of which may play a role in degradation of host glycoproteins or extracellular matrix, and many of which are associated with surface expression [112]. A few of these are known virulence factors, including the neuraminidases and the hyaluronate lyase [113,114]. Neuraminidases cleave sialic from host surfaces, particularly in the liver and the kidney, and thus, may significantly impede the host's ability to efficiently recover from an infection. Injected neuraminidase is toxic to mice, and *nanA* mutant strains are more efficiently cleared from the lung [115]. Immunization with NanA could extend the life of mice [13]. Hyaluronate lyase is predicted to be a surface-bound protein in the pneumococcus, contrary to its secreted status in several other organisms. It degrades hyaluronic acid, a component of basement membrranes and connective tissue; a *hya* mutant exhibited virulence in a mouse bacteremia model [114].

One less-characterized member of the hydrolase surface protein group is SpuA [116], a pullanase which has an alpha-1,6-glucanohydrolase activity that could be involved in scavenging carbohydrate or in uncovering receptors for adhesion. None of the hydrolytic class of proteins has been fully tested for their ability to elicit protective antibody, but some could prove useful as components of a multivalent protein vaccine.

G. PavA

Among the more suitable vaccine candidates are the newly described adhesins. Antibodies to adhesins may limit colonization and carriage in the nasopharynx, and may decrease invasiveness by interfering with adhesion in the lung or middle ear. One newly defined adhesin is pneumococcal adhesion and virulence (PavA), which appears to be present at the bacterial cell surface, even though it lacks any known signals for transport or for surface attachment [117].

H. PhtA, B, C, and D

A family of histidine triad proteins, designated as PhtA, B, C, and D, are also potential vaccine candidates [31]. Their exact function unknown, these proteins are surface-exposed and may be surface-attached through a lipoprotein attachment site. Antibodies to PhtA and PhtD are found in human convalescent sera, and rabbit antisera raised to recombinant proteins protect in passive immunization experiments in mice. Some of the recombinant proteins elicit immunity against systemic challenge with pneumococci [31]. An additional histidine triad protein, PhpB, is initially a 79-kDa protein that is processed to a 20-kDa protein which has a putative human complement C3-proteolytic activity. Antibodies elicited by the 79-kDa recombinant protein protect CBA/N mice against death and bacteremia, and reduce nasopharyngeal colonization, but immunization with the 20-kDa portion of the PhpA protein does not protect mice [118].

I. PiuA and PiaA

PiuA and PiaA are lipoproteins that form as components of iron uptake transporters of *S. pneumoniae*. PiuA and PiaA are antigenically cross-reactive, and immunity to these pro-teins is reactive with pneumococci of nine different *S. pneumoniae* serotypes. Immunity to PiuA and PiaA protects mice, and immunity to both PiuA and PiaA is more protective than immunity to either protein alone [119].

J. IgA1 Protease

IgA1 protease is a cell surface-associated enzyme of *S. pneumoniae* that cleaves human IgA1, but not IgA2. IgA1 is the IgA isotype most common in human secretions. It is assumed that cleaving human IgA1 improves the ability of pneumococci to successfully colonize the human host [120,121]. Pneumococcal IgA1 protease does not cleave mouse IgA. IgA1 protease is highly variable [1,121], suggesting that human protective responses to IgA1 protease have selected for variability in the structure of IgA1 protease. Animal tests of this potential vaccine antigen await the development of an IgA knockout mouse expressing transgenic human IgA1 under the control of the mouse promoter for the IgA in murine secretions. Determining the possible usefulness of IgA1 as a vaccine antigen will depend in part on whether or not it contains any highly cross-reactive protection-eliciting epitopes.

IV. COMBINATION PROTEIN VACCINES

Virtually all of the pneumococcal proteins under consideration as vaccine antigens are directly or indirectly involved in the pathogenesis of pneumococcal disease. Mutagenesis of some combinations of virulence factor genes, for example those encoding pneumolysin and either PspA or PspC [141], or PspA and PspC [25], has been shown to synergistically attenuate the pneumococcal virulence in animal models, implying that the respective proteins function independently in the pathogenic process. Such results suggest that immunization with combination of these antigens might provide additive protection. Moreover, the individual antigens differ in their capacity to protect against various *S. pneumoniae* strains [17,99]. Thus a combined pneumococcal protein vaccine may elicit a higher degree of protection against a wider variety of strains than any single antigen. To date, only a limited number of combination experiments have been performed. The combination of pneumolysoid PdB and PspA clearly provides enhanced protection against systemic infection and pneumonia [15,24], whereas the combination of PspA and PsaA provides additive protection against carriage [14]. Thus the present data suggest that, for elicitation of protection against sepsis, pneumonia, and carriage, a vaccine containing PspA, pneumolysoid, and PsaA might work well. As additional antigens are examined, some may be found to be of significant value for use in new vaccine formulations.

V. PNEUMOCOCCAL PROTEIN AS POSSIBLE CARRIERS FOR POLYSACCHARIDES

Pneumococcal proteins could be used in combination with PS–protein conjugates or as carriers for conjugation of pneumococcal polysaccharides. By including cross-reactive protection-eliciting proteins to a vaccine containing pneumococcal polysaccharides or polysaccharide–protein conjugates, the spectrum of protection elicited by the polysaccharide and conjugate vaccines could be broadened. Preparing pneumococcal polysaccharide conjugates using pneumococcal proteins rather than proteins of other species, such as diphtheria or tetanus toxoid, should also have an advantage in terms of anamnestic responses elicited by a pneumococcal infection. If the vaccine stimulates T-cell memory that can be boosted upon infection, a better anamnestic antibody response may be achieved than when the carrier in the vaccine is not presented by infecting pneumococci. The speed with which anamnestic antibody is elicited is probably especially critical in the most susceptible human hosts, because it is in individuals with rapidly progressing disease that death is most likely to occur.

Using pneumococcal proteins as carriers for pneumococcal polysaccharides could also lead to the development of a "hybrid" vaccine containing three or four of the most common polysaccharides conjugated to the three or four most promising cross-reactive proteins. By limiting the number of different polysaccharide–protein conjugates, it may be possible to help control the vaccine's cost.

Pneumolysin [98] and PspA have both been successfully used as carriers for immune responses to polysaccharides in animals. Detoxified pneumolysin mutant PdB conjugated to capsular 9F polysaccharide elicited protection against fatal infection in infant mice challenged with capsular type 19 pneumococci [122]. A conjugate containing PspA and capsular type 14 polysaccharide was immunogenic in mice and elicited good titers of antibodies to the both the polysaccharide and to PspA (Mond, Lees, and Briles, unpublished results). Although conjugated to polysaccharide, PspA was still able to elicit protective immunity. Mice immunized with

the PspA–PN14 conjugate were protected against otherwise lethal challenge with the highly virulent capsular type 2 strain (D39) of *S. pneumoniae* (Figure 3).

VI. PROTECTION AGAINST CARRIAGE

It is assumed that to achieve herd immunity against the pneumococcus, it will be important to protect against carriage of pneumococci in the nasopharynx. Immunization to prevent carriage should also protect the immunized individual against invasive disease. Because invasion is invariably thought to be preceded by at least a short duration of carriage [123], protection against carriage should prevent the opportunity for invasion. Whether immunity to carriage is elicited by mucosal or systemic immunization, it is expected that there will also be high levels of systemic antibody, which should also protect against invasive disease [124,125].

Intramuscular immunization with appropriate pneumococcal proteins may also protect against carriage. However, mouse studies indicate that mucosal immunization may be more effective at preventing carriage than systemic immunization. In the mouse, mucosal immunization elicited better protection against carriage than systemic immunization, although the systemic immunization elicited higher serum titers of IgG antibody. In the mouse, mucosal antibody was detected by intranasal, but not by systemic, immunization [125].

VII. MUCOSAL IMMUNIZATION WITH WHOLE, KILLED VACCINE

In an effort to develop a pneumococcal vaccine for developing countries, the use of killed pneumococci for intranasal immunization has been investigated [126]. The rationale for this approach is that no preparation of isolated antigen, conjugated antigen, or bacterial DNA would be required, thus permitting the vaccine to be produced at relatively low cost and, therefore, perhaps more accessible to children in these countries. By using a nonencapsulated pneumococcus as immunogen, it is hoped to maximize the immune responses to the cross-reactive somatic antigens [126]. The earliest studies of this type were conducted in the first third of the 20th century, and demonstrated that parenteral immunization with nonencapsulated killed pneumococci could elicit protection against systemic infection with encapsulated virulent organisms [127]. Bull and McKee demonstrated in 1929 that intranasal immunization of rabbits with whole killed pneumococci could protect against carriage and invasion through the nasal route [128]. More recent studies in mice demonstrate that immunization of mice mucosally with heat-killed pneumococci elicits mucosal and systemic antibody that protects against systemic infection [129] and against nasopharyngeal carriage [130]. Alcohol-killed pneumococci are more immunogenic than those killed by heat. Immunization with alcohol-killed pneumococci protects rodents against carriage and invasive disease [126]. Malley et al. prepared their heat-killed vaccine using nonencapsulated pneumococci that were also autolysin negative [126]. The absence of the autolytic activity facilitates reproducible

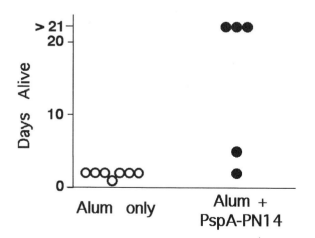

Figure 3 Immunity to PspA elicited by PspA–PN14 conjugate. CBA/N mice were immunized on days 1, 14, and 28 with 1.2 µg of PspA–PN14 conjugate on alum or with alum alone. Fourteen days after the last boost, they were challenged i.v. with 250 CFU of capsular type 2 strain D39. The greater protection of the PspA-PN14 immunized mice was significant at $P = 0.018$ by comparison of days to death using a two tailed Wilcoxon two-sample rank test.

growth and harvesting of the bacteria, because autolysis is largely avoided [101].

VIII. SUMMARY

In the last 20 years, the approach to pneumococcal vaccination has evolved from a single focus on the polysaccharide antigen to the multiple approach that now includes the cell surface and cell-released protein antigens of the pneumococcus. This evolution in thinking has also extended to the use of mucosal immunization, as well as the possibility of using the mucosal route for immunization with killed pneumococci. It is likely that one or more of these new immunization strategies will play a role in the control of the pneumococcus in the future.

REFERENCES

1. Lomholt H. Evidence for recombination and an antigenically diverse immunoglobulin A1 protease among strains of *Streptococcus pneumoniae*. Infect Immun 1995; 63:4238–4243.
2. Briles DE, et al. Immunity to *Streptococcus pneumoniae*. In: Cunningham M, Fujinami RS, eds. Effect of Microbes on the Immune System. Philadelphia: Lippincott-Raven, 2000:263–280.
3. Briles DE, et al. Antipneumococcal effects of C-reactive protein and monoclonal antibodies to pneumococcal cell wall and capsular antigens. Infect Immun 1989; 57:1457–1464.
4. Weiser JN, et al. Decoration of lipopolysaccharide with phosphorylcholine: a phase-variable characteristic of *Haemophilus influenzae*. Infect Immun 1997; 65:943–950.
5. Lysenko ES, et al. Bacterial phosphorylcholine decreases susceptibility to the antimicrobial peptide LL-37/hCAP18 expressed in the upper respiratory tract. Infect Immun 2000; 68:1664–1671.
6. Szalai AJ, et al. Human C-reactive protein is protective against *Streptococcus pneumoniae* infection in transgenic mice. J Immunol 1995; 155:2557–2563.
7. Weiser JN, et al. Phosphorylcholine on the lipopolysaccharide of *Haemophilus influenzae* contributes to persistence in the respiratory tract and sensitivity to serum killing mediated by C-reactive protein. J Exp Med 1998; 187:631–640.
8. Tomasz A. Choline in the cell wall of a bacterium: novel type of polymer-linked choline in pneumococcus. Science 1967; 57:694–697.
9. Brundish DE, Baddiley J. Pneumococcal C-substance, a ribitol teichoic acid containing choline phosphate. Biochem J 1968; 110:573–582.
10. Briles DE, et al. Mouse IgG3 antibodies are highly protective against infection with *Streptococcus pneumoniae*. Nature 1981; 294:88–90.
11. Goebel WF, Adams MH. The immunological properties of the heterophile antigen and somatic polysaccharide of pneumococcus. J Exp Med 1943; 77:435–449.
12. Briles DE. Pneumococcal diversity: considerations for new vaccine strategies with an emphasis on pneumococcal surface protein A (PspA). Clin Microbiological Rev 1998; 11:645–657.
13. Mond JJ, et al. Inability of mice with defect in B-lymphocyte maturation to respond to phosphocholine on immunogenic carriers. J Exp Med 1977; 146:1138–1142.
14. Briles DE, et al. Intranasal immunization of mice with a mixture of the pneumococcal proteins PsaA and PspA is highly protective against nasopharyngeal carriage of *Streptococcus pneumoniae*. Infect Immun 2000; 68:796–800.
15. Ogunniyi AD, et al. Immunization of mice with combinations of pneumococcal virulence proteins elicits enhanced protection against challenge with *Streptococcus pneumoniae*. Infect Immun 2000; 68:3028–3033.
16. Paton JC, Ferrante A. Inhibition of human polymorphonuclear leukocyte respiratory burst, bactericidal activity, and migration by pneumolysin. Infect Immun 1983; 41:1212–1216.
17. McDaniel LS, et al. Monoclonal antibodies against protease sensitive pneumococcal antigens can protect mice from fatal infection with *Streptococcus pneumoniae*. J Exp Med 1984; 160:386–397.
18. McDaniel LS, et al. Use of insertional inactivation to facilitate studies of biological properties of pneumococcal surface protein A (PspA). J Exp Med 1987; 165:381–394.
19. Walker JA, et al. Molecular cloning, characterization, and complete nucleotide sequence of the gene for pneumolysin, the sulfhydryl-activated toxin of *Streptococcus pneumoniae*. Infect Immun 1987; 55:1184–1189.
20. Lock RA, et al. Comparative efficacy of pneumococcal neuraminidase and pneumolysin as immunogens protective against *Streptococcus pneumoniae*. Microb Pathog 1988; 5: 461–467.
21. Berry AM, et al. Contribution of autolysin to virulence of *Streptococcus pneumoniae*. Infect Immun 1989; 57:2324–2330.
22. Tart RC, et al. Truncated *Streptococcus pneumoniae* PspA molecules elicit cross-protective immunity against pneumococcal challenge in mice. J Infect Dis 1996; 173:380–386.
23. Briles DE, et al. Immunization of humans with rPspA elicits antibodies, which passively protect mice from fatal infection with *Streptococcus pneumoniae* bearing heterologous PspA. J Infect Dis 2000; 182:1694–1701.
24. Briles DE, et al. The potential for using protein vaccines to protect against otitis media caused by *Streptococcus pneumoniae*. Vaccine 2001; 19:S87–S95.
25. Balachandran P, et al. The role of pneumococcal surface protein C (PspC) in nasopharyngeal carriage and pneumonia and its ability to elicit protection against carriage of *Streptococcus pneumoniae*. Infect Immun 2002; 70:2526–2534.
26. Stryker LM. Variations in the pneumococcus induced by growth in immune serum. J Exp Med 1916; 24:49–68.
27. Wood WB, Smith MR. The inhibition of surface phagocytosis by the capsular "slime layer" of pneumococcus type III. J Exp Med 1949; 90:85–99.
28. Watson DA, Musher DM. Interruption of capsule production in *Streptococcus pneumoniae* serotype 3 by insertion of transposon Tn916. Infect Immun 1990; 58:3135–3138.
29. Magee AD, Yother J. Requirement for capsule in colonization by *Streptococcus pneumoniae*. Infect Immun 2001; 69: 3755–3761.
30. Zysk G, et al. Detection of 23 immunogenic pneumococcal proteins using convalescent-phase serum. Infect Immun 2000; 68:3740–3743.
31. Adamou JE, et al. Identification and characterization of a novel family of pneumococcal proteins that are protective against sepsis. Infect Immun 2001; 69:949–958.
32. Wizemann TM, et al. Use of a whole genome approach to identify vaccine molecules affording protection against Streptococcus pneumoniae infection. Infect Immun 2001; 69:1593–1598.
33. Crain MJ, et al. Pneumococcal surface protein A (PspA) is serologically highly variable and is expressed by all clinically important capsular serotypes of *Streptococcus pneumoniae*. Infect Immun 1990; 58:3293–3299.
34. Nabors GS, et al. Immunization of healthy adults with a single recombinant pneumococcal surface protein A (PspA)

variant stimulates broadly cross-reactive antibodies. Vaccine 2000; 18:1743–1754.

35. Hollingshead SK, et al. Diversity of PspA: mosaic genes and evidence for past recombination in *Streptococcus pneumoniae*. Infect Immun 2000; 68:5889–5900.

36. Yother J, Briles DE. Structural properties and evolutionary relationship of PspA, a surface protein of *Streptococcus pneumoniae*, as revealed by sequence analysis. J Bacteriol 1992; 174:601–609.

37. Jedrzejas MJ, et al. Production and characterization of the functional fragment of pneumococcal surface protein A. Arch Biochem Biophys 2000; 373:116–125.

38. McDaniel LS, et al. Localization of protection-eliciting epitopes on PspA of *Streptococcus pneumoniae* between amino acid residues 192 and 260. Microb Pathog 1994; 17:323–337.

39. Yother J, White JM. Novel surface attachment mechanism for the *Streptococcus pneumoniae* protein PspA. J Bacteriol 1994; 176:2976–2985.

40. McDaniel LS, et al. Comparison of the PspA sequence from *Streptococcus pneumoniae* EF5668 to the previously identified PspA sequence from strain Rx1 and ability of PspA from EF5668 to elicit protection against pneumococci of different capsular types. Infect Immun 1998; 66:4748–4754.

41. Tu A-HT, et al. Pneumococcal surface protein A (PspA) inhibits complement activation by *Streptococcus pneumoniae*. Infect Immun 1999; 67:4720–4724.

42. Hakansson A, et al. Characterization of the binding of human lactoferrin to pneumococcal surface protein A (PspA). Infect Immun 2001; 69:3372–3381.

43. Talkington DF, et al. A 43-kilodalton pneumococcal surface protein, PspA: isolation, protective abilities, and structural analysis of the amino-terminal sequence. Infect Immun 1991; 59:1285–1289.

44. Briles DE, et al. PspA, a protection-eliciting pneumococcal protein: immunogenicity of isolated native PspA in mice. Vaccine 1996; 14:858–867.

45. McDaniel LS. Immunization with a plasmid expressing pneumococcal surface protein A (PspA) can elicit protection against fatal infection with *Streptococcus pneumoniae*. Gene 1997; 188:279–284.

46. Bosarge JR, et al. Genetic immunization with the region encoding the alpha-helical domain of PspA elicits protective immunity against *Streptococcus pneumoniae*. Infect Immun 2001; 69:5456–5463.

47. McDaniel LS, et al. Analysis of a surface protein of *Streptococcus pneumoniae* recognized by protective monoclonal antibodies. Microb Pathog 1986; 1:519–531.

48. Dee TH, et al. Immunologic studies in pneumococcal disease. J Lab Clin Med 1977; 89:1198–1207.

49. Giebink GS, et al. Alterations in serum opsonic activity and complement levels in pneumococcal disease. Infect Immun 1980; 29:1062–1066.

50. Winkelstein JA, et al. The role of the capsular polysaccharide in the activation of the alternative pathway by the pneumococcus. J Immunol 1976; 116:367–370.

51. Winkelstein JA, Tomasz A. Activation of the alternative complement pathway by pneumococcal cell wall teichoic acid. J Immunol 1978; 120:174–178.

52. Hummell DS, et al. Activation of the alternative complement pathway by pneumococcal lipoteichoic acid. Infect Immun 1985; 47:384–387.

53. Stephens CG, et al. Classical and alternative complement pathway activation by pneumococci. Infect Immun 1977; 17:296–302.

54. Briles DE, et al. PspA and PspC: their potential for use as pneumococcal vaccines. Microb Drug Resist 1997; 3:401–408.

55. Neeleman C, et al. Resistance to both complement activation and phagocytosis in type 3 pneumococci is mediated by

binding of complement regulatory protein factor H. Infect Immun 1999; 67:4517–4524.

56. Abeyta M. 1999. Ph.D Thesis. University of Alabama at Birmingham.

57. Briles DE, et al. Systemic and mucosal protective immunity to pneumococcal surface protein A. N Y Acad Sci USA 1996; 797:118–126.

57a. Ren B, et al. Both family 1 and family 2 PspAs can inhibit complement deposition and confer virulence to a capsular 3 serotype *Streptococcus pneumoniae*. Infect Immun 2003; 71:75–85.

58. Ravetch JV. Fc receptors. Curr Opin Immunol 1997; 9:121–125.

59. Jansen WTM, et al. Use of highly encapsulated *Streptococcus pneumoniae* strains in a flow-cytometric assay for assessment of the phagocytic capacity of serotype-specific antibodies. Clin Diagnost Lab immunol 1998; 5:703–710.

60. Overweg K, et al. The putative proteinase maturation protein A of Streptococcus pneumoniae is a conserved surface protein with potential to elicit protective immune responses. Infect Immun 2000; 68:4180–4188.

61. Arulanandam BP, et al. Intranasal vaccination with pneumococcal surface protein A and IL-12 augments antibody-mediated opsonization and protective immunity against *Streptococcus pneumoniae* Infection. Infect Immun 2001; 69:6718–6724.

62. Hammerschmidt S, et al. Identification of pneumococcal surface protein A as a lactoferrin-binding protein of *Streptococcus pneumoniae*. Infect Immun 1999; 67:1683–1687.

63. Vorland LH. Lactoferrin: a multifunctional glycoprotein. Apmis 1999; 107:971–981.

64. Masson PL, et al. Lactoferrin, an iron-binding protein in neutrophilic leukocytes. J Exp Med 1969; 130:643–658.

65. Crichton RR. Proteins of iron storage and transport. Adv Protein Chem 1990; 40:281–363.

66. Tai SS, et al. Hemin utilization is related to virulence of Streptococcus pneumoniae. Infect Immun 1993; 61:5401–5405.

67. Bullen JJ, Griffiths E. Iron and Infection. 2d ed. New York: John Wiley and Sons, 1999:1–515.

68. Rainard P. Activation of the classical pathway of complement by binding of bovine lactoferrin to unencapsulated Streptococcus agalactiae. Immunology 1993; 79:648–652.

69. Kijlstra A, Jeurissen SH. Modulation of classical C3 convertase of complement by tear lactoferrin. Immunology 1982; 47:263–270.

70. Veerhuis R, Kijlstra A. Inhibition of hemolytic complement activity by lactoferrin in tears. Exp Eye Res 1982; 34:257–265.

71. Rapola S, et al. Natural development of antibodies to pneumococcal surface protein A, pneumococcal surface adhesin A, and pneumolysin in relation to pneumococcal carriage and acute otitis media. J Infect Dis 2000; 182:1146–1152.

72. Samukawa T, et al. Immune response to surface protein A of Streptococcus pneumoniae and to high-molecular-weight outer membrane protein A of Moraxella catarrhalis in children with acute otitis media. J Infect Dis 2000; 181:1842–1845.

73. Virolainen A, et al. Human antibodies to pneumococcal surface protein A, PspA. Ped Infect Dis J 2000; 19:134–138.

74. Simell B, et al. Pneumococcal carriage and otitis media induce salivary antibodies to pneumococcal surface adhesin A, pneumolysin, and pneumococcal surface protein A in children. J Infect Dis 2001; 183:887–896.

75. McCool TL, et al. The Immune Response to Pneumococcal Proteins during Experimental Human Carriage. J Exp Med 2002; 195:359–365.

76. Brooks-Walter A, et al. The pspC gene encodes a second pneumococcal surface protein homologous to the gene en-

coding the protection-eliciting PspA protein of *Streptococcus pneumoniae* [abstr]. ASM Annual Meeting, 1997: 35.

77. Hammerschmidt S, et al. SpsA, a novel pneumococcal surface protein with specific binding to secretory immunoglobulin A and secretory component. Mol Microbiol 1997; 25: 1113–1124.

78. Rosenow C, et al. Contribution of novel choline-binding proteins to adherence, colonization and immunogenicity of *Streptococcus pneumoniae*. Mol Microbiol 1997; 25:819–829.

79. Brooks-Walter A, et al. The pspC gene of *Streptococcus pneumoniae* encodes a polymorphic protein PspC, which elicits cross-reactive antibodies to PspA and provides immunity to pneumococcal bacteremia. Infect Immun 1999; 67:6533–6542.

80. Hammerschmidt S, et al. Species-specific binding of human secretory component to SpsA protein of streptococcus pneumoniae via a hexapeptide motif [In Process Citation]. Mol Microbiol 2000; 36:726–736.

81. Zhang JR, et al. The polymeric immunoglobulin receptor translocates pneumococci across human nasopharyngeal epithelial cells. Cell 2000; 102:827–837.

82. Cheng Q, et al. Novel purification scheme and functions for a C3-binding protein from Streptococcus pneumoniae. Biochemistry 2000; 39:5450–5457.

83. Janulczyk R, et al. Hic, a novel surface protein of streptococcus pneumoniae that interferes with complement function. J Biol Chem 2000; 275:37257–37263.

84. Dave S, et al. PspC, a pneumococcal surface protein, binds human factor H. Infect Immun 2001; 69:3435–3437.

85. Jarva H, et al. Streptococcus pneumoniae Evades Complement Attack and Opsonophagocytosis by Expressing the pspC Locus-Encoded Hic Protein That Binds to Short Consensus Repeats 8-11 of Factor H. J Immunol 2002; 168:1886–1894.

86. Iannelli F, et al. Allelic variation in the highly polymorphic locus pspC of Streptococcus pneumoniae. Gene 2002; 284:63–71.

87. Paton JC, et al. Effect of immunization with pneumolysin on survival time of mice challanged with *Streptococcus pneumoniae*. Infect Immun 1983; 40:548–552.

88. Rossjohn J. The molecular mechanism of pneumolysin, a virulence factor from Streptococcus pneumoniae. J Mol Biol 1998; 284:449–461.

89. Paton JC, et al. The contribution of pneumolysin to the pathogenicity of *Streptococcus pneumoniae*. Trends in Microbiology 1996; 4:103–106.

90. Paton JC, et al. Activation of human complement by the pneumococcal toxin pneumolysin. Infect Immun 1984; 43: 1085–1087.

91. Mitchell TJ, et al. Complement activation and antibody binding by pneumolysin via a region of the toxin homologous to a human acute-phase protein. Mol Microbiol 1991; 5:1883–1888.

92. Houldsworth S, et al. Pneumolysin stimulates production of tumor necrosis factor alpha and Interleukin-1b by human mononuclear phagocytes. Infect Immun 1994; 62:1501–1503.

93. Benton K, Briles DE. Pneumolysin facilitates pneumococcal sepsis by interfering with an antipneumococcal inflammatory response. ASM Abstracts 1994; 1994:104.

94. Feldman C, et al. Pneumolysin induces the salient histologic features of penumococcal infection in the rat lung in vivo. Am J Respir Cell Mol Biol 1992; 5, 416–423.

95. Berry AM, et al. Reduced virulence of a defined pneumolysin-negative mutant of *Streptococcus pneumoniae*. Infect Immun 1989; 57:2037–2042.

96. Berry AM, et al. Effect of defined point mutations in pneumolysin gene on the virulence of *Streptococcus pneumoniae*. Infect Immun 1995; 63:1969–1974.

97. Rubins JB, et al. Distinct roles for pneumolysin's cytotoxic and complement activities in pathogenesis of pneumococcal pneumonia. Am J Respir Crit Care Med 1996; 153:1339–1346.

98. Paton JC, et al. Purification and immunogenicity of genetically obtained pneumolysin toxoids and their conjugation to *Streptococcus pneumoniae* type 19F polysaccharide. Infect Immun 1991; 59:2297–2304.

99. Alexander JE, et al. Immunization of mice with pneumolysin toxoid confers a significant degree of protection against at least nine serotypes of *Streptococcus pneumoniae*. Infect Immun 1994; 62:5683–5688.

100. Musher DM, et al. Protection against bacteremic pneumococcal infection by antibody to pneumolysin. J Infect Dis 2001; 183:827–830.

101. Balachandran P, et al. The Autolytic Enzyme LytA of *Streptococcus pneumoniae* Is Not Responsible For Releasing Pneumolysin. J Bacteriol 2001; 183:3108–3116.

102. Dintilhac A, et al. Competence and virulence of S. pneuminiae: Adc and PsaA mutants exhibit a requirement for Zn and Mn resulting from inactivation of metal permeases. Mol Microbiol 1997; 25:727–739.

103. Berry AM, Paton JC. Sequence heterogeneity of PsaA, a 37-kilodalton putative adhesin essential for virulence of *Streptococcus pneumoniae*. Infect Immun 1996; 64:5255–5262.

104. Marra A, et al. In vivo characterization of the psa genes from Streptococcus pneumoniae in multiple models of infection. Microbiology 2002; 148:1483–1491.

105. Tseng HJ, et al. Virulence of Streptococcus pneumoniae: PsaA mutants are hypersensitive to oxidative stress. Infect Immun 2002; 70:1635–1639.

106. Lawrence MC, et al. The crystal structure of pneumococcal surface antigen PsaA reveals a metal-binding site and a novel structure for a putative ABC-type binding protein. Structure 1998; 6:1553–1561.

107. Weiser JN, Kapoor M. Effect of intrastrain variation in the amount of capsular polysaccharide on genetic transformation of Streptococcus pneumoniae: implications for virulence studies of encapsulated strains. Infect Immun 1999; 67:3690–3692.

108. Mosser JL, Tomasz A. Choline-containing teichoic acid as a structural component of pneumococcal cell wall and its role in sensitivity to lysis by an autolytic enzyme. J Biol Chem 1970; 245:287–298.

109. Lock RA, et al. Comparative efficacy of autolysin and pneumolysin as immunogens protecting mice against infection by Streptococcus pneumoniae. Microb Pathog 1992; 12:137–143.

110. Berry AM, et al. Effect of insertional inactivation of the genes encoding pneumolysin and autolysin on the virulence of *Streptococcus pneumoniae* type 3. Microb Pathog 1992; 12: 87–93.

111. Canvin JR, et al. The role of pneumolysin and autolysin in the pathology of pneumoniae and septicemia in mice infected with a type 2 pneumococcus. J Infect Dis 1995; 172: 119–123.

112. Tettelin H, et al. Complete genome sequence of a virulent isolate of Streptococcus pneumoniae. Science 2001; 293:498–506.

113. Paton JC, et al. Molecular analysis of putative pneumococcal virulence proteins. Microbial Drug Resistance 1997; 3:3–10.

114. Berry AM, J. Paton C. Additive attenuation of virulence of *Streptococcus pneumoniae* by mutation of the genes encoding pneumolysin and other putative pneumococcal virulence proteins. Infect Immun 2000; 68:133–140.

115. Mitchell TJ. Virulence factors and the pathogenesis of disease caused by Streptococcus pneumoniae. Res Microbiol 2000; 151:413–419.

116. Bongaerts RJ, et al. Antigenicity, expression and molecular characterization of surface-locaed pullulunase of Streptococcus pneumoniae. Infection and Immunity 2000; 68:7141–7143.

117. Holmes AR, et al. The pavA gene of Streptococcus pneumoniae encodes a fibronectin-binding protein that is essential for virulence. Mol Microbiol 2001; 41:1395–1408.

118. Zhang Y, et al. Recombinant PhpA protein, a unique histidine motif-containing protein from Streptococcus pneumoniae, protects mice against intranasal pneumococcal challenge. Infect Immun 2001; 69:3827–3836.

119. Brown JS, et al. Immunization with components of two iron uptake ABC transporters protects mice against systemic Streptococcus pneumoniae infection. Infect Immun 2001; 69:6702–6706.

120. Lomholt H. Molecular biology and vaccine aspects of bacterial immunoglobulin A1 proteases. APMIS Suppl 1996; 104 (Supplement 62):5–28.

121. Wani JH, et al. Identification, cloning, and sequencing of the immunoglobulin A1 protease gene of *Streptococcus pneumoniae*. Infect Immun 1996; 64:3967–3974.

122. Lee C-J, et al. Protection in infant mice from challenge with *Streptococcus pneumoniae* type 19F by immunization with a type 19F polysaccharide-pneumolysoid conjugate. Vaccine 1994; 12:875–877.

123. Gray BM, et al. Epidemiologic studies of *Streptococcus pneumoniae* in infants: acquisition, carriage, and infection during the first 24 months of life. J Infect Dis 1980; 142:923–933.

124. Bergquist C, et al. Intranasal vaccination of humans with recombinant cholera toxin B subunit induces systemic and local antibody responses in the upper respiratory tract and the vagina. Infect Immun 1997; 65:2676–2684.

125. Wu H-Y, et al. International immunization of mice with PspA (pneumococcal surface protein A) can prevent intranasal carriage and infection with *Streptococcus pneumoniae*. J Infect Dis 1997; 175:839–846.

126. Malley R, et al. Intranasal immunization with killed unencapsulated whole cells prevents colonization and invasive disease by capsulated pneumococci. Infect Immun 2001; 69:4870–4873.

127. Tillett WS. Active and passive immunity to pneumococcus infection induced in rabbits by immunization with R pneumococci. J Exp Med 1928; 48:791–804.

128. Bull CG, McKee CM. Respiratory immunity in rabbits: VII resistance to intranasal infection in the absence of demonstrable antibodies. Am J Hyg 1929; 9:490–499.

129. Hvalbye BK, et al. Intranasal immunization with heat-inactivated Streptococcus pneumoniae protects mice against systemic pneumococcal infection. Infect Immun 1999; 67:4320–4325.

130. Wu H-Y, et al. Establishment of a Streptococcus pneumoniae nasopharyngeal model of pneumococcal carriage in adult mice. Microb Pathogen 1997; 23:127–137.

40

Polysaccharide-Based Conjugate Vaccines for Enteric Bacterial Infections: Typhoid Fever, Nontyphoidal Salmonellosis, Shigellosis, Cholera, and *Escherichia coli* O157

Shousun C. Szu, John B. Robbins, Rachel Schneerson, Vince Pozsgay, and Chiayung Chu
National Institutes of Child Health and Human Development, National Institutes of Health, Bethesda, Maryland, U.S.A.

I. INTRODUCTION

Although a variety of vaccines to prevent typhoid fever and cholera (caused by *Vibrio cholerae* O1) are licensed in many countries, there are no licensed vaccines against nontyphoidal *Salmonella*, *Shigella*, *V. cholerae* O139, and *Escherichia coli* O157. We investigated the protective antigens and the host components that confer immunity against this latter important group of diseases to devise safe and effective vaccines [1]. The long experience with vaccines composed of either inactivated or attenuated strains of bacterial pathogens was based largely upon Pasteur's idea for vaccine development: that convalescence from disease induces immunity. But inactivated or attenuated strains of bacteria are not good immunogens when administered in a clinically acceptable form, and convalescence from many enteric infections, such as shigellosis, does not reliably confer a high degree of immunity of long duration [2].

We have exploited the *similarities* in the pathogenesis of and immunity to enteric and respiratory pathogens for the development of enteric vaccines. The surface polysaccharides (PS) of many bacterial pathogens are both essential virulence factors and protective antigens, including the capsular polysaccharides (CP) of respiratory pathogens such as pneumococci, *Haemophilus influenzae* type b, and meningococci, and the Vi CP of the enteric pathogen *Salmonella enterica* serovar *typhi* (*S. typhi*) [3–5]. For most other Gram-negative enteric pathogens, the O-specific polysaccharide (O-SP) domain of their lipopolysaccharides (LPS), including nontyphoidal *Salmonella*, *Shigella*, *V. cholerae*, *E. coli*, etc., serves the same role as a CP [4,6]. Surface PS shields the bacterium from the protective actions of serum complement (lysis for Gram-negatives and opsonophagocytic killing by polymorphonuclear leukocytes). A critical level of serum IgG antibodies to these surface PS confers immunity to diseases by initiating these protective actions. Serum IgG anti-

PS transudes onto the surface of respiratory or intestinal epithelium, where it induces complement-mediated lysis of the inoculum containing the pathogen [7,8].

II. *S. TYPHI* AND OTHER ENTERIC FEVERS

A. *S. Typhi*

Three types of typhoid vaccines are currently licensed: parenterally administered inactivated whole cell vaccines [9,10], orally administered attenuated *S. typhi* strain Ty21a [11], and parenterally administered CP Vi vaccine [12–14a]. These three vaccines confer ca. 70% protection in older children and adults. In children less than 5 years of age, these vaccines are either poorly immunogenic and protective (e.g., Vi), or insufficient data are available to draw conclusions about their efficacy (e.g., Ty21a) [14b]. Notably, it has been shown that in some endemic areas, the highest incidence of typhoid may be seen in children <5 years of age [15].

S. typhi is covered by the Vi CP, which serves as a virulence attribute. An early-generation Vi PS vaccine candidate was prepared in the early 1950s, which involved treatment with 1 N acetic acid at 100°C for 24 hr. This early Vi vaccine failed to protect volunteers against experimental challenge with *S. typhi* [16], and it was subsequently discovered that the harsh treatment with acid denatured the Vi. Vi prepared by modern technology results in a nondenatured PS product that is safe, easily standardized, and, following administration of a single dose, confers immunity to typhoid fever for subjects living in areas of high incidence (albeit only to individuals over the age of 5 years). In double-blinded, randomized, controlled trials in areas of high endemicity, Vi elicited 65–75% efficacy in Nepal, South Africa, and China [12–14a]. The efficacy declined to 55% over 3 years of follow-up, paralleling the decline in Vi antibody levels [13]. Vi is licensed in more than 80 countries and has been highly successful in reducing the incidence of typhoid (H. H. Yang, personal communication).

Although Vi is immunogenic in older children and adults, it does not elicit protective levels of antibodies in infants and young children, nor does it give a booster response (age-related and T-cell-independent). Reinjection of Vi in adults was safe, but it only restored Vi antibody levels to the peak postprimary injection levels [17]. These deficiencies were overcome by applying the discoveries of investigators at the Rockefeller Institute in the 1920s and 1930s [18], who showed that the immunogenicity of pneumococcal type 3 CP could be increased by binding these substances to a protein to form a conjugate. The *H. influenzae* type b CP was the first conjugate to be clinically useful, and its widespread introduction has virtually eliminated this most common cause of meningitis in infants and children [5]. Accordingly, the conjugate technology was adapted to the pneumococcus, meningococcus, *S. typhi*, and *Shigella*.

Vi is a linear homopolymer of $(1–4)\alpha$-D-galaturonic acid, C3-*O*-acetylated, and C2-*N*-acetylated; it has no vicinal hydroxyls; and its carboxyl is relatively inaccessible [20,21]. Nevertheless, a safe and highly immunogenic Vi conjugate was devised, which elicited high levels of IgG antibodies and provided memory for booster responses in 2- to 5-year-olds [20–23]. In a randomized, double-blinded, placebo-controlled trial in the Mekong Delta region of Vietnam, involving about 5000 vaccinees and an equal number of controls, the Vi conjugate elicited 91.1% protection over 27 months of active surveillance [24]. With additional passive surveillance for 19 months, there have been 17 cases in the controls and three in the vaccinees [25]. Over the ensuing 19 months, the efficacy declined slightly to 82% (91.1% vs. 82%, $P < 0.2$). The efficacy for the whole study period (46 month) is 89%. This efficacy is among the highest reported for any typhoid vaccine and was achieved in an age group for which there was no effective vaccine. Based upon the antibody data of the whole study period, we estimate the protective level of IgG anti-Vi to be about 0.35 g/mL (the titer of the younger age group at 46 months after immunization) [25]. It is a safe prediction that the Vi conjugate will be close to 100% protective after one injection in individuals older than 5 years.

The Efficacy of Vi-rEPA in 2- to 5-Year-Old Children in Vietnam Was Determined by Active (1–27 Months) and Passive Surveillance (28–46 Months)

	Vaccinees	Placebos	Efficacy
1–27 months	5991	6017	
Typhoid fever ($n =$)	5	56	91.1%
28–46 months	5383	5420	
Typhoid fever ($n =$)	3	17	82.3%
0–46 months	5991	6017	
Typhoid fever ($n =$)	8	73	89.0%
	91.5% vs. 89.0%	82.3%	NS

The immunogenicity of the Vi conjugate at lower dosages or administered to infants concurrently with DTP is under study. Should the Vi conjugate induce levels of IgG anti-Vi comparable to those in the 2- to 5-year-olds, this new typhoid vaccine could be incorporated into the World Health Organization's Expanded Program on Immunization schedule, which targets routine vaccination [26].

B. Nontyphoidal *Salmonella* Conjugates

The TAB vaccine, composed of inactivated *S. typhi*, *S. paratyphi* A, and *S. paratyphi* B, was removed as a licensed product because of the lack of data on the efficacy of the paratyphoid components and the frequent and severe adverse reactions observed. Currently, there are no licensed vaccines to prevent nontyphoidal *Salmonella* infections, including paratyphoid fevers [27,28]. *Salmonella* groups A, B, and D share the same LPS backbone [29]:

$$2\text{-}\alpha\text{-}\text{D-Man}p\text{-}(1 \rightarrow 4)\text{-}\alpha\text{-}\text{L-Rha}p\text{-}(1 \rightarrow 3)\text{-}\alpha\text{-}\text{D-Gal}p(1 \rightarrow$$

According to the Kauffman–White scheme, the backbone is designated as factor 12. The serogroup specificity lies on the 3,6-dideoxyhexoses branch linked $(1\rightarrow3)$ to the mannose:paratose for group A (factor 2) [30], abequose for group B (factor 4), and tyvelose for group D (factor 9) [30]. The rhamnose is partially *O*-acetylated at C3 for *S. paratyphi* A [31]. The galactose for group B linked $(1–6)$ with glucose (factor 1) and abequose is partially *O*-acetylated at C2 (factor 5) [29].

1. *S. Paratyphi* A Conjugate Vaccine

S. typhi and *S. paratyphi* A are inhabitants and pathogens of humans only, and can be considered as clones. The second most common *Salmonella* infection in the southeast Asia is *S. paratyphi* A. In the 1990s, approximately one-tenth of *Salmonella* cases in Indonesia, India, and Vietnam were *S. paratyphi* A. There is an increase of *S. paratyphi* A infections in the southwest region of China. This region had a high incidence of typhoid prior to the implementation of massive immunization with Vi in 1997. *S. paratyphi* A has become the most common *Salmonella* infection in this region (private communication).

The LPS of *S. paratyphi* A has two *O*-acetyls that are essential for the immunogenicity of the O-SP. Removal of the *O*-acetyls eliminated the immunogenicity of the O-SP [32]. The O-SP and tetanus toxoid conjugated vaccines were prepared using schemes that preserved the *O*-acetyl groups [32]. The immunogenicity data from Phase I and Phase II studies in Vietnamese adults and children are shown [33]:

IgG LPS Antibodies Elicited *S. paratyphi* A O-SP–TT Conjugate

Age (years)	Number of injections	n	IgG anti-LPS (ELISA units)			
			0 day	42 days	70 days	180 days
18–44	One	20	1.47	18.5	—	6.00
13–17	One	108	1.69	15.1	—	7.05
2–4	One	63	0.91	19.3	11.7	3.47
2–4	Two[a]	47	0.77	16.7	11.9	4.08

[a]The second dose was injected 42 days after the first dose.

There were no significant adverse reactions. After one injection, 75% of adults, 85% of teenagers, and 90% of young children responded with more than a fourfold rise of IgG anti-LPS. After 6 months, the antibody levels were approximately 3.8–4 times higher than the preimmune levels. The bactericidal titer was roughly related to the IgG anti-LPS level: the absorption of specific LPS removed most of the bactericidal activities. An efficacy trial in a highly endemic area is being planned.

2. *S. Typhimurium* Conjugates

The most common *Salmonella* infection in developed countries is caused by *S. typhimurium*. In 2001, the National *Salmonella* Center in the Netherlands reported an increase in *S. typhimurium* H8380 phage-type DT104 isolations from humans [34–36]. The DT104 strains were resistant to ampicillin, chloramphenicol, streptomycin, sulphonamides, and tetracyclines. Strains were also found to be resistant to fluoroquinolones, trimethoprim, and ciprofloxacin. Most cases were in 0- to 5-year-olds and the clinical course of the DT104 infection was severe with many unusual extraintestinal complications [37].

The *S. typhimurium* infection of mice is a suitable animal model. Serum LPS antibodies, whether actively induced or passively administered, confer protection to mice [38]. Monoclonal antibodies identified the abequose side chain (factor 4) as the most important protective epitope [39]. We prepared conjugate vaccines with the O-SP purified from an *O*-acetyl negative strain of *S. typhimurium* TML (O:4,12) linked to cholera toxin or tetanus toxoid [40]. In outbred young mice injected subcutaneously without adjuvant, the conjugates elicited antibodies: reinjection induced booster responses of both IgG and IgM anti-LPS. Most mice produced group B-specific antibodies (abequose or factor 4). Passive administration of conjugate-induced anti-LPS antibodies conferred protection.

About half of the disease isolates contain another antigenic epitope (factor 5): the *O*-acetyl in glucose. The cross-reaction between the *O*-acetyl-positive and *O*-acetyl-negative strains is limited. For example, antibodies raised against factors O4,05 do not cross-react with the O:4,12 strains [40]. Vaccines containing both *O*-acetyl-positive and *O*-acetyl-negative LPS may be necessary for the optimal protection against *S. typhimurium* infections. The complexity of the group B O-SP of *S. typhimurium* will require a surveillance of this pathogen prior to any efficacy trial.

III. SHIGELLA

An estimated 200 million people worldwide suffer from shigellosis with 650,000 deaths annually [41,42]. The highest incidence, morbidity, and mortality occur in children 1–4 years of age [43]. In developed countries, attendance at day care centers and chronic care institutions poses a major risk factor for sporadic cases and small outbreaks. *Shigella* is the most frequent cause of *dysentery* (diarrhea with gross blood and mucus in stools) in developing countries. Dysentery often results in stunted growth [44]. Because of the low infectious dose (~100 organisms), person-to-person transmission is frequent in young children and in overcrowded living conditions. Antibiotics can shorten the duration of fecal excretion but treatment has become increasingly difficult due to the multiantimicrobial resistance of *Shigella*. For these reasons, the World Health Organization (WHO) has assigned a high priority to the development of a vaccine against shigellosis [41].

The genus *Shigella*, Gram-negative nonmotile bacilli that do not ferment lactose, includes groups A (*Shigella dysenteriae*), B (*S. flexneri*), C (*S. boydii*), and D (*S. sonnei*) [44]. From the taxonomic perspective, some contend that *Shigella* and *E. coli* can be considered members of the same genus based on their DNA homology [43,45].

Parenterally injected inactivated *Shigella* vaccines elicited serum antibodies but did not prevent shigellosis. But whole cell vaccines administered once or twice intramuscularly to humans elicit low levels of IgG anti-LPS of short duration [46,47a,47b].

The LPS of *Shigella* is both an essential virulence factor and a protective antigen. The virulence of *Shigella* requires a full expression of their LPS. The outer domain of LPS, the O-SP, shields the bacterium against the protective action of serum complement [48]. Serum O-SP antibody is required to initiate protection against complement actions [49]. Shigellosis confers LPS-specific immunity of limited duration [48]. A significant correlation was shown between the level of serum IgG LPS antibodies and the resistance to shigellosis among Israeli soldiers [49]. Seroepidemiological data provide evidence of serum IgG O-SP antibody-mediated immunity to *Shigella* [50]. The rarity of shigellosis in newborns and young infants and middle-aged and older adults argues for serum IgG O-SP antibody-mediated immunity. Much of this IgG antibody is elicited by cross-reacting bacteria, as shown by serum IgG anti-LPS in most adults, even in countries such as Sweden where shigellae such as *S. dysenteriae* type 1 have not been present during this century [50,51]. Ashkenazi et al. [52a], Shears [52b], and Passwell et al. [53] have shown a similar age-related development of serum IgG anti-LPS for *S. sonnei*. These "natural" antibodies may explain in part why both newborns, young infants, and adults are relatively immune to shigellosis.

It is hypothesized that IgG LPS antibodies inactivate the *Shigella* inoculum as it reaches the intestine. Once the organism has multiplied and becomes intracellular, vaccine-induced serum IgG anti-LPS is ineffectual. A randomized, double-blind, vaccine-controlled study showed that the *S. sonnei* rEPA elicited 74% protection ($P = 0.001$) in Israel Defense Forces recruits [54,55].

Cases occurred in three companies about 3 months after vaccination. This immunization also conferred 43% ($P = 0.04$) protection in one company against an outbreak occurring 1–17 days following vaccination. This preliminary observation suggests that our *Shigella* conjugates might be of value in controlling epidemics. Efficacy in this study was correlated with the level of conjugate vaccine-induced serum IgG anti-LPS [55].

Culture-Proven Infection in Israel Army Recruits Following Vaccination with *S. sonnei* Conjugates

	Vaccine groups					
	S. sonnei rEPA		EcSf 2A-2 and meningococci		Percent efficacy	
Cohort	*n*/total	%	*n*/total	%	*P*	95% CI
A	1/32	3.1	7/48	14.6	0.135	75
B	0/32	0	3/48	6.2	0.271	100
C	3/115	2.6	13/72	18.1	0.073	65
Total	4/179	2.2	23/168	13.7	0.006	84 (28–100)
D	15/127	11.8	40/93	20.7 (2–82)	0.039	43

The safety and the immunogenicity of similar *Shigella* conjugates were demonstrated in children of ages 4–7 and 1–4 years in Israel [56]. The fold rise in anti-LPS was similar in adults and children, but the level of anti-LPS elicited by the conjugates was lower in young children:

Age-Related Serum IgG Geometric Mean (GM) Anti-LPS Responses in Vaccines Elicited by O-Specific PS Conjugates

	Age of vaccinees					
	Adults		4–7 years		1–4 years	
Conjugate	Pre	Post	Pre	Post	Pre	Post
S. sonnei rEPA	1.64	48.0	0.32	8.05	0.16	2.86
S. flexneri 2a rEPA	6.28	113.0	1.25	48.0	0.59	40.0

The table above compares the GM of IgG anti-LPS 2 weeks following the second injection of *Shigella* O-SP conjugates in studies undertaken in adults, 5- to 7-year-olds, and 1- to 4-year-olds.

The O-SP of *S. dysenteriae* type 1 is a tetrasaccharide repeating unit: 3)-α-L-Rha*p*-(1→3)-α-L-Rha*p*-(1→2)-α-D-Gal*p*-(1→3)-α-D-Glc*p*NAc-(1→. This saccharide is a hapten and must be conjugated to a protein to induce serum antibodies. The O-SP of *S. dysenteriae* type 1 (natural product) was bound to human serum albumin by multiple point attachment (O-SP–HSA) [57]. Saccharides, corresponding to the O-SP, have been synthesized including tetrasaccharides, octasaccharides, dodecasaccharides, and hexadecasaccharides with a spacer at their reducing end, bound to the protein by single point attachment: the molar ratios of the saccharides to HSA ranged from 4 to 24. In mice, except the tetramer, conjugates of the octamer, dodecamer, and hexadecamer elicited IgG LPS antibodies after the second injection, a statistically significant rise (booster) after the third injection, and higher levels than those vaccinated with O-SP–HSA ($P = 0.0001$). The highest GM levels of IgG

anti-LPS were elicited by the hexadecamer with nine chains or 9 mol of saccharide/HSA (15.5 ELISA units) followed by the octamer with 20 chains (11.1 ELISA units) and the dodecamer with 10 chains (9.52 ELISA units).

The superior immunogenicity of the conjugate prepared with the synthetic saccharides may be explained by assuming that there is a ratio and saccharide-to-protein length that permit optimal stimulation of B cells and T cells [58]. Polysaccharides or their degradation products are comparatively heterogenous and have not allowed such precise synthesis as has been achieved with synthetic saccharides. Clinical trials of *S. dysenteriae* type 1 conjugates prepared with synthetic saccharides are planned.

IV. *V. CHOLERAE* O1 AND O139 CONJUGATE VACCINES

In the United States, the parenteral *V. cholerae* whole cell vaccine was withdrawn because of frequent adverse reactions and short duration of protection. Although the vast majority of clinical infections worldwide are caused by *V. cholerae* O1, in some parts of Asia, 5–20% of cases are caused by serogroup O139; strains of both serogroups can secrete cholera toxin. *V. cholerae* O1 has two LPS types, designated as Inaba and Ogawa, composed of a linear homopolymer α1→2 linked perosamine glycerol-tetronic acid [59]. Serotype Ogawa, in addition, has a methyl group on its C2 at the nonreducing terminal saccharide. *V. cholerae* O139 has a CP composed of a hexasaccharide repeating unit that consists of a trisaccharide backbone and two branches [60]. Our vaccine program for cholera is based upon the following:

A) The causative agent is confined to the intestinal lumen. Bacteremia and systemic complications such as fever or shock are rarely encountered in cholera patients.

B) The severe watery diarrhea of cholera gravis is largely mediated by cholera toxin and the disease can be mimicked by feeding the purified protein to volunteers. But neither serum nor intestinal secretory antitoxin confers long-lived protection to cholera in humans [61].

C) Only the level of serum vibriocidal antibodies has been correlated with resistance to cholera caused by V. cholerae O1: the attack rate varies inversely with the serum vibriocidal titer and is rare in individuals with a titer of >1:160 [62].

D) Most serum vibriocidal activities from convalescent sera can be absorbed by LPS for V. cholerae O1, or by CP for V. cholerae O139 [63].

E) Newborns and infants, independent of breast feeding, have a low attack rate of cholera than older children, suggesting that maternally derived serum IgG confer immunity [64].

A. Inaba and Ogawa Serotypes of *V. Cholerae* Serogroup O1

V. cholerae O1 Inaba conjugates made with hydrazine-treated LPS were evaluated in adult volunteers and the level of serum IgG anti-LPS was compared with that elicited in parenteral whole cell killed cholera vaccine containing 4×10^9 mL^{-1} serotypes Inaba and Ogawa [65–67]. Both conjugates and the cellular vaccine elicited vibriocidal antibodies. The correlation coefficient between IgG anti-LPS (ELISA) and 2-mercaptoethanol (2-ME)-resistant vibriocidal antibodies was 0.81 ($P < 0.0004$) and vibriocidal activities were absorbed by LPS.

B. Serogroup O139

The CP from *V. cholerae* O139 was not immunogenic. A conjugate synthesized with CP from O139 was prepared with the mutant diphtheria toxin, DT-H21G [68,69]. Mice injected with conjugates elicited vibriocidal antibodies toward *V. cholerae* O139, but not serotype O1. Treatment with 2-ME reduced (~ 4-fold) but did not eliminate their vibriocidal activity, indicating that much of this activity was mediated by IgG anti-CP.

We have also inspected convalescent sera from *V. cholerae* O1 patients in Mexico and *V. cholerae* O139 patients in Thailand. The vibriocidal activities for both serotypes were specific toward the surface PS and largely mediated by IgM; the vibriocidal activities were nearly all removed by treatment with 2-ME. The whole cell oral vaccine mimics the pathway of the disease and also induced more IgM than IgG. Conjugate vaccines elicited IgG vibriocidal antibodies that persist longer and can better penetrate into the intestinal fluid than IgM. The evaluation of these conjugates in endemic areas is being planned.

V. *E. COLI* O157

In 2001, ~ 70,000 people in the United States were infected with *E. coli* O157, up from 20,000 cases in 1999 [70–72]. The natural reservoirs of *E. coli* O157 are in cattle, sheep, and deer. Cattle can be infected with the organism for a period from 1 week to 1 month without symptoms. Contaminated beef hamburgers, dairy products, water, vegetable, and fruits are common sources of *E. coli* O157. The ingested infectious dose may be as low as a few hundred organisms. *E. coli* O157 can cause severe clinical disease including hemorrhagic colitis and hemolytic uremic syndrome (HUS) in 5–10% of infected pediatric patients; a subset of HUS patients experiences severe kidney damage. We propose that bactericidal antibodies against the O157 O-SP will lyse the inoculum in the jejunum. The O-SP of *E. coli* O157 consists of four neutral sugars:

$$\rightarrow 3)\text{-}\alpha\text{-}\text{D-Gal}p\text{Nac-}(1 \rightarrow 2)\text{-}\alpha\text{-}\text{D-Per}p\text{Nac-}(1 \rightarrow 3)\text{-}\alpha\text{-L}$$
$$\text{-Fuc}p\text{-}(1 \rightarrow 4)\text{-}\beta\text{-}\text{D-Glc}p\text{-}$$

where perosamine (4,6-dideoxy-L-mannosamine) is the immunodominant sugar and is found in many cross-reacting organisms [73,74]. The O-SP was conjugated to protein by several schemes. A Phase I evaluation of these investigational vaccines was conducted in healthy adults at Carolina Medical Center (Charlotte, NC) [75,76]. The conjugates were safe and elicited statistically significant rises of IgG anti-LPS levels at 4 weeks and up to 26 weeks following

ing vaccination: 80% responded with at least a fourfold rise in the anti-LPS IgG level within 1 week, and 100% responded at 6 weeks. These sera precipitated in immunodiffusion with LPS from *E. coli* O157 but not with LPS from *E. coli* O55 or strain K-12, indicating that the antibodies are directed against the O-SP region and not the core region of the LPS. Postvaccination sera had bactericidal activity [76]:

IgG LPS Antibodies Elicited in Adult Volunteers by *E. coli* O157 O-SP–rEPA Conjugates

	Anti-LPS IgG (GM, ELISA units)			
Conjugate	Preimmune	1 week	4 weeks	26 weeks
O-SP–rEPA	0.47	7.93	61.9	32.8
DeALPS–rEPA[a]	0.51	5.73	46.3	31.2
DeALPS–rEPAv	0.54	4.12	36.6	33.1

[a]DeALPS LPS was prepared by treatment with anhydrous hydrazine. (From Ref. 76.)

There were 29 volunteers in each group; each volunteer received one injection containing 25 μg of PS. A high-titer postvaccination serum was used as standard and assigned a value of 100 ELISA units. The postimmune sera were bactericidal and their titer was related to their content of IgG anti-LPS as measured by ELISA. Currently, the safety and the immunogenicity of O-SP–rEPA are being evaluated in 2- to 5-year-old children. Preliminary results showed that conjugate vaccine is safe and induces more than a 10-fold rise of IgG anti-LPS 6 months after the first injection; booster responses were detected after reinjection.

The anti-LPS bactericidal activity from the conjugate vaccines could theoretically release Shiga toxin [77]. Accordingly, we synthesized conjugates of *E. coli* O157 O-SP bound to the nontoxic B subunit of Shiga toxin 1 (Stx1B). We modified our conjugation scheme to retain the immunogenicity of the Stx1B and to accommodate the smaller molecular weight of Stx1B (7300 kDa). The conjugates elicited both neutralizing antitoxin (titer 1/10,000) and induced the bacteriolysis of *E. coli* O157 [78].

Clinical isolates of *E. coli* O157 from HUS patients mostly contain the gene that encodes Stx2 [79]. Furthermore, from our experience with cholera toxin conjugates, the immunogenicity of holotoxin provided higher neutralization activity than the B-subunits. Thus, a recombinant nontoxic Stx2 as the carrier protein will be more desirable [80].

VI. SUMMARY

The surface PS of respiratory and enteric bacterial pathogens are essential virulence factors and protective antigens. These CP or O-SP exert their virulence by shielding the bacteria from complement. A critical (protective) level of antibodies, most importantly of the IgG isotype, confers immunity to these pathogens by killing the inoculum. Protein conjugates of these PS enhance the immunogenicity and prolong the duration of antibody synthesis. This approach to develop vaccines has provided the first vaccine for typhoid that protects young (2- to 5-year-old) children, and preliminary data indicate that O-SP conjugates will prevent shigellosis. Conjugate vaccines are also being developed to prevent *E. coli* O157 and *V. cholerae* disease. Preliminary clinical data show these conjugates to be safe and immunogenic. We are enthusiastic about the potential of synthetic saccharides to replace the natural product for conjugate vaccines.

REFERENCES

1. Robbins JB, et al. Perspective: hypothesis: serum IgG antibody is sufficient to confer protection against infectious diseases by inactivating the inoculum. J Infect Dis 1995; 171:1387–1398.
2. Robbins JB, et al. Hypothesis for vaccine development: protective immunity to enteric diseases caused by nontyphoidal *Salmonellae* and *Shigella* may be conferred by serum IgG antibodies to the O-specific polysaccharide of their lipopolysaccharides. Can Infect Dis 1992; 15:346–361.
3. Szu SC, et al. Vi capsular polysaccharide–protein conjugates for prevention of typhoid fever. J Exp Med 1987; 166:1510–1524.
4. Robbins JB, et al. O-specific polysaccharide–protein conjugates for prevention of enteric bacterial diseases. In: Levine MM, Woodrow GC, Paper JB, Cobol GS, eds. New Generation Vaccines. New York: Marcel Dekker, 1997: 803–815.
5. Robbins JB, et al. Prevention of systemic infections, especially meningitis, caused by *Haemophilus influenzae* type b: impact on public health and implications for other polysaccharide-based vaccines. JAMA 1996; 276:1181–1185.
6. Szu SC, et al. Development of O-specific polysaccharide–protein conjugates is based upon the protective effect of serum vibriocidal antibodies against cholera. Bull Inst Pasteur 1995; 93:269–272.
7. Bull DM, et al. Studies on human intestinal immunoglobulin A. Gastroenterology 1971; 60:370–380.
8. Ahrenstedt O, et al. Enhanced production of complement components in the small intestines of patients with Crohn's Disease. N Engl J Med 1990; 322:1345–1349.
9. Engels EA. Typhoid fever vaccines: a meta-analysis of studies on efficacy and toxicity. Br Med J 1998; 316:110–116.
10. Parry CM, et al. Typhoid fever. N Engl J Med 2002; 347: 1770–1782.
11. Levine MM. Duration of efficacy of Ty21a, attenuated *Salmonella typhi* live oral vaccine. Vaccine Suppl 1999; 17:S22–S27.
12. Acharya IL, et al. Prevention of typhoid fever in Nepal with the Vi capsular polysaccharide of *Salmonella typhi*: a preliminary report one year after immunization. N Engl J Med 1987; 317:1101–1104.
13. Klugman KP, et al. Protective activity of Vi capsular polysaccharide vaccine against typhoid fever. Lancet 1987; ii: 1165–1169.
14a. Yang HH, et al. Efficacy trial of Vi polysaccharide vaccine against typhoid fever in southwestern China. Bull World Health Organ 2001; 79:625–631.
14b. Simanjuntak C, et al. Oral immunisation against typhoid fever in Indonesia with Ty21a vaccine. Lancet 1991; 338: 1055–1059.
14c. Cryz SJ Jr, et al. Safety and immunogenicity of *Salmonella*
typhi Ty21a vaccine in young Thai children. Infect Immun 1993; 61:1149–1151.
15. Sinha A, et al. Typhoid fever in children aged less than 5 years. Lancet 1999; 354:734–737.
16. Robbins JD, Robbins JB. Reexamination of the protective role of the capsular polysaccharide (Vi antigen) of *Salmonella typhi*. J Infect Dis 1984; 150:436–449.
17. Keitel WA, et al. Clinical and serological responses following primary and booster immunization with *Salmonella typhi* Vi capsular polysaccharide vaccines. Vaccine 1994; 12: 195–199.
18. Goebel WF. Chemo-immunological studies on conjugated carbohydrate–proteins: XII. The immunochemical properties of an artificial antigen containing cellobiuronic acid. J Exp Med 1938; 68:469–484.
19. Gilman RH, et al. Relative efficacy of blood, urine, rectal swab, bone-marrow, and rose-spot cultures for recovery of *Salmonella typhi* in typhoid fever. Lancet 1975; 1:1211–1213.
20. Szu SC, et al. Vaccines for prevention of enteric bacterial infections caused by *Salmonellae*. In: Cabello F, ed. The Biology of *Salmonella*. New York: Plenum Press, 1993:361–371.
21. Szu SC, et al. Laboratory and preliminary clinical characterization of Vi capsular polysaccharide–protein conjugate vaccines. Infect Immun 1994; 62:4440–4444.
22. Szu SC, et al. Relation between structure and immunologic properties of the Vi capsular polysaccharide. Infect Immun 1991; 59:4555–4561.
23. Kossaczka Z, et al. Safety and immunogenicity of Vi conjugate vaccines for typhoid fever in adults, teenagers, and 2- to 4-year-old children in Vietnam. Infect Immun 1999; 67:5806–5810.
24. Lin FY, et al. The efficacy of a *Salmonella typhi* Vi conjugate vaccine in two- to five-year-old children. N Engl J Med 2001; 344:1263–1269.
25. Lanh MN, et al. Duration of efficacy and persistence of antibodies against typhoid fever 28–46 months following a trial of a Vi conjugate vaccine (Vi-rEPA) in 2 to 5 years old. N Engl J Med. Submitted for publication.
26. Saha SK, et al. Typhoid fever in Bangladesh: implications for vaccination policy. Pediatr Infect Dis J 2001; 20:521–524.
27. Syverton JT, et al. Typhoid and paratyphoid A in immunized military personnel. JAMA 1946; 131:507–514.
28. Chalker RB, Blaser MJ. A review of human salmonellosis: III. Magnitude of *Salmonella* infection in the United States. Rev Infect Dis 1988; 10:111–124.
29. Hellerqvist CG, et al. Structural studies on the O-specific side-chain of the cell-wall lipopolysaccharide from *Salmonella typhimurium* 395 MS. Carbohydr Res 1968; 8:43–55.
30. Kabat EA, Mayers MM. Experimental Immunochemistry. 2d ed. Springfield: Charles Thomas, 1961:256–267.
31. Hellerqvist CG, et al. Structural studies on the O-specific side-chains of the cell-wall lipopolysaccharide from *Salmonella paratyphi* A var. durazzo. Acta Chem Scand 1971; 25:955–961.
32. Konadu E, et al. Synthesis, characterization, and immunological properties in mice of conjugates composed of detoxified lipopolysaccharide of *Salmonella paratyphi* A bound to tetanus toxoid, with emphasis on the role of O-acetyls. Infect Immun 1996; 64:2709–2715.
33. Konadu E, et al. Phase 1 and phase 2 studies of *Salmonella enterica* serovar paratyphi A O-specific polysaccharide-tetanus toxoid conjugates in adults, teenagers, and 2- to 4-year-old children in Vietnam. Infect Immun 2000; 68:1529–1534.
34. Zaidi E, et al. Non-typhoidal *Salmonella* bacteremia in children. Pediatr Infect Dis J 1999; 18:1073–1077.

35. Fisher IST, et al. International outbreak of *Salmonella typhimurium* DT104—update from Enter-net. Eurosurveillance Wkly 2002; 5:010809.

36. Threlfall EJ, et al. Multiresistant *Salmonella typhimurium* DT104 and *Salmonella* bacteraemia. Lancet 1998; 352:287–288.

37. Ankobiah WA, Salehi F. *Salmonella* lung abscess in a patient with acquired immunodeficiency syndrome. Chest 1991; 100:591.

38. Svenson SB, Lindberg AA. Artificial *Salmonella* vaccines: *Salmonella typhimurium* O-antigen-specific oligosaccharide–protein conjugates elicit protective antibodies in rabbits and mice. Infect Immun 1981; 32:490–496.

39. Colwell DE, et al. Monoclonal antibodies to *Salmonella* lipopolysaccharide: anti-O-polysaccharide antibodies protect C3H mice against challenge with virulent *Salmonella typhimurium*. J Immunol 1984; 133:950–957.

40. Watson DC, et al. Protection of mice against *Salmonella typhimurium* with an O-specific polysaccharide–protein conjugate vaccine. Infect Immun 1992; 60:4679–4686.

41. Kotloff KL, et al. Global burden of *Shigella* infections: implications for vaccine development and implementation of control strategies. Bull World Health Organ 1999; 77:651–666.

42. Centers for Disease Control. Shigellosis in day care centers. Morb Mortal Wkly Rep 1992; 41:440–442.

43. Taylor DV, et al. Clinical and microbiological features of *Shigella* and enteroinvasive *Escherichia coli* infections detected by DNA hybridization. J Clin Microbiol 1988; 26:1362–1366.

44. Henry FJ, et al. Dysentery, not watery diarrhoea, is associated with stunting in Bangladeshi children. Hum Nutr Clin Nutr 1987; 41C:243–249.

45. Ørskov I, et al. Serology, chemistry, and genetics of 0 and K antigens in *Escherichia coli*. Bacteriol Rev 1977; 41:667–710.

46. Robbins JB, et al. Hypothesis for vaccine development: serum IgG LPS antibodies confer protective immunity to non-typhoidal *Salmonella* and *Shigellae*. Clin Infect Dis 1992; 15:346–361.

47a. DuPont HL, et al. Immunity in Shigellosis: II. Protection induced by oral live vaccine or primary infection. J Infect Dis 1972; 125:12–16.

47b. Mel DM, et al. Live oral *Shigella* vaccine: vaccination schedule and the effect of booster dose. Acta Microbiol Acad Sci Hung 1974; 21:109–114.

48. Liang-Takasaki C-J, et al. Complement activation by polysaccharide of lipopolysaccharide: an important virulence determinant of *Salmonellae*. Infect Immun 1983; 41:563–569.

49. Cohen D, et al. Serum antibodies to lipopolysaccharide and natural immunity to shigellosis in an Israeli military population. J Infect Dis 1988; 157:1068–1071.

50. Lindberg AA, et al. The humoral antibody response to *Shigella dysenteriae* type 1 as determined by ELISA. Bull World Health Organ 1984; 62:597–606.

51. Ferreccio C, et al. Epidemiologic patterns of acute diarrhea and endemic *Shigella* infections in children in a poor periurban setting in Santiago, Chile. Am J Epidemiol 1991; 136:614–627.

52a. Ashkenazi S, et al. Recent trends in the epidemiology of *Shigella* species in Israel. Clin Infect Dis 1993; 17:897–899.

52b. Shears P. *Shigella* infections. Ann Trop Med Parasitol 1996; 90:105–114.

53. Passwell JH, et al. *Shigella* lipopolysaccharide antibodies in pediatric populations. Pediatr Infect Dis J 1995; 14:859–865.

54. Taylor DN, et al. Synthesis, characterization, and clinical evaluation of conjugate vaccines composed of the O-specific polysaccharides of *Shigella dysenteriae* type 1, *Shigella flexneri* type 2a, and *Shigella sonnei* (*Plesiomonas shigel-*

loides) bound to bacterial toxoids. Infect Immun 1993; 61:3678–3687.

55. Cohen D, et al. Double-blind vaccine-controlled randomised efficacy trial of an investigational *Shigella sonnei* conjugate vaccine in young adults. Lancet 1997; 349:156–159.

56. Ashkenazi S, et al. Safety and immunogenicity of *Shigella sonnei* and *Shigella flexneri* 2a O-specific polysaccharide conjugates in children. J Infect Dis 1999; 179:1565–1568.

57. Pozsgay V, et al. Protein conjugates of synthetic saccharides elicit higher levels of serum IgG lipopolysaccharide antibodies in mice than do those of the O-specific polysaccharide from *Shigella dysenteriae* type 1. Proc Natl Acad Sci USA 1999; 96:5194–5197.

58. Anderson PW, et al. Effect of oligosaccharide chain length, exposed terminal group, and hapten loading on the antibody response of human adults and infants to vaccines consisting of *Haemophilus influenzae* type b capsular antigen terminally coupled to the diphtheria protein CRM197. J Immunol 1989; 142:2464–2468.

59. Kenne L, et al. Structural studies of *Vibrio cholerae* O-antigen. Carbohydr Res 1982; 100:341–349.

60. Knirel YA, et al. Structure of the capsular polysaccharide of *Vibrio cholerae* O139 synonym Bengal containing D-galactose-4,5-cyclophosphate. Eur J Biochem 1995; 232:391–396.

61. Finkelstein RA. Cholera. In: Germainer R, ed. Bacterial Vaccines. New York: Academic Press, 1984:107–136.

62. Mosley WH, et al. The 1968–1969 cholera-vaccine trial in rural East Pakistan. Effectiveness of monovalent Ogawa and Inaba vaccines and a purified Inaba antigen, with comparative results of serological and animal protections test. J Infect Dis 1970; 121:S1–S9.

63. Finkelstein RA. Vibriocidal antibody inhibition (VAI) analysis: a technique for the identification of the predominant vibriocidal antibodies in serum and for the detection and identification of *Vibrio cholerae* antigens. J Immunol 1962; 89:264–271.

64. Clemens JD, et al. Field trial of oral cholerae vaccines in Bangladesh: evaluation of anti-bacterial and anti-toxic breast-milk immunity in response to ingestion of the vaccines. Vaccine 1990; 8:469–472.

65. Gupta RK, et al. Synthesis, characterization and some immunological properties of conjugates composed of the detoxified lipopolysaccharide of *Vibrio cholerae* O1 serotype Inaba bound to cholera toxin. Infect Immun 1966; 60:3201–3208.

66. Neoh SH, Rowley D. The antigens of *Vibrio cholerae* involved in the vibriocidal action of antibody and complement. J Infect Dis 1970; 121:505–513.

67. Szu SC, et al. Induction of serum vibriocidal antibodies by O-specific polysaccharide–protein conjugate vaccines for prevention of cholera. In: Wachsmuth IK, Blake PA, Olsvik O, eds. *Vibrio cholerae*. Washington, DC: American Society of Microbiologists, 1994:381–394.

68. Kossaczka Z, et al. *Vibrio cholerae* O139 conjugate vaccines: synthesis and immunogenicity of *V. cholerae* O139 capsular polysaccharide conjugates with recombinant diphtheria toxin mutant in mice. Infect Immun 2000; 68:5037–5043.

69. Kossaczka Z, Szu SC. Evaluation of synthetic schemes to prepare immunogenic conjugates of *Vibrio cholerae* O139 capsular polysaccharide with chicken serum albumin. Glycoconj J 2000; 17:425–433.

70. Committee on Infectious Diseases, American Academy of Pediatrics: 2000 Red Book. Elk Grove Village, IL: American Academy of Pediatrics, 2000.

71. Waterborne outbreak of gastroenteritis associated with a contaminated municipal water supply, Walkerton, Ontario, May–June, 2000. Can Commun Dis Rep 2000; 26:170–173.

72. Michino H, et al. Massive Outbreak of *Escherichia coli* O157:H7 infection in schoolchildren in Sakai City, Japan, 1996 associated with consumption of white radish sprouts. Am J Epidemiol 1996; 150:787.

73. Perry MB, et al. The structure of the antigenic lipopolysaccharide O-chains produced by *Salmonella urbana* and *Salmonella godesberg*. Carbohydr Res 1986; 156:107–122.

74. Aleksic S, et al. A biotyping scheme for Shiga-like toxin-producing *Escherichia coli* O157 and a list of serological cross-reactions between O157 and other Gram-negative bacteria. Zentralbl Bakteriol 1992; 276:221–230.

75. Konadu E, et al. Preparation, characterization, and immunological properties in mice of *Escherichia coli* O157 O-specific polysaccharide–protein conjugate vaccines. Infect Immun 1994; 62:5048–5054.

76. Konadu E, et al. Investigational vaccine for *Escherichia coli* O157: phase 1 study of O157 O-specific polysaccharide–*Pseudomonas aeruginosa* recombinant exoprotein A (rEPA) conjugates in adults. J Infect Dis 1998; 177:383–387.

77. O'Brien AD, LaVeck GD. Purification and characterization of a *Shigella dysenteriae* 1-like toxin produced by *Escherichia coli*. Infect Immun 1983; 40:675–683.

78. Konadu E, et al. Syntheses and immunologic properties of *Escherichia coli* O157 O-specific polysaccharide and Shiga toxin 1B subunit conjugate in mice. Infect Immun 1999; 67:6191–6193.

79. Tarr PI, Neill MA. *Escherichia coli* O157:H7. Gastroentrol Clin North Am 2001; 30:735–751.

80. Oku Y, et al. Purification and some properties of a Vero toxin from a human strain of *Escherichia coli* that is immunologically related to Shiga-like toxin II (VT2). Nucri OATG 1898; 6:113–122.

41

Attenuated Strains of *Salmonella enterica* serovar Typhi as Live Oral Vaccines Against Typhoid Fever

Myron M. Levine, James Galen, Carol O. Tacket, Eileen M. Barry, Marcela F. Pasetti, and Marcelo B. Sztein
University of Maryland School of Medicine, Baltimore, Maryland, U.S.A.

I. TARGET POPULATIONS

Typhoid fever is exceedingly uncommon in modern industrialized countries where populations are served by treated, bacteriologically monitored water supplies and by sanitation that removes human fecal waste. In contrast, in less-developed countries where populations commonly lack such amenities, typhoid fever is often endemic and, from the public health perspective, typically constitutes the most important enteric disease problem of school-age children [1]. Systematic clinical, epidemiological, and bacteriological surveillance for typhoid fever carried out in relation to field trials of the efficacy of candidate vaccines has provided more precise data on the incidence of typhoid in many populations [2–9]. The incidence rates recorded were much higher than predicted based on nonsystematic surveillance. Systematic household and health center-based surveys have also demonstrated a surprisingly high frequency of bacteremic (but in general clinically mild) typhoid infection among febrile infants and toddlers in endemic areas [10,11].

Besides school-age children in less-developed countries, travelers [12] and clinical microbiologists [13] represent other groups at increased risk of developing typhoid fever. Among U.S. travelers, the risk is highest in the Indian subcontinent [12,14]. Because of increased exposure to *Salmonella enterica* serovar Typhi (*S.* Typhi), clinical microbiologists, even in industrialized countries, constitute a high-risk group [13,15].

II. MULTIRESISTANT *S.* Typhi STRAINS

Since 1990, strains of *S.* Typhi resistant to most of the antimicrobials that previously were clinically effective have spread aggressively throughout the Middle East, the Indian subcontinent, and Southeast Asia [16–18]. The few antibiotics that remain effective against these multiresistant strains, such as ciprofloxacin and ceftriaxone, are relatively expensive and not readily available in rural areas of less-developed countries. The dissemination of these multiresist-ant *S.* Typhi strains in many less-developed countries constitutes a public health crisis that has rekindled interest in the development of improved oral typhoid vaccines [19].

III. CURRENTLY LICENSED LIVE ORAL TYPHOID VACCINE Ty21a

Ty21a, an attenuated strain of *S.* Typhi that is safe and protective as a live oral vaccine, was developed in the early 1970s by the chemical mutagenesis of pathogenic *S.* Typhi strain Ty2 [20]. The characteristic mutations in this strain include an inactivation of *galE* (which encodes UDP-galactose-4-epimerase, an enzyme involved in LPS synthesis) and an inability to express Vi capsular polysaccharide. Whereas Ty21a has been remarkably well tolerated in placebo-controlled clinical trials, it is not clear precisely what mutations are responsible for the stable, attenuated phenotype of this vaccine.

Ty21a provides significant protection without causing adverse reactions. Results of three double-blind, placebo-controlled studies that utilized active surveillance to assess the reactogenicity of Ty21a in adults and children show that adverse reactions are not observed significantly more often in vaccinees than placebo recipients for any symptom or sign [9,21,22]. In large-scale efficacy field trials with Ty21a, involving approximately 530,000 schoolchildren in Chile and 32,000 in Egypt, and approximately 20,000 subjects from 3 years of age to adults in Indonesia, passive surveillance failed to identify vaccine-attributable adverse reactions [2,3,5,9,23].

Notably, results of controlled field trials of Ty21a emphasize that the formulation of the vaccine, the number of doses administered, and the spacing of the doses markedly influence the level of protection that can be achieved [1–5,9,24,25]. In the first field trial of Ty21a in Alexandria, Egypt, 6- to 7-year-old schoolchildren received three doses of vaccine (suspended in a diluent) on Monday, Wednesday, and Friday of 1 week [24]; to neutralize gastric acid, the children chewed a 1.0-g tablet of $NaHCO_3$ several minutes before ingesting the vaccine or placebo. During the 3 years of surveillance, 96% protective efficacy against bacteriologically confirmed typhoid fever was observed [24].

A more recent formulation that has been a commercial product since the mid-1980s consists of lyophilized vaccine in enteric-coated, acid-resistant capsules. In a randomized, placebo-controlled field trial in Santiago, Chile, three doses of this enteric-coated formulation given within 1 week provided 67% efficacy during the first 3 years of follow-up [3] and 62% protection over 7 years of follow-up [26]. Four doses of Ty21a in enteric-coated capsules given within 8 days are significantly more protective than two or three doses [25]. When Ty21a was licensed in the United States by the Food and Drug Administration in late 1989, it was with a recommended schedule of four doses given at an every-other-day interval; other countries use a three-dose immunization schedule.

In the mid-1980s, the Swiss Serum and Vaccine Institute (currently Berna Biotech) succeeded in preparing for large-scale field trials a "liquid suspension" formulation of Ty21a that was amenable to large-scale manufacture. The new formulation consists of two packets: one containing a dose of lyophilized vaccine and the other containing a buffer. Contents of the two packets are mixed in a cup containing 100 ml of water and the suspension is then ingested by the subject to be vaccinated. A fourth field trial was initiated in Santiago, Chile [3] and a parallel trial was carried out in Plaju, Indonesia [9] to compare directly this new liquid formulation (that somewhat resembles what was used in the Alexandria, Egypt field trial) with the enteric-coated capsule formulation. Vaccine administered as a liquid suspension was superior to vaccine in enteric-coated capsules. In the Santiago trial, the difference was highly significant. Ty21a given as a liquid suspension protected young children as well as older children [2]. In previous trials with enteric-coated vaccine, young children were not as well protected as older children [5]. The "liquid formulation," which is now available in a number of countries, is not only superior in efficacy to the enteric-coated capsule formulation but is more practical for administering vaccine to toddlers and preschool children. Although there are no field trial data to document the efficacy of Ty21a in children below 3 years of age, nevertheless, the liquid formulation is well tolerated and strongly immunogenic in toddlers and preschool children [27,28]. In contrast, an attempt to prepare a liquid suspension of Ty21a by emptying the contents of an enteric-coated capsule into a mixture of milk containing 0.5 g of $NaHCO_3$ resulted in an ineffective mixture that was poorly immunogenic [29]. Despite its pioneering role and positive attributes, recognized drawbacks of Ty21a include the lack of a molecular basis for its attenuation, relatively modest immunogenicity, and, most importantly, the need to administer at least three spaced doses in order to confer protection.

IV. CORRELATES OF PROTECTION OF LIVE TYPHOID VACCINES

Although Ty21a is only modestly immunogenic and requires three or four spaced doses to elicit protection, the efficacy is surprisingly long-lasting, enduring for 5–7 years [26]. Two immunological assays were found to correlate with the protection conferred by different formulations and immunization schedules of Ty21a in field trials. These include serum IgG O antibody seroconversions [4] and enumeration of gut-derived IgA O antibody-secreting cells (ASCs) detected among peripheral blood mononuclear cells (PBMCs) [30]. The identification of these measurements as immunological correlates of protection provides an invaluable tool for use in early clinical trials of new attenuated S. Typhi strains as possible live oral vaccines.

V. NEW GENERATIONS OF ATTENUATED S. Typhi AS LIVE ORAL VACCINES

Investigators in various laboratories worldwide have undertaken to engineer new candidate vaccine strains that are as well tolerated as Ty21a yet are more immunogenic, such that a single oral dose will elicit protective immunity. One attempt was made to increase the immunogenicity of Ty21a by restoring its ability to express Vi antigen [31]. Following other strategies (Table 1), candidate vaccine strains have been prepared by inactivating genes encoding various biochemical pathways [32,33], global regulatory systems [34], heat shock proteins [35], other regulatory genes [36,37], and putative virulence properties [38,39]. An elucidation of the sequence of the complete genome of wild-type S. Typhi strain CT 18 has provided an important resource for the development of attenuated S. Typhi strains.

The relative attenuating potential of various mutations has typically been assessed by feeding S. Typhimurium strains harboring these mutations to mice and by observing the result, in comparison with isogenic wild-type strains. Regrettably, the behavior of attenuated S. Typhimurium strains in mice has not proven to be reliable for predicting the behavior of homologous S. Typhi mutants in humans. There exist several examples where specific mutations that successfully attenuate S. Typhimurium for mice failed to adequately attenuate S. Typhi for humans [32,40,41]. These observations underscore the critical importance of careful clinical trials. The availability of the complete S. Typhi genome sequence has assisted in the identification of target sites to introduce attenuating mutations [42,43].

A. Vi-Positive Ty21a

A derivative of Ty21a was constructed by introducing viaB, which encodes the enzymes required for the synthesis of Vi polysaccharide, from wild-type strain Ty2 into the chromosome of Ty21a and by demonstrating the expression of Vi capsular polysaccharide [44]. Tacket et al. [31] fed this Vi-positive Ty21a strain with buffer to healthy North American adults in single liquid suspension doses containing 5×10^5, 5×10^7, and 5×10^9 colony-forming units (cfu); an additional group of subjects received three 5×10^9 cfu doses and buffer (every-other-day interval between the doses). The Vi-positive variant was well tolerated and most subjects who received three doses developed rises in serum IgG antibodies and IgA ASCs against S. Typhi O antigen. However, no

Table 1 Attenuating Mutations Present in Recombinant Strains of *S.* Typhi that Have Been Evaluated in Clinical Trials as Candidate Live Oral Vaccines

Mutated gene	Vaccine strain	Wild-type parent	Clinical phenotype	Immunogenicity phenotype	References
galE, via	EX645	Ty2	Not attenuated	Immunogenic	[32]
aroA, purA	541Ty	CDC 1080	Overly attenuated	Poorly immunogenic	[46,48]
aroA, purA, Vi-negative*	543Ty	CDC 1080	Overly attenuated	Poorly immunogenic	[46,48]
aroC, aroD	CVD 906	ISP 1820	Insufficiently attenuated	Immunogenic	[40]
aroC, aroD	CVD 908	Ty2	Attenuated (but silent bacteremias at high dosage levels)	Highly immunogenic	[41,49,50]
aroC, aroD, htrA	CVD 908-*htrA*	Ty2	Attenuated	Immunogenic	[35,57,58]
aroC, aroD, htrA, P_{tac}–*tviA*	CVD 909	Ty2	Attenuated	Immunogenic	[63]
aroA, aroD	PBCC 211	CDC 1080	Insufficiently attenuated	Immunogenic	[64]
aroA, aroD, htrA,	PBCC 222	CDC 1080	Insufficiently attenuated at high dosage levels	Poorly immunogenic at well-tolerated dosage levels	[64]
cya, crp	X3927	Ty2	Insufficiently attenuated	Immunogenic	[34,41,70]
cya, crp, cdt	X4073	Ty2	Attenuated	Immunogenic	[34,61,65,70]
cya, crp, cdt	X8110	ISP 1820	Attenuated (but silent bacteremias at high dosage levels)	Weakly immunogenic	[66]
phoP/phoQ	Ty800	Ty2	Attenuated	Immunogenic	[62]
phoP/phoQ, aroA	Ty445	CDC 1080	Overly attenuated	Poorly immunogenic	[67]
aroC, ssaV	ZH9	Ty2	Attenuated	Immunogenic	[39]

subject manifested rises in serum IgG anti-Vi or exhibited ASCs that secrete IgA anti-Vi [31].

B. 541Ty and 543Ty

Hoiseth and Stocker [45] and Edwards and Stocker [46] popularized the concept of making auxotrophic mutants of *Salmonella* with inactivations of genes encoding enzymes in the aromatic amino acid biosynthesis pathway. These mutations render the *Salmonella* nutritionally dependent on substrates (*para*-aminobenzoic acid and 2,3-dihydroxybenzoate) that are not available in sufficient quantity in mammalian tissues; as a consequence, the vaccine remains viable but is severely inhibited in its ability to proliferate.

Edwards and Stocker [46] constructed prototype strains 541Ty and 543Ty (a Vi-negative variant of 541Ty) from CDC 1080, a wild-type strain obtained from the collection of the Centers for Disease Control. It may be of some relevance that the pathogenicity of this strain had never been directly tested in volunteers. In contrast, most other investigators have started with wild-type strain Ty2, the parent of Ty21a [20], in their attempts to engineer new attenuated strains. The pathogenicity of Ty2 has been established in volunteer studies [47].

Strains 541Ty and 543Ty also harbor a deletion mutation in *purA*, which results in a specific requirement for adenine (or an assimilable compound such as adenosine) [46]. A third mutation in *hisG*, leading to a histidine requirement, does not affect virulence but provides an additional biochemical marker to clearly differentiate the vaccine strain from wild *S.* Typhi. Strains 541Ty and 543Ty were quite well

tolerated in dosages up to 5×10^{10} cfu in Phase I studies but were notably less immunogenic than Ty21a in stimulating humoral antibody responses [48]. For example, only 11% of subjects developed serum IgG anti-O antibodies [48].

C. Attenuated *S.* Typhi Strain CVD 908

The first vaccine strain that proved to be well tolerated and impressively immunogenic following administration of a single oral dose in Phase I clinical trials in humans is strain CVD 908 [41,49], which harbors precise deletion mutations in *aroC* and *aroD* [50]. CVD 908 was the first engineered *S.* Typhi vaccine candidate shown to be highly immunogenic yet well tolerated. At a well-tolerated dose of 5×10^7 cfu, 92% of CVD 908 recipients manifested IgG O antibody seroconversions and showed evidence of priming of the intestinal immune system (IgA ASCs) [49]. Moreover, vaccinees exhibited lymphoproliferative responses and their PBMCs were shown to secrete cytokines (in particular gamma interferon) upon exposure to *S.* Typhi flagella [51]. CVD 908 also stimulates cytotoxic lymphocytes that recognize targets (Epstein–Barr virus-immortalized prevaccination B lymphocytes) expressing *S.* Typhi antigens on their surface [52].

One possible drawback observed in the Phase I clinical trials with CVD 908 is that 50% of subjects who ingested this vaccine strain at a dose of 5×10^7 cfu and 100% of subjects who received a 5×10^8 cfu dose manifested silent vaccinemias wherein vaccine organisms were recovered from blood cultures collected at one or more time points between days 4 and 8 after vaccination. The blood cultures were collected systematically in these individuals within hours after they ingested the vaccine and then on days 2, 4, 5, 7, 8, 10, 14, 20, 27, and 60. No blood cultures from any vaccinee were positive prior to day 4 nor after day 8. The vaccinemias appeared to have no clinical consequence (e.g., they were not associated with fever) and they were short-lived, spontaneously disappearing without the use of antibiotics. There is a precedent for the licensure and mass use in public health of live vaccine strains that cause short-lived vaccinemia. For example, viremia occurs in many recipients of attenuated rubella vaccine strain RA27/3 [53] or attenuated poliomyelitis vaccine (mostly serotype 2 component) [54,55]. Thus, if licensure of CVD 908 was to be pursued, sufficient empirical data would have to be generated to document that the vaccinemias are not associated with any untoward reactions, as was done for the licensure of attenuated rubella and oral polio vaccines. Pursuing an alternative strategy, it was decided to introduce additional mutations into CVD 908 to yield a derivative that would remain well tolerated and immunogenic yet would not manifest vaccinemias.

D. CVD 908-*htrA*

Chatfield et al. [35] found that the inactivation of *htrA*, a gene encoding a stress protein that functions as a serine protease, attenuates wild-type *S*. Typhimurium in the mouse model. Moreover, mice immunized orally with Δ*htrA S.* Typhimurium are protected against subsequent challenges with a lethal dose of wild-type *S.* Typhimurium. Levine et al. [56] thereupon introduced a deletion mutation into the *htrA* of CVD 908, resulting in strain CVD 908-*htrA*. Tacket et al. [57] fed CVD 908-*htrA* as a single dose to three groups of subjects who ingested 5×10^7 cfu ($n = 7$), 5×10^8 cfu ($n = 8$), or 5×10^9 cfu ($n = 7$). The CVD 908-*htrA* strain was as well tolerated as the CVD 908 parent. Only 1 of 22 subjects developed a low-grade fever, which was detected by routine surveillance and was not associated with any complaints of malaise. However, 2 of 22 subjects developed loose stools [57]; mild diarrhea had not been observed in any recipient of CVD 908 [41,49]. The immune response elicited by CVD 908-*htrA* was excellent: 20 of 22 individuals manifested

significant rises in serum IgG O antibody, and in 100% of subjects, gut-derived IgA antibody-secreting cells were detected, which made antibody to O antigen (Table 2). These responses are virtually identical to what was observed in Phase I clinical trials in subjects immunized with comparable doses of CVD 908. The one striking difference was with respect to vaccinemias. Whereas vaccinemias were detected in 12 of 18 subjects who received a 5×10^7 or 5×10^8 cfu dose of CVD 908, no vaccinemias were detected in any of the 22 individuals who ingested well-tolerated, highly immunogenic $5 \times 10^{7-9}$ cfu doses of CVD 908-*htrA* ($P < 0.001$).

CVD 908-*htrA* was then evaluated in a Phase II randomized, placebo-controlled clinical trial in a larger number of adult North American subjects to assess the clinical acceptability and immunogenicity of a lyophilized formulation of the vaccine administered following reconstitution. Dosage levels of 5×10^7 and 5×10^8 cfu were evaluated [58]. There were no differences in the rates of side effects among recipients of either the high dose, the low dose, or the placebo during 21 days of follow-up. The vaccine strain was immunogenic at both dosage levels, although responses were stronger in recipients of the higher dose [58,59].

Vaccine strain ACAM 948-CVD was derived from wild-type Ty2 by introducing the identical mutations as found in CVD 908-*htrA*. The difference between these strains is that in the construction of ACAM 948-CVD, only bacteriological media devoid of animal products were used. ACAM 948-CVD is in early clinical trials.

E. Strain CVD 909, A Further Derivative of CVD 908-*htrA* that Constitutively Expresses Vi Capsular Antigen

From the results of two large-scale field trials, it is known that parenteral administration of nondenatured purified Vi polysaccharide confers a moderate level of protection against typhoid fever (55% vaccine efficacy over 3 years of follow-up) by stimulating serum Vi antibodies [6,7,60]. Results of other field trials show that attenuated strain Ty21a, which lacks Vi capsular polysaccharide, also confers

Table 2 Leading Live Oral Typhoid Vaccine Candidates Based on Results of Early (Phase I or II) Trials Assessing the Clinical, Immunological, and Bacteriological Response of Adult Volunteers Following Ingestion of a Single Dose of Vaccine

| Vaccine strain and dosage (cfu) | Formulation | Number of subjects | Positive cultures | | Fever | | | Immunological responses | | References |
			Stool	Blood	≥38.2	≥39.5	Diarrhea	Serum IgG O antibody	IgA O ASCs	
CVD 908-*htrA* (10^{7-9})	Freshly harvested	22	17 (77%)	0	1 (5%)	0	2 (9%)	20 (91%)	22 (100%)	[57]
CVD 908-*htrA* (10^{7-8})	Lyophilized	78	48 (62%)	0	1 (1%)	0	5 (6.8%)	37 (47%)	68 (78%)	[71]
Ty800 (10^{7-10})	Freshly harvested	11	10 (91%)	0	0	0	1 (9%)	6 (55%)	10 (91%)	[62]
χ4073 (10^{7-9})	Freshly harvested	10	3 (30%)	0	0	0	0	9 (90%)	9 (90%)	[61]
ZH9 (10^{7-9})	Frozen in glycerol	9	3 (33%)	0	0	0	0	5 (56%)	6 (67%)	[39]

a moderate level of protection and achieves this by eliciting cell-mediated and humoral immune responses other than the stimulation of Vi antibodies [3,5,26]. Levine et al. [4] hypothesized that a live oral vaccine may achieve a much higher level of protection against typhoid fever if it stimulated anti-Vi antibody, in addition to stimulating antibody responses to other antigens and eliciting cell-mediated immunity. Regrettably, the new generation of attenuated *S.* Typhi vaccine strains—exemplified by strains such as CVD 908, CVD 908-*htrA*, Ty800, and X4073, which are well tolerated and more immunogenic than Ty21a in eliciting serum O and H antibodies [41,49,57,61,62]—only rarely stimulate serum Vi antibodies in subjects. Because Vi expression is highly regulated and appears to be turned off when *S.* Typhi gains its intracellular niche, Wang et al. [63] engineered CVD 909, a further derivative of CVD 908-*htrA* that constitutively expresses Vi. CVD 909 was constructed by replacing the native promoter of *tviA* with the strong constitutive promoter P_{tac}. Constitutive expression of Vi was thereby achieved. In mice immunized mucosally (intranasally) with a single dose of vaccine, CVD 909 stimulated a significantly higher GMT of serum Vi antibodies than CVD 908-*htrA* [63].

F. Derivatives of Wild-Type Strain CDC 1080 with Mutations in *aro* and *htrA*

Deletions were introduced in *aroA* and *aroD* (encoding enzymes in the aromatic biosynthetic pathway) in wild-type strain CDC 1080 to produce vaccine candidate PBCC 211. Three different formulations of PBCC 211 were tested in Phase I clinical trials [64]. Among subjects who ingested either of two lyophilized formulations, a proportion developed fever. At the highest dosage levels tested, some vaccinees manifested silent self-limited vaccinemias on days 4–5 after ingesting a single dose of vaccine [64]. A deletion in *htrA* was introduced into strain PBCC 211 to derive vaccine strain PBCC 222 [64]. A lyophilized formulation of PBCC 222 contained in sachets was tested in Phase I clinical trials in subjects who received dosage levels of 10^7–10^9 cfu [64]. No vaccinemias were detected in recipients of this further derivative but some who ingested the highest dosage level developed fever, chills, and headache, leading to abandonment of further clinical trials.

G. Strains with Mutations in *cya,crp* or *cya,crp,cdt*

Curtiss et al. demonstrated that in *Salmonella*, *cya* (encoding adenylate cyclase) and *crp* (cyclical AMP receptor protein) constitute a global regulatory system that affects many genes and operons. They showed that an *S.* Typhimurium strain that harbors deletions in *cya* and *crp* [34] is attenuated compared to its wild-type parent, and that oral immunization protects mice against challenge with virulent *S.* Typhimurium.

Curtiss et al. constructed vaccine candidate strain χ3927, a *cya,crp* double mutant of *S.* Typhi strain Ty2 . In Phase I clinical trials, Tacket et al. [41] demonstrated that χ3927 was attenuated compared to wild type but insufficiently so to serve as a live oral vaccine in humans because

occasional subjects developed high fever and typhoidlike symptoms. Several subjects also manifested vaccinemias. In order to achieve a greater degree of attenuation, Kelly et al. [65] introduced into the *cya,crp* mutant a third deletion mutation in *cdt*, a gene that affects the dissemination of *Salmonella* from gut-associated lymphoid tissue to deeper organs of the reticuloendothelial system such as the liver, spleen, and bone marrow. The resultant *cya,crp,cdt* triple mutant strain χ4073 was fed to healthy adult North Americans, with buffer, in single doses containing 5×10^5, 5×10^6, 5×10^7, or 5×10^8 cfu. The strain was well tolerated except for one individual in the 5×10^6 cfu group who developed diarrhea [61]. No subjects manifested vaccinemia. Four of five subjects who ingested 5×10^8 cfu exhibited significant rises in serum IgG O antibody and had ASCs that made IgA O antibody [61] (Table 2).

The *cya,crp,cdt* mutant strain χ8110, derived from wild-type strain ISP 1820, was fed to volunteers at dosage levels of 10^5, 10^6, 10^7, and 10^8 cfu [66]. No subjects developed fever, one of four who ingested the highest dosage level developed diarrhea, and two of eight who received 10^{7-8} cfu manifested vaccinemia [66].

H. Strains with Mutations in *phoP/phoQ*

Hohmann et al. [62,67] constructed two candidate *S.* Typhi strains harboring deletions in *phoP/phoQ*. Strain Ty445, which also harbors a deletion in *aroA*, was found to be overly attenuated and only minimally immunogenic [67]. In contrast, strain Ty800, a derivative of Ty2 deleted only in *phoP/phoQ*, was generally well tolerated and immunogenic when evaluated in dosage levels from 10^7 to 10^{10} cfu in a small Phase I clinical trial involving 11 subjects [62] (Table 2). At the highest dosage level, one of three vaccinees developed diarrhea (10 loose stools). It is difficult to compare the immune responses of subjects who received Ty800 with those observed in recipients of CVD 908-*htrA* and χ4073 because some of the immunological assay techniques were different and, even where the same assay was used (e.g., IgA ASCs that make O antibody), considerable variation is known to occur between laboratories. Nevertheless, for purposes of comparison, the data from the clinical trial with Ty800 are summarized in Table 2 along with data from clinical trials involving comparable dosage levels of CVD 908-*htrA*, χ4073, Ty800, and ZH9.

I. Strain ZH9 with Mutations in *aroC* and *ssaV*

Salmonella Pathogenicity Island 2 (SPI 2) encodes a type III secretion system that is necessary for *S.* Typhimurium to manifest full pathogenicity in the mouse model [68,69]. *S.* Typhimurium strains harboring deletions in SPI 2 do not manifest a full-blown systemic infection and show a diminished ability to replicate in macrophages. SPI 2, which is activated under intracellular conditions, translocates effector proteins from the vacuole containing the *Salmonella* across the vacuolar membrane to the cytosol of the host cell (e.g., macrophages). *ssaV* forms part of the SSP 2 secreton, the needlelike bacterial structure that transports proteins across the inner and outer bacterial membranes. *S. enterica* derivatives harboring mutations in *ssaV* are crippled in their ability to secrete SPI 2 effector proteins. Deletion mutations in *aroC* and *ssaV* were introduced in wild-type strain *S.* Typhi strain Ty2 to derive vaccine candidate ZH9 [39].

In a small Phase I clinical trial that included nine adult subjects, ZH9 was well tolerated and elicited anti-Typhi immune responses in the majority of vaccinees (Table 2). The vaccine strain was recovered from stool cultures in only three subjects.

J. Mixing and Matching of Attenuating Mutations

If current leading vaccine candidate strains such as CVD 908-*htrA*, χ4073, Ty800, and ZH9 encounter difficulties in the course of Phase II or III clinical trials, a careful review of the clinical and serological data should provide critical feedback to allow investigators to engineer new vaccine candidates that incorporate different combinations of attenuating mutations. The goal would be to choose attractive new combinations of mutations based on the clinical, bacteriological, and immunological data generated in previous trials.

VI. FUTURE USE OF LIVE ORAL TYPHOID VACCINES

Ideally, an attenuated strain constituting the live oral vaccine of the future will be so well tolerated that it will be possible to administer the vaccine routinely to infants as well as to immunocompromised subjects with AIDS or other immune deficiencies. On the other hand, the ideal live vaccine will be so immunogenic that a single dose will confer a high level of long-term protection that will endure throughout childhood, including during the usual peak risk for typhoid fever during the period of 5–19 years of age. With such properties, it will be possible to pursue the control of typhoid by a strategy involving routine immunization of infants within the Expanded Program on Immunization schedule, perhaps supplemented by school-based immunization campaigns.

An alternative epidemiological approach to control endemic typhoid fever would be to institute only school-based immunization programs. Because peak incidence of typhoid fever in most endemic areas occurs in school-age children 5–19 years of age, and because this is a "captive" population, it should be possible in the future to design control programs to incorporate school-based immunization with a single-dose oral vaccine. Field experiences with Ty21a support such an approach. Even using multiple dose regimens of Ty21a, Ferreccio et al. [5] reported the practicality of school-based immunization in a field trial in 230,000 school children that compared two-dose, three-dose, and four-dose regimens (all within 8 days) of Ty21a. Moreover, Olanratmanee et al. [28] observed a herd immunity effect in geographically separate areas of metropolitan Santiago when large-scale use of Ty21a was carried out in the course of field trials in other areas of the city. Practicality will be

greatly enhanced with the advent of a single-dose live oral vaccine, and herd immunity effects should be even more pronounced with a vaccine that exhibits greater efficacy than Ty21a.

REFERENCES

1. Levine MM, et al. Typhoid vaccines come of age. Pediatr Infect Dis J 1989; 8:374–381.
2. Black RE, et al. Efficacy of one or two doses of Ty21a *Salmonella typhi* vaccine in enteric-coated capsules in a controlled field trial. Chilean Typhoid Committee. Vaccine 1990; 8:81–84.
3. Levine MM, et al. Comparison of enteric-coated capsules and liquid formulation of Ty21a typhoid vaccine in randomised controlled field trial. Lancet 1990; 336:891–894.
4. Levine MM, et al. Progress in vaccines against typhoid fever. Rev Infect Dis 1989; 11(suppl 3):S552–S567.
5. Levine MM, et al. Large-scale field trial of Ty21a live oral typhoid vaccine in enteric-coated capsule formulation. Lancet 1987; 1:1049–1052.
6. Acharya VI, et al. Prevention of typhoid fever in Nepal with the Vi capsular polysaccharide of *Salmonella typhi*. A preliminary report. N Engl J Med 1987; 317:1101–1104.
7. Klugman K, et al. Protective activity of Vi polysaccharide vaccine against typhoid fever. Lancet 1987; 2:1165–1169.
8. Lin FY, et al. The efficacy of a *Salmonella typhi* Vi conjugate vaccine in two- to-five-year-old children. N Engl J Med 2001; 344:1263–1269.
9. Simanjuntak C, et al. Oral immunisation against typhoid fever in Indonesia with Ty21a vaccine. Lancet 1991; 338:1055–1059.
10. Ferreccio C, et al. Benign bacteremia caused by *Salmonella typhi* and *paratyphi* in children younger than 2 years. J Pediatr 1984; 104:899–901.
11. Sinha A, et al. Typhoid fever in children aged less than 5 years. Lancet 1999; 354:734–737.
12. Mermin JH, et al. Typhoid fever in the United States, 1985–1994: changing risks of international travel and increasing antimicrobial resistance. Arch Intern Med 1998; 158:633–638.
13. Blaser MJ, et al. *Salmonella typhi*: the laboratory as a reservoir of infection. J Infect Dis 1980; 142:934–938.
14. Ryan CA, et al. *Salmonella typhi* infections in the United States, 1975–1984: increasing role of foreign travel. Rev Infect Dis 1989; II:1–8.
15. Blaser MJ, Lofgren JP. Fatal salmonellosis originating in a clinical microbiology laboratory. J Clin Microbiol 1981; 13:855–858.
16. Gupta A. Multidrug-resistant typhoid fever in children: epidemiology and therapeutic approach. Pediatr Infect Dis 1994; 13:124–140.
17. Rowe B, et al. Spread of multiresistant *Salmonella typhi*. Lancet 1990; 336:1065–1066.
18. Mermin JH, et al. A massive epidemic of multidrug-resistant typhoid fever in Tajikistan associated with consumption of municipal water. J Infect Dis 1999; 179:1416–1422.
19. Ivanoff B, et al. Vaccination against typhoid fever: present status. Bull World Health Organ 1994; 72:957–971.
20. Germanier R, Furer E. Isolation and characterization of *galE* mutant Ty21a of *Salmonella typhi*: a candidate strain for a live oral typhoid vaccine. J Infect Dis 1975; 141:553–558.
21. Levine MM, et al. The efficacy of attenuated *Salmonella typhi* oral vaccine strain Ty21a evaluated in controlled field trials. In: Holmgren J, Lindberg A, Molly R, eds. Development of Vaccines and Drugs Against Diarrhea. Lund, Sweden: Studentlitteratur, 1986:90–101.

22. Black R, et al. Immunogenicity of Ty21a attenuated *Salmonella typhi* given with sodium bicarbonate or in enteric-coated capsules. Dev Biol Stand 1983; 53:9–14.

23. Wahdan MH, et al. A controlled field trial of live oral typhoid vaccine Ty21a. Bull World Health Organ 1980; 58:469–474.

24. Wahdan MH, et al. A controlled field trial of live *Salmonella typhi* strain Ty21a oral vaccine against typhoid: three year results. J Infect Dis 1982; 145:292–296.

25. Ferreccio C, et al. Comparative efficacy of two, three, or four doses of Ty21a live oral typhoid vaccine in enteric-coated capsules: a field trial in an endemic area. J Infect Dis 1989; 159:766–769.

26. Levine MM, et al. Duration of efficacy of Ty21a, attenuated *Salmonella typhi* live oral vaccine. Vaccine 1999; 17(suppl 2): S22–S27.

27. Cryz SJ Jr, et al. Safety and immunogenicity of *Salmonella typhi* Ty21a vaccine in young Thai children. Infect Immun 1993; 61:1149–1151.

28. Olanratmanee T, et al. Safety and immunogenicity of *Salmonella typhi* Ty21a liquid formulation vaccine in 4- to 6-year old Thai children. J Infect Dis 1992; 166:451–452.

29. Murphy JR, et al. Immunogenicity of *Salmenella typhi* Ty21a vaccine for young children. Infect Immun 1991; 59:4291–4293.

30. Kantele A. Antibody-secreting cells in the evaluation of the immunogenicity of an oral vaccine. Vaccine 1990; 8:321–326.

31. Tacket CO, et al. Lack of immune response to the Vi component of a Vi-positive variant of the *Salmonella typhi* live oral vaccine strain Ty21a in human studies. J Infect Dis 1991; 163: 901–904.

32. Hone DM, et al. A *galE via* (Vi antigen-negative) mutant of *Salmonella typhi* Ty2 retains virulence in humans. Infect Immun 1988; 56:1326–1333.

33. Wang JY, et al. Construction, genotypic and phenotypic characterization, and immunogenicity of attenuated Δ*guaBA* *Salmonella enterica* serovar *typhi* strain CVD 915. Infect Immun 2001; 69:4734–4741.

34. Curtiss R III, Kelly SM. *Salmonella typhimurium* deletion mutants lacking adenylate cyclase and cyclic AMP receptor protein are avirulent and immunogenic. Infect Immun 1987; 55:3035–3043.

35. Chatfield SN, et al. Evaluation of *Salmonella typhimurium* strains harbouring defined mutations in *htrA* and *aroA* in the murine salmonellosis model. Microb Pathog 1992; 12:145–151.

36. Miller SI, et al. A two-component regulatory system (*phoP phoQ*) controls *Salmonella typhimurium* virulence. Proc Natl Acad Sci USA 1989; 86:5054–5058.

37. Pickard D, et al. Characterization of defined *ompR* mutants of *Salmonella typhi*: *ompR* is involved in the regulation of Vi polysaccharide expression. Infect Immun 1994; 62:3984–3993.

38. Miller SI, et al. The PhoP virulence regulon and live oral *Salmonella* vaccines. Vaccine 1993; 11:122–125.

39. Hindle Z, et al. Characterization of *Salmonella enterica* derivatives harboring defined *aroC* and *Salmonella Pathogenicity* Island 2 type III secretion system (*ssaV*) mutations by immunization of healthy volunteers. Infect Immun 2002; 70: 3457–3467.

40. Hone DM, et al. Evaluation in volunteers of a candidate live oral attenuated *S. typhi* vector vaccine. J Clin Invest 1992; 90:1–9.

41. Tacket CO, et al. Comparison of the safety and immunogenicity of *aroC*, *aroD* and *cya*, *crp Salmonella typhi* strains in adult volunteers. Infect Immun 1992; 60:536–541.

42. Parkhill J, et al. Complete genome sequence of a multiple drug resistant *Salmonella enterica* serovar Typhi CT18. Nature 2001; 413:848–852.

43. Wain J, et al. Unlocking the genome of the human typhoid bacillus. Lancet Infect Dis 2002; 2:163–170.

44. Cryz SJ Jr, et al. Construction and characterization of a Vi-positive variant of the *Salmonella typhi* live oral vaccine strain Ty21a. Infect Immun 1989; 57:3863–3868.

45. Hoiseth S, Stocker BAD. Aromatic-dependent *Salmonella typhimurium* are non-virulent and effective as live vaccines. Nature 1981; 292:238–239.

46. Edwards MF, Stocker BAD. Construction of *aroA his pur* strains of *Salmonella typhi*. J Bacteriol 1988; 170:3991–3995.

47. Hornick RB, et al. Typhoid fever; pathogenesis and immunologic control. N Engl J Med 1970; 283:686–691, 739–746.

48. Levine MM, et al. Safety, infectivity, immunogenicity and in vivo stability of two attenuated auxotrophic mutant strains of *Salmonella typhi*, 541Ty and 543Ty, as live oral vaccines in man. J Clin Invest 1987; 79:888–902.

49. Tacket CO, et al. Clinical acceptability and immunogenicity of CVD 908 *Salmonella typhi* vaccine strain. Vaccine 1992; 10:443–446.

50. Hone DM, et al. Construction of genetically-defined double *aro* mutants of *Salmonella typhi*. Vaccine 1991; 9:810–816.

51. Sztein MB, et al. Cytokine production patterns and lymphoproliferative responses in volunteers orally immunized with attenuated vaccine strains of *Salmonella typhi*. J Infect Dis 1994; 170:1508–1517.

52. Sztein MB, et al. Cytotoxic T lymphocytes after oral immunization with attenuated vaccine strains of *Salmonella typhi* in humans. J Immunol 1995; 155:3987–3993.

53. Balfour HH, et al. Rubella viremia and antibody responses after rubella vaccination and reimmunization. Lancet 1981; 1:1078–1080.

54. Horstmann DM, et al. Viremia in infants vaccinated with oral poliovirus vaccine (Sabin). Am J Hyg 1964; 79:47–63.

55. Melnick JL, et al. Free and bound virus in serum after administration of oral poliovirus vaccine. Am J Epidemiol 1966; 84:329–342.

56. Levine MM, et al. Attenuated *Salmonella* as live oral vaccines against typhoid fever and as live vectors. J Biotechnol 1995; 44:193–196.

57. Tacket CO, et al. Safety of live oral *Salmonella typhi* vaccine strains with deletions in *htrA* and *aroC aroD* and immune response in humans. Infect Immun 1997; 65:452–456.

58. Tacket CO, et al. Phase 2 clinical trial of attenuated *Salmonella enterica* serovar Typhi oral live vector vaccine CVD 908-*htrA* in U.S. volunteers. Infect Immun 2000; 68:1196–1201.

59. Salerno-Goncalves R, et al. Concomitant induction of CD4(+) and CD8(+) T cell responses in volunteers immunized with *Salmonella enterica* serovar Typhi strain CVD 908-*htrA*. J Immunol 2003; 170:2734–2741.

60. Klugman KP, et al. Immunogenicity, efficacy and serological correlate of protection of *Salmonella typhi* Vi capsular polysaccharide vaccine three years after immunization. Vaccine 1996; 14:435–438.

61. Tacket CO, et al. Safety and immunogenicity in humans of an attenuated *Salmonella typhi* vaccine vector strain expressing plasmid-encoded hepatitis B antigens stabilized by the ASD balanced lethal system. Infect Immun 1997; 65:3381–3385.

62. Hohmann EL, et al. *phoP/phoQ*-deleted *Salmonella typhi* (Ty800) is a safe and immunogenic single-dose typhoid fever vaccine in volunteers. J Infect Dis 1996; 173:1408–1414.

63. Wang JY, et al. Constitutive expression of the Vi polysaccharide capsular antigen in attenuated *Salmonella enterica* serovar *typhi* oral vaccine strain CVD 909. Infect Immun 2000; 4647–4652.

64. Dilts DA, et al. Phase I clinical trials of *aroA aroD* and *aroA aroD htrA* attenuated *S. typhi* vaccines: effect of formulation on safety and immunogenicity. Vaccine 2000; 18:1473–1484.

65. Kelly SM, et al. Characterization and protective properties of attenuated mutants of *Salmonella cholerasuis*. Infect Immun 1992; 60:4881–4890.

66. Frey SE, et al. Bacteremia associated with live attenuated chi8110 *Salmonella enterica* serovar *typhi* ISP1820 in healthy adult volunteers. Clin Immunol 2001; 101:32–37.

67. Hohmann EL, et al. Evaluation of a *phoP/phoQ*-deleted, *aroA*-deleted live oral *Salmonella typhi* vaccine strain in human volunteers. Vaccine 1996; 14:19–24.

68. Hensel M, et al. Genes encoding putative effector proteins of the type III secretion system of *Salmonella* Pathogenicity Island 2 are required for bacterial virulence and proliferation in macrophages. Mol Microbiol 1998; 30:163–174.

69. Shea JE, et al. Identification of a virulence locus encoding a second type III secretion system in *Salmonella typhimurium*. Proc Natl Acad Sci USA 1996; 93:2593–2597.

70. Curtiss R III, et al. Recombinant *Salmonella* vectors in vaccine development. Dev Biol Stand 1994; 82:23–33.

71. Tacket CO, et al. Phase 2 clinical trial of attenuated *Salmonella enterica* serovar Typhi oral live vector vaccine CVD 908-*htrA* in U.S. volunteers. Infect Immun 2000; 68:1196–1201.

42

Vaccines Against Lyme Disease

Mark S. Hanson *

MedImmune, Inc., Gaithersburg, Maryland, U.S.A.

Robert Edelman

University of Maryland School of Medicine, Baltimore, Maryland, U.S.A.

I. INTRODUCTION

In this chapter, we review the progress of Lyme disease (LD) vaccine development, the licensure in 1998 of the first human LD vaccine, the removal of that vaccine from the market in 2002, and the scientific and marketing challenges that lie ahead for the next generation of LD vaccines.

A. An Overview of Lyme Disease

Lyme disease, or Lyme borreliosis, presents as a multisystemic inflammatory disease with protean manifestations in humans and domestic animals [1]. The disease is caused by *Borrelia burgdorferi* sensu lato [2], a spirochete transferred from a diversity of wild mammals or birds to humans and animals by the bite of *Ixodes* spp. ticks. The taxonomic grouping *B. burgdorferi* sensu lato is subdivided into at least 10 species based on DNA–DNA reassociation and biochemical analyses [3]. In this chapter, *B. burgdorferi* sensu lato will be referred to as "Bb" for simplicity, unless otherwise specified. The three species of Bb that have been isolated from humans and well known to cause human disease are *B. burgdorferi* sensu stricto, isolated in North America and Europe, and *B. garinii* and *B. afzelii*, isolated in Europe and Asia including Japan and Taiwan. These three species may have different clinical presentations [1,4]. Many additional related species circulate in environmental reservoirs, and newer evidence suggests that at least some of them may also infect humans [5,6].

Certain manifestations of the clinical entity now called LD has been known in Europe for more than a century (reviewed in Ref. 7). First recognized clinically in the United States in the 1970s [8], LD is currently the most commonly reported tick-borne disease in the North America and Europe [1,9]. Currently, about 15,000 cases are reported each year in the United States, although the annual incidence is undoubtedly higher [9,10].

After Bb-infected tick saliva is deposited into the skin, Bb proliferates and causes a macular skin rash called erythema migrans within several days at the site of the tick bite. Constitutional symptoms may occur. The organism then enters the blood, circulating for days to weeks, during which time it disseminates to the joints, heart, brain, and other organs. Weeks or months later, meningitis, facial palsy, heart block, or migratory musculoskeletal pain may develop. Episodes of frank oligoarticular arthritis, encephalopathy, polyneuropathy, or acrodermatitis may occur months or years after the infection [1].

The early manifestations of LD, such as erythema migrans, are readily treated by oral antibiotics. By contrast, many patients with late LD, particularly those having arthritis and nervous system symptoms, must be treated with lengthy regimens of oral or parenteral antibiotics, and some of these patients fail therapy altogether [11]. About 10% of individuals with chronic arthritis, particularly those patients with HLA-DRB1*0401 or related alleles, are refractory to multiple courses of antibiotics and may have persistent joint inflammation [1,12,13].

Serology is used to confirm the clinical diagnosis of Lyme borreliosis [1]. *B. burgdorferi* infection in humans induces specific IgM and IgG antibodies detected by enzyme-linked immunosorbent assay (ELISA), IFA, and Western immunoblot [14], with antibodies to P41/FlaB and OspC antigens among the most prevalent.

Current affiliation: NIAID Scientific Program, LTS Corporation, Bethesda, Maryland, U.S.A.

B. Outer Surface Proteins of *B. burgdorferi* as Vaccine Targets

The earliest Bb antigens characterized were proteins presumed to be on the Bb outer surface membrane based on immunofluorescence and were termed "outer surface proteins" (Osp). OspA through OspF are lipoproteins having covalently attached fatty acids. The term *Osp* is sometimes used collectively for all Bb lipoproteins. OspA was the first of these [15] and is the most abundant membrane protein expressed in vitro by the majority of Bb isolates. OspA proteins are similar across each Bb species (>98% identity within *B. burgdorferi* sensu stricto and *B. afzelii*) [16]. OspB is somewhat less abundant than OspA and is structurally more variable [17,18]. OspC proteins are the most heterogeneous, often sharing only 70–80% identity between strains of a particular Bb species [19]. OspC is the most abundant membrane protein in cultures of many *B. afzelii* and *B. garinii* isolates. At least three additional distinct proteins have been designated "Osp," including OspD, OspE, and OspF. OspA promotes spirochetal adherence to tick gut and colonization of the vector [20]. The functions of the other Osp are less well understood.

II. JUSTIFICATION FOR LYME DISEASE VACCINES

There are many reasons to develop and utilize vaccines against LD. First, considerable morbidity is associated with *B. burgdorferi* infection [1]. Second, areas exist in the United States and Europe where 1–3% of a population are infected annually, and the infection seems to be growing in range and intensity [9,21,22]. Third, substantial costs result from multiple and unnecessary diagnostic tests, lengthy oral and parenteral antibiotic treatment regimens, loss of work and school, diminished quality of life, decline of tourism and real estate values in endemic communities, and a widespread fear of acquiring the disease. Fourth, practical and environmentally safe methods of tick control are not available [23], and wildlife (deer) management seems futile [24]. Fifth, personal protection, which includes wearing light-colored clothes, tucking pants into socks, applying tick repellents to skin, applying acaracides to clothes, and promptly removing ticks (nymphal ticks are difficult to detect on the body and clothes), has not reduced the incidence of LD [9,25]. Sixth, the infection can be difficult to diagnose, particularly early LD [26], and although uncommon, patients with chronic LD, who are seronegative and thus go untreated, can also be found [27]. Finally, treatment failures of chronic Lyme arthritis and neuroborreliosis are not uncommon [11].

III. RATIONALE AND EXPERIMENTAL VACCINE DEVELOPMENT

A. Naturally Acquired Immunity to *B. burgdorferi*

If a naturally acquired infection by a pathogenic organism induces robust protective immunity, it is likely that a vaccine against that infectious agent would be similarly protective. In human LD, naturally acquired immunity has not been formally demonstrated [33]. On the contrary, repeated Bb infection of patients treated for early LD has been reported [34], although the frequency of such reinfections is unknown.

B. Initial Studies of Active and Passive Immunity

The first evidence that vaccines will protect mammals was provided by the studies of Johnson et al. [35] who demonstrated that a single injection of a thimerosal-treated, whole cell Bb vaccine protected hamsters in a dose-dependent fashion against cultured Bb-inoculated 30 days after vaccination. In a companion study, hamsters passively immunized with immune rabbit serum were protected against challenge with 1000, 50% infective doses of Bb [28]. Because Bb-infected hamsters developed circulating antibodies that protected recipient hamsters against subsequent challenge but not against established infection [36], and because immune serum infused 18 hr after inoculation of Bb did not prevent infection, early vaccine development with OspA focused on immunoprophylaxis rather than immunotherapy of LD [29].

C. Immunity to Tick-Borne *B. burgdorferi*

The efficiency of Bb transmission between tick and vertebrate hosts correlates with the duration of attachment of the infected *Ixodes* tick [43]. Although *Ixodes scapularis* ticks feed for 3–11 days, few infectious Bb spirochetes are transmitted to mammals during the first 2 days [37,43]. Transmission increases dramatically thereafter. The 37°C temperature, shift in pH, and unknown nutrients in the imbibed blood activate Bb in the midgut of the tick, which then multiply and pass to the salivary glands. In Europe and Asia, where *I. ricinus* and *I. persulcatus* transmit *B. burgdorferi* sensu stricto, *B. garinii*, and *B. afzelii*, transmission may begin during the first day of tick attachment [38].

The adaptation of Bb as it cycles between its tick and vertebrate hosts involves the expression of many internal and surface-associated molecules [31]. For example, Bb spirochetes in the midguts of unfed ticks express OspA, but the burst of spirochete replication on tick feeding is accompanied by an upregulation of other proteins, in particular OspC, and a loss of OspA [31,32]. This helps explain the more robust antibody response to OspC than to OspA during early LD [13]. Conversely, OspA-negative Bb in vertebrate hosts become OspA-positive after they infect feeding ticks [32].

A seminal discovery, that Bb are destroyed within the midgut of ticks feeding on passively [39] or actively immunized mice [40–42], has molded our concept of how vaccine-induced immunity may protect against LD. Passive immunization with antiserum from rabbits hyperimmunized against cultured Bb protects mice against tick-transmitted spirochetal infection only when the antibody is administered within 24–48 hr after tick attachment [39], the initial lag period before spirochetes are deposited into the skin of the host [37,43]. Passive antibody administered 3 days after tick attachment does not protect mice [39]. This type of immunity, essentially a passive immunization of the vector by the serum of the vaccinated host, is probably uniquely effective against pathogens such as Bb that reside in a metabolically inactive state in the midgut of an arthropod vector that feeds for several days. Most Bb spirochetes lose OspA expression during transmission from ticks in parallel with their loss of vulnerability to OspA antiserum [44]. For Bb, this has been described as "transmission-blocking immunity." Malaria vaccinologists have used the same terminology to describe the reverse process when the mosquito's acquisition of gametocytes from a parasitic host is blocked. The effectiveness of this novel mechanism of protection depends on the maintenance of circulating Bb antibodies at protective levels in mammals during tick transmission season.

B. burgdorferi expresses OspC during transmission from ticks and during early infection in mammals, and may be vulnerable to OspC immunity at both vector and host stages. Supporting this hypothesis, an OspC monoclonal antibody (mAb) that prevents tick-borne Bb infection of mice also blocks the migration of blood meal-activated Bb from the tick gut to the salivary glands [45]. OspC may be another target of transmission-blocking antibody. Successful therapy of Bb-infected mice with OspC antibody has also been reported [46].

Additional antigenic targets against tick-borne Bb undoubtedly exist. Mice infected by tick bite with Bb strain B31, then administered a curative regimen of tetracycline 30 days postinfection, were immune to subsequent reinfection by tick-borne Bb B31 for 10 months. Immunity occurred in the absence of OspA antibodies and did not correlate with OspC antibody levels [47].

1. Cross-Protection Among *B. burgdorferi* Senso Lato

Studies evaluating the passive immunization of irradiated hamsters with Bb polyvalent antiserum [48], severe combined immune-deficient mice with OspA mAbs [49], or immune-competent mice with OspA or decorin-binding protein A (DbpA) hyperimmune serum [50] suggested that monovalent subunit vaccines may be effective against only cultured isolates within a single Bb species, but not between species. OspC cross-protection is even more restricted. Active immunization with OspC from one *B. burgdorferi* sensu stricto isolate failed to protect mice against challenge with other cultured Bb sensu stricto isolates [51]. Cross-protective immunity among *B. burgdorferi* senso lato has been successful in some tick-borne challenge studies [52] but not all [53]. The murine immune response to Bb infection protected against reinfection challenge with homologous, but not heterologous, *B. burgdorferi* sensu lato species [54]. From the foregoing experiments, we predict that an antigen from the three major clinically relevant Bb species will be required for a Lyme vaccine to be effective worldwide. Such a trivalent OspA vaccine has, in fact, protected mice against challenge with a wild population of ticks harboring infections with *B. burgdorferi* sensu stricto, *B. afzelii*, and *B. garinii* [55].

D. Borreliacidal Antibody

The observations that passive transfer of immune antiserum, but not immune cells, protected scid mice from Bb challenge provided evidence that immunity is antibody-mediated. In vitro assays have been developed for detecting and quantifying functional antibodies having borreliacidal [56] or growth-inhibiting [17,57] properties. The Bb form surface blebs and lyse within 30 min to 2 hr [17] after exposure to immune sera or mAb in the presence [17,56] or absence [58] of complement. Remarkably, Bb can be directly killed in vitro even by Fab fragments of borreliacidal antibodies [57], a vulnerability shared by few other pathogens. Opsonizing antibody, with subsequent phagocytosis and intracellular killing, may also contribute to protection [61]. Cell-mediated immunity is insufficient for protection; in fact, CMI mechanisms, including pro-inflammatory cytokines and CD4 + T cell mediation, seem to enhance destructive arthritis [62]. Antibodies against OspA are the best characterized. A key mechanism of protection results from the development of high-titered antibodies to a conformational epitope in the C-terminal end of OspA [63]. The protective epitope is identified by the murine mAb LA-2 in competitive inhibition enzyme immunoassays [64]. A good correlation exists between LA-2-equivalent antibody titers and a bactericidal assay [65].

Antibodies against OspC also can protect against Bb infection. Although some studies have failed to detect borreliacidal activity for OspC antibodies [45,46,66], others have been successful [67].

E. Preclinical Development of Lyme Disease Subunit Vaccines

Recombinant proteins expressed in *Escherichia coli* have been the focus of LD vaccine development efforts because it is expensive or impractical to purify vaccine antigens from Bb cultures. Table 1 lists the Bb antigens examined as targets for protective immunity. Most works have concentrated on the OspA lipoprotein and, to a lesser extent, on OspB and OspC lipoproteins. Many preclinical studies in mouse models of human Lyme borreliosis [29,30,63,68] documented that an OspA vaccine was feasible. The lipoprotein OspA initially developed by Connaught Laboratories (now Aventis Pasteur) [69] and SmithKline Beecham (now GlaxoSmithKline, GSK) [42] provided promising first-generation Lyme vaccines for humans [70,71], as discussed in "Clinical Development of Human Lyme Disease Vaccines" below.

IV. CLINICAL DEVELOPMENT OF CANINE LYME DISEASE VACCINES

A. Canine Whole Cell Vaccine

Spurred by the veterinary need and by the early success of an experimental thimerosal-inactivated whole cell vaccine candidate [35], a "chemically inactivated" whole cell vaccine comprised of a proprietary strain of Bb adjuvanted with a proprietary polymer-based system was developed for dogs (Lymevax® *B. burgdorferi* Bacterin; Ft. Dodge Laboratories, Ft. Dodge, IA). Based on its favorable safety profile, the U.S. Department of Agriculture gave Lymevax conditional license in 1990 and full licensure in 1992. The vaccine has been popular and is used widely by veterinarians and dog owners, particularly in Lyme-endemic areas in the United States.

Table 1 Protective Immunity Associated with *B. burgdorferi* Antigens

Antigen									
Properties[b]			Expression pattern[c]			*B. burgdorferi* inoculum protection[a]			
Name	Mass kDa (M_r)	Type	Culture	Tick	Host	Cultured	Tick-borne	Host-adapted	References
OspA	31	Lip	Yes	Yes	No	Yes	Yes	No	[52,68]
OspB	34	Lip	Yes	Yes	No	Yes	Yes	—	[52,68]
OspC	22	Lip	Yes	Yes	Yes	Yes	Yes	—	[51,131]
OspD	28	Lip	Yes	—	—	No	—	—	[66]
OspE	19	Lip	Yes	—	Yes	No	No	—	[41]
OspF	29	Lip	Yes	—	Yes	Partial	Partial	—	[41]
Arp (ErpT)	37	(Lip)	Yes	No	(Yes)	No	No	—	[127,132]
BmpA (P39)	39	(Lip)	Yes	—	(Yes)	No	No	—	[131,133]
DbpA	20	Lip	Yes	No	Yes	Yes	No	Partial	[50,122]
DbpB	18	(Lip)	Yes	—	Yes	Partial	—	—	[50]
Lp6.6	6.6	(Lip)	Yes	—	(No)	No	—	—	[134]
VlsE	34 (45)	Lip	Yes	—	(Yes)	—	No	—	[135]
VraA	52 (70)	(Lip)	Yes	—	(Yes)	Partial	—	—	[119]
P21	21	(Lip)	No	No	Yes	—	No	—	[126]
P37 (BBK50)	37	(Lip)	No	Yes	Yes	No	No	—	[118,136]
P47 (BBK32)	40 (47)	(Lip)	No	Yes	Yes	Partial	Partial	—	[118,136]
P37-42	37	(Lip)	—	—	(Yes)	No	—	—	[132]
P30	30	Peri	Yes	—	(Yes)	—	No	—	[137]
P55	55	Peri	Yes	—	(Yes)	—	No	—	[138]
P83	83	Peri	Yes	—	(Yes)	No	—	—	[66]
FlaB	41	Peri	Yes	Yes	Yes	No	—	—	[68]
Oms66 (P66)	66	TM	Yes	—	(Yes)	No	—	Partial	[121]

Lip = confirmed (or putative) lipoprotein; Peri = periplasmic; TM = transmembrane.

[a] Protection of actively immunized mice from experimental infection by cultured spirochetes, infected ticks, or tissues (skin, blood) from infected donors.

[b] Apparent mass (M_r) is indicated when differing substantially from predicted mass (in kDa).

[c] Predominant phenotype independent of modulation. (—) No data reported. ( ) Indirect evidence (seroconversion).

1. Immunogenicity and Protective Efficacy

Two years after conditional licensure, a laboratory-based immunogenicity and efficacy trial of Lymevax in dogs was reported [72]. Only 1 (3%) of 30 vaccinated dogs developed lameness compared to 15 (63%) of 24 control dogs, a statistically significant result. The favorable laboratory results were confirmed by a field study conducted in three veterinary practices in New York and Connecticut among 1969 vaccinated and 4498 control dogs [73]. Lymevax prevented 78% of clinically apparent cases of Lyme borreliosis, although the study was unblinded and potentially biased.

2. Safety

Serious adverse reactions or immune-mediated diseases were not detected in any of the 1969 dogs vaccinated with Lymevax and followed in some instances for 20 months. Despite this safety profile, laboratory results have raised the possibility of autoimmune reactions to components of the whole cell Bb vaccine. Severe destructive arthritis was evoked by vaccinating inbred hamsters with a whole cell preparation of formalin-inactivated Bb in alum or Freund's incomplete adjuvant, and then by challenging the hamsters with the homologous strain of Bb via syringe before high levels of protective borreliacidal antibody developed [74]. The destructive arthritis in hamsters was induced by the interaction of vaccine-specific T lymphocytes with viable spirochetes and not dead spirochetes [75]. It is unclear if this hamster model mimics the arthritis seen in other animal models or human LD.

Theoretical concerns of molecular mimicry have been raised by the antigenic cross-reactivity and the protein sequence homology that exist between non-OspA Bb antigens and human tissues [76,77]. The risk of destructive immune-mediated reactions by whole cell vaccines has helped to fuel the development of subunit Osp vaccines for both dogs and humans. Nonetheless, a second-killed Bb bacterin, the bivalent Galaxy® Lyme (Schering Plough Animal Health), has been licensed and marketed in the United States and Canada for canine use.

B. Canine OspA and OspB Subunit Vaccines

Immunization with several recombinant OspA or OspB vaccine formulations, singly and in combination, designed for dogs appear safe, immunogenic, and protective [78]. OspA was superior to OspB, and QS-21, a purified saponin component, was superior to alum at eliciting functional antibody response [79]. Although QS-21 formulations are promising, they have not been licensed. A recombinant OspA-containing bacterial extract, Recombitek™ Lyme

(Merial, Ltd.), has been licensed and marketed in the United States and Canada for dogs.

V. CLINICAL DEVELOPMENT OF HUMAN LYME DISEASE VACCINES

A. OspA Vaccines

1. LYMErix™ (GlaxoSmithKline)

Clinical Trials. The GSK rOspA vaccines initially tested in rhesus monkeys [80] performed well in Phase I and Phase II clinical trials conducted in adults [64,65] and later in children [83–85].

The pivotal efficacy trial of the LYMErix vaccine was conducted by Steere et al. [70] at 31 clinical sites during the winter of 1995. The study involved 10,936 volunteers between 15 and 70 years of age who were at risk of acquiring LD. Volunteers were randomized into two groups, with 5469 participants receiving one to three injections of vaccine (at 0, 1, and 12 months) and 5467 volunteers receiving a placebo. Volunteers were followed up in a blinded fashion for 20 months. Cases of LD were confirmed by cultures of skin lesions, polymerase chain reaction (PCR) tests, or serological tests.

In the first year, after two injections, 22 persons in the vaccine group and 43 in the placebo group contracted definite LD ($P = 0.009$). Vaccine efficacy was 49%. In volunteers followed up for 20 months, by which time they had received the third injection of vaccine, 16 vaccine recipients and 66 placebo recipients contracted LD ($P < 0.001$), and vaccine efficacy was 76%. The efficacy of the vaccine in preventing asymptomatic infection was 83% after two injections, and 100% after three injections. Antibody levels to the protective epitope of OspA (LA-2-equivalent antibody [64,65,86]) were measured in 938 participants followed at one study site (Yale University). At 1 month after the second injection, 95% of the vaccinees had positive test results for LA-2-equivalent antibody; 1 month after the third injection, 99% had positive test results associated with a marked anamnestic response to OspA. The higher protective antibody titers after three injections were associated with greater protective efficacy after three injections. Based largely on this pivotal trial, the LYMErix vaccine was licensed by the Food and Drug Administration (FDA) on December 28, 1998. The Public Health Service's Advisory Committee on Immunization Practice (ACIP) [87] and the Committee on Infectious Diseases of the American Academy of Pediatrics have published specific recommendations for vaccine use [88].

Limitations of LYMErix. Many unresolved issues surround the use and safety of the LYMErix vaccine. They include the durability of protection, a shortened schedule for primary immunization, an approved schedule of booster doses, the cost-effectiveness of vaccinating against LD, the use of LYMErix in persons younger than 15 years of age and older than 70 years of age, confusing serological cross-reactions engendered by the vaccine, and, most importantly, the possible induction of arthritis and post-LD syndrome in genetically susceptible persons.

Alternative primary vaccine schedules and booster doses. Data indicate that a 0–1–6 months primary immunization schedule [81] and a 0–1–2 months schedule [82] both result in high-enough antibody levels 1 month after the third vaccination to provide protective immunity for 1 year in >90% of vaccinees. Although this antibody level is achieved with the currently approved three-dose primary immunization schedule and the two shorter schedules, levels decay rapidly. In an open-label continuation trial, individuals from the LYMErix Phase III trial received booster doses of vaccine at 24 and 36 months after the three-dose primary series. Data supplied by GSK in a safety letter show no adverse impact on vaccine safety associated with administration of a fourth or fifth dose [89].

Cost effectiveness. Several pharmacoeconomic studies of the LD vaccine have been published [90–92]. The authors of two studies conclude that economic benefits will be greatest when vaccination is used based on individual risk, particularly in persons whose probability of contracting LD is >1% annually [90,92]. All studies conclude that the vaccine should not be used universally. The Institute of Medicine (IOM) report estimates that it would cost more than US$100,000 per QALY (cost per quality-adjusted life-year) saved if the vaccine were given "to resident infants born in, and immigrants of any age to, geographically defined high risk areas" [91]. In fact, the IOM report ranked the LD vaccine among the lowest priority for vaccine development. Lyme anxiety has fueled a virtual epidemic of overdiagnosis and overtreatment of LD and, until recently, has helped drive public demand for the vaccine [93,94].

Pediatric trials. The safety and immunogenicity of LYMErix have been evaluated through pediatric trials in Europe and the United States [83–85]. Trials in the Czech Republic administering LYMErix to children 5–15 years of age on a 0–1–2 months schedule [83], or children 2–5 years old administered a more preferred two-dose schedule at 0 and 1 months, demonstrated that the 15- and 30-μg doses of LYMErix were well tolerated and immunogenic [84]. The 38-μg dose produced antibody levels predictive of protection in 100% of children at 2 months, and protective levels persisted in 93% of the cohort for 6 months (one tick season).

The third pediatric trial was multicenter, double-blind, placebo-controlled, and randomized; it involved 4087 children 4–18 years of age vaccinated at 17 clinical sites in the United States [85]. This large trial employed the 0–1–12 months schedule approved for use in adults. As in European children, the vaccine was safe and highly immunogenic, with 100% of U.S. children attaining a presumptively protective antibody level by 1 month after the third injection. LYMErix induced threefold higher antibody titers in these children and adolescents than in adults previously tested [70]. No efficacy trials in children have been reported. In the fall of 1999, GSK filed a supplement for the use of LYMErix in children <14 years old, which was pending before the FDA until the vaccine was withdrawn by GSK on February 25, 2002 [95].

Safety

Commonly reported adverse events. A summary of adverse reactions to LYMErix was published in the Physicians' Desk Reference [96]. Clinical trials involved 6478 individuals who received a total of 18,047 doses, including 5469 vaccinated individuals who participated in the randomized, placebo-controlled Phase III trial [70]. LYMErix was generally well tolerated, with pain at the injection site being the most common adverse event (AE), reported more often in vaccine than placebo recipients. These local inflammatory reactions were usually mild, generally resolved spontaneously, and did not increase with subsequent injections.

In all trials combined, systemic reactions occurred in up to 40% of individuals, with headache and fatigue being the most frequent. Most systemic symptoms were rated as mild, spontaneously resolved within 72 hr, and, like local reactions, did not increase with subsequent vaccinations [96]. There were no significant differences in the incidence of clinical arthritis or musculoskeletal inflammation. The original cohort of vaccinees from the Phase III LYMErix trial has shown no pattern of late-onset vaccine-related serious AEs after 36 months of follow-up [89].

As with any biological product or drug, previously unrecognized AEs may occur during postlicensure use in a larger number of individuals [97]. Therefore AEs reported to the Vaccine Adverse Event Reporting System (VAERS) during the first 19 months of the vaccine's licensure were evaluated for unexpected patterns in age, gender, time to onset, dose number, and clinical characteristics [98]. Over 1,400,000 vaccine doses were distributed, and 905 AEs were reported to VAERS. Except for the 22 hypersensitivity reactions, the AEs reported to VAERS were consistent with AEs noted during the Phase III clinical trial.

Uncommon adverse events—evidence for induction of arthritis. There is a theoretical, albeit serious, concern that an OspA-based vaccine for LD might induce chronic inflammatory arthritis in genetically susceptible individuals through a molecular mimicry mechanism [13,62,99,100]. The arguments for [1,89] and against [101] molecular mimicry have been published. To summarize, antibiotic-resistant arthritis is a chronic inflammatory joint disease that follows Bb infection in ~10% of patients [102]. Major histocompatibility complex (MHC) class II HLA-DR4 alleles are associated with an increased risk of chronic antibiotic-refractory arthritis. During the treatment-resistant phase of the disease, these individuals often develop high titers of IgG antibodies against OspA, especially the C-terminal epitope of OspA [13]. This epitope is present in LYMErix vaccine. This immunodominant T-cell epitope of OspA (OspA$_{165-173}$) and human lymphocyte function-associated antigen 1 (hLFA-1$\alpha_{L332-340}$) cross-react [99]. HLA-DR4-positive patients with chronic Lyme arthritis, but not HLA-DR4-negative patients or HLA-DR4-positive persons without chronic arthritis, mount a strong T-cell response against hLFA-1 [99]. T cells that react to (OspA$_{165-173}$) are concentrated in the joints of these patients and react with HLFA-1 [104]. In theory, when hLFA-1$\alpha_{L332-340}$ is processed and presented by the HLA-DRB1*0401 molecule, this self-peptide may behave as a partial agonist for such OspA-reactive T cells [100].

However suggestive, this example of epitope mimicry cannot yet be considered definitive. First, there is the lack of an adequate rodent model. HLA-DRB1*0401 transgenic mice injected with OspA responded primarily to the relevant OspA$_{165-173}$, but developed no signs of arthritis [99]. Second, although intense expression of LFA-1 on T cells

among patients with antibiotic treatment-resistant arthritis exists, it is yet unclear if MHC class II molecules in the synovial lesions actually present the LFA-1$\alpha_{L332-340}$ peptide [103]. Finally, there are no clues as to what precipitates an inflammatory response several months after the borrelial infection [101].

Possible Lyme vaccine-associated chronic arthritis was reported recently in two children and two adults [105]. There were spectra of changes including severe polyarthritis. Such clinical reports need to be confirmed by long-term follow-up of vaccinated individuals as high-priority studies. A more detailed analysis of the theoretical concern of autoimmune induction in vaccinees has been published [89].

Another theoretical safety problem is that the rOspA vaccine may prime some vaccinees to develop arthritis after they receive an infected tick bite, particularly if protective borreliacidal antibodies have waned or have never developed.

Litigation. Both class action and individual lawsuits have been filed against GSK alleging that "LYMErix™ effectively introduces high levels of OspA into the blood stream and places HLA-DR4-positive recipients (who make up 30% of the general population) at risk of developing the autoimmune reaction of treatment-resistant Lyme arthritis" [89]. The complaint charges that GSK should advise the general population and physicians to have patients undergo blood testing to assure that they are HLA-DR4-negative before the administration of LYMErix. This suit alleges that the vaccine itself may cause the "autoimmune condition" of "treatment-resistant Lyme arthritis," so the caution printed in the package insert against administering the vaccine to individuals with a history of treatment-resistant Lyme arthritis is inadequate [97]. It must be recognized that about 1.4 million doses of vaccine have been distributed, representing some 400,000 vaccinees, and except for four suggestive cases, all self-limiting and inconsequential in the long run [105], there are no documented cases of vaccine-induced chronic arthritis to substantiate the risk narrated in the complaint: "risk of a chronic, degenerative, and incurable autoimmune disease." Nevertheless, many clinicians are reluctant in the current legal climate to recommend LYMErix for their patients who meet the criteria for its administration.

GlaxoSmithKline initiated a large, FDA-mandated Phase IV study to address unanswered questions about LYMErix-induced arthritis. As of February 2001, only 15% of the targeted 25,000 subjects were enrolled [106]. The target number will not be reached, as GSK removed LYMErix from the market on February 25, 2002 because of dwindling sales, undoubtedly influenced by the concerns presented above.

Effect of LYMErix on Serological Diagnosis. The OspA vaccine confounds well-established serological test results by inducing a positive reaction in ELISA assays containing whole Bb organisms [107]. As expected, most persons develop the expected 31-kDa OspA band in response to the vaccine. But some individuals, particularly after multiple doses, unexpectedly develop antibodies reactive with other Bb antigens in their IgG Western blots, such as to 66-, 41-, 31-, and 21-kDa antigens [107]. Some of these Western blot patterns are broad enough to satisfy the criteria for Bb infection and the diagnosis of LD. These confusing serological results reported after rOspA vaccination have several theoretical explanations, from induction of cross-reactivity to laboratory artifact. An investigational ELISA utilizing recombinant chimeric *Borrelia* proteins devoid of OspA has distinguished persons naturally infected with Bb from OspA vaccinees [108]. Recently, an ELISA based on the Bb peptide *VlsE* C6 was approved by the FDA to differentiate between cases of natural Bb infections and rOspA vaccinees (C6 Bb [Lyme] ELISA; Immunogenics, Cambridge, MA).

2. ImuLyme™ (Aventis Pasteur)

Two formulations of a lipidated OspA vaccine [69] were studied by Connaught Laboratories (now Aventis Pasteur) in two Phase I trials [59,60]. No preclinical animal studies of the exact human formulation have been reported, although the vaccine prototype was safe and protective in rodents [69]. Two or three 10-µg doses of unabsorbed or alum-absorbed formulations injected at 0, 1, and 6 months were equally safe. The vaccines were immunogenic in 92% of vaccinees. Serum borreliacidal activity nearly disappeared within 5 months, although it was restimulated in all 12 vaccinees tested 1 month after the 6-month booster [59].

In a preliminary report of a Phase II dose-seeking study, two injections of placebo or of 1-, 5-, 10-, or 30-µg doses of the nonadjuvanted lipidated OspA vaccine were administered to 330 adult volunteers [109]. The ELISA seroconversion rates in volunteers varied as a function of vaccine dose, and ranged from 2.4% (1-µg dose) to 97.6% (30-µg dose). Borreliacidal titers were not reported. Both vaccine injections and all vaccine doses were equally safe with minimal side effects observed.

Two efficacy trials of the Connaught Laboratories rOspA vaccine have been conducted [71,110]. The larger trial was conducted in 10,305 persons aged 18–92 years old enrolled at 14 U.S. study sites in five states endemic for LD. Volunteers received two doses of either 30 µg of ImuLyme or placebo given 1 month apart; 7515 volunteers also received a booster dose at 12 months. The volunteers were observed for two tick transmission seasons. Clinical cases were confirmed by serology but not by culture or PCR. The incidence of asymptomatic seroconversion was not determined. The efficacy of the vaccine was 68% in the first year of the study, and 92% in the second year among subjects who received the third injection; persons immunized twice were not protected during the second transmission season. The vaccine was well tolerated. There was no significant increase in the frequency of arthritis or neurological events in vaccine recipients, including persons with and without a prior history of LD.

The second efficacy trial [110], a subset of the larger trial [71], was conducted on 1634 persons (adolescents to 80 years old) recruited at one site in New York State. Vaccine efficacy was 40% during the first year and 37% during the second year. Vaccine efficacy was absent among persons older than 60 years. The reasons for the lower protective efficacy in this single-site study compared to the multisite study are unclear.

Aventis Pasteur filed an application for license with the FDA in 1998 for its ImuLyme vaccine, but the vaccine has not been marketed.

3. Live Recombinant Bacille Calmette–Guérin OspA (MedImmune, Inc., Gaithersburg, MD)

A Phase I clinical trial was designed to determine the feasibility of using rBCG as a live bacterial vaccine vector for the outer surface protein A (OspA) of *B. burgdorferi* and as model for other vaccines based on a rBCG vector. Investigators at MedImmune, Inc. developed a rBCG vaccine expressing OspA as a membrane-associated lipoprotein. The rBCG OspA vaccine was safe and immunogenic in several animal species, and protective in a mouse model of Lyme borreliosis [111]. One intradermal injection (0.1 ml) of rBCG OspA was administered to 24 healthy adult volunteers sequentially at one of four dose levels, using a dose escalation design. All volunteers were initially negative for PPD skin test and OspA antibody, and they were monitored for 2 years after immunization. Localized, resolving ulcerations typical of BCG vaccination were observed. Thirteen of 24 vaccinees, principally in the two highest dose groups, converted their PPD skin tests from negative to positive, but notably, none of the 24 volunteers developed OspA antibody [112]. The manufacturer has discontinued the vaccine.

B. OspC Multivalent Vaccines (Baxter)

The first reported Phase I trial of an OspC vaccine was sponsored by Baxter (formerly Immuno AG) [113]. The trial was performed in 80 volunteers from the Åland Islands (Finland), a population at high risk of contracting LD (>1% incidence per year). Half of the volunteers were seropositive for Bb, and they received three vaccinations at dose levels of 25 or 50 µg. Seronegative volunteers received dose levels of 10, 25, or 50 µg. The vaccine was adjuvanted with aluminum and was pentavalent in design, comprised of recombinant OspC proteins from one strain of *B. burgdorferi* sensu stricto and two strains each from *B. afzelii* and *B. garinii*. Recombinant OspC was expressed as a nonlipoprotein form in the yeast *Pichia pastoris*. The vaccine appeared to be safe and well tolerated at all dose levels. Mild and moderate local and systemic AEs occurred in a dose-dependent manner. Antibody responses were similarly dose-dependent, and seroconversion against the five component antigens was observed in 95% or greater of the formerly seronegative volunteers receiving the highest dose level.

To determine the antigenic composition necessary for the formulation of a pan-European Lyme vaccine, the *ospC* genes of approximately 300 Bb isolates were analyzed for restriction fragment length polymorphisms to estimate the extent of OspC heterogeneity. Sera from several thousand patients with a variety of LD syndromes, and representing 16 European countries, were screened to determine the most clinically relevant OspC serotypes. These analyses predicted that a cocktail of OspC antigens from 14 Bb strains, including two from *B. burgdorferi*, six from *B. afzelii*, and six from *B. garinii*, would provide at least 80% coverage of the most clinically relevant Bb strains. A Phase II trial testing the safety and preliminary efficacy of this 14-valent OspC vaccine formulation has been completed and its data are being analyzed (Dr. Noel Barrett, Baxter, personal communication).

VI. NEXT-GENERATION VACCINES

A. Evaluation of New Subunit Vaccines for Lyme Disease

Much effort has been spent identifying and characterizing the structural and antigenic constituents of Bb. Many of these proteins identified as potential diagnostic antigens, membrane components, or colonization and dissemination factors have also been evaluated as experimental vaccines, usually in mice (Table 1). Their effectiveness as vaccine antigens provides some of the best pieces evidence of their surface exposure on live spirochetes. Direct or indirect evidence indicates that most of these proteins are expressed by Bb in mammalian hosts, and some also in the feeding tick. The functions of most of these antigens are obscure. Bb proteins that bind decorin (DbpA and DbpB), fibronectin (P47/BBK32), and glycosaminoglycans (Bgp) appear to have a role in the adherence of Bb to mammalian extracellular matrix [114–116]. Other than OspA, OspB, and OspC, few of these newer proteins have been successful vaccines. Vaccination with some of these antigens kill Bb in ticks, but only two of these antigens, OspF [117] and P47(BBK32) [118], partially protect mice against tick-borne Bb [41,118]. These two antigens plus VraA and DbpB protect mice against challenge with cultured Bb [119], although the immunity conferred by DbpB is inconsistent [50,119]. Cultured Bb are killed by DbpA antibodies, and spirochetes are killed during the early stages of infection after subcutaneous injection into vaccinated mice [50]. DbpA antibodies also have borreliacidal activity with strain cross-reactivity rivaling that of OspA. However, tick-borne Bb expresses little DbpA, presumably until entering the mammalian host, and transmission-blocking immunity is ineffective [120]. Most Bb anti-gens tested for vaccine effectiveness are biochemically confirmed or presumptive lipoproteins except for one outer membrane-spanning protein (Oms66), which conferred partial immunity against host-adapted Bb [121].

B. Multicomponent and Chimeric Protein Vaccines

Hypothetically, a combination vaccine composed of Bb antigens upregulated in the tick and in the mammalian host will enhance transmission-blocking immunity and will supplement mammalian-stage immunity against infection or disease. The model combining antigens from multiple stages of infection has its origin in malaria vaccine development. Validation of this approach for Bb has just begun. A combination vaccine comprised of vector-stage OspA and mammalian-stage DbpA was much more effective than either OspA or DbpA alone at protecting mice from cultured Bb, and mice were better protected against heterologous Bb

isolates [122]. OspA–DbpA vaccines remain to be tested against tick-borne Bb.

Vaccination of mice with a DNA plasmid expressing a OspA–OspC chimeric fusion elicited antibodies to both proteins, but protective antibodies appeared to be primarily against OspA, suggesting that further refinement of this strategy is required [123].

C. Genomics

The complete nucleotide sequence of the large linear chromosome of Bb sensu stricto strain B31 and 17 of its 21 plasmids was reported in 1997, and these genomic data were subsequently refined further, including the sequencing of the additional plasmids [124,125]. The relatively small Bb genome has several striking features. First, no homologs of surface proteins, virulence factors, or vaccine antigens from other pathogens are yet recognizable in the Bb genome. Second, the Bb genome encodes at least 132 presumptive lipopoteins, more than any other bacterium to date. Much work remains to screen for vaccine candidates among the additional members of this class of membrane proteins. Third, the existence of multiple paralogs of several lipoprotein genes (such as the *VlsE* locus), either clustered or distributed on multiple plasmids, suggests several potential mechanisms for antigenic variation.

D. Challenges of *B. burdorferi* Antigenic Modulation and Phenotypical Heterogeneity

B. burdorferi adapts to the different environments encountered during transmission through the tick vector by changes that include alteration of its surface protein phenotype and consequent antigenic modulation. OspA and OspC are the prototypes of such modulated antigens. Additional temporal or tissue-specific gene expression by Bb also occurs during the infection of mammalian hosts [126,127]. One example is the lipoprotein Arp (ErpT), which is an antigenic target for the resolution of Lyme arthritis in mice, but Arp antibodies do not alter carditis [118]. Another example is DbpA, which is expressed by the majority of Bb, infecting heart tissues of mice, but is expressed by few spirochetes in ear tissues [128].

An important, emerging issue affecting vaccine design and interpretation of data in vaccinated animal models is the striking heterogeneity of Bb phenotypes. As discussed in "Immunity to Tick-Borne *B. burgdorferi*," initial observations on antigen expression by tick-stage Bb using immunohistochemistry suggested that the spirochete population shifts from expressing OspA to OspC during transmission [31,44]. However, substantial heterogeneity exists within the Bb population at each stage of transmission, including many spirochetes expressing either both OspA and OspC or neither antigen [129]. Another immunohistochemical study has recently detected a heterogeneous expression of protective antigens OspC and DbpA in mice at various sites of disseminated Bb infection [128]. These studies suggest that second-generation vaccines will require either: 1) identification of a new antigenic target that is both constitutively expressed at multiple stages of Bb transmission and infection and is serologically conserved; or 2) different antigens, each inducing immunity against its unique antigenic target expressed at different stages of transmission and infection. Lastly, Bb phenotypical heterogeneity is also present in vitro, even for cloned Bb isolates [122,130], suggesting that partial protection against challenges with cultured Bb need to be reinterpreted; such vaccine candidates may be effective in combination with other antigens.

VII. CONCLUSION

Less than 20 years elapsed between the 1982 report of the identification and isolation of *B. burgdorferi* and the licensure and marketing in the United States of a prophylactic vaccine against this pathogen. However, the evolving understanding of the agent's antigenic complexity, the elucidation of the unique and unanticipated mechanism of protection of the first-generation vaccine, and the progress on determining LD immunopathogenesis have fueled concerns about autoimmune reactions to the OspA antigen. Such concerns have combined to limit the acceptance of LYMErix and have lead to its withdrawal from the marketplace. Second-generation polyvalent OspC vaccines may overcome some of these concerns, but the precise antigenic components required for efficacy are uncertain. The development of the next generation of novel-antigen or multiantigen LD vaccines is in its infancy.

REFERENCES

1.   Steere AC. Lyme disease. N Engl J Med 2001; 345:115–125.
2.   Benach JL, et al. Spirochetes isolated from the blood of two patients with Lyme disease. N Engl J Med 1983; 308: 740–742.
3.   Wang G, et al. Molecular typing of *Borrelia burgdorferi* sensu lato: taxonomic, epidemiological, and clinical implications. Clin Microbiol Rev 1999; 12:633–653.
4.   van Dam AP, et al. Different genospecies of *Borrelia burgdorferi* are associated with distinct clinical manifestations of Lyme borreliosis. Clin Infect Dis 1993; 17:708–717.
5.   Strle F. Lyme borreliosis in Slovenia. Zentralbl Bakteriol 1999; 289:643–652.
6.   James AM, et al. *Borrelia lonestari* infection after a bite by an *Amblyomma americanum* tick. J Infect Dis 2001; 183: 1810–1814.
7.   Anderson JF, Magnarelli LA. A tick-associated disease originally described in Europe, but named after a town in Connecticut. Am Entomol 1994; 217–227.
8.   Steere AC, et al. Lyme arthritis: an epidemic of oligoarticular arthritis in children and adults in three Connecticut communities. Arthritis Rheum 1977; 20:7–17.
9.   Orloski KA, et al. Surveillance for Lyme disease—United States, 1992–1998. Morb Mortal Wkly Rep CDC Surveill Summ 2000; 49:1–11.
10. Coyle BS, et al. The public health impact of Lyme disease in Maryland. J Infect Dis 1996; 173:1260–1262.
11. Klempner MS, et al. Two controlled trials of antibiotic treatment in patients with persistent symptoms and a history of Lyme disease. N Engl J Med 2001; 345:85–92.
12. Steere AC, et al. Association of chronic Lyme arthritis with HLA-DR4 and HLA-DR2 alleles. N Engl J Med 1990; 323:219–223 [published erratum appears in N Engl J Med Jan 10 1991; 324(2):129].
13. Kalish RA, et al. Early and late antibody responses to full-length and truncated constructs of outer surface protein A of *Borrelia burgdorferi* in Lyme disease. Infect Immun 1995; 63:2228–2235.
14. Dressler F, et al. Western blotting in the serodiagnosis of Lyme disease. J Infect Dis 1993; 167:392–400.
15. Barbour AG, et al. Lyme disease spirochetes and ixodid tick spirochetes share a common surface antigenic determinant defined by a monoclonal antibody. Infect Immun 1983; 41: 795–804.
16. Will G, et al. Sequence analysis of OspA genes shows homogeneity within *Borrelia burgdorferi* sensu stricto and *Borrelia afzelii* strains but reveals major subgroups within the *Borrelia garinii* species. Med Microbiol Immunol (Berl) 1995; 184:73–80.
17. Sadziene A, et al. A bactericidal antibody to *Borrelia burgdorferi* is directed against a variable region of the OspB protein. Infect Immun 1994; 62:2037–2045.
18. Shoberg RJ, et al. Identification of a highly cross-reactive outer surface protein B epitope among diverse geographic isolates of *Borrelia* spp. causing Lyme disease. J Clin Microbiol 1994; 32:489–500.
19. Jauris-Heipke S, et al. Molecular analysis of genes encoding outer surface protein C (OspC) of *Borrelia burgdorferi* sensu lato: relationship to OspA genotype and evidence of lateral gene exchange of OspC. J Clin Microbiol 1995; 33:1860–1866.
20. Pal U, et al. Inhibition of *Borrelia burgdorferi*–tick interactions in vivo by outer surface protein A antibody. J Immunol 2001; 166:7398–7403.
21. Hanrahan JP, et al. Incidence and cumulative frequency of endemic Lyme disease in a community. J Infect Dis 1984; 150:489–496.
22. Fahrer H, et al. The prevalence and incidence of clinical and asymptomatic Lyme borreliosis in a population at risk. J Infect Dis 1991; 163:305–310.
23. Curran KL, et al. Reduction of nymphal *Ixodes dammini* (Acari: Ixodidae) in a residential suburban landscape by area application of insecticides. J Med Entomol 1993; 30:107–113.
24. Deblinger RD, et al. Reduced abundance of immature *Ixodes dammini* (Acari: Ixodidae) following incremental removal of deer. J Med Entomol 1993; 30:144–150.
25. Shadick NA, et al. Determinants of tick-avoidance behaviors in an endemic area for Lyme disease. Am J Prev Med 1997; 13:265–270.
26. Barbour AG, Fish D. The biological and social phenomenon of Lyme disease. Science 1993; 260:1610–1616.
27. Dattwyler RJ, et al. Seronegative Lyme disease. Dissociation of specific T- and B-lymphocyte responses to *Borrelia burgdorferi* [see comments]. N Engl J Med 1988; 319:1441–1446.
28. Johnson RC, et al. Passive immunization of hamsters against experimental infection with the Lyme disease spirochete. Infect Immun 1986; 53:713–714.
29. Fikrig E, et al. Protection of mice against the Lyme disease agent by immunizing with recombinant OspA. Science 1990; 250:553–556.
30. Simon MM, et al. Recombinant outer surface protein a from *Borrelia burgdorferi* induces antibodies protective against spirochetal infection in mice. J Infect Dis 1991; 164:123–132.
31. Schwan TG, et al. Induction of an outer surface protein on *Borrelia burgdorferi* during tick feeding. Proc Natl Acad Sci USA 1995; 92:2909–2913.
32. Schwan TG, Piesman J. Temporal changes in outer surface proteins A and C of the Lyme disease-associated spirochete, *Borrelia burgdorferi*, during the chain of infection in ticks and mice. J Clin Microbiol 2000; 38:382–388.
33. Edelman R. Perspective on the development of vaccines against Lyme disease. Vaccine 1991; 9:531–532.
34. Nowakowski J, et al. Culture-confirmed infection and re-

infection with *Borrelia burgdorferi*. Ann Intern Med 1997; 127:130–132.

35. Johnson RC, et al. Active immunization of hamsters against experimental infection with *Borrelia burgdorferi*. Infect Immun 1986; 54:897–898.

36. Schmitz JL, et al. Passive immunization prevents induction of Lyme arthritis in LSH hamsters. Infect Immun 1990; 58: 144–148 [published erratum appears in N Engl J Med Feb 1993; 61(2):791].

37. Piesman J. Dynamics of *Borrelia burgdorferi* transmission by nymphal *Ixodes dammini* ticks. J Infect Dis 1993; 167: 1082–1085.

38. Kahl O, et al. Risk of infection with *Borrelia burgdorferi* sensu lato for a host in relation to the duration of nymphal *Ixodes ricinus* feeding and the method of tick removal. Zentralbl Bakteriol 1998; 287:41–52.

39. Shih CM, et al. Short report: mode of action of protective immunity to Lyme disease spirochetes. Am J Trop Med Hyg 1995; 52:72–74.

40. Fikrig E, et al. Elimination of *Borrelia burgdorferi* from vector ticks feeding on OspA-immunized mice. Proc Natl Acad Sci USA 1992; 89:5418–5421.

41. Nguyen TP, et al. Partial destruction of *Borrelia burgdorferi* within ticks that engorged on OspE- or OspF-immunized mice. Infect Immun 1994; 62:2079–2084.

42. Telford SR III, et al. Efficacy of human Lyme disease vaccine formulations in a mouse model. J Infect Dis 1995; 171:1368–1370.

43. Piesman J, et al. Duration of tick attachment and *Borrelia burgdorferi* transmission. J Clin Microbiol 1987; 25:557–558.

44. de Silva AM, et al. *Borrelia burgdorferi* OspA is an arthropod-specific transmission-blocking Lyme disease vaccine. J Exp Med 1996; 183:271–275.

45. Gilmore RD Jr, Piesman J. Inhibition of *Borrelia burgdorferi* migration from the midgut to the salivary glands following feeding by ticks on OspC-immunized mice. Infect Immun 2000; 68:411–414.

46. Zhong W, et al. Therapeutic passive vaccination against chronic Lyme disease in mice. Proc Natl Acad Sci USA 1997; 94:12533–12538.

47. Piesman J, et al. Duration of immunity to reinfection with tick-transmitted *Borrelia burgdorferi* in naturally infected mice. Infect Immun 1997; 65:4043–4047.

48. Lovrich SD, et al. Seroprotective groups of Lyme borreliosis spirochetes from North America and Europe. J Infect Dis 1995; 170:115–121.

49. Schaible UE, et al. Immune sera to individual *Borrelia burgdorferi* isolates or recombinant OspA thereof protect SCID mice against infection with homologous strains but only partially or not at all against those of different OspA/ OspB genotype. Vaccine 1993; 11:1049–1054.

50. Hanson MS, et al. Active and passive immunity against *Borrelia burgdorferi* decorin-binding protein A (DbpA) protects against infection. Infect Immun 1998; 66:2143–2153.

51. Probert WS, et al. Immunization with outer surface protein (Osp) A, but not OspC, provides cross-protection of mice challenged with North American isolates of *Borrelia burgdorferi*. J Infect Dis 1997; 175:400–405.

52. Telford SR III, et al. Protection against antigenically variable *Borrelia burgdorferi* conferred by recombinant vaccines. J Exp Med 1993; 178:755–758.

53. Golde WT, et al. The Lyme disease vaccine candidate outer surface protein A (OspA) in a formulation compatible with human use protects mice against natural tick transmission of *B. burgdorferi*. Vaccine 1995; 13:435–441.

54. Barthold SW. Specificity of infection-induced immunity among *Borrelia burgdorferi* sensu lato species. Infect Immun 1999; 67:36–42.

55. Gern L, et al. Immunization with a polyvalent OspA vaccine protects mice against *Ixodes ricinus* tick bites infected by *Borrelia burgdorferi* ss, *Borrelia garinii* and *Borrelia afzelii*. Vaccine 1997; 15:1551–1557.

56. Lovrich SD, et al. Borreliacidal activity of sera from hamsters infected with the Lyme disease spirochete. Infect Immun 1991; 59:2522–2528.

57. Sadziene A, et al. In vitro inhibition of *Borrelia burgdorferi* growth by antibodies. J Infect Dis 1993; 167:165–172.

58. Schmitz JL, et al. Depletion of complement and effects on passive transfer of resistance to infection with *Borrelia burgdorferi*. Infect Immun 1991; 59:3815–3818.

59. Keller D, et al. Safety and immunogenicity of a recombinant outer surface protein A Lyme vaccine. JAMA 1994; 271:1764–1768.

60. Padilla ML, et al. Characterization of the protective *Borrelia*cidal antibody response in humans and hamsters after vaccination with a *Borrelia burgdorferi* outer surface protein A vaccine. J Infect Dis 1996; 174:739–746.

61. Benach JL, et al. Interactions of phagocytes with the Lyme disease spirochete: role of the Fc receptor. J Infect Dis 1984; 150:497–507.

62. Lengl-Janssen B, et al. The T helper cell response in Lyme arthritis: differential recognition of *Borrelia burgdorferi* outer surface protein A in patients with treatment-resistant or treatment-responsive Lyme arthritis. J Exp Med 1994; 180:2069–2078.

63. Schaible UE, et al. Monoclonal antibodies specific for the outer surface protein A (OspA) of *Borrelia burgdorferi* prevent Lyme borreliosis in severe combined immunodeficiency (scid) mice. Proc Natl Acad Sci USA 1990; 87:3768–3772.

64. Van Hoecke C, et al. Evaluation of the safety, reactogenicity and immunogenicity of three recombinant outer surface protein (OspA) Lyme vaccines in healthy adults. Vaccine 1996; 14:1620–1626.

65. Van Hoecke C, et al. Clinical and immunological assessment of a candidate Lyme disease vaccine in healthy adults: antibody persistence and effect of a booster dose at month 12. Vaccine 1998; 16:1688–1692.

66. Probert WS, LeFebvre RB. Protection of C3H/HeN mice from challenge with *Borrelia burgdorferi* through active immunization with OspA, OspB, or OspC, but not with OspD or the 83-kilodalton antigen. Infect Immun 1994; 62: 1920–1926.

67. Rousselle JC, et al. Borreliacidal antibody production against outer surface protein C of *Borrelia burgdorferi*. J Infect Dis 1998; 178:733–741.

68. Fikrig E, et al. Roles of OspA, OspB, and flagellin in protective immunity to Lyme borreliosis in laboratory mice. Infect Immun 1992; 60:657–661.

69. Erdile LF, et al. Role of attached lipid in immunogenicity of *Borrelia burgdorferi* OspA. Infect Immun 1993; 61:81–90.

70. Steere AC, et al. Vaccination against Lyme disease with recombinant *Borrelia burgdorferi* outer-surface lipoprotein A with adjuvant. N Engl J Med 1998; 339:209–215.

71. Sigal LH, et al. A Vaccine consisting of recombinant *Borrelia burgdorferi* outer-surface protein A to prevent Lyme disease. N Engl J Med 1998; 339:216–222.

72. Kazmierczak JJ, Sorhage FE. Current understanding of *Borrelia burgdorferi* infection, with emphasis on its prevention in dogs. J Am Vet Med Assoc 1993; 203:1524–1528.

73. Levy SA, et al. Performance of a *Borrelia burgdorferi* bacterin in borreliosis-endemic areas. J Am Vet Med Assoc 1993; 202:1834–1838.

74. Lim LC, et al. Development of destructive arthritis in vaccinated hamsters challenged with *Borrelia burgdorferi*. Infect Immun 1994; 62:2825–2833.

75. Lim LC, et al. *Borrelia burgdorferi*-specific T lymphocytes

induce severe destructive Lyme arthritis. Infect Immun 1995; 63:1400–1408.

76. Aberer E, et al. Molecular mimicry and Lyme borreliosis: a shared antigenic determinant between *Borrelia burgdorferi* and human tissue. Ann Neurol 1989; 26:732–737.

77. Sigal LH. Cross-reactivity between *Borrelia burgdorferi* flagellin and a human axonal 64,000 molecular weight protein. J Infect Dis 1993; 167:1372–1378.

78. Coughlin RT, et al. Protection of dogs from Lyme disease with a vaccine containing outer surface protein (Osp) A, OspB, and the saponin adjuvant QS21. J Infect Dis 1995; 171:1049–1052.

79. Ma J, et al. Impact of the saponin adjuvant QS-21 and aluminium hydroxide on the immunogenicity of recombinant OspA and OspB of *Borrelia burgdorferi*. Vaccine 1994; 12:925–932.

80. Philipp MT, et al. The outer surface protein A (OspA) vaccine against Lyme disease: efficacy in the rhesus monkey. Vaccine 1997; 15:1872–1887.

81. Van Hoecke C, et al. Alternative vaccination schedules (0, 1, and 6 months versus 0, 1, and 12 months) for a recombinant OspA Lyme disease vaccine. Clin Infect Dis 1999; 28:1260–1264.

82. Schoen RT, et al. Safety and immunogenicity profile of a recombinant outer-surface protein A Lyme disease vaccine: clinical trial of a 3-dose schedule at 0, 1, and 2 months. Clin Ther 2000; 22:315–325.

83. Feder HM Jr, et al. Immunogenicity of a recombinant *Borrelia burgdorferi* outer surface protein A vaccine against Lyme disease in children. J Pediatr 1999; 135:575–579.

84. Beran J, et al. Reactogenicity and immunogenicity of a Lyme disease vaccine in children 2–5 years old. Clin Infect Dis 2000; 31:1504–1507.

85. Sikand VK, et al. Safety and immunogenicity of a recombinant *Borrelia burgdorferi* outer surface protein A vaccine against Lyme disease in healthy children and adolescents: a randomized controlled trial. Pediatrics 2001; 108:123–128.

86. Golde WT, et al. Reactivity with a specific epitope of outer surface protein A predicts protection from infection with the Lyme disease spirochete, *Borrelia burgdorferi*. Infect Immun 1997; 65:882–889.

87. Centers for Disease Control and Prevention. Recommendations for the use of Lyme disease vaccine. Morb Mortal Wkly Rep 1999; 48(RR-7):1–25.

88. American Academy of Pediatrics Committee on Infectious Diseases. Prevention of Lyme disease. Pediatrics 2000; 105:142–147.

89. Rahn DW. Lyme vaccine: issues and controversies. Infect Dis Clin North Am 2001; 15:171–187.

90. Meltzer MI, et al. The cost effectiveness of vaccinating against Lyme disease. Emerg Infect Dis 1999; 5:321–328.

91. Institute of Medicine. Vaccines for the 21st Century: A Tool for Decision Making. Washington, DC: National Academy Press, 1999:1–476.

92. Shadick NA, et al. The cost-effectiveness of vaccination against Lyme disease. Arch Intern Med 2001; 161:554–561.

93. Shapiro ED, Gerber MA. Lyme disease. Clin Infect Dis 2000; 31:533–542.

94. Sigal LH. Misconceptions about Lyme disease: confusions hiding behind ill-chosen terminology. Ann Intern Med 2002; 136:413–419.

95. Anonymous. Lyme disease vaccine is taken off market. Washington Post A February 27, 2002; 10.

96. Physicians' Desk Reference. Montvale, NJ: Medical Economics Company, Inc., 2002:1592–1596.

97. Braun MM, Ellenberg SS. Descriptive epidemiology of adverse events after immunization: reports to the Vaccine Adverse Event Reporting System (VAERS), 1991–1994. J Pediatr 1997; 131, 529–535.

98. Lathrop SL, et al. Adverse event reports following vaccination for Lyme disease: December 1998–July 2000. Vaccine 2002; 20:1603–1608.

99. Gross DM, et al. Identification of LFA-1 as a candidate autoantigen in treatment-resistant Lyme arthritis. Science 1998; 281:703–706.

100. Trollmo C, et al. Molecular mimicry in Lyme arthritis demonstrated at the single cell level: LFA-1 alpha L is a partial agonist for outer surface protein A-reactive T cells. J Immunol 2001; 166:5286–5291.

101. Benoist C, Mathis D. Autoimmunity provoked by infection: how good is the case for T cell epitope mimicry? Nat Immunol 2001; 2:797–801.

102. Steere AC, et al. Treatment of Lyme arthritis. Arthritis Rheum 1994; 37:878–888.

103. Akin E, et al. Expression of adhesion molecules in synovia of patients with treatment-resistant Lyme arthritis. Infect Immun 2001; 69:1774–1780.

104. Meyer AL, et al. Direct enumeration of *Borrelia*-reactive CD4 T cells ex vivo by using MHC class II tetramers. Proc Natl Acad Sci USA 2000; 97:11433–11438.

105. Rose CD, et al. Arthritis following recombinant outer surface protein A vaccination for Lyme disease. J Rheumatol 2001; 28:2555–2557.

106. FDA LYMErix study to test potential genetic marker for adverse events. Pink Sheet February 5, 2001; 63(3).

107. Molloy PJ, et al. Detection of multiple reactive protein species by immunoblotting after recombinant outer surface protein A Lyme disease vaccination. Clin Infect Dis 2000; 31, 42–47.

108. Gomes-Solecki MJ, et al. Recombinant assay for serodiagnosis of Lyme disease regardless of OspA vaccination status. J Clin Microbiol 2002; 40:193–197.

109. Marks DH, et al. Clinical studies in humans of outer surface protein A (OspA) vaccine for Lyme disease. VIth International Conference on Lyme Borreliosis, Bologna, Italy, June 19–22, 1994.

110. Wormser GP, et al. Efficacy of an OspA vaccine preparation for prevention of Lyme disease in New York State. Infection 1998; 26:208–212.

111. Stover CK, et al. Protective immunity elicited by recombinant bacille Calmette–Guérin (BCG) expressing outer surface protein A (OspA) lipoprotein: a candidate Lyme disease vaccine. J Exp Med 1993; 178:197–209.

112. Edelman R, et al. Safety and immunogenicity of recombinant bacille Calmette–Guérin (rBCG) expressing *Borrelia burgdorferi* outer surface protein A (OspA) lipoprotein in adult volunteers: a candidate Lyme disease vaccine. Vaccine 1999; 17:904–914.

113. Eder G, et al. A candidate OspC Lyme disease vaccine under clinical investigation. Zentralbl Bakteriol 1999; 289:688–689.

114. Guo BP, et al. Decorin-binding adhesins from *Borrelia burgdorferi*. Mol Microbiol 1998; 30:711–723.

115. Probert WS, et al. Mapping the ligand-binding region of *Borrelia burgdorferi* fibronectin-binding protein BBK32. Infect Immun 2001; 69:4129–4133.

116. Parveen N, Leong JM. Identification of a candidate glycosaminoglycan-binding adhesin of the Lyme disease spirochete *Borrelia burgdorferi*. Mol Microbiol 2000; 35:1220–1234.

117. Lam TT, et al. Outer surface proteins E and F of *Borrelia burgdorferi*, the agent of Lyme disease. Infect Immun 1994; 62:290–298.

118. Fikrig E, et al. Arthropod- and host-specific *Borrelia burgdorferi* bbk32 expression and the inhibition of spirochete transmission. J Immunol 2000; 164:5344–5351.

119. Labandeira-Rey M, et al. VraA (BBI16) protein of *Borrelia burgdorferi* is a surface-exposed antigen with a repetitive motif that confers partial protection against experimental Lyme borreliosis. Infect Immun 2001; 69:1409–1419.

120. Hagman KE, et al. Decorin-binding protein A (DbpA) of *Borrelia burgdorferi* is not protective when immunized mice are challenged via tick infestation and correlates with the lack of DbpA expression by *B. burgdorferi* in ticks. Infect Immun 2000; 68:4759–4764.

121. Exner MM, et al. Protection elicited by native outer membrane protein Oms66 (p66) against host-adapted *Borrelia burgdorferi*: conformational nature of bactericidal epitopes. Infect Immun 2000; 68:2647–2654.

122. Hanson MS, et al. Evidence for vaccine synergy between *Borrelia burgdorferi* decorin-binding protein A and outer surface protein A in the mouse model of Lyme borreliosis. Infect Immun 2000; 68:6457–6460.

123. Wallich R, et al. DNA vaccines expressing a fusion product of outer surface proteins A and C from *Borrelia burgdorferi* induce protective antibodies suitable for prophylaxis but not for resolution of Lyme disease. Infect Immun 2001; 69:2130–2136.

124. Fraser CM, et al. Genomic sequence of a Lyme disease spirochaete, *Borrelia burgdorferi*. Nature 1997; 390:580–586.

125. Casjens S, et al. A bacterial genome in flux: the twelve linear and nine circular extrachromosomal DNAs in an infectious isolate of the Lyme disease spirochete *Borrelia burgdorferi*. Mol Microbiol 2000; 35:490–516.

126. Das S, et al. Temporal pattern of *Borrelia burgdorferi* p21 expression in ticks and the mammalian host. J Clin Invest 1997; 99:987–995.

127. Fikrig E, et al. *Borrelia burgdorferi* erpT expression in the arthropod vector and murine host. Mol Microbiol 1999; 31:281–290.

128. Patel NK, et al. Immunohistochemical analysis of lipoprotein antigens expressed by *Borrelia burgorferi* during persistent infection of mice provides insights into the pathogenesis of Lyme disease. Mod Pathol 2000; 13:171A.

129. Ohnishi J, et al. Antigenic and genetic heterogeneity of *Borrelia burgdorferi* populations transmitted by ticks. Proc Natl Acad Sci USA 2001; 98:670–675.

130. Fingerle V, et al. Differential expression of outer surface proteins A and C by individual *Borrelia burgdorferi* in different genospecies. Med Microbiol Immunol (Berl) 2000; 189:59–66.

131. Gilmore RD Jr, et al. Outer surface protein C (OspC), but not P39, is a protective immunogen against a tick-transmitted *Borrelia burgdorferi* challenge: evidence for a conformational protective epitope in OspC. Infect Immun 1996; 64:2234–2239.

132. Feng S, et al. Lyme arthritis resolution with antiserum to a 37-kilodalton *Borrelia burgdorferi* protein. Infect Immun 2000; 68:4169–4173.

133. Barthold SW, et al. Protective and arthritis-resolving activity in sera of mice infected with *Borrelia burgdorferi*. Clin Infect Dis 1997; 25(Suppl 1):S9–S17.

134. Lahdenne P, et al. Molecular characterization of a 6.6-kilodalton *Borrelia burgdorferi* outer membrane-associated lipoprotein (lp6.6) which appears to be downregulated during mammalian infection. Infect Immun 1997; 65:412–421.

135. Liang FT, et al. C-terminal invariable domain of *VlsE* may not serve as target for protective immune response against *Borrelia burgdorferi*. Infect Immun 2001; 69:1337–1343.

136. Fikrig E, et al. *Borrelia burgdorferi* P35 and P37 proteins, expressed in vivo, elicit protective immunity. Immunity 1997; 6:531–539.

137. Das S, et al. Characterization of a 30-kDa *Borrelia burgdorferi* substrate-binding protein homologue. Res Microbiol 1996; 147:739–751.

138. Feng S, et al. P55, an immunogenic but nonprotective 55-kilodalton *Borrelia burgdorferi* protein in murine Lyme disease. Infect Immun 1996; 64:363–365.

43

Oral B Subunit–Killed Whole-Cell Cholera Vaccine

Jan Holmgren
Gothenburg University, Gothenburg, Sweden

Charlotta Bergquist
SBL Vaccines AB, Stockholm, Sweden

I. INTRODUCTION

Diarrheal diseases remain a leading global health problem. It has been estimated that $(3–5)\times10^9$ episodes of diarrhea, resulting in approximately 4 million deaths, occur annually in developing countries with the highest incidence and severity in children below the age of 5 years [1,2]. About half of these diarrheas are caused by bacteria that produce one or more enterotoxins. Cholera, resulting from infection with *Vibrio cholerae* bacteria, is the most severe of these "enterotoxic enteropathies," while infection with enterotoxigenic *Escherichia coli* (ETEC) is causing the largest number of cases [3,4].

Vibrio cholerae of serogroup O1 is the prototype for the enterotoxin-producing bacteria and was first isolated by Robert Koch in 1884. *V. cholerae* O1 can appear as either of two main different serotypes, Inaba and Ogawa. Until the beginning of the 20th century all examined *V. cholerae* O1 isolates were of the same "classical" biotype. In 1906, however, vibrios of a new biotype, El Tor, were isolated, and for many years vibrios of either the classical or El Tor biotype were isolated from cholera cases.

During the early part of the 19th century, cholera started to spread from its likely ancient home in Bengal, and since then seven major pandemics have been described that have affected large parts of the world. The latest pandemic that took its departure from Celebes in 1961 has spread to and become endemic in many countries in Asia and Africa. Beginning in 1991 cholera has also reappeared as a significant health problem throughout most of South and Central America for the first time in more than 100 years [5]. The causative agent in Latin America appears to be identical to the seventh pandemic O1 El Tor organisms isolated from Asia and Africa.

Since 1993, as yet limited to a few countries in Southeast Asia, a new *V. cholerae* serogroup, O139 Bengal, has been found to cause a variable percentage, usually below 5%, of all cholera cases. If increasing, and even worse, if also spreading to other areas, this new organism may cause yet another major cholera pandemic in parallel with the still ongoing seventh *V. cholerae* O1 El Tor pandemic.

When an epidemic strikes an area where hygiene is poor and health care is not adequate the results can be disastrous, as happened during the refugee crisis in Goma, Zaire, in 1994. An estimated 58,000–80,000 cases and 23,800 deaths occurred within 1 month [6]. Although in endemic areas the highest incidence of cholera is seen in children below 5 years of age, still approximately two-thirds of all *V. cholerae* O1 cases occur in older children and adults in these areas [3,7]. When, on the other hand, cholera has spread to new countries, all age groups have been affected to the same degree. This pattern is probably due to that natural immunity normally develops by age in endemic countries, which is lacking in newly attacked nonendemic areas [8].

The total number of cholera cases annually in the world is uncertain because several affected countries do not monitor or report the disease accurately, in part due to surveillance difficulties but also for fear of economic and social consequences [9]. According to WHO, perhaps only 5–10% of cholera cases are reported. The recent outbreaks of *V. cholerae* O1 in Latin America as well as of *V. cholerae* O139 in Asia have probably resulted in a substantially increased number of cholera cases in the last 5 years. Therefore, the often cited figures of 3–5 million cases and 120,000–200,000 deaths from cholera annually may well be significant underestimates of the present situation.

A cholera-like syndrome can also be seen in some infections with enterotoxigenic *E. coli* (ETEC). ETEC is the most common bacterial cause of diarrhea in developing countries, accounting for an estimated 400 million cases annually. Although many episodes are relatively mild, a sufficient number of cases are severe and it is estimated that disease caused by ETEC is responsible for 300,000–500,000 deaths a year among children under 5 years of age [2]. In addition, ETEC is also the most common cause of traveler's diarrhea isolated in one-third to one-half of these episodes [10].

The disease caused by enterotoxin-producing bacteria such as *V. cholerae* and ETEC is characterized by watery stools without blood and mucus [4]. In most cases, cholera is characterized by acute, profuse watery diarrhea lasting for one or a few days. In a substantial proportion, however, cholera causes dehydrating disease, and in its extreme manifestations, cholera is one of the most rapidly fatal infectious illnesses known. Within 3–4 hr of the onset of symptoms, a previously healthy person may become hypotensive and may die within 6–8 hr. More commonly, fatal cases progress to hypovolemic shock within 6–12 hr with death following in the next one to several days of dehydrating disease. The most severe cholera cases can purge as much as 15–25 L of water and electrolytes per day, and the mortality rate in severe, nontreated cholera is 30–50%. Persons of blood group O are known to have increased risk of developing severe cholera (cholera gravis) when infected [9].

ETEC disease may vary from mild diarrhea to severe cholera-like disease and is often accompanied by nausea, vomiting, abdominal cramps, anorexia, and more often than in cholera also with significant fever [3,4].

The recommended primary treatment for cholera and ETEC today is with simple, oral rehydration solutions containing salts and glucose, which will save lives when properly administered. If the patient is severely dehydrated on arrival to the treatment center, is unable to drink, or if the rate of fluid loss by diarrhea exceeds what can be compensated by oral rehydration, aggressive intravenous fluid rehydration is necessary. With effective rehydration treatment, the case fatality rate may go down to below 1% even in severe cases of cholera. Antibiotics can be used to shorten the duration of cholera disease and decrease the risk for further spread of the infection. WHO recommends that antibiotics be used only in the treatment of cholera cases with signs of severe dehydration. Whenever possible the sensitivity of the cholera isolate to antibiotics should be assessed. Antibiotics are not indicated in the treatment of milder cases of cholera or for mass prophylaxis and should not be used in the treatment of ETEC diarrhea [9].

In general, vaccines are considered useful tools for controlling bacterial infectious diseases. Effective vaccines, if available and widely used, could prevent a substantial part of the morbidity and mortality in cholera and ETEC infections in developing countries [11]. However, until very recently, no sufficiently effective vaccines for use in humans against either cholera or ETEC diarrhea, or for that matter, other enteric infections, have been available. Thus, previous parenteral cholera vaccines induced at most 50% protection with a duration of only 3 to at most 6 months [12], and vaccines against ETEC and other enterotoxin-producing bacteria have been lacking completely.

The limitations in the protection induced by the previous cholera vaccines could probably to a large part be explained by the parenteral administration route used and in part also by their composition. In cholera infection, both the bacteria and the toxin they produce exert their action locally in the gut. In accordance with this, local mucosal immunity is of critical importance for protection. The parenteral cholera vaccines have been found to give rise to little, if any immune response locally in the gut in individuals who have not been immunologically primed by previous natural exposure to *V. cholerae*. Also, in the previously primed host, the injection route has been found to be much less efficient than oral immunization [13,14]. In addition, the parenteral cholera vaccines did not stimulate any antitoxic immunity.

Recently, however, the situation has changed for the better with regard to vaccine development against both cholera and ETEC diarrhea. New cholera vaccines are under development, and two oral vaccines are already registered internationally. (See also chapter by Kaper in this volume.) One of these vaccines, which is described in further detail in this chapter, consists of killed whole *V. cholerae* O1 cells in combination with recombinantly produced binding (B) subunit of cholera toxin. This vaccine, which is given in two or three doses in a bicarbonate buffer, is well tolerated and confers a high level (85%) protection against cholera for 6 months [15], and the level of protection is still about 50% three years after immunization in vaccinees who were aged 5 years or older at the time of vaccination [16]. Because of its documented ability to also protect against diarrhea caused by ETEC strains producing cholera-like toxin [17,18], the recombinant cholera B subunit-killed whole cell (BS-WC) vaccine is also registered for use for prophylactic vaccination against ETEC diarrhea. (See also Svennerholm et al., this volume).

II. MECHANISMS OF IMMUNITY

The development of the oral BS-WC cholera vaccine has to a large extent been based on new insights into the mechanisms of disease and immunity in cholera and related enterotoxin-induced diarrheas gained over the past 30 years [19]. The main findings guiding the modern cholera vaccine development may be summarized as follows:

(1) The pathogenesis of cholera was shown to critically depend on bacterial colonization associated with toxin production and action locally in the small intestine;

(2) Therefore, either or both of antibacterial and antitoxic immunity capable of preventing these events were found to protect against disease;

(3) Both antibacterial and antitoxic immunity were found to depend mainly if not exclusively on locally (mucosally) produced antibodies of the secretory IgA (SIgA) type, and it was shown that intestinal antibacterial and antitoxic antibodies can cooperate synergistically in protection against disease by interfering with the two most important separate pathogenic events in the gut, i.e., colonization and toxin action.

(4) To stimulate a protective gut mucosal immune response comprising both intestinal antibacterial

and antitoxic antibodies, and for longer-lasting protection also local immunological memory, vaccination by the oral route was found to be superior to parenteral vaccination.

A. Toxins and Antitoxic Immunity

As stated, the major pathogenic mechanisms of both *V. cholerae* and other enterotoxigenic bacteria include initial bacterial colonization of the small intestine followed by the elaboration of enterotoxin(s) that through specific mechanisms can induce electrolyte and water secretion resulting in diarrhea [19–21]. These enterotoxins, which have a cytotonic rather than cytotoxic effect on the intestinal epithelium, are believed to stimulate secretion, primarily from the crypt cells in the upper part of the small intestine, by inducing increased formation of cyclic AMP and/or cyclic GMP in the epithelial cells. Cholera toxin (CT) is the prototype enterotoxin and is produced by most *V. cholerae* O1 bacteria of either the classical or El Tor biotype. CT with identical structure to O1 El Tor CT is also formed by the novel *V. cholerae* O139 serogroup [22]. Cholera toxin consists of five identical B subunits forming a ring structure into which a single toxic-active (A) subunit is noncovalently inserted. The toxin binds to cells by each B subunit interacting with a binding receptor identified as a specific glycolipid, the ganglioside GM1 [20]. Binding allows for the translocation into the cell interior of the A subunit, which then through an enzymatic reaction couples ADP-ribose to a subunit of adenylate cyclase and thus causes increased formation and accumulation of cAMP in exposed cells [14]. ETEC bacteria may produce either or both of a heat-labile enterotoxin (LT) and a heat-stable enterotoxin (ST) [19,21]. Of these, LT is closely related to CT with a similar 5B:1A subunit structure and strong structure homology and immunological cross-reactivity in both the A and B subunits [19,23,24]. ST, on the other hand, is of low molecular weight and completely unrelated to LT or CT in structure and function.

Studies in experimental animals have shown a direct correlation between protection against CT-induced fluid secretion and intestinal synthesis of SIgA antibodies and also between protection and the number of SIgA antitoxin-producing cells in the intestine [19]. A protective role of SIgA antitoxin has also been clearly indicated by the direct correlation in breast-fed children in Bangladesh of a reduced risk of developing disease even upon infection with *V. cholerae* O1 and the ingestion of mother's milk with SIgA antitoxin antibodies above a certain level [25]. Furthermore, as will be discussed below, vaccine-induced antitoxic immunity associated with intestinal SIgA antitoxin production in a large field trial in Bangladesh has been shown to confer significant protection against both cholera and diarrhea caused by LT-producing ETEC.

The identification of the AB subunit structure of CT and LT and the roles of the different subunits in pathogenesis and immunity suggested that the isolated CT or LT B subunits (CTB or LTB) could be useful vaccine components to induce protective antitoxic immunity. This notion was further strengthened by findings in animals showing that immunization with highly purified CTB or LTB gave rise to toxin-

neutralizing antibodies that could fully protect against disease also by live challenge in the gut [26,27]. Furthermore, the B subunit pentamers have been found to be particularly well suited as oral immunogens because they are stable in the intestinal milieu and capable of binding to the intestinal epithelium, including the M-cells of the Peyer's patches, properties that are very important for stimulating mucosal immunity and local immunological memory [28].

B. Colonization Factors and Antibacterial Immunity

The best correlate between protection and naturally acquired immunity in cholera is the level of serum vibriocidal antibodies, which in populations living in cholera endemic areas increase by age in an almost parallel manner to decreased susceptibility to cholera infection and disease [7,12]. However, there is no direct correlation between vibriocidal antibody and protection, especially not after vaccination. Thus, for instance, extremely high vibriocidal antibody levels can be achieved in serum after immunization with parenteral cholera vaccines, but the protection is low because little mucosal immunity is evoked. In contrast, the new oral cholera vaccines whether consisting of killed whole-cell vibrios together with cholera B subunit or of live attenuated vaccine strains induce substantially lower levels of vibriocidal antibodies in serum than achieved with parenteral vaccines, yet provide stronger and more long-lasting protection.

It is well established that *V. cholerae* O1 lipopolysaccharide (LPS) is the predominant antigen inducing protective antibacterial immunity against experimental cholera caused by O1 bacteria [13]. Recent studies have suggested that when it comes to protection against *V. cholerae* O139, immunity is also to a large extent provided by specific antibodies to (O139) LPS. Most of the vibriocidal antibodies in serum are directed against *V. cholerae* LPS, and the extent to which the vibriocidal antibody levels reflect protection probably relates to the degree these antibodies reflect the levels of locally produced, protective IgA antibodies against *V. cholerae* LPS in the intestine.

In *V. cholerae* O1 bacteria of the classical biotype, a toxin-coregulated pilus (TCP) has been shown to be of importance for colonization of the small intestine [29]. There is evidence that also for *V. cholerae* O1 El Tor and O139, an antigenically distinct form of TCP is in an analogous way important for colonization and disease [30]. In addition, *V. cholerae* bacteria have been found to express several other fimbrial structures. One of these is the mannose-sensitive hemagglutinin (MSHA), which is found on O1 El Tor and O139 *V. cholerae* but not on O1 bacteria of classical biotype, and which can mediate bacterial attachment to epithelial cells [31]. The role of these other attachment factors for colonization and infection in humans, however, remains to be defined.

The identification of TCP as an important colonization factor on *V. cholerae* suggests that it should be possible to raise protective antibacterial immunity also against these fimbrial antigens. Indeed, in experimental systems both monoclonal antibodies and polyclonal antisera against

TCP can protect against infection and disease [32]. However, following natural infection, little if any anti-TCP immunity develops. Therefore, as an overall conclusion, it remains to be defined whether mucosal immune responses against TCP and other surface antigens on *V. cholerae* can add significantly to the protective action mediated by antibodies to O1 LPS antigen.

An important observation guiding the design of new cholera vaccines has concerned the cooperation between antitoxic and antibacterial immune mechanisms in protection. Either of the two main protective antibodies against cholera which, as mentioned above, are directed against the cell wall LPS and CTB, can confer strong protection against disease by inhibiting bacterial colonization and toxin binding, respectively [13]. When present together in the gut these antibodies have been shown to have a strongly synergistic protective effect [33].

C. Immunological Memory

The acute local antibody response to the oral BS-WC cholera vaccine in unprimed individuals normally lasts for up to 6 months [34,35]. However, in accordance with studies in animals showing almost lifelong gut mucosal immunological memory after oral vaccination with CT [36] it has been shown that a long-lasting immunological memory is also induced in humans by the oral vaccine [37–39].

Thus, healthy Swedish volunteers who received a booster vaccination 5 years after an initial two-dose cholera vaccination responded with significantly higher antitoxin and antibacterial serum IgG and IgA antibody levels than previously unvaccinated controls [37]. In another study, the frequencies of CTB-specific antibody-secreting cells (ASCs) extracted from duodenal mucosal biopsies of vaccinated Swedish volunteers were found to be considerably higher after the second than after the first vaccine dose, and the response to a third booster dose at 5 months fully matched that after the second dose at 2 weeks [39]. Furthermore, circulating ASCs, known to mainly be derived from and reflect the gut mucosal immune response, were higher after either of the second and third vaccine doses than after the first vaccine dose [39]. Almost identical results were obtained in Swedish volunteers given a booster dose 10 months after either two or three initial vaccinations [38].

Taken together, these studies suggest that the oral BS-WC cholera vaccine induces a very long-lasting immunological memory. A stronger and faster immune response than after an initial vaccination can be obtained by a booster vaccination given at any time from 2 weeks up to at least 5 years after the primary immunization. Furthermore, in individuals who have received a fully immunizing two-dose regimen, a single booster immunization given even 5 years later evokes an apparently maximal gut mucosal immune response to the vaccine.

III. COMPOSITION OF VACCINE

The oral killed BS-WC cholera vaccine (registered under the trademark Dukoral®, SBL Vaccin, Sweden) consists of killed whole *V. cholerae* O1 cells and recombinantly produced CTB. A detailed description of the vaccine composition is given in Table 1. A total of 1×10^{11} heat-killed or formalin-killed *V. cholerae* O1 bacterial cells, comprising both the Inaba and Ogawa serotypes and the classical and El Tor biotypes, are supplied as a suspension mixed with CTB in phosphate-buffered saline. The vaccine is taken together with a bicarbonate buffer provided in the registered vaccine product as a single-dose dry salt preparation, which is dissolved in water and mixed with the vaccine before administration in order to protect the CTB component against stomach acidity.

Table 1 Composition and Recommended Administration of Oral B Subunit–Killed Whole-Cell Cholera Vaccine

Each dose of vaccine suspension (3 ml) contains:	
Whole-cell component:	
V. cholerae O1 Inaba classic strain (heat inactivated)	2.5×10^{10} vibrios
V. cholerae O1 Inaba El Tor strain (formalin inactivated)	2.5×10^{10} vibrios
V. cholerae O1 Ogawa classic strain (heat inactivated)	2.5×10^{10} vibrios
V. cholerae O1 Ogawa classic strain (formalin inactivated)	2.5×10^{10} vibrios
B subunit component:	
Recombinant CTB	1 mg

The vaccine is produced by SBL Vaccin, Sweden, and currently registered in some 20 countries worldwide under the trade name Dukoral. For immunization, the 3-ml vaccine solution is emptied into a glass of sodium hydrogen carbonate solution and drunk (the buffer salts are supplied in the vaccine package as effervescent granules, which should be dissolved in a glass of cool water, approx. 150 ml; the whole volume is used for vaccinees older than 6 years of age, for younger children only half the volume, ca. 75 ml, is used but still with the full 3-ml dose of vaccine). The recommended primary vaccination comprises two doses of vaccine for adults and children over the age of 6 years and three doses of vaccine to children from 1 to 6 years of age. Doses should be administered at intervals of 1–6 weeks. For maintaining a continuous protection, a booster dose is recommended for adults and children above the age of 6 years after 2 years; children below 6 years of age should receive a booster dose after 6 months.

The first-generation oral cholera vaccine contained CTB subunits purified from CT produced in a fermentor by the wild-type strain 569B. This method made the preparation of this extensively purified component laborious and relatively expensive [40]. These drawbacks were overcome by the development of an efficient recombinant overexpression system for the large-scale production of CTB [41]. These latter procedures now yield more than 1 g of highly purified CTB per liter of fermentor culture even in 1000-L fermentations, which is approximately 100-fold better than the yield obtained with the early nonrecombinant production and isolation of CTB. Since there is no CTA subunit gene present in the production strain used, no active toxin can be formed, which makes the purification processes further efficient and cheaper [41]. No differences have been found in the function of recombinantly produced CTB and toxin-derived CTB as a vaccine component. Immunological and functional studies, including immunogenicity studies in both animals and humans, have not been able to demonstrate any differences in the two molecules or in the immune response they evoke [41,42]. Moreover, the results from an efficacy field trial in Peru with vaccine containing the recombinantly produced CTB [43] were fully consistent with the efficacy results obtained in Bangladesh with first-generation vaccine containing native CTB [15].

IV. PROTECTION AGAINST CHOLERA

The first evidence for protective efficacy of a killed oral BS-WC vaccine was seen in a challenge study in North American volunteers in the early 1980s [44]. Immunization with oral killed *V. cholerae* WC vaccine, alone or given with CTB, was evaluated. Vaccinees, who had received three doses of either vaccine, and unvaccinated controls were challenged with 1×10^6 *V. cholerae* O1 El Tor organisms to determine the protective efficacy of the vaccines. The combination vaccine provided 64% protection ($p < 0.01$), and the whole cell vaccine without any B subunit provided 56% protection ($p < 0.05$). In addition, illnesses in vaccinees were milder than in controls, and both vaccines gave 100% protection

against more severe disease. This substantial level of protection against challenge with a dose of *V. cholerae* that caused cholera in nearly 90% of controls suggested that these vaccines might provide at least as high a level of protection if given to the population of an endemic area. This prediction has then been tested and confirmed in three large field trials with the combined oral BS-WC cholera vaccine.

The first of these field trials was conducted in Bangladesh in 1985–1990 [15,16,45,46]. The study included nearly 90,000 volunteers 2–65 years of age, and surveillance for cholera was conducted during a 5-year period. The volunteers received three doses of BS-WC vaccine, WC only vaccine, or *E. coli* K12 placebo. The results of the study are summarized in Tables 2 and 3. The overall short-term (4–6 months) protection with the BS-WC vaccine was 85% [15]. The protection in children aged 2–5 years was 100% during this period but declined to 38% for the entire first year and 47% for the second year [Table 2] [46]. Adults were very well protected by the BS-WC vaccine for the first 2 years, 78% and 63% protective efficacy for the first and second year, respectively, while a decline was seen during the third year, 41% protective efficacy [46]. It was also shown that two doses were sufficient for protection giving 77% and 70% protection during the first and second year, respectively (data reanalyzed by SBL, unpublished) [16].

The WC vaccine without any B subunit also provided significant short-term as well as long-term protection against cholera in adults (Table 3). However, the short-term protection, 58% for the initial 4- to 6-month period, was significantly lower than the 85% efficacy of the combined BS-WC vaccine during the same period. This added short-term protection seen with the BS-WC vaccine supports the existence of an independent immunogenic effect of the B subunit component in this vaccine. Indeed, if for calculation of the protective efficacy of the B subunit component one estimates a protective efficacy of BS-WC in comparison with WC by looking at the WC groups as "placebo," the protective efficacy of the B subunit over the WC component was 73% during this period. The BS-WC vaccine continued to be significantly more protective than the WC-alone vaccine for the first 9 months after vaccination. Thereafter, however, the overall efficacy was similar, approximately 55% during the

Table 2 Protection Against Cholera by the Oral B Subunit–Killed Whole-Cell (BS/WC) Vaccine in the Bangladesh Field Trial

Follow-up period	Protective efficacy % (95% confidence interval)		
	All ages	Children 2–5 years	Adults and children > 5 years
4–6 months	85 (56–95)	100	76
First year	64 (50–74)	38	78
Second year	52 (30–76)	47	63
Third year	19 (nil–46)	Nil	41

Source: Ref. 46.

Table 3 Protection Against Cholera by the Oral Whole-Cell Only (WC) Vaccine in the Bangladesh Field Trial

Follow-up period	Protective efficacy % (95% confidence interval)		
	All ages	Children 2–5 years	Adults and children > 5 years
4–6 months	58 (14–79)	35	71
First year	56 (39–76)	31	67
Second year	55 (33–69)	24	73
Third year	41 (7–62)	2	61

Source: Ref. 46.

second year of follow-up and 20–40% during the third year. The protective contribution of the B subunit component appeared to be particularly strong with regard to short-term protection in children less than 5 years of age at the time of vaccination: in contrast to the 100% protective efficacy of the BS-WC vaccine the WC-alone vaccine only provided 35% protection in this age group during the same period [46]. Thus, children 2–5 years were very well protected by the BS-WC vaccine during the first 6 months, but protection declined thereafter, whereas the WC-alone vaccine did not confer sufficient protection to the young children although it protected older children and adults well.

The second randomized, placebo-controlled field vaccine efficacy trial was conducted among Peruvian military personnel in 1992, quite soon after cholera first appeared in Peru (1991) [43]. There were many differences compared with the previous Bangladesh trial; for example, the Peru trial included only high-risk blood group adults who were not exposed to cholera previously, administration of two doses of vaccine only, the use of recombinant CTB rather than native CTB in the vaccine, the fact that all cholera was caused by El Tor biotype, a much smaller population ($n = 1500$), and a very high attack rate in the placebo group. Even so, however, the results of 5 months of follow-up showed 85% protective efficacy (95% confidence interval being 36–97%; $p = 0.004$ for comparison with the placebo group), which is strikingly similar to the short-term efficacy in the Bangladesh trial.

A third large field trial was also conducted in Peru [47]. It resembled the Bangladesh trial in that it was a large trial (17,000 subjects) and a target population 2–65 years of age. In this study, two primary vaccinations were given to all subjects regardless of age, followed by a third booster dose after 1 year. In contrast to the Bangladesh study, there was active surveillance for cholera and very few cases of cholera seeking treatment at a hospital during the first year of surveillance. The outcome of this study was also in contrast to what was seen previously in that no protection was seen during the first year of surveillance. However, during the second year, when there were also more hospitalized cases,

there was 60% protection against cholera (78% against hospitalized cases), which is in agreement with the results of the Bangladesh trial. The study has been criticized and several possible explanations for this outcome have been proposed [48], including the use of active surveillance for detection of cholera cases with nearly exclusively mild cases during the first year.

V. CROSS-PROTECTIVE EFFICACY AGAINST ENTEROTOXIGENIC *ESCHERICHIA COLI*

There is ample evidence from preclinical studies that antibodies to CTB can effectively neutralize *E. coli* LT, and that antitoxic immunity induced by either CT or CTB can protect against LT ETEC diarrhea [49].

The first evidence that oral immunization with CTB also provides significant cross-protection against disease caused by LT-producing ETEC in humans was demonstrated in the Bangladesh field trial [17]. The protective efficacy against ETEC diarrhea during the first three months after vaccination, a period in which there was much ETEC disease including strains that produce LT with or without ST, was 67%. Protection was stronger against severe dehydrating disease (86%) than against milder illness (54%). It was not possible to determine the protective efficacy for the following 6 months as there were no ETEC cases, and when the next ETEC season started, 9 months after the last vaccination, no protection was evident. There were no age-dependent differences in protection. Thus, in endemic areas, a good, short-term cross-protection against LT-ETEC disease by the oral BS-WC cholera vaccine, specifically mediated by the CTB component, was shown.

As ETEC is the single most common cause of traveler's diarrhea, it was of interest to study protection in travelers as well. This has been done in two randomized, placebo-controlled studies. The first, and most convincing of these studies, was done on Finnish travelers going to Morocco [18]. In this study, a protective efficacy of 60% was seen against LT-producing ETEC. A second travelers' study was conducted among U.S. students going to Mexico [50]. The design of this study differed from the Finnish study in that the U.S. students were vaccinated immediately after arrival in Mexico, while the Finnish tourists were vaccinated before departure. Most diarrhea cases occurred during the first two weeks after arrival, when the vaccine could not be expected to protect. When considering only cases occurring more than 7 days after the second vaccination there was 50% (CI: 14–71%) protection against all ETEC diarrhea. The conclusions of the study were that sufficient protection can only be achieved if the vaccine is taken before departure, so that the second dose is taken at least 1 week before arrival, and under these conditions the protection seen in this study supports the previous findings.

VI. VACCINE SAFETY AND USE IN RISK GROUPS

A. Overall Vaccine Safety

The oral BS-WC vaccine is generally considered very safe and has been extensively tested in clinical trials involving approximately 240,000 volunteers. No serious adverse events have been associated with vaccination. The most commonly reported adverse events in association with vaccination are mild gastrointestinal symptoms such as abdominal discomfort or pain, loose stools, or diarrhea. In all placebo-controlled trials the frequencies of adverse events, 0–24% of the studied populations, are similar in the vaccine and placebo groups. Both endemic and nonendemic populations have been included in clinical trials, but no differences in adverse reaction rates can be seen [42,51–53].

It has also been suggested that the symptoms are caused by the bicarbonate buffer given together with the vaccine [54]. When the vaccine was given together with a decreased amount of buffer the rate of symptoms decreased, but the antibody responses to CTB also decreased. This implies that although the buffer may be responsible for some gastrointestinal symptoms, it is required for maximum immunogenicity of the vaccine.

In addition to the clinical trials, over 1,000,000 doses of the vaccine have been sold in Sweden and Norway since 1992. During these years the Swedish and Norwegian Medical Products Agencies have received a total of 45 reports describing 63 adverse reactions, which is considered a very low number considering the large number of doses sold.

B. Children

The safety and immunogenicity aspects of the oral BS-WC cholera vaccine are very well documented for children from 1 to 2 years of age. Protection has been studied in children from 2 years and up, and several additional studies have addressed the safety and immunogenicity of the vaccine in children from 1 year of age [15,16,45–47,51,53,55–57]. In total over 5300 children aged 1–5 years have received the vaccine in clinical trials with strict active surveillance of adverse reactions. In some trials both children and adults have been included, and there is no indication of age-related adverse events.

C. Pregnant and Breast-Feeding Women

Considering the number of volunteers included in the large field trials with the BS-WC vaccine and the exclusion of pregnancy only by interviews and inspection it could be assumed that an unknown number of pregnant women came to be included. Although an individual follow-up of these women was not done on a systematic basis, there were no reports of pregnancy-related complications or complications in the newborns that were linked to the intake of the vaccine. The experience from Scandinavia, where more than 1,000,000 doses of BS-WC vaccine (Dukoral) have been sold to adults of both sexes, also supports the safety of the vaccine in pregnant women. The Adverse Drug Reaction (ADR) reporting system in Sweden is well developed through the Medical Product Agency (MPA) and there are no ADR reports related to pregnancy or postpartum conditions. In addition, there are no reports of any increased rate of malformation even following cholera infection in the literature. The previous parenteral cholera vaccine was studied in pregnant women and no increase in complications in pregnancy after vaccination was found [58]. Thus, it is extremely unlikely that the oral BS-WC cholera vaccine should have any negative effect when given during pregnancy. The vaccine has been given to a large number of breast-feeding women in several different studies, and no adverse events in relation to breast-feeding have been reported [59,60].

D. Immunocompromised and HIV-Infected Individuals

There is a wide range of conditions leading to a deficient immune response to infections and vaccinations, with varying degrees of severity. Most of these conditions have not been studied in relation to oral cholera vaccines or cholera disease. However, the immune responses to oral BS-WC cholera vaccine in a group of IgA-deficient patients were studied in relation to vaccination, and it was found that the vaccine caused no adverse reactions and the intestinal IgG and IgM responses to the vaccine in this group were significantly higher than in subjects with normal IgA levels [61]. The potential risk that vaccination of patients with IgA deficiency combined with concurrent gut disease might lead to aggravated disease, due to the absence of anti-inflammatory IgA, has not been confirmed in clinical trials [62].

Three trials have been undertaken with the oral BS-WC cholera vaccine (Dukoral) in HIV-infected subjects in Sweden, Brazil, UK, and Kenya [63–65]. All three trials addressed immunogenicity and safety. The conclusion of these trials with regard to safety is that the vaccine does not cause any other side effects in HIV-infected than in healthy subjects and that there is no HIV disease progression. In general, killed vaccines are not considered a risk to HIV-infected individuals. Today, WHO recommends use of all vaccines included in the Expanded Program of Vaccination (EPI) in HIV-positive individuals, with the exception of BCG and yellow fever vaccines, which should not be given to patients with AIDS [66]. Protective efficacy after oral BS-WC cholera vaccination has not been studied specifically in HIV-infected individuals. However, at least one report has stated that there is a higher risk ratio for mortality due to cholera in HIV-infected than in uninfected individuals, which underlines the importance of cholera vaccines that are functional also in this group [67].

VII. PUBLIC HEALTH INDICATIONS AND EXPERIENCE

The main indication for vaccination against cholera is protection of the population at risk in endemic areas. At least 120,000 persons, and probably significantly more, die each year from cholera, reflecting a failure of health system infrastructure and difficulties in implementation of control measures. Nearly 120 countries have reported indigenous cases of cholera since 1991; almost half of them have reported cases for at least 5 out of the past 8 years. Therefore, WHO has recently concluded [9] that although the establishment of adequate personal hygiene, food safety, and sanitation are the mainstay of cholera control, in the short-term drastic improvements in these fields are difficult to achieve in most cholera endemic areas, and there is therefore an urgent need for efficient vaccines as an additional public health tool for cholera prevention. Compared with the parenteral vaccine, the now internationally available cholera vaccines represent significant improvements in terms of protective efficacy duration of protection, safety, and ease of administration [9]. There is an especially high public health need of such vaccines for use in emergency situations with high-risk populations, such as refugees in primitive camps and urban slum residents. WHO emphasizes that the use of cholera vaccines should always be preemptive before an outbreak has started and not reactive as a method of trying to contain an already ongoing epidemic, and that vaccination should always be combined with other preventional control measures currently recommended by WHO. There is also a place for cholera vaccination in civilian and military personnel traveling to highly endemic areas [9].

A. Attractive Public Health Features of B Subunit–Killed Whole-Cell Vaccine

Results from Phase III efficacy trials do not automatically predict the effectiveness of the same vaccine under conditions of public health use. As opposed to the typical randomized, placebo-controlled efficacy trial, assessment of the public health effectiveness should take into account the impact by vaccination on the population at large, including both vaccinated people and those who for various reasons are not reached by the vaccination. The perceived value of the vaccine and its overall community acceptability are therefore important components in addition to efficacy in determining the public health effectiveness of a given vaccine. Whereas these latter aspects might tend to lower the effectiveness in comparison with the efficacy measured under the more idealized conditions of a placebo-controlled Phase III field trial, the routine public health use of vaccine may also elevate effectiveness above the level expected from efficacy trials through at least two different mechanisms. One of these is the beneficial effects of the so-called "herd immunity" in populations were vaccine coverage is high.

Another less well recognized factor is the generally much higher risk of infection and disease among people who elect to not participate in vaccine trials than among participants [68]. These people may well accept to be vaccinated in public health programs with vaccine that is perceived to be valuable and have few and mild adverse reactions.

The oral BS-WC cholera vaccine has several attractive features for public health use. It has, as described above, an excellent safety profile, does not require a strict cold chain by being stable also at temperatures at or above 30°C (although cold storage is recommended by the manufacturer), and is easy to administer. The BS-WC cholera vaccine is the only internationally registered vaccine with documented efficacy against cholera in endemic countries and is also the only vaccine available with documented protective activity against ETEC diarrheal disease. Consistent with these features and the importance of cholera and ETEC as enteric pathogens in a country like Bangladesh, in addition to their disease-specific efficacy in the Bangladesh field trial, both the BS-WC and the WC vaccines substantially reduced the overall diarrheal morbidity among those vaccinated, resulting in a 51% and 32% reduction in admissions for severe watery diarrhea in the BS-WC and WC vaccinated groups, respectively, as compared with the placebo group during the first year after vaccination [69]. The latter finding provides ample evidence of the public health application potential of the BS-WC cholera vaccine in settings found not only in Bangladesh but also in many other countries, where cholera, ETEC, and other enterotoxic diarrheal diseases account for a large number of life-threatening watery diarrheas and where adequate treatment facilities in rural areas often are scarce [70].

In the first year of follow-up after vaccination in Bangladesh, there was also a dramatic effect of both the BS-WC and WC vaccines as compared with placebo on total mortality [69]. Thus, overall mortality rates were 26% lower in the BS-WC group and 23% lower in the WC group during the first year. Among women vaccinated at ages > 15 years those who received BS-WC had 45% fewer deaths ($p < 0.01$) and those who received WC had 33% fewer deaths ($p < 0.05$) than placebo recipients. Several additional findings suggested that this reduction in overall mortality was a specific effect rather than a statistical coincidence: (1) the effect was restricted to the high-cholera season, (2) it was correlated with deaths associated with or preceded by diarrheal disease according to "verbal autopsy" reports by household members, and (3) as mentioned, it was limited to the underprivileged group of women rather than children participating in the study [69]. The effect on total mortality was restricted to the first year. The results suggest that even in a "well-treated" area such as the field site in Matlab there may be a significant number of hidden cholera and severe ETEC diarrhea deaths that might be averted by effective cholera and/or ETEC vaccination programs.

One special aspect studied in the Bangladesh field trial of oral cholera vaccines was the association between breast-feeding and the risk of severe cholera among children under 36 months of age [71]. The results showed that overall, breast-feeding was associated with a 70% reduction of the risk of developing clinical severe cholera and exclusive breast-feeding during infancy appeared to be associated with nearly 100% protection against severe cholera. Furthermore, maternal vaccination with either the BS-WC or WC oral cholera vaccine was associated with a 50% reduced risk of their nonvaccinated children to develop severe cholera. These results raised a possibility that vaccination of mothers may provide protection to their young children in endemic settings by either or both of two potential mechanisms, i.e., interrupting maternal–child transmission of cholera and/or increasing the specific immune protecting potential of the mothers' breast milk.

B. WHO Recommendations and Vaccination Experiences in High-Risk Groups

For public health use, WHO concludes that owing to its low efficacy and short duration of protection, use of the old parenteral vaccine is not recommended. Among the new-generation cholera vaccines, WHO concludes that convincing protection in field situations has been demonstrated only with the BS-WC vaccine. The oral BS-WC cholera vaccine is currently the only cholera vaccine on the WHO list of prequalified vaccines. This means that the vaccine may be used by other organizations, e.g., United Nations agencies. WHO has concluded [9] that the vaccine is safe, lacks any significant adverse reactions, is well tolerated by HIV-positive individuals, and can be given safely to both pregnant and lactating women.

For vaccination of populations at immediate risk of a cholera epidemic, the BS-WC vaccine is recommended by WHO [9]. A special WHO expert group issued specific recommendations on the use of oral cholera vaccines in emergency situations and in very high risk populations as follows: "The oral BS-WC cholera vaccine should be considered among the tools to prevent cholera in populations believed to be at risk of a cholera epidemic within 6 months and not experiencing a current epidemics. Such high-risk populations may include, but are not limited to, refugees and urban slum residents" [74]. The group emphasized that cholera vaccine should be considered only for preemptive use, not reactively as a method of containing an outbreak once it has started. Further, vaccination to prevent cholera outbreaks should be undertaken only in conjunction with other prevention and control measures currently recommended by WHO, and intervention studies should be performed to establish the role cholera vaccination can play in cholera control programs [9,74].

C. Vaccination Campaigns in High-Risk Groups

The oral killed BS-WC cholera vaccine has been used in a mass-vaccination study in refugee camps in Uganda, which was conducted by Groupe Européen d'Expertise en Epidémiologie Pratique (EPICENTRE), Paris, in cooperation with Médecins Sans Frontières, France [72,73]. The primary objective was to assess the feasibility of a mass cholera vaccination campaign in refugee camps, and it was not designed to determine the protective efficacy of the vaccine. The refugees represented about 55% of the total district population and were spread over 35 different settlements. Approximately 27,000 adults and children above 1 year of age were immunized with the oral BS-WC cholera vaccine.

The general conclusion of the study was that mass vaccination of refugee camps in sub-Saharan Africa is feasible. All vaccinations were carried out within 1 month. One year after vaccination there was an outbreak of cholera in the non-vaccinated settlements. There were 358 cases of cholera in the area, but none occurred in the vaccinated settlements. The data collected are not suitable for valid calculations of protective efficacy of the vaccine, but the organizers of the study conclude that "the results of this study are strongly in favor of a protective effect of the BS-WC cholera vaccine, both against *V. cholerae* and other infectious agents responsible of diarrheal disease."

Following a cholera epidemic in the Comores island, near Madagascar (particularly in the Anjouan island close to Mayotte), the French authorities decided to initiate a vaccination campaign against cholera for the whole population of Mayotte including illegal immigrants. The official decision to carry out a vaccination campaign was made in early October 2000 for implementation on site from November 1 and terminating December 15 before the school holidays, the beginning of Ramadan, and the rainy season. In spite of a very tight time schedule, 64% of the population (93,000 people) was vaccinated. Since this campaign, two cases of cholera have been identified in Mayotte: one in a woman who had not been vaccinated, and the other in a woman who had received only one vaccine dose.

D. Locally Produced Whole-Cell Vaccine in Viet Nam

By technology transfer, a simplified version of the killed WC vaccine (without the B subunit) has been locally produced, tested, and licensed in Viet Nam. The production cost of this vaccine has been estimated to be US$0.20 per dose. In a large-scale, open (not placebo-controlled) field trial conducted in more than 22,000 households in the central coastal city of Hue, persons aged over 1 year were allocated in alternate households to receive two doses of vaccine or no vaccine (67,000 persons in each group). During an outbreak of El Tor cholera that occurred 8–10 months after vaccination, significant protection (66%; $p < 0.01$) was noted among the persons who received the two-dose vaccine regimen, and protection was similar for children aged 1–5 years (68%) and for older persons (66%) [75].

Since 1997, in an area of Viet Nam endemic for cholera, a second-generation bivalent WC vaccine, containing serogroup O139 in addition to O1 [76], has been tested in a large-scale, randomized, double-blind, placebo-controlled effectiveness trial. Results from this study have not been analyzed, but in a preceding Phase II trial the vaccine was shown to be safe and to give rise to vibriocidal antibodies against both the O139 and O1 serogroups. The anti-O1 vibriocidal antibody levels achieved were comparable to those elicited by the Swedish-registered BS-WC vaccine (Dukoral) tested side by side with the locally produced vaccine.

These findings give encouragement to the notion that an inexpensive, locally produced effective oral cholera vaccine may be within reach for the limited health care budget of poor countries with endemic cholera.

VIII. CONCLUSIONS

Many studies in Europe, Asia, Africa, North America, and Latin America have shown that the BS-WC vaccine is safe and immunogenic in both children and adults in cholera-endemic as well as nonendemic countries, stimulating protective gut mucosal immune responses to the CTB and WC vaccine components. A good protective efficacy of the vaccine has been demonstrated, being 85% for the first 6 months after vaccination in both endemic and nonendemic populations, and remaining at or above 60% for at least 2 years in vaccinated adults and children above 5 years of age. In children below age 5, the short-term efficacy is very high (100% for the first 6 months when tested in a field trial in Bangladesh) but of shorter duration than in older children and adults. Based on these data the recommended primary vaccination comprises two doses of vaccine for adults and children over the age of 6 years and three doses of vaccine to children from 1 to 6 years of age. Doses should be administered at intervals of 1–6 weeks. For maintaining a continuous protection, a booster dose after 2 years is recommended for adults and children above the age of 6 years; children below 6 years of age should receive a booster dose after 6 months. The BS-WC cholera vaccine also offers short-term protection against ETEC diarrhea, for which there is currently no other vaccine available, and has been found to substantially reduce overall diarrhea morbidity in areas where cholera and ETEC diarrheas are common.

REFERENCES

1. Committee on Issues and Priorities for New Vaccine Development. The burden of disease resulting from diarrhea. New Vaccine Development: establishing Priorities. Vol. 2. Diseases of importance in developing countries. Washington, DC: National Academy Press, 1986:159–169.
2. Davey S. State of the World's Vaccines and Immunization. World Health Organisation, 1996.
3. Black RE. The epidemiology of cholera and enterotoxigenic *E. coli* diarrheal disease. In: Holmgren J, Lindberg A, Möllby R, eds. 11th Nobel Conference, Stockholm. Lund: Studentlitteratur, 1986; 23–32.
4. Farthing M, Keusch G. Global Impact and Patterns of Intestinal Infection: Enteric Infection. Mechanisms, Manifestations and Management. London: Chapman and Hall, 1989:3–12.
5. Blake PA. Historical perspectives on pandemic cholera. In: Wachsmuth IK, Blake PA, Olsvik O, eds. *Vibrio cholerae* and Cholera: Molecular to Global Perspectives. Washington: ASM Press, 1994:293–295.
6. Goma Epidemiology Group. Public health impact of Rwandan refugee crisis: what happened in Goma, Zaire, in July, 1994? Lancet 1995; 345:339–344.
7. Mosley WH, et al. The relationship of vibriocidal antibody titre to susceptibility to cholera in family contacts of cholera patients. Bull World Health Organ 1968; 38:777–785.
8. Tauxe RV, et al. The Latin American epidemic. In: Wachsmuth IK, Blake PA, Olsvik O, eds. *Vibrio cholerae* and Cholera: Molecular to Global Perspectives. Washington: ASM Press, 1994:321–344.
9. WHO. Cholera vaccines. WHO position paper. Wkly Epidemiol Rec 2001; 76:117–124.
10. Black RE. Epidemiology of travelers' diarrhea and relative importance of various pathogens. Rev Infect Dis 1990; 12: S73–S79.
11. Black RE. Epidemiology of diarrheal disease: implications for control by vaccines. Vaccine 1993; 11:100–106.
12. Feeley J, Gangarosa E. Field trials of cholera vaccines. In: Ouchterlony O, Holmgren J, eds. Cholera and Related Diarrheas. 43rd Nobel Symposium. Stockholm. Basel: Karger, 1978:204–210.
13. Holmgren J, Svennerholm AM. Cholera and the immune response. Prog Allergy 1983; 33:106–119.
14. Svennerholm AM, et al. Mucosal antitoxic and antibacterial immunity after cholera disease and after immunization with a combined B subunit–whole cell vaccine. J Infect Dis 1984; 149:884–893.
15. Clemens JD, et al. Field trial of oral cholera vaccines in Bangladesh. Lancet 1986; 2:124–127.
16. Clemens JD, et al. Field trial of oral cholera vaccines in Bangladesh: results from three-year follow-up. Lancet 1990; 335:270–273.
17. Clemens JD, et al. Cross-protection by B subunit–whole cell cholera vaccine against diarrhea associated with heat-labile toxin-producing enterotoxigenic *Escherichia coli*: results of a large-scale field trial. J Infect Dis 1988; 158:372–377.
18. Peltola H, et al. Prevention of travellers' diarrhea by oral B-subunit/whole-cell cholera vaccine. Lancet 1991; 338:1285–1289.
19. Holmgren J, Svennerholm A-M. Bacterial enteric infections and vaccine development. In: McDermott RP, Elson CO, eds. Mucosal Immunology, Gastroenterology Clinics of North America. W B Saunders, 1992:283.
20. Holmgren J. Actions of cholera toxin and the prevention and treatment of cholera. Nature 1981; 292:413–417.
21. Guerrant RL. Microbial toxins and diarrheal disease: introduction and overview. In: Evered D, Whelan J, eds. Microbial Toxins and Diarrheal Disease. London: Pitman, 1985:1.
22. Waldor MK, Mekalanos JJ. Emergence of a new cholera pandemic: molecular analysis of virulence determinants in *Vibrio cholerae* O139 and development of a live vaccine prototype. J Infect Dis 1994; 170:278–283.
23. Dallas WS, Falkow S. Amino acid sequence homology between cholera toxin and *Escherichia coli* heat-labile toxin. Nature 1980; 288:499–501.
24. Sixma TK, et al. Crystal structure of a cholera toxin-related heat-labile enterotoxin from *E. coli*. Nature 1991; 351:371–377.
25. Glass RI, et al. Protection against cholera in breast-fed children by antibodies in breast milk. N Engl J Med 1983; 308:1389–1392.
26. Holmgren J, et al. Development of improved cholera vaccine based on subunit toxoid. Nature 1977; 269:602–604.
27. Pierce NF, et al. Procholeragenoid: a safe and effective antigen for oral immunization against experimental cholera. Infect Immun 1983; 40:1112–1118.
28. Neutra MR, Kraehenbuhl JP. The role of transepithelial transport by M cells in microbial invasion and host defense. J Cell Sci Suppl 1993; 17:209–215.
29. Taylor RK, et al. Use of phoA gene fusions to identify a pilus colonization factor coordinately regulated with cholera toxin. Proc Natl Acad Sci USA 1987; 84:2833–2837.
30. Voss E, et al. The toxin-coregulated pilus is a colonization factor and protective antigen of *Vibrio cholerae* El Tor. Microb Pathog 1996; 20:141–153.
31. Jonson G, et al. Identification of a mannose-binding pilus on *Vibrio cholerae* El Tor. Microb Pathog 1991; 11:433–441.
32. Osek J, et al. Protection against *Vibrio cholerae* El Tor infection by specific antibodies against mannose-binding hemagglutinin pili. Infect Immun 1992; 60:4961–4964.
33. Svennerholm AM, Holmgren J. Synergistic protective effect in rabbits of immunization with *Vibrio cholerae* lipopolysaccharide and toxin/toxoid. Infect Immun 1976; 13:735–740.

34. Kilhamn J, et al. Kinetics of local and systemic immune responses to an oral cholera vaccine given alone or together with acetylcysteine. Clin Diagn Lab Immunol 1998; 5:247–250.

35. Svennerholm AM, et al. Local and systemic antibody responses and immunological memory in humans after immunization with cholera B subunit by different routes. Bull World Health Organ 1984; 62:909–918.

36. Lycke N, Holmgren J. Long-term cholera antitoxin memory in the gut can be triggered to antibody formation associated with protection within hours of an oral challenge immunization. Scand J Immunol 1987; 25:407–412.

37. Jertborn M, et al. Five-year immunologic memory in Swedish volunteers after oral cholera vaccination. J Infect Dis 1988; 157:374–377.

38. Jertborn M, et al. Immunological memory after immunization with oral cholera B subunit–whole-cell vaccine in Swedish volunteers. Vaccine 1994; 12:1078–1082.

39. Quiding M, et al. Intestinal immune responses in humans. Oral cholera vaccination induces strong intestinal antibody responses and interferon-gamma production and evokes local immunological memory. J Clin Invest 1991; 88:143–148.

40. Tayot JL, et al. Receptor-specific large-scale purification of cholera toxin on silica beads derivatized with lysoGM1 ganglioside. Eur J Biochem 1981; 113:249–258.

41. Sanchez J, Holmgren J. Recombinant system for over-expression of cholera toxin B subunit in *Vibrio cholerae* as a basis for vaccine development. Proc Natl Acad Sci USA 1989; 86:481–485.

42. Jertborn M, et al. Safety and immunogenicity of an oral recombinant cholera B subunit–whole cell vaccine in Swedish volunteers. Vaccine 1992; 10:130–132.

43. Sanchez JL, et al. Protective efficacy of oral whole-cell/recombinant-B-subunit cholera vaccine in Peruvian military recruits. Lancet 1994; 344:1273–1276.

44. Black RE, et al. Protective efficacy in humans of killed whole-vibrio oral cholera vaccine with and without the B subunit of cholera toxin. Infect Immun 1987; 55:1116–1120.

45. Clemens JD, et al. Field trial of oral cholera vaccines in Bangladesh: results of one year of follow-up. J Infect Dis 1988; 158:60–69.

46. van Loon FP, et al. Field trial of inactivated oral cholera vaccines in Bangladesh: results from 5 years of follow-up. Vaccine 1996; 14:162–166.

47. Taylor DN, et al. Two-year study of the protective efficacy of the oral whole cell plus recombinant B subunit cholera vaccine in Peru. J Infect Dis 2000; 181:1667–1673.

48. Clemens JD, et al. Misleading negative findings in a field trial of killed, oral cholera vaccine in Peru. J Infect Dis 2001; 183:1306–1308.

49. Pierce NF. Protection against challenge with *Escherichia coli* heat-labile enterotoxin by immunization of rats with cholera toxin/toxoid. Infect Immun 1977; 18:338–341.

50. Scerpella EG, et al. Safety, immunogenicity, and protective efficacy of the whole-cell/recombinant B subunit (WC/rBS) oral cholera vaccine against travelers' diarrhea. J Travel Med 1995; 2:22–27.

51. Clemens JD, et al. B subunit–whole cell and whole cell-only oral vaccines against cholera: studies on reactogenicity and immunogenicity. J Infect Dis 1987; 155:79–85.

52. Jertborn M, et al. Evaluation of different immunization schedules for oral cholera B subunit–whole cell vaccine in Swedish volunteers. Vaccine 1993; 11:1007–1012.

53. Taylor DN, et al. Safety, immunogenicity, and lot stability of the whole cell/recombinant B subunit (WC/rCTB) cholera vaccine in Peruvian adults and children. Am J Trop Med Hyg 1999; 61:869–873.

54. Sanchez JL, et al. Safety and immunogenicity of the oral, whole cell/recombinant B subunit cholera vaccine in North American volunteers. J Infect Dis 1993; 167:1446–1449.

55. Concha A, et al. Safety and immunogenicity of oral killed whole cell recombinant B subunit cholera vaccine in Barranquilla. Colombia. Bull Pan Am Health Organ 1995; 29:312–321.

56. Begue RE, et al. Immunogenicity in Peruvian volunteers of a booster dose of oral cholera vaccine consisting of whole cells plus recombinant B subunit. Infect Immun 1995; 63:3726–3728.

57. Begue RE, et al. Community-based assessment of safety and immunogenicity of the whole cell plus recombinant B subunit (WC/rBS) oral cholera vaccine in Peru. Vaccine 1995; 13:691–694.

58. Freda V. A preliminary report on typhoid, tetanus and cholera immunization during pregnancy. Am J Obstet Gynecol 1956; 71:1134–1136.

59. Jertborn M, et al. Saliva, breast milk, and serum antibody responses as indirect measures of intestinal immunity after oral cholera vaccination or natural disease. J Clin Microbiol 1986; 24:203–209.

60. Clemens JD, et al. Field trial of oral cholera vaccines in Bangladesh: evaluation of anti-bacterial and anti-toxic breast-milk immunity in response to ingestion of the vaccines. Vaccine 1990; 8:469–472.

61. Friman V, et al. Intestinal and circulating antibody-forming cells in IgA-deficient individuals after oral cholera vaccination. Clin Exp Immunol 1994; 95:222–226.

62. Nilssen DE, et al. B-cell activation in duodenal mucosa after oral cholera vaccination in IgA deficient subjects with or without IgG subclass deficiency. Scand J Immunol 1993; 38:201–208.

63. Eriksson K, et al. Intestinal antibody responses to oral vaccination in HIV-infected individuals. AIDS 1993; 7:1087–1091.

64. Ortigao-de-Sampaio MB, et al. Increase in plasma viral load after oral cholera immunization of HIV-infected subjects. AIDS 1998; 12:F145–F150.

65. Lewis DJ, et al. Immune response following oral administration of cholera toxin B subunit to HIV-1-infected UK and Kenyan subjects. AIDS 1994; 8:779–785.

66. WHO. EPI vaccines in HIV-infected individuals. Available at http://www.who.int/vaccines-diseases/diseases/HIV.shtml.

67. Rey JL, et al. HIV seropositivity and cholera in refugee children from Rwanda. AIDS 1995; 9:1203–1204.

68. Clemens JD, et al. Nonparticipation as a determinant of adverse health outcomes in a field trial of oral cholera vaccines. Am J Epidemiol 1992; 135:865–874.

69. Clemens JD, et al. Impact of B subunit killed whole-cell and killed whole-cell-only oral vaccines against cholera upon treated diarrheal illness and mortality in an area endemic for cholera. Lancet 1988; 1:1375–1379.

70. Sack DA, et al. Swedish Agency for Research Cooperation with Developing Countries. Prospects for public health benefits in developing countries from new vaccines against enteric infections. J Infect Dis 1991; 163:503–506.

71. Clemens JD, et al. Breast feeding and the risk of severe cholera in rural Bangladeshi children. Am J Epidemiol 1990; 131:400–411.

72. Dorlencourt F, et al. Effectiveness of mass vaccination with WC/rBS cholera vaccine during an epidemic in Adjumani district, Uganda. Bull World Health Organ 1999; 77:949–950.

73. Legros D, et al. Mass vaccination with a two-dose oral cholera vaccine in a refugee camp. Bull World Health Organ 1999; 77:837–842.

74. WHO. Potential use of oral cholera vaccines in emergency situations. Report of a WHO meeting, 12–13 May 1999. http://www.who.int/emc. World Health Organization, 1999.

75. Trach DD, et al. Field trial of a locally produced, killed, oral cholera vaccine in Vietnam. Lancet 1997; 349:231–235.

76. Naficy AB, et al. Cost of immunization with a locally produced, oral cholera vaccine in Viet Nam. Vaccine 2001; 19:3720–3725.

44

Attenuated *Vibrio cholerae* Strains as Live Oral Cholera Vaccines and Vectors

James B. Kaper and Carol O. Tacket
University of Maryland School of Medicine, Baltimore, Maryland, U.S.A.

I. INTRODUCTION

The first cholera vaccine developed in the 19th century consisted of live whole *Vibrio cholerae* organisms injected parenterally. This vaccine was quickly abandoned. An ideal modern cholera vaccine should possess a number of characteristics regarding safety, efficacy, and practicality. In our view, an ideal cholera vaccine would (1) be well tolerated in all age groups; (2) protect high-risk groups (including young children and persons of blood group O); (3) require only a single dose; (4) be administered orally for practicality and for better stimulation of the intestinal immune system; (5) stimulate both anticolonizing and antitoxic immunity; (6) confer a high level of protection (>80% efficacy) that would endure for at least 5 years; (7) begin protecting within a few days of administering the single oral dose (important for use in explosive outbreak situations); (8) be available in a simple formulation that would retain potency when stored in tropical climates and would facilitate mass vaccination, including vaccination of young children; and (9) be inexpensive.

We think that live, attenuated *V. cholerae* vaccine strains administered orally offer the best possibility for meeting all of the above characteristics. The rationale for the use of attenuated *V. cholerae* strains as live oral cholera vaccines is based on several observations which have been extensively reviewed elsewhere [1–3]:

1. A single clinical infection due to wild-type *V. cholerae* O1 confers significant protection against cholera upon subsequent exposure to wild-type *V. cholerae* O1.
2. Although many virulence properties contribute to the pathogenesis of cholera, the in vivo expression of cholera enterotoxin is a prerequisite for the profuse purging of voluminous rice water stools that is a characteristic of cholera gravis.
3. The critical protective immunity to cholera is antibacterial rather than antitoxic in nature, although in

the short term, antitoxic immunity may synergistically enhance antibacterial immunity.
4. The degree of stimulation of serum vibriocidal antibody following ingestion of a live oral cholera vaccine or following infection with wild-type *V. cholerae* O1 constitutes the best correlate of antibacterial immunity in the intestine.
5. The critical antigen or combination of antigens that provide protective immunity in humans has not been definitively identified.

The development of live attenuated vaccines to prevent cholera has been greatly aided by the application of recombinant DNA technology. The major virulence factor of *V. cholerae* is cholera enterotoxin, which is responsible for the large volume of watery diarrhea that is the hallmark of this disease [1]. Before the development of recombinant DNA technology, many attempts were made to attenuate *V. cholerae* O1 using chemical mutagenesis to derive a strain that produced the nontoxic yet immunogenic B subunit of the cholera toxin (CTB) but not the A subunit (CTA), which is the enzymatically active portion of the toxin (reviewed in Ref. 2). This chapter will review recent progress in the development of live oral cholera vaccine strains and *V. cholerae* vector strains. Additional background on the epidemiology, pathogenesis, and immunogenicity of *V. cholerae* can be found in Chapter 43.

II. EARLY GENERATIONS OF RECOMBINANT ATTENUATED CHOLERA VACCINE CANDIDATES

The basic methods involved in developing live recombinant vaccines against cholera have been to clone and to characterize genes encoding specific virulence factors, to mutate these genes in vitro using recombinant techniques, and then to reintroduce the mutated genes into wild-type *V. cholerae* via homologous recombination. The crucial common mutation in the early and later generations of attenuated cholera vaccines is the deletion of genetic sequences encoding the *ctxA* gene encoding the cholera enterotoxin A subunit which is responsible for the ADP-ribosylating activity of the holotoxin. A number of such vaccines have been constructed by investigators at the Center for Vaccine Development at the University of Maryland and at the Harvard University [1,3–5].

The first generation recombinant cholera vaccines were generated from wild-type El Tor strain N16961 and classical strain 395. These vaccine candidates, strain JBK70 from N16961 and strains CVD 101 and 395N1 from 395, were markedly attenuated compared to the wild parent strain and were highly immunogenic [6,7]. When volunteers who were immunized with a single dose of 10^6 JBK70 were challenged with the virulent parent strain, significant protection was observed [6]. Diarrhea occurred in 7 of 8 unimmunized controls but in only 1 of 10 vaccinees, a vaccine efficacy of 89%. This level of efficacy was equivalent to that seen following sequential experimental infections with wild-type El Tor strains. Interestingly, JBK70 produced neither the A nor B subunits of cholera toxin, so this challenge study demonstrated the importance of antibacterial immunity in the absence of antitoxic immunity.

Despite the high levels of immunity engendered by these three vaccine candidates, they were unexpectedly reactogenic. Approximately one-half of the recipients of JBK70, CVD 101, and 395N1 suffered adverse reactions such as mild diarrhea, malaise, nausea, vomiting, abdominal cramps, low-grade fever, and headache [6,7]. These strains never caused severe or even moderate diarrhea but were nonetheless not studied further because of these reactions. These results were surprising since it was previously believed that cholera toxin was the only diarrheagenic factor produced by *V. cholerae*. Two hypotheses were proposed to explain this response [6]. The first hypothesis was that a previously unknown enterotoxin was responsible for the diarrhea in the absence of cholera toxin (CT). The second hypothesis was that avid colonization by the attenuated *V. cholerae* strain in the proximal small bowel, a site where only low numbers of bacteria are found in healthy North Americans, would somehow disturb the normal balance of secretion and absorption resulting in diarrhea and other symptoms.

To investigate the hypothesis that a previously undescribed enterotoxin was responsible for the reactogenicity, reactogenic *V. cholerae* vaccine candidates were tested for enterotoxic activity in rabbit ileal tissue mounted in Ussing chambers. Two candidate toxins, Zot (zonula occludens toxin) and Ace (accessory cholera enterotoxin), were discovered that possessed enterotoxic properties, and the genes for these factors were found to be located immediately upstream of the *ctx* gene in a 4.5-kb region called the "core region" of the Ctx genetic element (reviewed in Ref. 1). This region was subsequently shown to encode a filamentous bacteriophage [8], and at least the *zot* gene is essential for phage morphogenesis, suggesting that Zot and Ace may have dual functions. To address the hypothesis that the putative Zot and Ace toxins were responsible for the reactogenicity of the

attenuated *V. cholerae* O1 strains, a derivative of wild-type El Tor strain E7946 was constructed with the *ace*, *zot*, and *ctxA* genes deleted and the *ctxB* gene was cloned under the control of the *ctx* promoter and inserted into the *hlyA* gene encoding the El Tor hemolysin. Although the resulting strain, CVD 110, provided excellent vibriocidal and antitoxic immune responses in volunteers, it caused mild to moderate diarrhea in 7 of 10 vaccinees (which was accompanied by malaise, nausea, and low-grade fever) and was therefore unacceptably reactogenic [9].

III. RECOMBINANT ATTENUATED *V. CHOLERAE* O1 CLASSICAL STRAIN CVD 103-HgR

The first recombinant *V. cholerae* vaccine strain to be well tolerated yet highly immunogenic and protective was strain CVD 103, derived from the classical Inaba *V. cholerae* O1 strain 569B. This parent strain colonized the intestine at lower levels than other toxigenic *V. cholerae* strains and was reported to lack a Shiga-like toxin activity that was possibly involved in vaccine reactogenicity. CVD 103 was derived from 569B by deletion of the *ctxA* subunit [10], and a further derivative was constructed by inserting genes encoding resistance to mercury (*mer*) into the chromosomal *hlyA* locus. The mercury resistance provides a marker to readily differentiate the vaccine strain from wild-type *V. cholerae*. The resulting strain, CVD 103-HgR, exhibits many of the characteristics of an ideal cholera vaccine and is now licensed and sold in numerous countries under the trade names Orochol® and Mutacol®.

CVD 103-HgR has been extensively studied in a number of randomized, placebo-controlled, double-blind phase I and phase II clinical trials involving more than 7000 subjects in countries in Asia, Latin America, Africa, Europe, and North America (reviewed in Refs. 1, 4, 11, and 12). The safety and immunogenicity of this vaccine have been demonstrated in subjects as young as 3 months and as old as 65 years of age, including subjects infected with the human immunodeficiency virus (HIV) [13,14]. In all studies, neither diarrhea nor any other adverse reaction occurred significantly more often in vaccinees than in placebo recipients. Several efficacy studies have been conducted in which subjects were vaccinated with CVD 103-HgR and then challenged along with unvaccinated controls with virulent toxigenic *V. cholerae* O1 strains. A single dose of CVD 103-HgR provided significant protection against challenge with classical Inaba, classical Ogawa, El Tor Inaba, or El Tor Ogawa strains [3,4,15,16]. In a multicenter, randomized, double-blind, placebo-controlled efficacy trial of a single dose of classical CVD 103-HgR against challenge with virulent El Tor strain N16961, moderate or severe diarrhea (>3 L) was seen in 9 of 23 placebo recipients vs. 1 of 28 vaccinees (91% efficacy). When mild diarrhea was assessed, 21 of 23 placebo recipients and 5 of 28 vaccinees had any diarrhea (mild to severe) (80% efficacy) [15]. Another trial demonstrated that protection is evident as early as 8 days after vaccination and lasts for at least 6 months (the shortest and longest intervals tested) [17]. The single-dose efficacy and rapid onset of protection are attractive advantages of the live cholera vaccine CVD 103-HgR compared to killed whole cell cholera vaccines.

The efficacy of CVD 103-HgR against natural challenge in a cholera-endemic country was studied in a randomized, double-blind, placebo-controlled field trial involving 67,508 pediatric and adult subjects in Indonesia [18]. A single dose of vaccine did not confer significant long-term protection over the 4-year observation period (13.5% vaccine efficacy overall), but individuals of blood group O, who are at highest risk for severe diarrhea, were modestly protected by the vaccine ($p = 0.06$, vaccine efficacy = 45%). Unfortunately, too few cases (5 in controls, 2 in vaccinees) occurred in the first 4 months of follow-up to assess whether CVD 103-HgR provided short-term protection similar to the short-term duration of previous clinical trials involving North American volunteers. The most likely explanation for the poor efficacy in subjects in the developing world is their lower postvaccination vibriocidal titers compared to titers in North American volunteers. Diminished immunogenicity of live oral vaccines given to subjects living in developing countries compared to subjects in industrialized countries has also been observed with both oral polio and rotavirus vaccines. In order to achieve high seroconversion rates of vibriocidal antibody in Indonesian children, it was necessary to give a dose of CVD 103-HgR 10-fold higher (5×10^9 CFU) than the dose (5×10^8 CFU) that is consistently immunogenic in North Americans and Europeans (reviewed in Refs. 4 and 12). Potential explanations for the diminished immunogenicity include small bowel overgrowth [19] and heavy infection with intestinal helminthes [20].

Although the protective efficacy of a single dose of CVD 103-HgR in individuals living in developing countries has not been established, the significant protective immunity demonstrated in challenge studies involving North American volunteers offers strong evidence that this vaccine will protect individuals from noncholera-endemic countries in North America and Europe who travel to cholera-endemic countries. The vaccine is manufactured by Berna Biotech Ltd., Berne, Switzerland, and over 500,000 doses have been distributed worldwide. It is available in a convenient formulation consisting of two aluminum foil sachets, one containing lyophilized vaccine (and aspartame as sweetener) and the other containing buffer (to protect the vaccine strain from gastric acid). The two sachets are mixed in a cup containing 100 ml of water, and the resultant suspension is swallowed. *V. cholerae* CVD 103-HgR is also available in a combination vaccine with attenuated *Salmonella* Typhi vaccine strain Ty21a, and antibody responses resulting from coadministration of the two vaccines were comparable in frequency and magnitude to those levels seen in previous studies using each vaccine alone [21].

IV. RECOMBINANT ATTENUATED *V. CHOLERAE* O1 EL TOR VACCINE STRAINS

The current predominant O1 biotype throughout the world is the El Tor biotype, and the attenuated *V. cholerae* CVD 103-HgR vaccine strain belongs to the classical biotype of *V. cholerae* O1. As discussed above, this classical vaccine provided strong protective immunity against experimental challenge with toxigenic El Tor Inaba or Ogawa strains. Although an El Tor vaccine strain may initially appear to be more desirable than a classical strain given the predominance of the El Tor biotype, there is compelling evidence, both from epidemiological and volunteer studies, that infection with the classical biotype is a more powerful immunizing experience than infection with the El Tor biotype. Clemens et al. [22] studied cholera in Bangladesh during a time in which both classical and El Tor biotypes were causing disease. Over a 42-month observation period, 2214 initial episodes of cholera were recorded in the study population. Seven of these individuals had a second episode of cholera. An initial infection with a classical strain provided 100% protection against a second episode of cholera due to either classical or El Tor strains. In contrast, an initial infection with El Tor provided only 30% protection against a second El Tor episode and no protection whatsoever against subsequent classical biotype disease. (However, a recent examination of cholera in Bangladesh over a 33-year period suggests that classical and El Tor strains protect equally well and that initial infection with an Ogawa strain offers less protection than infection with an Inaba strain [23]). In studying short-term protection in North American volunteers infected with wild-type *V. cholerae* O1 strains, an initial infection with a classical strain led to 100% protection upon subsequent challenge, whereas an initial infection with an El Tor strain led to ca. 90% protection [2]. The reasons for the differences in protection induced by El Tor and classical strains are unknown. The regulation of *ctx* and the *tcp* gene encoding the essential toxin co-regulated pilus (TCP) colonization factor differs between the two biotypes in response to environmental conditions. The TCP from El Tor and classical strains shares only 82% protein sequence homology of the major pilin subunit [24]. Support for the importance of TCP sequence differences in biotype-specific protection comes from animal studies using passive immunization against El Tor or classical TCP preparations. However, in humans, infection with either El Tor or classical strains leads to little or no immune response against either form of TCP, although TCP is clearly essential for intestinal colonization and generation of a protective immune response against other antigens [25]. A mannose-sensitive hemagglutinin (MSHA) expressed by O1 El Tor and the related O139 strains, but not by classical strains, was originally proposed to be important in intestinal colonization and biotype-specific protection. However, in a volunteer trial using an isogenic *V. cholerae* O139 strain in which the gene encoding MSHA was mutated, intestinal colonization was not affected by the deletion of MSHA [26]. Mannose-sensitive hemagglutinin may play a role in environmental survival rather than in disease in the human intestine. Despite the lack of certainty as to the critical differences between El Tor and classical biotypes, a variety of attenuated El Tor vaccine candidates have been prepared using molecular genetic techniques similar to those employed in construction of classical candidates, and these candidates are in various stages of clinical evaluation.

Vaccine candidate CVD 111 was derived from the toxigenic El Tor O1 strain N16117 using methods similar to those used to construct CVD 110 [27]. In previous volunteer studies, this parent strain was not as virulent as other wild-type El Tor challenge strains. The *ctxA*, *ace*, *zot*, and *hlyA* genes were deleted, and the *ctxB* gene expressed from the *ctx* promoter along with the *mer* genes was inserted into the hlyA locus to generate CVD 111. When tested in volunteers, CVD 111 caused mild diarrhea in 3 of 25 volunteers (12%) at a dose of 10^8 CFU [27]. The seroconversion rate for both vibriocidal and antitoxin responses was 92% after a single dose. When challenged 7 weeks after vaccination, 3 (16.7%) of 18 vaccinees and 7 (87.5%) of 8 controls developed diarrhea, a vaccine efficacy of 80.9%. A bivalent CVD 103-HgR/CVD 111 vaccine has been evaluated in Phase II trials in Peru and Panama and was found to be safe and immunogenic [28,29].

V. cholerae IEM101 is an O1 El Tor Ogawa strain that was isolated from a river water sample in China. It naturally lacks *ctxAB*, *ace*, and *zot* genes but contains *tcp* genes encoding the TCP pilus [30]. In volunteer trials in China, this strain colonized well, no diarrhea, fever, or other side effects occurred, and serum vibriocidal antibodies were engendered. This strain has subsequently been modified to express a genetically detoxified derivative of cholerae toxin [31] as well as heterologous antigens such as fragment C of tetanus toxin and tracheal colonization factor from *Bordetella pertussis* [32]. To date, no human efficacy data have been reported for this strain.

V. cholerae strain 638 is an attenuated O1 El Tor Ogawa strain developed by investigators in Cuba who deleted the *ctx*, *zot*, and *ace* genes as well as the *hap* gene encoding a hemagglutinin/protease (HAP) possibly involved in the reactogenicity of earlier *V. cholerae* vaccine strains. In an initial phase I study, this vaccine engendered significant vibriocidal antibody titers and mild diarrhea in 4 of 42 vaccinees upon vaccination [33]. No challenge studies of protective efficacy have been reported.

Peru-15 is an El Tor Inaba strain created from a wild-type *V. cholerae* O1 strain (C6709) isolated in Peru in 1991. It was constructed by deleting the 4.5-kb core element containing *ctx*, *ace*, and *zot* as well as the RS I element and attRS sequences flanking the core element. In addition, the *ctxB* gene was cloned under the control of the *htpG* heat-shock promoter and inserted into the chromosomal *recA* gene, thereby inactivating this gene involved in homologous recombination. The attenuated strain resulting from these initial genetic manipulations was called Peru-3. When tested in volunteers at doses of 4×10^6 and 1×10^8 CFU, Peru-3 stimulated significant vibriocidal antibody responses in 5 of 6 vaccinees and mild diarrhea in 2 of 6 [34]. A spontaneous nonmotile mutant of Peru-3 was isolated and designated Peru-15 [35]; the nonmotile mutant was better tolerated in volunteers than the Peru-3 parent. A recent randomized, placebo-controlled clinical trial enrolled 59 North American volunteers who received 2×10^8 CFU of Peru-15 or placebo [36]. Recipients of the vaccine and placebo had similar rates of symptoms, except for headaches, which were more frequently reported by vaccinees on days 0 and 3 ($p = 0.002$ and 0.05, respectively), and abdominal cramps, which did

not reach statistical significance. Ninety-seven percent of vaccinees mounted significant vibriocidal antibody responses and 28% mounted significant antitoxin responses. After challenge with wild-type El Tor strain N16961, 5 (42%) of the 12 placebo recipients and none of the 24 vaccinees had moderate or severe diarrhea (>3 kg diarrheal stool) (protective efficacy 100%). When mild diarrhea was included, 7 (58%) of 12 placebo recipients and 1 (4%) of 24 vaccinees had any diarrhea (protective efficacy 93%). Further clinical studies of Peru-15 are underway.

V. LIVE ATTENUATED VACCINE CANDIDATES AGAINST *V. CHOLERAE* O139

Before 1992, cholera was exclusively associated with *V. cholerae* of the O1 serogroup. However, in late 1992, epidemic cholera caused by a *V. cholerae* strain of a serogroup other than O1 appeared in India and Bangladesh. The serogroup associated with this new epidemic was designated O139. By late 1993, the O139 serogroup had largely displaced O1 as the principal cause of cholera in Bangladesh and Calcutta, India, although by 1995, O1 had returned as the predominant serogroup in these countries [37]. In contrast to the expected epidemiology of O1 *V. cholerae* in cholera-endemic countries, in which the attack rates are highest in young children and decrease in older age groups, indicating acquisition of immunity in adults after repeated antigenic contact, the attack rate for the initial O139 outbreak was higher in adults than in children, suggesting that antibacterial and antitoxic immunity engendered by *V. cholerae* O1 did not confer cross protection against disease due to *V. cholerae* O139 [38]. Subsequent animal studies supported the lack of cross protection between these two serogroups. Thus vaccination against *V. cholerae* O139 will require new vaccines that contain O139 antigens.

V. cholerae O139 strains are very similar to O1 El Tor strains in numerous phenotypic and genetic traits [38]. However, O139 differs from O1 in that a different lipopolysaccharide (LPS) antigen and a capsular polysaccharide not found in O1 strains is expressed by O139 strains. At the molecular level, the O139 clone appears to have arisen by the substitution of ca. 22 kb of DNA encoding the O1 LPS with a unique 35-kb region involved in the expression of the O139 LPS and capsular polysaccharide [39]. The experience gained from construction of attenuated O1 vaccine candidates provided the basis for the rapid development of live attenuated vaccine candidates for the prevention of cholera due to *V. cholerae* O139.

CVD 112 is an O139 vaccine candidate constructed from wild-type O139 strain AI1837 by deleting the core region containing the *ctxAB*, *zot*, and *ace* genes and inserting the *ctxB* and *mer* genes into the *hlyA* locus, analogous to CVD 110 [40]. CVD 112 was fed to volunteers in doses of 10^6 and 10^8 CFU with buffer. At the lower dose, no adverse reactions such as diarrhea, headache, nausea, fever, or abdominal cramps occurred among 6 recipients. At the higher dose, 3 of 6 volunteers passed a few small volume diarrheal stools without any accompanying symptoms. Five weeks after vaccination, 8 vaccinees and 15 unvaccinated control subjects were challenged with wild-type O139 strain AI1837. Diarrhea occurred in 1 vaccinee and 12 control subjects after challenge. The vaccine efficacy of 84% was remarkably similar to protection conferred by primary wild-type infection with AI1837 against subsequent challenge (80%) [41].

Bengal-3 is another promising attenuated O139 vaccine candidate constructed from the wild-type O139 strain MO10. Like CVD 112, the core element containing *ctxAB*, *ace*, and *zot* genes was deleted along with the flanking RSI and attRSI sequences. The *ctxB* gene was cloned under the control of the *htpG* heat-shock promoter and inserted into the chromosomal *recA* gene [42]. A spontaneous, nonmotile derivative of Bengal-3 was isolated which lacked flagella and was designated Bengal-15 [43]. In initial clinical trials, one of four volunteers who received 10^7 CFU of Bengal-3 and none of 10 recipients of 6×10^6 or 10^8 CFU of Bengal-15 experienced diarrhea upon vaccination [43]. In a challenge study, diarrhea occurred in 1 of 7 Bengal-15 vaccinees and 6 of 7 unimmunized controls, a vaccine efficacy of 83% [43].

A different approach to an attenuated live vaccine against O139 *V. cholerae* was pursued by Favre et al. [44]. Rather than attenuate a wild-type O139 strain, these authors used the O1 vaccine strain CVD 103-HgR as a vector for O139 antigens, specifically the short core-linked O139 polysaccharide (SOPS) and the highly polymerized capsular polysaccharide (CPS). A derivative of CVD 103-HgR was constructed which lacked *rfbAB* genes necessary for expression of the O1 LPS. The cloned genes encoding the O139 polysaccharides were then incorporated into the chromosome of the CVD 103-HgR derivative. The resulting strain, CH25, expressed both O139 SOPS and CPS and stimulated high levels of anti-SOPS and anti-CPS serum antibodies when injected intramuscularly into rabbits. No clinical trials of this vaccine candidate have yet been reported, but if clinical results are promising, the extensive safety record accumulated for CVD 103-HgR and the fact that it has already been licensed by regulatory agencies in several countries should speed the development of such a hybrid vaccine.

VI. ATTENUATED *V. CHOLERAE* AS A LIVE VECTOR FOR EXPRESSION OF HETEROLOGOUS ANTIGENS

A variety of foreign antigens have been expressed in attenuated *V. cholerae* vaccine strains including Shiga toxin (Stx) B subunit [45], fragment C of tetanus toxin [32], tracheal colonization factor of *B. pertussis* [32], *Shigella sonnei* O antigen [46], the immunogenic portion of *Clostridium difficile* toxin A [47], the Intimin colonization factor of enterohemorrhagic *Escherichia coli* [48], hepatitis B middle surface antigen [49], gp120 from HIV [50], and the serine-rich *Entamoeba histolytica* protein [51]. No human studies have yet been reported with any of these constructs, but protective immunity has been demonstrated in a rabbit model against challenge with *C. difficile* toxin A [51] and Stx holotoxin [45] and in an intranasal mouse model against challenge with tetanus toxin and *B. pertussis* [32].

To develop optimal *V. cholerae*-vectored vaccines, a number of variables such as choice of promoter, integration

site, and location for heterologous antigen expression within the *V. cholerae* cell have been studied, but extensive comparisons of the relative importance of these variables have not yet been conducted. Most studies have used *E. coli* promoters including P_{tac} [45,48,52], P_{trc} [53], P_{slt} [53], P_{lpp} [51], and P_{nirB} [32], but two *V. cholerae* promoters have also been used, the iron-regulated P_{irgA} promoter and the heat-shock promoter P_{htpG} [52,54]. A comparison was made among the constitutively expressed P_{tac} and the in vivo-induced P_{irgA} and P_{htpG} in the attenuated *V. cholerae* strain Peru-2 [52], and it was found that P_{tac} elicited the most prominent specific antibodies in vivo despite the fact that P_{tac} and P_{irgA} expressed equivalent amounts of the antigen in vitro. Regarding integration site of the heterologous antigen gene, most studies have used multicopy plasmids, which usually yield higher antigen expression but are not as stable as chromosomal integration. Ryan et al. [51] have developed a balanced lethal plasmid system for expression of heterologous antigens in *V. cholerae* involving the *glnA* gene in which the chromosomal *glnA* gene copy is deleted and is complemented by a complete *glnA* gene on the plasmid vector. There has been relatively little investigation into the advantages or disadvantages of different cellular locations, i.e., cytoplasmic, periplasmic, or extracellular, of heterologous antigens expressed in *V. cholerae*, nor has there been much investigation of different mechanisms by which noncytoplasmic locations might be achieved. The efficient extracellular secretion of CT via a type II secretion system has led to the construction of CTB fusion proteins with epitopes from hepatitis B middle surface antigen [49], gp120 from HIV [50], and the serine-rich *E. histolytica* protein [51] to allow expression and secretion of these epitopes. However, this system is limited by the small size of the epitope that can be attached while still allowing secretion of the fusion protein. Another approach for extracellular secretion of heterologous antigens from *V. cholerae* utilizes the hemolysin export system of *E. coli*. Ryan et al. [47] used the HlyA export system to export a 720 amino acid portion of *C. difficile* toxin A fused to the HlyA protein and demonstrated that for some but curiously not all strains of *V. cholerae*, the majority (70%) of the fusion protein was found in the supernatant.

VII. CONCLUSIONS

At the present time, there is no ideal cholera vaccine that can provide long-term protection to individuals from both industrialized and developing countries in a single dose formulation. The live attenuated vaccine that is furthest along in development is CVD 103-HgR, which solidly protected North Americans against experimental challenge but which failed in a field trial in Indonesia. It is not known whether the result of the Indonesian field trial was an aberration, possibly because of the low attack rate for cholera during the surveillance period or other reasons. A second field trial of CVD 103-HgR, possibly comparing a one- and two-dose regimen, is needed. There is precedence for a cholera vaccine providing protection in one field setting but not in another. For example, the killed whole cell B subunit vaccine gave 86% protection in one two-dose field trial in children and adults in Peru, yet 0% protection in a separate two-dose trial in military recruits in Peru [55,56].

Beyond the unanswered questions specific to CVD 103-HgR, there are additional questions that apply to any live attenuated *V. cholerae* vaccine. For example, can volunteer trials in North Americans reliably predict the success of trials conducted in cholera-endemic countries? Volunteer trials in North Americans are probably most relevant in predicting immunization success for travelers or military personnel from industrialized countries. The higher levels of microbial flora in the proximal small bowels of individuals in developing countries compared to levels in individuals in industrialized countries could present a substantial barrier to replication of a live vaccine in this critical intestinal site. In addition, preexisting antibodies to *V. cholerae* in individuals in cholera-endemic countries could inhibit replication of a live vaccine. Moreover, the mechanism responsible for the mild diarrhea induced in some North American volunteer who received early *ctx*-negative *V. cholerae* vaccine strains is unknown. It is conceivable that these highly immunogenic vaccine strains which were discarded because of their reactogenicity might have been well tolerated and effective among residents of endemic countries.

Another important unanswered question concerns the identity of the antigens required to raise a protective immune response. Clearly, the LPS plays a major role in protective immunity, as demonstrated by the apparent lack of immunity to *V. cholerae* O139 in adults who were presumably immune to *V. cholerae* O1. But additional as-yet-unidentified protein antigens are likely to contribute to protective immunity. Additional questions concern the need for a combined O1 and O139 vaccine. In the early 1990s, some predicted that the emergence of *V. cholerae* O139 was the start of the eighth pandemic of cholera. However, O139 did not spread widely and it is currently present in only a minority of cholera patients in Bangladesh and eastern India. A formulation for worldwide use containing both O1 and O139 would increase production costs of a vaccine that would be marginally profitable in any circumstance. A larger question concerns the fundamental nature of the emergence of the O139 serogroup. How did this novel organism emerge in the early 1990s? Could another novel and lethal serogroup of *V. cholerae* emerge in the future? Such questions continue to challenge us more than a century after the development of the first cholera vaccine.

REFERENCES

1. Kaper JB, et al. Cholera. Clin Microbiol Rev 1995; 8:48–86.
2. Levine MM, Pierce NF. Immunity and vaccine development. In: Barua D, Greenough WB III, eds. Cholera. New York: Plenum Medical Book Co., 1992:285–327.
3. Levine MM, Kaper JB. Live oral vaccines against cholera: an update. Vaccine 1993; 11:207–212.
4. Kaper JB, et al. New and improved vaccines against cholera. Part i: Attenuated *Vibrio cholerae* O1 and O139 strains as live oral cholera vaccines. In: Levine MM, Woodrow GC, Kaper JB, Cobon GS, eds. New Generation Vaccines. New York: Marcel Dekker, 1997:447–458.
5. Waldor MK, Mekalanos JJ. Progress toward live-attenuated cholera vaccines. In: Kiyono H, Ogra PL, McGhee JR, eds.

6. Mucosal Vaccines. San Diego: Academic Press, 1996:229–240.
6. Levine MM, et al. Volunteer studies of deletion mutants of *Vibrio cholerae* O1 prepared by recombinant techniques. Infect Immun 1988; 56:161–167.
7. Herrington DA, et al. Toxin, toxin-coregulated pili, and the toxR regulon are essential for *Vibrio cholerae* pathogenesis in humans. J Exp Med 1988; 168:1487–1492.
8. Waldor MK, Mekalanos JJ. Lysogenic conversion by a filamentous phage encoding cholera toxin. Science 1996; 272:1910–1914.
9. Tacket CO, et al. Safety and immunogenicity of live oral cholera vaccine candidate CVD 110, a *ΔctxA Δzot Δace* derivative of El Tor Ogawa *Vibrio cholerae*. J Infect Dis 1993; 168:1536–1540.
10. Ketley JM, et al. Construction of genetically-marked *Vibrio cholerae* O1 vaccine strains. FEMS Microbiol Lett 1993; 111: 15–22.
11. Levine MM, Tacket CO. Live oral vaccines against cholera. In: Ala'Aldeen DAA, Hormaeche CE, eds. Molecular and Clinical Aspects of Bacterial Vaccine Development. New York: John Wiley & Sons, Ltd., 1995:233–258.
12. Campbell JD, Kaper JB. Vaccines against *Vibrio cholerae*. Bacterial Vaccines. In: Ellis RW, Brodeur BR, eds. Landes Bioscience, 2003:339–349.
13. Lagos R, et al. Palatability, reactogenicity and immunogenicity of engineered live oral cholera vaccine CVD 103-HgR in Chilean infants and toddlers. Pediatr Infect Dis J 1999; 18:624–630.
14. Perry RT, et al. A single dose of live oral cholera vaccine CVD 103-HgR is safe and immunogenic in HIV-infected and HIV-noninfected adults in Mali. Bull World Health Organ 1998; 76:63–71.
15. Tacket CO, et al. Randomized, double-blind, placebo-controlled, multicentered trial of the efficacy of a single dose of live oral cholera vaccine CVD 103-HgR in preventing cholera following challenge with *Vibrio cholerae* O1 El Tor Inaba three months after vaccination. Infect Immun 1999; 67: 6341–6345.
16. Levine MM, et al. Safety, immunogenicity, and efficacy of recombinant live oral cholera vaccines, CVD 103 and CVD 103-HgR. Lancet 1988; 2:467–470.
17. Tacket CO, et al. Onset and duration of protective immunity in challenged volunteers after vaccination with live oral cholera vaccine CVD 103-HgR. J Infect Dis 1992; 166:837–841.
18. Richie EE, et al. Efficacy trial of single-dose live oral cholera vaccine CVD 103-HgR in North Jakarta, Indonesia, a cholera-endemic area. Vaccine 2000; 18:2399–2410.
19. Lagos R, et al. Effect of small bowel bacterial overgrowth on the immunogenicity of single-dose live oral cholera vaccine CVD 103-HgR. J Infect Dis 1999; 180:1709–1712.
20. Cooper PJ, et al. Albendazole treatment of children with ascariasis enhances the vibriocidal antibody response to the live attenuated oral cholera vaccine CVD 103-HgR. J Infect Dis 2000; 182:1199–1206.
21. Cryz SJ Jr, et al. Safety and immunogenicity of a live oral bivalent typhoid fever (*Salmonella typhi*: Ty21a) cholera (*Vibrio cholerae* CVD 103-HgR) vaccine in healthy adults. Infect Immun 1995; 634:1336–1339.
22. Clemens JD, et al. Biotype as determinant of natural immunising effect of cholera. Lancet 1991; 337:883–884.
23. Longini IM Jr, et al. Epidemic and endemic cholera trends over a 33-year period in Bangladesh. J Infect Dis 2002; 186: 246–251.
24. Rhine JA, Taylor RK. TcpA pilin sequences and colonization requirements for O1 and O139 *Vibrio cholerae*. Mol Microbiol 1994; 13:1013–1020.
25. Hall RH, et al. Immunogenicity of *Vibrio cholerae* O1 toxin-

coregulated pili in experimental and clinical cholera. Infect Immun 1991; 59:2508–2512.

26. Tacket CO, et al. Investigation of the roles of toxin-coregulated pili and mannose- sensitive hemagglutinin pili in the pathogenesis of *Vibrio cholerae* O139 infection. Infect Immun 1998; 66:692–695.

27. Tacket CO, et al. Volunteer studies investigating the safety and efficacy of live oral El Tor *Vibrio cholerae* O1 vaccine strain CVD 111. Am J Trop Med Hyg 1997; 56:533–537.

28. Taylor DN, et al. Evaluation of a bivalent (CVD 103-HgR/CVD 111) live oral cholera vaccine in adult volunteers from the United States and Peru. Infect Immun 1997; 65:3852–3856.

29. Taylor DN, et al. Expanded safety and immunogenicity of a bivalent, oral, attenuated cholera vaccine, CVD 103-HgR plus CVD 111, in United States military personnel stationed in Panama. Infect Immun 1999; 67:2030–2034.

30. Liu YQ, et al. A natural vaccine candidate strain against cholera. Biomed Environ Sci 1995; 8:350–358.

31. Fontana MR, et al. IEM101, a naturally attenuated *Vibrio cholerae* strain as carrier for genetically detoxified derivatives of cholera toxin. Vaccine 2000; 19:75–85.

32. Chen I, et al. A recombinant live attenuated strain of *Vibrio cholerae* induces immunity against tetanus toxin and *Bordetella pertussis* tracheal colonization factor. Infect Immun 1998; 66:1648–1653.

33. Benitez JA, et al. Preliminary assessment of the safety and immunogenicity of a new CTXφ-negative, hemagglutinin/protease-defective El Tor strain as a cholera vaccine candidate. Infect Immun 1999; 67:539–545.

34. Taylor DN, et al. Development of a live, oral, attenuated vaccine against El Tor cholera. J Infect Dis 1994; 170:1518–1523.

35. Kenner JR, et al. Peru-15, an improved live attenuated oral vaccine candidate for *Vibrio cholerae* O1. J Infect Dis 1995; 172:1126–1129.

36. Cohen MB, et al. Randomized, controlled human challenge study of the safety, immunogenicity, and protective efficacy of a single dose of Peru-15, a live attenuated oral cholera vaccine. Infect Immun 2002; 70:1965–1970.

37. Faruque ASG, et al. Changing epidemiology of cholera due to *Vibrio cholerae* O1 and O139 Bengal in Dhaka, Bangladesh. Epidemiol Infect 1996; 116:275–278.

38. Albert MJ. *Vibrio cholerae* O139 Bengal. J Clin Microbiol 1994; 32:2345–2349.

39. Comstock LE, et al. Cloning and sequence of a region encoding surface polysaccharide of *Vibrio cholerae* O139 and characterization of the insertion site in the chromosome of *Vibrio cholerae* O1. Mol Microbiol 1996; 19:815–826.

40. Tacket CO, et al. Initial clinical studies of CVD 112 *Vibrio cholerae* O139 live oral vaccine: safety and efficacy against experimental challenge. J Infect Dis 1995; 172:883–886.

41. Morris JG Jr, et al. Clinical and immunologic characteristics of *Vibrio cholerae* O139 Bengal infection in North American volunteers. J Infect Dis 1995; 171:903–908.

42. Waldor MK, Mekalanos JJ. Emergence of a new cholera pandemic: molecular analysis of virulence determinants in *Vibrio cholerae* O139 and development of a live vaccine prototype. J Infect Dis 1994; 170:278–283.

43. Coster TS, et al. Safety, immunogenicity and efficacy of live attenuated *Vibrio cholerae* O139 vaccine prototype. Lancet 1995; 345:949–952.

44. Favre D, et al. Construction and characterization of a potential live oral carrier-based vaccine against *Vibrio cholerae* O139. Infect Immun 1996; 64:3565–3570.

45. Acheson DWK, et al. Protective immunity to Shiga-like toxin I following oral immunization with Shiga-like toxin I B-subunit-producing *Vibrio cholerae* CVD 103-HgR. Infect Immun 1996; 64:355–357.

46. Viret JF, et al. Expression of *Shigella sonnei* lipopolysaccharide in *Vibrio cholerae*. Mol Microbiol 1996; 19:949–963.

47. Ryan ET, et al. Protective immunity against *Clostridium difficile* toxin A induced by oral immunization with a live, attenuated *Vibrio cholerae* vector strain. Infect Immun 1997; 65:2941–2949.

48. Butterton JR, et al. Coexpression of the B subunit of Shiga toxin 1 and EaeA from enterohemorrhagic *Escherichia coli* in *Vibrio cholerae* vaccine strains. Infect Immun 1997; 65:2127–2135.

49. Schodel F, et al. Synthesis in *Vibrio cholerae* and secretion of hepatitis B virus antigens fused to *Escherichia coli* heat-labile enterotoxin subunit B. Gene 1991; 99:255–259.

50. Backstrom M, et al. Insertion of a HIV-1-neutralizing epitope in a surface-exposed internal region of the cholera toxin B-subunit. Gene 1994; 149:211–217.

51. Ryan ET, et al. Oral immunization with attenuated vaccine strains of *Vibrio cholerae* expressing a dodecapeptide repeat of the serine-rich *Entamoeba histolytica* protein fused to the cholera toxin B subunit induces systemic and mucosal antiamebic and anti-*V. cholerae* antibody responses in mice. Infect Immun 1997; 65:3118–3125.

52. John M, et al. In vitro and in vivo analyses of constitutive and in vivo-induced promoters in attenuated vaccine and vector strains of *Vibrio cholerae*. Infect Immun 2000; 68:1171–1175.

53. Acheson DWK, et al. Comparison of Shiga-like toxin I B-subunit expression and localization in *Escherichia coli* and *Vibrio cholerae* by using *trc* or iron-regulated promoter systems. Infect Immun 1993; 61:1098–1104.

54. Butterton JR, et al. Heterologous antigen expression in *Vibrio cholerae* vector strains. Infect Immun 1995; 63:2689–2696.

55. Taylor DN, et al. Two-year study of the protective efficacy of the oral whole cell plus recombinant B subunit cholera vaccine in Peru. J Infect Dis 2000; 181:1667–1673.

56. Sanchez JL, et al. Protective efficacy of oral whole-cell/recombinant-B-subunit cholera vaccine in Peruvian military recruits. Lancet 1994; 344:1273–1276.

45

Novel Vaccines Against Tuberculosis

Robert J. Wilkinson and Douglas B. Young
Imperial College of Science, Technology and Medicine, London, England

I. INTRODUCTION

In the 5 years that have elapsed since the second edition of this book, extraordinary and encouraging advances have been made in the field of mycobacteriology. This updated and revised chapter is thus written with the advantage of the whole genome sequence of *Mycobacterium tuberculosis* [1] and the recent completion of the human genome project [2]. Novel analytic techniques now permit comparison of the entire genome, transcriptome, and proteome of bacilli from varying sources grown under differing conditions [3–5]. The difficulties of achieving genetic recombination in *M. tuberculosis* have been overcome. The emphasis now has shifted rapidly from the purely microbiological characterization of recombinant strains to their cellular microbiological characterization in model systems [6–8] and use of such strains as potential vaccines [9]. Tuberculosis was among the first diseases to be shown to be potentially preventable by DNA vaccination [10,11]: subsequent research has also revived interest in the potential for therapeutic vaccination [12]. The analysis of novel rare immunodeficiencies predisposing to mycobacterial infection has greatly clarified human immune resistance to *M. tuberculosis* [13–16]. Lastly, and of greatest clinical significance, the evolution of highly active multidrug regimes to treat HIV infection is potentially of major significance to the 8% of tuberculosis patients co-infected with this virus and to countless millions of other HIV-infected persons who have latent tuberculosis infection.

How well has this explosion in basic knowledge translated into clinical practice? In the United States, the incidence of tuberculosis progressively fell during the 1990s [17]. Nowhere else in the world was this true. No new first line drugs were introduced, and the coexistence of HIV and tuberculosis particularly in Africa has contributed to epidemic tuberculosis [18]. Acquired multiple drug resistance in *M. tuberculosis* has become increasingly prevalent [19], contributing to the fear that the implementation of directly observed chemotherapy (DOTS) alone will be insufficient to control tuberculosis [20]. In 1997, new cases of TB were es-timated to be 7.96 million and an estimated 1.87 million people died of TB: a case fatality rate of 23% [21]. Never has there been a greater need for an improved or additional vaccine.

II. BACILLE CALMETTE–GUÉRIN VACCINE

There is a vaccine against tuberculosis that is effective in animals and in humans and which is safe and inexpensive. This vaccine, bacille Calmette–Guérin (BCG), has been evaluated in a series of clinical trials and is currently administered to around 100 million newborn children each year as part of the WHO Expanded Program for Immunization (EPI). What can be learnt from this story and why is it necessary to improve upon BCG?

Calmette and Guérin derived BCG, after 13 years of continuous laboratory passage on deficient media, from an initially virulent isolate of *Mycobacterium bovis*, a member of the pathogenic *M. tuberculosis* complex. The resulting isolate was avirulent in mice, guinea pigs, and humans and was found (and continues to be found) to be effective as an experimental vaccine in animals. By contrast, the efficacy of BCG in humans has been under continuous debate. Bacille Calmette–Guérin has been found to confer a high degree of protection in some trials; for example, in the United Kingdom, the incidence of tuberculosis in the vaccinated group was reduced by 77% when compared to the control group [22]. However, in other trials, the efficacy has been close to zero, most notably in South India (reviewed by Ref. 23). Variations between trials reflect the differences in the ability of BCG to protect adults against pulmonary tuberculosis, as the vaccine has consistently shown significant protective efficacy against the disseminated forms of tuberculosis that are a major cause of childhood mortality [24]. This feature justifies the vaccine's inclusion in the EPI. Bacille Calmette–Guérin also confers protection against leprosy [25]. However, the same trial concluded that revaccination with BCG did not improve its efficacy against tuberculosis. In addition, the limited data available suggest that the efficacy of BCG vaccination wanes over time.

The reasons for the variations in efficacy have been discussed in extensive detail [23]. There are a number of genetically distinct substrains of BCG, all of which were maintained by further continuous passage until the advent of lyophilization in 1961 [5], raising the possibility that differences in immunogenicity between strains might contribute to the varying efficacy of BCG worldwide. The route of administration and efficacy of immunizing technique have not been rigorously evaluated. A widely favored hypothesis is that saprophytic mycobacteria, which are more common in the environment and water supply in warmer climates, may influence the results of the trials [26]. Thus sensitization by environmental mycobacteria could reverse the immunological benefits conferred by BCG vaccination. Conversely, sensitization by environmental mycobacteria might immunize in the same way as BCG [27], effectively equilibrating responses in control and trial groups.

An alternative hypothesis to account for the variations in trial results is based on recent genomic analysis of BCG strains. Using the genome of the sequenced H37Rv strain of *M. tuberculosis* as a template, it has been possible to identify genetic regions that are missing from various substrains of the original BCG vaccine [5,28]. In addition to regions absent from all *M. bovis* isolates, five regions encompassing 38 open reading frames were found to have been deleted from some or all BCG substrains. By a process of forensic genomics, a chronology for the occurrence of the deletions leading from *M. tuberculosis* to BCG could be drawn up [5]. It is also the case that some genes, contained in regions designated RvD1 and RvD2, are absent from H37Rv but found in *M. bovis* and BCG [29]. Further, in BCG Pasteur, there are two tandemly duplicated regions, DU1 and DU2 [30]. The potential contribution of these genetic differences between BCG and *M. tuberculosis* to the virulence of the latter is not yet clear. However, it is possible that the sequential loss of genes during subculture of BCG substrains has been accompanied by a parallel decline in their protective ability. Calmette [31] was always of the impression that isolates of BCG, which caused regional lymphadenopathy and extensive scar formation, were better vaccines.

Experience with BCG thus holds a number of important lessons for any future TB vaccine program. Firstly, BCG does demonstrate that it is indeed possible to use a vaccine to confer protection against TB. A caveat, however, is that an immunization protocol capable of inducing protection in one population group, whether defined by age or geography, may be ineffective in a different population. A central lesson from the BCG story has been the limitations in understanding protective immunity against tuberculosis. The effect of vaccination has been evaluated solely on the basis of long-term follow-up and monitoring of disease incidence. Unless some short-term measure of potential protective efficacy in humans can be established, future tuberculosis vaccines may follow BCG into decades of controversy and uncertainty.

III. IMMUNOLOGICAL MECHANISMS AND CORRELATES OF PROTECTION

Tuberculosis is a chronic disease, often difficult to diagnose, which can have a long incubation period of years or decades. Experimental infection of humans, an ethical option when studying some readily curable infectious diseases [32], is difficult to envisage in tuberculosis given that the therapy even of fully drug-sensitive asymptomatic infection involves months of treatment. Thus vaccine trials would benefit enormously if reliable correlates of protective immunity could be established.

A. Experimental Models

1. Effector Function

In the last decade, experiments in gene knockout mice have delineated some of the crucial host regulatory and effector pathways necessary to contain tuberculosis in this animal. Broadly speaking, two effector pathways necessary to control the replication of *M. tuberculosis* have emerged. Activation of infected mononuclear phagocytes to kill resident intracellular bacilli is the predominant pathway. The second pathway involves the lysis of infected phagocytes, thus facilitating uptake of bacilli by competent phagocytes or the induction of apoptosis of infected phagocytes with concomitant destruction of the bacteria.

The monokine tumor necrosis factor-α (TNF-α) is essential for bactericidal granuloma formation [33]. Mice with a disruption of the gene encoding the p55 TNF-α receptor (TNFR1) rapidly develop disseminated infection as do mice which overexpress the soluble TNFR1 [34,35]. Deletion of the gene for interferon-γ (IFN-γ) markedly increases susceptibility to tuberculosis via a mechanism involving inducible nitric oxide (NO) [36–38]. Production of IFN-γ is, in turn, dependent on the production of interleukin (IL)-12. Deletion of the gene encoding secreted IL-12p40 results in mice that are unable to control mycobacterial growth [39] (Figure 1).

2. T Cell Subsets

T cell responses are accepted to be quantitatively most relevant to protection against mycobacterial infection as the antibody response, with a few interesting exceptions [40,41], is thought to be ineffective. The regulatory T cell subsets required to control murine tuberculosis have been extensively researched. There is an obligate requirement for the CD4$^+$ subset of T cells [42]. In mice, there is also evidence that the phenotypic separation of CD4$^+$ T cells into IFN-γ secreting type 1 and IL-4 (IL-10 and IL-13) secreting type 2 cells is of relevance. It is widely assumed that type 2 cells, which downregulate the type 1 response and favor IgG1 and IgE production, are nonprotective. However, mice that are unable to make either IL-4 or IL-10 are no more resistant to tuberculosis [43]. Thus type 1 responses are necessary for protection, but the absence of type 2 responses does not improve resistance. The CD4$^+$ response is thought to be mediated largely by antigen presentation via MHC Class II

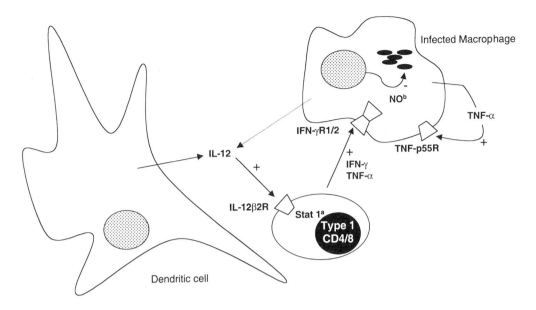

Figure 1 Key protective pathways in murine and human tuberculosis. (a) Only of proven significance in human. (b) Only of proven significance in mice.

molecules, as MHC Class II β chain knockout mice are unable to control growth even of the attenuated BCG vaccine strain [44].

There also appears to be a role for MHC Class I restricted T cells, as mice lacking β₂ microglobulin (a component of the MHC Class I molecule) are highly susceptible to intravenous *M. tuberculosis* infection [45]. However, the precise phenotype of MHC Class I restricted T cells involved is more debatable as the degree of susceptibility of the β₂ microglobulin knockout animals is not reproduced in mice lacking the gene for CD8 [42] or in those which lack CD1d (which also requires β₂ microglobulin to present antigen to CD8⁺ T cells) [46]. Mice which lack either perforin, an effector of the granule exocytosis pathway, or CD95 (Fas) ligand, an effector of apoptosis, are also able to control initial infection [47,48]. Some effect of deletion of the genes for CD8, perforin, and CD95L is observed, however, as the infection progresses [42,49]. The inability to attribute a special effector role unique to CD8⁺ cells has led some to suggest that CD8⁺ T cells contribute to IFN-γ production [50,51]. Alternatively, antigen may be available for recognition by Class I restricted cells earlier in infection [52] or on cells which only express the more widely distributed MHC Class I molecule.

B. Humans

Epidemiological surveys suggest that *M. tuberculosis* latently infects 32% of the world's population, and it is estimated that 7.96 million new cases of active disease occurred in 1997 [21]. From these figures, it can be inferred that around 90% of latently infected people will remain free of disease for life. Thus the immune mechanisms that control *M. tuberculosis* are, in most humans, efficient. In the minority who do

develop disease, however, there is a pronounced role for the immune response in contributing to pathology. It thus follows that the immune response in persons who develop tuberculosis must be qualitatively or quantitatively different from those who remain infected but healthy. Dissecting this paradox between pathology and protection has been at the center of human tuberculosis research.

1. Effector Function

When defining the protective response in man, the most informative analyses have been of very small numbers of patients with severe recurrent atypical mycobacterial or *Salmonella* infections. Such individuals have been shown to have mutations in the IL-12- and IFN-γ-driven type 1 cytokine pathway (Table 1). Thus in a way that is analogous to the situation in mice with selective gene deletions, there appears to be an obligate requirement for the type 1 pathway in human antimycobacterial defense (Figure 1).

The evidence for a direct role for reactive nitrogen intermediates (RNI) in human defense is less compelling than in the mouse. Induction of the iNOS (*NOS1*) gene has been documented in cells from the lungs of human tuberculosis patients [55], as has the accumulation of nitrite in *M. tuberculosis*-stimulated cultures of alveolar macrophages [56]. However, in the latter study, NO synthase inhibitors inhibited the production of RNI by alveolar macrophages but did not significantly affect the intracellular growth of *M. tuberculosis*. Recently, the 19-kDa antigen-mediated suppression of intracellular *M. tuberculosis* in human cells was shown to be RNI-independent, whereas in mice, clear evidence that this effect was RNI-dependent was shown [57].

Recently, the first convincing evidence for the role of TNF-α in containing latent infection in humans has also been provided by informal reporting of side effects of

Table 1 Novel Genetic Immunodeficiency Syndromes which Predispose to Mycobacterial Infection

Molecule	Phenotype	Mutation	Reference
IFN-γ receptor I	Severe atypical mycobacterial infection	Point mutation at nucleotide 395 that introduces a stop codon	16
IFN-γ receptor II	*Mycobacterium fortuitum* and *M. avium* infection	Homozygous dinucleotide deletion at nucleotides 278 and 279, resulting in a premature stop codon	53
IL-12p40	BCG and *S. enteritidis* infection	Large homozygous deletion	54
IL-12β1 receptor subunit	Severe mycobacterial and salmonella infections	A variety of missense and deletion mutations	15, 54
Stat 1	Disseminated BCG or *M. avium* infection	Point mutation at nucleotide position 2116	13

infliximab [58]. Infliximab is a humanized antibody against TNF-α that is used in the treatment of Crohn's disease and rheumatoid arthritis. Out of 147,000 patients treated with infliximab, 70 developed tuberculosis within a median of 12 weeks, some after as few as 3 or 4 infusions. Whether this is a true increase over background incidence can be argued, but the trials of infliximab were carried out in countries with a low incidence of tuberculosis, in the order of 10/100,000. The disease pattern was predominantly (57%) postprimary and extrapulmonary, strongly suggesting that TNF-α prevents endogenous reactivation. These data therefore powerfully support a role for TNF-α in containing latent infection.

Are humans and mice therefore similar with important roles in the protective response for IFN-γ, IL-12, and TNF-α (Figure 1)? Do measurements of the in vitro cytokine response of stimulated cells from larger numbers of patients with tuberculosis and healthy *M. tuberculosis*-infected subjects support this conclusion? Before reviewing such studies, it is important to point out that they rely predominantly on sampling of responses of peripheral blood mononuclear cells (PBMC), and that these may not always accurately reflect events at the site of infection. Lymphocyte IL-2 production is increased in both tuberculous pleural fluid and bronchoalveolar lavage of patients with pulmonary tuberculosis by comparison with PBMC, for example [59,60], and IFN-γ mRNA is increased about 60-fold in pleural fluid mononuclear cells of patients with tuberculous pleuritis over that in their PBMC [61]. Sequestration and local activation of lymphocyte replication may contribute to the lower level of IL-2 in *M. tuberculosis* antigen-stimulated PBMC from patients by comparison with control subjects [62–64].

Responses Favoring Macrophage Activation. *IFN-γ.* It seems logical that a deficit of IFN-γ production by PBMC may characterize patients with pulmonary tuberculosis, and some reports do indeed document a reduction in IFN-γ production in patients when stimulating with PPD or a 30-kDa antigen [65], *M. tuberculosis* [64], or the recombinant 10-, 38-, or 65-kDa antigens [66]. This is not always been observed, however. No reduction in the frequency of IFN-γ secreting cells in the blood of patients by comparison with healthy BCG-vaccinated controls was detected when PBMC were stimulated with *M. tuberculosis* soluble extract or the recombinant 19- and 38-kDa antigens [67]. It has more

recently been shown that the frequency of IFN-γ secreting cells responding to the antigen early-secreted antigenic target-6 (ESAT-6) is high in untreated patients with tuberculosis and that this frequency tends to fall after effective antituberculous chemotherapy [68]. These apparent discrepancies may be due to the selection of control subjects, the extent of disease of the patients, the choice of antigen, and the potentially confounding effects of chemotherapy.

In an attempt to resolve some of these points, a recent large study placed greater emphasis on the definition of groups with various *M. tuberculosis* sensitization within households of tuberculosis cases and, in particular, on the responses of children with primary infection. In response to culture filtrate antigens of *M. tuberculosis*, IFN-γ production was found to be highest in skin test positive children with primary disease and in adults with latent infection [69]. The lowest response was in cases of far-advanced disease. Thus while bulk IFN-γ secretion in response to culture filtrate did not discriminate *M. tuberculosis*-infected healthy subjects from those with early disease, progression to advanced disease was associated with a decreased IFN-γ response (Figure 2). Therefore differences in the cellular phenotype (e.g., memory vs. short-lived effector cells), antigenic specificity, or rate of loss of IFN-γ producing T cells between those who remain healthy and those who progress may be crucial. The dynamics of IFN-γ producing cells during infection are also almost certainly more complex than originally suspected.

IL-12. Interleukin-12 is a monocyte/macrophage-derived cytokine which favors the differentiation of IFN-γ producing T cells [70]. Its active form is a p70 heterodimer formed from inducible p40 and constitutively expressed p35 chains. The p40 chain can also associate with a p19 chain to form IL-23 whose biological spectrum of activity appears similar to IL-12p70 [71]. Interleukin-12 would be expected to favor a protective role in tuberculosis. In humans, small amounts of IL-12 have been demonstrated in tuberculous pleural effusions [72], and an increased frequency of IL-12 producing cells has been demonstrated in patients with tuberculosis [73]. Interleukin-12 production is best stimulated by phagocytosis of intact *M. tuberculosis* organisms [74], but it has also been shown that ligation of the surface-expressed TLR2 toll-like receptor by lipoproteins of *M. tuberculosis* added to cultures of mononuclear phagocytes

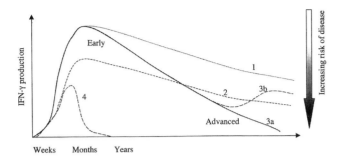

Figure 2 Possible dynamics of CD4 mediated IFN-γ production at various stages in the natural history of tuberculosis infection. The curves are idealized representations of induced IFN-γ production in various groups over time based on data that are largely cross-sectional in nature. Curve 1 represents natural infection accompanied by lifelong freedom from disease. Curve 2 represents BCG vaccination. This intervention may prime sufficient response to decrease the risk of severe or advanced disease in children, but, over time, its efficacy is known to wane. Curve 3 is the disease curve. Curve 3b shows the effect of chemotherapy, which tends to increase the IFN-γ response, although some differences from healthy controls persist even after successful chemotherapy. Curve 4 represents tuberculosis infection in patients already infected by HIV. This is a pernicious combination and the risk of disease is very high.

can induce IL-12p40 [75]. The most potent IL-12p40 inducing lipoprotein, the 19-kDa antigen, has also been shown to trigger the death of intracellular mycobacteria in human cells by a mechanism that is RNI-independent [57]. These findings are, in turn, not easy to reconcile with the observation that expression of the 19-kDa gene in *Mycobacterium smegmatis* inhibits IL-12p40 induction by the recombinant bacteria [76]. In addition, the 19-kDa antigen has recently been reported to deactivate the antigen-presenting function of murine cells by decreasing the expression of MHC Class II by a TLR2-dependent mechanism [77].

Despite these paradoxes, a significant area of consensus in studies on the 19-kDa lipoprotein is that its immunomodulatory activity requires it to be acylated, as recombinant nonacylated 19 kDa does not show these effects. Acylation affects the intracellular trafficking of the 19 kDa directing it to the MHC Class I pathway [78], and it is possible that such differential trafficking may account for some of the diverse effects seen in various systems. One approach to untangling this complex interaction would be the generation of recombinant *M. tuberculosis* that does not express the 19 kDa. In conjunction with complementation of such a recombinant with wild-type and site-directed mutagenized forms of the 19-kDa gene lacking acylation or glycosylation motifs, such an approach would allow dissection of this interaction in the context of the immune response to the whole bacillus.

Interferon-γ Inducing Factor. Interferon-γ inducing factor, or IL-18, is synergistic with IL-12 in IFN-γ induction in mice and humans [79,80]. Deletion of the IL-18 gene decreases the granulomatous response to *M. tuberculosis* but has no effect on the survival of mice or the replication of

mycobacteria [81]. The available evidence in humans suggests that IL-18 does have a role in promoting type 1 activation, but that its constitutive production is increased by IFN-γ in a positive feedback loop in turn dependent on intact IL-12 function [82–84].

TNF-α. Tumor necrosis factor-α is produced by monocytes in response to intact *M. tuberculosis* and to both protein and nonprotein antigens [61,63,85–87]. The observation that orderly (as opposed to necrotic) granuloma formation is accompanied by the highest expression of mRNA for TNF-α supports a protective role [88], as do the findings relating to this cytokine's neutralization in vivo by infliximab [58]. However, TNF-α is also associated with the fever and weight loss characteristic of tuberculosis, leading to the suggestion that this cytokine may be associated with pathology [89–91]. Serum TNF-α levels transiently rise at the onset of antituberculous chemotherapy, and this rise is accompanied by a fall in Karnofsky score [92]. The production of TNF-α is downregulated by both IL-10 and transforming growth factor-β (TGF-β) [93] and can also be specifically downregulated by the drug thalidomide, which has been proposed as an immunomodulatory therapy [90].

Responses Favoring Macrophage Deactivation. Given that evidence is accruing that a type 1 cytokine response is protective, is there evidence that a type 2 response is deleterious?

IL-4. A marked antibody response associated with depression of antigen-specific lymphocyte proliferation occurs in active tuberculosis [94,95]. Interleukin-4 promotes antibody production and antagonizes the effects of IFN-γ. Antigen-specific (as opposed to mitogen-induced) IL-4 secretion in tuberculosis has only been demonstrated in T cell clones [96] and in stimulated PBMC by the highly sensitive enzyme-linked immunospot (ELISPOT) assay [67]. In the latter study, the frequency of IL-4 producing cells was increased in tuberculosis patients by comparison with control subjects, although the number of IL-4 secreting cells was very small. It has been demonstrated that very small amounts of IL-4 can markedly bias innate responses to *M. tuberculosis* [97]. However, IL-4 is generally undetectable by conventional ELISA [65,66,98,99] in tuberculosis, which is in marked contrast to other conditions where there is established and significant type 2 activation such as atopic asthma or helminth infection. Using a highly sensitive nested RT-PCR, both IL-4 message and its splice variant IL-4δ2 were detected in PBMC from tuberculosis patients [100]. However, others have found no IL-4 or IL-5 gene expression in bronchoalveolar lavage cells, pleural fluid, or lymph nodes from patients with tuberculosis [59,61,98].

Transforming Growth Factor-β (TGF-β). Transforming growth factor-β mediates a predominantly immunosuppressive and macrophage deactivating response during tuberculosis. Transforming growth factor-β downmodulates both T cell responses [101] and macrophage activation [102]; neutralization of TGF-β enhances T cell responses to mycobacterial antigens [65]. Macrophages in tuberculous granulomas and monocytes from tuberculous patients (but not healthy subjects) express TGF-β1 [103]. Furthermore, some mycobacterial proteins and lipoarabinomannan induce TGF-β secretion by monocytes [87]. Transforming growth factor-β also induces IL-1Ra [104] and IL-10 [105]. Naturally occurring inhibitors of TGF-β, decorin and latency associated peptide (LAP), reverse depressed T cell functions in peripheral blood mononuclear cells (PBMC) from patients with pulmonary tuberculosis [106]. Recently, an enhanced murine antimycobacterial response to a recombinant BCG expressing LAP has also been reported [107].

IL-10. The suppression of proliferation and assistance for antibody production may also be partly accounted for by IL-10, which deactivates macrophages and downregulates type 1 cytokine responses. Expression of MHC Class II molecules on antigen-presenting cells is also suppressed by IL-10 [108,109]. Anti-IL-10 neutralizing antibody is effective in reversing depressed cell proliferation in HIV-infected patients with tuberculosis [110]. In addition, IL-10 downregulates *M. tuberculosis*-induced type 1 responses and CTLA-4 expression [111]. Interleukin-10 is released spontaneously by PBMC from tuberculosis patients (perhaps reflecting macrophage activation), and additional increments due to PPD stimulation are only consistently demonstrable in untreated patients [99]. The above evidence suggests that IL-10 has an important downregulatory role. However, IL-10 did not enhance the growth of *Mycobacterium avium* in human macrophages [112]. Furthermore, levels of IL-10 in supernatants of PBMC stimulated by 30-kDa antigen or PPD were not increased in patients by comparison with controls [65].

Overall, the most available evidence suggests that the classical Th1/Th2 dichotomy as defined by terminally differentiated murine T cell clones [113] is not clearly observed in human tuberculosis. The overwhelming majority of responding T cells are of the type 1 or type 0 and not type 2 phenotype. The suppression of the type 1 response that does occur may be more readily attributable to the overproduction of downregulatory cytokines by monocytes and macrophages.

2. T Cell Subsets

The protective function of CD4⁺ cells in containing latent infection can be indirectly inferred from the high risk of tuberculosis conferred by HIV infection. This risk, although increased at all stages of HIV infection, is highest in persons with the lowest CD4⁺ counts. It is also worth pointing out, however, that cavitating pulmonary tuberculosis is a less common disease form in advanced HIV infection, implying that a competent CD4⁺ T cell response is also necessary for the characteristic clinical syndrome to develop. Thus CD4⁺ T cell responses contribute to pathogenesis as well as to protection.

Numerous studies have identified multiple antigenic targets that induce the proliferation of, and IFN-γ production from, CD4⁺ cells. There is hierarchy in the stimulatory capacity of individual antigens: particularly potent molecules are found among the secreted antigens, with the Antigen 85 complex and ESAT-6 being prominent [95,114]. In addition, certain "somatic" antigens are also highly immunogenic, particularly the heat-shock proteins [115]. At the level of individual peptide epitopes, some

peptides are able to restimulate cells from a high proportion of individuals with varying HLA Class II types. Such "permissive" peptide recognition has been shown in the better-characterized cases to be due to the ability of peptide to bind with high affinity to multiple HLA-DR molecules [94,116]. Interestingly, in another instance, this ability appears to be conferred by peptide presentation in the context of the less polymorphic HLA-DQ molecule [117].

Because of the findings in the murine system, there has also been attention to the possibility that CD8⁺ T cells may contribute to human defense. Such T cells may contribute because of their unique effector function, timing, or ability to recognize infected cells which are not "seen" by the CD4⁺ subset. Initial studies confirmed that, in addition to conventional responses restricted by MHC Class I molecules, CD1-restricted and MHC-unrestricted CD8⁺ responses can be detected [118–121]. Subsequent studies have defined a number of T cell epitopes [122–125]. A general conclusion from these studies is that the frequency of CD8⁺ cells is low, much lower than the frequency of CD4⁺ cells. Most studies have used IFN-γ production as a measure of the CD8⁺ cell response. However, in one case, tetramer analysis did reveal a slightly higher frequency of peptide-specific cells and potentially interesting evidence of functional heterogeneity in the CD8⁺ population [122].

Whether CD8⁺ cells contribute in a unique way to human defense remains conjectural. An important aspect of the early interaction between infected mononuclear phagocytes and *M. tuberculosis* is that the bacillus manipulates the phagosome that it resides in, preventing the normal maturation of this organelle into an acidic, hydrolytic compartment [126]. In this way, degradation and presentation of peptides via MHC Class II may be crucially delayed allowing the bacillus a "window" to establish intracellular replication before the immune onslaught. The ability of CD8⁺ cells to recognize infected targets by way of alternative antigen-presenting pathways may provide an important adjunct to the MHC Class II-restricted response. It has been postulated that antigens can traffic out of the phagosome into the cytoplasm [127] and are thus potentially available for presentation via MHC Class I, and intracellular trafficking of glycolipid antigens makes them available for presentation by CD1 molecules [128].

Alternatively CD8⁺ cells may have some unique effector function. A great deal of interest has been stimulated by the derivation from infected healthy donors of CD1-restricted CD8⁺ and CD4⁻CD8⁻ double-negative human T cell clones. These clones recognize a variety of hydrophobic mycobacterial lipids in the context of CD1, a relatively nonpolymorphic MHC Class I molecule [129]. Additional evidence of functional dichotomy was presented by the finding that CD8⁺ clones lysed infected cells via the granule exocytosis pathway and thereby reduced the growth of bacteria. By contrast, the CD4⁻CD8⁻ double negative clones triggered lysis via the ligation of Fas by Fas ligand, but this did not reduce mycobacterial viability [118]. The antimicrobial, and thus unique effector, function of the CD8⁺ cells was ascribed to granulysin, a mediator of the granule exocytosis pathway [130]. However, it has subsequently been shown that granulysin is also associated with CD4⁺

cells in leprosy lesions [131] and is produced by *M. tuberculosis*-specific MHC Class II restricted CD4$^+$ T cells [132]. In addition, the latter study showed the CD8$^+$-mediated growth restriction of *M. tuberculosis* within infected cells to be uninfluenced by inhibitors of the granule–exocytosis pathway. As CD1-restricted T cells remain to be demonstrated at appreciable frequencies in the peripheral blood of infected subjects, their quantitative significance and unique function therefore remain open to question. The recent successful assembly of human CD1d-glycolipid tetramers should allow this question to be answered definitively [133].

There has also been considerable work on the human γδ TCR T cell response. These cells are known to expand in response to both proteins and nonpeptide ligands of mycobacterial origin [134,135]. γδ cells can be cytolytic and produce IFN-γ and accumulate at disease sites [136,137]. A possibility is that γδ cells play a part in early infection [138].

IV. POTENTIAL APPLICATION OF NOVEL TUBERCULOSIS VACCINES

A. Replace Neonatal Bacille Calmette–Guérin

The ideal vaccine would be of greater overall efficacy than BCG such that the latter would be replaced. The vaccine should be administered as a single dose at birth and go on to confer lifelong protection against disease. This is an ambitious goal as no single candidate in animal models has yet to clearly surpass the efficacy of BCG, although some combinations are promising. Perhaps it is not realistic to conceive a single "magic bullet," but rather to consider whether a new vaccine could be given in addition to BCG in order to augment the latter's partial efficacy.

B. Boost Preexisting Immunity in Late Adolescence

The peak incidence of tuberculosis is in young adults, in the 20–30 year age group, with pulmonary disease as the most common presentation. Adult tuberculosis usually results from the reactivation of latent tuberculosis infection (LTBI), although in some circumstances, reinfection contributes [139,140]. Therefore when BCG fails to prevent adult tuberculosis, this could be due to failure to control LTBI or to a gradual decline in the BCG-induced resistance to repeated reinfection episodes. To prevent reinfection, it would be necessary for a new vaccine to be superior to BCG in its ability to protect against initial challenge. The T cell response required to maintain latency in humans is very poorly characterized, and the requirements for a vaccine that would improve the immune control of LTBI are largely unknown. To address this area, there is a need for longitudinal study of healthy *M. tuberculosis*-infected subjects in addition to current patient-centered investigations. One major problem in this respect has been the accurate identification of individuals who are actually infected, as the PPD skin test has important limitations in specificity. Blood-based assays, which rely on antigens of greater species specificity, may offer a route around this problem [116,141]. If the responses maintaining LTBI can be better defined, a boost strategy could be targeted towards adolescents who would have received neonatal BCG vaccination and subsequently exposed to challenge with *M. tuberculosis*. The available data suggest that revaccination with BCG at this age confers no additional protection [25] and, in contrast to neonatal vaccination, there are no ethical questions related to withholding BCG as part of a vaccine trial. Given the high incidence of disease in early adulthood, this might therefore offer the best opportunity for early vaccination trials in humans.

C. Disease-Modifying or Transmission-Blocking Vaccines

The fact that BCG reduces the incidence of miliary and meningeal disease in infants suggests that vaccines may also impact disease severity. If host and bacillary determinants of disease severity (as opposed to correlates of protection) could be ascertained, it might be a basis for designing a third type of vaccine that would lessen clinical symptoms without completely preventing disease. It may be possible to impact transmission of tuberculosis if the immune intervention reduced the number of sputum smear positive patients, for example. The most transmissible form of tuberculosis, cavitating pulmonary disease, is associated with most extensive tissue damage, suggesting that the induction of immunopathology by *M. tuberculosis* may be subject to positive evolutionary selection [142]. The underlying immunopathological mechanisms are poorly understood, but it is conceivable that immune modulation of this event could contribute to decreased transmission. Such a vaccine may be useful for disease control within populations, but might present difficulties in relation to diagnosis of individual patients since the diagnosis of tuberculosis usually relies mainly on detection of bacilli in the sputum.

D. Immunotherapeutic Vaccines

Early studies of the chemotherapeutic action of antituberculous drugs established that, while initial bacillary counts fall precipitously, treatment of less than 6 months duration is associated with an unacceptably high relapse rate. This phenomenon is attributed to "persisting" organisms, which, by virtue of not dividing, are insensitive to drug action. In humans with active tuberculosis, quantitative and qualitative changes in the immune response occur during treatment, encouraging the view that immunomodulation should be possible [99]. Such modulation would undoubtedly be beneficial if the duration of treatment could be shortened and also of potential impact when there is drug resistance. There is experimental evidence of therapeutic vaccine efficacy in mice [12]. In leprosy, addition of immunotherapy with *Mycobacterium w* vaccine to multidrug therapy benefits multibacillary leprosy patients by increasing the rate of bacillary clearance [143]. However, this is at the cost of an increased risk of upgrading reactions. In leprosy, these immunopathological reactions are of considerable clinical significance. Less well recognized, but known since the adverse experience of Robert Koch with tuberculin, is the upgrading reaction which can occur in tuberculosis [144].

The risk of inducing immunopathology therefore has to be carefully weighed against likely therapeutic advantage. More knowledge of the correlates of pathology, as distinct from protection, in human tuberculosis is also required.

V. THE FRAMEWORK FOR VACCINE EVALUATION AND DEVELOPMENT

Vaccines are, in general, produced and marketed by large pharmaceutical companies. There are anxieties within the private sector regarding the likely financial yield of developing a new tuberculosis vaccine since such a product would be predominantly used in resource-poor environments. While the massive health benefits that would accrue from a successful vaccine do not preclude justifying a relatively high unit vaccine cost, at present, tuberculosis vaccine development is not a major priority for big pharmaceutical companies. There is commendable work from smaller biotech companies [145–147], but it is likely that the major impetus for vaccine development will have to come from the public sector.

Development of new vaccines will require effort not only from research scientists, but also from epidemiologists and clinicians. Considerable momentum towards developing and testing novel vaccines in humans has built up in the last few years. Following wide consultation which included the WHO, the International Union Against Tuberculosis and Lung Disease (IUALTD), and the Food and Drugs Administration, the NIH has issued a "blueprint" for tuberculosis vaccine development [148]. A specific commitment to evaluation of novel vaccines in aerosol-infected mice and guinea pigs was made and over a hundred candidates and combinations have been tested [149]. The European Community has also recognized the need for a wide-ranging approach to preclinical research with the establishment of a TB Vaccine Cluster [150] which includes a primate model for testing of novel vaccines [151]. Human tuberculosis vaccine research units have also been created which will facilitate the Phase I/II clinical testing of promising candidates. Identification of appropriate high-incidence areas for future efficacy trials and establishment of suitable long-term clinical and epidemiological support for such ventures are a priority. Importantly, ethical approval for studies should be obtained both in the country in which the trial will take place (likely resource-poor) and also from the country in which the vaccine originated (likely resource-rich). It is important to appreciate that, even in high-incidence areas, Phase III trials will need to include many tens of thousands of participants and, because the efficacy of BCG is known to vary by geographical region, parallel trials may need to be established in different parts of the world. The need for longstanding international collaboration and expense is therefore clear.

VI. VACCINE CANDIDATES

It has already been noted that many new candidate vaccines have already been produced. This section cannot therefore be comprehensive: we have used candidates to illustrate principles (Table 2). There is no clear rationale at this stage

Table 2 Novel Vaccine Candidates with Protective Efficacy in Small Animal Models

Vaccine	Model	Reference
Live vaccines		
BCG overexpressing Ag85B	Guinea pig	9
M. tuberculosis leuD auxotroph	Mouse	156
M. tuberculosis trpD auxotroph	Mouse	157
Protein subunit vaccines		
M. tuberculosis culture filtrate	Mouse	163, 165
M. tuberculosis culture filtrate	Guinea pig	185
Ag85B (Rv1886c)	Mouse	186
	Guinea pig	164
ESAT-6 (Rv3875)	Mouse	186
Ag85B/ESAT-6 fusion	Mouse	171
38-kDa antigen (PstS1; Rv0934)	Mouse	187
Mtb8.4 (Rv1174c)	Mouse	146
DNA vaccines		
Ag85A (Rv3804c)	Mouse	11
	Guinea pig	188
Ag85B (Rv1886c)[a]	Mouse	179
M. leprae Hsp60[b]	Mouse	10
ESAT-6 (Rv3875)	Mouse	179
38-kDa antigen (PstS1; Rv0934)[c]	Mouse	175
PstS3 (Rv0928)	Mouse	189
MPT64 (Rv1980c)	Mouse	179
Mtb39A (Rv1196)	Mouse	145
MPT63 (Rv1926c)	Mouse	190
MPT83 (Rv2873)	Mouse	190
MTB41 (Rv0915c)	Mouse	191
Mtb8.4 (Rv1174c)	Mouse	146
Combination vaccines		
MPT63/ESAT-6 DNA + vaccinia boost	Mouse	182
Ag85A DNA + protein boost	Mouse	178
Ag85B DNA + BCG boost	Mouse	184

[a] Other investigators found Ag85B to be ineffective as a DNA vaccine [11,178].
[b] DNA vaccination with the corresponding *M. tuberculosis* gene (Rv0440) induced immunopathology [180].
[c] Other investigators found no protection with PstS1 DNA [189].

for the design of the optimal tuberculosis vaccine. Bacille Calmette–Guérin provides a precedent to indicate that vaccination with a live mycobacterium can confer protection, but considerations related to safety, manufacture, and distribution favor a nonliving subunit formulation. This approach requires identification of relevant antigens and selection of appropriate delivery systems. It is not clear whether priority should be given to formulations designed to induce a prolonged memory response per se or whether the aim should be to set up a strong initial response that would be boosted by natural exposure to infection and environmental organisms.

A. Live Vaccines

Experience with BCG provides a precedent for tuberculosis vaccines based on live attenuated mycobacteria, and the improvement of the existing BCG vaccine represents one general approach to the generation of new vaccine candidates. New tools for genetic manipulation of mycobacteria provide an opportunity to refine the live vaccine strategy of Calmette and Guérin by addition of genes to BCG or by targeted removal of genes from initially virulent *M. tuberculosis* [152].

1. Modified Strains of Bacille Calmette–Guérin

Bacille Calmette–Guérin has been engineered to express recombinant mammalian cytokines designed to augment immunogenicity or decrease immunopathology, for example [107,153]. The addition of the listeriolysin gene has been shown to enhance the ability of BCG antigens to traffic into the cytoplasm and thereby to induce a $CD8^+$ T cell response [154]. Particularly promising results have been generated by the overexpression of antigen 85B carried on a multicopy episomal plasmid in recombinant BCG [9]. However, the in vivo stability of such plasmid-bearing strains was not assessed: for bacteria, the possession of plasmid often reduces fitness, especially under immune pressure.

One possible reason for the incomplete efficacy of BCG is that it lacks "protective" antigens present in *M. tuberculosis*. Comparison of the genomes of *M. tuberculosis* and BCG identified a 9.5-kb region, designated RD1, that has been deleted from all strains of BCG [5,28]. RD1 encodes two antigens (ESAT-6 and CFP-10) that are highly immunogenic and prominent immune targets in *M. tuberculosis*-infected humans [141,155]. Further, there is some evidence that ESAT-6-specific $CD8^+$ T cells may contribute to the immune maintenance of latency in humans [119,124]. Selective reintroduction of the genes for ESAT-6 and CFP-10 into BCG is an attractive concept. In pursuing this as a vaccine strategy, it would be important to ensure that adding back RD1 products does not increase virulence. A second caveat is that the specific diagnostic advantage conferred by the use of these antigens would be lost.

2. Attenuation of *M. tuberculosis*

Several laboratories have generated novel attenuated strains by deletion of genes from *M. tuberculosis*. Three strategies have been pursued. The first involves the introduction of auxotrophic mutations that render the bacteria dependent on exogenous growth factors that are in limited supply. Successful examples include the derivation of attenuated strains dependent on leucine [156] and tryptophan [157]. A second approach is to inactivate *M. tuberculosis* genes analogous to those involved in virulence in other bacterial pathogens. An interesting recent example is the construction of a *phoP* attenuated mutant, based on the knowledge of the key role of this regulator in pathogenic *Salmonella* [158]. The third strategy for identification of attenuated strains exploits the technique of signature-tagged transposon mutagenesis (STM). This involves screening of a library of transposon mutants to identify clones selectively lost during murine infection. The STM approach has identified attenuated mutants with defects in biosynthesis of cell-wall lipids [159,160]. Decreased persistence within tissues and altered patterns of tissue dissemination has been described for several attenuated variants of *M. tuberculosis* or *Mycobacterium marinum* [6–8,161], further indicating that the technology of mycobacterial attenuation is now well established.

Whether any of these mutants could function as vaccine candidates still requires empirical analysis. Aside from the overriding need for safety, the properties required for an improved live vaccine strain are unknown; interactions with antigen-presenting cells, the precise mode of death, and duration of persistence within the host are all likely to influence vaccine efficacy. Information from the current round of trial and error screening of novel attenuated strains, together with progress in understanding of the cellular microbiology of mycobacterial infection, may ultimately allow the design of rational selection procedures for improved live vaccines.

B. Protein Subunit Vaccines

Two criteria have been used to identify *M. tuberculosis* antigens for incorporation into programs for subunit vaccine development. The first is the ability to elicit a strong recall response in man or experimental animals exposed to *M. tuberculosis* infection. The response is assessed primarily in terms of the release of IFN-γ from antigen-specific $CD4^+$ T cells. While this represents a realistic strategy to identify antigens available for T cell recognition, it will (like BCG) tend to reproduce rather than augment the natural immune response. Amplification of naturally subdominant responses represents a potentially interesting alternative approach [162], particularly in the context of postexposure vaccination.

A second common criterion for antigen selection is their identification in the supernatant of in vitro cultures. The presence of proteins secreted by actively dividing bacilli may be one factor in determining the superior protective efficacy of live as compared to killed mycobacteria. This idea is supported by experiments from several laboratories demonstrating successful vaccination with culture filtrate preparations [163–165]. However, live mycobacteria also require immunogenic proteins that are not secreted such as the small heat-shock protein Acr or 16-kDa antigen [166]. Given this protein's putative role in stabilizing cellular structures during conditions of stress such as those found in the "immune" granuloma, it may be an important target of T cells maintaining immunity during persistent infection [94].

Several purified protein antigens have been shown to induce protective immunity following immunization in appropriate adjuvant (Table 2). The most extensively studied are antigen 85B (Ag85B) and ESAT-6. Ag85B is a member of the antigen [85] complex, a set of three closely related proteins which function as mycolyl transferases and are the most abundant protein components in culture filtrate preparations [167]. Early secreted antigenic target-6 is a low molecular weight protein antigen, present in culture filtrates of *M. tuberculosis* but absent from BCG [168]. Early secreted antigenic target-6 is a member of a *M. tuberculosis* gene family comprising several prominent immunogens [169], including CFP-10 which is encoded by the adjacent gene and is also deleted from BCG [170]. Since any single protein may be insufficiently immunogenic, the use of fusion proteins could be important for future subunit vaccine development [171].

Subunit vaccination with purified proteins requires delivery of the protein in adjuvant in order to generate a strong immune response. Unfortunately, the adjuvants currently licensed for use in humans generally optimize the antibody rather than the T cell responses, although novel preparations such as the SBAS2 adjuvant or microspheres [172,173] may be useful in moving mycobacterial protein subunit candidates into clinical trials.

C. DNA Vaccines

DNA-based vaccines are considered to be potentially revolutionary due to their ease of production, low cost, long shelf life, lack of requirement for a cold chain, and ability to induce good T cell responses. However, there are concerns about the potential for mutagenesis and the induction of autoimmunity. Despite this, a number of phase 1 trials in humans are underway and, in the case of falciparum malaria, completed phase 1 studies with exciting early evidence of efficacy are available [32,174].

DNA vaccination against tuberculosis has proved effective in small animal models using some [10,11,175], but not all, antigens [176,177]. Two examples from DNA vaccine studies highlight the potential importance of fine antigenic specificity in the protective response. Firstly, Ag85A, but not Ag85B, is effective when administered as a DNA vaccine [11,178]. Interestingly, when antigen 85B is delivered to guinea pigs either as a subunit or overexpressed in a recombinant BCG, it is an effective vaccine [9,164] and protection has also been reported using an alternative Ag85B DNA formulation [179]. Thus the form of vaccination and host species are also crucial for any given antigen. The second instance indicating a potential contribution of fine specificity to the immune response in tuberculosis concerns the very closely related Hsp60 molecules of *Mycobacterium leprae* and *M. tuberculosis*. DNA vaccination using Hsp60 of *M. leprae* is effective in mice both as a prophylactic and an immunotherapeutic vaccine [10,12]. The vaccine efficacy could not, however, be reproduced using a DNA construct encoding the closely related Hsp60 gene of *M. tuberculosis* [180]. Further, rather than clearing persistent infection when administered as a therapeutic vaccine, as had been shown for the *M. leprae* Hsp60 [12], the *M. tuberculosis* homologue was found to induce necrotizing bronchointerstitial pneumonia. It is intriguing to consider the heterologous protection apparently associated with the *M. leprae* antigen in light of the protective efficacy of BCG vaccination against leprosy [25]. Might the immune response to an *M. leprae* gene

protect against tuberculosis, and the minor sequence differences between the Hsp60 molecules be immunologically crucial, contributing to the protection/pathology paradox in this instance?

D. Combination Vaccines

Vaccinia virus has also been used as a delivery system for mycobacterial antigens [181,182]. This live vector has the advantage of proven safety and efficacy in the context of the smallpox eradication program. The combination of three vaccinations of plasmid DNA containing MPT63 and ESAT-6 plus one "boost" with a recombinant *Vaccinia* construct expressing the same antigens induced protection against intraperitoneal infection of mice close to that conferred by BCG [182]. Protection was attributed to increased antigen-specific CD4$^+$ IFN-γ producing T cells induced by this vaccination protocol. Similarly, injection of Ag85A DNA-primed mice with purified Ag85A protein in adjuvant increased the protective efficacy of the DNA vaccine against an intravenous *M. tuberculosis* challenge: again, the response was CD4$^+$-mediated [178]. However, there is at least one report of a theoretically elegant prime–boost strategy using ESAT-6 in which there was no enhancement above the protection provided by individual subunits [183]. Perhaps of greatest interest is that sequential immunization with antigen Ag85B-expressing DNA followed by BCG was more effective than BCG immunization alone. In this case, depletion of the CD8$^+$ T cells in the immunized mice impaired protection in their spleens, indicating that this improved efficacy was partially mediated by CD8$^+$ T cells [184]. This last study suggests a clear and ethical way ahead for trials of novel vaccines in humans. It would seem entirely reasonable to propose a comparative trial of BCG against BCG plus another vaccine.

VII. STRATEGIES FOR VACCINE EVALUATION

A. Testing in Animal Models

While success or failure of any given vaccine candidate in a traditional animal model for tuberculosis will not necessarily predict similar behavior in humans, scientists and public health officials agree that evidence of effectiveness in experimental animal models is a crucial factor in selecting vaccine candidates for entry into clinical trials. Mice and guinea pigs have been used extensively for evaluation of new tuberculosis vaccines. More expensive models in rabbits, cattle, and nonhuman primates are available for further characterization of promising candidates.

1. Mice

The mouse, apart from being least costly, is an invaluable model for investigation of the genetics and the immunology of the host response to tuberculosis [192]. Mice are, however, relatively resistant to tuberculosis; they have a low degree of skin test reactivity to tuberculin and show an almost complete absence of caseation and fibrosis, histopathological hallmarks of human tuberculosis.

2. Guinea Pigs

Guinea pigs are innately susceptible to low-dose infection with virulent *M. tuberculosis* and display at least some of the necrotic pathology found in immunocompetent humans. Their exquisite sensitivity to tuberculosis infection provides an experimental window of sufficient width to allow ranking different vaccines according to their individual protective efficacies [149].

3. Rabbits

Rabbits are relatively resistant to *M. tuberculosis* but display an intermediate type of susceptibility to *M. bovis*, similar to human susceptibility to *M. tuberculosis*. In an additional parallel with human disease, infection of rabbits with virulent *M. bovis* frequently produces pulmonary cavities as a result of the liquefaction of caseous foci and subsequent extracellular multiplication of tubercle bacilli [193]. This feature renders the rabbit model particularly interesting, presenting the opportunity to study the pathology largely responsible for flooding the lungs of infected humans and thereby via sputum of the immediate environment, with massive numbers of bacteria.

4. Cattle

Tuberculosis in cattle and in farmed deer is of considerable economic significance [194], and efforts to develop a new vaccine against human tuberculosis are paralleled by attempts to develop diagnostic agents and vaccine control strategies for bovine tuberculosis [195–197]. Given the relationship between the respective infectious agents, *M. tuberculosis* and *M. bovis*, it may be that the prevention of human and bovine tuberculosis can be achieved using similar vaccines. Therefore vaccine trials in cattle can be considered a relevant animal model for human tuberculosis, given the fact that the endpoint of this model will be the reduction of transmission in a naturally susceptible host system.

5. Nonhuman Primates

Establishment of experimental tuberculosis in nonhuman primates provides an opportunity to study protective and pathological mechanisms with close resemblance to those in humans [198]. Bacille Calmette–Guérin vaccination has been characterized in rhesus and cynomologous monkeys, and studies have been initiated with new candidates [151]. It should be borne in mind that nonhuman primate models are relatively poorly standardized, however, and ethical and financial aspects of such research dictate that it should be reserved for the end stages of preclinical evaluation.

In each of these model systems, challenge with virulent mycobacteria can be by parenteral injection or, in an attempt to mimic the natural route of infection, by aerosol. Measuring the reduction of bacterial load in target tissues, particularly in the lung and spleen, at a specified time after challenge is the most widely accepted readout system to assess protection in the above animal models, although there is increasing recognition that the effect of vaccination on longer-term pathological changes is important in the comprehensive analysis of a new candidate. Typically, BCG vac-

cination results in a reduction of approximately 10-fold in bacterial numbers in mice and up to 5-log reduction in guinea pigs. The slow growth rate of mycobacteria makes the standard determination of colony forming units both labor-intensive and time-consuming and thus unsuitable for high throughput screening of the large numbers of vaccine candidates discussed above. Recently, reporter gene technology has been applied to mycobacteria with luciferase-expressing mycobacteria allowing the measurement of luminescence in organ homogenates as a rapid endpoint for vaccine evaluation [199]. Extension of the use of such bacteria into simple whole blood-based assays in humans also has considerable potential as a surrogate of protective immunity that makes no assumptions of the detailed nature of this response [200]. An alternative surrogate for colony forming units (CFU) is the use of precisely quantitated PCR: both the RNA for some genes and DNA content are closely related to CFU [91,201,202].

B. Clinical Trials in Humans

There are general logistic and ethical issues related to tuberculosis vaccine trials that will determine the type of vaccine that can be tested and may therefore have an important influence on more immediate research strategies. It is important that these issues begin to be addressed now, rather than waiting till vaccine candidates have already reached the stage of field evaluation. Clinical evaluation of any new tuberculosis vaccine will follow the general path of vaccine testing, starting off with phase I safety trials in a small group of healthy volunteers. This will be followed by phase II trials in a larger population to establish a preliminary estimate of protection and parameters such as induction of appropriate immune responses, dose response, and possible interaction with preexisting tuberculous infection. Phase III trials, finally, will establish the overall efficacy and the incidence of adverse effects in a large study group.

1. Preinfection Trials

In testing a vaccine designed to replace BCG, an important ethical problem would arise in relation to any side-by-side comparison. In light of the proven efficacy of BCG in prevention of childhood forms of tuberculosis, it is difficult to envisage the withdrawal of BCG as part of a trial design. A comparative trial may therefore be impossible in children from developing countries, the most important group of future users for a new tuberculosis vaccine. Comparative trials may be possible by focusing on high-risk groups in countries such as the United States, where BCG is not used. A prerequisite for such trials would be the further development and field applicability of specific tests to distinguish vaccination from infection in order to avoid compromise of existing control strategies. Even in high-incidence areas, TB case rates rarely exceed 250/100,000 of the population, imposing a requirement for large study populations and long follow-up periods for vaccine trials. The key readout period for a new vaccine would be when the neonatal target group reaches adulthood, representing a minimum 20-year trial period.

2. Postinfection Trials

An antireactivation vaccine might be simpler to evaluate. By administration to a high-risk young adult cohort, a trial period in the region of several years could be envisaged. Evaluation of a transmission-blocking vaccine, measured by a reduction in the number of smear-positive cases, would require the development of improved diagnostic tools for smear-negative tuberculosis. For any live vaccine formulation, safety concerns related to use in HIV-positive individuals would require detailed consideration.

The point has already been made that, in the absence of an understanding of the factors responsible for variable results with BCG, a series of trials in different populations of BCG will be necessary. There is a moderate genetic influence on susceptibility to tuberculosis [203], and the tuberculin reaction following BCG vaccination is under stronger influence [204,205]. Therefore individuals may also vary in their response to vaccination. Identification of genes involved in determining susceptibility to mycobacterial infection has been an area of revived interest that might provide new insight relevant to vaccine design and testing [206].

3. Immunotherapeutic Vaccination

Control of TB by immunomodulation has been a long-standing scientific goal. After the discovery of the tubercle bacillus in 1882, Robert Koch devoted his efforts to the development of an immunotherapeutic vaccine. In some patients, the results were disastrous, with the induction of pathogenic responses leading to death, dramatically illustrating that the immune response also mediates the pathology of tuberculosis. However, one new tuberculosis vaccine has already undergone clinical trials. *Mycobacterium vaccae* is an environmental mycobacterium, which in some trials showed dramatic effects, including prolonged survival of HIV-positive tuberculosis patients [207–210]. However, the initial promise of *M. vaccae* as an immunotherapeutic vaccine has not been upheld by more recent randomized clinical trials [211,212].

VIII. CONCLUDING COMMENTS

The goal of tuberculosis vaccine development has frustrated several generations of enthusiastic research. Nevertheless, there has been considerable progress and Phase I/II trials in humans can be anticipated in the near future. Whether this optimism can be translated into improved efficacy will take much longer to ascertain. In the meantime, the availability of genetic tools for mycobacteria and the development of novel immunization strategies remain to be important objectives. The magnitude of the public health problem requires international coordination of translational effort and is a problem that cannot be put to one side.

REFERENCES

1. Cole S, et al. Deciphering the biology of *Mycobacterium tuberculosis* from the complete genome sequence. Nature 1998; 393:537–544.

2. Lander ES, et al. Initial sequencing and analysis of the human genome. Nature 2001; 409:860–921.

3. Jungblut PR, et al. Comparative proteome analysis of *Mycobacterium tuberculosis* and *Mycobacterium bovis* BCG strains: towards functional genomics of microbial pathogens. Mol Microbiol 1999; 33:1103–1117.

4. Wilson M, et al. Exploring drug-induced alterations in gene expression in *Mycobacterium tuberculosis* by microarray hybridization. Proc Natl Acad Sci USA 1999; 96:12833–12838.

5. Behr MA, et al. Comparative genomics of BCG vaccines by whole-genome DNA microarray. Science 1999; 284:1520–1523.

6. Stewart GR, et al. Overexpression of heat-shock proteins reduces survival of *Mycobacterium tuberculosis* in the chronic phase of infection. Nat Med 2001; 7:732–737.

7. McKinney JD, et al. Persistence of *Mycobacterium tuberculosis* in macrophages and mice requires the glyoxylate shunt enzyme isocitrate lyase. Nature 2000; 406:735–738.

8. Ramakrishnan L, et al. Granuloma-specific expression of Mycobacterium virulence proteins from the glycine-rich PE-PGRS family. Science 2000; 288:1436–1439.

9. Horwitz MA, et al. Recombinant bacillus Calmette–Guérin (BCG) vaccines expressing the *Mycobacterium tuberculosis* 30-kDa major secretory protein induce greater protective immunity against tuberculosis than conventional BCG vaccines in a highly susceptible animal model. Proc Natl Acad Sci USA 2000; 97:13853–13858.

10. Tascon R, et al. Vaccination against tuberculosis by DNA injection. Nat Med 1996; 2:888–892.

11. Huygen K, et al. Immunogenicity and protective efficacy of a tuberculosis DNA vaccine. Nat Med 1996; 2:893–898.

12. Lowrie DB, et al. Therapy of tuberculosis in mice by DNA vaccination. Nature 1999; 400:269–271.

13. Dupuis S, et al. Impairment of mycobacterial but not viral immunity by a germline human STAT1 mutation. Science 2001; 293:300–303.

14. Altare F, et al. Inherited interleukin 12 deficiency in a child with bacille Calmette–Guérin and *Salmonella enteritidis* disseminated infection. J Clin Invest 1998; 102:2035–2040.

15. Jong R, et al. Severe mycobacterial and salmonella infections in interleukin-12 receptor-deficient patients. Science 1998; 280:1435–1438.

16. Newport MJ, et al. A mutation in the interferon-gamma-receptor gene and susceptibility to mycobacterial infection. N Engl J Med 1996; 335:1941–1949.

17. Talbot EA, et al. Tuberculosis among foreign-born persons in the United States, 1993–1998. JAMA 2000; 284:2894–2900.

18. Johnson JL, Ellner JJ. Adult tuberculosis overview: African versus Western perspectives. Curr Opin Pulm Med 2000; 6:180–186.

19. Espinal MA, et al. Global trends in resistance to antituberculosis drugs. World Health Organization–International Union against Tuberculosis and Lung Disease Working Group on Anti-Tuberculosis Drug Resistance Surveillance. N Engl J Med 2001; 344:1294–1303.

20. De Cock KM, Chaisson RE. Will DOTS do it? A reappraisal of tuberculosis control in countries with high rates of HIV infection. Int J Tuberc Lung Dis 1999; 3:457–465.

21. Dye C, et al. Consensus statement. Global burden of tuberculosis: estimated incidence, prevalence, and mortality by country. WHO Global Surveillance and Monitoring Project. JAMA 1999; 282:677–686.

22. Hart PD, Sutherland I. BCG and vole bacillus vaccines in the prevention of tuberculosis in adolescence and early adult life. Br Med J 1977; 2:293–295.

23. Bloom BR, Fine PEM. The BCG experience: implications for future vaccines against tuberculosis. In: Bloom BR, ed.

Tuberculosis: Pathogenesis, Protection and Control. Washington, DC: American Society for Microbiology, 1994:531–557.

24. Colditz GA, et al. Efficacy of BCG vaccine in the prevention of tuberculosis. meta-analysis of the published literature. JAMA 1994; 271:698–702.

25. Karonga prevention trial group. Randomised controlled trial of single BCG, repeated BCG, or combined BCG and killed *Mycobacterium leprae* vaccine for prevention of leprosy and tuberculosis in Malawi. Lancet 1996; 348:17–24.

26. Black GF, et al. Patterns and implications of naturally acquired immune responses to environmental and tuberculous mycobacterial antigens in northern Malawi. J Infect Dis 2001; 184:322–329.

27. Palmer CE, Long MW. Effects of infection with atypical mycobacteria on BCG vaccination and tuberculosis. Am Rev Respir Dis 1966; 94:553–568.

28. Mahairas GG, et al. Molecular analysis of genetic differences between *Mycobacterium bovis* BCG and virulent *M. bovis*. J Bacteriol 1996; 178:1274–1282.

29. Gordon SV, et al. Identification of variable regions in the genomes of tubercle bacilli using bacterial artificial chromosome arrays. Mol Microbiol 1999; 32:643–655.

30. Brosch R, et al. Comparative genomics uncovers large tandem chromosomal duplications in *Mycobacterium bovis* BCG Pasteur. Yeast 2000; 17:111–123.

31. Calmette A. L'infection bacillaire et la tuberculose chez l'homme et chez les animaux. Paris: Masson et Cie, 1920.

32. Wang R, et al. Induction of antigen-specific cytotoxic T lymphocytes in humans by a malaria DNA vaccine. Science 1998; 282:476–480.

33. Kindler V, et al. The inducing role of tumor necrosis factor in the development of bactericidal granulomas during BCG infection. Cell 1989; 56:731–740.

34. Garcia I, et al. High sensitivity of transgenic mice expressing soluble TNFR1 fusion protein to mycobacterial infections: synergistic action of TNF and IFN-gamma in the differentiation of protective granulomas. Eur J Immunol 1997; 27:3182–3190.

35. Flynn JL, et al. Tumor necrosis factor-alpha is required in the protective immune response against *Mycobacterium tuberculosis* in mice. Immunity 1995; 2:561–572.

36. MacMicking JD, et al. Identification of nitric oxide synthase as a protective locus against tuberculosis. Proc Natl Acad Sci USA 1997; 94:5243–5248.

37. Cooper A, et al. Disseminated tuberculosis in interferon-g gene-disrupted mice. J Exp Med 1993; 178:2243–2247.

38. Flynn J, et al. An essential role for Interferon-g in resistance to *Mycobacterium tuberculosis* infection. J Exp Med 1993; 178:2249–2254.

39. Cooper AM, et al. Interleukin 12 (IL-12) is crucial to the development of protective immunity in mice intravenously infected with *Mycobacterium tuberculosis*. J Exp Med 1997; 186:39–45.

40. Teitelbaum R, et al. A mAb recognizing a surface antigen of *Mycobacterium tuberculosis* enhances host survival. Proc Natl Acad Sci USA 1998; 95:15688–15693.

41. Vordermeier HM, et al. Increase of tuberculous infection in the organs of B cell-deficient mice. Clin Exp Immunol 1996; 106:312–316.

42. Mogues T. The relative importance of T cell subsets in immunity and immunopathology of airborne *Mycobacterium tuberculosis* infection in mice. J Exp Med 2001; 193:271–280.

43. North RJ. Mice incapable of making IL-4 or IL-10 display normal resistance to infection with *Mycobacterium tuberculosis*. Clin Exp Immunol 1998; 113:55–58.

44. Ladel CH, et al. Immune response to *Mycobacterium bovis* bacille Calmette Guérin infection in major histocompati-

bility complex class I- and II-deficient knock-out mice: contribution of CD4 and CD8 T cells to acquired resistance. Eur J Immunol 1995; 25:377–384.

45. Flynn JL, et al. Major histocompatibility complex class I-restricted T cells are required for resistance to *Mycobacterium tuberculosis* infection. Proc Natl Acad Sci USA 1992; 89:12013–12017.

46. Behar SM, et al. Susceptibility of mice deficient in CD1D or TAP1 to infection with *Mycobacterium tuberculosis*. J Exp Med 1999; 189:1973–1980.

47. Laochumroonvorapong P, et al. Perforin, a cytotoxic molecule which mediates cell necrosis, is not required for the early control of mycobacterial infection in mice. Infect Immun 1997; 65:127–132.

48. Cooper AM, et al. The course of *Mycobacterium tuberculosis* Infection in the lungs of mice lacking expression of either perforin- or granzyme-mediated cytolytic mechanisms. Infect Immun 1997; 65:1317–1320.

49. Turner J. CD8- and CD95/95L-dependent mechanisms of resistance in mice with chronic pulmonary tuberculosis. Am J Respir Cell Mol Biol 2001; 24:203–209.

50. Caruso AM, et al. Mice deficient in CD4 T cells have only transiently diminished levels of IFN-gamma, yet succumb to tuberculosis. J Immunol 1999; 162:5407–5416.

51. Tascon R, et al. Protection against *Mycobacterium tuberculosis* infection by CD8$^+$ T cells requires the production of interferon-g. Infect Immun 1998; 66:830–834.

52. van Pinxteren LA, et al. Control of latent *Mycobacterium tuberculosis* infection is dependent on CD8 T cells. Eur J Immunol 2000; 30:3689–3698.

53. Dorman SE, Holland SM. Mutation in the signal-transducing chain of the interferon-g receptor and susceptibility to mycobacterial infection. J Clin Invest 1998; 101:2364–2369.

54. Altare F, et al. Impairment of mycobacterial immunity in human interleukin-12 receptor deficiency. Science 1998; 280:1432–1435.

55. Nicholson S, et al. Inducible nitric oxide synthase in pulmonary alveolar macrophages from patients with tuberculosis. J Exp Med 1996; 183:2293–2302.

56. Rich EA, et al. *Mycobacterium tuberculosis* (MTB)-stimulated production of nitric oxide by human alveolar macrophages and relationship of nitric oxide production to growth inhibition of MTB. Tuber Lung Dis 1997; 78:247–255.

57. Thoma-Uszynski S, et al. Induction of direct antimicrobial activity through mammalian toll-like receptors. Science 2001; 291:1544–1547.

58. Keane J, et al. Tuberculosis associated with infliximab, a tumor necrosis factor alpha- neutralizing agent. N Engl J Med 2001; 345:1098–1104.

59. Robinson DS, et al. Evidence for a Th1-like bronchoalveolar T cell subset and predominance of Interferon-gamma gene activation in pulmonary tuberculosis. Am J Respir Crit Care Med 1994; 149:989–993.

60. Shimokata K, et al. Cytokine content in pleural effusion. Comparison between tuberculous and carcinomatous pleurisy. Chest 1991; 99:1103–1107.

61. Barnes P, et al. Cytokine production at the site of disease in human tuberculosis. Infect Immun 1993; 61:3482–3489.

62. Toossi Z, et al. Defective interleukin 2 production and responsiveness in human pulmonary tuberculosis. J Exp Med 1986; 163:1162–1172.

63. Schauf V, et al. Cytokine gene activation and modified responsiveness to interleukin-2 in the blood of tuberculosis patients. J Infect Dis 1993; 168:1056–1059.

64. Johnson BJ, et al. Cytokine gene expression by cultures of human lymphocytes with autologous *Mycobacterium tuberculosis*-infected monocytes. Infect Immun 1994; 62:1444–1450.

65. Hirsch CS, et al. Cross-modulation by transforming growth factor beta in human tuberculosis: suppression of antigen-driven blastogenesis and interferon gamma production. Proc Natl Acad Sci USA 1996; 93:3193–3198.

66. Mehra V, et al. Immune response to recombinant mycobacterial proteins in patients with tuberculosis infection and disease. J Infect Dis 1996; 174:431–434.

67. Surcel H-M, et al. T_h1/T_h2 profiles in tuberculosis based on proliferation and cytokine response of blood lymphocytes to mycobacterial antigens. Immunology 1994; 81:171–176.

68. Lalvani A, et al. Enumeration of T cells specific for RD1-encoded antigens suggests a high prevalence of latent *Mycobacterium tuberculosis* infection in healthy urban Indians. J Infect Dis 2001; 183:469–477.

69. Ellner JJ, et al. Correlates of protective immunity to *Mycobacterium tuberculosis* in humans. Clin Infect Dis 2000; 30(suppl 3):S279–S282.

70. Trinchieri G. Interleukin-12: a proinflammatory cytokine with immunoregulatory functions that bridge innate resistance and antigen-specific adaptive immunity. In: Paul WE, Fathman CG, Metzger H, eds. Annual Review of Immunology. Vol. 13. Palo Alto: Annual Reviews Inc, 1995: 251–276.

71. Oppmann B, et al. Novel p19 protein engages IL-12p40 to form a cytokine, IL-23, with biological activities similar as well as distinct from IL-12. Immunity 2000; 13:715–725.

72. Zhang M, et al. Interleukin 12 at the site of disease in tuberculosis. J Clin Invest 1994; 93:1733–1739.

73. Munk ME, et al. Increased numbers of interleukin-12 producing cells in human tuberculosis. Infect Immun 1996; 64: 1078–1080.

74. Fulton SA, et al. Interleukin-12 production by human monocytes infected with *Mycobacterium tuberculosis*: role of phagocytosis. Infect Immun 1996; 64:2523–2531.

75. Brightbill HD, et al. Host defense mechanisms triggered by microbial lipoproteins through toll-like receptors. Science 1999; 285:732–736.

76. Post FA, et al. The 19 kDa lipoprotein of *Mycobacterium tuberculosis* inhibits *Mycobacterium smegmatis* induced cytokine production by human macrophages in vitro. Infect Immun 2001; 69:1433–1439.

77. Noss EH, et al. Toll-like receptor 2-dependent inhibition of macrophage class II MHC expression and antigen processing by 19-kDa lipoprotein of *Mycobacterium tuberculosis*. J Immunol 2001; 167:910–918.

78. Neyrolles O, et al. Lipoprotein access to MHC Class I presentation during infection of murine macrophages with live mycobacteria. J Immunol 2001; 166:447–457.

79. Okamura H, et al. Cloning of a new cytokine that induces IFN-gamma production by T cells. Nature 1995; 378:88–91.

80. Micallef MJ, et al. Interferon-g-inducing factor enhances T helper 1 cytokine production by stimulated human T cells: synergism with Interleukin-12 for Interferon-g production. Eur J Immunol 1996; 26:1647–1651.

81. Sugawara I, et al. Role of interleukin-18 (IL-18) in mycobacterial infection in IL-18-gene-disrupted mice. Infect Immun 1999; 67:2585–2589.

82. Vankayalapati R, et al. T cells enhance production of IL-18 by monocytes in response to an intracellular pathogen. J Immunol 2001; 166:6749–6753.

83. Vankayalapati R, et al. Production of interleukin-18 in human tuberculosis. J Infect Dis 2000; 182:234–239.

84. Garcia VE, et al. IL-18 promotes type 1 cytokine production from NK cells and T cells in human intracellular infection. J Immunol 1999; 162:6114–6121.

85. Moreno C, et al. Lipoarabinomannan from *Mycobacterium tuberculosis* induces the production of tumour necrosis factor from human and murine macrophages. Clin Exp Immunol 1989; 76:240–245.

86. Aung H, et al. Induction of monocyte expression of tumor necrosis factor alpha by the 30-kD alpha antigen of *Mycobacterium tuberculosis* and synergism with fibronectin. J Clin Invest 1996; 98:1261–1268.

87. Dahl KE, et al. Selective induction of transforming growth factor beta in human monocytes by lipoarabinomannan of *Mycobacterium tuberculosis*. Infect Immun 1996; 64:399–405.

88. Bergeron A, et al. Cytokine patterns in tuberculous and sarcoid granulomas: correlations with histopathologic features of the granulomatous response. J Immunol 1997; 159: 3034–3043.

89. Kaplan G. Cytokine regulation of disease progression in leprosy and tuberculosis. Immunobiology 1994; 191:564–568.

90. Tsenova L, et al. A combination of thalidomide plus antibiotics protects rabbits from mycobacterial meningitis-associated death. J Infect Dis 1998; 177:1563–1572.

91. Wilkinson RJ, et al. An increase in expression of a *M. tuberculosis* mycolyl transferase gene (fbpB) occurs early after infection of human monocytes. Mol Microbiol 2001; 39:813–821.

92. Bekker LG, et al. Selective increase in plasma tumor necrosis factor-alpha and concomitant clinical deterioration after initiating therapy in patients with severe tuberculosis. J Infect Dis 1998; 178:580–584.

93. Chantry D, et al. Modulation of cytokine production by transforming growth factor-beta. J Immunol 1989; 142:4295–4300.

94. Wilkinson RJ, et al. Human T and B cell reactivity to the 16 kDa alpha crystallin protein of *Mycobacterium tuberculosis*. Scand J Immunol 1998; 48:403–409.

95. Huygen K, et al. Specific lymphoproliferation, gamma interferon production, and serum immunoglobulin G directed against a purified 32 kDa mycobacterial protein antigen (P32) in patients with active tuberculosis. Scand J Immunol 1988; 27:187–194.

96. Agrewala JN, Wilkinson RJ. Differential regulation of Th1 and Th2 cells by p91-110 and p21-40 peptides of the 16kDa a-crystallin antigen of *Mycobacterium tuberculosis*. Clin Exp Immunol 1998; 104:392–397.

97. Wilkinson RJ, et al. Influence of polymorphism in the genes for the interleukin 1 receptor antagonist and interleukin IL-1b on tuberculosis. J Exp Med 1999; 189:1863–1874.

98. Lin Y, et al. Absence of a prominent Th2 cytokine response in human tuberculosis. Infect Immun 1996; 64:1351–1356.

99. Wilkinson RJ, et al. Peptide specific response to *M. tuberculosis*: clinical spectrum, compartmentalization, and effect of chemotherapy. J Infect Dis 1998; 178:760–768.

100. Seah GT, et al. Type 2 cytokine gene activation and its relationship to extent of disease in patients with tuberculosis. J Infect Dis 2000; 181:385–389.

101. Toossi Z, et al. Induction of transforming growth factor beta 1 by purified protein derivative of *Mycobacterium tuberculosis*. Infect Immun 1995; 63:224–228.

102. Hirsch CS, et al. Enhancement of intracellular growth of *Mycobacterium tuberculosis* in human monocytes by transforming growth factor-beta 1. J Infect Dis 1994; 170:1229–1237.

103. Toossi Z, et al. Enhanced production of TGF-beta by blood monocytes from patients with active tuberculosis and presence of TGF-beta in tuberculous granulomatous lung lesions. J Immunol 1995; 154:465–473.

104. Zavala F, et al. HIV predominantly induces IL-1 receptor antagonist over IL-1 synthesis in human primary monocytes. J Immunol 1995; 155:2784–2793.

105. Maeda H, et al. TGF-b enhances macrophage ability to produce IL-10 in normal and tumor-bearing mice. J Immunol 1995; 155:4926–4932.

106. Hirsch CS, et al. In vitro restoration of T cell responses in

tuberculosis and augmentation of monocyte effector function against *Mycobacterium tuberculosis* by natural inhibitors of transforming growth factor beta. Proc Natl Acad Sci USA 1997; 94:3926–3931.

107. Marshall BG, et al. Enhanced antimycobacterial response to recombinant *Mycobacterium bovis* BCG expressing latency-associated peptide. Infect Immun 2001; 69:6676–6682.

108. Malefyt de Waal R, et al. Interleukin 10 (IL-10) inhibits cytokine synthesis by human monocytes: an autoregulatory role of IL-10 produced by monocytes. J Exp Med 1991; 174:1209–1220.

109. Kennedy MK, et al. Interleukin-12 regulates the proliferation of Th1, but not Th2 or Th0, clones. Eur J Immunol 1994; 24:2271–2278.

110. Zhang M, et al. T cell cytokine responses in persons with tuberculosis and human immunodeficiency virus infection. J Clin Invest 1994; 94:2435–2442.

111. Gong J-H, et al. Interleukin-10 downregulates *Mycobacterium tuberculosis*-induced Th1 responses and CTLA-4 expression. Infect Immun 1996; 64:913–918.

112. Shiratsuchi H, et al. Evidence against a role for interleukin-10 in the regulation of growth of *Mycobacterium avium* in human monocytes. J Infect Dis 1996; 173:410–417.

113. Mosmann TR, Coffman RL. Th1 and Th2 cells: different patterns of lymphokine secretion lead to different functional properties. Annu Rev Immunol 1989; 7:145–173.

114. Arend SM, et al. Detection of active tuberculosis infection by T cell responses to early- secreted antigenic target 6-kDa protein and culture filtrate protein 10. J Infect Dis 2000; 181:1850–1854.

115. Zugel U, Kaufmann SH. Role of heat shock proteins in protection from and pathogenesis of infectious diseases. Clin Microbiol Rev 1999; 12:19–39.

116. Jurcevic S, et al. T cell responses to a mixture of *Mycobacterium tuberculosis* peptides with complementary HLA-DR binding profiles. Clin Exp Immunol 1996; 105:416–421.

117. Pathan AA, et al. Direct ex vivo analysis of antigen-specific IFN-gamma-secreting CD4 T cells in *Mycobacterium tuberculosis*-infected individuals: associations with clinical disease state and effect of treatment. J Immunol 2001; 167:5217–5225.

118. Stenger S, et al. Differential effects of cytolytic T cell subsets on intracellular infection. Science 1997; 276:1684–1687.

119. Lalvani A, et al. Human cytolytic and Interferon-g secreting CD8+ T lymphocytes specific for *Mycobacterium tuberculosis*. Proc Natl Acad Sci USA 1998; 95:270–275.

120. Wilkinson RJ, et al. 38000 MW Antigen specific MHC Class I restricted interferon-g secreting CD8+ T cells in healthy contacts of tuberculosis. Immunology 1998; 95:585–590.

121. Lewinsohn DM, et al. Characterization of human CD8+ T cells reactive with *Mycobacterium tuberculosis*-infected antigen-presenting cells. J Exp Med 1998; 187:1633–1640.

122. Smith SM, et al. Human CD8+ CTL specific for the mycobacterial major secreted antigen 85A. J Immunol 2000; 165:7088–7095.

123. Klein MR, et al. HLA-B*35-restricted CD8 T cell epitopes in the antigen 85 complex of *Mycobacterium tuberculosis*. J Infect Dis 2001; 183:928–934.

124. Pathan AA, et al. Identification of a novel HLA class I restricted epitope in *M. tuberculosis*: high frequencies of circulating peptide-specific IFN-g secreting CD8+ cytotoxic T lymphocytes in a healthy exposed contact. Eur J Immunol 2000; 30:2713–2721.

125. Mohagheghpour N, et al. CTL response to *Mycobacterium tuberculosis*: identification of an immunogenic epitope in the 19-kDa lipoprotein. J Immunol 1998; 161:2400–2406.

126. Russell DG. *Mycobacterium tuberculosis*: here today, and here tomorrow. Nat Rev Mol Cell Biol 2001; 2:569–577.

127. Teitelbaum R, et al. Mycobacterial infection of macrophages results in membrane-permeable phagosomes. Proc Natl Acad Sci USA 1999; 96:15190–15195.

128. Schaible UE, et al. Intersection of group I CD1 molecules and mycobacteria in different intracellular compartments of dendritic cells. J Immunol 2000; 164:4843–4852.

129. Ulrichs T, Porcelli SA. CD1 proteins: targets of T cell recognition in innate and adaptive immunity. Rev Immunogenet 2000; 2:416–432.

130. Stenger S, et al. An antimicrobial activity of cytolytic T cells mediated by granulysin. Science 1998; 282:121–125.

131. Ochoa MT, et al. T-cell release of granulysin contributes to host defense in leprosy. Nat Med 2001; 7:174–179.

132. Canaday DH, et al. CD4(+) and CD8(+) T cells kill intracellular *Mycobacterium tuberculosis* by a perforin and Fas/Fas ligand-independent mechanism. J Immunol 2001; 167:2734–2742.

133. Karadimitris A, et al. Human CD1d-glycolipid tetramers generated by in vitro oxidative refolding chromatography. Proc Natl Acad Sci USA 2001; 98:3294–3298.

134. Constant P, et al. Stimulation of human gd T cells by nonpeptidic mycobacterial ligands. Science 1994; 264:267–270.

135. Boom WH, et al. Characterization of a 10- to 14-kilodalton protease-sensitive *Mycobacterium tuberculosis* H37Ra antigen that stimulates human gamma delta T cells. Infect Immun 1994; 62:5511–5518.

136. Lang F, et al. Early activation of human Vg9Vd2 T cell broad cytotoxicity and TNF production by nonpeptidic mycobacterial ligands. J Immunol 1995; 154:5986–5994.

137. Sanchez-Garcia J, et al. Antigen driven shedding of l-selectin from human gd T cells. Immunology 1996; 89:213–219.

138. Ladel CH, et al. Protective role of gamma/delta T cells and alpha/beta T cells in tuberculosis. Eur J Immunol 1995; 25:2877–2881.

139. Caminero JA, et al. Exogenous reinfection with tuberculosis on a European island with a moderate incidence of disease. Am J Respir Crit Care Med 2001; 163:717–720.

140. van Rie A, et al. Exogenous reinfection as a cause of recurrent tuberculosis after curative treatment. N Engl J Med 1999; 341:1174–1179.

141. Lalvani A, et al. Rapid detection of *M. tuberculosis* infection by enumeration of antigen-specific T cells. Am J Respir Crit Care Med 2001; 15:824–828.

142. Young DB. A postgenomic perspective. Nat Med 2001; 7:11–13.

143. Zaheer SA, et al. Addition of immunotherapy with *Mycobacterium w* vaccine to multi-drug therapy benefits multibacillary leprosy patients. Vaccine 1995; 13:1102–1110.

144. Chambers ST, et al. Paradoxical expansion of intracranial tuberculomas during chemotherapy. Lancet 1984; 2:181–184.

145. Dillon DC, et al. Molecular characterization and human T-cell responses to a member of a novel *Mycobacterium tuberculosis* mtb39 gene family. Infect Immun 1999; 67:2941–2950.

146. Coler RN, et al. Vaccination with the T cell antigen Mtb 8.4 protects against challenge with *Mycobacterium tuberculosis*. J Immunol 2001; 166:6227–6235.

147. Lodes MJ, et al. Serological expression cloning and immunological evaluation of MTB48, a novel *Mycobacterium tuberculosis* antigen. J Clin Microbiol 2001; 39:2485–2493.

148. Ginsberg AM. A proposed national strategy for tuberculosis vaccine development. Clin Infect Dis 2000; 30(suppl 3):S233–S242.

149. Orme IM, et al. Tuberculosis vaccine development: recent progress. Trends Microbiol 2001; 9:115–118.

150. http://www.pasteur.fr/recherche/EC_TBvaccine/.

151. Langermans JA, et al. Divergent effect of bacillus Calmette–Guérin (BCG) vaccination on *Mycobacterium tuberculosis* infection in highly related macaque species: implications for

primate models in tuberculosis vaccine research. Proc Natl Acad Sci USA 2001; 98:11497–11502.

152. Glickman MS, Jacobs WR Jr. Microbial pathogenesis of *Mycobacterium tuberculosis*: dawn of a discipline. Cell 2001; 104:477–485.

153. Wangoo A, et al. Bacille Calmette–Guérin (BCG)-associated inflammation and fibrosis: modulation by recombinant BCG expressing interferon-gamma (IFN-gamma). Clin Exp Immunol 2000; 119:92–98.

154. Hess J, et al. *Mycobacterium bovis* bacille Calmette–Guérin strains secreting listeriolysin of *Listeria monocytogenes*. Proc Natl Acad Sci USA 1998; 95:5299–5304.

155. Skjot RL, et al. Comparative evaluation of low-molecular-mass proteins from *Mycobacterium tuberculosis* identifies members of the ESAT-6 family as immunodominant T-cell antigens. Infect Immun 2000; 68:214–220.

156. Hondalus MK, et al. Attenuation of and protection induced by a leucine auxotroph of *Mycobacterium tuberculosis*. Infect Immun 2000; 68:2888–2898.

157. Smith DA, et al. Characterization of auxotrophic mutants of *Mycobacterium tuberculosis* and their potential as vaccine candidates. Infect Immun 2001; 69:1142–1150.

158. Perez E, et al. An essential role for *pho*P in *Mycobacterium tuberculosis* virulence. Mol Microbiol 2001; 41:179–187.

159. Cox JS, et al. Complex lipid determines tissue-specific replication of *Mycobacterium tuberculosis* in mice. Nature 1999; 402:79–83.

160. Camacho LR, et al. Identification of a virulence gene cluster of by signature-tagged transposon mutagenesis. Mol Microbiol 1999; 34:257–267.

161. Pethe K, et al. The heparin-binding haemagglutinin of *M. tuberculosis* is required for extrapulmonary dissemination. Nature 2001; 412:190–194.

162. Olsen AW, et al. Efficient protection against *Mycobacterium tuberculosis* by vaccination with a single subdominant epitope from the ESAT-6 antigen. Eur J Immunol 2000; 30: 1724–1732.

163. Andersen P. Effective vaccination of mice against *Mycobacterium tuberculosis* infection with a soluble mixture of secreted mycobacterial proteins. Infect Immun 1994; 62: 2536–2544.

164. Horwitz MA, et al. Protective immunity against tuberculosis induced by vaccination with major extracellular proteins of *Mycobacterium tuberculosis*. Proc Natl Acad Sci USA 1995; 92:1530–1534.

165. Roberts A, et al. Characteristics of protective immunity engendered by vaccination of mice with purified culture filtrate protein antigens of *Mycobacterium tuberculosis*. Immunology 1995; 85:502–508.

166. Yuan Y, et al. The 16-kDa alpha-crystallin (Acr) protein of *Mycobacterium tuberculosis* is required for growth in macrophages. Proc Natl Acad Sci USA 1998; 95:9578–9583.

167. Wiker HG, Harboe M. The antigen 85 complex: a major secretion product of *Mycobacterium tuberculosis*. Microbiol Rev 1992; 56:648–661.

168. Harboe M, et al. Evidence for occurrence of the ESAT-6 protein in *Mycobacterium tuberculosis* and virulent *Mycobacterium bovis* and for its absence in *Mycobacterium bovis* BCG. Infect Immun 1996; 64:16–22.

169. Weldingh K, Andersen P. Immunological evaluation of novel *Mycobacterium tuberculosis* culture filtrate proteins. FEMS Immunol Med Microbiol 1999; 23:159–164.

170. Berthet FX, et al. A *Mycobacterium tuberculosis* operon encoding ESAT-6 and a novel low-molecular-mass culture filtrate protein (CFP-10). Microbiology 1998; 144:3195–3203.

171. Weinrich Olsen A, et al. Protection of mice with a tuberculosis subunit vaccine based on a fusion protein of antigen 85B and ESAT-6. Infect Immun 2001; 69:2773–2778.

172. Stoute JA, et al. A preliminary evaluation of a recombinant circumsporozoite protein vaccine against Plasmodium falci-

parum malaria. RTS,S Malaria Vaccine Evaluation Group. N Engl J Med 1997; 336:86–91.

173. Vordermeier H-M, et al. Synthetic delivery systems for tuberculosis vaccines: immunological evaluation of the *M. tuberculosis* 38kDa protein entrapped in biodegradable PLG microparticles. Vaccine 1995; 13:1576–1582.

174. Le TP, et al. Safety, tolerability and humoral immune responses after intramuscular administration of a malaria DNA vaccine to healthy adult volunteers. Vaccine 2000; 18: 1893–1901.

175. Zhu X, et al. Functions and specificity of T cells following nucleic acid vaccination of mice against *M. tuberculosis* infection. J Immunol 1997; 158:5921–5926.

176. Erb K, et al. Identification of potential CD8+ T-cell epitopes of the 19 kDa and AhpC proteins from *Mycobacterium tuberculosis*. No evidence for CD8+ T-cell priming against the identified peptides after DNA-vaccination of mice. Vaccine 1998; 16:692–697.

177. Yeremeev VV, et al. The 19-kD antigen and protective immunity in a murine model of tuberculosis. Clin Exp Immunol 2000; 120:274–279.

178. Tanghe A, et al. Improved immunogenicity and protective efficacy of a tuberculosis DNA vaccine encoding Ag85 by protein boosting. Infect Immun 2001; 69:3041–3047.

179. Kamath AT, et al. Co-immunization with DNA vaccines expressing granulocyte-macrophage colony-stimulating factor and mycobacterial secreted proteins enhances T-cell immunity, but not protective efficacy against *Mycobacterium tuberculosis*. Immunology 1999; 96:511–516.

180. Turner OC, et al. Lack of protection in mice and necrotizing bronchointerstitial pneumonia with bronchiolitis in guinea pigs immunized with vaccines directed against the hsp60 molecule of *Mycobacterium tuberculosis*. Infect Immun 2000; 68:3674–3679.

181. Zhu X, et al. Vaccination with recombinant Vaccinia viruses protects mice against *Mycobacterium tuberculosis* infection. Immunology 1997; 92:6–9.

182. McShane H, et al. Enhanced immunogenicity of CD4(+) T-cell responses and protective efficacy of a DNA-modified Vaccinia virus Ankara prime-boost vaccination regimen for murine tuberculosis. Infect Immun 2001; 69:681–686.

183. Mollenkopf HJ, et al. Protective efficacy against tuberculosis of ESAT-6 secreted by a live *Salmonella typhimurium* vaccine carrier strain and expressed by naked DNA. Vaccine 2001; 19:4028–4035.

184. Feng CG, et al. Priming by DNA immunization augments protective efficacy of *Mycobacterium bovis* bacille Calmette–Guérin against tuberculosis. Infect Immun 2001; 69:4174–4176.

185. Pal PG, Horwitz MA. Immunization with extracellular proteins of *Mycobacterium tuberculosis* induces cell-mediated immune responses and substantial protective immunity in a guinea pig model of pulmonary tuberculosis. Infect Immun 1992; 60:4781–4792.

186. Brandt L, et al. ESAT-6 subunit vaccination against *Mycobacterium tuberculosis*. Infect Immun 2000; 68:791–795.

187. Falero-Diaz G, et al. Intranasal vaccination of mice against infection with *Mycobacterium tuberculosis*. Vaccine 2000; 18:3223–3229.

188. Baldwin SL, et al. Evaluation of new vaccines in the mouse and guinea pig model of tuberculosis. Infect Immun 1998; 66:2951–2959.

189. Tanghe A, et al. Immunogenicity and protective efficacy of tuberculosis DNA vaccines encoding putative phosphate transport receptors. J Immunol 1999; 162:1113–1119.

190. Morris S, et al. The immunogenicity of single and combination DNA vaccines against tuberculosis. Vaccine 2000; 18:2155–2163.

191. Skeiky YA, et al. T cell expression cloning of a *Mycobacterium tuberculosis* gene encoding a protective antigen asso-

ciated with the early control of infection. J Immunol 2000; 165:7140–7149.

192. Orme IM. The immunopathogenesis of tuberculosis: a new working hypothesis. Trends Microbiol 1998; 6:94–97.

193. Bishai WR, et al. Virulence of *Mycobacterium tuberculosis* CDC1551 and H37Rv in rabbits evaluated by Lurie's pulmonary tubercle count method. Infect Immun 1999; 67: 4931–4934.

194. Krebs JR, et al. Badgers and bovine TB: conflicts between conservation and health. Science 1998; 279:817–818.

195. Rhodes SG, et al. Antigen recognition and immunomodulation by gamma delta T cells in bovine tuberculosis. J Immunol 2001; 166:5604–5610.

196. Vordermeier HM, et al. Effective DNA vaccination of cattle with the mycobacterial antigens MPB83 and MPB70 does not compromise the specificity of the comparative intradermal tuberculin skin test. Vaccine 2000; 19:1246–1255.

197. Rhodes SG, et al. Antigen specificity in experimental bovine tuberculosis. Infect Immun 2000; 68:2573–2578.

198. Walsh GP, et al. The Philippine cynomolgus monkey (*Macaca fasicularis*) provides a new nonhuman primate model of tuberculosis that resembles human disease. Nat Med 1996; 2:430–436.

199. Snewin VA, et al. Assessment of immunity to mycobacterial infection with luciferase reporter constructs. Infect Immun 1999; 67:4586–4593.

200. Kampmann B, et al. Evaluation of human antimycobacterial immunity using recombinant reporter mycobacteria. J Infect Dis 2000; 182:895–901.

201. Hellyer TJ, et al. Quantitative analysis of mRNA as a marker for viability of *Mycobacterium tuberculosis*. J Clin Microbiol 1999; 37:290–295.

202. Desjardin LE, et al. Comparison of the ABI 7700 system (TaqMan) and competitive PCR for quantification of IS6110 DNA in sputum during treatment of tuberculosis. J Clin Microbiol 1998; 36:1964–1968.

203. Pasvol G, Wilkinson RJ. Host genetics and susceptibility to infection. In: Guerrant RL, Walker DH, Weller PF, eds. Tropical Infectious Disease: Principles, Pathogens, and Practice. Vol. 1. Philadelphia: Churchill Livingstone, 1999:88–100.

204. Sepulveda RL, et al. Evaluation of tuberculin reactivity in BCG immunised siblings. Am J Respir Crit Care Med 1994; 149:620–624.

205. Sepulveda RL, Heiba IM, Navarrete C, Elston RC, Gonzalez B, Sorensen RU. Tuberculin reactivity after newborn BCG immunisation in mono- and dizygotic twins. Tuberc Lung Dis 1994; 75:138–143.

206. Hill AV. The genomics and genetics of human infectious disease susceptibility. Annu Rev Genomics Hum Genet 2001; 2:373–400.

207. Stanford JL, et al. A modern approach to the immunotherapy of tuberculosis. Bull Int Union Against Tuberc Lung Dis 1990; 65:27–29.

208. Stanford JL, Stanford CA. Immunotherapy of tuberculosis with *Mycobacterium vaccae* NCTC 11659. Immunobiology 1994; 191:555–563.

209. Onyebujoh PC, et al. Immunotherapy with *Mycobacterium vaccae* as an addition to chemotherapy for the treatment of pulmonary tuberculosis under difficult conditions in Africa. Respir Med 1995; 89:199–207.

210. Rook G, Stanford J. Adjuvants, endocrines and conserved epitopes; factors to consider when designing "therapeutic vaccines". Int J Immunopharmacol 1995; 17:91–102.

211. Johnson JL, et al. Randomized controlled trial of *Mycobacterium vaccae* immunotherapy in non-human immunodeficiency virus-infected Ugandan adults with newly diagnosed pulmonary tuberculosis. The Uganda-Case Western Reserve University Research Collaboration. J Infect Dis 2000; 181: 1304–1312.

212. Durban Immunotherapy Trial Group. Immunotherapy with *Mycobacterium vaccae* in patients with newly diagnosed pulmonary tuberculosis: a randomised controlled trial. Lancet 1999; 354:116–119.

46
New Approaches to Influenza Vaccine

John J. Treanor
University of Rochester School of Medicine, Rochester, New York, U.S.A.

James C. King
University of Maryland School of Medicine, Baltimore, Maryland, U.S.A.

Kenneth M. Zangwill
University of California, Los Angeles, School of Medicine, and Harbor-UCLA Medical Center, Torrance, California, U.S.A.

I. INTRODUCTION

A. Significance and Magnitude of Influenza

Influenza epidemics are regularly associated with excess rates of pneumonia- and influenza-associated hospitalizations [1,2]. Both influenza A (H3N2 and H1N1) and B can cause severe illness [3], although the highest mortality rates in recent years have generally been seen during years with significant H3 virus activity [4]. Complications and deaths from influenza are of particular concern in those with certain high-risk medical conditions, including adults and children with cardiovascular and pulmonary conditions, or those requiring regular medical care because of chronic metabolic, renal, blood, or immune diseases [5]. Influenza may cause more severe disease and increased hospitalization rates in individuals with human immunodeficiency virus infection [6,7] or iatrogenic immunosuppression [8], and women in the second or third trimesters of pregnancy [9]. Influenza is increasingly recognized as an important health problem in young children. Rates of influenza-related hospitalizations are particularly high in healthy children under 2 years of age, in whom rates approach those of older children with high-risk conditions [10,11]. In addition, a high rate of secondary complications, particularly otitis media and pneumonia, occur in children with influenza infection [12].

Although the impact of influenza has been extensively documented in terms of death and hospitalization, it is important to recognize the impact of influenza illness even in young, healthy individuals. A typical case of influenza, on average, is associated with 5–6 days of restricted activity, 3–4 days of bed disability, and about 3 days lost from work or school [13,14]. The average number of medical visits for cases in which medical attention was sought is between 1.1 and 3.6 visits, depending on year of the outbreak and age of the patient. Influenza is also associated with significant lost workplace productivity [15]. Therefore development and implementation of more effective control measures for influenza represents an important research and health policy priority.

B. Immune Responses Involved in Protection

1. Serum Antibody

Infection with influenza virus stimulates antibody to the viral envelope glycoproteins hemagglutinin (HA) and neuraminidase (NA), as well as to the structural matrix (M) and nucleoprotein (NP) proteins. Some individuals may develop antibody to the matrix-2 (M2) protein as well [16]. Serum IgM, IgA, and IgG antibody to HA appear within 2 weeks of inoculation of virus [17], and anti-NA antibodies parallel anti-HA antibodies [18]. Peak antibody responses are seen 4–7 weeks after infection and slowly decline thereafter; titers can still be detected years after infection even without re-exposure.

Antibody to HA can be measured by hemagglutination–inhibition (HAI) tests, enzyme-linked immunosorbent assay (ELISA), and neutralization of virus infectivity [19]. Anti-hemagglutinin antibody protects against both disease and infection with the homologous virus [20]. Serum HAI titers of 1:40 or greater, or serum neutralizing titers of 1:8 or greater, are associated with protection against infection [21]; HAI titers of 1:20 or 1:10 are associated with lesser degrees of protection [22]. Among the elderly, a serum HAI antibody titer above 1:80 may be required for protection [23,24]. Protection in clinical studies is primarily strain specific but some protection is present against strains showing antigenic drift within a subtype, depending on the degree of drift [25,26]. Antibody which is present in low quantity, or which is primarily directed against a heterologous strain of influenza, may not prevent infection but may modify the severity of illness.

Antibody to NA can be measured by NA inhibition (NI) or ELISA. In contrast to anti-HA, anti-NA antibody does not neutralize virus infectivity but instead reduces efficient release of virus from infected cells, resulting in decreased plaque size in vitro [27] and reductions in virus shedding in vivo [28,29]. Observations on the relative protection of those with anti-N2 antibody during the A/Hong Kong/68 (H3N2) pandemic [18,30], as well as experimental challenge studies in humans [31], show that anti-NA antibody does not prevent infection but does protect against disease, diminishes severity of illness and decreases virus shedding [32]. Passive transfer studies in mice suggest that antibody to the M2 protein of influenza A viruses may have a similar effect to that of anti-NA antibody [33,34].

2. Local Immunity

Because the replication of influenza virus in humans is restricted to epithelial cells of the respiratory tract, it is reasonable to expect that immune responses with a mucosal site of action would be highly effective at preventing infection. Studies in a variety of systems confirm the importance of mucosal immunity in protection against influenza. Studies in mice and ferrets have emphasized the importance of local IgA antibody in resistance to infection, particularly in protection of the upper respiratory tract. Polymeric IgA is specifically transported into the nasal secretions of mice and protects against nasal challenge. Protection could be abrogated by intranasal administration of antiserum against IgA but not IgM or IgG [35]. Limited studies have demonstrated significant mucosal responses to influenza virus infection in humans, with development of both HA-specific IgA and IgG in nasal secretions. Nasal HA-specific IgG is predominantly IgG$_1$, and correlates well with serum levels, suggesting that nasal IgG originates by passive diffusion from the systemic compartment [36]. Nasal HA-specific IgA is predominantly polymeric and mostly IgA$_1$, suggesting local synthesis. Studies in humans suggest that protective immunity induced by influenza virus infection is predominantly mediated by local HA-specific IgA [31,37]. Thus methods to induce mucosal immunity are being pursued.

3. Cellular Immunity

Influenza-virus-infected cells can be lysed by antibody in the presence of complement, by antibody-dependent cellular cytotoxicity [38], or by the action of cytotoxic T (Tc) lymphocytes. Generally, Tc lymphocytes express CD8 and are restricted by class I. Such cells may recognize either HA, or internal proteins such as M, NP, or PB2 [39]. Therefore Tc lymphocytes may be subtype specific, or in the case of those that recognize internal proteins, may be broadly cross-reactive, e.g., lysing cells infected with influenza A but not influenza B virus [40–42]. Class II restricted cells may exhibit cytotoxic activity similar to class I restricted cells [41].

Adoptive transfer experiments show that virus-specific Tc lymphocytes mediate recovery from influenza virus infection in animal models [43–48], including both HA-specific and cross-reactive Tc. Virus-specific prechallenge class I restricted Tc lymphocytes correlate with reductions in the duration and level of virus replication in adults with low levels of serum HA and NA antibody following experimental challenge with influenza A virus [49]. The significance of Tc directed against internal viral proteins in protection against severe disease in humans is unclear, as the internal virus proteins were shared between viruses causing the pandemics of 1957 and 1968 and the viruses in circulation immediately prior to these pandemics [50,51]. However, memory Tc lymphocyte responses may play a role in ameliorating the severity of disease and speeding recovery following infection, as suggested by the finding of more severe influenza in individuals with severe defects in cell mediated immunity [8]. For these reasons, there is interest to improve the ability of influenza vaccines to induce Tc, in addition to antibody.

C. Inactivated Influenza Vaccine

The most effective measure available for the control of influenza is the annual administration of inactivated influenza vaccines. Chemically inactivated influenza virus vaccines first licensed in the United States in 1943, consisting of formalin-inactivated whole virions grown in embryonated chicken eggs, showed a protective efficacy of 70% in healthy adults [52]. Although there have been advances in the techniques for producing vaccine, the basic vaccine strategy remains the same. The zonal gradient centrifuge, which can remove reactogenic contaminants, allows more efficient production of more highly purified vaccines [53]. Treatment of whole virus with solvents to create "split" vaccines, or detergents to create "subunit" vaccines, results in vaccines that cause fewer adverse reactions, particularly fever, compared to whole-cell vaccine [54]. Efficiency of vaccine production has also been improved through techniques that create high-yield reassortant strains that contain HA and NA genes from currently circulating influenza viruses and remaining genes from a master strain adapted for high yield from hens' eggs [55]. The current vaccine is generally formulated as a trivalent preparation, containing influenza A (H1N1, H3N2) and influenza B viruses thought most likely to cause disease in the upcoming season based on epidemiological and antigenic analysis of currently circulating strains. Since the late 1970s, vaccine has been standardized to contain at least 15 g of each hemagglutinin (HA) antigen as assessed by single radial immunodiffusion (SRID) [56].

Influenza vaccine is generally very well tolerated in adults. A randomized, double-blind, prospective study in over 800 healthy working adults [57] documented rates of arm soreness of 64% in vaccine recipients compared to 24% in placebo recipients. Only 3% rated arm soreness as severe. Rates of mild local soreness following inactivated influenza vaccine in the range of 60–80% have been documented in other, similar studies [58–60]. Local side effects are slightly more common in women than in men [57].

Systemic reactions, including malaise, flu-like illnesses, and fever, are relatively uncommon. For example, in the large randomized study of influenza vaccine in working adults, systemic complaints, such as fever (6% in both placebo and vaccine recipients) and malaise (17.5% in placebo and 16.0% in vaccine), were seen at equal rates in vaccine and placebo recipients. In other studies, rates of transient, low-grade fever have varied from 2% to 10% of recipients [58–61]. In these studies, rates of systemic effects immediately following vaccination are only marginally increased above baseline [61]. Whole virus and split product vaccines are similarly reactogenic in adults [62], but whole virus vaccines are associated with fever in children [63], and should not be used in those under 12 years of age. Fever occurs in approximately 8–50% of vaccinated children and may be associated with other systemic symptoms such as myalgia, arthralgia, headache, and malaise, but not respiratory symptoms [64]. Severe, life-threatening, immediate hypersensitivity reactions to parenteral inactivated vaccine have been rare. Although the vaccine is grown in eggs, most individuals with "egg allergy" can be safely immunized [65].

During the 1976 National Immunization Program against swine influenza, 45 million persons received influenza vaccine. In the first 4–6 weeks after vaccination, an excess rate of Guillain–Barré syndrome (GBS) occurred among vaccinees as compared with persons who did not receive the vaccine [66]. The estimated risk of acquiring GBS during that vaccination program was 1 in 100,000 vaccinations; the mortality for those with GBS was 5% (i.e., 1 in 2,000,000 vaccinations), and another 5–10% had some residual neurologic abnormality [66]. The relationship between inactivated influenza vaccines other than the Swine/New Jersey/76 vaccine and GBS is less clear cut. National surveillance conducted since 1976 has generally not identified increased rates of this syndrome following vaccination [67]. However, slight increases in the risk of GBS were seen following the 1992–1993 and 1993–1994 vaccines, representing an excess of approximately 1 case per million persons vaccinated [68].

Increases in HAI antibody are seen in about 90% of recipients of vaccine [62,69,70]. A single dose of vaccine elicits seroconversion in individuals who have been previously vaccinated or who have experienced prior infection with a related subtype, but a two-dose schedule is required in unprimed individuals [63,71]. Primed individuals generally respond with antibody that recognizes a broader range of antigenic variants than do unprimed individuals [72]. Serum antibodies peak between 2 and 4 months after vaccination but quickly fall to near baseline before the next influenza season [73]. Mucosal anti-influenza antibodies are not efficiently generated by parenteral inactivated influenza parenteral vaccine [74,75]. Cytotoxic T lymphocyte or cellular immune responses have been reported after administration of parenteral inactivated influenza vaccine [76].

Adults who generally mount decreased responses to inactivated influenza vaccine include the elderly [77–79], those with renal disease [80], and transplant recipients [81–83]. The responsiveness to influenza vaccination in human immunodeficiency virus (HIV)-infected individuals is related to the degree of immunosuppression [84,85]. The immune activation associated with influenza immunization may transiently stimulate HIV replication [86], but the clinical significance of these observations is unclear. Most patients with chronic lung disease respond reasonably well to vaccination, and steroids at doses commonly used to treat reactive airways disease do not appear to preclude vaccine responses [87,88].

Inactivated influenza vaccine is effective in the prevention of influenza A in controlled studies conducted in young adults, with levels of protection of 70–90% when there is a good antigenic match between vaccine and epidemic viruses [26,89,90]. In the most recent randomized controlled trial [91], the efficacy of TIV for preventing culture proven influenza A illness in adults was 76% (95% C.I. 58–87%) for H1N1 and 74% (95% C.I. 52–86%) for H3N2. A subanalysis of efficacy in children in this trial demonstrated efficacy of 91% and 77% in preventing symptomatic, culture-positive influenza A H1N1 and A H3N2 illness respectively compared to placebo [92]. Vaccination of young adults is also associated with decreased absenteeism from work or school [93]. Two studies have demonstrated a reduction in otitis media in children who received TIV. In Finland, children less than 3 years of age who received TIV had an 83% reduction in influenza-associated otitis media and 36% reduction of all otitis media during the subsequent influenza season [94]. In North Carolina, a 41% reduction in acute otitis media was demonstrated in 6–30-month old children attending day care after receiving parenteral TIV [95].

Few prospective trials of protective efficacy have been conducted in high-risk populations. In one placebo-controlled prospective trial in an elderly population, inactivated vaccine was approximately 58% effective in preventing laboratory-documented influenza [96]. In addition, numerous retrospective case control studies are available, which have documented the effectiveness of inactivated influenza vaccines in the elderly [5,97–103]. Vaccine is protective against influenza- and pneumonia-related hospitalization in the elderly, and is accompanied by a decrease in all-cause mortality [104]. However, the protective efficacy of vaccination appears to be lower in individuals over age 65 than in younger adults. Vaccine has also been shown to be protective in limited studies in other high-risk groups, including those with HIV infection [105].

D. Economics of Influenza Vaccination in Adults and Children

The potential economic benefits of influenza vaccination are often underappreciated among clinicians and policy makers. This is due in part to confusion over the economic terms used in such studies, the specific methodologies used to assess economic impact, and the context of cost analyses. The economic impact of a vaccination program can be presented as the cost per outcome of interest such as episodes of pneumonia prevented or life saved (cost-effectiveness), general net cost savings or loss per person vaccinated (cost–benefit analysis), or cost per quality-adjusted life year (QALYs, cost-utility analysis). Economic analyses may include direct costs (which include expenses associated with disease, care for the ill, or prevention) and/or indirect costs (which include unpaid goods or services such as lost wages or extra caregiving). They must also be understood in the context of the "perspective" (from the view of the individual, the health-care payer, e.g., direct costs only) or from society as a whole (direct and indirect costs) and with the target population and morbidities in mind (adult vs. pediatric groups; low-risk vs. high-risk for influenza). Most studies of children and healthy adults have included indirect and direct costs, whereas those of the elderly usually have only included direct costs. Some studies have included information over several influenza seasons, which allows for stratified results for those seasons in which the vaccine strain may or may not match the circulating strain. The magnitude of the economic impact depends on several factors including the assumed level of vaccine efficacy, coverage, and cost, disease incidence, herd immunity, age of the vaccine recipient, and inclusion of future medical costs with years of life gained [106–108]. Ultimately, use of such analyses is tailored to local or national needs and prevailing societal value systems for prioritization of available resources.

1. Adults

In general, influenza vaccination appears to be most cost-effective among the elderly (i.e., those ≥65 years of age) and those at high risk of complications of infection, regardless of age. In elderly populations, vaccination has consistently

been shown to be cost-effective or cost saving, due in large part to the higher risk of incurring substantial health care costs related to influenza complications in this age group. The cost savings per vaccine in studies in the elderly varied from as little as $1 to nearly $250 [109–111], and often resulted in savings of millions of dollars [110–113]. Details of selected studies are noted in Table 1.

Stratified analyses of the elderly, based on the presence of underlying medical conditions, are conflicting: One study reported cost savings, over a 6-year period, for the elderly regardless of whether concomitant comorbid conditions were present [109] and the other reported, over a 9-year period, that vaccination of the low-risk elderly group would incur net costs to the health maintenance organization (HMO), although vaccination of all the elderly (regardless of risk) would be cost saving [111]. In addition, one study from Hong Kong found that vaccination of the elderly would not be cost saving, due likely to exclusion of the prevention of influenza-related hospitalizations because of congestive heart failure (CHF) and other respiratory conditions and the relatively small amount of saved productivity earnings through vaccination since wages are substantially lower in Hong Kong compared to the United States [114]. A comprehensive analysis of clinical preventive services recommended by the U.S. Public Health Service noted that vac-

Table 1 Selected Economic Analyses of Influenza Vaccination in Adults

Study	Main effectiveness result	Main economic result	Comments
Healthy adults <65 years of age			
Nichol, 2001 [118]	12% less workdays missed, 6% less ILI	Average $14 savings/ vaccinee (95% C.I.: $33 savings–$2 cost)	Direct and indirect costs, simulation model
Muennig, 2001 [117]	Not reported	$13 savings/vaccinee	Direct costs only, decision analysis model
Bridges, 2000 [116]	34%, 42%, 32% less ILI, MD visits, lost workdays, respectively (when vaccine strain matched community strain)	$66 cost/vaccinee (poor strain match); $11 cost/vaccinee (good strain match)	Direct and indirect costs, randomized trial over two seasons
Nichol, 1995 [93]	35%, 52%, 24% less URI, days of URI-associated missed work, MD visits, respectively	$47 savings/vaccinee	Direct and indirect costs, randomized trial over one season
Riddiough, 1983 [113]	Not reported	$64 and $23 cost/year healthy life gained for 25–44 and 45–64 years, respectively	Direct costs only, simulation model
Seniors ≥65 years of age			
Nichol, 1998 [109]	39%, 27% less hospitalized pneumonia or CHF, respectively; 50% less all-cause mortality	$73 savings/vaccinee	Direct costs only, staff model HMO over six influenza seasons
Nichol, 1994 [110]	48–57% less hospitalization for pneumonia and influenza; 39–54% less all-cause mortality	$21–235 savings/vaccinee according to year	Direct medical hospitalization costs in staff model HMO over three seasons
Mullooly, 1994 [111]	Effectiveness for prevention of influenza and pneumonia: 30% and 40%, high-risk and all elderly, respectively	$6.1 savings/high-risk vaccinee; $1.1 savings/ any vaccine	Direct costs in one HMO over nine seasons
Riddiough, 1983 [113]	Not reported	Cost savings/year healthy life gained	Direct costs only, simulation model

cination of the elderly against influenza is more cost-effective than many other interventions including screening for high cholesterol and breast cancer [115].

Among healthy working adult populations less than 65 years of age, economic data generally support routine vaccination, if the vaccine strain matches the strain circulating in the community. All studies that include direct and indirect costs, except for one [116], report net savings to society [93,106,113,117]. The range of cost savings to society was approximately $14–47 per vaccinee. A recent study reported that vaccination of working adults was cost saving (average nearly $14 per vaccinee over a 6-year period) and was predicted to be so 95% of the time using up to 10,000 Monte Carlo simulations—a multivariate technique that allows for simultaneous variance of several variables to estimate the probability distribution of the cost–benefit [118]. The most important cost driver in these studies is the indirect costs avoided through prevention of missed work by vaccination. Selected data are summarized in Table 1.

However, one study using data from a randomized trial over two seasons, reported net societal cost of $11 per vaccinee in a year in which the vaccine strain matches the community strain [116]; this value was $66 per vaccinee in the unmatched year. Another study from Hong Kong also concluded that routine vaccination of adults was not cost saving, but the wages in that country are somewhat low compared to the United States (depressing indirect costs benefits of vaccination) and illnesses expected to be worsened following influenza infection (CHF, respiratory disease) were not included in the direct costs assessments [114]. In 1983, the U.S. Congress Office of Technology Assessment determined that routine influenza vaccination of persons 15–24, 25–44, and 45–64 years of age was cost-effective at $181, $64, and $23 per year of healthy life gained, respectively. If productivity gains were included in the analysis for adults 15–44 years, then 25–50% of the costs associated with vaccination would be offset [113]. A meta analysis of influenza vaccination of healthy adults performed by the Cochrane Center group did not reveal it to be cost-effective, but the authors did not include loss of productivity because of illness [119].

The generally favorable economic impact of vaccination of healthy adults results in large part because of prevention of work absenteeism and increased productivity, unlike the elderly among whom reduced utilization of healthcare resources by vaccination is the important cost driver. The economic data, coupled with the significant impact of adult influenza vaccination on health, make a compelling case for annual vaccination of all adults against influenza.

2. Children

The cost implications of influenza vaccination in children have been analyzed using pediatric influenza morbidity data. Two reports evaluated this issue in preschool and school-aged children, respectively [120,121]. These cost–benefit studies included direct and indirect costs, and considered two different vaccine delivery scenarios: (1) a health provider's office during normal work hours, and (2) a more flexible setting that does not require parents to miss work to vaccinate their child (e.g., community-based settings such as day-care centers, schools, or supermarkets). Vaccination was cost saving for each age group, in either scenario. The net savings ranged from $1–21 per vaccine recipient for the preschool age group and $4–35 for the older children (Table 2). In both studies, the largest proportion of savings was attributed to prevention (by vaccination) of indirect costs incurred with disease. However, the cost savings for each study were likely underestimated because (1) the school-aged group study did not include savings associated with prevention of influenza-associated otitis media and hospitalization and (2) the preschool study did not include prevention of day-care transmission.

Another study reported a cost-effectiveness analysis using prospective data collected during a 2-year, randomized trial of a live, intranasal influenza vaccine among children 15–71 months of age [122]. This study found that routine vaccination was cost-effective assuming a vaccine price of $20, resulting in $19–30 per febrile influenza-like illness day prevented, and was cost saving to society when vaccination is performed in the flexible setting defined above (Table 2). When given in the health provider's office, the societal cost-

Table 2 Economic Evaluations of Routine Influenza Vaccination of U.S. Children

| Study | Vaccine cost[a] | Vaccination in physician offices | | Vaccination in community-based setting | |
		Societal perspective[b]	Health Payer perspective[c]	Societal perspective	Health Payer perspective
Luce, 2001 [122]	$20	$30 cost/febrile ILI day avoided	$19 cost/febrile ILI day avoided	Cost saving	$19 cost/febrile ILI day avoided
White, 1999 [121]	$10, $4[d]	$4 savings/vaccinee	$6 cost/vaccinee	$35 savings/vaccinee	Not cost savings
Cohen, 2000 [120]	$10	$1 savings/vaccinee	$15 cost/vaccine	$21 savings/vaccinee	$15 cost/vaccine
Riddiough, 1983 [113]	$11	$258, $196 cost/year healthy life gained for 1–3 and 3–14 years, respectively			
Dayan, 2001 [123]	$10	For children 0–15 years (direct and indirect costs): savings of $10/vaccinee and $57 savings/influenza episode averted (study performed in Argentina)			

[a] Cost is sum of estimated vaccine price and costs associated with its administration.
[b] Direct and lost productivity costs included.
[c] Direct medical costs only.
[d] In this study, the vaccine cost was $10 in the "physician offices" setting and $4 in the "community-based" setting.

effectiveness was $30 per influenza-like illness prevented with greater cost-effectiveness noted from the health payer perspective. Another analysis from Argentina concluded that immunization of high-risk children 6 months to 15 years of age with the inactivated vaccine would be cost saving to society at approximately $10 per vaccinated child, a societal savings of $57 per influenza case averted [123]. This study also showed, using Monte Carlo simulation, that vaccination was cost saving 64% of the time over 1000 trials, with the following variables subjected to variation: vaccine efficacy, vaccine price, incidence of infection, and number of days lost by a parent. These economic benefits favorably compare to immunization against pediatric disease of high incidence and relatively low morbidity, such as varicella and rotavirus diarrhea [124,125].

E. Indications and Usage

The main goal of the current strategy for use of influenza vaccine is to reduce complications by targeting individuals at highest risk of influenza-related hospitalizations or death. Table 3 lists those groups for whom annual influenza vaccination is currently recommended [126], including the elderly and adults and children with chronic conditions known to increase the risk of influenza complications. The age at which annual vaccination is recommended has been lowered from 65 to 50. The rationale for this recommendation is to achieve higher vaccination rates in nonelderly individuals with high-risk conditions, a large proportion of whom are between 50 and 65 years old.

The Advisory Committee on Immunization Practices (ACIP) has recommended that practitioners consider annual influenza vaccine for all children 6–23 months of age [127], mostly to prevent medically attended illnesses and complications such as otitis media. An additional benefit of widespread vaccination of young children could be reductions in rates of influenza in other groups, because children play an important role in the propagation of influenza epidemics in a community [22]. There is relatively little direct evidence supporting the use of influenza vaccine to prevent transmission, but in one study mass vaccination of school-age children resulted in reduced rates of influenza in teachers and parents compared to a control community where children were not vaccinated [128]. In addition, it has been observed that influenza-related mortality rates among the elderly have increased in Japan, coincident with discontinuation of that country's policy of universal vaccination of school children [129]. Targeting of children for annual influenza immunization could reduce the impact of influenza in the whole community.

II. OPPORTUNITIES TO IMPROVE CURRENT VACCINES

The performance of inactivated influenza vaccines could be improved by enhancing the level and duration of systemic immune responses (particularly in elderly and high-risk subjects), augmenting mucosal responses, and stimulating cellular immune responses. Two features of the current in-

activated vaccines are important to keep in mind while considering the development of new or improved vaccines. First, although the current vaccine is very well tolerated, concern about side effects is one factor that is frequently cited as a reason why individuals choose not to receive influenza vaccine. In addition, successful implementation of vaccine strategies will necessarily expose large numbers of recipients to potential side effects. Therefore any new influenza vaccine must be very safe, and significant increases in local or systemic reactinogenicity over that seen with current vaccine would probably be unacceptable. Second, the current vaccine is relatively inexpensive, and is cost-effective and possibly cost saving. These types of considerations will become increasingly important as large health care providers make decisions about covered benefits.

III. IMPROVED PARENTERAL INFLUENZA VACCINES

A. High-Dose Vaccine

Within the relatively narrow dose range feasible using standard technology inactivated vaccines, there is a fairly flat dose–response curve [62,71,130,131], but improved purification techniques have allowed exploration of much higher doses. In young adults, highly purified hemagglutinins have been administered at doses as high as 405 μg without significant adverse events. Administration of 405 μg of monovalent H1 antigen, or trivalent vaccine containing 135 μg of each antigen was well tolerated and associated with twofold to fourfold higher geometric mean HAI and neutralizing antibody titers 4 weeks after vaccination, compared to standard doses [132]. Improved nasal secretion antibody responses with high-dose vaccines were also seen [132]. Elderly subjects have manifested a more flattened dose response curve than young adults [133,134], but the efficacy of very high doses of HA in this population remains to be evaluated.

B. Neuraminidase Vaccines

The infection-permissive nature of anti-NA immunity has stimulated interest in NA-based vaccines that could provide clinical protection yet allow subclinical infection that would elicit other immune responses to the virus. Purified NA antigens induce NA antibody and prevent death in lethal mouse models of influenza [32,135–137]. Because the neuraminidase appears to undergo antigenic drift at a slower rate than hemagglutinin, a neuraminidase or neuraminidase-supplemented inactivated vaccine may induce better protection against drifted viruses than does standard inactivated vaccine [138]. Preliminary results in the human challenge model suggest that neuraminidase-supplemented vaccines may be more efficacious than standard vaccine in protection against an antigenic variant [139].

C. Vaccines Produced in Alternative Substrates

Production of inactivated influenza vaccines in embryonated hen's eggs has practical drawbacks, including: (1) the expense and difficulty in ensuring the availability of sufficient numbers of hens in the compressed time frame in which influenza vaccine is prepared, and (2) the potential for antigenically variant influenza A viruses to be selected during the process of developing strains for vaccine production, which grow well in eggs. Direct polymerase chain reaction (PCR) amplification of viruses in nasal secretions has documented that the HA of the major population of virus shed from the nasopharynx of infected humans is identical to that isolated in MDCK cells, and significantly different from that isolated in eggs. Antigenic differences of this type have been documented for H3N2, H1N1, and influenza B viruses [140–147]. Alterations in CTL epitopes have also been described [148]. Although these differences may amount to only a few amino acids, the MDCK-cell-grown virus appears to be more effective than egg-grown virus as an inactivated vaccine for protection of experimental animals [149,150]. Thus current inactivated influenza vaccines grown in eggs may not exhibit optimal antigenic representation of the viruses that are infecting humans.

For these reasons, mammalian cell culture for growth of influenza viruses for vaccine production is being explored [151]. The main technical challenges have been to develop mammalian cell lines suitable for use as vaccine production substrates [152], and to optimize culture techniques to obtain maximal yields. Vaccine generated in Vero cells induces serum antibody responses to the same extent as standard vaccine in mice [153]. Recently, human studies showed that at similar doses a candidate MDCK cell grown vaccine generated antibody titers similar to those generated by egg-grown vaccines [154].

Recombinant DNA techniques to generate vaccine antigen expressed in cells also allow control over the sequence of the HA used. Hemagglutinin antigens generated in insect cells by recombinant baculoviruses have been evaluated in young adults and elderly community dwelling adults over the age of 65 years [155–157]. Administration of recombinant HA vaccine stimulated HA-specific serum antibody in both young and older adults. Antibody responses to higher doses of 90 or 135 μg of H3 vaccine antigen occurred with greater frequency and resulted in higher titers of antibody than did subvirion vaccine. Antibody responses to both the H1 and H3 antigens when a bivalent vaccine containing 45 μg of each antigen was administered were similar to those when the monovalent vaccines were separately administered at doses of 45 μg each. Similar results were seen for neutralizing and HA-specific IgG ELISA antibody. In one trial of A/Beijing/89 (H3) vaccine in healthy adults, subjects were followed during the subsequent influenza season for ascertainment of influenza-like illnesses [155], and although not designed as an efficacy trial, preliminary evidence of protection was reported. These results suggest that the known differences in glycosylation in insect as compared to mammalian cells [158] do not affect the generation of a functional antibody response in primed individuals; however, confirmation awaits studies in children.

D. Adjuvants and Alternative Formulations

Generally, adjuvants used with influenza vaccine have consisted of agents that directly modify the immune response, such as the squalene derivative MF59, monophosphoryl lipid A (MPL), the purified soap-bark derivatives Quil A or QS-21, dihydroepiandosterone (DHEA) [159], or cytokines such as IL-2 or thymosin [160]; or consist of attempts to physically modify the vaccine to improve antigen presentation, such as formulation in liposomes [161,162], or multimeric complexes such as ISCOMs (immunostimulating complexes) [163,164]. Combinations of both approaches are frequently applied.

In healthy adults, MF-59-adjuvanted vaccine is well tolerated and results in slightly higher GMT rises than standard subunit vaccine [165,166]. This vaccine has also been well tolerated and induced somewhat higher titered serum antibody responses in the elderly than does standard split-product vaccine [167,168]. Formulation of hemagglutinin into ISCOMS with the adjuvant Quil A improved antibody and CTL responses in Phase I studies in humans [169,170]. Formulation of HA into liposomes with the *Escherichia coli* heat labile toxin (HLT) has been evaluated for intranasal immunization, but such virosomes are also effective adjuvants for parenteral immunization [171].

E. Transcutaneous and Dermal Immunization

Two transcutaneous immunization approaches have recently been described for influenza. When influenza antigen is directly applied to hydrated skin in the form of a patch for several hours, antigen penetrates the stratum corneum to reach antigen-presenting cells [172]. In a second approach, antigen is applied to the skin using a powder vehicle such as trehalose delivered via gene gun device [173]. Both approaches require the use of powerful adjuvants for optimal responses to elicit systemic antibody, cytotoxic T-lymphocytes, and mucosal antibodies.

IV. INTRANASAL APPROACHES TO VACCINATION

A. Cold-Adapted Influenza Vaccines (CAIV)

Live virus vaccines for influenza, which have been intensively evaluated in humans, offer several potential advantages over parenteral inactivated vaccines, including induction of a mucosal immune response that closely mimics that induced by natural influenza virus infection [174]. In addition, the potential superiority of such vaccines in protection of the upper respiratory tract [175] might be useful in immunization strategies to limit transmission of influenza. In practical terms, the nasal, rather than parenteral, route of administration might be more acceptable to patients, particularly in certain age groups.

A key requirement for the development of attenuated influenza vaccines is the ability to rapidly attenuate new antigenic variants. The most widely used approach takes advantage of the segmented nature of the influenza virus genome to generate reassortant viruses in which the gene segments encoding attenuation are derived from a well-characterized master donor vaccine virus, and the gene segments encoding the HA and NA are derived from the new antigenic variant [176,177] (Figure 1). In the past,

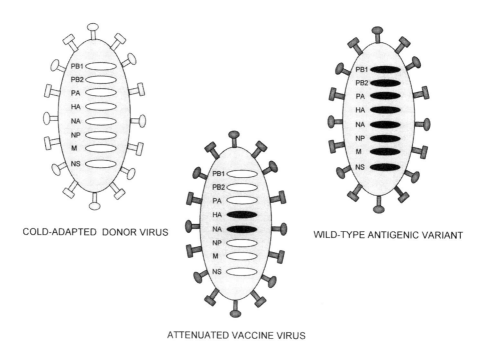

COLD-ADAPTED DONOR VIRUS   WILD-TYPE ANTIGENIC VARIANT

ATTENUATED VACCINE VIRUS

Figure 1 New influenza antigenic variants can be rapidly attenuated by genetic reassortment with a well-characterized master attenuated vaccine virus. The attenuated vaccine master virus donates the gene segments encoding attenuation, while the epidemic virus donates the genes encoding the antigenically variant HA and NA in the construction of a live attenuated reassortant vaccine virus.

extensive studies were performed to evaluate the use of temperature-sensitive [178] or avian [179] influenza viruses as donors of attenuating genes. However, these approaches were not successful, either because of genetic instability [180] or unreliable attenuation [181,182]. Importantly, such deficiencies in the safety profile of these approaches to live attenuated influenza vaccine were only detected when studies were performed in young children, who are generally most susceptible to infection by the vaccine viruses.

The most promising master donor viruses are cold-adapted influenza A/Ann Arbor/6/60 (H2N2) and B/Ann Arbor 1/66 strains [183]. The process of cold adaptation refers to the repetitive passage of a virus at gradually decreasing temperature until a virus is isolated that efficiently replicates at a low temperature at which the replication of the original wild-type virus is significantly restricted [184]. During this process, additional mutant phenotypes are frequently acquired. The cold-adapted influenza viruses demonstrate three such phenotypes: (1) the cold-adapted (*ca*) phenotype, defined as the ability to replicate efficiently at 25°C, a restrictive temperature for wild-type influenza viruses; (2) the temperature-sensitive (*ts*) phenotype, defined as significant (>2 log10) restriction of virus replication at 38–39°C; and the attenuation (*att*) phenotype, defined as restricted replication in the lower respiratory tract of experimental animals.

Genetic analysis of the cold-adapted A/Ann Arbor/6/60 virus has demonstrated multiple mutations in all six of the so-called "internal" or non-HA or NA gene segments, and analysis of single gene reassortants has shown that at least

three of these gene segments (PB1, PB2, and PA) participate in the attenuation of the virus in animals and humans (Table 4) [185,186]. The basis of attenuation of the B/AnnArbor/6/66 virus has been less completely worked out. Mutations in five of the six internal gene segments have been described [187], and analysis of laboratory-derived revertant viruses has implicated the PA gene segment as playing an important role in attenuation [188,189].

1. Safety

A large number of monovalent *ca* A/AA/6/60 and B/AA/6/66 reassortant influenza viruses have been evaluated in young adults, children, and elderly subjects, and found to be reliably attenuated and immunogenic (reviewed in Ref. 190). Bivalent or trivalent CAIV has also been well tolerated in adults [91,191–195]. Adults who receive bivalent or trivalent CAIV have had the following statistically significant excess symptoms compared to placebo recipients in the immediate period following vaccination: runny nose or coryza, sore throat, lethargy, headache, and muscle ache (Table 5) [91,191–195]. However, when considering these studies in aggregate, nasal symptoms (runny nose, nasal congestion or coryza) and sore throat were the most frequently identified adverse symptoms in these studies. No severe reactions have been consistently attributed to CAIV.

Bivalent and trivalent CAIV have been safe and well tolerated in children [92,196–206]. As seen in Table 5, the following symptoms have occasionally been found to be significantly more common within 7–11 days after vaccina-

Table 3 Target Groups to Receive Annual Trivalent, Inactivated Influenza Vaccine

Individuals at high risk for influenza-related complications
- Age 50 years or older.
- Adults and children who have chronic disorders of the pulmonary or cardiovascular systems, including asthma.
- Residents of chronic-care facilities that house persons of any age who have chronic medical conditions
- Adults and children who have required medical follow-up or hospitalization during the preceding year because of chronic metabolic diseases (including diabetes mellitus), renal dysfunction, hemoglobinpathies, or immunosuppression (including immunosuppression by medication or by HIV virus).
- Children and teenagers (6 months to 18 years) who are receiving long-term aspirin therapy and therefore might be at risk for developing Reye syndrome after influenza.
- Women who will be in the second or third trimester of pregnancy during the influenza season. (Please note that some experts prefer to administer influenza vaccine beyond the first trimester to avoid coincidental association with spontaneous abortion, which is common during this trimester, and because vaccines have traditionally been avoided during this trimester.)

Individuals who can transmit influenza to those at high risk
- Physicians, nurses, and other health care personnel in both hospital and outpatient-care settings, including emergency responses workers.
- Employees of nursing homes and chronic-care facilities who have contact with patients or residents.
- Employees of assisted living and other residences for persons in groups at high risk.
- Individuals who provide home care to persons in high-risk groups.
- Household members (including children) of person in high-risk groups.

Other groups to consider
- Breastfeeding is not a contraindication for influenza vaccine.
- Travelers
  - Travel to the tropics
  - Travel with large tourist groups
  - Travel in the Southern Hemisphere from April through September
- General population: any person for whom influenza illness might be problematic (e.g., individuals who provide essential services, students, or other persons in dormitories or institutional setting depending on vaccine availability.)

Source: Centers for Disease Control and Prevention. Prevention and control of influenza: recommendations of the Advisory Committee on Immunization Practices (ACIP). MMWR 2001; 50(RR-4):1–45.

tion in young children (under 8 years of age) who received multivalent CAIV compared to placebo: low-grade fever, runny nose or coryza, cough, headache, chills, vomiting, and abdominal pain. All symptoms resolved without sequelae. However, when considering all the pediatric studies in aggregate, no consistent symptom was seen significantly more commonly in CAIV compared to placebo recipients. Nasal symptoms (runny nose, nasal congestion, or coryza) were more frequently observed in CAIV recipients in only 3 of 12 pediatric studies cited in Table 3. In older children, 11 to < 16 years of age, sore throat was observed slightly more frequently in CAIV recipients than in inactivated influenza

Table 4 Genetic Basis of Attenuation of the Cold-Adapted (*ca*) A/Ann Arbor/6/60 Virus

| Gene segment from the *ca* A/AA/6/60 Virus | Phenotype of single gene reassortants with respect to: | | | Sequence of gene product | | |
	Temperature sensitivity (*ts*)	Cold adaptation (*ca*)	Attenuation (*att*)	Amino acid position	*Wt* A/AA/6/60 virus	*ca* A/AA/6/60 virus
PB2	*ts*	*wt*	*att*	265	Asn	Ser
PB1	*ts*	*wt*	*att*	391	Lys	Glu
				457	Glu	Asp
				581	Glu	Gly
				661	Ala	Thr
PA	*wt*	*ca*	*att*	613	Lys	Glu
				715	Leu	Pro

Source: Refs. 185 and 186.

Table 5 Reactogenicity of Multivalent CAIV in Adults and Children

Trial	Ages of participants	No. CAIV/No. placebo recipients	Days followed after vaccination	Fever	Runny nose/ Nasal congestion/ Coryza	Sore throat
Adult Trials						
Jackson et al. [191]	65 to 75 years	100/100	7	—	—	13%
Keitel et al. [194]	18 to 40 years	11/10	7	—	NA	NA
Edwards et al. [91]	1 to 65 years[a]	1733/3477[b]	4	—	6%	11%
Treanor et al. [195]	18 to 45 years	103/36	7	—	—	—
Nichol et al. [193]	18 to 64 years	3041/1520	7	—	18%	10%
King et al. [192]	18 to 58 years	27/27	10	—	34%	—
Pediatric Trials						
Neuzil et al. [92]	1 to <6 years	144/330[c]	4	—	11%	—
	6 to <11 years	247/497[c]	4	—	—	—
	11 to <16 years	209/382[c]	4	—	—	6%
Belshe et al. [196]	15 to 71 months (first dose only)	1070/532	10	4%	11%	—
Belshe et al. [197]	27 to 73 months	917/441 (2nd year of above)	10	—	—	—
Zangwill et al. [198]	12 to 36 months	Dose 1:400/100	10	—	7%	—
		Dose 2: 400/100	10	—	—	—
King et al. [199]	18–71 months	234/122[d]	10	—	—	—
King et al. [200]	1–7 years	25/25	10	—	—	—
Sweirkosz et al. [201]	2–22 months	Dose 1: 17/5	11	—	—	NA
		Dose 2: 15/3	11	—	—	NA
Belshe et al. [202]	6 months to 3 years	32/17	11	—	—	NA
Gruber et al. [203]	6 months to 2 years	50/19	10	—	—	NA
Gruber et al. [204]	6 to 18 months	47/44	10	—	—	NA
Wright et al. [205]	12 to 37 months	18/4	10	—	—	NA
Gruber et al. [206]	2 months to 3 years	1126/1017	7	—	—	—

The percentages below each adverse event column represent statistically significant increases in events compared to placebo groups. Negative (−) signs represent no statistical difference between CAIV and placebo recipients and NA signifies not assessed in that report. The parentheses under the trial column is the reference number.

[a] Eighty five of the subjects were >16 years of age.

[b] There were 4120 doses of intranasal CAIV and 8380 doses of nasal placebo given to the study participants. The 1733 intranasal CAIV recipients received intramuscular saline in year 1 and intramuscular monovalent influenza B vaccine in years 2–5. Of the 3477 nasal placebo recipients, 1738 received saline intramuscularly in year 1 and intramuscular monovalent inactivated influenza B vaccine in years 2–5 and 1739 received TIV for years 1–5. The latter two groups comprise the placebo group to compare to CAIV recipients.

[c] Doses of vaccine. In this subanalysis of Ref. 91, 791 total children under 16 years of age participated. See footnote [b] for dosing assignments.

[d] Includes doses of 10^{4-7} $TCID_{50}$; 63 children received 10^7 $TCID_{50}$.

vaccines [92]. CAIV has been demonstrated to be safe in infants 2 to 6 months of age [207].

Safety has also been demonstrated in high-risk individuals who would not be able to tolerate even minor lower respiratory tract inflammation. No significant vaccine-related adverse events have been seen in studies of children with cystic fibrosis [208,209] or asthma [210,211], and vaccinated children with asthma have not experienced significant changes in FEV1, use of beta adrenergic rescue medications or asthma symptom scores compared to placebo recipients [211]. CAIV has been well tolerated in adults with or chronic obstructive airway disease [212–214]. Vaccine is well tolerated in the elderly, although in one study vaccine recipients had a 13% excess of sore throats compared to those who received placebo [191].

Young children with advanced HIV infection have difficulty clearing influenza virus from the respiratory tract, and there have been several reports of very prolonged virus shedding in highly immunosuppressed individuals [215], including children with AIDS. Although CAIV is not intended for use in individuals with HIV, such persons could be inadvertently vaccinated. Small numbers of adults with relatively asymptomatic HIV infection have received CAIV [192]. There was a 30% excess reporting of runny nose/congestion compared to placebo recipients but no lower respiratory tract illnesses were observed in this group. No excess or prolonged CAIV virus shedding was detected in HIV-infected compared to non-HIV-infected CAIV recipients. No significant changes in blood CD4 counts or quantitative HIV RNA levels after vaccination with CAIV were detected in HIV-infected adults who received CAIV compared to those who received placebo. This was followed by a study in which 23 children, 1–8 years of age, with relatively asymptomatic human immunodeficiency infection, received triva-

Decrease in activity/lethargy	Cough	Wheezing	Headache	Muscle ache	Chills	Vomit	Irritability	Abdominal pain
–	–	NA	–	–	–	NA	NA	NA
NA	NA	NA	NA	NA	NA	NA	NA	NA
5%	–	NA	3%	2%	–	NA	NA	NA
NA	–	NA	NA	–	–	NA	NA	NA
–	–	NA	–	–	–	NA	NA	NA
NA	–	NA	–	–	NA	–	NA	–
–	–	NA	NA	NA	NA	NA	NA	NA
–	–							
–	–							
–	–	–	–	–	–	2%	–	1.6%
–	–	–	–	–	–	–	–	NA
–	–	NA	7%	–	–	–	–	NA
–	–	–	–	–	–	–	–	
NA	–	–	NA	NA	NA	NA	–	NA
–	–	NA	–	–	–	–	–	NA
NA	–	NA	NA	NA	NA	NA	NA	NA
NA	NA	NA	NA	NA	NA	NA	NA	NA
NA	–	NA	NA	NA	NA	NA	NA	NA
NA	–	NA	NA	NA	NA	NA	NA	NA
NA	67%	NA	NA	NA	NA	NA	NA	NA
NA	–	NA	NA	NA	NA	NA	NA	NA

lent CAIV [200]. In that study, CAIV was safe and well tolerated compared to placebo in these children. Importantly, no increased frequency, excess quantity, or prolonged shedding of the trivalent CAIV vaccine viruses were detected in HIV-infected compared to non-HIV-infected children of similar age, nor were significant differences observed in peripheral blood quantitative HIV RNA levels or CD4 counts.

Although vaccinated adults and children shed CAIV, transmission to susceptible contacts is rare. No transmission of CAIV from vaccine recipients to susceptible contacts was detected in studies of young children in day-care-like settings where CAIV and placebo recipients played together for up to 8 hr a day for 7–10 days after vaccination [177,216]. In the largest study [217], 197 children between 8 and 36 months of age were randomized to intranasally receive trivalent CAIV or placebo, and vaccine virus shedding was assessed for 21 days after vaccination. Although 80% of CAIV recipients shed at least one vaccine strain, for a mean of 7.6 days, trans-

mission was detected in only one placebo recipient, for an estimated transmission rate of 1.75% (95% upper bound of 8%). Vaccine virus recovered from vaccinated volunteer subjects have all retained the attenuated phenotype and genotype [217,218].

2. Immunogenicity

The immunogenicity of cold-adapted reassortant vaccines in children, adults, and the elderly correlates with replication of cold-adapted vaccines in the upper respiratory tract, and hence their immunogenicity is influenced by the susceptibility of the host at the time of vaccination. Therefore the frequency and magnitude of immune responses to vaccination is highest in young children, intermediate in adults, and lowest in elderly subjects who have been repeatedly infected with influenza viruses throughout their lifetimes. Mucosally administered *ca* vaccine is generally more effective than parenterally administered inactivated influenza vaccine at inducing nasal HA-specific IgA, while inactivated vaccine usually induces higher titered serum HAI and HA-specific IgG antibody [219].

The serum and mucosal HA-specific antibody responses in children in several studies are shown in Table 6 [198,199, 201,202,204,206,209,220]. Most susceptible children demonstrate measurable serum and mucosal antibody responses. For example, nasal vaccine strain-specific IgA responses were detected in 50% of susceptible children who received A/H3N2 CAIV [221]. Post-CAIV-vaccination secretory antibody persists for up to or beyond a year in children. A study of trivalent CAIV administered to children 15–71 months of age demonstrated mucosal IgA strain specific responses of 62–85% [222]. In contrast, vaccination with bivalent or trivalent CAIV in unscreened adults generally results in a low proportion of more than fourfold rises in serum strain specific influenza antibody [91,194,195] and relatively lower rates of mucosal responses [223]. Even in those prescreened to have low prevaccination vaccine-specific influenza antibody, the rates of serum antibody responses to intranasal CAIV in adults and the elderly are low [195,224].

Cytotoxic T lymphocyte responses to live CAIV have been measured in adults who intranasally received CAIV [76,225]. Although not extensively studied, limited data suggest that cold-adapted influenza vaccines may induce antibody and cytotoxic T cells (Tc) with more broadened recognition within a subtype than seen after inactivated vaccine as well [226,227]. However, these responses have been more difficult to measure in young children [228].

There may be interference between components of multivalent cold-adapted vaccines [192,196,199,201,204,220]. However, interference can be overcome by administering a second dose of multivalent CAIV within 1–2 months after the first dose [196,201]. This may reflect development of immunity to the dominant virus with the first dose of a multivalent vaccine, allowing the weaker component to replicate upon a second dose. A similar situation has been well described for multivalent live poliovirus vaccine [229].

3. Efficacy and Effectiveness

CAIV was efficacious in the prevention of influenza in a 2-year, randomized placebo-controlled trial conducted in 1314 children aged 15–74 months in the United States [196]. Efficacy against culture confirmed influenza illness in the first year of this trial was 95% (95% C.I., 88%–97%) against influenza A/H3N2 and 91% (95% C.I., 79%–96%) for influenza B. In the second year of the trial, the H3 component of the vaccine (A/Wuhan/93) was not a close match with the predominant H3 virus that season, A/Sydney/95. Nevertheless, the efficacy of CAIV against this variant was 86% (95% C.I., 75%–92%) [197], suggesting that CAIV can induce protective immunity against drift variants. Overall, the efficacy of intranasal trivalent CAIV to prevent any influenza illness during the 2-year period of surveillance in this field study was 92% (95% C.I. 88%–94%). Although some CAIV recipients developed culture-documented influenza infection, the spectrum of influenza illnesses were milder compared to influenza illnesses in placebo recipients. There were

fewer febrile illnesses, fewer days of fever, and fewer cases of influenza associated otitis media in CAIV recipients who did contract influenza illness compared to placebo recipients.

The efficacy in children determined in this trial is consistent with the results of earlier trials using monovalent or bivalent vaccines. In a subset analysis of a large field trial of bivalent CAIV [92], efficacy against culture positive A/ H1N1 influenza illness was 96% (95% C.I., 67%–99%) and was 68% (95% C.I., 1%–90%) against A/H3N2 illness in 791 children less than 16 years of age. This favorably compared to parenteral trivalent inactivated vaccine where the efficacy against A/H1N1 was 91% and A/H3N2 was 77%. In another, smaller study in children 6–18 months old, efficacy against H3N2 culture positive illness was 65% for children 6–18 months of age who received monovalent H3N2 CAIV or bivalent (H3N2 + H1N1) CAIV compared to those that intranasally received placebo or monovalent A/H1N1 CAIV [204].

Efficacy of trivalent cold-adapted influenza vaccine against naturally acquired influenza in adults has not been directly demonstrated. However, efficacy of trivalent CAIV was demonstrated in an experimental infection study in which adults were given either trivalent live intranasal CAIV, parenteral trivalent inactivated influenza vaccine, or placebo and then experimentally infected with wild-type influenza A/H1N1, A/H3N2, or B viruses [195]. The combined efficacy in preventing laboratory-documented influenza illness because of the three wild-type influenza strains was 85% for the CAIV and 71% for the inactivated vaccine. These data are consistent with observations from other experimental infection studies conducted with monovalent CAIV in which protection against challenge with wild-type virus was at least equal to and sometimes better than that provided by inactivated vaccine [37,175,230,231]. In addition, in a large, 5-year field trial in Nashville [91], the efficacy of bivalent CAIV was 85% (95% C.I., 70%–92%) against A/H1N1 illness and 58% (95% C.I., 29%–75%) against A/ H3N2 illness. This efficacy against influenza illness was similar to that induced by parenteral trivalent inactivated vaccine which was 76% against H1N1 illness and 74% against H3N2 illness.

The potential utility of trivalent CAIV in adults has been demonstrated in an effectiveness trial where the endpoints were not influenza virus specific. In this study, performed in 4561 healthy working adults [193], effectiveness in preventing severe febrile respiratory illness of any cause during the influenza season was 29%. Of note, this trial was conducted in a year when the antigenic match between the vaccine virus (A/Wuhan) and the predominant epidemic virus (A/Sydney) was not close.

No studies of the protective efficacy of *ca* vaccine alone have been conducted in the elderly, an age group in which immunogenicity may be reduced. However, the combination of local live attenuated influenza vaccine and parenteral inactivated vaccine administered together resulted in an approximately 60% decrease in cases of laboratory confirmed influenza in an elderly nursing home population, compared to inactivated vaccine alone [232].

The mechanism of protection induced by cold-adapted vaccine has mostly been evaluated in experimental infection

Table 6 Serologic Responses to Multivalent CAIV (trivalent A/H1N1, A/H3N2, and B=T-CAIV, bivalent A=B-CAIV)

Trial	Ages	Vaccine and dose (TCID$_{50}$)	Prevaccination seronegative to A/H3N2	Prevaccination seronegative to A/H1N1	Prevaccination seronegative to B	All subjects to A/H3N2	All subjects to A/H1N1	All subjects to B
Adult Trials								
Treanor et al. [195]	18–45 years	10^7 T-CAIV	39	29	10	33	23	3
Keitel et al. [194]	18–40 years[a]	10$^{7.1}$ T-CAIV						
		Dose 1:				24[b]	67[b]	10[b]
		Dose 2:				33	86	19
King et al. [192]	18–58 years	10^7 T-CAIV				4	0	4
Edwards et al. [91]	1–65 years	10$^{6-7.6}$ B-CAIV				14	34	NA
Pediatric Trials								
Edwards et al. [220]	12 to 37 months	10$^{6.5}$ B-CAIV	33	75	NA			
Sweirkotz et al. [201]	2 to 22 months	10^7 T-CAIV						
		Dose 1:	88	12	18			
		Dose 2:	93	80	67			
Zangwill et al. [198]	12 to 36 months	10^7 T-CAIV						
		Dose 1:	NA	NA	NA	53–85	17–74	42–70
		Dose 2:	99–100	42–94	96–100	65–72	37–88	64–72
King et al. [200]	18 to 71 months	10^7 T-CAIV	90	16	50	40	13	25
Belshe et al. [196]	15 to 71 months	10^7 T-CAIV						
		Dose 1:	92	16	88			
		Dose 2:	99	61	96			
King et al. [199]	1 to 7 years	10^7 T-CAIV						
		Dose 1:	100	67	100	16	52	48
		Dose 2:	100	94	89	17	71	42
Belshe et al. [202]	6 months to 3 years	10$^{4.4-5}$ T-CAIV	71	59	47	44	31	38
Gruber et al. [204]	6 to 18 months	10$^{6.2}$ B-CAIV	97	45	NA			
Gruber et al. [206]	≤6 months	10^7 B-CAIV	70	65	NA			
	7–18 months		87	80				
	>18 months to 3 years		92	80				

All serologic responses represent more than fourfold rises pre- to postvaccination measured by hemagglutination inhibition assay except where indicated.
[a] Subjects were selected who had "low" prevaccination titers to at least one of the three vaccine strains.
[b] Serology performed = neutralizing antibody.
[c] Four separate lots of T-CAIV assessed.

studies. Cold-adapted vaccine is protective in these experiments in the absence of significant serum HAI responses, suggesting that the main protective effect is via induction of mucosal antibodies. However, protection can be demonstrated in some circumstances in the absence of detectable mucosal responses [233], and the specific levels of mucosal antibody required for protection are unknown. In addition, the role that induction of cellular immune responses plays in the protective effect has not been elucidated.

B. Other Live Viral Vaccines

The development of techniques for direct genetic engineering of specific mutations in the genome of influenza A and B viruses [234–236] has provided a tool to generate live influenza vaccine candidates. Because these viruses can now be entirely constructed from plasmid DNA [237,238], any nonlethal mutation in any gene can be incorporated (Figure 2). Directly introduced mutations at several sites have been shown to result in attenuation. These include replacement of the 3′ and 5′ ends of a gene segment of influenza A virus by the corresponding regions of an influenza B virus [239], manipulation of the stalk of the NA [240,241], and placement of avian-like sequences into the PB2 gene [242,243]. One intriguing approach has been complete or partial deletion of the NS1 protein [244]. These viruses manifest significantly reduced replication in systems in which the type I interferon system is intact, implicating the NS1 protein as an interferon

antagonist. Complete or partial NS1-deleted viruses provide excellent protection against homologous wild-type influenza virus in mice [245], and are being developed as possible second-generation vaccines.

C. Intranasal Inactivated Influenza Vaccines

Studies in humans conducted over many years have shown that nasopharyngeal administration of inactivated vaccines by nose drops or aerosol can stimulate production of local antibody in primed individuals [246–250]. However, the simple administration of soluble antigen to this mucosal surface is inefficient, requiring relatively large amounts of antigen to induce mucosal immune responses. Therefore attenuation has focused on ways to enhance the immunogenicity of mucosal inactivated vaccine, basically by increasing uptake by mucosal antigen-presenting cells. Strategies used have included mucosal adjuvants, incorporation of HA and other antigens into particulate formulations, or both.

Bacterial enterotoxins, such as cholera toxin (CT), have been extensively evaluated as mucosal adjuvants for influenza and other vaccines. However, these toxins are far too reactogenic in man for routine use, as even a few microgram quantities can induce cholera diarrhea if they reach the intestine. Initial studies showing a potential adjuvant effect of purified B subunit [251,252] were complicated by the presence of residual amounts of holotoxin [253], and it became more clear that the holotoxin was responsible for the major-

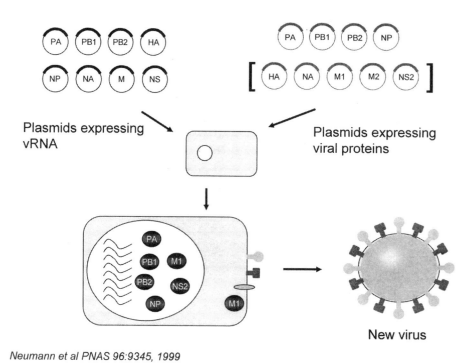

Neumann et al PNAS 96:9345, 1999

Figure 2 Generation of new attenuated viruses by direct manipulation of the viral genome. Cells are simultaneously transfected with plasmids expressing each of the eight virion RNAs and with plasmids expressing, at a minimum, the viral polymerase (PA, PB1, and PB2) and nucleoproteins. Transfection of the plasmids shown in brackets is not required but increases the efficiency of recovery of transfectants. (From Ref. 238.)

ity of the adjuvant effect [254]. Further development has focused on engineering mutations designed to reduce or eliminate toxicity while retaining adjuvanticity into CT or the highly-related heat-labile toxin (LT) of *E. coli.* Two types of mutations have been described: mutations that block the enzymatically active (ADP-ribosylating) site (e.g., LTK63 or LTR172) and mutations that block the protease activation site (e.g., LTG192) [255].

In animal models, LT-adjuvanted intranasal vaccine has provided protection against infection with antigenically distinct strains of virus [256,257]. The mechanism of protection is B-cell dependent and appears to be the result of the induction of nonneutralizing HA-specific mucosal antibody after nasal but not parenteral administration [258]. Similar observations have been made with transcutaneous vaccination (see below).

The largest experience in humans with intranasal inactivated influenza vaccine has been with HA formulated in phosphatydylcholine liposomes coadministered with mutant LT. In prelicensure studies, this vaccine was well tolerated in adults, children, and the elderly, and induced strong nasal anti-HA IgA responses in adults [259]. Responses were less strong in the elderly, but the vaccine exceeded European licensing guidelines for serum antibody in all age groups [260]. In addition, the vaccine protected adults and children and reduced the frequency of otitis media in otitis-prone children [261,262]. However, this vaccine was later withdrawn from the market after multiple reports suggesting an association between administration of vaccine and subsequent development of Bell's palsy. These observations were consistent with studies in rodents showing that the strong avidity of enterotoxins for GM1 gangliosides present on neuronal cells of the olfactory bulb can result in colocalization of toxin and antigen in neural tissue [263]. Thus intranasal administration of enterotoxins could potentially result in low level neural toxicity.

Additional adjuvants or alternative formulations that do not include enterotoxins are currently being evaluated in humans with inactivated influenza vaccine for intranasal immunization. These include liposomes [264], proteosomes (mixtures of influenza HA and outer membrane proteins of group B *N. meningitidis*) [265] (see the chapter on Proteosomes) and the use of the MF59 oil-in-water adjuvant intranasally [266] (see the chapter on MF59 adjuvant). Each of these studies has shown induction of serum HAI responses in a minority of recipients, with detectable nasal IgA responses in 50–70% of subjects.

V. POLYNUCLEOTIDE VACCINES

Immunization of mice with DNA encoding HA, as well as the internal M and NP proteins of influenza A, induces long-lived humoral and cellular immune responses [267,268] that are protective against viral infection and disease. Immunization of African Green monkeys with DNA encoding a combination of three HAs and other influenza virus genes induced serum antibody against all three HAs [269]. However, studies in humans of influenza DNA vaccines have not yielded impressive responses.

VI. VACCINES FOR PANDEMIC INFLUENZA

Pandemics, a defining characteristic of the epidemiology of influenza, occurred in 1918 (550,000 U.S. deaths), 1957 (70,000 U.S. deaths), and 1968 (38,000 U.S. deaths). The mechanisms of pandemic influenza have been extensively considered and reviewed [270]. It is considered inevitable that a new pandemic will occur in the future. This concern was heightened with the recent epidemic of A/Hong Kong/157/97 (H5N1) influenza on the island of Hong Kong that killed six people [271,272]. This epidemic represented the first documented natural infection of humans with H5 influenza viruses, and represents direct transmission of the avian virus from birds to humans in live poultry markets. Subsequently, two cases of human infection with avian H9N1 viruses in Hong Kong have also been recognized [273].

The first strategy for control of a pandemic would be the use of a traditional egg-grown inactivated influenza vaccine. However, use of highly pathogenic viruses for vaccine production would require stringent infection control procedures to prevent contamination of vaccine workers or release of the virus into the environment. In addition, some avian influenza viruses are highly lethal to eggs. To circumvent these problems, one approach to generate vaccines for H5N1 utilizes the nonpathogenic, but antigenically related A/Duck/Singapore/57 (H5N2) virus. This virus is antigenically similar to the A/Hong Kong/157/97 virus but does not have the highly cleavable HA and would not pose an agricultural risk or risk to humans. However, conventional inactivated vaccine generated from this virus was poorly immunogenic in humans, and induced antibody to the Duck/Singapore virus that did not cross react well with the Hong Kong virus [274]. Subsequent studies have suggested that the immunogenicity of the Duck Singapore vaccine can be significantly enhanced with the MF59 adjuvant.

Baculovirus-expressed HA of the A/HK was also evaluated. Because generation of this vaccine did not require handling live influenza virus, special containment facilities were not needed, and a candidate vaccine representing the authentic A/HK HA could be quite rapidly generated. This vaccine was also poorly immunogenic, requiring doses of 90 µg to generate significant neutralizing titers in most recipients [275]. Other approaches to vaccination against H5 that were tested in animal models but not in humans included attenuation of the pathogenicity of the virus by genetically deleting the HA cleavage site, and the use of a cold-adapted H5 reassortant virus as either a nonpathogenic seed for generation of an inactivated vaccine, or as a live vaccine [276], and DNA vaccination [277].

The experience in confronting the H5 outbreak underscores some of the difficulties that will be encountered in dealing with vaccine development for the next pandemic. No vaccine was available for testing, the optimal dose and timing of vaccination was not known, and it was not clear which tests of immune response should be used to assess immunogenicity. To be better prepared, there is interest in developing and testing pilot vaccine representing likely candidates for the next pandemic virus. Several such viruses can be identified based on current surveillance. These include avian viruses of the H5 and H7 subtype, possibly the H9 viruses, and H2 influenza viruses, and Phase I studies of pilot lots of vaccine for some of these viruses are in progress. The logistics of vaccine delivery are also generating much discussion. One economic analysis suggested that in a pandemic setting, the economic impact to society would range from $71 to 167 billion, but that a vaccine delivery policy that strives to prevent the largest number of deaths (>65 years of age) would not be as economically advantageous as targeting those 0–64 years of age as a group, regardless of risk [278]. The continued threat of pandemics and the re-emergence of new influenza viruses ensure that the topic of influenza vaccine will continue to be of great interest in the years to come.

REFERENCES

1. Glezen WP. Serious morbidity and mortality associated with influenza epidemics. Epidemiol Rev 1982; 4:24–44.
2. Perrotta DM, et al. Acute respiratory disease hospitalizations as a measure of impact of epidemic influenza. Am J Epidemiol 1985; 122:468–476.
3. Blaine WB, et al. Severe illness with influenza B. Am J Med 1980; 68:181–189.
4. Simonsen L, et al. The impact of influenza epidemics on mortality: introducing a severity index. Am J Pub Health 1997; 87:1944–1950.
5. Barker WH, Mullooly JP. Impact of epidemic type A influenza in a defined adult population. Am J Epidemiol 1980; 112:798–813.
6. Safrin S, et al. Influenza in patients with human immunodeficiency virus infection. Chest 1990; 98:33–37.
7. Neuzil KM, et al. Influenza-associated morbidity and mortality in young and middle-aged women. JAMA 1999; 281:901–907.
8. Whimbey E, et al. Influenza A virus infection among hospitalized adult bone marrow transplant recipients. Bone Marrow Transplant 1994; 13:437–440.
9. Neuzil KM, et al. The impact of influenza on acute cardiopulmonary hospitalizations in pregnant women. Am J Epidemiol 1998; 148:1094–1102.
10. Neuzil KM, et al. The effect of influenza on hospitalizations, outpatient visits, and courses of antibiotics in children. N Engl J Med 2000; 342:225–231.
11. Izurieta HS, et al. Influenza and the rates of hospitalization for respiratory disease among infants and young children [see comments]. N Engl J Med 2000; 342:232–239.
12. Silberry GK. Complications of influenza infection in children. Pediatr Ann 2000; 29:683–690.
13. Schoenbaum SC. Impact of influenza in persons and populations. In: Brown LE, Hampson AW, Webster RG, eds. Options for the Control of Influenza III. New York: Elsevier Science BV, 1996:17–25.
14. SKavet J. A perspective on the significance of pandemic influenza. Am J Pub Health 1977; 67:1063–1070.
15. Keech M, et al. The impact of influenza and influenza-like illness on productivity and healthcare resource utilization in a working population. Occup Med 1998; 48:85–90.
16. Black RA, et al. Antibody response to the M2 protein of influenza A virus expressed in insect cells. J Gen Virol 1993; 74:143–146.
17. Murphy BR, et al. Secretory and systemic immunologic response in children infected with live attenuated influenza A virus. Infect Immun 1982; 36:1102–1108.
18. Murphy BR, et al. Association of serum antineuraminidase antibody with resistance to influenza in man. N Engl J Med 1972; 286:1329–1332.
19. Virelizier J-L. Host defenses against influenza virus: the role of anti-hemagglutinin antibody. J Immunol 1975; 115:434–439.
20. Murphy BR, Clements ML. The systemic and mucosal immune response of humans to influenza A virus. Curr Top Microbiol Immunol 1989; 146:107–116.
21. Hobson D, et al. The role of serum haemagglutination-inhibiting antibody in protection against challenge infection with influenza A2 and B viruses. J Hyg 1972; 70:767–777.
22. Fox JP, et al. Influenza virus infections in Seattle families, 1975–1979: II. Pattern of infection in invaded households and relation of age and prior antibody to occurrence of infection and related illness. Am J Epidemiol 1982; 116:228–242.
23. Arden NH, et al. The roles of vaccination and amantadine prophylaxis in controlling an outbreak of influenza A(H3N2) in a nursing home. Arch Intern Med 1988; 148:865–868.
24. Betts RF, et al. A comparison of the protective benefit of influenza (FLU) vaccine in reducing hospitalization of patients infected with FLU A or FLU B. Clin Infect Dis 1993; 17:573 (A257).
25. Foy HM, et al. Single-dose monovalent A 2 -Hong Kong influenza vaccine. Efficacy 14 months after immunization. JAMA 1971; 217:1067–1071.
26. Meiklejohn G, Eickhoff TC, Graves PIJ. Antigenic drift and efficacy of influenza virus vaccines, 1976–1977. J Infect Dis 1978; 138:618–624.
27. Webster RG, et al. Protection against lethal influenza with neuraminidase. Virology 1988; 164:230–237.
28. Schulman JL, et al. Protective effects of specific immunity to viral neuraminidase on influenza virus infection of mice. J Virol 1968; 2:778–786.
29. Schulman JL, et al. Protective effects of hemagglutinin and neuraminidase antigens on influenza virus: distinctiveness of hemagglutinin antigens of Hong Kong-68 virus. J Virol 1968; 2:778.
30. Monto AS, Kendal AP. Effect of neuraminidase antibody on Hong Kong influenza. Lancet 1973; 7804:623–625.
31. Clements ML, et al. Serum and nasal wash antibodies associated with resistance to experimental challenge with influenza A wild-type virus. J Clin Microbiol 1986; 24:157–160.
32. Johansson BE, et al. Infection-permissive immunization with influenza virus neuraminidase prevents weight loss in infected mice. Vaccine 1993; 11:1037–1039.
33. Treanor JJ, et al. Passively transferred monoclonal antibody to the M2 protein inhibits influenza A virus replication in mice. J Virol 1990; 64:1375–1377.
34. Mozdzanowska K, et al. Treatment of influenza virus-infected SCID mice with nonneutralizing antibodies specific for the transmembrane proteins matrix 2 and neuraminidase reduces the pulmonary virus titer but fails to clear the infection. Virology 1999; 254:138–146.
35. Renegar KB, Small PAJ. Passive transfer of local immunity to influenza virus by IgA antibody. J Immunol 1991; 146:1972–1978.
36. Wagner DK, et al. Analysis of immunoglobulin G antibody responses after administration of live and inactivated influenza A vaccine indicates that nasal wash immunoglobulin G is a transudate from serum. J Clin Microbiol 1987; 25:559–562.
37. Clements ML, et al. Resistance of adults to challenge with influenza A wild-type virus after receiving live or inactivated virus vaccine. J Clin Microbiol 1986; 23:73–76.
38. Hashimoto G, et al. Antibody-dependent cell-mediated cytotoxicity against influenza virus-infected cells. J Infect Dis 1983; 148:785–794.
39. Fleischer B, et al. Recognition of viral antigens by human influenza A virus-specific T lymphocyte clones. J Immunol 1985; 165:2800–2804.

40. Braciale TJ. Immunologic recognition of influenza virus-infected cells. II. Expression of influenza A matrix protein on the infected cell surface and its role in recognition by cross-reactive cytotoxic T cells. J Exp Med 1977; 146:673–689.

41. Yewdell JW, Hackett CJ. The specificity and function of T lymphocytes induced by influenza A viruses. In: Krug R, ed. The Influenza Viruses. New York: Plenum Press, 1989:361–429.

42. Jameson J, et al. Human cytotoxic T-lymphocyte repertoire to influenza A viruses. J Virol 1998; 72:8682–8689.

43. Lin Y-L, Askonas BA. Biologic properties of an influenza A virus-specific killer T cell clone. Inhibition of virus replication in vivo and induction of delayed-type hypersensitivity reactions. J Exp Med 1981; 154:225–234.

44. Lukacher AE, et al. In vivo effector function of influenza virus-specific cytotoxic T lymphocyte clones is highly specific. J Exp Med 1984; 160:814–826.

45. Taylor PM, Askonas BA. Influenza nucleoprotein-specific cytotoxic T-cell clones are protective in vivo. Immunology 1986; 58:417–420.

46. Yap KL, et al. Transfer of specific cytotoxic T lymphocytes protects mice inoculated with influenza virus. Nature 1978; 273:238–239.

47. MacKenzie CD, et al. Rapid recovery of lung histology correlates with clearance of influenza virus by specific CD8 + cytotoxic cells. Immunology 1989; 67:375–381.

48. Reiss CS, Schulman JL. Cellular immune responses of mice to influenza virus infection. Cell Immunol 1980; 56:502–506.

49. McMichael AJ, et al. Cytotoxic T-cell immunity to influenza. N Engl J Med 1983; 309:13–17.

50. Treanor J, et al. Nucleotide sequence of the avian influenza A/Mallard/NY/6750 virus polymerase genes. Virus Res 1989; 14:257–270.

51. Treanor JJ, Murphy B. Genes involved in the restriction of replication of avian influenza A viruses in primates. Kurstak E, ed. Virus Variability, Epidemiology, and Control. Vol. 2. New York, New York: Plenum Publishing, 1990:159–176.

52. Francis T Jr, et al. Protective effect of vaccination against influenza A. Proc Soc Exp Biol Med 1944; 55:104–105.

53. Peck FB Jr. Purified influenza vaccine. JAMA 1968; 10:2277–2282.

54. Wright PF, et al. Summary of clinical trials of influenza vaccine II. J Infect Dis 1976; 134:633–638.

55. Kilbourne ED, et al. Correlated studies of a recombinant influenza-virus vaccine. I. Derivation and characterization of virus and vaccine. J Infect Dis 1971; 124:449–462.

56. Wood JM. Standardization of inactivated influenza vaccine. In: Nicholson KG, Webster RG, Hay AJ, eds. Textbook of Influenza. London: Blackwell Science, Ltd, 1998:333–345.

57. Nichol KL, et al. Side effects associated with influenza vaccination in healthy working adults. A randomized, placebo-controlled trial. Arch Intern Med 1996; 156:1546–1550.

58. Scheifele DW, et al. Evaluation of adverse events after influenza vaccination in hospital personnel. Can Med Assoc J 1990; 142:127–130.

59. Aoki FY, et al. Effects of acetaminophen on adverse effects of influenza vaccination in health care workers. Can Med Assoc J 1993; 149:1425–1430.

60. al-Mazrou A, et al. Comparison of adverse reactions to whole-virion and split-virion influenza vaccines in hospital personnel. Can Med Assoc J 1991; 145:213–218.

61. Margolis KL, et al. Frequency of adverse reactions after influenza vaccination. Am J Med 1990; 88:27–30.

62. LaMontagne JR, et al. Summary of clinical trials of inactivated influenza vaccine—1978. Rev Infect Dis 1983; 5:723–736.

63. Wright PF, Thompson J, Vaughn WT, Folland DS, Sell SHW, Karzon DT. Trials of influenza A/New Jersey/76 virus vaccine in normal children: an overview of age-related an-

tigenicity and reactogenicity. J Infect Dis 1977; 136:S731–S741.

64. Gross PA, et al. A controlled double-blind comparison of reactogenicity, immunogenicity, and protective efficacy of whole-virus and split-product influenza vaccines in children. J Infect Dis 1977; 136:623–632.

65. Bierman CW, et al. Safety of influenza vaccination in allergic children. J Infect Dis 1977; 136:S652–S655.

66. Schonberger LB, et al. Guillan–Barre syndrome following vaccination in the national influenza immunization program, United States, 1976–1977. Am J Epidemiol 1979; 110:105–123.

67. Kaplan JE, et al. Guillain–Barre syndrome in the United States, 1979–1980 and 1980–1981. Lack of an association with influenza vaccination. JAMA 1982; 248:698–700.

68. Lasky T, et al. The Guillan–Barre syndrome and the 1992–1993 and 1993–1994 influenza vaccines. N Engl J Med 1998; 339:1797–1802.

69. Cate TR, et al. Reactogenicity, immunogenicity, and antibody persistence in adults given inactivated influenza virus vaccines—1978. Rev Infect Dis 1983; 5:737–747.

70. Quinnan GV, et al. Serologic responses and systemic reactions in adults after vaccination with monovalent A/USSR/77 and trivalent A/USSR/77, A/Texas/77, B/Hong Kong/72 influenza vaccines. Rev Infect Dis 1983; 5:748–757.

71. Wright PF, et al. Antigenicity and reactogenicity of influenza A/USSR/77 virus vaccine in children—a multicentered evaluation of dosage and toxicity. Rev Infect Dis 1983; 5:758–764.

72. Levandowski RA, et al. Antibody responses to influenza B viruses in immunologically unprimed children. Pediatrics 1991; 88:1031–1036.

73. Lerman SJ, et al. Antibody decline in children following A/New Jersy/76 influenza virus immunization. J Pediatr 1980; 96:271–274.

74. Zahradnik JM, et al. Immune responses in serum and respiratory secretions following vaccination with a live cold-recombinant (CR35) and inactivated A/USSR/77 (H1N1) influenza virus vaccine. J Med Virol 1983; 11:277–285.

75. Bokstad KA, et al. Parenteral vaccination against influenza does not induce a local antigen-specific immune response in the nasal mucosa. J Infect Dis 2002; 185:878–884.

76. Ennis FA, et al. Antibody and cytotoxic T lymphocyte responses of humans to live and inactivated influenza vaccines. J Gen Virol 1982; 58:273–281.

77. Powers DC, Belshe RB. Effect of age on cytotoxic T lymphocyte memory as well as serum and local antibody responses elicited by inactivated influenza vaccine. J Infect Dis 1993; 197:584–592.

78. Nicholson KG, et al. Immunogenicity of inactivated influenza vaccine in residential homes for elderly people. Age Ageing 1992; 21:182–188.

79. Remarque EJ, et al. Improvement of the immunoglobulin subclass response to influenza vaccine in elderly nursing-home residents by the use of high-dose vaccines. Vaccine 1993; 11:649–654.

80. Pabico RC, et al. Influenza vaccination of patients with glomerular diseases: effects on creatinine clearance, urinary protein excretion, and antibody response. Ann Intern Med 1974; 81:171–177.

81. Pabico RC, et al. Antibody response to influenza vaccination in renal transplant patients: correlation with allograft function. Ann Intern Med 1976; 85:431–436.

82. Stiver HG, et al. Impaired serum antibody response to inactivated influenza A and B vaccine in renal transplant recipients. Infect Immun 1977; 16:738–741.

83. Kumar SS, et al. Influenza vaccination in renal transplant recipients. JAMA 1978; 239:840–842.

84. Nelson KE, et al. The influence of human immunodeficiency

virus (HIV) infection on antibody responses to influenza vaccines. Ann Intern Med 1988; 109:383–388.

85. Kroon FP, et al. Antibody response after influenza vaccination in HIV-infected individuals: a consecutive 3-year study. Vaccine 2000; 18:3040–3049.

86. O'Brien WA, et al. Human immunodeficiency virus-type 1 replication can be increased in peripheral blood of seropositive patients after influenza vaccination. Blood 1995; 86: 1082–1089.

87. Kubiet MA, et al. Serum antibody response to influenza vaccine in pulmonary patients receiving corticosteroids. Chest 1996; 110:367–370.

88. Park CL, et al. Influenza vaccination of children during acute asthma exacerbation and concurrent prednisone therapy. Pediatrics 1996; 98:196–200.

89. Meiklejohn G. Viral respiratory disease at Lowry Air Force Base in Denver, 1952–1982. J Infect Dis 1983; 148:775–783.

90. Ruben FL. Prevention and control of influenza: role of vaccine. Am J Med 1987; 82:31–33.

91. Edwards KM, et al. A randomized controlled trial of cold-adapted and inactivated vaccines for the prevention of influenza A disease. J Infect Dis 1994; 169:68–76.

92. Neuzil KM, et al. Efficacy of inactivated and cold-adapted vaccines against influenza A infection, 1985 to 1990: the pediatric experience. Pediatr Infect Dis J 2001; 20:733–740.

93. Nichol KL, et al. The effectiveness of vaccination against influenza in healthy, working adults. N Engl J Med 1995; 333:889–893.

94. Heikkinen T, et al. Influenza vaccination in the prevention of acute otitis media in children. Am J Dis Child 1991; 145:445–448.

95. Clements DA, et al. Influenza A vaccine decreases the incidence of otitis media in 6- to 30- month old children in day care. Arch Pediatr Adolesc Med 1995; 149:1113–1117.

96. Govaert TM, et al. The efficacy of influenza vaccination in elderly individuals. A randomized double-blind placebo-controlled trial. JAMA 1994; 272:1956–1961.

97. Paul WS, et al. Acute respiratory illness among immunized and nonimmunized patients with high-risk factors during a split season of influenza A and B. J Infect Dis 1988; 157:633–639.

98. Ruben FL, et al. Influenza in a partially immunized population: effectiveness of killed Hong Kong vaccine against infection with the England strain. JAMA 1974; 230:863–866.

99. Patriarca PA, Weber JA, Parker RA, Hall WN, Kendal AP, Bregman DJ, Schonberger LB. Efficacy of influenza vaccine in nursing homes: reduction in illness and complications during an influenza A (H3N2) epidemic. JAMA 1985; 253: 1136–1139.

100. Saah AJ, et al. Influenza vaccine and pneumonia mortality in a nursing home population. Arch Intern Med 1986; 146: 2353–2357.

101. Patriarca PA, et al. Risk factors for outbreaks of influenza in nursing homes: a case-control study. Am J Epidemiol 1986; 124:114–119.

102. Gross PA, et al. Association of influenza immunization with reduction in mortality in an elderly population: a prospective study. Arch Intern Med 1988; 148:562–565.

103. Betts RF, et al. Inactivated influenza vaccine reduces frequency and severity of illness in the elderly. 24th Interscience Conference on Antimicrobial Agents and Chemotherapy, Washington, DC. American Society for Microbiology, 1984.

104. Fedson DS, et al. Clinical effectiveness of influenza vaccination in Manitoba. JAMA 1993; 270:1956–1961.

105. Tasker SA, et al. Efficacy of influenza vaccination in HIV-infected persons: a randomized, double-blind, placebo-controlled trial. Ann Intern Med 1999; 131:430–433.

106. Postma MJ, et al. Pharmacoeconomics of influenza vacci-

nation for healthy working adults. Drugs 2002; 62:1013–1024.

107. Perez-Tirse J, Gross PA. Review of cost–benefit analyses of influenza vaccine. Pharmacoeconomics 1992; 2:198–206.

108. Edmunds WJ, et al. Evaluation of the cost-effectiveness of vaccination programmes: a dynamic perspective. Stat Med 1999; 18:3263–3282.

109. Nichol KL, et al. Benefits of influenza vaccination for low-, intermediate-, and high-risk senior citizens. Arch Intern Med 1998; 158:1769–1776.

110. Nichol KL, et al. The efficacy and cost-effectiveness of vaccination against influenza among elderly persons living in the community. N Engl J Med 1994; 331:778–784.

111. Mullooly JP, et al. Influenza vaccination programs for elderly persons: cost-effectiveness in a health maintenance organization. Ann Intern Med 1994; 121:947–952.

112. Maucher JM, Gambert SR. Cost-effective analysis of influenza vaccination in the elderly. Age 1990; 13:3–9.

113. Riddiough MA, et al. Influenza vaccination: cost-effectiveness and public policy. JAMA 1983; 249:3189–3195.

114. Fitzner KA, et al. Cost-effectiveness study on influenza prevention in Hong Kong. Health Policy 2001; 56:215–234.

115. Coffield AB, et al. Priorities among recommended clinical preventive services. Am J Prev Med 2001; 21:1–9.

116. Bridges CB, et al. Effectiveness and cost–benefit of influenza vaccination of healthy working adults: A randomized controlled trial [see comments]. JAMA 2000; 284:1655–1663.

117. Muennig PA, Khan K. Cost-effectiveness of vaccination versus treatment of influenza in healthy adolescents and adults. Clin Infect Dis 2001; 33:1879–1885.

118. Nichol KL. Cost–benefit analysis of a strategy to vaccinate healthy working adults against influenza. Arch Intern Med 2001; 161:749–759.

119. Demicheli V, et al. Prevention and early treatment of influenza in healthy adults. Vaccine 2000; 18:957–1030.

120. Cohen GM, Nettleman MD. Economic impact of influenza vaccination in preschool children. Pediatrics 2000; 106:973–976.

121. White T, et al. Potential cost savings attributable to influenza vaccination of school-aged children. Pediatrics 1999; 103: e73.

122. Luce BR, et al. Cost-effectiveness analysis of an intranasal influenza vaccine for the prevention of influenza in healthy children. Pediatrics 2001; 108:E24.

123. Dayan GH, et al. Cost-effectiveness of influenza vaccination in high-risk children in Argentina. Vaccine 2001; 19:4204–4213.

124. Tucker AW, et al. Cost-effectiveness analysis of a rotavirus immunization program for the United States. JAMA 1998; 279:1371–1376.

125. Lieu TA, et al. Cost-effectiveness of a routine varicella vaccination program for US children. JAMA 1994; 271:375–381.

126. CDC. Prevention and control of influenza: Recommendations of the Advisory Committee on Immunization Practices (ACIP). MMWR 2001; 50:1–32.

127. CDC. Prevention and control of influenza: recommendations of the advisory committee on immunization practices. MMWR 2002; 51(RR03):1–31.

128. Monto AS, et al. Modification of an outbreak of influenza in Tecumseh, Michigan. J Infect Dis 1970; 122:16–25.

129. Reichert TA, et al. The Japanese experience with vaccinating schoolchildren against influenza. N Engl J Med 2001; 344: 889–896.

130. Mostow RA, et al. Studies on inactivated influenza vaccine II effect of increasing dosage on antibody response and adverse reactions in man. Am J Epidemiol 1970; 92:248–256.

131. Goodeve A, et al. A graded-dose study of inactivated, surface antigen influenza B vaccine in volunteers: reactogenicity, an-

tibody response and protection to challenge virus infection. J Hyg 1983; 90:107–115.

132. Keitel WA, et al. High doses of purified influenza A virus hemagglutinin significantly augment serum and nasal secretion antibody responses in healthy young adults. J Clin Microbiol 1994; 32:2468–2473.

133. Palache AM, et al. Antibody response after influenza immunization with various vaccine doses: a double-blind, placebo-controlled, multi-centre, dose-response study in elderly nursing home residents and young volunteers. Vaccine 1993; 11:3–9.

134. Gross PA, et al. Immunization of elderly people with high doses of influenza vaccine. J Am Geriatr Soc 1988; 36:209–212.

135. Johansson BE, et al. Purified influenza virus hemagglutinin and neuraminidase are equivalent in stimulation of antibody response but induce contrasting types of immunity to infection. J Virol 1989; 63:1239–1246.

136. Johansson BE, Kilbourne ED. Comparative long-term effects in a mouse model system of influenza whole virus and purified neuraminidase vaccines followed by sequential infections. J Infect Dis 1990; 162:800–809.

137. Johansson BE, Kilbourne ED. Programmed antigenic stimulation: kinetics of the immune response to challenge infections of mice primed with influenza inactivated whole virus or neuraminidase vaccine. Vaccine 1991; 9:330–333.

138. Johansson BE. Immunization with influenza A virus hemagglutinin and neuraminidase produced in recombinant baculovirus results in a balanced and broadened immune response superior to conventional vaccine. Vaccine 1999; 17:2073–2080.

139. Schiff G, et al. Phase 2 clinical evaluation of an influenza A virus recombinant N2 neuraminidase, Options for the control of influenza IV, Crete, 2000.

140. Robertson JS, et al. Structural changes in the haemagglutinin which accompany egg adaptation of an influenza A (H1N1) virus. Virology 1987; 160:31–37.

141. Robertson JS, et al. The hemagglutinin of influenza B virus present in clinical material is a single species identical to that of mammalian cell-grown virus. Virology 1990; 179:35–40.

142. Robertson JS, et al. Sequence analysis of the haemagglutinin (HA) of influenza A (H1N1) viruses present in clinical material and comparison with the HA of laboratory-derived virus. J Gen Virol 1991; 72:2671–2677.

143. Rocha EP, et al. Comparison of 10 influenza A (H1N1 and H3N2) haemagglutinin sequences obtained directly from clinical specimens to those of MDCK cell- and egg-grown viruses. J Gen Virol 1993; 74:2513–2518.

144. Wang M, et al. Extensive heterogeneity in the hemagglutinin of egg-grown influenza viruses from different patients. Virology 1989; 171:275–279.

145. Katz JM, et al. Direct sequencing of the HA gene of influenza (H3N2) reveals sequence identity with mammalian cell-grown virus. J Virol 1990; 64:1808–1811.

146. Katz JM, Webster RG. Antigenic and structural characterization of multiple subpopulations of H3N2 influenza virus from an individual. Virology 1988; 165:446–456.

147. Katz JM, Webster RG. Amino acid sequence identity between the HA1 of influenza A (H3N2) viruses grown in mammalian and primary chick kidney cells. J Gen Virol 1992; 73:1159–1165.

148. Terajima M, et al. High-yield reassortant influenza vaccine production virus has a mutation at an HLA-A 2.1-restricted CD8+ CTL epitope on the NS1 protein. Virology 1999; 259:135–140.

149. Katz JM, Webster RG. Efficacy of inactivated influenza A virus (H3N2) vaccines grown in mammalian cells or embryonated eggs. J Infect Dis 1989; 160:191–198.

150. Wood JM, et al. Influenza A(H1N1) vaccine efficacy in animal models is influenced by two amino acid substitutions in the hemagglutinin molecule. Virology 1989; 171:214–221.

151. Govorkova EA, et al. Replication of influenza A viruses in a green monkey continuous cell line (Vero). J Infect Dis 1995; 172:250–253.

152. Levandowski RA. Regulatory perspective in the United States on cell cultures for production of inactivated influenza virus vaccines. Dev Biol Stand 1999; 98:171–175; discussion 197.

153. Bruhl P, et al. Humoral and cell-mediated immunity to vero cell-derived influenza vaccine. Vaccine 2000; 19:1149–1158.

154. Halperin SA, et al. Safety and immunogenicity of a trivalent, inactivated, mammalian cell culture-derived influenza vaccine in healthy adults, seniors, and children. Vaccine 2002; 20:1240–1247.

155. Powers DC, et al. Influenza A virus vaccines containing purified recombinant H3 hemagglutinin are well-tolerated and induce protective immune responses in healthy adults. J Infect Dis 1995; 171:1595–1598.

156. Treanor JJ, et al. Evaluation of a recombinant hemagglutinin expressed in insect cells as an influenza vaccine in young and elderly adults. J Infect Dis 1996; 173:1467–1470.

157. Lakey DL, et al. Recombinant baculovirus influenza A hemagglutinin vaccines are well tolerated and immunogenic in healthy adults. J Infect Dis 1996; 174:838–841.

158. Luckow VA, Summers MD. Trends in the development of baculovirus expression vectors. Biotechnology 1988; 6:47–55.

159. Daynes RA, Araneo BA. The development of effective vaccine adjuvants employing natural regulators of T-cell lymphokine production in vivo. Ann N Y Acad Sci 1994; 730:144–161.

160. Gravenstein S, et al. Augmentation of influenza antibody response in elderly men by thymosin alpha one: a double-blind placebo-controlled clinical study. J Am Geriatr Soc 1989; 37:1–8.

161. el Guink N, et al. Intranasal immunization with proteoliposomes protects against influenza. Vaccine 1989; 7:147–151.

162. Kaji M, et al. Phase I clinical tests of influenza MDP-virosome vaccine (KD-5382). Vaccine 1992; 10:663–667.

163. Sundquist B, et al. Influenza virus ISCOMs: biochemical characterization. Vaccine 1988; 6:44–48.

164. Lovgren K, et al. An experimental influenza subunit vaccine (ISCOM): induction of protective immunity to challenge infection in mice after intranasal or subcutaneous administration. Clin Exp Immunol 1990; 82:435–439.

165. Podda A. The adjuvanted influenza vaccines with novel adjuvants: experience with the MF59-adjuvanted vaccine. Vaccine 2001; 19:2673–2680.

166. Menegon T, et al. Influenza vaccines: antibody responses to split virus and MF59-adjuvanted subunit virus in an adult population. Eur J Epidemiol 1999; 15:573–576.

167. De Donato S, et al. Safety and immunogenicity of MF59-adjuvanted influenza vaccine in the elderly. Vaccine 1999; 17:3094–3101.

168. Minutello M, et al. Safety and immunogenicity of an inactivated subunit influenza virus vaccine combined with MF59 adjuvant emulsion in elderly subjects, immunized for three consecutive influenza seasons. Vaccine 1999; 17:99–104.

169. Ennis FA, Thipphawong J, et al. Augmentation of human influenza A virus-specific cytotoxic T lymphocyte memory by influenza vaccine and adjuvanted carriers (ISCOMS). Virology 1999; 259:256–261.

170. Rimmelzwaan GF, et al. A randomized, double-blind study in young healthy adults comparing cell mediated and humoral immune responses induced by influenza ISCOM vaccines and conventional vaccines. Vaccine 2000; 19:1180–1187.

171. Schaad UB, et al. Comparison of immunogenicity and safety of a virosome influenza vaccine with those of a subunit influenza vaccine in pediatric patients with cystic fibrosis. Antimicrob Agents Chemother 2000; 44:1163–1167.

172. Hammond SA, et al. Transcutaneous immunization: T cell responses and boosting of existing immunity. Vaccine 2001; 19:2701–2707.

173. Chen D, et al. Epidermal powder immunization induces both cytotoxic T-lymphocyte and antibody responses to protein antigens of influenza and hepatitis B Viruses. J Virol 2001; 65:11630–11640.

174. Johnson PR, et al. Immunity to influenza A virus infection in young children: a comparison of natural infection, live cold-adapted vaccine, and inactivated vaccine. J Infect Dis 1986; 154:121–127.

175. Clements ML, et al. Advantage of live attenuated cold-adapted influenza A virus over inactivated vaccine for A/Washington/80 (H3N2) wild-type virus infection. Lancet 1984; 1:704–708.

176. Chanock RM, Murphy BR. Use of temperature-sensitive and cold-adapted mutant viruses in the immunoprophylaxis of acute respiratory tract disease. Rev Infect Dis 1980; 2:421–432.

177. Wright PF, Karzon DT. Live attenuated influenza vaccines. Prog Med Virol 1987; 34:70–88.

178. Murphy BR, et al. Temperature-sensitive mutants of influenza virus. XV. The genetic and biologic characterization of a recombinant influenza virus containing two *ts* lesions produced by mating two complementing, single lesion *ts* mutants. Virology 1978; 88:231–243.

179. Murphy BR, et al. Avian-human reassortant influenza A viruses derived by mating avian and human influenza A viruses. J Infect Dis 1984; 150:841–850.

180. Tolpin MD, et al. Genetic factors associated with loss of the temperature-sensitive phenotype of the influenza A/Alaska/77-*ts*-1A2 recombinant during growth in vivo. Virology 1981; 112:505–517.

181. Steinhoff MC, et al. Comparison of live, attenuated cold-adapted and avian-human influenza A/Bethesda/85 (H3N2) reassortant virus vaccines in infants and children. J Infect Dis 1990; 162:394–401.

182. Steinhoff MC, et al. The A/Mallard/6750/78 avian-human, but not the A/Ann Arbor/6/60 cold-adapted, influenza A/Kawasaki/ (H1N1) reassortant virus vaccine retains partial virulence for infants and children. J Infect Dis 1991; 165:1023–1028.

183. Maassab HF. Biologic and immunologic characteristics of cold-adapted influenza virus. J Immunol 1969; 102:728–732.

184. Maassab HF, DeBorde DC. Development and characterization of cold-adapted viruses for use as live virus vaccines. Vaccine 1985; 3:335–369.

185. Snyder MH, et al. Four viral genes independently contribute to attenuation of live influenza A/Ann Arbor/6/60 (H2N2) cold-adapted reassortant virus vaccines. J Virol 1988; 62:488–495.

186. Subbarao EK, et al. The attenuation phenotype conferred by the M gene of the influenza A/Ann Arbor/6/60 cold-adapted virus (H2N2) on the A/Korea/82 (H3N2) reassortant virus results from a gene constellation effect. Virus Res 1992; 25:37–50.

187. DeBorde DC, et al. Sequence comparison of wild-type and cold-adapted B/Ann Arbor/1/66 influenza virus genes. Virology 1988; 163:429–443.

188. Donabedian AM, et al. Genetics of cold-adapted B/Ann Arbor/1/66 influenza virus reassortants: the acidic polymerase (PA) protein gene confers temperature sensitivity and attenuated virulence. Microbiol Pathol 1987; 3:97–108.

189. Donabedian AM, et al. A mutation in the PA protein gene of cold-adapted B/Ann Arbor/1/66 influenza virus associated with reversion of temperature sensitivity and attenuated virulence. Virology 1988; 163:444–451.

190. Murphy BR. Use of live, attenuated cold-adapted influenza A reassortant virus vaccines in infants, children, young adults, and elderly adults. Infect Dis Clin Pract 1993; 2:176–181.

191. Jackson LA, et al. Safety of a trivalent live attenuated intranasal vaccine, FluMist, administered in addition to parenteral trivalent inactivated influenza vaccine to seniors with chronic medical conditions. Vaccine 1999; 17:1905–1909.

192. King JC, et al. Comparison of the safety, vaccine virus shedding, and immunogenicity of influenza virus vaccine, trivalent, types A and B, live cold-adapted, administered to human immunodeficiency virus (HIV)-infected and non-HIV-infected adults. J Infect Dis 2000; 181:725–728.

193. Nichol KL, et al. Effectiveness of live, attenuated intranasal influenza virus vaccine in healthy, working adults: a randomized controlled trial. JAMA 1999; 282:137–144.

194. Keitel WA, et al. Trivalent attenuated cold-adapted influenza virus vaccine: reduced viral shedding and serum antibody responses in susceptible adults. J Infect Dis 1993; 167:305–311.

195. Treanor JJ, et al. Evaluation of trivalent, live, cold-adapted (CAIV-T) and inactivated (TIV) influenza vaccines in prevention of virus infection and illness following challenge of adults with wild-type influenza A (H1N1), A (H3N2), and B viruses. Vaccine 1999; 18:899–906.

196. Belshe RB, et al. The efficacy of live attenuated cold-adapted trivalent, intranasal influenza virus vaccine in children. N Engl J Med 1998; 358:1405–1412.

197. Belshe RB, et al. Efficacy of vaccination with live attenuated, cold-adapted, trivalent, intranasal influenza virus vaccine against a variant (A/Sydney) not contained in the vaccine. J Pediatr 2000; 136:168–175.

198. Zangwill KM, et al. Prospective, randomized, placebo-controlled evaluation of the safety and immunogenicity of three lots of intranasal trivalent influenza vaccine among young children. Pediatr Infect Dis J 2001; 20:740–746.

199. King JC Jr, Belshe RB, et al. Safety and immunogenicity of low and high doses of trivalent live cold-adapted influenza vaccine administered intranasally as drops or spray to healthy children. J Infect Dis 1998; 177:1394–1397.

200. King JC Jr, et al. Safety, vaccine virus shedding and immunogenicity of trivalent, cold-adapted, live attenuated influenza vaccine administered to human immunodeficiency virus-infected and noninfected children. Pediatr Infect Dis J 2001; 20:1124–1131.

201. Swierkosz EM, et al. Multidose, live attenuated, cold-recombinant, trivalent influenza vaccine in infants and young children. J Infect Dis 1994; 169:1121–1124.

202. Belshe RB, et al. Immunization of infants and young children with live attenuated trivalent cold-recombinant influenza A H1N1, H3N2, and B vaccine. J Infect Dis 1992; 165:727–732.

203. Gruber WC, et al. Comparison of monovalent and trivalent live attenuated influenza vaccines in young children. J Infect Dis 1993; 168:53–60.

204. Gruber WC, et al. Evaluation of live attenuated influenza vaccines in children 6–18 months of age: safety, immunogenicity, and efficacy. J Infect Dis 1996; 173:1313–1319.

205. Wright PF, et al. Simultaneous administration of live attenuated influenza A vaccines representing different serotypes. Vaccine 1985; 3:305–308.

206. Gruber WC, et al. Evaluation of bivalent live attenuated influenza A vaccines in children 2 months to 3 years of age: safety, immunogenicity and dose–response. Vaccine 1997; 15:1379–1384.

207. Clements ML, et al. Effective immunization with live attenuated influenza A virus can be achieved in early infancy. Pediatric Care Center. J Infect Dis 1996; 173:44–51.

208. King JC Jr, et al. Comparison of live and inactivated influenza vaccine in high risk children. Vaccine 1987; 5:234–238.

209. Gruber WC, et al. Comparison of live attenuated and inactivated influenza vaccines in cystic fibrosis patients and their families: results of a 3-year study. J Infect Dis 1994; 169:241–247.

210. Miyazaki C, et al. Immunization of institutionalized asthmatic children and patients with psychomotor retardation using live attenuated cold-adapted reassortment influenza A H1N1, H3N2, and B vaccines. Vaccine 1993; 11:853–858.

211. Redding G, et al. Safety and tolerability of cold-adapted influenza virus vaccine in children and adolescents with asthma. Pediatr Infect Dis J 2002; 21:44–48.

212. Gorse GJ, et al. Safety of and serum antibody response to cold-recombinant influenza A and inactivated trivalent influenza virus vaccines in older adults with chronic diseases. J Clin Microbiol 1986; 24:336–342.

213. Gorse GJ, et al. Local and systemic antibody responses in high-risk adults given live attenuated and inactivated influenza A virus vaccines. J Clin Microbiol 1988; 26:911–918.

214. Atmar RL, et al. Effect of live attenuated, cold recombinant (CR) influenza virus vaccines on pulmonary function in healthy and asthmatic adults. Vaccine 1990; 8:217–224.

215. Klimov AI, et al. Prolonged shedding of amantadine-resistant influenzae A viruses by immunodeficient patients: detection by polymerase chain reaction-restriction analysis. J Infect Dis 1995; 172:1352–1355.

216. Wright PF, et al. Clinical experience with live, attenuated vaccines in children. In: Kendal AP, Patriarca PA, eds. Options for the control of influenza. New York: Alan R Liss, 1986:243–253.

217. Vesikari T, et al. A randomized, double-blind, placebo-controlled trial of the safety, transmissibility and phenotypic stability of a live, attenuated, cold-adapted influenza virus vaccine (CAIV-T) in children attending day care, 41st ICAAC, Chicago, IL. ASM press, 2001.

218. Cha TA, et al. Genotypic stability of cold-adapted influenza virus vaccine in an efficacy clinical trial. J Clin Microbiol 2000; 38:839–845.

219. Beyer WEP, et al. Cold-adapted live influenza vaccine versus inactivated vaccine: systemic vaccine reactions, local and systemic antibody response, and vaccine efficacy: a meta-analysis. Vaccine 2002; 20:1340–1353.

220. Edwards KM, et al. In vitro production of anti-influenza virus antibody after simultaneous administration of H3N2 and H1N1 cold-adapted vaccines in seronegative children. Vaccine 1986; 4:50–54.

221. Johnson PR, et al. Comparison of long-term systemic and secretory antibody responses in children given live attenuated or inactivated influenza A vaccine. J Med Virol 1985; 17:325–335.

222. Boyce TG, et al. Mucosal immune response to trivalent live attenuated intranasal influenza vaccine in children. Vaccine 1999; 18:82–88.

223. Clements ML, Murphy BR. Development and persistence of local and systemic antibody responses in adults given live attenuated or inactivated influenza A virus vaccine. J Clin Microbiol 1986; 23:66–72.

224. Powers DC, et al. In elderly persons live attenuated influenza A virus vaccines do not offer an advantage over inactivated virus vaccine in inducing serum or secretory antibodies or local immunologic memory. J Clin Microbiol 1991; 29:498–505.

225. Ennis FA, et al. HLA restricted virus-specific cytotoxic T-lymphocyte responses to live and inactivated influenza vaccines. Lancet 1981; 2:887–891.

226. Gorse GJ, Belshe RB. Enhancement of anti-influenza A virus cytotoxicity following influenza A vaccination in older, chronically ill adults. J Clin Microbiol 1990; 28:2539–2550.

227. Clover RD, et al. Comparison of heterotypic protection against influenza A/Taiwan/86 (H1N1) by attenuated and inactivated vaccines to A/Chile/83-like viruses. J Infect Dis 1991; 163:300–304.

228. Mbawuike IN, et al. Cytotoxic T lymphocyte responses of infants after natural infection or immunization with live cold-recombinant or inactivated influenza A virus vaccine. J Med Virol 1996; 50:105–111.

229. Robertson HE, et al. Community-wide use of a balanced trivalent oral poliovirus vaccine (Sabin). Can J Public Health 1962; 53:179–181.

230. Keitel WA, et al. Cold-recombinant influenza B/Texas/1/84 virus vaccine: attenuation, immunogenicity, and efficacy against homotypic challenge. J Infect Dis 1990; 161:22–26.

231. Clements ML, et al. Evaluation of the infectivity, immunogenicity, and efficacy of live cold-adapted influenza B/Ann Arbor/1/86 reassortant virus in adult volunteers. J Infect Dis 1990; 161:869–877.

232. Treanor JJ, et al. Protective efficacy of combined live intranasal and inactivated influenza A virus vaccines in the elderly. Ann Intern Med 1992; 117:625–633.

233. Belshe RB, et al. Correlates of immune protection induced by live attenuated, cold-adapted, trivalent, intranasal influenza virus vaccine. J Infect Dis 2000; 181:1133–1137.

234. Enami M, et al. Introduction of site-specific mutations into the genome of influenza virus. Proc Natl Acad Sci USA 1990; 87:3802–3805.

235. Luytjes W, et al. Amplification, expression, and packaging of a foreign gene by influenza virus. Cell 1989; 59:1107–1113.

236. Barclay WS, Palese P. Influenza B viruses with site-specific mutation introduced into the HA gene. J Virol 1995; 69:1275–1279.

237. Fodor E, et al. Rescue of influenza A virus from recombinant DNA. J Virol 1999; 73:9679–9682.

238. Neumann G, et al. Generation of influenza A viruses entirely from cloned cDNAs. Proc Natl Acad Sci USA 1999; 96:9345–9350.

239. Muster T, et al. An influenza A virus containing influenza B virus 5′ and 3′ noncoding regions on the neuraminidase gene is attenuated in mice. Proc Natl Acad Sci 1991; 88:5177–5181.

240. Castrucci MR, et al. Attenuation of influenza A virus by insertion of a foreign epitope into the neuraminidase. J Virol 1992; 66:4647–4653.

241. Castrucci MR, Kawaoka Y. Biologic importance of neuraminidase stalk length in influenza A viruses. J Virol 1993; 67:759–764.

242. Subbarao EK, et al. Sequential addition of temperature-sensitive missense mutations into the PB2 gene of influenza A transfectant viruses can effect an increase in temperature sensitivity and attenuation and permits the rational design of a genetically engineered live influenza A virus vaccine. J Virol 1995; 69:5969–5977.

243. Parkin NT, et al. Genetically engineered live attenuated influenza A virus vaccine candidates. J Virol 1997; 71:2772–2778.

244. Palese P, et al. Learning from our foes: a novel vaccine concept for influenza virus. Arch Virol Suppl 1999; 15:131–138.

245. Talon J, et al. Influenza A and B viruses expressing altered NS1 proteins: A vaccine approach. Proc Natl Acad Sci USA 2000; 97:4309–4314.

246. Waldman RH, et al. Influenza antibody in human respiratory secretions after subcutaneous or respiratory immunization with inactivated virus. Nature 1968; 216:594–595.

247. Waldman RH, et al. Influenza antibody response following aerosol administration of inactivated virus. Am J Epidemiol 1970; 91:575–584.

248. Kasel JA, et al. Antibody responses in nasal secretions and serum of elderly persons following local or parenteral administration of inactivated influenza virus vaccine. J Immunol 1969; 102:555–562.

249. Fulk RV, et al. Antibody responses in serum and nasal secretions according to age of recipient and method of administration of A2/Hong Kong/68 inactivated influenza virus vaccine. J Immunol 1970; 104:8–13.

250. Wright PF, et al. Secretory immunological response after intranasal inactivated influenza A virus vaccinations: evidence for immunoglobulin A memory. Infect Immun 1983; 40:1092–1095.

251. Hirabayashi Y, et al. Comparison of intranasal inoculation of influenza HA vaccine combined with cholera toxin B subunit with oral or parenteral vaccination. Vaccine 1990; 8: 243–248.

252. Tamura S, et al. Effectiveness of cholera toxin B subunit as an adjuvant for nasal influenza vaccination despite pre-existing immunity to CTB. Vaccine 1989; 7:503–505.

253. Wilson AD, et al. Adjuvant action of cholera toxin and pertussis toxin in the induction of IgA antibody response to orally administered antigen. Vaccine 1993; 11:113–118.

254. Wilson AD, et al. Whole cholera toxin and B subunit act synergistically as an adjuvant for the mucosal immune responses of mice to keyhole limpet haemocyanin. Scand J Immunol 1990; 31:443–451.

255. Pizza M, et al. Mucosal vaccines: non toxic derivatives of LT and CT as mucosal adjuvants. Vaccine 2001; 19:2534–3541.

256. Tamura S, et al. Cross-protection against influenza virus infection afforded by trivalent inactivated vaccines inoculated intranasally with cholera toxin B subunit. J Immunol 1992; 149:981–988.

257. Tamura SI, et al. Superior cross-protective effect of nasal vaccination to subcutaneous inoculation with influenza hemagglutinin vaccine. Eur J Immunol 1992; 22:477–481.

258. Tumpey TM, et al. Mucosal delivery of inactivated influenza vaccine induces B-cell-dependent heterosubtypic cross-protection against lethal influenza A H5N1 virus infection. J Virol 2001; 75:5141–5150.

259. Gluck U, et al. Phase 1 evaluation of intranasal virosomal influenza vaccine with and without Escherichia coli heat-labile toxin in adult volunteers. J Virol 1999; 73:7780–7786.

260. Gluck R, et al. Safety and immunogenicity of intranasally administered inactivated trivalent virosome-formulated influenza vaccine containing Escherichia coli heat-labile toxin as a mucosal adjuvant. J Infect Dis 2000; 181:1129–1132.

261. Marchisio P, et al. Efficacy of intranasal virosomal influenza vaccine in preventing acute otitis media in children, Options for the control of influenza IV, Crete, 2000.

262. Crovari P, et al. The efficacy of intranasal inactivated trivalent influenza vaccine in children and adults, Options for the Control of Influenza IV, Crete, 2000.

263. van Ginkel FW, et al. Cutting Edge: the mucosal adjuvant cholera toxin redirects vaccine proteins into olfactory tissues. J Immunol 2000; 165:4778–4782.

264. Babai I, et al. A novel influenza subunit vaccine composed of liposome-encapsulated haemagglutinin/neuraminidase and IL-2 or GM-CSF II Induction of TH1 and TH2 responses in mice. Vaccine 1999; 17:1239–1250.

265. Treanor J, et al. Phase I evaluation of an intranasal proteosome-influenza vaccine in healthy adults, Fourth Annual Conference on Vaccine Research, Washington DC, 2000.

266. Boyce TG, et al. Safety and immunogenicity of adjuvanted and unadjuvanted subunit influenza vaccines administered intranasally to healthy adults. Vaccine 2000; 19:217–226.

267. Ulmer JB, et al. Heterologous protection against influenza by injection of DNA encoding a viral protein. Science 1993; 259:1745–1749.

268. Robinson HL, et al. Protection against a lethal influenza virus challenge by immunization with a haemagglutinin-expressing plasmid DNA. Vaccine 1993; 11:957–960.

269. Donnelly JJ, et al. Preclinical efficacy of a prototype DNA vaccine: enhanced protection against antigenic drift in influenza virus. Nat Med 1995; 1:583–587.

270. Horimoto T, Kawaoka Y. Pandemic threat posed by avian influenza A viruses. Clin Microbiol Rev 2001; 14:129–149.

271. Claas ECJ, et al. Human influenza A H5N1 related to a highly pathogenic avian influenza virus. Lancet 1998; 351: 472–477.

272. Yuen KY, et al. Clinical features and rapid viral diagnosis of human disease associated with avian influenza A H5N1 virus. Lancet 1998; 351:467–471.

273. Peiris M, et al. Human infection with influenza H9N2. Lancet 1999; 354:916–917.

274. Nicholson KG, et al. Evaluation of two doses of either subunit- or MF-59 adjuvanted subunit influenza Duck/Singapore-Q/F119-3/97 (H5N3) vaccine in healthy adults, Second International Conference on Influenza and Other Respiratory Viruses, Cayman Islands, 1999.

275. Treanor JJ, et al. Safety and immunogenicity of a recombinant hemagglutinin vaccine for H5 influenza in humans. Vaccine 2001; 19:1732–1737.

276. Li S, et al. Recombinant influenza A virus vaccines for the pathogenic human A/Hong Kong/97 (H5N1) viruses. J Infect Dis 1999; 179:1132–1138.

277. Kodihalli S, et al. DNA vaccine encoding hemagglutinin provides protective immunity against H5N1 influenza virus infection in mice. J Virol 1999; 73:2094–2098.

278. Meltzer MI, et al. The economic impact of pandemic influenza in the United States: priorities for intervention. Emerg Infect Dis 1999; 5:659–671.

47

Chimeric Vaccines Against Japanese Encephalitis, Dengue, and West Nile

Konstantin V. Pugachev, Thomas P. Monath, and Farshad Guirakhoo
Acambis, Inc., Cambridge, Massachusetts, U.S.A.

Japanese encephalitis (JE) and dengue (DEN) viruses are two of the most important human pathogens within the *Flavivirus* genus of the *Flaviviridae* family. This group of small RNA viruses includes approximately 70 members, 38 of which have been associated with human illnesses. The West Nile (WN) virus is an important emerging pathogen recently introduced into the Western Hemisphere. In addition to the *Flavivirus* genus, the *Flaviviridae* family also includes the *Pestivitus* genus, which encompasses several veterinary pathogens of worldwide economic impact, such as bovine viral diarrhea virus (BVDV) and classical swine fever virus (CSFV), and the *Hepacivirus* genus, represented by only one member, hepatitis C virus (HCV), which is yet another extremely important human pathogen. Although currently grouped together, recent studies have shown that pestiviruses and HCV differ significantly from representatives of the *Flavivirus* genus in terms of their life cycle, genome organization, processing of viral proteins, etc. (reviewed in Refs. [1a,1b,3]). Therefore, the approaches to vaccine development discussed below may not be easily applied to these viruses. In the following pages, we will refer to members of the *Flavivirus* genus only as flaviviruses.

With a few exceptions, flaviviruses are mostly arboviruses, transmitted by mosquitoes and ticks (reviewed in Ref. [1]). Based on immunological cross-reactivity and genome sequence similarity, different flaviviruses are grouped into four distinct complexes (Table 1): the YF complex (contains only YF virus); the JE complex [JE, WN, St. Louis encephalitis (SLE), Kunjin (KUN), and Murray Valley encephalitis (MVE) viruses]; the dengue complex that includes the four steroviruses of DEN (types 1–4), and the TBE complex [TBE, Langat (LGT), Powassan, and Louping ill viruses] [1]. Because of the lack of effective antiviral drugs and obstacles in vector control programs, prevention through vaccination of people living in or traveling to endemic and epidemic areas is the most effective weapon in fighting these devastating illnesses. No licensed vaccines against dengue fever and WN encephalitis exist. The vaccines, currently available against

JE can be improved in terms of their efficacy, manufacturing cost, and use of acceptable cell substrates by applying the tools of molecular biology. Several molecular approaches, as well as the classic approaches currently being explored to create new DEN and JE vaccines have recently been reviewed [2]. This chapter will focus on the construction of live attenuated vaccines generated by one new approach, ChimeriVax™ technology.

I. FLAVIVIRUS ORGANIZATION AND REPLICATION

Flavivirions are spherical particles of roughly 50 nm in diameter (Figure 1A). The genome, which is a single-stranded RNA molecule of positive polarity of about 11,000 nucleotides (nt) in length, encompasses a long open reading frame (ORF) flanked by 5′ and 3′ untranslated terminal regions (UTRs), ~120 and 500 nt in length, respectively. The ORF encodes a polyprotein precursor which is cleaved co- and posttranslationally to generate individual viral proteins. The proteins are encoded in the order: C–prM/M–E–NS1–NS2A/2B–NS3–NS4A/4B–NS5, where C (core), prM/M (premembrane/membrane), and E (envelope) are the structural proteins, i.e., the components of viral particles, and NS are the nonstructural proteins necessary for intracellular virus replication (reviewed in Ref. [3]) (Figure 1B).

Upon infection of cells and translation of genomic RNA, the processing of the polyprotein starts with translocation of the prM portion into the lumen of endoplasmic reticulum (ER) of infected cells, followed by translocation of E and NS1 portions as directed by the hydrophobic anchor-signal tails of C, M, and E proteins, respectively. The amino-termini of prM, E, and NS1 are generated after cleavages by cellular signalase located on the luminal side of the ER membrane, and the resulting individual proteins remain carboxy-terminally anchored in the membrane. It is still unclear which protease is responsible for the NS1/NS2A

Table 1 Major Serocomplexes of Flavivirus Human Pathogens[a]

Serocomplex (by name of prototype virus)	Viruses	Principal vector
Yellow fever (YF)	YF virus	Mosquito
Japanese Encephalitis (JE)	JE, St. Louis encephalitis (SLE), West Nile (WN), Murray Valley encephalitis (MVE), Kunjin (KUN) viruses, etc.	Mosquito
Dengue (DEN)	DEN types 1–4 viruses	Mosquito
Tick-borne encephalitis (TBE)	TBE (Russian spring–summer encephalitis and Central European encephalitis), Omsk hemorrhagic fever, Langat (LGT) viruses, etc.	Tick

[a] Based on phylogenetic analysis of E protein sequences, the serocomplexes generally share 40–44% of amino acid sequence (46–53% between the JE and DEN serocomplexes), while the homologies between species within serocomplexes are higher, 62–96%.
Source: Ref. 1.

cleavage. Most of the remaining cleavages in the nonstructural region are carried out by the viral NS2B/NS3 serine protease, with the exception of the N-terminus of NS4B formed by the signalase. The viral protease is also responsible for generating the C-terminus of the mature C protein found in progeny virions (C_{vir}). Newly synthesized genomic RNA molecules and the C protein form a dense spherical nucleocapsid, which becomes surrounded by cellular membrane in which are embedded the E and prM proteins (Figure 1A). The mature M protein is produced by cleavage of prM shortly prior to virus release by cellular furin or a similar protease [4]. In addition to M, small amounts of residual uncleaved prM can often be found on the virion surface [5]. Among the NS proteins, NS1 remains an enigma. It appears to be essential for viral RNA amplification [6,7], but it is also secreted from cells and could be involved in virus spread and pathogenesis in the host. The prM (but not M), E, and NS1 of most flaviviruses are glycosylated.

E, the major protein of the envelope, is the principal target for neutralizing antibodies. The crystal structure of the ectodomain of E has been resolved [8]. This milestone significantly advanced our understanding of the function of the E protein, such as putative receptor recognition and fusion of viral and cell membranes during infection, and also elucidated the locations of antibody-binding epitopes. The virus-specific cytotoxic T-lymphocyte (CTL) response is the other key attribute of immunity. Multiple CD8[+] and CD4[+] CTL clones have been characterized in both humans and mice that recognize specific epitopes in many flavivirus structural and NS proteins (reviewed in Refs. [1] and [9]; [10,11]). The CTL responses are primarily directed against E and NS3 of DEN [12–15], NS3, NS4A, and NS4B of WN, KUN, and MVE viruses [1], as well as E of the JE virus (but not NS1) expressed in poxvirus vectors [16].

II. ENEMIES AND A FRIEND

A. Japanese Encephalitis Virus

In Asia, JE is a grave neurological disease of children with a case-fatality rate ranging from 5% to 40%. Three billion people are estimated to live in endemic regions. In the last 25 years, the incidence has intensified in certain countries, and the disease has extended its geographical range to previously unaffected areas of Asia and northern Australia [17,18]. More than 35,000 JE cases are reported officially each year, of which 5000–10,000 are fatal. A high proportion of survivors suffer from neurological and psychological sequelae. The virus is transmitted from infected animals, mainly domestic pigs, to humans by *Culex* mosquitoes. A mouse brain-derived, formalin-inactivated vaccine (Biken, Japan) is available internationally, and has significantly reduced disease rates in Japan, Republic of Korea, Taiwan, Sri Lanka, and parts of Thailand and Vietnam. The vaccine is 91% effective [19] and is administered in two primary doses, one booster at 1 year and subsequent boosters every 3 years. It has been associated with 0.6% rate of allergic reactions in adults, sometimes severe [17], and it is costly to manufacture. A live, cell culture-derived vaccine (attenuated SA14-14-2 strain produced in primary hamster kidney cells) is used in China. Although inexpensive and quite effective, it requires two doses for full protection [20] and has not been licensed for use outside China [17].

B. Dengue

Dengue is a global public health problem occurring mostly in tropical regions of the world. Over 2 billion people in tropical Asia, Africa, Australia, and the Americas are at risk of infection. Annually, up to 100 million cases of dengue

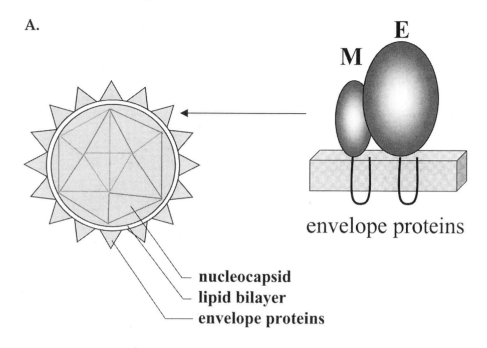

A.

E
M

envelope proteins

nucleocapsid
lipid bilayer
envelope proteins

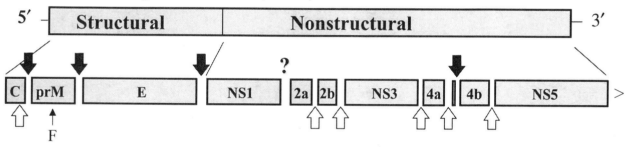

B. **Flavivirus genomic RNA, ~11,000 nucleotides**

5′ | Structural | Nonstructural | 3′

C | prM | E | NS1 | 2a | 2b | NS3 | 4a | 4b | NS5

?

F

⬆ **Host signalase** ⇧ **NS2b/NS3 serine protease**

Figure 1 Flavivirus structure. A. Organization of the virion. Each viral particle contains a nucleocapsid composed of one genomic RNA molecule and the capsid protein C. Nucleocapsid is surrounded by a lipid membrane with embedded membrane M and envelope E proteins. B. Organization of the genome. The positive-sense RNA molecule encodes a long open reading frame, which is translated into a polyprotein precursor. Most of the individual viral proteins are produced by cleavages of the polyprotein by the cellular signalase (black arrows) and the viral NS2B/NS3 protease (open arrows). The prM protein (precursor for M) is cleaved by furin-like protease shortly prior to virus release (F). The C protein generated by the signalase cleavage ($C_{intracellular}$) can only be found inside infected cells. Virions contain a carboxy-terminally truncated form of C (C_{vir}) that is generated by the viral protease and lacks the signal peptide for prM.

fever and 450,000 cases of the more severe form of the disease, dengue hemorrhagic fever (DHF)/dengue shock syndrome (DSS), occur [1,21]. The majority of DHF/DSS cases occur in young children living in Asia, who suffer a case-fatality rate of 1–10%, depending on the quality of supportive medical care. The virus is transmitted to humans by *Aedes aegypti* mosquitoes. Dengue strains constitute a separate antigenic complex among flaviviruses. Four antigenically related, but distinct serotypes of DEN (types 1–4)

are recognized by cross-neutralization tests. The amino acid homology between the four serotypes is 63–68% (and up to 77% in the E protein), compared with 44–51% between DEN and other flaviviruses [1,22–24]. Infected individuals become protected against homotypic infection, probably for life, but cross-protection between serotypes is short, lasting for less than 12 weeks [25]. Therefore, repetitive infections with different serotypes occur. Epidemiological data indicate that the majority of cases of DHF/DSS occur in patients who have previously encountered one of the serotypes, and became superinfected with a different serotype. This led to the emergence of the theory of immune enhancement of heterologous serotype infection because of the antibody-dependent enhancement of virus replication [26,27] and exacerbation of symptoms by preexisting cellular immunity [9,28]. Both virus-specified and host-related factors may influence the severity of the disease, because only a small subset of persons with secondary infections develops DHF (~3%). Alternatively, DHF may be caused by particularly virulent strains [29,30], and it has been suggested that anti-NS1 antibodies may cross-react with fibrinogen, thrombo-cytes, and endothelial cells triggering hemorrhage [31]. It is generally accepted that a dengue vaccine must be tetravalent, capable of inducing a robust protective immunity against all four serotypes simultaneously.

C. West Nile Virus

The virus is widespread and prevalent in Africa, Middle East, some European and former USSR countries, India, and Indonesia, and has caused sporadic outbreaks of encephalitis in humans and horses (reviewed in Ref. [1]). In humans, the infection is typically self-limited, accompanied by mild flu-like symptoms that usually go unnoticed. Infection of the central nervous system (CNS) happens infrequently (roughly in 1 out of 300 infections), principally in the elderly. The transmission cycle of WN virus includes *Culex* mosquitoes and primarily birds, while humans and horses develop low viremias, insufficient for further transmission to mosquitoes.

Recent WN encephalitis outbreaks have been documented in traditionally endemic regions, such as in Romania, Democratic Republic of the Congo, southern Russia, and Israel, with 200–800 reported human cases and a 15% case-fatality rate in patients with encephalitis. But in 1999, the WN virus unexpectedly emerged for the first time in the Western Hemisphere, in North America. It debuted in the United States, in Queens, NY (and surrounding areas), resulting in 62 confirmed cases, including 7 deaths. The disease then reemerged in New York City in 2000, with 18 cases and 2 deaths. During 2000 and 2001, the virus successfully invaded nearly the entire eastern one-third of the country, causing deaths as far south as the state of Georgia. Based on nucleotide sequence data, the U.S. virus appears to have come from Israel, but the means is unknown. An intriguing feature of the virus in the United States is its high mortality in wild birds (e.g., crows and blue jays), which is conspicuously absent in the Old World, ironically facilitating its epidemiological surveillance in the United States (reviewed in Ref. [32]).

As with other flaviviruses, there is no specific antiviral drug treatment. Currently, there is no licensed WN vaccine for humans. All WN strains belong to a single serotype and are similar at the nucleotide sequence level, which should simplify the development of a vaccine with broad protection. There were hopes that the inactivated Biken JE vaccine (marketed in the United States as JE-VAX®, Aventis-Pasteur) could provide cross-protection from WN. However, recent studies have suggested that no detectable cross-reac-

tivity could be elicited in human volunteers vaccinated with JE-VAX® [33]. Besides the necessity of a new human WN vaccine, there is a need for a veterinary horse vaccine. Recently, Fort Dodge received a Department of Agriculture (USDA) approval to market their formalin inactivated vaccine for horses, and is developing a DNA vaccine using technology developed at the Centers for Disease Control (Ft. Collins, CO).

D. Yellow Fever 17D—A Friend

The YF virus is the prototype member of the *Flavivirus* genus. Yellow fever was first clinically recognized in the seventeenth century and remained one of the most dreaded diseases in tropical areas of the world until the twentieth century, when an effective vaccine was finally developed. The symptoms of this highly lethal hemorrhagic fever transmitted to humans by *Aedes* mosquitoes include fever, hepatic, renal, and myocardial injury, hemorrhage, prostration, and shock. Today, due to the incomplete vaccination coverage, YF still affects approximately 200,000 persons a year, mainly in tropical South America and Africa, and continues to be a threat to people traveling to these regions [1,34]. Wild-type YF virus, strain Asibi, was first isolated in 1927 by inoculation of a rhesus monkey with blood of a patient in Ghana. In 1937, Theiler and Smith [35] reported the successful attenuation of this virus by multiple passages in mouse and chick embryo tissues that yielded the 17D vaccine strain. Since its development more than 60 years ago, the 17D vaccine has been administered to over 400 million people, with a remarkable history of safety and efficacy [36]. Yellow fever vaccines are currently manufactured in several countries (United Kingdom, Germany, France, United States, Russia, Brazil, Senegal, and Colombia) in embryonated chicken eggs under standards established by the World Health Organization (WHO) (Brazil uses a substrain of 17D called 17DD). The vaccine is well tolerated, with very few, usually mild, side effects (injection site pain, redness, headache, etc.) After vaccination, a low viremia is detectable during the first few days, not exceeding 2 $\log_{10}$ plaque-forming units (PFU) per milliliter. Because of a low viremia in vaccinated individuals and the fact that, in contrast to wild-type virus, the 17D virus does not replicate well in mosquitoes, vaccination cannot lead to dissemination of 17D in nature. Serious postvaccination complications (such as encephalitis or classical YF symptoms) are extremely rare. Vaccination is contraindicated in persons with immune deficiency disorders or taking immunosuppressive medications [34]. Because of the vulnerability of infants, the vaccine is not recommended in children under 9 months of age. Pregnancy is another contraindication. Congenital infection has been shown to occur (albeit at low rate, 1–2%), although not clearly associated with any harm to the fetus [34]. The period of onset of immunity is short. Ninety percent of vaccinees develop protective levels of YF neutralizing antibodies by day 10, and 99% by day 30 after vaccination. The immunity appears to be lifelong after a single dose. All the above features of the 17D vaccine are surrogate characteristics of an ideal vaccine, and validate the use of YF 17D virus in the construction of novel genetically engineered vaccines against other flavivirus diseases.

III. INFECTIOUS CLONES OF FLAVIVIRUSES: THE TOOL

Since it was first successfully implemented some 20 years ago for bacteriophage Qβ [37] and poliovirus [38], infectious cDNA clones of RNA-containing viruses have become an invaluable tool for studying the mechanisms of viral replication and pathogenesis, as well as for developing modern, genetically engineered vaccines. An infectious cDNA clone is a DNA copy of a viral RNA genome, which is stably cloned (most frequently in bacteria), and can be easily manipulated in vitro. Various mutations can be introduced, and parts of genomes from different viruses can be swapped. To initiate virus replication, the cDNA template is converted to RNA via in vitro transcription, and appropriate substrate cells are transfected with the RNA transcripts. Alternatively, the infectious clone can be engineered in such a way that cells can be directly transfected with plasmid DNA. The DNA is then transcribed in the nucleus, and the resulting RNA exits into the cytoplasm to start normal virus replication cycle. The construction of a first flavivirus infectious clone was reported in 1989 for YF virus, strain 17D [39], followed by several strains of DEN types 1, 2, and 4 [40–45], JE [46], TBE [47], LGT [48], MVE [49], KUN [50], and WN [51] viruses. Construction of infectious clones is a very complicated task accompanied by many technical hurdles. Because of the toxicity of some flavivirus cDNA regions for *Escherichia coli*, it is sometimes difficult to assemble a stable full-length clone in one bacterial plasmid. Therefore researchers have to resort to splitting viral sequence into two [39,46] or three [52] pieces cloned in separate plasmids, which have to be ligated prior to in vitro transcription.

IV. PREHISTORY OF ChimeriVax™

A. Dengue Intertypic Chimeras

The construction of the very first live flavivirus chimera was reported in 1991 by Bray and Lai of the National Institutes of Health (NIH; Bethesda, MD). They were able to replace the entire structural region, the C–prM–E genes, in the infectious clone of DEN4 (wild-type strain 814669) with the corresponding C–prM–E cassettes from DEN1 [Western Pacific strain (WP)] and DEN2 [New Guinea C (NGC), a laboratory strain neurovirulent for mice] [53]. Upon transfection of simian LLC-MK₂ cells with in vitro RNA transcripts, the DEN4/DEN1 and DEN4/DEN2 chimeras were readily recovered and grew to peak titers of 5×10^6 and 10^5 PFU/mL, respectively. The DEN4/DEN2 virus grew slower and produced smaller plaques compared to its parent NGC virus. Suckling (3-day-old) mice inoculated intracerebrally (i.c.) with both the neuroadapted DEN2 NGC and the chimeric DEN4/DEN2 viruses developed encephalitis and died. There was, however, a 3- to 5-day delay in death caused by the chimera, while both the DEN1 WP and DEN4/DEN1 viruses were not neurovirulent. Later, other chimeras between DEN4 and DEN2 were successfully generated, containing the prM–E cassette (without C) or only NS1 gene from DEN2 in place of the corresponding genes in the DEN4 backbone [54]. Both the prM–E and NS1 chimeras grew efficiently in mosquito C6/36 cells (10^6 and 2×10^7 PFU/mL, respectively). However, it is intriguing that attempts to produce a chimera containing all four DEN2 C–prM–E–NS1 genes failed [54]. A DEN4/DEN3 chimera containing the C–prM–E genes from a wild-type DEN3 strain CH53489 was also obtained and shown to replicate to a high titer in mosquito C6/36 cells (10^6 PFU/mL) [55].

These studies indicated that the engineering of live intertypic dengue chimeras by replacement of the structural proteins (as well as NS1) is possible. Further genetic analysis of these and other similar chimeras based on the DEN4 background yielded valuable information on genetic determinants of neurovirulence of DEN viruses in mice [54–56]. Next, the ability of these viruses to replicate efficiently in nonhuman primates and to induce a protective immunity (precluding replication of corresponding wild-type DEN viruses upon challenge) was addressed [57]. Both the DEN4/DEN1$_{C–prM–E}$ and DEN4/DEN2$_{prM–E}$ chimeras inoculated subcutaneously (s.c.) into rhesus monkeys (4 animals per virus; 3×10^5 PFU per dose) induced detectable short-lived viremias in half and all inoculated monkeys, respectively, as well as respective homologous type-specific neutralizing antibodies. Antibody titers ranged from 1.640 to 1:1,280 in most animals, which was similar to titers observed in control animals inoculated with the wild-type parents. After challenge at 66 days postimmunization with corresponding wild-type DEN viruses (DEN1 or DEN2), no viremia could be detected in the majority of immunized monkeys, while it was pronounced in all unimmunized animals. Similarly, monkeys immunized with a mixture of the two chimeras (DEN4/DEN1$_{C–prM–E}$ and DEN4/DEN2$_{prM–E}$) developed high titers of both DEN1- and DEN2-specific neutralizing antibodies (generally ranging between 1:320 and 1:640). Animals were solidly protected from challenge with both wild-type DEN1 and DEN2, even despite the fact that the DEN4/DEN2 chimera clearly outgrew the DEN4/DEN1 chimera in the doubly immunized animals as evidenced by the analysis of postimmunization viremias [57]. These data confirmed the theoretical possibility of constructing a tetravalent dengue vaccine composed of chimeric viruses based on the genetic background of one flavivirus. In this particular case, the DEN4 genetic background was used, which may sensitize vaccinees to DEN4-primed DHF. On the other hand, the backbone of these viruses was a pathogenic virus. Thus some of the created chimeras might be pathogenic for humans per se. In addition, they may be efficiently transmitted in nature by mosquitoes. The latter two issues were recently addressed by the introduction of various nonlethal deletions into the 5′ and 3′ UTRs of the DEN4 infectious clone. This resulted in an array of variants with altered characteristics in terms of plaque morphology and reduced growth rates in simian and/or mosquito cell cultures, or in *Aedes* mosquitoes [58,59]. Some of the 3′-UTR deletions, such as the deletions of nt 303–183 and 172–113 (numbering from the 3′ end of the genome), resulted in a marked reduction of viremia in rhesus monkeys compared to wild-type DEN4. Nevertheless, those variants were able to induce high DEN4 neutralizing antibody titers (geometric mean titers of 1:334 and 1:115, respectively, compared to 1:337 for wild-type virus) [59].

Another possibility to create a safer backbone could be the introduction of attenuating point mutations affecting functions of the nonstructural genes [60]. However, the theoretical disadvantage of this approach is that the mutations could back-mutate more easily than defined deletions, returning the virus to its original virulent phenotype. In any case, the vector virus, DEN4 containing 3′-UTR deletions has recently been tested in humans, and appeared to be both safe and immunogenic (Durbin, A., presentation at Annual Meeting, Am. Soc. Trop. Med. Hyg., Atlanta GA, Nov. 13, 2001).

Recently, scientists from the CDC (Fort Collins, CO) and Mahidol University (Bangkok, Thailand) have adopted the above strategy to design a different set of intertypic DEN chimeras [61]. They chose the PDK-53 strain of DEN2 as a backbone, which offers several principal advantages over the wild-type DEN4 backbone. This virus is one of the four attenuated DEN vaccine candidates (DEN1 PDK13, DEN2 PDK-53, DEN3 PGMK-30/FRhL-3, and DEN4 PDK-48) that were originally obtained at Mahidol University [62] by multiple passages of wild-type isolates in primary dog kidney cells or PGMK/FRhL cells for DEN3. These empirically derived vaccines are currently being tested in a tetravalent formulation by Aventis-Pasteur (Lyon, France). The DEN2 PDK-53 candidate vaccine has the lowest infectious dose in humans (only 5 vs. 10,000 PFU for DEN1 PDK-13 virus, for example), is highly immunogenic, and appears to have a satisfactory safety profile. In contrast to its wild-type parent DEN2 strain 16681, its replication is restricted in *Aedes albopictus* C6/36 cells [42] and *A. aegypti* mosquitoes [63]). Thus this attenuated DEN2 backbone appears to be superior to the DEN4 backbone described above in terms of safety. In addition, attenuation determinants of the PDK-53 virus have been identified that are responsible for its small-plaque phenotype, temperature-sensitivity, reduced replication in C6/36 cells, and low neurovirulence in newborn mice [64]. The three major attenuation markers (C to T change at nt 57 in the 5′ UTR, Gly to Asp amino acid change at NS1-53, and Glu to Val change at NS3-250) were mapped outside the structural protein region. Because all the attenuating mutations in the DEN2 PDK53 vector reside outside the structural region, it should be possible to construct chimeras containing the C–prM–E region from any heterologous donor dengue serotype or strain, and expect that the nonstructural genes of the vector would confer acceptable properties of safety and immunogenicity. Chimeras with the donor genes, for example, of either the DEN1 attenuated strain PDK-13 or its wild-type parent, DEN1 strain 16007 [61] would have a good potential as safe vaccine candidates. Three variants of the chimera containing the structural genes from the wild-typeDEN1 were immunogenic in 3-week-old outbred ICR mice (10^4 PFU/dose; mean titers of anti-DEN1 neutralizing antibodies ranging between 1:40 and 1:160 after primary immunization and 1:2560–1:10,240 after secondary boost). Interestingly, however, the other variants with the structural genes from the attenuated DEN1 strain appeared to be significantly less immunogenic. Chimeras based on this backbone for the other three serotypes are being constructed. Some concerns about whether this genetic background will potentiate DHF in vaccinees encountering DEN

viruses in nature still remain. It is also impossible to examine the potential of these viruses to lead to DHF in any models other than humans. Therefore clinical field trials will be the ultimate test.

B. Chimeras Between Unrelated Flaviviruses

The construction of the intertypic DEN chimeras described above was a major breakthrough and stimulated experimentation with other flaviviruses. However, it did not guarantee that viable chimeras between unrelated flaviviruses from different serocomplexes could be made. The first report on the construction of a viable chimera between two distinct flaviviruses, a mosquito-borne DEN4 and a tick-borne TBE virus, was published by Pletnev and coworkers in 1992 [65]. The same DEN4 genetic background described above was used (DEN4 wild-type strain 814669). A construct containing the prM-E genes from a highly virulent Russian isolate of TBE (Far Eastern subtype, strain Sofjin) readily yielded viable virus following transfection of LLC-MK$_2$ cells. The DEN4/TBE$_{prME}$ chimera grew to a titer of 10^8 PFU/mL in these cells, which was ~1000 times greater than the parental DEN4 virus, but replicated ~100 times less efficiently than DEN4 in mosquito C6/36 cells (a peak titer of roughly 10^4 PFU/mL). A chimera containing the TBE C–prM–E genes was also viable, but crippled in terms of its replication compared to the prM–E chimera. The latter fact could be attributed to a number of possible reasons, including the inefficient encapsidation of the hybrid genomic RNA by the TBE-specific C protein, the disruption of viral RNA cyclization essential for viral RNA synthesis [66], and the inefficient cleavage at the C-terminus of the TBE-specific C protein by the DEN4-specific viral protease that generates the mature form of C (C$_{vir}$; see Figure 1B) [67,68]. Attempts to generate other chimeras containing TBE-specific prM–E–NS1 or E–NS1 cassettes, or singly C, E, or NS1 genes, also did not result in viable viruses [65]. As discussed above, the DEN4/DEN2$_{NS1}$ chimera was viable [54]. Therefore in contrast to closely related DEN types, it appears that NS1 is not easily interchangeable between distant flaviviruses. This is not surprising if NS1 is a component of a very delicate RNA replication complex that could be highly restrained in terms of structural compatibility of all participating proteins. Recent data from trans-complementation studies in vitro seem to support this point of view. Specifically, the YF virus with an engineered in-frame deletion of the entire NS1 gene could not replicate in cells expressing DEN2-specific NS1 protein. However, replication of the deletion mutant in these cells was restored in selected variants, each containing a specific mutation in NS4A protein, one of the components of the viral replicase [7].

The DEN4/TBE$_{prM–E}$ chimera remained highly neurovirulent for both suckling and adult BALB/c mice, causing 100% mortality at the doses tested (10^2 and 10^3 PFU, respectively) [65]. Surprisingly, the chimera completely lost its neuroinvasiveness (the ability to invade the brain upon peripheral inoculation). It induced protective immunity in mice [65,69].

In hopes to obtain a better, less neurovirulent TBE vaccine candidate, viable DEN4-based chimeras containing the prM–E genes from LGT virus (wild-type TP21 and its attenuated E5 derivative strains) were constructed. LGT is a member of the TBE serocomplex and provides strong cross-protection against TBE, but has been associated with very rare cases of human illness [70]. Attempts to generate other chimeric variants containing the LGT-specific C–prM–E, NS1–NS2A, NS1–NS2A–NS2B–part of NS3, and NS2B–NS3 cassettes failed, again suggesting that the prM–E genes are easily interchangeable while the others are not. Interesting peculiarities were observed with these DEN4/LGT$_{prM–E}$ chimeras compared to the DEN4/TBE$_{prM–E}$ virus. They could only be produced by transfection of mosquito C6/36 cells, but not of simian LLC-MK$_2$ cells, and initially they grew well only in these mosquito cells (peak titer of up to 10^6 PFU/mL). In contrast, the DEN4, LGT E5, and LGT TP21 parents replicated efficiently in both LLC-MK$_2$ and Vero cells (titers of 6–9 $\log_{10}$ PFU/mL). The chimerization resulted in approximately 6000-fold reduction of neurovirulence of both TP21 and E5. Both chimeras were completely

nonneuroinvasive in outbred Swiss mice as well as in more susceptible immunodeficient SCID mice [70,71]. It was recently shown that the DEN4/TP21 chimera induced barely detectable viremia in inoculated rhesus monkeys but, nevertheless, was highly immunogenic in this model at all tested doses (10^3, 10^5, or 10^7 PFU). It did not replicate in nonhematophagous mosquitoes *Toxorhynchites splendens*, which are highly permissive for DEN viruses [72].

V. CHIMERIVAX™ VACCINES

A. ChimeriVax™-JE

Early reports on the construction of intertypic dengue chimeras and DEN4/TBE were a prelude to the ChimeriVax™ technology (illustrated in Figure 2), the essence of which is the use of the best characterized and safest flavivirus backbone available, that of the YF 17D vaccine. It started with the work of Chambers and coworkers, who

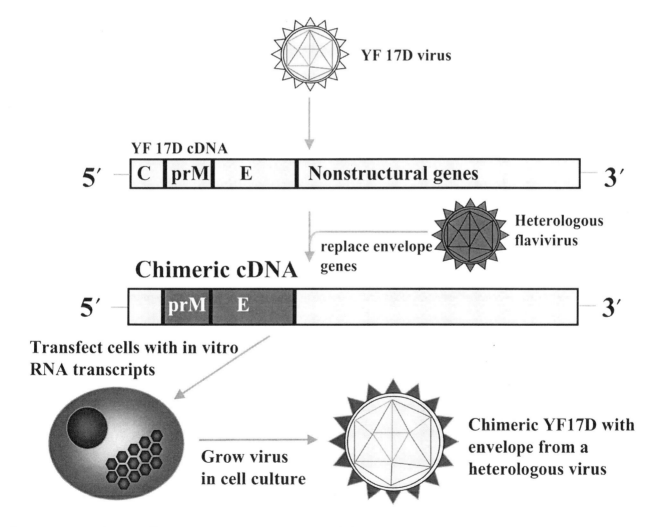

Figure 2 The ChimeriVax™ technology. The prM–E genes of the YF 17D virus are replaced with their analogs from a heterologous flavivirus. The C/prM junction is at the signalase cleavage site (see Figure 1B). Chimeric virus is produced following transfection of appropriate culture cells. Its new envelope induces a robust protective immunity in inoculated animals against the heterologous virus infection/pathology.

succeeded in the construction of first YF 17D chimeras containing the prM–E genes (but not C–prM–E) from either a virulent strain of JE virus, Nakayama, or the attenuated JE vaccine strain SA14-14-2 [73]. The chimeric viruses were obtained by transfection of simian Vero cells and had the antigenic specificity of JE virus (i.e., were neutralized by anti-JE specific antibodies but not by anti-YF antibodies). They efficiently replicated in several simian, human, mouse, and mosquito cell cultures. Similar to the YF17D parent, the YF/JE-Nakayama chimera remained neurovirulent for 3-week-old ICR mice. In contrast to its parent Nakayama, it was not neuroinvasive in ICR mice and was only partially neuroinvasive in C57/BL6 mice, indicating that a significant degree of attenuation had been attained by chimerization. Most importantly, the YF/JE-SA14-14-2 chimera (as well as the SA14-14-2 donor strain) was completely avirulent in mice by both i.c. and i.p. routes, even at the highest tested i.c. dose of 6 log$_{10}$ PFU. This indicated that the use of the SA14-14-2-specific envelope provided an additional degree of attenuation. Later, we investigated relative contribution of each of the 10 amino acid differences between the SA14-14-2-specific and Nakayama-specific E protein to the attenuation. The results showed that E to K mutation at E138 had a dominant attenuating effect, but multiple simultaneous reversions in at least three distinct clusters were required to restore the high neurovirulence of YF/JE-Nakayama virus [74]. The YF/JE-SA14-14-2 virus was subsequently chosen as a primary candidate chimeric JE vaccine designated ChimerVax™-JE and was further evaluated in cell culture and mouse model [75] (Table 2).

The ChimeriVax™-JE virus grew to titers in excess of 7 log$_{10}$ PFU/mL in Vero cells, a cell line acceptable for human vaccine production. C57/BL6 mice immunized s.c. with 10^3 PFU (or more) of the chimera were solidly protected from subsequent i.p. challenge with 158 LD50 doses of the virulent JE strain IC-37. The virus was completely avirulent in adult ICR mice by the i.c. route, despite efficient replication in mouse brains reaching a peak titer of 6 log$_{10}$ PFU/g of brain tissue on day 6 postinoculation, which then declined to undetectable levels by day 12. The neurovirulence test in infant mice was found to be a sensitive marker of the attenuated phenotype of ChimeriVax™-JE. Infant mice (3–5 days old) were sensitive to i.c. inoculation, but became

resistant to the virus around 7 days of age, at which point the mortality rate was 40% (at a dose of 10^4 log$_{10}$ PFU). For comparison, 66% of 8-day-old mice were killed by only 1.4 log$_{10}$ PFU of YF 17D, and thus, ChimeriVax™-JE was significantly less neurovirulent in this model than the commercial YF vaccine. The chimera was also found to be highly genetically stable, which is an important feature of a candidate vaccine. All putative attenuating SA14-14-2-specific mutations were preserved after 18 passages in cell culture or six brain-to-brain passages in mice, and there was no increase in neurovirulence [75].

The ChimeriVax™-JE virus was then extensively tested in a nonhuman primate model for its safety and immunogenicity [76,77] (Tables 2 and 3). Undiluted ChimeriVax™-JE as well as YF 17D virus were inoculated i.c. into rhesus macaques, followed by observation of clinical signs, viremia measurements, clinical laboratory tests, as well as pathological examination of the brain, spinal cord, and extraneural organs. Low, similar viremias were observed in all monkeys inoculated with YF 17D or ChimeriVax™-JE. ChimeriVax™-JE caused no clinical signs, while some monkeys inoculated with YF 17D developed transient mild encephalitis. Neither hematological or biochemical serum abnormalities, nor histopathologic changes in liver, spleen, kidney, heart, or adrenal glands were detected, demonstrating the lack of ChimeriVax™-JE-induced pathology. Lesion scores in all animals that received ChimeriVax™-JE were statistically significantly lower compared to YF 17D. Upon peripheral (s.c.) inoculation, all monkeys also developed low, self-limited viremias, similar to those induced by the YF 17D vaccine (Table 2). The low level of viremia suggested that the likelihood of neuroinvasion as well as the capacity of the host to serve as a source of infection for blood-feeding mosquitoes is low.

To demonstrate protective properties of ChimeriVax™-JE in nonhuman primates, an efficient challenge model had to be first developed that relied on the i.c. inoculation of rhesus monkeys with a large dose of a wild-type JE virus (~5 log$_{10}$ PFU of IC37 strain) [76], because these animals do not develop illness after parenteral inoculation. Because natural infection occurs by intradermal injection of small doses of virus, this challenge model is a very severe test of vaccine efficacy.

Table 2 Attenuation/Safety Phenotype of ChimeriVax™/JE in Animal Models as Compared to YF 17D [32,75–78]

Virus	Lack of mouse neurovirulence[a]		Pathogenicity in rhesus monkeys				Replication in mosquitoes[d]			
	Adult mice	Suckling mice	Illness score[b]	Brain lesion score[b]	Peak viremia[c]	Duration of viremia[c], Days	Culex		Aedes	
							IT	OF	IT	OF
ChimeriVax™/JE	>6.0	4.9	0	0.29	1.84	3.3	0	0	3.6	0
YF 17D	1.67	0.4	1	1.17	1.93	2.7	0	0	4.4	0

[a] i.c. LD$_{50}$ in log$_{10}$ pfu.
[b] Mean values after i.c. inoculation; scoring methods described in Refs. [76,77].
[c] Mean values after s.c. inoculation (log$_{10}$ pfu/mL for viremia).
[d] Titers in mosquitoes in log$_{10}$ pfu/mosquito; IT, intrathoracic inoculation; OF, infection by oral feeding; in comparison, JE virus strains (both wild-type and vaccine SA14-14-2) grew to titers of ~6 log$_{10}$ pfu/mosquito in both species by either route [78].

All animals immunized s.c. with graded doses of Chi-meriVax™-JE (varying from 2 to 5.3 $\log_{10}$ PFU) developed high titers of neutralizing antibodies (Table 3) [76,77]. They were solidly protected from i.c. challenge with wild-type JE virus, judged by the absence of viremia and clinical encephalitis (except for one monkey which turned out to be pregnant; whether pregnancy played a role is unknown, but it is a contraindication for YF 17D vaccination). These results provided strong evidence that ChimeriVax™-JE had a very good potential as a safe and robust human vaccine.

Three Phase I/II clinical trials of ChimeriVax™-JE vaccine have been carried out in healthy adult volunteers. It was demonstrated that the vaccine is well tolerated and fully immunogenic after a single inoculation of 4 or 5 $\log_{10}$ PFU of the virus. In one trial, subjects with or without prior immunization against YF were vaccinated with Chi-meriVax™-JE. All 24 subjects (100%) developed JE virus-specific neutralizing antibodies. Interestingly, the mean neutralizing antibody titers were higher in the YF-immune subjects, indicating that anti-YF vector immunity (e.g., T-cell-mediated immunity to the YF-specific nonstructural proteins) did not preclude, and indeed may have enhanced, immune responses to the envelope proteins of this YF-based chimeric vaccine. In another trial, 10 subjects vaccinated with ChimeriVax™-JE 9 months earlier, and 10 control subjects were challenged with one standard dose of forma-lin-inactivated JE vaccine (noninfectious JE antigen repre-senting a surrogate for exposure to live virus). The vaccinated subjects responded with a significant rise in JE-specific neutralizing antibody titers (mean titers were 20- and 100-fold higher on days 7 and 14 postchallenge, respectively, compared to prechallenge titers), while none of the control subjects developed antibodies by day 7, and only 2 out of 10 had any detectable antibody response within the 30-day observation period [differences in titers between the treat-ment groups were statistically significant on all study days ($P<0.001$)]. Thus a strong anamnestic immune response, which is an important prerequisite of vaccine effectiveness, was observed in the vaccinated subjects.

Finally, the concern about whether ChimeriVax™-JE can infect insects feeding on the blood of vaccinees was addressed. The YF 17D vaccine lost its ability to infect mosquitoes in the process of its attenuation. In contrast to the JE SA14-14-2 parent virus, ChimeriVax™-JE was un-able to infect *Aedes* and *Culex* mosquitoes by oral feeding and replicated poorly following direct intrathoracic inoc-ulation (Table 2), suggesting that the restricted mode of replication is specified by the YF 17D nonstructural proteins [78]. Together with the fact of low viremias in vaccinees, these data make the possibility of uncontrolled spread of chimeras in nature very unlikely.

B. ChimeriVax-DEN Tetravalent Vaccine

The first viable YF 17D/DEN chimera was constructed by Chambers and coworkers using the prM–E genes from PUO-218 strain of DEN2 virus isolated from a case of dengue fever in Thailand [79]; this construct became ChimeriVax™-DEN2. Interestingly, initial attempts to pro-duce a similar chimera by a group from Brazil failed [80]. Close examination of the cloning strategies used by the two groups revealed that the latter initially followed the ap-proach of Pletnev and coworkers for the DEN4/TBE chi-mera. They attempted to fuse the 5′ end of the DEN2 prM gene with the 3′ end of the YF C gene at the C_{virion}/$C_{intracellular}$ cleavage site and thus, the signal peptide for prM was DEN2-specific, whereas Chambers et al. retained the YF-specific signal sequence (Figure 1B). Our working hypothesis to explain this phenomenon is that the length of the signal peptide makes a principal difference. While the YF and TBE parental viruses both contain a 20-amino acid-long signal, the DEN2 and DEN4 parents contain a shorter, 14-amino acid signal. Thus it appears that when the DEN4-backbone is used to create a chimera, the short DEN4-specific signal can be replaced with the long TBE-specific signal, resulting in a viable chimera (DEN4/TBE). How-ever, when the long YF-specific signal is replaced with the short one of DEN2 (Brazilian group), no viable recombi-nant virus can be recovered. It is possible that the replace-ment of a long signal with a short one renders the C_{vir}/C_{int} cleavage site inaccessible for the viral NS2B–NS3 protease, possibly because it becomes buried inside the ER mem-

Table 3 Immunogenicity of ChimeriVax™/JE in Rhesus Monkeys: Animals Were Immunized with Different Graded Doses of the Chimera and Later Challenged I.C. with Wild-Type JE Virus [76,77]

Dose of virus ($\log_{10}$ pfu)[a]	Postimmunization antibody titer[b]	Post-challenge antibody titer[b]	Postchallenge illness[c]	Postchallenge mortality[c]
2.0	1280	7241	0	0
3.0	1076	8611	0	0
4.0	905	6089	0	0
4.3	806	1800	1 (33%)	1 (33%)
5.0	640	10,240	0	0
5.3	1613	14,000	0	0
Mock	<10	<20	6 (100%)	6 (100%)

[a] 3–6 animals per group.

[b] Mean JE-specific neutralizing antibody titers.

[c] Number of animals (%).

brane. Cleavage at this site was shown to be critical for virus replication [67,68]. When the YF-specific signal is preserved in YF/DEN2 chimera (Chambers' approach), the virus is viable. Consistent with this view, when we experimentally replaced the YF-specific signal with the short DEN2-specific signal in the ChimeriVax™-DEN2 virus, viability was lost (C. Miller and J. Arroyo, Acambis Inc., unpublished data). The Brazilian group eventually succeeded when the Chambers' approach was implemented [80]. A third group engineered another YF 17D/DEN2 chimera and demonstrated that it induced robust CD8+ T-cell response directed against the DEN2-specific prM–E envelope proteins in immunized mice [81].

Recently, we reported the construction of the three additional YF 17D/DEN chimeras, ChimeriVax™-DEN1, 3, and 4 containing the prM–E cassettes from wild-type DEN1 PUO 359 (isolated in 1980 in Thailand), DEN3 PaH881/88 (Thailand-1988), and DEN4 1228 (Indonesia-1978) strains [52]. These viruses were recovered after the transfection of Vero cells, and efficiently replicated in this vaccine substrate cell line to similar titers of ~7.5 log$_{10}$ PFU/mL (except for DEN3 chimera which produced 10-fold lower titers). They demonstrated the same low neurovirulence profile described above for ChimeriVax™-JE in that they were completely avirulent in adult outbred ICR mice (inoculated i.c. at doses of up to 6 log$_{10}$ PFU) and significantly less neurovirulent in suckling mice, compared to the YF 17D parent (which is lethal for mice of all ages inoculated by the i.c. route) [52,79]. No increase in mouse neurovirulence was observed after the DEN2 chimera was passaged 18 times in Vero cells, suggesting its genetic stability and safety profile [79].

The four DEN chimeras were then evaluated in rhesus monkeys for their safety, as judged by the levels of induced viremia, and protective efficacy, judged by the levels of

corresponding DEN-specific neutralizing antibodies and protection against challenge [52,79]. Monkeys inoculated s.c. with one dose of these chimeric viruses as monovalent (~4 log$_{10}$ PFU) or tetravalent (5.3 log$_{10}$ PFU total) formulations developed brief viremia with magnitudes similar to that of YF 17D (mean peak titers of 0.7–1.65 log$_{10}$ PFU/mL), but significantly lower than those of their parent wild-type viruses (2.2–4.9 log$_{10}$ PFU/mL). They produced neutralizing antibodies of expected type-specificities. Interestingly, in one experiment in which graded doses of ChimeriVax™-DEN2 were administered (2, 3, 4, and 5 log$_{10}$ PFU/dose), animals from the lowest-dose group had viremia similar in magnitude and duration (although slightly delayed) to the other groups (mean peak titer of ~1.5 log$_{10}$ PFU/mL and mean duration of ~4 days). Similar levels of neutralizing antibodies were produced (mean titer of ~1:320 across all groups on day 30), indicating that the vaccine may be effective even at a dose as low as 2 log$_{10}$ PFU [79]. Sixty-two days postimmunization, these animals were challenged by the s.c. route with 5.0 log$_{10}$ PFU of a wild-type DEN2 virus. No viremia was detected in any of the vaccinated groups, demonstrating the effectiveness of immunization, whereas all animals in the placebo control group developed high viremia of the challenging virus. Importantly, a strong anamnestic response was observed after challenge of ChimeriVax™-DEN2-vaccinated animals, with an increase in mean neutralizing antibody titers of about 10-fold.

Because the final dengue vaccine will contain all four chimeras, the behavior of these viruses after being administered as a tetravalent mixture is of critical importance. Ideally, all four components should replicate equally well and induce uniform immune response to all four dengue serotypes. This is not an easy goal because rates of replication in vivo can be different for these viruses, and because they presumably target the same cells and tissues of the body,

Table 4 Properties of Tetravalent ChimeriVax™-DEN Vaccine in YF-Immune or Nonimmune Rhesus Monkeys [52][a]

YF immune monkeys?	Dose[b]	Viremia after first dose[c]	Neutralizing antibody titers after first dose			Neutralizing antibody titers after second dose[d]	Viremia after second dose
			Specificity	Day 30	Day 180		
NO (Experiment 1, 6 animals)	5.3	1.5/3.3	DEN1	160	142	640	0
			DEN2	1015	905	1810	
			DEN3	80	127	452	
			DEN4	32	71	359	
NO (Experiment 2, 6 animals)	5.4	2.4/4.7	DEN1	180	ND	ND	ND
			DEN2	1280			
			DEN3	36			
			DEN4	63			
YES (Experiment 2, 3 animals)	5.4	1.3/1.5	DEN1	254	ND	ND	ND
			DEN2	1016			
			DEN3	350			
			DEN4	80			

[a] All entries are mean values of each parameter. Characteristics of individual chimeras administered monovalently have also been studied extensively [52,79].
[b] log$_{10}$ pfu of tetravalent mixture composed of almost equal amounts of each chimera.
[c] Peak titer (log$_{10}$ pfu/mL)/duration of viremia (days).
[d] Day 30 after second dose.

they may interfere with each other. In this regard, in our first published experiment with the tetravalent ChimeriVax™-DEN candidate, we observed that ChimeriVax™-DEN2 induced noticeably higher viremia in rhesus monkeys inoculated with a mixture of equal amounts of the four chimeras (4.7 $\log_{10}$ PFU of each virus, 5.3 $\log_{10}$ PFU total dose) compared to the other three [52]. The animals seroconverted to all four DEN serotypes after first inoculation, although the neutralizing anti-DEN2 titers in the sera were higher (mean titers on day 180 postvaccination of 1:142, 1:905, 1:127, and 1:71 against DEN1 through DEN4, respectively) (Table 4). Nevertheless, a second inoculation with the tetravalent mixture resulted in higher and more uniform titers (1:640, 1:1810, 1:452, and 1:359, respectively) demonstrating that a two-dose immunization regimen can be a good alternative to achieve the same goal [52]. No viremias were detected in these animals after the boost, indicating that the primary immunization was already completely protective.

The issue of antivector immunity was also addressed in these experiments [52,79]. For example, vaccinia recombinants expressing JE virus genes (NYVAC-JEV) failed to induce JE-neutralizing antibody response in vaccinia virus-immune volunteers [82]. The mechanism of antivector immunity in the case of ChimeriVax™ viruses would involve CTL responses against YF 17D nonstructural proteins or cytolytic antibodies against YF 17D NS1. In our studies, no statistically significant difference was observed in the levels of DEN-specific neutralizing antibodies in YF virus-immune and nonimmune monkeys that received the tetravalent ChimeriVax™-DEN vaccine (or only DEN2 chimera) (see Experiment 2 in Table 4). These data together with those obtained from ChimeriVax™-JE clinical trials indicate that antivector immunity will not be a significant factor limiting the practical use of chimeric vaccines or vice versa.

C. ChimeriVax™-WN

ChimeriVax™-WN has been constructed using the prM–E genes from the New York-1999 strain that was introduced into the Northern Hemisphere just 2 years ago. The chimeric virus was recovered from the supernatant of transfected Vero cells and replicated to titers in the excess of 7 $\log_{10}$ PFU/mL in this culture [32]. Based on the extensive knowledge of attenuating residues in the closely related JE virus, a number of attenuating mutations were introduced singly or in different combinations into its wild-type envelope in order to obtain a safer, more attenuated virus. The wild-type chimera, as well as variants with additional mutations, were examined in mice with the result that the original construct was highly attenuated. Thus it is possible that no additional attenuation of this virus will be necessary.

The virus was also tested in horses and was shown to elicit WN-specific neutralizing antibodies and protection against challenge (J. Arroyo and R. Bowen, unpublished data).

VI. CONCLUSION

The recent advances of molecular biology opened doors to the development of principally new recombinant flavivirus

vaccines currently championed in terms of their high promise by chimeric vaccine candidates, particularly ChimeriVax™ vaccines that were constructed based on one of the most effective and safest vaccines available, YF 17D. The accumulating body of evidence demonstrates their high replication efficiency, the highly attenuated phenotype in animal models (as well as in humans), robust immunogenicity and protective efficacy, and high genomic stability. Other important issues, such as the effect of antivector immunity and infectivity for mosquitoes, were addressed. The opportunity that we now have to help save lives of thousands of people worldwide with these new vaccines is breathtaking.

REFERENCES

1. Monath TP, Heinz FX. Flaviviruses. In: Fields BN, Knipe DM, Howley PM, Chanock RM, Melnick JL, Monath TP, Roizman B, Straus SE, eds. Fields Virology. 3rd ed. Philadelphia: Lippincott-Raven Publishers, 1996:961–1034.

1a. Thiel H-J, et al. Pestiviruses. In: Fields BN, Knipe DM, Howley PM, Chanock RM, Melnick JL, Monath TP, Roizman B, Straus SE, eds. Fields Virology. 3rd ed. Philadelphia: Lippincott-Raven Publishers, 1996:1059–1073.

1b. Lindenbach BD, Rice CM. Flaviviridae: the viruses and their replication. In: Knipe DM, Howley PM, Griffin DE, Lamb RA, Martin MA, Roizman B, Straus SE, eds. Fields Virology. 4th ed. Philadelphia: Lippincott Williams and Wilkins, 2001:991–1041.

2. Kinney RM, Huang CYH. Development of new vaccines against dengue fever and Japanese encephalitis. Intervirology 2001; 44:176–197.

3. Rice CM. Flaviviridae: the viruses and their replication. In: Fields BN, Knipe DM, Howley PM, Chanock RM, Melnick JL, Monath TP, Roizman B, Straus SE, eds. Fields Virology. 3rd ed. Philadelphia: Lippincott-Raven Publishers, 1996:931–959.

4. Stadler K, et al. Proteolytic activation of tick-borne encephalitis virus by furin. J Virol 1997; 71:8475–8481.

5. Russell PK, et al. Chemical and antigenic structure of flaviviruses. In: Schlesinger RW, ed. The Togaviruses: Biology, Structure, Replication. New York: Academic Press, 1980:503–529.

6. Muylaer IR, et al. Genetic analysis of the yellow fever virus NS1 protein: identification of a temperature-sensitive mutation which blocks RNA accumulation. J Virol 1997; 71:291–298.

7. Lindenbach BD, Rice CM. Genetic interaction of flavivirus nonstructural protein NS1 and NS4A as a determinant of replicase function. J Virol 1999; 73:4611–4621.

8. Rey FA, et al. The envelope glycoprotein from tick-borne encephalitis virus at 2 Å resolution. Nature 1995; 375:291–298.

9. Kurane I, Ennis FA. Immunity and immunopathology in dengue virus infections. Semin Immunol 1992; 4:121–127.

10. Gagnon SJ, et al. Identification of two epitopes on the dengue 4 virus capsid protein recognized by a serotype-specific and a panel of serotype-cross-reactive human CD4$^+$ cytotoxic T-lymphocyte clones. J Virol 1996; 70:141–147.

11. Green S, et al. Recognition of dengue virus NS1–NS2a proteins by human CD4$^+$ cytotoxic T lymphocyte clones. Virology 1997; 234:383–386.

12. Bukowski JF, et al. Dengue virus-specific cross-reactive CD8$^+$ human cytotoxic T lymphocytes. J Virol 1989; 63:5086–5091.

13. Kurane I, et al. Dengue virus-specific, human CD4$^+$CD8-cytotoxic T-cell clones: multiple patterns of virus cross-reactivity recognized by NS3-specific T-cell clones. J Virol 1991; 65:1823–1828.

14. Livingston PG, et al. Recognition of envelope protein by dengue virus serotype-specific human CD4$^+$CD8-cytotoxic T-cell clones. J Virol 1994; 68:3283–3288.

15. Rothman AL, et al. Dengue virus protein recognition by virus-specific murine CD8$^+$ cytotoxic T lymphocytes. J Virol 1993; 67:801–806.

16. Konishi E, et al. Poxvirus-based Japanese encephalitis vaccine candidates induce virus-specific CD8$^+$ cytotoxic T lymphocytes in mice. Virology 1997; 2270:353–360.

17. World Health Organization. Wkly Epidemiol Rec No 44 1998; 73:337–344.

18. Tsai TF. New initiatives for the control of Japanese encephalitis by vaccination: minutes of the WHO/CVI meeting, Bangkok, Thailand, 13–15 October 1998. Vaccine 2000; 18:1–25.

19. Hoke C, et al. Protection against Japanese encephalitis by inactivated vaccines. New Engl J Med 1988; 319:608–614.

20. Hennessy S, et al. Effectiveness of live-attenuated Japanese encephalitis vaccine (SA14-14-2): a case-control study. Lancet 1996; 347:1583–1586.

21. Monath TP. Dengue—the risk to developed and developing countries. Proc Natl Acad Sci USA 1994; 91:2395–2400.

22. Deubel V, et al. Nucleotide sequence and deduced amino acid sequence of the nonstructural proteins of dengue-2 virus, Jamaica: comparative analysis of the full-length genome. Virology 1988; 165:234–244.

23. Hahn YS, et al. Nucleotide sequence of dengue-2 RNA and comparison of the encoded proteins with those of other flaviviruses. Virology 1988; 162:167–180.

24. Mason PW, et al. Sequence of the dengue-1 virus genome in the region encoding the three structural proteins and the major nonstructural protein NS1. Virology 1987; 161:262–267.

25. Sabin AB. Research on dengue during World War II. Am J Trop Med Hyg 1952; 1:30–50.

26. Halstead SB, et al. Observations related to pathogenesis of dengue related to pathogenesis of dengue hemorrhagic fever: IV. Relation of disease severity to antibody response and virus recovered. Yale J Biol Med 1970; 42:311–328.

27. Halstead SB. Pathogenesis of dengue: challenge to molecular biology. Science 1988; 239:476–481.

28. Halstead SB. Antibody, macrophage, dengue virus infection, shock and hemorrhage: a pathogenetic cascade. Rev Infect Dis 1989; 11:S830–S839.

29. Leitmeyer KC, et al. Dengue virus structural differences that correlate with pathogenesis. J Virol 1999; 73:4738–4747.

30. Murgue B, et al. Dengue virus inhibits human hematopoietic progenitor growth in vitro. J Infect Dis 1997; 175:1497–1501.

31. Falconar AK. The dengue virus nonstructural-1 protein (NS1) generates antibodies to common epitopes on human blood clotting, integrin/adhesin proteins and binds to human endothelial cells: potential implications in haemorrhagic fever pathogenesis. Arch Virol 1996; 142:897–916.

32. Monath TP, et al. West Nile virus vaccine. Curr Drug Trends-Infect Disord 2001; 1:37–50.

33. Kanesa-Thasan N, et al. Absence of protective neutralizing antibodies to West Nile virus in subjects following vaccination with Japanese encephalitis or dengue vaccines. Am J Trop Med Hyg. In press.

34. Monath TP. Yellow fever: an update. Lancet 2001; 1:11–20.

35. Theiler M, Smith HH. The effect of prolonged cultivation in vitro upon the pathogenicity of yellow fever virus. J Exp Med 1937; 65:767–786.

36. Monath TP. Yellow fever. In: Plotkin S, Orenstein W, eds. Vaccines. 3rd ed. Philadelphia: WB Saunders, 1999:815–879.

37. Taniguchi T, et al. Qβ DNA-containing hybrid plasmids giving raise to Qβ phage formation in the bacterial host. Nature 1978; 274:2293–2298.

38. Racaniello VR, Baltimore D. Cloned poliovirus cDNA is infectious in mammalian cells. Science 1981; 214:916–919.

39. Rice CM, et al. Transcription of infectious yellow fever RNA from full-length cDNA templates produced by in vitro ligation. New Biol 1989; 1:285–296.

40. Lai C-J, et al. Infectious RNA transcribed from stably cloned full-length cDNA of dengue type 4 virus. Proc Natl Acad Sci USA 1991; 88:5139–5143.

41. Kapoor M, et al. Synthesis and characterization of an infectious dengue virus type-2 RNA genome (New Guinea C strain). Gene 1995; 162:175–180.

42. Kinney RM, et al. Construction of infectious cDNA clones for dengue 2 virus: strain 16681 and its attenuated vaccine derivative, strain PDK-53. Virology 1997; 230:300–308.

43. Polo S, et al. Infectious RNA transcripts from full-length dengue virus type 2 cDNA clones made in yeast. J Virol 1997; 71:5366–5374.

44. Gualano RC, et al. Identification of a major determinant of mouse neurovirulence of dengue virus type 2 using stably cloned genomic cDNA. J Gen Virol 1998; 79:437–446.

45. Pur B, et al. Construction of a full-length infectious clone for dengue 1 virus Western Pacific, 74 strain. Virus Genes 2000; 20:57–63.

46. Sumiyoshi H, et al. Infectious Japanese encephalitis virus RNA can be synthesized from in vitro-ligated cDNA templates. J Virol 1992; 66:5425–5431.

47. Mandl CW, et al. Infectious cDNA clones of tick-borne encephalitis virus European subtype prototypic strain Neudoerfl and high virulence strain Hypr. J Gen Virol 1997; 78: 1049–1057.

48. Pletnev AG. Infectious cDNA clone of attenuated Langat tick-borne flavivirus (strain E5) and a 3′ deletion mutant constructed from it exhibit decreased neuroinvasiveness in immunodeficient mice. Virology 2001; 282:288–300.

49. Hurrelbrink RJ, et al. Characterization of infectious Murray Valley encephalitis virus derived from a stably cloned genome-length cDNA. J Gen Virol 1999; 80:3115–3125.

50. Khromykh AA, Westaway EG. Completion of Kunjin virus RNA sequence and recovery of an infectious RNA transcripts from stably cloned full-length cDNA. J Virol 1994; 68:4580–4588.

51. Yamshchikov VF, et al. An infectious clone of the West Nile flavivirus. Virology 2001; 281:294–304.

52. Guirakhoo F, et al. Construction, safety, and immunogenicity in nonhuman primates of a chimeric yellow fever-dengue virus tetravalent vaccine. J Virol 2001; 75:7290–7304.

53. Bray M, Lai CJ. Construction of intertypic chimeric dengue viruses by substitution of structural protein genes. Proc Natl Acad Sci USA 1991; 88:10342–10346.

54. Bray M, et al. Genetic determinants responsible for acquisition of dengue type 2 virus mouse neurovirulence. J Virol 1998; 72:1647–1651.

55. Chen W, et al. Construction of intertypic chimeric dengue viruses exhibiting type 3 antigenicity and neurovirulence for mice. J Virol 1995; 69:5186–5190.

56. Kawano H, et al. Genetic determinants of dengue type 4 virus neurovirulence for mice. J Virol 1993; 67:6567–6575.

57. Bray M, et al. Monkeys immunized with intertypic chimeric dengue viruses are protected against wild-type virus challenge. J Virol 1996; 70:4162–4166.

58. Cahour A, et al. Growth-restricted dengue virus mutants containing deletions in the 5′ noncoding region of the RNA genome. Virology 1995; 207:68–76.

59. Men R, et al. Dengue type 4 virus mutants containing deletions in the 3′ noncoding region of the RNA genome: analysis of growth restriction in cell culture and altered viremia pattern and immunogenicity in rhesus monkeys. J Virol 1996; 70:3930–3937.

60. Pethel M, et al. Mutational analysis of the octapeptide sequence motif at the NS1–NS2A cleavage junction of dengue type 4 virus. J Virol 1992; 66:7225–7231.

61. Huang CY, et al. Chimeric dengue type 2 (vaccine strain

PDK-53)/dengue type 1 virus as a potential candidate dengue type 1 virus vaccine. J Virol 2000; 74:3020–3028.

62. Bhamarapravati N, Yoksan S. Live attenuated tetravalent vaccine. In: Gubler DJ, Kuno G, eds. Dengue and Dengue Hemorrhagic Fever. Wallingford, UK: CAB International, 1997:367–377.

63. Khin MM, et al. Infection, dissemination, transmission, and biological attributes of dengue-2 PDK53 candidate vaccine virus after oral infection in *Aedes aegypti*. Am J Trop Med Hyg 1994; 51:849–864.

64. Butrapet S, et al. Attenuation markers of a candidate dengue type 2 vaccine virus, strain 16681 (PDK-53), are defined by mutations in the 5′ noncoding region and nonstructural proteins 1 and 3. J Virol 2000; 74:3011–3019.

65. Pletnev AG, et al. Construction and characterization of chimeric tick-borne encephalitis/dengue type 4 viruses. Proc Natl Acad Sci USA 1992; 89:10532–10536.

66. Khromykh AA, et al. Essential role of cyclization sequences in flavivirus RNA replication. J Virol 2001; 75:6719–6728.

67. Yamshchikov VF, Compans RW. Regulation of the late events in flavivirus protein processing and maturation. Virology 1993; 192:38–51.

68. Amberg SM, Rice CM. Mutagenesis of the NS2B–NS3-mediated cleavage site in the flavivirus capsid protein demonstrates a requirement for coordinated processing. J Virol 1999; 73:8083–8094.

69. Pletnev AG, et al. Chimeric tick-borne encephalitis and dengue type 4 viruses: effects of mutations on neurovirulence in mice. J Virol 1993; 67:4956–4963.

70. Pletnev AG, Men R. Attenuation of the Langat tick-borne flavivirus by chimerization with mosquito-borne flavivirus dengue type 4. Proc Natl Acad Sci USA 1998; 95:1746–1751.

71. Pletnev AG, et al. Chimeric Langat/Dengue viruses protect mice from heterologous challenge with the highly virulent strains of tick-borne encephalitis virus. Virology 2000; 274:26–31.

72. Pletnev AG, et al. Tick-borne Langat/mosquito-borne dengue flavivirus chimera, a candidate live attenuated vaccine for protection against disease caused by members of the tick-borne encephalitis virus complex: evaluation in rhesus monkeys and in mosquitoes. J Virol 2001; 75:8259–8567.

73. Chambers TJ, et al. Yellow fever/Japanese encephalitis chimeric viruses: construction and biological properties. J Virol 1999; 73:3095–3101.

74. Arroyo J, et al. Molecular basis for attenuation of neurovirulence of a yellow fever Virus/Japanese encephalitis virus chimera vaccine (ChimeriVax-JE). J Virol 2001; 75:934–942.

75. Guirakhoo F, et al. Immunogenicity, genetic stability, and protective efficacy of a recombinant, chimeric yellow fever–Japanese encephalitis virus (ChimeriVax-JE) as a live, attenuated vaccine candidate against Japanese encephalitis. Virology 1999; 257:363–372.

76. Monath TP, et al. Recombinant, chimaeric live, attenuated vaccine (ChimeriVax) incorporating the envelope genes of Japanese encephalitis (SA14-14-2) virus and the capsid and nonstructural genes of yellow fever (17D) virus is safe, immunogenic and protective in non-human primates. Vaccine 1999; 17:1869–1882.

77. Monath TP, et al. Chimeric yellow fever virus 17D-Japanese encephalitis virus vaccine: dose-response effectiveness and extended safety testing in rhesus monkeys. J Virol 2000; 74:1742–1751.

78. Bhatt TR, et al. Growth characteristics of the chimeric Japanese encephalitis virus vaccine candidate, ChimeriVax-JE (YF/JE SA14-14-2), in *Culex tritaeniorhynchus*, *Aedes albopictus*, and *Aedes aegypti* mosquitoes. Am J Trop Med Hyg 2000; 62:480–484.

79. Guirakhoo F, et al. Recombinant chimeric yellow fever-dengue type 2 virus is immunogenic and protective in non-human primates. J Virol 2000; 74:5477–5485.

80. Caufour PS, et al. Construction, characterization and immunogenicity of recombinant yellow fever 17D-dengue type 2 viruses. Virus Res 2001; 79:1–14.

81. van Der Most RG, et al. Chimeric yellow fever/dengue virus as a candidate dengue vaccine: quantitation of the dengue virus-specific CD8 T-cell response. J Virol 2000; 74:8094–8101.

82. Kanesa-thasan N, et al. Safety and immunogenicity of NYVAC-JEV and ALVAC-JEV attenuated recombinant Japanese encephalitis virus–poxvirus vaccines in vaccinia-nonimmune and vaccinia-immune humans. Vaccine 2000; 19:483–491.

48

Challenges and Current Strategies in the Development of HIV/AIDS Vaccines

Chad A. Womack and Barney S. Graham
National Institute of Allergy and Infectious Diseases, National Institutes of Health, Bethesda, Maryland, U.S.A.

Margaret A. Liu
Transgene Inc., Strasbourg, France

I. CHALLENGES AND PROSPECTS FOR THE DEVELOPMENT OF HIV/AIDS VACCINES

Not since the Black Death of Europe during the middle ages has an infectious disease caused a global public health crisis on the same scale as the human immunodeficiency virus type 1 (HIV-1) pandemic. The acquired immune deficiency syndrome (AIDS), first described in the early 1980s, has reached the far corners of the globe, and has now become the leading cause of death for many populations throughout the developing world. According to recent UNAIDS estimates, at least 40 million adults and children have been infected with HIV-1, the virus that causes AIDS, and it is estimated that approximately 14,000 new infections occur daily or roughly 5 million new infections annually. The global burden of HIV/AIDS is most notable in Sub-Saharan Africa where over 70% of all infections have occurred and where the prevalence of HIV-1 has risen above 25% of the adult population in some countries within the southern region of Sub-Saharan Africa. Current projections indicate that while the epidemics in countries such as Botswana and the Republic of South Africa may have already peaked, having already reached saturation levels in at-risk populations, the next phase of the pandemic is rapidly expanding in other countries. For instance, recent reports indicate that Nigeria, Ethiopia, India, China, and Russia, nations with very large populations, are now experiencing burgeoning epidemics

that will likely have a serious regional impact on the epidemiology of the HIV/AIDS pandemic. These countries, which are now in the early growth phase of their respective epidemics, will likely experience a rapid increase in HIV incidence inevitably followed by a growing number of AIDS cases over the next decade. Even with serious efforts toward HIV/AIDS prevention and the effective implementation of public health measures, populations within these countries and their respective surrounding geographical regions are going to experience an increasing burden of disease that will be unprecedented in magnitude compared to any other single cause. To compound the problem, over 95% of HIV infections occur in resource-poor settings without ready access to antiretroviral treatment (ART) and where formidable challenges to the effective delivery and monitoring of ART still remain. In short, the HIV/AIDS pandemic represents the most serious infectious disease threat to global public health in history, and requires the urgent development of an effective vaccine that can control the epidemic spread of infection and can reduce the global burden of HIV/AIDS-related disease.

A. Challenges for Vaccine Development

Despite two decades of intense biomedical research into the biology of HIV and the pathogenesis of HIV/AIDS, basic questions regarding the underlying immunopathogenic mechanisms and determinants of effective antiviral immunity still remain. With the exception of those rare individuals harboring genetic mutations within genes expressing viral coreceptors (i.e., delta-32 CCR5), immunological correlates of protection in humans remain unknown or controversial. There are also inherent biological properties of HIV that make vaccine development a daunting task. Although not the focus of this chapter, it is important to note some of these

The authors wish to respectfully dedicate this chapter to Dr. Mary Lou Clements. Dr. Clements wrote the chapter for the previous edition of this book, and many of the studies reported here were influenced by her work prior to her untimely death on September 2, 1998 caused by the SwissAir 111 accident.

key factors including: (a) HIV's ability to establish molecular latency and persist in reservoirs of long-lived CD4$^+$ T cells; (b) its ability to infect immunopriviliged sites, such as the brain and eyes, that are relatively sequestered from immune responses; (c) its cellular tropism and preference to infect HIV-specific CD4$^+$ T lymphocytes, creating the potential for vaccine-induced CD4$^+$ T cells to provide a conduit rather than a barrier to infection; (d) its unprecedented ability to generate a diverse population of genetically distinct yet related strains (termed viral quasi-species); (e) structural features of the envelope that limit the effectiveness of neutralizing antibodies; and (f) its subsequent ability to evade vigorous attack mediated by both the humoral and cellular arms of antiviral immunity. These concepts have been reviewed elsewhere in more depth [1–6].

B. Prospects for Achieving Vaccine-Induced Immunity

Despite the discouraging news of expanding epidemics and the many biological challenges imposed by HIV, vaccine-induced immunity may be possible. First, prospective analyses of HIV transmission in sero-discordant couples in Uganda indicate that heterosexual transmission is relatively inefficient [7]. On average, several hundred exposures are required to cause one infection in settings of sexual transmission [8] or needle stick injuries [9]. Therefore, vaccines that induce even a modest improvement in antiviral defenses may have a profound impact on the transmissibility of HIV. Second, based on an analysis of HIV isolates in acute infection, most individuals are infected with a very small infectious inoculum of limited genotypic and phenotypic diversity [10,11]. This improves the chances that even modest preexisting vaccine-induced immunity could prevent or modify infection. In addition, there are examples of natural antiviral immunity from studies of highly exposed, uninfected commercial sex workers [12,13] and long-term nonprogressor [14,15] populations. Most importantly, there are also many examples of passive protection and vaccine-induced immunity in nonhuman primate models of lentivirus infection [16–28].

II. CLINICAL TRIALS OF HUMAN IMMUNODEFICIENCY VIRUS VACCINES

During the course of the last 15 years, there have been more than 30 HIV/AIDS vaccine concepts evaluated in more than 50 clinical trials that have involved approximately 12,500 volunteers. Most of these studies were small Phase I trials to determine the initial safety and immunogenicity profile of a particular approach. During this process, selected approaches that have prompted evaluation in larger-scale Phase II and Phase III studies emerged. This chapter will examine the rationale and merits of the three major "generations" of HIV vaccine approaches that have advanced to the stage of Phase II/III clinical evaluation, and will also describe newer concepts and combinations in the vaccine pipeline being evaluated in or considered for Phase I testing.

A. First-Generation Approaches—Envelope Glycoprotein Antigens

Initial approaches in the mid to late 1980s to produce vaccine antigens focused on recombinant protein subunit products based on safety and available technology. Most products were based on envelope glycoproteins, gp120 or gp160, because of their functional importance for virus attachment and entry, and as primary targets for neutralizing antibody. Recombinant subunit gp160 or gp120 has been produced in insects, yeast, or mammalian cells [29–33]; however, CHO-derived rgp120 emerged as the most immunogenic of the early subunit vaccines [32,33]. Several properties of subunit proteins limited the utility of this approach. For instance, serum antibody titers induced by gp120 products have a short half-life (<6 months), and although they can be boosted, the titers generally achieve their peak level after the third or fourth injections. Repeated boosting does not prolong the half-life significantly.

The rgp120 formulated in alum and produced by Genentech, the parent company of VaxGen, has progressed to Phase III efficacy evaluation in two trials. One study in the United States, Puerto Rico, and the Netherlands utilized VanGen B/B derived from HIV clade B strains LAI (one of the original T-cell line-adapted viruses) and GNE8 (a primary R5 isolate) enrolled 5108 gay and bisexual men and 309 women at high-risk of HIV infection. The other study, which is ongoing, utilizes VanGen B/E derived from HIV clade B LAI and clade E primary R5 isolate strain A244, and has thus far enrolled approximately 2500 injection drug users in Bangkok, Thailand. The participants received vaccine at 0, 1, 6 months, then an additional four booster injections at 6 month intervals. Preliminary results for the B/B study were announced at the Keystone meeting in March 2003. Overall there was no efficacy, with a 5.7% infection rate among vaccinees and 5.8% in placebo recipients. However, subset analyses suggested there may be evidence of protection among selected groups with the most extreme high-risk exposures. Although the subgroups are small, these data have stimulated additional analysis. Data from the Thailand study should be announced near the end of 2003.

The major concern about the immunogenicity of monomeric gp120 is that it can only elicit antibody and CD4$^+$ T-cell responses, and those antibodies are very type-specific, typically failing to neutralize commonly transmitted primary R5 HIV-1 isolates [34]. However, the advantage of these types of vaccine products lie in their safety. The ongoing Phase III trial analysis will hopefully teach us about the breadth, magnitude, and properties of envelope-specific antibody needed to protect against HIV-1. Further, the process of performing Phase III trials has also provided a number of lessons that will be valuable in future HIV vaccine efficacy trials (as discussed at the end of this chapter).

B. Second-Generation Approaches— Recombinant Poxvirus Vectors with or Without Recombinant Envelope Boosting

The eradication of smallpox using replication-competent attenuated vaccinia was one of the greatest achievements of medical science. This legacy of vaccine efficacy and the development of technology to express recombinant genes from poxviruses [35,36] (Chapter 29) led to the development of recombinant poxviruses as potential vaccine candidates for other pathogens. Importantly, the delivery of the vaccine by a vector allows the endogenous production and processing of the antigen, thereby promoting MHC class I epitope presentation and CD8$^+$ T-cell induction. Poxvirus vectors that express *gag* induce the production of pseudovirions from infected cells [37–39], and may have some immunological advantages that can be optimized by altering vector construction [40,41]. Early studies, beginning in the late 1980s, utilized live recombinant vaccinia [42,43], and they were indeed able to consistently induce long-lived CD8$^+$ cytotoxic T lymphocyte (CTL) responses in vaccinia-naive subjects [44–46]. However, concerns over the safety of replication-competent vaccinia, diminished immunogenicity caused by prior vaccinia seropositivity, and product supply issues prompted an evaluation of alternative recombinant poxvirus approaches.

Canarypox was the recombinant poxvirus vector that became available in the mid 1990s and was evaluated in a series of clinical trials. Canarypox is grown and manufactured in chicken embryo fibroblasts (CEFs) but is replication-incompetent in mammalian cells. Therefore, it can deliver its recombinant genes to the cytoplasm, where it provides all the machinery necessary for gene expression, but is unable to propagate itself to cause primary disease and has been proven safe even in profoundly immunocompromised animals. These vectors were produced by Aventis-Pasteur (formerly Pasteur-Merieux-Connaught) and studies were performed by French and U.S. investigators in the AIDS Vaccine Evaluation Group (AVEG) and the Walter Reed Army Institute of Research (WRAIR).

The constructs included a series of products that expressed gp160 (vCP125); gp120, gp41 (transmembrane), *gag*, and protease (vCP205); vCP205 plus selected epitopes from *nef* and *pol* (vCP300); vCP300 plus E3L and K3L genes from vaccinia that inhibit dsRNA; and interferon-inducible protein kinase, PKR; and that inhibited the apoptosis of the infected cell (vCP1452). More than 1000 subjects have been enrolled in studies of recombinant canarypox vectors expressing the HIV genes. The evaluation of these products has included dose ranging, a variety of injection schedules, combined administration by parenteral and mucosal routes, and combination with rgp120 envelope products. Some phase II studies have been conducted in developing countries with groups at relatively higher risk for HIV infection.

The data from these studies have shown canarypox vectors to be well tolerated at doses above 10^7 pfu, although local and systemic immunogenicity increased at the higher doses. The HIV-specific antibody response after recombinant canarypox immunization alone is weak, but subsequent boosting with purified recombinant envelope subunit protein induces HIV-specific antibody titers of the same or higher magnitude and quality as three or four inoculations of the purified recombinant envelope subunit protein alone [47,48]. The sequence of recombinant canarypox priming, followed by envelope subunit protein boosting, results in a slightly longer antibody half-life than immunization with purified protein alone. The HIV-specific CD8$^+$ CTL can be detected in fresh PBMCs from subjects immunized with recombinant canarypox virus vectors, and in a subset of individuals, the activity is detectable for > 2 years. The activity detected in classical ^{51}Cr release assays requires 2 weeks of in vitro stimulation and is detected in about 20% of subjects at any given time point [47–51]. Although these responses may be of marginal strength, recombinant canarypox-induced CTLs have been shown to lyse target cells infected with primary R5 HIV-1 isolates from multiple clades [52]. In addition, CD8$^+$ CTL effectors have been isolated from rectal mucosa (McElrath et al., unpublished observations), and both classical MHC class I-restricted cytolytic activity and nonlytic CD8$^+$-mediated HIV-1 suppression have been demonstrated in recipients of recombinant canarypox vaccines [53].

A pair of studies, performed by the HIV Vaccine Trials Network (HVTN), evaluated vCP1452 in combination with VaxGen rgp120 B/B at U.S. (HVTN 203) and international sites (HIVNET 026 was performed in Haiti, Brazil, and Trinidad and Tobago). The primary objective of these studies was to determine a correlate of immunity and to define whether T-cell immunogenicity could be elicited and measured at a high-enough frequency to conduct a specially designed efficacy trial (HVTN 501). To qualify for that particular study design, a frequency of about 30% was required. Unfortunately, this frequency of vaccine-induced CTL response was not achieved, and the HVTN 501 efficacy trial initially designed with vCP1452 was cancelled. However, there are still plans to perform a more conventional efficacy trial in Thailand using a recombinant canarypox (vCP1521) constructed like vCP205, but with the envelope gene derived from a clade E HIV isolate.

This trial will include booster injections of the VaxGen B/E rgp 120 and will evaluate protection from heterosexual HIV transmission, and should therefore answer some of the questions raised in the subset analysis of the initial rgp120 Phase III study.

C. Third-Generation Approaches—More Potent Gene Delivery Vehicles Alone or in Combination with DNA Vaccination

As the focus shifted away from monomeric envelope subunit vaccines in the mid 1990s, the development of several new strategies for the induction of strong CD8$^+$ CTL responses emerged while recombinant canarypox vectors were being actively investigated in clinical trials. This effort has culminated in a series of successful vaccine studies utilizing the SHIV macaque model. These studies have helped to form the basis for the current paradigm that a sufficiently high vaccine-induced CD8$^+$ CTL can control lentivirus infection. These studies utilized either recombinant modified vaccinia Ankara (rMVA) or replication-incompetent recombinant adenovirus (rAd) alone or in combination with deoxyribonucleic acid (DNA) immunization [24–28,54], and have provided a direction for the next series of large-scale clinical trials. In particular, there is interest in combinations of DNA priming followed by MVA [26,54] (Chapter 34) or rAd [27] boosting as a potent mechanism for inducing high levels of HIV-specific CD8$^+$ CTL responses.

The initial product concept being advanced into clinical trials by the NIAID Vaccine Research Center (VRC)—a new intramural program on the campus of the National Institutes of Health focused on the development of an HIV/AIDS vaccine—is based on the following basic assumptions: (a) CD8$^+$ CTL can control infection, but an antibody to the envelope will be critical for preventing infections and achieving sterilizing immunity; (b) it is essential to induce a broad immune response against a large number of epitopes; and (c) the vaccine should represent the major subtypes of viruses causing new HIV infections worldwide. The leading VRC vaccine candidate includes envelope constructs [55] as well as a *gag/pol/nef* fusion gene [56], thereby representing the majority of the HIV genome. The envelope genes are derived from viruses in clades A, B, and C, representing the subtypes causing nearly 90% of new HIV infections worldwide. The vaccine includes a cocktail of four DNA plasmids given as a series of priming injections followed by a booster injection of four replication-incompetent recombinant adenoviruses expressing a matching set of genes. All the genes have been codon-modified to reduce the content of AT-rich regions that inhibit nuclear export of message, allowing high levels of rev-independent protein expression. The DNA is delivered intramuscularly by a needleless injection system, Biojector®, that sprays the injectate into the muscle in a pattern that improves the overall gene expression. The combination of DNA priming and rAd boosting is the most potent vaccine regimen discovered to date for the induction of CD8$^+$ CTL responses.

The development of DNA vaccines is reviewed in Chapter 33, and replication-competent recombinant adenovirus vectors are discussed in Chapter 30. However, the rAd being used in the VRC vaccine approach and an approach being promoted by Merck and Co., Inc. utilize a replication-defective virus, a vehicle for gene delivery borrowed from the gene therapy field. The rAd vectors are produced by inserting the recombinant genes of interest into the E1 gene cassette of the adenovirus genome and by producing the rAd particles in a cell line that constitutively expresses complementary E1 genes (PER.C6 or 293-ORF6). In addition, portions of the E3 or E4 region are removed from the vector genome to make room for larger recombinant genes.

The extensive clinical experience of utilizing rAd vectors provides some advantages to this approach. Hundreds of patients have already been treated with rAd vectors as gene therapy for cancer, cardiovascular diseases, cystic fibrosis, and other diseases. Many of the hurdles that have faced the development of gene therapy turn out to be ideal properties for vector-based gene delivery of vaccine antigens. These include: (a) relatively transient expression; (b) lack of integration into host cell genome; and (c) induction of immune responses to the recombinant gene products. Although intravascular injection of rAd has been associated with a highly publicized case of fatal outcome in an 18-year-old patient with a rare liver condition at the University of Pennsylvania (Reuters Health Information, January 26, 2001), when given intradermally or intramuscularly, rAd vectors have been well tolerated at high doses. Importantly, the delivery of recombinant genes is efficient and immuno-

genic. This may be due to the nature of rAd production, which can achieve extremely high yields of concentrated particles, allowing the delivery of a 10- to 100-fold higher particle dose above currently available recombinant poxvirus candidates. Because this is a nonreplicating gene delivery vehicle, the effective dose delivered correlates with the overall level of recombinant gene expression and subsequent immune response.

The major challenges for the implementation of rAd vectors for vaccines include the technical aspects of building a stable vector and overcoming preexisting immunity to the adenovirus vector. Current candidate vaccines are produced using an adenovirus serotype 5 (Ad5) packaging system; Ad5 seroprevalence is high throughout the world. However, significant progress has been made to develop alternative serotype packaging systems that should overcome any problems associated with preexisting adenovirus immunity.

III. FUTURE CONCEPTS IN THE PIPELINE FOR HUMAN IMMUNODEFICIENCY VIRUS VACCINE CLINICAL TRIALS

A. New Deoxyribonucleic Acid Vaccine Approaches

As noted above and in Chapter 33, bacterial DNA plasmids are being explored as a method of gene delivery and immunization in many HIV vaccine concepts. In addition to the use of DNA for priming individuals prior to boosting with recombinant virus vectors, DNA plasmids encoding HIV-derived genes are being used as a primer for subsequent envelope subunit protein administration and are being given in combination with plasmids encoding an IL-2–Ig fusion protein as an adjuvant [25]. Because of the versatility of DNA vaccine construction and the relative ease in manufacturing, new concepts in antigen design are being investigated using this delivery approach. For example, antigens designed by investigators at Epimmune Inc. include a series of T-cell epitopes from a variety of HIV-1 subtypes, relevant for major HLA class I supertypes (groups of MHC class I haplotypes that process and present identical epitopes) [57]. An artificial gene encoding the relevant epitopes is designed to facilitate the processing of individual epitopes and is delivered by DNA plasmids. Poor delivery or immunogenicity is the major challenge for DNA vaccines being developed for HIV. Although this modality allows enormous flexibility in design, immunogenicity in humans has been marginal. Efforts to improve delivery and expression are ongoing and include the use of specialized delivery devices as mentioned above under the VRC program, adjuvants such as the nonionic block copolymer (CRL1005) [27], or attachment to poly(lactide-coglycolide) (PLG) microparticles [58].

B. Synthetic Peptides

Using peptides as immunogens is an attractive approach because: (a) they are safe; (b) large quantities can be prepared relatively inexpensively; (c) they are made synthetically and are therefore free of contaminating host materials;

(d) immune responses to precise specificities can be induced; (e) multiple epitopes with desirable immunogenic properties can easily be combined in a single formulation; and (f) theoretically, they can be presented through either the MHC class I or II pathways. There are, however, major limitations of the peptide vaccine approach, which include the following: (a) the breadth of antigenic sites within a given formulation may be too narrow; (b) conformational epitopes are difficult to represent; and (c) historically, peptides have not been as immunogenic as more complex antigens. Several approaches have been taken to produce peptide immunogens as candidate AIDS vaccines. First, peptides based on the V3 loop sequence from one or multiple HIV-1 strains have been covalently linked to an oligolysine backbone and formulated with alum for intramuscular injection, or in poly(DL-lactide-coglycolide) microspheres for mucosal administration. Unfortunately, products based on this technology have not been immunogenic in humans [59]. Another approach has been to synthesize a hybrid linear peptide consisting of helper T-cell, B-cell, and CTL epitopes formulated in incomplete Freund's adjuvant [60,61]. Although this approach was found to be immunogenic in humans, the product as formulated in incomplete Freund's adjuvant as a strong emulsion caused sterile abscess formation in some participants; thus, the trial was stopped prematurely. New formulations are currently in development, and other groups have made peptide–lipid conjugates. Initial studies of a *gag*-based peptide were disappointing (unpublished observations), but newer formulations have shown more promise and are being studied in early phase clinical trials [62].

C. Live Recombinant Virus Vectors

Live recombinant viruses as expression vectors for HIV-1 gene products hold several attractions: (a) immunogens are presented in the context of natural infection (i.e., oligomeric glycoprotein is expressed in infected cell membranes, with native conformation and glycosylation patterns); (b) antigens are processed by and presented in the context of MHC class I molecules leading to CTL responses; (c) multiple antigens, diverse strain specificities, or immune modifiers may be simultaneously expressed; (d) administration by percutaneous or mucosal routes is relatively simple; and (e) production and delivery are inexpensive. Live bacterial vectors have similar advantages although the posttranslational processing of viral protein will differ from that of mammalian processes, and the induction of MHC class I-restricted CTL may be less efficient. An advantage of bacterial vectors is that the constituents of the vector may provide additional adjuvant properties. Each approach offers unique advantages and disadvantages often related to the tropism and virulence of the parent vector. Further, preexisting immunity is an additional challenge that these types of approaches must face.

Adenovirus vectors have several desirable features, including feasibility of oral delivery with gut replication, induction of systemic and mucosal immunity after a single oral dose, and a record of safe use for the prevention of respiratory diseases in the U.S. military (the reader is referred to an excellent discussion on the development of a

live attenuated recombinant adenovirus vaccine for HIV in Chapter 30). Other viral vectors that have been investigated include polio [63–65], influenza [66], rhinovirus [67,68], and hepatitis B [69,70] chimeras. These vectors are of interest because of their ability to induce mucosal immune responses. Their major limitations are the amount of foreign genome that can be accommodated and the virulence properties of the parent vector.

D. Live Recombinant Bacterial Vectors

Several approaches utilizing bacterial vectors have been developed as approaches for HIV/AIDS vaccines. Attenuated *Salmonella* has been developed as a vaccine vehicle to deliver recombinant HIV antigens [71,72] or recombinant plasmid DNA, and are being introduced into clinical testing (discussed in detail in Chapter 32). Recombinant bacille Calmette–Guérin (BCG) constructs that express HIV-1 *gag*, *pol*, and *env* gene products have also been developed. These products can induce antibody, helper T-cell, and CTL responses in mice [73,74] and macaques [75]. Some future improvements of BCG vectors may include the coexpression of selected recombinant cytokine genes [76]. *Listeria monocytogenes* is mentioned here as another potential live recombinant bacterial vector, but its development has advanced only to the level of testing in small animal models [77,78]. As previously mentioned, the potential virulence of the parent organism and prior immunity to the vector should be underscored as major concerns for safety and immunogenicity, respectively, in the development of live vector approaches.

E. Replication-Defective Virus-Based Vectors or Gene Delivery Vehicles

There is a diverse array of defective virus-based vectors and gene delivery vehicles being developed as candidate HIV vaccines, but only the ones likely to reach clinical trials in the short term will be emphasized here. A vaccine expressing *gag* from a HIV-1 clade C isolate in a Venezuelan equine encephalitis (VEE) virus vector is being prepared for clinical testing and has been described in Chapter 31. The advantage of this vector as well as one derived from Sindbis virus, another alphavirus, lies in their unique abilities to target [79,80] specialized antigen presentation cells. Adeno-associated virus (AAV) [81,82], retroviruses [83], and recombinant replication-defective herpes simplex virus (HSV) [84,85] are mentioned as approaches that may provide a more prolonged antigen expression than the other gene delivery approaches discussed, but concerns about integration may limit their entry into clinical trials of preventive HIV vaccines.

F. Replication-Defective Fungi-Based and Bacteria-Based Vectors or Gene Delivery Vehicles

Heat-killed recombinant *Saccharomyces cerevisiae* is a novel approach for delivering vaccine antigens that may enter clinical trial evaluation within the next year. The yeast particles express HIV antigens and, when phagocytized by dendritic cells, that antigen is available for presentation in both class I and class II MHC molecules [86]. A similar approach has been suggested for *Brucella abortus* [87], but has only been tested in rodents to date.

G.   New Subunit Protein Vaccines

As noted, one of the critical needs in HIV vaccine development is to find ways of eliciting broadly neutralizing antibodies against primary CCR5 utilizing HIV isolates. One of the leading concepts for accomplishing that goal is to produce oligomeric envelope structures. Several groups have made oligomeric envelope proteins that mimic envelope structures more likely to exist in vivo [88–90]. The product from Chiron Corporation, derived from a primary HIV isolate SF162 and based on a V2-deleted gp140 envelope construct, is being prepared for clinical evaluation. In addition to producing oligomeric structures, a number of groups are pursuing methods to present a "receptor-triggered" envelope conformation to the immune system. Recently, a CD4–gp120 env single-chain fusion protein has been shown to elicit some degree of neutralizing antibody responses in mice and Rhesus macaques [91]. However, the extent to which those responses are directed against viral gp120 targets versus human CD4 epitopes contained within the fusion construct remains to be determined. Another controversial vaccine approach has involved the use of tat protein as an immunogen. GlaxoSmithKline has developed a nef–tat fusion protein being evaluated in clinical trials in combination with a monomeric rgp120 protein. This product and tat-protein-only vaccine concepts [92] are currently being evaluated in clinical trials. However, no data as of yet are available for review.

H.   Strategies for Vaccine Adjuvants and Delivery Systems

The adjuvant component of a vaccine can determine the composition, magnitude, and duration of the immune response to the antigenic component of the vaccine formulation. These concepts are being applied in HIV vaccine development and are topics discussed in more detail elsewhere [93] and in other chapters of this book. Of particular note has been the advancement of cytokine adjuvants in HIV vaccine evaluation. Granulocyte–macrophage colony-stimulating factor (GM-CSF) has been delivered with canarypox vectors, and clinical studies are in the planning phase for using IL-2–Ig plasmid in combination with the VRC plasmids expressing *gag/pol/nef* and multiclade envelope genes [94], and IL-12 in combination with a peptide cocktail.

IV.   CONSIDERATIONS FOR PHASE III TRIAL DESIGN WITH VACCINES THAT CONTROL, RATHER THAN PREVENT, INFECTION

With the current generation of vaccines being developed that are based largely on the induction of CD8$^+$ CTL responses,

it is possible that efficacy will be manifest by controlling, rather than preventing, infection. Animal models of vaccine protection from lentivirus challenge using the kinds of approaches being studied in current clinical trials have indicated that this type of approach may be successful [24–28]. It is hoped that in natural settings of HIV transmission where relatively low inoculum and transmission efficiency occur, studies of vaccines based solely on the induction of CD8$^+$ CTL may achieve some level of sterilizing immunity. However, for the design of efficacy trials, the assumption will be made that the HIV vaccines currently being tested will control, rather than prevent, infection.

This raises a number of issues that have not existed for the efficacy evaluation of vaccines for other infectious diseases. One practical issue raised is the length of follow-up period required for a study in which research questions are asked concerning disease progression, rather than the absence or presence of infection. Subsequent endpoints might include: (a) the magnitude of the peak in viral load during acute infections and the viral load set point during early-established infection; (b) the slope of the CD4$^+$ T cell counts; or (c) the length of time-to-treatment according to predetermined criteria. Another practical consideration is the mechanism for diagnosing and distinguishing HIV infection from vaccination. Most of the current vaccines will be complex in that they will likely induce responses to multiple genes. Therefore, serological assays will not be sufficient to readily distinguish between infection and vaccine-induced responses. This means that gene-based diagnostics will be necessary on a regular basis to detect HIV infection in its early stages. Another major consideration in the organization of efficacy trials for a partially effective vaccine is the standardization and maintenance of sexual risk reduction counseling, and the accurate monitoring of sexual risk-taking activities. This will require enormous time and resources, but will be essential for interpreting the outcome of the study. Increasing HIV infection risk among vaccinees could mask the impact of vaccination.

Of equal importance in the design and management of efficacy trials for HIV vaccines will be the provision of ART for subjects who become infected during the trial period. One reason for providing ART as part of the study is to make it possible to use time-to-treatment as a study endpoint. Another reason is to standardize the treatment regimens so that control of viremia can be a longer-term endpoint for the study. There are also ethical considerations, as the efficacy trials will be performed in both developed and developing countries simultaneously, and access to ART for subjects who need it will not be equal if it is not provided as part of the study. This will incur significant expenses and will add a layer of complexity at trial sites required to diagnose and manage the initial stages of HIV infection.

If the vaccine's greatest impact is on the viral load of persons subsequently infected (despite vaccination), then a potential measurement of efficacy could be the reduction of secondary transmission [95]. Designing studies within or between communities to assess the rates of spread to those not participating in these studies will be necessary to determine these types of population effects, and are not a standard element of prelicensure vaccine evaluation. It is intriguing to consider the implication of recently published studies on other sexually transmitted diseases, showing vaccine-induced protection of human papilloma virus [96] and herpes simplex virus [97], on the approach to trial design. These studies highlight the ability of parenterally administered vaccines to protect women from HPV and HSV, and suggest that gender-specific efficacy trials should be considered for HIV vaccine evaluation. This type of subject selection also provides a mechanism to evaluate the secondary spread to male partners of female subjects who become infected despite vaccination.

The evaluation of "breakthrough" infections in Phase II and Phase III studies will be another critical part of defining the efficacy of HIV vaccines, and will require a level of detailed analysis of virus genotypes and host immune responses that has never been attempted on this large a scale for any other pathogen. For vaccines that control, rather than prevent, infection, it will be important to determine the specificity and breadth of immune responses necessary for control and to define the thresholds that allow immune escape and disease progression. For vaccines that only prevent a subset of virus strains from infecting the vaccinated host, it will be important to determine which viruses were excluded and why. This may be best accomplished in areas where diverse strains of HIV are responsible for multiple concurrent epidemics, where the chances for exposure to viruses that could escape preexisting immunity would be the highest.

Our aim in this chapter was to highlight some of the major challenges that exist for HIV vaccine development, and to provide a conceptual context for organizing and ranking the current products advancing to clinical trials. This discussion is by no means exhaustive. Interested readers are referred to other chapters contained in this volume and recent reviews that provide more detail. Human immunodeficiency virus is a formidable opponent and will take sustained, intense, and thoughtful effort to overcome. Although there are many biological and logistic obstacles remaining, we believe that vaccine development remains the best hope of controlling the HIV/AIDS pandemic, and that advancing new product concepts to Phase III testing is the next critical step in the process.

Internet sites for updates of ongoing clinical trials for HIV vaccines: http://www.iavi.org/trialsdb/basicsearch-form.asp; http://www.hvtn.org/trials; and http://vrc.nih.gov/clintrials/clinslides.htm.

REFERENCES

1. Graham BS. Clinical trials of HIV vaccines. Annu Rev Med 2002; 53:207–221.
2. Johnson WE, Desrosiers RC. Viral persistence: HIV's strategies of immune system evasion. Annu Rev Med 2002; 53:499–518.
3. Blankson JN, Persaud D, Siliciano RF. The challenge of viral reservoirs in HIV-1 infection. Annu Rev Med 2002; 53:557–593.
4. Gandhi RT, Walker BD. Immunologic control of HIV-1. Annu Rev Med 2002; 53:149–172.
5. Gaschen B, et al. Diversity considerations in HIV-1 vaccine selection. Science 2002; 296:2354–2360.

6. Douek DC, et al. HIV preferentially infects HIV-specific CD4$^+$ T cells. Nature 2002; 417:95–98.
7. Quinn TC, et al. Viral load and heterosexual transmission of human immunodeficiency virus type 1. Rakai Project Study Group. N Engl J Med 2000; 342:921–929.
8. Gray RH, et al. Probability of HIV-1 transmission per coital act in monogamous, heterosexual, HIV-1-discordant couples in Rakai, Uganda. Lancet 2001; 357:1149–1153.
9. Geberding JL. Incidence and prevalence of human immunodeficiency virus, hepatitis B virus, hepatitis C virus, and cytomegalovirus among health care personnel at risk for blood exposure: final report from a longitudinal study. J Infect Dis 1994; 170:1410–1417.
10. Wolinsky SM, et al. Selective transmission of human immunodeficiency virus type-1 variants from mothers to infants. Science 1992; 255:1134–1137.
11. Wolfs TF, et al. HIV-1 genomic RNA diversification following sexual and parenteral virus transmission. Virology 1992; 189:103–110.
12. Fowke KR, et al. Resistance to HIV-1 infection among persistently seronegative prostitutes in Nairobi, Kenya. Lancet 1996; 348:1347–1351.
13. Rowland-Jones S, et al. HIV-specific cytotoxic T-cells in HIV-exposed but uninfected Gambian women. Nat Med 1995; 1:59–64.
14. Wagner R, et al. Molecular and functional analysis of a conserved CTL epitope in HIV-1 p24 recognized from a long-term nonprogressor: constraints on immune escape associated with targeting a sequence essential for viral replication. J Immunol 1999; 162:3727–3734.
15. Migueles SA, Connors M. The role of CD4(+) and CD8(+) T cells in controlling HIV infection. Curr Infect Dis Rep 2002; 4:461–467.
16. Prince AM, et al. Prevention of HIV infection by passive immunization with HIV immunoglobulin. AIDS Res Hum Retrovir 1991; 7:971–973.
17. Emini EA, et al. Prevention of HIV-1 infection in chimpanzees by gp120 V3 domain-specific monoclonal antibody. Nature 1992; 355:728–730.
18. Putkonen P, et al. Prevention of HIV-2 and SIV$_{sm}$ infection by passive immunization in cynomolgus monkeys. Nature 1991; 352:436–438.
19. Van Rompay KK, et al. Passive immunization of newborn rhesus macaques prevents oral simian immunodeficiency virus infection. J Infect Dis 1998; 177:1247–1259.
20. Shibata R, et al. Neutralizing antibody directed against the HIV-1 envelope glycoprotein can completely block HIV-1/SIV chimeric virus infections of macaque monkeys. Nat Med 1999; 5:204–210.
21. Mascola JR, et al. Protection of macaques against pathogenic simian/human immunodeficiency virus 89.6PD by passive transfer of neutralizing antibodies. J Virol 1999; 73:4009–4018.
22. Baba TW, et al. Human neutralizing monoclonal antibodies of the IgG1 subtype protect against mucosal simian–human immunodeficiency virus infection. Nat Med 2000; 6:200–206.
23. Mascola JR, et al. Protection of macaques against vaginal transmission of a pathogenic HIV-1/SIV chimeric virus by passive infusion of neutralizing antibodies. Nat Med 2000; 6:207–210.
24. Seth A, et al. Immunization with a modified vaccinia virus expressing simian immunodeficiency virus (SIV) Gag–Pol primes for an anamnestic Gag-specific cytotoxic T-lymphocyte response and is associated with reduction of viremia after SIV challenge. J Virol 2000; 74:2502–2509.
25. Barouch DH, et al. Control of viremia and prevention of clinical AIDS in rhesus monkeys by cytokine-augmented DNA vaccination. Science 2000; 290:486–492.
26. Amara RR, et al. Control of a mucosal challenge and pre-

vention of AIDS by a multiprotein DNA/MVA vaccine. Science 2001; 292:69–74.

27. Shiver JW, et al. Replication-incompetent adenoviral vaccine vector elicits effective anti-immunodeficiency-virus immunity. Nature 2002; 415:331–335.

28. Rose NF, et al. An effective AIDS vaccine based on live attenuated vesicular stomatitis virus recombinants. Cell 2001; 106:539–549.

29. Dolin R, et al. The safety and immunogenicity of a human immunodeficiency virus type 1 (HIV-1) recombinant gp160 candidate vaccine in humans. NIAID AIDS Vaccine Clinical Trials Network. Ann Intern Med 1991; 114:119–127.

30. Keefer MC, et al. Safety and immunogenicity of Env 2–3, a human immunodeficiency virus type 1 candidate vaccine, in combination with a novel adjuvant, MTP-PE/MF59. AIDS Res Hum Retrovir 1996; 12:683–693.

31. Belshe RB, et al. Safety and immunogenicity of a fully gly-cosylated recombinant gp160 human immunodeficiency virus type 1 vaccine in subjects at low risk of infection. J Infect Dis 1993; 168:1387–1395.

32. Graham BS, et al. Safety and immunogenicity of a candidate HIV-1 vaccine in healthy adults: recombinant glycoprotein (rgp) 120-A randomized, double-blind trial. Ann Intern Med 1996; 125:270–279.

33. Belshe RB, et al. Neutralizing antibodies to HIV-1 in sero-negative volunteers immunized with recombinant gp120 from the MN strain of HIV-1. NIAID AIDS Vaccine Clinical Trials Network. JAMA 1994; 272:475–480.

34. Berman PW, et al. Development of bivalent (B/E) vaccines able to neutralize CCR5-dependent viruses from the United States and Thailand. Virology 1999; 265:1–9.

35. Moss B. Vaccinia virus: a tool for research and vaccine de-velopment. Science 1991; 252:1662–1667.

36. Panicali D, Paoletti E. Construction of poxvirus as cloning vectors: insertion of the thymidine kinase gene from herpes simplex virus into the DNA of infectious vaccinia virus. Proc Natl Acad Sci USA 1982; 79:4927–4931.

37. Haffar O, et al. Human immunodeficiency virus-like, non-replicating, gag–env particles assemble in a recombinant vac-cinia virus expression system. J Virol 1990; 64:2653–2659.

38. Shioda T, Shibuta H. Production of human immunodeficiency virus (HIV)-like particles from cells infected with recombinant vaccinia viruses carrying the gag gene of HIV. Virology 1990; 175:139–148.

39. Spearman P, et al. Identification of human immunodeficiency virus type 1 Gag protein domains essential to membrane binding and particle assembly. J Virol 1994; 68:3232–3242.

40. Fang ZY, et al. Expression of vaccinia E3L and K3L genes by a novel recombinant canarypox HIV vaccine vector enhances HIV-1 pseudovirion production and inhibits apoptosis in human cells. Virology 2001; 291:272–284.

41. Fang ZY, et al. Efficient human immunodeficiency virus (HIV)-1 Gag–Env pseudovirion formation elicited from mam-malian cells by a canarypox HIV vaccine candidate. J Infect Dis 1999; 180:1122–1132.

42. Graham BS, et al. Vaccination of vaccinia-naive adults with human immunodeficiency virus type 1 gp160 recombinant vaccinia virus in a blinded, controlled, randomized clinical trial. J Infect Dis 1992; 166:244–252.

43. Cooney EL, et al. Enhanced immunity to human immunode-ficiency virus (HIV) envelope elicited by a combined vaccine regimen consisting of priming with a vaccinia recombinant expressing HIV envelope and boosting with gp160 protein. Proc Natl Acad Sci USA 1993; 90:1882–1886.

44. Corey L, et al. Cytotoxic T cell and neutralizing antibody responses to HIV-1 envelope with a combination vaccine re-gimen. J Infect Dis 1998; 177:301–309.

45. Hammond SA, et al. Comparative clonal analysis of human immunodeficiency virus type 1 (HIV-1)-specific CD4$^+$ and CD8$^+$ cytolytic T lymphocytes isolated from seronegative humans immunized with candidate HIV-1 vaccines. J Exp Med 1992; 176:1531–1542.

46. El-Daher N, et al. Persisting human immunodeficiency virus type 1 gp160-specific human T lymphocyte responses includ-ing CD8$^+$ cytotoxic activity after receipt of envelope vaccines. J Infect Dis 1993; 168:306–313.

47. Clements-Mann ML, et al. HIV-1 immune responses induced by canarypox (ALVAC)-gp160 MN, SF-2 rgp120, or both vaccines in seronegative adults. J Infect Dis 1998; 177:1230–1246.

48. Evans TG, et al. A canarypox vaccine expressing multiple HIV-1 genes given alone or with rgp120 elicits broad and durable CD8$^+$ CTL responses in seronegative volunteers. J Infect Dis 1999; 180:290–298.

49. Belshe RB, et al. Induction of immune responses to HIV-1 by canarypox virus (ALVAC) HIV-1 and gp120 SF-2 recombi-nant vaccines in uninfected volunteers. AIDS 1998; 12:2407–2415.

50. Salmon-Ceron D, et al. Safety and immunogenicity of a live recombinant canarypox virus expressing HIV type 1 gp120 MN tm/gag/protease LAI (ALVAC-HIV, vCP205) followed by a p24E-V3 MN synthetic peptide (CLTB-36) administered in healthy volunteers at low risk for HIV infection. AIDS Res Hum Retrovir 1999; 15:633–645.

51. Belshe RB, et al. Safety and immunogenicity of a canarypox-vectored human immunodeficiency virus type 1 vaccine with or without gp120: a phase 2 study in higher- and lower-risk volunteers. J Infect Dis 2001; 183:1343–1352.

52. Ferrari G, et al. Clade B-based HIV-1 vaccines elicit cross-clade cytotoxic T lymphocyte reactivities in uninfected vo-lunteers. Proc Natl Acad Sci USA 1997; 94:1396–1401.

53. Castillo RC, et al. Resistance to human immunodeficiency virus type 1 in vitro as a surrogate of vaccine-induced pro-tective immunity. J Infect Dis 2000; 181:897–903.

54. Hanke T, et al. Development of a DNA–MVA/HIVA vaccine for Kenya. Vaccine 2002; 20:1995–1998.

55. Chakrabarti BK, et al. Modifications of the human immuno-deficiency virus envelope glycoprotein enhance immunoge-nicity for genetic immunization. J Virol 2002; 76:5357–5368.

56. Huang Y, et al. Human immunodeficiency virus type 1-specific immunity after genetic immunization is enhanced by modification of Gag and Pol expression. J Virol 2001; 75:4947–4951.

57. Altfeld MA, et al. Identification of novel HLA-A2-restricted HIV-1-specific CTL epitopes predicted by the HLA-A2 supertype peptide-binding motif. J Virol 2001; 75:1301–1311.

58. O'Hagan D, et al. Induction of potent immune responses by cationic microparticles with adsorbed human immunodefi-ciency virus DNA vaccines. J Virol 2001; 75:9037–9043.

59. Lambert JS, et al. A Phase I safety and immunogenicity trial of UBI microparticulate monovalent HIV-1 MN oral peptide immunogen with parenteral boost in HIV-1 seronegative human subjects. Vaccine 2001; 19:3033–3042.

60. Palker TJ, et al. Polyvalent human immunodeficiency virus synthetic immunogen comprised of envelope gp120 T helper cell sites and B cell neutralization epitopes. J Immunol 1989; 142:3612–3619.

61. Ahlers JD, et al. Candidate HIV type 1 multideterminant cluster peptide–P18MN vaccine constructs elicit type 1 helper T cells, cytotoxic T cells, and neutralizing antibody, all using the same adjuvant immunization. AIDS Res Hum Retrovir 1996; 12:259–272.

62. Gahery-Segard H, et al. Multiepitopic B- and T-cell responses induced in humans by a human immunodeficiency virus type 1 lipopeptide vaccine. J Virol 2000; 74:1694–1703.

63. Porter DC, et al. Immunization of mice with poliovirus

replicons expressing the C-fragment of tetanus toxin protects against lethal challenge with tetanus toxin. Vaccine 1997; 15:257–264.

64. Porter DC, et al. Encapsidation of genetically engineered poliovirus minireplicons which express human immunodeficiency virus type 1 Gag and Pol proteins upon infection. J Virol 1993; 67:3712–3719.

65. Crotty S, et al. Protection against simian immunodeficiency virus vaginal challenge by using Sabin poliovirus vectors. J Virol 2001; 75:7435–7452.

66. Muster T, et al. Mucosal model of immunization against human immunodeficiency virus type 1 with a chimeric influenza virus. J Virol 1996; 69:6678–6686.

67. Arnold GF, et al. Chimeric rhinoviruses as tools for vaccine development and characterization of protein epitopes. Intervirology 1996; 39:72–78.

68. Zhang A, et al. A disulfide-bound HIV-1 V3 loop sequence on the surface of human rhinovirus 14 induces neutralizing responses against HIV-1. J Biol Chem 1999; 380:365–374.

69. Grene E, et al. Relationship between antigenicity and immunogenicity of chimeric hepatitis B virus core particles carrying HIV type 1 epitopes. AIDS Res Hum Retrovir 1997; 13:41–51.

70. Koletzki D, et al. Mosaic hepatitis B virus core particles allow insertion of extended foreign protein segments. J Gen Virol 1997; 78:2053–2059.

71. Cattozzo EM, et al. Expression and immunogenicity of V3 loop epitopes of HIV-1, isolates SC and WMJ2, inserted in *Salmonella flagellin.* J Biotechnol 1997; 56:191–203.

72. Hone DM, et al. Optimization of live oral *Salmonella*–HIV-1 vaccine vectors for the induction of HIV-specific mucosal and systemic immune responses. J Biotechnol 1996; 44:203–207.

73. Aldovini A, Young RA. Humoral and cell-mediated immune responses to live recombinant BCG–HIV vaccines. Nature 1991; 351:479–482.

74. Stover CK, et al. New use of BCG for recombinant vaccines. Nature 1991; 351:456–460.

75. Leung NJ, et al. The kinetics of specific immune responses in rhesus monkeys inoculated with live recombinant BCG expressing SIV Gag, Pol, Env, and Nef proteins. Virology 2000; 268:94–103.

76. Murray PJ, et al. Manipulation and potentiation of antimycobacterial immunity using recombinant bacille Calmette–Guérin strains that secrete cytokines. Proc Natl Acad Sci USA 1996; 93:934–939.

77. Frankel FR, et al. Induction of cell-mediated immune responses to human immunodeficiency virus type 1 gag protein by using *Listeria monocytogenes* as a live vaccine vector. J Immunol 1995; 155:4775–4782.

78. Lieberman J, Frankel FR. Engineered *Listeria monocytogenes* as an AIDS vaccine. Vaccine 2002; 20:2007–2010.

79. Caley IJ, et al. Humoral, mucosal, and cellular immunity in response to a human immunodeficiency virus type 1 immunogen expressed by a Venezuelan equine encephalitis virus vaccine vector. J Virol 1997; 71:3031–3038.

80. Davis NL, et al. A viral vaccine vector that expresses foreign genes in lymph nodes and protects against mucosal challenge. J Virol 1996; 70:3781–3787.

81. Manning WC, et al. Genetic immunization with adeno-associated virus vectors expressing herpes simplex virus type 2 glycoproteins B and D. J Virol 1997; 71:7960–7962.

82. Liu X, et al. Selective Rep–Cap gene amplification as a mechanism for high-titer recombinant AAV production from stable cell lines. Mol Ther 2000; 2:394–403.

83. Irwin MJ, et al. Direct injection of a recombinant retroviral vector induces human immunodeficiency virus-specific immune responses in mice and nonhuman primates. J Virol 1994; 68:5036–5044.

84. Hocknell PK, et al. Expression of human immunodeficiency virus type 1 gp120 from herpes simplex virus type 1-derived amplicons results in potent, specific, and durable cellular and humoral immune responses. J Virol 2002; 76:5565–5580.

85. Murphy CG, et al. Vaccine protection against simian immunodeficiency virus by recombinant strains of herpes simplex virus. J Virol 2000; 74:7745–7754.

86. Stubbs AC, et al. Whole recombinant yeast vaccine activates dendritic cells and elicits protective cell-mediated immunity. Nat Med 2001; 7:625–629.

87. Lapham C, et al. *Brucella abortus* conjugated with a peptide derived from the V3 loop of human immunodeficiency virus (HIV) type 1 induces HIV-specific cytotoxic T-cell responses in normal and in CD4[+] cell-depleted BALB/c mice. J Virol 1996; 70:3084–3092.

88. Yang X, et al. Improved elicitation of neutralizing antibodies against primary human immunodeficiency viruses by soluble stabilized envelope glycoprotein trimers. J Virol 2001; 75: 1165–1171.

89. Schulke N, et al. Oligomeric and conformational properties of a proteolytically mature, disulfide-stabilized human immunodeficiency virus type 1 gp140 envelope glycoprotein. J Virol 2002; 76:7760–7776.

90. Srivastava IK, et al. Purification and characterization of oligomeric envelope glycoprotein from a primary R5 subtype B human immunodeficiency virus. J Virol 2002; 76:2835–2847.

91. Fouts T, et al. Crosslinked HIV-1 envelope–CD4 receptor complexes elicit broadly cross-reactive neutralizing antibodies in rhesus macaques. Proc Natl Acad Sci USA 2002; 99:11842–11847.

92. Fanales-Belasio E, et al. HIV-1 Tat-based vaccines: from basic science to clinical trials. DNA Cell Biol 2002; 21:599–610.

93. Graham BS, Karzon DT. AIDS vaccine development. Merigan TC, Bartlett JG, Bolognesi D, eds. Textbook of AIDS Medicine. 2d ed. Baltimore: Williams and Wilkins, 1998; 42: 689–724.

94. Barouch DH, et al. Potent CD4[+] T cell responses elicited by a bicistronic HIV-1 DNA vaccine expressing gp120 and GM-CSF. J Immunol 2002; 168:562–568.

95. Chakraborty H, et al. Viral burden in genital secretions determines male-to-female sexual transmission of HIV-1: a probabilistic empiric model. AIDS 2001; 15:621–627.

96. Koutsky LA, et al. A controlled trial of a human papillomavirus type 16 vaccine. N Engl J Med 2002; 347:1645–1651.

97. Stanberry LR, et al. Glycoprotein-D-adjuvant vaccine to prevent genital herpes. N Engl J Med 2002; 347:1652–1661.

49

Vaccine Strategies to Prevent Dengue Fever

Niranjan Kanesa-thasan
U.S. Army Medical Research Institute of Infectious Diseases, Fort Detrick, Maryland, U.S.A.

J. Robert Putnak
Walter Reed Army Institute of Research, Silver Spring, Maryland, U.S.A.

David W. Vaughn
Military Infectious Diseases Research Program, Fort Detrick, Maryland, U.S.A.

Dengue viruses cause classic dengue fever, an acute nonspecific febrile illness, and dengue hemorrhagic fever (DHF) [1]. The principal mosquito vector for dengue, *Aedes aegypti*, infests much of the tropics and subtropics. Unchecked expansion of vector mosquitoes over the past three decades has resulted in explosive spread of dengue viruses [2]. Dengue fever is consequently the most common arthropod-borne viral infection of humans, with over 50 million cases annually [3]. In some regions, such as the in Caribbean and South America, dengue fever has reappeared after an absence of several decades [4]. Of newer and greater concern is increasing incidence of DHF in areas where multiple dengue viruses circulate simultaneously or in sequence [5].

Flavivirus vaccines have proved effective to reduce or prevent disease from yellow fever, Japanese encephalitis (JE), and tick-borne encephalitis (TBE) viruses [6,7]. However, a licensed dengue vaccine remains elusive, and vector control and the use of personal protective measures are mainstays to prevent dengue disease. Readily available, safe, and effective dengue vaccines are urgently needed for global use, and the World Health Organization actively promotes their development [8]. This review will discuss new replicating and nonreplicating dengue vaccines (Table 1). Since the last review [9], investigational tetravalent dengue vaccines have transitioned to clinical trials. This acceleration of development suggests that the prospects for expanded clinical testing and fielding of new dengue vaccines are bright.

I. DENGUE VIRUSES

Dengue viruses are 40- to 50-nm enveloped spherical virions with a core of single-strand positive-sense RNA complexed with nucleocapsid protein [10]. The viral genomes are 11 kilobases in length and encode three structural proteins [capsid (C), membrane (prM, M), and envelope (E) proteins] and five nonstructural proteins (NS1, NS2a/b, NS3, NS4a/b, and NS5). The viruses preferentially infect cells of reticuloendothelial lineage, particularly macrophages and dendritic cells [11]. These antigen-presenting cells may be important in dengue pathogenesis, as they may be essential for direction of primary immune responses. After binding to cellular receptors, viruses *enter* the cytoplasm where their RNA is released from the nucleocapsid, translated, and transcribed [12]. Maturation of virions occurs in the cytoplasm, with assembly in the endoplasmic reticulum; progeny viruses bud into intracellular vesicles and are released from the cell surface [13]. Both structural and nonstructural viral proteins are expressed on the surface of the infected cell.

There are four serotypes of dengue viruses: dengue-1, -2, -3, and -4. These four dengue viruses are members of a single antigenic complex in the family Flaviviridae and share 60–80% sequence homology [14]. Despite significant genetic diversity among virus strains, both among and within different serotypes, there is good congruence between traditional serological classification of dengue isolates and classification based on genetic relatedness.

Dengue virus infections cause a spectrum of disease, ranging from asymptomatic infections to infections complicated by hemorrhage, shock, and death. Classical dengue fever is commonly encountered in adults and older children, presenting as a self-limited incapacitating acute illness with fever, muscle pains, headache, and an occasional rash [15]. Dengue viruses have proved to be a major cause of febrile illness among U.S. troops and travelers in dengue-endemic tropical areas [16,17]. In younger children, however, dengue

Table 1 Current Status of Dengue Vaccines

Vaccines	Developers	No. tetravalent candidates	Clinical trials	Commercial partner
Replicating				
Live attenuated	Mahidol; WRAIR	2	Phase 2	Yes (2)
Infectious clones	NIH; CDC; NMRC/FDA/WRAIR	2	Phase 2 (NIH)	Yes
Vectored vaccines	Acambis	1	Phase 1	Yes
Nonreplicating				
Recombinant	NMRC; others	1	NT[a]	No
Nucleic acid	NMRC; WRAIR	0	NT (planned)	No
Inactivated	WRAIR	0	NT	No

Abbreviations used: Mahidol, Mahidol University, Bangkok, Thailand; WRAIR, Walter Reed Army Institute of Research, Silver Spring, MD, USA; NIH, National Institutes of Health, Bethesda, MD, USA; CDC, Centers for Disease Control and Prevention, Fort Collins, CO, USA; NMRC, Naval Medical Research Command, Silver Spring, MD, USA; FDA, Food and Drug Administration, Bethesda, MD, USA; Acambis Inc, Cambridge, MA, USA.
[a]NT, not tested or results not available.

virus infection may result in mild illness associated only with upper respiratory symptoms.

Illness may be complicated in <1% of all cases of dengue by DHF, manifested by plasma leakage that can lead to a bleeding diathesis (positive tourniquet test), frank hemorrhage (e.g., spontaneous petechiae, gastrointestinal bleeding, epistaxis), or shock. Dengue hemorrhagic fever is a potential outcome of dengue virus infection that currently cannot be predicted. However, individuals with preexisting antibody from an earlier dengue virus infection who experience a secondary dengue virus infection have been shown to be at 100-fold increased risk for DHF [18]. Anamnestic antibody responses to dengue viruses are commonly found in individuals with DHF, along with evidence of enhanced cellular responses (increased γ-IFN, T-cell activation markers) [19,20]. In areas where dengue is endemic, DHF predominantly occurs in children and is fatal in about 0.5–5% of cases. However, DHF may be seen in adults when there is introduction of a new dengue virus into a community decades after transmission of another virus serotype [21].

II. IMMUNITY TO DENGUE VIRUSES

Infection with dengue virus of one serotype results in apparent lifelong monotypic immunity against that serotype, but not against any other serotype [22]. Thus, separate infections with all four dengue viruses are theoretically possible in a single host. Following infection, antibody and cell-mediated immune responses develop over several days. Appearance of IgM and IgG antibodies detectable by enzyme immunoassay, and of neutralizing antibodies detectable by plaque assay, coincides with cessation of fever and decrease in viremia [23]. Neutralizing antibodies may persist for decades [24]. Cell-mediated immune responses are evident during the acute phase of illness; both T-cell activation and cytokine release (TNF-α, IL-1, IL-6, and γ-IFN) have been documented [25]. These features may help to eliminate infected cells and hence decrease viral burden following infection.

Several dengue virus antigens (components of the dengue virus that induce protection against subsequent infection) have been implicated in the generation of both humoral and cell-mediated responses [26]. Attempts to stimulate immune responses mimicking those that follow natural infection with dengue virus have focused on E protein, the major surface protein of the dengue virion that contains the dominant antigens for eliciting neutralizing antibody responses [27]. B-cell epitopes that stimulate nonneutralizing antibodies are found on other structural proteins (prM, M) and nonstructural protein 1 (NS1). There may also be a protective role for these antibodies that may serve to limit virus replication after infection.

Protection from infection with dengue viruses (defined as prevention of virus replication and/or generation of host responses to virus) has been attributed to the presence of neutralizing antibodies to dengue virus [28]. Maternally derived neutralizing antibody appears to protect infants against infection until approximately 6 months of age [29]; additionally, monkeys are protected against challenge following transfer of immune sera [30]. In practice, development of neutralizing antibodies at a titer ≥1:10 following infection has been used as a surrogate marker for protective immunity to dengue viruses.

The role of cell-mediated immune responses in protection against infection or disease with dengue viruses is uncertain. Adaptive T-cell responses may ameliorate or abort progression to disease, and thus may be closely associated with recovery from infection. Recent hospital-based studies run from the Armed Forces Research Institute of Medical Sciences laboratory in Bangkok suggest the importance of cellular responses for disease manifestations and for long-term protection from subsequent exposure to dengue viruses [31–37]. Responses to antigens implicated in the generation of cell-mediated immunity, such as NS3 and NS5 nonstructural proteins, may restrict virus replication; the resulting diminution in viral burden lessens disease duration. Importantly, cell-mediated responses may provide some cross-reactive immunity as T-cell epitopes may be conserved across all four dengue virus serotypes [38].

The issue of protection against dengue virus infection is further complicated by the potential for subneutralizing concentrations of cross-reactive antibody to promote virus replication (antibody-dependent enhancement) [39]. In addition, increased and/or unregulated cell-mediated immune responses may play a role in the pathogenesis of DHF in some cases of secondary dengue [40]. A vaccine that stimulates an inadequate or altered humoral immune response, or that leads to an exaggerated cell-mediated immune response following infection, may have potential untoward consequences. Conversely, a successful vaccine will stimulate balanced humoral and cellular immunity that protects against but does not enhance the severity of dengue virus infection. A central observation that patient viremia titer is associated with disease outcome [41] suggests that vaccines that keep virus replication below a given threshold may suffice to prevent disease [42,43]. Evaluation of protection against viremia will be aided by new methods that rapidly quantitate viral burden in natural and experimental infection [44].

During the first half of the 20th century, wild-type dengue viruses were administered to volunteers to better understand the vector biology and the pathophysiology of dengue fever and to assess the protective efficacy of candidate dengue vaccines [45,46]. With a better understanding of dengue pathogenesis, dengue challenge studies in a few adult volunteers in a controlled setting have been revisited using GMP-produced dengue challenge viruses (M. Mammen, personal communication). Immunological evaluation showed the following (J. Scherer, personal communication): (1) volunteers that developed clinical illness had the greatest amount of immune activation, (2) immune activation was detectable before the development of clinical symptoms, and (3) activated T cells were detectable after clinical illness resolved.

III. DENGUE VACCINE DEVELOPMENT

An effective dengue virus vaccine would protect children residing in endemic areas as well as travelers to endemic or epidemic areas to include tourists, business travelers, expatriates, and military personnel. In many endemic regions, three or even four dengue viruses may cocirculate or circulate sequentially, resulting in multiple possible exposures and the potential for reinfection with different viruses. Hence, a dengue vaccine would have to contain appropriate viral antigens to confer long-term protection against infection with all four dengue viruses, or provide immunity that inhibits viral replication shortly after infection (infection-permissive immunity). It must protect against development of clinical illness and particularly against onset of severe dengue including DHF. A dengue vaccine that is capable of protecting 80% or more of recipients against clinical diseases due to any of the four viruses without predisposing to enhanced disease would certainly be considered a success.

The ideal dengue vaccine will be safe, immunize with one dose, stimulate neutralizing antibody in over 90% of recipients, protect against all dengue viruses, be efficacious in children, be stable, and be inexpensive. However, successful dengue vaccine development has been hindered by the lack of animal models of disease and known, reliable indicators of attenuation of the dengue virus. In the past, empirical testing established if a candidate vaccine was adequate for further testing. Recent advances in possible new animal models and

in molecular dissection of the viral genome may bypass these obstacles [47]. Challenge studies in a few adult volunteers in a controlled setting will further accelerate our understanding of dengue pathophysiology and will enable us to down-select available dengue vaccine candidates before launching large-scale Phase 3 vaccine field trials involving tens of thousands of children in dengue-endemic areas.

IV. REPLICATING DENGUE VACCINES

These vaccines include live attenuated dengue viruses, derived either empirically by classical methods in tissue culture or using genetic engineering of infectious clones. The former are the best-established approaches to dengue vaccine development. In addition, vectored viruses offer an alternative strategy for delivery and amplification of selected dengue genes in vivo.

A. Live Attenuated Dengue Vaccines

Most viral vaccines licensed in the United States are live-attenuated virus vaccines (yellow fever, measles, mumps, rubella, polio, adenovirus 4, adenovirus 7, varicella, influenza) that offer the possibility of single dose vaccination. Dr. Albert Sabin developed the Army's first dengue live attenuated dengue vaccine (LAV) via serial passage of dengue-1 in mouse brain. The vaccine became attenuated after seven passages and protected volunteers from homotypic challenge [46,48]. Wisseman and colleagues expanded this work using the dengue-1 MD-1 vaccine strain [49]. Subsequently, a plaque-picked, temperature sensitive mutant of dengue-2 virus isolated in Puerto Rico (PR-159/S1) was developed as a vaccine during the 1970s [50,51]. The seroconversion rate for dengue-2 PR-159/S1 was 61% in flavivirus naive volunteers, but 90% in volunteers who had previously received yellow fever vaccine [52].

During the 1980s, vaccine development efforts focused on dengue viruses serially passaged in primary dog kidney (PDK) cells, a nonpermissive cell line. The Mahidol University in Thailand and the Walter Reed Army Institute of Research (WRAIR) in the United States selected several candidate attenuated live vaccines for clinical evaluation. Increasing viral passage in PDK cells was associated with diminished reactogenicity, decreased viremia, and lower antibody responses [9,53]. The principal symptoms of headache and muscle pain after vaccination were generally mild and transient, while signs of systemic illness, such as fever, were infrequent. Crucially, both centers discovered that combining two or more dengue strains into a single vaccine results in no apparent increase in reactogenicity over that observed with monovalent vaccines.

At the WRAIR, a series of pilot studies identified six monovalent dengue vaccines suitable for advanced development: dengue-1 45AZ5 at either PDK 20 (passage level 20 in PDK cells) or PDK 27, dengue-2 S16803 PDK 50, dengue-3 CH53489 PDK 20, and dengue-4 341750 at PDK 20 or PDK [6]. Subsequent Phase 1 trials allowed empiric down-selection from 18 candidate tetravalent formulations [53a,53b]. A single best formulation was identified for expanded clinical testing, formulation #17 comprised of dengue-1 PDK 27, dengue-2, dengue-3, and dengue-4 PDK 6 (Sun et al., personal communication). Vaccine protective efficacy was demonstrated in rhesus monkeys where 18 of 20 animals were protected from monovalent challenge following vaccination with dengue-1 PDK 20, dengue-2, dengue-3, and dengue-4 PDK [20]. Challenge experiments in human subjects are under way. In total, safety and immunogenicity of at least one dose of tetravalent vaccine has been evaluated in 145 volunteers, including some with previous partial immunity to flaviviruses [53b,54].

The Mahidol University group led by Dr Natth Bhamarapravati has successfully developed alternate live vaccines with attenuated dengue-1, -2, -3, and -4 viruses [55]. These viruses were tested singly and in combination and were found to be safe and immunogenic in Thai volunteers [56,57]. The success of the Mahidol dengue vaccine program has led to commercial development with Aventis Pasteur (AvP). Testing of this vaccine in monovalent and tetravalent preparations was completed using flavivirus-naïve American volunteers at the WRAIR and revealed unexpected interference by dengue-3 virus in the tetravalent vaccine [58,59]. After reformulation, the tetravalent vaccine is being evaluated in Phase 2 trials in children in Thailand (J. Lang, 50th Annual Meeting of the American Society of Tropical Medicine and Hygiene, November 2001, Atlanta, GA) (59a).

B. Live Infectious Clone Dengue Vaccines

A successful attenuated dengue virus vaccine must retain the ability to infect in order to establish a protective immune response. Attenuated viruses have been obtained empirically, but the critical mutations have not been fully identified [60]. The availability of full length, infectious cDNA clones for dengue-4 [61], dengue-2 [62], dengue-1 [63], and recently dengue-3 (Bangti Zhao, personal communication) opens exciting possibilities for development of genetically engineered dengue vaccines that are either more attenuated or have increased genetic stability. These attempts include attenuated infectious clones, molecularly attenuated deletion mutants, and chimeric dengue virus vaccines. Although, in many cases, these approaches remain empirical because of our limited understanding of the mechanism(s) of attenuation for flaviviruses and the mutations responsible, they have significantly advanced our understanding of virus replication and may suggest future vaccine development strategies.

1. Infectious Clones of Live Attenuated Dengue Vaccine

One strategy is to clone naturally attenuated variants from wild virus populations ("swarms") or from existing laboratory-attenuated vaccines to create safer vaccines. Infectious clones offer the advantages of consistent starting materials for vaccine production, separation of the vaccine virus from potential adventitious agents present in cell substrates, and the provision of a starting point for site-directed mutagenesis and chimeric viruses. Theoretical disadvantages include a reduced number of virus "quasispecies" that may reduce immune responses among heterogeneous human populations and a lack of certainty that cloned viruses based on a "consensus sequence" truly represent the attenuated vaccine virus.

The WRAIR, working with the NMRC and the FDA, has produced infectious clones from traditionally attenuated (PDK cell passaged) vaccine viruses. Full-length infectious clones of dengue-1 45AZ5 PDK 20, dengue-2 S16803 PDK 50, dengue-3 CH53489 PDK 20, and dengue-4 341750 PDK 20 have been produced. The infectious clones of the dengue-1 and dengue-2 vaccine viruses were evaluated in rhesus monkeys and performed similarly to the vaccine viruses from which they were derived in terms of viremia and elicited neutralizing antibodies (M. Mammen, personal communication).

2. Molecularly Attenuated Vaccine Viruses

Another approach has been to engineer mutations that might be expected to limit the replicational capability of flaviviruses in the host, for example, by modification of crucial cis- and trans-acting elements such as replicases, proteases and their recognition sites, and transcriptional and translational regulatory elements. The National Institutes of Health produced a full-length infectious clone of dengue-4 [61]. Using this strategy, various deletion mutations in the 3' noncoding region were introduced to attenuate the virus for man while maintaining adequate growth in Vero cells [64]. Compared with the original dengue 4 parent viruses, several viable deletion mutant viruses have altered phenotypes in vitro and in vivo; some may also have an altered host range as evidenced by their variably restricted replication in mammalian or mosquito cells. The 3' deletion dengue-4 vaccine has been administered to more than 100 volunteers at the Johns Hopkins University [65]. Thus far, the dengue-4 vaccine is safe and immunogenic with minimal reactogenicity.

FDA researchers produced a mutant dengue-2 virus with properties that suggest it may be attenuated for humans [66]. The mutations consist of three changes to the stem and loop structure at the far 3' end of the genome (a small portion of that stem and loop structure was replaced with the sequence from West Nile virus). A dengue-1 construct protects monkeys from viremia when challenged with wild-type dengue-1. Immunogenicity has been comparable to wild-type dengue-1 virus infection, while viremia has been delayed and greatly reduced, suggesting that there may be reduced reactogenicity in human recipients (MP Mammen, Jr., personal communication). All MutF vaccine recipients were protected from challenge a year (3/3) and 17 months (2/2) following a single dose [67]. A Phase 1 clinical study of dengue-1 MutF vaccine candidate is planned.

3. Intertypic Chimeric Vaccine Viruses

Yet another and possibly even more novel approach has been to make chimeric dengue virus vaccines by using an attenuated infectious cDNA clone as a carrier or backbone for the structural antigen genes from the other three virus serotypes. Chimeric viruses derived from the full-length dengue-4 cDNA infectious clone, which had been substituted with either dengue-1 or dengue-2 structural genes, elicited serotype-specific antibodies in rhesus monkeys and conferred protection against challenge with the homologous virus (i.e., the structural protein donor) [68]. As one approach to a tetravalent dengue vaccine, the NIH plans to create three intertypic chimeras replacing structural genes (prM and E) of the backbone virus with corresponding structural genes of the other serotypes [68]. It is expected that growth characteristics in cell culture and replication in humans will mimic the attenuated backbone vaccine virus, while the neutralizing antibody response will be directed against the new prM and E proteins expressed on the virus surface.

The CDC laboratory in Ft. Collins has produced an infectious clone of the Mahidol/AvP dengue-2 vaccine virus [69]. The CDC uses the dengue-2 vaccine virus infectious clone as the backbone (and dengue-2 component) to produce intertypic chimeric viruses for dengue-1, -3, and -4 [70]. Improved immunogenicity in mice was seen using the structural genes (C-prM-E) from wild-type viruses rather than vaccine viruses, and rhesus monkey studies are planned.

C. Vectored Dengue Vaccines

Work by Oravax (now Acambis) with a yellow fever–JE virus chimera, suggests that flavivirus chimeras offer a viable vaccine approach [71–73] (see Monath chapter in this volume). Acambis, backed by AvP, has subsequently developed chimeric dengue vaccine viruses using the infectious clone of the yellow fever 17D vaccine virus as the backbone. Chimeric viruses presenting the structural genes of dengue-1 through dengue-4 are immunogenic in monkeys with minimal viremia [74]. The monovalent vaccines each protect rhesus monkeys from challenge with wild-type homotypic dengue viruses. A Phase 1 trial of dengue-2 chimera is in progress following successful completion of the JE chimera clinical study [75]. Current concerns about the chimeric approach center around the consequences of producing incomplete immunity, i.e., immunity for the structural proteins for dengue-1 through -4 but only nonstructural protein-directed

immunity to the single dengue or yellow fever backbone virus.

Vaccinia vectors have been extensively utilized for expression of dengue genes and several recombinant viruses have been tested as vaccines in animal models [76–79]. Recently, novel highly attenuated strains of vaccinia virus (NYVAC, MVA) [80,81] or poxviruses with a host range limited to nonhuman species (ALVAC) [82] have been engineered to express flavivirus genes. Studies of the NYVAC and ALVAC recombinant vaccines with inserted JE structural genes were carried out in monkeys and humans [83,84]. The data from these trials revealed that the potency of these vectored vaccines was limited, particularly in vaccinia-immune individuals.

V. NONREPLICATING DENGUE VACCINES

The nonreplicating vaccines are a diverse group including recombinant subunit vaccines, nucleic acid vaccines, and inactivated virus vaccines (Table 1). Several investigators have developed candidate recombinant subunit or inactivated dengue vaccines that have demonstrated at least partial efficacy in mice and in nonhuman primates (Table 2). Among the most promising is a purified inactivated vaccine (PIV) vaccine for dengue-2 virus, which induced "sterile immunity" in some rhesus macaques following the administration of two doses (Putnak et al., manuscript in reparation). Vaccination with nucleic acid sequences encoding protective epitopes is another promising approach [85], which has been used to immunize experimentally against flaviviruses such as St. Louis encephalitis [65], JE [66], and dengue [86] (Table 2). None of these vaccines has yet progressed to clinical trials, although the dengue-1 DNA vaccine developed at Naval Medical Research Command (NMRC) and the dengue-2 PIV developed at WRAIR are awaiting clinical evaluation.

Table 2 Preclinical Results with Nonreplicating Dengue Vaccine Candidates

Vaccine (dengue virus types)	Antigen composition	Induces neutralizing antibody	Induces T-cell responses	Protects mice	Protects monkeys
E. coli subunit (1–4)	E (B domain)	Yes	NT[a]	Yes (dengue-2)	NT
Baculovirus subunit (4)	80% E	Yes	Yes	Yes	No
Baculovirus subunit (2)	E + MBP	Yes	NT	NT	NT
Baculovirus subunit (2)	100% E aggregates	Yes	NT	Yes	No
Yeast subunit (2)	VLPs	Yes	NT	NT	NT
Mammalian cell subunit (2)	VLPs	Yes	NT	Yes	NT
Nucleic acid (1)	prM-E (92–100%)	Yes	NT	NT	Yes (partial)
Nucleic acid (1)	prM-E + CpG DNA	Yes	NT	NT	Yes (partial)
Nucleic acid (2)	prM-E + LAMP	Yes	Yes	NT	NT
Nucleic acid (2)	prM-E + GM-CSF	Yes	Yes	NT	NT
Nucleic acid (2)	prM-E (100%)	Yes	Yes	NT	Yes (partial)
Purified inactivated (2)	Whole virions	Yes	NT	Yes	Yes

Abbreviations used: E, envelope; prM, premembrane; MBP, maltose-binding protein; VLPs, viruslike particles; CpG, cytosine–guanine dinucleotides; LAMP, lysosome-associated membrane protein; GM-CSF, granulocyte, monocyte, colony-stimulating factor.
[a]NT, not tested or results not available.

Although concerns about the ability to produce large amounts of recombinant or inactivated materials in a highly immunogenic form have largely been overcome [87], other concerns about the long-term safety and efficacy of non-replicating vaccines remain. These relate to the duration of protective immunity, the ability to elicit effective cell-mediated immune responses (see dengue immunology section), and perhaps most importantly, the potential risk for enhanced disease once neutralizing antibody levels decline. Despite these concerns, viable roles for recombinant and inactivated vaccines remain, e.g., for protection during short-term travel to endemic areas, as alternatives to live vaccines and to supplement the immune responses generated by live or vectored vaccines. The high degree of structural and antigenic conservation among dengue viruses suggests that common strategies for vaccine development may be successful.

A. Recombinant Dengue Vaccines

Recombinant subunit dengue vaccines have been produced from structural proteins C, prM, and E and nonstructural (NS) proteins NS1, NS2A, NS2B, and NS3, expressed in a variety of systems, including *E. coli*, insect, yeast, and mammalian cells. Attempts to express full-length dengue antigens in *E. coli* in an immunogenic form were unsuccessful and have now largely been abandoned [88]. However, the successful expression in *E. coli* of a truncated version of dengue E protein (the approximately 110 amino acid B domain) fused to maltose-binding protein has been reported [89], and a tetravalent vaccine made using this approach was immunogenic for mice [90].

Insect cells may be more efficient than *E. coli* for expressing near-full-length dengue antigens because these cells are natural hosts for the virus. In particular, recombinant baculovirus has been used to produce dengue E subunit antigens in *Spodoptera frugiperda* (Sf9) insect cells [91–94]. These antigens, truncated at the C terminus to remove the hydrophobic membrane anchor domain, are secreted from Sf9 cells in a soluble form. However, mixed results have been obtained with soluble baculovirus-expressed dengue subunit antigens in animal models. An unpurified dengue-4 E antigen vaccine, while immunogenic and protective in mice, failed to protect rhesus monkeys against viremia [95]. Another crude dengue-2 E antigen fused to maltose binding protein conferred partial protection to mice but was not tested in monkeys [96,97]. More highly purified baculovirus-expressed E antigen preparations also conferred little or no protection against virus challenge [98] (Putnak, unpublished results). A full-length dengue-2 E protein formed large, intracellular aggregates, which were partially purified by detergent lysis and size exclusion chromatography [99]. Mice immunized with this particulate antigen with alum adjuvant made high-titer dengue-2 virus-neutralizing antibodies and were protected against virus challenge. This suggests that particle-based baculovirus-expressed dengue subunit vaccines may be equivalent or superior to soluble vaccines, at least in mice.

Recently, expression of the dengue virus structural gene antigens in yeast has been reported to produce 30-nm, viruslike particles, which induced virus-neutralizing antibodies in rabbits [100]. However, studies of the protective efficacy of this immunogen in mice and nonhuman primates have not been reported. Recombinant subunit flavivirus antigens produced in mammalian cells have demonstrated utility for making effective vaccines [101]. Expression of the prM and E genes of dengue-2 virus in Chinese hamster ovary cells gave rise to secreted, viruslike particles, which immunized and partially protected mice against a nonlethal challenge [102]. These vaccines have not been tested yet in primates.

Current results with subunit vaccines in animal models are promising, but more work is required in the areas of protein purification and the identification of safe and effective adjuvants before the full potential of recombinant subunit vaccines can be realized. Future development of subunit vaccines also remains uncertain without a good animal disease model to help assess the risk of DHF. Subunit vaccines may be further improved by the addition of NS1 and NS3 antigens, which may provide additional protective epitopes. However, multicomponent, tetravalent vaccines may eventually prove to be too expensive to produce.

B. Nucleic Acid Dengue Vaccines

Initial dengue nucleic vaccines, made by cloning dengue-2 prM gene with 92% of the E gene (prM-92% E) into two different plasmid expression vectors, proved immunogenic in mice [86]. There was a positive correlation between neutralizing antibody titers and the levels of expression of the E antigen *in vitro*. Coadministration of the vaccine with pUC 19 plasmid DNA containing immunostimulatory CpG sequences elicited higher antibody titers and conferred partial protection to 3-week-old mice [103]. A dengue-1 DNA vaccine was tested using different gene inserts, including prM-92% E, prM-80% E, prM-100% E, and 80% E gene without prM [104]. Expression of the prM-100% E construct resulted in the formation of extracellular, viruslike particles and induced the highest and most persistent neutralizing antibody titers in mice. Similar results were also reported for a dengue-2 prM-100% E vaccine [105].

Subsequently, the dengue-1 prM-100% E vaccine was evaluated in rhesus macaques that received up to four 1-mg doses of vaccine administered intramuscularly (im) or intradermally (id) with or without CpG DNA [106]. The im route conferred more rapid seroconversion, higher and more persistent antibody titers, and partial protection against viremia upon virus challenge compared to id doses. Protection correlated with the presence of neutralizing antibodies; cell-mediated responses were not apparent in vaccinated animals. The CpG DNA had no effect. A parallel experiment with the DEN-1 prM-100% E vaccine in *Aotus* monkeys yielded similar results, except the im and id routes were comparable [107]. In both models, an anamnestic antibody response was observed after virus challenge, indicating a lack of sterile immunity.

To improve cellular immune responses, dengue-2 prM-100% E DNA was codelivered with lysosome-associated membrane protein (LAMP) trafficking sequences (which increase E antigen processing and presentation through the MHC class II pathway) or a plasmid expressing mouse granulocyte macrophage colony-stimulating factor (GM-CSF)

[108]. The vaccine with LAMP induced more rapid and higher rates of seroconversion and higher neutralizing antibody titers in mice than vaccine alone. Supplementing the vaccine with GM-CSF also resulted in significantly higher seroconversion rates and increased neutralizing antibody titers.

The gene gun is an alternate delivery device for delivery of DNA vaccines that uses compressed helium to deliver DNA coated onto gold microspheres to the epidermis. Effective immunization can be completed with microgram rather than milligram amounts of DNA, and may be more efficiently targeted to antigen-presenting cells of the dermis. The gene gun has been used recently to deliver dengue-2 prM-100% E DNA vaccine to mice and rhesus monkeys (Putnak R, manuscript in preparation). Mice vaccinated by gene gun made high-titer neutralizing antibody responses following inoculation with a single 0.5-µg dose, and good CTL responses following two 0.5-µg doses. In rhesus monkeys, two 2-µg doses of DNA delivered by gene gun resulted in universal seroconversion, and 2 of 3 vaccinated animals were protected against viremia after virus challenge 1 month following the second dose. However, none of the protected animals demonstrated sterile immunity.

C. Inactivated Dengue Vaccines

There are several licensed inactivated whole virus vaccines, such as inactivated polio vaccine (IPV), which are safe and effective. Recently, a formalin-inactivated vaccine candidate made in mammalian cells was developed for dengue-2 virus [109]. This vaccine, which is highly purified and formulated with alum, elicited high-titer virus-neutralizing antibodies in mice and protected them against virus challenge. In rhesus monkeys, two 7.5-µg doses elicited high-titer virus-neutralizing antibodies and conferred nearly complete protection against viremia [87]. Dengue PIV vaccine lots have also been produced for the other serotypes (Putnak, unpublished results). If they are as immunogenic as the dengue-2 PIV, it should be possible to use this approach for producing a tetravalent vaccine for dengue.

However, as with inactivated RSV and measles vaccines, questions relating to duration of immunity and the possible potentiation of immune enhancement must still be addressed [110]. In the event of an inadequate CD8 memory T-cell response, vaccinees could be at increased risk for enhanced disease should neutralizing antibodies fall below protective levels. However, these are only theoretical concerns and there are assays that can be used for measuring T-cell activation and cytotoxic T-cell memory in Phase 1 trials of candidate vaccines.

An inactivated or other nonreplicating vaccine could also serve to boost antibody levels once cellular immunity has been established using a live or nucleic acid-based vaccine. Recent recommendations for polio have established a precedent for the combined use of live-attenuated vaccine and IPV to prevent that disease. Such a strategy was reported for dengue-2 virus, where vaccination with prM-E DNA followed by boosting with a recombinant E protein (B domain) subunits elicited better immune responses in mice than the DNA vaccine alone [111].

VI. CONCLUSION

Following successes with live attenuated 17D yellow fever vaccine, formalin-inactivated JE and TBE vaccines, and cell-culture-derived JE vaccine, decades of efforts to develop live attenuated dengue vaccines may be nearing a conclusion. Two empirically derived attenuated tetravalent dengue vaccines are in Phase 2 clinical testing in the United States and in Thailand, and their pace toward licensure seems to be accelerating with the entry of commercial partners. The availability of dengue–yellow fever chimeras (Chimerivax, Acambis) may alter the equation by providing a third option based on a different live vaccine technology. The maturation of these candidates will expedite development of standardized viremia and antibody assays, further evaluation of protective responses in dengue infection, and promote investment in field study sites.

Moreover, the advent of novel molecular techniques to express viral subunit proteins and to construct infectious clones has also led to rapid exploration of dozens of candidate vaccines. While few candidates have advanced to the clinic, an enormous amount of information on dengue virus biology and immunology has been gained in the process. New viruses derived from infectious viral clones hold promise as stable live vaccines, if proven effective. Results with dengue nucleic acid vaccines are encouraging, but more work is needed to demonstrate tetravalent seroconversion and protection in animals and safety in clinical trials. The future possibility of licensed dengue vaccines seems assured, with first- and second-generation candidates entering into clinical testing.

REFERENCES

1. Innis BL. Dengue and dengue hemorrhagic fever. In: Porterfield JS, ed. Kass Handbook of Infectious Diseases: Exotic Virus Infections. London: Chapman and Hall, 1995:103–146.
2. Monath TP. Dengue: the risk to developed and developing countries. Proc Natl Acad Sci U S A 1994; 91:2395–2400.
3. Anonymous. Dengue Haemorrhagic Fever: Diagnosis, Treatment, Prevention and Control. 2d ed. Geneva: World Health Organization, 1997.
4. Gubler DJ. Dengue and dengue hemorrhagic fever. Clin Microbiol Rev 1998; 11:480–496.
5. Guzman MG, Kouri G. Dengue: an update. Lancet Infect Dis 2002; 2:33–42.
6. Hoke CH Jr, et al. Protection against Japanese encephalitis by inactivated vaccines. N Engl J Med 1988; 319:608–614.
7. Kunz C. Tick-borne encephalitis in Europe. Acta Leiden 1992; 60:1–14.
8. Chambers TJ, et al. Vaccine development against dengue and Japanese encephalitis: report of a World Health Organization meeting. Vaccine 1997; 15:1494–1502.
9. Kanesa-thasan N, et al. New and improved vaccines for dengue, Japanese encephalitis, and yellow fever viruses. In: Levine MM, Woodrow GC, Kaper JB, Cobon GS, eds. New Generation Vaccines. New York: Marcel, 1997:587–606.
10. Henchal EA, Putnak JR. The dengue viruses. Clin Microbiol Rev 1990; 3(4):376–396.
11. Wu SJ, et al. Human skin Langerhans cells are targets of dengue virus infection. Nat Med 2000; 6:816–820.

12. Putnak JR, et al. A putative cellular receptor for dengue viruses [news; comment]. Nat Med 1997; 3:828–829.

13. Hase T, et al. Morphogenesis of flaviviruses. Subcell Biochem 1989; 15:275–305.

14. Kuno G, et al. Phylogeny of the genus Flavivirus. J Virol 1998; 72:73–83.

15. Rigau-Perez JG, et al. Dengue and dengue haemorrhagic fever. Lancet 1998; 352:971–977.

16. Kanesa-thasan N, et al. Dengue serotypes 2 and 3 in US forces in Somalia. Lancet 1994; 343:678.

17. Trofa AF, et al. Dengue fever in US military personnel in Haiti. JAMA 1997; 277:1546–1548.

18. Halstead SB. Pathogenesis of dengue: challenges to molecular biology. Science 1988; 239:476–481.

19. Kurane I, et al. Activation of T lymphocytes in dengue virus infections. High levels of soluble interleukin 2 receptor, soluble CD4, soluble CD8, interleukin 2, and interferon-gamma in sera of children with dengue. J Clin Invest 1991; 88:1473–1480.

20. Rothman AL, Ennis FA. Immunopathogenesis of dengue hemorrhagic fever. Virology 1999; 257:1–6.

21. Bravo JR, et al. Why dengue haemorrhagic fever in Cuba? 1. Individual risk factors for dengue haemorrhagic fever/dengue shock syndrome (DHF/DSS). Trans R Soc Trop Med Hyg 1987; 81:816–820.

22. Sabin AB, et al. Research on dengue during World War II. Am J Trop Med Hyg 1952; 1:30–50.

23. Vaughn DW, et al. Dengue in the early febrile phase: viremia and antibody responses. J Infect Dis 1997; 176:322–330.

24. Halstead SB. Etiologies of the experimental dengues of Siler and Simmons. Am J Trop Med Hyg 1974; 23:974–982.

25. Green S, et al. Early immune activation in acute dengue illness is related to development of plasma leakage and disease severity. J Infect Dis 1999; 179:755–762.

26. Schlesinger JJ, et al. New approaches to flavivirus vaccine development. Biotechnology 1992; 20:289–307.

27. Chang GJ. Molecular biology of dengue viruses. In: Gubler DJ, Kuno G, eds. Dengue and Dengue Hemorrhagic Fever. New York: CAB International, 1997:175–198.

28. Innis BL. Antibody responses to dengue virus infection. In: Gubler DJ, Kuno G, eds. Dengue and Dengue Hemorrhagic Fever. Cambridge: CAB International, 1997:221–243.

29. Kliks SC, et al. Evidence that maternal dengue antibodies are important in the development of dengue hemorrhagic fever in infants. Am J Trop Med Hyg 1988; 38:411–419.

30. Halstead SB. In vivo enhancement of dengue virus infection in Rhesus monkeys by passively transferred antibody. J Infect Dis 1979; 140:527–533.

31. Green S, et al. Dengue virus-specific human CD4+ T-lymphocyte responses in a recipient of an experimental live-attenuated dengue virus type-1 vaccine—bulk culture proliferation, clonal analysis, and precursor frequency determination. J Virol 1993; 67:5962–5967.

32. Green S, et al. Early CD69 expression on peripheral blood lymphocytes from children with dengue hemorrhagic fever. J Infect Dis 1999; 180:1429–1435.

33. Green S, et al. Elevated plasma interleukin-10 levels in acute dengue correlate with disease severity. J Med Virol 1999; 59: 329–334.

34. Mathew A, et al. Predominance of HLA-restricted cytotoxic T-lymphocyte responses to serotype-cross-reactive epitopes on nonstructural proteins following natural secondary dengue virus infection. J Virol 1998; 72:3999–4004.

35. Mathew A, et al. Impaired T cell proliferation in acute dengue infection. J Immunol 1999; 162:5607–5615.

36. Gagnon SJ, et al. T cell receptor Vbeta gene usage in Thai children with dengue virus infection. Am J Trop Med Hyg 2001; 64:41–48.

37. Libraty DH, et al. Differing influences of virus burden and

38. immune activation on disease severity in secondary dengue-3 infections. J Infect Dis 2002; 185:1697–1703.

38. Kurane I, et al. Dengue virus-specific human T cell clones. Serotype crossreactive proliferation, interferon gamma production, and cytotoxic activity. J Exp Med 1989; 170:763–775.

39. Morens DM. Antibody-dependent enhancement of infection and the pathogenesis of viral disease. Clin Infect Dis 1994; 19:500–512.

40. Cardosa MJ. Dengue haemorrhagic fever: questions of pathogenesis. Curr Opin Infect Dis 2000; 13:471–475.

41. Vaughn DW, et al. Dengue viremia titer, antibody response pattern, and virus serotype correlate with disease severity. J Infect Dis 2000; 181:2–9.

42. Endy TP, et al. Spatial and temporal circulation of dengue virus serotypes: a prospective study of primary school children in Kamphaeng Phet, Thailand. Am J Epidemiol 2002; 156:52–59.

43. Mangada MM, et al. Dengue-specific T cell responses in PBMCs obtained prior to secondary dengue virus infections in Thai schoolchildren. J Infect Dis 2002; 185:1697–1703.

44. Houng HH, et al. Development of a fluorogenic RT-PCR system for quantitative identification of dengue virus serotypes 1–4 using conserved and serotype-specific 3' noncoding sequences. J Virol Methods 2001; 95:19–32.

45. Ashburn PM, Craig CF. Experimental investigations regarding the etiology of dengue fever. J Infect Dis 1907; 4: 440–475.

46. Sabin AB. Recent advances in our knowledge of dengue and sandfly fever. Am J Trop Med Hyg 1955; 4:198–207.

47. Johnson AJ, Roehrig JT. New mouse model for dengue virus vaccine testing. J Virol 1999; 73:783–786.

48. Sabin AB, Schlesinger RW. Production of immunity to dengue with virus modified by propagation in mice. Science 1945; 101:640–642.

49. Wisseman CL Jr, et al. Attenuated living type 1 dengue vaccines. Am J Trop Med Hyg 1963; 12:620–623.

50. Eckels KH, et al. Isolation of a temperature-sensitive dengue-2 virus under conditions suitable for vaccine development. Infect Immun 1976; 14:1221–1227.

51. Bancroft WH, et al. Dengue-2 vaccine: virological, immunological, and clinical responses of six yellow fever-immune recipients. Infect Immun 1981; 31:698–703.

52. Scott RM, et al. Dengue 2 vaccine: dose response in volunteers in relation to yellow fever immune status. J Infect Dis 1983; 148:1055–1060.

53. Edelman R, et al. A live attenuated dengue-1 vaccine candidate (45AZ5) passaged in primary dog kidney cell culture is attenuated and immunogenic for humans. J Infect Dis 1994; 170:1448–1455.

53a. Edelman R, et al. Phase 1 trial of 16 formulations of a tetravalent live-attenuated dengue vaccine. Am J Trop Med Hyg. Submitted.

53b. Sun W, et al. Vaccination of human volunteers with monovalent and tetravalent live-attenuated dengue vaccine candidates. Am J Trop Med Hyg. Submitted.

54. Kanesa-thasan N, et al. A phase I study of the WRAIR tetravalent live attenuated dengue vaccine in flavivirus-immune adult volunteers. 5th Annual Conference on Vaccine Research, Baltimore, MD, May 2002.

55. Bhamarapravati N, Yoksan S. Live attenuated tetravalent dengue vaccine. In: Gubler DJ, Kuno G, eds. Dengue and Dengue Hemorrhagic Fever. New York: CAB International, 1997:367–377.

56. Bhamarapravati N, Yoksan S. Study of bivalent dengue vaccine in volunteers. Lancet 1989; 1:1077.

57. Bhamarapravati N, Yoksan S. Live attenuated tetravalent dengue vaccine. Vaccine 2000; 18(suppl 2):44–47.

58. Vaughn DW, et al. Testing of a dengue 2 live-attenuated

vaccine (strain 16681 PDK 53) in ten American volunteers. Vaccine 1996; 14:329–336.

59. Kanesa-thasan N, et al. Safety and immunogenicity of attenuated dengue virus vaccines (Aventis Pasteur) in human volunteers. Vaccine 2001; 19:3179–3188.

59a. Sabchareon A, et al. Safety and immunogenicity of tetravalent live-attenuated dengue vaccines in Thai adult volunteers: role of serotype concentration, ratio, and multiple doses. Am J Trop Med Hyg 2002; 66:264–272.

60. Butrapet S, et al. Attenuation markers of a candidate dengue type 2 vaccine virus, strain 16681 (PDK-53), are defined by mutations in the 5′ noncoding region and nonstructural proteins 1 and 3. J Virol 2000; 74:3011–3019.

61. Lai CJ, et al. Infectious RNA transcribed from stably cloned full-length cDNA of dengue type 4 virus. Proc Natl Acad Sci U S A 1991; 88:5139–5143.

62. Kapoor M, et al. Synthesis and characterization of an infectious dengue virus type-2 RNA genome (New Guinea C strain). Gene 1995; 162:175–180.

63. Puri B, et al. Construction of a full length infectious clone for dengue-1 virus Western Pacific, 74 strain. Virus Genes 2000; 20:57–63.

64. Men R, et al. Dengue type 4 virus mutants containing deletions in the 3′ noncoding region of the RNA genome: analysis of growth restriction in cell culture and altered viremia pattern and immunogenicity in rhesus monkeys. J Virol 1996; 70:3930–3937.

65. Durbin AP, et al. Attenuation and immunogenicity in humans of a live dengue virus type-4 vaccine candidate with a 30 nucleotide deletion in its 3′-untranslated region. Am J Trop Med Hyg 2001; 65:405–413.

66. Zeng L, et al. Identification of specific nucleotide sequences within the conserved 3′-SL in the dengue type 2 virus genome required for replication. J Virol 1998; 72:7510–7522.

67. Markoff L, et al. Derivation and characterization of a dengue type 1 host range-restricted mutant virus that is attenuated and highly immunogenic in monkeys. J Virol 2002; 76:3318–3328.

68. Bray M, et al. Monkeys immunized with intertypic chimeric dengue viruses are protected against wild-type virus challenge. J Virol 1996; 70:4162–4166.

69. Kinney RM, et al. Construction of infectious cDNA clones for dengue 2 virus: strain 16681 and its attenuated vaccine derivative, strain PDK-53. Virology 1997; 230:300–308.

70. Huang CY, et al. Chimeric dengue type 2 (vaccine strain PDK-53)/dengue type 1 virus as a potential candidate dengue type 1 virus vaccine. J Virol 2000; 74:3020–3028.

71. Guirakhoo F, et al. Immunogenicity, genetic stability, and protective efficacy of a recombinant, chimeric yellow fever–Japanese encephalitis virus (ChimeriVax-JE) as a live, attenuated vaccine candidate against Japanese encephalitis. Virology 1999; 257:363–372.

72. Monath TP, et al. Recombinant, chimaeric live, attenuated vaccine (ChimeriVax) incorporating the envelope genes of Japanese encephalitis (SA14-14-2) virus and the capsid and nonstructural genes of yellow fever (17D) virus is safe, immunogenic and protective in non-human primates. Vaccine 1999; 17:1869–1882.

73. Monath TP, et al. Chimeric yellow fever virus 17D-Japanese encephalitis virus vaccine: dose–response effectiveness and extended safety testing in rhesus monkeys. J Virol 2000; 74:1742–1751.

74. Guirakhoo F, et al. Recombinant chimeric yellow fever-dengue type 2 virus is immunogenic and protective in non-human primates. J Virol 2000; 74:5477–5485.

75. Monath TP, et al. Clinical proof of principle for ChimeriVax: recombinant live, attenuated vaccines against flavivirus infections. Vaccine 2002; 20:1004–1018.

76. Fonseca BAL, et al. Recombinant vaccinia viruses co-expressing dengue-1 glycoproteins prM and E induce neutralizing antibodies in mice. Vaccine 1994; 12:279–285.

77. Falgout B, et al. Immunization of mice with recombinant vaccinia virus expressing authentic dengue virus nonstructural protein NS1 protects against lethal dengue virus encephalitis. J Virol 1990; 64:4356–4363.

78. Hahn YS, et al. Expression of the structural proteins of dengue 2 virus and yellow fever virus by recombinant vaccinia viruses. Arch Virol 1990; 115:251–265.

79. Zhao BT, et al. Expression of dengue virus structural proteins and nonstructural protein NS1 by a recombinant vaccinia virus. J Virol 1987; 61:4019–4022.

80. Tartaglia J, et al. NYVAC: A highly attenuated strain of vaccinia virus. Virology 1992; 188:217–232.

81. Men R, et al. Immunization of rhesus monkeys with a recombinant of modified vaccinia virus Ankara expressing a truncated envelope glycoprotein of dengue type 2 virus induced resistance to dengue type 2 virus challenge. Vaccine 2000; 18:3113–3122.

82. Salmon-Ceron D, et al. Safety and immunogenicity of a live recombinant canarypox virus expressing HIV type 1 gp120 MN MN tm/gag/protease LAI (ALVAC-HIV, vCP205) followed by a p24E-V3 MN synthetic peptide (CLTB-36) administered in healthy volunteers at low risk for HIV infection. AGIS Group and L'Agence Nationale de Recherches sur Le Sida. AIDS Res Hum Retroviruses 1999; 15:633–645.

83. Raengsakulrach B, et al. Safety, immunogenicity, and protective efficacy of NYVAC-JEV and ALVAC-JEV recombinant Japanese encephalitis vaccines in rhesus monkeys. Am J Trop Med Hyg 1999; 60:343–349.

84. Kanesa-thasan N, et al. Safety and immunogenicity of NYVAC-JEV and ALVAC-JEV attenuated recombinant Japanese encephalitis virus–poxvirus vaccines in vaccinia-nonimmune and vaccinia-immune humans. Vaccine 2001; 19:483–491.

85. Wolff JA, et al. Long-term persistence of plasmid DNA and foreign gene expression in mouse muscle. Hum Mol Genet 1992; 1:363–369.

86. Kochel T, et al. Inoculation of plasmids expressing the dengue-2 envelope gene elicit neutralizing antibodies in mice. Vaccine 1997; 15:547–552.

87. Putnak R, et al. Development of a purified, inactivated, dengue-2 virus vaccine prototype in Vero cells: immunogenicity and protection in mice and rhesus monkeys. J Infect Dis 1996; 174:1176–1184.

88. Putnak R. Progress in the development of recombinant vaccines against dengue and other arthropod-borne flaviviruses. In: Kurstak E, ed. Modern Vaccinology. New York: Plenum Medical, 1994:231–252.

89. Simmons M, et al. Evaluation of the protective efficacy of a recombinant dengue envelope B domain fusion protein against dengue 2 virus infection in mice. Am J Trop Med Hyg 1998; 58:655–662.

90. Simmons M, et al. Short report: antibody responses of mice immunized with a tetravalent dengue recombinant protein subunit vaccine. Am J Trop Med Hyg 2001; 65:159–161.

91. Putnak R, et al. Dengue-1 virus envelope glycoprotein gene expressed in recombinant baculovirus elicits virus-neutralizing antibody in mice and protects them from virus challenge. Am J Trop Med Hyg 1991; 45:159–167.

92. Feighny R, et al. Purification of native dengue-2 viral proteins and the ability of purified proteins to protect mice. Am J Trop Med Hyg 1992; 47:405–412.

93. Delenda C, et al. Analysis of C-terminally truncated dengue 2 and dengue 3 virus envelope glycoproteins: Processing in insect cells and immunogenic properties in mice. J Gen Virol 1994; 75:1569–1578.

94. Zhang YM, et al. Immunization of mice with dengue struc-

tural proteins and nonstructural protein NS1 expressed by baculovirus recombinant induces resistance to dengue virus encephalitis. J Virol 1988; 62:3027–3031.

95. Eckels KH, et al. Immunization of monkeys with baculovirus–dengue type-4 recombinants containing envelope and nonstructural proteins: evidence of priming and partial protection. Am J Trop Med Hyg 1994; 50:472–478.

96. Delenda C, et al. Protective efficacy in mice of a secreted form of recombinant dengue-2 virus envelope protein produced in baculovirus infected insect cells. Arch Virol 1994; 139:197–207.

97. Staropoli I, et al. Dengue virus envelope glycoprotein can be secreted from insect cells as a fusion with the maltose-binding protein. J Virol Methods 1996; 56:179–189.

98. Velzing J, et al. Induction of protective immunity against dengue virus type 2: comparison of candidate live attenuated and recombinant vaccines. Vaccine 1999; 17:1312–1320.

99. Smucny JJ, et al. Murine immunoglobulin G subclass responses following immunization with live dengue virus or a recombinant dengue envelope protein. Am J Trop Med Hyg 1995; 53:432–437.

100. Sugrue RJ, et al. Expression of the dengue virus structural proteins in *Pichia pastoris* leads to the generation of virus-like particles. J Gen Virol 1997; 78:1861–1866.

101. Heinz FX, et al. Recombinant and virion-derived soluble and particulate immunogens for vaccination against tickborne encephalitis. Vaccine 1995; 13:1636–1642.

102. Konishi E, Fujii A. Dengue type 2 virus subviral extracellular particles produced by a stably transfected mammalian cell line and their evaluation for a subunit vaccine. Vaccine 2002; 20:1058–1067.

103. Porter KR, et al. Protective efficacy of a dengue 2 DNA vaccine in mice and the effect of CpG immuno-stimulatory motifs on antibody responses. Arch Virol 1998; 143:997–1003.

104. Raviprakash K, et al. Immunogenicity of dengue virus type 1 DNA vaccines expressing truncated and full length envelope protein. Vaccine 2000; 18:2426–2434.

105. Konishi E, et al. A DNA vaccine expressing dengue type 2 virus premembrane and envelope genes induces neutralizing antibody and memory B cells in mice. Vaccine 2000; 18:1133–1139.

106. Raviprakash K, et al. Dengue virus type 1 DNA vaccine induces protective immune responses in rhesus macaques. J Gen Virol 2000; 81(Pt 7):1659–1667.

107. Kochel TJ, et al. A dengue virus serotype-1 DNA vaccine induces virus neutralizing antibodies and provides protection from viral challenge in Aotus monkeys. Vaccine 2000; 18:3166–3173.

108. Raviprakash K, et al. Synergistic neutralizing antibody response to a dengue virus type 2 DNA vaccine by incorporation of lysosome-associated membrane protein sequences and use of plasmid expressing GM-CSF. Virology 2001; 290:74–82.

109. Putnak R, et al. Immunogenic and protective response in mice immunized with a purified, inactivated, dengue-2 virus vaccine prototype made in fetal rhesus lung cells. Am J Trop Med Hyg 1996; 55:504–510.

110. Openshaw PJ, et al. Immunopathogenesis of vaccine-enhanced RSV disease. Vaccine 2001; 20(suppl 1):S27–S31.

111. Simmons M, et al. Characterization of antibody responses to combinations of a dengue-2 DNA and dengue-2 recombinant subunit vaccine. Am J Trop Med Hyg 2001; 65:420–426.

50

Vaccination Against the Hepatitis C Viruses

Michael Houghton
Chiron Corporation, Emeryville, California, U.S.A.

Sergio Abrignani
Chiron S.r.l., Siena, Italy

I. THE HEPACIVIRUS GENUS

Hepatitis C viruses (HCV) are classified as members of the Hepacivirus genus within the Flaviviridae family [1] and are positive-stranded RNA viruses containing genomes of approximately 10,000 nucleotides [2]. The genomes encode a polyprotein precursor of about 3000 aa that is cleaved co- and post-translationally to yield a variety of virion and nonstructural (NS) proteins (Figure 1) [3]. Translation is mediated through an internal ribosome entry site (IRES) situated within the 5′ untranslated region (UTR) of the RNA genome [4]. Recently, a −2/+1 ribosomal frame-shift has been observed to occur around aa11 of the C protein resulting in the synthesis of the F protein. The sequence of the F protein is partially conserved within the genus but its function is unknown [5,6]. However, the basic charged character of the F protein may also imply a nucleocapsid-like function. Unfortunately, HCV cannot be grown efficiently or reproducibly in cell culture, and limiting viral levels in infected individuals has rendered large-scale purification of virus unfeasible. This has meant that information on the structure of the virion is largely derived from expression studies with cloned cDNAs. Such studies have revealed co-translational processing of the polyprotein precursor via host signalase to yield the presumptive structural proteins [the nucleocapsid (C) and envelope glycoproteins gpE1 and gpE2] [7–9]. gpE1 and gpE2 have been shown to translocate into the lumen of the er where they remain tightly anchored in the form of a noncovalently bound heterodimer [10–12]. Deletion of the C-terminal transmembrane anchor regions (TMR) of either gpE1 or gpE2 results in secretion of the respective ectodomain from cDNA-transfected cells via the golgi apparatus, although this is an inefficient process in the case of gpE1 [8,13]. The nucleocapsid is also cleaved by host signal peptide peptidase to yield a smaller species (p19 or p21) which appears to be the form found within virions cir-culating in the bloodstream [14,15]. C has the ability to self-associate into core particles [16] and is phosphorylated [17].

A large variety of NS proteins are thought to be processed downstream of the structural protein region (Figure 1) [3]. p7 is processed through the action of host signalase [18] and in the related pestiviruses has been shown to be required for virion assembly and/or secretion [19]. Further downstream proteins are processed from the precursor polyprotein through the action of viral-encoded proteases encoded by NS genes 2, 3, and 4a [20–22]. The NS proteins associate together on the er to form a viral replication complex and various individual functions have been assigned (Figure 1). The 3′ UTR region comprises a 3′-terminal 98 nt region that is highly conserved, which is located immediately downstream from a short pyrimidine-rich tract. The latter is preceded by a more variable region immediately downstream of the polyprotein precursor terminator codon [23,24].

Being RNA viruses encoding error-prone RNA replicases that lack the proofreading abilities of host DNA polymerase, the HCV genomes and encoded proteins are highly variable. The 5′ and 3′ UTRs are highly conserved as is the C gene and encoded nucleocapsid protein, but the rest of the viral genes/proteins exhibit considerable heterogeneity (Table 1) [25].

In addition, the N-terminal 30 aa of gpE2 (E2HVR1) is hypervariable and using the chimpanzee infection model, it has been shown to contain antibody-binding viral neutralizing epitopes that are under considerable selective pressure [26–31]. At least six different basic genotypes have been distinguished phylogenetically along with numerous subtypes (Figure 2), with type 1 being the most common genotype in the United States, China, and Japan, and it being also common in Europe (Figure 3). Unfortunately, due to the lack of an in vitro virus-neutralizing antibody assay, the number of serotypes is unknown. Recent progress in developing mouse infection models may facilitate further studies

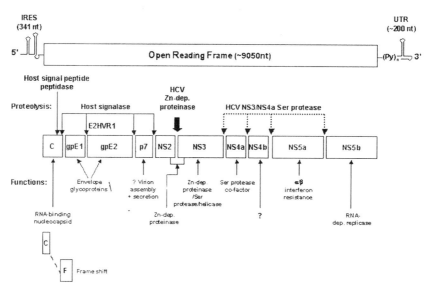

Figure 1 Organization of the HCV genome and encoded proteins.

Table 1

Coding region	Isolate	89.8–99.0	
	Genotype	71.1–79.4	} 0.9%
	Group	64.2–70.2	
C	Isolate	93.5–99.7	
	Genotype	81.5–91.1	
	Group	76.8–86.6	
E1	Isolate	88.9–98.4	
	Genotype	61.8–76.9	
	Group	52.1–67.2	
E2/NS1	Isolate	84.6–98.5	
	Genotype	66.7–76.1	
	Group	60.5–69.1	
NS2	Isolate	84.8–99.5	
	Genotype	65.0–75.8	} 0.5%
	Group	53.8–64.5	
NS3	Isolate	89.5–99.0	
	Genotype	73.1–81.4	
	Group	66.8–73.4	
NS4a	Isolate	85.2–100.0	
	Genotype	70.4–88.9	
	Group	56.2–77.8	
NS4b	Isolate	89.1–99.9	
	Genotype	70.5–82.5	
	Group	62.5–70.9	
NS5a	Isolate	89.1–99.0	
	Genotype	62.4–76.7	
	Group	56.6–67.9	
NS5b (total)	Isolate	92.0–99.2	
	Genotype	74.8–83.7	} 1.0%
	Group	67.5–73.8	
NS5b (1093 bp)	Isolate	93.7–99.2	
	Genotype	75.6–85.3	
	Group	67.2–76.0	
NS5b (222 bp)	Isolate	89.2–99.5	
	Genotype	67.1–82.9	
	Group	57.2–72.1	

in this important area [32]. It has been estimated that there are around 170 million HCV carriers worldwide [33].

II. NATURAL IMMUNITY AND IMMUNE CORRELATES

Recent studies in the chimpanzee challenge model and of multiply-exposed humans have demonstrated that there is significant natural immunity against HCV. In one chimpanzee study [34], an animal was infected by intrahepatic administration of an infectious RNA derived from HCV strain HCV-1 (of the 1a subtype). This subtype is the most common clade in the United States (Figure 3). Following resolution of the ensuing acute infection and disappearance of viremia, the animal was shown to be resistant to an intravenous rechallenge with homologous virus. No viremia was observed following rechallenge, indicating that sterilizing immunity was generated by the original infection. When rechallenged subsequently with a heterologous 1a strain, the animal experienced very transient, minimal viremia unlike the substantial viremia observed in control animals. Resolution of the infection in the rechallenged animal was confirmed by showing the subsequent absence of viral RNA from the blood and liver. Furthermore, when rechallenged again with a heterologous 1b strain, the most common clade worldwide (Figure 3), only a transient viremia was observed prior to disappearance of the virus from plasma and the liver [34]. Very similar results were obtained in separate chimpanzee studies in which animals were challenged and then rechallenged i.v. with different infectious viral inocula. Only transient viremia occurred when animals that recovered initially from a 1a infection were rechallenged with either a heterologous 1a strain or a heterologous 1b strain [35,36]. Additional chimpanzee studies indicate the existence of cross-protective immunity between HCV types 1

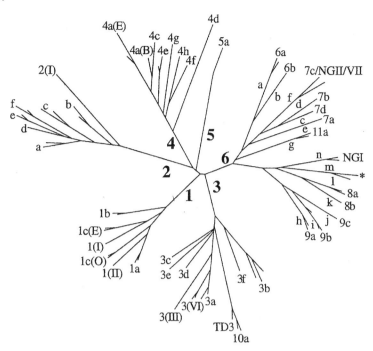

Figure 2 Phylogenetic analysis of nucleotide sequences from part of the HCV NS5b region amplified from HCV-infected blood donors and patients from several countries. (From Ref. 140.)

and 3 (A. Weiner, unpublished). The latter HCV type is commonly found in intravenous drug users (IVDUs).

Similar findings have also been reported in a prospective study of IVDUs from the United States. Strikingly, the incidence of persistent viremia in IVDUs who had recovered from a previous infection was 12× lower than that in IVDUs who had not experienced a previous infection, as shown using multivariate analyses [37]. As seen in the chimpanzee studies, peak viral loads were substantially higher (by almost 2 logs) in the first-time infections as compared with the re-infections [37]. Also, HIV co-infection produced persistent HCV infection in all cases, indicating the role of the immune response in HCV recovery [37]. Intriguingly, it has now been shown that HIV patients co-infected with HCV have lowered peripheral immune responses to HCV as compared with patients with HCV monoinfections, even in the absence of severe CD4$^+$ T-cell depletion [38].

Collectively, these chimpanzee and human data provide evidence for the existence of significant immunity to HCV and, importantly, for the existence of cross-protective immunity within and between commonly occurring HCV clades. It is important to note, however, that not all re-infections were resolved without progressing to chronicity (3/9 became chronically infected [37]), indicating that natural immunity to HCV is not complete and not as effective as for the hepatitis A and B viruses. It should also be mentioned that earlier studies in the chimpanzee model have concluded a lack of protective immunity to HCV [39]. This apparent contradiction may be due to the earlier studies measuring immunity more in terms of sterilizing immunity, rather than the ability to prevent the development of chronic infection, as in the more recent studies.

It was first noted that early and broad MHC class II-restricted CD4$^+$ T helper responses to HCV are associated with recovery from acute, symptomatic infections of man (Figure 4) [40,41]. Subsequently, using the valuable chimpanzee model again, it was shown that recovery could occur in the absence of any antibody to the viral envelope glycoproteins but in the presence of an early and broad MHC class I-restricted CD8$^+$ cytotoxic lymphocyte (CTL) response to the virus [42]. This association of HCV-specific CD4$^+$ T helper and CD8$^+$ CTL responses with resolution of acute infection has been confirmed in many human studies [43–48], although the relative importance of each type of cellular immune response is unknown at present. A recent study sheds further light on the potential mechanism of recovery from clinically asymptomatic, acute infections of man. Shortly following infection, activated HCV-specific CD8$^+$ T cells appeared in the peripheral blood that were associated with an increase in serum alanine aminotransferease (ALT) levels (signifying liver damage), and with a small decrease in viral RNA levels. These activated CD8$^+$ cells did not secrete gamma interferon. Shortly afterwards, a 5-log reduction in viral load occurred commensurate with the appearance of HCV-specific, gamma interferon-secreting CD8$^+$ cells with a nonactivated phenotype (CD38-negative). This large reduction in viral load was not accompanied by an increase in serum ALT levels, suggesting that a noncytolytic, viral clearance mechanism mediated by gamma interferon might be operative (Figure 5) [47]. This conclusion is consistent with the demonstrated anti-HCV activity of gamma interferon in cell cultures containing HCV replicons [49]. In contrast, individuals who develop chronic, persistent infection show weaker cellular immune responses to the viruses that are not

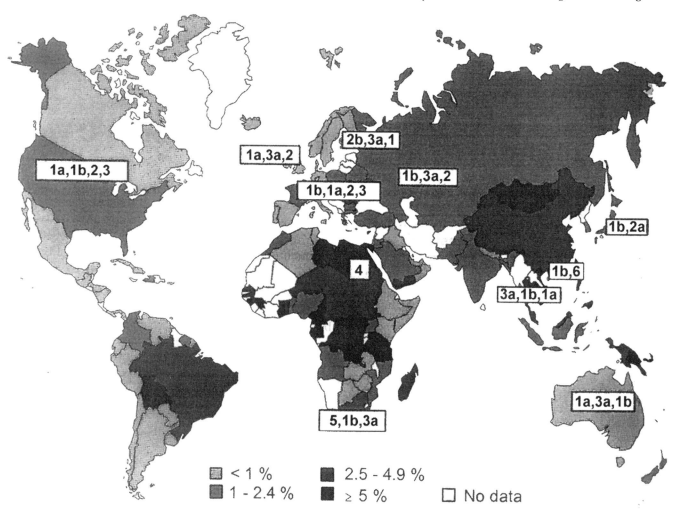

Figure 3 Approximate HCV prevalence and genotype distribution. (From Ref. 141.)

maintained over time (Figure 4) [43–47,50] and that have dysfunctional CD8$^+$ T-cell effector functions [51–53].

The association of HCV-specific, cellular immune responses with recovery is further reinforced by data from several studies showing that memory T-cell responses to the virus can be detected in long-term convalescent individuals [50], in nonviremic and HCV antibody-negative, healthy family members of HCV patients [54], and in other individuals who lack HCV antibody and RNA but who may have been exposed to the virus earlier [55]. However, further work is necessary to define the relative roles of HCV-specific CD4$^+$ and CD8$^+$ T-cell responses in protection as well as the mechanism of action.

The kinetics of induction of HCV-specific T-cell responses to multiple epitopes may be crucial in determining the outcome of infection, because the ability of the virus to mutate and thus evade CD8$^+$ T-cell responses has been demonstrated convincingly in the chimpanzee model [56]. The latter study suggests that if a multispecific T-cell response is made early in infection, then it is harder for the virus to mutate several epitopes simultaneously and, therefore, more likely to result in resolution of infection. Host and

viral factors involved in determining the breadth, strength, kinetics, and decline [51,52] of HCV-specific cellular immune responses will deserve much attention in the future. In this regard, certain MHC class I and II alleles are associated with recovery in humans [57–59].

The role of anti-envelope antibody in resolution of HCV infection is unclear at present. Initially, it was found that nearly all chronically infected humans have significant antibodies to gpE1 and gpE2, as measured in ELISA assays, and that there was not a clear relationship between the induction of these antibodies and resolution of acute infection [60]. These findings were extended in other studies showing that in man and chimpanzees, it was more likely to find anti-envelope antibody (as measured in ELISA assays) in chronically infected individuals than in resolvers of acute infection [61–63]. This contrasts with the situation found for many infectious agents, e.g., the hepatitis B virus, where anti-envelope antibody is a strong correlate of immunity. It should be noted, however, that a true in vitro, viral-neutralizing antibody assay has not been developed, due to the lack of a reliable cell culture system for HCV, and so the presence, level, and affinity of neutralizing antibody cannot be easily

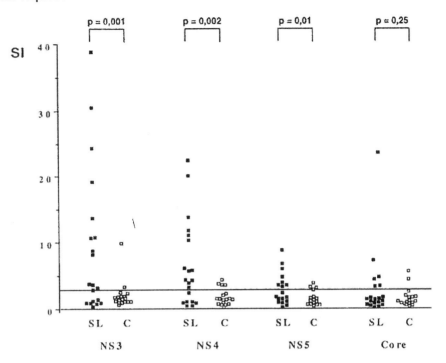

Figure 4 Proliferative CD4$^+$ T-cell response of the first sample in the acute phase of disease to recombinant HCV proteins (HCV–NS3, –NS4, –NS5, and –core) of peripheral blood mononuclear cells (PBMCs) from 38 patients with acute hepatitis C. Patients are grouped according to the final outcome of disease in self-limited hepatitis C (SL, $n = 20$) and patients with chronic evolution (C, $n = 18$). Results are shown as SI–^{3}H-thymidine incorporation of antigen-stimulated PBMCs (cpm)/unstimulated control (cpm). Values ≥ 3 are considered significant. All patients with self-limited disease displayed a significant proliferative T-cell response against at least one of the viral proteins, while patients with chronic evolution mounted no or only transient antiviral T-cell responses. NS3 and NS4 revealed the most frequent and most vigorous responses. In four patients, the proliferative response against NS5 was not tested in the first sample. (From Ref. 40.)

monitored. However, the presence of neutralizing antibody has been demonstrated using the chimpanzee model. Serum derived from a patient was shown capable of neutralizing the infectivity of virus taken from the same patient, 2 years earlier. However, the same viral inoculum could not be neutralized using serum from the patient obtained many years later [64]. The infectivity of various viral inocula in chimpanzees was also shown to be inversely proportional to the level of immune complexes, providing further evidence for the existence of neutralizing antibody [65]. Additional evidence for the generation of neutralizing antibody comes from several studies showing the efficacy of human Ig preparations, derived from numerous donors, in preventing the transmission of HCV following blood transfusion [66], liver transplantation [67], and between sexual partners [68]. Chimpanzees that received human Ig prior to experimental viral challenge also showed a clear inhibition of acute hepatitis and viremia throughout the lifetime of the antibodies [69]. When combined with clinical evidence for worse HCV-associated disease in hypogammaglobulinemics [70,71], the combined data clearly suggest that HCV infection does induce neutralizing antibody.

Why then is there a lack of correlation between anti-envelope antibody and the outcome of infection? Several possibilities exist; firstly, it has been shown that antisera raised against the N-terminal region of gpE2, the so-called

E2 hypervariable region 1 (E2HVR1), can neutralize the infectivity of homologous virus in the chimpanzee model [30]. Preliminary studies have reported that the early induction of anti-E2HVR1 may correlate with resolution of acute infection in humans [72,73]. Many studies have also suggested that this region mutates readily in response to the specific, humoral immune response, thus evading the binding of anti-E2HVR1 [27,29,31]. If this is a principal neutralizing domain of the virus, then it is possible to imagine how the virus might evade the antibody response. This might also explain the apparent, protective efficacies of complex human Ig preparations, if they contain highly plural anti-E2HVR1 antibodies.

A second theory revolves around the observation that infectious HCV virus has a very low density in sucrose gradients (~1.06 g/ml) [74] and that this fraction contains low-density lipoproteins that can bind and mask the virus, at least partially, from the action of neutralizing antibody [75,76]. A third possibility is that HCV may be transmitted between adjacent hepatocytes in the liver because giant, multinucleated hepatocytes are observed in the HCV-infected liver. In conclusion, the role of anti-envelope antibody in the protective immune response is poorly defined at present, although it is most likely a complex situation. While it is well established that humans and experimentally infected chimpanzees can resolve acute infections in the absence of de-

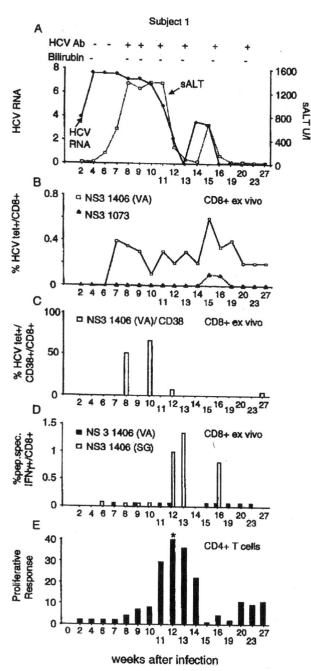

Figure 5 HCV-specific T-cell responses in subject I during asymptomatic, resolving acute HCV infection. (A) Course of infection. (B) Percentage of CD8$^+$ lymphocytes that were tetramer-positive at each time point. CD8$^+$ T-cell responses were tested directly ex vivo using HLA-A2 tetramers complexed with five different HLA-A2 restricted epitopes. CD8$^+$ T-cell responses against two epitopes [NS3 1073 and NS3 1406 (VA)] were detectable. (C) Percentage of NS3 1406 (VA)-specific CD8$^+$ T cells expressing the activation marker CD38. (D) Percentage of CD8$^+$ T cells that produce IFN-γ in response to HCV NS3 1406 (VA) (black bars) and NS3 1406 (SG) (white bars). (E) Proliferative CD4$^+$ T-cell responses against core, NS3, NS4, and NS5 are shown as the sum of all positive stimulation indices. *Sum of all specific stimulation indices is 56. (From Ref. 47.)

tectable anti-envelope antibody, but in the presence of early and broad T-cell responses, this does not rule out a role for neutralizing antibodies in the protective immune response in all individuals.

III. VACCINE STRATEGIES

A. Aims

In view of the current knowledge regarding protective immune responses to HCV, many investigators are focusing on vaccines capable of priming specific, broad cellular immune responses, including both MHC class II-restricted CD4$^+$ 1 helper responses as well as MHC class I-restricted CD8$^+$ responses. Conventionally, it has proven difficult to achieve the latter through the use of soluble proteins combined with adjuvants, although there has been recent progress in this area using recombinant HCV proteins combined with the ISCO Ms adjuvant. Therefore most activities designed to achieve the priming of CD8$^+$ T cells to the virus have centered around the use of DNA vaccines, using either bacterial plasmids or various viral vectors. In this way, HCV proteins are synthesized endogenously within the cytosol where they can then be processed within the proteosome and the resulting peptides are transported to the cell surface in association with MHC class I antigens, thus stimulating CD8$^+$ T-cell responses. In addition, some groups have also aimed at priming anti-envelope antibody responses via protein or DNA immunization involving either the gpE1/gpE2 heterodimer or either envelope glycoprotein alone. Other strategies have centered around creating a consensus E2HVR1 peptide that can prime broadly cross-reactive, neutralizing antibody. Due to the lack of a system for propagating HCV in vitro, the prospect of using a killed or attenuated HCV viral vaccine is unfeasible at present.

B. Adjuvanted, Recombinant HCV Protein Vaccines

A vaccine comprising the recombinant gpE1/gpE2 heterodimer combined with an oil/water microemulsified adjuvant has been tested for efficacy in the chimpanzee model [77–79]. The heterodimer was derived from HeLa cells infected with a recombinant vaccinia virus expressing a C–gpE1–gpE2–p7–NS2′ gene cassette derived from the HCV-1 strain (1a clade). Following cleavage by host signalase in the er, gpE1 and gpE2 translocate into the lumen of the er where they remain associated together and tightly anchored via type 1 transmembrane domains located at the C termini of both molecules [7–13]. Following extraction in nonionic detergent and affinity purification using GNA-lectin (that specifically binds the high mannose chains found on the heterodimer), the purified subunit proteins were used to immunize naïve chimpanzees along with the adjuvant. Generally, 30–40 μg of the subunits were administered intramuscularly (i.m.) on approximately months 0, 1, and 6, and a homologous viral challenge was given i.v., 2–3 weeks after the third immunization. Encouragingly, of seven animals receiving the vaccine, five were completely protected against the challenge, with no signs of viral infection in any of the assays, including sensitive RT-PCR assays for viral RNA (Figure 6) [77]. These five apparently sterilized animals were the highest responders to the vaccine in terms of elicited titers of anti-gpE1/gpE2 [77]. Sterilization did not correlate with antibody titers to E2HVR1 but did correlate with the titer of antibodies that block the binding of recombinant E2 to the CD81 ligand [80]. The latter has been shown to bind intact virus and could be involved in the receptor for HCV [81]. In addition, the two lowest responders

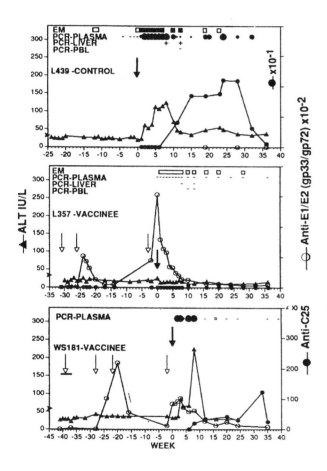

Figure 6 HCV-1 challenge of vaccinated and control chimpanzees. Control and immunized chimpanzees (L, Laboratory for Experimental Medicine and Surgery in Primates; W.S., White Sands) were challenged with ≈ 10 CID50 of HCV-1. The presence (solid boxes) or absence (open boxes) of hepatocyte ultrastructural changes observed in the electron microscope (EM) is indicated. The approximate relative levels of HCV-1 RNA detected in plasma using reverse transcriptase (RT)-PCR assays are reflected by sizes of the shaded circles (open circles denote borderline positives; minus signs denote undetectable levels). The results of RT-PCR assays of liver and PBL extracts are recorded as either + or −. The arrows in the ALT axes indicate the mean + 3.75 SD of prechallenge values; open vertical arrows denote time of subunit vaccine administration, and the solid vertical arrow denotes viral challenge on week 0. IU/L, international units per liter. (From Ref. 77.)

that became infected following challenge eventually resolved the acute infection without becoming chronic carriers (Figure 6) [77–79]. In contrast, most control animals become chronically infected following viral challenge [77–79]. Given that the prime, practical goal of an HCV vaccine would be to prevent the development of chronic infection following exposure to the virus, this study provided much encouragement for the development of an effective vaccine challenge [77,79].

This work has now been extended to address the key question of whether the vaccine protects against experimental challenge with a heterologous 1a viral strain. Initial data were derived from three vaccinees, previously protected against homologous viral challenge, that were then re-boosted with vaccine prior to rechallenge with the HCV-H strain (another member of the 1a clade common in the United States). While sterilization was not achieved, two of the three animals exhibited an amelioration of the acute infection followed by resolution [78,79]. Using additional chimpanzees, including five naïve animals that had not been challenged with HCV previously, it has been shown that out of a cumulative total of 10 vaccinees challenged with the heterologous HCV-H strain, while all 10 animals experienced acute infections, only 1 developed chronic, persistent infection. In contrast, most control animals challenged with HCV-H become chronic carriers (7/9; $P = 0.005$; M. Houghton, unpublished). Interestingly, the single carrier of HCV-H generated in the vaccine group actually elicited the highest anti-gpE1/gpE2 antibody titer of the group, indicating that such antibodies alone are not sufficient for protection [77–80]. Presumably, vaccine-mediated T-cell responses and/or the host's immune response to HCV replication following challenge are also involved in the protection observed.

Another group has also immunized a chimpanzee with insect cell-derived recombinant gpE1 and gpE2 (from HCV strain N2), in addition to a peptide spanning the E2HVR1 (from HCV strain #6). gpE1 and gpE2 were each expressed and purified separately and lacked the C-terminal transmembrane anchors. The E2HVR1 peptide was conjugated to keyhole limpet hemocyanin and Freund's adjuvant was employed to augment immune responses. Their conclusion, from a series of immunizations and challenges with HCV strain #6 in the same animal, was that sterilization was dependent on high anti-E2HVR1 titers rather than anti-gpE2 or anti-gpE1 titers [82,83]. The outcome of challenging with other viral strains was not reported, however. It should also be noted that insect-derived gpE2 (truncated at the C terminus) has been shown to bind poorly to a putative HCV receptor, CD81, as compared with gpE2 derived from mammalian cells [80]. The latter group also showed that the full-length gpE1/gpE2 heterodimer, derived from mammalian cells, bound to CD81 with high affinity as did intracellular forms of gpE2, truncated at the C terminus. However, secreted forms of gpE2 were not effective at binding CD81. Because deglycosylation of secreted gpE2 restored CD81-binding activity, it appears that the addition of complex carbohydrate during secretion either masks the CD81-binding site or changes the conformation to an inactive form [84]. The physiological significance of these findings is unclear at present, because the method of HCV virion secretion and the nature of the virion carbohydrate are unknown.

Intracellular, C-terminally truncated forms of gpE2 have been shown to be immunogenic in human volunteers, although efficacy in the chimpanzee challenge model has not yet been demonstrated (M. Houghton, unpublished). However, the gpE1/gpE2 heterodimer is generally considered to be a more native reflection of the HCV virion than either ectodomain alone and, as mentioned above, has demonstrable prophylactic efficacy in the chimpanzee. Therefore recombinant gpE1/gpE2 represents an encouraging human vaccine candidate.

Some work has been directed to the synthesis of viral-like particles (VLPs) by expressing the structural genes in different cells. In insect cells, expression of the C-gpE1–gpE2 gene cassette has been reported to result in the generation of 40–60-nm VLPs within cytoplasmic cysternae [85]. Following partial purification, these VLPs appear to be immunogenic in small animals and, as such, represent a potential vaccine candidate for humans [86]. Similar-sized VLPs have been observed in the process of budding into the lumen of the er, following expression of the same gene cassette in mammalian cells using a Semliki Forest viral vector [87]. HCV gene expression was observed to induce convoluted membranes or membranes similar to those seen in infected livers

[87]. However, some viral or host factor is limiting the release of the VLPs into the lumen and from being secreted into the cell media [87].

Because the E2HVR1 region of gpE2 has been shown to possess viral neutralizing epitopes and to be highly mutable, attempts have been made to select for a cross-reacting version using phage display of mimotopes. Rabbit antisera raised against one mimotype was highly cross-reactive with the E2HVR1 of many viral isolates and reacted to discontinuous epitopes [88]. Such mimotypes or consensus E2HVR1 peptides may be valuable components of an HCV vaccine. In this regard, a consensus E2HVR1 peptide sequence has been fused to the B subunit of cholera toxin and expressed in plants through the use of a tobacco mosaic viral vector. Crude extracts were then administered intranasally to mice, which then generated cross-reactive E2HVR1 antibodies that were capable of capturing virions [89].

Recombinant C protein is also being studied as a potential component of an HCV vaccine for several reasons. Firstly, broad HCV-specific CD4$^+$ and CD8$^+$ T-cell responses, including those of the C protein, are associated with recovery from HCV infection [42–44,46,47]. Secondly, the C protein is the most conserved HCV polypeptide and contains CD4$^+$ and CD8$^+$ epitopes that are highly conserved among the different HCV genotypes, which should therefore facilitate the generation of cross-protective immu-

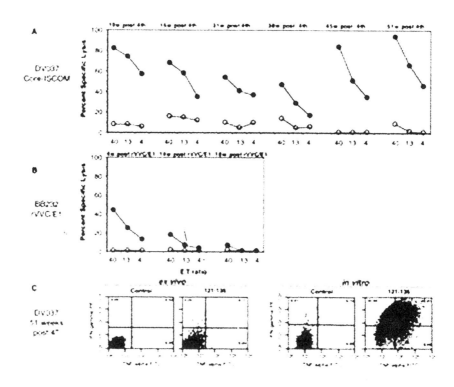

Figure 7 Longevity of the CTL responses primed by vaccination with recombinant HCV core in ISCOMs adjuvant. Peripheral blood mononuclear cells from rhesus macaques DV037 (A) and BB232 (B) were restimulated in vitro with the epitopic peptide 121–135. After CD8$^+$ enrichment, cells were tested for cytotoxic activity against autologous B-LCLs sensitized with the epitopic peptide 121–135 (●) or an irrelevant peptide (○). (C) Freshly isolated PBMCs from DV037 51 weeks after its last immunization (two left panels) or in vitro restimulated PBMCs from the same time point (two right panels) were restimulated for 12 hr with peptide 121–135 or a control peptide and stained for surface CD8 and intracellular IFN-γ and TNF-α. Lymphocytes were gated by side vs. forward scatter light and then for CD8-PerCP. Plots show log fluorescence intensity for TNF-α-FITC and IFN-γ-PE. (From Ref. 94.)

nity [90,91]. Thirdly, recombinant C protein has been shown to self-assemble into particles [16] with concomitant high immunogenicity in animal models. Substantial CD4$^+$ T-cell priming and high anti-C antibody titers have been obtained in mice and sheep [92,93].

In general, immunization with adjuvanted polypeptide subunits does not result in cross-priming, a process in which the antigen is deposited within the cytosol of antigen-presenting cells and processed peptides then placed on the MHC class I-presentation pathway, resulting in stimulation of CD8$^+$ CTLs. However, through the use of the ISCOM adjuvant, a particulate adjuvant comprising cholesterol, phospholipid, and naturally occurring saponins, it has been possible to prime strong CD8$^+$ CTL activity (and CD4$^+$ activity) in rhesus macaques, using a recombinant C antigen derived from *E. coli* (Figure 7) [94]. Cytotoxic lymphocytes to at least two epitopes were identified. This approach is a promising and practical option for the development of an HCV vaccine capable of priming cross-reactive HCV-specific T-cell responses associated with protection.

There are numerous CD4$^+$ and CD8$^+$ epitopes that are conserved among the different HCV genotypes. These reside within the various HCV-encoded virion and nonstructural proteins [90,91,95]. The inclusion of a multiplicity of these epitopes will facilitate the vaccine-mediated generation of broad cellular immune responses to the virus, which could then result in the elicitation of cross-protective immunity against different HCV genotypes. One such approach involves the assembly of "HCV polytope vaccines" consisting of a consecutive sequence of these conserved HCV T-cell epitopes, in the form of a recombinant polypeptide or DNA vaccine. Focusing the immune response on a collection of highly conserved epitopes that can be presented by diverse human MHC class I and class II antigens may optimize the generation of strong, cross-protective immunity and possibly avoid the "dilution" of the immune response to variable, more mutable HCV epitopes.

Other approaches being explored to generate cellular immune responses include the fusion of recombinant HCV proteins with bacterial pore-forming toxoids. Certain detoxified bacterial toxoids have the ability to induce pore-mediated endocytosis in antigen-presenting cells, thus resulting in the generation of strong CD8$^+$ and CD4$^+$ T-cell responses to the toxoid and fused HCV moiety [96]. Electrically mediated uptake of synthetic HCV peptides has also been reported to result in priming of reactive CTLs in electroporated Balb/c mice [97]. Host heat-shock proteins are known to be good mediators of CD8$^+$ MHC I-restricted immune responses to associated foreign protein sequences [98]. As such, this approach may be applicable to the development of HCV vaccines, provided that harmful, auto-immune responses are not generated. Another intriguing avenue of research involves the use of influenza-based virosomes to deposit recombinant HCV proteins or synthetic HCV peptides on the MHC class I pathway, resulting in the generation of viral-specific CD8$^+$ CTLs. Comprising liposomes with influenza hemagglutinin and neuraminidase on the surface, these VLPs allow fusion with the membrane of antigen-presenting cells and the subsequent deposition of the HCV moiety in the cytosol. This then facilitates associ-ation of peptides with MHC class I molecules and TAP-mediated transfer to the surface of the cell where priming of reactive CTLs occurs [99].

C. HCV DNA Vaccines

The discovery that naked DNA or RNA administered i.m. or i.d. results in expression of encoded antigens and the elicitation of specific humoral and cellular immune responses has opened up a new area of vaccinology [100–103]. Advantages of using a DNA vaccine relate to the ease and cost of manufacture, the gene-mediated synthesis in vivo of native and often complex protein structures (that would otherwise be difficult to produce in the form of recombinant proteins), good stability (that renders the use of DNA vaccines particularly suitable to the needs of developing countries), and the ready ability to employ multiple genes, gene cassettes, or plasmids to elicit broad immune responses against heterogeneous pathogens such as HIV, HCV, and malaria, for example. Another important feature relates to the ability of DNA vaccines to stimulate CD8$^+$ MHC class I-restricted CTL responses via the endogenous synthesis of proteins de novo in the cytosol. Disadvantages, however, can include a weaker potency as compared with other vaccine formulations as well as safety issues revolving around their potential to integrate into the host genome, thereby increasing the risks of mutagenesis and carcinogenesis.

Additional safety issues may also be of concern, depending on the infectious agent under study. In the case of HCV, relatively long-term expression of the C gene has been reported to exert multiple pathogenic, oncogenic, and regulatory functions in transfected cells and animals. Its role in inducing steatosis and hepatocellular carcinoma in transgenic mice has been documented [104,105], as has its ability to co-promote cellular transformation in vitro [106]. There have been numerous other reports demonstrating the ability of the C gene product to bind to a member of the TNF-alpha superfamily [107], modulate apoptosis [108], induce oxidative stress [109,110], activate cellular and viral promoters [111], and affect other regulatory functions [112]. While the pathogenic significance of these findings in infected humans, if any, remains to be determined, it may be prudent in the meantime to omit the C gene from a potential HCV DNA vaccine (although the intermittent use of a recombinant C polypeptide subunit vaccine is unlikely to pose such a safety risk). Similarly, the 5′ terminal region of the NS3 gene (encoding the protease domain) has been linked with transformation of cells and carcinogenesis in nude mice [113].

Most of the work performed so far with HCV DNA vaccines has been performed in small animals, with very little done using nonhuman primates. This is important because, while most DNA vaccines are immunogenic in mice and other small animals, such results are harder to reproduce in higher animals. Furthermore, even the rhesus macaque is a questionable model for immunogenicity of DNA vaccines in humans. Many studies have immunized mice with plasmids expressing the envelope genes of HCV, generally using the immediate-early CMV promoter and intron to achieve high expression levels. Accordingly, the generation of humoral and cellular immune responses to gpE2 has been widely reported, including cross-reactive anti-gpE2 antibodies between subtypes 1a and 1b [114–120]. The use of a DNA vaccine encoding intracellular forms of gpE2, rather than secreted forms, has been emphasized in order to elicit anti-gpE2 antibodies capable of preventing the interaction between gpE2 and CD81, the latter being a candidate HCV receptor [84]. Boosting DNA-primed mice with recombinant gpE2 has been reported to elicit higher anti-gpE2 titers than repeated DNA or protein immunizations [121]. Immunogenicity of gpE2 DNA vaccines has also been demonstrated in rhesus macaques [118].

As with DNA vaccines targeting other infectious agents, the mode of injection drastically alters the immune response. Administration of a gpE2 DNA vaccine by gene gun, in which DNA is physically administered intraepithelially on gold microparticles, resulted in anti-gpE2 titers that were 100× higher than if delivered by needle, i.m. [120]. This increase in vaccine potency should translate to the use of lower doses in humans, thus lessening safety concerns.

Other methods to improve the potency of DNA vaccines include the application of an electric field at the site of DNA injection (so-called "electroporation"). In the case of a gpE2 DNA vaccine, electroporation led to 10-fold increases in expression levels and in concomitant anti-gpE2 responses. The latter also included cross-reactive anti-E2HVR1 antibodies that were not obtained without the use of electroporation. This technique also resulted in significant increases in gpE2-specific CD4$^+$ T helper and CD8$^+$ CTL responses [122]. However, the potential of electroporation to increase the rate of integration of the DNA vaccine into the host genome remains to be evaluated.

Other improvements include the formulation of DNA vaccines into particles, thereby increasing the uptake by antigen-presenting dendritic cells with corresponding increases in immunogenicity [123]. Lipid formulations of DNA that result in improved transfection efficiency in vivo as well as better uptake by dendritic cells have been shown to be part of an encouraging immunization regimen for rhesus macaques against SHIV challenge and have applications to HCV and other infectious diseases [124].

Only one small HCV DNA vaccine study in the chimpanzee model has been reported so far. In an attempt to optimize immunogenicity, the ectodomain of gpE2 (aa 384–715) was fused to the CD4 C-terminal, transmembrane region (TMR) that facilitated sequestration of the encoded gpE2 glycoprotein to the outer cell surface, rather than being anchored in the lumen of the er via the use of the homologous TMR. Ten milligrams of DNA were administered using a bioinjector into the quadriceps of two animals on weeks 0, 9, and 23, followed by experimental challenge with homologous, monoclonal virus 3 weeks later. Humoral and cellular immune responses to the vaccine were observed in only one animal, but following challenge, viremia was lowered as compared with a control animal and hepatitis occurred earlier, as a result of the primed immunity. Importantly, both vaccinees resolved their acute infections quickly, whereas the control, unvaccinated animal became chronically infected following viral challenge. This result is promising, but further studies are warranted due to the small number of animals and because one of the vaccinees had

already experienced an experimental HCV infection, prior to vaccination, that would have conferred immunity [125].

In order to recapitulate the broad T-cell responses associated with protective immunity against HCV infection, many groups are investigating DNA vaccines capable of priming HCV-specific CD4$^+$ and CD8$^+$ T-cell responses to many HCV gene products. A DNA vaccine encoding NS3, NS4, and NS5 not only primed broad and specific antibodies, CD4$^+$ T helper and CD8$^+$ CTL responses, but also conferred protection to the immunized BAL B/c mice against challenge with syngeneic, SP2/0 myeloma cells expressing NS5 [126]. Co-expression of the GM-CSF cytokine gene has also been shown to augment cellular immune responses to these NS gene products when administered as a bicistronic plasmid to Buffalo rats [127].

Many studies have been conducted with DNA vaccines containing the HCV C gene, as this encodes the most conserved viral protein and is known to contain important T-cell epitopes. Immunogenicity in mice has been reported [128–131] and, in addition, the co-administration of either IL2 or GM-CSF has been shown to augment humoral and cellular immune responses to C in mice [129]. On the contrary, co-immunization with a plasmid expressing IL4 resulted in the elicitation of a Th0 phenotype and a concomitant suppression of C-specific CTLs [129]. The use of transgenic mice expressing human HLA-A2.1 has also shown the ability of NS3 DNA vaccines to induce specific CTLs to the same immunodominant epitope observed in humans [132].

Finally, it is also noteworthy that defective RNA vaccines have been shown to be very effective at protecting against flaviviral infections [133]. Conferring good protective immunity in the absence of integration into the host genome, this approach has great promise for HCV and other infectious diseases.

D. HCV Vaccines Using Disabled Viral or Bacterial Vectors

The use of a defective or attenuated viral or bacterial vector to deliver vaccines has several potential advantages. Firstly, a wide tropism of the host vector leads to the efficient delivery of the vaccine genes and encoded antigens. Preferably, this tropism includes antigen-presenting cells leading to a very effective priming of the immune response, thereby requiring only one immunization for long-lasting immunity. The use of a vector already used as a vaccine itself offers further obvious advantages with respect to manufacturing, distribution, and user acceptance. Finally, many vectors allow the insertion of multiple genes thus facilitating the induction of a broad, cross-protective immune response, particularly useful against heterogeneous agents such as HCV.

One such promising approach for HCV has been the use of an attenuated rabies viral vector into which either the HCV gpE1–gpE2–p7 gene cassette was inserted, or just the ectodomain of gpE2 linked to the CD4, C-terminal TMR, and cytoplasmic domain. In the case of the latter construction, recombinant rabies virions were produced that actually contained the hybrid gpE2 within the virion. Virions expressing gpE1–gpE2–p7 were immunogenic in mice eliciting CTL responses to gpE2 [134]. Similarly, defective Semliki Forest virions containing the HCV NS3 gene produced long-lasting NS3-specific CTLs after one immunization in mice transgenic for human HLA-A2.1 [135]. As observed in HCV-infected patients, the immune response was directed to one immunodominant epitope within NS3. Defective, recombinant adenoviruses expressing the HCV C–gpE1–gpE2 gene cassette have also been shown to prime HCV-specific CTLs in mice immunized i.m., although the induction of anti-gpE1/gpE2 antibodies required further immunization with purified gpE1/gpE2 glycoproteins [136]. Replication-defective adenoviruses expressing C and gpE1 also primed long-lasting, specific CTL responses in mice [137]. Recombinant canary pox viruses, expressing an HCV gene cassette containing C–gpE1–gpE2–p7–NS2–NS3, elicited HCV-specific humoral and cellular immune responses in mice, although the optimum immunization regimen required first priming with a plasmid DNA expressing the HCV genes prior to boosting with the recombinant canary pox virus [138].

Attenuated *Salmonella typhimurium* transformed with a plasmid expressing the HCV NS3 gene has also been shown to elicit NS3-specific CTLs in mice transgenic for human HLA-A2.1. The bacterium was administered orally and the resulting CTL responses persisted for at least 10 months [139].

IV. SUMMARY

Recent studies in man and in the chimpanzee model provide evidence for significant natural immunity to HCV infection. Broad and early HCV-specific CD4$^+$ and CD8$^+$ T-cell responses are associated with recovery from acute infections. In contrast, chronic evolvers have a delayed, weaker T-cell response that deteriorates further with the onset of chronicity. The virus also mutates readily to evade both specific CD8$^+$ CTLs as well as neutralizing antibodies directed to the hypervariable region in gpE2. Chimpanzee challenge studies, using recombinant envelope glycoprotein vaccines, have demonstrated prophylactic efficacy and the feasibility of protecting against the development of chronic infection following experimental challenge with both homologous and heterologous viral strains. The application of broad technologies to HCV vaccination should result in effective vaccines which, although may not be 100% effective, should be very useful in lowering substantially the current incidence of HCV infection with its ensuing clinical sequelae. Vaccine immunotherapy, especially as an adjunct to antiviral treatment regimens, deserves clinical investigation.

REFERENCES

1. Robertson B, et al. Classification, nomenclature, and database development for hepatitis C virus (HCV) and related viruses: proposals for standardization. International Committee on Virus Taxonomy. Arch Virol 1998; 143(12):2493–2503.

2. Houghton M. Hepatitis C Viruses. In: Fields BN, Knipe PM, Howley PM, eds. Fields Virology. 3rd ed. Philadelphia: Lippincott-Raven Publishers, 1996:1035–1058.

3. Reed KE, Rice CM. Overview of hepatitis C virus genome structure, polyprotein processing, and protein properties. Curr Top Microbiol Immunol 2000; 242:55–84.

4. Rijnbrand R, et al. The influence of downstream protein-coding sequence on internal ribosome entry on hepatitis C virus and other flavivirus RNAs. RNA 2001; 7(4):585–597.

5. Walewski JL, et al. Evidence for a new hepatitis C virus antigen encoded in an overlapping reading frame. RNA 2001; 7 (5):710–721.

6. Xu Z, et al. Synthesis of a novel hepatitis C virus protein by ribosomal frameshift. EMBO J 2001; 20(14):3840–3848.

7. Hijikata M, et al. Gene mapping of the putative structural region of the hepatitis C virus genome by in vitro processing analysis. Proc Natl Acad Sci USA 1991; 88(13):5547–5551.

8. Spaete RR, et al. Characterization of the hepatitis C virus E2/NS1 gene product expressed in mammalian cells. Virology 1992; 188(2):819–830.

9. Grakoui A, et al. Expression and identification of hepatitis C virus polyprotein cleavage products. J Virol 1993; 67(3):1385–1395.

10. Ralston R, et al. Characterization of hepatitis C virus envelope glycoprotein complexes expressed by recombinant vaccinia viruses. J Virol 1993; 67(11):6753–6761.

11. Dubuisson J, et al. Formation and intracellular localization of hepatitis C virus envelope glycoprotein complexes expressed by recombinant vaccinia and Sindbis viruses. J Virol 1994; 68(10):6147–6160.

12. Dubuisson J. Folding, assembly and subcellular localization of hepatitis C virus glycoproteins. Curr Top Microbiol Immunol 2000; 242:135–148.

13. Michalak JP, et al. Characterization of truncated forms of hepatitis C virus glycoproteins. J Gen Virol 1997; 78(Pt 9):2299–2306.

14. Hussy P, et al. Hepatitis C virus core protein: carboxy-terminal boundaries of two processed species suggest cleavage by a signal peptide peptidase. Virology 1996; 224(1):93–104.

15. Yasui K, et al. The native form and maturation process of hepatitis C virus core protein. J Virol 1998; 72(7):6048–6055.

16. Kunkel M, et al. Self-assembly of nucleocapsid-like particles from recombinant hepatitis C virus core protein. J Virol 2001; 75(5):2119–2129.

17. Shih CM, et al. Modulation of the trans-suppression activity of hepatitis C virus core protein by phosphorylation. J Virol 1995; 69(2):1160–1171.

18. Lin C, et al. Processing in the hepatitis C virus E2-NS2 region: identification of p7 and two distinct E2-specific products with different C termini. J Virol 1994; 68(8):5063–5073.

19. Harada T, et al. E2-p7 region of the bovine viral diarrhea virus polyprotein: processing and functional studies. J Virol 2000; 74:9498–9506.

20. Grakoui A, et al. Characterization of the hepatitis C virus-encoded serine proteinase: determination of proteinase-dependent polyprotein cleavage sites. J Virol 1993; 67(5):2832–2843.

21. Grakoui A, et al. A second hepatitis C virus-encoded proteinase. Proc Natl Acad Sci USA 1993; 90(22):10583–10587.

22. Hijikata M, et al. Two distinct proteinase activities required for the processing of a putative nonstructural precursor protein of hepatitis C virus. J Virol 1993; 67(8): 4665–4675.

23. Tanaka T, et al. Structure of the 3′ terminus of the hepatitis C virus genome. J Virol 1996; 70(5):3307–3312.

24. Kolykhalov AA, et al. Identification of a highly conserved sequence element at the 3′ terminus of hepatitis C virus genome RNA. J Virol 1996; 70(6):3363–3371.

25. Tokita H, et al. The entire nucleotide sequences of three hepatitis C virus isolates in genetic groups 7–9 and com-

parison with those in the other eight genetic groups. J Gen Virol 1998; 79(Pt 8):1847–1857.

26. Weiner AJ, et al. Variable and hypervariable domains are found in the regions of HCV corresponding to the flavivirus envelope and NS1 proteins and the pestivirus envelope glycoproteins. Virology 1991; 180(2):842–848.

27. Weiner AJ, et al. Evidence for immune selection of hepatitis C virus (HCV) putative envelope glycoprotein variants: potential role in chronic HCV infections. Proc Natl Acad Sci USA 1992; 89(8):3468–3472.

28. Kato N, et al. Humoral immune response to hypervariable region 1 of the putative envelope glycoprotein (gp70) of hepatitis C virus. J Virol 1993; 67(7):3923–3930.

29. Kato N, et al. Genetic drift in hypervariable region 1 of the viral genome in persistent hepatitis C virus infection. J Virol 1994; 68(8):4776–4784.

30. Farci P, et al. Prevention of hepatitis C virus infection in chimpanzees by hyperimmune serum against the hypervariable region 1 of the envelope 2 protein. Proc Natl Acad Sci USA 1996; 93(26):15394–15399.

31. Farci P, et al. The outcome of acute hepatitis C predicted by the evolution of the viral quasispecies. Science 2000; 288 (5464):339–344.

32. Mercer DF, et al. Hepatitis C virus replication in mice with chimeric human livers. Nat Med 2001; 7(8):927–933.

33. WHO. Hepatitis C: global prevalence. WHO Wkly Epidemiol Rec 1997; 72:341–344.

34. Weiner AJ, et al. Intrahepatic genetic inoculation of hepatitis C virus RNA confers cross-protective immunity. J Virol 2001; 75(15):7142–7148.

35. Bassett SE, et al. Protective immune response to hepatitis C virus in chimpanzees rechallenged following clearance of primary infection. Hepatology 2001; 33(6):1479–1487.

36. Major ME, et al. Previously infected and recovered chimpanzees exhibit rapid responses that control hepatitis C virus replication upon rechallenge. J Virol 2002; 76(13):6586–6595.

37. Mehta SH, et al. Protection against persistence of hepatitis C. Lancet 2002; 359(9316):1478–1483.

38. Lauer GM, et al. Human immunodeficiency virus type 1-hepatitis C virus coinfection: intraindividual comparison of cellular immune responses against two persistent viruses. J Virol 2002; 76(6):2817–2826.

39. Farci P, et al. Lack of protective immunity against reinfection with hepatitis C virus. Science 1992; 258(5079):135–140.

40. Diepolder HM, et al. Possible mechanism involving T-lymphocyte response to non-structural protein 3 in viral clearance in acute hepatitis C virus infection. Lancet 1995; 346 (8981):1006–1007.

41. Gerlach JT, et al. Recurrence of hepatitis C virus after loss of virus-specific CD4(+) T-cell response in acute hepatitis C. Gastroenterology 1999; 117(4):933–941.

42. Cooper S, et al. Analysis of a successful immune response against hepatitis C virus. Immunity 1999; 10(4):439–449.

43. Missale G, et al. Different clinical behaviors of acute hepatitis C virus infection are associated with different vigor of the anti-viral cell-mediated immune response. J Clin Invest 1996; 98(3):706–714.

44. Tsai SL, et al. Detection of type 2-like T-helper cells in hepatitis C virus infection: implications for hepatitis C virus chronicity. Hepatology 1997; 25(2):449–458.

45. Rosen HR, et al. Frequencies of HCV-specific effector CD4+ T cells by flow cytometry: correlation with clinical disease stages. Hepatology 2002; 35(1):190–198.

46. Lechner F, et al. Analysis of successful immune responses in persons infected with hepatitis C virus. J Exp Med 2000; 191(9):1499–1512.

47. Thimme R, et al. Determinants of viral clearance and per-

sistence during acute hepatitis C virus infection. J Exp Med 2001; 194(10):1395–1406.

48. Gruner NH, et al. Association of hepatitis C virus-specific CD8+ T cells with viral clearance in acute hepatitis C. J Infect Dis 2000; 181(5):1528–1536.

49. Frese M, et al. Interferon-gamma inhibits replication of subgenomic and genomic hepatitis C virus RNAs. Hepatology 2002; 35(3):694–703.

50. Takaki A, et al. Cellular immune responses persist and humoral responses decrease two decades after recovery from a single-source outbreak of hepatitis C. Nat Med 2000; 6(5):578–582.

51. Lechner F, et al. CD8+ T lymphocyte responses are induced during acute hepatitis C virus infection but are not sustained. Eur J Immunol 2000; 30(9):2479–2487.

52. Gruener NH, et al. Sustained dysfunction of antiviral CD8+ T lymphocytes after infection with hepatitis C virus. J Virol 2001; 75(12):5550–5558.

53. Wedemeyer H, et al. Impaired effector function of hepatitis C virus-specific CD8+ T cells in chronic hepatitis C virus infection. J Immunol 2002; 169(6):3447–3458.

54. Scognamiglio P, et al. Presence of effector CD8+ T cells in hepatitis C virus-exposed healthy seronegative donors. J Immunol 1999; 162(11):6681–6689.

55. Koziel MJ, et al. Hepatitis C virus-specific cytolytic T lymphocyte and T helper cell responses in seronegative persons. J Infect Dis 1997; 176(4):859–866.

56. Erickson AL, et al. The outcome of hepatitis C virus infection is predicted by escape mutations in epitopes targeted by cytotoxic T lymphocytes. Immunity 2001; 15(6):883–895.

57. Thursz M, et al. Influence of MHC class II genotype on outcome of infection with hepatitis C virus. The HENCORE Group. Hepatitis C European Network for Cooperative Research. Lancet 1999; 354(9196):2119–2124.

58. Thio CL, et al. HLA-Cw*04 and hepatitis C virus persistence. J Virol 2002; 76(10):4792–4797.

59. Harcourt G, et al. Effect of HLA class II genotype on T helper lymphocyte responses and viral control in hepatitis C virus infection. J Viral Hepatitis 2001; 8(3):174–179.

60. Chien DY, et al. Persistence of HCV despite antibodies to both putative envelope glycoproteins. Lancet 1993; 342 (8876): 933.

61. Lesniewski R, et al. Antibody to hepatitis C virus second envelope (HCV-E2) glycoprotein: a new marker of HCV infection closely associated with viremia. J Med Virol 1995; 45 (4):415–422.

62. Bassett SE, et al. Viral persistence, antibody to E1 and E2, and hypervariable region 1 sequence stability in hepatitis C virus-inoculated chimpanzees. J Virol 1999; 73(2):1118–1126.

63. Prince AM, et al. Significance of the anti-E2 response in self-limited and chronic hepatitis C virus infections in chimpanzees and in humans. J Infect Dis 1999; 180(4):987–991.

64. Farci P, et al. Prevention of hepatitis C virus infection in chimpanzees after antibody-mediated in vitro neutralization. Proc Natl Acad Sci USA 1994; 91(16):7792–7796.

65. Hijikata M, et al. Equilibrium centrifugation studies of hepatitis C virus: evidence for circulating immune complexes. J Virol 1993; 67(4):1953–1958.

66. Knodell RG, et al. Development of chronic liver disease after acute non-A, non-B post-transfusion hepatitis. Role of gamma-globulin prophylaxis in its prevention. Gastroenterology 1977; 72(5 Pt 1):902–909.

67. Feray C, et al. Incidence of hepatitis C in patients receiving different preparations of hepatitis B immunoglobulins after liver transplantation. Ann Intern Med 1998; 128(10):810–816.

68. Piazza M, et al. Sexual transmission of the hepatitis C virus and efficacy of prophylaxis with intramuscular immune se-

rum globulin. A randomized controlled trial. Arch Intern Med 1997; 157(14):1537–1544.

69. Krawczynski K, et al. Effect of immune globulin on the prevention of experimental hepatitis C virus infection. J Infect Dis 1996; 173(4):822–828.

70. Bjoro K, et al. Hepatitis C infection in patients with primary hypogammaglobulinemia after treatment with contaminated immune globulin. N Engl J Med 1994; 331(24):1607–1611.

71. Christie JM, et al. Clinical outcome of hypogammaglobulinaemic patients following outbreak of acute hepatitis C: 2 year follow up. Clin Exp Immunol 1997; 110(1):4–8.

72. Allander T, et al. Patients infected with the same hepatitis C virus strain display different kinetics of the isolate-specific antibody response. J Infect Dis 1997; 175(1):26–31.

73. Zibert A, et al. Epitope mapping of antibodies directed against hypervariable region 1 in acute self-limiting and chronic infections due to hepatitis C virus. J Virol 1997; 71(5):4123–4127.

74. Bradley D, et al. Hepatitis C virus: buoyant density of the factor VIII-derived isolate in sucrose. J Med Virol 1991; 34(3):206–208.

75. Thomssen R, et al. Association of hepatitis C virus in human sera with beta-lipoprotein. Med Microbiol Immunol (Berlin) 1992; 181(5):293–300.

76. Thomssen R, et al. Density heterogeneities of hepatitis C virus in human sera due to the binding of beta-lipoproteins and immunoglobulins. Med Microbiol Immunol (Berlin) 1993; 182(6):329–334.

77. Choo QL, et al. Vaccination of chimpanzees against infection by the hepatitis C virus. Proc Natl Acad Sci USA 1994; 91(4):1294–1298.

78. Houghton M, et al. Prospects for prophylactic and therapeutic hepatitis C virus vaccines. Princess Takamatsu Symp 1995; 25:237–243.

79. Houghton M, et al. Development of an HCV Vaccine. In: Rizzetto M, Purcel RH, Gerin JL, Verme G, eds. Viral Hepatitis and Liver Disease, Proceedings of the IX Triennial International Symposium on Viral Hepatitis and Liver Disease. Vol. 1996. Rome, Italy: Edizioni Minerva Med, 1996:656–659.

80. Rosa D, et al. A quantitative test to estimate neutralizing antibodies to the hepatitis C virus. cytofluorimetric assessment of envelope glycoprotein 2 binding to target cells. Proc Natl Acad Sci USA 1996; 93(5):1759–1763.

81. Pileri P, et al. Binding of hepatitis C virus to CD81. Science 1998; 282(5390):938–941.

82. Esumi M, et al. Experimental vaccine activities of recombinant E1 and E2 glycoproteins and hypervariable region 1 peptides of hepatitis C virus in chimpanzees. Arch Virol 1999; 144(5):973–980.

83. Goto J, et al. Prevention of hepatitis C virus infection in a chimpanzee by vaccination and epitope mapping of antiserum directed against hypervariable region 1. Hepatol Res 2001; 19(3):270–283.

84. Heile JM, et al. Evaluation of hepatitis C virus glycoprotein E2 for vaccine design: an endoplasmic reticulum-retained recombinant protein is superior to secreted recombinant protein and DNA-based vaccine candidates. J Virol 2000; 74(15):6885–6892.

85. Baumert TF, et al. Hepatitis C virus structural proteins assemble into viruslike particles in insect cells. J Virol 1998; 72(5):3827–3836.

86. Lechmann M, et al. Hepatitis C virus-like particles induce virus-specific humoral and cellular immune responses in mice. Hepatology 2001; 34(2):417–423.

87. Blanchard E, et al. Hepatitis C virus-like particle morphogenesis. J Virol 2002; 76(8):4073–4079.

88. Roccasecca R, et al. Mimotopes of the hyper variable region

1 of the hepatitis C virus induce cross-reactive antibodies directed against discontinuous epitopes. Mol Immunol 2001; 38(6):485–492.

89. Nemchinov LG, et al. Development of a plant-derived subunit vaccine candidate against hepatitis C virus. Arch Virol 2000; 145(12):2557–2573.

90. Lamonaca V, et al. Conserved hepatitis C virus sequences are highly immunogenic for CD4(+) T cells: implications for vaccine development. Hepatology 1999; 30(4):1088–1098.

91. Wentworth PA, et al. Identification of A2-restricted hepatitis C virus-specific cytotoxic T lymphocyte epitopes from conserved regions of the viral genome. Int Immunol 1996; 8(5):651–659.

92. Acosta Rivero N, et al. In vitro self-assembled HCV core virus-like particles induce a strong antibody immune response in sheep. Biochem Biophys Res Commun 2002; 290(1):300–304.

93. Alvarez-Obregon JC, et al. A truncated HCV core protein elicits a potent immune response with a strong participation of cellular immunity components in mice. Vaccine 2001; 19(28-29):3940–3946.

94. Polakos NK, et al. Characterization of hepatitis C virus core-specific immune responses primed in rhesus macaques by a nonclassical ISCOM vaccine. J Immunol 2001; 166(5):3589–3598.

95. Urbani S, et al. Identification of immunodominant hepatitis C virus (HCV)-specific cytotoxic T-cell epitopes by stimulation with endogenously synthesized HCV antigens. Hepatology 2001; 33(6):1533–1543.

96. Moriya O, et al. Induction of hepatitis C virus-specific cytotoxic T lymphocytes in mice by immunization with dendritic cells treated with an anthrax toxin fusion protein. Vaccine 2001; 20(5-6):789–796.

97. Uno-Furuta S, et al. Induction of virus-specific cytotoxic T lymphocytes by in vivo electric administration of peptides. Vaccine 2001; 19(15-16):2190–2196.

98. Planelles L, et al. DNA immunization with *Trypanosoma cruzi* HSP70 fused to the KMP11 protein elicits a cytotoxic and humoral immune response against the antigen and leads to protection. Infect Immun 2001; 69(10):6558–6563.

99. Hunziker IP, et al. In vitro studies of core peptide-bearing immunopotentiating reconstituted influenza virosomes as a non-live prototype vaccine against hepatitis C virus. Int Immunol 2002; 14(6):615–626.

100. Wolff JA, et al. Direct gene transfer into mouse muscle in vivo. Science 1990; 247:1465–1468.

101. Tang DC, et al. Genetic immunization is a simple method for eliciting an immune response. Nature 1992; 356(6365):152–154.

102. Williams WV, et al. Genetic infection induces protective in vivo immune responses. DNA Cell Biol 1993; 12(8):675–683.

103. Ulmer JB, et al. Heterologous protection against influenza by injection of DNA encoding a viral protein. Science 1993; 259(5102):1745–1749.

104. Moriya K, et al. The core protein of hepatitis C virus induces hepatocellular carcinoma in transgenic mice. Nat Med 1998; 4(9):1065–1067.

105. Moriya K, et al. Hepatitis C virus core protein induces hepatic steatosis in transgenic mice. J Gen Virol 1997; 78 (Pt 7):1527–1531.

106. Ray RB, et al. Hepatitis C virus core protein cooperates with ras and transforms primary rat embryo fibroblasts to tumorigenic phenotype. J Virol 1996; 70(7):4438–4443.

107. Matsumoto M, et al. Hepatitis C virus core protein interacts with the cytoplasmic tail of lymphotoxin-beta receptor. J Virol 1997; 71(2):1301–1309.

108. Ray RB, et al. Suppression of apoptotic cell death by hepatitis C virus core protein. Virology 1996; 226(2):176–182.

109. Moriya K, et al. Oxidative stress in the absence of inflammation in a mouse model for hepatitis C virus-associated hepatocarcinogenesis. Cancer Res 2001; 61(11):4365–4370.

110. Okuda M, et al. Mitochondrial injury, oxidative stress, and antioxidant gene expression are induced by hepatitis C virus core protein. Gastroenterology 2002; 122(2):366–375.

111. Ray RB, et al. Transcriptional regulation of cellular and viral promoters by the hepatitis C virus core protein. Virus Res 1995; 37(3):209–220.

112. Ray RB, et al. Transcriptional repression of p53 promoter by hepatitis C virus core protein. J Biol Chem 1997; 272(17): 10983–10986.

113. Sakamuro D, et al. Hepatitis C virus nonstructural protein NS3 transforms NIH 3T3 cells. J Virol 1995; 69(6):3893–3896.

114. Saito T, et al. Plasmid DNA-based immunization for hepatitis C virus structural proteins: Immune responses in mice. Gastroenterology 1997; 112:1321–1330.

115. Tedeschi V, et al. A specific antibody response to HCV E2 elicited in mice by intramuscular inoculation of plasmid DNA containing coding sequences for E2. Hepatology 1997; 25(2):459–462.

116. Inchauspe G, et al. DNA vaccination for the induction of immune responses against hepatitis C virus proteins. Vaccine 1997; 15(8):853–856.

117. Fournillier A, et al. Expression of noncovalent hepatitis C virus envelope E1–E2 complexes is not required for the induction of antibodies with neutralizing properties following DNA immunization. J Virol 1999; 73(9):7497–7504.

118. Forns X, et al. DNA immunization of mice and macaques with plasmids encoding hepatitis C virus envelope E2 protein expressed intracellularly and on the cell surface. Vaccine 1999; 17(15-16):1992–2002.

119. Gordon EJ, et al. Immune responses to hepatitis C virus structural and nonstructural proteins induced by plasmid DNA immunizations. J Infect Dis 2000; 181(1):42–50.

120. Nakano I, et al. Immunization with plasmid DNA encoding hepatitis C virus envelope E2 antigenic domains induces antibodies whose immune reactivity is linked to the injection mode. J Virol 1997; 71(9):7101–7109.

121. Song MK, et al. Enhancement of immunoglobulin G2a and cytotoxic T-lymphocyte responses by a booster immunization with recombinant hepatitis C virus E2 protein in E2 DNA-primed mice. J Virol 2000; 74(6):2920–2925.

122. Zucchelli S, et al. Enhancing B- and T-cell immune response to a hepatitis C virus E2 DNA vaccine by intramuscular electrical gene transfer. J Virol 2000; 74(24):11598–11607.

123. O'Hagan D, et al. Induction of potent immune responses by cationic microparticles with adsorbed HIV DNA vaccines. J Virol 2001; 75(19):9037–9043.

124. Caulfield MJ, et al. Sustained peptide-specific gamma interferon T-cell response in rhesus macques immunized with human immunodeficiency virus gag DNA vaccines. J Virol 2002; 76(19):10038–10043.

125. Forns X, et al. Vaccination of chimpanzees with plasmid DNA encoding the hepatitis C virus (HCV) envelope E2 protein modified the infection after challenge with homologous monoclonal HCV. Hepatology 2000; 32(3):618–625.

126. Encke J, et al. Genetic immunization generates cellular and humoral immune responses against the nonstructural proteins of the hepatitis C virus in a murine model. J Immunol 1998; 161(9):p4917–p4923.

127. Cho JH, et al. Enhanced cellular immunity to hepatitis C virus nonstructural proteins by codelivery of granulocyte macrophage-colony stimulating factor gene in intramuscular DNA immunization. Vaccine 1999; 17(9-10):1136–1144.

128. Tokushige K, et al. Expression and immune response to hepatitis C virus core DNA-based vaccine constructs. Hepatology 1996; 24(1):14–20.

129. Geissler M, et al. Enhancement of cellular and humoral immune responses to hepatitis C virus core protein using DNA-based vaccines augmented with cytokine-expressing plasmids. J Immunol 1997; 158(3):1231–1237.

130. Shirai M, et al. An epitope in hepatitis C virus core region recognized by cytotoxic T cells in mice and humans. J Virol 1994; 68(5):3334–3342.

131. Lagging LM, et al. Immune responses to plasmid DNA encoding the hepatitis C virus core protein. J Virol 1995; 69 (9):5859–5863.

132. Brinster C, et al. Different hepatitis C virus nonstructural protein 3 (Ns3)-DNA-expressing vaccines induce in HLA-A2.1 transgenic mice stable cytotoxic T lymphocytes that target one major epitope. Hepatology 2001; 34(6):1206–1217.

133. Mandl CW, et al. In vitro-synthesized infectious RNA as an attenuated live vaccine in a flavivirus model. Nat Med 1998; 4(12):1438–1440.

134. Siler CA, et al. Live and killed rhabdovirus-based vectors as potential hepatitis C vaccines. Virology 2002; 292(1):24–34.

135. Brinster C, et al. Hepatitis C virus non-structural protein 3-specific cellular immune responses following single or combined immunization with DNA or recombinant Semliki Forest virus particles. J Gen Virol 2002; 83(Pt 2):369–381.

136. Seong YR, et al. Immunogenicity of the E1E2 proteins of hepatitis C virus expressed by recombinant adenoviruses. Vaccine 2001; 19(20–22):2955–2964.

137. Bruna-Romero O, et al. Induction of cytotoxic T-cell response against hepatitis C virus structural antigens using a defective recombinant adenovirus. Hepatology 1997; 25(2): 470–477.

138. Pancholi P, et al. DNA prime-canarypox boost with polycistronic hepatitis C virus (HCV) genes generates potent immune responses to HCV structural and nonstructural proteins. J Infect Dis 2000; 182(1):18–27.

139. Wedemeyer H, et al. B. Oral immunization with HCV-NS3-transformed Salmonella: induction of HCV-specific CTL in a transgenic mouse model. Gastroenterology 2001; 121(5): 1158–1166.

140. Simmonds P. Hepatitis C Virus Genotypes. In: Liang TJ, Hoofnagle JH, eds. Hepatitis C. Academic Press, 2000:53–70.

141. Ebeling F. Epidemiology of the hepatitis C virus. Vox Sang 1998; 74(Suppl 2):143–146.

51
Live Vaccine Strategies to Prevent Rotavirus Disease

Richard L. Ward
Children's Hospital Medical Center, Cincinnati, Ohio, U.S.A.

H. Fred Clark and Paul A. Offit
The Children's Hospital of Philadelphia and the University of Pennsylvania School of Medicine, Philadelphia, Pennsylvania, U.S.A.

Roger I. Glass
National Center for Infectious Diseases, Centers for Disease Control and Prevention, Atlanta, Georgia, U.S.A.

I. WORLDWIDE IMPORTANCE OF AN EFFECTIVE ROTAVIRUS VACCINE

Diarrheal diseases are among the most common illnesses of mankind, and the first or second most common cause of death, hospitalization, and doctor visits among children worldwide [1,2]. They almost always result from infection and, over the past three decades, more than 25 different infectious agents have been identified as etiological agents of diarrheal diseases. For most children, episodes of diarrhea are self-limited, the disease is mild, and recovery occurs within several days. However, in some children, the disease can be severe, progressively leading to dehydration, hospitalization, and death. Of the many diarrheal illnesses, rotavirus has been identified to be the most common cause of severe diarrhea in children.

Several key features define the epidemiology of rotavirus diseases and suggest approaches to the prevention and control of the disease with vaccines [3]. First, infections are universal and all children worldwide are infected in their first 3 years of life. This suggests that improvements in food and water sanitation are unlikely to alter the incidence of disease; therefore, other approaches are necessary. First infections with rotavirus that occur several months after birth are often associated with severe diarrhea. Immunity to the disease develops after the first infection, so second infections are usually not associated with illness and the incidence of rotavirus disease diminishes with increasing age [4]. Despite global efforts to diminish the severity of diarrhea through the use of oral rehydration, diarrhea related to rotavirus remains a major cause of hospitalization and death.

Global interest in the development of rotavirus vaccines has been driven by the burden of fatal disease in developing countries (Figure 1) and the burden of rotavirus diseases on medical and societal costs in industrialized countries [5,6]. In developing countries, rotavirus is estimated to cause 450,000–600,000 deaths each year (Figure 2). This represents about 5% of the 12,000,000 deaths worldwide annually among children <5 years of age, or about one death per 270 children born worldwide (ca. 135,000,000 births per year) [7]. In both developed and industrialized countries, rotavirus accounts for between 20% and 60% of hospitalizations for diarrhea, and recent surveys suggest that one child in every 30–120 will be hospitalized for rotavirus diarrhea before their fifth birthday. In the United States, efforts to include a rotavirus vaccine in the national immunization schedule were prompted by estimates that rotavirus diarrhea results in 600,000 doctor or emergency room visits, 55,000 hospitalizations, and 20–40 deaths each year [6]. The cost of this illness has been estimated to exceed US$400 million in medical expenses and more than US$1 billion when societal costs (e.g., parents' lost work time) are included.

II. THE ROTAVIRUS PARTICLE AND ITS ROUTE OF PATHOGENESIS

Conventional electron microscopy revealed the rotavirus particle as a double-shelled structure with icosahedral symmetry [8,9]. The outer shell is composed of two proteins, VP4 and VP7, which form capsomeres that radiate from the inner

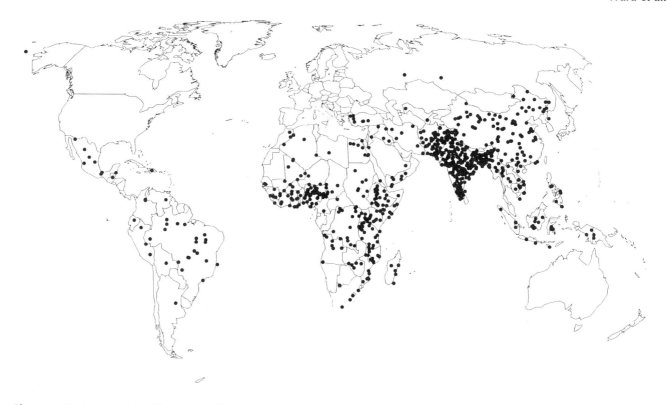

Figure 1 Estimated global distribution of annual deaths due to rotavirus diarrhea in children under 5 years of age. (From Glass RI, et al. Nat Med 1997; 3:1324–1325.)

capsid comprising the major structural protein VP6 [10]. This inner shell surrounds a core containing 11 segments of double-stranded RNA and three additional structural proteins: VP1, VP2, and VP3. A much greater definition was obtained using cryoelectron microscopy (Figure 3). With this technique, it was revealed that the rotavirus core is surrounded by a third protein shell composed of VP2, thus establishing the mature rotavirus particle as triple-layered

[11,12]. These particles appear to be ca. 75 nm in diameter, but the 60 VP4 dimers anchored to the VP6 intermediate shell extend by an additional 11–12 nm beyond the surface of the outer shell, thus making the entire particle ca. 100 nm in diameter.

The replication cycle of rotavirus is activated by the cleavage of the VP4 protein by trypsinlike proteases, but its VP5* and VP8* products remain virus-associated [13]. After

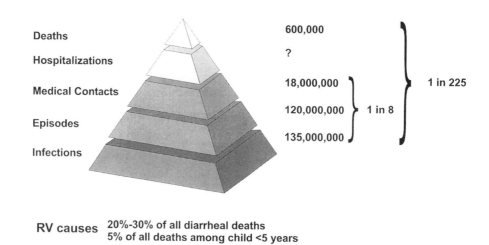

Figure 2 Estimated annual global burden of rotavirus infections, episodes of serious disease, and deaths.

attachment to receptors via VP8*, the virion passes into the cytoplasm where the outer capsid proteins are removed [14]. This stimulates the VP1 transcriptase to synthesize 11 viral mRNAs that are capped by VP3 and translated into six structural proteins and six nonstructural proteins (NSP1–NSP6) [10]. Viral assembly begins when the full complement of 11 plus-sense mRNA accumulates within the precursor particles containing several structural and nonstructural rotavirus proteins [15]. These particles mature stepwise by the addition of the capsid layers and the removal of non-structural proteins, the final event occurring within the rough endoplasmic reticulum [16].

Rotavirus replication in its host occurs primarily, if not solely, in the mature enterocytes at the tips of the intestinal villi [17]. Thus, the transmission of this virus may be strictly fecal–oral. Following infection of calves and piglets, the cells at the villus tips become denuded (Figure 4), which results in the shortening and stunting of the villi [18]. In the underlying lamina propria, mononuclear cell infiltration is observed. Similar responses have been observed in infected children [8,19]. It has been proposed that the gastrointestinal symptoms of vomiting and diarrhea associated with rotavirus infection are due to the loss of the mature villus enterocytes and the retarded differentiation of the uninfected immature enterocytes [17,20]. Recently, it was reported that the nonstructural NSP4 protein of rotavirus can induce diarrhea in infant mice after intraperitoneal inoculation

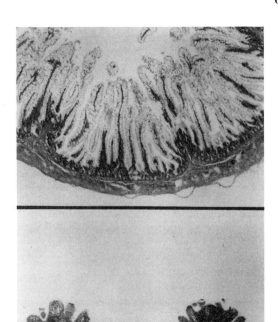

Figure 4 (Top) Normal histological appearance of the ileum from an 8-day-old gnotobiotic piglet. Normal mature vacuolate absorptive cells cover the villi. (Bottom) Ileum from an 8-day-old gnotobiotic piglet after oral inoculation with the virulent human rotavirus strain Wa. Severe atrophy and early crypt hyperplasia are evident. (From Dr. L. A. Ward, Ohio Agricultural Research and Development Center, The Ohio State University, Wooster, OH.)

[21,22], possibly by the activation of a calcium-dependent signal transduction pathway [23]. Whether NSP4 acts as an enterotoxin and stimulates gastroenteritis in humans remains to be determined.

III. NATURAL ROTAVIRUS INFECTION PROTECTS AGAINST SUBSEQUENT ROTAVIRUS DISEASE

Rotavirus infection of animals or humans has been shown in numerous studies to be highly protective against subsequent rotavirus illnesses. In one of the earliest studies, it was found that neonates infected with the rotavirus during the first 2 weeks of life were protected against severe rotavirus disease but were not protected against rotavirus reinfection [24]. More recent studies on protection after neonatal rotavirus infection conducted in India provided similar conclusions [25,26]. Symptomatic or asymptomatic rotavirus infection of young children has been reported in multiple studies to provide at least partial, and sometimes complete, protection against subsequent rotavirus illness. For example, in one of

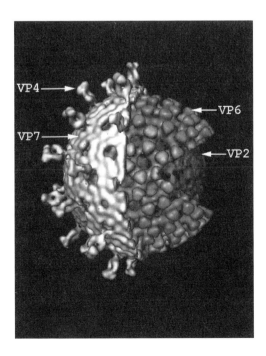

Figure 3 Computer-generated image of the triple-layered rotavirus particle. The cutaway diagram shows the outer capsid composed of VP4 spikes and VP7 layer, intermediate VP6 layer, and inner VP2 layer surrounding the core containing 11 double-stranded RNA segments and VP1 and VP3 proteins. (From Dr. B. V. V. Prasad, Baylor College of Medicine.)

the most recent studies, it was found that subjects followed from birth to 2 years of age often have two or more rotavirus infections during this period, but the severity of rotavirus-associated illness plummeted as the infection number increased [4]. This occurred even though there were several rotavirus serotypes that circulated within the study population during the evaluation period. The interpretation of this and similar observations has led to divergent approaches in rotavirus vaccine development as will be discussed. Regardless of the approach used, it is universally agreed upon that the protection elicited by natural rotavirus infection provides both a rationale for the development of live, orally deliverable rotavirus vaccine candidates and a standard against which to evaluate the effectiveness of these vaccines.

IV. DEVELOPMENT OF ATTENUATED ROTAVIRUSES AS VACCINE CANDIDATES

Within a few years after the discovery of human rotaviruses and the recognition that they are the primary cause of severe gastroenteritis in young children, clinical trials evaluating rotavirus vaccine candidates were already underway [17]. The first candidates evaluated in young children were animal rotavirus strains. The use of animal rotaviruses, or the Jennerian approach, has continued, either directly or indirectly, in the development of several of the current live rotavirus vaccine candidates. This approach is based on the finding that, although animal rotaviruses have been found to infect humans [27], the transmission of rotavirus diseases from animals to humans still appears to be relatively uncommon, probably due, at least in part, to natural genetic barriers. Furthermore, when animal rotavirus strains are developed for use as human vaccine candidates, they are passed in cell culture—a procedure that should cause them to be further attenuated. The prediction that cell culture-grown animal rotaviruses are attenuated has been supported by clinical trial results in that vaccine candidates developed from animal rotaviruses have caused few, if any, symptoms typically associated with rotavirus diseases after administration to young children [17,28].

The first rotavirus isolated in cell culture was also the first to be evaluated in clinical trials. This bovine virus (NCDV), attenuated by >260 passages in cell culture, produced no adverse effects when administered to newborn calves [29]. Likewise, when prepared for human use, this virus (RIT 4237) produced no disease in young children, even when administered at a dose of 10^8 TCID$_{50}$ [30]. Administration of the vaccine during initial efficacy trials conducted in Finland resulted in serum antibody responses in 50–70% of children aged 5–12 months and was associated with >80% protection against clinically significant rotavirus disease [31,32]. When evaluated in subsequent trials, particularly those conducted in settings of developing countries, the administration of this candidate vaccine resulted in less protection and its development was discontinued [33–35].

The development and evaluation of another bovine rotavirus and a simian rotavirus followed soon after the initial studies with RIT 4237. The bovine strain (WC3),

isolated from a calf in Pennsylvania, was evaluated in humans after 12 passages in cell culture. Following the administration of 10^7 pfu to several hundred young children in immunogenicity and efficacy trials in both developed and developing countries, between 70% and 100% developed serum rotavirus antibody responses [36]. However, efficacy was inconsistent and even insignificant in two of four studies [37–39]. The simian (rhesus) rotavirus strain MMU 18006 (rhesus rotavirus, RRV) was evaluated at doses of 10^4–10^5 pfu in >1000 young children after nine passages in primary or secondary monkey kidney cells and seven passages in diploid fetal rhesus monkey lung cells [17]. This vaccine typically induced self-limited febrile responses in approximately one-third of vaccinees >5 months of age, but in only a small fraction of younger infants [40–42]. MMU 18006 was highly immunogenic and induced serum rotavirus antibody responses in nearly every vaccinee. However, its ability to stimulate protection against subsequent rotavirus disease was, like the other candidates, inconsistent [34,43–48]. Based on these inconsistencies, both the WC3 and RRV vaccine candidates were modified to include gene segments encoding at least one of two neutralization proteins (i.e., VP7 and VP4) derived from different serotypes of human rotaviruses. The rationale for this, and results of clinical trials in which these "reassortant" vaccine candidates have been evaluated, will be described in detail in the "Development of Attenuated Rotaviruses as Vaccine Candidates" and the "Design, Production, and Clinical Evaluation of Live Rotavirus Vaccine Candidates Developed from Evidence that Neutralizing Antibody Is the Essential Effector of Protection." The only other animal strain developed for evaluation as a vaccine candidate in humans was derived from a lamb. This vaccine, which has been administered to >1000 children in China [49], will also be described in a subsequent section.

The other rotaviruses developed for use as live virus vaccine candidates have all been derived from infected humans. Because humans are the natural hosts for these strains, it has been suggested that the immune responses they stimulate in infected humans, even after growth in cell culture, may be greater and more consistent than those elicited after the administration of animal strains. Furthermore, because the protection they produce will be directed against rotaviruses that also naturally infect humans, it has also been postulated that they may stimulate greater protection against these strains than that elicited by vaccination with animal rotaviruses. Although several live rotavirus vaccine candidates derived from human strains are under evaluation, the general validity of these suggestions has not yet been determined. However, it is clear that not all vaccines derived from human rotavirus strains elicit greater protection in immunized subjects than that found after immunization with animal strains [50,51].

Several of the human rotavirus strains that have been developed and evaluated as vaccine candidates were obtained from neonates. Neonatal rotavirus infections are typically endemic in some hospital settings and do not normally cause disease in this population. Although these neonatal strains are often readily distinguishable from the circulating community strains responsible for illnesses in older subjects, this is not always the case. Studies reported over a decade ago suggested that the VP4 proteins of neonatal strains belonged to the P[6] genotype [52,53], but this distinguishing feature has vanished with multiple reports of P[6] community strains and non-P[6] neonatal strains. Therefore, it is unclear whether the absence of disease in infected neonates is due to the strains causing the infections, or to the innate resistance of full-term newborns to rotavirus disease. Even so, several neonatal strains have been developed as rotavirus vaccine candidates based on the suggestion that they might be naturally attenuated and based on reports that they elicit at least partial protection against clinically significant rotavirus disease [24–26]. Although neonatal strains continue to be evaluated as vaccine candidates, as will be discussed below, the first examined (i.e., strain M37) stimulated poor immune responses and no protection against subsequent rotavirus diseases after administration to young children [50,51].

The other human rotaviruses that have been developed as vaccine candidates were derived from community strains. Initial trials with several of these strains suggested that they might be insufficiently attenuated, even after 16 passages in cultured cells [54]. Some community strains were further attenuated by cold adaptation, but this resulted in a significant reduction in their immunogenicities [54]. Interest in attenuating a virulent human rotavirus for use as a vaccine candidate was revived following a report that an initial symptomatic or asymptomatic infection with a circulating community strain resulted in 100% protection against subsequent rotavirus diseases over a 2-year period [55]. Although a vaccine (i.e., strain 89-12) derived from one of the subjects infected with this virus was not fully attenuated, even after 33 passages in cell culture, 94% of young children administered the vaccine developed rotavirus antibody responses [56]. After an individual virus within the passage 33 preparation was isolated and passed several more times in the cell culture, it appeared to be further attenuated without a measurable reduction in its immunogenicity [57]. The new preparation is being extensively evaluated in clinical trials. A listing of the live rotavirus vaccine candidates that have been evaluated in clinical trials and their current status is presented in Table 1.

V. THEORIES REGARDING THE EFFECTORS OF PROTECTION AFTER LIVE ROTAVIRUS INFECTION

The mechanism of protection against rotavirus diseases following a live virus infection has been examined in humans and, more extensively, in animal model studies. However, the outcome of these studies has left open a crucial question: Is neutralizing antibody (NA) the only significant effector of protection after these live rotavirus infections? The lack of a definitive answer to this question has led to two distinctly different approaches in the development of live rotavirus vaccine candidates that persist today. If NA is essential for protection, it is expected that a live rotavirus vaccine should contain multiple strains of rotavirus with serotype-specific epitopes to protect against rotaviruses belonging to the numerous serotypes that have been identified. If, on the other hand, effectors of protection other than classical NA play important roles in the prevention of rotavirus diseases, it is possible that vaccination with a single strain of rotavirus may be sufficient to protect against illnesses due to infections with numerous distinct serotypes. The vaccine candidates being developed and evaluated today are direct outcomes of these contrasting opinions regarding the crucial importance of NA in protection. Studies that support each of the two approaches will be presented below along with the results of efficacy trials in which each approach was utilized.

Before listing these studies, three points should be noted. The first is that intestinal NA is generally accepted as an important effector of protection after live rotavirus infection if it is present in sufficient titer. The only conflict concerns the roles of other effectors. The second is that even though distinct serotypes of rotaviruses have been defined based on differences in NA against the VP4 and VP7 proteins generated after the hyperimmunization of animals, some NA epitopes are shared between serotypes [17]. Thus, it is possible that protection against multiple rotavirus serotypes will be generated by vaccination with a single strain of rotavirus through NA produced against these shared epitopes. The third is that even when the background studies and clinical trial results have been presented, questions regarding the better approach will remain, at least until candidate

Table 1 Live Rotavirus Vaccine Candidates that Have Been Evaluated in Clinical Trials

Vaccine candidate	Type of vaccine	Status of vaccine
RIT 4237	Single-strain bovine virus	Discontinued
WC3	Single-strain bovine virus	Developed into reassortants
RRV	Single-strain simian virus	Developed into reassortants
LLR	Single-strain lamb virus	Being evaluated
M37	Single-strain neonatal virus	Discontinued
RV3	Single-strain neonatal virus	Being evaluated
I321	Single-strain neonatal virus	Being evaluated
116E	Single-strain neonatal virus	Being evaluated
89-12	Single-strain infant virus	Being evaluated
RRV-TV (Rotashield™)	Tetravalent reassortant viruses	Withdrawn from U.S. market
WC3-QV (RotaTeq™)	Quintavalent reassortant viruses	Being evaluated

vaccines representative of each have been thoroughly compared in efficacy trials, possibly head to head.

VI. EVIDENCE THAT NEUTRALIZING ANTIBODY IS AN ESSENTIAL EFFECTOR OF PROTECTION AGAINST ROTAVIRUS DISEASE IN HUMANS INDUCED BY LIVE ROTAVIRUS INFECTION

It has been established that antirotavirus antibody bathing the gut in adequate concentration is protective against rotavirus diseases [58]. However, it is impractical to provide meaningful passive protection for the duration of susceptibility in a young child. Therefore, it is necessary to actively immunize to provide adequate protection. Rotavirus immunization or natural infection induces a broad range of circulating and secretory antibody responses as well as cell-mediated immune responses [59]. Attempts to correlate levels of serotype-specific serum NA with the specificity of protection following immunization have failed [30,31,60–62]. However, clues regarding the role of serotype specificity in the protection against rotavirus diseases have been derived from epidemiological evidence, vaccination/challenge studies in animals, and experimental vaccination of infants.

It has frequently been stated that the only severe rotavirus infection is the first infection [24,55]. This suggests the possibility that serotype cross-reactive antibodies provide adequate protection against all rotavirus serotypes. However, there have been severe rotavirus disease episodes recorded in children, and even adults, with demonstrated serological evidence of prior rotavirus infection [63,64]. Although second episodes of severe human disease caused by the same serotype have been reported, second clinical infections in infants have more often been associated with serotypes different from the first [4,65]. Thus, the epidemiological evidence regarding the importance of NA in protection against rotavirus diseases is equivocal.

Published differences in conclusions concerning the importance of rotavirus serotype in protective immunity from vaccination/challenge experiments in animals have also never been resolved. Early studies revealed cross-protection between simian and murine rotavirus serotypes in mice [66,67]. Other studies showed cross-protection between bovine rotavirus and human serotype rotavirus in calves [68] and in piglets [69]. The latter studies supported the use of bovine rotavirus in the first extensive vaccination studies in infants. However, contrasting evidence was also obtained in vaccination/challenge studies in domestic animals. Cross-protection studies with distinct bovine serotypes in calves and with distinct porcine serotypes in swine revealed only serotype-specific immune protection against virus challenge [36].

Evidence regarding the importance of NA in the protection against rotavirus, which is of most importance to pediatric practice, is that obtained from clinical trials in infants. The first vaccine trials in infants were performed with bovine strain RIT 4237, which is serotypically unrelated to human rotaviruses. This vaccine provided protection against human rotavirus diseases in several early trials but failed in later trials [31,33,70]. Subsequently, trials with another bovine rotavirus strain (WC3) also showed inconsistent protection against human diseases [37–39]. Other clinical trials based on an assumption of heterotypical protection were conducted in infants with the simian RRV strain. RRV is related to a common human rotavirus serotype (G3; see below). It protected against rotavirus diseases in certain trials in which the natural challenge was not predominately G3, but failed to protect in others [48,71,72].

The common thread of experience with these three animal rotavirus vaccines was that they often protected against heterotypical human rotaviruses, but the unexplained inconsistency of this protection rendered them inadequate for universal application. However, recognizing the apparent clinical safety of these animal rotaviruses, attempts were made to enhance their protective efficacy by incorporating into them viral genes encoding outer capsid neutralization proteins of common human rotavirus serotypes. The resulting "reassortant" rotavirus vaccines, both those of simian RRV and bovine WC3 origin, have been consistently protective in infant clinical trials, with some quantitative variability. Therefore, empirical evidence that vaccine candidates of animal rotavirus origin need to be reassorted with human serotype rotaviruses to provide consistent protection represents the most definitive evidence of the importance of human serotype-specific antigenic stimulation for maximal efficacy. The specific and distinct contributions of the heterotypical and homotypical antigen-specific immune responses to the protection of the infant host are not yet well understood. Nevertheless, extensive clinical trial experience suggests that a combination of the responses to serotype-heterotypical and serotype-homotypical antigenic determinants contributes to effective protective immunity induced by reassortant rotavirus vaccines.

VII. DESIGN, PRODUCTION, AND CLINICAL EVALUATION OF LIVE ROTAVIRUS VACCINE CANDIDATES DEVELOPED FROM EVIDENCE THAT NEUTRALIZING ANTIBODY IS THE ESSENTIAL EFFECTOR OF PROTECTION

The outer capsid proteins of rotavirus, VP4 and VP7, determine the specificity of the NA response and thereby establish serotype. Orally administered NA directed against either VP4 or VP7 is protective in experimental animals [73,74]. The importance of NA in active immunity after immunization or natural infection is less clearly defined, but is presumed to play a role. The NA response, most easily measured in the serum, is assumed to represent the most accurate available indicator of the "take," magnitude, and specificity of immune responses leading to protection against rotavirus disease in the intestine.

A. VP7 Surface Protein

Early studies established that NA in hyperimmune serum was directed primarily against VP7 [75]. Neutralization assays conducted with hyperimmune serum separated rotaviruses into at least 14 serotypes [76,77]. VP7 serotypes are termed G (glycoprotein) types and rotavirus strains are considered to belong to different G types when a ≥20-fold difference in titer is detected in cross-neutralization tests using polyclonal antisera. Ten of 14 G types have been identified in humans [10]. G types 1–4 and 9 are the major human serotypes [78], but serotypes G8 [79] and G5 [80] are regionally important. G1 is the most frequently detected rotavirus in infected humans [78], but it is impossible to predict which serotype will predominate at a given time or in a particular location. G types 3 and 4 have commonly been detected in animals, but the animal isolates may be distinguished from the human strains [81]. G types 1, 2, and 9 have been found almost exclusively in humans [10].

The sequence of VP7 for each of the 14 G types has been determined [82]. A comparison of the VP7 sequences has enabled the detection of regions that are divergent among serotypes and could be involved in encoding serotype-specific epitopes [83]. It is noteworthy that VP7 sequences are highly conserved among rotaviruses belonging to the same G type, even among strains separated in the time and location of isolation [84]. This indicates that rotavirus evolution may be slow. Studies of monoclonal antibody-selected escape mutants have identified epitopes in VP7 responsible for evoking NA [83–86], the most predominant of which are located in regions designated A (aa 87–99), B (aa 145–150), and C (aa 211–223) [84].

B. VP4 Surface Protein

VP4 protrudes from the outer capsid in the form of 60 spikes [87–89]. Activation of rotavirus infectivity is associated with trypsin cleavage into two components, VP5* (60 kDa) and VP8* (28 kDa) [82], and both components remain attached to the virion. VP4 also induces NA, and VP4 serotypes are termed P types (protease-sensitive). Greater NA responses may be directed against VP4 than VP7 following oral immunization or natural infection [90]. VP4 molecules possess both serotype-specific and cross-reactive antigenic sites. Serotype-specific sites reside primarily on the smaller VP8* component, whereas the larger VP5* component contains mostly cross-reactive sites [91].

Because of extensive cross-reactivity, it has proven very difficult to develop a complete classification of rotavirus VP4 types by serology alone. No battery of polyclonal hyperimmune antisera or monoclonal antibodies that adequately characterizes most VP4 types has been produced. Therefore, a supplementary system of classification of P types by gene sequencing, which has allowed identification of at least 20 P "genotypes," has evolved. In practice, the P serotype (when known) is indicated by an open number whereas the genotype is indicated by a bracketed number (e.g., P1a[8]) [17]. Most rotaviruses of human origin include P1a[8] VP4 coupled with G1, G3, or G4 VP7, or P1b[4] VP4 coupled with G2 VP7 [92], but recently, an increasing number of differing combinations have been detected. Although it is assumed that VP4 contributes to cross-protection between different rotavirus serotypes through its cross-reactive epitopes, this has not been experimentally demonstrated.

C. Reassortant Rotavirus Vaccine Candidates

1. Primate × Human Reassortant Rotaviruses

The G3 simian RRV strain was highly immunogenic in infants but irregularly protective against diseases [48,71,72]. It was postulated that the addition of human VP7 serotype specificity to RRV by gene reassortment might yield an improved vaccine [93]. RRV reassortants containing VP7 genes from G1, G2, and G4 human rotaviruses were, therefore, generated, and these reassortants, along with RRV, were combined into the tetravalent RRV (RRV-TV) vaccine. Safety profiles of the reassortants were similar to RRV, with fevers in infants sometimes observed 3–5 days after inoculation [94]. RRV reassortants tested individually or in combination exhibited immune response rates (serum IgA or serum NA to RRV) in ≥80% of recipients. However, the NA response rates to human serotypes G1, G2, G3, or G4 were consistently <50% and normally <20% [62,95].

When the RRV-G1 and RRV-G2 monovalent vaccine strains were tested for efficacy in Finland, each was equally effective even though natural challenge was almost exclusively with G1 strains [96]. A comparative efficacy trial of RRV and RRV-G1 conducted in Rochester, NY in 1987 found that RRV provided protection against G1 natural challenge (66%) that was nearly as effective as that provided by the G1 reassortant (77%). Two years earlier, RRV had provided no protection against G1 natural challenge at this site. No explanation was established for this discrepant result [61]. In a study with the complete RRV-TV vaccine conducted in Peru, in which G1 and G2 rotaviruses were circulating, there was no significant protection against either serotype [97]. Upon reanalysis using a more precise scoring system for disease, significant levels of protection were induced by RRV-TV when only more severe cases of rotavirus diarrhea were considered [98]. In a similar study in Brazil, three doses of RRV-TV provided 57% protection against G1 rotavirus challenge but other serotypes were not circulating [99].

In five other efficacy trials, RRV-TV was uniformly protective, commonly preventing approximately 50% of all rotavirus disease and ≥70% of "severe" rotavirus infections [34,94,101–103]. Three of these trials involved a comparison of RRV-TV with the monovalent RRV-G1 vaccine. In one large U.S. trial [100], the natural challenge was primarily G1 rotavirus, and RRV-TV and the monovalent vaccine were equally protective. In another large U.S. trial [101], the natural challenge viruses in year 1 were also G1, and RRV-TV and monovalent RRV-G1 vaccine provided similar protection. In the second year of this trial, 35% of the challenge viruses were not G1, and only the RRV-TV vaccinees exhibited protection against these non-G1 rotaviruses. A trial conducted in the southwestern United States involved natural challenge primarily of G3 strains [34]. In the first year, the RRV-TV vaccine provided 53% protection against all cases of G3 rotavirus disease, whereas the monotypic RRV-G1 vaccine provided only 20% protection. Results of these last two studies suggest that protection with RRV or its reassortants was at least partially serotype-specific even though no correlation was found with serotype-specific NA titers [62,103]. Because of its ability to consistently elicit good protection against rotavirus disease in vaccinated infants and its low reactogenicity in this population during prelicensure studies, RRV-TV was licensed and marketed in the United States beginning in 1998. Unfortunately, postlicensure surveillance indicated an association between RRV-TV vaccination and intussusception (bowel blockage), and the vaccine was withdrawn [104].

2. Bovine × Human Reassortant Viruses

The first vaccine reassortant using a bovine rotavirus genome was constructed to include the VP7 gene from human rotavirus G1 strain WI79 in the genome of the WC3 bovine rotavirus. When administered orally at a dose of $10^{7.3}$ pfu, this reassortant retained the excellent safety characteristics of its WC3 parent. Two doses administered to infants induced NA responses of G1 specificity from 22% [61] to 55% [105], but this incidence was less than the nearly 100% NA response to WC3 (represented by the VP4 of the reassortant). Surprisingly, when the mirror image reassortant (human rotavirus VP4 P1a included in the WC3 rotavirus genome) was tested, the NA responses were again predominantly against the WC3 parent [54,106]. A mixture of both single gene reassortants induced vigorous NA responses to both parent viruses. However, a double NA gene reassortant was also constructed, bearing both human G1 and P1a genes within an otherwise WC3 virus genome. When administered to infants, the immune response to this reassortant was disappointing (<50% developed NA responses to either WC3 or the human strain). This suggested that a virus with two human rotavirus outer capsid proteins was less immunogenic in humans than rotaviruses with a single human surface protein accompanied by a nonhuman rotavirus surface protein. The reason for this is unknown.

Two efficacy studies conducted with the univalent human G1 reassortant revealed high levels of protection against circulating G1 strains. Administration of two doses in an initial trial of 77 infants produced 100% protection [61]. In a subsequent trial involving 312 infants given three doses of vaccine or placebo, efficacy was 64% against all rotavirus diarrheal diseases and 87% against clinically significant rotavirus diarrhea [107]. The use of this vaccine in these two studies also produced >50% reduction in all episodes of severe diarrhea, total days of diarrheal illness, and diarrhea episodes requiring the attention of a physician. Serological studies of a subset of the infants given three doses of vaccine in these trials revealed the development of G1 serotype-specific neutralizing antibodies at an incidence of 70% (H. F. Clark, unpublished results).

Serotype G2 and G3 reassortants on a WC3 background were next constructed. Because human serotype VP4 responses also potentially contribute to protective immunity, reassortants of serotypes G1, G2, G3, and P1a, all at a titer of approximately 10^7 pfu, were combined into a quadrivalent human bovine reassortant rotavirus vaccine (QHBRV). The QHBRV was evaluated in a placebo-controlled, multicenter study in the United States after the administration of three oral doses of vaccine or placebo to 439 infants [108]. No adverse effects were associated with vaccination and the response rates were approximately 90% for rotavirus IgA antibody and 57% for G1 NA. The vaccine was 75% efficacious against all rotavirus diseases (G1 and G3 strains) and 100% against severe rotavirus disease.

In order to include all of the traditionally prevalent human rotavirus G types in the vaccine, a single gene reassortant was created with a G4 VP7 protein on a WC3 rotavirus background. This reassortant was added to the QHBRV to yield a quintavalent vaccine, now designated RotaTeq™. This vaccine candidate is currently being tested in expanded efficacy trials and in very large safety trials, both in the United States and internationally.

VIII. EVIDENCE THAT THE NEUTRALIZING ANTIBODY IS NOT AN ESSENTIAL EFFECTOR OF PROTECTION AGAINST ROTAVIRUS DISEASE IN HUMANS INDUCED BY LIVE ROTAVIRUS INFECTION

Evidence that NA is not the only product of the adaptive immune system responsible for the prevention of rotavirus diseases has been provided from three types of studies. These include studies on immunity after natural or experimental rotavirus infection of both animals and humans, studies associated with vaccination of humans with live rotaviruses, and studies with animals using experimental rotavirus vaccines. Initial studies on experimental infection of piglets and calves suggested that NA was a critical component of protection against diseases following subsequent rotavirus challenge [109–111]. Later studies, however, indicated the opposite (i.e., mechanisms other than NA appeared to be important in protection) [68,112,113]. For example, an avirulent strain of bovine rotavirus produced little or no NA against a virulent challenge strain in gnotobiotic calves, yet provided excellent protection against rotavirus disease following challenge [112]. A subsequent study conducted with mice showed no correlation between either serum NA or rotavirus IgG titers following experimental infection with homologous or heterologous rotavirus strains and the protection against murine rotavirus shedding [114]. In contrast, there was an excellent correlation between serum and stool rotavirus IgA titers and protection in this model [115,116].

Studies in naturally infected humans have also suggested that NA is not the only effector of protection. In 1983, Bishop et al. [24] reported, for the first time, that neonatal rotavirus infections are protective against severe disease following subsequent rotavirus exposure. The serotypes of the neonatal strains and the rotaviruses circulating in the community during that period were dissimilar. Later reports have also generally found neonatal rotavirus strains to be distinctly different from circulating strains, yet provide protection against rotavirus illness. For example, Aijaz et al. [26] reported that approximately one-third of neonates born in the Bangalore region of southern India between 1988 and 1994 became infected with G10P[11] rotaviruses. During that period, there was a sharp reduction in the incidence of rotavirus-induced infantile gastroenteritis from 45.3% to

1.8% among hospitalized children with diarrhea. These G10P[11] strains appeared to have only two gene segments of human rotavirus origin (both nonstructural protein genes) and the remainder appeared to be derived from bovine rotaviruses. Furthermore, these strains were not found in children with rotavirus diarrhea, thus suggesting a possible association between neonatal rotavirus infections and a decline in disease incidence due to heterotypical rotaviruses. During the same period, G9P[11] rotavirus strains were isolated from neonates in the New Delhi region of India. These strains also appeared to be human × bovine rotavirus reassortants and neonates infected with these strains experienced 46% fewer attacks of rotavirus diseases than infants without neonatal rotavirus infections [25].

As already noted, natural rotavirus infections in older infants have been reported to provide substantial protection against subsequent rotavirus disease, particularly against severe disease. When repeat illnesses do occur, they are often, but not always, caused by rotavirus serotypes that are different from those responsible for the first infection, thus suggesting that NA plays some role in protection following these first infections. However, there is also evidence that NA is not solely responsible for the observed protection. In a study with Bangladeshi children, it was found that subjects who experienced clinically significant rotavirus diseases had substantially less rotavirus-specific NA at the time of their illnesses than age-matched well children [117]. Interestingly, multivariate logistic regression models demonstrated that only NA titers to heterotypical rotaviruses were independently associated with protection against rotavirus disease. These data suggested that immunity to rotavirus disease might be mediated by factors other than NA. More recently, in a study conducted in Mexico, it was reported that although repetitive rotavirus infections occurred in a cohort of infants followed from birth to 2 years of age, the severity of their illnesses, particularly moderate-to-severe illnesses, decreased dramatically with subsequent rotavirus infections [4]. In fact, no moderate-to-severe rotavirus illnesses were found after the second infection even though the four major G serotypes of human rotavirus (i.e., G1–G4) were each well represented within the circulating rotavirus strains found during the study period. Although titers of NA to different rotavirus serotypes have been reported to broaden with sequential infection, these results can be interpreted to suggest that protection, at least against more severe rotavirus diseases, was not strictly serotype-specific.

Studies on the vaccination of humans with live rotaviruses have provided mixed signals regarding the importance of NA in the protection against rotavirus disease. The first rotavirus vaccine candidate, the bovine RIT 4237 strain, was highly efficacious when first evaluated in Finland, particularly against severe disease, even though it was serotypically unrelated to circulating rotavirus strains [28,31,32]. Likewise, the first trial with the WC3 bovine rotavirus vaccine candidate conducted in Philadelphia found it also to be efficacious against heterotypical rotaviruses [37]. Neither of these bovine strains was, however, consistently protective against rotavirus diseases and the evaluation of both as single-strain vaccine candidates was discontinued. Based on results of clinical trials with WC3, this candidate vaccine was

modified to contain genes for VP4 and VP7 proteins from human rotaviruses by reassortant formation. These WC3 reassortants, which are expected to produce NA against multiple serotypes of human rotaviruses, are being actively evaluated as a vaccine candidate. A similar outcome was found in clinical trails with the rhesus rotavirus vaccine candidate, and it, too, was modified by reassortment with human rotaviruses to create the tetravalent RRV (RRV-TV) vaccine. Although RRV-TV contained genes encoding VP7 proteins belonging to the major G types of human rotavirus (i.e., G1–G4), <20% of vaccinees administered three doses of RRV-TV typically developed rises in NA to prototype human rotaviruses belonging to any of these G types [100,101]. Furthermore, no correlation was found between titers of serum NA to specific G types and protection against rotaviruses belonging to these G types [103]. In spite of this, RRV-TV consistently elicited about 50% protection against all rotavirus disease and >70% protection against severe disease.

Studies conducted with nonliving subunit rotavirus vaccine candidates in experimental animal models have clearly shown that protection against rotavirus shedding after challenge is not dependent on classical NA. These studies have been conducted primarily with mice and have utilized several different immunogens, adjuvants, and routes of vaccine delivery. In this model, active immunity is against fecal rotavirus shedding rather than against rotavirus disease because mice are susceptible to rotavirus diarrhea for only their first 14 days of life, too short a time period in which to develop active immunity. Using this adult mouse model, it was found that intranasal administration of either of three types of subunit vaccines [i.e., psoralen-inactivated, double-layered (dl) rotavirus particles; viruslike particles (VLPs) composed of only the rotavirus VP2 and VP6 proteins; or an *Escherichia coli*-expressed chimeric murine rotavirus VP6 protein], along with a powerful mucosal adjuvant, elicited nearly complete protection against murine rotavirus shedding [118–120]. All three immunogens lacked the VP4 and VP7 rotavirus neutralization proteins and were, therefore, unable to elicit classical NA. Although protection could not be associated with measurable NA, it was also found that immunization of mice with triple-layered, inactivated rotavirus particles containing VP4 and VP7 was more effective than the dl particles, but only if they were homotypical relative to the challenge strain [118]. These results implied that protection was not dependent on NA in this model but was enhanced by its presence. Additional studies with these immunogens administered to mice by intramuscular or oral routes have provided similar conclusions [118,119,121].

IX. DEVELOPMENT OF LIVE ROTAVIRUS VACCINE CANDIDATES BASED ON THE HYPOTHESIS THAT THE NEUTRALIZING ANTIBODY IS NOT THE ONLY EFFECTOR OF PROTECTION

If effectors of protection other than NA are induced by live rotavirus immunization, it is important to establish their identities, their duration of production, and their effectiveness in the prevention of rotavirus infection and disease. Studies using the adult mouse model have implicated CD8 T cells in the resolution of rotavirus infection and, possibly, in the protection against reinfection [122–124]. CD4 T cells clearly play indirect roles in rotavirus immunity by providing helper functions for B-cell and CD8 T-cell development and have been suggested to provide direct effector roles in mice as well [125,126]. Finally, anti-VP6 IgA has been reported to protect mice against rotavirus shedding [127]. Because the epitopes responsible for stimulating protective T cells and non-NA could potentially reside on any structural—and, possibly, nonstructural—rotavirus protein, they might have little association with rotavirus serotype. Furthermore, effectors stimulated by any group A rotavirus may protect against many, if not all, group A rotaviruses. This has led to the development of several vaccine candidates consisting of single rotavirus strains.

The bovine rotavirus vaccine candidates, RIT 4237 and WC3, and the simian RRV vaccine candidate were the first to be developed, but the evaluation of all three was discontinued due to inconsistent efficacy. Neonatal strain M37 was also developed, evaluated, and discarded due to poor immunogenicity and lack of efficacy [50,51]. However, several live, single-strain, rotavirus vaccine candidates remain under active development. These include one animal (lamb) strain, three neonatal strains, and one strain obtained from a symptomatically infected child. The G10P[12] lamb strain was developed at the Lanzhou Institute in China and has been administered to ca. 20,000 children with no evidence of side effects [49]. It has been reported that inoculation with this lamb strain can stimulate NA against multiple human G types in >50% of vaccinees. However, these observed increases in antibody titers against heterotypical strains may be a reflection of the older-than-usual ages of the vaccinees and the likelihood that many had experienced previous natural rotavirus infections. The ability of this vaccine strain to elicit protection in previously uninfected infants is unknown.

The neonatal strains under development as vaccine candidates have all been reported to elicit substantial protection against subsequent rotavirus disease. The first is a G3P2A[6] strain that was endemic in neonatal nurseries in Melbourne, Australia from 1975 to 1980 [128]. This vaccine candidate has been reported to be safe and moderately immunogenic after administration to children (35–58% seroconverted). Furthermore, vaccinees in a recent Phase II trial were protected against a circulating G1P1A[8] strain when they demonstrated a rotavirus immune response following vaccination [49]. The other two neonatal strains were obtained from subjects in India. In the 1980s, researchers in New Delhi and Bangalore routinely identified rotavirus infections among newborns that remained in the hospital for three or more days postdelivery [25,129]. These infections were not associated with diarrhea but the neonates shed viruses for up to 10 days, developed robust immune responses, and were protected against diarrhea upon reinfection. When further examined, these neonatal strains were found to have gene segments of both human and animal rotaviruses that appeared to have reassorted in nature [130–

132]. The G9P[10] strain from New Delhi, 116E, contained 10 genes from a human rotavirus and a single gene, VP4, from a bovine rotavirus. In contrast, the G10P[10] strain from Bangalore, I321, was primarily of bovine rotavirus origin but contained two nonstructural genes from a human rotavirus. When vaccine preparations of these strains were evaluated in small Phase I trials with either adults or previously infected children in the United States, they appeared to be safe and partially immunogenic (D. I. Bernstein, R. L. Ward, unpublished results). Further plans to develop these vaccine candidates are underway in India.

The vaccine candidate developed from a rotavirus that caused symptomatic infection was obtained during an efficacy trial of the bovine rotavirus WC3. When WC3 was evaluated in Cincinnati during the 1988–1989 rotavirus season, it had no significant impact on the development of subsequent rotavirus illnesses [38,55]. In contrast, children with either symptomatic or asymptomatic natural rotavirus infection during the first year were fully protected against rotavirus diseases during the following year and only 2 of 60 even had detectable asymptomatic reinfections. In contrast, of the 82 subjects not infected during the first year, 9 had symptomatic and 20 had asymptomatic infections in the second year [55]. Exposure to a variety of serotype G1 rotavirus strains circulating during this second year was based on their RNA electropherotypes. All rotavirus isolates from ill subjects obtained during the first year were also serotype G1, but surprisingly, these were essentially indistinguishable from one another based on electropherotype. Therefore, the protection elicited against multiple G1 strains during year 2 was induced almost solely by infections with a single rotavirus strain in year 1. It followed, therefore, that if attenuation of this G1[P8] strain did not ablate its protective capacity, it should make an excellent vaccine candidate, at least against serotype G1 strains. Furthermore, if the protection that it stimulates is at least partially through mechanisms other than NA, it may be broadly protective as a single-strain rotavirus vaccine. Consequently, rotavirus from the stool of one ill subject from the 1989 trial was developed as a vaccine candidate and designated 89-12. Attenuation of strain 89-12 was performed by 33 passages in cultured monkey kidney cells.

When the 89-12 rotavirus vaccine candidate was evaluated for safety and immunogenicity in adults, in previously infected children, and, finally, in infants, it was found to be generally safe and highly immunogenic [133]. It was then tested for efficacy in healthy infants aged 10–16 weeks at four centers in the United States [56]. Two doses of either 10^5 focus-forming units or placebo were administered to 108 or 107 subjects, respectively. Low-grade fever after the first dose was the only side effect more common in vaccinees than placebo recipients (21 vs. 5 subjects; $P = 0.001$). An immune response to rotavirus was detected in 94% of vaccinees and in only 4% of the placebo recipients. During the first rotavirus season, rotavirus disease was detected in 18 placebo recipients and two vaccinees (efficacy: 89%). Ten placebo recipients but no vaccinees presented for medical care associated with rotavirus disease. In the second year, efficacy decreased to 59% but only one case of severe rotavirus gastroenteritis was found in vaccinees, whereas 10 severe cases were found in placebo recipients. The overall efficacy for the 2 years was 76% against any rotavirus gastroenteritis, 84% against severe disease, and 100% against very severe rotavirus G1 disease. Because G1 rotaviruses predominated during both years, the efficacy against heterotypical rotaviruses was not determinable. This vaccine candidate has been further attenuated by additional cell culture passages [57] and the new preparation is being extensively evaluated in larger trials and in countries where non-G1 community strains are typically isolated.

X. VACCINE STRATEGIES NOT UTILIZING LIVE ROTAVIRUSES

Because live virus vaccines have potential disadvantages such as side effects due to insufficient attenuation, adverse reactions associated with viral replication, or insufficient efficacies against rotavirus disease, nonliving rotavirus vaccine candidates are being developed. None, however, has been administered to humans and, at this time, only two candidates are being actively evaluated in animal model studies. These are viruslike particles and recombinant VP6 proteins. The VLPs being evaluated are composed of baculovirus-expressed VP2/VP6 proteins as well as those that additionally contain one or both outer capsid neutralization proteins. Challenge studies conducted with the adult mouse model have shown that intranasal inoculation with the VP2/VP6 particles along with a powerful mucosal adjuvant stimulated nearly complete protection against murine rotavirus shedding [119]. Similar studies conducted with *E. coli*-expressed chimeric VP6 proteins of murine or human rotavirus origin found that these immunogens elicited nearly complete protection of mice against murine rotavirus shedding after either intranasal or oral immunization [120]. These combined studies clearly established that protection was not dependent on NA in this model system. In contrast to the results found in mice, intranasal immunization of gnotobiotic piglets with the VP2/VP6 VLPs and adjuvant did not elicit protection against shedding or diarrheal illness induced by a virulent human rotavirus [134]. However, when this method of immunization was used in piglets following oral administration of an attenuated strain of human rotavirus, it did stimulate substantial protection against the virulent human strain [135]. Viruslike particles have also been administered parenterally to rabbits along with adjuvants and were found to elicit substantial protection against lapine rotavirus shedding, particularly if they contained one or more outer capsid proteins, even if these proteins were from a different serotype than the challenge strain [136]. If humans are protected by these nonliving vaccine candidates as well as mice and rabbits, they offer promise as second-generation rotavirus vaccines.

ACKNOWLEDGMENTS

We thank Harry Greenberg (Stanford University) and Osamu Nakagomi (Akita University) for their critical reading of this chapter and their helpful suggestions.

REFERENCES

1. Bern C, et al. The magnitude of the global problem of diarrhoeal disease: a ten year update. Bull World Health Organ 1992; 70:705–714.
2. Murray CJ, Lopez AD. Global mortality, disability, and the contribution of risk factors: global burden of disease study. Lancet 1997; 349:1436–1442.
3. Glass RI, et al. The epidemiology of rotavirus diarrhea in the United States: surveillance and estimates of disease burden. J Infect Dis 1996; 174(suppl 1):S5–S11.
4. Velazquez FR, et al. Rotavirus infection in infants as protection against subsequent infections. N Engl J Med 1996; 335:1022–1028.
5. Institute of Medicine. The prospects of immunizing against rotavirus. New Vaccine Development: Diseases of Importance in Developing Countries. Vol. 2. Washington, DC: National Academy Press, 1986:D13-1–D13-12.
6. Tucker AW, et al. Cost-effectiveness analysis of a rotavirus immunization program for the United States. JAMA 1998; 279:1371–1376.
7. Parashar UD, et al. Global illness and deaths caused by rotavirus disease in children. Emerging Infect Dis 2003; 9:565–571.
8. Holmes IH, et al. Infantile enteritis viruses: morphogenesis and morphology. J Virol 1975; 16:937–943.
9. Martin ML, et al. Ultrastructure of infantile gastroenteritis virus. Virology 1975; 68:146–153.
10. Estes MK. Rotaviruses and their replication. In: Knipe DM, Howley PM, Griffin DE, Lamb RA, Martin MA, Roizman B, Straus SE, eds. Fields Virology. 4th ed. Philadelphia: Lippincott, Williams and Wilkins, 2001:1747–1785.
11. Prasad BVV, Chiu W. Structure of rotavirus. Curr Top Microbiol Immunol 1994; 185:9–29.
12. Shaw AL, et al. Three-dimensional visualization of the rotavirus hemagglutinin structure. Cell 1993; 74:693–701.
13. Arias CF, et al. Trypsin activation pathway of rotavirus infectivity. J Virol 1996; 70:5832–5839.
14. Cuadras MA, et al. Rotaviruses induce an early membrane permeabilization of MA104 cells and do not require a low intracellular Ca^{2+} concentration to initiate their replication cycle. J Virol 1997; 71:9065–9074.
15. Patton JT. Rotavirus replication. Curr Top Microbiol Immunol 1994; 185:107–127.
16. Clarke ML, et al. Membrane binding and endoplasmic reticulum retention sequences of rotavirus VP7 are distinct: role of carboxy-terminal and other residues in membrane binding. J Virol 1995; 69:6473–6478.
17. Kapikian AZ, et al. Rotaviruses. In: Knipe DM, Howley PM, Griffin DE, Lamb RA, Martin MA, Roizman B, Straus SE, eds. Fields Virology. 4th ed. Philadelphia: Lippincott, Williams and Wilkins, 2001:1787–1833.
18. Greenberg HB, et al. Rotavirus pathology and pathophysiology. Curr Top Microbiol Immunol 1994; 185:255–283.
19. Suzuki H, Konno T. Reovirus-like particles in jejunal mucosa of a Japanese infant with acute infectious non-bacterial gastroenteritis. Tohoku J Exp Med 1975; 115:199–221.
20. Davidson GP, et al. Human rotavirus enteritis induced in conventional piglets: intestinal structure and transport. J Clin Invest 1977; 60:1402–1409.
21. Ball JM, et al. Age-dependent diarrhea induced by a rotaviral nonstructural glycoprotein. Science 1996; 272:101–104.
22. Zhang M, et al. Mutations in rotavirus nonstructural glycoprotein NSP4 are associated with altered virus virulence. J Virol 1998; 72:3666–3672.
23. Tian P, et al. The rotavirus nonstructural glycoprotein NSP4 mobilizes Ca^{2+} from the endoplasmic reticulum. J Virol 1995; 69:5763–5772.
24. Bishop RF, et al. Clinical immunity after neonatal rotavirus

infection. A prospective longitudinal study in young children. N Engl J Med 1983; 309:72–76.

25. Bhan MK, et al. Protection conferred by neonatal rotavirus infection against subsequent rotavirus diarrhea. J Infect Dis 1993; 168:282–287.

26. Aijaz S, et al. Epidemiology of symptomatic human rotaviruses in Bangalore and Mysore, India, from 1988 to 1994 as determined by electropherotype, subgroup and serotype analysis. Arch Virol 1996; 141:715–726.

27. Nakagomi O, Nakagomi T. Interspecies transmission of rotaviruses studied from the perspective of genogroup. Microbiol Immunol 1993; 37:337–348.

28. Vesikari T. Clinical trials of live oral rotavirus vaccines: the Finnish experience. Vaccine 1993; 11:255–261.

29. Mebus CA, et al. Neonatal calf diarrhea: results of a field trial using a reo-like virus vaccine. Vet Med Small Anim Clin 1972; 67:173–174.

30. Vesikari T, et al. Immunogenicity and safety of live oral attenuated bovine rotavirus vaccine strain RIT 4237 in adults and young children. Lancet 1983; 2:807–811.

31. Vesikari T, et al. Clinical efficacy of the RIT 4237 live attenuated bovine rotavirus vaccine in infants vaccinated before a rotavirus epidemic. J Pediatr 1985; 107:189–194.

32. Vesikari T, et al. Protection of infants against rotavirus diarrhoea by RIT 4237 attenuated bovine rotavirus strain vaccine. Lancet 1984; 1:977–981.

33. Hanlon P, et al. Trial of an attenuated bovine rotavirus vaccine (RIT4237) in Gambian infants. Lancet 1987; 1:1342–1345.

34. Santosham M, et al. Efficacy and safety of high-dose rhesus–human reassortant rotavirus vaccine in Native American populations. J Pediatr 1997; 131:632–663.

35. Vesikari T, et al. Efficacy of two doses of RIT 4237 bovine rotavirus vaccine for prevention of rotavirus diarrhoea. Acta Pediatr Scand 1991; 80:173–180.

36. Clark HF. Rotavirus vaccines. In: Plotkin SA, Mortimar EA, eds. Vaccines. Philadelphia: WB Saunders Company, 1988:517–525.

37. Clark HF, et al. Protective effect of WC3 vaccine against rotavirus diarrhea in infants during a predominantly serotype 1 rotavirus season. J Infect Dis 1988; 158:570–587.

38. Bernstein DI, et al. Evaluation of WC3 rotavirus vaccine and correlates of protection in healthy infants. J Infect Dis 1990; 162:1055–1062.

39. Georges-Courbot MC, et al. Evaluation of the efficacy of a low passage bovine rotavirus (strain WC3) vaccine in children in Central Africa. Res Virol 1991; 142:405–411.

40. Losonsky GA, et al. Safety, infectivity, transmissibility, and immunogenicity of rhesus rotavirus vaccine (MMU 18006) in infants. Pediatr Infect Dis 1986; 5:25–29.

41. Perez-Schael I, et al. Reactogenicity and antigenicity of the rhesus rotavirus vaccine MMU 18006 in Venezuelan children. J Infect Dis 1987; 155:334–337.

42. Vesikari T, et al. A comparative trail of rhesus monkey (RRV-1) and bovine (RIT 4237) oral rotavirus vaccines in young children. J Infect Dis 1986; 153:832–839.

43. Flores J, et al. Protection against severe rotavirus diarrhoea by rhesus rotavirus vaccine in Venezuelan infants. Lancet 1987; 1:882–884.

44. Rennels M, et al. Preliminary evaluation of the efficacy of rhesus rotavirus vaccine strain MMU 18006 in young children. Pediatr Infect Dis J 1986; 5:587–588.

45. Perez-Schael I, et al. Prospective study of diarrheal diseases in Venezuelan children to evaluate the efficacy of rhesus rotavirus vaccine. J Med Virol 1990; 30:219–229.

46. Rennels M, et al. An efficacy trial of the rhesus rotavirus vaccine in Maryland. Am J Dis Child 1990; 144:601–604.

47. Vesikari T, et al. Rhesus rotavirus candidate vaccine: clinical trial in children vaccinated between 2 and 5 months of age. Am J Dis Child 1990; 144:285–289.

48. Christy C, et al. Field trial of rhesus rotavirus vaccine in infants. Pediatr Infect Dis J 1988; 7:645–650.

49. Global Alliance for Vaccines and Immunization (GAVI). GAVI Task Force for R&D Rotavirus Vaccine Agenda Meeting: Minutes and Summary of the Meeting. Geneva: World Health Organization, May 14–15, 2001.

50. Vesikari T, et al. Evaluation of the M37 human rotavirus vaccine in 2- to 6-month-old infants. Pediatr Infect Dis J 1991; 10:912–917.

51. Flores J, et al. Comparison of reactogenicity and antigenicity of M37 rotavirus vaccine and rhesus-rotavirus-based quadrivalent vaccine. Lancet 1990; 2:330–334.

52. Flores J, et al. Conservation of the fourth gene among rotaviruses recovered from asymptomatic newborn infants and its possible role in attenuation. J Virol 1986; 60:972–979.

53. Gorziglia M, et al. Conservation of amino acid sequence of VP8 and cleavage region of 84-kDa outer capsid protein among rotaviruses recovered from asymptomatic neonatal infection. Proc Natl Acad Sci 1986; 83:7039–7043.

54. Clark HF, et al. The development of multivalent bovine rotavirus (strain WC3) reassortant vaccine for infants. J Infect Dis 1996; 174(suppl):S73–S80.

55. Bernstein DI, et al. Protection from rotavirus reinfection: 2-year prospective study. J Infect Dis 1991; 164:277–283.

56. Bernstein DI, et al. Efficacy of live, attenuated, human rotavirus vaccine 89-12 in infants: a randomised placebo-controlled trial. Lancet 1999; 354:287–290.

57. Vesikari T, et al. Reactogenicity and immunogenicity of a human rotavirus vaccine (HRV), given as primary vaccination to healthy infants aged 6 to 12 weeks. Conference on Vaccines for Enteric Diseases VED 2001, Tampere, Finland, September 12–14, 2001.

58. Offit PA, Clark HF. Protection against rotavirus-induced gastroenteritis in a murine model by passively acquired gastrointestinal but not circulating antibodies. J Virol 1985; 54:58–64.

59. Offit PA. Host factors associated with protection against rotavirus disease: the skies are clearing. J Infect Dis 1996; 174(suppl 1):S59–S64.

60. Madore HP, et al. Field trial or rhesus rotavirus or human–rhesus rotavirus reassortant vaccine of VP7 serotype 3 or 1 specificity in infants. J Infect Dis 1992; 166:235–243.

61. Clark HF, et al. Immune protection of infants against rotavirus gastroenteritis by a serotype 1 reassortant of bovine rotavirus WC3. J Infect Dis 1990; 161:1099–1104.

62. Ward RL, Bernstein DI. Lack of correlation between serum rotavirus antibody titers and protection following vaccination with reassortant RRV vaccines. Vaccine 1995; 13:1226–1232.

63. Champsaur H, et al. Rotavirus carriage asymtomatic infection, and disease in the first two years of life: II. Serological response. J Infect Dis 1984; 149:675–682.

64. Clark HF, et al. Diverse serological response to rotavirus infection of infants in a single epidemic. Pediatr Infect Dis 1985; 4:626–631.

65. Friedman MG, et al. Two sequential outbreaks of rotavirus gastroenteritis: evidence for symptomatic and asymptomatic reinfections. J Infect Dis 1988; 158:814–822.

66. Sheridan JF, et al. Prevention of rotavirus-induced diarrhea in neonatal mice born to dams immunized with empty capsids of simian rotavirus SA-11. J Infect Dis 1984; 149:434–438.

67. Bartz CR, et al. Prevention of murine rotavirus infection with chicken egg yolk immunoglobins. J Infect Dis 1980; 142:439–441.

68. Wyatt RG, et al. Rotaviral immunity in gnotobiotic calves: heterologous resistance to human virus induced by bovine virus. Science 1979; 203:548–550.

69. Zissis G, et al. Protection studies in colostrum-deprived piglets of a bovine rotavirus vaccine candidate using human

rotavirus strains for challenge. J Infect Dis 1983; 148:1061–1068.

70. De Mol P, et al. Failure of live, attenuated and rotavirus vaccine [letter]. Lancet 1986; 2:108.

71. Gothefors L, et al. Prolonged efficacy of rhesus rotavirus vaccine in Swedish children. J Infect Dis 1989; 159, 753–757.

72. Santosham M, et al. A field study of the safety and efficacy of two candidate rotavirus vaccines in a Native American population. J Infect Dis 1991; 163:483–487.

73. Offit PA, et al. Reassortant rotaviruses containing structural proteins vp3 and vp7 from different parents induce antibodies protective against each parental serotype. J Virol 1986; 60:491–496.

74. Hoshino Y, et al. Independent segregation of two antigenic specificities (VP3 and VP7) involved in neutralization of rotavirus infectivity. Proc Natl Acad Sci 1985; 82:8701–8704.

75. Kalica AR, et al. Genes of human (strain Wa) and bovine (strain UK) rotaviruses that code for neutralization and subgroup antigens. Virology 1981; 112:385–390.

76. Hoshino Y, et al. Serotypic similarity and diversity of rotaviruses of mammalian and avian origin as studies by plaque reduction neutralization. J Infect Dis 1984; 149:694.

77. Hoshino Y, Kapikian AZ. Classification of rotavirus VP4 and VP7 serotypes. Arch Virol Suppl 1996; 12, 99–111.

78. Gentsch JR, et al. Review of G and P typing results from a global collection of rotavirus strains: implications for vaccine development. J Infect Dis 1996; 174(suppl):S30–S36.

79. Cunliffe NA, et al. Rotavirus G and P types in children with acute diarrhea in Blantyre, Malawi, from 1997–1998; predominance of novel P[6]G8 strains. J Med Virol 1999; 57:308–312.

80. Gouvea V, et al. Rotavirus serotypes G5 associated with diarrhea in Brazilian children. J Clin Microbiol 1994; 32:1408–1409.

81. Nishikawa K, et al. Rotavirus VP7 neutralization epitopes of serotype 3 strains. Virology 1989; 171:503–515.

82. Mattion NM, et al. The rotavirus proteins. In: Kapikian AZ ed. Viral Infections of the Gastrointestinal Tract. New York: Marcel Dekker, 1994:169–249.

83. Green KY, et al. Comparison of the amino acid sequences of the major neutralizing protein of four human rotavirus serotypes. Virology 1987; 160:153.

84. Dyall-Smith M, et al. Location of the major antigenic sites involved in rotavirus serotype-specific neutralization. Proc Natl Acad Sci 1986; 83:3465.

85. Green KY, et al. Prediction of human rotavirus serotype by nucleotide sequence analysis of the VP7 protein gene. J Virol 1988; 62:1819.

86. Flores J, et al. A dot hybridization assay for distinction of rotavirus serotypes. J Clin Microbiol 1989; 27:29.

87. Prasad BV, et al. Localization of VP4 neutralization sites in rotavirus by three-dimensional cryo-electron microscopy. Nature 1990; 343:476–479.

88. Prasad BV, et al. Three-dimensional structure of rotavirus. J Mol Biol 1988; 199:269–275.

89. Yeager M, et al. Three-dimensional structure of rhesus rotavirus by cryoelectron microscopy and image reconstruction. J Cell Biol 1990; 110:2133–2134.

90. Flores J, et al. Reactogenicity and antigenicity of two human–rhesus rotavirus reassortant vaccine candidates serotypes 1 and 2 in Venezuelan infants. J Clin Microbiol 1989; 27:512.

91. Larralde G, et al. Serotype-specific epitope(s) present on the VP8 unit of rotavirus VP4. J Virol 1991; 65:3213–3218.

92. Desselberger U, et al. Rotavirus epidemiology and surveillance. In: Chadwick D, Goode JA, eds. Gastroenteritis Viruses. Chichester: Novartis Foundation Symposium, 2001:125–152.

93. Midthun K, et al. Reassortant rotaviruses as potential live rotavirus vaccine candidates. J Virol 1985; 53:949–954.

94. Joensuu J, et al. Symptoms associated with rhesus–human reassortant rotavirus vaccine in infants. Pediatr Infect Dis J 1998; 17:334–340.

95. Wright PF, et al. Simultaneous administration of two human–rhesus rotavirus reassortant strains of VP7 serotype 1 and 2 specificity to infants and young children. J Infect Dis 1991; 164:271–276.

96. Vesikari T, et al. Protective efficacy against serotype 1 rotavirus diarrhea by live oral rhesus–human reassortant rotavirus vaccines with human rotavirus VP7 serotype 1 or 2 specificity. Pediatr Infect Dis J 1992; 11:535–542.

97. Lanata CF, et al. Safety, immunogenicity, and protective efficacy of one and three doses of the tetravalent rhesus rotavirus vaccine in infants in Lima, Peru. J Infect Dis 1996; 174:268–275.

98. Linhares AC, et al. Immunogenicity, safety and efficacy of tetravalent rhesus–human, reassortant rotavirus vaccine in Belém, Brazil. Bull World Health Organ 1996; 74:491–500.

99. Linhares AC, et al. Reappraisal of the Peruvian and Brazilian lower titer tetravalent rhesus–human reassortant rotavirus vaccine efficacy trials: analysis by severity of diarrhea. Pediatr Infect Dis J 1999; 18:1001–1006.

100. Rennels MB, et al. Safety and efficacy of high-dose rhesus–human reassortant rotavirus vaccines—Report of the National Multicenter Trial. Pediatrics 1996; 97:7–13.

101. Bernstein DI, et al. Evaluation of Rhesus rotavirus monovalent and tetravalent reassortant vaccines in US children. JAMA 1995; 273:1191–1196.

102. Perez-Schael I, et al. Efficacy of the rhesus rotavirus-based quadrivalent vaccine in infants and young children in Venezuela. N Engl J Med 1997; 337(17):1181–1187.

103. Ward RL, et al. Serologic correlates of immunity in a tetravalent reassortant rotavirus vaccine trial. J Infect Dis 1997; 176:570–577.

104. Murphy TV, et al. Intussusception among infants given an oral rotavirus vaccine. N Engl J Med 2001; 344:564–572.

105. Clark HF, et al. Serotype 1 reassortant of bovine rotavirus WC3, strain WI79-9, induces a polytypic antibody response in infants. Vaccine 1990; 8:327–332.

106. Clark HF, et al. WC3 reassortant vaccines in children. Arch Virol Suppl 1996; 12:187–198.

107. Treanor J, et al. Evaluation of the protective efficacy of a serotype 1 bovine–human rotavirus reassortant vaccine in infants. Pediatr Infect Dis J 1995; 14:301–307.

108. Clark HF, et al. Preliminary evaluation of safety and efficacy of quadrivalent human–bovine reassortant rotavirus vaccine. Pediatr Res 1995; 37:172.

109. Gaul SK, et al. Antigenic relationships among some animal rotaviruses: virus neutralization in vitro and cross-protection in piglets. J Clin Microbiol 1982; 16:494–503.

110. Murakami Y, et al. Prolonged excretion and failure of cross-protection between distinct serotypes of bovine rotavirus. Vet Microbiol 1986; 12:7–14.

111. Woode GN, et al. Antigenic relationships among some bovine rotaviruses: serum neutralization and cross-protection in gnotobiotic calves. J Clin Microbiol 1983; 18:358–364.

112. Woode GN, et al. Protection between different serotypes of bovine rotavirus in gnotobiotic calves: specificity of serum antibody and coproantibody responses. J Clin Microbiol 1987; 25:1052–1058.

113. Bridger JC, Oldham G. Avirulent rotavirus infections protect calves from disease with and without inducing high levels of neutralizing antibody. J Gen Virol 1987; 68:2311–2317.

114. Ward RL, et al. Evidence that active protection following oral immunization of mice with live rotavirus is not dependent on neutralizing antibody. Virology 1992; 188:57–66.

115. McNeal MM, et al. Active immunity against rotavirus infec-

tion in mice is correlated with viral replication and titers of serum rotavirus IgA following vaccination. Virology 1994; 204:642–650.

116. Feng N, et al. Comparison of mucosal and systemic humoral immune responses and subsequent protection in mice orally inoculated with a homologous or a heterologous rotavirus. J Virol 1994; 68:7766–7773.

117. Ward RL, et al. Evidence that protection against rotavirus diarrhea after natural infection is not dependent on serotype-specific neutralizing antibody. J Infect Dis 1992; 166:1251–1257.

118. McNeal MM, et al. Antibody-dependent and -independent protection following intranasal immunization of mice with rotavirus particles. J Virol 1999; 73:7565–7573.

119. O'Neal CM, et al. Rotavirus virus-like particles administered intranasally induce protective immunity. J Virol 1997; 71:8707–8717.

120. Choi AH-C, et al. Antibody-independent protection against rotavirus infection of mice stimulated by intranasal immunization with chimeric VP4 or VP6 protein. J Virol 1999; 73: 7574–7581.

121. McNeal MM, et al. Stimulation of local immunity and protection in mice by intramuscular immunization with triple- or double-layered particles and QS-21. Virology 1998; 243:158–166.

122. Franco MA, Greenberg HB. Role of B cells and cytotoxic T lymphocytes in clearance of and immunity to rotavirus infection in mice. J Virol 1995; 69:7800–7806.

123. McNeal MM, et al. Effector functions of antibody and CD8$^+$ cells in resolution of rotavirus infection and protection against reinfection in mice. Virology 1995; 214:387–397.

124. Franco MA, et al. CD8$^+$ T cells can mediate almost complete short-term and partial long-term immunity to rotavirus in mice. J Virol 1997; 71:4165–4170.

125. McNeal MM, Rae MN, Ward RL. Evidence that resolution of rotavirus infection in mice is due to both CD4 and CD8 cell-dependent activities. J Virol 1997; 71:8735–8742.

126. McNeal MM, et al. CD4 T cells are the only lymphocytes needed to protect mice against rotavirus shedding after in-

tranasal immunization with a chimeric VP6 protein and the adjuvant LT(R192G). J Virol 2002; 76:560–568.

127. Burns JW, et al. Protective effect of rotavirus VP6-specific IgA monoclonal antibodies that lack neutralizing activity. Science 1996; 272:104–107.

128. Barnes GL, et al. Phase I trial of a candidate rotavirus vaccine (RV3) derived from a human neonate. J Pediatr Child Health 1997; 33:300–304.

129. Sukumaran M, et al. Exclusive asymptomatic neonatal infections by human rotavirus strains having subgroup I specificity and "long" RNA electropherotype. Arch Virol 1992; 126:239–251.

130. Das BK, et al. Characterization of the G serotype and genogroup of New Delhi newborn rotavirus strain 116E. Virology 1993; 197:99–107.

131. Das M, et al. Both surface proteins (VP4 and VP7) of an asymptomatic neonatal rotavirus strain (I321) have high levels of sequence identity with the homologous proteins of a serotype 10 bovine rotavirus. Virology 1993; 194:374–379.

132. Gentsch J, et al. Similarity of the VP4 protein of human rotavirus strain 116E to that of the bovine B223 strain. Virology 1993; 194:424–430.

133. Bernstein DI, et al. Safety and immunogenicity of live, attenuated human rotavirus vaccine 89-12. Vaccine 1998; 16:381–387.

134. Yuan L, et al. Intranasal administration of 2/6-rotavirus-like particles with mutant *Escherichia coli* heat-labile toxin (LT-R192G) induces antibody-secreting cell responses but not protective immunity in gnotobiotic pigs. J Virol 2000; 74:8843–8853.

135. Yuan L, Iosef C, Azevedo MP, Kim Y, Quan Y, Geyer A, Nguyen TV, Chang K-O, Saif LJ. Protective immunity and antibody-secreting cell responses elicited by combined oral attenuated Wa human rotavirus and intranasal Wa 2/6 VLPs with mutant *Escherichia coli* heat-labile toxin in gnotobiotic pigs. J Virol 2001; 75:9229–9238.

136. Ciarlet M, et al. Subunit rotavirus vaccine administered parenterally to rabbits induces active protective immunity. J Virol 1998; 72:9233–9246.

52

Vaccines Against Respiratory Syncytial Virus and Parainfluenza Virus Types 1–3

James E. Crowe, Jr.
Vanderbilt University Medical Center, Nashville, Tennessee, U.S.A.

Peter L. Collins and Brian R. Murphy
National Institute of Allergy and Infectious Diseases, National Institutes of Health, Bethesda, Maryland, U.S.A.

I. INTRODUCTION

Respiratory syncytial virus (RSV) and parainfluenza virus types 1, 2, and 3 (PIV1, PIV2, and PIV3) are responsible for more than 40% of viral respiratory tract disease leading to hospitalization of infants and children. For this reason, there is a need to develop vaccines effective against these viruses. Because RSV and PIV3 cause severe lower respiratory tract disease in early infancy, vaccines for these viruses must be effective in immunologically immature recipients who have circulating maternal antibodies. To date, several strategies for immunization against disease caused by these viruses have been explored including peptide vaccines, inactivated or subunit vaccines, vectored vaccines (e.g., vaccinia-RSV or adenovirus-RSV recombinants), and live-attenuated virus vaccines. The most promising approaches are summarized in Table 1. The status of these approaches is reviewed. In addition, the immunologic basis for the disease potentiation seen in vaccinees immunized with formalin-inactivated RSV during subsequent RSV infection is reviewed. The efficacy of immunization in the presence of maternal antibodies is discussed.

II. VACCINE DEVELOPMENT FOR RESPIRATORY SYNCYTIAL VIRUS

A. General Considerations

Respiratory syncytial virus, a single-stranded negative-sense RNA virus of the Paramyxoviridae family, is the leading viral agent of severe lower respiratory tract disease in the pediatric population. This virus is also a major cause of respiratory disease in the elderly, especially in nursing home patients [1,2]. Respiratory syncytial virus causes pneumonia and bronchiolitis and is unusual in its ability to infect very young infants despite the presence of maternally acquired serum antibodies. A number of significant obstacles have hindered the development of an RSV vaccine. First, because the peak incidence of severe RSV disease is in 2-month-old infants, immunization should be initiated within the first month of life so that protective levels of immunity are achieved by 2 months of age [3,4]. Because most infants in the first months of life possess maternally acquired anti-RSV serum antibodies, the results obtained from evaluation of experimental vaccines in older seronegative subjects cannot be directly extrapolated to the very young infant. Maternally acquired antibodies suppress the immunogenicity of subunit and vectored RSV vaccines parenterally administered through a poorly defined immunologic mechanism termed antibody-mediated immune suppression [5–8].

Passively acquired antibodies can decrease the infectivity and the immunogenicity of live-attenuated viral vaccines that are parenterally administered, such as live-attenuated measles virus vaccines. Measles vaccine virus is sensitive to neutralization by passively acquired antibodies, and therefore its administration must be delayed until the level of maternal antibody has decreased to a level that does not interfere with replication of the vaccine virus. The loss of infectivity of a live virus vaccine mediated by passive serum antibodies can be circumvented by administration of the vaccine by a mucosal route [9], as has been successfully accomplished for polioviruses. Passively acquired serum antibodies have limited access to the respiratory or gastro-intestinal mucosa and, therefore, infection and immunization via mucosal surfaces can proceed despite the presence of antibodies in the serum. However, in breast-fed infants, antibodies in breast milk may influence the infectivity of mucosally administered vaccines. Immunization or infection in the

Table 1 Respiratory Syncytial Virus and Parainfluenza Virus Type 3 Vaccines that Have Been Tested in Clinical Trials

Vaccine type	Designation or type	Preclinical testing	Status of clinical trials	References describing clinical trials
Respiratory Syncytial Virus				
Formalin-inactivated RSV (1960s)	FI-RSV, Lot 100	Induced antibodies with high ELISA titer but low neutralizing activity, partially protective in rodents; retrospective studies showed enhanced pulmonary histopathology	In Phase I trials, induced antibodies with high ELISA titer but low neutralizing activity; poor protective efficacy; severe adverse events, 2 deaths. Studies terminated.	[20,21]
Live-attenuated mutants, biologically derived (1960s to present)	*ts* mutants *cp*-RSV *cpts* mutants	Attenuated, immunogenic, and protective; some were genetically stable	Multiple Phase I trials completed, ongoing[a]	[62,94,95,98,113]
Live-attenuated mutants, recombinantly derived (current trials)	Multiple combined point mutations, deletions, insertions, and other alterations; chimeric viruses	Increased level of attenuation compared to biologically derived viruses; immunogenic and protective	Multiple Phase I trials completed, ongoing	Unpublished
Live *wt* RSV given IM (1970s)	Live RSV	Immunogenic; protective against lower respiratory tract infection in seronegative rodents	Poor immunogenicity; lack of protective efficacy in children with maternal RSV-specific antibodies. Studies terminated.	[61]
Purified F glycoprotein (1980s to present)	PFP-1, PFP-2	Induced antibodies with high ELISA titer but low neutralizing activity; some rodent studies showed enhanced histopathology	Moderately immunogenic in Phase I trials in seropositive subjects, including high-risk children and the elderly; under evaluation for maternal immunization	[37–48]
Purified recombinant RSV G protein fragment fused to a streptococcal G protein fragment (current trials)	BBG2Na	Immunogenic and protective	Phase I completed	[70]
Parainfluenza Virus Type 3				
Bovine PIV3 (1990s to present)	BPIV3	Attenuated, immunogenic and protective	Phase I completed[a]	[143–145]
Live-attenuated mutant (1990s to present)	*cp*-45	Attenuated, immunogenic and protective; genetically stable	Phase I, II completed[a]	[161]

[a] The use of biologically derived, live-attenuated mutants is likely to be superseded by the improved, related recombinantly derived mutants, with the possible exception of PIV3 *cp*45.

presence of passively acquired antibodies can be protective even when high levels of serum neutralizing antibodies are not induced [10]. The mechanism for such protection is not well defined, but cellular immunity is implicated based on the finding that CD4+ and CD8+ T cells contribute to protection in a mouse model of RSV passive/active immunization [11].

A second obstacle to immunization against RSV is that immunity induced by infection with wild-type RSV itself does not completely protect against reinfection. Multiple upper respiratory infections occurring throughout life are a hallmark of this virus. Although subsequent infections typically are partially restricted by host immunity, severe disease can occur during the second infection [3]. Animal models suggest RSV infection may have immunosuppressive effects that thwart induction of immunologic memory in the respiratory tract [12]. Protection against disease caused by RSV in the lower respiratory tract can be achieved, but two or more infections are often required. Therefore immunization against RSV, like that against poliovirus, likely will require multiple doses of vaccine to achieve the level of immunity needed to prevent serious disease.

Third, the immune response to the F glycoprotein of RSV is reduced in the very young infant independent of the immunosuppressive effect of maternal antibodies [13]. This reduced immune response of the infant is also seen for the antibody response to the influenza A virus hemagglutinin protein [14] and to the PIV3 hemagglutinin–neuraminidase protein [15].

The fourth obstacle to RSV vaccine development is that circulating field strains exhibit an antigenic dimorphism. Two antigenic subgroups designated A and B have been defined that are approximately 25% antigenically related by reciprocal cross-neutralization analysis [3,6,16]. Second infections by RSV are often caused by virus belonging to the heterologous subgroup, indicating that antigenic diversity is responsible in part for the high frequency of second infections, and more importantly, for lower respiratory disease upon second infection [3,17]. An effective RSV vaccine should protect against disease caused by virus of either subgroup.

Fifth, during vaccine trials in the 1960s, immunization of infants and young children with an inactivated RSV vaccine unexpectedly primed for enhanced RSV disease during subsequent natural infection (discussed in more detail later in this chapter) [18,19]. This observation, in the context of comparable observations for inactivated measles virus vaccine, dictated that vaccine development for RSV should proceed with great caution.

In summary, a successful RSV vaccine will (1) immunize very young immunologically immature infants even in the presence of maternally acquired serum antibodies, (2) induce a level of resistance to disease in the lower respiratory tract comparable to or greater than that of primary infection with wild-type virus, (3) induce resistance to both subgroup A and B strains of RSV, and (4) immunize without potentiating RSV disease during subsequent natural infection.

B. Nonreplicating Antigens

1. Inactivated Virus Vaccine and Disease Potentiation

Inactivated RSV is not currently being considered as a vaccine candidate, but an understanding of the unexpected disease potentiation observed in the formalin inactivated RSV (FI-RSV) vaccine recipients during subsequent natural infection is important for RSV vaccine development in general. Recent observations, in the context of the previous observations in the 1960s and 1970s, have permitted the formulation of a plausible mechanism for disease potentiation seen in the FI-RSV vaccinees or reproduced in experimental animals receiving FI-RSV or subunit vaccines (discussed below). We previously summarized the literature on this subject [20]; the major findings are summarized here.

Two main factors are thought to have contributed to enhanced disease in FI-RSV vaccinees. First, FI-RSV failed to induce a high level of resistance to RSV replication. FI-RSV vaccinees developed a high titer of serum antibodies to the F glycoprotein as determined by enzyme-linked immunosorbent assay (ELISA), but these antibodies had a low level of neutralizing activity and likely had insufficient antiviral activity in vivo. Interestingly, immunization of cattle with inactivated bovine RSV (BRSV) also led to dissociation between ELISA binding to F protein (high titer) and virus neutralization (low titer) in vaccinated animals [21]. In contrast, live virus BRSV immunization of cattle induces a high level of neutralizing antibodies. In addition, it is unlikely that appreciable amounts of secretory antibodies were induced in the respiratory tract of the FI-RSV infant vaccinees because the FI-RSV vaccine was given parenterally. Thus, with local and systemic humoral immunity to RSV being largely deficient in FI-RSV vaccinees, pulmonary RSV replication was not restricted in the vaccinees during subsequent natural infection. Pulmonary RSV replication may then have provided the stimulus for immune mediators to cause enhanced disease. It is also unlikely that FI-RSV induced a CD8 + T cell response, which is also known to contribute to resistance to RSV in experimental animals.

The second factor postulated to be involved in the enhanced disease in the vaccinees was a state of heightened CD4 + T cell activity induced by immunization with FI-RSV. This mechanism was previously suggested by the increased lymphocyte proliferative response of peripheral blood lymphocytes of FI-RSV human vaccinees to RSV antigens. Studies in rodents demonstrated that the mechanism underlying the disease potentiation in FI-RSV immunized animals was completely dependent on Th2 type CD4 + T cells. This dependence of disease potentiation on Th2 T cells contrasts with the predominantly Th1 T cell response to RSV infection. Thus the imbalances in the immune response of FI-RSV immunized mice outlined above were accompanied by another imbalance, an altered ratio of T-helper subsets present in the pulmonary inflammatory cell infiltrate. Pathologic effects in some rodent studies were shown to be mediated by oligoclonal lymphocyte responses [22].

Considering the quantitative and qualitative differences in the cellular immune responses to infection or FI-RSV noted in both humans and rodents, we suggest that in the infant recipients of the FI-RSV vaccine a heightened CD4 + T cell response occurred at the sites of RSV replication in the bronchioles and alveoli. Thus the enhanced disease in vaccinees was a Th2 CD4 + T-cell-mediated pulmonary delayed-type hypersensitivity reaction. These observations with FI-RSV have important implications for the development of RSV vaccines. It is reasonable to predict that to be useful in RSV immunoprophylaxis, immunogens will have to induce (1) both serum and mucosal antibodies with high neutralizing activities and (2) a cellular immune response similar to that induced by infection with wild-type RSV, and dissimilar from that induced by FI-RSV.

2. Respiratory Syncytial Virus Subunit Vaccine

The major protective antigens of RSV, the fusion (F), and attachment (G) glycoproteins that induce neutralizing and protective antibodies [3,23], are the target antigens for inclusion in an RSV subunit vaccine. Initial studies found that rodents could be successfully immunized with purified F or G glycoprotein antigens and protected against wild-type RSV challenge [24,25]. The F or G glycoproteins used in these studies were purified by physical techniques from virions, by immunoaffinity chromatography from insect cells infected with an F-glycoprotein recombinant baculovirus, or from lysates obtained from RSV-infected mammalian cell culture [24,26–28], and they were protective in rodents [28,29]. However, the protection observed was incomplete in that significant resistance to virus replication was observed only in the lower respiratory tract, while the challenge virus efficiently replicated in the upper respiratory tract [28,29]. This pattern of resistance differed from that induced by prior infection with RSV, which provided complete protection of both sites of the respiratory tract. These findings suggest that immunization against RSV is most effective when administered by the mucosal route. Studies in mice using topically applied F glycoprotein coadministered with cholera toxin or with the B subunit of cholera toxin (CTB) demonstrated protective efficacy for the upper respiratory tract, while simultaneous parenteral administration of F and mucosal immunization with F and CTB induced a level of efficacy similar to that induced by live virus infection [30]. Other investigators examined the feasibility of using the purified fraction 21 of *Quillaja saponaria* (QS-21) as an adjuvant with purified F glycoprotein and found that use of this adjuvant in immunization of mice (as compared with immunization using aluminum hydroxide and F) induced an immune response characterized by higher IgG2a antibody levels, higher neutralizing antibody titers, and decreased neutrophil infiltration of the lungs [31]. Further evaluation of this formulation will be necessary to determine its stability and its effect in infection-permissive hosts.

Disease potentiation in rodents, as indicated by enhanced pulmonary histopathology, was not observed in initial studies of F-protein immunized animals following RSV challenge; however, subsequent studies raised concern about aberrant immune responses to immunization with nonreplicating antigens (reviewed in Refs. 20 and 32). The unusual pattern of antibody response of FI-RSV human vaccinees (antibodies against the F glycoprotein that exhibited high titers of ELISA binding antibodies but low neutralizing activity) was subsequently observed in rodents immunized with either FI-RSV or with purified F glycoprotein [29,33]. In contrast, the neutralizing activity of RSV F-specific antibodies induced by infection of rodents RSV recombinant vaccinia virus expressing the RSV F glycoprotein was similar to that induced by wild-type RSV infection [34]. These observations strongly suggest that purification of the F glycoprotein resulted in altered immunogenicity, perhaps by disrupting conformationally dependent neutralizing epitopes present in the protein. Furthermore, immunization with purified F glycoprotein produced in mammalian or insect cells was shown to result in enhanced pulmonary histopathology in cotton rats challenged with RSV 3–6 months following immunization [33]. The pattern and magnitude of the cellular infiltration and the pattern of cytokine mRNA expression in the lungs of these RSV-challenged animals was

similar to that present in FI-RSV immunized RSV-challenged cotton rats [32,33,35]. Despite efficient induction of ELISA antibody in rodents, the purified F subunit vaccine was poorly immunogenic in seronegative chimpanzees. The purified F subunit vaccine candidate induced only low levels of serum neutralizing antibodies (~1:50) in young seronegative chimpanzees after three doses [36]. This finding in chimpanzees suggests that subunit vaccines likely would be weakly immunogenic in seronegative humans. Maternally acquired antibodies also likely would further diminish the immunogenicity of parenterally-administered subunit vaccines.

A series of clinical safety and immunogenicity studies has been performed in seropositive adults and children using different formulations of the purified F glycoprotein vaccines (designated PFP-1 or PFP-2) [37–42]. The vaccines were observed to be safe in seropositive subjects. The immunogenicity of the F subunit vaccine in humans was poor when used at a single dose of 5 or 20 µg [37,39]. However, when seropositive individuals received two doses of 50 µg, 100% responded by ELISA to the F glycoprotein and 70% responded with significant rise in titer of RSV-neutralizing antibodies [42]. These findings suggest that the purified F subunit vaccine might be useful as a vaccine for boosting the antibody levels of previously infected patients, especially those with underlying diseases that place them at high risk for severe RSV disease. Such patients include the elderly or individuals with cystic fibrosis, bronchopulmonary dysplasia, cardiovascular disease, or immunodeficiencies. The subunit vaccine might represent a more immunogenic vaccine for boosting the immunity of these subjects than would live virus vaccines, which are highly restricted in replication in seropositive subjects [43]. Trials have been conducted in several of these high-risk populations. Piedra et al. [44] conducted a double-blind, placebo-controlled study in 17 RSV-seropositive cystic fibrosis (CF) patients 12 months to 8 years of age using the PFP-2 vaccine candidate at a dose of 50 µg purified protein, compared with 17 patients administered saline placebo. The PFP-2 vaccine caused mild local reactions and induced a significant neutralizing antibody response in two-thirds of the vaccinees and a significant RSV F glycoprotein ELISA antibody response in most of the vaccinees. In a follow-up study, 29 of those 34 CF children who participated in the previous study were enrolled in an open label study, in which a second vaccine administration was found to be safe [45]. Groothuis et al. [46] performed a small, blinded study using a 50 µg dose of the PFP-2 vaccine in 10 RSV-seropositive patients with bronchopulmonary disease over a year of age, compared with 11 matched vaccinees receiving influenza vaccine. PFP-2 vaccine appeared to be safe and moderately immunogenic by serologic response in that population.

Two trials have been conducted with this RSV subunit vaccine candidate in the elderly, a high-risk adult population. A dose of 50 µg PFP-2 was found to be safe and moderately immunogenic in healthy older adults (60–80 years old) in an outpatient study comparing 33 vaccinees and 31 saline placebos [47]. A subsequent open label study in 37 frail institutionalized persons over age 65 showed that this vaccine was well tolerated without significant side effects. The vaccine was less immunogenic in this population, with only 53% of vaccinees mounting a greater than or equal to fourfold increase in IgG antibody titer to the F protein [48].

Studies with a novel recombinant RSV chimeric FG subunit vaccine were conducted in parallel with those of the F subunit vaccine described above. This vaccine consisted of a purified FG chimeric protein in which the anchor regions of the F (COOH-terminal) and G (NH$_2$-terminal) glycoproteins were deleted, and the two ectodomains of the proteins were expressed as a fusion protein with F sequences being at the NH$_2$-terminal end of the chimera [49]. This FG protein was expressed in insect cells by a recombinant baculovirus, and the FG protein, which was secreted into the medium, was purified by immunoaffinity chromatography. The FG subunit vaccine had several properties in common with purified F subunit vaccine. First, immunization with FG glycoprotein was protective in rodents, with protection largely confined to the lungs [34,50,51]. Second, the serum antibodies that were induced had a high ELISA titer but low neutralizing activity [34]. Third, enhanced pulmonary histopathology was observed in RSV FG-immunized cotton rats following RSV challenge [34]. Immunization of African green monkeys with FG glycoprotein did not induce enhanced pulmonary histopathology upon challenge, although the vaccine was weakly immunogenic and only marginally protective in the lower respiratory tract in these studies [52]. In addition, it was found that the immunogenicity of the G component of the FG vaccine was very low [34]. When FG glycoprotein was intranasally administered to mice with cholera toxin B (CTB) as a mucosal adjuvant, local IgA and IgG antibodies against RSV were induced in the respiratory tract of mice and protection of the upper respiratory tract was observed [53]. It is now recognized that the source of CTB used in these studies almost certainly contained minute quantities of contaminating cholera toxin, which would have been responsible for adjuvant activity. Cholera toxin B purified from recombinant sources that does not contain contaminating holotoxin does not exhibit adjuvant activity for coadministered antigens. The feasibility and safety of this FG chimera approach will require further evaluation.

Studies of the immune response to the FG subunit vaccine expanded previous studies of F subunit vaccine in two important ways. First, studies of cell-mediated immunity induced by FG demonstrated that CD4+ T cells were efficiently induced by immunization with FG, but CD8+ cytotoxic T cells were not [54–56]. Second, rodent studies demonstrated that antibodies induced by FG had low neutralizing activity in vitro and had low functional activity in vivo; that is, they failed to provide passive protection. Increased pulmonary histopathology was not observed in the passively immunized animals following RSV challenge, suggesting that antibody was not the major mediator of the inflammatory response. Rather, the histopathology observed in the FG-immunized, RSV-challenged animals appears to be mediated by T cells.

Another RSV subunit vaccine candidate is a recombinant fusion protein, designated BBG2Na, consisting of a central conserved domain of the RSV attachment (G) protein (amino acid residues 130–230) fused to the C-terminus

of the albumin-binding domain (BB) of streptococcal protein G [57]. This construct contains five linear B cell epitopes that map to residues 152–163, 165–172, 171–187 (two overlapping epitopes), and 196–204. Passive transfer of antibody and peptide immunization studies suggested that each of the epitopes is protective [58]. The vaccine candidate itself was previously shown to protect the upper and lower respiratory tracts of mice against intranasal RSV challenge [57]. In mice, CD4+ T cells induced by parenteral immunization with this protein fragment mediated protection of the upper respiratory tract against infection [59]. Neonatal rodent responses to this vaccine candidate were not inhibited by the presence of RSV maternal antibodies [60]. Safety trials using the BBG2Na vaccine candidate in healthy young adults have been initiated [61].

In summary, four major characteristics of current formulations of RSV F and FG subunit vaccines make them unlikely to be successful vaccines in seronegative humans. First, the poor immunogenicity of these vaccines in seronegative chimpanzees suggests that it will be difficult to deliver a sufficient number of doses in the neonatal period, when virus protein antigens are least immunogenic in humans, to induce a protective level of immunity. Second, the antibodies that are induced by such vaccines generally have a low level of functional activity in vivo that likely will not protect vaccinees. Third, maternally acquired serum antibodies can be expected to significantly suppress the immune response to parenterally administered vaccines. Fourth, the humoral and cellular immune responses to immunization with the RSV subunit vaccines are very similar to those induced by the deleterious FI-RSV vaccine. This similarity suggests that immunization of humans with an RSV subunit vaccine might result in disease potentiation, as was seen with FI-RSV. However, the safety profile of BBG2Na and its ability to induce neutralizing antibody and CD4+ T cell responses, in the context of the known immunogenicity of RSV G protein in young infants [62], suggest that continued cautious evaluation of this immunogen is warranted. While subunit RSV vaccines might not be ideal immunogens in young infants, they might prove useful in protecting older high-risk subjects against RSV lower respiratory tract disease.

3. Other Approaches

Synthetic peptide, anti-idiotype antibodies, and immunostimulating complex (ISCOM) formulated RSV vaccines are being developed as candidate vaccines [63–66]. Bacterial expression of RSV F protein has been developed using *Staphylococcus xylosus*, a nonpathogenic coagulase-negative gram-positive bacterium present on the skin [36]. Other investigators have generated an RSV G glycoprotein produced in *Salmonella* that was found to induce neutralizing antibodies in cotton rats [67]. The major drawback associated with the expression of viral glycoproteins in prokaryotes is the general lack of posttranslational folding and processing that may result in the expression of antigens lacking critical neutralization epitopes. Sufficient information on the safety, immunogenicity, and efficacy of these preparations is not available at this time to determine if they offer an advantage over the more extensively evaluated subunit vaccines. Furthermore, the phenomenon of immune-mediated disease potentiation means that any non-replicating, subunit-type vaccine must of necessity be developed with considerable caution. Plasmid DNA immunization with vectors encoding a DNA copy of the RSV F [68] or G [69] protein has been moderately immunogenic in rodent studies. This strategy is of interest because expression of viral proteins from similar vectors has been demonstrated to persist for several months in animal studies. Prolonged expression of vaccine antigens in vivo might circumvent the suppressive effects of maternal antibodies. However, the safety, immunogenicity, and feasibility of DNA immunization in human infants are unknown.

Immunization with live RSV administered by a parenteral route is another unusual approach that has been tested. A live RSV vaccine parenterally administered was evaluated for efficacy in a double-blind, placebo-controlled field trial in 510 children 6–47 months of age [70]. The rationale for that study was that intramuscular administration of a live respiratory virus that does not cause viremia or spread to the respiratory tract would be safe because immunization would be without direct risk of causing respiratory tract disease. The immunization might result in a dual response to native antigens present in the whole virus and possibly to antigens expressed by abortively infected cells outside the respiratory tract. Only 68 of 98 initially seronegative children (as determined by ELISA assay) developed antibody to RSV. Most of the 30 initially seronegative children who did not develop antibody were less than 12 months old, which suggested that levels of maternal antibody that could not be detected by ELISA inhibited replication of the vaccine virus. That trial did not demonstrate any benefit of the attenuated RSV vaccine after 2 years of follow up [70].

C. Live Virus Vaccines

1. Vectored Vaccines

Vaccinia virus, a live-attenuated virus vaccine previously used to prevent smallpox in humans, was used as a model to evaluate the immunogenicity and protective efficacy of a viral vector expressing RSV antigens. Vaccinia virus (strain WR)-RSV (vac-RSV) recombinants expressing each of the RSV proteins (except the polymerase L) were evaluated separately in BALB/c mice and cotton rats to determine the immunogenicity of each antigen and its contribution to resistance to intranasal RSV challenge [23]. These studies showed that the G and F glycoproteins were the only proteins that induced detectable RSV-neutralizing antibodies [71]. Each glycoprotein independently induced a high level of RSV-neutralizing antibodies and long-lasting resistance to RSV challenge, with F appearing to be somewhat more immunogenic than G. The N and M2-1 proteins also independently induced resistance to RSV challenge, and further analysis with the vac-M2 recombinant showed that MHC class I-restricted CD8+ CTLs mediated this protection [72,73]. In contrast to the durable resistance associated with G and F, the CTL-mediated resistance induced by vac-N and vac-M2 was transient and waned completely by 45

days after immunization. These observations suggest that RSV-specific CTL can play a role in restricting reinfection in the short term, but antigens that induce neutralizing antibodies (i.e., F and G) are the more important ones to include in a vectored vaccine.

Although the initial evaluation of vac-RSV recombinants in rodents and monkeys was encouraging [72,74], intradermal immunization of seronegative chimpanzees with vac-F and vac-G provided only low to moderate levels of serum neutralizing antibodies, inconsistent resistance in the lower respiratory tract, and no resistance in the upper respiratory tract [75,76]. More recently, the MVA strain of vaccinia virus was used to construct recombinants expressing the RSV F, G, or both glycoproteins [77]. The MVA strain is highly defective in producing infectious virus in most mammalian cells and undergoes only a single cycle of replication in human cells. Thus it is a much safer vector than replication-competent vaccinia virus strains and offers the possibility of topical administration. MVA-RSV recombinants were highly immunogenic when inoculated intranasally into RSV-naive mice and were effective in boosting immunity conferred by previous intranasal infection with an attenuated strain of RSV. However, evaluation in rhesus monkeys of comparable MVA-PIV3 recombinants expressing the HN or F glycoproteins showed that the recombinants were much more sensitive to immunosuppression by passively administered serum antibodies compared to a live-attenuated PIV3 virus [78]. Because infants and young children characteristically possess maternally derived PIV3- and RSV-specific serum antibodies, the MVA-based recombinants likely would be insufficiently immunogenic as pediatric vaccines.

Adenovirus has also been evaluated as a vector for expressing RSV antigens. Initial studies in rodents, ferrets, and dogs demonstrated that topical administration of adenovirus (ad)-RSV recombinant viruses was immunogenic and protective in both the upper and the lower respiratory tracts [79–81]. However, the ad-RSV did not appear to be immunogenic in a seronegative chimpanzee, despite three sequential immunizations with ad-4, ad-5, and ad-7 RSV F recombinant viruses [81]. Thus construction of a recombinant vector that expressed high levels of RSV antigen in vitro was not sufficient to provide an effective RSV vaccine.

More recently, an attenuated version of PIV3 was evaluated as a vector for RSV antigens. The specific vector was a cDNA-derived human PIV3 (HPIV3) vaccine candidate called rB/HPIV3 [82]. This virus was a chimera consisting of a bovine PIV3 (BPIV3) backbone in which the BPIV3 HN and F genes were replaced by their counterparts from HPIV3 (see Section III.B.2). Thus rB/HPIV3 combines the F and HN major protective antigen genes of HPIV3 with the BPIV3 backbone, which is attenuated in primates due to a natural host-range restriction. The RSV G or F glycoproteins were inserted singly or together into the promoter-proximal position of rB/HPIV3, and recombinants were made representing both RSV antigenic subgroups [83,84]. The chimeric rB/HPIV3-RSV viruses efficiently replicated in vitro and expressed high levels of the RSV G and F glycoproteins. When inoculated into the respiratory tract of rhesus monkeys, the rB/HPIV3-RSV chimeras were somewhat more attenuated than their rB/HPIV3 parent, presumably due to the presence of the insert, but nonetheless were highly immunogenic against both RSV and HPIV3. Thus these rB/HPIV3-RSV viruses have properties that make them attractive candidates as a bivalent pediatric vaccine against RSV and HPIV3. This strategy has the advantage that the vector itself is a needed vaccine rather than simply being a carrier. The attenuation phenotype conferred by the BPIV3 backbone is very stable (see Section III.B.2). Coimmunization against RSV and PIV3 is appropriate and desirable because they cause disease in the same age group, and the natural tropism of PIV3 for the respiratory tract makes it well suited for use as a vector/vaccine for intranasal administration. In addition, the vectored vaccine is free of infectious RSV.

Recombinant vesicular stomatitis virus (VSV) also has been evaluated as a vector to express the RSV G and F glycoprotein genes, each added singly as an additional gene (VSV-RSV-G and VSV-RSV-F viruses) or in place of the VSV G gene (VSVΔG-RSV-G and VSVΔG-RSV-F viruses) [85]. The VSVΔG-RSV viruses were infectious only when grown in the presence of VSV G expressed in *trans*, and thus represent a replication-defective vector that can undergo only a single round of infection in vivo. When evaluated as a live vaccine intranasally administered to mice, each of the viruses induced resistance to RSV challenge. However, the levels of RSV-specific serum antibodies that were induced were low, particularly for the VSVΔG-RSV viruses, and immunogenicity and efficacy studies in primates will be needed to determine whether these new vectors constitute an advance over vaccinia virus and adenovirus vectors. Vesicular stomatitis virus is a virus to which the young infant is not normally exposed, and it does not represent a needed pediatric vaccine. These considerations, together with the lack of experience with the administration of VSV to humans, pose obstacles to its development as a pediatric vaccine vector.

2. Live Attenuated Respiratory Syncytial Virus Vaccines

Live-attenuated RSV vaccines are attractive candidates for use as a pediatric RSV vaccine for a number of reasons. First, a live, topical RSV vaccine likely would stimulate an immune response similar to that of wild-type RSV infection, including the induction of serum and mucosal antibodies and the stimulation of cellular and innate immunity that are important as antiviral effectors [86–88]. Second, topical administration reduces the inhibitory effects of maternally derived serum antibodies on infection and immunogenicity of an RSV vaccine, as has been demonstrated in rodents and chimpanzees [9–11] and in recent clinical studies [62]. Third, while immunization of experimental animals with nonreplicating RSV vaccines such as purified proteins or formalin-inactivated virus can prime for enhanced RSV disease upon subsequent RSV exposure [33], this effect has not been observed with natural RSV infection [62]. Indeed, the balanced, protective immune response associated with live RSV infection supports its use as the first, priming immunization in the young infant.

The host immune response to a single infection with wild-type RSV typically provides incomplete protection against reinfection, particularly in the young infant in whom the immune response is reduced due to immunological immaturity and to the immunosuppressive effect of RSV-specific maternal antibodies on the antibody response to RSV. Therefore it is reasonable to anticipate that the same will be true of a live-attenuated RSV vaccine. It will likely be necessary to administer such a vaccine two or three times during the first year of life, probably as a mixture of viruses representing both RSV subgroups (A and B) and HPIV3. The optimal schedule and dose will need to be determined by experimentation.

Several programs, starting as early as the 1960s, employed conventional approaches to develop a live-attenuated RSV vaccine. Attenuated viruses were sought using techniques such as extensive passage in vitro at suboptimal low temperature to select cold-adapted (*ca*) mutants or mutagenizing virus and selecting temperature sensitive (*ts*) mutants [89–92]. The goal was to produce mutants that retain the ability to replicate efficiently in cell culture under permissive conditions (reduced temperature in the case of *ts* and *ca* mutants), thereby permitting efficient vaccine production, but that would be attenuated in vivo. These studies were impeded by the difficulty of manipulating RSV due to unstable infectivity and relatively poor growth in vitro, the uncontrolled, random nature of the attenuation methods, the lack of a convenient experimental animal for RSV disease, and the complexity involved in the clinical evaluation of a pediatric vaccine.

Recent progress has been obtained in work to generate highly attenuated genetically stable mutant viruses begun at the National Institute of Allergy and Infectious Diseases (NIAID). Initial studies evaluated the level of attenuation, genetic stability, and efficacy in seronegative juvenile chimpanzees of three *ts* mutants of the subgroup A wild-type virus RSV A2, designated *ts*-1, *ts*-1-NG1, and *ts*-4 [76]. These mutants had been prepared previously by one (*ts*-1, *ts*-4) or two (*ts*-1NG1) rounds of chemical mutagenesis [93]. Each of the *ts* mutants was restricted in replication in the lower respiratory tract of the chimpanzee, but retained the capacity to induce significant rhinorrhea. In addition, each of the three *ts* mutants underwent partial reversion to a non-*ts* phenotype during replication in a minority of the chimpanzees. Data obtained with the *ts*-1, *ts*-1-NG1, and *ts*-4 viruses in chimpanzees [76] were entirely congruent with that from clinical trials with *ts*-1 in seronegative human infants [94], in whom the virus also demonstrated residual reactogenicity and low levels of genetic instability. These studies showed that the seronegative chimpanzee was appropriate to serve as a model for the rapid evaluation of attenuation level and genetic stability of the next generation of live-attenuated RSV vaccines that are more attenuated than *ts*-1, *ts*-1-NG1, and *ts*-4.

A cold-passaged (*cp*) RSV mutant, designated *cp*-RSV, was developed in the 1960s by 52 passages at low temperature in bovine cell culture [95]. The *cp*-RSV virus was not significantly *ca* or *ts*, but was completely attenuated for seropositive adults and children. However, *cp*-RSV retained the capacity to cause upper respiratory disease in seronegative infants and thus was insufficiently attenuated. Cp-RSV was then subjected to chemical mutagenesis and the resulting virus suspension was screened to identify *ts* derivatives [96]. The two *ts* mutants with the lowest in vitro shutoff temperature (the cpts-248 and cpts-530 mutants) replicated less efficiently in the chimpanzee nasopharynx and caused less rhinorrhea than their cp-RSV parent and were 1000-fold restricted in replication in the trachea compared to wild-type RSV. The cpts-248 and cpts-530 progeny viruses also exhibited a greater degree of stability of the *ts* phenotype in nude mice and in chimpanzees than the previously studied *ts*-1 virus. The cpts-248 and cpts-530 viruses were thought likely to be incompletely attenuated for fully susceptible seronegative human infants and young children, based on data from seronegative chimpanzees. Therefore each virus was subjected to a second round of chemical mutagenesis and mutants were selected for increased *ts* phenotype [10,97]. Mutants designated cpts-248/955, cpts-248/404, cpts-530/1009, and cpts-530/1030, each with an in vitro shutoff temperature (i.e., the lowest temperature at which ≥100-fold reduction in plaquing efficiency is observed) of approximately 37 °C, were selected for further evaluation. The cpts-248/955 virus was more restricted in replication in chimpanzees than its parental viruses cp-RSV and cpts-248 (J. Crowe et al, unpublished observations). Clinical trials revealed that cpts-248/955 was attenuated in seropositive adults and children but retained virulence for seronegative infants and was transmissible to contacts [98]. Importantly, the *ts* phenotype of this mutant was observed to be stable even when replicating to high titers in seronegative infants. Thus, this virus was the first to demonstrate that a high level of genetic stability of an RSV *ts* mutant in the fully susceptible human infant could be achieved. Subsequent clinical studies in seronegative infants with cpts-530/1009 [98] showed that it, too, was phenotypically stable but was insufficiently attenuated, and preclinical data for cpts-530/1030 were similar.

The cpts-248/404 virus appeared to be somewhat more attenuated in the seronegative chimpanzee and thus suitable for evaluation in 1–2-month-old RSV-naive infants, the target age for an RSV vaccine [62]. This vaccine virus replicated in the nasopharynx to similar levels in older seronegative infants and in the 1–2-month-old infants, who possess substantial titers of maternally derived RSV-specific antibodies. This finding indicated that maternal antibody does not significantly inhibit the replication of the attenuated virus. More than 80% of vaccinees were infected and shed from 10^3 to 10^5 PFU of vaccine virus per milliliter of nasal wash. This level of virus replication was sufficient for immunization, because the majority of infants were not infected with a second vaccine dose given 1 month later. In addition, more than 80% of vaccinees had a significant rise in RSV-specific IgA. Interestingly, the antibody response to the G protein was more frequent and of greater magnitude than that to the F protein. Thus although there is speculation that G has antigenic properties when administered in the absence of other RSV antigens that contribute to priming for immune-enhanced RSV disease in rodents [99], it probably would be ill advised to delete this antigen from a pediatric vaccine. More than 70% of vaccinees experienced brief nasal congestion

that interfered with sleep and feeding following the initial immunization and that appeared coincident with the peak of virus shedding, indicating that the virus needs to be further attenuated. In addition, virus recovered on several days from a single vaccinee exhibited a partial loss of the *ts* and attenuation phenotypes. Although this revertant virus did not become a predominant species and remained significantly attenuated, it would be desirable to achieve a greater level of phenotypic stability.

Given the difficulty in obtaining an appropriately attenuated, phenotypically stable vaccine virus by conventional biological methods, the studies shifted to using recombinantly derived RSV as the substrate for producing a live-attenuated vaccine. Recombinant wild-type RSV strain A2 can be produced entirely from cDNA by the intracellular coexpression of a complete positive-sense copy of RSV genomic RNA and the RSV N, P, L, and M2-1 proteins from transfected plasmids (Fig. 1) [100]. This recombinant wild-type virus was confirmed to be virulent in seronegative chimpanzees and thus was an appropriate substrate for the development of attenuated derivatives.

To identify attenuating mutations for insertion into recombinant RSV, the biologically-derived cp-RSV and cpts-RSV mutants described above were sequenced in their entirety, and the contribution of the mutations identified to the *ts* and attenuation phenotypes was evaluated by introduction into the wild-type recombinant virus. Sequence analysis showed that the cp-RSV mutant had five nucleotide substitutions in the N, F, and L genes that each gave rise to an amino acid change, and the introduction of all five mutations into wild-type recombinant RSV reconstituted the attenuation phenotype [101,102]. Sequence analysis of the cpts-248, cpts-530, cpts-248/404, cpts-530/1009, and cpts-530/1030 viruses showed that the singly and doubly mutagenized viruses each contained one and two point mutations, respectively, that independently conferred *ts* and attenuation phenotypes [103–107]. Each of the mutations involved an amino acid substitution in the L polymerase protein with the exception of one of the mutations in cpts-248/404, which involved a single nucleotide change in the transcription gene-start signal of the M2 gene. Biologically derived viruses such as cpts-248/404 and cpts-530/1009 were then reconstructed in recombinant form, which reconstituted the authentic *ts* and attenuation phenotypes and confirmed that the attenuating mutations had been correctly and completely identified. The recombinant version of the cpts-248/404 virus was then modified by the introduction of one of the attenuating mutations from the cpts-530/1030 virus, resulting in a recombinant virus called cp248/404/1030 that was more *ts* and more attenuated than cpts-248/404. This recombinant virus represents a promising new RSV vaccine candidate [108]. This work demonstrated that the recombinant recovery method (also called "reverse genetics") can indeed be used to place predetermined changes into infectious virus to obtain new combinations of attenuating mutations and to obtain incremental increases in the *ts* and attenuation phenotypes. It also is noteworthy that, while each of the amino acid changes in the biologically derived mutants was due to a single nucleotide change and thus could revert to the wild-type assign-

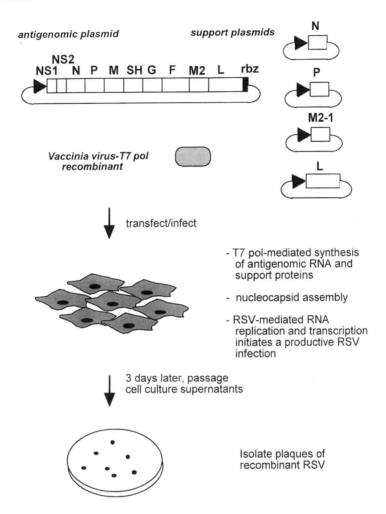

Figure 1 Production of infectious recombinant RSV from cloned cDNAs. The antigenomic plasmid contains a cloned cDNA of the complete RSV genome, with the viral genes shown as boxes. This cDNA is flanked on the upstream, left side by the promoter for T7 RNA polymerase (filled triangle) and on the downstream, right side by sequence encoding a self-cleaving ribozyme (rbz, filled box). Transcription by T7 RNA polymerase yields the positive sense replicative intermediate RNA, the antigenome: the strategy of synthesizing the antigenome rather than the negative-sense genome is to avoid hybridization with the positive-sense RNAs produced by the support plasmids. The four support plasmids contain cDNAs encoding the RSV N, P, M2-1, and L proteins under the control of T7 RNA polymerase. The antigenomic and support plasmids are transfected into cultured cells that are also infected with a vaccinia virus recombinant expressing T7 RNA polymerase. Co-expression of the antigenomic RNA and the N, P, M2-1, and L proteins results in the assembly of a viral nucleocapsid, which includes the RSV polymerase and is the minimum unit of infectivity. This nucleocapsid is replicated and transcribed by the RSV polymerase, thereby producing progeny genome and antigenome as well as expressing all of the genes. This launches a productive infection that results in the production of infectious recombinant virus. Following a three-day incubation, the clarified cell culture supernatant fluid is passaged onto a fresh monolayer and viral plaques are isolated and propagated. Production of recombinant PIV, such as PIV3, follows the same strategy except that only three support plasmids are required, namely N, P, and L: the PIVs lack an equivalent to the RSV M2-1 protein.

ment in a single step, in many cases it was possible to introduce the attenuating amino acid assignments into recombinant virus using two nucleotide differences per codon relative to wild type. This modification might greatly reduce the frequency of reversion and thus provide greater genetic stability.

Another source of attenuating RSV mutations has been the deletion of nonessential genes. Surprisingly, five RSV genes can be deleted or silenced individually and in certain combinations without the loss of infectivity in vitro [109–115]. For example, the genes encoding the NS1 and NS2

nonstructural proteins can be deleted individually or together, resulting in viruses that replicate only slightly less efficiently than wild-type RSV in Vero cell culture. Recent work suggests that the function of NS1 and NS2 is to coordinately antagonize the interferon type I-mediated antiviral state [116]. Deletion of the gene encoding the small hydrophobic SH surface protein, whose function is unknown, results in a virus that replicates as efficiently in vitro as wild-type. Remarkably, the G glycoprotein gene also can be deleted without much effect on the ability of the virus to replicate in Vero cell culture [115], although this particular deletion mutant likely would not be useful for vaccine purposes because G is one of the major protective antigens. Finally, deletion or silencing of the M2-2 open reading frame (ORF), which is the second, downstream ORF of the M2 mRNA, resulted in a virus in which the balance between transcription versus RNA replication appeared to be shifted, such that transcription is increased and RNA replication is decreased. This provided the novel phenotype of increased antigen expression concomitant with attenuation, a phenotype that might be highly desirable for vaccine purposes. When evaluated in chimpanzees and compared to the *cpts*-248/404 virus, the order of increasing attenuation of these gene-deletion viruses was: ΔSH < ΔNS2 < *cpts*-248/404 < ΔNS1 < ΔM2-2 [117,118]. Thus these gene deletions represent promising attenuating mutations for vaccine purposes, either on their own or in combination with point mutations previously described. For example, a virus consisting of the *cpts*-248/404/1030 backbone mentioned above together with the deletion of the SH gene was more attenuated and resulted in a lower level of virus shedding in seronegative children compared to *cpts*-248/404, and represents a promising vaccine candidate (R. Karron, unpublished data). An advantage of a gene deletion is that it is likely to be phenotypically highly stable.

Another method of attenuation is based on the naturally occurring host range restriction of bovine RSV (BRSV) in primates. Bovine RSV and human RSV (HRSV) are closely related viruses that share considerable antigenic cross-reactivity as measured with pooled human antibodies or HRSV F-specific monoclonal antibodies [119]. Bovine RSV has been considered for use as a live vaccine against human RSV (HRSV). Immunization of cotton rats with BRSV provided partial resistance to HRSV challenge [120]. However, BRSV strain A51908 did not replicate to a detectable level in seronegative chimpanzees and failed to induce resistance to challenge with HRSV [121], indicating that BRSV was overattenuated in primates. To reduce the host range restriction and improve antigenic cross-reactivity with HRSV, a recombinant version of BRSV was modified so that the HRSV counterparts replaced the BRSV G and F genes. This chimeric rBRSV/A2 virus replicated to very low levels in chimpanzees and did not induce significant protection against HRSV challenge [121]. This finding indicated that the introduction of the HRSV glycoproteins provided some improvement in growth, but that the rBRSV/A2 chimeric virus remained overattenuated. The next step will be to replace additional BRSV genes in rBRSV/A2 with the HRSV counterparts to improve the growth of the chimeric virus and achieve a satisfactory level of immunogenicity.

A successful live-attenuated RSV vaccine should induce protection against viruses of either antigenic subgroup A or B. Attempts to produce a satisfactorily attenuated subgroup B vaccine candidate by conventional methods have not been successful so far [113,122,123], and a reverse genetics system for subgroup B has not yet been developed. Therefore the existing subgroup A strain A2 recombinant virus was modified so that its G and F glycoprotein genes were replaced by those of the subgroup B strain B1 virus [24]. The resulting AB virus, bearing the major antigenic determinants of subgroup B in the A2 backbone, replicated like a wild-type virus in cell culture and chimpanzees. Because nearly all of the available attenuating mutations identified for the A2 strain lie outside the G and F genes, they can be directly inserted into the A2 backbone of the A/B chimeric virus. The glycoprotein swap had very little effect on virus growth; therefore it is likely that the same attenuated backbone can be used for the subgroup A and B vaccine viruses. For example, an AB chimeric virus that was constructed with the backbone of the *cpts*-248/404/1030 vaccine candidate described above possessed the same shut-off temperature as *cpts*-248/404/1030 and exhibited a similar, high degree of attenuation in chimpanzees [124]. A second approach to making a subgroup B vaccine is to express the G protein of subgroup B as a supernumerary gene inserted into the subgroup A strain A2 genome [125]. Because G is highly divergent between the subgroups, whereas F is relatively well conserved, this single chimeric virus expressing the G proteins of both subgroups and the F protein of subgroup A alone could serve as a bivalent vaccine against both subgroups.

3. Future Directions

The ability to introduce predetermined changes into infectious RSV via a cloned DNA intermediate provides the means to produce novel, improved vaccine candidates and to fine-tune their level of attenuation. A critical feature of this strategy was to develop a menu of mutations that attenuate in vivo but have little or minimal effect on virus growth in vitro. The present menu, including non-*ts* point mutations, *ts* point mutations, gene deletions, and host range determinants, has been used to produce a number of promising recombinantly derived vaccine candidates that are in clinical trials or in preparation. Other methods of attenuation also are available, such as inserting additional sequence or genes into the genome, which has the effect of reducing the efficiency of virus growth [126], or rearrangement of the viral genome so that the expression of the various proteins is suboptimal and growth efficiency is reduced [127]. However, these methods appear to reduce growth in vitro as well as in vivo, and hence might interfere with vaccine production to an unacceptable level.

The ability of reverse genetics to derive viruses that are more attenuated than *cpts*-248/404 suggests that it will be possible to produce vaccine candidates that are sufficiently attenuated for use as pediatric vaccines. It remains to be seen whether such viruses will be able to induce a satisfactory level of protective immunity in the very young infant. The ability of *cpts*-248/404 to confer a high degree of resistance to a second vaccine dose suggests that effective immunity can be achieved in the young infant, at least for the short term [62]. Additional immunizations or restricted natural infection in the context of the maturing immune response might result in increased, longer-lived protection.

It might also be possible to produce an RSV vaccine that is "better than nature" with regard to the balance between immunogenicity and attenuation. The ΔM2-2 virus is one example because it has a higher intrinsic level of transcription per genome compared to wild-type RSV and thus provides a higher level of antigen expression. Another way to increase the level of expression of the protective antigens would be to move their genes to be promoter-proximal [128] or to manipulate the encoded mRNAs to be more efficiently translated. The expression of cytokines or chemokines from one or more genes inserted into RSV offers another way to attenuate virus replication and to boost and alter the immune response [129,130] although additional care might be needed to demonstrate the safety of such a vaccine. It might also be possible to improve vaccine virus by eliminating features that have been suggested to enhance pathogenesis or interfere with the host immune response. For example, deletion of the NS1 and NS2 interferon antagonists might improve the immune response. In addition, the G glycoprotein is expressed in part as a secreted form that might mimic a protein vaccine in priming for enhanced immunopathology [131], and G contains a CX3C-like domain that might function as a chemokine antagonist [132]. Either of these features could be removed from vaccine virus by reverse genetics. In addition, we still do fully not understand why RSV can infect young infants despite the presence of moderate titers of RSV-neutralizing serum antibody, nor why the immune response to RSV is relatively inefficient in blocking reinfection. Hopefully, answers will be obtained in future work and used to improve RSV immunoprophylaxis.

Respiratory syncytial virus is a significant cause of respiratory tract disease in adults and, in particular, the elderly, where its impact approaches that of nonpandemic influenza virus [133]. A vaccine virus that is appropriately attenuated for young infants likely will be overattenuated for adults, based on an evaluation of the above-mentioned *cpts*-248/404 virus in both age groups [43,62]. Therefore it also is important to define a second group of live-attenuated vaccine candidates, such as ΔNS2, that are somewhat less attenuated than *cpts*-248/404 and are appropriate for evaluation in the elderly.

III. VACCINE DEVELOPMENT FOR HPIV1, HPIV2, AND HPIV3

A. General Considerations

HPIV1, HPIV2, and HPIV3 cause severe respiratory tract disease that leads to hospitalization of infants and young children [134]. HPIV1, HPIV2, and HPIV3 are distinct serotypes, and significant cross-neutralization or cross-protection is not seen following primary infection. In a long-term study in infants and children over a 20-year period, HPIV1, HPIV2, and HPIV3 were identified as etiologic agents responsible for 6.0%, 3.2%, and 11.5%, respectively, of hospitalizations for respiratory tract disease [134], accounting in total for slightly less than that caused by RSV. Respiratory syncytial virus and PIV3 cause significant illness within the first 4 months of life whereas most of the illness caused by HPIV1 and HPIV2 occurs after 6 months of age. A likely immunization sequence employing live-attenuated RSV and HPIV vaccines would be administration of RSV and HPIV3 vaccines together as a combined vaccine that would be given two or more times, with the first dose administered at or before 1 month of age, followed by a bi-

valent HPIV1 and HPIV2 vaccine at 4 and 6 months of age. The protective antigens of the PIVs are the hemagglutinin-neuraminidase (HN) glycoprotein (the attachment protein) and the fusion (F) glycoprotein, both of which induce neutralizing antibodies [134]. Because the PIVs, like RSV, cause repeat infection of humans, resistance against these viruses in humans may be best achieved by the induction of an immune response consisting of antibodies, both serum and mucosal, and cell-mediated immunity [134,135].

The PIV gene order is 3′ leader-N-P-M-F-HN-L-5′ trailer [134]. The 3′ end of genomic RNA and its full-length positive-sense replicative intermediate antigenomic RNA contains promoter elements that direct RNA synthesis. The genes are bordered by short conserved gene-start and gene-end signals that guide the polymerase during sequential transcription. The nucleocapsid-associated proteins are composed of the nucleocapsid protein (N), the phosphoprotein (P), and the large polymerase (L). The internal matrix protein (M) and the major protective antigens, the F and HN, are the envelope-associated proteins. The PIV P gene gives rise to additional, accessory proteins (designated C, C′, Y1, Y2, V, D, and X) that vary in occurrence among the different PIVs [134].

Previously tested, inactivated PIV vaccines were not sufficiently immunogenic to be protective in humans [136], but disease potentiation was not observed in these clinical studies as it had been for RSV. However, disease potentiation has recently been observed following wild-type PIV3 challenge of rodents previously immunized with either formalin- or UV-inactivated PIV3 vaccines [137]. Therefore as is the case for RSV and measles virus, there are concerns that nonreplicating vaccines such as purified proteins might be associated with immune-mediated disease potentiation. Other factors impede the development of PIV subunit vaccines including the weak immunogenicity of purified proteins in immunologically naive subjects and the need for the codevelopment of a safe adjuvant that is effective in humans, including the young infant [138]. There have been few recent studies on inactivated or subunit vaccines [139], and this summary of new vaccines will focus on the live or vectored PIV vaccine candidates under active study. The extensive safety record of live-attenuated measles and mumps virus vaccines, together with the experience with experimental live RSV vaccines, suggests that it is unlikely that immunization with a live-attenuated HPIV vaccine would be followed by disease potentiation.

B. Live Virus Vaccines

1. Vaccines Whose Attenuation Is Based on Host Range

Bovine PIV3 (BPIV3) was chosen as a candidate live-attenuated virus vaccine to protect against infection with HPIV3 for several reasons. First, antigenic analysis using monoclonal antibodies and postinfection sera from rodents and primates indicated that the surface glycoproteins of the BPIV3 and HPIV3 are about 25% related by reciprocal cross-neutralization [140]. The majority of the antigenic sites recognized by humans undergoing infection with HPIV3 also were recognized by sera of monkeys and chimpanzees following infection with BPIV3 [141]. This high degree of relatedness revealed by antigenic analysis is consistent with the relatively high degree of sequence relatedness between the HN and F glycoproteins of BPIV3 and HPIV3 (77% and 80% identity, respectively) [142]. Second, infection of cotton rats or monkeys with BPIV3 induced resistance to subsequent challenge infection with HPIV3 [140]. The replication of the two different strains of BPIV3 that were tested was restricted 100- to 1000-fold in rhesus monkeys or chimpanzees, but was sufficient to induce moderate levels of serum neutralizing antibodies to HPIV3 [140]. It seems likely that many of the sequence differences between BPIV3 and HPIV3 are a result of evolution and adaptation in their respective hosts. This principle forms the basis for natural host range restriction. This mechanism of attenuation based on host range is analogous to that of vaccinia virus (the vaccine virus for prevention of smallpox), which was much less virulent in humans than smallpox virus but, nonetheless, provided excellent protection against smallpox. This approach to immunization against viral pathogens has been termed the "Jennerian" approach. The combined properties of restriction of replication and induction of a protective immune response to HPIV3 in nonhuman primates made the BPIV3 a promising candidate for use as a live virus vaccine.

BPIV3 was restricted in replication, poorly infectious, and avirulent in both seropositive children and adults [143,144]. However, BPIV3 was highly infectious for seronegative vaccinees when administered at a dose of $10^{4.0}$ or $10^{5.0}$ TCID$_{50}$ and was nonreactogenic at these doses. BPIV3 infected 92% of HPIV3-seronegative children; 92% developed a serum hemagglutination inhibiting (HAI) antibody response to BPIV3 and 61% to HPIV3. Additional studies indicated that the live BPIV3 vaccine is attenuated, infectious, immunogenic, poorly transmissible, and phenotypically stable, and it is continuing to be evaluated as a candidate vaccine in infants and children [145].

An investigation has been initiated into the genetic basis of attenuation of BPIV3 using reverse genetics. A chimeric recombinant human–bovine parainfluenza virus type 3 (PIV3) virus (rHPIV3-N$_B$) was constructed in which the nucleoprotein (N) ORF of HPIV3 was replaced by its counterpart from BPIV3 [82]. rHPIV3-N$_B$ was restricted in replication in rhesus monkeys to a similar extent as its BPIV3 parent, showing that the BPIV3 N protein is a determinant of the host range restriction of replication, i.e., the attenuation phenotype, of BPIV3 in primates [146]. There are 79 differences out of a total of 515 amino acids between the N proteins of human PIV3 and BPIV3 [147]. Many of these 79 amino acid differences likely contribute to the host range attenuation phenotype of rHPIV3-N$_B$. Because of this, it is anticipated that the attenuation phenotype of rHPIV3-N$_B$ will be stable following prolonged replication in vivo, and preliminary findings indicate that this is so [144]. The HN and F genes of BPIV3 also have been shown to contribute to its attenuation for primates [82]. Because BPIV3 is only 25% antigenically related to HPIV3 [141], its immunogenicity against HPIV3 would be improved if it could be modified to express the protective F and HN antigens of HPIV3.

rHPIV3-N$_B$, which combines the antigenic determinants of HPIV3 with the host range restriction and attenuation phenotype of BPIV3, represents such a virus. In nonhuman primates, it induced a level of resistance to HPIV3 challenge that was indistinguishable from that conferred by immunization with HPIV3. Thus in the process of analyzing the genetic basis of attenuation of BPIV3 for primates, a promising vaccine candidate, rHPIV3-N$_B$, was generated, and this analysis identified chimerization of human and bovine PIV3 viruses as a novel method to produce an attenuated HPIV3 vaccine.

A second vaccine candidate based on the host range attenuation of BPIV3 for primates was constructed. rBPIV3 was recovered from cDNA and was used to construct a BPIV3/HPIV3 chimeric virus, designated rB/HPIV3, in which the F and HN genes of BPIV3 were replaced with their HPIV3 counterparts [82,148]. The F and HN genes were exchanged as pairs because of the known requirement for the presence of homologous F and HN proteins of parainfluenza viruses for full functional activity [149–151] and because the two proteins together constitute the PIV3 neutralization antigens. rB/HPIV3 replicated in vitro as efficiently as its parental viruses, and it replicated in the upper respiratory tract of rhesus monkeys to the same level as that of its BPIV3 parent [82,83]. Thus introduction of the HPIV3 F and HN genes into the BPIV3 backbone was insufficient alone to alter its attenuation phenotype. Immunization of rhesus monkeys with rB/HPIV3 induced a higher level of antibody to HPIV3 than did immunization with BPIV3, consistent with the presence of the homologous HPIV3 glycoproteins in rB/HPIV3. Furthermore, rB/HPIV3 conferred a level of protection against replication of HPIV3 challenge in the upper and lower respiratory tract that was statistically indistinguishable from that conferred by previous infection with wild-type HPIV3. Thus rB/HPIV3 and rHPIV3-N$_B$ represent promising new PIV3 vaccine candidates, and studies with them are planned in humans. A possible advantage of rB/HPIV3 over rHPIV3-N$_B$ is that it possesses all of the BPIV3 genes other than HN and F, so that if more than one BPIV3 gene is involved in the host range restriction of replication of BPIV3 for primates, rB/HPIV3 should be even more phenotypically stable than rHPIV3-N$_B$. Conversely, a potential advantage of rHPIV3-N$_B$ over rB/HPIV3 is that it possesses all of the HPIV3 antigens except N, and thus might induce a cell-mediated response that would more closely resemble that of HPIV3. Studies of safety (attenuation), immunogenicity, and protective efficacy in humans will be needed to resolve these issues.

The close antigenic relatedness between Sendai virus and HPIV1 suggested that Sendai virus could be used as a Jennerian vaccine to protect against HPIV1. Mice immunized with HPIV1 were partially protected against a lethal dose of Sendai virus [152]. Similarly, African green monkeys immunized with Sendai virus were protected against experimental challenge with HPIV1 infection [153]. However, these studies did not evaluate the level of replication of Sendai virus and HPIV1 in the upper and lower respiratory tract of the primates, and it was unclear whether Sendai virus would be satisfactorily attenuated for primates. A subsequent study showed that Sendai virus is not significantly restricted in its replication in the upper and lower respiratory tract of African green monkeys and chimpanzees compared to HPIV1 [154], suggesting that it is an unlikely vaccine candidate for use in humans.

2. Live-Attenuated Human Parainfluenza Virus Vaccines

Live-attenuated mutants of HPIV3 are also being developed. A wild-type strain of HPIV3, designated strain JS, was cultivated in primary monkey kidney tissue culture at low temperatures for 45 passages and mutants were selected after 12, 18, or 45 passages and designated HPIV3cp12, HPIV3cp18, or HPIV3cp45, according to their cold-passage level [155]. Three phenotypic markers were acquired during the process of low temperature passage: cold-adaptation (ca), i.e., the ability to replicate efficiently at 25 °C; temperature sensitivity (ts), i.e., restriction of growth at 40 °C in tissue culture; and attenuation (att), restricted replication in hamsters [155,156]. The HPIV3 cpPIV3 mutants protected hamsters against HPIV3 challenge [157], and each of the three cp mutant viruses was attenuated in seronegative rhesus monkeys [158]. The level of temperature-sensitivity of the cp mutants directly correlated with the degree of attenuation in monkeys, with the HPIV3cp12 being the least ts and the least attenuated, whereas the HPIV3cp45 mutant was the most ts and the most attenuated. Data derived from the evaluation of the HPIV3cp12, HPIV3cp18, and HPIV3cp45 viruses in rhesus monkeys indicated that HPIV3cp45 was the most promising of the three cp mutants because it was the most restricted in replication in the lower respiratory tract and its ts phenotype was the most stable following replication in vivo. The HPIV3cp45 mutant was also the only one of the three cold-passaged viruses that possessed both ts and non-ts mutations contributing to the attenuation phenotype in rhesus monkeys, suggesting that the HPIV3cp45 virus had acquired a greater number of attenuating mutations compared to the HPIV3cp12 and HPIV3cp18 mutants [159].

The HPIV3cp45 virus was highly restricted in replication in both the upper and lower respiratory tract of the chimpanzee compared to the JS wild-type parent virus and the animals were highly resistant to wild-type HPIV3 challenge [160]. The HPIV3cp45 virus present in the respiratory tract secretions of chimpanzees retained the ts phenotype, but some decrease in the level of temperature sensitivity was observed in the virus isolated in tissue culture (referred to as isolates). In other words, the input HPIV3cp45 vaccine virus was more restricted in plaque formation at 38°C than the HPIV3cp45 isolates, but all the isolates were ts at 40°C. Stability of the attenuation phenotype was demonstrated by the administration of an isolate of HPIV3cp45 (ts at 39°C), obtained after 10 days of replication in a chimpanzee, to two additional chimpanzees. This chimpanzee-passaged HPIV3cp45 virus was attenuated in both the upper and lower respiratory tracts, indicating that the attenuation phenotype of the HPIV3cp45 virus was stable following replication in chimpanzees, despite the decrease in temperature sensitivity. These results provided the basis on which to proceed to clinical trials in humans.

The HPIV3cp45 mutant was evaluated in a randomized, placebo-controlled, double-blind trial in 114 children 6 months to 10 years of age [161]. The cp45 vaccine was well tolerated when given intranasally to HPIV3 seropositive or seronegative children. A cp45 vaccine dose of 10^4 or 10^5 $TCID_{50}$ infected 86% of seronegative vaccinees, 83% of whom shed virus at a mean peak titer of $10^{2.2}$ pfu/mL. Virus present in the respiratory specimens retained the ts phenotype, and each of 86 cp45 isolates tested retained both the ts and ca phenotypes. A single dose of 10^5 $TCID_{50}$ induced a serum HAI antibody response in 81% of vaccinees; the geometric mean titer achieved was 1:32. These studies indicate that the HPIV3cp45 vaccine is satisfactorily attenuated, infectious, immunogenic, and phenotypically stable. Further evaluation of this promising vaccine candidate is underway.

To characterize the genetic basis for the ts, ca, and att phenotypes of this promising vaccine candidate, a recombinant HPIV3cp45 (rHPIV3cp45) virus was constructed that contained all fifteen HPIV3cp45-specific mutations identified by sequence analysis [159,162]. rHPIV3cp45 was indistinguishable from the biologically derived HPIV3cp45 on the basis of plaque size, level of temperature sensitivity, cold-adaptation, level of replication in the upper and lower respiratory tract of hamsters, and ability to protect hamsters from subsequent wild-type HPIV3 challenge. A series of recombinant viruses was constructed containing individual HPIV3cp45 mutations or combinations of several mutations. Analysis of these recombinant viruses revealed that multiple HPIV3cp45 mutations distributed throughout the genome contribute to the ts, ca, and att phenotypes [162]. Each of the three amino acid substitutions in the L polymerase protein of HPIV3cp45 independently confers the ts and att phenotypes, but not the ca phenotype [163]. In addition to the mutations in the L gene, at least one other mutation in the 3'-N region (i.e., including mutations in the leader, in the gene start cis-acting sequence of N, and in the N coding region) contributes to the ts phenotype. A recombinant virus containing all the HPIV3cp45 mutations except those in L was more ts than HPIV3cp45, illustrating the complex nature of this phenotype. The ca phenotype of HPIV3cp45 also is a complex composite phenotype reflecting contributions of at least three separate genetic elements, namely mutations within the 3'N region, the L protein, and the CMFHN region. The att phenotype, which is the most relevant for vaccine purposes, was found to be a composite phenotype due to both ts and non-ts mutations. Attenuating ts mutations are in L, and non-ts attenuating mutations are located in C and F. The presence of multiple ts and non-ts attenuating mutations in cp45 likely contributes to the high level of attenuation and phenotypic stability of this promising vaccine candidate.

A live-attenuated HPIV1 vaccine candidate was generated by modification of the extensively studied HPIV3cp45 vaccine candidate using the techniques of reverse genetics [164,165]. Promising vaccine candidates had not been developed for HPIV1, and a reverse genetics system was not available for HPIV1 until very recently [166]. It was found that the HN and F glycoproteins of HPIV3 could be replaced with those from HPIV1, and an rHPIV3-1 chimeric virus was recovered that possesses a wild-type phenotype for replication in vitro and in vivo [167]. Next, the HN and F glycoproteins of the HPIV3cp45 candidate vaccine virus were replaced with those of HPIV1. This created a live-attenuated HPIV1 vaccine candidate, termed rHPIV3-1cp45, which contained the attenuated background of the rHPIV3cp45 vaccine virus together with the HN and F protective antigens of HPIV1. The chimeric rHPIV3-1cp45 virus was more restricted in replication in hamsters than HPIV3cp45, indicating that the introduction of the heterologous HPIV1 HN and F proteins into HPIV3 had an attenuating effect (i.e., attenuation due to chimerization) that was additive to that conferred by the 12 HPIV3cp45 mutations present in rHPIV3-1cp45. rHPIV3-1cp45 was immunogenic and protective against challenge with wild-type HPIV1 in hamsters. This virus shows sufficient promise that it should be evaluated further as a candidate live-attenuated vaccine strain for the prevention of severe lower respiratory tract disease caused by HPIV1 in infants and young children.

The same strategy as described above for the rHPIV3-1 chimeric virus was used to develop a live-attenuated HPIV2 vaccine virus, but a recombinant chimeric HPIV3–HPIV2 virus carrying the full-length HPIV2 glycoproteins in a wild-type HPIV3 backbone could not be recovered [167]. This difficulty was presumably due to incompatibility between the HPIV2 glycoproteins and the HPIV3 internal proteins, and might reflect the more distant relatedness between HPIV3 and HPIV2 than between HPIV1 and HPIV3 [134]. However, viable HPIV3-HPIV2 chimeric viruses were recovered when chimeric HN and F ORFs rather than complete HPIV2 F and HN ORFs were used to construct the full-length cDNA. One recovered virus, designated rHPIV3-2CT, in which the HPIV2 F and HN ectodomains and transmembrane domains were fused to their HPIV3 counterpart F and HN cytoplasmic domains, replicated efficiently in vitro. Thus it appears that only the cytoplasmic tail of the HN or F glycoprotein or both of HPIV3 were required for successful recovery of HPIV3-HPIV2 chimeric viruses. Although rHPIV3-2CT replicated efficiently in vitro, it was moderately to highly attenuated for replication in the respiratory tract of hamsters, African green monkeys (AGMs), and chimpanzees. This unexpected finding indicated that chimerization of the HN and F proteins of HPIV2 and HPIV3 itself specified a strong attenuation phenotype in vivo. Despite this attenuation, these viruses were highly immunogenic and protective against challenge with HPIV2 wild-type virus in hamsters and AGMs, and they represent promising candidates for clinical evaluation as a vaccine against HPIV2.

Although antigenic chimeric viruses provide a strategy for the rapid generation of new vaccine candidates, there might be a price to pay for their use. As indicated above, the epidemiology of RSV and HPIV1, HPIV2, and HPIV3 suggests that it would be optimal to administer vaccines in a sequential schedule with RSV and HPIV3 vaccines given before HPIV1 or HPIV2 vaccines. Should cross-protection between an HPIV3 and an HPIV3-1 vaccine occur, this would complicate a scheme of sequential immunization with a HPIV3 vaccine followed by an HPIV3-1 vaccine. We found that prior infection with HPIV3 moderately decreased the replication, immunogenicity, and efficacy of an rHPIV3-1 vaccine candidate [135]. This resistance to replication of HPIV3-1 likely was mediated by T cells directed against the shared internal PIV3 proteins of the two viruses, and in hamsters the resistance had waned within 4 months. The magnitude and duration of cell-mediated immunity to HPIV3 in primates and in young human vaccines is unknown. Thus a sequential immunization protocol using HPIV3-1 and HPIV3-2 antigenic chimeric vaccines in HPIV3 immune persons might pose potential problems for the infectivity and immunogenicity of these vaccines. A successful vaccine against HPIV1 and HPIV2 might require the development of attenuated human HPIV1 and HPIV2 vaccine viruses using the recently described reverse genetics systems for each of these viruses [166,168,172].

3. Use of Human Parainfluenza Viruses as Vectors

The limitations of the use of vaccinia or MVA viruses as vectors for RSV protective antigens was discussed above, as was the usefulness of attenuated HPIV3 viruses as vectors for the RSV F and G protective antigens. Human PIV3-based vectors, either based on attenuation specified by mutations present in HPIV3cp45 or host range sequences present in BPIV3, have also been used as vectors to express the HA protective antigen of measles virus, resulting in a bivalent vaccine virus against HPIV3 and measles viruses [169,170]. The HPIV3/HPIV1 antigenic chimeric virus described above, designated rHPIV3-1, in which the HN and F proteins of wild-type HPIV3 were replaced by their HPIV1 counterparts, was used as a vector to express the HN protein of HPIV2 to generate a single virus capable of inducing immunity to both HPIV1 and HPIV2 [171]. The HPIV2 HN ORF was expressed from an extra gene cassette, under the control of HPIV3 cis-acting transcription signals, inserted between the F and HN genes of rHPIV3-1. The recombinant derivative, designated rPIV3-1.2HN, was readily recovered and exhibited a level of in vitro growth similar to that of its parental virus. The rPIV3-1.2HN virus was restricted in replication in both the upper and lower respiratory tract of hamsters compared to rPIV3-1, identifying an in vivo attenuating effect of the HPIV2 HN insert. In hamsters, rPIV3-1.2HN elicited serum antibodies to both HPIV1 and HPIV2 and induced resistance against challenge with wild-type HPIV1 or HPIV2. Thus rPIV3-1.2HN, a virus solely attenuated by the insertion of the HPIV2 HN gene, functioned as a live-attenuated bivalent vaccine candidate against both HPIV1 and HPIV2.

REFERENCES

1. Falsey AR, Walsh EE. Humoral immunity to respiratory syncytial virus infection in the elderly. J Med Virol 1992; 36:39–43.
2. Falsey AR, et al. Respiratory syncytial virus and influenza A infections in the hospitalized elderly. J Infect Dis 1995; 172:389–394.
3. Collins PL, Murphy BR. Respiratory syncytial virus. In: Knipe DM, Howley PM, Griffin DE, Martin MA, Lamb RA, Roizman B, Straus SE, eds. Fields Virology. 4th ed.

Vol. 1. Philadelphia: Lippincott Williams and Wilkins, 2001:1443–1485.

4. Crowe JE Jr. Immune responses of infants to infection with respiratory viruses and live attenuated respiratory virus candidate vaccines. Vaccine 1998; 16:1423–1432.

5. Murphy BR, et al. Passive transfer of respiratory syncytial virus (RSV) antiserum suppresses the immune response to the RSV fusion (F) and large (G) glycoproteins expressed by recombinant vaccinia viruses. J Virol 1988; 62:3907–3910.

6. Murphy BR, Chanock RM. The immunobiology of RSV. In: Meigner B, Murphy B, Ogra P, eds. Animal Models of Respiratory Syncytial Virus Infections. Lyon, France: Merieux Foundation, 1991:25–30.

7. Crowe JE Jr. Host responses to respiratory virus infection and immunization. Curr Top Microbiol Immunol 1999; 236:191–214.

8. Crowe JE Jr. Influence of maternal antibodies on neonatal immunization against respiratory viruses. Clin Infect Dis 2001; 33:1720–1727.

9. Murphy BR, et al. Immunosuppression of the antibody response to respiratory syncytial virus (RSV) by pre-existing serum antibodies: partial prevention by topical infection of the respiratory tract with vaccinia virus-RSV recombinants. J Gen Virol 1989; 70:2185–2190.

10. Crowe JE Jr, et al. Cold-passaged, temperature-sensitive mutants of human respiratory syncytial virus (RSV) are highly attenuated, immunogenic, and protective in seronegative chimpanzees, even when RSV antibodies are infused shortly before immunization. Vaccine 1995; 13:847–855.

11. Crowe JE Jr, et al. Passively acquired antibodies suppress humoral but not cell-mediated immunity in mice immunized with live attenuated respiratory syncytial virus vaccines. J Immunol 2001; 167:3910–3918.

12. Chang J, Braciale TJ. Respiratory syncytial virus infection suppresses lung CD8+ T-cell effector activity and peripheral CD8+ T-cell memory in the respiratory tract. Nat Med 2002; 8:54–60.

13. Murphy BR, et al. Effect of age and preexisting antibody on serum antibody response of infants and children to the F and G glycoproteins during respiratory syncytial virus infection. J Clin Microbiol 1988; 24:894–898.

14. Clements ML, et al. Effective immunization with live attenuated influenza A virus can be achieved in early infancy. J Infect Dis 1996; 173:44–51.

15. Karron RA, et al. Evaluation of a live attenuated bovine parainfluenza type 3 vaccine in two-to six-month-old infants. Pediatr Infect Dis J 1996; 15:650–654.

16. Hendry RM, et al. Strain-specific serum antibody responses in infants undergoing primary infection with respiratory syncytial virus. J Infect Dis 1988; 157:640–647.

17. Muelenaer PM, et al. Group-specific serum antibody responses in children with primary and recurrent respiratory syncytial virus infections. J Infect Dis 1991; 164:15–21.

18. Kapikian AZ, et al. An epidemiologic study of altered clinical reactivity to respiratory syncytial (RS) virus infection in children previously vaccinated with an inactivated RS virus vaccine. Am J Epidemiol 1969; 89:405–421.

19. Kim HW, et al. Respiratory syncytial virus disease in infants despite prior administration of antigenic inactivated vaccine. Am J Epidemiol 1969; 89:422–434.

20. Murphy BR, et al. An update on approaches to the development of respiratory syncytial virus (RSV) and parainfluenza virus type 3 (PIV3) vaccines. Virus Res 1994; 32:13–36.

21. Ellis JA, et al. Bovine respiratory syncytial virus-specific immune responses in cattle following immunization with modified-live and inactivated vaccines. Analysis of the specificity

22. Varga SM, et al. Immunopathology in RSV infection is mediated by a discrete oligoclonal subset of antigen-specific CD4(+) T cells. Immunity 2001; 15:637–646.

23. Connors M, et al. Respiratory syncytial virus (RSV) F, G, M2 (22K), and N proteins each induce resistance to RSV challenge, but resistance induced by M2 and N proteins is relatively short-lived. J Virol 1991; 65:1634–1637.

24. Wathen MW, et al. Immunization of cotton rats with the human respiratory syncytial virus F glycoprotein produced using a baculovirus vector. J Infect Dis 1989; 159:255–264.

25. Walsh EE. Subunit vaccines for respiratory syncytial virus. In: Meigner B, Murphy B, Ogra P, eds. Animal Models of Respiratory Syncytial Virus Infections. Lyon, France: Merieux Foundation, 1991:109–114.

26. Levine S, et al. The envelope proteins from purified respiratory syncytial virus protect mice from intranasal virus challenge. Proc Soc Exp Biol Med 1989; 190:349–356.

27. Routledge EG, et al. The purification of four respiratory syncytial virus proteins and their evaluation as protective agents against experimental infection in BALB/c mice. J Gen Virol 1988; 69:293–303.

28. Walsh EE, et al. Immunization with glycoprotein subunits of respiratory syncytial virus to protect cotton rats against viral infection. J Infect Dis 1987; 155:1198–1204.

29. Murphy BR, et al. Immunization of cotton rats with the fusion (F) and large (G) glycoproteins of respiratory syncytial virus (RSV) protects against RSV challenge without potentiating RSV disease. Vaccine 1989; 7:533–540.

30. Walsh EE. Mucosal immunization with a subunit respiratory syncytial virus vaccine in mice. Vaccine 1993; 11:1135–1138.

31. Hancock GE, et al. Formulation of the purified fusion protein of respiratory syncytial virus with the saponin QS-21 induces protective immune responses in Balb/c mice that are similar to those generated by experimental infection. Vaccine 1995; 13:391–400.

32. Murphy BR, et al. Current approaches to the development of vaccines effective against parainfluenza and respiratory syncytial viruses. Virus Res 1988; 11:1–15.

33. Murphy BR, et al. Enhanced pulmonary histopathology is observed in cotton rats immunized with formalin-inactivated respiratory syncytial virus (RSV) or purified F glycoprotein and challenged with RSV 3-6 months after immunization. Vaccine 1990; 8:497–502.

34. Connors M, et al. Cotton rats previously immunized with a chimeric RSV FG glycoprotein develop enhanced pulmonary pathology when infected with RSV, a phenomenon not encountered following immunization with vaccinia-RSV recombinants or RSV. Vaccine 1992; 10:475–484.

35. Graham BS, et al. Priming immunization determines T helper cytokine mRNA expression patterns in lungs of mice challenged with respiratory syncytial virus. J Immunol 1993; 151:2032–2040.

36. Crowe JE Jr. Current approaches to the development of vaccines against disease caused by respiratory syncytial virus (RSV) and parainfluenza virus (PIV). A meeting report of the WHO Programme for Vaccine Development. Vaccine 1995; 13:415–421.

37. Tristram DA, et al. Comparative immunogenicity of two respiratory syncytial virus (RSV) fusion (F) protein vaccines in 12–30 m children. The 32nd Interscience Conference on Antimicrobial Agents and Chemotherapy, Anaheim, CA, October 11–14, 1992, Anaheim, CA: 1992:125.

38. Tristram DA, et al. Immunogenicity and safety of respiratory syncytial virus subunit vaccine in seropositive children 18–36 months old. J Infect Dis 1993; 167:191–195.

39. Belshe RB, et al. Immunogenicity of purified F glycoprotein

of respiratory syncytial virus: clinical and immune responses to subsequent natural infection in children. J Infect Dis 1993; 168:1024–1029.

40. Welliver RC, et al. Respiratory syncytial virus-specific cell-mediated immune responses after vaccination with a purified fusion protein subunit vaccine. J Infect Dis 1994; 170:425–428.

41. Tristram DA, et al. Second-year surveillance of recipients of a respiratory syncytial virus (RSV) F protein subunit vaccine, PFP-1: evaluation of antibody persistence and possible disease enhancement. Vaccine 1994; 12:551–556.

42. Paradiso PR, et al. Safety and immunogenicity of a subunit respiratory syncytial virus vaccine in children 24 to 48 months old. Pediatr Infect Dis J 1994; 13:792–798.

43. Gonzalez IM, et al. Evaluation of the live attenuated cpts 248/404 RSV vaccine in combination with a subunit RSV vaccine (PFP-2) in healthy young and older adults. Vaccine 2000; 18:1763–1772.

44. Piedra PA, et al. Purified fusion protein vaccine protects against lower respiratory tract illness during respiratory syncytial virus season in children with cystic fibrosis. Pediatr Infect Dis J 1996; 15:23–31.

45. Piedra PA, et al. Sequential annual administration of purified fusion protein vaccine against respiratory syncytial virus in children with cystic fibrosis. Pediatr Infect Dis J 1998; 17:217–224.

46. Groothuis JR, et al. Safety and immunogenicity of a purified F protein respiratory syncytial virus (PFP-2) vaccine in seropositive children with bronchopulmonary dysplasia. J Infect Dis 1998; 177:467–469.

47. Falsey AR, Walsh EE. Safety and immunogenicity of a respiratory syncytial virus subunit vaccine (PFP-2) in ambulatory adults over age 60. Vaccine 1996; 14:1214–1218.

48. Falsey AR, Walsh EE. Safety and immunogenicity of a respiratory syncytial virus subunit vaccine (PFP-2) in the institutionalized elderly. Vaccine 1997; 15:1130–1132.

49. Wathen MW, et al. Characterization of a novel human respiratory syncytial virus chimeric FG glycoprotein expressed using a baculovirus vector. J Gen Virol 1989; 70:2625–2635.

50. Oien NL, et al. Vaccination with a heterologous respiratory syncytial virus chimeric FG glycoprotein demonstrates significant subgroup cross-reactivity. Vaccine 1993; 11:1040–1048.

51. Wathen MW, et al. Vaccination of cotton rats with a chimeric FG glycoprotein of human respiratory syncytial virus induces minimal pulmonary pathology on challenge. J Infect Dis 1991; 163:477–482.

52. Kakuk TJ, et al. A human respiratory syncytial virus (RSV) primate model of enhanced pulmonary pathology induced with a formalin-inactivated RSV vaccine but not a recombinant FG subunit vaccine. J Infect Dis 1993; 167:553–561.

53. Oien NL, et al. Induction of local and systemic immunity against human respiratory syncytial virus using a chimeric FG glycoprotein and cholera toxin B subunit. Vaccine 1994; 12:731–735.

54. Brideau RJ, et al. Protection of cotton rats against human respiratory syncytial virus by vaccination with a novel chimeric FG glycoprotein. J Gen Virol 1989; 70:2637–2644.

55. Brideau RJ, Wathen MW. A chimeric glycoprotein of human respiratory syncytial virus termed FG induces T-cell mediated immunity in mice. Vaccine 1991; 9:863–864.

56. Nicholas JA, et al. Cytolytic T-lymphocyte responses to respiratory syncytial virus: effector cell phenotype and target proteins. J Virol 1990; 64:4232–4241.

57. Power UF, et al. Induction of protective immunity in rodents by vaccination with a prokaryotically expressed recombinant fusion protein containing a respiratory syncytial virus G protein fragment. Virology 1997; 230:155–166.

58. Power UF, et al. Identification and characterisation of multiple linear B cell protectopes in the respiratory syncytial virus G protein. Vaccine 2001; 19:2345–2351.

59. Plotnicky-Gilquin H, et al. CD4(+) T-cell-mediated antiviral protection of the upper respiratory tract in BALB/c mice following parenteral immunization with a recombinant respiratory syncytial virus G protein fragment. J Virol 2000; 74:3455–3463.

60. Brandt C, et al. Protective immunity against respiratory syncytial virus in early life after murine maternal or neonatal vaccination with the recombinant G fusion protein BBG2Na. J Infect Dis 1997; 176:884–891.

61. Power UF, et al. Safety and immunogenicity of a novel recombinant subunit respiratory syncytial virus vaccine (BBG2Na) in healthy young adults. J Infect Dis 2001; 184:1456–1460.

62. Wright PF, et al. Evaluation of a live, cold-passaged, temperature-sensitive, respiratory syncytial virus vaccine candidate in infancy. J Infect Dis 2000; 182:1331–1342.

63. Palomo C, et al. Induction of a neutralizing immune response to human respiratory syncytial virus with anti-idiotypic antibodies. J Virol 1990; 64:4199–4206.

64. Trudel M, et al. Protection of BALB/c mice from respiratory syncytial virus infection by immunization with a synthetic peptide derived from the G glycoprotein. Virology 1991; 185:749–757.

65. Trudel M, et al. Synthetic peptides corresponding to the F protein of RSV stimulate murine B and T cells but fail to confer protection. Arch Virol 1991; 117:59–71.

66. Trudel M, et al. Initiation of cytotoxic T-cell response and protection of Balb/c mice by vaccination with an experimental ISCOMs respiratory syncytial virus subunit vaccine. Vaccine 1992; 10:107–112.

67. Martin-Gallardo A, et al. Expression of the G glycoprotein gene of human respiratory syncytial virus in Salmonella typhimurium. J Gen Virol 1993; 74:453–458.

68. Li X, et al. Protection against respiratory syncytial virus infection by DNA immunization. J Exp Med 1998; 188:681–688.

69. Andersson C, et al. Protection against respiratory syncytial virus (RSV) elicited in mice by plasmid DNA immunisation encoding a secreted RSV G protein-derived antigen. FEMS Immunol Med Microbiol 2000; 29:247–253.

70. Belshe RB, et al. Parenteral administration of live respiratory syncytial virus vaccine: results of a field trial. J Infect Dis 1982; 145:311–319.

71. Olmsted RA, et al. Expression of the F glycoprotein of respiratory syncytial virus by a recombinant vaccinia virus: comparison of the individual contributions of the F and G glycoproteins to host immunity. Proc Natl Acad Sci USA 1986; 83:7462–7466.

72. Connors M, et al. Resistance to respiratory syncytial virus (RSV) challenge induced by infection with a vaccinia virus recombinant expressing the RSV M2 protein (Vac-M2) is mediated by CD8 + T cells, while that induced by Vac-F or Vac-G recombinants is mediated by antibodies. J Virol 1992; 66:1277–1281.

73. Kulkarni AB, et al. Cytotoxic T cells specific for a single peptide on the M2 protein of respiratory syncytial virus are the sole mediators of resistance induced by immunization with M2 encoded by a recombinant vaccinia virus. J Virol 1995; 69:1261–1264.

74. Olmsted RA, et al. Evaluation in non-human primates of the safety, immunogenicity and efficacy of recombinant vaccinia viruses expressing the F or G glycoprotein of respiratory syncytial virus. Vaccine 1988; 6:519–524.

75. Collins PL, et al. Evaluation in chimpanzees of vaccinia virus recombinants that express the surface glycoproteins of human respiratory syncytial virus. Vaccine 1990; 8:164–168.

76. Crowe JE Jr, et al. A comparison in chimpanzees of the immunogenicity and efficacy of live attenuated respiratory syncytial virus (RSV) temperature-sensitive mutant vaccines and vaccinia virus recombinants that express the surface glycoproteins of RSV. Vaccine, 1993, 1395–1404.

77. Wyatt LS, et al. Priming and boosting immunity to respiratory syncytial virus by recombinant replication-defective vaccinia virus MVA. Vaccine 1999; 18:392–397.

78. Durbin AP, et al. Comparison of the immunogenicity and efficacy of a replication-defective vaccinia virus expressing antigens of human parainfluenza virus type 3 (HPIV3) with those of a live attenuated HPIV3 vaccine candidate in rhesus monkeys passively immunized with PIV3 antibodies. J Infect Dis 1999; 179:1345–1351.

79. Collins PL, et al. Evaluation of the protective efficacy of recombinant vaccinia viruses and adenoviruses that express respiratory syncytial virus glycoproteins. In: Brown F, Chanock RM, Ginsberg HS, Lerner RA, eds. Vaccines 90. Cold Spring Harbor, NY: Cold Spring Harbor Laboratory Press, 1990:79–84.

80. Hsu KH, et al. Efficacy of adenovirus-vectored respiratory syncytial virus vaccines in a new ferret model. Vaccine 1994; 12:607–612.

81. Hsu KH, et al. Immunogenicity of recombinant adenovirus-respiratory syncytial virus vaccines with adenovirus types 4, 5, and 7 vectors in dogs and a chimpanzee. J Infect Dis 1992; 166:769–775.

82. Schmidt AC, et al. Bovine parainfluenza virus type 3 (BPIV3) fusion and hemagglutinin-neuraminidase glycoproteins make an important contribution to the restricted replication of BPIV3 in primates. J Virol 2000; 74:8922–8929.

83. Schmidt AC, et al. Recombinant bovine/human parainfluenza virus type 3 (B/HPIV3) expressing the respiratory syncytial virus (RSV) G and F proteins can be used to achieve simultaneous mucosal immunization against RSV and HPIV3. J Virol 2001; 75:4594–4603.

84. Schmidt AC, et al. Mucosal immunization of rhesus monkeys against respiratory syncytial virus subgroups A and B and human parainfluenza virus type 3 using a live cDNA-derived vaccine based on a host range-attenuated bovine parainfluenza virus type 3 vector backbone. J Virol 2002; 76:1089–1099.

85. Kahn JS, et al. Replication-competent or attenuated, nonpropagating vesicular stomatitis viruses expressing respiratory syncytial virus (RSV) antigens protect mice against RSV challenge. J Virol 2001; 75:11079–11087.

86. Hussell T, Openshaw PJ. Intracellular IFN-gamma expression in natural killer cells precedes lung CD8+ T cell recruitment during respiratory syncytial virus infection. J Gen Virol 1998; 79:2593–2601.

87. Srikiatkhachorn A, Braciale TJ. Virus-specific CD8+ T lymphocytes downregulate T helper cell type 2 cytokine secretion and pulmonary eosinophilia during experimental murine respiratory syncytial virus infection. J Exp Med 1997; 186:421–432.

88. Waris ME, et al. Priming with live respiratory syncytial virus (RSV) prevents the enhanced pulmonary inflammatory response seen after RSV challenge in BALB/c mice immunized with formalin-inactivated RSV. J Virol 1997; 71:6935–6939.

89. Tolley KP, et al. Identification of mutations contributing to the reduced virulence of a modified strain of respiratory syncytial virus. Vaccine 1996; 14:1637–1646.

90. Broughan JH, et al. Biochemical characterizations of two temperature-sensitive and attenuated strains of respiratory syncytial virus subgroup B. J Virol 1997; 71:4962–4970.

91. Randolph VB, et al. Attenuated temperature–sensitive respiratory syncytial virus mutants generated by cold adaptation. Virus Res 1994; 33:241–259.

92. Herlocher ML, et al. Immunological properties of plaque purified strains of live attenuated respiratory syncytial virus (RSV) for human vaccine. Vaccine 1999; 17:172–181.

93. Chanock RM, Murphy BR. Past efforts to develop safe and effective RSV vaccines. In: Meigner BB, Murphy B, Ogra P, eds. Animal Models of Respiratory Syncytial Virus Infections. Lyon, France: Merieux Foundation, 1991:35–42.

94. Wright PF, et al. Evaluation of a live, attenuated respiratory syncytial virus vaccine in infants. J Pediatr 1976; 88:931–936.

95. Friedewald WT, et al. Low-temperature-grown RS virus in adult volunteers. JAMA 1968; 203:690–694.

96. Crowe JE Jr, et al. Satisfactorily attenuated and protective mutants derived from a partially attenuated cold-passaged respiratory syncytial virus mutant by introduction of additional attenuating mutations during chemical mutagenesis. Vaccine 1994; 12:691–699.

97. Crowe JE Jr, et al. A further attenuated derivative of a cold-passaged temperature-sensitive mutant of human respiratory syncytial virus retains immunogenicity and protective efficacy against wild-type challenge in seronegative chimpanzees. Vaccine 1994; 12:783–790.

98. Karron RA, et al. Evaluation of two live, cold-passaged, temperature-sensitive respiratory syncytial virus (RSV) vaccines in chimpanzees, adults, infants and children. J Infect Dis 1997; 176:1428–1436.

99. Hancock GE, et al. Generation of atypical pulmonary inflammatory responses in BALB/c mice after immunization with the native attachment (G) glycoprotein of respiratory syncytial virus. J Virol 1996; 70:7783–7791.

100. Collins PL, et al. Production of infectious human respiratory syncytial virus from cloned cDNA confirms an essential role for the transcription elongation factor from the 5′ proximal open reading frame of the M2 mRNA in gene expression and provides a capability for vaccine development. Proc Natl Acad Sci USA 1995; 92:11563–11567.

101. Connors M, et al. A cold-passaged, attenuated strain of human respiratory syncytial virus contains mutations in the F and L genes. Virology 1995; 208:478–484.

102. Whitehead SS, et al. Recombinant respiratory syncytial virus (RSV) bearing a set of mutations from cold-passaged RSV is attenuated in chimpanzees. J Virol 1998; 72:4467–4471.

103. Crowe JE Jr, et al. Acquisition of the ts phenotype by a chemically mutagenized cold-passaged human respiratory syncytial virus vaccine candidate results from the acquisition of a single mutation in the polymerase (L) gene. Virus Genes 1996; 13:269–273.

104. Firestone CY, et al. Nucleotide sequence analysis of the respiratory syncytial virus subgroup A cold-passaged (cp) temperature sensitive (ts) cpts-248/404 live attenuated virus vaccine candidate. Virology 1996; 225:419–422.

105. Juhasz K, et al. The two amino acid substitutions in the L protein of cpts530/1009, a live-attenuated respiratory syncytial virus candidate vaccine, are independent temperature-sensitive and attenuation mutations. Vaccine 1999; 17:1416–1424.

106. Juhasz K, et al. The temperature-sensitive (ts) phenotype of a cold-passaged (cp) live attenuated respiratory syncytial virus vaccine candidate, designated cpts530, results from a single amino acid substitution in the L protein. J Virol 1997; 71:5814–5819.

107. Whitehead SS, et al. A single nucleotide substitution in the transcription start signal of the M2 gene of respiratory syncytial virus vaccine candidate cpts248/404 is the major determinant of the temperature-sensitive and attenuation phenotypes. Virology 1998; 247:232–239.

108. Whitehead SS, et al. Addition of a missense mutation present in the L gene of respiratory syncytial virus (RSV) cpts530/

1030 to RSV vaccine candidate cpts248/404 increases its attenuation and temperature sensitivity. J Virol 1999; 73:871–877.

109. Bermingham A, Collins PL. The M2-2 protein of human respiratory syncytial virus is a regulatory factor involved in the balance between RNA replication and transcription. Proc Natl Acad Sci USA 1999; 96:11259–11264.

110. Bukreyev A, et al. Recombinant respiratory syncytial virus from which the entire SH gene has been deleted grows efficiently in cell culture and exhibits site-specific attenuation in the respiratory tract of the mouse. J Virol 1997; 71:8973–8982.

111. Jin H, et al. Respiratory syncytial virus that lacks open reading frame 2 of the M2 gene (M2-2) has altered growth characteristics and is attenuated in rodents. J Virol 2000; 74:74–82.

112. Jin H, et al. Recombinant respiratory syncytial viruses with deletions in the NS1, NS2, SH, and M2-2 genes are attenuated in vitro and in vivo. Virology 2000; 273:210–218.

113. Karron RA, et al. Respiratory syncytial virus (RSV) SH and G proteins are not essential for viral replication in vitro: clinical evaluation and molecular characterization of a cold-passaged, attenuated RSV subgroup B mutant. Proc Natl Acad Sci USA 1997; 94:13961–13966.

114. Teng MN, Collins PL. Altered growth characteristics of recombinant respiratory syncytial viruses which do not produce NS2 protein. J Virol 1999; 73:466–473.

115. Teng MN, et al. Contribution of the respiratory syncytial virus G glycoprotein and its secreted and membrane-bound forms to virus replication in vitro and in vivo. Virology 2001; 289:283–296.

116. Schlender J, et al. Bovine respiratory syncytial virus nonstructural proteins NS1 and NS2 cooperatively antagonize alpha/beta interferon-induced antiviral response. J Virol 2000; 74:8234–8242.

117. Teng MN, et al. Recombinant respiratory syncytial virus that does not express the NS1 or M2-2 protein is highly attenuated and immunogenic in chimpanzees. J Virol 2000; 74:9317–9321.

118. Whitehead SS, et al. Recombinant respiratory syncytial virus bearing a deletion of either the NS2 or SH gene is attenuated in chimpanzees. J Virol 1999; 73:3438–3442.

119. Beeler JA, et al. Neutralization epitopes of the F glycoprotein of respiratory syncytial virus: effect of mutation upon fusion function. J Virol 1989; 63:2941–2950.

120. Piazza FM, et al. Bovine respiratory syncytial virus protects cotton rats against human respiratory syncytial virus infection. J Virol 1993; 67:1503–1510.

121. Buchholz UJ, et al. Chimeric bovine respiratory syncytial virus with glycoprotein gene substitutions from human respiratory syncytial virus (HRSV): effects on host range and evaluation as a live-attenuated HRSV vaccine. J Virol 2000; 74:1187–1199.

122. Crowe JE Jr, et al. Live subgroup B respiratory syncytial virus vaccines that are attenuated, genetically stable, and immunogenic in rodents and nonhuman primates. J Infect Dis 1996; 173:829–839.

123. Crowe JE Jr, et al. The live attenuated subgroup B respiratory syncytial virus vaccine candidate RSV 2B33F is attenuated and immunogenic in chimpanzees, but exhibits partial loss of the ts phenotype following replication in vivo. Virus Res 1999; 59:13–22.

124. Whitehead SS, et al. Replacement of the F and G proteins of respiratory syncytial virus (RSV) subgroup A with those of subgroup B generates chimeric live attenuated RSV subgroup B vaccine candidates. J Virol 1999; 73:9773–9780.

125. Jin H, et al. Recombinant human respiratory syncytial virus (RSV) from cDNA and construction of subgroup A and B chimeric RSV. Virology 1998; 251:206–214.

126. Bukreyev A, et al. Recovery of infectious respiratory syncytial virus expressing an additional, foreign gene. J Virol 1996; 70:6634–6641.

127. Wertz GW, et al. Gene rearrangement attenuates expression and lethality of a nonsegmented negative strand RNA virus. Proc Natl Acad Sci USA 1998; 95:3501–3506.

128. Flanagan EB, et al. Moving the glycoprotein gene of vesicular stomatitis virus to promoter–proximal positions accelerates and enhances the protective immune response. J Virol 2000; 74:7895–7902.

129. Bukreyev A, et al. Interferon gamma expressed by a recombinant respiratory syncytial virus attenuates virus replication in mice without compromising immunogenicity. Proc Natl Acad Sci USA 1999; 96:2367–2372.

130. Bukreyev A, et al. Effect of coexpression of interleukin-2 by recombinant respiratory syncytial virus on virus replication, immunogenicity, and production of other cytokines. J Virol 2000; 74:7151–7157.

131. Johnson TR, et al. Priming with secreted glycoprotein G of respiratory syncytial virus (RSV) augments interleukin-5 production and tissue eosinophilia after RSV challenge. J Virol 1998; 72:2871–2880.

132. Tripp RA, et al. CX3C chemokine mimicry by respiratory syncytial virus G glycoprotein. Nat Immunol 2001; 2:732–738.

133. Gessner BD. The cost-effectiveness of a hypothetical respiratory syncytial virus vaccine in the elderly. Vaccine 2000; 18:1485–1494.

134. Chanock RM, et al. Parainfluenza viruses. Knipe DM, Howley PM, Griffin DE, Martin MA, Lamb RA, Roizman B, Straus SE, eds. Fields Virology. 4th ed. Vol. 1. Philadelphia: Lippincott Williams and Wilkins, 2001:1341–1379.

135. Tao T, et al. A live attenuated recombinant chimeric parainfluenza virus (PIV) candidate vaccine containing the hemagglutinin-neuraminidase and fusion glycoproteins of PIV1 and the remaining proteins from PIV3 induces resistance to PIV1 even in animals immune to PIV3. Vaccine 2000; 18:1359–1366.

136. Chin J, et al. Field evaluation of a respiratory syncytial virus vaccine and a trivalent parainfluenza virus vaccine in a pediatric population. Am J Epidemiol 1969; 89:449–463.

137. Ottolini MG, et al. Enhanced pulmonary pathology in cotton rats upon challenge after immunization with inactivated parainfluenza virus 3 vaccines. Viral Immunol 2000; 13:231–236.

138. Murphy BR, Chanock RM. Immunization against viral diseases. Knipe DM, Howley PM, Griffin DE, Martin MA, Lamb RA, Roizman B, Straus SE, eds. Fields Virology. Vol. 1. Philadelphia: Lippincott Williams and Wilkins, 2001: 435–468.

139. Ewasyshyn M, et al. Prospects for a parainfluenza virus vaccine. Pediatr Pulmonol Suppl 1997; 16:280–281.

140. van Wyke Coelingh KL, et al. Attenuation of bovine parainfluenza virus type 3 in nonhuman primates and its ability to confer immunity to human parainfluenza virus type 3 challenge. J Infect Dis 1988; 157:655–662.

141. van Wyke Coelingh KL, et al. Antibody responses of humans and nonhuman primates to individual antigenic sites of the hemagglutinin-neuraminidase and fusion glycoproteins after primary infection or reinfection with parainfluenza type 3 virus. J Virol 1990; 64:3833–3843.

142. Suzu S, et al. Nucleotide sequence of the bovine parainfluenza 3 virus genome: the genes of the F and HN glycoproteins. Nucleic Acids Res 1987; 15:2945–2958.

143. Clements ML, et al. Evaluation of bovine, cold-adapted human, and wild-type human parainfluenza type 3 viruses in adult volunteers and in chimpanzees. J Clin Microbiol 1991; 29:1175–1182.

144. Karron RA, et al. A live attenuated bovine parainfluenza virus type 3 vaccine is safe, infectious, immunogenic, and phenotypically stable in infants and children. J Infect Dis 1995; 171:1107–1114.

145. Lee MS, et al. Antibody responses to bovine parainfluenza virus type 3 (PIV3) vaccination and human PIV3 infection in young infants. J Infect Dis 2001; 184:909–913.

146. Bailly JE, et al. A recombinant human parainfluenza virus type 3 (PIV3) in which the nucleocapsid N protein has been replaced by that of bovine PIV3 is attenuated in primates. J Virol 2000; 74:3188–3195.

147. Bailly JE, et al. Sequence determination and molecular analysis of two strains of bovine parainfluenza virus type 3 that are attenuated for primates. Virus Genes 2000; 20:173–182.

148. Haller AA, et al. Expression of the surface glycoproteins of human parainfluenza virus type 3 by bovine parainfluenza virus type 3, a novel attenuated virus vaccine vector. J Virol 2000; 74:11626–11635.

149. Hu XL, et al. Functional interactions between the fusion protein and hemagglutinin–neuraminidase of human parainfluenza viruses [published erratum appears in J Virol 1992; 66:5176. J Virol 1992; 66:1528–1534.

150. Deng R, et al. Localization of a domain on the paramyxovirus attachment protein required for the promotion of cellular fusion by its homologous fusion protein spike. Virology 1995; 209:457–469.

151. Tanabayashi K, Compans RW. Functional interaction of paramyxovirus glycoproteins: identification of a domain in Sendai virus HN which promotes cell fusion. J Virol 1996; 70:6112–6118.

152. Sangster M, et al. Human parainfluenza virus type 1 immunization of infant mice protects from subsequent Sendai virus infection. Virology 1995; 212:13–19.

153. Hurwitz JL, et al. Intranasal Sendai virus vaccine protects African green monkeys from infection with human parainfluenza virus-type one. Vaccine 1997; 15:533–540.

154. Skiadopolous MH, et al. Sendai virus, a murine parainfluenza virus type 1 (PIV1) replicates to a level similar to human PIV1 in the upper and lower respiratory tract of African green monkeys and chimpanzees. Virology 2002; 297:153–160.

155. Belshe RB, Hissom FK. Cold adaptation of parainfluenza virus type 3: induction of three phenotypic markers. J Med Virol 1982; 10:235–242.

156. Crookshanks FK, Belshe RB. Evaluation of cold-adapted and temperature-sensitive mutants of parainfluenza virus type 3 in weanling hamsters. J Med Virol 1984; 13:243–249.

157. Crookshanks-Newman FK, Belshe RB. Protection of weanling hamsters from experimental infection with wild-type parainfluenza virus type 3 (para 3) by cold-adapted mutants of para 3. J Med Virol 1986; 18:131–137.

158. Hall SL, et al. Cold-passaged human parainfluenza type 3 viruses contain ts and non-ts mutations leading to attenuation in rhesus monkeys. Virus Res 1992; 22:173–184.

159. Stokes A, et al. The complete nucleotide sequence of two cold-adapted, temperature-sensitive attenuated mutant vaccine viruses (cp12 and cp45) derived from the JS strain of human parainfluenza virus type 3 (PIV3). Virus Res 1993; 30:43–52.

160. Hall SL, et al. A cold-adapted mutant of parainfluenza virus type 3 is attenuated and protective in chimpanzees. J Infect Dis 1993; 167:958–962.

161. Karron RA, et al. A live human parainfluenza type 3 virus vaccine is attenuated and immunogenic in healthy infants and children. J Infect Dis 1995; 172:1445–1450.

162. Skiadopoulos MH, et al. Identification of mutations contributing to the temperature-sensitive, cold-adapted, and attenuation phenotypes of the live-attenuated cold-passage 45 (cp45) human parainfluenza virus 3 candidate vaccine. J Virol 1999; 73:1374–1381.

163. Skiadopoulos MH, et al. Three amino acid substitutions in the L protein of the human parainfluenza virus type 3 cp45 live attenuated vaccine candidate contribute to its temperature-sensitive and attenuation phenotypes. J Virol 1998; 72:1762–1768.

164. Tao T, et al. Recovery of a fully viable chimeric human parainfluenza virus (PIV) type 3 in which the hemagglutinin–neuraminidase and fusion glycoproteins have been replaced by those of PIV type 1. J Virol 1998; 72:2955–2961.

165. Skiadopoulos MH, et al. Generation of a parainfluenza virus type 1 vaccine candidate by replacing the HN and F glycoproteins of the live-attenuated PIV3 cp45 vaccine virus with their PIV1 counterparts. Vaccine 1999; 18:503–510.

166. Newman JT, et al. Sequence analysis of the Washington/1964 strain of human parainfluenza virus type 1 (HPIV1) and recovery and characterization of wild-type recombinant HPIV1 produced by reverse genetics. Virus Genes 2002; 24:77–92.

167. Tao T, et al. Replacement of the ectodomains of the hemagglutinin–neuraminidase and fusion glycoproteins of recombinant parainfluenza virus type 3 (PIV3) with their counterparts from PIV2 yields attenuated PIV2 vaccine candidates. J Virol 2000; 74:6448–6458.

168. Kawano M, et al. Recovery of infectious human parainfluenza type 2 virus from cDNA clones and properties of the defective virus without V-specific cysteine-rich domain. Virology 2001; 284:99–112.

169. Durbin AP, et al. Human parainfluenza virus type 3 (PIV3) expressing the hemagglutinin protein of measles virus provides a potential method for immunization against measles virus and PIV3 in early infancy. J Virol 2000; 74:6821–6831.

170. Skiadopoulos MH, et al. A chimeric human–bovine parainfluenza virus type 3 expressing measles virus hemagglutinin is attenuated for replication but is still immunogenic in rhesus monkeys. J Virol 2001; 75:10498–10504.

171. Tao T, et al. Construction of a live-attenuated bivalent vaccine virus against human parainfluenza virus (PIV) types 1 and 2 using a recombinant PIV3 backbone. Vaccine 2001; 19:3620–3631.

172. Skiadopoulos MH, et al. The genome length of human parainfluenza virus type 2 follows the rule of six, and recombinant viruses recovered from non-polyhexameric-length antigenomic cDNAs contain a biased distribution of correcting mutations. J Virol 2003; 77:270–279.

53

Developing a Vaccine Against Epstein–Barr Virus

Denis Moss and Mandvi Bharadwaj
University of Queensland, Herston, Queensland, Australia

I. INTRODUCTION

There is a strong scientific and commercial focus on developing vaccines and immunotherapeutic strategies for the treatment of Epstein–Barr virus (EBV)-associated diseases. This increased interest is due to a deeper understanding of the immune variables that control EBV infection and an appreciation of the biology of this potentially oncogenic virus [1,2]. Epstein–Barr virus, discovered in 1964 by Epstein and colleagues, is a human gamma herpesvirus that infects over 90% of the world's population. It is a double-stranded DNA virus encoding approximately 100 proteins [3]. Primary infection most commonly occurs during childhood and is generally asymptomatic, resulting in a lifelong viral latency in B cells. In developed countries, primary infection is sometimes delayed until adolescence and then results in clinical infectious mononucleosis (IM) (commonly called as "glandular fever"). This clinical manifestation occurs in about 50% of adolescents experiencing primary EBV infection (typically following kissing) and is characterized by fatigue, pharyngitis, fever, cervical lymphadenopathy, and splenomegaly. The major target of EBV infection is apparently the B lymphocyte, although a role for squamous epithelial cells cannot be unequivocally discounted. During primary infection (Figure 1), colonization of the lymphoid system occurs through virus-driven expansion of infected B cells that selectively express six latent EBV nuclear antigens (EBNAs 1–4, 6, -LP) and latent membrane proteins (LMPs 1, 2A, and 2B) [4,5]. These latently infected B cells maintain a lifelong virus carrier state and constitute the reservoir on which viral persistence depends. Viral shedding into the oropharynx is another feature of primary EBV infection and arises from expression of the "lytic switch" protein BZLF1 [6], which launches the productive cycle cascade. Lytic and structural proteins gp85, BMLF1, BMRF1, BHRF1, and gp350 are also a feature of virus replication [7].

II. EPSTEIN–BARR VIRUS-ASSOCIATED CANCERS

Epstein–Barr virus is presently the most prolific viral contributor to the development of human lymphomas [8]. It is strongly linked to several human malignancies including Burkitt's lymphoma (BL), a common form of childhood cancer in areas of Africa and Papua New Guinea, nasopharyngeal carcinoma (NPC), a tumor of epidermoid origin most prevalent in southern China, posttransplant lymphoproliferative disease (PTLD) in transplant recipients, and certain types of Hodgkin's disease (HD) common in western countries and characterized by the presence of mononuclear Hodgkin and multinuclear Reed–Sternberg (RS) cells. Recent evidence also suggests that some T-cell lymphomas [9], gastric carcinomas [10], oral hairy leukoplakia [11], and breast cancer [12] may also be linked to EBV.

Epstein–Barr virus-associated diseases are best classified by the degree of latent EBV antigen expression in vivo (Figure 1). Latency III diseases (IM and PTLD) are characterized by the expression of the full array of EBV latent antigens (EBNAs 1–6 and LMP1, LMP2A, and LMP2B). In NPC and HD, which are classified as latency II diseases, the latent gene expression is limited to EBNA 1, LMP1, and/or LMP2A/B. and in some cases of NPC the lytic protein, BARF1 may also be expressed [13]. Endemic BL biopsies exhibit the classical features of latency I with the expression of a single EBV protein, EBNA 1.

III. IMMUNE RESPONSE TO EBV

Although many details of the cell–virus relationship that occur during primary infection remain obscure, there is now convincing evidence that EBV-specific cytotoxic T cells (CTLs) are of prime importance in controlling the expansion

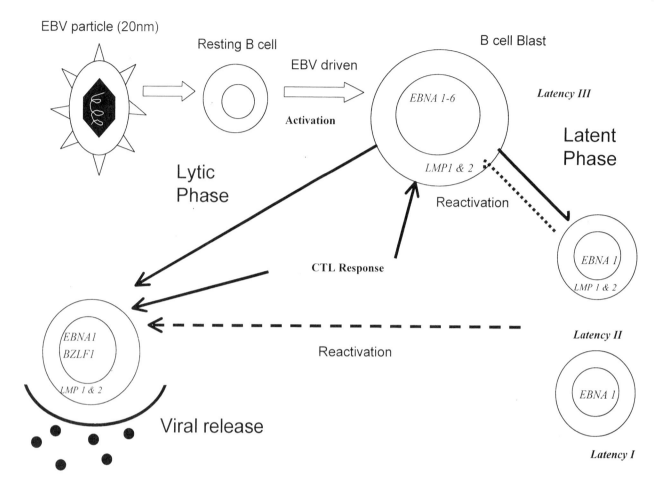

Figure 1 A model of EBV and B cell interactions depicting the different levels of viral antigen expression in infected B cells associated with the different latency phenotypes in EBV-associated diseases and stages of immunological intervention by CTLs.

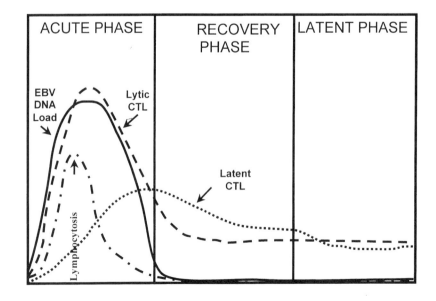

Figure 2 The figure represents the CTL response to the latent and lytic epitopes in the different phases of EBV infection and its relation to the viral load and lymphocytosis in healthy virus carriers.

of latently infected B cells and reducing viral load by targeting peptide epitopes (processed antigens) expressed on infected B cells (Figure 2). During acute infection this response is directed toward peptide epitopes encoded within the EBV latent (EBNA 2–6, LMP1 and 2) and lytic/structural (BZLF, BARF1, BMLF, gp350/340) proteins presented in association with molecules of the major histocompatibility complex (MHC) on infected B cells. This T-cell response is generally virus-specific, class I-restricted (CD8$^+$ α/β CTL) although CD4$^+$, class II-restricted CTLs have also been described [5]. A higher number of precursor CTLs are generally found to epitopes during acute infection compared to the latent infection in healthy virus carriers.

Analysis of CTL responses in a large panel of healthy virus carriers screened for reactivity to latent antigens revealed a marked predominance of reactivity toward epitopes within EBNA 3, 4, and 6 [14–16], while CTL responses to other latent proteins (LMP1 and 2 and EBNA 2) were less frequently detected. An interesting feature of EBV-specific CTL responses in healthy virus carriers is that certain class I alleles (predominantly the B alleles) such as HLA-B7, -B8, -B27, -B35, and -B44 commonly present immunogenic peptide epitopes encoded within the EBV latent proteins, whereas weaker activity is observed through other alleles such as HLA A1, A3, and A24. It is also relevant that there is no class I processing of EBNA 1 due to a glycine–alanine (GAr) repeat that has an inhibitory effect on the endogenous processing of this antigen [17].

IV. LESSONS FROM ANIMAL MODELS

A. Murine Models

Murine models present a potentially important tool to study the efficacy of EBV immunotherapeutics. First, combined immunodefficient (SCID) mice that lack mature B and T cells provided an in vivo model that demonstrated the efficacy of adoptive transfer of CTLs to control EBV-associated lymphoma [18–20] paving the path for clinical trials of adoptive immunotherapy using CD8$^+$ CTL in PTLD patients [21]. Second, transgenic mice expressing chimeric human and murine class I domains are a useful and convenient method of quantifying and optimizing CTL responses to epitopes restricted by diverse HLA alleles [16,22]. Third, MHV-68 is a naturally occurring herpes virus of wild rodents and represents a potential model of both latent and lytic EBV infection. The virus offers an opportunity to study the acute lytic phase of a gamma herpesvirus infection as it readily replicates in epithelial cells both in vivo and in vitro [23].

B. Primate Models

It is unfortunate that there is no model of EBV infection in animals that entirely reproduces the cell–virus relationships seen in symptomatic primary infection in humans and on which vaccine-formulation decisions could be based. However, a potential model for testing vaccine formulations might involve primates infected with either EBV or closely related viruses. Three species of new-world monkeys that can be experimentally infected have been studied. Cotton top tamarins (*Saguinus oedipus oedipus*) inoculated with high-titered EBV develop multiple B-cell lymphomas. Several studies using this model have demonstrated that purified or recombinant gp350 formulated with various adjuvants or delivered by live vectors induce virus-neutralizing gp350 antibodies and in some cases have shown protection from tumor development after high-dose EBV challenge [24,25]. However, there is some doubt about the relevance of this result because immunoblotting and immunochemical studies have suggested that latent rather than replicative antigens are expressed in these tumors [26], thus indicating a cell-mediated rather than antibody-mediated mechanism of protection. Other primate models include the common marmoset (*Callithrix jaccus*), which presents a rather ill defined IM-like syndrome, and the owl monkey (*Aotus trivirgatus*), which is susceptible to EBV-induced lymphomas [27,28].

However, none of these models are ideal as there is no demonstrable asymptomatic virus persistence and/or replication in these primate models. Furthermore, the route of experimental challenge in these models is generally intraperitoneal and the virus–cell relationships established in human mucosal surfaces might be quite different. Moreover, although the lymphomas in this model have some features in common to those of PTLD, symptoms associated with acute primary EBV infection are not seen.

Perhaps the best primate model is that based on infection of rhesus monkeys with the rhesus lymphocryptovirus (LCV). This virus, which shares significant sequence homology with EBV, reproduces many of the key events associated with primary EBV infection when these primates are infected orally. Moreover, this model appears to be relevant to vaccine formulation because resistance to a second challenge following primary infection is observed [29]. Although, this model is likely to prove expensive when used to screen potential formulations, it may provide an excellent system for demonstrating final confirmation of the efficacy of a formulation before human trials.

V. STRATEGIES FOR EBV VACCINE DEVELOPMENT

The latency phenotypes have determined to a large extent the available strategies in developing vaccines to EBV-associated diseases. Thus, in the case of the latency III diseases (IM and PTLD) there are available the complete array of latent antigens as potential targets (EBNAs 1–6 and LMP1, LMP2A, and LMP2B). In contrast, fewer available targets are expressed in latency II (NPC and HD) or latency I diseases (BL).

A. Development of a Vaccine to Latency III Diseases

Commercial considerations have meant that the focus of attention in developing a vaccine to EBV has been dominated by IM. However, it should be pointed out that a successful vaccine to IM would be effective in reducing the incidence of disease in individuals most at risk of developing

PTLD (EBV seronegative graft recipients). Infectious mononucleosis affects an estimated 250,000 young adults in the United States and Europe annually. Approximately 90% of adults in the United States have been infected with EBV and between 35% and 50% of young adults will develop IM when exposed to EBV for the first time [30].

1. Potential for an Attenuated EBV Vaccine

One of the earliest and most successful methods of creating vaccines has been the use of live, attenuated forms of the pathogen. This approach evokes both humoral and cellular immunity because the full repertoire of viral proteins is presented in the same quantity and context as in the virulent form. This method has proven successful in developing the chickenpox vaccine, currently the only herpesvirus vaccine licensed by the FDA. However, in the case of EBV, the potential oncogenicity of the virus precludes its use particularly in the case of the IM. Another obstacle toward developing such an attenuated vaccine is the absence of an efficient in vitro culture system capable of yielding the quantities of virus required for a commercially viable vaccine [31].

2. Potential of Recombinant-Based EBV Vaccine

The membrane proteins of EBV have been targeted as potential vaccine candidates for IM. Three glycoproteins with similar antigenic determinants have been found: gp340/350 (of molecular weight 340,000–350,000 Da), gp220 (220,000–270,000 Da), and gp85 (85,000 Da). Most attention has focused on gp340/350, because it includes the main neutralizing determinants of the virus [31,32]. Various formulations of gp340/350, either presented as a subunit protein or expressed from recombinant viral vectors, have shown protection against challenge in the tamarin model of EBV infection [33]. The mechanism of protection in this primate model is not yet clear, but it seems likely that it is mediated either by antibody- and/or cell-mediated responses [34]. The importance of the cell-mediated response has gained further support by the observation of CTL epitopes within gp340/350 [35].

3. Cytotoxic T-Cell Epitope-Based Vaccines

An alternative approach to vaccine development is based on formulations that exploit defined CTL epitopes. Here the aim is not to prevent primary infection per se but to limit those events occurring immediately postinfection, namely, virus replication in the oropharynx and/or the expansion of virus-transformed B cells within the lymphoid pool. There is circumstantial evidence that establishment of such a CTL response against the EBV nuclear antigens (EBNA 2–6) may prevent symptoms of IM [36] and PTLD [manuscript in preparation]. As a first step to developing a CTL-epitope-based vaccine, we have conducted a Phase I clinical trial based on a single epitope. Healthy EBV seronegative HLA B8 volunteers were vaccinated with a formulation consisting of the synthetic peptide FLRGRAYGL from EBNA 3 with tetanus toxoid and emulsified in the water-in-oil adjuvant, Montanide ISA 720. To date this vaccine preparation has been well tolerated and no serious adverse events have been recorded. Furthermore, although not specifically designed to yield any statistically relevant data in regard to protection, it is interesting that all vaccinated individuals recorded a detectable CTL response and no individuals experienced a clinical seroconversion [Bharadwaj, Elliott, Lawrence, Suhrbier, and Moss, manuscript in preparation].

An EBV vaccine based on CTL epitopes will need to incorporate protective determinants restricted by a range of class I MHC to provide cover for all human populations. In considering this selection, it should also be borne in mind that the response seen during natural primary infection may be different from the immunogenic potential of CTL epitopes delivered in an effective formulation. For example, a hierarchy of HLA-A2-restricted CTL responses was established in acute IM and in healthy seropositive individuals and the relative immunogenicity of these epitopes assessed in HLA-A2 transgenic mice. When analyzed using the ELISPOT assay of interferon-γ release there was no obvious correlation between the strength of the response seen to individual epitopes in transgenic mice and that seen in healthy seropositive individuals or during acute IM. This is an important observation and serves to highlight the difference in responses seen as a result of natural infection and that deliverable by a formulation in which all of the epitopes are presented to the immune system at the same concentration and at the same site. It might thus be possible to boost protective responses to individual epitopes in a vaccine preparation to levels not seen in naturally infected individuals [16]. Since the virus encodes 100 latent and lytic proteins, it may be necessary to restrict the choice of proteins to those for which there is a priori evidence of immune-mediated protection from the clinical consequences of primary EBV infection by dominant CTL epitopes. Indeed, independent evidence suggests a limited role for epitopes within lytic antigens [36].

As with any subunit vaccine, critical decisions need to be reached not only on the choice of immunogen but on the means of delivering a comparatively large number of CTL epitopes that might be needed to span the MHC diversity seen in man. Although formally this requirement might be satisfied by mixing peptide epitopes, technical and regulatory considerations are likely to restrict the use of this approach. An alternative approach under active consideration is to make use of a technical advance [37] in which minimal EBV CTL epitopes are encoded in a recombinant or synthetic polyepitope protein. The constituent epitopes are processed and presented on the cell surface and can efficiently activate CTL responses [37,38]. Thus, for example, it might be possible to link an array of dominant CTL epitopes from EBV latent proteins as a polyepitope, either formulated in an adjuvant capable of inducing a CTL response or injected directly as purified DNA.

B. Vaccine Strategies for Latency I and II Diseases

Epstein–Barr virus vaccines directed against BL, NPC, and HD are conceptually different from latency III diseases because the malignant cells do not express the immunodominant latent antigens. Moreover, in the case of BL, escape mechanisms enable them to evade CTL recognition by (1) downregulating the processing of proteins and adhesion molecules [39] and (2) the observation that the only protein expressed, EBNA 1, is devoid of class I CTL epitopes [17]. Protection from the long-term consequences of these tumors would ideally require a vaccine that either conferred sterile immunity, thereby preventing establishment of the long-term latent EBV infection, or a therapeutic vaccine based on tumor antigens. Thus, an effective vaccine against BL appears to have limited chance of success and it may be necessary to either target non-EBV tumor antigens or to use an approach that shifted the phenotype of BL to either latency II or III.

Both NPC and HD share certain features that offer some hope that a successful therapeutic vaccine might be developed. A number of studies have shown that most NPCs retain detectable EBV-specific T-cell surveillance, indicating that CTL dysfunction is an unlikely reason for the outgrowth of this tumor [40]. Furthermore, immunohistochemical analysis of fresh biopsies and laboratory-established tumor lines indicate that malignant cells in both NPC and HD express normal levels of HLA class I and TAP-1 and TAP-2 [41,42]. Because NPC and HD may express both LMP1 and 2, conceptually a polytope vaccine including these epitopes may be the preferred strategy. However, it should be borne in mind that although NPC is classified as a latency II disease, there has been no unequivocal evidence of LMP2 expression in this malignancy. Furthermore, the recent observation that NPC cells express BARF1 should provide impetus to the definition of CTL epitopes within this protein and to incorporation of these epitopes within a polytope formulation [13].

VI. EPSTEIN–BARR VIRUS VACCINE TRIALS

There have been three EBV Phase I vaccine trials to date. The first was conducted in China in 1995 using a recombinant vaccinia vector gp220/350 [43] in three distinct human populations: EBV-positive adults preexposed to vaccinia virus, EBV-positive children not preexposed to vaccinia virus, and EBV-negative infants not exposed to the vaccinia virus. The vaccination resulted in (1) no significant impact on the level of EBV antibody in the adults, (2) an increase in the level of EBV-neutralizing antibody titers in the vaccinated children, while antibodies to the viral capsid antigen remained the same, (3) development of membrane antigen antibodies with neutralizing properties in vitro in all vaccinated infants. The second Phase I clinical trial conducted by Aviron [44] demonstrated safety and immunogenicity for a subunit vaccine containing the gp220/350 surface glycoprotein. The trial was a randomized, double-blind study containing 67 healthy adult participants. The study indicated that the vaccine was tolerated and safe. Evidence of an immune response was shown by laboratory tests from participant sera [32]. A third Phase 1 clinical trial of a peptide vaccine with an EBNA 3 epitope (FLRGRAYGL) was conducted at the Queensland Institute of Medical Research

(QIMR), Australia. As mentioned previously, no adverse reactions to date were noted and CTLs were induced [Bharadwaj, Elliott, Lawrence, Suhrbier, and Moss, unpublished].

VII. FUTURE TRIALS

Aviron has announced the initiation of a new Phase 2 clinical trial of an EBV vaccine. This randomized, double-blind trial has enrolled 79 individuals aged 18–45 years. The study is being conducted at two universities in Belgium. On the other hand, the EBV unit at QIMR, Australia, is currently working on the development of a CTL-based polytope vaccine in collaboration with CSL Limited.

VIII. FUTURE DIRECTIONS

Much of the groundwork regarding the immune control of EBV infection has been developed to the point where application to clinical situations has become a reality. However, there remain many intriguing basic scientific questions. Foremost among these are the factors that define the focusing and dominance of the CTL response to certain EBV proteins. The two extremes of this immunodominance are the EBNA 3, 4, and 6 proteins on the one hand and EBNA 1 on the other. Although the definition of the lytic response is still in its relative infancy, there is an early indication that there may also be a focused response to particular lytic cycle proteins. It will be fascinating to determine whether this dominance distribution is a function either of protein concentration or of the kinetics of induction, or is influenced by differences in the efficiency with which different proteins are processed. Of course, in the case of EBNA 1, there is likely to be keen interest in defining the mechanism(s) whereby this protein evades HLA class I processing. It remains something of an enigma how EBNA 1-specific CTLs can be activated and whether they perform any useful function. A full definition of the mechanism of the GAr-mediated inhibitory effect may lead to strategies to inhibit its function, and this in turn could find application in the control of EBV-associated malignancies. Now that it is possible to quantitatively define CTL responses using tetramer and ELISPOT technology [16,45,46], it will be possible to consider the relative importance of individual CTL responses in the control of EBV infection. As with antibody responses, it is likely that all CTL responses may not be protective, nor should we assume that the quantitatively abundant responses serve any useful role in vivo. One early approach to unraveling this problem may be to define the induction and decay of CTL responses in various EBV-associated diseases as has been done in the case of IM. For example, there is still no clear view of the distribution of responses seen in NPC and HD patients before and after treatment. Indeed, there is still a degree of uncertainty regarding the magnitude of the response to epitopes within the LMP proteins in both these groups of patients compared with normal healthy individuals.

Furthermore, it will be most important to define the response in those individuals who undergo a clinically silent seroconversion. It is not clear, for instance, whether such individuals experience a relatively early protective response or whether their response is more or less focused than those undergoing an acute infection. It is possible that a subclinical infection might be characterized by a broad response to multiple T-cell epitopes compared with the more focused response seen in acute infection [36].

REFERENCES

1. Rickinson AB. Targeting human tumours with antigen-specific cytotoxic T-cells. Br J Cancer 1999; 80:51–56.
2. Moss DJ, et al. The immunology of Epstein–Barr virus infection. Philos Trans R Soc 2000; 356:475–488.
3. Niederman JC, Evans AS. Epstein–Barr Virus. Viral Infections of Humans: Epidemiology and Control. New York: Plenum, 1997:253–283.
4. Kieff E. Epstein–Barr virus and its replication. In: Fields BN, Knipe DM, Howley PM, eds. Field's Virology. Philadelphia: Lippincott-Raven, 1996:2343–2396.
5. Rickinson AB, Moss DJ. Human cytotoxic T lymphocyte responses to Epstein–Barr virus infection. Annu Rev Immunol 1997; 15:405–431.
6. Speck SH, et al. Reactivation of Epstein–Barr virus: regulation and function of the BZLF1 gene. Trends Microbiol 1997; 5:399–405.
7. Edson CM, Thorley-Lawson DA. Epstein–Barr virus membrane antigens: characterization, distribution, and strain differences. J Virol 1981; 39:172–184.
8. Klein G. EBV and B cell lymphomas. In: Medveczky PG, Friedman H, Bendinelli M, eds. Herpesviruses and Immunity. New York: Plenum, 1998:165–190.
9. Chiang AK, et al. Nasal T/natural killer (NK)-cell lymphomas are derived from Epstein–Barr virus-infected cytotoxic lymphocytes of both NK- and T-cell lineage. Int J Cancer 1997; 73:332–338.
10. Shibata D, Weiss LM. Epstein–Barr virus-associated gastric adenocarcinoma. Am J Pathol 1992; 140:769–774.
11. Webster-Cyriaque J, et al. Hairy leukoplakia: an unusual combination of transforming and permissive Epstein–Barr virus infections. J Virol 2000; 74:7610–7618.
12. Bonnet M, et al. Detection of Epstein–Barr virus in invasive breast cancers. J Natl Cancer Inst 1999; 91:1376–1381.
13. Decaussin G, et al. Expression of BARF1 gene encoded by Epstein–Barr virus in nasopharyngeal carcinoma biopsies. Cancer Res 2000; 60:5584–5588.
14. Khanna R, et al. Localization of Epstein–Barr virus cytotoxic T cell epitopes using recombinant vaccinia: implications for vaccine development. J Exp Med 1992; 176:169–176.
15. Murray RJ, et al. Identification of target antigens for the human cytotoxic T cell response to Epstein–Barr virus (EBV): implications for the immune control of EBV-positive malignancies. J Exp Med 1992; 176:157–168.
16. Bharadwaj M, et al. Contrasting Epstein–Barr virus-specific cytotoxic T cell responses to HLA A2-restricted epitopes in humans and HLA transgenic mice: implications for vaccine design. Vaccine 2001; 19:3769–3777.
17. Levitskaya J, et al. Inhibition of antigen processing by the internal repeat region of the Epstein–Barr virus nuclear antigen-1. Nature 1995; 375:685–688.
18. Mosier DE, et al. Transfer of a functional human immune system to mice with severe combined immunodeficiency. Nature 1988; 335:256–259.
19. Veronese ML, et al. Lymphoproliferative disease in human peripheral blood mononuclear cell-injected SCID mice. I. T lymphocyte requirement for B cell tumor generation. J Exp Med 1992; 176:1763–1767.
20. Boyle TJ, et al. Adoptive transfer of cytotoxic T lymphocytes for the treatment of transplant-associated lymphoma. Surgery 1993; 114:218–225.
21. Rooney CM, et al. Use of gene-modified virus-specific T lymphocytes to control Epstein–Barr-virus-related lymphoproliferation. Lancet 1995; 345:9–13.
22. Ishioka GY, et al. Utilization of MHC class I transgenic mice for development of minigene DNA vaccines encoding multiple HLA-restricted CTL epitopes. J Immunol 1999; 162:3915–3925.
23. Nash AA, Sunil-Chandra NP. Interactions of the murine gammaherpesvirus with the immune system. Curr Opin Immunol 1994; 6:560–563.
24. Finerty S, et al. Protective immunization against Epstein–Barr virus-induced disease in cottontop tamarins using the virus envelope glycoprotein gp340 produced from a bovine papillomavirus expression vector. J Gen Virol Feb 1992; 73:449–453.
25. Epstein MA, et al. Protection of cottontop tamarins against Epstein–Barr virus-induced malignant lymphoma by a prototype subunit vaccine. Nature 1985; 318:287–289.
26. Young LS, et al. Epstein–Barr virus gene expression in malignant lymphomas induced by experimental virus infection of cottontop tamarins. J Virol 1989; 63:1967–1974.
27. Shope T, et al. Malignant lymphoma in cottontop marmosets after inoculation with Epstein–Barr virus. Proc Natl Acad Sci USA 1973; 70:2487–2491.
28. Epstein MA, et al. Pilot experiments with EB virus in owl monkeys (Aotus trivirgatus). II EB virus in a cell line from an animal with reticuloproliferative disease. Int J Cancer 1973; 12:319–332.
29. Moghaddam A, et al. An animal model for acute and persistent Epstein–Barr virus infection. Science 1997; 276:2030–2033.
30. National Center for Infectious Diseases. Epstein–Barr Virus and Infectious Mononucleosis. http://www.cdc.gov/ncidod/diseases/ebv.htm
31. Arrand JR. Prospects for a vaccine against Epstein–Barr virus. Cancer J 1992; 5:188–193.
32. Herpesvirus infections. The Jordan Report: Accelerated Development of Vaccine. 18–23. http://www.niaid.nih.gov/publications/pdf/jordan.pdf
33. Morgan AJ. Epstein–Barr virus vaccines. Vaccine 1992; 10:563–571.
34. Wilson AD, et al. The major Epstein–Barr virus (EBV) envelope glycoprotein gp340 when incorporated into Iscoms primes cytotoxic T-cell responses directed against EBV lymphoblastoid cell lines. Vaccine 1999; 17:1282–1290.
35. Khanna R, et al. EBV structural antigens, gp350 and gp85, as targets for ex vivo virus-specific CTL during acute infectious mononucleosis: potential use of gp350/gp85 CTL epitopes for vaccine design. J Immunol 1999; 162:3063–3069.
36. Bharadwaj M, et al. Longitudinal dynamics of antigen-specific CD8 + cytotoxic T lymphocytes following primary Epstein–Barr virus infection. Blood 2001; 98:2588–2589.
37. Thomson SA, et al. Minimal epitopes expressed in a recombinant polyepitope protein are processed and presented to CD8 + cytotoxic T cells: implications for vaccine design. Proc Natl Acad Sci USA 1995; 92:5845–5849.
38. Thomson SA, et al. Recombinant polyepitope vaccines for the delivery of multiple CD8 cytotoxic T cell epitopes. J Immunol 1996; 157:822–826.
39. Moss DJ, et al. Immune regulation of Epstein–Barr virus (EBV): EBV nuclear antigen as a target for EBV-specific T cell lysis. Semin Immunopathol 1991; 13:147–156.
40. Moss DJ, et al. Epstein–Barr virus specific T-cell response in nasopharyngeal carcinoma patients. Int J Cancer 1983; 32:301–305.

41. Khanna R, et al. Molecular characterization of antigen-processing function in nasopharyngeal carcinoma (NPC): evidence for efficient presentation of Epstein–Barr virus cytotoxic T-cell epitopes by NPC cells. Cancer Res 1998; 58:310–314.

42. Lee SP, et al. Antigen presenting phenotype of Hodgkin Reed–Sternberg cells: analysis of the HLA class I processing pathway and the effects of interleukin-10 on Epstein–Barr virus-specific cytotoxic T-cell recognition. Blood 1998; 92:1020–1030.

43. Gu SY, et al. First EBV vaccine trial in humans using recombinant vaccinia virus expressing the major membrane antigen. Dev Biol Stand 1995; 84:171–177.

44. Aviron announces initiation of phase 2 clinical trial with Epstein–Barr virus vaccine Mountain View, CA, October 25, 2000. http://www.aviron.com/press/102500.html

45. Callan MF, et al. T cell selection during the evolution of CD8 + T cell memory in vivo. Eur J Immunol 1998; 28:4382–4390.

46. Tan LC, et al. A re-evaluation of the frequency of CD8 + T cells specific for EBV in healthy virus carriers. J Immunol 1999; 162:1827–1835.

54
Cytomegalovirus Vaccines

David I. Bernstein
Cincinnati Children's Hospital Medical Center, Cincinnati, Ohio, U.S.A.

Stanley A. Plotkin
University of Pennsylvania and Wistar Institute of Anatomy and Biology, Philadelphia, and Aventis Pasteur Corporation, Doylestown, Pennsylvania, U.S.A.

I. INTRODUCTION

The human cytomegalovirus (HCMV) causes the most prevalent maternal infection transmitted to the fetus, often with adverse consequences for the unborn child. Those consequences may be severe or mild, starkly evident at birth or becoming manifest later in life. Because of those sometimes subtle late effects in infancy and childhood, one of us has called HCMV the "changeling demon" [1].

In general, postnatal HCMV infection is quite common throughout the world, with seroprevalence rates of 50–90%. Seroprevalence is inversely related to socioeconomic level, but directly related to the intensity of contact between toddlers, who acquire HCMV in day care. Most HCMV infections produce few, if any, symptoms in healthy individuals, but occasionally infection can produce a mononucleosis-like illness. Human cytomegalovirus is also a leading cause of morbidity and occasional mortality in immunocompromised children and adults, particularly HIV-infected individuals and transplant recipients. More recently, there has been concern regarding the possible role of HCMV in atherosclerosis [2] and autoimmune disease [3]. The availability of antivirals and intravenous immunoglobulins has led to a decreased incidence of HCMV diseases in some of these high-risk populations, but such modalities provide incomplete or no protection, depending on the population at risk. In view of the limitation of available measures for preventing HCMV disease, an effective vaccine against HCMV would be highly desirable.

II. CLINICAL MANIFESTATIONS

A. Congenital Infection

Severe congenital infections with HCMV were first recognized in the early 1900s when they were termed cytomegalic inclusion disease (CID). Human cytomegalovirus is the most common congenital infection with 0.2–2.5% of newborns infected in utero ($\approx$40,000 infants in the United States), and the most common infectious cause of congenital abnormalities. Severe disease is seen in about 10% of congenitally infected infants and is characterized by intrauterine growth retardation, hepatosplenomegaly, jaundice, a rash often described as "blueberry muffin"-like, and severe central nervous system involvement including microcephaly, intracranial calcifications, and chorioretinitis. Laboratory abnormalities include thrombocytopenia, elevated liver function levels, and hemolytic anemia. Most infants severely affected at birth develop significant neurologic sequelae with a mortality of 4–37%. The most common sequelae of congenital HCMV is progressive sensorineural hearing disease which can be seen in both infants who are symptomatic or asymptomatic at birth [4,5]. The precise number of affected infants born annually in the United States is unknown, but the estimate by Fowler et al. [6], is about 8000 infants. Cost–benefit analysis have suggested that an estimated $834 million would be saved annually by immunization, assuming complete immunization of all women ages 15–24 years with a moderately priced vaccine [7].

Important distinctions have been drawn between congenital infection which follows a primary maternal infection and that which results from an infection in a previously infected mother [6,8–16,16a]. Transmission to the fetus occurs in about 30–50% of pregnancies complicated by a primary HCMV infection during pregnancy compared to about 1% following recurrent infection. Initial reports suggested that severe sequelae were almost exclusively seen following pregnancies complicated by primary HCMV infection [6,9]. For example, Fowler et al. [6] found that sequelae occurred in 25% of 125 infants with congenital infection following primary CMV infection during pregnancy but in only 8% of 64 infants with congenital infection born to mothers who were HCMV seropositive prior to pregnancy. More importantly, none of the infected infants born to seropositive mothers developed severe sequelae; defined as bilateral hearing loss or mental retardation (an I.Q. of <70). These sequelae occurred only among infants born to mothers who had a primary infection during pregnancy. Such observations suggest that maternal immunity to HCMV prior to pregnancy prevents the majority of severe sequelae associated with congenital infection and form an important argument for the feasibility of developing HCMV vaccines to prevent congenital HCMV disease.

Other reports [12–15] and, especially recent observations [16–18], suggest that symptomatic congenital infection and permanent neurologic sequelae are not as rare in infants of women with preconceptional immunity as previously thought. For example, Boppana et al. [17] recently reported that 8 out of 47 infants with symptomatic congenital HCMV infections were born to mothers with a confirmed nonprimary or recurrent HCMV infection. They caution, however, that the type of maternal infection could only be categorized in 43% of the 47 pregnancies evaluated. Clearly symptomatic congenital infection can occur after nonprimary or recurrent maternal infections but the extent of the risk is not clear. Determining whether these infections are due to reactivated virus in the mother or reinfections has significant implications for the development of vaccines. Recent evidence based on the antibody response to the amino terminal region of glycoprotein H suggests that reinfection may account for a substantial portion of symptomatic congenitally infected infants born to women with preconceptional immunity [19].

B. HCMV Infections in Immunocompromised Individuals

Bone marrow and solid organ transplant patients are both at risk to develop HCMV disease [20–23]. Depending on the serostatus of the donor and recipient and the level of immunosuppression, the onset of most active HCMV infections is from 2 weeks up to several months after transplantation. The mortality rate remains at about 5% even with available therapies. Besides the direct effects of infection, HCMV also increases immunosuppression, elevating the risk for fungal and other infections, and increases the risk for organ rejection, and/or organ dysfunction [23]. The risk of HCMV disease is least in kidney, followed by heart and liver transplants (8–35%), while the highest risk is in pancreas (50%) and lung or lung–heart transplants (50–80%] [21]. The most common clinical manifestations include fever, pneumonitis, hepatitis, leukopenia, gastroenteritis, and encephalitis. Bone marrow transplant recipients who are seropositive or who are seronegative and receive bone marrow from a seropositive donor are at equal risk to develop HCMV disease. In contrast, among patients receiving solid organ transplants, the risk of developing HCMV disease is highest among those who are seronegative prior to transplant and receive an organ from a seropositive donor. However, HCMV disease also occurs among recipients who are seropositive prior to transplant. In such patients, HCMV infection may occur as a result of reactivation of the patient's own virus or reinfection with HCMV strains introduced via the transplanted organ.

Recent improvements in diagnostic assays including polymerase chain reaction, and antigen (pp65) detection, and the availability of prophylactic (ganciclovir, acyclovir, and hyperimmune HCMV serum) and therapeutic drugs (ganciclovir, cidofovir, and foscarnet) have dramatically changed the way HCMV infections are approached in transplant recipients [22].

Human cytomegalovirus is also an important cause of opportunistic infection in HIV-infected individuals [24–26]. In this population, HCMV retinitis is the most common disease manifestation, but gastrointestinal manifestations including oral ulcers, esophagitis, colitis and cholecystitis, pulmonary involvement, and central nervous system involvement are also seen. The advent of highly active antiretroviral therapy has decreased the incidence of HCMV disease by decreasing the profound immunosuppression that leads to HCMV reactivation and disease but continued attention to this important pathogen is required [25].

III. MICROBIOLOGY

Cytomegaloviruses are the principal members of the betaherpesvirus subgroup of the Herpesviradae family. Cytomegalovirus is an enveloped virus with a large icosohedral capsid surrounded by a tegument. The double-stranded DNA genome of HCMV is approximately 235 kb in size. The unique long sequence, U_L, and the unique short sequence, U_S, of HCMV are flanked by repetitive sequences that are inverted relative to each other allowing for the presence of four isomeric forms. The replication of CMV is slow, at least 24 hr, and replication is highly species-specific. In vitro, human fibroblasts show the greatest susceptibility to infection while in vivo fibroblasts, epithelial cells, macrophages, smooth muscle, and endothelial cells can support replication [27]. The macrophage is the probable major site of latency, together with other cells of myeloid derivation [28–30].

The purified virus contains 30–40 polypeptides including seven capsid proteins, perhaps as many as 60 glycoproteins (8 major), and 25 proteins making up the tegument or matrix [27,31,32]. The most prominent glycoproteins are found as complexes. gB, encoded by UL 55, is the major envelope glycoprotein and appears as a heterodimer of two cleaved products, 93 and 55 kDa in size [31,32]. It plays a critical role in virus entry and is the most important target for neutralizing antibody. The gH, gL, and gO complex, UL75, UL115, and UL 74, respectively, also play an important role in virus entry. Recently, four distinct gB and two distinct gH genotypes have been observed which are useful in epidemiologic studies [33–39].

IV. IMMUNOLOGY

Protection from CMV infections is multifactorial. Innate, humoral, and cell-mediated immunity all contribute to protection. Initial studies suggesting a role for innate immunity came from mouse experiments showing that animals deficient in functional natural killer (NK) cells were more susceptible to CMV. Later, Cmv-1, the gene that controls the initial splenic replication of murine CMV (MCMV) was identified and linked to NK cell activity [40]. Most recently, the definitive evidence linking NK cell activity to protection form MCMV infections was provided when the NK cell subset and receptor, Klra8, that confers susceptibility was identified [41–43]. The MCMV-susceptible mouse strains were found to lack Klra8 while all resistant strains carried it [42].

Evidence linking protection to antibody comes from several sources. Mouse studies have found that passive transfer of antibody can provide protection from a lethal infection [44 45] Furthermore, by using the guinea pig model of congenital infection two groups have showed that passive transfer of antibody can protect the fetus from a lethal infection [46,47]. Further support for a role of antibody in protection comes from neonatal transfusion studies [48,49]. These studies showed that premature newborns born of HCMV seronegative mothers developed symptomatic CMV infections following transfusion, but that the premature newborns born to HCMV seropositive mothers remained asymptomatic after receiving the same blood products. These observations indicate that maternal antibody modulates HCMV infection. The role of antibody in protection following organ transplantation is less clear except for kidney transplants where passive immunization does not protect against infection but decreases the severity of disease in seronegative recipients of kidneys from seropositive donors [50]. For review of the many studies evaluating HCMV immune globulin, immune serum globulin, antivirals, and combinations of these strategies, the reader is referred to the comprehensive review by King [51].

The proteins that appear to induce the most consistent antibody response include glycoproteins gB(UL55), and gH(UL75), the tegument proteins pp150 (UL32), the matrix protein pp65 (UL83), and the nonstructural DNA binding phosphoprotein pp52 (UL44) [52]. Neutralizing antibody is primarily induced by gB, 60–70%, followed by gH [1,53,54].

The critical role of cell-mediated immunity and protection from CMV is documented by animal and human studies. Perhaps, the best evidence is the fact that the depletion of T-cell responses following HIV infections or transplants leads to severe HCMV disease. Early mouse studies demonstrated that suppression of T cell function lead to reactivation and dissemination of MCMV [55,56], while adoptive transfer studies confirmed a role for CD8$^+$ cytotoxic T-lymphocyte (CTL) in protection [57,58]. Similarly, in transplant patients, a correlation between recovery of the cytotoxic T cell response and recovery from HCMV infections has been identified [59,60], while adoptive transfer of CD8$^+$ cytotoxic T clones were able to reconstitute the cellular immune response to HCMV and possible provide protection [61]. A role for CD4$^+$ T cells has also been proposed [62,63].

In humans, several targets for the CD8$^+$ CTL response to HCMV have been identified. The predominate target is p65 (UL83), although responses to IE1 (UL123), pp150 (UL32), and gB (UL55) have been identified [64–67].

V. ANIMAL MODELS

The lack of an animal model in which HCMV replicates has hindered the development of an HCMV vaccine. Thus most animal models utilize species-specific CMV strains that are

similar, but not identical, to HCMV. More recently, HCMV has been utilized in SCID and nude mouse models [68 69] but thus far, these have little relevance to vaccine evaluation. Animal models of CMV include mouse, guinea pig, rat, and rhesus monkey [70–73]. Murine CMV models have provided important insights into the immunology and pathogenesis of CMV, but differences in placental structure severely limit its use for evaluating congenital CMV. Primate models would be of interest for studying congenital CMV, but the cost and ubiquity of natural simian CMV infection makes these studies difficult. Thus the guinea pig has become the model of choice for initial investigation of vaccines for congenital infection because the placental structure of the guinea pig is similar to that of humans [74], and the cost of study is reasonable.

Guinea pig CMV (gpCMV) infection of the pregnant guinea pig produces a maternal infection that can be lethal or cross the placenta to induce fetal resorption, fetal death, or fetal growth retardation, depending on the challenge dose and time of virus challenge in relation to pregnancy [71]. The primary infection of a pregnant animal typically produces a vertical transmission rate of 40–80%, similar to that in women following a primary HCMV infection. Several groups have used this model to explore the protection provided by live virus, killed and subunit vaccines [75–77].

This model was also used to examine the protective effect of gpCMV antibody alone, because it is not clear if a CMV vaccine will need to induce cell-mediated immune responses or whether the antibody alone would provide protection by neutralization or other mechanisms. Thus these studies have significant implications for the choice of proteins to include in a subunit or vectored vaccine. In two recent studies, passive transfer of high titered antibody to pregnant CMV challenge dams provided significant protection against pup mortality but results on protection from infection differed [46,47]. From these studies, it appears that a vaccine that primarily induces neutralizing antibody (such as subunit gB) would be an effective vaccine. Whether the addition of other proteins that are more likely to induce CTLs would provide additional benefit is unclear, but can be tested in this model [78].

Two recent vaccine evaluations using the guinea pig model of congenital infection provide further evidence for

Table 1 Effect of gpCMV Immunization on Pregnancy Outcome in Guinea Pigs Following gpCMV Challenge

	Control	Immunized
Glycoprotein Immunization		
Litters	11	15
Liveborn pups	21/48 (44%)	54/63 (86%)[a]
Infected pups	27/47 (57%)	26/63 (41%)
Infected liveborn pups	16/20 (80%)	24/54 (44%)[a]
gB Immunization		
Litters	6	7
Liveborn pups	13/23 (57%)	21/22 (95%)[a]
Infected pups	12/23 (52%)	4/22 (18%)[a]

[a] $p \leq 0.01$.

the utility of a subunit gB vaccine (Table 1). In one study, the purified homolog of HCMV gB was used to immunize guinea pigs [76], while in the other, purified gpCMV glycoprotein consisting mostly of gB was used [77]. Both studies combined gB with complete Freund's adjuvant, followed by incomplete Freund's adjuvant. Vaccination decreased pup mortality, shortened maternal viremia, and decreased infection rates in pups.

VI. VACCINES

The main public health objective of an HCMV vaccine is to prevent symptomatic congenital HCMV disease. This can be accomplished by preventing HCMV infection of pregnant women, by modifying the infection so that virus is not passed to the fetus, or by modifying the fetal infection so that it does not induce disease. A secondary objective is to provide HCMV immunity and limit the number of HCMV infected individuals prior to a time when they might become immunosuppressed as a result of transplantation, HIV infection, etc.

The neurological consequences of congenital HCMV are at least equal to several other pathogens for which vaccines are available, including rubella, H. flu meningitis, and pneumococcal meningitis. Thus there is an unmet need that has been recognized for many years [79,80]. Delays in vaccine development are attributed to the difficulty and cost of evaluating HCMV vaccine efficacy, the lack of a correlate of protection, and the concern regarding persistence of live virus, and possible reactivation of live vaccine virus, as well as the lack of priority given to HCMV vaccines by vaccine companies. Approaches to HCMV vaccines have included primarily live attenuated vaccines, subunit and killed vaccines, DNA vaccines, and vectored vaccines.

A. Subunit Vaccines

Much of the interest in subunit HCMV vaccines has centered on glycoprotein B (gB) because gB (UL55) is the major target of neutralizing antibodies [53,81–83]. Antibodies to gB are thought to represent 60–70% of the HCMV-specific neutralizing antibody response [53], with the majority of this response directed to the AD1 region of the protein (residues 560–635), also known as the principal neutralizing domain [82]. In addition to neutralizing antibody response, several laboratories have reported that gB can elicit major histocompatibility complex (MHC)-restricted, CD8$^+$ cytotoxic lymphocyte responses, and proliferative CD4$^+$ T cell responses following natural infection[84]. However, as discussed in Section 4, the dominant CTL target for HCMV is the pp65 phosphoprotein (UL83 gene product) [85].

Most recently, results of two large human trials evaluating a subunit gB vaccine developed by Chiron Corporation (Emeryville, CA) and combined with an oil-in-water-based adjuvant, MF59 have been reported [86,87]. The HCMV gB vaccine is derived from Chinese hamster ovary cells that have been stably transfected with the coding sequence of HCMV Towne strain gB, except that the membrane spanning domain was deleted to facilitate secretion of HCMV gB and the single protease cleavage site was mutagenized [88]. The resulting uncleaved protein is 807 aa in length with 19 putative N-linked glycosylation sites. The adjuvant, MF59, is a squalene in water emulsion that induces higher antibody titers than alum alone [86,87], which is the only approved adjuvant for human vaccines in the United States. MF59 has been used by Chiron in over 7000 individuals, including the recently published trial of their genital herpes subunit glycoprotein D herpes simplex virus vaccine [89].

In the two recent human trials, the HCMV gB vaccine plus 10.75 mg dose of MF59 was shown to be safe and immunogenic. Evaluations included vaccine regimens of 0, 1, and 2 months, 0, 1, and 4 months, and 0, 1, and 6 months; doses of HCMV gB between 5 and 100 µg; and a comparison of alum vs. MF59. Immunization at 0, 1, and 6 months induced the highest level of antibody with neutralizing and gB enzyme-linked immunosorbent assay (ELISA) antibody titers that were higher than natural infection [86,87]. An optimal HCMV gB dose, between 5 and 30 µg, was detected and groups receiving MF59 developed higher titers compared to alum gB recipients.

Subunit gB vaccines remain a viable candidate for further evaluation, either alone or combined with other vaccine strategies, designed to induce CTL responses such as canarypox expressing pp65 (discussed later). Other HCMV glycoproteins, including gH (UL75) and the gM (UL100)/gN (UL73) complex, are also targets for neutralizing antibody [90,91] and may need to be considered more strongly for inclusion in a vaccine, given the recent reports of the heterogenicity of gB and gH [33–39], especially as it pertains to congenital infection [38,39]. Thus if gB and/or gH heterogeneity contribute to reinfection, then inclusion of several other proteins that elicit neutralizing antibody may be necessary.

B. Live Attenuated

1. Towne

The Towne strain vaccine was developed in the mid-1970s by multiple passages of an isolate from a congenitally infected infant in human fibroblast cells. Towne vaccine remains the most widely evaluated HCMV vaccine [92]. The first clinical trial utilized pass 125 (MRC-5 cells) in healthy male subjects [93]. Infection was not seen following intranasal administration, but following subcutaneous inoculation, all seronegative volunteers seroconverted. Transient local reactions, including erythema and induration, beginning in the second week and lasting about 1 week, occurred in more than half of the recipients. Systemic signs and symptoms, however, were not seen. Subsequent studies supported the safety and immunogenicity of the vaccine when given subcutaneously. Other important aspects of the vaccine include its inability to establish latency [94], inability to be isolated after immunization (including attempts from urine, saliva, and blood), and its ability to induce antibody, lymphoproliferative (CD4$^+$) responses, and CD8$^+$ cytolytic responses.

Studies of Towne vaccine were also performed in renal transplant recipients because of the known risk associated with transplant, especially when an HCMV seronegative recipient receives a kidney from a seropositive donor. Three

Table 2 Comparative Results of Three Blinded Trials of Towne Vaccine in Seronegative Renal Transplant Patients Who Received Kidneys from Seropositive Donors

Trial	n	Rate of all CMV disease (%)		Rate of severe CMV disease (%)		Reduction of severe disease in vaccinated compared with placebo (%)
		V	P	V	P	
Pennsylvania	67	39	55	6	35	84
Minnesota	35	33	43	5 (10)[a]	36	87
Multicentric	61	38	59	0	17	100
All	163	37	54	3	29	89

[a] A 10% rate was reported in the original publication, but this includes one case that occurred subsequent to pancreatic transplant after a renal transplant free of CMV disease. Without that case, the incidence was 5%.

P, patients given placebo; V, patients given vaccine.

Source: Ref. 1.

placebo-controlled, randomized studies revealed that Towne vaccine did not prevent HCMV infection but modified the severity of disease with severe disease reduced by 85% [95–97] (Table 2). A unique challenge study conducted in 1989 [98] provided further evidence for the protection offered by Towne vaccine (Table 3). In this study, healthy HCMV seronegative Catholic priests were either immunized with vaccine, or not immunized and then challenged with a range of doses of the Toledo strain of HCMV, a low passage isolate that retained virulence [99]. Vaccinated subjects were protected from infection compared to unimmunized controls but were not protected as well as those who were naturally immune prior to challenge with Toledo.

In a study of women naturally exposed to HCMV from their infant shedding HCMV in day care, Towne vaccine did not provide protection from infection, whereas those women with prior natural infection were protected from reinfection [100]. However, in this study, one dose of Towne vaccine induced neutralizing antibody titers that were 10- to 20-fold less than after wild-type infection. In a subsequent trial, using a different lot of Towne vaccine, neutralizing titers was comparable to natural infection [101]. As the latest trial did not measure protection, it is unclear if a more potent Towne or other attenuated HCMV vaccine would provide better protection.

Furthermore, evidence for the utility of attenuated live virus vaccines comes from recent studies using a temperature-sensitive, replication-defective MCMV [102] or an attenuated MCMV, RV7, that contains a deletion of 7.7 kb spanning portions of MCMV HindIII-J and -I [103]. RV7 replication was similar to wild-type MCMV in vitro but RV7 failed to replicate in target organs of immunocompetent BALB/c mice or severe combined immunodeficient mice [103,104]. Following immunization with RV7 protection against a virulent salivary gland, passaged virus was seen following parenteral, as well as mucosal, routes of challenge [104].

2. Recombinant Towne/Toledo

An ideal live HCMV vaccine might combine the safety profile of Towne vaccine and the immunogenicity of wild-type HCMV. If the Towne strain is overattenuated because

of extensive mutations acquired during the 125 passages, then perhaps, replacing defined regions of the Towne genome with the corresponding region from a wild-type virus could modify this overattenuation. Indeed, researchers at Aviron (Mountain View, CA) have chosen this approach and are using the Toledo strain, a low passage isolate that had been previously characterized and used as the wild-type challenge in studies of Towne vaccine [98,99], as the wild-type virus donor. They initially characterized the genetic differences between Towne and Toledo, and identified deletions in the Towne vaccine strain including the UL/b′ sequence, which is at the right edge of the unique long segment of the HCMV genome of Toledo and wild-type isolates [105]. They then constructed a set of four vaccine candidates (Figure 1).

Vaccine candidates were constructed by cotransfection of overlapping cosmid clones so that every region of the

Table 3 Challenge with Low-Passage Toledo Strain CMV in Seronegative, Seropositive, and Towne-Vaccinated Participants [98,99]

Dose	(# Positive/# Inoculated)		
	10^3 PFU	10^2 PFU	10 PFU
Seronegative			
Illness	ND	2/2	4/4
Laboratory abnormalities[a]	ND	2/2	4/4
Infection	ND	2/2	4/4
Naturally seropositive			
Illness	3/5	0/5	0/2
Laboratory abnormalities	5/5	0/5	0/2
Infection	3/5	1/5	1/2
Vaccinated			
Illness	ND	1/7	0/5
Laboratory abnormalities	ND	3/7	1/5
Infection	ND	4/7	0/5

[a] Laboratory abnormalities include evidence of lymphocytosis, thrombocytopenia, or hepatitis.

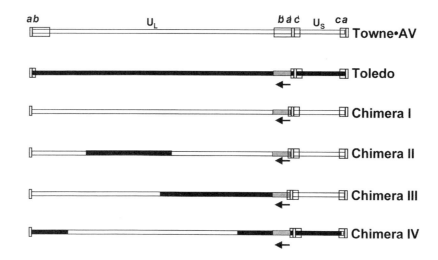

Figure 1 CMV chimeric strains prepared by recombination of the Towne attenuated virus and the low passage virulent Toledo virus. Open lines represent portions of the Towne genome and solid lines portions of the Toledo genome. The Ulb′ region is shown as the gray portion at the right edge of the unique long segment. It has been found in all clinical isolates but in the reverse orientation compared to the Toledo strain and the chimeras, thus allowing differentiation between vaccine and clinical isolates.

Towne genome was replaced in at least one candidate vaccine [106]. For safety reasons, the genome of each cosmid is primarily derived from the genome of the Towne strain ($\approx 70\%$) and each still contains at least one of the defined Towne deletions. In order to increase the immunogenicity, each construct also contains a Toledo replacement for at least one of the defined Towne deletions and in addition the UL/b′ region of Toledo. Gene products of UL/b′ are targets of the humoral immune response. Because the UL/b′ of Toledo is in reverse orientation to wild-type HCMV, this can also serve as a marker, allowing differentiation between vaccine and wild-type HCMV.

Phase I clinical trials of these four vaccine candidates have begun in HCMV seropositive adults. Only subsequent clinical trials in seronegatives can determine whether the right balance between safety and immunogenicity has been achieved in any of the four candidates.

C. Canarypox Recombinants

Canarypox virus is considered to be a good candidate vector for recombinant vaccines. Canarypox can accommodate large amounts of foreign DNA, which can be expressed in infected mammalian cells [107]. Canarypox and other fowl-pox viruses productively infect avian cells but do not produce infectious virus in mammalian cells, providing a safety factor not seen in vaccinia virus. The canarypox infection of mammalian cells results in transcription and translation of early genes including genes that are inserted downstream of early promoters, thus inducing both humoral cell-mediated immune response to the inserted gene product.

Recombinant canarypox expressing the glycoprotein B of HCMV Towne strain was initially evaluated in mice and guinea pigs. Immunization appeared to be safe and induced neutralizing antibodies and CD8$^+$ CTL responses [108]. Vaccination of HCMV seronegative humans with this vac-

cine, however, failed to induce significant gB ELISA or neutralizing antibody [109]. In later experiments, this gB expressing vector was shown to prime for the induction of a booster response following subsequent Towne vaccination as discussed below [109].

Because one of the main advantages to vectored vaccines is the induction of CTLs, there is still interest in using canarypox as a vector for expressing major CTL targets such as pp65. Indeed, recent evaluations of canarypox expressing pp65 showed that it induced HCMV-specific CD8$^+$ CTL, helper T lymphocyte, and antibodies [110]. The CTLs were elicited after only two vaccinations and were still detectable 12 and 26 months after vaccination (Figure 2).

D. Prime Boost

The rationale for evaluating prime boost strategies with canarypox was largely developed by HIV researchers in the hope of achieving antibody and cell-mediated immune responses that were higher than with either vaccine alone [111]. In the initial report evaluating HCMV prime boost strategies, Adler et al. [109] showed that priming with two doses of canarypox expressing HCMV gB induced only a weak response but primed for a subsequent boost by live attenuated Towne CMV vaccine. Subjects primed with the canarypox HCMVgB developed higher neutralization and gB ELISA titers that developed sooner and lasted longer than in Towne recipients who had first received a canarypox expressing a rabies protein. In a subsequent trial [112], the effect of priming with two doses of canarypox HCMVgB followed by two doses of the subunit HCMVgB vaccine with the adjuvant MF59 or the combination of canarypox HCMVgB plus simultaneous HCMVgB/MF59 did not have an advantage over immunization with three doses of gB/MF59. Neutralization and ELISA gB titers, lymphoproliferative, and γ interferon response were all equivalent after

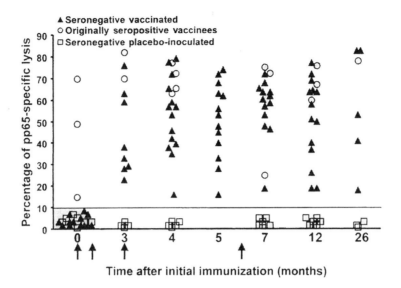

Figure 2 Kinetics of phosphoprotein 65 (pp65)-specific cytotoxic T cell activity of 25 subjects after initial immunization with canarypox–cytomegalovirus pp65. Pp65-specific lysis at an effector-to-target ratio of 25:1 (E:T of 30:1 for subjects 9, 27, 32, 33, and 38 at month 5). pp65-specific lysis was considered to be significant at 10%. (Reprinted with permission from *The Journal of Infectious Diseases*. From Ref. 110.)

the final dose of vaccine. Thus it appears that the potent combination of gB and MF59 induces substantial levels of antibody and cell-mediated immune responses to HCMV gB that were not enhanced by previous or simultaneous canarypox HCMVgB immunizations.

E. DNA and Other Vaccine Approaches

Several approaches to creating an HCMV vaccine have not yet reached clinical trials, to our knowledge. DNA vaccines, or genetic immunization, has become a popular concept but initial optimism stemming from small animal evaluations have been tempered by the poorer immunogenicity seen in larger mammals including man. Several studies have reported both cell-mediated and humoral responses to DNA immunization with either CMV gB or pp65 plasmids in mice and guinea pigs [113–116]. In one study, immunization with a plasmid expressing the MCMV immediate early gene (IE1), the major CD8 CTL target provided some but incomplete protection against a lethal MCMV infection and more consistent protection against a sublethal MCMV challenge [116]. In another report, the same group evaluated plasmids encoding MCMV homologs of HCMV, including the tegument (M32, M48, M56, M82, M83, M69, and M99), capsid (M85 and M86), and nonstructural antigens IE1-pp89 and M84. Only pp89 and M84, a nonstructured protein that shows homology with HCMV UL83-pp65, provided protection [117].

Several vectors, including adenovirus and vaccinia, were also used to deliver CMV genes [118–120]. A recombinant adenovirus gene expressing gB was found to be immunogenic when given intranasally [119] and vaccinia expressing the dominant CTL target of mice, pp89, protected animals from a lethal challenge through a CD8$^+$ T lymphocyte response [120]. Using synthetic peptides spanning the IE1 epitope of pp89, other investigators were also able to elicit protective

CD8$^+$ T cell responses [121]. The use of plant expression systems has paved the way for the delivery of oral vaccines through edible transgenic plants. Recently, a research group expressed the HCMVgB in tobacco plants as a model system [122]. They found that transformed plants produced antigenic gB at levels of 70–146 mg/mL extracted protein.

Because of the probable importance of CTL induction to protection from CMV disease, the use of CMV peptide vaccination with CTL epitopes of pp65 is also being explored [123,124]. Lipid modification at the amino terminal of one peptide produced a vaccine that did not require the use of adjuvant [123]. More recently, using a new approach, positional scanning synthetic combinatorial libraries, researchers were able to modify the HLA-A* 0201 pp65 (495–503) epitope to enhance activity [124]. The fusion of a promiscuous tetanus Th epitope to the pp65 CTL epitope produced an even more robust response [125]. Peptide vaccines are limited because of the requirement of HLA allele-specific peptide motifs; however, estimates made by using epitopes from two CMV proteins suggested that this approach is feasible, even for a diverse, multiethnic populations [126].

Another intriguing approach for CMV immunization is the use of dense bodies, defective noninfectious enveloped particles as vaccine candidates. Pepperl et al. [127] recently reported that immunization with dense bodies without adjuvant, induced both humoral and CTL responses. Titers of neutralizing antibody were similar to those seen in convalescent human sera.

VII. CONCLUSIONS

The major obstacle to the development of a vaccine against HCMV is the lack of a defined correlate of protection. The available evidence points in two directions: i.e., both antibody and cellular immunity play a role. Fortunately, experimental vaccines have been developed that stimulate either humoral or cellular responses, and both prior natural infection and live virus vaccination have been shown to protect against CMV disease to some degree. Future clinical trials will determine which immune responses, and accordingly, which vaccines offer the best protection against fetal disease or disease acquired after immunosuppression. It may be that prevention of viremia will be easier to accomplish than prevention of infection. In that regard, it should be noted that we have little information concerning mucosal immune responses to CMV.

REFERENCES

1. Plotkin SA. Vaccination against cytomegalovirus, the changeling demon. Pediatr Infect Dis J 1999; 18(4):313–325.
2. High KP. Atherosclerosis and infection due to *Chlamydia pneumoniae* or cytomegalovirus: weighing the evidence. Clin Infect Dis 1999; 28(4):746–749.
3. Newkirk MM, et al. Autoimmune response to U1 small nuclear ribonucleoprotein (U1 snRNP) associated with cytomegalovirus infection. Arthritis Res 2001; 3(4):253–258.
4. Williamson WD, et al. Progressive hearing loss in infants with asymptomatic congenital cytomegalovirus infection. Pediatrics 1992; 90(6):862–866.
5. Fowler KB, et al. Progressive and fluctuating sensorineural hearing loss in children with asymptomatic congenital cytomegalovirus infection. J Pediatr 1997; 130(4):624–630.
6. Fowler KB, et al. The outcome of congenital cytomegalovirus infection in relation to maternal antibody status. N Engl J Med 1992; 326(10):663–667.
7. Porath A, et al. Effectiveness and cost benefit of a proposed live cytomegalovirus vaccine in the prevention of congenital disease. Rev Infect Dis 1990; 12(1):31–40.
8. Grant S, et al. A prospective study of cytomegalovirus infection in pregnancy. I. Laboratory evidence of congenital infection following maternal primary and reactivated infection. J Infect 1981; 3(1):24–31.
9. Stagno S, et al. Congenital cytomegalovirus infection: the relative importance of primary and recurrent maternal infection. N Engl J Med 1982; 306(16):945–949.
10. Stagno S, et al. Primary cytomegalovirus infection in pregnancy. Incidence, transmission to fetus, and clinical outome. J Am Med Assoc 1986; 256(14):1904–1908.
11. Griffiths PD, Baboonian C. A prospective study of primary cytomegalovirus infection during pregnancy: final report. Br J Obstet Gynaecol 1984; 91(4):307–315.
12. Ahlfors K, et al. Secondary maternal cytomegalovirus infection causing symptomatic congenital infection. N Engl J Med 1981; 305(5):284.
13. Peckham CS, et al. Cytomegalovirus infection in pregnancy: preliminary findings from a prospective study. Lancet 1983; 1(8338):1352–1355.
14. Ahlfors K, et al. Congenital cytomegalovirus infection and disease in Sweden and the relative importance of primary and secondary maternal infections. Preliminary findings from a prospective study. Scand J Infect Dis 1984; 16(2):129–137.
15. Casteels A, et al. Neonatal screening for congenital cytomegalovirus infections. J Perinat Med 1999; 27(2):116–121.
16. Ahlfors K, et al. Report on a long-term study of maternal and congenital cytomegalovirus infection in Sweden. Review of prospective studies available in the literature. Scand J Infect Dis 1993; 31(5):443–457.
16a. Fowler KB, et al. Maternal immunity and prevention of congenital cytomegalovirus infection. JAMA 2003; 289: 1008–1011.
17. Boppana SB, et al. Symptomatic congenital cytomegalovirus infection in infants born to mothers with preexisting immunity to cytomegalovirus. Pediatrics 1999; 104(1 Pt 1): 55–60.
18. Ahlfors K, et al. Secondary maternal cytomegalovirus infection—a significant cause of congenital disease. Pediatrics 2001; 107(5):1227–1228.
19. Boppana SB, et al. Intrauterine transmission of cytomegalovirus to infants of women with preconceptional immunity. N Engl J Med 2001; 344(18):1366–1371.
20. Hibberd PL, Snydman DR. Cytomegalovirus infection in organ transplant recipients. Infect Dis Clin North Am 1995; 9(4):863–877.
21. van der Bij W, Speich R. Management of cytomegalovirus infection and disease after solid-organ transplantation. Clin Infect Dis 2001; 33(suppl 1):S32–S37.
22. Hebart H, et al. Management of cytomegalovirus infection after solid-organ or stem-cell transplantation. Current guidelines and future prospects. Drugs 1998; 55(1):59–72.
23. Paya CV. Indirect effects of CMV in the solid organ transplant patient. Transpl Infect Dis 1999; 1:8–12.
24. Jacobson MA. Current management of cytomegalovirus disease in patients with AIDS. AIDS Res Hum Retrovir 1994; 10(8):917–923.
25. Drew WL. Cytomegalovirus infection in patients with AIDS. Clin Infect Dis 1992; 14(2):608–615.
26. Whitley RJ, et al. Guidelines for the treatment of cytomegalovirus diseases in patients with AIDS in the era of potent antiretroviral therapy: recommendations of an international panel. International AIDS Society-USA. Arch Intern Med 1998; 158(9):957–969.
27. Mocarski ES, Courcelle CT. Cytomegaloviruses and their replication. In: Knipe DM, Howley PM, eds. Fields Virology. 4th ed. Philadelphia: Lippincott, Williams and Wilkins, 2001:2629–2673.
28. Hahn G, et al. Cytomegalovirus remains latent in a common precursor of dendritic and myeloid cells. Proc Natl Acad Sci USA 1998; 95(7):3937–3942.
29. Minton EJ, et al. Human cytomegalovirus infection of the monocyte/macrophage lineage in bone marrow. J Virol 1994; 68(6):4017–4021.
30. Soderberg-Naucler C, Nelson JY. Human cytomegalovirus latency and reactivation—a delicate balance between the virus and its host's immune system. Intervirology 1999; 42(5–6):314–321.
31. Britt WJ, Mach M. Human cytomegalovirus glycoproteins. Intervirology 1996; 39(5–6):401–412.
32. Spaete RR, et al. Human cytomegalovirus structural proteins. J Gen Virol 1994; 75(Pt 12):3287–3308.
33. Chou SW, Dennison KM. Analysis of interstrain variation in cytomegalovirus glycoprotein B sequences encoding neutralization-related epitopes. J Infect Dis 1991; 163(6):1229–1234.
34. Meyer-Konig U, et al. Intragenic variability of human cytomegalovirus glycoprotein B in clinical strains. J Infect Dis 1998; 177(5):1162–1169.
35. Fries BC, et al. Frequency distribution of cytomegalovirus envelope glycoprotein genotypes in bone marrow transplant recipients. J Infect Dis 1994; 169(4):769–774.
36. Rasmussen L, et al. Cytomegalovirus gB genotype distribution differs in human immunodeficiency virus-infected patients and immunocompromised allograft recipients. J Infect Dis 1997; 175(1):179–184.
37. Rasmussen L. Molecular pathogenesis of human cytomegalovirus infection. Transpl Infect Dis 1999; 1(2):127–134.
38. Bale JF Jr, et al. Intrauterine cytomegalovirus infection and glycoprotein B genotypes. J Infect Dis 2000; 182(3):933–936.
39. Boppana SB, et al. Intrauterine transmission of cytomega-

lovirus to infants of women with preconceptional immunity. N Engl J Med 2001; 344(18):1366–1371.

40. Scalzo AA, et al. The effect of the Cmv-1 resistance gene, which is linked to the natural killer cell gene complex, is mediated by natural killer cells. J Immunol 1992; 149(2):581–589.

41. Brown MG, et al. Vital involvement of a natural killer cell activation receptor in resistance to viral infection. Science 2001; 292(5518):934–937.

42. Lee SH, et al. Susceptibility to mouse cytomegalovirus is associated with deletion of an activating natural killer cell receptor of the C-type lectin superfamily. Nat Genet 2001; 28(1):42–45.

43. Daniels KA, et al. Murine cytomegalovirus is regulated by a discrete subset of natural killer cells reactive with monoclonal antibody to Ly49H. J Exp Med 2001; 194(1):29–44.

44. Farrell HE, Shellam GR. Protection against murine cytomegalovirus infection by passive transfer of neutralizing and non-neutralizing monoclonal antibodies. J Gen Virol 1991; 72(Pt 1):149–156.

45. Shanley JD, et al. Modification by adoptive humoral immunity of murine cytomegalovirus infection. J Infect Dis 1981; 143(2):231–237.

46. Bratcher DF, et al. Effect of passive antibody on congenital cytomegalovirus infection in guinea pigs. J Infect Dis 1995; 172(4):944–950.

47. Chatterjee A, et al. Modification of maternal and congenital cytomegalovirus infection by anti-glycoprotein β antibody transfer in guinea pigs. J Infect Dis 2001; 183(11):1547–1553.

48. Yeager AS, et al. Prevention of transfusion-acquired cytomegalovirus infections in newborn infants. J Pediatr 1981; 98(2):281–287.

49. Adler SP, et al. Cytomegalovirus infections in neonates acquired by blood transfusions. Pediatr Infect Dis 1983; 2(2):114–118.

50. Snydman DR. Cytomegalovirus immunoglobulins in the prevention and treatment of cytomegalovirus disease. Rev Infect Dis 1990; 12(suppl 7):S839–848.

51. King SM. Immune globulin versus antivirals versus combination for prevention of cytomegalovirus disease in transplant recipients. Antivir Res 1999; 40(3):115–137.

52. Greijer AE, et al. Molecular fine-specificity analysis of antibody responses to human cytomegalovirus and design of novel synthetic-peptide-based serodiagnostic assays. J Clin Microbiol 1999; 37(1):179–188.

53. Britt WJ, et al. Induction of complement-dependent and -independent neutralizing antibodies by recombinant-derived human cytomegalovirus gp55-116 (gB). J Virol 1988; 62(9):3309–3318.

54. Urban M, et al. Glycoprotein H of human cytomegalovirus is a major antigen for the neutralizing humoral immune response. J Gen Virol 1996; 77(Pt 7):1537–1547.

55. Gardner MB, et al. Induction of disseminated virulent cytomegalovirus infection by immunosuppression of naturally chronically infected wild mice. Infect Immun 1974; 10(4):966–969.

56. Jordan MC, et al. Immunosuppression reactivates and disseminates latent murine cytomegalovirus. J Gen Virol 1977; 37(2):419–423.

57. Reddehase MJ, et al. CD8-positive T lymphocytes specific for murine cytomegalovirus immediate-early antigens mediate protective immunity. J Virol 1987; 61(10):3102–3108.

58. Holtappels R, et al. Experimental preemptive immunotherapy of murine cytomegalovirus disease with CD8 T-cell lines specific for ppM83 and pM84, the two homologs of human cytomegalovirus tegument protein ppUL83 (pp65). J Virol 2001; 75(14):6584–6600.

59. Quinnan GV, et al. Cytotoxic T cells in cytomegalovirus infection: HLA-restricted T-lymphocyte cytotoxic responses correlate with recovery from cytomegalovirus infection in bone-marrow-transplant recipients. N Engl J Med 1982; 207:7–13.

60. Reusser P, et al. Cytomegalovirus (CMV)-specific T cell immunity after renal transplantation mediates protection from CMV disease by limiting the systemic virus load. J Infect Dis 1999; 180(2):247–253.

61. Walter EZ, et al. Reconstitution of cellular immunity against cytomegalovirus in recipients of allogeneic bone marrow by transfer of T-cell clones from the donor. N Engl J Med 1995; 333(16):1038–1044.

62. Erlich KS, et al. Effects of L3T4+ lymphocyte depletion on acture murine cytomegalovirus infection. J Gen Virol 1989; 70(Pt 2):1765–1771.

63. Sester M, et al. Levels of virus-specific CD4 T cells correlate with cytomegalovirus control and predict virus-induced disease after renal transplantation. Transplantation 2001; 71(9):1287–1294.

64. Wills MR, et al. The human cytotoxic T-lymphocyte (CTL) response to cytomegalovirus is dominated by structural protein pp65: frequency, specificity, and T-cell receptor usage of pp65-specific CTL. J Virol 1996; 70(11):7569–7579.

65. Boppana SB, Britt WJ. Recognition of human cytomegalovirus gene products by HCMV-specific cytotoxic T cells. Virology 1996; 222(1):293–296.

66. Borysiewicz LK, et al. Human cytomegalovirus-specific cytotoxic T cells. Relative frequency of stage-specific CTL recognizing the 72-kD immediate early protein and glycoprotein B expressed by recombinant vaccinia viruses. J Exp Med 1988; 168(3):919–931.

67. Gyulai Z, et al. Cytotoxic T lymphocyte (CTL) responses to human cytomegalovirus pp65, 1E1-Exon4, gB, pp150, and pp28 in healthy individuals: reevaluation of prevalence of 1E1-specific CTLs. J Infect Dis 2000; 181(5):1537–1546.

68. Mocarski ES, et al. Human cytomegalovirus in a SCID-hu mouse: thymic epithelial cells are prominent targets of viral replication. Proc Natl Acad Sci USA 1993; 90(1):104–108.

69. Pari GS, et al. Generation of a nude mouse tumor model for in vivo replication of human cytomegalovirus. J Infect Dis 1998; 177(3):523–528.

70. Kern ER. Animal models for cytomegalovirus infection: murine CMV. In: Zak O, Sande MA, eds. Handbook of Animal Models of Infection: Experimental Models in Antimicrobial Chemotherapy. New York: Academic Press, 1999:927–934.

71. Bernstein DI, Bourne N. Animal models for cytomegalovirus infection: guinea-pig. CMV Handbook of Animal Models of Infection: Experimental Models in Antimicrobial Chemotherapy. New York: Academic Press, 1999:935–941.

72. Stals FS. Animal models for cytomegalovirus infection: rat. CMV. Handbook of Animal Models of Infection: Experimental Models in Antimicrobial Chemotherapy. New York: Academic Press, 1999:943–950.

73. Lockridge KM, et al. Pathogenesis of experimental rhesus cytomegalovirus infection. J Virol 1999; 73(11):9576–9583.

74. Enders AC. A comparative study of the fine structure of the trophoblast in several hemochorial placentas. Am J Anat 1965; 116:29–68.

75. Bia FJ, et al. Vaccination for the prevention of maternal and fetal infection with guinea pig cytomegalovirus. J Infect Dis 1980; 142(5):732–738.

76. Harrison CJ, et al. Reduced congenital cytomegalovirus (CMV) infection after maternal immunization with a guinea pig CMV glycoprotein before gestational primary CMV infection in the guinea pig model. J Infect Dis 1995; 172(5):1212–1220.

77. Bourne N, et al. Preconception immunization with a cyto-

megalovirus (CMV) glycoprotein vaccine improves pregnancy outcome in a guinea pig model of congenital CMV infection. J Infect Dis 2001; 183(1):59–64.

78. Schleiss MR, et al. Immunogenicity evaluation of DNA vaccines that target guinea pig cytomegalovirus proteins glycoprotein B and UL83. Vir Immunol 2000; 13(2):155–167.

79. Yow MD. Congenital cytomegalovirus disease: a NOW problem. J Infect Dis 1989; 159(2):163–167.

80. Yow MD, Demmler GJ. Congenital cytomegalovirus disease—20 years is long enough. N Engl J Med 1992; 326(10): 702–703.

81. Britt WJ, et al. Cell surface expression of human cytomegalovirus (HCMV) gp55–116 (gB): use of HCMV-recombinant vaccinia virus-infected cells in analysis of the human neutralizing antibody response. J Virol 1990; 64(3):1079–1085.

82. Ohlin M, et al. Fine specificity of the human immune response to the major neutralization epitopes expressed on cytomegalovirus gp58/116 (gB), as determined with human monoclonal antibodies. J Virol 1993; 67(2):703–710.

83. Marshall GS, et al. Antibodies to recombinant-derived glycoprotein B after natural human cytomegalovirus infection correlate with neutralizing activity. J Infect Dis 1992; 165(2): 381–384.

84. Gyulai Z, et al. Cytotoxic T lymphocyte (CTL) responses to human cytomegalovirus pp65, 1E1-Exon4, gB, pp150, and pp28 in healthy individuals: reevaluation of prevalence of 1E1-specific CTLs. J Infect Dis 2000; 181(5):1537–1546.

85. Wills MR, et al. The human cytotoxic T-lymphocyte (CTL) response to cytomegalovirus is dominated by structural protein pp65: frequency, specificity, and T-cell receptor usage of pp65-specific CTL. J Virol 1996; 70(11):7569–7579.

86. Pass RF, et al. A subunit cytomegalovirus vaccine based on recombinant envelope glycoprotein B and a new adjuvant. J Infect Dis 1999; 180(4):970–975.

87. Frey SE, et al. Effects of antigen dose and immunization regimens on antibody responses to a cytomegalovirus glycoprotein B subunit vaccine. J Infect Dis 1999; 180(5):1700–1703.

88. Spaete RR. A recombinant subunit vaccine approach to HCMV vaccine development. Transplant Proc 1991; 23(3 suppl 3):90–96.

89. Corey L, et al. Recombinant glycoprotein vaccine for the prevention of genital HSV-2 infection: two randomized controlled trials. Chiron HSV Vaccine Study Group. J Am Med Assoc 1999; 282(4):331–340.

90. Simpson JA, et al. Neutralizing monoclonal antibodies that distinguish three antigenic sites on human cytomegalovirus glycoprotein H have conformationally distinct binding sites. J Virol 1993; 67(1):489–496.

91. Mach M, et al. Complex formation by human cytomegalovirus glycoproteins M (gpUL100) and N (gpUL73). J Virol 2000; 74(24):11881–11892.

92. Marshall GS, Plotkin SA. Progress toward developing a cytomegalovirus vaccine. Infect Dis Clin North Am 1990; 4(2):283–298.

93. Plotkin SA, et al. Clinical trials of immunization with the Towne 125 strain of human cytomegalovirus. J Infect Dis 1976; 134(5):470–475.

94. Plotkin SA, Huang ES. Cytomegalovirus vaccine virus (Towne strain) does not induce latency. J Infect Dis 1985; 152(2):395–397.

95. Plotkin SA, et al. Towne-vaccine-induced prevention of cytomegalovirus disease after renal transplants. Lancet 1984; 1(8376):528–530.

96. Balfour HH Jr. Prevention of cytomegalovirus disease in renal allograft recipients. Scand J Infect Dis Suppl 1991; 80:88–93.

97. Plotkin SA, et al. Multicenter trial of Towne strain attenuated virus vaccine in seronegative renal transplant recipients. Transplantation 1994; 58(11):1176–1178.

98. Plotkin SA, et al. Protective effects of Towne cytomegalovirus vaccine against low-passage cytomegalovirus administered as a challenge. J Infect Dis 1989; 159(5):860–865.

99. Quinnan GV Jr, et al. Comparative virulence and immunogenicity of the Towne strain and a nonattenuated strain of cytomegalovirus. Ann Intern Med 1984; 101(4):478–483.

100. Adler SP, et al. Immunity induced by primary human cytomegalovirus infection protects against secondary infection among women of childbearing age. J Infect Dis 1995; 171(1): 26–32.

101. Adler SP, et al. Safety and immunogenicity of the Towne strain cytomegalovirus vaccine. Pediatr Infect Dis J 1998; 17(3):200–206.

102. Gill TA, et al. Replication-defective mutants of mouse cytomegalovirus protect against wild-type virus challenge. J Med Virol 2000; 62(2):127–139.

103. Cavanaugh VJ, et al. Murine cytomegalovirus with a deletion of genes spanning HindIII-J and -I displays altered cell and tissue tropism. J Virol 1996; 70(3):1365–1374.

104. MacDonald MR, et al. Mucosal and parenteral vaccination against acute and latent murine cytomegalovirus (MCMV) infection by using an attenuated MCMV mutant. J Virol 1998; 72(1):442–451.

105. Cha TA, et al. Human cytomegalovirus clinical isolates carry at least 19 genes not found in laboratory strains. J Virol 1996; 70(1):78–83.

106. Mocarski ES Jr, Kemble GW. Recombinant cytomegaloviruses for study of replication and pathogenesis. Intervirology 1996; 39(5–6):320–330.

107. Plotkin SA, et al. The safety and use of canarypox vectored vaccines. Dev Biol Stand 1995; 165–170.

108. Gonczol E, et al. Preclinical evaluation of an ALVAC (canarypox)-human cytomegalovirus glycoprotein B vaccine candidate. Vaccine 1995; 13(12):1080–1085.

109. Adler SP, et al. A canarypox vector expressing cytomegalovirus (CMV) glycoprotein B primes for antibody responses to a live attenuated CMV vaccine (Towne). J Infect Dis 1999; 180(3):843–846.

110. Berencsi K, et al. A canarypox vector-expressing cytomegalovirus (CMV) phosphoprotein 65 induces long-lasting cytotoxic T cell responses in human CMV-seronegative subjects. J Infect Dis 2001; 183(8):1171–1179.

111. Tartaglia J, et al. Canarypox virus-based vaccines: primeboost strategies to induce cell-mediated and humoral immunity against HIV. AIDS Res Hum Retrovir 1998; 14: S291–298.

112. Bernstein DI, et al. Effect of Previous or Simultaneous Immunization with Canarypox Expressing Cytomegalovirus (CMV) Glycoprotein B (gB) on Response to Subunit gB vaccine plus MF59 in Healthy CMV Seronegative Adults. J Infect Dis 2002; 185:686–690.

113. Pande H, et al. Direct DNA immunization of mice with plasmid DNA encoding the tegument protein pp65 (ppUL83) of human cytomegalovirus induces high levels of circulating antibody to the encoded protein. Scand J Infect Dis Suppl 1995; 99:117–120.

114. Endresz V, et al. Induction of human cytomegalovirus (HCMV)-glycoprotein B (gB)-specific neutralizing antibody and phosphoprotein 65 (pp65)-specific cytotoxic T lymphocyte responses by naked DNA immunization. Vaccine 1999; 27(1):50–58.

115. Endresz V, et al. Optimization of DNA immunization against human cytomegalovirus. Vaccine 2001; 19(28–29):3972–3980.

116. Gonzalez Armas JC, et al. DNA immunization confers protection against murine cytomegalovirus infection. J Virol 1996; 70(11):7921–7928.

117. Morello CS, et al. Suppression of murine cytomegalovirus (MCMV) replication with a DNA vaccine encoding MCMV

M84 (a homolog of human cytomegalovirus). J Virol 2000; 74(8):3696–3708.

118. Berencsi K, et al. Murine cytotoxic T cell response specific for human cytomegalovirus glycoprotein B (gB) induced by adenovirus and vaccinia virus recombinants expressing gB. J Gen Virol 1993; 74(Pt 11):2507–2512.

119. Marshall GS, et al. An adenovirus recombinant that expresses the human cytomegalovirus major envelope glycoprotein and induces neutralizing antibodies. J Infect Dis 1990; 162(5):1177–1181.

120. Jonjic S, et al. A nonstructural viral protein expressed by a recombinant vaccinia virus protects against lethal cytomegalovirus infection. J Virol 1988; 62(5):1653–1658.

121. Del Val M, et al. Protection against lethal cytomegalovirus infection by a recombinant vaccine containing a single nonameric T-cell epitope. J Virol 1991; 65(7):3641–3646.

122. Tackaberry ES, et al. Development of biopharmaceuticals in plant expression systems: cloning, expression and immunological reactivity of human cytomegalovirus glycoprotein B (UL55) in seeds of transgenic tobacco. Vaccine 1999; 17(23–24):3020–3029.

123. Diamond DJ, et al. Development of a candidate HLA A*0201 restricted peptide-based vaccine against human cytomegalovirus infection. Blood 1997; 90(5):1751–1767.

124. La Rosa C, et al. Enhanced immune activity of cytotoxic T-lymphocyte epitope analogs derived from positional scanning synthetic combinatorial libraries. Blood 2001; 97(6): 1776–1786.

125. La Rosa C, et al. Fusion peptides provide powerful T-help (Th) to stimulate CMV-specific cellular immunity in a transgenic mouse model (8th) International CMV Workshop, Monterey, CA, May 20–25, 112.

126. Longmate J, et al. Population coverage by HLA class-I restricted cytotoxic T-lymphocyte epitopes. Immunogenetics 2001; 52(3-4):165–173.

127. Pepperl S, et al. Dense bodies of human cytomegalovirus induce both humoral and cellular immune responses in the absence of viral gene expression. J Virol 2000; 74(13):6132–6146.

55

Herpes Simplex Vaccines

Richard J. Whitley
University of Alabama at Birmingham, Birmingham, Alabama, U.S.A.

I. INTRODUCTION

Our knowledge of the pathogenesis, natural history, treatment, and molecular biology of herpes simplex virus (HSV) and its resultant infections has increased dramatically over the past decade. These advances, in part, paralleled the development of antiviral drugs that are selective and specific inhibitors of viral replication. The unequivocal establishment of the value of antiviral therapy has had a major impact on altering the severity of human disease and has major implications for long-range control of HSV infections. Nevertheless, no studies have indicated that therapy interrupts transmission of infection. Furthermore, some clinical diseases (e.g., herpes simplex encephalitis and neonatal HSV infections) are still associated with significant mortality and morbidity despite antiviral therapy. Even with the rapidly evolving knowledge of the molecular biology of HSV, the development of a successful vaccine—either subunit or live attenuated—has eluded the biomedical investigator. The past decade has witnessed increasing insight into viral gene structure and function, particularly those genes responsible for latency, virulence, and host immune responses. Such advances have been recently summarized [1]. Our current level of biomedical knowledge sets a stage for the application of molecular biology to the evaluation of human disease, the development of genetically engineered vaccines, and the potential for the development of antiviral therapeutics predicated upon newly identified site-specific molecular targets [2,3].

The development of an HSV vaccine has attracted the interest of investigators for the better part of the 20th century. The goal of producing a vaccine that protects against HSV disease has not been fully realized, as compared to other vaccines described in this book. In large part, the unique properties of HSV—especially its ability to become latent and reactivate—and its human biology make the potential success of a vaccine more difficult to achieve than with many other viral pathogens. This chapter will review the unique problems of HSV infections and consider approaches that have been developed historically. Further,

initial success with subunit vaccines, albeit limited, and the application of genetically engineered HSV to treatment of human disease will be described.

II. HISTORY

Herpes simplex virus infections of humans have been documented since ancient Greek times [4–6]. Records of human HSV infections began with descriptions of cutaneous spreading lesions thought to be of herpetic etiology, particularly in the writings of Hippocrates, as reviewed [6,7]. Scholars of Greek civilization defined the word "herpes" to mean creep or crawl in reference to the spreading nature of the skin lesions [4,5]. The Roman scholar Herodotus associated mouth ulcers and lip vesicles with fever and defined this association as "herpes febrilis" [8]. Likely, many of these original observations reiterated Galen's deduction that the appearance of such lesions was an attempt by the body to rid itself of evil humors, and, perhaps, led to the name of "herpes excretins" [4]. However, these original descriptions of skin lesions probably bare little resemblance to later reports of the 19th and 20th century [8].

As noted by Wildy [4], Shakespeare described recurrent labial lesions. As he wrote in *Romeo and Juliet*, Queen Mab, the midwife of the fairies, stated: "O'er ladies lips, who straight on kisses dream, which oft the angry Mab with blisters plagues, because their breaths with sweetmeats tainted are."

In the 18th century, Astruc, physician to the King of France, drew the appropriate correlation between herpetic lesions and genital infection [9]. By the early 19th century, the vesicular nature of lesions associated with herpetic infections was well ascertained. However, it was not until 1893 that Vidal specifically recognized human transmission of HSV infections [4].

Observations from the early 20th century brought an end to the early imprecise descriptive era of HSV infections. First, histopathologic studies described the multinucleated giant cells associated with herpesvirus infections [10]. Second, the unequivocal infectious nature of HSV was recognized by Lowenstein in 1919 [11]. He experimentally demonstrated that virus retrieved from the lesions of humans with HSV keratitis or the vesicles of patients with HSV labialis produced lesions on the rabbit cornea. These corneal lesions were similar to that encountered in humans with HSV eye infection. Furthermore, the vesicle fluid from patients with herpes zoster failed to reproduce similar dendritic lesions in the rabbit eye model. In fact, these observations were actually attributed to earlier investigations by Grüter who performed virtually identical experiments around 1910 but did not report them until much later [12].

Reports between 1920 and the early 1960s focused on the biologic manifestations of these viruses as well as the natural history of human disease. During these four decades, the host range of HSV infections was expanded to include a variety of laboratory animals, chick embryos, and, ultimately, in vitro cell culture systems. Expanded animal studies demonstrated that transmission of human virus to the rabbit resulted not only in corneal disease but also could lead to infections of either the skin or central nervous system [13], as reviewed [7,14–16].

Host immune responses to HSV were reported initially in the early 1930s. The first studies were performed by Andrews and Carmichael who defined the presence of HSV neutralizing antibodies in the serum of previously infected adults [17]. Subsequently, some of these patients developed recurrent labial lesions, albeit less severe than those associated with the initial episode. This observation led to the recognition of a unique biologic property of HSV, namely, the ability of these viruses to recur in the presence of humoral immunity—a characteristic known as reactivation of latent infection. Only individuals with neutralizing antibodies developed these recurrent vesicular lesions, a paradoxical finding given the classical lessons of such infectious diseases as measles and rubella whereby antibodies were normally associated with protection from subsequent episodes of disease. By the late 1930s it was well recognized that infants with severe stomatitis, who shed a virus thought to be HSV [18], subsequently developed neutralizing antibodies during the convalescent period [19]. Later in life, some of these children had recurrent lesions of the lip.

The medical literature of the 1940s and 1950s was replete with descriptions of disease entities such as primary and recurrent infections of mucous membranes and skin (e.g., gingivostomatitis, herpes labialis and genitalis, herpetic whitlow or eczema herpeticum) [20], keratoconjunctivitis [21], neonatal HSV infection, visceral HSV infections of the immunocompromised host, and HSV encephalitis [22]. The clinical spectrum of HSV infections subsequently was expanded to include Kaposi's varicella-like eruption and severe and prolonged recurrent infections of the immunocompromised host.

Significant laboratory advances have provided a foundation for the application of molecular biology to the study of human disease and, no less, vaccine development. These advances include, among others, 1) detection of antigenic differences between HSV-1 and -2 [6,23–25]; 2) proven antiviral therapy for virtually all manifestations of HSV disease [26–36]; 3) application of restriction endonuclease

technology to HSV strains in order to show epidemiologic relatedness [37]; 4) definition of type-specific antigens allowing the development of serologic assays that distinguish HSV-1 from HSV-2 [38,39]; 5) the characterization of the replication of HSV, its resultant gene products, and the biologic properties of some of these products [1]; and 6) the attenuation of HSV through genetic engineering and the subsequent expression of foreign genes, providing technology for the development of new vaccines [40].

III. THE INFECTIOUS AGENT

Herpes simplex virus, types 1 and 2, are members of a family of large DNA viruses that contain centrally located, linear, double-stranded DNA. All of the herpesviruses consist of similar structural elements arranged in concentric layers [1,41,42]. Other members of the human herpesvirus family include cytomegalovirus, varicella-zoster virus, Epstein–Barr virus, human herpes virus 6, 7, and 8. Human herpesvirus 8 is also known as Kaposi Sarcoma virus. The DNA of HSV has a molecular weight of approximately 100 million and encodes for about 80 polypeptides, an increasing number of which have biologic functions that are understood. The genome consists of two components, a unique long and unique short region which can invert upon themselves, allowing for the coexistence of four isomers in virus suspensions [1,42,43]. The genomic arrangement of HSV-1 and -2 indicates that a number of genes are collinear with reasonable, but not identical, matching of base pairs.

Viral DNA is packaged inside a protein structure known as the capsid, which confers icosapentahedral symmetry to the virus. The capsid consists of 162 capsomers and is surrounded by a tightly adherent membrane known as the tegument [44]. An envelope loosely surrounds the capsid and tegument, consisting of glycoproteins, lipids, and polyamines. The envelope glycoproteins are primarily responsible for the induction of humoral immune responses.

The replication of HSV is characterized by the expression of three gene classes: alpha (immediate early), beta (early), and gamma (late) genes, respectively, although there is some overlap between of each of these classes. These genes are expressed temporally and in a cascade fashion [1,45,46]. Several observations are relevant as it relates to the replication of HSV for vaccine development. First, although herpesvirus genes carry transcriptional and translational signals similar to those of other DNA viruses, the mRNAs arising from the vast majority of genes are not spliced [47,48]. Second, the information density is lower than that encoded in the genes of smaller viruses [1,48], permitting insertion and deletion of genes into the HSV genome without significant alteration of the genomic structure. This property provides an opportunity to genetically engineer HSV as either a vaccine or a vector for the delivery of foreign antigens [40]. In this later circumstance, expression of foreign genes in HSV could provide an endogenous adjuvant or be useful for gene therapy. Finally, replication requires the expression of a viral coded protein, α-transinducing factor, a potentially unique target for antivirals or antigen for vaccines [1]. The replication of HSV appears under the control of alpha genes of which there are five. The beta gene products include the enzymes necessary for viral replication, such as HSV thymidine kinase, as well as the regulatory proteins. These genes require functional alpha gene products for expression. The onset of expression of beta genes products coincides with the decline in the rate of expression of alpha genes and an irreversible shut-off of host cellular macromolecular protein synthesis [45,49]. This latter event equates with cell death. Structural proteins are usually of the gamma gene class [45, 50]. The gamma gene products are heterogeneous and are differentiated from beta genes solely by the requirement for viral DNA for maximum expression of their genes.

Assembly of virus begins in the nucleus with formation of empty capsids, insertion of DNA, and acquisition of the envelope as the capsid buds through the inner lamella of the nuclear membrane. Further maturation of envelope glycoproteins occurs in the endoplasmic reticulum. Eleven glycoproteins have been described; these are gB, gC, gD, gE, gG, gH, gI, gJ, gK, gL, and gM [1,51]. The biologic properties of some of these glycoproteins have been identified [15,49]. For example, gD is related to viral infectivity and is the most potent inducer of neutralizing antibodies. Glycoprotein B (gB) is required for infectivity. These two glycoproteins have been utilized extensively in subunit vaccines which have been developed for human experimentation. Glycoprotein C (gC) binds to the C3b component of complement while gE binds to the Fc portion of IgG. In addition, it appears as though a deletion in gC enhances viral pathogenicity [52]. Glycoprotein G (gG) provides antigenic specificity to HSV and, therefore, results in an antibody response which allows for the distinction between HSV-1 and -2 [38]. Glycoprotein I interacts with gE at the Fc receptor [53,54]. The importance of these glycoproteins for vaccine development cannot be overemphasized. Considerable antigenic cross-reactivity exists between HSV-1 and -2.

IV. HOST VIRUS INTERACTION

In considering the development of vaccines directed against HSV, some understanding of the induced pathology and its implications on the modulation of the biology of human disease is relevant. The pathogenesis of HSV infections can best be understood through knowledge of the events of replication and establishment of latency in both animal models and humans. Infection is initiated by contact of the virus with mucosal surfaces or abraded skin. The fundamental principle of the pathogenesis of human infections is that transmission occurs by intimate personal contact, resulting in viral replication at the mucosal surfaces of initial infection. With viral replication at the site of infection, either an intact virion or, more simply, the naked capsid enters the nerve termini and is carried by retrograde axonal flow to the dorsal root ganglia where, after several cycles of viral replication, latency is established [55]. These events have been demonstrated in a variety of animal models, as reviewed [56]. After latency is established, reactivation can occur with a proper provocative stimulus (i.e., stress, menstruation, fever, exposure to ultraviolet light, etc.), and virus is transported anterograde down the axon to replicate at

mucocutaneous sites, appearing as skin vesicles or mucosal ulcers.

Viral replication can lead to systemic disease such as disseminated neonatal HSV infection with multi-organ involvement, or, very rarely, multi-organ disease of pregnancy and, infrequently, dissemination in severely immunosuppressed patients. Presumably, widespread organ involvement is the consequence of viremia in a host not capable of limiting replication to mucosal surfaces. It is unlikely that an HSV vaccine will prevent infection; however, disease, particularly multisystem disease, must be prevented or ameliorated for a vaccine to be considered successful. Recently completed vaccine trials support this concept.

Infection with HSV-1 is commonly transmitted to the oropharynx by direct contact of a susceptible individual with infected secretions (such as virus contained in labial vesicular fluid) [57–59]. Thus initial replication of virus occurs in the oropharyngeal mucosa; the trigeminal ganglion becomes colonized and harbors latent virus. Acquisition of HSV-2 infection is usually the consequence of transmission via genital routes. Under these circumstances, virus replicates in the vaginal tract or on penile skin sites with colonization of the sacral ganglia. For uncertain reasons, HSV-1 infection, when symptomatic, recurs more frequently in the oropharyngeal area, and HSV-2, when symptomatic, recurs more frequently in the genital area [60].

Operative definitions for the type of infection are of relevance. For individuals susceptible to HSV infections, namely, those without pre-existing antibodies, first exposure to either HSV-1 or -2 results in primary infection. The epidemiology and clinical characteristics of primary infection are distinctly different than that associated with recurrent infection. This subject has been reviewed extensively [7,14,15,61,62]. During primary infection of the genital tract or oropharynx, viral replication persists for nearly 2 weeks and disease for 3 weeks. After the establishment of latency, reactivation of HSV is known as recurrent infection. During recurrent symptomatic infection, viral replication persists for 24–48 hr and total disease lasts 7 to 10 days. Reactivation of infection leads to recurrent skin vesicular lesions such as HSV labialis or recurrent HSV genitalis. Individuals with pre-existing antibodies to one type of HSV can experience a first infection with the opposite virus type at the same or different site. This occurrence is known as an initial infection rather than primary. An example of an initial infection would be those individuals who have pre-existing HSV-1 antibodies, acquired after HSV gingivostomatitis, who, then, acquire a genital HSV-2 infection. The natural history of an initial infection more closely resembles recurrent infection. Pre-existing antibodies to HSV-1 appear to have an ameliorative effect on disease associated with HSV-2 infection [63]. Both initial and primary infections have also been named first-episode infection. Importantly, shedding of virus can be either symptomatic or asymptomatic. Indeed, transmission occurs more frequently during periods of asymptomatic shedding. Reinfection with the same strain of HSV can occur, albeit exceedingly uncommon [64,65]. This occurrence is defined as exogenous reinfection.

Ideally, vaccines directed against HSV should prevent infection as well as disease. However, it is unlikely that such a vaccine will uniformly confer protection from infection, as discussed below in the context of a recently completely clinical trial. Thus a vaccine should significantly alter the clinical manifestations of primary disease and, perhaps, the frequency and severity recurrent infection. In so doing, it is anticipated that transmission of infection will be decreased.

V. ANIMAL MODELS OF HSV VACCINE DEVELOPMENT

Numerous animal models have been used to study the pathogenesis of HSV infections, especially latency, antiviral therapeutics, and vaccines. Potential HSV vaccines have been evaluated in rodents (mice, guinea pigs, rabbits, etc.) and subhuman primates. Selection of the animal model system for vaccine evaluation is relevant. The animal species, virus type, route of infection, state of immune competence, and specific viral challenge strain all influence disease pathogenesis and, synonymously, the evaluation of a vaccine. Disease progression alone can be selectively modulated by the specific strain of the animal selected. The route and site of inoculation of virus become especially important in distinguishing one disease state from another and its prevention.

When HSV-1 is inoculated by the ocular route, encephalitis (virulence) and/or latency ensue, as reviewed [66]. The eye route of infection has been best utilized to study latency. Endpoints of virulence and latency, however, have distinct differences for predicting human disease. Following ocular inoculation after corneal scarification, replication of virus in the eye peaks within 48 hr and declines over the next 6 days. Virus appears in the trigeminal ganglia approximately 1 day after inoculation with peak replication occurring between 4 and 6 days. Subsequently, if the inoculum of virus is large enough and/or a virulent strain of virus is used, brain infection follows invasion of the trigeminal ganglia. Fortunately, while the trigeminal ganglion is routinely infected following human eye infection [67,68], subsequent invasive brain infection is an exceedingly uncommon event, if ever having occurred.

Mice, particularly the hairless mouse [69], rabbits and guinea pigs with abraded or punctured skin have been used to study virus replication and pathogenesis of HSV-1, and to evaluate both antiviral therapies and vaccines. While in each model the nature of the lesions, their duration, and histopathology parallel human infection, there are notable differences, particularly the lack of recurrent lesions similar to those seen in people.

Type 2 genital infections have been studied best in the guinea pig model. Intravaginal inoculation of HSV into female Hartley guinea pigs appears the most predictive of all the animal models for human disease [70]. Reasons for these inconsistencies include endogenous host defenses, the artificial nature of infection, and viral strain differences. Moreover, these animals tend to suffer from continual recurrences of lesions; however, retrieval of HSV from these lesions is most variable. Models of life-threatening disease have been developed for both HSV-1 and -2. Intranasal inoculation of HSV-1 or -2 in young (3 weeks of age) Balb/c mice leads to central nervous system and visceral (usually lung) disease which may be predictive for neonatal HSV infection. However, inoculation of older mice with similar quantities of either virus may lead to no evidence of disease or, if so, encephalitis but certainly not overwhelming multiorgan disease. Direct intracerebral inoculation of virus is an unnatural route of infection even for the study of either antiviral therapeutics or vaccine efficacy.

Accurate and predictive models of human HSV encephalitis have been described in a rabbit model [71–73]. Virus is inoculated directly into the olfactory bulb or upon abraded nasal epithelium over nerves from the olfactory bulb; it can be traced along the olfactory tract to the anterior-frontal region of the rabbit brain where it causes focal infection, as compared to the diffuse pancortical infection which follows infection by the murine ocular route. The region of the rabbit brain involved correlates with the temporal lobe of humans. Immunosuppression following subclinical infection can result in focal reactivation [73].

Primate models have been utilized to study vaccines. These animals have been thought to more closely approximate that which is encountered in humans; however, the disease pathogenesis varies for each primate species. Specifically, the Aotus monkey (*Aotus trivirgatus* or *nancymani*) is exquisitely sensitive to HSV and, therefore, serves as a useful model for assessment of attenuated live vaccines but is, perhaps, less amenable to protection studies. The demonstration of safety in the Aotus model provides confidence of safety before introducing such a vaccine into humans [74]. In contrast, the owl monkey is far less susceptible to HSV and, therefore, may more closely resemble humans.

VI. HOST IMMUNE RESPONSES

A. Primary HSV Infection

Local control mechanisms of viral spread aim to neutralize the infectious agent and lead to viral clearance. Following primary HSV infection, the initial, local immunological responses involve both nonspecific defense mechanisms, namely, interferons (IFNs) alpha and beta, activated natural killer (NK) cells, and macrophages, as well as HSV-specific responses, such as cytotoxic T cells [75].

In response to a viral infection, the initial cellular response is synthesis and secretion of type I IFNs (alpha and beta). Interferons induce an antiviral state in infected and surrounding cells. The antiviral activity is modulated in part by IFN-mediated activation of cellular enzymes such as 2′–5′ oligoadenylate synthetase (2′–5′ AS) and double-stranded RNA-dependent protein kinase, as well as intracellular signaling molecules by activation of the JAK/STAT kinase pathway. More specific to HSV infection, IFN-α appears to inhibit immediate-early (IE) gene expression [76]. Thus the antiviral mechanism directly affects transactivation of the IE responsive element necessary for synthesis of viral proteins.

In addition to antiviral activity, IFNs are potent immunomodulators. As such, they mediate macrophage and NK cell activation, activate cytotoxic T cells (CTLs), induce MHC class I (in the case of IFN-α and IFN-β) or MHC class II (in the case of IFN-γ) antigens, stimulate cytokine secretion, and induce local inflammation. IFN-γ may aid the control of HSV infection. Evidence that γδ T cells, NK cells, CD4+ T cells, and possibly neurons produce IFN-γ and TNF in response to HSV infection in the nervous system has been reported. IFN-γ down regulates proliferation of CD4+ Th2 cells, responsible for inducing Ig isotype B-cell switching from IgA to IgG, thereby exerting a major effect on humoral immune responses [77].

NK cells lyse pathogen-infected cells before virus-specific T-cell immunity is generated and constitute a first line of defense against infection. In vitro and in vivo experiments have demonstrated that NK cells protect from HSV challenge in a murine model [78]. Severe herpetic disease has correlated with low in vitro NK activity in newborns, as well as in a patient lacking NK cells [79]. NK cell involvement is also supported by direct evidence of resolution of herpetic disease in humans. Other mononuclear cells, such as macrophages, are recruited to the site of infection and, upon activation, release immune cell mediators such as IFN-γ and interleukins. Macrophages play a major role in mediating antibody-dependent cellular toxicity for viral clearance and antigen presentation [80].

An important aspect of immune responses to HSV infections is the maturation of dendritic cells (DCs) at the site of infection. Mucosal immunity is generated by DCs, such as Langerhans cells (LCs), which contribute to disease resolution because of their antigen-presenting capacity to CTLs [81]. Langerhans cells migrate to the site of infection, where they process viral antigens for presentation to both naïve and primed T cells [82]. Langerhans cells produce IFNs and other cytokines, express MHC class II antigens, and interact closely with CTLs in genital mucosa.

As infection progresses, virus-specific immune responses are detected. On days 4 and 5 post infection, HSV-specific CD4+ Th1 lymphocytes are detected in genital lymph nodes and in smaller numbers in peripheral blood; they can subsequently be found in the genital mucosa [83].

Humoral immune responses rapidly follow initial HSV infection. The predominant mucosal antibodies are of the IgA isotype, being secreted by plasma cells. These antibodies can be detected as early as day 3 following infection, peaking within the first 6 weeks after disease onset, and are followed by the appearance of IgG1 and IgG3 subclasses of antibodies, which are typically found following viral infections. HSV-specific IgA antibodies are present for at least 6 weeks, gradually decreasing to undetectable levels. IgM-secreting B cells have also been detected in secretions of the female genital mucosa [84]. Shorter periods of viral shedding in women with primary genital herpes have been positively correlated with the presence of secretory IgA in vaginal secretions [78].

B. Recurrent HSV Infection

Although immunosuppression enhances the frequency of reactivation, there is no proof that the immune system exerts any influence on reactivation at the level of the ganglia [85]. Repeated subclinical episodes of HSV excretion may be a source of antigenic stimulation leading to long-term HSV-specific immune memory [80]. In recurrent HSV-2 infections,

NK and HSV-specific CD4+ cells are detected earlier than CD8+ cells in genital lesions [77]. CD4+ T cells, and more recently, CD8+ T cells have been highlighted as major mediators of viral clearance from mucocutaneous lesions in recurrent episodes [75,86,87]. Low IFN-γ titers in vesicle fluid have been associated with a shorter time to the next recurrence in patients with frequent recurrences. T-cell proliferation is decreased in these patients in comparison to patients with less frequent recurrences [80].

Inasmuch as the involvement of cytokines has been studied, IFN-γ has been reported to have a role in viral clearance from mucocutaneous sites, whereas altered cytokine production appears to correlate with recurrence [88].

As with primary HSV infection, a shorter duration of viral shedding occurs in women with recurrent genital herpes who have detectable secretory IgA in vaginal secretions [78]. IgA, IgG1, and IgG3 antibodies have been found in the sera of all patients with recurrent HSV-2 episodes, while IgM and IgG4 antibodies were detected in 70–80% of these patients. However, there does not appear to be a clear correlation between humoral immune responses and disease prognosis [89].

Table 1 summarizes the immune responses to primary versus recurrent herpes infection.

C. Persistence of Immune Responses

The host's immune responses persist and partially control HSV disease; recurrent episodes are generally less severe and of shorter duration over the years, perhaps due to progressive enhancement of long-term immunity [90]. Furthermore, some degree of cross-protection exists between HSV-1 and HSV-2. Additionally, newborns are partially protected by maternal antibodies [91]. Finally, HSV-specific T-cell infiltrates are detected in herpetic lesions during early disease resolution [75].

Studies indicate that persistent cell-mediated immune responses are more important than humoral immune responses in the resolution of HSV disease [92]. NK cells, macrophages, and T lymphocytes as well as cytokines such as IFN-α and IFN-γ, IL-2, and IL-12 all have central roles in resolving HSV disease [93]. HSV-specific CD4+ and CD8+ cells are detected in lesions from recurrent episodes, indicating their potential role in controlling HSV disease [75,86]. By contrast, agammaglobulinemic patients do not experience more severe or more frequent herpetic recurrences than the general population [94]. Furthermore, several vaccine trials have demonstrated that the presence of neutralizing antibodies to HSV glycoproteins does not provide protection against HSV infection or disease.

D. Correlation of Immune Response with Disease

Vaccine development, in general, requires the correlation of disease with host immune responses. The development of a vaccine to prevent HSV infections is no exception. Nevertheless, efforts to precisely incriminate that arm of the host response responsible for disease have remained elusive. Humoral immunity to HSV infection has been evaluated

Table 1

Primary infection

Local response

Early nonspecific response interferon (IFN)-α and IFN-β, natural killer (NK) cells, macrophages (3 to 4 hr after infection, appearance of viral glycoproteins as targets for ADCC). Mucosal dendritic cells are MHC class II antigen presenting cells, acting as antigen-presenting cells. Herpes simplex virus (HSV) infection induces maturation of these cells that produce high levels of type I IFN. From days 4 to 5: HSV-specific CD4$^+$ Th1 appear in genital lymph nodes, then in the genital mucosa. Cervical immunoglobulin A (IgA) antibodies to several HSV-2 glycoproteins and IgG responses follow.

Systemic response

From 2 weeks: detection of IgG to HSV glycoproteins in primary HSV-2 infected patients. IgA and IgG types of HSV-specific antibodies are maintained for at least 6 weeks. IgG responses increase in the first year after primary infection and are detected in all genital herpes patients.

Recurrent infection

Local response

Twelve to 24 hr after appearance of recurrent lesions: HSV-specific CD4$^+$ and CD8$^+$ cells, as well as macrophages are detected, with predominance of CD4$^+$ cells.

Systemic response

Frequent subclinical reactivations may maintain relatively high frequencies of HSV-specificity memory T cells. CD8$^+$ cells have been recently proposed as being a critical component in recurrent disease resolution.

Source: From Ref. 275.

exhaustively in disease pathogenesis. Polyclonal antibodies have been used to alter disease lethality, particularly in the newborn mouse or to limit progression of both neurologic and ocular disease [95–99]. Monoclonal antibodies to selected specific infected cell polypeptides, especially the envelope glycoproteins gB and gD, confer protection from lethality [100–102]. Importantly, gD2 is a known target of neutralizing antibodies, antibody-dependent cell-mediated cytotoxicity, and CD4 and CD8 T-cell-mediated responses [103–106]. As a consequence, this antigen has been a prime component of subunit vaccines.

Efforts to correlate the frequency recurrences with immune responses have failed to identify any specific humoral response to specified polypeptides [92,107,108]. Thus further efforts focused, in large part, on cell-mediated immune responses. As noted, lymphocyte blastogenetic responses are demonstrable within 4 to 6 weeks after the onset of infection and sometimes as early as 2 weeks [109–116]. With recurrences, boosts in blastogenic responses occur; however, these responses, as after primary infection, decrease with time. Nonspecific blastogenic responses do not correlate with a history of recurrences. HSV-1 and -2 are cross-reactive in these assays.

Lymphokine production has been incriminated in the pathogenesis of frequently recurrent genital and labial HSV infection. Notably, several investigators have recognized a decrease in both gamma interferon production and natural killer cells during disease prodrome [117–119]. Nevertheless, there are no reproducible data from selected populations to confirm these observations. The relevance of lymphokine expression in vaccine development can be assessed only in prospective field trials.

Host response of the newborn to HSV must be defined separately from that of older individuals. Immaturity of host

defense mechanisms is a cause of the increased severity of some infectious agents in the fetus and the newborn. Factors that must be considered in defining the host response of the newborn include also the mode of transmission of the agent (viremia versus mucocutaneous infection without blood-borne spread), time of acquisition of infection, and the potential of increased virulence of certain strains, although this last point remains purely speculative. Two broad issues are of relevance; these are protection of the fetus by transplacental antibodies and definition of host responses of the newborn. Transplacentally acquired neutralizing antibodies either prevent or ameliorate infection in exposed newborns as do antibody-dependent cell-mediated cytotoxicity [120–122]. Importantly, pre-existing antibodies, indicative of prior infection, significantly decrease the transmission of infection from pregnant women to their offspring [123]. This observation provides a strong rationale for the development of an HSV vaccine.

Humoral IgG and IgM responses have been well characterized. Infected newborns produce IgM antibodies specific for HSV, as detected by immunofluorescence, within the first 3 weeks of infection. These antibodies increase rapidly in titer during the first 2 to 3 months, and they may be detectable for as long as 1 year after infection. The most reactive immunodeterminants are the surface viral glycoproteins, particularly gD. Humoral antibody responses have been studied using contemporary immunoblot technology and the patterns of response are similar to those encountered in adults with primary infection [116,124]. The quantity of neutralizing antibodies is lower in babies with disseminated infection [116,121].

Cellular immunity has been considered to be important in the host response of the newborn. The T-lymphocyte proliferative response to HSV infections is delayed in newborns compared to older individuals [116]. Most infants studied in a recent evaluation had no detectable T-lymphocyte responses to HSV 2 to 4 weeks after the onset of clinical symptoms [111,116,125]. The correlation between these delayed responses may be of significance in evaluating the outcome to neonatal HSV infection. Specifically, if the response to T-lymphocyte antigens in children who have disease localized to the skin, eye, or mouth at the onset of disease is significantly delayed, disease progression may occur at a much higher frequency than babies with a more appropriate response [116,126].

Infected newborns have decreased production of IFN-α in response to HSV when compared to adults with primary HSV infection [116] The importance of the IFN generation on the maturation of host responses, particularly the elicitation of NK-cell responses, remains to be defined [127,128] Lymphocytes from infected babies have decreased responses to IFN-γ during the first month of life [116,128,129]. These data taken together would indicate that the newborn has a poorer immune response than older children and adults. Antibodies plus complement and antibodies mixed with killer lymphocytes, monocytes, macrophages, or polymorphonuclear leukocytes will lyse HSV-infected cells in vitro [130]. Antibody-dependent cell-mediated cytotoxicity has been demonstrated to be an important component of the development of host immunity to infection [131]. However, the total population of killer lymphocytes of the newborn seems to be lower than that found in older individuals, and monocytes and macrophages of newborns are not as active as those of adults [132–137]. These findings are supported by animal model data.

VII. CRITERIA FOR EVALUATION OF HUMAN HERPESVIRUS VACCINES

The development of an efficacious HSV vaccine is very much needed as best defined by disease burden. In the United States alone, over 100 million individuals are infected by HSV-1 and at least 40 to 60 million individuals have been infected by HSV-2. Annually, a minimum of 2500 cases of neonatal herpes and 3000 cases of herpes simplex encephalitis results in significant morbidity and mortality despite efficacious antiviral therapy. Furthermore, because HSV results in genital ulcerative disease, the risk of acquisition of human immunodeficiency virus (HIV) is significantly increased [138].

An ideal vaccine should induce immune responses adequate to prevent infection. If primary infection was prevented, the colonization of the sensory ganglia would not occur and, therefore, no source of virus for either subsequent recurrences or transmission would exist. No one knows today if such ideal objectives can be met. In fact, it is open to discussion whether the criteria of success for candidate vaccines should be one or any combination of the following effects: abrogation or mitigation of primary clinical episodes, prevention of the colonization of the ganglia, suppression or reduction of the frequency and/or of the severity of recurrences, reduction of the shedding (duration and/or quantity) of the virus during primary, recurrent episodes, reduction of asymptomatic shedding (frequency, duration,

quantity), and/or prevention of person-to-person transmission (either vertical or horizontal). These issues must be weighed in the context of the age of the target population, the duration of the desired results. Arguably, fundamental to a successful vaccine is the last point—namely, its ability to prevent person-to-person transmission in order to interrupt the ongoing HSV epidemic. To illustrate the difficulty of achieving such an end, overt clinical recurrences may only be apparent in approximately 20% of HSV-infected individuals, resulting in a large reservoir of unknowingly infected individuals who may intermittently excrete virus in the absence of symptoms and transmit it to intimate partners. Further complicating the issue, HSV DNA has been detected by polymerase chain reaction (PCR) in the genital secretions of women without either lesions or evidence of infectious virus [139], usually threefold more frequently than infectious virus. Subsequent person-to-person transmission has been documented from infected mothers to their newborns. The persistent detection of HSV DNA implies that HSV is a more chronic infection than previously thought and a more difficult vaccine target.

Prospective clinical trials, a time consuming and expensive exercise, will be required to appropriately define the true utility of an HSV vaccine. For these reasons, it is of the utmost importance to determine which factors are protective against HSV infection (humoral versus cell-mediated immunity, local immunity versus systemic immunity, antibody-dependent cell-mediated cytotoxicity versus cytotoxic T cells) such that markers can be developed to expedite the evaluation of vaccines in humans [74].

The rationale for an HSV vaccine is threefold. First, exogenous re-infection is exceedingly uncommon in the immune competent host. Second, many more individuals are infected by HSV than experience either clinical recurrences or shed virus. Finally, transplacental antibodies significantly decrease the risk of infection in the newborn exposed to HSV at the time of delivery. Taken together, these facts strongly suggest that a properly designed vaccine could be efficacious.

VIII. HERPES SIMPLEX VIRUS VACCINE DEVELOPMENT

Two of the more promising HSV vaccines represent entirely different theoretical approaches. The first is based on either microorganisms or cell lines producing gB or gD2 for use as subunit vaccines in combination with an adjuvant. The second is a genetically engineered live, attenuated vaccine from which putative neurovirulence sequences have been removed. Each of these approaches has been evaluated extensively in animal model studies and to varying extents in human investigations. While these vaccines are exciting, much prior effort has been devoted to vaccine development. These latter studies will be reviewed first.

Extrapolating protection from animal model systems to humans has not been possible because there are no markers of protection comparable to neutralizing antibodies for other viral diseases [140–147]. While initial HSV vaccine efforts were oriented toward the prevention of recurrent infections and, therefore, were considered therapeutic vaccines, more recent efforts have been devoted to the prevention of infection following exposure to an infected partner.

The approaches to HSV vaccine development include the utilization of 1) wild-type virus; 2) inactivated or killed virus; 3) subunit vaccines; and 4) genetically engineered vaccines.

A. Wild-Type Virus

Numerous clinicians attempted to alter the pattern of recurrences by inoculation of autologous virus, of virus from another infected individual or, in one set of experiments, of virus recovered from an experimentally infected rabbit [148–150]. The consequences were obvious with lesions appearing at the site of inoculation in as many as 40% to 80% of volunteers [151–153]. Despite the appearance of lesions and the evaluation of only a very limited number of patients, the efficacy of such an approach was reported in the literature. Furthermore, these studies failed to utilize controls [153–155]. In some cases, inoculation led to recurrences [149,150, 156,157]. In large part, live viruses were abandoned on the grounds that many patients did not develop lesions at the site of inoculation and, therefore, it was not perceived that the patient had an "adequate take" [158–160]. At the present time, inoculation of either autologous or heterologous virus is unacceptable.

B. Inactivated (or Killed) Virus

Killed virus vaccines have been studied in a variety of animal model systems, often with good results, as reviewed [161–163]. Unfortunately, when these vaccines were administered to HSV-infected individuals to alleviate recurrences, most studies failed to include an appropriate control group. Under such circumstances, significant bias was introduced because patients may experience 30% to 70% decrease in the frequency of recurrences as well as improvement in severity, simply from having received placebo [164–169].

The initial inactivated vaccines were derived from phenol-treated infected animal tissues [158–160]. Because of the possibility that administration of animal proteins might lead to demyelination, these vaccines did not attract much biomedical attention. Instead, ultraviolet light inactivation of purified virus derived from tissue culture replaced phenol inactivation. Over the past two decades, numerous reports in the literature suggested either the success or failure of these approaches. As reviewed [162], viral antigen obtained from amniotic or allantoic fluid, chorioallantoic membranes, chick cell cultures, sheep kidney cells, rabbit kidney cells and inactivated either by formalin, ultraviolet light, or heat led to a series of vaccine studies in thousands of patients [164, 170–193]. With one exception [170], each of these studies reported significant improvement in as many as 60% to 80% of patients [184–186,192].

As these studies progressed several important observations were made. First, despite repeated inoculations, antibody titers (as measured by neutralization or complement fixation) remained unchanged in the majority of patients [173,180,194] or only demonstrated slight increases [171,

191]. Second, while these efforts reported few side effects, some authors noted concern that, in patients with keratitis, autoimmune phenomena might make the herpetic disease worse [181,189,195–197]. Placebo-controlled studies utilizing inactivated vaccines were few, as reviewed [168,197–199]. The results were widely discrepant, even when the same vaccine was utilized, a finding most discouraging. A conclusion from these investigations was that there may be some initial benefit for patients with recurrent infection; however, long-term benefit could not be established. The only prospective study of prevention of HSV infections by vaccination was performed by Anderson et al. in children of an orphanage [199]. In this study 10 children received vaccine and 10 the placebo; yet, HSV stomatitis developed in an equal number of patients on long-term follow-up.

C. Subunit Vaccines

Subunit vaccines evolved out of attempts to remove viral DNA and eliminate the potential for cellular transformation, to enhance antigenic concentration and induce a stronger immunity, and, finally, to exclude any possibility of residual live virus contamination [200]. Available subunit vaccines have been prepared from a variety of methods combining antigen extraction from infected cell lysates by detergent and subsequent purification. The immunogenicity of vaccines derived from all of the envelope glycoproteins, free of viral DNA, has been demonstrated in animals [62, 201–203]. The results of studies in humans are conflicting. While one vaccine was reported to decrease recurrences in infected patients, the study design did not employ a placebo control [204]; thus no conclusions of efficacy can be drawn. Vaccination with envelope glycoproteins does not protect uninfected sexual partners of individuals with genital HSV infection [205,206].

More recently, specific subunit vaccines have arisen out of the cloning of specific glycoproteins in either yeast or Chinese hamster ovary cell systems [166,207,208], as well as by other methods [209–211].

Subunit vaccines have been studied in a variety of animal model systems including mice [212–218], guinea pigs [219–224], and rabbits [225]. Neutralizing antibodies can be detected in these systems in varying amounts, and in some systems ELISA antibodies as well [226]. In these systems the quantity of neutralizing antibody correlated with the degree of protection upon challenge. Challenge in the experimental systems has been studied in mice [212–215,218,226–228], rabbits [225,229–231], and guinea pigs [219,221,222,231]. Each of these systems utilized a variety of different routes of challenge as well as dosages. Challenge included skin, lip abrasion, intravaginal inoculation, intradermal ear pinna inoculation, intradermal injection, foot pad challenge, intraperitoneal, ocular, or subcutaneous. Thus interpretation of these results is extremely difficult. While there are many conflicting animal model studies, in general, the subunit vaccines elicited a degree of protection as evidenced by amelioration of morbidity and reduction in mortality in the immunized animals. Nevertheless, several injections were required to induce protection and must include adjuvant as well. The necessity for an appropriate adjuvant has been recently emphasized [232,233]. Protection in the rodent is significantly easier than in higher primate species. This may be especially the case as the HSV is not indigenous to rodent species and, thus, protection studies may be totally irrelevant when evaluating human responses.

Vaccination of primates, specifically rhesus monkeys [225], chimpanzee [201,225], and cebus monkeys [228] can induce neutralizing antibodies, leading to an amnestic response following subsequent injection months later. The significance of the protection in these animals remains unclear for human experimentation.

Subunit vaccines have been evaluated in humans. Both HSV-1 and -2 antigens have been prepared in human diploid cells, Chinese hamster ovary cells, and chicken embryo fibroblasts for vaccine purposes. Several studies have reported evidence of improvement [204,234,235]. Other studies suggested very little benefit [201,205,206].

Several human subunit vaccine trials have now been completed. One of the earliest human vaccine experiences was with an early Merck Sharpe and Dohme [228] glycoprotein envelope subunit vaccine [205,206,236]. This vaccine was produced by purification of the envelope glycoproteins. In a Phase IIA study, carried out in sexual partners of patients known to have genital herpes, the number of individuals developing herpetic infection was nearly equal between placebo and vaccine recipients; thus vaccination failed to provide any benefit at all.

More recently, a series of clinical trials have evaluated the Chiron Corporation gB2 and gD2 and SmithKline Beecham gD2 subunit vaccines in humans. Both vaccines incorporated either a single glycoprotein or both in combination with adjuvants unique to each company. From a developmental perspective, important lessons were learned. Extensive rodent experiments, utilizing the guinea pig and murine genital herpes models demonstrated that either combined gB and gD or gD-2, with a Freund's adjuvant, completely protected against both primary and spontaneous recurrent disease following intravaginal viral inoculation [221]. However, complete Freund's adjuvant is not acceptable for human administration. Thus alternative adjuvants were explored, including Chiron Corporation MF59 and a proprietary SmithKline Beecham adjuvant. Both afforded a high level of protection from HSV disease [208,232]. An important finding from these preclinical studies was that the quantity of neutralizing antibody elicited by immunization and the total HSV antibody titer (as measured by ELISA) were higher after vaccination than following natural infection and, furthermore, that these antibody titers correlated with protection from disease [221,237].

Data from the largest series of vaccinated individuals with the Chiron Corporation construct failed to demonstrate significant long-term prevention of infection in susceptible sexual partners, although initial benefit was apparent for the first 5 months [238]. In this trial, there was a 50% reduction in the rate of infection among HSV seronegative women during this short window. The overall efficacy of the vaccine for 1 year following a 6-month vaccination period was 9%. The vaccine had no *apparent* effect on the frequency of recurrences [239]. No further vaccine studies are planned for this construct. Of note, the

adjuvant for these studies was MF59, a potent inducer of Th-2 responses.

Another series of clinical trials utilizing gD2 [SmithKline Beecham (now Glaxo SmithKline)] have been reported. Here, the adjuvant was alum plus monophosphoryl lipid A, a potent inducer of Th-1 responses. In these studies, women who were seronegative for both HSV-1 and -2 were protected from both disease (72% efficacy) and infection (43% efficacy). However, in individuals seropositive for HSV-1, irrespective of sex, and seronegative men, no significant clinical benefit could be demonstrated. Thus the two Phase III efficacy studies suggest that the GSK candidate genital herpes vaccine (gD/Alum/MPL) may be effective in preventing HSV-1 or -2 genital herpes disease in a subset of volunteers, i.e., women who were HSV-1 and -2 seronegative (HSV1-/2-) prior to vaccination. However, these studies were neither designed nor powered to assess efficacy in HSV1-/2- exclusively in women and therefore did not meet their primary endpoints of overall efficacy. Consequently, a double-blind, randomized, controlled Phase III study is currently planned to assess the prophylactic efficacy of gD/Alum/MPL vaccine in the prevention of genital herpes disease in young HSV1-/2- sexually active women.

D. Live Vaccines

Live vaccines, in general, are considered preferable to killed or subunit vaccines because they are more likely to induce a broad range of immune responses to the expressed gene products and, therefore, provide a high level of protection as has been the case with numerous viral pathogens such as measles, mumps, and rubella. Furthermore, as these vaccines replicate in the recipient, the resulting immunity should be longer lasting. Moreover, they usually require smaller doses of antigen and, therefore, should be more economical. Several approaches to live virus vaccines have been attempted. These include HSV mutants, heterologous herpesviruses, antigens expressed in non-HSV viral vectors, and genetically engineered viruses.

1. Herpes Simplex Virus Mutants

It was recognized very early in biologic laboratory investigations that virulence varied significantly among wild-type HSV isolates. Conceivably, one could use the least virulent wild-type HSV as a vaccine, but reversion from nonpathogenic to pathogenic strains easily occurs following serial passages either in cell culture or animal hosts. This lack of genetic stability is unacceptable for potential human vaccines [237,240].

2. Heterologous Herpesvirus Vaccines

While considered for other herpesvirus infections, such as Marek's disease, the utilization of heterologous herpesvirus for humans is considered untenable medically or ethically.

3. Antigens Expressed in Live, Non-HSV Vectors

Vaccinia virus has been proposed as a vector for delivering antigens to animals or humans [241]. The principle of inserting foreign genes into a vaccinia vector has been exploited for the expression of the gD and gB genes of HSV [242–248]. Significant concern has been raised over the utilization of vaccinia as a vector for delivering foreign antigens. In large part this concern stems from the occurrence of vaccinia gangrenosum and disseminated vaccinia in individuals who were vaccinated to prevent smallpox. As such, this major concern for adverse effects has led to decreased interest in utilizing vaccinia as a vector in the prevention of HSV, although this virus has become of increased importance with the threat of bioterrorism. Furthermore, immune memory in individuals who have previously received vaccinia may prevent recognition of any foreign gene insert. Likely, the use of canary pox as a vector will be attempted.

Adenoviruses have also been proposed as expression vectors, on the grounds that they might be safer than vaccinia [249].

4. Genetically Engineered Herpes Simplex Viruses

Molecular biology makes it possible to modify, almost at will, the genome of large DNA viruses and construct genetically engineered attenuated live viruses [40]. Utilizing the technology developed by Post and Roizman [250,251], recombinant HSVs were constructed as a prototype of HSV vaccines [252]. These vaccines were engineered with the objective that they should be attenuated, whether for primary inoculation or potential reactivation of latent virus; protect against HSV-1 or HSV-2 infections; provide serological markers of immunization distinct from wild-type infections; and serve as vectors to express immunogens of other human pathogens.

The construction of these viruses was based on the use of an HSV-1 [HSV-1(F)] as a backbone. The genome was deleted in the domain of the viral thymidine kinase (TK) gene and in the junction region between the unique long and short sequences in order to excise some of the genetic loci responsible for neurovirulence and to create convenient sites and space within the genome for insertion of other genes. Last, an HSV-2 DNA fragment encoding the HSV-2 glycoproteins D, G, and I was inserted in place of the internal inverted repeat. The purpose of type 2 genes was to broaden the spectrum of the immune response and to create a chimeric pattern of antibody specificities as a serological marker of vaccination. The resulting recombinant, designated as R7017, had no TK activity and, therefore, would be resistant to acyclovir. Therefore another recombinant was created, designated R7020, by insertion of the TK gene next to the HSV-2 DNA fragment. As this virus expresses TK, it is susceptible to antiviral chemotherapy with acyclovir. When analyzed by restriction enzyme digestion, the DNA of the recombinants shows typical patterns which enable their unambiguous identification.

When evaluated in rodent models, the two constructs appeared considerably attenuated in their pathogenicity and ability to establish latency and were capable of inducing protective immunity. The recombinants did not regain virulence, nor did they change DNA restriction enzyme cleavage patterns when subjected serial passages in the mouse brain [252]. It is remarkable that the TK deleted virus R7017 behaved similarly to the TK expressing virus R7020, be-

cause the deletion of this gene was thought to attenuate the virus.

These results were corroborated by studies in owl monkeys (*Aotus trivirgatus*) [253]. While 100 PFU of wild-type viruses administered by peripheral routes was fatal to the monkeys, recombinants given by various routes in amounts at least 10^5-fold greater were innocuous or produced mild infections, even in the presence of immunosuppression by total lymphoid irradiation [252].

Unfortunately, human studies with this vaccine were disappointing. The maximum dose of vaccine administered was 10^5 PFU which elicited only mild immunogenicity even with the administration of two doses [253]. In many respects, the R7020 construct was overly attenuated. However, as noted below, this virus is now being studied for gene therapy of adenocarcinoma metastases from the colon to the liver. Regardless, these same principles of genetic engineering have been applied to newer generation of newer constructs. The recent identification of a neurovirulence gene, identified as $\gamma_1 34.5$, provided a marker for genetic engineering [254]. The deletion of the two copies of this gene and genes $U_L 55$ and 56, genes associated with nuclear associated proteins, results in an attenuated candidate vaccine that is currently undergoing evaluation in animal models. Importantly, engineered viruses have been evaluated for gene therapy of malignancy and, therefore, can also be assessed for the ability to induce host immune responses.

An alternative strategy for attenuation is under investigation by Knipe and colleagues.

5. Genetically Engineered Replication Attenuated HSV

Background. Genetically engineered HSV have mainly been assessed for the treatment of human glioblastoma multiforme. These constructs have included mutations in the viral genes thymidine kinase, DNA polymerase, ribonucleotide reductase, and $\gamma_1 34.5$ [255–261]. Each of these studies sought to optimize the therapeutic index in the treatment of gliomas by exploring therapies with different types of genetically engineered HSV constructs. While virtually any alteration of HSV ameliorates neurovirulence, only the deletions in the $\gamma_1 34.5$ gene consistently demonstrate safety and efficacy in animal models. Tumoricidal effects in vitro and in vivo in multiple glioma models (mouse, rat, and human glioma cell lines, human glioma explants) are demonstrable. In vivo models include tumor reduction in subrenal capsule and flank subcutaneous implants but, more importantly, increased survival and some tumor cures in intracranial implant models. These effects are reproducible in vivo for both immune deficient animals (nude, *scid* mice) [255,256,260,261] as well as immune competent models (rats and mice) [258,259,262–264].

Animal Model Studies. Studies in animal models of gliomas of various constructs of HSV (engineered viruses deleted in $\gamma_1 34.5$) have been performed. These studies demonstrate the following principles: 1) the time course of infection (quantitative virology and PCR) represents impaired replication with limited spread of virus across the brain using marker genes (*lacZ* under an ICP6 promoter) with HSV antibody staining [258,259,263,265]; 2) two selected mutations appear to avoid second-site mutations with reversion to wild-type phenotype ($\gamma_1$34.5 and ribonucleotide reductase deletions) [266]; 3) the retention of the native HSV TK allows for acyclovir susceptibility [261]; 4) the safety of these constructs was established in susceptible primates (*Aotus*) [266]; and 5) HSV could be used in successful vector genes [264,267,268], as reviewed [269].

Indeed, one construct, namely, G207 [255], demonstrated an adequate safety profile in both cell culture as well as in animal models [270,271] and was efficacious in several tumor models in vivo [255–261]. This candidate therapeutic is deleted in both copies of the $\gamma_1$34.5 gene as well as ribonucleotide reductase. Sufficient quantities of virus were produced under GMP conditions in a Phase I study in humans with recurrent glioblastomas, as described below.

Numerous other constructs have been developed, including cytokine/chemokine genes, enzymes, and receptors [272]. These constructs will be detailed below in the description of our accomplishments. However, other investigators have taken the approach of altering host recognition of HSV by deleting the α-47 gene and, thereby, avoiding host MHC-I processing. The potential utility of this approach remains to be established.

Clinical Experience with Intratumoral HSV in Glioma Patients. The leading genetically engineered HSV candidate for the treatment of glioblastomas is G207, a conditionally replicating HSV mutant, as described above. G207 was evaluated in a Phase I safety trial for patients with recurrent malignant gliomas, failing standard therapy, and with a lesion greater than 1 cm in diameter [273]. A total of 21 patients were recruited and received escalating doses of G207, beginning at 1×10^6 and in cohorts of three to a final dose of 3×10^9 PFU at five intratumoral sites. While adverse events were noted in several patients, no toxicity or adverse event was unequivocally ascribed to G207 administration. Importantly, no patient developed herpes simplex encephalitis. Host seroconversion to HSV was documented in one of five seronegative volunteers. Two volunteers have survived greater than 3 years with stable Kornofsky scores. These data provide the basis for a Phase I B and II clinical trials, recently approved by the FDA, for further dose escalation after tumor debridement or administration of concomitant radiotherapy.

An HSV deleted in both copies of the $\gamma_1$34.5 gene, mutant 1716, and expressing *lacZ* under the control of the latency associated transcript was studied in Scotland in a similar population. In this trial, a total of nine patients were evaluated at one of three doses of virus, beginning at 1×10^3 and escalating by a factor of 10 to 1×10^5 [274]. As in the U.S. study, there were no reports of significant adverse events directly attributable to virus administration. Four of the nine patients were alive 14–24 months after injection. Of note, the maximum amount of virus administered in this trial was four logs lower than that of the study performed in the United States. These promising studies have led to Phase II trials in both the United States and the United Kingdom.

Although the two trials utilized different genetically engineered constructs and doses of virus for administration, the demonstration of safety following intratumoral inocula-

tion is truly remarkable and paves the way for the evaluation of genetically engineered HSV in Phase II trials. Importantly, future studies should address the extent and magnitude of viral replication in the tumor as well as the host response in much more detail.

Follow-Up Investigations. In studies in Europe and the United States, Phase II investigations of genetically engineered HSV for the treatment of brain tumors are currently in progress. Second-generation constructs that express the cytokine IL-12 will be in human investigations in the immediate future. This later construct will assuredly induce an enhanced effect within the tumor bed. Such studies will provide the groundwork for using a similar construct as a vaccine to prevent HSV infections.

IX. CONCLUSION

Within the last several years focused efforts on developing vaccines for HSV infections as well as gene therapy have led to creative potential candidates. These vaccines have entered human investigations. These studies should indicate the potential efficacy of these vaccines. We have learned for example that seronegative individuals at high-risk for infection represent ideal candidates for participation in vaccine trials, while individuals with frequent recurrences probably do not offer the opportunity for complete suppression of symptomatic disease. As a consequence, vaccination should be scheduled for a time prior to exposure of the offending pathogen. For a vaccine designed to prevent HSV-2 infections, this would be early in adolescence prior to the onset of sexual activity.

Adequate methodology has not always been applied to previously performed evaluations of HSV vaccines. The current and future studies are to be randomized, double-blind, placebo-controlled, with a sufficient number of volunteers for appropriate statistical analyses to comply with proper trial drugs. Interim analyses predicated on results obtained during the performance of the trial will guarantee the ethical nature of the trial design. After enrollment into a prospective clinical trial, the diversity of clinical HSV diseases, the lack of predictability of patterns of recurrence, will mandate a very careful prospective evaluation for both symptomatic and asymptomatic evidence of infection in vaccine recipients, including the use of PCR. On both clinical and laboratory levels, detailed evaluations will have to determine the presence or absence of subsequent wild-type infection.

Nevertheless, the intellectual and scientific challenges posed by the development of a vaccine to prevent HSV infections are extremely rewarding. Hopefully, within the next several years the results of excellent clinical trials will help establish the value or failure of such an approach.

ACKNOWLEDGMENT

Studies performed by the author and herein reported were initiated and supported under a contract (NO1-AI-65306, NO1-AI-15113, NO1-AI-62554) with the Development and

Applications Branch of the National Institute of Allergy and Infectious Diseases (NIAID), a Program Project Grant (PO1 AI 24009), by grants from the General Clinical Research Center Program (RR-032) and the State of Alabama.

REFERENCES

1. Roizman B, Sears AE. Herpes simplex viruses and their replication. In: Fields BN, Knipe DM, Howley PM, Chanock RM, Melnick JL, Monath TP, Roizman B, Straus SE, eds. Fields Virology. Philadelphia: Lippincott-Raven Publishers, 1996:2231–2295.
2. Elion GB, et al. Selectivity of action of an antiherpetic agent, 9-(2-hydroxyethoxymethyl) guanine. Proc Natl Acad Sci USA 1977; 74:5716–5720.
3. Schaeffer HJ, et al. 9-(2-hydroxyethoxymethyl) guanine activity against viruses of the herpes group. Nature 1978; 272:583–585.
4. Wildy P. Herpes: History and classification. In: Kaplan AS, ed. The Herpesviruses. New York: Academic Press, 1973:1–25.
5. Beswick TS. The origin and the use of the word herpes. Med Hist 1962; 6:214.
6. Nahmias AJ, Dowdle WR. Antigenic and biologic differences in herpesvirus hominis. Prog Med Virol 1968; 10:110–159.
7. Whitley RJ. Herpes simplex virus. In: Knipe DM, Howley RM, Grriffin D, Lamb R, Martin M, Straus SE, eds. Fields Virology. 4th ed. New York: Lippincott Williams and Wilkins, 2001:2461–2509.
8. Mettler C. History of Medicine. Hill (Blakiston), New York: McGraw, 1947.
9. Hutfield DC. History of herpes genitalis. Br J Vener Dis 1966; 42:263–268.
10. Unna PG. The Histopathology of the Diseases of the Skin. In: Clay WF, ed. New York: MacMillan, Co., 1886. Walker N, Translator.
11. Lowenstein A. Aetiologische untersuchugen uber den fieberhaften, herpes. Munch Med Wochenschr 1919; 66:769–770.
12. Gruter W. Experimentelle und Klinische untersuchungen uber den sogenannten herpes comea. Ber Dtsch Ophthalmol Ges 1920; 42:162.
13. Doerr R. Sitzungs berichte der gesellschaft der schweizerischen. Klin Monatsbl Augenheilkd 1920; 65:104.
14. Nahmias AJ, Roizman B. Infection with herpes simplex viruses 1 and 2. N Engl J Med 1973; 289:667–674, 719–725, 781–789.
15. Corey L, Spear P. Infections with herpes simplex viruses. N Engl J Med 1986; 314:686–691.
16. Naib ZM, et al. Relation of cytohistopathology of genital herpesvirus infection to cervical anaplasia. Cancer 1973; 33:1452–1463.
17. Andrews CH, Carmichael EA. A note on the presence of antibodies to herpesvirus in post-encephalitic and other human sera. Lancet 1930; 1:857–858.
18. Dodd K, et al. Herpetic stomatitis. J Pediatr 1938; 12:95.
19. Burnet FM, Williams SW. Herpes simplex: New point of view. Med J Aust 1939; 1:637–640.
20. Seidenberg S. Zur Aetiologic det Pustulosis vacciniformis acuta. Schweiz Z Pathol Bakteriol 1941; 4:398.
21. Gallardo E. Primary herpes simplex keratitis: clinical and experimental study. Arch Ophthalmol 1943; 30:217.
22. Smith MG, et al. Isolation of the virus of herpes simplex and the demonstration of intranuclear inclusions in a case of acute encephalitis. Am J Pathol 1941; 17:55–68.
23. Lipschutz B. Untersuchugen uber die atiologie der krakheiten der herpesgruppe (herpes zoster, herpes genitalis, and herpes febrilis). Arch Dermatol Syph 1921; 136:428–482.
24. Plummer G. Serological comparison of the herpesviruses. Br J Exp Pathol 1964; 45:135.
25. Schneweis KE, Nahmias AJ. Antigens of herpes simplex virus types 1 and 2—Immunodiffusion and inhibition passive hemagglutination studies. Z Immunitaetsforsch Exp Klin Immunol 1971; 141:471–487.
26. Whitley RJ, et al. Adenine arabinoside therapy of biopsy proved herpes simplex encephalitis: National Institute of Allergy and Infectious Diseases Collaborative Antiviral Study. N Engl J Med 1977; 297:289–294.
27. Corey L, et al. A trial of topical acyclovir in genital herpes simplex virus infections. N Engl J Med 1982; 306:1313–1319.
28. Bryson YJ, et al. Treatment of first episodes of genital herpes simplex virus infection with oral acyclovir: A randomized double-blind controlled trial in normal subjects. N Engl J Med 1983; 308:916–921.
29. Corey L, et al. Intravenous acyclovir for the treatment of primary genital herpes. Ann Intern Med 1983; 98:914–921.
30. Corey L, et al. Treatment of primary first episode genital herpes simplex virus infections with acyclovir: Results of topical, intravenous, and oral therapy. J Antimicrob Chemother 1983; 12:79–88.
31. Saral R, et al. Acyclovir prophylaxis of herpes simplex virus infections: a randomized, double-blind, controlled trial in bone-marrow-transplant recipients. N Engl J Med 1981; 305:63–67.
32. Meyers JD, et al. Multicenter collaborative trial of intravenous acyclovir for treatment of mucocutaneous herpes simplex virus infection in immunocompromised host. Ann J Med 1982; 73:229–235.
33. Whitley RJ, et al. Vidarabine therapy of neonatal herpes simplex virus infection. Pediatrics 1980; 66:495–501.
34. Whitley RJ. Approaches to therapy of viral infections. In: Barness L, ed. Advances in Pediatrics. Vol. 34. Illinois: Year Book Medical Publishers, 1987:89–110.
35. Dorsky DI, Crumpacker CS. Drugs five years later: acyclovir. Ann Intern Med 1987; 107:859–874.
36. Goldsmith S, Whitley RJ. Antiviral therapy. In: Gorbach SL, Bartlett JG, Blacklow NR, eds. Infectious Diseases in Medicine and Surgery. Philadelphia: W.B. Saunders Company, 1991:288–306.
37. Buchman TG, et al. Restriction endonuclease fingerprinting of herpes simplex DNA: A novel epidemiological tool applied to a nosocomial outbreak. J Infect Dis 1978; 138:488–498.
38. Roizman B, et al. Identification and preliminary mapping with monoclonal antibodies of a herpes simplex virus 2 glycoprotein lacking a known type 1 counterpart. Virology 1984; 133:242–247.
39. Johnson RE, et al. A semi epidemiologic survey of the prevalence of herpes simplex virus type 2 infection in the United States. N Engl J Med 1989; 321:7–12.
40. Roizman B, Jenkins FJ. Genetic engineering of novel genomes of large DNA viruses. Science 1985; 229:1208–1214.
41. Nahmias A, Norrid B. Herpes simplex viruses 1 and 2: Basic and clinical aspects. Dis-Mon 1979; 25:1–49.
42. Roizman B. The organization of herpes simplex virus genomes. Annu Rev Genet 1979; 13:25–57.
43. Hayward GS, et al. Anatomy of herpes simplex virus DNA. Evidence for four populations of molecules that differ in the relative orientations of their long and short components. Proc Natl Acad Sci USA 1975; 72:4243–4247.
44. Frenkel N, et al. Isolation of a new herpesvirus from human $CD4^+$ T cells. Proc Natl Acad Sci USA 1990; 87:748–752.
45. Roizman B, Furlong D. The replication of herpesviruses. In:

Fraenkel-Conrat H, Wagner RR, eds. Comprehensive Virology. Vol. 3. New York: Plenum Publishing, 1974:229–403.

46. Honess RW, Roizman B. Regulation of herpesvirus macromolecular synthesis. Cascade regulation of the synthesis of three groups of viral proteins. J Virol 1974; 14:8–19.

47. Wagner EK. Individual HSV transcript: Characterization of specific genes. In: Roizman B, ed. The Herpesviruses. Vol. 3. New York: Plenum Publishing Company, 1985:45.

48. Kristie TM, Roizman B. The binding of the major regulatory protein, alpha 4 to the promoter-regulatory domains of herpes simplex virus 1 genes. Proceedings from the UCLA/ICN Symposium on Transcriptional Regulation. New York: Alan R. Liss, Inc., 1986:415–422.

49. Spear PG. Glycoproteins specified by herpes simplex virus. In: Roizman B, ed. The Herpesviruses. Vol. 3. New York: Plenum Publishing, 1984:315–356.

50. Lagunoff M, Roizman B. The regulation of synthesis and properties of the protein product of open reading frame P of the herpes simplex virus 1 genome. J Virol 1995; 69:3615–3623.

51. Ward PL, Roizman B. Herpes simplex genes the blueprint of a successful human pathogen. Trend Genet 1994; 10:267–274.

52. Centifanto-Fitzgerald YM, et al. Ocular disease pattern induced by herpes simplex virus is genetically determined by a specific region of viral DNA. J Exp Med 1982; 155:475–489.

.53. Longnecker R, et al. Identification of a novel herpes simplex virus 1 glycoprotein gene within a gene cluster dispensable for growth in cell culture. Proc Natl Acad Sci USA 1987; 84:4303–4307.

54. Richman DD, et al. Identification of a new glycoprotein of herpes simplex virus type 1 and genetic mapping of the gene that codes for it. J Virol 1986; 57:647–655.

55. Cook ML, Stevens JG. Pathogenesis of herpetic neuritis and ganglionitis in mice: evidence of intra-axonal transport of infection. Infect Immun 1973; 7:272–288.

56. Hill TJ. Herpes simplex virus latency. In: Roizman B, ed. The Herpesviruses. Vol. 3. New York: Plenum Publishing, 1985: 175–240.

57. Lafferty WE, et al. Herpes simplex virus type 1 as a cause of genital herpes: impact on surveillance and prevention. J Infect Dis 2000; 181:1454–1457.

58. Nilson A, Myrmel H. Changing trends in genital herpes simplex virus infection in Bergen, Norway. Acta Obstet Gynecol Scand 2000; 79:693–696.

59. Vyse AJ, et al. The burden of infection with HSV-1 and HSV-2 in England and Wales: implications for the changing epidemiology of genital herpes. Sex Transm Dis 2000; 76: 183–187.

60. Lafferty WE, et al. Recurrences after oral and genital herpes simplex virus infection. Influence of site of infection and viral type. N Engl J Med 1987; 316:1444–1449.

61. Corey L. The diagnosis and treatment of genital herpes. JAMA 1982; 248:1041–1049.

62. Mertz GJ, et al. Herpes simplex virus type 2 glycoproteins-subunit vaccine: tolerance and humoral and cellular responses in humans. J Infect Dis 1984; 150:242–249.

63. Rattray MC, et al. Recurrent genital herpes among women: symptomatic versus asymptomatic viral shedding. Br J Vener Dis 1978; 54:262–265.

64. Sakaoka H, et al. Demonstration of either endogenous recurrence or exogenous reinfection by restriction endonuclease cleavage analysis of herpes simplex virus from patients with recrudescent genital herpes. J Med Virol 1995; 46:387–396.

65. Lakeman AD, et al. Analysis of DNA from recurrent genital herpes simplex virus isolates by restriction endonuclease digestion. J Sex Transm Dis 1986; 13:61–66.

66. Kern ER. Animal models as assay systems for the development of antivirals. In: DeClerque E, Walker RT, eds. Antiviral Drug Development: a Multi-Disciplinary Approach. New York: Plenum Press, 1987:149–172.

67. Kirchner H. Immunobiology of infection with herpes simplex virus. In: Milnick JL, ed. Monographs in Virology. Vol. 13. Basel: Karger, 1982:1–104.

68. Knotts FB, et al. Pathogenesis of herpetic encephalitis in mice after ophthalmic inoculation. J Infect Dis 1974; 130:16–27.

69. Underwood GE, Weed SD. Recurrent cutaneous herpes simplex in hairless mice. Infect Immun 1974; 10:471–474.

70. Stanberry LR, et al. Genital herpes in guinea pigs: Pathogenesis of the primary infection and description of recurrent disease. J Infect Dis 1982; 146:397–404.

71. Schlitt M, et al. A rabbit model of focal herpes simplex encephalitis. J Infect Dis 1986; 153:732–735.

72. Schlitt M, et al. Mortality in an experimental focal herpes encephalitis: relationship to seizures. Brain Res 1988; 440: 293–298.

73. Stroop WG, Schaefer DC. Production of encephalitis restricted to the temporal lobes by experimental reactivation of herpes simplex virus. J Infect Dis 1986; 153:721–731.

74. Meignier B, et al. In vivo behavior of genetically engineered herpes simplex viruses R7017 and R7020: II. Studies in immunocompetent and immunosuppressed owl monkeys (Aotus trivirgatus). J Infect Dis 1990; 162:313–321.

75. Posavad CM, et al. Tipping the scales of herpes simplex virus reactivation: The important responses are local. Nat Med 1998; 4:381–382.

76. De Stasio PR, Taylor MW. Specific effect of interferon on the herpes simplex virus type 1 transactivation event. J Virol 1990; 64:2588–2593.

77. Holterman AX, et al. An important role for major histocompatibility complex class I-restricted T cells, and a limited role for gamma interferon, in protection of mice against lethal herpes simplex virus infection. J Virol 1999; 73:2058–2063.

78. Mester JC, et al. The immunobiology of herpes simplex virus. In: Stanberry LR, ed. Genital and Neonatal Herpes. New York: John Wiley and Sons Ltd, 1996:49–91.

79. Biron CA, Byron KS, Sullivan JL. Severe herpesvirus infections in an adolescent without natural killer cells. N Engl J Med 1989; 320:1731–1735.

80. Lopez C, et al. Immunity to herpesvirus infections in humans. In: Roizman B, Whitley RJ, Lopez C, eds. The Human Herpesviruses. New York: Raven Press, 1993:397–425.

81. Stumbles PA, et al. Dendritic cells and mucosal macrophages. In: Ogra P, Mestecky J, Lamm M, Strober W, McGhee JR, eds. Mucosal Immunology. New York: Academic Press, 1998:397–412.

82. Rouse BT, et al. DNA vaccines and immunity to herpes simplex virus. Curr Top Microbiol Immunol 1998; 226:69–78.

83. Milligan GN, Bernstein DI. Analysis of herpes simplex virus-specific T cells in the murine female genital tract following infection with herpes simplex virus type 2. Virology 1995; 212:481–489.

84. Murphy BR. Mucosal immunity to viruses. In: Ogra P, Mestecky J, Lamm M, Strober W, McGhee JR, eds. Mucosal Immunology. New York: Academic Press, 1998:695–707.

85. Dasheshia M, et al. Herpes simplex virus latency and the immune response. Curr Opin Microbiol 1998; 1:430–435.

86. Koelle DM, et al. Clearance of HSV-2 from recurrent genital lesions correlates with infiltration of HSV-specific cytotoxic T lymphocytes. J Clin Invest 1998; 101:1500–1508.

87. Posavad CM, et al. Severe genital herpes infections in HIV-infected individuals with impaired herpes simplex virus-

specific CD8$^+$ cytotoxic T lymphocyte responses. Proc Natl Acad Sci USA 1997; 94:10289–10294.

88. Stanberry LR, et al. Prospects for control of herpes simplex virus disease through immunization. Clin Infect Dis 2000; 30:549–566.

89. Hashido M, Kawana T. Herpes simplex virus-specific IgM, IgA and IgG subclass antibody responses in primary and nonprimary genital herpes patients. Microbiol Immunol 1997; 41:415–420.

90. Benedetti JK, Zeh J, Corey L. Clinical reactivation of genital herpes simplex virus infection decreases in frequency over time. Ann Intern Med 1999; 131:14–20.

91. Whitley RJ, et al. Herpes simplex virus. Clin Infect Dis 1998; 26:541–555.

92. Bernstein DI, Stanberry LR. Herpes simplex virus vaccines. Vaccine 1999; 17:1681–1689.

93. Rinaldo CR, Torpey DJ. Cell-mediated immunity and immunosuppresion in herpes simplex virus infection. Immunodeficiency 1993; 5:33–90.

94. Krause PR, Straus SE. Herpesvirus vaccines. Development, controversies and applications. Infect Dis Clin North Am 1999; 13:61–81.

95. Davis WB, et al. Ocular infection with herpes simplex virus type 1: prevention of acute herpetic encephalitis by systemic administration of virus specific antibody. J Infect Dis 1979; 140:534–540.

96. Kapoor AK, et al. Pathogenesis of herpes simplex virus in B-cell suppressed mice: the relative role of cell-mediated and humoral immunity. J Gen Virol 1982; 61:127–131.

97. McKendall RR, et al. Host defense in herpes simplex infection of the nervous system: Effect of antibody in disease and viral spread. Infect Immun 1979; 23:305–311.

98. Oakes JE, Lausch RN. Role of Fc fragments in antibody-mediated recovery from ocular and subcutaneous herpes simplex virus infection. Infect Immun 1981; 33:109–114.

99. Oakes JE, Rosemond-Horubeak H. Antibody-mediated recovery for subcutaneous herpes simplex virus type 2 infection. Infect Immun 1978; 21:489–495.

100. Balachandran N, et al. Protection against lethal challenge of Balb/c mice by passive transfer of monoclonal antibodies to five glycoproteins in herpes simplex virus type 2. Infect Immun 1982; 37:1132–1137.

101. Dix RD, et al. Use of monoclonal antibody directed against herpes simplex virus glycoproteins to protect mice against acute virus-induced neurological disease. Infect Immun 1981; 34:192–199.

102. Rector JT, et al. Use of monoclonal antibodies for analysis of antibody-dependent immunity to ocular herpes simplex virus type 1 infection. Infect Immun 1982; 38:168–174.

103. Minson AC, et al. An analysis of the biological properties of monoclonal antibodies against glycoprotein D of herpes simplex virus and identification of amino acid substitutions that confer resistance to neutralization. J Gen Virol 1986; 67:1001–1013.

104. Heber-Katz E, et al. Overlapping T cell antigenic sites on a synthetic peptide fragment from herpes simplex virus glycoprotein D, the degenerate MHC restriction elicited, and functional evidence of antigen-Ia interaction. J Exp Med 1988; 167:275–287.

105. Johnson RM, et al. Herpes simplex virus glycoprotein D is recognized as antigen by CD4 and CD8 lymphocytes from infected mice: characterization to T cell clones. J Immunol 1990; 145:702–710.

106. Zarling JM, et al. Human cytotoxic T cells clones directed against herpes simplex virus infected cells. J Immunol 1986; 136:4669–4673.

107. Kahlon J, et al. Human antibody response to herpes simplex virus specified polypeptides following primary and recurrent infection. J Clin Microbiol 1985; 23:725–730.

108. Bernstein DI, et al. Antibody response to type-common and type-unique epitopes of herpes simplex virus polypeptides. J Med Virol 1985; 15:251–263.

109. Rasmusse LE, et al. Lymphocyte interferon production and transformation after herpes simplex infections in humans. J Immunol 1974; 112:728–736.

110. Corey L, et al. Cellular immune response in genital herpes simplex virus infection. N Engl J Med 1978; 299:986–991.

111. Pass RF, et al. Specific lymphocyte blastogenic responses in children with cytomegalovirus and herpes simplex virus infections acquired early in infancy. Infect Immun 1981; 34: 166–170.

112. Russell AS. Cell-mediated immunity to herpes simplex virus in man. Am J Clin Pathol 1973; 60:826–830.

113. Russell AS. Cell-mediated immunity to herpes simplex virus in man. J Infect Dis 1974; 129:142–146.

114. Shillitoe EJ, et al. Sequential changes in T and B lymphocyte responses to herpes simplex virus in man. Scand J Immunol 1978; 7:357–366.

115. Starr SE, et al. Stimulation of human lymphocytes by herpes simplex virus antigens. Infect Immun 1975; 11:109–112.

116. Sullender WM, et al. Humoral and cell-mediated immunity in neonates with herpes simplex virus infection. J Infect Dis 1987; 155:28–37.

117. Cunningham AL, Merigan TC. Alpha interferon production appears to predict time of recurrence of herpes labialis. J Immunol 1983; 130:2397–2400.

118. Overall JC Jr, et al. Viral-induced leukocyte interferon in vesicle fluid from lesions of recurrent herpes labialis. J Infect Dis 1981; 143:543–547.

119. Sheridan JF, et al. Immunity to herpes simplex virus type 2: IV. Impaired lymphokine production during recrudescence correlates with an imbalance in T-lymphocyte subsets. J Immunol 1982; 129:326–331.

120. Kohl S, et al. Neonatal antibody-dependent cellular cytotoxic antibody levels are associated with the clinical presentation of neonatal herpes simplex virus infection. J Infect Dis 1989; 160:770–776.

121. Yeager AS, et al. Relationship of antibody to outcome in neonatal herpes simplex infections. Infect Immun 1980; 29:532–538.

122. Prober CG, et al. Low risk of herpes simplex virus infections in neonates exposed to the virus at the time of vaginal delivery to mothers with recurrent genital herpes simplex virus infections. N Engl J Med 1987; 316:240–244.

123. Brown ZA, et al. Neonatal herpes simplex virus infection in relation to asymptomatic maternal infection at the time of labor. N Engl J Med 1991; 324:1247–1252.

124. Kahlon J, Whitley RJ. Antibody response of the newborn after herpes simplex virus infection. J Infect Dis 1988; 158:925–933.

125. Rasmussen L, Merigan TC. Role of T-lymphocytes in cellular immune responses during herpes simplex virus infection in humans. Proc Natl Acad Sci USA 1978; 75:3957–3961.

126. Chilmonczyk BA, et al. Characterization of the human newborn response to herpesvirus antigen. J Immunol 1985; 134: 4184–4188.

127. Bryson YJ, et al. Deficiency of immune interferon production by leukocytes of normal newborns. Cell Immunol 1980; 55:191–200.

128. Kohl S, Harmon MW. Human neonatal leukocyte interferon production and natural killer cytotoxicity in response to herpes simplex virus. J Interferon Res 1983; 3:461–463.

129. Burchett SK, et al. Ontogeny of neonatal mononuclear cell transformation and interferon gamma production after herpes simplex virus stimulation. Clin Res 1986; 34:129.

130. Rouse BT. Immunobiology and prophylaxis of human herpesvirus infections. In: Roizman B, Lopez C, eds. The Herpesviruses. Vol. 4. New York: Plenum Press, 1985:103.

131. Kohl S, et al. Normal function of neonatal polymorphonuclear leukocytes in antibody-dependent cellular cytotoxicity to herpes simplex virus infected cells. J Pediatr 1981; 98:783–785.

132. Armerding D, Rossiter H. Induction of natural killer cells by herpes simplex virus type 2 in resistant and sensitive inbred mouse strains. Immunobiology 1981; 158:369–379.

133. Hirsch MS, et al. Macrophages and age-dependent resistance to herpes simplex virus in mice. J Immunol 1970; 104:1160–1165.

134. Kohl S, et al. Human neonatal and maternal monocyte-macrophage and lymphocyte mediated antibody dependent cytotoxicity to herpes simplex infected cells. J Pediatr 1978; 93:206–210.

135. Kohl S, et al. Protection of neonatal mice against herpes simplex viral infection by human antibody and leukocytes from adults, but not neonatal humans. J Immunol 1981; 127:1273–1275.

136. Lopez C, et al. Marrow dependent cells depleted by 89Sr mediate genetic resistance to herpes simplex virus type 1 infection in mice. Infect Immun 1980; 28:1028–1032.

137. Trofatter KF, et al. Growth of type 2 herpes simplex virus in newborn and adult mononuclear leukocytes. Intervirology 1979; 2:117–123.

138. Wald A, Link K. Risk of human immunodeficiency virus infection in herpes simplex virus type 2-seropositive persons: a meta-analysis. J Infect Dis 2002; 185:45–52.

139. Wald A, et al. Acyclovir suppresses asymptomatic shedding of HSV-2 in the genital tract. N Eng J Med 1995; 326: 770.

140. Parks WP, Rapp R. Prospects for herpes virus vaccination: safety efficacy considerations. Prog Med Virol 1975; 21:188–206.

141. Wise TG, et al. Herpes simplex virus vaccines. J Infect Dis 1977; 136:706–711.

142. Allen WP, Rapp F. Concept review of genital herpes vaccines. J Infect Dis 1982; 145:413–421.

143. Moreschi GI, Ennis FA. Prevention and treatment of HSV infections. In: Nahmias AJ, Dowdle WR, Schinazi RF, eds. Human Herpesviruses: An Interdisciplinary Perspective. North Holland, Amsterdam: Elsevier, 1982:441.

144. Meignier B, Roizman B. Herpes simplex virus vaccines. Antiviral Res 1985; 1:259–265.

145. Corey L. Laboratory diagnosis of herpes simplex virus infections. Principles guiding the Simplex Virus, Pathogenesis, Immunobiology and Control. Berlin: Springer Verlag, 1992: 137–158.

146. Burke RL. Contemporary approaches to vaccination against HSV. In: Rouse BT, ed. Herpes Simplex Virus, Pathogenesis, Immunobiology and Control. Berlin: Springer Verlag, 1992:137–158.

147. Burke RL. Development of a herpes simplex virus subunit glycoprotein vaccine for prophylactic and therapeutic use. Rev Infect Dis 1991; 13:S906–S911.

148. Nicolau S, et al. Quelques caracteres de l'herpes experimental chez l'homme. C R Soc Biol 1923; 89:779–781.

149. Nicolau S, Banciu A. Herpes recidivant experimental chez l'homme. C R Soc Biol 1924; 90:138–140.

150. Paulian D. Le virus herpetique et la sclerose laterale amyotrophique. Bull Acad Med Roum 1932; 107:1462–1467.

151. Tessier P, et al. L'inoculabilité de l'herpès: presence du virus keratogene dans les lesions. C R Soc Biol 1922; 87:648.

152. Tessier P, et al. L' inoculabilité de l'herpès chez les e encéphalitiques. C R Soc Biol 1923; 88:255.

153. Macher E. Zur behandlung des chronisch-rezidivierenden herpes simplex (treatment of chronic recurrent herpes simplex). Z Hautkr Geschlechtskr 1957; 23:18–22.

154. Goldman L. Reactions by autoinoculation for recurrent herpes simplex. Arch Dermatol 1961; 84:1025.

155. Panscherewski D, Rhode B. Zuar serologie und therapie des herpes simplex recidivans. Hautarzt 1962; 13:275–278.

156. Lazar MP. Vaccination for recurrent herpes simplex infection: initiation of a new disease site following the use of unmodified material containing the live virus. Arch Dermatol 1956; 73:70.

157. Blank H, Haines HG. Experimental human reinfection with herpes simplex virus. J Invest Dermatol 1973; 61:223–225.

158. Biberstein H, Jessner M. Experiences with herpin in recurrent herpes simplex together with a review and analysis of the literature on the use of CNS substance as a virus-antigent-carrier. Dermatology 1958; 117:267–287.

159. Brain RT. Biological therapy in virus diseases. Br J Dermatol Syph 1936; 48:21–26.

160. Frank SB. Formalized herpes therapy and deneutralizing substance in herpes simplex. J Invest Dermatol 1938; 1:267–282.

161. Hall MJ, Katrak K. The quest for a herpes simplex virus vaccine: background and recent development. Vaccine 1986; 4:138–150.

162. Merignier B. Vaccination against herpes simplex virus infections. In: Roizman B, Lopez C, eds. The Herpesviruses, Immunobiology and Prophylaxis of Human Herpesvirus Infections. New York: Plenum Press, 1985:265–269.

163. Dix RD. Prospects for vaccine against herpes simplex virus type 1 and type 2. Progr Med Virol 1987; 34:89–128.

164. Jawetz E, et al. Studies on herpes simplex virus: VI. Observations on patients with recurrent herpetic lesions injected with herpes viruses of their antigens. Am J Med Sci 1955; 229:477–485.

165. Steppert A. Zur Behandlung des rezidivierenden herpes simplex (treatment of recurrent herpes simplex). Wien Klin Wochenschr 1956; 68:452–453.

166. Berman PW, et al. Detection of antibodies to herpes simplex virus with a continuous cell line expressing cloned glycoprotein D. Science 1983; 222:524–527.

167. Kern AB, Schiff BL. Smallpox vaccinations in the management of recurrent herpes simplex: a controlled evaluation. J Invest Dermatol 1959; 33:99–102.

168. Kern AB, Schiff BL. Vaccine therapy in recurrent herpes simplex. Arch Dermatol 1964; 89:844–845.

169. Vallee G. Traitement de l'herpes current par le vaccin anti-poliomyelitique Sabin. Thesis, University of Paris, 1980.

170. Nagler FPO. A herpes skin test reagent from amniotic fluid. Aust J Exp Biol Med Sci 1946; 24:103–105.

171. Soltz-Szots J. New methods of specific vaccination in recurrent herpes simplex. Hautartz 1960; 11:465–467.

172. Fanta D, et al. Problems and treatment of recurrent herpes simplex. Z Hautkr 1974; 49:597–606.

173. Henocq E, et al. Essai de therapeutique de l'herpes recidivant par un vaccin prepare en culture cellulaire et inactive par les rayons ultra-violets: II. Essais cliniques. Semain des Hospitaux de Paris 1964; 40:1474–1480.

174. Degos R, Touraine R. Traitement de l'herpes recidivant par un vaccin specifique. Bull Soc Fr Dermatol Syph 1964; 71: 161.

175. Santoianni P. Relapsing herpes simplex: treatment with specific vaccine. Minerva Dermatol 1966; 41:30–36.

176. Henocq E. Current status of the anti-herpetic vaccine. Therapeutique 1972; 48:485–488.

177. Macotela-Ruiz E. Antiherpetic vaccine and ointment with 5-iodo-2-deoxyuridine in cutaneous-mucous recurrent herpes simplex: comparative results. Prense Med Mex 1973; 38:362–367.

178. Baron A, et al. Corneal herpes. Treatment with specific vaccines. Bull Soc Ophthalmol Fr 1966; 66:137–142.

179. Bruckner R. First personal experiences with the antiherpes vaccine. Ophthalmologe 1970; 161:104–107.

180. Bubola D, Mancosu A. Clinical and immunological research

on 30 patients affected by recurring herpes after specific vaccination. Ital Dermatol 1967; 108:107–122.

181. Pouliquen Y, et al. Directions for use of antiherpetic vaccine in ophthalmologic practice. Arch Ophthalmol 1966; 26:565–686.

182. Chapin HB, et al. The value of tissue culture vaccine in the prophylaxis of recurrent attacks of herpetic keratitis. Am J Ophthalmol 1962; 54:255–265.

183. Hull RN, Peck FB Jr. Vaccination against herpesvirus infections. PAHO, Sci Publ 1967; 147:266–275.

184. Nasemann T. Die behandlung der infektionen durch das Herpes simplex virus. Ther Ggw 1965; 104:294–309.

185. Nasemann T. Recent therapeutic methods for various herpes simplex infections. Arch Klin Exp Dermatol 1970; 237:234–237.

186. Nasemann T, Schaeg G. Herpes simplex virus. type II: microbiology and clinical experiences with attenuated vaccine. Hautarzt 1973; 24:133–139.

187. Schmersahl P, Rudiger G. Results of treatment with the herpes simplex antigen Lupidon H. resp. Lupidon G. Z Hautkr 1975; 50:105–112.

188. Kitagawa K. Therapy of herpes simplex with heat inactivated herpes simplex hominis type 1 and type 2. Z Hautkr 1973; 48:533–535.

189. Schneider J, Rohde B. Antigen therapy of recurring herpes simplex with herpes simplex vaccine LUPIDON H and G. Z Haut Geschlechtskr 1972; 47:973–980.

190. Weitgasser H. New possibilities of herpes simplex therapy in the dermatological practice. Hautarzt 1973; 24:298–301.

191. von Rodovsky J, et al. Preventive treatment of recurring herpes with a formaldehyde vaccine made of rabbit kidney cells. Dermatol Monatsschr 1971; 157:701–708.

192. Dundarov S, et al. Immunotherapy with inactivated polyvalent herpes vaccines. Dev Biol Stand 1982; 52:351–358.

193. Shubladze AK, et al. Mechanism of specific vaccine therapy in ocular herpes simplex. Vopr Virusol 1978; 1:63–68.

194. Remy W, et al. Antibody titers-curse in patients with recurring herpes simplex virus infections under vaccination with heat-inactivated herpes viruses. Z Hautkr 1975; 51:103–107.

195. Henocq E, et al. Table ronde sur l'herpes recidivant. Rev Med 1967; 8:695–720.

196. Lepine P, de Rudder J. Essai de therapeutique de l'herpes recidivant par un vaccin prepare en culture cellulaire et inactive par les rayons ultra-violets: I. Preparation du vaccin et essais d'immunisation sur l'animal. Sem Ther (Paris) 1964; 40:469–474.

197. Soltz-Szots J. Therapy of recurrent herpes simplex. Z Haut Geschlechtskr 1971; 46:267–272.

198. Weitgasser H. Controlled clinical study of the herpes antigens LUPIDON H and LUPIDON G. Z Hautkr 1977; 52:625–628.

199. Anderson SG, et al. An attempt to vaccinate against herpes simplex. Aust J Exp Biol Med Sci 1950; 28:579–584.

200. Fenyves A, Strupp L. Heat-resistant infectivity of herpes simplex virus revealed by viral transfection. Intervirology 1982; 17:222–228.

201. Cappel R, et al. Efficacy of a nucleic acid free submit vaccine. Arch Virol 1980; 65:12–23.

202. Skinner GR, et al. Prepubertal vaccination of mice against experimental infection of the genital tract with type 2 herpes simplex virus. Arch Virol 1980; 64:329–338.

203. Cappel R, et al. Immune response to a DNA free herpes simplex vaccine in man. Arch Virol 1982; 73:61–67.

204. Skinner GR, et al. Preparation and immunogenicity of vaccine Ac NFU1 (S-) MRC towards the prevention of herpes genitalis. Br J Vener Dis 1982; 58:381–386.

205. Ashley R, et al. Detection of asymptomatic herpes simplex virus infections after vaccination. J Virol 1987; 61:264–268.

206. Zarling JM, et al. Herpes simplex virus (HSV) specific proliferative and cytotoxic T-cell responses in humans immunized with an HSV type glycoprotein subunit vaccine. J Virol 1988; 62:4481–4485.

207. Berman PW, et al. Protection from genital herpes simplex virus type 2 infection by vaccination with cloned type 1 glycoprotein D. Science 1985; 227:1490–1492.

208. Burke RL, et al. Development of herpes simplex virus subunit vaccine. In: Lerner RA, Ginsberg H, Chanock RM, Brown F, eds. Vaccines 89: Modern Approaches to New Vaccines Including Prevention of AIDS. Cold Springs Harbor, New York: Cold Springs Harbor Laboratory, 1989:377–382.

209. Watson RJ, et al. Herpes simplex virus type 1 glycoprotein D gene: nucleotide sequence and expression in *Escherichia coli.* Science 1983; 218:381–384.

210. Weis JH, et al. An immunologically active chimaeric protein containing herpes simplex virus type 1 glycoprotein D. Science 1983; 302:72–74.

211. Eisenberg RJ, et al. Synthetic glycoprotein D-related peptides protect mice against herpes simplex virus challenge. J Virol 1985; 56:1014–1017.

212. Klein RJ, et al. Efficacy of a virion envelope herpes simplex virus against experimental skin infections in hairless mice. Arch Virol 1981; 68:73–80.

213. Kitces EN, et al. Protection from oral herpes simplex virus infection by a nucleic acid-free virus vaccine. Infect Immun 1977; 16:955–960.

214. Kutinova L, et al. Immunogenicity of subviral herpes simplex virus preparation: protection of mice against intraperitoneal infection with live virus. Acta Virol 1980; 24:391–398.

215. Slichtova V, et al. Immunogenicity of subviral herpes simplex virus type 1 preparation: protection of mice against intradermal challenge with type 1 and type 2 viruses. Arch Virol 1980; 66:207–214.

216. Dix RD, Mils J. Acute and latent herpes simplex virus neurological disease in mice immunized with purified virus-specific glycoproteins gB or gD. J Med Virol 1985; 17:9–18.

217. Lasky LA, et al. Protection of mice from lethal herpes-simplex virus-infection by vaccination with a secreted form of cloned glycoprotein-D. Bio-Technology 1984; 2:527.

218. Meignier B, et al. Immunization of experimental animals with reconstituted glycoprotein mixtures of herpes simplex virus 1 and 2: protection against challenge with virulent virus. J Infect Dis 1987; 155:921–930.

219. Thornton B, et al. Herpes simplex vaccine using cell membrane associated antigen in an animal model. Dev Biol Stand 1982; 50:201–206.

220. Kutinova L, et al. Subviral herpes simplex vaccine. Dev Biol Stand 1982; 52:313–319.

221. Stanberry LR, et al. Vaccination with recombinant herpes simplex virus glycoproteins: protection against initial and recurrent genital herpes. J Infect Dis 1987; 155:914–920.

222. Stanberry LR, et al. Preinfection prophylaxis with herpes simplex virus glycoprotein immunogens: factors influencing efficacy. J Gen Virol 1989; 70:3177–3185.

223. Wachsman M, et al. Protection of guinea pigs from primary and recurrent herpes simplex virus (HSV) type 2 cutaneous disease with vaccinia virus recombinants expressing HSV glycoprotein D. J Infect Dis 1987; 155:1188–1197.

224. Yoshino K, et al. Efficacy of intradermal administration of herpes simplex virus subunit vaccine. Microbiol Immunol 1982; 26:753–757.

225. Cappel R, et al. Antibody and cell-mediated immunity to a DNA free herpes simplex subunit vaccine. Dev Biol Stand 1979; 43:381–385.

226. Hilfenhaus J, Moser H. Prospects for a subunit vaccine

against herpes simplex virus infections. Behring-Inst Mitt 1981; 69:45.

227. Skinner G, et al. Preparation and efficacy of an inactivated subunit vaccine (NFUIBHK) against type 2 Herpes simplex virus infection. Med Microbiol Immunol 1978; 166:119–132.
228. Hilleman MR, et al. Subunit herpes simplex virus vaccine. In: Nahmias AJ, Dowdle WR, Schinazi RF, eds. The Human Herpesviruses: An Interdisciplinary Perspective. North-Holland, Amsterdam: Elsevier, 1982:503–506.
229. Carter CA, et al. Experimental ulcerative herpetic keratitis: IV. Preliminary observations on the efficacy of a herpes simplex subunit vaccine. Br J Ophthalmol 1981; 65:679–682.
230. Rajcani J, et al. Restriction of latent herpes virus infection in rabbits immunized with subviral herpes simplex virus vaccine. Acta Virol 1980; 24:183–193.
231. Scriba M. Vaccination against herpes simplex virus. animal studies on the efficacy against acute, latent, and recurrent infection. In: Sundmacher R, ed. Herpetische Augenkrankungen. Munich: Springer-Verlag (Bergmann), 1981:67–72.
232. Sanchez-Pescador L, et al. The effect of adjuvants on the efficacy of a recombinant herpes simplex virus glycoprotein vaccine. J Immun 1988; 141:1720–1727.
233. Thomson TA, et al. Comparison of effects of adjuvants on efficacy of virion envelope herpes simplex virus vaccine against labial infection of BALB/c mice. Infect Immun 1983; 41:556–562.
234. Skinner GR, et al. Early experience with "antigenoid" vaccine Ac NFUI(S-) MRC towards prevention or modification of herpes genitalis. Dev Biol Stand 1982; 52:333–344.
235. Straus SE, et al. Placebo-controlled trial of vaccination with recombinant glycoprotein D of herpes simplex virus type 2 for immunotherapy of genital herpes. Lancet 1994; 343:1460–1463.
236. Mertz GJ, et al. Double-blind, placebo-controlled trial of a herpes simplex virus type 2 glycoprotein vaccine in persons at high risk for a genital herpes infection. J Infect Dis 1990; 161:653–660.
237. Kaerner HC, et al. Genetic variability of herpes simplex virus: development of a pathogenic variant during passaging of a nonpathogenic herpes simplex virus type 1 virus strain in mouse brain. J Virol 1983; 46:83–93.
238. Corey L, et al. Recombinant glycoprotein vaccine for the prevention of genital HSV-2 infection: two randomized controlled trials. Chiron HSV Vaccine Study Group. JAMA 1999; 28:331–340.
239. Langenberg AG, et al. A prospective study of new infections with herpes simplex virus type 1 and type 2. Chiron HSV Vaccine Study Group. N Engl J Med 1999; 341:1432–1438.
240. Thompson RL, Stevens J. Replication at body temperature selects a neurovirulent herpes simplex virus type 2. Infect Immun 1983; 41:855–857.
241. Smith GL, et al. Infectious vaccinia virus recombinants that express hepatitis B virus surface antigen. Nature 1983; 302:490–495.
242. Paoletti E, et al. Construction of live vaccines using genetically engineered poxviruses: biological activity of vaccinia virus recombinants expressing the hepatitis B virus surface antigen and the herpes simplex virus glycoprotein D. Proc Natl Acad Sci USA 1984; 81:193–197.
243. Cremer KJ, et al. Vaccinia virus recombinant expressing herpes simplex virus type 1 glycoprotein D prevents latent herpes in mice. Science 1985; 228:737–740.
244. Wachsman M, et al. Expression of herpes simplex virus glycoprotein D on antigen presenting cells infected with vaccinia recombinants and protective immunity. Biosci Rep 1988; 8:323–334.
245. Cantin EM, et al. Expression of herpes simplex virus 1 glycoprotein B by a recombinant vaccinia virus and protection of mice against lethal herpes simplex virus infection. Proc Natl Acad Sci USA 1987; 84:59.
246. Willey DE, et al. Herpes simplex virus type 1-vaccinia virus recombinant expressing glycoprotein B. Protection from acute and latent infection. J Infect Dis 1988; 158:1382–1386.
247. Paoletti E, Panicali D. Genetically engineered pox viruses as live recombinant vaccines. Modern Approaches to Vaccines-Molecular and Clinical Basis of Virus Virulence and Immunospecificity. Cold Spring Harbor, New York: Cold Spring Harbor Laboratory, 1984:295–299.
248. Smith GL, et al. Vaccinia virus recombinants expressing genes from pathogenic agents have potential as live vaccines. Modern Approaches to Vaccines-Molecular and Clinical Basis of Virus Virulence and immunospecificity. Cold Spring Harbor, New York: Cold Spring Harbor Laboratory, 1984:213–317.
249. McDermott MR, et al. Protection of mice against lethal challenge with herpes simplex virus by vaccination with an adenovirus vector expressing HSV glycoprotein B. Virology 1989; 169:244–247.
250. Post LE, Roizman B. A generalized technique for deletion of specific genes in large genomes: alpha gene 22 of herpes simplex virus 1 is not essential for growth. Cell 1981; 25:227–232.
251. Mocarski ES, et al. Molecular engineering of the herpes simplex virus genome: insertion of a second L–S junction into the genome causes additional genome inversions. Cell 1980; 22:243–255.
252. Meignier B, et al. In vivo behavior of genetically engineered herpes simplex virus R7017 and R7020. Construction and evaluation in rodents. J Infect Dis 1988; 158:602–614.
253. Cadoz M, et al. Phase 1 trial of R7020: A live attenuated recombinant herpes simplex (HSV) candidate vaccine. In: 32nd Interscience Conference on Antimicrobial Agents and Chemotherapy. Anaheim, CA, 1992 October 11–14.
254. Chou J, et al. Mapping of herpes simplex virus-1 neurovirulence to gamma$_1$ 34.5, a gene nonessential for growth in culture. Science 1990; 250:1262–1266.
255. Martuza RL, et al. Experimental therapy of human glioma by means of a genetically engineered virus mutant. Science 1991; 252:854–856.
256. Markert JM, et al. Reduction and elimination of encephalitis in an experimental glioma therapy model with attenuated herpes simplex mutants that retain susceptibility to acyclovir. Neurosurgery 1993; 32:597–603.
257. Boviatsis EJ, et al. Antitumor activity and reporter gene transfer into rat brain neoplasms inoculated with herpes simplex virus vectors defective in thymidine kinase or ribonucleotide reductase. Gene Ther 1994; 1:323–331.
258. Jia WW, et al. Selective destruction of gliomas in immunocompetent rats by thymidine kinase-defective herpes simplex virus 1.6. J Natl Cancer Inst 1994; 86:1209–1215.
259. Kaplitt MB, et al. Mutant herpes simplex virus induced regression of tumors growing in immunocompetent rats. J Neuro-Oncol 1994; 19:137–147.
260. Mineta T, et al. Treatment of malignant gliomas using ganciclovir-hypersensitive, ribonucleotide reductase-deficient herpes simplex viral mutant. Cancer Res 1994; 54:3963–3966.
261. Chambers R, et al. Comparison of genetically engineered herpes simplex viruses for the treatment of brain tumors in a scid mouse model of human malignant glioma. Proc Natl Acad Sci USA 1995; 92:1411–1425.
262. Mineta T, et al. CNS tumor therapy by attenuated herpes simplex viruses. Gene Ther 1994; 1(Suppl 1):S78.
263. Boviatsis EJ, et al. Long-term survival of rats harboring brain neoplasms treated with ganciclovir and a herpes simplex virus vector that retains an intact thymidine kinase gene. Cancer Res 1994; 54:5745–5751.
264. Parker J, et al. Engineered herpes simplex virus expressing

interleukin 12 in the treatment of experimental murine tumors. Proc Natl Acad Sci USA 2000; 97:2208–2213.

265. Boviatsis EJ, et al. Gene transfer into experimental brain tumors mediated by adenovirus, herpes simplex virus, and retrovirus vectors. Hum Gene Ther 1994; 5:183–191.

266. Yazaki T, et al. Treatment of human malignant meningiomas by G207, a replication-competent multimutated herpes simplex virus 1. Cancer Res 1995; 55:4752–4756.

267. Andreansky S, et al. Treatment of intracranial gliomas in immunocompetent mice using herpes simplex viruses that express murine interleukins. Gene Ther 1998; 5:121–130.

268. Fong IW. Hair loss associated with lamivudine. Lancet 1994; 344:1702.

269. Chung S-M, et al. The use of a genetically engineered herpes simplex virus (R7020) with ioning radiation for experimental hepatoma. Gene Ther 2002; 9:75–80.

270. Sundaresan P, et al. Attenuated, replication-competent herpes simplex virus type 1 mutant G207: safety evaluation in mice. J Virol 2000; 74:3832–3841.

271. Hunter WD, et al. Attenuated, replication-competent herpes simplex virus type 1 mutant G207: safety evaluation of intracerebral injection in nonhuman primates. J Virol 1999; 73:6319–6326.

272. Markert JM, et al. Genetically engineered HSV in the treatment of glioma: a review. Rev Med Virol 2000; 10:17–30.

273. Markert JM, et al. Conditionally replicating herpes simplex virus mutant, G207 for the treatment of malignant glioma: results of a Phase I trial. Gene Ther 2000; 7:867–874.

274. Rampling R, et al. Toxicity evaluation of replication-competent herpes simplex virus (ICP 34.5 null mutant 1716) in patients with recurrent malignant glioma. Gene Ther 2000; 7:859–866.

275. Whitley RJ, Miller RL. Immunologic approach to herpes simplex virus. Viral Immunol 2001; 14:111–118.

56

Vaccines for Hantaviruses, Lassa Virus, and Filoviruses

Connie Schmaljohn and Alan Schmaljohn
U.S. Army Medical Research Institute for Infectious Diseases, Frederick, Maryland, USA

Joseph B. McCormick
University of Texas Health Science Center at Houston School of Public Health, Brownsville, Texas, USA

Gary J. Nabel
National Institute of Allergy and Infectious Diseases, National Institutes of Health, Bethesda, Maryland, USA

I. VACCINES AGAINST HANTAVIRUSES

A. Hantaviruses and Hantaviral Diseases

The genus *Hantavirus*, family Bunyaviridae, contains more than 20 viruses, including those causing hemorrhagic fever with renal syndrome (HFRS) or hantavirus pulmonary syndrome (HPS) [1]. Each distinct hantavirus is generally carried by a single rodent host species, although spillover of viruses into other rodents and rare species-jumping events has been observed [2–5]. Genetically closely related rodents carry closely related hantaviruses, reflecting coevolution or cospeciation of hantaviruses and rodents, probably over hundreds of thousands of years [3,6]. Because of this close association of the viruses and hosts, hantaviral diseases are geographically restricted to the range of the rodent carrying a particular virus. For this reason, HFRS, which is caused by hantaviruses carried by Old World rodents, is found in the eastern hemisphere, whereas HPS, which is caused by viruses carried by New World rodents, is found in the western hemisphere. An exception to this generality is Seoul virus, an etiologic agent of HFRS, carried by rats (*Rattus norvegicus* or *Rattus rattus*). Although rats are native to the Old World they, along with Seoul virus, have been distributed worldwide over the past few centuries, mostly as passengers on cargo ships.

Rodents carrying hantaviruses show no detrimental signs of infection, and where studied, the viruses persist in the presence of high levels of neutralizing antibodies [7–10]. The characteristics of and mechanism by which persistence is maintained has not been determined for many hantavirus–

rodent host pairs [11]. Hantavirus transmission usually results from inhalation of virus contained in rodent excreta [12,13]. Biting has also been suggested to be a frequent mode of transmission among rodents [14].

Rodent control is an effective way of preventing HFRS or HPS; however, it is not always possible or practical to avoid exposure to hantavirus-carrying rodents. Highly effective drugs or therapeutics are not available for HFRS or HPS; consequently, vaccines are the most rational approach to controlling hantaviral diseases. HFRS is a much more common disease than HPS. Whereas less than 1000 cases of HPS have been observed in North and South America since the discovery of HPS in 1993 (http://www.cdc.gov/ncidod/diseases/hanta), 60,000 to 150,000 cases of HFRS are reported each year [15]. Of these, the majority is found in China, with the rest occurring throughout western Russia, other parts of Europe, and Scandinavia [15].

Four hantaviruses are known to cause HFRS. Hantaan virus (HTNV), carried by *Apodemus agrarius* (striped field mice), and Dobrava virus (DOBV), carried by *Apodemus flavicollis* (yellow-necked mice), cause severe HFRS in Asia and in Europe, respectively, with mortality rates from 4% to 15% [15]. Puumala virus (PUUV), carried by *Clethrionomys glareolus* (bank voles) causes HFRS in Europe, European Russia, and Scandinavia. Puumala virus infection is usually not fatal (1–2% mortality) [16]. Seoul virus (SEOV) is most prevalent in China and Korea, but has also been associated with HFRS found in other parts of the Eurasian continent [16,17]. Although SEOV infections can be fatal, generally, SEOV causes a disease with lower mortality than that associated with HTNV [18].

Four hantaviruses are known to cause HPS in North America: Sin Nombre (SNV), New York, Bayou, and Black Creek Canal viruses. Sin Nombre virus, carried by *Peromyscus maniculatus* (deer mice) was the first pathogenic New World hantavirus described [19] and has caused most of the ~ 320 known cases of HPS in North America. Hantavirus pulmonary syndrome has been observed in 31 states in the United States with a mortality rate of approximately 37%. In South America and Central America, several hantaviruses have been associated with HPS [20]. Andes virus (ANDV), carried by *Oligoryzomys longicaudatus* (long-tailed pygmy rice rat), was identified in southern Argentina in 1995 and was later shown to be a prevalent cause of HPS in Chile [20]. Andes virus is the only hantavirus shown to be transmitted from person to person, causing secondary HPS [21–23].

B. Protective Immunity to Hantaviruses

The large number of hantaviruses that are potentially pathogenic for humans, and their genetic and antigenic diversity, pose a challenge for developing a comprehensive vaccine (Figure 1). Assessing cross-protection among hantaviruses has been difficult because, except for ANDV, hantaviruses are not known to be pathogenic for animals. The discovery that ANDV causes a disease in hamsters that is very similar to human HPS [24] provides an opportunity for studying protection from ANDV challenge; however, for other hantaviruses, protective immunity can only be gauged by the ability to prevent infection of a challenge virus. Typically, this is done by measuring viral antigens in target organs after challenge, and/or comparing antibody responses before and after challenge [25–29]. Such studies suggest that it may be possible to generate cross-protective immunity among the more closely related viruses, e.g., HTNV, SEOV, and DOBV viruses, but not against the more distantly related viruses [27,30]. If the hamster studies can be extrapolated to indicate that the ~ 80% amino acid sequence homologies of HTNV,

SEOV, and DOBV are sufficient to elicit cross-protective immunity, but that the ~ 65% homologies of PUUV and these other HFRS-causing viruses are insufficient, then none of the HFRS-causing hantaviruses could serve as a basis for an HPS vaccine (Figure 1). The amino acid sequence homologies of the known HPS-causing hantaviruses, however, suggest that a single vaccine component could offer cross-protective immunity to HPS.

Protection from infection is primarily mediated by neutralizing antibodies, as indicated by the ability of passively transferred immune sera to prevent infection by various hantaviruses in laboratory rodents [25,31,32]. In humans, a strong neutralizing antibody response has been linked to a better chance for survival of HPS [33]. Although a neutralizing antibody response alone appears to be sufficient for preventing infection with hantaviruses, cell-mediated responses have also been measured and found to offer cross-protective immunity in mice [34–36]. Cell-mediated immunity in humans has been documented by isolating T-cell clones from the blood of hantavirus-infected individuals [37–39]. The cell-mediated immune response to hantaviral infection is thought to be involved in pathogenesis. Inflammatory responses, particularly those associated with certain cytokines including tumor necrosis factor (TNF-α) and gamma interferon, are thought to be major contributors to the increased vascular permeability that is characteristic of both syndromes [40–44].

C. Conventional Vaccine Approaches

Because HPS is so rare, commercial vaccine development has not yet been actively pursued. In contrast, HFRS is a significant infectious disease problem in Asia, and several inactivated-virus vaccines have been developed and tested. A Korean vaccine, Hantavax®, is modeled after the commercially successful Biken vaccine for Japanese encephalitis. This vaccine was originally produced in suckling rats, but now consists of brain preparations from suckling mice

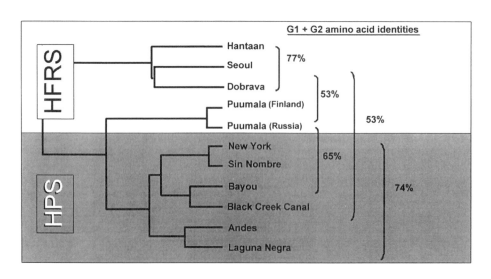

Figure 1 The phylogenetic basis of antigenic differences among hantaviruses.

infected with Hantaan virus. The vaccine is formulated with aluminum hydroxide adjuvant and is given by intramuscular injection. A clinical study of the original rat brain-derived vaccine demonstrated that 89% of the 456 volunteers who received one dose of vaccine, and 99% of 336 who received two doses of vaccine, seroconverted as determined by indirect fluorescent antibody test (IFAT) on infected, fixed cells. Neutralizing antibodies were not reported. A subsequent study showed that 97% of 64 volunteers given two doses of the mouse-brain-derived vaccine developed antibodies to HTNV detectable by ELISA or IFA and 75% had neutralizing antibodies. At 1 year after vaccination, neutralizing antibodies were no longer detected and a booster vaccination resulted in neutralizing antibodies in only 50% of the volunteers [45]. In another study of Hantavax in 30 volunteers, 76% developed antibodies detectable by ELISA and 33% developed low levels of neutralizing antibodies [46]. Antibody responses to individual HTNV proteins were not reported for these volunteers, but the discordance between ELISA and neutralizing antibodies might reflect a stronger response to the nucleocapsid protein than to the envelope glycoproteins of HTNV. Although controlled efficacy studies of the vaccine have not been reported, the incidence of HFRS in Korea has dropped since the introduction of the vaccine in 1990. Of course, other factors may also have contributed to the decline in cases of HFRS such as rodent population fluctuations or improved living conditions. Thus, proactive studies are still needed to validate the vaccine's effectiveness.

Rodent-brain-derived vaccines have also been developed and given to more than a million people in The People's Democratic Republic of Korea (North Korea). Although few details are available, one such vaccine reportedly consists of brain suspensions (from HTNV-infected suckling rats or hamsters) prepared by heating at 56°C for 30 min and mixing with protamine sulfate and coal powder [47]. Two doses of the vaccine, given to more than 1000 individuals, resulted in antibodies detected by IFA in 75% of recipients.

Both suckling mouse brain (SMB)-derived and cell-culture-derived inactivated vaccines for HFRS have been tested in China. A vaccine for HFRS caused by HTNV is prepared from virus-infected primary Mongolian gerbil (*Meriones unguiculatus*) kidney cells (MGKC). Virus is recovered and concentrated from whole-cell preparations by filtration. Beta-propiolactone (BPL; 0.025%) was chosen for inactivating infectivity because when compared to formalin, BPL treatment resulted in higher levels of hemagglutinating antigen, indicating better preservation of the envelope proteins [48]. Aluminum hydroxide (0.5 mg/mL) is added as an adjuvant. Three doses of vaccine given to two groups of 12 volunteers at intervals of 0, 7, and 28 days or 0, 28, and 60 days resulted in low levels of neutralizing antibodies to HTNV (GMT ~ 50) in all but one of the volunteers [49]. A booster vaccination given at 1 year resulted in a two- to threefold increase in antibodies titers as compared to those measured after the primary series [49].

A vaccine for HFRS caused by SEOV is prepared in primary golden hamster kidney cells (GHKC). Infected cells are harvested 9–10 days after infection and the whole-cell preparations treated with 0.025% formalin to inactivate infectivity. The vaccine is formulated with aluminum hy-droxide (0.5 mg/mL) adjuvant. Three doses of the vaccine were tested in 10 volunteers and two doses in 2 volunteers with intervals of 0, 1, and 3 weeks. All of the volunteers developed neutralizing antibodies in a focus reduction test, although titers were low, ranging from 1:10 to 1:160 [50].

The HTNV and SEOV cell-culture-derived vaccines and an SMB-derived inactivated vaccine were compared in more than 100,000 individuals in China. Each vaccine was given as a primary series of three intramuscular inoculations according to the specifications of the manufacturer followed by a boost at 1 year. The HTNV-MGKC vaccine was given at 0, 1, and 2 weeks. The SEOV-GHKC vaccine was given at 0, 2, and 4 weeks. The HTNV-SMB vaccine was given at 0, 2, and 4 weeks [51]. Evaluation of antibody responses in some of the recipients after the primary series of vaccinations revealed the SEOV vaccine to more effectively elicit neutralizing antibodies (~80% of volunteers) compared to the other two vaccines (~50–60% of volunteers). Of approximately 40,000 recipients of each vaccine, 4 who received the SEOV vaccine and 7 who received the HTNV vaccine developed HFRS during the 4 years after vaccination. Although this was apparently not a randomized study, and it is not clear how controls were chosen, there were many more cases of HFRS in each control group, with incidence as high as ~150 cases per 100,000 population in the first year after vaccination [51].

Because both of the monovalent vaccines elicited no or low cross-neutralizing antibodies to the heterotypic virus (HTNV or SEOV), efforts to develop a bivalent HTV-SEOV vaccine have been made. Two such vaccines have been tested in humans in China, one prepared in GHKC and one in MGKC. Three inoculations with the MGKC-derived vaccine elicited neutralizing antibodies to HTNV or SEOV in 88% or 96% of 81 volunteers [49].

The MGKC-derived vaccine was further tested in more than 1000 individuals in two regions of China [51,52]. About 10% of the recipients were screened for neutralizing antibodies after the primary series of vaccinations. Approximately 87% had neutralizing antibodies to HTNV and 96% to SEOV; however, the geometric mean titers were less than 15. A similar study with the GHKC-derived vaccine produced nearly the same results [51]. Further studies are in progress to evaluate the protective efficacies of these vaccines.

D. Recombinant DNA-Based Vaccine Approaches

None of the vaccines produced in Asia has been licensed for use outside their country of origin, and it is not likely that any will. The inherent problems associated with rodent-brain-derived vaccines, such as concerns about allergic encephalitis and potential prion-mediated diseases, make this approach unattractive. Cell-culture-derived hantavirus vaccines suffer from production problems associated with maintaining certified cells in acceptable substrates, purification, and inactivation of infectious virus, and formulation with adjuvant. In addition, because hantaviruses grow slowly and only to low titer, such vaccines would likely be expensive if produced under conditions mandated in many countries. To avoid these problems, recombinant DNA approaches have been the preferred method of vaccine development for HFRS outside of Asia.

Several recombinant DNA vaccine approaches have been evaluated in animals. These include the following: baculovirus-derived expression products [25,53], E. coli-expression products [28], chimeric and mosaic hepatitis B core antigens [54,55], packaged Sindbis replicons and DNA-launched Sindbis replicons [56], and naked DNA [27,57,58]. A comparison of the protective properties of these vaccine candidates in various models was reviewed recently elsewhere [51]. To date, only one recombinant DNA-based vaccine has been tested in humans. A recombinant vaccinia virus (VACV) was engineered from the Connaught strain of VACV to express both the M and S gene segments of HTNV [26]. The M segment, which encodes the two envelope glycoproteins (G1 and G2), was chosen to elicit neutralizing antibodies. The S segment, which encodes the nucleocapsid (N), was included because of earlier studies that demonstrated that vaccination with baculovirus-derived N elicited protective immunity to infection in hamsters [25]. The vaccine was tested in Phase I and Phase II clinical trials [59]. Neutralizing antibody responses (geometric mean titer, 160) were found in 72% of the 43 VACV-naive volunteers who received two doses of vaccine by subcutaneous inoculation in the Phase II trial. However, only 26% of the 47 VACV-immune volunteers developed neutralizing antibodies to HTNV after two vaccinations (geometric mean titer 24). Evaluation of lymphocyte proliferative responses to HTNV, SNV, and VACV of Phase I volunteers demonstrated a cross-reactive response with SNV and indicated that VACV-naive individuals had more vigorous responses than VACV-immune individuals [59]. The outcome of the study indicated that unlike experiments in hamsters [25], in which preexisting immunity to VACV was not an obstacle to successful vaccination, preexisting immunity to VACV in humans interfered with the ability of the vaccine to elicit a neutralizing antibody response.

Of the potential vaccine platforms assessed so far, DNA vaccines appear to be closest to further evaluation in humans. Comparing HTNV and SEOV M segment DNA vaccines delivered by gene gun to the recombinant VACV M + S vaccine in rhesus macaques demonstrated that the DNA vaccines elicited higher amounts of and longer-lasting neutralizing antibody responses than did the VACV vaccine [27]. Unlike results in hamsters, however, only low levels of cross-neutralizing antibodies to heterotypic virus (HTNV or SEOV) were observed. These results are similar to those observed in humans inoculated with the monovalent, cell-culture-derived Chinese vaccines. Further studies are needed to define more fully the minimal complement of hantaviral genes needed for vaccine efficacy in areas where more than one hantavirus causes disease.

II. TOWARD A HUMAN LASSA FEVER VACCINE

A. The Public Health Problem of Lassa Fever

Lassa fever is a viral hemorrhagic fever caused by an Arenavirus, first described in West Africa in the 1950s, although the virus was not isolated until 1969 [60,61].

Arenaviruses produce mostly silent, persistent infection in rodents. The principal risk to humans from Lassa virus is that the natural host, a small African rat, Mastomys natalensis, has successfully adapted to a peridomestic life in village houses in West Africa [62]. Exposure to the virus is therefore frequent, and with the human population growth in the endemic area over the last 50 years, the opportunities for human exposure to this virus, and thus risk of disease, have increased. Among the hemorrhagic fevers, Lassa fever affects by far the largest number of people, creating a geographic patchwork of endemic foci encompassing a population of ~ 180 million from Guinea to eastern Nigeria.

The lymphocytic choriomeningitis virus (LCMV) and Lassa virus (LASV) complex viruses are monophyletic with three distinct lineages, one of which contains Lassa, Mopeia, and Mobala viruses [63]. Mopeia comes from southern Africa and Mobala from central Africa, and both are carried by related Mastomys species [64]. Both can infect humans, but are apparently unable to cause significant clinical disease. Experimental infection of nonhuman primates (NHPs) with Mopeia virus is also silent. Mopeia virus has been proposed as a potential live-attenuated Lassa vaccine, and it is effective as such in NHPs.

In some areas of West Africa 50% of domestic rodents may be Mastomys [62]. Because Lassa virus is transmitted vertically in these rodents, infection of local populations of rodents tends to cluster. Thus, human infections tend also to be focal with periodic familial or village clusters against a background of single infections that make up the bulk of endemic disease. Over 200,000 Lassa virus infections are estimated to occur annually, with several thousand deaths [62,65–67]. Lassa fever occurs in all age groups and sexes and antibody prevalence increases with age. This is compatible with viral transmission to humans in and around the homes where the Mastomys live. Estimates of antibody prevalence range from 4–6% in Guinea to 15–20% in Nigeria, though in some villages in Sierra Leone, as many as 60% of the population have evidence of past infection. Among hospitalized patients, the mortality is 17% if untreated. In endemic areas, Lassa fever may account for 10–16% of all adult medical admissions and about 30% of adult deaths. Lassa fever also affects children, with higher mortality in infants [68,69].

Person-to-person spread of Lassa virus occurs within homes as well as in hospitals where the main problems have been inadequate disinfection and direct contact with infected blood and contaminated needles. The nosocomial epidemics can be devastating, resulting in deaths of patients and health care workers [70,71].

Lassa fever is an increasing threat that now affects West African communities outside of the broad area of rural endemicity. Indeed, urban Lassa fever in West Africa has been increasing in frequency [71]. In early 2000, hospital epidemics occurred in large towns in Nigeria, the most populous country in Africa. Since 1990, severe social disruption from conflicts and terror campaigns in Sierra Leone and Liberia have resulted in displacement of up to 2,000,000 people—25% of the population of the area—with a substantial increase in the already large number of Lassa fever cases and deaths. Lassa fever is the exotic hemorrhagic fever most likely to infect returning travelers. In the year 2000, four cases imported into Europe [72] died due to delay in diagnosis and in instituting antiviral therapy (ribavirin). Increased cases in non-West Africans have been seen since 2000 among United Nations peacekeeping efforts in Sierra Leone [73].

B. The Disease

Lassa fever begins insidiously, after an incubation period of 7–18 days, with fever, weakness, malaise, and severe head-ache—usually frontal—and a painful sore throat [74]. Up to a third of hospitalized Lassa fever patients progress to a prostrating illness 6 to 8 days after onset of fever, usually with persistent vomiting and diarrhea. Bleeding is seen in only 15–20% of patients, limited primarily to the mucosal surfaces or occasionally conjunctival hemorrhages or gastrointestinal or vaginal bleeding. Severe pulmonary edema and adult respiratory distress syndrome is common in fatal cases with gross head and neck edema, pharyngeal stridor, and hypovolemic shock. Case fatality in hospitalized patients is about 16%, albeit higher in some Nigerian outbreaks and in pregnant women in the third trimester (30–70% depending on the quality of obstetric care) [75]. Lassa fever may result in long-term sequelae. For example, nearly 30% of patients with Lassa fever suffer unilateral or bilateral deafness [76]. About half of the patients show a near or complete recovery by 3–4 months after onset, but the other half continue with significant sensorineural deafness, which after about a year will be permanent [76].

C. Molecular Biology of Lassa Virus

Like all arenaviruses, Lassa virus is an enveloped, pleomorphic, membrane virus with a mean diameter of 110–130 nm [1]. It contains two segments of single-stranded RNA, tightly associated with a nucleocapsid protein of molecular weight 65,000–72,000. The large strand of ambisense RNA, of molecular weight $(2.0–3.2) \times 10^6$, encodes the viral polymerase and a zinc-binding RING protein [77]. The small RNA ambisense single-strand, molecular weight about $(1.1–1.6) \times 10^6$, encodes the glycoprotein precursor (GPC) and the nucleoprotein (N). The genome is enclosed in a membrane bearing two glycosylated proteins of molecular weights of about 34,000–44,000 (G1) and 54,000–72,000 (G2), derived from GPC by posttranslational cleavage. Antigenic cross-reactivity by monoclonal antibodies occurs at least at one epitopic site across all known arenaviruses, but more cross-reactivity occurs between more geographically proximal viruses [78].

D. The Immunology of Lassa Fever

This rodent virus is handled quite differently by the immune systems of rodents and primates. In rodents, persistent infection ensues with little effect on the rodent. In humans, clearance of Lassa and LCM viruses depends primarily on cytotoxic T cells, while neutralizing antibodies are associated with clearance of viremia due to the South American arenaviruses [79]. There appears to be a brisk B-cell response with a classic primary IgG and IgM antibody response to Lassa

virus early in the illness. Development of antibody, however, does not coincide with viral clearance, and high viremia and high IgG and IgM titers often coexist in both humans and primates [80]. Indeed, virus may persist in the serum and urine of humans for several weeks after infection, and possibly in occult sites, such as renal tubules, for longer.

Neutralizing antibodies to Lassa virus are rarely detected in the serum of patients at the beginning of convalescence, and in most people and in experimentally infected monkeys, they are never detectable by a classical plaque reduction–neutralization assay. In a minority of patients, some low-titer serum neutralizing activity may be observed several months after resolution of the disease, but only by using a fixed-serum varying-virus dilution assay (log neutralization assay) [81]. Passive protection from Lassa virus has been demonstrated in animals given selected antiserum but only at the time or soon after inoculation with virus. While there have been anecdotal reports on the clinical effectiveness of Lassa immune plasma, controlled clinical trials with human convalescent plasma containing high-titer antibodies have shown no protective effect. Thus, the clearance of Lassa virus appears to be independent of antibody formation, and presumably depends on the CMI response.

E. Prevention of Lassa Fever: Why a Vaccine?

Lassa virus is acquired in the community either from infected rodents or from people. Rodent to human infection is highly associated with indiscriminate food storage, and practices such as catching, cooking, and eating rodents [62]. Person-to-person spread of Lassa virus in households is common, and in villages, risk of infection is associated with direct contact with someone during the acute phases of illness. Preventing rodent/human contact will eliminate the bulk of the primary cases, and if these are prevented, then person-to-person spread will be eliminated. Control could be largely achieved by improving living conditions, food storage, education, and general hygiene in the community.

Direct contact between virus-contaminated articles and surfaces and cuts and scratches on bare hands and feet may be the most important and consistent mode of transmission in endemic areas. The sporadic pattern of human infection in households suggests that aerosol is not a mode of transmission. Rodent control can reduce the risk of Lassa fever considerably, but rodent control on the scale needed in rural West Africa is unlikely [82]. Similarly, economic development that might lead to improvements in housing, food storage, and education is unlikely to ensue soon in conflict ravaged West Africa. On the contrary, Lassa fever cases continue to increase with displacement of large populations throughout the endemic areas in Liberia and Sierra Leone and in parts of Nigeria. An effective vaccine could be a useful control measure, assuming that it could be delivered in face of the social upheaval affecting endemic areas.

F. Is a Vaccine Feasible?

Data from human observations in the field show that immunity is achievable, as a single infection with Lassa virus provides long-term protective immunity against future disease. A second clinical attack of Lassa fever has never been documented despite more than 13 years of continuous observation in a single endemic area (J. B. McCormick, unpublished data). People living or working in conditions where repeated exposure could be expected do have periodic rises in Lassa-virus-specific antibody titers, but no disease [62,83].

There is an excellent precedent for Lassa vaccine in Argentina, where a successful vaccine for AHF has now undergone Phase III studies, and is in use in the endemic area of Argentina, where it has all but eliminated the disease [84]. This is a live-attenuated vaccine, designated Candid1.

G. Options for a Vaccine

1. Live-Attenuated Vaccine

Approaches to vaccines to Lassa virus began in the 1980s. Soon after its isolation, it was shown that Mopeia virus provides monkeys with full protection against fatal Lassa virus challenge [85]. However, data on Mopeia virus are limited, and the virus is classified as BSL3, mostly because of "guilt by association." In many ways it is an ideal "natural" vaccine, but concerns for safety have not yet allowed us to consider Mopeia a valid option and there are currently no other live candidates in sight [86,87].

2. Killed Whole Virus Vaccine Candidates

A killed vaccine was tried in nonhuman primates and found to offer no protection at all [88]. Vaccination of primates with inactivated (gamma irradiated) whole Lassa virus resulted in antibody responses to both envelope proteins, and a brisk booster response after challenge, but all animals died with serum viral titers equal to unvaccinated controls (Table 1). This disappointing experience further emphasizes that protection depends on the ability to elicit a robust T-cell response.

3. Genetically Engineered Virus Vaccine Candidates

The first genetically engineered vaccines appeared in the early 1980s. S segment sequences of the Lassa virus genome were expressed as a fusion protein in *Escherichia coli* [89]. The Lister strain of vaccinia virus was used to express the nucleocapsid gene of Lassa virus. Guinea pigs vaccinated with the recombinant virus were protected against challenge of 10^2 of Lassa virus, whereas control animals died [90]. This recombinant, however, did not protect primates. It was not until the glycoprotein was expressed in vaccinia that both guinea pigs and primates were uniformly protected [91]. The protection resulting from vaccination with the recombinant virus vaccines did not correlate with the levels of prechallenge serum antibodies, suggesting that a CMI response is a critical component of protective immunity to Lassa fever [92,93].

A broader study of protection was performed with a range of recombinant vaccinia viruses expressing NP, GPC, and combinations of these proteins [87,92]. The studies were performed using 44 nonhuman primates: 28 *Macaca mulatta* (rhesus) and 16 *Macaca fascicularis* (cynomolgus). The recombinant vaccinia viruses expressed S-segment Lassa structural proteins derived from the Josiah strain of Lassa virus, namely: (1) the full-length glycoprotein (V-LSG), (2) the nucleoprotein (V-LSN), (3) full-length glycoprotein and nucleoprotein in the same construct (V-LSG/N), and (4) single glycoproteins (V-LSG1, residues 1–296, and V-LSG2, deletion of residues 67–234) [87]. Two animals were "vaccinated" with Mopeia virus, which, as it produces no symptoms in humans or in monkeys, was used as a live-attenuated positive control; both animals "vaccinated" with Mopeia were protected. All animals were challenged subcutaneously with 10^3 to 10^4 plaque-forming units (PFU) of the Josiah strain of Lassa virus. After Lassa virus challenge, all unvac-

Table 1 Antibody and Viremia in Primates Vaccinated with Inactivated Lassa Vaccine and Challenged with 10^4 Lassa Virus

	Antibody to Lassa virus				
	Vaccinated			Unvaccinated	
Day post vaccine					
0	0	0	0	0	0
14	64	16	256	0	0
35	32	32	128	0	0
71	64	64	256	0	0
101	64	64	64	0	0
108	256	64	64	0	0
Day post challenge					
4	256	64	256	0	0
8	1024	256	1024	0	0
10	4096	1024	4096	0	4
12	4096	4096	4096	64	256
Peak viremia after challenge (all animals died)					
Viremia	6.1	5.7	5.2	6.1	6.1

cinated animals died (0% survival) (Table 2), whereas 9 of 10 animals vaccinated with full S segment proteins survived (90% survival). Although no animals that received full-length glycoprotein alone had high-titer antibody before challenge, 8 of 9 survived (89%). In contrast, all animals vaccinated with nucleoprotein developed high-titer antibody but 8 of 11 died (27% survival). No animals vaccinated with single glycoproteins (G1 or G2) survived challenge but all those that received both single glycoproteins (G1 + G2) at separate sites survived, showing that both glycoproteins are independently important in protection [87]. Neither group of survivors had demonstrable antibody after vaccination and before challenge.

These data show that the GPC gene is necessary and sufficient to protect primates against a large parenteral challenge dose. Still, we conclude that antibody, even to the Lassa glycoprotein, plays a minor, if any, role in clearance of infection and protection in nonhuman primates and probably humans [86,87].

H. Specificity of the Vaccine

Amino acid sequence comparisons between the nucleoproteins and glycoproteins reveal that the G2 envelope glycoprotein is more conserved among arenaviruses than the internal nucleoprotein [94]. Monoclonal antibody mapping of the glycoproteins of African arenaviruses also show that the G2 is more conserved than G1. Indeed there is a conserved B-cell epitope on G2 across all of the known African arenaviruses including the protective Mopeia virus, and most South American arenaviruses studied [78]. This may not be of as much consequence to vaccine design as it first appears because the variation at the level of the glycoprotein is much less, and we know that it is the antiglycoprotein CTL response that protects. Variation between Mopeia and Lassa viruses in glycoprotein sequences ranges from 20 to 25%; nevertheless, Mopeia protects in nonhuman

primates against Lassa challenge [87]. Fortunately, it may turn out that the protective CTL epitopes are relatively well conserved throughout the continent. Because there is no evolutionary pressure on the virus to evade the primate immune system, we can hope that a single vaccine strain will be adequate for the entire endemic region.

I. Candidates for a Human-Use Lassa Vaccine

It is likely that a Lassa fever vaccine could be developed with an acceptable safety and efficacy profile. However, the vaccinia format is no longer tenable because of potential side effects, particularly in Africa, where HIV prevalence is high.

The population to be served is poor, so a Lassa virus vaccine must be cheap, easily and safely administered, and stable. Because we have now clearly shown that a recombinant vaccine bearing the glycoprotein affords protection, the first issue is the delivery format for this protein. There are several options. A nonpathogenic vaccine such as Mopeia should work very well, but safety issues are likely to impede its development. The attraction of the live-attenuated vaccine approach is that a single immunization, as with the 17D yellow fever vaccine, might well provide protection for many years, particularly among persons living in endemic areas who might receive natural boosts to immunity. Given the remoteness and mobility of the target population, this is a highly desirable property for any vaccine candidate.

Candidate-killed vaccines have been ineffective, and without other innovations, are excluded from consideration. Attenuated poxviruses, such as the Canarypox virus [92], an avian virus that does not replicate in mammalian cells, remain a possibility, but the question is whether the immunogenicity will be sufficient, and how many doses might be needed to achieve protection.

A Lassa fever vaccine requires new approaches. DNA vaccines would offer much in the way of low-cost, stable

Table 2 Results of Lassa Vaccine Experiments in Nonhuman Primates

Virion protein expression	Vaccine	Survivors/Total	Protection (%)	Peak viremia	Median day of death (range)
None	NYBH Vaccinia	0/3	0	6.7	15 (15–19)
	None	0/7			12 (10–15)
Single glycoproteins	V-LSG1	0/2	0	6.9	15 (14–16)
	V-LSG2	0/2		6.8	12.5 (12–13)
Full glycoprotein	V-LSG	6/7	89	4.6	21[a]
	V-LSG1 + V-LSG2	2/2			
Nucleoprotein	V-LSN	3/11	27	9	11.5 (9–13)
Full S-segment	Mopeia Virus	2/2	90	2.2	11[a]
	V-LSG + V-LSN	5/6		1.7	
	V-LSG/N	2/2		7	
Total		20/44			

V-LSG1 = Lassa virus glycoprotein 1.
V-LSG2 = Lassa virus glycoprotein 2.
V-LSG = Lassa virus complete glycoprotein (1 and 2).
V-LSN = Lassa nucleoprotein.
[a] These two animals were challenged 488 and 700 days post vaccination. All protected animals were challenged between 38 and 354 days post vaccination. Diminution of survival with duration of interval, $p = 0.034$.

vaccines, but several booster doses might be needed. Another approach is to use the 17D strain of yellow fever virus as a vehicle, without losing yellow fever antigenicity, because the population at risk for Lassa fever is also exposed to yellow fever. For the long term, a yellow fever/Lassa fever chimera vaccine for use in EPI in West Africa is a very attractive solution. The cDNA clone of yellow fever virus could also be used as a vehicle for delivering Lassa virus DNA. This chimera might be a very interesting and very practical model for the future of vaccines, particularly for populations in developing countries. Yellow fever chimera vaccines are already undergoing trials for Japanese encephalitis and dengue [95,96]. However, these last two diseases are caused by flaviviruses, and the chimeras replace the yellow fever E proteins with the proteins of the related virus. A yellow fever/Lassa chimera requires a different approach, that of inserting an additional gene. Still another approach, involving a replication-defective alphavirus that carries genes of both Lassa and Ebola, has shown preliminary promise in guinea pigs [97].

J. Target Population

The population at risk encompasses most of the population of West Africa to Nigeria, of the order of 200 million or more by the time we have a vaccine in place. The people most at risk are the poorest of the rural inhabitants and health care workers, who should be the first people offered the vaccine. Because the epidemiological profile of Lassa fever is similar to that for yellow fever, long-term objectives should envisage inclusion of a Lassa vaccine in EPI for West Africa. However, decisions such as these will depend largely on the format of the final vaccine, particularly the recommended schedule for booster shots.

Recently, aid workers including UN personnel and NGO employees have been infected in West Africa. Consequently, travelers to the region who expect to venture outside the strict confines of the major cities should be considered targets for vaccination. Finally, laboratory staff in any country likely to receive specimens from Lassa-virus-infected patients, staff caring for sick returning travelers from Lassa endemic regions, or those working with Lassa virus in research capacity, would also benefit from a future licensed vaccine. Indeed, the existence of an effective vaccine should allow the virus to be downgraded to BSL3, because at that point it would not only be treatable but preventable.

K. Economics and Clinical Trials

The economic and political obstacles to producing an effective Lassa fever vaccine far outweigh the practical and scientific obstacles. The fear of biological warfare and manipulation of the hemorrhagic fever viruses, including Lassa virus, to produce weapons has spurred some publicly funded research. The fact remains, however, that there is not a credible market for a Lassa fever vaccine, despite the endemic disease burden and risk to travelers and laboratory workers.

Among the viral hemorrhagic fevers, Lassa fever along with hantaviruses afflicts the greatest number of victims and represents an emerging disease that could threaten larger communities. Although development of an effective and safe vaccine is scientifically feasible, obstacles to Lassa fever vaccine development are more economic than scientific. The challenge is to overcome these obstacles.

III. VACCINES AGAINST FILOVIRUSES

A. Filoviruses and Filovirus Disease

Filoviruses (from the Latin *filum*: thread, as in *filament*) are distinctively pleomorphic, threadlike viral particles, measuring 78–80 nm in diameter with median lengths of ca. 790 nm (Marburg virus) to 970 nm (Ebola virus) [98]. One of the families in the viral order Mononegavirales, filoviruses contain nonsegmented, negative-stranded RNA genomes of about 19 kb. In the most recent taxonomy [1], the constellation of distinct but related viruses known as Marburg virus is considered a single species, and given the abbreviation MARV; Ebola viruses (EBOV) are even more diverse and divided into four species, with corresponding abbreviations for the species called Zaire (ZEBOV), Sudan (SEBOV), Cote d'Ivoire (CIEBOV), and Reston (REBOV). Most remarkable about filoviruses is the high mortality rate of the hemorrhagic fever that ensues upon infection: case fatality rates have been as high as 88% (ZEBOV), 67% (MARV), and 53% (SEBOV). This, together with the demonstrated potential for airborne infection [99,100], and the concern that at least one of these viruses (MARV) was carried to an advanced form of weaponization [101,102], have raised the alarm about their potential uses as weapons of mass casualty and terror, and have underscored the need for antiviral therapies and preventive vaccines [103].

The first documented and characterized filovirus outbreak occurred in 1967 consequent to Ugandan nonhuman primates imported to Marburg, Germany [104]. Ebola virus was recognized in 1976, and subsequent recorded outbreaks of both viruses were sporadic. More recently, whether due to increased incidence or better surveillance, outbreaks of human disease are typically observed almost every year in sub-Saharan Africa [105]. Infections are transmitted through close contact with fluids or tissues from infected patients or monkeys, or by accidental exposure to infected instruments. A reservoir host in which filoviruses reside between outbreaks has not been identified, although small mammals, especially bats, have been incriminated [106].

Among the seven viral genes, the glycoprotein (GP) undergoes abundant N- and O-glycosylation cleavage by furinlike enzymes to two molecules called GP1 (N terminal) and GP2 (C terminal) [107]. Glycoprotein is the only protein known to be present on the surface of viral particles and infected cells, and thus has received attention as the logical candidate for cell receptor interactions and viral tropisms [108–110], antibody mediated protection [111–114], and critical pathways of virus entry and egress [109,110,115]. VP35 has been described as an interferon antagonist, a functional analog of proteins found in such diverse viruses as influenza and vaccinia, and which appear to increase viral virulence in some hosts [116]. NP is a nucleoprotein with observed molecular mass (M_r) of ca. 100 kDa, and VP40 is a matrix protein essential for viral formation and budding [115]. With all species of EBOV but not MARV, the genome encodes and produces in abundance a truncated and partially frame-shifted variant of GP known as soluble GP (sGP); its role in EBOV biology remains an enigma, as does its relevance to immunity [107,117].

B. Animal Models of Filovirus Infection and Immunity

In terms of experimental infections by any of several routes, the known filoviruses are extraordinarily virulent for NHPs, usually exceeding 90% mortality, though typical manifestations of disease and times to death may vary between NHP species [100,118–121]. In NHPs, lethal doses tend to equate with infectious doses, which in turn are more numerous than the plaque-forming units conventionally measured in cell culture. By comparison, human susceptibility is difficult to judge from fragmented epidemiological data; in general, humans appear only marginally less susceptible than NHP, with the exception of REBOV, which is highly virulent in NHP but has not been associated with human disease. Guinea pigs are typically vulnerable to infection but not to death when infected with primary filovirus isolates, but several Marburg and Ebola viruses have been rendered lethal for guinea pigs by serial passage in this species [104,111,117,119]. Mice are even more refractory to lethal infection, and only ZEBOV has been adapted to lethal infection of immunocompetent mice [122]. From the capacity of several Ebola and Marburg viruses to cause lethal infection in severe combined immunodeficient (SCID) mice, it was inferred that any innate immunity to filoviruses in mice is not absolute, and that resistance to disease and death require adaptive immune responses in this species [122]. Several other animal species, including bats, can be infected by ZEBOV [106], but much remains unknown about potential host ranges of these viruses.

Filoviruses are relatively promiscuous in their binding and entry into numerous cell types in vitro, with only lymphocytes being wholly refractory [110,123], yet filovirus infections of mice, monkeys, and humans indicate substantial biases in the cells and tissues affected. Whether by virtue of higher receptor affinities (and/or unidentified coreceptors), or less specific phagocytic properties, it is striking that both Marburg and Ebola viruses preferentially infect cells of the monocyte–macrophage lineage early in infection [104,107,121]. What marks lethal infections is that viral infection proceeds to high levels (e.g., 10^8 PFU/mL in blood, and higher in some organs) unchecked by an effective immune response [104,124], with death some 7–16 days (typically shorter in NHPs) after onset of febrile disease. Endothelial cell infection is prominent late in infection, as are infections of liver and other organs; but disease manifestations differ sufficiently among human cases in a single outbreak, among different filoviruses, and among animal models for a given filovirus, that a universal pathogenetic pathway has eluded description. Interferon was suggested as a potential therapeutic approach in mice [122] but only delayed death in NHP [125]. VP35 was found to act as an interferon antagonist [116], fitting into a pattern of viral evasion of host innate immunity established previously with influenza virus and its interferon antagonist NS1. The mechanism by which host interferon responses may affect resistance is unclear, and host factors that affect viral replication in different cells or host species also remain to be identified.

1. Immune Responses in Animal Models

As with most infectious diseases, protection against filoviruses is thought to involve both innate and adaptive immune responses, the former perhaps crucial in the fate of nonimmune persons [124,126] and animals, the latter more the target of vaccine technology. Current knowledge of the roles of cellular and humoral immunity to filoviruses is at best an incomplete guide to the kinds and specificities of responses to be evoked by effective filovirus vaccines. Experimental transfers of sera or monoclonal antibodies, derived from convalescent or hyperimmunized animals, into naive (unvaccinated) animals, have yielded mixed results that ultimately do support a significant role for antibodies. For MARV, sera from guinea pigs—elicited by nonlethal infection or by vaccination with killed virus in adjuvant—was able to protect nonimmune guinea pigs [104,127]; moreover, murine monoclonal antibodies were moderately efficacious in guinea pigs [111]. For ZEBOV, certain murine monoclonal antibodies reactive with GP were proven capable of preventing lethal infection (in a murine disease model) in both prophylactic and therapeutic regimens, and the data suggested complex requirements of specificity, affinity, and perhaps isotype for optimal antibody effectiveness [112]. A human monoclonal antibody showed some efficacy against ZEBOV in guinea pigs [114]. In NHPs, the protection afforded by transferred antibodies has been more difficult to demonstrate, with reports of significant success [128] opposed by others that showed only a delay in viremia and death [125]. With both MARV [104] and EBOV [129], plasma or whole blood from convalescent patients has been used during outbreaks in attempts to mitigate disease in the later victims of the outbreak; the treatments were interpreted as harmless and arguably helpful, but were confounded by small sample sizes, patient selection criteria, and an observed tendency for mortality rates to decrease during filovirus outbreaks. A further complicating factor in filovirus vaccine development strategies is that no reliable laboratory correlate has been identified for the protective effects of antibodies: the term "neutralizing antibody" has proven wholly inadequate to describe events either in vitro or in vivo [112,117,118,127]. ZEBOV data affirm a longstanding observation with many viruses, namely, that some antibodies may lack any demonstrable neutralizing activity in vitro but nonetheless mediate protection in vivo. Except for a provocative assertion of protection by nonneutralizing anti-VP40 antibodies with Marburg virus [130], it appears that protective antibodies against filoviruses are directed against GP, and that, absent the discovery of particularly effective subpopulations, such antibodies by themselves may be inadequate to afford robust protection.

Although far from understood, the role for T cells in immunity to filoviruses appears to be highly significant. In the murine model for ZEBOV, it was shown that CTLs are elicited by DNA- or RNA-based vaccines that contain NP [131,132] and that NP-specific CTL adoptively transferred into naive mice protected them against ZEBOV [132]. Similarly, the other internal or non-surface antigens of Ebola virions (VP40, VP35, VP30, VP24) were also proven capable of protecting against Ebola virus, and characteristic of T-cell responses, different antigens were shown more or less effective in different inbred strains of mice [133]. With MARV, the role of T cells was inferred from the capacities of NP and VP35 to protect guinea pigs [118,134], and from the capacity of NP to evoke incomplete protection in NHP [118]. In trials to determine which filoviral antigens are most effective in inducing protective immunity, GP has remained a principal candidate. That GP is a likely target not only for antibodies but also for T cells is supported by data obtained from mice [131,135] and by T-cell proliferation induced in NHPs and measured against sGP antigen [136].

Efficacy studies of Marburg virus vaccines in experimental animals have raised a notable caveat. In both guinea pigs and NHP, a minor proportion of vaccinated animals not only remained susceptible to lethal infection, but died earlier than unvaccinated controls, an accelerated but ineffectual immune response apparently exacerbating disease (reviewed in Ref. 119; see also Ref. 118). These observations underscore a need for caution in vaccine development, a lesson learned long ago with inactivated vaccines for another member of Mononegavirales, respiratory syncytial virus [137]. However, before despairing for the prospects of a safe vaccine, it should be noted that the altered disease course was only observed in the context of a viral infection that is nearly 100% lethal in unvaccinated animals. Some manifestation of "immune enhancement" is not unique to MARV, as incomplete immunity mediated either by antibodies or T cells has been shown previously in several models of viral disease to be potentially harmful. Similar observations of "early deaths" in vaccinated animals have not been reported with EBOV.

2. Antigenic Diversity of Filoviruses

Vaccine research to date has centered largely on the Zaire species of Ebola virus and on the Marburg virus clade that includes Popp and Musoke isolates. There exists very little serologic cross-reactivity between EBOV and MARV, and no cross-protection between these viruses has been observed. The emphasis on ZEBOV derives from its having the highest mortality rates among all filoviruses in humans, and from the experimental convenience that lethal animal models are well established for this virus in NHP, guinea pigs, and mice. However, the ability of a vaccine for ZEBOV to protect against the Sudan species (SEBOV), which has also caused major human outbreaks with high mortalities, is unknown. In particular, the GP molecule, incriminated as a principal target of protective immune responses, shares only 50% sequence identity between ZEBOV and SEBOV (Figure 2), and serological differences between these viruses are substantial [1,112]. Even for Marburg virus, where all isolates are considered a single species taxonomically, both polyclonal and monoclonal antibodies

underscore the substantial antigenic differences in GP between the Musoke and Ravn strains, imparted by 22% nonidentity in GP protein sequences [127]. The degree to which conserved epitopes [112] can be exploited to construct broadly protective vaccines versus a requirement for antigenically complex vaccines for both EBOV and MARV remains to be determined.

C. Conventional Vaccine Approaches

1. Killed Vaccines

From the earliest attempts to develop classical vaccines for filoviruses, it was suggested that vaccination was feasible, yet potentially difficult. In particular, formalin-inactivated viruses evoked protective immunity in half or more vaccinated guinea pigs, with both ZEBOV [138] and MARV [119]. In subsequent studies, it was shown that purified and irradiated MARV, given in adjuvant, could evoke robust immunity in guinea pigs [127,139]. Cursory examinations of killed ZEBOV vaccines in NHPs illustrated little protective efficacy [140]. Combined with the obvious hazards of producing such vaccines, these results did little to encourage further development of killed filovirus vaccines.

2. Live Vaccines

Although laboratory animals that survive filovirus infection are typically protected against lethal infection with the same isolate or a closely related virus [122,139], live-attenuated vaccines for filoviruses have not been considered widely as a safe alternative for human use. However, the recent capacity to recover infectious Ebola virus from cloned DNA and thereby insert attenuating mutations rationally and perhaps irreversibly into filoviruses [141,142] renders a live vaccine approach feasible.

D. Recombinant DNA Vaccines

1. Subunit Vaccines Derived from Recombinant DNA Technology

Relatively little has been reported on the vaccine potential of individual filovirus antigens prepared first by recombinant DNA technology and then used as experimental vaccines. For MARV, some efficacy was noted with NP but not VP40 in guinea pigs [134]. The GP molecule was produced as a truncated soluble product (its C-terminal membrane anchor removed) by recombinant baculoviruses in lepidopteran cells; this antigen, together with adjuvant, was sufficient to protect most but not all guinea pigs from lethal challenge [127,139]. It was also found that the GP made in insect cells, though abundantly glycosylated, differed in its carbohydrates from the native GP made in mammalian cells [127]. EBOV vaccine efforts have largely bypassed subunit strategies in favor of other approaches [117]. As an alternative way to prepare recombinant antigen and present it to the immune system, it was recently found that viruslike particles, resembling ZEBOV or MARV both physically and antigenically, could be produced from mammalian cells in vitro; minimally, these particles required and contained both GP and VP40 [115].

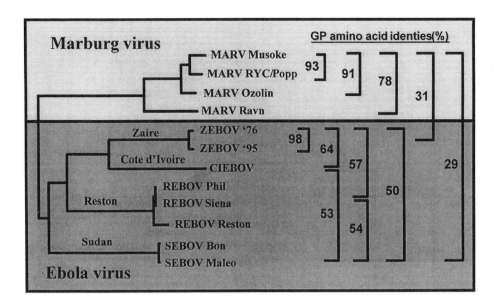

Figure 2 The phylogenetic basis of antigenic differences among filoviruses. Trees were determined from glycoprotein (GP) gene sequences. GP amino acid identities are approximations from BLASTP pairwise comparisons of translated GP genes. Marburg virus is considered a single species within its genus, while the Ebola virus genus is taxonomically divided into four species (see text, "Filoviruses and Filovirus Disease").

2. Gene-Based Vaccination

A series of reports indicated that the filovirus GP molecule could serve as a protective antigen in guinea pigs or mice, and that efficacy could be achieved using any of several vaccine strategies that involved production of the antigen within the cells of vaccinated animals. Thus, recombinant GP expressed by recombinant vaccinia virus was shown to confer incomplete protection against ZEBOV [143]; GP expressed by alphavirus replicons was shown to protect against lethal MARV challenge [111,118] or ZEBOV [144]; and GP delivered as DNA plasmid was shown to protect against ZEBOV [131,135] and MARV [139] in guinea pigs or mice. When other proteins were examined, it was shown that MARV NP or VP35 delivered via alphavirus replicons could protect most guinea pigs [118], whereas the capacity of ZEBOV NP to protect guinea pigs was either negative [143,144] or equivocal [135]. In mice, where EBOV but not MARV virus could be tested in lethal challenge models, it was found that either replicon or DNA vaccines could protect, and that protective antigens included GP, NP, VP40, VP35, VP30, and VP24 [131–133,144].

The more rigorous tests of filovirus vaccine efficacies are in NHPs, the only known species for which primary isolates of filoviruses are generally even more lethal than in humans. Encouragingly, it was found that a replicon-based vaccine for MARV, whether comprised of GP or a mixture of GP and NP, afforded robust protection (no detectable viremia, no disease) in six of six cynomolgus macaques inoculated with a relatively high dose (8000 PFU) of the prototype MARV strain, Musoke. By itself, NP elicited only incomplete protection, i.e., two of three animals survived but were viremic and symptomatic [118]. An identical vaccination

protocol using a replicon expressing Ebola GP, with similar serological indices of successful vaccination (Hevey, unpublished), resulted in no protection from viremia or death in cynomolgus macaques infected with 1000 PFU Ebola virus [140]. While DNA vaccines containing GP protected the majority of monkeys from MARV (C. Schmaljohn, unpublished), neither DNA vaccines nor vaccinia recombinants proved efficacious against ZEBOV, affirming the apparently greater difficulty of protecting cynomolgus macaques from ZEBOV [140] as compared either to MARV in this primate species, or to ZEBOV in rodents.

3. Prime-Boost Vaccination in Nonhuman Primates

More recently, an alternative experimental approach has been used to vaccinate monkeys successfully against ZEBOV, providing new cause for optimism [136]. Cynomolgus macaques were vaccinated three times, at 4-week intervals, with a DNA-based vaccine that contained GP antigen genes from ZEBOV, SEBOV, and ICEBOV along with the NP antigen from ZEBOV. Animals were then "boosted" 12 weeks after the last DNA vaccination with 10^{10} PFU of a defective adenovirus that expressed only ZEBOV GP. Twelve weeks later, after a substantial rise in antibody levels (ELISA) had been demonstrated, macaques were inoculated intraperitoneally with approximately 6 PFU of ZEBOV. Four of four vaccinated animals survived this challenge, while all four unvaccinated animals either died or were killed while symptomatic. Further studies are in progress to reconcile and explain the differences in outcomes with different vaccine approaches. Additional efforts are designed to define the mechanisms of protection and relevant immune correlates for human studies, as well as to define efficacy with respect to viral challenge dose, route of infection, and breadth of protection against different viral isolates.

E. Prospects for Human Vaccines

Vaccine discovery efforts with filoviruses suggest that safe and effective vaccines are achievable. Based on progress to date, the National Institutes of Health is proceeding toward a Phase 1 human safety/immunogenicity trial of a DNA-based vaccine for Ebola virus. Marburg virus vaccine candidates are also advancing through the necessary production and regulatory steps required for human trials. In either case, because controlled human trials are neither feasible nor ethical, vaccine licensure for human use will face a relatively new and daunting challenge: the requirement that efficacy in humans be unambiguously inferred from animal efficacy data. Understanding the nature of protective immune responses will be among the requirements for this task.

IV. SUMMARY: VACCINES FOR VIRAL HEMORRHAGIC FEVERS

"Viral hemorrhagic fevers" is a collective term that is often used to simplify discussion of a highly diverse group of agents largely unfamiliar to and rarely encountered by Western medicine. As illustrated in this chapter for an important subset of these agents (hantaviruses, arenaviruses, and filoviruses), the diseases caused by these viruses are usually febrile, often deadly, but not always hemorrhagic [103]. Moreover, the antigenic structures, predominant forms of immunity required, and pathogenetic mechanisms of different viral hemorrhagic fevers are so divergent as to prevent their reduction to a single medical or vaccine problem. Recently, many have awakened to an unprecedented need to be vigilant about the natural or malevolent emergence of these viruses in society [103]. Fortunately, as shown in this chapter, much progress has already been made toward human vaccines for these viruses. Still, vaccines for hantaviruses, arenaviruses, and filoviruses remain largely untested or unproven in humans, and none is licensed for use in the United States. Adequate resources and commitment, required to bring vaccine discovery efforts to the full fruition of licensure, were previously lacking, and it remains unclear whether the recent surge in interest will be sustained.

ACKNOWLEDGMENTS

The views, opinions and/or findings contained in this report are those of the authors and should not be construed as an official Department of the Army position, policy, or decision unless so designated by other documentation.

REFERENCES

1. van Regenmortel MHV, et al. Seventh Report of the International Committee on Taxonomy of Viruses. Academic Press, 2000.

2. Monroe MC, et al. Genetic diversity and distribution of *Peromyscus*-borne hantaviruses in North America [published erratum appears in Emerg Infect Dis 1999 Mar–Apr;5(2):314]. Emerg Infect Dis 1999; 5:75–86.

3. Plyusnin A, Morzunov SP. Virus evolution and genetic diversity of hantaviruses and their rodent hosts. Curr Top Microbiol Immunol 2001; 256:47–75.

4. Nichol ST. Genetic analysis of hantaviruses and their host relationships. In: Saluzzo JF, Dodet B, eds. Emergence and Control of Rodent-Borne Viral Diseases. Paris: Elsevier Press, 1999 (In press).

5. Sanchez AJ, et al. Genetic identification and characterization of limestone canyon virus, a unique *Peromyscus*-borne hantavirus. Virology 2001; 286:345–553.

6. Schmaljohn C, Hjelle B. Hantaviruses: a global disease problem. Emerg Infect Dis 1997; 3:95–104.

7. Arikawa J, et al. Epizootiological studies of hantavirus infection among urban rats in Hokkaido, Japan: evidences for the persistent infection from the sero-epizootiological surveys and antigenic characterizations of hantavirus isolates. J Vet Med Sci 1994; 56:27–32.

8. Kariwa H, et al. Modes of Seoul virus infections: persistency in newborn rats and transiency in adult rats. Arch Virol 1996; 141:2327–2338.

9. Lee H, et al. Antibody response to Hantaan virus, the etiologic agent of Korean hemorrhagic fever, after inoculation in experimental animal. Korean J Virol 1981; 11:7–11.

10. Tanishita O, et al. Persistent infection of rats with haemorrhagic fever with renal syndrome virus and their antibody responses. J Gen Virol 1986; 67(Pt 12):2819–2824.

11. Meyer BJ, Schmaljohn CS. Persistent hantavirus infections: characteristics and mechanisms. Trends Microbiol 2000; 8:61–67.

12. Lee HW, et al. Intraspecific transmission of Hantaan virus, etiologic agent of Korean hemorrhagic fever, in the rodent *Apodemus agrarius*. Am J Trop Med Hyg 1981; 30:1106–1112.

13. Lee HW, Johnson KM. Laboratory-acquired infections with Hantaan virus, the etiologic agent of Korean hemorrhagic fever. J Infect Dis 1982; 146:645–651.

14. Glass G, et al. Association of intraspecific wounding with hantaviral infection in wild rats (*Rattus norvegicus*). Epidemiol Infect 1988; 101:459–472.

15. Lee HW. Epidemiology and pathogenesis of hemorrhagic fever with renal syndrome. In: Elliott RM ed. The Bunyaviridae. New York: Plenum Press, 1996:253–267.

16. Clement J, et al. The hantaviruses of Europe: from the bedside to the bench. Emerg Infect Dis 1997; 3:205–211.

17. Clement J, et al. Spread of hantavirus infections in Europe [letter; comment]. Lancet 1996; 347:771771.

18. Lee HW, van der Groen G. Hemorrhagic fever with renal syndrome. Prog Med Virol 1989; 36:62–102.

19. Ksiazek TG, et al. Identification of a new North American hantavirus that causes acute pulmonary insufficiency. Am J Trop Med Hyg 1995; 52:117–123.

20. Enria DA, et al. Clinical manifestations of New World hantaviruses. Curr Top Microbiol Immunol 2001; 256:117–134.

21. Padula PJ, et al. Hantavirus pulmonary syndrome outbreak in Argentina: molecular evidence for person-to-person transmission of Andes virus. Virology 1998; 241:323–330.

22. Enria D, et al. Hantavirus pulmonary syndrome in Argentina. Possibility of person to person transmission. Medicina 1996; 56:709–711.

23. Wells RM, et al. An unusual hantavirus outbreak in southern Argentina: person-to-person transmission? Hantavirus Pulmonary Syndrome Study Group for Patagonia. Emerg Infect Dis 1997; 3:171–174.

24. Hooper JW, et al. A lethal disease model for hantavirus pulmonary syndrome. Virology 2001; 289:6–14.

25. Schmaljohn CS, et al. Antigenic subunits of Hantaan virus expressed by baculovirus and vaccinia virus recombinants. J Virol 1990; 64:3162–3170.

26. Schmaljohn CS, et al. Preparation of candidate vaccinia-vectored vaccines for haemorrhagic fever with renal syndrome. Vaccine 1992; 10:10–13.

27. Hooper JW, et al. DNA vaccination with the Hantaan virus M gene protects hamsters against three of four HFRS hantaviruses and elicits a high-titer neutralizing antibody response in rhesus monkeys. J Virol 2001; 75:8469–8477.

28. Lundkvist A, et al. Characterization of Puumala virus nucleocapsid protein: identification of B-cell epitopes and domains involved in protective immunity. Virology 1996; 216:397–406.

29. Xu X, et al. Immunity to hantavirus challenge in *Meriones unguiculatus* induced by vaccinia-vectored viral proteins. Am J Trop Med Hyg 1992; 47:397–404.

30. Chu Y-K, et al. A vaccinia-vectored Hantaan virus vaccine protects hamsters from challenge with Hantaan and Seoul viruses, but not Puumala virus. J Virol 1995; 69:6417–6423.

31. Arikawa J, et al. Protective role of antigenic sites on the envelope protein of Hantaan virus defined by monoclonal antibodies. Arch Virol 1992; 126:271–281.

32. Zhang X, et al. Characteristics of passive immunity against hantavirus infection in rats. Arch Virol 1989; 105:235–246.

33. Bharadwaj M, et al. Humoral immune responses in the hantavirus cardiopulmonary syndrome. J Infect Dis 2000; 182:43–48.

34. Asada H, et al. Cross-reactive immunity among different serotypes of virus causing haemorrhagic fever with renal syndrome. J Gen Virol 1989; 70(Pt 4):819–825.

35. Asada H, et al. Cell-mediated immunity to virus causing haemorrhagic fever with renal syndrome: generation of cytotoxic T lymphocytes. J Gen Virol 1988; 69:2179–2188.

36. Asada H, et al. Role of T lymphocyte subsets in protection and recovery from Hantaan virus infection in mice. J Gen Virol 1987; 68:1961–1969.

37. Ennis FA, et al. Hantavirus pulmonary syndrome: CD8+ and CD4+ cytotoxic T lymphocytes to epitopes on Sin Nombre virus nucleocapsid protein isolated during acute illness. Virology 1997; 238:380–390.

38. Van Epps HL, et al. Human memory cytotoxic T-lymphocyte (CTL) responses to Hantaan virus infection: identification of virus-specific and cross-reactive CD8(+) CTL epitopes on nucleocapsid protein. J Virol 1999; 73:5301–5308.

39. Van Epps H, et al. Long-lived human memory T lymphocyte responses to a hantavirus causing hemorrhagic fever with renal syndrome. 2001. Submitted.

40. Linderholm M, et al. Elevated plasma levels of tumor necrosis factor (TNF)-alpha, soluble TNF receptors, interleukin (IL)-6, and IL-10 in patients with hemorrhagic fever with renal syndrome, J Infect Dis 1996; 173:38–43.

41. Mori M, et al. High levels of cytokine-producing cells in the lung tissues of patients with fatal hantavirus pulmonary syndrome. J Infect Dis 1999; 179:295–302.

42. Temonen M, et al. Cytokines, adhesion molecules, and cellular infiltration in nephropathia epidemica kidneys: an immunohistochemical study. Clin Immunol Immunopathol 1996; 78:47–55.

43. Huang C, et al. Hemorrhagic fever with renal syndrome: relationship between pathogenesis and cellular immunity. J Infect Dis 1994; 169:868–870.

44. Peters CJ, et al. Spectrum of hantavirus infection: hemorrhagic fever with renal syndrome and hantavirus pulmonary syndrome. Annu Rev Med 1999; 50:531–545.

45. Cho HW, Howard CR. Antibody responses in humans to an inactivated hantavirus vaccine (Hantavax). Vaccine 1999; 17:2569–2575.

46. Sohn YM, et al. Primary humoral immune responses to formalin inactivated hemorrhagic fever with renal syndrome vaccine (Hantavax): consideration of active immunization in South Korea. Yonsei Med J 2001; 42:278–284.

47. Kim RJ, et al. The special prevention of HFRS in P.D.R. of Korea. Chin Clin Exp Virol 1991; 4:487–492.

48. Zhu ZY, et al. Efficacy of inactivated vaccine containing cyto-hemagglutinin against epidemic hemorrhagic fever in rabbits. Chin Med J (Engl) 1989; 102:602–605.

49. Yu Y, et al. Inactivated cell-culture Hantavirus vaccine developed in China. In: Saluzzo JF, Dodet B, eds. Emergence and Control of Rodent-Borne Viral Diseases. Paris, France: Elsevier, 1999.

50. Song G, et al. Preliminary human trial of inactivated golden hamster kidney cell (GHKC) vaccine against haemorrhagic fever with renal syndrome (HFRS). Vaccine 1992; 10:214–216.

51. Hooper JW, Li D. Vaccines against hantaviruses. Curr Top Microbiol Immunol 2001; 256:171–191.

52. Dong GM, et al. Expanded human trial of the bivalent HFRS inactivated vaccine made from M gerbil kidney tissue culture. Chin J Microbiol Immunol 1998; 18:453–456.

53. Yoshimatsu K, et al. Protective immunity of Hantaan virus nucleocapsid and envelope protein studied using baculovirus-expressed proteins. Arch Virol 1993; 130:365–376.

54. Koletzki D, et al. Puumala (PUU) hantavirus strain differences and insertion positions in the hepatitis B virus core antigen influence B-cell immunogenicity and protective potential of core-derived particles. Virology 2000; 276:364–375.

55. Ulrich R, et al. Chimaeric HBV core particles carrying a defined segment of Puumala hantavirus nucleocapsid protein evoke protective immunity in an animal model. Vaccine 1998; 16:272–280.

56. Kamrud KI, et al. Comparison of the protective efficacy of naked DNA, DNA-based Sindbis replicon, and packaged Sindbis replicon vectors expressing Hantavirus structural genes in hamsters. Virology 1999; 263:209–219.

57. Bharadwaj M, et al. Intramuscular inoculation of Sin Nombre hantavirus cDNAs induces cellular and humoral immune responses in BALB/c mice. Vaccine 1999; 17:2836–2843.

58. Bucht G, et al. Modifying the cellular transport of DNA-based vaccines alters the immune response to hantavirus nucleocapsid protein. Vaccine 2001; 19:3820–3829.

59. McClain DJ, et al. Clinical evaluation of a vaccinia-vectored Hantaan virus vaccine. J Med Virol 2000; 60:77–85.

60. Buckley SM, et al. Isolation and antigenic characterization of Lassa virus. Nature 1970; 227:174174.

61. Buckley SM, Casals J. Lassa fever, a new virus disease of man from West Africa. 3. Isolation and characterization of the virus. Am J Trop Med Hyg 1970; 19:680–691.

62. McCormick JB, et al. A prospective study of the epidemiology and ecology of Lassa fever. J Infect Dis 1987; 155:437–444.

63. Bowen MD, et al. Genetic diversity among Lassa virus strains. J Virol 2000; 74:6992–7004.

64. Wulff H, et al. Isolation of an arenavirus closely related to Lassa virus from *Mastomys natalensis* in south-east Africa. Bull World Health Organ 1977; 55:441–444.

65. Fraser DW, et al. Lassa fever in the Eastern Province of Sierra Leone, 1970–1972. I. Epidemiologic studies. Am J Trop Med Hyg 1974; 23:1131–1139.

66. Tomori O, et al. Viral hemorrhagic fever antibodies in Nigerian populations. Am J Trop Med Hyg 1988; 38:407–410.

67. Yalley-Ogunro JE, et al. Endemic Lassa fever in Liberia. VI. Village serological surveys for evidence of Lassa virus activity in Lofa County, Liberia. Trans R Soc Trop Med Hyg 1984; 78:764–770.

68. Monson MH, et al. Pediatric Lassa fever: a review of 33 Liberian cases. Am J Trop Med Hyg 1987; 36:408–415.

69. Webb PA, et al. Lassa fever in children in Sierra Leone, West Africa. Trans R Soc Trop Med Hyg 1986; 80:577–582.

70. Fisher-Hoch SP, et al. Review of cases of nosocomial Lassa fever in Nigeria: the high price of poor medical practice. BMJ 1995; 311:857–859.

71. Monath TP, et al. A hospital epidemic of Lassa fever in Zorzor, Liberia, March–April 1972. Am J Trop Med Hyg 1973; 22:773–779.

72. Lassa fever, imported case, Netherlands. Wkly Epidemiol Rec 2000; 75:265265.

73. Lassa fever imported to England. Commun Dis Rep CDR Wkly 2000; 10:9999.

74. McCormick JB, et al. A case–control study of the clinical diagnosis and course of Lassa fever. J Infect Dis 1987; 155:445–455.

75. Price ME, et al. A prospective study of maternal and fetal outcome in acute Lassa fever infection during pregnancy. BMJ 1988; 297:584–587.

76. Cummins D, et al. Acute sensorineural deafness in Lassa fever. JAMA 1990; 264:2093–2096.

77. Salvato MS, et al. Biochemical and immunological evidence that the 11 kDa zinc-binding protein of lymphocytic choriomeningitis virus is a structural component of the virus. Virus Res 1992; 22:185–198.

78. Ruo SL, et al. Antigenic relatedness between arenaviruses defined at the epitope level by monoclonal antibodies. J Gen Virol 1991; 72:549–555.

79. Maiztegui JI, et al. Efficacy of immune plasma in treatment of Argentine haemorrhagic fever and association between treatment and a late neurological syndrome. Lancet 1979; 2:1216–1217.

80. Johnson KM, et al. Clinical virology of Lassa fever in hospitalized patients. J Infect Dis 1987; 155:456–464.

81. Jahrling PB. Protection of Lassa virus-infected guinea pigs with Lassa-immune plasma of guinea pig, primate, and human origin. J Med Virol 1983; 12:93–102.

82. Oldstone MBA. Viruses, Plagues, and History. New York: Oxford University Press, 1998:xi, 211.

83. Helmick CG, et al. No evidence for increased risk of Lassa fever infection in hospital staff. Lancet 1986; 2:1202–1205.

84. Maiztegui JI, et al. Protective efficacy of a live attenuated vaccine against Argentine hemorrhagic fever. AHF Study Group. J Infect Dis 1998; 177:277–283.

85. Kiley MP, et al. Protection of rhesus monkeys from Lassa virus by immunisation with closely related Arenavirus. Lancet 1979; 2:738738.

86. Fisher-Hoch SP, et al. Protection of rhesus monkeys from fatal Lassa fever by vaccination with a recombinant vaccinia virus containing the Lassa virus glycoprotein gene. Proc Natl Acad Sci U S A 1989; 86:317–321.

87. Fisher-Hoch SP, et al. Effective vaccine for Lassa fever. J Virol 2000; 74:6777–6783.

88. McCormick JB, et al. Inactivated Lassa virus elicits a non protective immune response in rhesus monkeys. J Med Virol 1992; 37:1–7.

89. Clegg JC, Oram JD. Molecular cloning of Lassa virus RNA: nucleotide sequence and expression of the nucleo-capsid protein gene. Virology 1985; 144:363–372.

90. Clegg JC, Lloyd G. Vaccinia recombinant expressing Lassa-virus internal nucleocapsid protein protects guineapigs against Lassa fever. Lancet 1987; 2:186–188.

91. Auperin DD, et al. Construction of a recombinant vaccinia virus expressing the Lassa virus glycoprotein gene and protection of guinea pigs from a lethal Lassa virus infection. Virus Res 1988; 9:233–248.

92. Auperin D. Construction and evaluation of recombinant virus vaccines for Lassa fever. In: Salvato MS ed. The Arenaviridae. New York: Plenum Press, 1993:259.

93. Morrison HG, et al. Protection of guinea pigs from Lassa fever by vaccinia virus recombinants expressing the nucleoprotein or the envelope glycoproteins of Lassa virus. Virology 1989; 171:179–188.

94. Auperin DD, McCormick JB. Nucleotide sequence of the Lassa virus (Josiah strain) S genome RNA and amino acid sequence comparison of the N and GPC proteins to other arenaviruses. Virology 1989; 168:421–425.

95. Arroyo J, et al. Molecular basis for attenuation of neuro-virulence of a yellow fever Virus/Japanese encephalitis virus chimera vaccine (ChimeriVax-JE). J Virol 2001; 75:934–942.

96. Guirakhoo F, et al. Viremia and immunogenicity in nonhuman primates of a tetravalent yellow fever–dengue chimeric vaccine: genetic reconstructions, dose adjustment, and antibody responses against wild-type dengue virus isolates. Virology 2002; 298:146–159.

97. Pushko P, et al. Individual and bivalent vaccines based on alphavirus replicons protect guinea pigs against infection with Lassa and Ebola viruses. J Virol 2001; 75:11677–11685.

98. Geisbert TW, Jahrling PB. Differentiation of filoviruses by electron microscopy. Virus Res 1995; 39:129–150.

99. Belanov EF, et al. [Survival of Marburg virus infectivity on contaminated surfaces and in aerosols]. Vopr Virusol 1996; 41:32–34.

100. Johnson E, et al. Lethal experimental infections of rhesus monkeys by aerosolized Ebola virus. Int J Exp Pathol 1995; 76:227–236.

101. Alibek K, Handelman S. Biohazard: The Chilling True Story of the Largest Covert Biological Weapons Program in the World, Told from the Inside by the Man Who Ran It. New York: Random House, 1999:xi, 319.

102. Miller J, et al. Germs: Biological Weapons and America's Secret War. New York: Simon and Schuster, 2001:382.

103. Borio L, et al. Hemorrhagic fever viruses as biological weapons: medical and public health management. JAMA 2002; 287:2391–2405.

104. Slenczka WG. The Marburg virus outbreak of 1967 and subsequent episodes. Curr Top Microbiol Immunol 1999; 235:49–75.

105. Leroy EM, et al. Re-emergence of Ebola haemorrhagic fever in Gabon. Lancet 2002; 359:712712.

106. Swanepoel R, et al. Experimental inoculation of plants and animals with Ebola virus. Emerg Infect Dis 1996; 2:321–325.

107. Feldmann H, Volchkov VE, Volchkova VA, Klenk HD. The glycoproteins of Marburg and Ebola virus and their potential roles in pathogenesis. Arch Virol Suppl 1999; 15:159–169.

108. Becker S, et al. The asialoglycoprotein receptor is a potential liver-specific receptor for Marburg virus. J Gen Virol 1995; 76:393–399.

109. Chan SY, et al. Folate receptor-alpha is a cofactor for cellular entry by Marburg and Ebola viruses. Cell 2001; 106:117–126.

110. Wool-Lewis RJ, Bates P. Characterization of Ebola virus entry by using pseudotyped viruses: identification of receptor-deficient cell lines. J Virol 1998; 72:3155–3160.

111. Hevey M, et al. Recombinant Marburg virus glycoprotein subunit vaccine protects guinea pigs from lethal infection. In: Brown F, Burton D, Doherty P, Mekalanos J, Norrby E, eds. Vaccines 97: Molecular Approaches to the Control

of Infectious Diseases. Cold Spring Harbor Laboratory Press, 1997.

112. Wilson JA, et al. Epitopes involved in antibody-mediated protection from Ebola virus. Science 2000; 287:1664–1666.

113. Maruyama T, et al. Ebola virus can be effectively neutralized by antibody produced in natural human infection. J Virol 1999; 73:6024–6030.

114. Parren PW, et al. Pre- and postexposure prophylaxis of Ebola virus infection in an animal model by passive transfer of a neutralizing human antibody. J Virol 2002; 76:6408–6412.

115. Bavari S, et al. Lipid raft microdomains: a gateway for compartmentalized trafficking of Ebola and Marburg viruses. J Exp Med 2002; 195:593–602.

116. Basler CF, et al. The Ebola virus VP35 protein functions as a type I IFN antagonist. Proc Natl Acad Sci U S A, 2000.

117. Wilson JA, et al. Ebola virus: the search for vaccines and treatments. Cell Mol Life Sci 2001; 58:1826–1841.

118. Hevey M, et al. Marburg virus vaccines based upon alphavirus replicons protect guinea pigs and nonhuman primates. Virology 1998; 251:28–37.

119. Ignatyev GM. Immune response to filovirus infections. Curr Top Microbiol Immunol 1999; 235:205–217.

120. Jahrling PB, et al. Passive immunization of Ebola virus-infected cynomolgus monkeys with immunoglobulin from hyperimmune horses. Arch Virol Suppl 1996; 11:135–140.

121. Ryabchikova EI, et al. An analysis of features of pathogenesis in two animal models of Ebola virus infection. J Infect Dis 1999; 179(Suppl 1):S199–S202.

122. Bray M. The role of the type I interferon response in the resistance of mice to filovirus infection. J Gen Virol 2001; 82:1365–1373.

123. Chan SY, et al. Distinct mechanisms of entry by envelope glycoproteins of Marburg and Ebola (Zaire) viruses. J Virol 2000; 74:4933–4937.

124. Leroy EM, et al. Human asymptomatic Ebola infection and strong inflammatory response. Lancet 2000; 355:2210–2215.

125. Jahrling PB, et al. Evaluation of immune globulin and recombinant interferon-alpha2b for treatment of experimental Ebola virus infections. J Infect Dis 1999; 179(suppl 51):S224–S234.

126. Leroy EM, et al. Early immune responses accompanying human asymptomatic Ebola infections. Clin Exp Immunol 2001; 124:453–460.

127. Hevey M, et al. Antigenicity and vaccine potential of Marburg virus glycoprotein expressed by baculovirus recombinants. Virology 1997; 239:206–216.

128. Kudoyarova-Zubavichene NM, et al. Preparation and use of hyperimmune serum for prophylaxis and therapy of Ebola virus infections. J Infect Dis 1999; 179(suppl 1):S218–S223.

129. Mupapa K, et al. Treatment of Ebola hemorrhagic fever with blood transfusions from convalescent patients. International Scientific and Technical Committee. J Infect Dis 1999; 179(suppl 1):S18–S23.

130. Razumov IA, et al. [Detection of antiviral activity of monoclonal antibodies, specific to Marburg virus proteins]. Vopr Virusol 2001; 46:33–37.

131. Vanderzanden L, et al. DNA vaccines expressing either the GP or NP genes of Ebola virus protect mice from lethal challenge. Virology 1998; 246:134–144.

132. Wilson JA, Hart MK. Protection from Ebola virus mediated by cytotoxic T lymphocytes specific for the viral nucleoprotein. J Virol 2001; 75:2660–2664.

133. Wilson JA, et al. Vaccine potential of Ebola virus vp24, vp30, vp35, and vp40 proteins. Virology 2001; 286:384–390.

134. Agafonov AP, et al. [The immunogenic properties of Marburg virus proteins]. Vopr Virusol 1992; 37:58–61.

135. Xu L, et al. Immunization for Ebola virus infection. Nat Med 1998; 4:37–42.

136. Sullivan NJ, et al. Development of a preventive vaccine for Ebola virus infection in primates. Nature 2000; 408:605–609.

137. Kapikian AZ, et al. An epidemiologic study of altered clinical reactivity to respiratory syncytial (RS) virus infection in children previously vaccinated with an inactivated RS virus vaccine. Am J Epidemiol 1969; 89:405–421.

138. Lupton HW, et al. Inactivated vaccine for Ebola virus efficacious in guinea pig model. Lancet 1980; 2:1294–1295.

139. Hevey M, et al. Marburg virus vaccines: comparing classical and new approaches. Vaccine 2001; 20:586–593.

140. Geisbert TW, et al. Evaluation in nonhuman primates of vaccines against Ebola virus. Emerg Infect Dis 2002; 8:503–507.

141. Neumann G, et al. Reverse genetics demonstrates that proteolytic processing of the Ebola virus glycoprotein is not essential for replication in cell culture. J Virol 2002; 76:406–410.

142. Volchkov VE, et al. Recovery of infectious Ebola virus from complementary DNA: RNA editing of the GP gene and viral cytotoxicity. Science 2001; 291:1965–1969.

143. Gilligan KJ, et al. Assessment of protective immunity conferred by recombinant vaccinia viruses to guinea pigs challenged with Ebola virus. In: Brown F, Burton D, Doherty P, Mekalanos J, Norrby E, eds. Vaccines 97: Molecular Approaches to the Control of Infectious Diseases. Cold Spring Harbor Laboratory Press, 1997.

144. Pushko P, et al. Recombinant RNA replicons derived from attenuated Venezuelan equine encephalitis virus protect guinea pigs and mice from Ebola hemorrhagic fever virus. Vaccine 2000; 19:142–153.

57

Development of a Vaccine to Prevent Infection with Group A Streptococci and Rheumatic Fever

Michael F. Good
The Queensland Institute of Medical Research, Brisbane, Queensland, Australia

P. J. Cleary
University of Minnesota, Minneapolis, Minnesota, U.S.A.

James Dale
University of Tennessee Health Science Center and the Veterans Affairs Medical Center, Memphis, Tennessee, U.S.A.

Vincent Fischetti, K. Fuchs, H. Sabharwal, and J. Zabriskie
Rockefeller University, New York, New York, U.S.A.

I. THE NEED FOR A VACCINE

Group A beta hemolytic streptococci (GABHS) cause a wide variety of infectious and postinfectious diseases ranging from the relatively benign to the very serious. Tissue-invasive forms of the disease, such as necrotizing fasciitis have a high mortality but are relatively uncommon. Pyoderma and pharyngitis are very common and can be debilitating but, in themselves, are not of major concern. Nevertheless, strep pharyngitis has been estimated to cost the U.S. economy up to $2 billion per annum. However, these conditions can give rise to serious postinfectious diseases, rheumatic fever (RF), rheumatic heart disease (RHD), and glomerulonephritis. Untreated, between 0.3% and 3% of streptococcal pharyngitis can lead to RF and this figure can increase to up to 50% among individuals who have experienced a previous episode of RF/RHD [1]. World Health Organization (WHO) estimates that of the approximate 50 million people who die every year, 500,000 die as a result of RF/RHD [2]. This number may be an underestimate.

GABHS only infects humans, and the factors responsible for its spread include the virulence of different strains, the proximity of individuals to each other (crowding), and the degree of pre-existing immunity. It is thought by some that RF/RHD only became common during the Industrial Revolution when very large groupings in towns and cities were formed. There is little way to reliably look back at early

civilizations and estimate the prevalence of these diseases. What is clear is that there has been, overall, a dramatic decrease in RF/RHD throughout the last century in developed countries. This decrease commenced prior to the discovery of sulfonamides and penicillin, and the use of antibiotics for primary and secondary prevention [3]. A blip in this pattern of decreasing incidence occurred in the United States in the mid-1980s, when there was an approximate 10-fold increase in the number of cases of RF reported in many states [4]. Coincident with this, there has been a resurgence of all serious streptococcal diseases, including sepsis with toxic shock and necrotizing fasciitis. This change in epidemiology has raised interest in vaccine development by several biotech and pharmaceutical companies, National Institutes of Health (NIH), and university research groups. Factors responsible for the increase in disease are not clear, but evidence pointed to the circulation of more virulent strains. It was of interest that a history of a preceding strep pharyngitis was found in only 33% of patients in one study [1].

The overall decline in the incidence of RF/RHD in the developed world has not been mirrored among individuals living in developing economy nations, nor of some indigenous groups living in developed countries. Australia's aboriginal population, for example, experienced the highest reported incidence of RF worldwide (up to 650/100,000 per year) while living alongside the non-Aboriginal population, which has one of the lowest incidence figures for RF [5].

The relative death rate for Australia's Aboriginal population compared to the non-Aboriginal population for RHD is 25 (Australian Bureau of Statistics). In developing countries, RHD is a very common cause for admission to hospital relative to other cardiac conditions. In India, for example, up to 50% of all cardiac admissions are for RHD [6], with similar statistics reported in many other developing countries [7].

Given that RF only ever follows a pharyngeal infection with GABHS and that antibiotics can provide both primary and secondary prevention [8,9], there is very good reason to believe that a vaccine that prevented infection with GABHS would also prevent RF. Compliance with antibiotic prophylaxis is variable with many recurrences with RF due to poor compliance, giving further impetus to the need to develop a vaccine. A vaccine that prevents GABHS infection will obviously prevent all strep-related pathology; however, one concern is that a vaccine might stimulate a host immune response that could provoke RF [10]. Although the pathogenesis of RF is not completely understood, it is widely believed that the disease is autoimmune in etiology. In preclinical studies, candidate vaccines must be screened for their ability to induce host-reactive antibodies and T cells. Obviously, clinical trials must also monitor the development of any potentially pathogenic auto-reactive immune responses.

As in all vaccine programs, the choice of immunogen(s), the route of administration, the method of delivery, and presentation of the immunogen, and the choice of adjuvant are all likely to be critical. This chapter aims to summarize some of the current approaches looking at three different potential immunogens: C5a peptidase, group A carbohydrate antigen, and various components of the M protein. Native, recombinant, synthetic, and vectored antigens are being developed, and parenteral and mucosal delivery routes are under investigation. It is essential to develop good correlates of protection; however, antibodies are believed to provide the likely mechanism of protection. One of the major challenges facing all approaches is to provide broad protection against the majority or all of the serotypes of GABHS present in the population. There is estimated to be over 150 different serotypes, based on the M protein, but the actual number of M protein sequence types is certainly much larger.

II. STREPTOCOCCAL C5a PEPTIDASE-SEROTYPE INDEPENDENT PROTECTION AGAINST *STREPTOCOCCUS PYOGENES*

GABHS are a moving target for M protein-based vaccines as the dominant serotypes in any given population are constantly changing with over 150 serotypes now recognized. This was most clearly demonstrated by Kaplan et al. [11], who reported nearly a complete shift from M1 to M6 strains responsible for pharyngitis over just a 6-month period in an isolated population. This observation indicates that a vaccine must contain multiple type-specific M epitopes, or peptide antigens that are antigenically conserved across serotype boundaries. One approach has been to focus vac-

cine development on the C5a peptidase, a large surface protein expressed by most, if not all, GAS serotypes. The discovery of C5a peptidase in 1985 suggested a new concept in bacterial pathogenesis [12]. It was proposed that surface-bound streptococcal C5a peptidase (SCPA) arms streptococci with the potential to destroy C5a chemotaxin at the bacterial surface, where it is formed by activation of the complement pathway, and to impede influxes of phagocytes at the initial loci of infection. C5a chemotaxin can be detected within 5 min following an inflammatory insult [13], and is therefore considered to be among the earliest initiators of a phagocytic response. Therefore, destruction of C5a is expected to delay phagocyte recruitment, providing GAS a window of time to replicate and adjust to their microchemical environment. Considerable support for this idea has accumulated over the past 15 years. In murine models, isogenic SCPA$^-$ streptococci are cleared more rapidly than parent SCPA$^+$ streptococci from subdermal sites of infection [15], and from the oral–nasal mucosa [15]. As predicted, infiltration of polymorphonuclear leukocytes PMNs and macrophages is more robust in response to SCPA$^-$ than SCPA$^+$ GABHS [14]. One surprising observation was that M protein had no measurable effect on the clearance of streptococci from the oral–nasal mucosa.

The intranasal infection model in mice was adapted to investigate whether immunization with recombinant SCPA influenced clearance of streptococci from throats of mice following infection. In initial experiments, mice were immunized without adjuvants by multiple intranasal inoculations with affinity purified SCPA protein that had been cloned from M49 streptococci [16]. Mice responded with strong serum IgA and IgM responses. Moreover, SCPA-specific secretory IgA (sIgA) was detected in saliva. Throat cultures following intranasal challenge of mice demonstrated that immunized animals cleared streptococci more rapidly than nonimmunized controls. Cross-protection against serotypes M2, M11, M1, and M6 was observed. An example of data is shown in Figure 1.

Four years ago, a collaboration between the team of Pat Cleary and Wyeth Lederle Vaccines was set up to develop a vaccine that would prevent colonization, pharyngitis, and carriage of GAS by children. Regulatory barriers were anticipated; therefore, the initial goal was to develop a traditional injectable vaccine. One of the first questions was whether parenterally administered antigen would produce protection against an intranasal challenge. The SCPA1 gene from an M1 streptococcal strain was cloned, genetically inactivated, and expressed in *Escherichia coli*. Again, protection studies made use of the intranasal infection model, except that CD1 mice were vaccinated by subcutaneous (SQ) injection with SCPA1 protein, mixed with adjuvants. Clearance of streptococci was assessed by daily throat swabs, or appraised quantitatively by viable bacterial counts in homogenized nasal tissue. Control mice were immunized with tetanus toxoid mixed with the same adjuvants. Figure 2 shows data from three experiments. Mice were immunized with recombinant SCPA1 or SCPA49 and then intranasally challenged with either serotype M1 or M49 streptococci. Immunization with either recombinant protein induced high titers of SCPA-specific serum IgG and these mice cleared

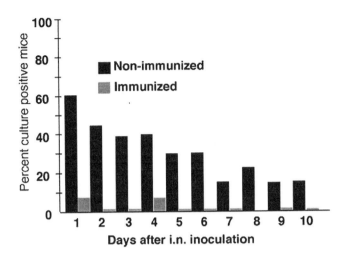

Figure 1 Clearance of M49 streptococci by mice that were intranasally immunized with recombinant SCPA49 protein [16]. Throat cultures were performed daily following intranasal inoculation of CD1 mice by strain CS101. Mice were immunized with a truncated form of SCPA49 (gray bars) or tetanus toxoid (black bars). Each experimental group contained 13 mice. (Data from P. Cleary.)

intranasally inoculated streptococci more efficiently than controls, which had been immunized with tetanus toxoid.

Until recently, it was assumed that protection was based on antibody that neutralized C5ase enzymatic activity. New experimental results, however, indicate that SCPA and SCPB proteins are also invasins, i.e., they promote ingestion of streptococci by epithelial cells. Moreover, SCPA is also a fibronectin binding protein. Rabbit anti-SCPA or anti-SCPB inhibits ingestion of GABHS and group B streptococci, respectively. These findings raised the possibility that antibody which inhibits invasion of epithelial could be as important as C5ase activity for more rapid clearance of streptococci from the oral–nasal mucosa.

Although GABHS are a far greater public health problem, β hemolytic forms of groups C and G streptococci are also associated with pharyngitis, and more rarely, sepsis and other serious complications [17]. Human β hemolytic iso-

lates of groups B, C, and G streptococci uniformly produce SCP protein [18–20]. A vaccine that also reduces the incidence of infection by these species would be especially attractive. Hill and colleagues were the first to demonstrate production of a C5ase enzyme by group B streptococci, then it was shown that all serotypes harbor a single *scpB* gene [19]. SCPB is 95–98% identical in amino acid sequence to SCPA. Franken et al. [21] recently showed that *scpB* resides on a 7-kb composite transposon in the chromosome of group B streptococci, which can be lost during cultivation in the laboratory, leaving behind a flanking insertion sequence (IS) element. Bovine strains rarely retain the transposon, and therefore, they fail to produce peptidase. It was postulated that a single peptidase protein could induce immune responses that would protect against these other species of β hemolytic streptococci. Cleary's laboratory reported that anti-SCPB antibody is opsonic in whole blood, and induces killing of group B streptococci by primary bone marrow macrophage [22]. Moreover, both opsonization and macrophage killing are serotype-independent. SCPB was also found to be an exceptional carrier protein when conjugated to serotype III capsular polysaccharide. Without a protein carrier, group B streptococcal capsular polysaccharides are virtually nonimmunogenic. Recent protection experiments clearly demonstrate that SQ vaccination of mice with SCPB induces serotype transparent protection against lung infection by this species (Cheng and Cleary, unpublished).

A safe vaccine with few side reactions is the goal of any development project. It was postulated that neither SCPB nor SCPA proteins are likely to induce an autoimmune response in humans or animals. In contrast to GABHS infection, autoimmune disease is never associated with group B streptococcal infections. This epidemiological observation strongly argues that neither SCPB nor SCPA will induce a pathogenic, tissue cross-reactive immune response. SCPA protein is now under intensive scrutiny for its potential to induce a tissue reactive immune response. Although still incomplete, studies to date have not observed autoimmune antibodies in rabbits or mice following vaccination with purified recombinant protein.

The failure of children to develop a protective immune response following pharyngitis or impetigo is not understood and questions whether any GABHS product will

		Percent positive cultures	
Vaccine Antigen	Challenge Strain	Tet-toxoid Control	Peptidase Immunized
SCPA1S512A	M1	23% (5)	8%
SCPA49S512A	M1	33% (5)	8%
SCPA49S512A	M49	58% (4)	8%

Figure 2 Parenteral vaccination with recombinant SCPA49 or SCPA1 peptidase enhances clearance of streptococci following intranasal infection. CD1 outbred mice were inoculated with recombinant antigen mixed with Alum and Monophosphoryl lipid A (Ribbi Inc.). Vaccinated mice were challenged with 1×10^9 CFU of log phase culture. The number in parentheses is the day cultures were taken after infection. Throat cultures with one β hemolytic colony were considered positive. (Data from P. Cleary.)

induce protection in children. Adults are thought to be more immune to infection, but they are not absolutely resistant to streptococcal disease as evidenced by occasional outbreaks of disease among military personnel. Healthy adults do not have high levels of type-specific antibody for multiple M proteins or other protein antigens. In a small study, more than 70% of saliva from adults contained measurable levels of SCPA-specific secretory sIgA and IgG [23]. This was in sharp contrast to sera obtained from children below 10 years old. Less than 15% of their saliva was found to contain SCPA-specific antibody. Measurements of SCPA-specific antibody in acute and convalescent sera also confirmed that children mount an antibody response to SCPA following infection, yet there is no evidence that these children are resistant to subsequent infection. It is not uncommon for children to have multiple infections by the same strain of streptococcus. Why don't they develop a protective immune response? One possible explanation is that streptococci suppressed the appropriate response or that children must be exposed multiple times to streptococcal proteins in order for sufficient a number of memory T cells or levels of specific antibody to be attained. Studies are in progress to evaluate the subclass of IgG, and antibody function with regard to neutralization of ingestion of streptococci by epithelial cells and to neutralization C5ase activity.

In conclusion, (1) intranasal immunization induces IgG and IgA responses, and reduces colonization by streptococci following intranasal infection; (2) subcutaneous injections of peptide with adjuvant induces a strong IgG response that speeds clearance of streptococci from the oral–nasal mucosa; (3) both intranasal and parental routes of administration of a single peptide induce protection against multiple serotypes.

III. GROUP A STREPTOCOCCAL CARBOHYDRATE

The general dogma for over 60 years has been that the broad-based immunity to group A streptococcal infections [24] which appears with increasing age is attributable to the presence of multiple type-specific antibodies in the serum of these individuals. Yet, as demonstrated by Dr. Lancefield's studies [25], the presence of multiple type-specific M protein antibodies in human sera is actually quite rare. In view of these observations, various groups looked for other antigens that might induce broad-based immunity and antibodies prepared against these antigens that might be both phagocytic and protective in an animal challenge model. A previous report [26] indicated that antibodies to the group A carbohydrate (GR A CHO) increased with age, antibodies were phagocytic for multiple type-specific streptococcal strains, and that specific removal of the antibody (leaving all others present in the serum) resulted in loss of phagocytosis. Furthermore, elution of the antibody from the N-acetyl glucosamine beads restored the majority of the phagocytic properties of the serum.

Several new questions have now been addressed: (1) whether these antibodies will passively protect in a mouse challenge model, (2) will active immunization with the GRA

CHO protect against a live streptococcal challenge, (3) do CHO antibodies increase with age and correlate with the presence or absence of group A streptococci in the throats of normal Mexican schoolchildren? Is there any evidence of cross-reactive antibodies induced by the GRA CHO?

1. Table 1 demonstrates that rabbit sera obtained from animals immunized with streptococcal group A CHO conjugated to TT were capable of significant passive protection against a lethal challenge mouse model using live group A streptococci.
2. Animals were actively immunized with streptococcal group A CHO-conjugated to TT subcutaneously with an average of four doses. Three different M^+ strains were used in these experiments, and the number of organisms needed to kill approximately 100% of the control animals is shown in Table 2. As can be seen, immunization with group A streptococcal CHO significantly decreased the number of deaths in immunized mice when compared to controls.
3. A study of 300 normal Mexican children has shown that the anti-CHO antibody titers increase with age, and these titers correlate with the presence or absence of group A colonization in the throat. The titers of other antistreptococcal antibodies were similar in both groups. In this study of children ages 5–14, it was determined that approximately 20% carried group A streptococci in their throats. Anticarbohydrate antibodies were measured in those children with positive Group A cultures and compared to those who had negative cultures. Figure 3A shows that the titers were twice as high in children with negative cultures when compared to children with positive cultures ($p < 0.003$). Figure 3B demonstrates that other antistreptococcal antibodies were equally divided between the two groups suggesting that the anticarbohydrate titers were uniquely increased in those children with negative throat cultures.

Finally, the question of whether the group A carbohydrate antibodies cross-reacted with human tissue was addressed. These questions were originally raised by Dudding and Ayoub [27], and expanded upon by Cunningham et al. [28]. Using human frozen tissue from organs known to be involved in cross-reactions between streptococcal antigens and human tissues, no evidence was found that anticarbohy-

Table 1 Passive Protection Test in Balb/c Mice Against Group A Streptococcus Type 6 (S43/46)

Serum	Colonies	Mice[a,b]
NRS	200–500	3/26b**,b
Group A CHO Ab	200–500	16/26

[a] Number of mice survived/injected.
[b] Similar protection was seen against Type 3 (D58/93/7).
**$p < 0.001$.
(Data from Sabharwal, Fuchs, and Zabriskie.)

Table 2 Active Immunization Studies with Group A Streptococcal CHO in Mice Challenged with Live Type 14 (S23) Streptococci[a]

Group	Adjuvant	Inoculum Range	Survived/Injected
CHO–TT Conjugate	Alum	$3–3.6 \times 10^5$	18/23[*,a]
TT	Alum	$3–3.6 \times 10^6$	5/22[*,a]

[a] Similar protection was seen against two other M[+] types.
[*]$p < 0.001$.
(Data from Sabharwal, Fuchs, and Zabriskie.)

drate antibodies were directed to these human antigens both by immunofluorescence and by enzyme-linked immunosorbent assays (ELISAs) using known human cytoskeletal antigens (data not shown).

In conclusion, the group A carbohydrate can elicit antibodies that are both phagocytic and protective against several different type-specific M[+] streptococcal strains. High titers of CHO antibodies are associated with decreased colonization of the throat by group A streptococci and the CHO antigen does not induce cross reactive antibodies to human tissue organs. For these reasons, a case can be put that group A streptococcal polysaccharide, is an excellent candidate for use as an immunogen in the prevention of GABHS infections.

IV. THE M PROTEIN

A. Structure and Function

Streptococcal M protein was identified over 70 years ago by Lancefield [29]. A review by Lancefield [30] clearly describes the studies carried out for nearly 35 years, defining this molecule as a major virulence factor for the streptococcus

due to its antiphagocytic property. In 1974, a comprehensive review by Fox [31] delineated studies since the Lancefield review and underscored the knowledge to that time of the structure, function, and immunochemistry of the M molecule.

The streptococcal M protein is probably one of the best-defined molecules among the known bacterial virulence determinants. Clearly, protective immunity to group A streptococcal infection is achieved through antibodies directed to the M protein [32,33], a major virulence factor present on the surface of all clinical isolates. M protein is a coiled-coil fibrillar protein composed of three major segments of tandem repeat sequences that extends nearly 60 nm from the surface of the streptococcal cell wall [32] (Figure 4). The A- and B-repeats located within the N-terminal half are antigenically variable among the >150 known streptococcal types with the N-terminal nonrepetitive region and A-repeats exhibiting hypervariability. The more C-terminal C-repeats, the majority of which are surface exposed, contain epitopes that are highly conserved among the identified M proteins [34]. Because of its antigenically variable N-terminal region, the M protein provides the basis for the Lancefield serological typing scheme for group A streptococci [32].

The M protein is considered as the major virulence determinant because of its ability to prevent phagocytosis when present on the streptococcal surface and thus, by this definition, all clinical isolates express M protein. This function may in part be attributed to the specific binding of complement factor H to both the conserved C-repeat domain [35] and the fibrinogen bound to the B-repeats [36], preventing the deposition of C3b on the streptococcal surface. It is proposed that when the streptococcus contacts serum, the factor H bound to the M molecule inhibits or reverses the formation of C3b,Bb complexes and helps to convert C3b to its inactive form (iC3b) on the bacterial surface, preventing C3b-dependent phagocytosis. Some studies have shown that antibodies directed to the B- and C-repeat regions of the M protein are unable to promote

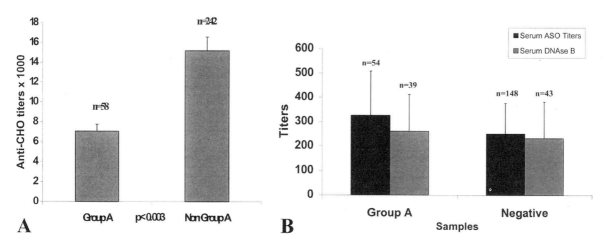

Figure 3 (A) Anti-CHO antibody titers in serum of children with positive and negative throat cultures from group A streptococci. Note the titers in the negative sera were twice as high as those with positive cultures. (B) Serum ASO and DNAse B titers in the same population. Note that there was no significant difference in the titers of the antibodies in the sera of the patients whose throat cultures were positive or negative for group A streptococci. (Data from Sabharwal, Fuchs, and Zabriskie.)

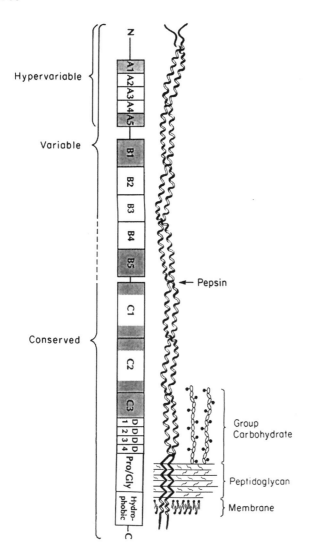

Figure 4 Proposed model of the M protein from M6 strain D471. The coiled-coil rod region extends about 60 nm from cell wall with a short nonhelical domain at the NH₂-terminus. The Pro/Gly-rich region of the molecule is found within the peptidoglycan. The membrane spanning segment is composed predominantly of hydrophobic amino acids and a short charged tail extends into the cytoplasm. Data suggests that the membrane anchor may be cleaved shortly after synthesis. The A-, B-, and C-repeat regions are indicated along with those segments containing conserved, variable, and hypervariable epitopes among heterologous M serotypes. Pepsin, designates the position of a pepsin susceptible site near the center of the molecule.

phagocytosis [37]. This may be the result of the ability of factor H to also control the binding of C3b to the Fc receptors on these antibodies, resulting in inefficient phagocytosis [38]. Antibodies directed to the hypervariable N-terminal region are opsonic, perhaps because they cannot be controlled by the factor H bound to the C-repeat region. Thus it appears that the streptococcus has devised a method to protect its conserved region from being used against itself by binding factor H to regulate the potentially opsonic

antibodies that bind to these regions. When this was found, Fischetti and coworkers reasoned that it could explain why even though adults are more resistant than children to streptococcal pharyngitis, they do get sporadic infections. If antibodies produced to the conserved region were in fact protective, then it would be expected that these antibodies would be protective to all serotypes encountered, because opsonic IgG is usually sterilizing (as is type-specific IgG). As this was not the case, it was suspected that another mechanism resulted in broad protection that could be occasionally breached.

B. Rationale for Multivalent N-Terminal M Protein-Based Vaccines

As well as being a major virulence factor of the organism and being able to confer resistance to phagocytosis, the M protein is a major protective antigen. Serum antibodies against M protein are opsonic and promote bactericidal killing of group A streptococci that are mediated by polymorphonuclear leukocytes [30]. Type-specific bactericidal antibodies that develop after natural infection correlate with protection against subsequent infection with the same serotype [30] and may persist for many years [25].

These seminal observations, which were largely those of Dr. Rebecca Lancefield, have served as the basis for M protein vaccine development for over 70 years. The overall goal of multivalent M protein-based vaccines is to approximate the type-specific protection induced following natural infection [25]. Early studies by Fox and his coworkers clearly demonstrated the protective efficacy in humans of highly purified M protein vaccines [39,40]. Volunteers that were immunized parenterally [39] or locally via the upper airway [40] were protected against challenge infections with the same serotype of group A streptococci.

M proteins contain protective (opsonic) epitopes and in some cases, human tissue cross-reactive epitopes [11]. Because of the theoretical possibility of inducing autoantibodies, a challenge has been to separate the protective epitopes from the autoimmune epitopes so that vaccine preparations would contain only protective M protein peptides. Multiple studies from several laboratories have shown that the epitopes contained in the hypervariable, type-specific N-terminus of the M proteins evoke antibodies with the greatest bactericidal activity and are least likely to cross-react with host tissues [41]. In addition, the majority of the autoimmune epitopes of M proteins that have been identified are located in the middle of the mature M proteins and are distinct from the type-specific, protective epitopes [11, 41]. These observations led investigators to focus on the N-terminal type-specific peptides of M proteins for inclusion in multivalent vaccines [42–44]. Synthetic and recombinant peptides as small as 10 amino acids have been shown to protect animals against subsequent challenge infections with the homologous serotype of group A streptococci [45].

The finding that small peptides from the M proteins could evoke bactericidal antibodies that were not cross-reactive with human tissue prompted investigators to identify methods of designing and formulating vaccines that contained protective epitopes from multiple M serotypes.

One approach has been to design fusion proteins that contain multiple N-terminal M peptides in tandem. The first of these was a trivalent synthetic peptide that was linked to an unrelated carrier [46]. Subsequent vaccines were produced by using recombinant techniques in which specific 5' regions of the *emm* genes were amplified by polymerase chain reaction (PCR) and linked together in-frame using unique restriction sites. Vaccines containing 4 [42], 6 [44], 8 [43], and now 26 [47] peptides from different M serotypes have been shown to evoke broadly opsonic antibodies in animals without evoking tissue cross-reactive antibodies. Other approaches are to combine N-terminal peptides with minimal C-repeat peptides. Two clinical trials designed to assess the safety and immunogenicity of the hexavalent [44] and 26-valent [47] vaccine are currently in progress (see below).

C. Defining a Minimal Conserved Epitope in the C-Repeat Region of the M Protein

The pathogenesis of RHD is believed to involve an autoimmune process. Studies have identified T cells in acute valvulitis lesions [48], and others have shown that such T cells can be stimulated by M protein peptides [49,50]. It has also been shown that human T-cell clones derived from the peripheral blood of individuals with or without a history of RF or signs of RHD and grown in response to a peptide from the conserved region of the M protein are able to react to myosin and an extract of human heart tissue [51]. These data suggest that while M protein-specific T cells may contribute to the pathogenesis of RHD, other factors are also required.

Given the evidence that the conserved region of the M protein can induce protection in animal models to GAS challenge [52,53], and that antibodies to conserved region peptides can be opsonic when a method based on a modification of Lancefield's original description is used [54], one approach to vaccine development has been to define minimal opsonic determinants on the conserved region of the M protein that do not stimulate T cells.

Because the M protein is conformational, it is critical that any minimal determinants are correctly folded in order to mimic native structure. A process was developed to display minimal M protein sequences within flanking non-GAS sequences designed to preserve the α-helical structure of the determinant [55]. Such peptides are referred to as "chimeric" peptides, and two such peptides, "J8" and "J14," were shown to be capable of inducing opsonic antibodies in mice without stimulating T cells to the conserved region ([56,57], and Batzloff and Good, submitted). Mice vaccinated with the chimeric peptides were able to withstand an otherwise lethal GAS challenge.

D. Combining Conserved and Serotypic Determinants

While a minimal conserved epitope can induce protection in mice against GABHS challenge [56] and can induce antibodies capable of opsonizing multiple strains of GABHS [58], it remains to be seen whether it will protect humans from GABHS and RF/RHD. We have no detailed knowl-

edge of how reliable the mouse model is for the human condition.

A theoretical concern is that antibodies to the minimal determinant are poorly opsonic compared with antibodies to the serotypic determinants [59,60]. Human antibodies specific for the conserved region taken from GAS-exposed volunteers can opsonize GABHS and there is a strong association between age-related acquisition of resistance to GABHS infection and age-related acquisition of serum antibodies to the conserved region of individuals living in highly endemic GABHS communities [61]. Nevertheless, short synthetic peptides may induce, in humans, antibodies of a different fine specificity and with less antibacterial efficacy. It could be argued that by combining a conserved epitope with a limited number of serotypic determinants representative of common strains, a more effective vaccine might result. The benefit of adding the serotypic determinants would be balanced by the drawback that strains that are common still vary between localities. Many of the strains from Thailand, for example, are "non-typeable" using reagents that can distinguish between strains common elsewhere. Strains that are common among the Australian Aboriginal population have been "typed" using a PCR approach [62] any many of these are "non-typeable" using serotypic reagents. The N-terminal peptides of seven of these common Aboriginal isolates were combined with the J14 minimal epitope using novel polymer chemistry [63]. The immunogen consisted of an alkane backbone and pendant side chains formed by the different epitopes. It is diagramatically illustrated in Figure 5. Outbred mice were vaccinated with the polymer and the sera of the mice contained antibodies against each of the individual epitopes. The sera were able to opsonize two different strains of GAS—one of which had an N-terminal sequence present on the vaccine and one which had an N-terminal sequence not present on the vaccine. Both strains had a conserved sequence identical to the epitope found on J14. These data suggested that both the N-terminal and C-terminal-specific antibodies contributed to the bactericidal activity of the serum. Following challenge with an otherwise lethal dose of either strain, the vaccinated mice demonstrated complete protection (Figure 6).

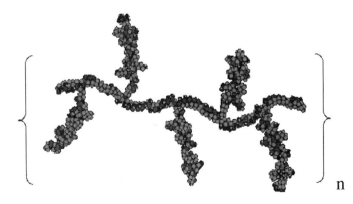

Figure 5 Space-filling model for "heteropolymer" immunogen consisting of alkane backbone and pendant side chains representing M protein epitopes. (From Refs. 63 and 56.)

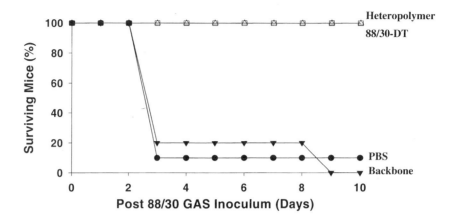

Figure 6 Heteropolymer with N-terminal and conserved peptide pendant side chains induces immunity to GABHS challenge (see Figure 5 and Ref. [56].)

While these data are promising, a potential drawback of this technology is that the polymerization technology cannot enable the ordering of the epitopes on the polymer to be defined. Thus it is expected that there would be batch-to-batch variation in the composition of the product which could affect immunogenicity. New polymer chemistries are being developed which will enable the production of a product with a defined order of epitopes on the polymer. Alternative approaches would be to produce a polymer as a recombinant protein or as a DNA vaccine with all epitopes joined head to tail (see above).

E. Toward a Mucosal Vaccine and Nontype-Specific Protection

Nearly 50% of children between the ages of 5 and 7 suffer from streptococcal infection each year. Furthermore, the siblings of a child with a streptococcal pharyngitis are 5 times more likely to acquire the organism than one of the parents. This decreased occurrence of streptococcal pharyngitis in adults might be explained by a nonspecific age-related host factor resulting in a decreased susceptibility to streptococci. Alternatively, protective antibodies directed to antigens common to a large number of GABHS serotypes might arise as a consequence of multiple infections or exposures experienced during childhood. This could result in an elevated response to conserved M protein epitopes. This latter hypothesis is partly supported by earlier studies on the immune response to the M protein, where it was found that the B-repeat domain (see Figure 4) was clearly immunodominant [64]. When rabbits were immunized with the whole M protein molecule, the first detectable antibodies were directed to the B-repeat region which rose steadily with time. It was only after repeated M protein immunization that antibodies were produced against the hypervariable A- and conserved C-repeat regions.

Unlike antibodies to the N-terminal region, antibodies directed to the exposed C-repeat region were not opsonic using the classical Lancefield methodology [37]. This result differed from data from Good's laboratory, but may be explained by differences in the technique of the opsonization assays used by the different laboratories. In any case, experiments were performed to explore whether mucosal antibodies to this conserved region of M protein could play a role in protection from infection. Taking advantage of the pepsin site in the center of the M molecule (separating the variable and conserved regions) (Figure 4), the recombinant M6 protein was cleaved and the N- and C-terminal fragments separated by SDS-PAGE and Western blotted. When the blots were reacted with different adult human sera, all adults tested had antibodies to the C-terminal conserved region while, as expected, only sera that were opsonic for the M6 organisms reacted with the N-terminal variable region [65,66,67]. Similar studies performed with M protein isolated from five different common serotypes (M3, M5, M6, M24, M29) revealed that sera from 10 of 17 adults tested did not have N-terminal-specific antibodies to these M types, while only two sera reacted with two serotypes and the remaining five sera with only one serotype. However, all sera tested reacted to the C-terminal fragment of the M molecule. Similar results were seen when salivary IgA from adults and children were tested in ELISA against the N- and C-terminal halves of the M6 molecule (V. Fischetti, unpublished data). Overall, this is further evidence that the relative resistance of adults to streptococcal pharyngitis is clearly not due to the presence of type-specific antibodies to multiple types, but may perhaps be a result of the presence of antibodies to conserved determinants.

From these findings, it was reasoned that an immune response to the conserved region of the M molecule might afford protection by inducing a mucosal response to prevent streptococcal colonization and ultimate infection. In view of the evidence that the conserved C-repeat epitopes of the M molecule are immunologically exposed on the streptococcal surface [34], it should be possible to generate mucosal antibodies that are reactive to the majority of streptococcal types using only a few distinct conserved region antigens for immunization.

1. Passive Protection

Secretory IgA (sIgA) is able to protect mucosal surfaces from infection by pathogenic microorganisms [68] despite the fact that its effector functions differ from those of serum-derived immunoglobulins [69]. When streptococci are administered intranasally to mice, they are able to cause death by first colonizing and then invading the mucosal barrier resulting in dissemination of the organism to systemic sites. Using this model Fischetti and coworkers first examined if secretory IgA (sIgA), delivered directly to the mucosa, plays a role in protecting against streptococcal infection. Live streptococci were mixed with affinity-purified M protein-specific sIgA or IgG antibodies and administered intranasally to the animals [70]. The results clearly showed that the anti-M protein sIgA protected the mice against streptococcal infection and death, whereas the opsonic serum IgG administered by the same route was without effect. This indicated that sIgA can protect at the mucosa, and may preclude the need for opsonic IgG in preventing streptococcal infection. These studies were also one of the first to compare purified, antigen-specific sIgA and serum IgG for passive protection at a mucosal site.

In another laboratory, passive protection against streptococcal pharyngeal colonization was also shown by the oral administration of purified lipoteichoic acid (LTA) but not deacylated LTA prior to oral challenge in mice [71]. The addition of anti-LTA by the same route also protected mice from oral streptococcal challenge. While several in vitro studies showed the importance of M protein [72–74] and LTA [75] in streptococcal adherence, these in vivo studies together with those presented above suggest that both M protein and LTA may play a key role in the colonization of the mouse pharyngeal mucosa. However, it is uncertain whether this is also true in humans.

2. Active Immunization with Conserved Region Peptides

To determine whether a local mucosal response directed to the conserved exposed epitopes of M protein can influence the course of mucosal colonization by group A streptococci, peptides corresponding to these regions were used as immunogens in a mouse model [66,67]. Overlapping synthetic peptides of the conserved region of the M6 protein were covalently linked to the mucosal adjuvant cholera toxin B subunit (CTB) and administered intranasally to mice in three weekly doses and boosted 30 days after the last dose with the peptide mixture. Ten days later, animals were challenged intranasally with live streptococci (either homologous M6 or heterologous M14) and pharyngeal colonization by the challenge organism was monitored for 10–15 days. Mice immunized with the peptide–CTB complex showed a significant reduction in colonization with either the M6 or M14 streptococci compared to mice receiving CTB alone [66,67] (Figure 7). Thus despite the fact that conserved region peptides were unable to evoke an opsonic antibody response in these studies [37], these peptides have the capacity to induce a local immune response capable of influencing the colonization of group A streptococci at the nasopharyngeal mucosa in this model system. These findings were the first to demonstrate protection against a heterologous serotype of group A streptococci with a vaccine consisting of the widely shared C-repeat region of the M6 protein.

Confirmation of these findings was later published independently using different streptococcal serotypes as the immunizing and challenge strains [76]. As mentioned above, in a separate study, Pruksakorn et al. [51] found, using a different criteria for streptococcal opsonization than previously published [25], that when a peptide derived from the conserved region of the M protein was administered to mice,

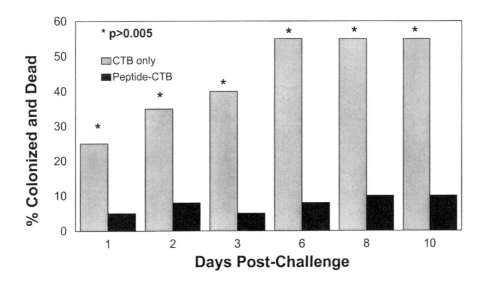

Figure 7   The extent of colonization of mice challenged with group A streptococci after oral immunization with M protein conserved region M6 peptides linked to CTB or CTB alone. Orally immunized mice were swabbed each day after challenge with M14 streptococci and plated on blood plates to determine the extent of colonization compared to mice vaccinated with CTB only. Plates showing group A streptococci were scored as positive.

it induced antibodies capable of opsonizing type 5 strepto-cocci and streptococci isolated from Aboriginal and Thai rheumatic fever patients. These findings were in sharp contrast to the earlier studies of Jones and Fischetti [37], who showed that antibodies to the conserved region of M protein were not opsonic. However, as the peptide reported by Quinn et al. [50] is similar to one of the peptides used by Bessen and Fischetti [65,67] in their mucosal protection studies (see above), the induction of serum IgG during mucosal immunization may offer added protection against streptococcal infection.

F. Vectoring the M Protein

To further verify the validity of using the M protein conserved region as a streptococcal vaccine, experiments were repeated in a vaccinia virus vector system. In these studies, the gene coding for the complete conserved region of the M6 molecule (from the pepsin site to the C-terminus, see Figure 4) was cloned and expressed in vaccinia virus producing the recombinant VVM6 virus [77,78]. Tissue culture cells infected with this virus were found to produce the conserved region of the M6 molecule. Animals immu-nized intranasally with only a single dose of recombinant virus were significantly protected from heterologous strep-tococcal challenge compared to animals immunized with wild-type virus (Figure 8). When the extent of colonization was examined in those animals immunized with wild-type or the VVM6 recombinant, the VVM6-immunized animals that exhibited positive swabs, showed a marked reduction in overall colonization compared to controls, indicating that mucosal immunization reduced the bacterial load on the mucosa in these animals. Animals immunized intradermally

with the VVM6 virus and challenged intranasally showed no protection.

The approaches described above proved that induction of a local immune response was critical for protection against streptococcal colonization and that the protection was not dependent upon an opsonic response as defined using the classical Lancefield method. However, in the event that the streptococcus was successful in penetrating the mucosa and establishing an infection, only then would type-specific antibodies be necessary to eradicate the organ-ism. This idea may perhaps explain why adults sporadically develop a streptococcal pharyngitis, i.e., a mucosal response may be breached when a large number of streptococci are encountered on the mucosal surface. The success of these strategies not only forms the basis of a broadly protective vaccine for the prevention of streptococcal pharyngitis but may offer insights for the development of other vaccines. For instance, a vaccine candidate previously shown by the parenteral route may prove to be successful by simply changing the site of immunization. Furthermore, these results emphasize the fact that in some cases antigens need to be presented to the immune system in a specific fashion to ultimately induce a protective response.

1. *Streptococcus gordonii* as a Vector

The importance of the C-terminal region in the attachment of surface proteins in gram-positive bacteria was previously demonstrated using the protein A from *Staphylococcus aureus* as a model system [79,80]. Surface proteins in gram-positive bacteria (which could number more than 20 in a single organism) are synthesized and exported at the septum, where new cell wall is also being produced and translocated to the surface [32,81]. Thus the C-terminal hydrophobic

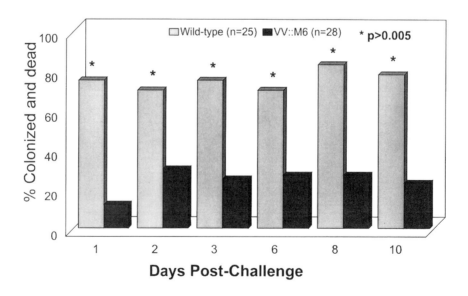

Figure 8 The extent of colonization of mice challenged with group A streptococci after oral immunization with recombinant vaccinia virus containing the gene for the whole conserved region of the M6 protein or vaccinia virus alone. Orally immunized mice were swabbed each day after challenge with M14 streptococci and plated on blood plates to determine the extent of colonization compared to mice vaccinated with wild-type vaccinia only. Plates showing group A streptococci were scored as positive.

domain and charged tail in these proteins function to control the export and anchoring process by acting as a temporary stop to position the LPXTG motif (the anchor motif common to >100 surface proteins on gram-positive bacteria [82]) precisely at the outer surface of the cytoplasmic membrane. This sequence motif, being an enzymatic recognition sequence, is cleaved resulting in the attachment of the surface-exposed segment of the protein to a cellular substrate [79]. This idea is supported by studies indicating that the C-terminal hydrophobic domain and charged tail are missing from the streptococcal surface M protein extracted from the cell wall [79,83].

Because the anchor region is highly conserved among a wide variety of surface molecules within several different gram-positive species, could it be fused to a foreign antigen and used to deliver the resulting fusion protein to the surface of a gram-positive bacterium, ultimately anchoring it to the cell? To answer this, the streptococcal M protein was employed in a model system.

Pozzi et al. [84,85] were the first to deliver a fusion protein to the surface of the gram-positive human oral commensal *S. gordonii*. The approach utilized a knowledge of the location of the surface-exposed and wall-associated regions of the fibrillar M protein [34,83]. Thus deleting the surface-exposed segment of the M molecule and replacing it in frame with the gene for a foreign protein (i.e., the E7 protein from human papillomavirus, consisting of 294 base pairs [85]), the fusion molecule could be presented on the bacterial cell surface and tightly anchored. Using this same strategy, a variety of protein antigens ranging from a few hundred to over 700 amino acids have now been successfully expressed on the surface of the human commensal *S. gordonii* ([85–88], and unpublished data).

To be certain that the expression of the recombinant molecule would be stable for many bacterial generations, the recipient *S. gordonii* was engineered such that the recombinant gene would be expressed from the chromosome under the control of an efficient resident promoter [84,85] (Figures 9 and 10). This strategy is one of the few in which the gene in question is chromosomally expressed. In contrast, most other reported live vaccine vector systems regulate their genes from high expression plasmids. Translocation of the recombinant molecule to the surface is assured by inclusion of the signal sequence and a short segment of the N-terminal region of the carrier M protein.

While the studies of Pozzi et al. [85] showed the feasibility of expressing a wide range of foreign proteins on the surface of gram-positive bacteria, an important question remained: would this mode of delivery induce an immune response, particularly a mucosal response in animals colonized by the recombinant organism? To answer this and to further verify the ability to deliver a diversity of proteins to the bacterial cell surface using this approach, Medaglini et al. [87] elected to express a 204-amino acid protein allergen from the white-faced hornet (Ag5.2) [89] on the surface of *S. gordonii*, essentially using the same methods described above [85,87] (see Figures 9 and 10). These studies clearly showed that mice colonized with the recombinant *S. gordonii* expressing the allergen were able to mount not only a mucosal response, but a serum IgG and T-cell response specifically to the allergen expressed on the *S. gordonii* cell surface.

Although still in development, the gram-positive commensal seems promising as a versatile live vector for vaccine delivery. Because the system induces both a mucosal and systemic immune response, it may be a more natural way of generating a protective response to a pathogen than systemic delivery alone. Although the animal studies indicate that this approach is feasible, human studies must be performed to determine if the same responses will be achieved. Early

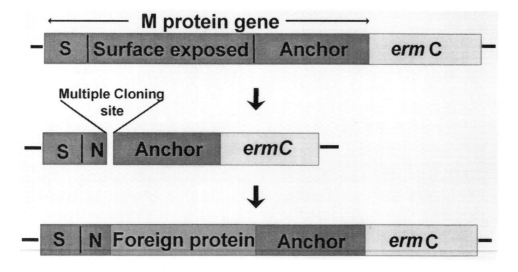

Figure 9 Engineering a fusion protein for surface expression. On a plasmid, the surface exposed region of the M protein is excised and replaced by a multiple cloning site. The foreign protein to be expressed on the bacterial surface is then inserted in frame in the multiple cloning site. The signal sequence (S) and a short segment of the M protein N-terminal sequence (N) is included in the construct to allow proper processing of the signal peptidase. The *erm*C antibiotic marker is used for selection of the construct.

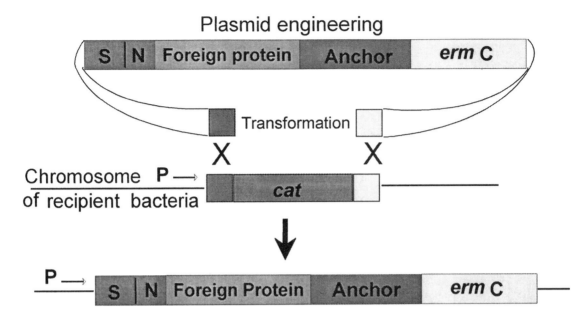

Figure 10 Insertion of the fusion protein into the gram-positive chromosome. A cassette is inserted in the chromosome of *S. gordonii* in front of a hi expression promoter selected at random. The cassette consists of a *cat* antibiotic reporter gene flanked by a short segment of the 5′ end of the signal sequence of the M protein gene (S) and the 3′ end by a short segment of the *erm*C marker. Because *S. gordonii* are naturally transformable, the linerarized plasmid inserts the M-protein fusion precisely in the chromosomal cassette in front of the promoter.

experiments show that when reintroduced into the human oral cavity, *S. gordonii* is capable of persisting for over 2 years [90]; therefore, it remains to be seen if the recombinant will perform similarly and induce an immune response to the fusion protein expressed on its surface. Although an immune response is in fact generated to commensal flora [91] even in humans ([92], and unpublished data), it is not a clearing response, however, it may be expected that the same would occur with the newly introduced recombinant strain.

G. Clinical Trials

1. Preclinical Evaluation of a 26-Valent M Protein-Based Vaccine

Current epidemiological data indicate that the majority of group A streptococcal infections in the United States are caused by relatively few serotypes. Surveillance of invasive disease conducted by the Centers for Disease Control and Prevention has shown that during 1998–2000, 19 serotypes accounted for 84% of the total isolates [93]. In ongoing studies to determine the serotype distribution of group A streptococci recovered from pediatric cases of pharyngitis in the United States, it was shown that 16 different serotypes accounted for 97% of all cases of pharyngitis [94]. These data indicate that a multivalent vaccine containing M protein fragments from a limited number of serotypes could potentially have a significant impact on the overall incidences of streptococcal infections within a population. Therefore, a 26-valent vaccine was designed to include N-terminal M peptides from epidemiologically important serotypes of group A streptococci. These include the serotypes commonly responsible for serious infections, uncomplicated pharyngitis in children, and the serotypes that are currently or historically associated with acute rheumatic fever. Based on this information, serotypes included in the 26-valent vaccine (Figure 11) account for 78% of all invasive infections, 80% of all cases of uncomplicated pharyngitis, and theoretically 100% of all "rheumatogenic" serotypes. Also included in the vaccine is a new protective antigen of group A streptococci (Spa) that is expressed by at least several serotypes [95]. Thus the 26-valent vaccine actually contains 27 distinct peptides.

The 26-valent vaccine consists of four component fusion proteins (Figure 11) that were mixed in equimolar ratios and formulated with alum to contain 400 μg of protein/dose. Three rabbits that received three intramuscular (IM) doses of the vaccine at 0, 4, and 16 weeks developed broadly opsonic antibodies that were not cross-reactive with human tissues. Antibody titers were determined by ELISA using serum obtained at 18 weeks against each of the purified recombinant dimeric peptide components of the vaccine. All preimmune titers were less than 200. Of the 81 immune serum titers determined (27 antigens × 3 rabbits), 69 titers (85%) increased by fourfold or greater. The vaccine elicited fourfold or greater increases in antibody levels against 25 of the 26 serotypes represented in the vaccine. To determine the functional activity of the M protein antibodies evoked by the 26-valent vaccine, in vitro opsonization and bactericidal tests were performed by using each of the 26 serotypes of group A streptococci. Opsonization assays were designed to determine the percentage of neutrophils that engulfed or

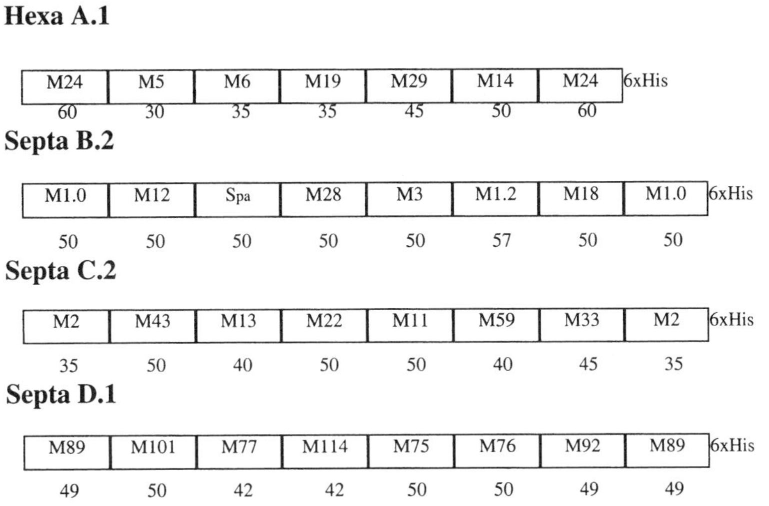

Hexa A.1

M24	M5	M6	M19	M29	M14	M24	6xHis
60	30	35	35	45	50	60	

Septa B.2

M1.0	M12	Spa	M28	M3	M1.2	M18	M1.0	6xHis
50	50	50	50	50	57	50	50	

Septa C.2

M2	M43	M13	M22	M11	M59	M33	M2	6xHis
35	50	40	50	50	40	45	35	

Septa D.1

M89	M101	M77	M114	M75	M76	M92	M89	6xHis
49	50	42	42	50	50	49	49	

Figure 11 Schematic diagram of the four recombinant fusion proteins contained in the 26-valent M protein-based vaccine. The number of amino acids contained in each M protein fragment is indicated below the M type. The four proteins are mixed in equimolar amounts and formulated with alum for intramuscular injection. M101 was formerly stNS5 and M114 was formerly st2967. The M13 is strain M13W, which has been newly designated as M94.

were associated with streptococci after rotation in nonimmune human blood that contained either preimmune or immune rabbit serum. The preimmune sera from all three rabbits resulted in ≤10% opsonization of each of the 26 serotypes tested, indicating that the donor blood used for these assays did not contain antibodies against the test organism and that each organism was fully resistant to opsonization in nonimmune blood. Using 30% opsonization in the presence of immune serum as a positive threshold result, 18 of the 26 serotypes (69%) were opsonized by at least one of three immune rabbit sera.

Bactericidal assays were also performed as an additional measure of the potential protective efficacy of the 26-valent vaccine. In these assays, each of the 26 serotypes of group A streptococci was rotated in nonimmune blood for 3 hr in the presence of either preimmune or immune rabbit sera. In all experiments, the test mixture containing preimmune serum resulted in growth of the organisms to eight generations or more, again indicating that the human blood did not contain opsonic antibodies against the test strains and that each organism was fully resistant to bactericidal killing in nonimmune blood. Using 50% reduction in growth (percent killing) after the 3-hr rotation in blood containing immune serum compared to the preimmune serum as a positive threshold, bactericidal activity was observed against 22 of the 26 serotypes tested. When the results of the opsonization and bactericidal assays were combined, 24 of the 26 serotypes (92%) tested were opsonized by the immune sera in one or both assays.

In summary, these results show that a highly complex 26-valent M protein-based vaccine was immunogenic in rabbits and evoked broadly opsonic antibodies against the vast majority of vaccine serotypes. This vaccine is now being tested in Phase I clinical trials to assess its safety and immunogenicity in normal adult volunteers (see below).

2. Clinical Experience with Multivalent Vaccines

There are currently two Phase I clinical trials in progress to determine the safety and immunogenicity of multivalent group A streptococcal vaccines. The first trial is under the direction of Karen Kotloff, and is being conducted at the Center for Vaccine Development at the University of Maryland. This is a dose-escalating study of a hexavalent vaccine [44] formulated in alum to contain either 50, 100, or 200 µg per dose. Each group of 8–10 adult volunteers is receiving three IM doses at 0, 4, and 16 weeks. The first two dose groups have been fully enrolled and have received the entire series of injections. Thus far, the vaccine has been well tolerated and is immunogenic. A complete analysis of the type-specific and opsonic antibody responses will be forthcoming after the completion of the 200-µg dose study, which is the target dose for this vaccine.

The second clinical trial is as a Phase I/II study to determine the safety and immunogenicity of the 26-valent vaccine described above [47]. This study is under the direction of Scott Haperin at the IWK Grace Health Center, Dalhousie University, Halifax, Canada. In the Phase I component of this study, 30 adult volunteers are receiving 400 µg of the 26-valent vaccine formulated with alum administered IM at 0, 4, and 16 weeks. The trial has been fully enrolled and is scheduled to be completed in 2002. Because the primary target population for this vaccine is preschool children, the Phase II trial will include two groups of 200 each, ages 3–6 and 10–14, who will receive 400 µg of the vaccine at 0, 4, and 16 weeks.

3. Toward Vaccine Trials with Recombinant *S. Gordonii*

Convinced that the use of a commensal bacteria as a vaccine delivery vehicle is a safe, effective, and inexpensive way to induce a mucosal response, a recombinant *S. gordonii* was prepared which contained the C-terminal half of the M protein containing the exposed conserved region of the molecule. This segment was similar to that used successfully in the vaccinia virus experiments (see above) [77]. *S. gordonii* expressing this conserved fragment of the M protein on its surface was used to successfully colonize for up to 12 weeks all of the 10 rabbits colonized. During this time, the animals raised a salivary IgA and serum IgG response to the intact M protein. The amount of M protein-specific sIgA was up to 5% of the total IgA in the saliva of these animals. Experiments revealed that conserved region-specific IgA and IgG induced by this method do not cross-react with human heart tissue as determined by immunofluorescence assay [96].

If proven to be successful, the commensal delivery system may be ideal for the developing countries. Being a live vector, it would be easy to administer and not likely require additional doses. Also, because gram-positive bacteria are stable for long periods in the lyophilized state, a cold chain would not be required. Early studies show that when reintroduced into the human oral cavity, *S. gordonii* is capable of persisting for over 2 years, and is transmitted to other members of the family [88]. For a developing country, this factor could be ideal considering that the whole population is rarely able to immunize. However, it remains to be seen if the recombinant will induce in humans a protective immune response to the M protein fragment expressed on its surface.

Because of the uncertainties of using *S. gordonii* in humans as a live vaccine vector system, safety trials were performed utilizing this organism delivered orally and nasally to adult volunteers. To be certain that the *S. gordonii* recovered were in fact the ones installed in the volunteers, two antibiotic resistance markers were introduced in the study strain (streptomycin and 5-fluro-2-deoxyuridine). Also, under the direction of Karen Kotloff, at the Center for Vaccine Development at the University of Maryland, over 100 volunteers were tested with differing doses of the marked *S. gordonii*, and in all, the vector was well tolerated with no observed adverse events. This result not only leads us to the use of this vector system for the delivery of the M protein conserved region, but sets the stage for the utilization of this vector system for a wide variety of protein antigens.

V. CONCLUSION

In this chapter, we have attempted to outline some of the different strategies being followed in an attempt to develop a vaccine to prevent infection with GABHS and subsequent pathology. The organism is relatively simple in its structure and life cycle, compared to some other organisms, such as the malaria parasite. Consequently, the number of strategies and vaccine candidates are more limited. This alone gives great hope. A challenge, however, and similarity with the malaria parasite, is that the greatest burden of disease is carried by people in the poorest parts of the world, making it more difficult to attract major funding from industry.

As in all areas of scientific discovery, there are the inevitable, yet healthy, differences of opinion regarding choice

of antigen and rationale for inclusion in a vaccine. The current clinical trials, either underway or planned, will shed important light on the approaches that we must focus on and hopefully convince philanthropic, government, and business organizations to invest in the development of this much-needed vaccine.

ACKNOWLEDGMENTS

The work of Dr. Cleary is supported in part by USPHS Grant AI20016. The work of Dr. Dale is supported by research funds from the Department of Veterans Affairs, USPH Grant A10085, and research funds from ID Biomedical Corporation, Bothell, WA. The work of Dr Fischetti is supported in part by USPHS Grant AI11822. The work of Dr Good is supported in part by grants from the NHMRC (Australia), National Heart Foundation (Australia), and the Prince Charles Hospital Research Foundation (Australia).

REFERENCES

1. Kumar RK, et al. Epidemiology of streptococcal pharyngitis, rheumatic fever, and rheumatic heart disease. In: Thomas D, ed. Rheumatic Fever. Washington, DC: American Registry of Pathology, Armed Forces Institute of Pathology, 1999:41–68.
2. The World Health Report, 1998. Office of World Health Reporting, World Health Organization, Geneva.
3. Stollerman GH. The return of rheumatic fever. Hosp Pract 1988; 23(11):100–113.
4. Kavey RE, Kaplan EL. Resurgence of acute rheumatic fever. Pediatrics 1989; 84(3):585–586.
5. Carapetis JR, et al. Acute rheumatic fever and rheumatic heart disease in the top end of Australia's Northern Territory. Med J Aust 1996; 164(3):146–149.
6. Vijaykumar M, et al. Incidence of rheumatic fever and prevalence of rheumatic heart disease in India. Int J Cardiol 1994; 43(3):221–228.
7. Michaud C, et al. Rheumatic heart disease. In: Jamieson DT, ed. Disease Control Priorities in Developing Countries: A Summary. Washington, DC: World Bank, 1993:221–232.
8. Wannamaker LW, et al. Prophylaxis of acute rheumatic fever by treatment of the preceding streptococcal infection with depot penicillin. Am J Med 1951; 10:673–695.
9. Stollerman GH, et al. Prophylaxis against group A streptococci in rheumatic fever. The use of single monthly injections of benzathine penicillin G. N Eng J Med 1955; 252:787–792.
10. Cunninghamm MW. Pathogenesis of group A streptococcal infections. Clin Microbiol Rev 2000; 13(3):470–511.
11. Kaplan EL, et al. Dynamic epidemiology of group A streptococcal serotypes associated with pharyngitis. Lancet 2001; 358:1334–1337.
12. Wexler D, et al. A streptococcal inactivator of chemotaxis: a new virulence factor specific to group A streptococci. Proc Natl Acad Sci USA 1985; 82:179–180.
13. Ivey CL, et al. Neutrophil chemoattractants generated in two phases during reperfusion of ischemic myocardium in the rabbit. J Clin Invest 1995; 95:2720–2728.
14. Ji Y, et al. C5a peptidase alters clearance and trafficking of group A streptococci by infected mice. Infect Immun 1996; 64:503–510.
15. Ji Y, et al. Impact of M49, Mrp, Enn, and C5a peptidase proteins on colonization of the mouse oral mucosa by *Streptococcus pyogenes*. Infect Immun 1998; 66:5399–5405.
16. Ji Y, et al. Intranasal immunization with C5a peptidase pre-

vents nasopharyngeal colonization of mice by the group A Streptococcus. Infect Immun 1997; 65:2080–2087.

17. Bisno AL, Stevens DL. Streptococcal infections of skin and soft tissues. N Engl J Med 1996; 334:240–245.

18. Hill HR, et al. Group B streptococci inhibit the chemotactic activity of the fifth component of complement. J Immunol 1988; 141:3551–3556.

19. Chmouryguina I, et al. Conservation of the C5a peptidase genes in group A and B streptococci. Infect Immun 1996; 64: 2387–2390.

20. Cleary PP, et al. Virulent human strains of group G streptococci express a C5a peptidase enzyme similar to that produced by group A streptococci. Infect Immun 1991; 59: 2305–2310.

21. Franken C, et al. Horizontal gene transfer and host specificity of beta-haemolytic streptococci: the role of a putative composite transposon containing scpB and lmb. Mol Microbiol 2001; 41:925–935.

22. Cheng Q, et al. Antibody against surface-bound C5a peptidase is opsonic and initiates macrophage killing of group B streptococci. Infect Immun 2001; 69:2302–2308.

23. O'Connor SP, et al. The human antibody response to streptococcal C5a peptidase. J Infect Dis 1990; 163:109–116.

24. Breese BB, Hall CB. Beta hemolytic streptococcal diseases. Boston: Houghton Mufflin, 1978.

25. Lancefield RC. Persistence of type specific antibodies in man following infection with group A streptococci. J Exp Med 1959; 110:271–292.

26. Salvadori LG, et al. Group A streptococcus-liposome ELISA antibody titers to group A polysaccharide and opsonophagocytic capabilities of the antibodies. J Infect Dis 1995; 171: 593–600.

27. Dudding BA, Ayoub EM. Persistence of streptococcal group A antibody in patinets with rheumatic valvular disease. J Exp Med 1968; 128:1081–1098.

28. Cunningham MW, et al. Human monoclonal antibodies reactive with antigens of the group A streptococcus and human heart. J Immunol 1988; 141:2760–2766.

29. Lancefield RC. The antigenic complex of *Streptococcus hemolyticus*: I. Demonstration of a type-specific substance in extracts of *Streptococcus hemolyticus*. J Exp Med 1928; 47:91–103.

30. Lancefield RC. Current knowledge of the type specific M antigens of group A streptococci. J Immunol 1962; 89:307–313.

31. Fox EN. M proteins of group A streptococci. Bacteriol Rev 1974; 38:57–86.

32. Fischetti VA. Streptococcal M protein: molecular design and biological behavior. Clin Microbiol Rev 1989; 2:285–314.

33. Bessen D, Fischetti VA. Vaccination against *Streptococcus pyogenes* infection. In: Levine M, Wood G, eds. New Generation Vaccines. New York: Marcel Dekker Inc., 1988a:599–609.

34. Jones KF, et al. Location of variable and conserved epitopes among the multiple serotypes of streptococcal M protein. J Exp Med 1985; 161:623–628.

35. Fischetti VA, et al. Location of the complement factor H binding site on streptococcal M6 protein. Infect Immun 1995; 63:149–153.

36. Horstmann RK, et al. Role of fibrinogen in complement inhibition by streptococcal M protein. Infect Immun 1992; 60: 5036–5041.

37. Jones KF, Fischetti VA. The importance of the location of antibody binding on the M6 protein for opsonization and phagocytosis of group A M6 streptococci. J Exp Med 1988; 167:1114–1123.

38. Ehlenberger AG, Nussenzweig V. Role of C3b and C3d receptors in phagocytosis. J Exp Med 1977; 145:357–371.

39. Fox EN, et al. Protective study with a group A streptococcal

M protein vaccine. Infectivity challenge of human volunteers. J Clin Invest 1973; 52:1885–1892.

40. Polly SM, et al. Protective studies with a group A streptococcal M protein vaccine: II. Challenge of volunteers after local immunization in the upper respiratory tract. J Infect Dis 1975; 131:217–224.

41. Dale JB. Group A streptococcal vaccines. Infect Dis Clin North Am 1999; 13:227–243.

42. Dale JB, et al. Recombinant tetravalent group A streptococcal M protein vaccine. J Immunol 1993; 151:2188–2194.

43. Dale JB, et al. Recombinant, octavalent group A streptococcal M protein vaccine. Vaccine 1996; 14:944–948.

44. Dale JB. Multivalent group A streptococcal vaccine designed to optimize the immunogenicity of six tandem M protein fragments. Vaccine 1999; 17:193–200.

45. Dale JB, Chiang EC. Intranasal immunization with recombinant group a streptococcal M protein fragment fused to the B subunit of *Escherichia coli* labile toxin protects mice against systemic challenge infections. J Infect Dis 1995; 171: 1038–1041.

46. Beachey EH, et al. Protective immunogenicity and T lymphocyte specificity of a trivalent hybrid peptide containing NH_2-terminal sequences of types 5, 6 and 24 M proteins synthesized in tandem. J Exp Med 1987; 166:647–656.

47. Hu MC, et al. Immunogenicity of a 26-valent group A streptococcal vaccine. Infect Immun 2002; 70:2171–2177.

48. Kemeny E, et al. Identification of mononuclear cells and T cell subsets in rheumatic valvulitis. Clin Immunol Immunopathol 1989; 52(2):225–237.

49. Guilherme L, et al. T-cell reactivity against streptococcal antigens in the periphery mirrors reactivity of heart-infiltrating T lymphocytes in rheumatic heart disease patients. Infect Immun 2001; 69(9):5345–5351.

50. Quinn A, et al. Induction of autoimmune valvular heart disease by recombinant streptococcal m protein. Infect Immun 2001; 69(6):4072–4078.

51. Pruksakorn S, et al. Towards a vaccine for rheumatic fever: identification of a conserved target epitope on M protein of group A streptococci. Lancet 1994; 344:639–642.

52. Bessen D, Fischetti VA. Influence of intranasal immunization with synthetic peptides corresponding to conserved epitopes of M protein on mucosal colonization by group A streptococci. Infect Immun 1988; 56(10):2666–2672.

53. Bronze MS, et al. Epitopes of group A streptococcal M protein that evoke cross-protective local immune responses. J Immunol 1992; 148(3):888–893.

54. Pruksakorn S, et al. Conserved T and B cell epitopes on the M protein of group A streptococci. Induction of bactericidal antibodies. J Immunol 1992; 149(8):2729–2735.

55. Relf WA, et al. Mapping a conserved conformational epitope from the M protein of group A streptococci. Pept Res 1996; 9(1):12–20.

56. Brandt ER, et al. New multi-determinant strategy for a group A streptococcal vaccine designed for the Australian Aboriginal population. Nat Med 2000a; 6(4):455–459.

57. Hayman WA, et al. Enhancing the immunogenicity and modulating the fine epitope recognition of antisera to a helical group A streptococcal peptide vaccine candidate from the M protein using lipid-core-peptide technology. Immunol Cell Biol 2002; 80:178–187.

58. Brandt ER, et al. Human antibodies to the conserved region of the M protein: opsonization of heterologous strains of group A streptococci. Vaccine 1997; 15(16):1805–1812.

59. Brandt ER, et al. Protective and nonprotective epitopes from amino termini of M proteins from Australian aboriginal isolates and reference strains of group A streptococci. Infect Immun 2000b; 68(12):6587–6594.

60. Hayman WA, et al. Mapping the minimal murine T cell and B cell epitopes within a peptide vaccine candidate from the

conserved region of the M protein of group A streptococcus. Int Immunol 1997; 9(11):1723–1733.

61. Brandt ER, et al. Opsonic human antibodies from an endemic population specific for a conserved epitope on the M protein of group A streptococci. Immunology 1996; 89(3): 331–337.

62. Gardiner D, et al. Vir typing: a long-PCR typing method for group A streptococci. PCR Methods Appl 1995; 4(5):288–293.

63. O'Brien-Simpson NM, et al. Polymerization of unprotected synthetic peptides: a view towards synthetic peptide vaccines. J Am Chem Soc 1997; 119:1183–1188.

64. Fischetti VA, Windels M. Mapping the immunodeterminants of the complete streptococcal M6 protein molecule: identification of an immunodominant region. J Immunol 1988; 141: 3592–3599.

65. Bessen D, Fischetti VA. Role of nonopsonic antibody in protection against group A streptococcal infection. In: Lasky L, ed. Technological Advances in Vaccine Development. New York: Alan R. Liss Inc., 1988b:493.

66. Bessen D, Fischetti VA. Influence of intranasal immunization with synthetic peptides corresponding to conserved epitopes of M protein on mucosal colonization by group A streptococci. Infect Immun 1988c; 56:2666–2672.

67. Bessen D, Fischetti VA. Synthetic peptide vaccine against mucosal colonization by group A streptococci: I. Protection against a heterologous M serotype with shared C repeat region epitopes. J Immunol 1990; 145:1251–1256.

68. Kiyono H, et al. The mucosal immune system: features of inductive and effector sites to consider in mucosal immunization and vaccine development. Reg Immun 1992; 4:54–62.

69. McGhee JR, et al. New perspectives in mucosal immunity with emphasis on vaccine development. Semin Hemat 1993; 30(4):3–15.

70. Bessen D, Fischetti VA. Passive acquired mucosal immunity to group A streptococci by secretory immunoglobulin A. J Exp Med 1988d; 167:1945–1950.

71. Dale JB, et al. Passive protection of mice against group A streptococcal pharyngeal infection by lipoteichoic acid. J Infect Dis 1994; 169:319–323.

72. Tylewska SK, et al. Binding selectivity of *Streptococcus pyogenes* and M-protein to epithelial cells differs from that of lipoteichoic acid. Curr Microbiol 1988; 16:209–216.

73. Alkan M, et al. Adherence of pharyngeal and skin strains of group A streptococci to human skin and oral epithelial cells. Infect Immun 1977; 18:555–557.

74. Caparon MG, et al. Role of M protein in adherence of group A streptococci. Infect Immun 1991; 59:1811–1817.

75. Beachey EH, Ofek I. Epithelial cell binding of group A streptococci by lipoteichoic acid on fimbriae denuded of M protein. J Exp Med 1976; 143:759–771.

76. Bronze MS, et al. Protective immunity evoked by locally administered group A streptococcal vaccines in mice. J Immunol 1988; 141:2767–2770.

77. Hruby DE, et al. Expression of streptococcal M protein in mammalian cells. Proc Natl Acad Sci USA 1988; 85:5714–5717.

78. Fischetti VA, et al. Protection against streptococcal phar-

yngeal colonization with a vaccinia: M protein recombinant. Science 1989; 244:1487–1490.

79. Schneewind O, et al. Sorting of protein A to the staphylococcal cell wall. Cell 1992; 70:267–281.

80. Schneewind O, et al. Cell wall sorting signals in surface proteins of gram-positive bacteria. EMBO J 1993; 12(12):4803–4811.

81. Cole RM, Hahn JJ. Cell wall replication in *Streptococcus pyogenes*. Science 1962; 135:722–724.

82. Fischetti VA, et al. Conservation of a hexapeptide sequence in the anchor region of surface proteins of Gram-positive cocci. Mol Microbiol 1990; 4:1603–1605.

83. Pancholi V, Fischetti VA. Isolation and characterization of the cell-associated region of group A streptococcal M6 protein. J Bacteriol 1988; 170:2618–2624.

84. Pozzi G, et al. Expression of M6 protein gene of *Streptococcus pyogenes* in *Streptococcus gordonii* after chromosomal integration and transcriptional fusion. Res Microbiol 1992a; 143: 449–457.

85. Pozzi G, et al. Delivery and expression of a heterologous antigen on the surface of streptococci. Infect Immun 1992b; 60:1902–1907.

86. Manca F, et al. The naive repertoire of human T helper cells specific for gp120. The envelope of glycoprotein of HIV. J Immunol 1991; 146:1964–1971.

87. Medaglini D, et al. Mucosal and systemic immune responses to a recombinant protein expressed on the surface of the oral commensal bacterium *Streptococcus gordonii* after oral colonization. Proc Natl Acad Sci USA 1995; 92:6868–6872.

88. Piard J-C, et al. Cell wall anchoring of the *Streptococcus pyogenes* M6 protein in various lactic acid bacteria. J Bacteriol 1997; 179:3068–3072.

89. King TP, et al. Immunochemical observations of antigen 5, a major venom allergen of hornets, yellowjackets and wasps. Mol Immunol 1987; 24:857–864.

90. Svanberg M, Westergren G. Persistence and spread of the orally-implanted bacterium *Streptococcus sanguis* between persons. Arch Oral Biol 1986; 31:1–4.

91. Shroff KE. Commensal enteric bacteria engender a self-limiting humoral mucosal immune response while permanently colonizing the gut. Infect Immun 1995; 63: 3904–3913.

92. Dougan G. The molecular basis for the virulence of bacterial pathogens: implications for oral vaccine development. Microbiology 1994; 140:215–224.

93. Schuchat A, et al. Active bacterial core surveillance of the emerging infections program network. Emerg Infect Dis 2001; 7:92–99.

94. S Shulman, et al. In U.S. Nationwide Streptococcal Pharyngitis Serotype Surveillance, Infectious Diseases Society of America 39th Annual Meeting, San Francisco, CA 2001, Abstr. No. 277, 87.

95. Dale JB, et al. New protective antigen of group A streptococci. J Clin Invest 1999; 103:1261–1268.

96. Zabriskie JB, et al. Heart-reactive antibody associated with rheumatic fever: characterization and diagnostic significance. Clin Exp Immunol 1970; 7:147–159.

58
Vaccines Against Group B *Streptococcus*

Morven S. Edwards and Carol J. Baker
Baylor College of Medicine, Houston, Texas, U.S.A.

Lawrence C. Paoletti
Brigham and Women's Hospital and Harvard Medical School, Boston, Massachusetts, U.S.A.

I. GROUP B STREPTOCOCCAL DISEASE BURDEN

A. Newborn and Young Infants

Group B *Streptococcus* (GBS) has been a leading cause of serious bacterial infection in neonates and young infants for more than a quarter of a century. Increased awareness of this important disease resulted in prompt initiation of empiric antimicrobial therapy for suspected cases of neonatal infection based on delineated risk factors, and has been associated with a very significant reduction of mortality and an improved the prognosis for infants with invasive GBS disease. During the 1990s, the overall case fatality rate was about 5%, but in prematurely born infants this is nearly 25%. Contemporary appraisal of the epidemiology of neonatal disease has affirmed that low birth weight and black ethnicity continue to be associated with enhanced risk for early-onset (age <7 days) neonatal disease and also has identified enhanced risk among infants born to Hispanic women [1]. The predominant serotypes of GBS currently causing neonatal and young infant disease are types Ia, III, and the new serotype which appeared in the 1990s, type V. Taken together, these three account for ~ 80% to 85% of invasive infections identified in a racially and ethnically diverse cohort from metropolitan areas in the United States [1].

Despite reduced case fatality rates, disease incidence was stable from the 1970s until the mid-1990s, when recommendations based on clinical trials demonstrated the efficacy of maternal intrapartum antibiotic prophylaxis (IAP) with intravenous penicillin G or ampicillin in preventing early-onset disease. Associated with the widespread implementation of consensus guidelines endorsed in 1996 by the American Academy of Pediatrics, the American College of Obstetricians and Gynecologists and the Centers for Disease Control and Prevention, there has been a substantial decline in the incidence of early-onset disease. Active, multistate, population-based surveillance has documented a 65% decrease in incidence from 1.7 cases per 1000 live births in 1993 to 0.6 per 1000 in 1998 [2]. Early-onset infection most commonly manifests as bacteremia, but ~ 6–7% of infants present with meningitis and a similar proportion with pneumonia. Maternal IAP has not decreased the number of late-onset (7–89 days of age) infant infections; the incidence persists at 0.3–0.5 cases per 1000 live births. Approximately one-fourth of infants with late-onset GBS disease present with meningitis and a substantial number of survivors (estimated at 20%) have neurological sequelae. Despite the widespread implementation of maternal IAP in the United States, it is projected that 2200 infants 0–6 days of age and 1400 infants 7–89 days of age will develop invasive GBS disease yearly and that 140 of these will have fatal infection.

B. Children

Group B streptococcal disease in children from 90 days to 14 years of age comprises a small but important portion of the total disease burden. A multistate active bacterial surveillance group tracking a population base of more than 12 million from 1993 expanding to 20 million in 1998 reported that 2% of cases of invasive GBS infections occurred in this age group, as opposed to 28% in the 0–90 days age group [2]. One-half of these patients were infants less than 6 months of age. The improved survival of extremely low birth weight infants, particularly those requiring long-term hospitalization in a neonatal intensive care unit, has extended the age of susceptibility for young infants beyond the classical definition for late-onset disease of 3 months. Many of these very late-onset infections manifest as bacteremia without a focus, and a benign outcome is typical. In children older than 6 months of age, the majority have an underlying condition predisposing to invasive infection, such as human immunodeficiency virus infection or a structural heart or central nervous system defect [3]. Taken as a group, the mortality rate for GBS disease in childhood is about 9% or nearly twice the case fatality in neonates.

C. Pregnant Women

Lower vaginal or rectal colonization with GBS is a risk factor for invasive infections in pregnant women as well as their neonates. The risk of intra-amniotic infection or chorioamnionitis is significantly higher for women with high-density [$>10^5$ colony-forming units (CFU) per mL] GBS vaginal colonization than for those with low-density colonization [4]. The advent of maternal IAP has had a small but significant impact upon invasive GBS disease, primarily bacteremia with or without endometritis or chorioamnionitis, among pregnant women, with a decline in incidence from 0.29 cases per 1000 deliveries in 1993 to 0.23 per 1000 in 1998 [2]. Despite this modest decline, there remains substantial morbidity attributable to GBS during pregnancy. Bacteremia accounted for approximately two-thirds of cases reported by investigators at the Centers for Diseases Control and Prevention; chorioamnionitis and endometritis each contributed 10% and septic abortion accounted for 7% of cases in the United States [2]. Among those for whom the outcome of pregnancy was known, 54% had infants who remained free from clinical illness, 17% had infants who had GBS disease but survived and 29% had spontaneous abortions, stillborn infants, or infants who had fatal invasive GBS infection.

D. Nonpregnant Adults

The diminished number of neonatal GBS infections has highlighted the substantial contribution to total disease burden of invasive GBS disease in adults. More than two-thirds of all invasive GBS disease in the United States now occurs in adults and most of these infections are unrelated to pregnancy [5]. Within the past decade, a 2- to 4-fold increase in the incidence of invasive GBS disease in nonpregnant adults has been documented [6,7]. Disease rates rise with advancing age and, in two recent reports, adults 65 years of age or older had GBS infection rates of 11.9 and 28.3 per 100,000 population, respectively [5,8]. Nursing-home residents are at particularly high risk. The age-adjusted annual incidence of GBS per 100,000 population among those 65 years of age and older was 72.3 for nursing home residents and 17.5 for community residents (relative risk, 4.1) [9]. As in neonates, disease rates were significantly higher in black compared with white adults (about 2-fold higher). Adults older than 65 years of age are projected to account for ~6900 cases of invasive GBS infections in the United States yearly, or more than one-half of the total number of adult cases, and for more than 60% of the total deaths attributable to invasive GBS infections [2].

The majority of adults have at least one underlying condition that presumably enhances susceptibility to invasive GBS infection [10]. Diabetes mellitus is the most common of these and 20–40% of nonpregnant adults developing invasive GBS infection have diabetes. A number of other conditions, including cirrhosis or other chronic liver disease, breast cancer, neurogenic bladder, and decubitus ulcer also are associated with significantly increased risk [5]. In one report, 49 of 51 episodes of GBS bacteremia in nonpregnant adults occurred in association with at least one underlying condition [6]. The aging of the population in the United States, together with improving treatments for such chronic diseases as diabetes mellitus, predict that GBS disease in nonpregnant adults will pose an ongoing and increasing proportion of the disease burden.

II. CLINICAL TRIALS WITH VACCINES FOR GBS

This following discussion is arranged chronologically from the earliest candidate vaccines [purified capsular polysaccharides (CPS) of GBS] to the development of more recent vaccine constructs (polysaccharide–protein conjugates). Clinical trials began with monovalent capsular polysaccharides for serotype III, followed by those for types Ia and II, based on the significant perinatal disease burden attributable to these serotypes in the 1970s and 1980s. With the availability of GBS conjugate vaccines, serotypes Ib and type V vaccines have also been evaluated in healthy adults. Recently, additional studies have been completed, including testing of the effect of an adjuvant or a second dose on the immune response to type III conjugate vaccine, and of a bivalent type II/III conjugate vaccine. Most of these candidate GBS vaccines were developed and prepared at the Channing Laboratory (Boston, MA).

A. GBS Capsular Polysaccharide Vaccines

The premise that antibodies against the capsular polysaccharides of GBS would be important in protective immunity was first suggested by Lancefield's observations in a mouse model of lethal infection. The first data indicating that CPS-specific antibodies were protective in human disease was reported by Baker and Kasper [11]. These investigators demonstrated that neonates at risk for invasive GBS disease (either early- or late-onset) were those born to women with very low concentrations of III CPS-specific antibodies in delivery sera. This initial observation was confirmed and extended by several others for serotypes Ia and Ib [12, 13]. Additional evidence implying the biologic importance of serum antibodies against GBS CPS antigens is the ability of these antibodies to promote opsonization of homologous capsular types for phagocytosis and killing by human polymorphonuclear leukocytes in vitro and to provide in vivo protection from lethal infection in several animal models. These data suggested that active immunization of pregnant women with GBS CPS antigens might elicit protective levels of antibodies, thus preventing infant GBS disease.

Initial characterization of the CPS antigens of GBS had employed hot acid extraction from whole organisms. This method was discovered to degrade terminal sialic acid moieties, rendering these antigens "incomplete." This was especially important for serotype III GBS, in which the terminal sialic acid moiety of the repeating side chain of the polysaccharide was found to dictate the tertiary structure of the molecule that defined the critical epitope for protection. Once "complete" Ia, II, and III CPS structures had been purified and characterized, their use as candidate vaccines in healthy adults was evaluated. Success was expected based on results with the multivalent pneumococcal polysaccharide vaccine, but while quite well tolerated GBS polysaccharides were variably immunogenic. It was discovered that the overwhelming majority of young healthy adults had low concentrations of CPS-specific antibodies in their preimmunization sera, and these low levels often predicted a poor immune response to immunization. In adults with low concentrations of CPS-specific antibodies prior to immunization with II CPS, 88% developed significant immune responses, but for Ia and III CPS, the response was 40% and 60%, respectively [14].

Despite these disappointing results, indicating the need for development of improved candidate GBS vaccines, an important study was conducted using type III polysaccharide vaccine. A total of 40 healthy pregnant women were immunized with purified III CPS at a mean of 31 weeks of gestation. Among the 25 women who developed an immune response, 90% had infants with presumably protective levels of III CPS-specific antibodies in their cord sera and the majority of sera from these infants promoted opsonophagocytosis and killing of type III GBS through age 3 months. These observations supported the concept that maternal immunization with a GBS vaccine could elicit potentially protective CPS-specific, IgG class antibodies that would be passively transferred to neonates and young infants to prevent GBS disease during the first 3 months of life [15].

B. GBS Type III CPS–Protein Conjugate Vaccine

The decision to begin GBS conjugate vaccine development with serotype III was based on the high proportion of disease caused by this serotype in neonates and young infants (currently estimated at 60%), and the abundance of data indicating that antibodies directed at the III CPS were protective against infant infection [11,12]. Strategies to improve the immunogenicity of the GBS CPS included the use of enzymatically derived oligosaccharides and of native polysaccharides as haptens. Conjugate vaccines prepared with III CPS oligosaccharides were highly immunogenic in animals and useful as reagents to study immune responses to a polymer that possesses conformationally dependent epitopes [16,17]. However, methods to derive III CPS oligosaccharides and the end-linking chemistry were inefficient, so these vaccines could not be made on a large scale. Conjugate vaccines using native type III CPS and tetanus toxoid (III–TT) with two different coupling chemistries [18,19] resulted in vaccines that were immunogenic in animals, elicited antibodies in adult mice that protected neonates from experimental challenge, and produced functionally active III CPS-specific IgG in mice, rabbits, and baboons [19–21]. To date, all GBS conjugate vaccines used in clinical trials have been developed by using the reductive amination coupling chemistry [19,22]. Issues of conjugate size, polysaccharide size and degree of polysaccharide–protein cross-linking all influence the immunogenicity and protective efficacy of III–TT con-

jugate vaccines [23]. These structural properties have been considerations in the vaccines formulated to date.

The first GBS conjugate vaccine for Phase 1 clinical trials was created by using purified III CPS with a M_r of approximately 200,000; aldehydes were formed on 26% of sialic acid residues before coupling to monomeric TT. This first III–TT conjugate vaccine was 56% carbohydrate and 44% protein, and was prepared at the Channing Laboratory (Boston, MA), under good laboratory practices (GLP) conditions [24]. As for all GBS conjugate vaccines, this first conjugate vaccine passed tests for general safety, microbial sterility, and pyrogenicity required by the Food and Drug Administration. A total of 60 healthy nonpregnant women, between 18 and 40 years of age, were randomized to receive a single intramuscular injection of III–TT conjugate at a dose containing of 58, 14.5, or 3.6 µg of III CPS or the unconjugated III CPS at a dose of 50 µg. Each vaccine and each dose of III–TT conjugate was well tolerated. The majority of women experienced no local symptoms or only tenderness at the injection site and a minority (25%) had soreness with arm movement. No more than 27% developed redness or swelling at the injection site and when this occurred, it was mild (<3 cm) in the majority, resolving within 72 hr after vaccine administration.

The geometric mean concentration (GMC) of III CPS-specific IgG in sera from the 30 recipients of the 58-µg dose of III–TT rose from 0.09 µg/mL before immunization to 4.89 µg/mL at 2 weeks after immunization. The III CPS-specific IgG GMC remained relatively unchanged 8 weeks after immunization (Table 1), and was 3.02 µg/mL 18 weeks later. The immunogenicity of III–TT was dose-dependent, with a substantially lower GMT in 8-week postimmunization sera from subjects who received the 3.6-µg dose than in sera from recipients of either of the two higher dosages. Proportional response rates (≥4-fold rises) 8 weeks after immunization were 97% in recipients of the highest dose but only 64% in those receiving the 3.6-µg dose. The group of women receiving unconjugated III CPS had significantly inferior immune responses (data not shown). Sera obtained before and 4 weeks after vaccination were tested for functional activity in an opsonophagocytic assay. A positive correlation ($r = 0.7$) was shown between killing of type III GBS by healthy adult polymorphonuclear leukocytes and the concentration of III CPS-specific IgG. The functional activity of III CPS-specific IgG also was examined by protection studies in mice. A pooled standard human reference serum (SHRS III) from five III–TT recipients (83.5 µg of III CPS-specific IgG) was administered intraperitoneally to pregnant dams. Among the 41 pups born to dams given SHRS III, 30 (73%) survived a usually lethal challenge of type III GBS, whereas each of the 11 pups born to a dam given normal human serum died [24]. Thus these Phase 1 trials demonstrated, in concept, the potential for GBS conjugate vaccines to prevent GBS disease in neonates and young infants through maternal immunization.

C. GBS Types Ia and Ib CPS Conjugate Vaccines

Two variables influence the number of aldehydes formed on GBS CPS, the size of the CPS (and thus the number of sialic

Table 1 Eight Weeks Postimmunization Response to GBS Conjugate Vaccines in Healthy Adults[a]

GBS vaccine (CPS dose in μg)	Number of subjects	Geometric mean concentration (μg/mL) of CPS-specific IgG, 95% CI and range			% with ≥4-fold increase in CPS-specific IgG by ELISA
III–TT (58)	30	4.53	[1.92–10.70]	(0.07–325.12)	97
III–TT (14.5)	15	2.72	[0.95–7.76]	(0.19–98.30)	87
III–TT (3.6)	15	1.1	[0.4–3.02]	(0.06–28.99)	64
Ia–TT (60)	30	26.2	[13.0–52.9]	(0.5–497.9)	93
Ia–TT (15)	15	18.3	[6.0–55.4]	(0.7–469.4)	80
Ia–TT (3.75)	15	1.9	[0.7–5.4]	(0.1–152.8)	80
Ib–TT (63)	30	12.9	[5.2–32.0]	(≤0.1–443.0)	78
Ib–TT (15.75)	15	11.1	[3.3–37.0]	(0.2–188.5)	80
Ib–TT (3.94)	15	2.9	[1.2–7.1]	(≤0.1–71.0)	47
II–TT (57)	30	34.3	[18.7–62.4]	(0.4–535)	97
II–TT (14.3)	13	29.5	[13.9–62.4]	(1.9–176)	100
II–TT (3.6)	15	11.2	[6.1–20.8]	(0.9–83.1)	87
V–TT (50)	15	8.2	[3.2–21.1]	(0.6–125)	93
V–CRM (50)	15	5.7	[2.2–14.9]	(0.2–435)	93
II/III–TT (3.6/12.5)	25	13.1	[5.6–30.6]	(0.4–571)	88

[a] *Source*: Refs. 24, 25, 27, 35, and 36.

acid residues) and the amount of sodium periodate added to the sialic acid oxidation reaction. Unlike other GBS capsular polysaccharides, types Ia and Ib have a $M_r > 800,000$. When the number of aldehydes created on these two GBS polysaccharides exceeded ~40%, the reductive amination coupling with TT resulted in the formation of insoluble gels. Preclinical lots of soluble type Ia–TT and Ib–TT conjugate vaccines were immunogenic in mice and rabbits, and prevented neonatal GBS disease in the maternal vaccination-neonatal mouse model [25].

On the basis of these preclinical data, type Ia–TT and Ib–TT conjugate vaccines were prepared with 25% and 9%, respectively, of sialic acid oxidation. Both vaccines were composed of 66% and 34% carbohydrate and protein, respectively. The Ia–TT conjugate contained 60 μg of CPS/0.5-ml dose, while Ib–TT conjugate contained 63 μg of CPS/0.5-ml dose. A total of 120 healthy, nonpregnant women, ages 18–40 years, were randomized to receive a single intramuscular dose of either type Ia–TT or type Ib–TT conjugate vaccine [25]. Thirty women received Ia–TT or Ib–TT at dosages of either 60 μg (type Ia) or 63 μg (type Ib) of the polysaccharide component, and 15 women each received 4-fold or 8-fold lower doses of each vaccine. In general, the vaccines were well tolerated; no serious adverse effects were observed. Most of the women receiving either the Ia–TT or Ib–TT conjugate vaccines at any dose had only mild tenderness at the injection site or no local symptoms or signs. Moderate pain or mild redness or swelling was observed in 40% and 38%, respectively, of recipients of the two highest vaccine doses.

Before vaccination, sera from each of the vaccine dose groups had low concentrations of Ia or Ib CPS-specific IgG (≤0.6 μg/mL) [25]. Among the recipients of the 60 μg Ia–TT conjugate vaccine dose, the Ia CPS-specific IgG GMC increased to 21.6 μg/mL 2 weeks after vaccination and peaked at 26.2 μg/mL 8 weeks later (Table 1). The 15-μg dose of Ia–TT conjugate evoked a GMC that did not differ significantly

from that in the sera from 60-μg-dose recipients, whereas the Ia CPS-specific IgG evoked by the lowest dose (3.75 μg) was significantly lower. Ninety-three percent of the 30 women who received the 60-μg dose of Ia–TT conjugate and 80% of those given the 15-μg dose had ≥4-fold increases in serum Ia CPS-specific IgG 8 weeks after vaccination (Table 1).

Recipients of the two higher doses of the Ib–TT conjugate vaccine had immune responses that did not differ significantly from each other, but evoked a significantly higher GMC of Ib CPS-specific IgG than the recipients of the 3.94-μg dose. The antibody responses to the two higher doses peaked 4–8 weeks after vaccination and changed little in the ensuing 18 weeks. In an analysis 2 years after vaccination, the Ib CPS-specific IgG GMC in sera from 13 recipients of the 63-μg dose was 10.7 μg/mL (range 0.26–147.7), indicating that this immune response was durable. When immunogenicity was analyzed by 4-fold increases in Ib CPS-specific IgG, 78% and 80% of recipients of the 63- and 15.75-μg doses, respectively, achieved these fold-rises.

When testing the functional activity of sera before and after immunization with these two conjugates by opsonophagocytic assay, there was a correlation between the concentration of Ia and Ib CPS-specific IgG and neutrophil-mediated killing by sera from recipients of type Ia TT ($r = 0.65$) and type Ib –TT ($r = 0.80$) vaccines. Taken together, the Phase 1 trials with these first three GBS serotypes—Ia, Ib, and III—documented consistently low reactogenicity, substantial immunogenicity, in vitro function of vaccine-induced specific antibodies, and a durable immune response.

D. GBS Type II CPS Conjugate Vaccine

GBS type II CPS contains sialic acid as one of two monosaccharide side chains in its seven-sugar repeating unit [26]. The relationship between the amount of sodium periodate added and the formation of aldehydes on sialic acid residues was found not to be direct, as had been observed with GBS types Ia, Ib, and III. This may be due to the proximity of sialic acid residues on the II CPS to the backbone sugars, unlike the other serotypes (Ia, Ib, III–VII) where sialic acid is two to three sugars away from the backbone. This structural difference demanded that a higher concentration of sodium periodate be added to create a sufficient number of aldehydes on the type II CPS for coupling to a protein carrier. To determine the degree of sialic acid oxidation that would yield immunogenic and efficacious conjugate vaccines, preclinical lots of II CPS–TT conjugate vaccines were prepared with CPS containing 31%, 57%, and 73% sialic acid oxidation. Immunogenicity and protective efficacy indicated that the II CPS prepared with 57% oxidation was the most consistently immunogenic and protective, results that prompted the preparation of II–TT conjugate vaccine for clinical trails with CPS containing 35% sialic acid oxidation [27]. GBS II–TT conjugate was composed of 51% carbohydrate and 49% protein. The choice to bottle the II–TT vaccine as a lyophilized multidose preparation was based on observations that lyophilized GBS oligosaccharide conjugates retained antigenic properties [28], and that this was a more conventional manner of bottling vaccines. The II–TT lyophilized vaccine used sucrose as the excipient to serve as a stabilizer and to add bulk to the mixture. When the multidose vial was reconstituted with saline containing 0.01% thimerosal, each 0.5-ml dose contained 57 µg of conjugate II CPS and 55 µg of TT. This vaccine was 95% protective in a mouse maternal vaccination-neonatal challenge model of GBS disease, a measure of GBS vaccine potency. This potency persisted 4 years after it was vialed [28], thus demonstrating the long-term stability of a lyophilized GBS conjugate vaccine.

The type GBS II–TT conjugate vaccine was well tolerated when given as a single intramuscular dose to 60 healthy, nonpregnant women between the ages of 18 and 45 years. Only one subject had systemic symptoms that were probably related to immunization. These symptoms consisted of low-grade fever, chills, and headache and resolved 36 hr after immunization. Most vaccine recipients experienced only mild or moderate pain at the injection sites, but a few had redness or swelling of < 3 cm in diameter. Before immunization the GMC of II CPS-specific IgG in sera from the three

groups of women receiving 4-fold decreasing vaccine doses was low (≤ 0.5 µg/mL) [27]. In sera from the 30 recipients of the highest II–TT dose (57 µg), the II CPS-specific IgG GMC increased to a peak of 47.1 µg/mL 2 weeks after immunization. Eight weeks after immunization, the II CPS-specific IgG GMC ranged from 11.2 to 34.3 µg/mL (Table 1), each representing a concentration that would ensure that adequate CPS-specific IgG would be available for placental transport. These II CPS-specific IgG responses were durable when assessed at 26 and 104 weeks after vaccination. Interestingly, the II–TT vaccine elicited substantial IgM- and IgA-specific antibody responses. For example, 8 weeks after immunization, the 3.6-µg dose elicited a II CPS-specific IgM GMC of 5.5 µg/mL (95% CI 3.0–10.2) and a IgA-specific GMC of 0.8 µg/mL (95% CI 0.4–1.5) (Table 2). The immunological explanation for this diversity of immunoglobulin isotype distribution in response to II–TT conjugate compared with type Ia, Ib, and III conjugate vaccines requires further study.

When the functional activity of sera from adults immunized with II–TT conjugate vaccine to promote opsonization, phagocytosis and killing of an opsonoresistant type II GBS strain before and 4 weeks later was studied, there was a significant increase from <0.3 mean $\log_{10}$ reduction in colony-forming units (CFU) to 0.9 $\log_{10}$. Also, there was a correlation between the concentration of II CPS-specific IgG and opsonophagocytic activity of sera from vaccine recipients, again indicative of the significant relationship between vaccine-induced antibodies and their in vitro functional activity.

E. GBS Type V CPS Conjugate Vaccines

Epidemiological studies during the 1970s and 1980s documented that virtually all invasive GBS infections in the United States were caused by serotypes Ia, Ib, II, and III. In the early 1990s, however, a new GBS serotype emerged [29–31]. Jelinkova and Motlova [32] first described the new type V GBS in the mid-1980s. With this finding of a new GBS serotype adding to the burden of serious GBS perinatal infections, the type V polysaccharide was purified and structurally characterized [33]. Type V polysaccharide has

Table 2 Isotype-Specific Immunogenicity of Type II and Type V GBS Conjugate Vaccines in Healthy Adults 8 Weeks After Immunization[a]

Vaccine (µg)	Number of subjects	ELISA	Geometric mean antibodies (µg/mL) by ELISA [95% CI] (Range)		
II–TT (3.6)	15	IgG	11.2	[6.1–20.8]	(0.9–83.1)
		IgM	5.5	[3.0–10.2]	(1.2–26.6)
		IgA	0.8	[0.4–1.5]	(0.3–2.8)
V–TT (50)	15	IgG	8.2	[3.2–21.1]	(0.6–125)
		IgM	17.8	[7.0–45.6]	(0.6–277)
		IgA	4.8	[1.8–12.4]	(0.4–97.9)
V–CRM (50)	15	IgG	5.7	[2.2–14.9]	(0.2–435)
		IgM	27.8	[14.8–52.4]	(4.8–182)
		IgA	7.2	[3.6–14.2]	(1.2–138)

[a] *Source*: Refs. 27 and 35.

structural uniqueness with respect to other GBS polysaccharides, but like the others, it possesses a side chain, which terminates with sialic acid [33]. This property meant that reductive amination could also be utilized to create a type V conjugate vaccine. GBS type V CPS conjugate vaccines were prepared with TT as the carrier protein and tested in rabbits and mice. Unlike the uncoupled V CPS, the V–TT conjugate induced type-specific antibodies in rabbits that opsonized the type V strain in vitro for killing by human polymorphonuclear leukocytes [34]. Like the other GBS serotypes, type V–TT conjugate vaccine also was superior to uncoupled type V CPS in protective efficacy against bacterial challenge to neonatal mice born to vaccinated dams [34].

Two lots of GBS type V conjugate vaccine were prepared for use in Phase 1 clinical trials. The first used TT as the carrier protein and was 76% carbohydrate and 14% protein, and the second cross-reactive material 197 (CRM_{197}, kindly provided by R. Rappuoli, IRIS, Siena, Italy) and was 73% carbohydrate and 17% protein. Both conjugate vaccines were prepared with purified type V CPS (173,000 M_r) that had of 18% of its sialic acid residues oxidated [35]. Like GBS II–TT conjugate, these type V conjugate vaccines were prepared as multidose lyophilized preparations with sucrose as the excipient.

Each of the type V conjugate vaccines was well tolerated by healthy, young adults [35]. Reactogenicity rates were comparable to other GBS conjugate vaccines and to each other. Thirty healthy, nonpregnant women, aged 18–45 years, were randomized to receive one of these type V conjugates. Sera from both groups of women had similarly low preimmunization concentrations of V CPS-specific IgG (GMC ≤ 0.2 μg/mL), and developed significant increases at each postvaccination interval through 26 weeks (Table 1). Type V–TT conjugate vaccine recipients had somewhat higher V CPS-specific IgG concentrations in their sera following immunization compared to the V–CRM group [e.g., GMC of 8.2 vs. 5.7 μg/mL at 8 weeks (Table 1)], but these differences were not statistically significant. Four-fold or greater increases in V CPS-specific IgG were observed in 93% of subjects in each conjugate vaccine group, and these increases persisted in 85% (V–TT) to 93% (V–CRM) of women 2 years later, indicating good durability of vaccine-induced antibodies. Thus in this pilot study in a small number of adults, both protein carriers appeared capable of providing the necessary T-cell help required for eliciting a response to the GBS type V CPS.

In contrast to results using type Ia–, Ib–, and III–TT conjugate vaccines but similar to those with II–TT conjugate vaccine, it was evident that a substantial proportion of the V CPS-specific antibodies produced after immunization with either V–TT or V–CRM were of isotypes other than IgG. Study participants had similarly low GMCs of V CPS-specific IgM and IgA GMCs in their pre-immunization sera. However, immunization induced a brisk V CPS-specific IgM and IgA response, and interestingly, the V CPS-specific IgM GMCs exceeded those for IgG (Table 2). Both groups of type V conjugate vaccine recipients had significant increases in V CPS-specific IgM and IgA 4 and 8 weeks after immunization, and these antibody levels persisted for 2 years. Further, recipients of V–CRM conjugate had substantially greater increases in V CPS-specific IgA than those who received V–TT conjugate, but this apparent difference was significant only at the 2-week interval.

Sera from V conjugate vaccine recipients before and 4 weeks after immunization were tested for in vitro functional activity against a relatively opsonoresistant type V GBS strain, G-106, in an opsonophagocytosis assay. The 4-week postvaccination sera from both groups of conjugate vaccine recipients promoted mean log_{10} reductions in type V CFU of 0.81 and 0.79 for GBS V–TT and V–CRM groups, respectively. There was no significant difference in the functional activity of antibodies induced by either of these conjugate vaccines.

F. GBS Type II–TT/III–TT Bivalent Vaccine

In moving toward the development and testing a multivalent GBS conjugate vaccine, a clinical trial was designed to determine whether the administration of two monovalent GBS conjugate vaccines, II–TT and III–TT, in a single syringe stimulated immune responses comparable to those elicited by either of the monovalent vaccines [36]. A Phase 2 randomized, double-blinded trial in 75 healthy adults between the age of 18 and 45 years was conducted. One group received II–TT (3.6 μg CPS/3.4 μg TT), another III–TT (12.5 μg CPS/16.1 μg TT), and the third the bivalent II–TT/III–TT (3.6 II μg CPS/12.5 III CPS/ 19.5 μg TT), each as a single 0.5-mL intramuscular dose. The choice of the concentration for each antigen in the bivalent vaccine was based on our earlier finding that at these concentrations nearly 90% of the volunteers receiving a single antigen showed a ≥4-fold increase in the specific IgG titers. Each vaccine was well tolerated. Mild injection site pain or redness was found in a minority of subjects and brief, mild systemic symptoms were noted in two (4%) III–TT conjugate vaccine recipients. Bivalent II/III–TT conjugate elicited increases in II or III CPS-specific IgG that were similar to those stimulated by the separate conjugate vaccine components. A ≥4-fold increase in II CPS-specific IgG was noted in 80% of sera from II–TT or bivalent vaccine recipients and in >90% of sera from subjects vaccinated with III–TT containing vaccine. Unexpectedly, 25% of III–TT subjects also developed ≥4-fold rises in II CPS-specific IgG, indicating immunologic cross-reactivity between the two structurally similar disaccharides in these two GBS CPSs. No immune interference from combining these vaccines was observed, results suggesting the feasibility of developing a multivalent GBS CPS-protein conjugate vaccine [36].

G. Booster Dose of GBS Type III Conjugate Vaccine

Each of the conjugate vaccines discussed above was prepared at the Channing Laboratory in Boston. However, to achieve the ultimate goal of evaluating the safety and immunogenicity of GBS conjugate vaccines in pregnant women, a GBS type III–TT vaccine prepared under GMP conditions was needed. In 1995, GMP lots of III–TT vaccine were prepared at the Salk Institute (Swiftwater, PA). These lots were prepared in multidose vials containing sucrose excipient. Approximately 30% of the sialic acid residues of III CPS were periodate oxidized to create reactive aldehydes as sites for coupling to tetanus toxoid (61% carbohydrate and 39% protein by weight for the first lot and 44% carbohydrate and 56% protein by weight for the second). The second vaccine lot was used in a trial designed to evaluate the effect of two doses of vaccine on immunogenicity [37].

A total of 36 healthy adults, aged 18–50 years and vaccinated previously with III–TT, were given a second 12.5-µg dose of III–TT conjugate 21 months later. The vaccine was well tolerated and there was no increase in the frequency with which local or systemic responses were observed with the booster dose. Four weeks after the second vaccine dose, the GMC of III CPS-specific IgG (8.4 µg/mL) was similar to that measured after the first dose (8.8 µg/mL), suggesting a lack of a "booster" effect. Of interest, a subset of 22% of the subjects who had undetectable III CPS-specific IgG levels (<0.5 µg/mL) before the first dose of III–TT conjugate exhibited a "booster" response to the second dose. This was defined as a ≥4-fold GMC of III CPS-specific IgG than after the initial immunization. Thus a second dose of GBS CPS conjugate vaccine may be required for adults previously "naïve" or "unprimed" to type III GBS CPS or to a related antigen. A second vaccine dose also might be useful to restore the initial peak III CPS-specific IgG serum levels in those previously responding to vaccination.

H. Alum as an Adjuvant for GBS Type III Conjugate Vaccine

Antibody response to GBS conjugate vaccines in healthy adults has been reported to be brisk, with peak serum levels achieved 4–8 weeks after administration of a single dose. In an effort to further improve the magnitude and proportion of immune responses to GBS conjugate vaccines, an adjuvant trial was conducted using III–TT conjugate. This vaccine was adsorbed to aluminum hydroxide gel in 0.9% saline (alum) that was prepared by the Massachusetts Public Health Laboratory (Jamaica Plain, MA), under good manufacturing practices (GMP) conditions using Alhydrogel 1.3% (aluminum hydroxide gel adjuvant) manufactured by Superfos Biosector (Vedbaek, Denmark) [37]. The rationale for choosing alum was based on its widespread use in human vaccines and its ability to improve the immunogenicity of GBS conjugate vaccines in mice [38] and baboons [20]. Thirty healthy adults, 18–50 years of age, received the III–TT vaccine adsorbed to alum. No increase in injection site pain, redness, or swelling was observed compared to III–TT conjugate without alum. Adsorption to alum did not improve the immune response to III-TT conjugate (12.5-µg dose of III CPS). Four weeks after immunization, the GMC for the 15 recipients of the III–TT with and without alum were 3.3 and 3.6 µg/mL, respectively. It is possible that because these human subjects were not immunologically naïve to tetanus, as are mice or baboons, the protein carrier is not suitable for adjuvancy. Children who received an 11-valent pneumococcal conjugate vaccine for which either diphtheria or TT was used as the protein carriers also have been reported to have no enhancement of immunogenicity with the addition of alum with vaccine [39].

I. Maternal Immunization with GBS Type III Conjugate Vaccine

Immunization during pregnancy is a strategy that takes advantage of the immunoresponsiveness of young healthy adults to provide protection passively for their immunologically immature infants. The value of this approach has been demonstrated globally with the eradication of tetanus neonatorum through widespread immunization of pregnant women with tetanus toxoid vaccine [40]. Polysaccharide conjugate vaccines also have been administered safely to women during pregnancy. For example, *Haemophilus influenzae* type b conjugate vaccines have been safely administered to pregnant women in the United States and in developing countries [41].

Two animal models have been used to gain a better understanding of placental transfer of GBS CPS-specific IgG after maternal immunization with III–TT. In a murine model of infection, female outbred CD-1 mice received two intraperitoneal injections of III–TT and subsequently were bred [42]. In sera from dams, CPS-specific IgG1 accounted for 83.2% of the total IgG, with a mean level of 9.1 ± 3.9 µg/mL. All of the 27 pups born to immunized dams survived challenge with a potentially lethal challenge of III GBS. In contrast, none of the 32 pups born to dams given placebo survived the GBS III challenge.

Because nonhuman primates produce antibodies which are structurally and functionally quite similar to those produced by humans, the III–TT vaccine was evaluated in a baboon model of infection. The GMC of III CPS-specific IgG increased from 0.9 to 7.5 µg/mL at delivery. Seven of nine baboons given the vaccine had ≥4-fold rises in antibody from the baseline level. The percent of III CPS-specific IgG transferred to their offspring ranged from 26% to 185% of the maternal values. The function of the maternal and neonatal antibodies was equivalent when assessed in an opsonophagocytosis assay.

A prospective Phase 1, randomized, double-blind, placebo-controlled trial recently was conducted to evaluate the safety and immunogenicity of III–TT vaccine in pregnant women. Thirty women, 18–45 years of age, received a single dose either of III–TT conjugate (12.5 µg) or placebo (0.9% saline) at a mean of 31 weeks of gestation [43]. The vaccine was well tolerated. Mild injection site pain occurred in 65% of vaccine and 10% of placebo recipients; no redness or swelling were observed in either group. All deliveries occurred beyond 37 weeks of gestation and each neonate was healthy and had normal Denver II developmental examinations at 6 months of age when the study concluded. The III CPS-specific IgG GMC in sera of the 20 women receiving III–TT conjugate was 0.18 µg/mL before immunization and 9.98 µg/mL 4 weeks later. The GMC remained stable at the time of delivery (mean 9.76 µg/mL). By contrast, placebo recipients received 0.06 µg/mL of III CPS-specific IgG before and 0.05 µg/mL in sera after "immunization." Vaccine recipients also developed immune response to the carrier protein, TT. The III CPS-specific IgG GMC in cord sera from infants whose mothers received vaccine was 7.48 µg/mL, reflecting 77% maternal delivery-cord III CPS-specific IgG transmission. The predominant IgG subclass of III

CPS-specific antibodies was IgG_2, as has been reported for *H. influenzae* type b conjugate maternal immunization [41]. Cord serum values remained elevated at 1 month (3.74 µg/ mL) and 2 months (2.16 µg/mL) of age. Infant sera also promoted opsonization, phagocytosis, and killing of type III GBS, with 1.4 and 1.5 log_{10} kill, respectively, at 1 and 2 months of age. These findings suggest that maternal immunization has the potential to prevent early- as well as late-onset GBS disease in infancy.

III. FUTURE VACCINE DIRECTIONS AND ISSUES

A. Formulation and Target Population

Although the principle that conjugation technology improves the immunogenicity of GBS CPSs has been established, several questions remain regarding formulation of an effective vaccine for use in the United States and elsewhere. Because five GBS serotypes (Ia, Ib, II, III, and V) are responsible for the majority of disease in the United States, a pentavalent vaccine appears to be warranted. That a multivalent GBS vaccine could confer protection against the serotypes included in the vaccine has been demonstrated in mice with a tetravalent CPS (Ia, Ib, II, and III) conjugate vaccine formulation [21]. How to vial five individually prepared conjugate vaccines is a technical challenge akin to that encountered by the developers of the 7-valent pneumococcal conjugate vaccine [44] and is a task best left to experienced manufacturers. However, the clinical studies summarized in the foregoing discussion suggest potential doses for each GBS serotype. Formulation of a vaccine is predicated on knowing the amount of specific antibody required to be protective. This is not known with certainty for GBS and is complicated in the case of neonatal disease by the necessity to predominately induce IgG class antibodies in pregnant women to assure passive protection to the infant. Clearly, the maternal levels must readily exceed the concentrations presumed to confer protection in the newborn, which from earlier studies are in the range of 1 µg/mL [45].

Generally, the amount of type-specific IgG elicited by GBS conjugate vaccines was dose-dependent. For types Ia–, Ib–, and III–TT conjugates there was no statistical difference in the amount of CPS-specific IgG elicited between 50–60 and 12–15 µg doses. It is possible that this latter dose range would be suitable for optimal immunogenicity. Type II–TT has been shown to be highly immunogenic (>10 µg/mL of II CPS-specific IgG) even at the lowest (3.6 µg) dose. It also induces II CPS-specific IgM and IgA [27]. Thus a relatively low dose (2–4 µg) could be included in a multivalent formulation. The amount of GBS type V–TT vaccine that would be included in a multivalent preparation will require further study [35].

Obviously, the formulation of a GBS conjugate vaccine will reflect the prevalence of GBS serotypes causing invasive disease in the country of its use. GBS colonization among pregnant women in Japan has been dominated by serotypes VI and VIII, which together accounted for 60% (44 out of 73) of isolates [46]. Although no clinical trials have been performed with type VI and VIII conjugate vaccines, pre-

clinical studies in mice with VI–TT and VIII–TT vaccines suggest that effective vaccines against these serotypes can be achieved [47].

B. GBS Protein-Based Vaccines

Not all GBS vaccine development focused on the CPS antigens. GBS possesses a number of surface-expressed proteins that have been tested as vaccine candidates or as carrier proteins for the CPSs. Indeed, even if GBS proteins cannot, by themselves, provide protection against GBS disease, a multivalent GBS CPS conjugate would benefit from using protein carriers of GBS origin rather than TT and CRM_{197} that are in widespread use in licensed vaccines. A review of GBS surface components with potential for use in vaccines has been published [48]. While all GBS protein antigens have shown promise in animal models of GBS disease, a correlation between low antibody to GBS proteins and susceptibility to disease in humans is lacking.

1. Alpha C Protein

Because the alpha C protein found in about 50% of clinical isolates of GBS and in 70% of nontype III GBS strains, this laddering protein is an attractive candidate for use in a GBS vaccine [49]. A III CPS conjugate vaccine prepared with a two-repeating unit alpha C protein conferred protection against GBS type III challenge in 95% of neonatal mice born to actively vaccinated dams, and 60% survival among pups challenged with a type Ia GBS strain containing the alpha C protein [49]. In addition, most (73%) of the pups born to mouse dams vaccinated with two-repeat alpha C protein alone survived lethal challenge with type Ia organisms, thus demonstrating the potential utility of this protein as an effective carrier for GBS CPS and an immunogen against alpha C protein-bearing GBS.

2. Beta C Protein

This trypsin-sensitive C protein is found on about 10% of GBS strains, predominantly those belonging to serotype Ib. GBS beta C protein induces protective antibodies in animals [50–52]. In addition to its being a good immunogen, this protein also has demonstrated characteristics of a thymus-dependent carrier for the type III CPS. A III CPS-beta C–protein conjugate elicited in mice protective antibodies against GBS strains bearing the type III antigen and beta C-proteins [53].

3. C5a Peptidase

Streptococcal C5a peptidase (SCPB) is a conserved surface protein among many strains of GBS [54]. Recently, Cheng and colleagues [55] showed that preincubation of GBS types Ia, Ib, II, III, and V with antibody to SCPB enhanced in vitro opsonic-mediated killing by mouse bone marrow-derived macrophages. Moreover, GBS type III CPS covalently coupled to SCPB by reductive amination induced high levels of both CPS-specific and SCPB-specific IgG that opsonized not only GBS type III, but types Ib and V as well [55], suggesting cross-serotype activity. Whether active immunization of female mice with coupled and uncoupled SCPB will result in cross-serotype protection remains to be determined.

4. Rib Protein

Found on GBS type III strains, Rib protein is structurally similar to, but antigenically separate from, the alpha C protein. Both proteins exhibit a laddering phenotype on sodium dodecyl sulfate-polyacrylamide gels and both are resistant to trypsin digestion [56]. Antiserum to this protein protected mice against GBS challenge, but only from GBS strains that did not contain the alpha C protein. A bivalent vaccine composed of Rib and alpha C proteins was protective [57].

5. Sip Protein

Another GBS surface protein, surface immunogenic protein (Sip), was recently shown to induce cross-serotype immunity in mice [58]. Monoclonal antibody to the 53-kDa protein of Sip revealed its presence on GBS strains representing all nine known serotypes [59]. Moreover, CD-1 mice actively immunized with recombinant Sip were protected against GBS infection with Ia, Ib, II, III, V, and VI and newborn mouse pups born to Sip-vaccinated dams were effectively protected against challenge with GBS serotypes Ia, Ib, II, III, and V [60]. These data suggest that cross-protective IgG to GBS may be able to be induced in animals by vaccination with a single surface protein common to all GBS serotypes. What remains to be determined is the prevalence of antibodies in sera from populations at risk for invasive GBS disease, and the effectiveness of Sip in inducing functionally active antibodies in humans.

IV. SUMMARY

Invasive GBS infection is a major health problem among infants, pregnant women, and nonpregnant adults, especially those beyond 65 years of age. The emergence of type V strains as a cause of a substantial proportion of invasive disease, especially that in nonpregnant adults, highlights the need for ongoing epidemiologic surveillance to correctly formulate a multivalent conjugate vaccine. However, the relative paucity of serotypes that contribute to human GBS disease by comparison, for example, with those documented to cause invasive pneumococcal infection, is an advantage for the development of GBS conjugate vaccines. In a recently published active statewide surveillance, Harrison and colleagues [61] determined the serotype distribution of invasive GBS isolates from over 500 infants, children, pregnant women, and adults. As with the pneumococcus, the serotype distribution differs between infants and adults. However, a pentavalent GBS vaccine, containing CPS from serotypes Ia, Ib, II, III, and V GBS would theoretically provide protection against more than 95% of the GBS isolates from both infants and adults.

The Phase 1 and 2 trials of monovalent GBS CPS–protein conjugate vaccines conducted to date and summarized in this chapter indicate the feasibility of developing a pentavalent GBS conjugate vaccine. The method for coupling to monomeric TT by reductive amination has gener-

ated custom vaccines of optimal immunogenicity. Each monovalent CPS–TT conjugate has been found safe, with only mild local reactions and on rare occasion, mild and time-limited systemic symptoms of less frequency than those associated with tetanus toxoid booster immunizations. These monovalent conjugates are highly immunogenic in healthy adults, with a ≥4-fold increase in CPS-specific IgG from baseline in 80% to 100% of subjects. The response to immunization is durable, persisting for at least 104 weeks. The dose dependence in the amount of CPS-specific IgG elicited indicates that the total CPS dose in a pentavalent vaccine is unlikely to exceed 50–75 μg. The main barrier to the development of a pentavalent GBS conjugate vaccine is the lack of a corporate partner willing to undertake the research and development necessary for approval by the Food and Drug Administration. The recent recognition that adults 65 years of age and older constitute the population with the greatest overall mortality caused by GBS may provide an opportunity to document efficacy first in this population because pregnancy with its attendant liability issues loom strong after a decades of outcry for a perinatal disease prevention strategy more practical than intrapartum antibiotic prophylaxis. Ultimately, the licensure and widespread use of a pentavalent GBS conjugate vaccine could result in thousands of lives saved annually in the United States alone.

ACKNOWLEDGMENTS

This work was supported in part by Contract #N01 AI-75236 from the National Institute of Allergy and Infectious Diseases of the National Institutes of Health.

REFERENCES

1. Zaleznik DF, et al. Invasive disease due to group B Streptococcus in pregnant women and neonates from diverse population groups. Clin Infect Dis 1999; 30: 276–281.
2. Schrag SJ, et al. Group B streptococcal disease in the era of intrapartum antibiotic prophylaxis. N Engl J Med 2000; 342:15–20.
3. Hussain SM, et al. Invasive group B streptococcal disease in children beyond early infancy. Pediatr Infect Dis J 1995; 14:278–281.
4. Krohn MA, et al. Maternal peripartum complications associated with vaginal group B streptococci colonization. J Infect Dis 1999; 179:1410–1415.
5. Farley MM, et al. Group B streptococcal disease in nonpregnant adults. Clin Infect Dis 2001; 33:556–561.
6. Muñoz P, et al. Group B Streptococcus bacteremia in nonpregnant adults. Arch Intern Med 1997; 157:213–216.
7. Farley MM, et al. A population-based assessment of invasive disease due to group B Streptococcus in nonpregnant adults. N Engl J Med 1993; 328:1807–1811.
8. Tyrrell GJ, et al. Invasive disease due to group B streptococcal infection in adults: results from a Canadian, population-based, active laboratory surveillance study—1996. J Infect Dis 2000; 182:168–173.
9. Henning KJ, et al. Invasive group B streptococcal disease in Maryland nursing home residents. J Infect Dis 2001; 183:1138–1142.

10. Jackson LA, et al. Risk factors for group B streptococcal disease in adults. Ann Intern Med 1996; 125:152–153.

11. Baker CJ, Kasper DL. Correlation of maternal antibody deficiency with susceptibility to neonatal group B streptococcal infection. N Engl J Med 1976; 294:753–756.

12. Baker CJ. Quantitative determination of antibody to capsular polysaccharide in infection with type III strains of group B Streptococcus. J Clin Invest 1977; 59:810–818.

13. Klegerman ME, et al. Estimation of the protective level of human IgG antibody to the type-specific polysaccharide of group B Streptococcus type Ia. J Infect Dis 1983; 148:648–655.

14. Baker CJ, Kasper DL. Group B streptococcal vaccines. Rev Infect Dis 1985; 7:458–467.

15. Baker CJ, et al. Immunization of pregnant women with a polysaccharide vaccine of group B Streptococcus. N Engl J Med 1988; 319:1180–1185.

16. Paoletti LC, et al. An oligosaccharide-tetanus toxoid conjugate vaccine against type III group B Streptococcus. J Biol Chem 1990; 265:18278–18283.

17. Paoletti LC, et al. Effects of chain length on the immunogenicity in rabbits of group B Streptococcus type III oligosaccharide–tetanus toxoid conjugates. J Clin Invest 1992; 89:203–209.

18. Lagergard T, et al. Synthesis and immunological properties of conjugates composed of group B Streptococcus type III capsular polysaccharide covalently bound to tetanus toxoid. Infect Immun 1990; 58:687–694.

19. Wessels MR, et al. Immunogenicity in animals of a polysaccharide–protein conjugate vaccine against type III group B Streptococcus. J Clin Invest 1990; 86:1428–1433.

20. Paoletti LC, et al. Immunogenicity of group B Streptococcus type III polysaccharide-tetanus toxoid vaccine in baboons. Infect Immun 1996; 64:677–679.

21. Paoletti LC, et al. Neonatal mouse protection against infection with multiple group B streptococcal (GBS) serotypes by maternal immunization with a tetravalent GBS polysaccharide–tetanus toxoid conjugate vaccine. Infect Immun 1994; 62:3236–3243.

22. Kasper D, et al. Glycoconjugate vaccines for the prevention of group B streptococcal infections. In: Norrby E., Brown F, Chanock RM, Ginsberg HS, eds. Vaccines 94, Modern Approaches to New Vaccines Including Prevention of AIDS. Cold Spring Harbor, NY: Cold Spring Harbor Laboratory Press, 1994:113–117.

23. Wessels MR, et al. Structural properties of group B streptococcal type III polysaccharide conjugate vaccines that influence immunogenicity and efficacy. Infect Immun 1998; 66:2186–2192.

24. Kasper DL, et al. Immune response to type III group B streptococcal polysaccharide–tetanus toxoid conjugate vaccine. J Clin Invest 1996; 98:2308–2314.

25. Baker CJ, et al. Safety and immunogenicity of capsular polysaccharide–tetanus toxoid conjugate vaccines for group B streptococcal types Ia and Ib. J Infect Dis 1999; 179:142–150.

26. Jennings HJ, et al. Structural determination of the capsular polysaccharide antigen of type II group B Streptococcus. J Biol Chem 1983; 258:1793–1798.

27. Baker CJ, et al. Use of capsular polysaccharide–tetanus toxoid conjugate vaccine for type II group B Streptococcus in healthy women. J Infect Dis 2000; 182:1129–1138.

28. Paoletti LC. Potency of clinical group B streptococcal conjugate vaccines. Vaccine 2001; 19:2118–2126.

29. Rench MA, Baker CJ. Neonatal sepsis caused by a new group B streptococcal serotype. J Pediatr 1993; 122:638–640.

30. Hervas JA, Benedi VJ. Neonatal sepsis caused by a new group B streptococcal serotype (type V). J Pediatr 1993; 123:839.

31. Greenberg DN, et al. Group B streptococcus serotype V. J Pediatr 1993; 123:494–495.

32. Jelinkova J, Motlova J. Worldwide distribution of two new serotypes of group B streptococci: type IV and provisional type V. J Clin Microbiol 1985; 21:361–362.

33. Wessels MR, et al. Structural determination and immunochemical characterization of the type V group B Streptococcus capsular polysaccharide. J Biol Chem 1991; 266:6714–6719.

34. Wessels MR, et al. Immunogenicity and protective activity in animals of a type V group B streptococcal polysaccharide-tetanus toxoid conjugate vaccine. J Infect Dis 1995; 171:879–884.

35. Paoletti LC, et al. Neonatal group B streptococcal disease: progress towards a multivalent maternal vaccine. The First Annual Conference on Vaccine Research, Washington, DC, Cold Spring Harbor, NY, 1996.

36. Baker CJ, et al. Safety and immunogenicity of a bivalent group B streptococcal conjugate vaccine for serotypes II and III. J Infect Dis 2003;188:66–73.

37. Paoletti LC, et al. Effects of alum adjuvant or a booster dose on immunogenicity during clinical trials of group B streptococcal type III conjugate vaccines. Infect Immun 2001; 69:6696–6701.

38. Guttormsen H-K, et al. Immunologic memory induced by a glycoconjugate vaccine in a murine adoptive lymphocyte transfer model. Infect Immun 1998; 66: 2026–2032.

39. Wuorimaa T, et al. Tolerability and immunogenicity of an eleven-valent pneumococcal conjugate vaccine in healthy toddlers. Pediatr Infect Dis J 2001; 20:272–277.

40. World Health Organization. Neonatal tetanus. Progress toward the global elimination of neonatal tetanus, 1990–1997. WHO website: www.who.int/vaccines-diseases/diseases/NeonatalTetanus.htm, accessed 3 November 2000.

41. Englund JA, et al. Transplacental antibody transfer following maternal immunization with polysaccharide and conjugate Haemophilus influenzae type b vaccines. J Infect Dis 1995; 171:99–105.

42. Paoletti LC, et al. Maternal antibody transfer in baboons and mice vaccinated with a group B streptococcal polysaccharide conjugate. J Infect Dis 2000; 181:653–658.

43. Baker CJ, Rench MA. Safety and immunogenicity of group B streptococcal (GBS) type III capsular polysaccharide (CPS)–tetanus toxoid (III–TT) conjugate vaccine in pregnant women. Clin Infect Dis 2001; 33:1151 (Abst. #370).

44. Rennels MB, et al. Safety and immunogenicity of heptavalent pneumococcal vaccine conjugated to CRM197 in United States infants. Pediatrics 1998; 101:604–611.

45. Baker CJ, et al. Role of antibody to native type III polysaccharide of group B Streptococcus in infant infection. Pediatrics 1981; 68:544–549.

46. Lachenauer CS, et al. Serotypes VI and VIII predominate among group B streptococci isolated from pregnant Japanese women. J Infect Dis 1999; 179:1030–1033.

47. Paoletti LC, et al. Synthesis and preclinical evaluation of glycoconjugate vaccines against group B Streptococcus types VI and VIII. J Infect Dis 1999; 180:892–895.

48. Paoletti LC, et al. Surface structures of group B Streptococcus important in human immunity. In: Fischetti VA, Novick RP, Ferretti JJ, Portnoy DA, Rood JI, eds. Gram-Positive Pathogens. Washington, DC: ASM Press, 2000: 137–153.

49. Gravekamp C, et al. Alpha C protein as a carrier for type III capsular polysaccharide and as a protective protein in group B streptococcal vaccines. Infect Immun 1999; 67: 2491–2496.

50. Fusco PC, et al. Bactericidal activity elicited by the beta C protein of group B streptococci contrasted with capsular polysaccharides. XIIIth Lancefield International Symposium on Streptococci and Streptococcal Diseases. 1996; 201.

51. Madoff LC, et al. Protection of neonatal mice from group B streptococcal infection by maternal immunization with beta C protein. Infect Immun 1992; 60:4989–4994.

52. Michel JL, et al. Cloned alpha and beta C-protein antigens of

group B streptococci elicit protective immunity. Infect Immun 1991; 59:2023–2038.

53. Madoff LC, et al. Maternal immunization of mice with group B streptococcal type III polysaccharide-beta C protein conjugate elicits protective antibody to multiple serotypes. J Clin Invest 1994; 94:286–292.

54. Suvorov AN, et al. C5a peptidase gene from group B streptococci. In: Dunny GM, Cleary PP, McKay LL, eds. Genetics and Molecular Biology of Streptococci, Lactococci, and Enterococci. Washington, DC: American Society for Microbiology, 1991:230–232.

55. Cheng Q, et al. Antibody against surface-bound C5a peptidase is opsonic and initiates macrophage killing of group B streptococci. Infect Immun 2001; 69:2302–2308.

56. Stalhammar-Carlemalm M, et al. Protein Rib: a novel group B streptococcal cell surface protein that confers protective immunity and is expressed by most strains causing invasive infections. J Exp Med 1993; 177:1593–1603.

57. Larsson C, et al. Protection against experimental infection with group B streptococcus by immunization with a bivalent protein vaccine. Vaccine 1999; 17:454–458.

58. Rioux S, et al. Localization of surface immunogenic protein on group B Streptococcus. Infect Immun 2001; 69: 5162–5165.

59. Brodeur BR, et al. Identification of group B streptococcal Sip protein, which elicits cross-protective immunity. Infect Immun 2000; 68:5610–5618.

60. Martin D, et al. Protection from group B streptococcal infection in neonatal mice by maternal immunization with recombinant Sip protein. Infect Immun 2002; 70:4897–4901.

61. Harrison LH, et al. Serotype distribution of invasive group B streptococcal isolates in Maryland: implications for vaccine formulation. J Infect Dis 1998; 177:998–1002.

59

Overview of Live Vaccine Strategies Against *Shigella*

Karen L. Kotloff and Eileen M. Barry
University of Maryland School of Medicine, Baltimore, Maryland, U.S.A.

Thomas L. Hale
Walter Reed Army Medical Center, Silver Spring, Maryland, U.S.A.

Philippe Sansonetti
Institut Pasteur, Paris, France

I. SIGNIFICANCE AND BURDEN OF *SHIGELLA* INFECTION

Shigella is a global infection that is notorious for disseminating rapidly in settings where there is overcrowding, inadequate sanitation, and insufficient supply of clean water. The spectrum of symptoms ranges from mild watery diarrhea to fulminant bacillary dysentery, characterized by bloody stools, high fever, prostration, cramps, and tenesmus. An array of severe intestinal and extra-intestinal complications can occur, such as hemolytic-uremic syndrome and a protein-losing enteropathy that contributes disproportionately to diarrhea-related malnutrition in young children. Most shigellosis results from endemic disease among children 1–5 years old living in developing countries, where it causes an estimated 163 million cases of diarrhea and 1 million deaths each year [1]. However, one serotype, *S. dysenteriae* 1, can cause devastating pandemics with high case fatality rates in all age groups. Shigellosis also occurs among persons living in industrialized countries [1], many of whom belong to known risk groups, such as travelers to endemic regions. High infectivity and antimicrobial resistance are factors that have enabled this bacterium to elude routine control measures. Widespread use of a safe and effective *Shigella* vaccine has long been considered a desirable strategy for combating this infection.

II. IMMUNITY TO *SHIGELLA*

A. Evidence for Protective Immunity

Demonstration, in several venues, that an initial wild-type *Shigella* infection prevents illness during subsequent exposure provides a strong argument for using a live, oral, attenuated vaccine approach [2–4]. The protection seen in field trials with noninvasive, attenuated *Shigella* vaccines offers additional hope that a live vaccine can succeed [5,6]. To date, approaches that have conferred clinical protection have not precluded intestinal colonization [5,6], although fecal excretion has been reduced [4].

B. Homotypic Versus Heterotypic Immunity

Vaccine development must take into consideration the antigenically distinct serotypes of *Shigella*. Groups A (*S. dysenteriae*), B (*S. flexneri*), and C (*S. boydii*) contain multiple serotypes [13, 6 (15 including subtypes) and 18, respectively], while Group D (*S. sonnei*) contains only a single serotype. Whereas type-specific immunity has been shown unequivocally in field and clinical settings, the data are conflicting as to whether cross-serotype or cross-species protection can be achieved. Monkeys fed wild-type *S. flexneri* 2a were fully protected when rechallenged with the same strain, but all monkeys became ill upon challenge with *S. sonnei* [4] and *S. flexneri* 6 [7]. A lack of heterologous protection was also seen in a field trial which measured the attack rate of shigellosis among recipients of a streptomycin-dependent *S. flexneri* 2a vaccine compared to unvaccinated controls [5]. However, with the exception of *S. flexneri* 4, the attack rate of non-vaccine strains was so low that heterologous immunity could not be assessed definitively.

In contrast, there is evidence both in humans [8] and in animals [9,10] that cross-protection can be induced among *S. flexneri* serotypes based on shared group and/or type-specific antigens on the O-polysaccharide molecule. Moreover, investigators conducting field trials in Romania [11] and in China [12] reported that the T_{32}-Istrati *S. flexneri* 2a vaccine provided both cross-species and cross-serotype protection. Additional investigation into this important area is necessary to guide vaccine development.

C. Specific Immunoprotective Responses

The examples of serotype-specific protection cited above are in agreement with the hypothesis that immunity is mediated by antibodies (serum or mucosal) directed against the LPS O-antigen [13,14]. The efficacy of parenteral *S. sonnei* O-antigen-specific polysaccharide conjugate vaccine in preventing *S. sonnei* disease among Israeli soldiers lends further support to this concept [15].

Immune responses to *Shigella* plasmid encoded outer membrane proteins (e.g., IpaA, B, C, and D and VirG/IcsA) are also encountered following wild-type infection [16,17]. In contrast to the O antigen, these peptides are shared among the four serogroups and thus could be exploited as a cross-protective vaccine antigen; however, a role in immunity has not been established.

The first line of defense must occur at the mucosa. The impact of mucosal immunity is illustrated by the efficacy of passively transferred type-specific oral immunoglobulin in preventing shigellosis [18], and perhaps the protective effects of breast feeding on disease severity in developing countries [19]. In volunteers, O-specific IgA antibody-secreting cells (ASCs) circulating in the bloodstream after vaccination are a measure of intestinal priming that has been correlated with vaccine efficacy [20,21].

Cell-mediated immune responses may also contribute to the defense against this intracellular pathogen. In animal models, IFN-γ production by NK cells seems to be an essential component of innate immunity to *Shigella* infection [22,23]. Up-regulation of IFN-γ production and expression of IFN-γ receptor are seen in the epithelium of rectal biopsies from Bangladeshi patients convalescing from shigellosis [24], and elevated levels are found in both serum and stool [25]. IFN-γ is the predominant cytokine produced by T cells in response to *Shigella* antigens, including highly purified Ipa proteins, following inoculation of volunteers with live attenuated *Shigella* vaccine candidates [26,27]. Nonetheless, prospective studies have not yet been performed in humans to correlate cell-mediated immune responses with protection.

III. RUPTURE, INVASION, AND INFLAMMATORY DESTRUCTION OF THE INTESTINAL EPITHELIUM BY *SHIGELLA*: AN EMERGING SCHEME

A. Genetic, Molecular, and Cellular Bases of the Invasive Phenotype: The Virulence Plasmid of *Shigella*

The invasive phenotype that characterizes *Shigella* pathogenesis encompasses several steps. First, the bacteria traverse the follicle-associated epithelium (FAC) located over mucosal lymphoid nodules, the inductive sites of the local

immune response [28]. Next, they are engulfed by phagocytic cells, particularly the resident macrophages located in the dome of the FAE [29]. Finally, the organisms invade the epithelial lining of the intestine through its basolateral pole and spread cell-to-cell [30].

In all *Shigella* serotypes, a 214-kb virulence plasmid carries most of the genes required for invasiveness [31,32]. A block of 30 kb corresponding to a pathogenicity island encodes a type III secretory system (TTSS, *mxi*-spa operons) and at least five effector proteins (*ipa* operon, IpaA-D, IpgD) that are secreted through this TTSS [33]. IpaB and IpaC form a pore in the cytoplasmic membrane of the target cell through which the bacterium injects its effector molecules [34]. IpaC induces a signaling cascade involving small GTPases of the Rho family, Cdc42 and Rac, that leads to actin nucleation and polymerization [35,36] and formation of localized filopodes and lamellipodes that entrap the bacterium. Injection of IpaA through the pore induces maturation of this entry focus by a complex process involving binding of IpaA to the head domain of vinculin, then bundling and depolymerization of actin filaments [37].

The *Shigella* virulence plasmid also contains *icsA/virG* which encodes a 120-kDa outer membrane protein that mediates actin-dependent motility of *Shigella* [38,39]. Once anchored to the outer membrane through its C-terminus, IcsA/VirG exposes its N-terminal characterized by a series of Glycine-rich repeats, three of which constitute the binding domain (C. Egile, unpublished) for N-WASP [40]. Binding of N-WASP to IcsA/VirG unleashes a process that results in an IcsA/VirG–N-WASP–Arp2/3 actin–nucleator complex. The association of monomeric actin (G-actin) with this complex is necessary and sufficient to cause actin nucleation/polymerization (F-actin) and to elicit the motility process of *Shigella* [41]. *Shigellae* then engage with components of the intermediate junctions and propel themselves via protrusions that are engulfed by adjacent cells [42]. Finally, the bacteria escape from the surrounding eukaryotic membrane into the cytoplasm of neighboring cells. Figure 1 summarizes this remarkable mechanism of epithelial colonization that is contained within the sanctuary of the intracellular environment.

The virulence plasmid of *Shigella* contains genes that encode about 15 additional proteins that are also secreted by the TTSS (i.e., IpaH, Osp, VirA proteins [32]). These genes are transcribed only when the TTSS is active, thus linking the delivery of the proteins mediating the early stage of invasion with subsequently injected proteins that are likely to modulate the behavior of infected cells [43].

B. Inflammatory Destruction of the Intestinal Epithelium

Shigella produce inflammation and destruction of the intestinal epithelium by several mechanisms that are illustrated in Figure 1. For one, macrophages that internalize *Shigellae* in the FAE undergo apoptotic death through a process that involves activation of Caspase-1 (a cysteine protease) by IpaB [44]. Pro-inflammatory cytokines such as IL-1β and IL-18 are released by dying macrophages [45]. The epithelial cell response to intracellular *Shigella* is also a major component

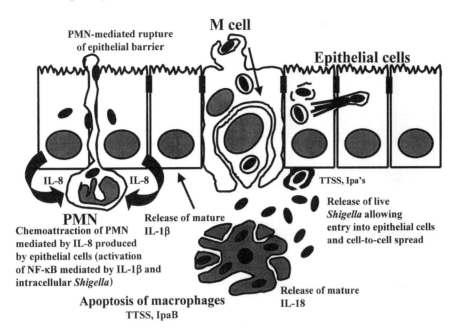

Figure 1 Rupture, invasion, and inflammatory destruction of the intestinal epithelium by *Shigella*: an emerging scheme. PMN: polymorphonuclear leukocyte; TTSS: type III secretion system.

of the inflammatory response, which includes secretion of IL-8 [46] and rapid, sustained activation of the pro-inflammatory transcription system NF-κB through a signaling cascade that involves cytosolic proteins of the Nod family, particularly Nod1 [41]. Inflammation in turn enhances invasion by disrupting the epithelial barrier and facilitating access of the bacteria to sites that permit epithelial invasion. Eventually this process leads to massive chemotaxis of neutrophils and bacterial killing, although at the cost of epithelial destruction [47]. Endotoxin (i.e., lipid A of *Shigella*) is necessary for the expression of the invasive phenotype and also contributes to the rupture and destruction of the epithelial lining, mostly through TNFα [46].

C. Role of Toxin in *Shigella* Pathogenesis

Shigella elaborate several toxins that contribute to virulence. *S. dysenteriae* type 1 is the only serotype that bears the chromosomal genes encoding the 70-kDa heterodimeric protein known as Shiga toxin. This potent cytotoxin also exhibits enterotoxigenic, neurotoxic, and pro-inflammatory properties [48] and has been implicated in the pathogenesis of hemolytic-uremic syndrome. Two enterotoxins have been identified in rabbit ileal loop and Ussing chamber studies as likely mediators of the watery diarrhea often seen in early shigellosis [49–51]. *Shigella* enterotoxin 1 (ShET1) is an iron-regulated, 55-kDa protein with a A_1–B_5 subunit configuration [51]. ShET1 is encoded by *set*, a chromosomal operon found almost exclusively in *S. flexneri* 2a [49]. *Shigella* enterotoxin 2 (ShET2) is a 62.8-kDa single-moiety protein that is encoded by *sen*, which is found in the invasion plasmid of nearly all *Shigella* serotypes [50]. Watery diarrhea could also result from inflammation and release of mediators such

as adenosine by colonic leukocytes [52], or by up-regulation of receptors such as Galanin-1 in inflamed epithelial cells [53].

D. Rational Construction of Live Attenuated *Shigella* Strains

The evolving understanding of the molecular pathogenesis of shigellosis is essential to the design of rational live-attenuated vaccines. For example, the organism's ability to traverse the FAE to reach the inductive sites of the mucosal immune system has been exploited to enhance the immunogenicity of vaccine candidates. The benefits of retaining triggers of macrophage apoptosis are less certain. On the one hand, this process generates a strong pro-inflammatory signal [54] that must be mitigated; on the other hand, apoptotic bodies of infected antigen-presenting cells are strongly immunogenic. Whereas preservation of epithelial cell invasiveness may enhance immunogenicity, elimination of cell-to-cell spread improves vaccine tolerance by minimizing the extent of the destructive intestinal lesion. The propensity for *Shigella* to cause watery diarrhea could be diminished with mutations in genes encoding enterotoxin synthesis. Clearly any *Shigella* vaccine formulation should be devoid of catalytically active Shiga toxin.

IV. MODELS FOR EVALUATION OF VACCINE CANDIDATES

A. Animal Models

The rhesus monkey model of shigellosis has been used extensively to assess the safety and efficacy of live oral vaccines.

The clinical and histologic response to intragastric inoculation closely mimics that seen during natural infection of humans, and diarrhea and dysentery are the principal clinical manifestations [55]. A disadvantage of this model is the frequent occurrence of *Shigella* infection among monkeys in captivity, which can render animals partially immune.

Small animal models have been developed for their practicality and lower cost. The Sereny test is a well-established model that measures the ability of *Shigella* inoculated into the conjunctival sac of animals (usually guinea pigs) to cause purulent keratoconjunctivitis [56]. Common practice is to demonstrate that a *Shigella* vaccine is Sereny negative before initiating Phase 1 trials. Nonetheless, some vaccines that are fully attenuated in the Sereny model have appeared reactogenic in humans. The model has also been adapted to assess vaccine efficacy [57].

The mouse intranasal challenge model can be used to evaluate the attenuation and protective efficacy of candidate vaccines. The simple columnar epithelium lining the tracheobronchial trees exquisitely is susceptible to invasion by *Shigellae* [23]. The lesions elicited by pulmonary *Shigella* infection are histologically similar to the colitis that characterizes shigellosis in primates and humans. The availability of inbred mouse strains and cytokine reagents allows the characterization of the immune response generated by *Shigella* vaccines on a molecular level, but intranasal challenge model, such as the Sereny test, can only hint at the complexity of a protective immune response in the human colon.

B. Volunteer Models for Vaccine Efficacy

Ultimately, the safety and efficacy of a *Shigella* vaccine must be determined by studies in humans. The experimental challenge model of *Shigella* in volunteers was developed in the 1960s [58] and its ability to detect protective efficacy has been validated using homologous strain re-challenge studies [3,4] which confirmed the immunizing ability of wild type that is observed in the field. Moreover, the *S. flexneri* 2a streptomycin-dependent vaccine which was efficacious in field trials [6] conferred significant protection in the volunteer challenge model (Table 1) [59]. In the 1990s, the *S. flexneri* 2a model was modified to administer the inoculum in sodium bicarbonate buffer rather than skim milk, which safely increased the attack rate and consistency of illness in control subjects and lowered the sample sizes necessary for an individual trial [4].

Table 1 Clinical and Immune Response of Adult Volunteers from Industrialized Countries to Wild-Type Infection and Live, Attenuated *Shigella flexneri* 2a Vaccine Candidates

Immunogen	*S. flexneri* 2a parent	Ref.	Dose (CFU)	Percent of subjects with adverse reactions	Anti-LPS response[a]		Protective efficacy vs. challenge
					IgA ASC (GM)	IgG antibody	
Wild type	245T	5	10^3	92%	92% (239)	50%	70%
			10^2	43%	71% (18)	29%	nd
SmD vaccines	245T	61	10^{10}	0-15%	nd	38%	49%[b]
EcSf2a-2	na	21, 56	10^9	0%	100% (59)	53%[c]	48%
			10^8	10%	100% (16)	19%	27%
			10^9	17%	93% (21)	35%[c]	0%
SC602	454	95, unpublished	10^6	60%	93% (154)	20%	nd
			10^4	20%[d]	66% (26)[d,e]	10%[d]	50%[d]
SFL1070	245T	87	10^9	44%	89% (10)	67%	nd
			10^8	0%	89% (5)	22%	nd
CVD 1203	245T	89	10^9	80%	100% (175)	46%	nd
			10^8	12%	91% (43)	45%	nd
			10^6	0%	60% (13)	30%	nd
CVD 1207	2457T	94	10^{10}	20%	100% (35)	17%	nd
			10^9	8%	64% (9)	17%	nd
			10^8	0%	67% (5)	0%	nd
			10^7	0%	100% (6)	0%	nd
			10^6	0%	0% (0.1)	14%	nd

Ref = reference; CFU = colony forming units; ASC = antibody secreting cells; GM = geometric mean per 10^6 peripheral blood mononuclear cells; SmD = streptomycin dependent; nd = not done; na = not applicable.
[a] Study-specific definitions of ASC responses were used. For serologic responses, values represent the percent of subjects with IgG antibody responses, defined as fourfold rises, with the exception of the SC602 study, which considered a threefold rise to be a response.
[b] Protection in field trial was 82–100% [5,6,61,62].
[c] The protective efficacy of these two trials combined was 36%.
[d] These values represent a composite of published and unpublished studies (see text).
[e] The geometric mean was 43 among volunteers who participated in the challenge trial.

V. LIVE *SHIGELLA* VACCINE STRAINS LACKING THE INVASIVE PHENOTYPE

A. Streptomycin-Dependent (SmD) Vaccines

Mel and coworkers developed SmD mutants of *S. sonnei* and *S. flexneri* by serial passage on streptomycin-containing media [60]. The basis of attenuation is now believed to be spontaneous deletion of virulence genes from the invasion plasmid (F. Noriega, unpublished). Monovalent and bivalent combinations of *S. flexneri* (serotypes 1, 2a, and 3) and *S. sonnei* were safe and protective (82–100% efficacy) when given (with buffer) to nearly 8000 adults and children in controlled field trials in Yugoslavia [6,61,62]. Both freshly harvested and lyophilized formulations were used. Vaccine was excreted by 90% of recipients, for a mean of 3 days [62]. However, drawbacks of these vaccines are recognized, including 1) the need for multiple (4 to 5) doses, and the large inocula ($2–6 \times 10^{10}$ CFU) required per dose (which affects cost) [5,6,61]; 2) the occurrence of vomiting and less often mild diarrhea (primarily after the first dose), which were minimized by giving gradually increasing inocula [5,6,61]; 3) the need for a booster dose at 1 year to maintain protection [62]; 4) occasional in vivo reversion to streptomycin-independence (without loss of attenuation) [63,64];and 5) equivocal efficacy in preventing endemic shigellosis among institutionalized children in the United States [65].

B. T$_{32}$-ISTRATI Strain

Romanian scientists used the Sereny test as a screening device to identify spontaneous avirulent mutants of *S. flexneri* 2a. After 32 passages on nutrient agar, a mutant was identified as consistently Sereny negative. This strain was designated T$_{32}$-Istrati, and it is now probably the most extensively tested live *Shigella* vaccine, having been administered to more than 60,000 individuals in Romania [66] and to more than 8000 subjects in China [12] between 1976 and 1980. The genetic basis of attenuation has since been shown to be a 32-MD deletion in the 140-MD plasmid of *S. flexneri* 2a [67]. This deletion eliminated the genes encoding the *Shigella* Ipa proteins and other virulence determinants such as *virF* (a positive regulator for *ipa* genes) and *virG/icsA*.

The Cantacuzino Institute of Bucharest manufactured T$_{32}$-Istrati under the trade name Vadizen as a liquid, refrigerated formulation that was administered with buffer as five oral doses increasing from 5×10^{10} to 2×10^{11} CFU at 3-day intervals. Open-label Romanian trials carried out in 131 children's collectives (32,000 subjects) and 7 adult collectives (5000 subjects) suggested 81% protection against *S. flexneri* 2a using historical data for comparison. These studies also reported 89% protection against heterologous *Shigella* species including *S. sonnei* [66].

Seven placebo-controlled studies involving 11,128 individuals 4–60 years of age were carried out at the Lanzhou Institute of Biological Products in China using an enteric-coated, refrigerated version of T$_{32}$-Istrati (without buffer). The vaccine was safe when administered in four doses of 2–4×10^{11} CFU (children received a lower dose) every third day. Most recipients excreted vaccine for 2 to 4 days after the last dose; interestingly, 7% excreted T$_{32}$-Istrati for 8 days. Efficacy was 85% against homologous disease and 63% against heterologous strains (*S. flexneri* 1b and *S. boydii* 1–6) [12].

C. FS Bivalent Vaccine

In 1987, Wang and coworkers at the Lanzhou Institute of Biological Products described a mutant *S. sonnei* virulence plasmid, designated S$_7$, that was used to construct a bivalent *S. flexneri*–*S. sonnei* (FS) vaccine based on T$_{32}$-Istrati [68]. *S. sonnei* is unique among *Shigella* species because the *rfb* locus, encoding the form I (smooth) O-polysaccharide of LPS, is carried on a 120-MD virulence plasmid. The S$_7$ plasmid was found in a spontaneously occurring, noninvasive mutant of *S. sonnei* that expressed the form I O-antigen [68,69]. The mutant plasmid fails to hybridize with probes containing the *ipa* genes or the *virF* regulatory locus for the invasive phenotype [70] and probably suffered a spontaneous deletion similar to the attenuating deletion in the T$_{32}$-Istrati virulence plasmid while retaining the form I encoding genes. The S$_7$ plasmid was tagged with Tn*5* (kanamycin resistance) and mobilized into T$_{32}$-Istrati using *E. coli* HU$_{735}$. Like the T$_{32}$-Istrati conjugal recipient, the FS hybrid is avirulent in HeLa cell invasion and Sereny tests. It protects rhesus monkeys against illness following challenge with both constituent strains. *S. sonnei* O-antigen expression is stable in vitro after 36 passages without kanamycin selection [68].

The FS vaccine was first evaluated in humans in a placebo-controlled trial using freshly harvested bacteria. At 3-day intervals, 34 volunteers received three ascending doses of $2–5 \times 10^{10}$ CFU without significant reactogenicity. Most recipients had fecal antibody responses recognizing *S. flexneri* 2a LPS (68%) and *S. sonnei* LPS (62%), with a twofold mean rise. In this and subsequent field trials, FS vaccine was found to be as safe as placebo and was excreted by 67–75% of vaccinees for 1–3 days.

During the 1990s, two double-blind, placebo-controlled efficacy trials of the FS vaccine were conducted in Changge City, China. A three-dose regimen using a lyophilized FS product was administered at $2–5 \times 10^{10}$ CFU to ca. 17,500 adults and children while 15,700 subjects received placebo. Passive surveillance for shigellosis was conducted for 5–6 months. Protective efficacy against *S. flexneri* 2a was 61–65% and against *S. sonnei* was 50–72%. Efficacy against heterologous *Shigella* spp. was 48–52% [71].

These data indicate that the noninvasive T$_{32}$-Istrati and FS hybrid vaccines are safe for Chinese adults and children and confer short-term efficacy against both homologous and heterologous serotypes. The immunological basis of heterologous protection is unclear, and the effect may be detectable only in large-scale trials. Nonetheless, the need for a three-dose regimen containing over 10-logs of live bacteria is a daunting logistical prospect for most developing countries although the 60% level of protection against shigellosis could have a positive public health impact. Additional trials of the FS vaccine specifically targeted to infants and toddlers could further define the public health application of this approach.

VI. HYBRID VACCINES

A. Bivalent *Salmonella* Typhi–*Shigella sonnei* Hybird Vaccine

In the 1980s, efforts to develop improved live *Shigella* vaccines included heterologous carrier strains designed to invade and proliferate within the intestine to more effectively deliver *Shigella* antigens to the local immune system, simulating the protective immune responses that follow natural infection. The *S. typhi*–*S. sonnei* hybrid (strain 5076-1C) utilizes an invasive attenuated mutant of *Salmonella enterica* serovar Typhi, strain Ty21a, to carry the form I *S. sonnei* plasmid and express *S. sonnei* O antigen. This vaccine offered the potential to protect against both typhoid fever and shigellosis. In volunteers, a lyophilized formulation of 5076-1C was well tolerated and in initial trials protected against experimental challenge [14]; however, the efficacy results could not be replicated with subsequent lots of vaccine and further testing was not done [3]. Chemical and immunoblot analyses of 5076-1C indicated that the O-polysaccharide of *S. sonnei* was transported to the cell surface without covalent linkage with the core lipid A of *S. typhi* perhaps accounting for its erratic immunogenicity [72].

B. *Escherichia coli* as a Carrier for *Shigella* Antigens

In the 1970s, a noninvasive *E. coli* carrier vaccine expressing *S. flexneri* 2a O-antigen on its surface was constructed [73]. Although the vaccine was safe and colonized the intestines of volunteers for several days, antibody responses to the type-specific O-antigen were meager and the vaccine did not confer protection against wild-type challenge. To enhance immunogenicity, second-generation *E. coli* carrier vaccine strains were constructed containing the invasion plasmid of *S. flexneri* 5 plus the chromosomal genes encoding *S. flexneri* 2a LPS [74]. These strains were invasive and expressed O-antigen but lacked full *Shigella* virulence [74]. An initial construct, designated EcSf2a-1, produced adverse reactions in subjects who ingested 10^9 CFU (with buffer), while at better tolerated doses (ca. 10^6 to 10^7 CFU), it did not protect against challenge [55]. A further attenuated aroD mutant was constructed and designated EcSf2a-2 [75]. Three oral doses of EcSf2a-2 over 1 week were well tolerated at doses up to ca. 10^9 CFU [55]. Although most recipients of ca. 10^9 CFU had immune responses, the vaccine conferred only 36% protection against challenge (Table 1). Subsequent studies attempted to improve safety by giving a lower, well-tolerated inoculum (7×10^8 CFU) and to enhance efficacy using a four-dose regimen. Unfortunately, immunogenicity was modest and vaccine efficacy was only 27% (Table 1) [20].

VII. ENTEROINVASIVE DELETION-MUTANTS OF *SHIGELLA*

Molecular engineering has enabled the development of live, oral *Shigella* vaccine candidates with precise, genetically defined mutations. The strains described below retain inva-

siveness but are attenuated by mutations which either induce auxotrophy for metabolites that are essential for survival of the bacteria in vivo, such as genes in the aromatic or purine metabolic pathways, or inactivate virulence factors, such as VirG/IcsA and the *Shigella* enterotoxins 1 and 2.

A. Aromatic Autotrophs

1. Auxotrophic *S. flexneri* Y Vaccine Candidates

Mutations in genes involved in aromatic amino acid synthesis pathway prevent intracellular bacteria from making folic acid de novo (Figure 2). If environmental sources are not available, the growth of the mutant is severely hindered [76]. Lindberg and coworkers applied this strategy to *Shigella* vaccine development, constructing strain SFL124 with a transposon-generated 1400-bp deletion in the *aroD* gene of virulent *S. flexneri* Y, strain SFL1 [77]. They postulated that a serotype Y strain might provide cross-protection against other *S. flexneri* serotypes as its O-polysaccharide shares tetrasaccharide repeating units with all other *S. flexneri* except serotype 6. SFL124 is invasive, Sereny negative, and protective in animal models. A dose of 10^9 CFU was given with buffer to adult volunteers living in Sweden [78] and Viet Nam [79], and to 9–14-year-old Vietnamese children (20–30 subjects per group) [80]. SFL124 appeared safe and elicited both primary and anamnestic immune responses. Regrettably, the ability of ΔaroD *S. flexneri* Y to confer homologous and heterologous immunity was never evaluated in humans.

2. Auxotrophic *S. flexneri* 2a Vaccine Candidates

A similar attenuating deletion was introduced into virulent *S. flexneri* 2a strain 2457T, resulting in the ΔaroD mutant SFL1070 [81]. When administered to 37 Swedish adults, SFL1070 exhibited a dose-dependent pattern of clinical tolerance, vaccine excretion, and immune responses [82]. Transient mild gastrointestinal symptoms occurred in 10–33% of subjects who received three doses of 10^5 to 10^8 CFU within 5 days. Vaccination with 10^9 CFU caused more severe symptoms (abdominal pain, watery diarrhea, or fever) in 44% of volunteers (Table 1). These results point to the importance of the inherent virulence of the parent strain in dictating the clinical tolerance of vaccines with identical attenuating lesions. The parent strain of SFL1070 is more pathogenic in humans than the SFL1 strain used to construct SFL124.

3. Auxotrophic *S. flexneri* 2a with a Deletion in *virG*

Noriega and coworkers attempted to enhance the attenuation conferred by aromatic auxotrophy by introducing a specific, in-frame deletion in the plasmid gene *virG* of ΔaroA *S. flexneri* 2a, resulting in double mutant ΔaroA, ΔvirG strain CVD 1203 [83]. These specific deletions were obtained in strain 2457T by allelic exchange of the modified genes for their wild-type counterparts using suicide vectors [83]. CVD 1203 was attenuated and protective in the Sereny model [83]. A Phase I study was conducted at the Center for Vaccine Development [84]. After a single dose of ca. 10^9, 10^8, or 10^6 CFU with buffer (10–11 subjects per group), brief clinical

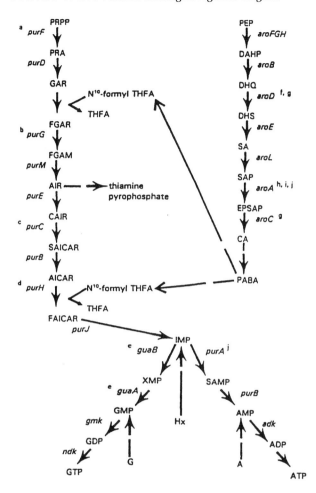

Figure 2 Purine de novo biosynthesis pathway and contribution of the aromatic metabolic pathway. Interrupted arrows illustrate pathways in which the individual steps are not represented. Enzymes are represented by their genes. Superscript letters represent selected published strains with a mutation of the gene involved in that reaction. Strains represented are: a: *purF1741*::Tn*10 S. dublin* SL5437 [85]; b: *purG876*::Tn*10 S. dublin* SL5436 [85]; c: *purC882*::Tn*10 S. dublin* SL5435 [85]; d: *purH887*::Tn*10 S. dublin* SL2975 [85]; e: Δ*guaBA S. flexneri* 2a CVD1204 and Δ*guaBA*, Δ*virG* CVD1205 [87]; f: *aroD25*::Tn*10 S. flexneri* Y SFL114 [77], SFL124 [79], *S. flexneri* 2a 1070 [82]; g: Δ*aroC*,Δ*aroD S. typhi* CVD908 [107]; h: *hisG46* DEL407, *aroA554*::Tn*10 S. typhimurium* SL3261 [76]; i: Δ*aroA S. flexneri* 2a CVD1201 and Δ*aroA*,Δ*virG* CVD1203 [83]; j: Δ*aroA*, Δ*hisG*, Δ*purA S. typhi* 541Ty [108]. PRPP: 5-phosphoribosyl-α-1-pyrophosphate; PRA: 5-phosphoribosylamine; GAR: 5′-phosphoribosyl-1-glycinamide; FGAR: 5′-phosphoribosyl-N-formylglycinamide; FGAM: 5′-phosphoribosyl-N-formylglycinamidine; AIR: 5′-phosphoribosyl-5-aminoimidazole; CAIR: 5′-phosphoribosyl-5-aminoimidazole-4-carboxylic acid; SAICAR: 5′-phosphoribosyl-4-(N-succinocarboxamide)-5-aminoimidazole; AICAR: 5′-phosphoribosyl-4-carboxamide-5-aminoimidazole; FAICAR: 5′-phosphoribosyl-4-carboxamide-5-formamidoimidazole; IMP: inosinic acid; Hx: hypoxanthine; G: guanine; A: adenine.

reactions (fever, diarrhea, and/or dysentery) occurred in 72%, 18%, and 0% of volunteers, respectively. Anti-LPS IgA ASC responses were dose-related, occurring even at doses of 10^6 CFU where illness was not seen (Table 1). A striking component of the reactogenicity observed with CVD 1203 was the occurrence of watery diarrhea in approximately 25% of those who receive 10^8 or 10^9 CFU [84]. This finding supports the hypothesis that deletion of genes involved in the production of *Shigella* enterotoxins may further attenuate *Shigella* vaccines.

B. Purine Auxotrophs

1. A Lineage of *S. flexneri* 2a Purine Auxotrophs: CVD 1204, CVD 1207, and CVD 1208

Stimulated by the observations of McFarland and Stocker on the attenuating effects of purine auxotrophy in the mouse model of *Salmonella* virulence [85], Noriega and coworkers constructed a new generation of *Shigella* vaccine candidates from *S. flexneri* 2a strain 2457T based on a mutation in the genes encoding two enzymes in the guanine nucleotide biosynthetic pathway, GMP synthetase (*guaA*) and IMP dehydrogenase (*guaB*) [86] (Figure 1). Using homologous recombinations with a suicide plasmid bearing the deleted alleles, they first created the Δ*guaBA* strain CVD 1204 [87]. Further mutations were added to this strain to find the optimal balance of safety and immunogenicity. To create CVD 1207 (Δ*guaBA*, Δ*virG*, Δ*sen*, Δ*set*), a second in-frame deletion was made in the plasmid gene *virG* [87]. The chromosomal mutation Δ*set* was accomplished with deletion of 85% of the subunit A [9]. A Δ*sen* cassette was constructed by fusing two 700-bp segments that included the N and C termini of *sen* minus 300 bp corresponding to the putative active site in the N-terminal region [9]. An *ars* operon, conferring resistance to arsenite, was cloned into the Δ*sen* to facilitate transfer of the mutated virulence plasmid to other *Shigella* vaccine strains and as a marker to distinguish CVD 1207 in the field [88]. Finally, Δ*guaBA*, Δ*sen*, Δ*set* strain CVD 1208 was derived by restoring wild-type *virG*. The lack of enterotoxic activity of CVD 1207 and 1208 was confirmed in Ussing chambers [9]. These strains appear highly attenuated and protective in the Sereny model [9]. Furthermore, when directly compared to Δ*aroA S. flexneri* 2a, the Δ*guaBA* strains are significantly less invasive for HeLa cells monolayers [87]. The mechanism for reduced invasiveness is unknown. The expression of IpaB and IpaC is not diminished, and the occurrence of other, spontaneous, metabolic mutations was ruled out by the recovery of the full invasive phenotype when the wild-type *guaBA* operon was reinstated.

2. Phase 1 Trial to Evaluate Δ*guaBA*,Δ*virG*,Δ*sen*, Δ*set* Strain CVD 1207

CVD 1207 was evaluated for safety and immunogenicity in volunteers at the Center for Vaccine Development (Table 1). Group of 3 to 12 subjects ingested CVD 1207 (with buffer) at one of five doses ranging from 10^6 to 10^{10} CFU. Vaccination was well tolerated at doses as high as 10^8 CFU. In comparison, one of 12 recipients of 10^9 CFU experienced mild diarrhea and another vomited once, and one of five recipients of 10^{10} CFU reported diarrhea and emesis. All recipients of 10^8 to 10^{10} CFU excreted vaccine, most for fewer than 3 days, although two subjects had positive stool cultures 14 days post-vaccination and were treated with ciprofloxacin. Dose-related IgA ASC anti-LPS responses were seen, with geometric mean peak values of 6.1 to 35.2 ASCs/10^6 PBMC among recipients of 10^7 to 10^{10} CFU.

CVD 1207 achieved a remarkable degree of attenuation of virulent Shigella compared with earlier invasive S. flexneri 2a recombinant strains. Moreover, when occasional adverse reactions did occur at very high inocula, neither fever nor dysentery was encountered. Nonetheless, it is conceivable that at well-tolerated doses, CVD 1207 may be insufficiently immunogenic after a single dose. Therefore clinical trials are ongoing to evaluate S. flexneri 2a purine auxotrophs with fewer attenuating mutations, such as CVD 1204 ($\Delta guaBA$) and CVD 1208 ($\Delta guaBA$, Δsen, Δset). These trials will also provide valuable information on the pathogenicity of Shigella enterotoxins in humans.

C. Shigella Fundamentally Attenuated with a Mutation in virG

1. S. flexneri 2a Harboring Deletions in virG/icsA and iuc (SC602)

Sansonetti and colleagues constructed a double mutant with deletions in both the virG/icsA gene and the iucA-iut chromosomal locus (encoding the aerobactin iron binding siderophore) from S. flexneri 2a strain 454. The iuc mutation was generated by recombination of iuc::Tn10 into the chromosome using phage P1 transduction. Spontaneous excision of the tetracycline resistance gene and the flanking regions including the iuc locus was selected by growth on fusaric acid medium. The virG gene was inactivated by double recombination with a kanamycin resistance-sucrose sensitivity (sacB) cartridge carrying flanking regions of virG. The selected clone, designated SC602, harbored a deletion of the entire virG gene along with substantial flanking sequences totaling 10 kb.

SC602 (lyophilized) was tested in a series of inpatient dose–response studies at the U.S. Army Medical Research Institute for Infectious Diseases (USAMRIID). In the first trial, test doses ranged from 10^4 to 10^8 CFU, with three vaccinees and three-unvaccinated controls per dose group. No subject who received 10^4 to 10^7 CFU developed diarrhea, but four had fever (23%), and one had a severe headache. However, two subjects who received 10^8 CFU experienced diarrhea, fever, and constitutional symptoms. Next, 15 volunteers were inoculated with 10^6 CFU, and nine (60%) experienced diarrhea, fever, and constitutional symptoms (Table 1). When 12 additional subjects ingested 10^4 CFU, only one had a significant symptom (diarrhea). The peak geometric mean anti-LPS IgA ASC response to 10^4 CFU was 18 per 10^6 PBMC. This dose was deemed clinically acceptable and immunogenic, and a challenge study was performed. The peak post-vaccination geometric mean anti-LPS IgA ASC count was 43 per 10^6 PBMC in the subset of vaccinees who participated in the challenge study (18 per 10^6 PBMC).

Eight weeks after vaccination with 10^4 CFU of SC602, seven vaccinees and seven naïve controls were challenged with 10^3 CFU of virulent S. flexneri 2a strain 2457T. Fever and/or severe shigellosis occurred in no vaccinees and in six controls (86%). However, three of the challenged vaccinees (43%) did experience mild diarrhea (overall protective efficacy 50%) (Table 1). Immune correlates of protection against any symptom of shigellosis in this challenge trial included >40 IgA ASC per 10^6 PBMC recognizing S. flexneri 2a LPS and ≥3-fold rise in serum IgA antibody against S. flexneri 2a LPS [21].

Next, the safety and immunogenicity of SC602 was evaluated in an outpatient trial at USAMRIID with 34 vaccinees and one control (T.S. Coster, unpublished). Vaccinees received either 2.6 or 5.6×10^4 CFU of SC602. Eight subjects (24%) experienced a measurable clinical reaction (fever or diarrhea). The vaccine was isolated from stools of all vaccinees, but shedding did not begin until 10 days post-vaccination in some. The mean duration of colonization was 12 days, and 5% of vaccinees exceeded 4 weeks [89]. All volunteers received ciprofloxacin 35 days after vaccination. Thereafter, another inpatient study was conducted at USAMRIID in which nine volunteers received the 4-log dose with similar results (D.E. Katz, unpublished). Three additional subjects received 10^3 CFU without reactions, all of whom excreted vaccine and had IgA ASC anti-LPS responses (10, 75, and 277 ASC per 10^6 PBMC).

In sum, approximately 20% of the 58 subjects who received 10^4 CFU of SC602 experienced diarrhea or fever of brief duration, and 10% had headaches or cramps of sufficient severity to modify normal activities. Significant IgA anti-LPS rises were seen in 66% of the 24 subjects who had ASC responses measured, and 58% of subjects had threefold or greater rises in serum anti-LPS IgA (Table 1). SC602 completely protected against severe shigellosis and offered partial protection against any illness. Phase 2 trials of the 4-log dose are being designed to determine consumer acceptance of the symptoms associated with vaccination. In light of the prolonged excretion, inadvertent spread of SC602 to household contacts will be carefully monitored in future trials.

In October of 2000, clinical trials of SC602 began in Bangladesh, an endemic area for S. flexneri 2a (A. Baqui and D. Isenbarger, unpublished). One inpatient and three outpatient trials were conducted in adult volunteers, followed by similar trials in children 8 to 10 years old, at a dose of 10^4, 10^5, or 10^6 CFU SC602 or placebo. Neither adults nor children experienced significant side effects, and SC602 was only rarely isolated from vaccinees. The final evaluation of SC602 in Bangladesh was a series of inpatient studies conducted in 12–36-month-old children who received escalating doses of 10^3 to 10^6 CFU. Diarrhea and/or fever occurred in a minority of subjects but was not dose related nor significantly more common in vaccinees than in placebo recipients. Neither vaccine excretion nor immune responses were detected.

The disappointing results of this attempt to use a minimally attenuated, live Shigella strain as a vaccine for children in the developing world suggests that safety and immunogenicity data from vaccine trials in adults of the developed world are not easily extrapolated to endemic areas. Perhaps lactoferrin in the intestines of milk-fed toddlers acted synergistically with the aerobactin (*iuc*) mutation to incapacitate the vaccine by depleting its iron stores. Maternal antibody, actively acquired immunity even at a young age, and small bowel bacterial overgrowth may also mitigate intestinal colonization with a small number of *Shigellae* even if the attenuation of the pathogen is minimal.

2. *S. sonnei* Attenuated Solely on the Basis of a Deletion Mutation in *virGIcsA* (WRSS1)

In the rabbit ileal loop model, deletion in *iuc* provides little additional attenuation of *S. flexneri* 2a above that seen by inactivating *virG* alone [90]. This finding prompted Hartman and Venkatesan to develop a *S. sonnei* vaccine candidate attenuated solely on the basis of a deletion in *virG*. To minimize the predilection of *S. sonnei* to spontaneously lose its virulence plasmid, they chose a wild-type strain that exhibited stability of the form I phenotype [91]. The *sacB* suicide vector pCVD422 was used to replace wild-type *virG* allele with *virG* possessing a 212-bp deletion. This strain, WRSS1, was fully attenuated in the Sereny model and induced protective immunity [91].

A Phase 1 trial was conducted at the Center for Vaccine Development in which volunteers were randomized, in a double-blind fashion, to receive either placebo (seven subjects) or vaccine with buffer (27 subjects) at a dose of ca. 10^3, 10^4, 10^5, or 10^6 CFU [27]. Self-limited illnesses (fever and mild diarrhea) occurred in 14%, 0%, 30%, and 33% of subjects in each ascending dose group, respectively. Subjective complaints (headache, abdominal cramps) were reported by 33% of vaccinees but no controls. Vaccination evoked vigorous IgA anti-LPS ASC responses, which often exceeded 100 per 10^6 PBMC. Geometric mean peak post-vaccination anti-LPS serum IgG and fecal IgA titers were also robust. For unknown reasons, the clinical, microbiologic, and immune responses in the 4-log dose group were weak. At all other doses, immune responses were similar in magnitude to those elicited by strains that prevent illness following experimental challenge [21], suggesting that WRSS1 may confer protective immunity.

Recent evidence indicates that knocking out the chromosomal and plasmid copies of the *S. flexneri msbB* genes that encode the full acyl-oxy-acylation of the lipid A induces a significant decrease in endotoxicity. As a consequence, the double-mutant has a diminished capacity to induce inflammatory destruction of the intestinal mucosa in a rabbit ligated intestinal loop model of infection [46]. Genetic attenuation of the endotoxin activity of currently available live attenuated vaccine candidates such as SC602 may eliminate residual reactogenicity, particularly the febrile component observed in some volunteers.

VIII. THE CONCEPT OF POLYVALENT *SHIGELLA* VACCINES

It is not realistic to attempt to protect against all 47 serotypes of *Shigella*. An analysis of serotype-specific disease burden suggests that five *Shigella* strains (*S. sonnei*, *S. dysenteriae* 1,

and *S. flexneri* 2a, 3a, and 6) are most critical to include in a potential vaccine [1]. *S. dysenteriae* comprises a small proportion of the endemic episodes, but the severe manifestations typical of serotype 1, which constitutes about 30% of *S. dysenteriae* isolates, argue for its inclusion. *S. sonnei* and *S. flexneri* are essential as they represent the most common causes of endemic shigellosis worldwide [1]. However, the variability (both geographic and temporal) of the 15 *S. flexneri* serotypes presents a logistical conundrum to vaccine developers. Accordingly, Noriega and coworkers discovered that a composite of three serotypes, *S. flexneri* 2a, 3a and 6, provides cross-protection against the remaining 12 *S. flexneri* serotypes [9]. The immunological rationale is that among these three serotypes there is a type- or group-specific antigen shared by each of the 15 *S. flexneri* serotypes. The functional activity of these serological cross reactions was shown in studies involving Sereny test challenge of mucosally immunized of guinea pigs [9].

Little is known about the immune response that can be generated by immunizing humans with multiple *Shigella* serotypes. Cooper and coworkers in the 1940s immunized children parenterally with a *S. flexneri* vaccine consisting of inactivated serotype II, III, and VII strains (later respectively known as serotypes 2, 3, and X) [92]. The sera from immunized children protected mice against challenge with the homologous wild-type strains [92]. Later, Formal and coworkers constructed attenuated strains by conjugating virulent *Shigella* with an Hfr$^+$ strain of *E. coli* K12. Two oral doses of a vaccine comprising *S. flexneri* 1b, 2a, and 3 plus *S. sonnei* protected monkeys against each homologous serotype [7]. Finally, Mel and coworkers immunized adults and children with bivalent vaccines containing SmD *S. flexneri* serotypes 2a and 3 [61], *S. flexneri* 1 and 2a, or *S. flexneri* 3 and *S. sonnei* [6]. These studies demonstrated in humans that oral delivery of two serotypes combined did not interfere with the immune response to the individual strains and suggest that protection against multiple *Shigella* serotypes with an oral polyvalent *Shigella* vaccine is feasible.

IX. *SHIGELLA* AS A LIVE VECTOR

A. *Shigella* Expressing Foreign Antigens

Attenuated *Shigella* are also attractive candidates to serve as live vector vaccines. These strains are delivered orally, colonize the FAE, and elicit a broad immune response that includes serum and mucosal antibodies, cell-mediated immune responses and a form of antibody-dependent cellular cytotoxicity [88,93]; moreover, *Shigella*, which share a high degree of homology with *E. coli*, are readily manipulated genetically. In theory, oral vaccines against a variety of infectious diseases can be developed by stable expression of foreign genes encoding protective antigens in a *Shigella* live vector strain.

Initial uses of *Shigella* as a live vector employed ΔaroD *S. flexneri* strain SFL 124 as a carrier for antigens from *S. dysenteriae* including shiga toxin B subunit and O-antigen determinants [94–96]. Such strains elicited immune responses in animal models against both *S. flexneri* and *S. dysenteriae* antigens. Additionally, attenuated strains of

Shigella have been used to express antigens from enterotoxigenic *E. coli* (ETEC) [97], VP of rotavirus [98], and the C3 epitope of VP1 of poliovirus [99]. Immunization with these strains elicited immune responses in animal models against both the heterologous antigen or epitope as well as the *Shigella* vector. Engineering of specialized stabilized plasmids has enabled reliable, high-level expression of multiple antigens from a single plasmid in attenuated *Shigella* strains. At the Center for Vaccine Development, investigators have used this system to express multiple different ETEC fimbriae as well as LT antigens in *ΔguaBA S. flexneri* vaccine strains that can elicit both serum and mucosal immune responses to the heterologous antigens as well as to the *Shigella* vector in animal models [100–102]. These systems demonstrate the possibility of constructing a multicomponent vaccine formulation capable of generating broad spectrum immunity against two important pathogens.

B. DNA Delivery

The ability of *Shigella* to invade eukaryotic cells and gain access to the cytoplasm has been exploited for the delivery of DNA vaccines. Sizemore and coworkers [103] used the marker protein β-galactosidase, driven by the CMV promoter, to show that mucosal administration of an attenuated strain of *Shigella* could deliver a DNA plasmid to the cytosol of a eukaryotic cell and elicit immune responses in a mouse model. Subsequently, investigators have used attenuated *Shigella* strains to deliver DNA plasmids encoding fragment C of tetanus toxin [104], measles virus H and F antigens [105,105A], and HIV gp120 [106]. In each case immune responses to the encoded antigen were generated in immunized animals.

X. CONCLUSIONS

The increasing knowledge of the *Shigella* genome has allowed investigators to target diverse genes for deletion mutations in an attempt to construct safe, attenuated oral *Shigella* vaccines. Experience suggests that the major impediment to creating a successful vaccine will be achieving safety in industrialized countries while retaining immunogenicity in developing countries. In the near future, it is expected that several promising vaccine candidates will reach Phase I clinical trials. The mutation or combination of mutations that demonstrates the best safety without compromising immunogenicity will likely be reproduced in other serotypes to form a polyvalent *Shigella* vaccine containing the most prevalent serotypes worldwide. It is possible that such a *Shigella* vaccine can also serve as a live vector vaccine to express antigens which confer protection against other relevant enteric pathogens.

REFERENCES

1. Kotloff KL, et al. Global burden of *Shigella* infections: implications for vaccine development and implementation. Bull WHO 1999; 77:651–656.
2. Ferreccio C, et al. Epidemiologic pattern of acute diarrhea and endemic *Shigella* infections in a poor periurban setting in Santiago, Chile. Am J Epidemiol 1991; 134:614–627.
3. Herrington DA, et al. Studies in volunteers to evaluate candidate *Shigella* vaccines: further experience with a bivalent *Salmonella typhi-Shigella sonnei* vaccine and protection conferred by previous *Shigella sonnei* disease. Vaccine 1990; 8:353–357.
4. Kotloff KL, et al. A modified *Shigella* volunteer challenge model in which the inoculum is administered with bicarbonate buffer: clinical experience and implications for *Shigella* infectivity. Vaccine 1995; 13:1488–1494.
5. Mel DM, et al. Studies on vaccination against bacillary dysentery: 3. Effective oral immunization against *Shigella flexneri* 2a in a field trial. Bull WHO 1965; 32:647–655.
6. Mel DM, et al. Studies on vaccination against bacillary dysentery: 6. Protection of children by oral immunization with streptomycin-dependent *Shigella* strains. Bull WHO 1971; 45:457–464.
7. Formal SB, et al. Protection of monkeys against experimental shigellosis with a living attenuated oral polyvalent dysentery vaccine. J Bacteriol 1966; 92:17–22.
8. Van de Verg LL, et al. Cross-reactivity of *Shigella flexneri* serotype 2a O antigen antibodies following immunization or infection. Vaccine 1996; 14:1062–1068.
9. Noriega FR, et al. Strategy for cross-protection among *Shigella flexneri* serotypes. Infect Immun 1999; 67:782–788.
10. Karnell A, et al. Auxotrophic live oral *Shigella flexneri* vaccine protects monkeys against challenge with *S. flexneri* of different serotypes. Vaccine 1992; 10:167–174.
11. Meitert T, et al. Efficiency of immunoprophylaxis and immunotherapy by live dysentery vaccine administration in children and adult collectivities. Arch Roum Pathol Exp Microbiol 1982; 41:357–369.
12. Bingrui W. Study on the effect of oral immunization of T32-Istrati strain against bacillary dysentery in field trials. Arch Roum Pathol Exp Microbiol 1984; 43:285–289.
13. Cohen D, et al. Prospective study of the association between serum antibodies to lipopolysaccharide O antigen and the attack rate of shigellosis. J Clin Microbiol 1991; 29: 386–389.
14. Black RE, et al. Prevention of shigellosis by a *Salmonella typhi–Shigella sonnei* bivalent vaccine. J Infect Dis 1987; 155:1260–1265.
15. Cohen D, et al. Double-blind vaccine-controlled randomised efficacy trial of an investigational *Shigella sonnei* conjugate vaccine in young adults. Lancet 1997; 349: 155–159.
16. Oaks EV, et al. Serum immune response to *Shigella* protein antigens in rhesus monkeys and humans infected with *Shigella* spp. Infect Immun 1986; 53:57–63.
17. Van de Verg LL, et al. Age-specific prevalence of serum antibodies to the invasion plasmid and lipopolysaccharide antigens of *Shigella* species in Chilean and North American populations. J Infect Dis 1992; 166:158–161.
18. Tacket CO, et al. Efficacy of bovine milk immunoglobulin concentrate in preventing illness after *Shigella flexneri* challenge. Am J Trop Med Hyg 1992; 47:276–283.
19. Clemens JD, et al. Breast feeding as a determinant of severity in shigellosis. Evidence for protection throughout the first three years of life in Bangladeshi children. Am J Epidemiol 1986; 123:710–720.
20. Kotloff KL, et al. Evaluation of the safety, immunogenicity and efficacy in healthy adults of four doses of live oral hybrid *Escherichia coli–Shigella flexneri* 2a vaccine strain EcSf2a-2. Vaccine 1995; 13:495–502.
21. Coster TS, et al. Vaccination against shigellosis with attenuated *Shigella flexneri* 2a strain SC602. Infect Immun 1999; 67:3437–3443.
22. Way SS, et al. An essential role for gamma interferon in

innate resistance to *Shigella flexneri* infection. Infect Immun 1998; 66:1342–1348.

23. Van de Verg LL, et al. Antibody and cytokine responses in a mouse pulmonary model of *Shigella flexneri* serotype 2a infection. Infect Immun 1995; 63:1947–1954.

24. Raqib R, et al. Local entrapment of interferon gamma in the recovery from *Shigella dysenteriae* type 1 infection. Gut 1996; 38:328–336.

25. Raqib R, et al. Cytokine secretion in acute shigellosis is correlated to disease activity and directed more to stool than to plasma. J Infect Dis 1995; 171:376–384.

26. Samandari T, et al. Production of IFN-gamma and IL-10 to *Shigella* invasions by mononuclear cells from volunteers orally inoculated with a Shiga toxin-deleted *Shigella dysenteriae* type 1 strain. J Immunol 2000; 164:2221–2232.

27. Kotloff KL, et al. Phase I evaluation of ΔvirG *Shigella sonnei* live, attenuated, oral vaccine strain WRSS1 in healthy adults. Infect Immun 2002; 70:2016–2021.

28. Sansonetti PJ, et al. OmpB (osmo-regulation) and icsA (cell-to-cell spread) mutants of *Shigella flexneri*: vaccine candidates and probes to study the pathogenesis of shigellosis. Vaccine 1991; 9:416–422.

29. Zychlinsky A, et al. *Shigella flexneri* induces apoptosis in infected macrophages. Nature 1992; 358:167–169.

30. Sansonetti PJ. Microbes and microbial toxins: paradigms for microbial–mucosal interactions. III. Shigellosis: from symptoms to molecular pathogenesis. Am J Physiol Gastrointest Liver Physiol 2001; 280:G319–G323.

31. Sansonetti PJ, et al. *Shigella sonnei* plasmids: evidence that a large plasmid is necessary for virulence. Infect Immun 1981; 34:75–83.

32. Buchrieser C, et al. The virulence plasmid pWR100 and the repertoire of proteins secreted by the type III secretion apparatus of *Shigella flexneri*. Mol Microbiol 2000; 38:760–771.

33. Sansonetti PJ. Rupture, invasion and inflammatory destruction of the intestinal barrier by *Shigella*, making sense of prokaryote–eukaryote cross-talks. FEMS Microbiol Rev 2001; 25:3–14.

34. Page AL, et al. Spa15 of *Shigella flexneri*, a third type of chaperone in the type III secretion pathway. Mol Microbiol 2002; 43:1533–1542.

35. Tran VN, et al. Bacterial signals and cell responses during *Shigella* entry into epithelial cells. Cell Microbiol 2000; 2:187–193.

36. Skoudy A, et al. CD44 binds to the *Shigella* IpaB protein and participates in bacterial invasion of epithelial cells. Cell Microbiol 2000; 2:19–33.

37. Bourdet-Sicard R, et al. Binding of the *Shigella* protein IpaA to vinculin induces F-actin depolymerization. EMBO J 1999; 18:5853–5862.

38. Makino S, et al. A genetic determinant required for continuous reinfection of adjacent cells on large plasmid in *S. flexneri* 2a. Cell 1986; 46:551–555.

39. Bernardini ML, et al. Identification of icsA, a plasmid locus of *Shigella-flexneri* that governs bacterial intra- and intercellular spread through interaction with F-actin. Proc Natl Acad Sci USA 1989; 86:3867–3871.

40. Miki H, et al. WAVE, a novel WASP-family protein involved in actin reorganization induced by Rac. EMBO J 1998; 17:6932–6941.

41. Egile C, et al. Activation of the CDC42 effector N-WASP by the *Shigella flexneri* IcsA protein promotes actin nucleation by Arp2/3 complex and bacterial actin-based motility. J Cell Biol 1999; 146:1319–1332.

42. Sansonetti PJ, et al. Cadherin expression is required for the spread of *Shigella flexneri* between epithelial cells. Cell 1994; 76:829–839.

43. Mavris M, et al. Regulation of transcription by the activity of the *Shigella flexneri* type III secretion apparatus. Mol Microbiol 2002; 43:1543–1553.

44. Chen Y, et al. A bacterial invasion induces macrophage apoptosis by binding directly to ICE. EMBO J 1996; 15:3853–3860.

45. Sansonetti PJ, et al. Caspase-1 activation of IL-1beta and IL-18 are essential for *Shigella flexneri*-induced inflammation. Immunity 2000; 12:581–590.

46. D'Hauteville H, et al. Two msbB genes encoding maximal acylation of lipid A are required for invasive *Shigella flexneri* to mediate inflammatory rupture and destruction of the intestinal epithelium. J Immunol 2002; 168:5240–5251.

47. Sansonetti PJ, et al. Interleukin-8 controls bacterial transepithelial translocation at the cost of epithelial destruction in experimental shigellosis. Infect Immun 1999; 67:1471–1480.

48. Thorpe CM, et al. Shiga toxins induce, superinduce, and stabilize a variety of C-X-C chemokine mRNAs in intestinal epithelial cells, resulting in increased chemokine expression. Infect Immun 2001; 69:6140–6147.

49. Noriega FR, et al. Prevalence of *Shigella* enterotoxin 1 among *Shigella* clinical isolates of diverse serotypes. J Infect Dis 1995; 172:1408–1410.

50. Nataro JP, et al. Identification and cloning of a novel plasmid-encoded enterotoxin of enteroinvasive *Escherichia coli* and *Shigella* strains. Infect Immun 1995; 633:4721–4728.

51. Fasano A, et al. *Shigella* enterotoxin 1: an enterotoxin of *Shigella flexneri* 2a active in rabbit small intestine in vivo and in vitro. J Clin Invest 1995; 95:2853–2861.

52. Sitaraman SV, et al. Neutrophil-epithelial crosstalk at the intestinal lumenal surface mediated by reciprocal secretion of adenosine and IL-6. J Clin Invest 2001; 107:861–869.

53. Matkowskyj KA, et al. Galanin-1 receptor up-regulation mediates the excess colonic fluid production caused by infection with enteric pathogens. Nat Med 2000; 6:1048–1051.

54. Zychlinsky A, Sansonetti PI. Apoptosis as a proinflammatory event: what can we learn from bacteria-induced cell death? Trends Microbiol 1997; 5:201–204.

55. Kotloff KL, et al. Safety, immunogenicity, and efficacy in monkeys and humans of invasive *Escherichia coli* K-12 hybrid vaccine candidates expressing *Shigella flexneri* 2a somatic antigen. Infect Immun 1992; 60:2218–2224.

56. Sereny B. Experimental keratoconjunctivitis shigellosa. Acta Microbiol Acad Sci Hung 1957; 4:367–376.

57. Hartman AB, et al. Small-animal model to measure efficacy and immunogenicity of *Shigella* vaccine strains. Infect Immun 1991; 59:4075–4083.

58. Levine MM, et al. Pathogenesis of *Shigella dysenteriae* 1 (Shiga) dysentery. J Infect Dis 1973; 127:261–270.

59. DuPont HL, et al. Immunity in shigellosis: II. Protection induced by oral live vaccine or primary infection. J Infect Dis 1972; 125:12–16.

60. Mel DM, et al. Studies on vaccination against bacillary dysentery: 2. Safety tests and reactogenicity studies on a live dysentery vaccine intended for use in field trials. Bull World Health Organ 1965; 32:637–645.

61. Mel DM, et al. Studies on vaccination against bacillary dysentery: 4. Oral immunization with live monotypic and combined vaccines. Bull WHO 1968; 39:375–380.

62. Mel DM, et al. Live oral *Shigella* vaccine: vaccination schedule and the effect of booster dose. Acta Microbiol Acad Sci Hung 1974; 21:109–114.

63. DuPont HL, et al. Immunity in shigellosis: I. Response of man to attenuated strains of *Shigella*. J Infect Dis 1972; 125:5–11.

64. Levine MM, et al. Shigellosis in custodial institutions: IV. In

vivo stability and transmissibility of oral attenuated streptomycin-dependent *Shigella* vaccines. J Infect Dis 1975;
131:704–707.

65. Levine MM, et al. Shigellosis in custodial institutions: V.
Effect of intervention with streptomycin-dependent *Shigella
sonnei* vaccine in an institution with endemic disease. Am J
Epidemiol 1976; 104:88–92.

66. Meitert T, et al. Vaccine strain *Sh. flexneri* T32-Istrati.
Studies in animals and in volunteers. Antidysentery immunoprophylaxis and immunotherapy by live vaccine Vadizen
(*Sh. flexneri* T32-Istrati). Arch Roum Pathol Exp Microbiol
1984; 43:251–278.

67. Xie G, et al. Study of the 140 Md plasmid DNA of T32-
Istrati vaccine strain. J Chin Microbiol Immunol 1989;
9:288–291.

68. Wang B, et al. Construction and characteristics of an attenuated *Shigella flexneri* 2a/*Shigella sonnei* bivalent vaccine. J Chin Microbiol Immunol 1987; 7:373–377.

69. Shong S, et al. The discovery of the large plasmid in a rough-
type strain of *Shigella sonnei*. J Biol Prod 1988; 1:13–16.

70. Liu W, Wang B-R. Studies on 120Md plasmid and its derivative plasmid in *Shigella sonnei*. J Chin Microbiol Immunol 1990; 10:205–208.

71. Tu G, et al. Double-blind field trial of oral live F2a-sonnei
(FS) dysentery vaccine. J Biol Prod 2002; 12:178–180.

72. Seid RC, et al. Unusual lipopolysaccharide antigens of
a *Salmonella typhi* oral vaccine strain expressing the *Shigella sonnei* form I antigen. J Biol Chem 1984; 259:9028–
9034.

73. Levine MM, et al. Studies with a new generation of oral
attenuated *Shigella* vaccine: *Escherichia coli* bearing surface antigens of *Shigella flexneri*. J Infect Dis 1977; 136:577–
582.

74. Formal SB, et al. Oral vaccination of monkeys with an
invasive *Escherichia coli* K-12 hybrid expressing *Shigella
flexneri* 2a somatic antigen. Infect Immun 1984; 46:465–
469.

75. Newland JW, et al. Genotypic and phenotypic characterization of an aroD deletion-attenuated *Escherichia coli*
K12-*Shigella flexneri* hybrid vaccine expressing *S. flexneri*
2a somatic antigen. Vaccine 1992; 10:766–776.

76. Hoiseth S, Stocker BAD. Aromatic-dependent *Salmonella
typhimurium* are non-virulent and effective as live vaccines.
Nature 1981; 292:238–239.

77. Lindberg AA, et al. Construction of an auxotrophic *Shigella flexneri* strain for use as a live vaccine. Microb Pathog
1990; 8:433–440.

78. Li A, Pal T, et al. Safety and immunogenicity of the live oral
auxotrophic *Shigella flexneri* SFL124 in volunteers. Vaccine
1992; 10:395–404.

79. Li A, et al. Safety and immunogenicity of the live oral
auxotrophic *Shigella flexneri* SFL124 in adult Vietnamese
volunteers. Vaccine 1993; 11:180–189.

80. Li A, et al. Immune responses in Vietnamese children after a
single dose of the auxotrophic, live *Shigella flexneri* Y
vaccine strain SFL124. J Infect 1994; 28:11–23.

81. Karnell A, et al. AroD deletion attenuates *Shigella flexneri*
strain 2457T and makes it a safe and efficacious oral vaccine
in monkeys. Vaccine 1993; 11:830–836.

82. Karnell A, et al. Safety and immunogenicity study of the
auxotrophic *Shigella flexneri* 2a vaccine SFL1070 with a
deleted aroD gene in adult Swedish volunteers. Vaccine
1995; 13:88–99.

83. Noriega FR, et al. Construction and characterization of
attenuated ΔaroA ΔvirG *Shigella flexneri* 2a strain CVD
1203, a prototype live oral vaccine. Infect Immun 1994; 62:
5168–5172.

84. Kotloff KL, et al. Safety, immunogenicity, and transmissibility in humans of CVD 1203, a live oral *Shigella flexneri*

2a vaccine candidate attenuated by deletions in aroA and
virG. Infect Immun 1996; 64:4542–4548.

85. McFarland WC, Stocker BA. Effect of different purine
auxotrophic mutations on mouse-virulence of a Vi-positive
strain of *Salmonella dublin* and of two strains of *Salmonella
typhimurium*. Microb Pathog 1987; 3:129–141.

86. Neuhard J, Nygaard P. *Escherichia coli* and *Salmonella
typhimurium*, cellular and molecular biology. In: Ingraham
JL, Low KB, Magasanik B, Schaechter M, Umbarger HE,
eds. Purines and PyrimidinesWashington, DC: American
Society for Microbiology, 1987:445–473.

87. Noriega FR, et al. Engineered ΔguaBA, ΔvirG *Shigella
flexneri* 2a strain CVD 1205: construction, safety, immunogenicity and potential efficacy as a mucosal vaccine.
Infect Immun 1996; 64:3055–3061.

88. Kotloff KL, et al. *Shigella flexneri* 2a strain CVD 1207, with
specific deletions in virG, sen, set, and guaBA, is highly
attenuated in humans. Infect Immun 2000; 68:1034–1039.

89. Teska JD, et al. Novel self-sampling culture method to
monitor excretion of live, oral *Shigella flexneri* 2a vaccine
SC602 during a community-based Phase 1 trial. J Lab Clin
Med 1999; 134:141–146.

90. Sansonetti PJ, Arondel J. Construction and evaluation of a
double mutant of *Shigella flexneri* as a candidate for oral
vaccination against shigellosis. Vaccine 1989; 7:443–450.

91. Hartman AB, Venkatesan MM. Construction of a stable
attenuated *Shigella sonnei* virG-vaccine strain, WRSS1, and
protective efficacy and immunogenicity in the guinea pig
keratoconjunctivitis model. Infect Immun 1998; 66:4572–
4576.

92. Cooper ML, et al. Studies in dysentery vaccination: VI.
Primary vaccination of children with polyvalent vaccines of
Shigella. J Immunol 1949; 61:209–219.

93. Lowell GH, et al. Antibody-dependent cell-mediated antibacterial activity: K lymphocytes, monocytes, and granulocytes are effective against *Shigella*. J Immunol 1980; 125:
2778–2784.

94. Ryd M, et al. Induction of a humoral immune response to a
Shiga toxin B subunit epitope expressed as a chimeric LamB
protein in a *Shigella flexneri* live vaccine strain. Microb
Pathog 1992; 12:399–407.

95. Klee SR, et al. Construction and characterization of
genetically-marked bivalent anti-*Shigella dysenteriae* 1
and anti-*Shigella flexneri* Y live vaccine candidates. Microb
Pathog 1997; 22:363–376.

96. Tzschaschel BD, et al. Towards a vaccine candidate against
Shigella dysenteriae: 1: Expression of the Shiga toxin B-
subunit in an attenuated *Shigella flexneri* aroD carrier
strain. Microb Pathog 1996; 21:277–288.

97. Noriega FR, et al. Further characterization of aroA, virG
Shigella flexneri 2a strain CVD 1203 as a mucosal *Shigella*
vaccine and as a live vector vaccine for delivering antigens of
enterotoxigenic *Escherichia coli*. Infect Immun 1996; 64:23–
27.

98. Loy AL, et al. Immune response to rotavirus VP4 expressed
in an attenuated strain of *Shigella flexneri*. FEMS Immunol
Med Microbiol 1999; 25:283–288.

99. Barzu S, et al. Immunogenicity of IpaC-hybrid proteins expressed in the *Shigella flexneri* 2a vaccine candidate SC602.
Infect Immun 1998; 66:77–82.

100. Altboum Z, et al. Attenuated *Shigella flexneri* 2a (guaBA
strain CVD 1204 expressing enterotoxigenic *Escherichia coli*
(ETEC) CS2 and CS3 fimbriae as a live mucosal vaccine
against *Shigella* and ETEC infection. Infect Immun 2001;
69:3150–3158.

101. Koprowski H, et al. Attenuated *Shigella flexneri* 2a vaccine
strain CVD 1204 expressing colonization factor antigen I
and mutant heat-labile enterotoxin of enterotoxigenic
Escherichia coli. Infect Immun 2000; 68:4884–4892.

102. Galen JE, et al. Optimization of plasmid maintenance in the attenuated live vector vaccine strain *Salmonella typhi* CVD 908-htrA. Infect Immun 1999; 67:6424–6433.

103. Sizemore DR, et al. Attenuated bacteria as a DNA delivery vehicle for DNA-mediated immunization. Vaccine 1997; 15:804–807.

104. Anderson RJ, et al. ΔguaBA attenuated *Shigella flexneri* 2a strain CVD 1204 as a *Shigella* vaccine and as a live mucosal delivery system for fragment C of tetanus toxin. Vaccine 2000; 18:2193–2202.

105. Fennelly GJ, et al. Mucosal DNA vaccine immunization against measles with a highly attenuated *Shigella flexneri* vector. J Immunol 1999; 162:1603–1610.

105a. Pasetti AMF, et al. Attenuated *Salmonella enterica* serovar Typhi and *Shigella flexneri* 2A strains mucosally deliver DNA vaccines encoding measles virus hemagglutinin, inducing specific immune responses and protection in cotton rats. J Virol 2003. In press.

106. Shata MT, Hone DM. Vaccination with a *Shigella* DNA vaccine vector induces antigen-specific CD8(+) T cells and antiviral protective immunity. J Virol 2001; 75:9665–9670.

107. Hone DM, et al. Construction of genetically-defined double aro mutants of *Salmonella typhi*. Vaccine 1991; 9:810–816.

108. Levine MM, et al. Safety, infectivity, immunogenicity and in vivo stability of two attenuated auxotrophic mutant strains of *Salmonella typhi*, 541Ty and 543Ty, as live oral vaccines in man. J Clin Invest 1987; 79:888–902. Against *Shigella flexneri* 2a in a field trial. Bull WHO 1965; 32:647–655.

60

Oral Inactivated Whole Cell B Subunit Combination Vaccine Against Enterotoxigenic *Escherichia coli*

Ann-Mari L. Svennerholm
Göteborg University, Göteborg, Sweden

Stephen J. Savarino
Naval Medical Research Center, Bethesda, Maryland, U.S.A.

I. INTRODUCTION

Enterotoxigenic *Escherichia coli* (ETEC) is one of the most common causes of diarrheal disease in the developing world [1]. In these areas, on an annual basis, ETEC results in an estimated 280–400 million diarrheal episodes in children under 5 years and an additional 100 million episodes in children aged 5–14 years [2,3]. Moreover, ETEC causes substantial disease in indigenous adults in developing countries, with the estimated number of cases per year in persons above 15 years exceeding 400 million [3]. Additionally, Western travelers who visit developing countries are frequently infected with ETEC, which is responsible for one-third to one-half of all diarrheal episodes in travelers to Africa, Asia, and Latin America [4].

Enterotoxigenic *E. coli* causes disease by colonizing the small intestine and elaborating a heat-labile (LT) or a heat-stable enterotoxin (ST) or both toxins [5]. The resulting illness usually lasts from 3 to 7 days and ranges from mild diarrhea without dehydration to severe cholera-like disease [1,3]. Although the illness is typically mild, it does result in an estimated 300,000–700,000 deaths per year, mostly in young children with more severe presentations [2,3]. Disease severity may partly be related to the toxin profile of the causative strain. A recent study found that ETEC producing ST alone or ST together with LT induced moderate or severe disease in a significantly higher proportion of episodes than LT only producing strains [6].

During the first 3 years of life, children in less-developed countries typically experience up to three separate episodes of ETEC diarrhea per year, after which the age-specific incidence of ETEC disease declines dramatically [1]. In Bangladeshi children under 5 years of age, ETEC diarrhea

has been associated with growth faltering [7]. Thus an effective vaccine that could reduce ETEC morbidity and mortality may have great public health utility, particularly for children in developing countries.

In regions of the world where ETEC is highly endemic, the aforementioned decline in ETEC diarrhea incidence as well as the decreased ratio of ETEC disease to infection with increasing age [6,8,9] are consistent with the notion that protective immunity develops with repeated ETEC infections. That adults from industrialized countries experience high attack rates of ETEC diarrhea when visiting areas where ETEC diarrhea is endemic [4] suggests that the lower incidence of ETEC disease in indigenous adults is due to acquired immunity rather than to other age-related host factors. Additional support for the induction of protective immunity against ETEC disease has been drawn from trials of the oral cholera toxin B subunit-whole cell (CTB-WC) cholera vaccine (see Chapter 59 this volume). Oral immunization with CTB, which is immunologically cross-reactive with the B subunit component of *E. coli* LT (LTB), afforded highly significant, albeit short lasting, protection against diarrhea caused by LT producing ETEC in Bangladesh [10]. Comparable levels of protection against LT ETEC disease (ranging from 50% to 80%) were also observed in controlled trials of the oral CTB-WC vaccine in Finnish travelers to Morocco [11] and U.S. travelers to Mexico [12]. In a recent pilot study, an oral ETEC vaccine was also shown to provide significant protection against ETEC disease in Austrian travelers visiting countries in Asia, Africa, and Latin America [13]. Together, these findings strongly support the notion that an effective ETEC vaccine is achievable. The design of such a vaccine should be based on the knowledge of mechanisms of ETEC disease and immunity.

II. PATHOGENIC MECHANISMS IN ENTEROTOXIGENIC *E. COLI* INFECTIONS

The critical virulence properties that contribute to the pathogenesis of ETEC diarrhea are the ability of bacteria to closely adhere to the mucosa of the proximal small intestine by means of colonization factors (CFs) and to elaborate enterotoxins that interact with enterocytes to yield electrolyte-rich watery secretions [5,14]. Clinical ETEC isolates are fairly diverse and comprise many different O:H serotypes, multiple antigenically distinct CF types, and three different toxin phenotypes (i.e., LT only, ST only, or LTST) [14–17]. The greatest diversity is in O and H serogroup expression. At least 70 different *E. coli* O groups have been found among clinical ETEC isolates [17]. Distribution of the different ETEC toxin profiles has differed considerably with time, population, and geographical area, although the proportion of ST only clinical isolates appears to have increased during recent years in children in endemic areas [6,15,17]. Thus until 5–10 years ago, the three toxin phenotypes were estimated to constitute approximately one-third each among clinical ETEC isolates [14,16], whereas epidemiological studies during recent years have found that around 50% of all clinical isolates produce ST only [6,17].

E. coli LT is similar to cholera toxin (CT) in that both toxins consist of a toxin-active A subunit attached to five B subunits that mediate binding to cell-membrane receptors. Both the LT A and B subunits cross-react immunologically with the corresponding CT subunits, although there are also unique A and B subunit epitopes on both toxins [16,18]. Immune responses against LT and CT are mainly directed against the B subunits [16]. Heat-stable enterotoxin a (STa) constitutes a family of closely related peptides that induce diarrhea both in humans and animals. There are two highly related STa congeners produced by ETEC, originally named for the source (STh, human; STp, porcine) from which the type strain was derived. Both are methanol-soluble peptides of 18 (STp) or 19 (STh) amino acids that activate guanylate cyclase C [19]. Both STa types are poorly immunogenic, but high titer polyclonal anti-STa sera or monoclonal antibodies can be obtained by immunization with conjugates consisting of STa coupled to a carrier protein [20].

Colonization of the small intestine is an important prerequisite for ETEC to cause disease [5,14]. All ETEC strains seem to possess distinct CFs. While most CFs display a fimbrial or fibrillar morphology, a few appear as structurally indistinct outer-membrane proteins (Table 1). At least 23 different CFs have been identified to date [14,21]. The best-characterized CFs are colonization factor antigens (CFA)/I, CFA/II, and CFA/IV. Whereas CFA/I is a homogenous protein, CFA/II consists of the three subcomponents CS1, CS2, and CS3; CS3 is usually expressed together with CS1 or CS2 [5,14]. Similarly, CFA/IV consists of CS4, CS5, and CS6. CS6, which is not a fimbrial antigen, is often expressed together with the fimbrial proteins CS4 or CS5. While prevalence of the different ETEC CFs shows considerable geographic variation [6,15,17,22–25], CFA/I, CFA/II, and CFA/IV are collectively expressed by as many as 40–80% of all clinical ETEC isolates in most surveys [6,14,23]. Surveys for additional putative CFs, e.g., PCFO159 (CS12),

Table 1 Colonization Factors Identified on ETEC Isolated in Endemic Areas and from Travelers

Most prevalent CFs (40–80%)		Less common CFs (10–25%)	
CFA/I		CS12	(PCFO159)
		CS14	(PCFO166)
CFA/II	(CS1 + CS3)	CS7	
	(CS2 + CS3)	CS17	
	(CS3)		
CFA/IV	(CS4 + CS6)		
	(CS5 + CS6)		
	(CS6)		

PCFO166 (CS14), CS7, CS17, and CFA/III (CS8), have shown that these factors are only expressed by 10–25% of all ETEC isolates [6,24,25]. In all epidemiological studies reported, a subset of ETEC has been found that does not express a CF [14], which may be due to the fact that assays were not used to detect all known CFs or that hitherto unidentified CFs are produced.

Accrual of more detailed data on temporal, geographic, and population-specific variations in CF prevalence is necessary because these represent the key somatic antigens for inclusion in any ETEC vaccine. Prospective studies that are presently in progress include a comparison of the distribution of CFs on ETEC isolated from children with diarrhea in endemic areas and from visitors to the same region who develop traveler's diarrhea (Svennerholm et al., unpublished data). Results from such studies may indicate whether one can extrapolate from studies of ETEC diarrhea in travelers to at-risk children living in the same country or vice versa.

Several of the different ETEC CFs have been shown to promote intestinal colonization, both in animal studies [26,27] and in human volunteers [28], indicating that they are indeed colonization factors. Volunteers ingesting CF-positive ETEC developed diarrhea, but individuals taking the isogenic CF-negative strain remained asymptomatic [29]. Furthermore, it has been shown that rabbits infected with CF-positive bacteria excreted the infecting strain in the stool for considerably longer time than rabbits receiving corresponding CF-negative mutants [26,27,30]. Similarly, patients infected with CF-positive ETEC strains had more frequent stools per day and longer duration of diarrhea than patients infected with CF-negative bacteria [29].

The various CFs are associated with a limited number of serogroups, some even with a single serotype [14]. Most LT only strains belong to serogroups that occur infrequently. Some CFs exclusively occur on strains producing ST, others exclusively on strains producing LT, and yet others on strains producing both toxin types [14]. Approximately 90% of the ETEC isolates that elaborate both LT and ST enterotoxins express known CFs, whereas such factors are found on about 60% of ST only strains [14]. Generally, only a small proportion of LT only strains bear the most prevalent CFs [5,14], i.e., CFA/I, CFA/II, and CFA/IV. Thus if a multivalent ETEC vaccine contained just CFA/I and the different subcomponents of CFA/II and CFA/IV, it could theoretically provide protection against 40–80% of the ETEC strains in most geographic areas. If an LT toxoid, such as the nontoxic B subunit component of LT (LTB) or CTB, was included in a multivalent vaccine, it might provide relatively broad protection against about 70–80% of ETEC strains worldwide. Inclusion of less frequent fimbrial antigens (e.g., CS7, CS12, CS14, and CS17) in a multivalent vaccine might expand the spectrum of coverage to greater than 80% of ETEC strains [14,16].

III. IMMUNE MECHANISMS AGAINST ENTEROTOXIGENIC *E. COLI*

The fact that both the bacteria and the toxins they produce are largely confined to the epithelial surface of the small intestine has suggested that antibodies produced locally in the small intestine should be the most important mediators of protective immunity [16,31]. These antibodies are mainly specific for the different CFs, LT, and other surface antigens. ST does not elicit neutralizing antibodies following natural infection. Thus, as shown in patients convalescing from ETEC diarrhea in Bangladesh, a majority responded with IgA antibody responses in intestinal lavage fluid [32] or IgA antibody-secreting cells in duodenal biopsies [33] against the CF of the infecting strain and against LT in those infected with LT only or LTST strains.

The assumption that intestinally produced antibodies may be protective against ETEC is based on studies in animals. Thus a highly significant correlation between the number of lamina propria cells producing anti-CF IgA antibodies and the diarrheal responses to challenge with ETEC producing the same CF has been observed [34]. Furthermore, intestinal infection with CF-positive ETEC, which is known to give rise to substantial mucosal anti-CF immune responses, has afforded significant protection against subsequent intestinal challenge with ETEC expressing the homologous but not heterologous CFs [26,27,30].

Antitoxic immunity is mainly mediated by locally produced antibodies against the B subunit of LT, although antibodies against the LT A subunit (LTA) have also been shown to have strong neutralizing capacity. Thus immunization with LT results in considerably higher levels of sIgA antibodies against LTB than against LTA in the small intestine. Induction of anti-LT immunity can provide solid protection not only against LT only, but also against LTST producing ETEC as shown in animal studies [31] and in clinical trials with the oral CTB-WC cholera vaccine [10–12]. This may suggest down-regulation of ST expression in LTST strains in vivo. The pentameric B subunits of CT and LT are very well suited as oral vaccine components due to their potent immunogenicity, lack of toxicity, and stability in the small intestine. Furthermore, they are capable of binding to the intestinal epithelium including the M-cells of the Peyer's patches, an important property for stimulating mucosal immunity [35]. Therefore either CTB or LTB may be suitable candidate antigens for providing anti-LT immunity.

The importance of anti-ST immunity for protection against ST producing *E. coli* seems to be modest. Infection with ST only ETEC provides solid protection against rein-fection by the same strain, but against heterologous ST only or LTST strains, only when the original challenge strain and the reinfecting strain share common CFs [26,27,30]. This suggests that ST immunity is not critical for preventing ST-induced diarrhea. By coupling *E. coli* STa to a carrier protein, e.g., LTB or bovine serum albumin either chemically or recombinantly, conjugates that give rise to ST neutralizing antibodies have been achieved [20,36,37]. However, all of these immunogenic conjugates have been toxic and elimination of their ST toxicity has resulted in failure to induce ST neutralizing antibodies. Although it may be possible to produce nontoxic ST conjugates that give rise to neutralizing ST antibodies locally in the small intestine, it is uncertain whether such antibodies would play an important protective role since comparatively large amounts of anti-ST antibodies will be required to provide neutralization of the small ST molecule [31].

Antibacterial immunity against ETEC may largely be ascribed to local gut immunity against the different CFs, although mucosal antibodies against the O antigens may play a protective role against O-group homologous ETEC [14,31]. The great diversity of O groups associated with human ETEC [1,5,17] does, however, place practical limits on the use of LPS as protective antigens against ETEC disease. Prospective epidemiological studies have provided indirect evidence that acquired immunity against ETEC is directed against the CFs [9], although corroborative evidence from sero-epidemiological studies is lacking [38]. Strong support for a protective role of anti-CF immunity has been obtained from studies in animals showing that antibodies against CFs are very effective in conferring passive protection against ETEC expressing the homologous CF. Furthermore, anti-CF antibodies have been shown to cooperate synergistically with anti-LT antibodies in conferring passive protection against experimental infection with LT-producing CF-positive ETEC [39]. Using a nonligated rabbit intestine model, it was demonstrated that an initial infection with CF-positive bacteria protected against subsequent infection with ETEC expressing the homologous CF [26,27,30]. Also in this model, evidence of synergistic cooperation between antitoxic and anti-CF immunity has been achieved [26].

Studies in human volunteers have also supported the importance of immunity against homologous CFs for protection. Thus an initial clinical infection with CF-positive ETEC elicits significant protection against CF-homologous rechallenge but not against challenge with ETEC strains expressing a heterologous CF [28,40]. These findings strongly support that immunity against the CFs is type-specific. However, recent studies have suggested that cross-protection against some of the CFs may occur. Several of the different CFs can be divided into two groups that share a high degree of primary amino acid sequence identity. The CFA/I-like group includes at least seven different CFs, each of which is largely composed of a major stalk-forming subunit, that share a high degree of overall amino acid sequence similarity with one another [14]. Other recently recognized CF groups include (1) CS5 and CS7, which share identical N-terminal amino acid sequences; (2) PCFO159 (CS12), PCFO20 (CS18), and CS20, whose major subunits share significant amino acid sequence similarity with one another and with the porcine ETEC CF 987P; and (3) CFA/III (CS8) and Longus (CS21), which are both type IV fimbriae [14]. Immunological cross-reactivity between the different fimbriae in the CFA/I group has been documented by immunoblot experiments suggesting the existence of common epitopes among these fimbriae [14]. The lack of immunological cross-reactivity in bacterial agglutination experiments, on the other hand, suggests that these common epitopes are not surface-expressed. However, they may be effective in vivo since experiments in animals have shown that a CF within the CFA/I-like group could both boost and prime immune responses against a heterologous CF within the same group [41]. Furthermore, patients living in an ETEC-endemic area, who most likely have been primed with different CFs, did not only mount an immune response against the CF of the infecting strain, but also against several different CFs of the homologous (CFA/I-like) group (Qadri et al., personal communication); such heterologous responses were, however, not observed in American volunteers infected with CFA/I-positive ETEC [42]. These findings leave open the possibility that immunization with an ETEC vaccine in an endemic population may induce immune responses against CFs that are not contained in the vaccine but are antigenically related to vaccine component CFs.

IV. DIFFERENT ETEC VACCINE CANDIDATES AND RATIONALE FOR AN INACTIVATED ETEC VACCINE

Based on the knowledge of the pathogenic and immune mechanisms in ETEC, an effective ETEC vaccine may be expected to evoke both anticolonization and antitoxic immunity locally in the intestine. The vaccine should contain the most prevalent CFs in highly immunogenic form in combination with a suitable enterotoxoid and induce gut secretory IgA antibodies against CFs and enterotoxin(s). Such immune responses are most efficiently evoked by oral or intraintestinal antigen administration [16,42]. Thus an ideal ETEC vaccine should be given orally and contain a combination of highly protective, yet nonreactogenic, bacterial and toxin antigens. Based on these considerations, different approaches for effective immunoprophylaxis against ETEC have been attempted. They include both live and inactivated candidate immunogens that in the vast majority of the cases are given orally along with acid-neutralizing buffer or incorporated into microcapsules (Table 2), or administration of preformed anti-CF antibodies, e.g., derived from the milk of hyperimmunized cows [43].

A. Live Bacteria

A number of different live bacterial vaccine candidates, either nontoxigenic derivatives of wild-type ETEC or attenuated heterologous carrier strains such as Shigellae or Salmonellae expressing the major CFs and producing an enterotoxoid, have been developed and will be described elsewhere in this volume (see Chapter 70). The potential

Table 2 Enterotoxigenic *E. coli* Vaccine Candidates Tested in Humans

Live
- Toxin-negative, CF-positive *Escherichia coli*
- Live vectors expressing different CFs (e.g., attenuated *Salmonella typhi*, *Shigella*, *Vibrio cholerae*)

Passive immunoprophylaxis
- Milk formulas containing anti-CF and/or anti-LT antibodies

Inactivated
- Enterotoxoids (LTB or CTB or LTBST)
- Purified colonization factors (CFs); alone or in microspheres
- Inactivated CF-positive *E. coli* (e.g., colicin-inactivated)
- Inactivated CF-positive *E. coli* together with enterotoxoid (rCTB-CF ETEC)

problem of coadministering several live strains with the risk of competition between strains in the intestine is a barrier to be overcome in the development of a live vaccine. Furthermore, the development of acquired ETEC immunity in persons living in ETEC-endemic areas may result in partial or complete protection against colonization, and hence effective immunization, by live ETEC vaccine strains. Thus it has been observed for other live oral candidate vaccines that considerably higher doses of bacteria are required for induction of significant immune responses in countries where the actual infection is endemic than in nonprimed populations, and that a vaccine dose that is protective in nonendemic areas fails to induce significant protection in a primed population [44]. High doses of a live vaccine may, however, even in endemic areas be reactogenic in those that have not been primed by natural exposure, e.g., very young infants and subjects that have been less exposed to ETEC during childhood. Therefore identification of a dose of live attenuated bacteria that is immunogenic and yet nonreactogenic in populations with different immune "preparedness" may be a difficult task.

B. Milk Formulas

Another approach that has been attempted is to immunize lactating animals with the key protective antigens and then to feed persons with antibodies derived from the milk or colostrum of the immunized cows or sows [43]. This approach obviously requires repeated administration of milk containing a suitable mixture of anti-CF, anti-LT, and perhaps also anti-ST antibodies during the entire period when the population is at risk of developing ETEC diarrhea.

C. Inactivated Vaccines

The third and perhaps most feasible current approach is to provide the key protective antigens in purified form or as expressed on inactivated bacteria.

1. *Purified fimbriae.* The most promising bacterial antigens for inclusion in an ETEC vaccine are those CFs that have the highest prevalence on ETEC

strains in different geographic areas, namely, CFA/I and the different subcomponents of CFA/II and CFA/IV and probably a few additional CFs. Monovalent vaccines consisting of purified CFA/I, CS1 + CS3, or CS6 have been tested in humans [28,45,46]. Efficient processes for preparation of purified CFs at a reasonable cost are still being worked out. Since purified CFs are very sensitive to proteolytic degradation in the stomach, incorporation of these antigens into biodegradable microspheres has been tried [29,46]. In one study, multiple high doses of microencapsulated CS1 + CS3 were given to human volunteers, but failed to confer significant protection against subsequent challenge with ETEC expressing the homologous CFs [29,46].

2. *Enterotoxoids.* Since the immunologically cross-reactive purified B subunits of CT and *E. coli* LT (CTB and LTB) are strongly immunogenic and lack toxicity, they are suitable candidate antigens to provide anti-LT immunity. Furthermore, LTB and CTB are particularly well suited as oral immunogens because they are stable in the gastrointestinal milieu, are capable of binding to the intestinal epithelium, and are effective in stimulating mucosal immunity, including local immunological memory [16]. Although CTB has afforded significant protection against *E. coli* LT disease in humans, an LT toxoid may be somewhat more effective than CTB in inducing protective anti-LT immunity. However, a suitable and cheap production method for CTB is available, making it the most attractive candidate LT toxoid to date. Thus a recombinant *Vibrio cholerae* strain, from which the genes for the toxic A subunit have been deleted and that overproduce CTB, has been constructed [47] and a simple method that allows purification of recombinant CTB (rCTB) of this strain has been developed [48]. Such rCTB is presently used for immunoprophylaxis against ETEC in the oral inactivated CTB-WC cholera vaccine (Dukoral®). Cholera toxin B may later be replaced by a more LT-like B subunit since the structural gene for CTB can be modified to encode B subunits that also contain LTB-specific epitopes [49].

3. *Inactivated whole cells.* The simplest approach to construct an inactivated ETEC vaccine is to prepare killed ETEC bacteria that express the most important CFs in immunogenic form on their surface. Such inactivated organisms may be combined with an appropriate toxoid component, e.g., CTB or LTB. Inactivation of the bacteria may be achieved by mild formalin treatment [50]. This procedure results in complete killing of bacteria without significant loss in antigenicity of the different CFs and O antigens. Formalin-inactivated bacteria retain 50–100% of the antigenicity of the CFs on the bacterial surface [14,16]. Furthermore, the fimbrial structure of the CFs as well as their capacity to bind to eukaryotic cell surfaces are retained. The CFs of the formalin-inactivated bacteria are more stable than purified fimbriae in that they retain their antigenicity even after incubation in human gastrointestinal secretions or in the human stomach/small intestine [31,50].

An alternative method to inactivate ETEC bacteria that does not damage protein antigens associated with the organisms was developed by Evans et al. [51]. The procedure involved the treatment of bacteria with colicin E2, a drug that enters the bacterial cell by means of receptors on sensitive *E. coli* strains. However, the issue of whether colicin E2 treatment could be relied on for reproducible inactivation of different *E. coli* strains for use in human vaccines was raised, and this approach has not been further developed.

V. ORAL INACTIVATED CTB-CF ETEC VACCINE

The ETEC vaccine that has been most extensively studied in clinical trials consists of different combinations of formalin-inactivated CF-expressing *E. coli* and CTB. In collaboration with SBL Vaccin, Stockholm, Sweden, an ETEC vaccine with the potential of providing broad protective coverage against ETEC disease in different countries has been developed [16,52,53]. The vaccine consists of a combination of CTB and formalin-inactivated *E. coli* bacteria that express CFA/I and different subcomponents of CFA/II and CFA/IV (CS1–CS5) as well as some of the O antigens that are commonly associated with ETEC [31]. The rationale for the design of this vaccine is indicated in Table 3.

A. Testing of a Prototype Vaccine

Initially, a prototype of this vaccine consisting of a mixture of killed *E. coli* expressing CFA/I, CS1, CS2, and CS3 together with CTB was tested. The CTB component was provided by adding the oral CTB-WC cholera vaccine to inactivated *E. coli* bacteria [52,53]. Strains that belonged to common ETEC groups (O6, O78, and O139) and expressed the different fimbriae in high concentrations were selected. The safety and immunogenicity of the prototype CTB-CF ETEC vaccine were studied in adult Swedish volunteers with promising results [52,53]. Thus as shown in studies of adult volunteers, the vaccine was safe and gave rise to significant IgA immune responses in intestinal lavages against CFA/I

Table 3 Rationale for the Design of the rCTB-CF ETEC Vaccine

- Synergy between antitoxic (anti-LT) and anticolonization immunity for protection against ETEC diarrhea
- CTB affords highly significant protection against ETEC LT and LTST disease in humans
- *E. coli* CFs are strongly protective against ETEC expressing homologous CFs in humans and animals
- Formalinized CF-positive *E. coli* are stable in the stomach and induce strong mucosal anti-CF immune responses
- Vaccine can be designed to include several CFs and recombinantly produced toxoid

and the different subcomponents of CFA/II as well as against CTB in a majority (70–90%) of the vaccines [51]. In most of the volunteers, intestinal immune responses were maximal after a second immunization. In some volunteers, there was even a decrease in CF response after the third as compared with the second dose [52]. The prototype ETEC vaccine also gave rise to significant increases in peripheral blood antibody-secreting cell (ASC) responses with specificity for CFA/I, CFA/II, and CTB in 85–100% of the volunteers [53]. Responses against the CFs were predominantly in IgA-producing cells suggesting that these cells were of mucosal origin. Antibody-secreting cell responses against CTB, on the other hand, were seen in both IgA and IgG cells but not in IgM. The results of these studies suggested that two oral immunizations are probably sufficient to induce optimal CF-specific immune response by the vaccine in immunologically naive volunteers.

B. Development of Methods for Assessing Mucosal Immune Responses for Use in Clinical Trials of ETEC Vaccine

Despite inducing significant intestinal lavage as well as peripheral blood ASC responses that were probably intestinally derived, the prototype-inactivated vaccine was relatively inefficient in eliciting serum antibody responses against the different CFs [52]. The CTB component, on the other hand, induced serum antibody responses that were comparable both in frequency and in magnitude to the responses in intestinal lavage fluid. Therefore the conventional approach of assessing immunogenicity of the vaccine as its capacity to induce serum antibody responses was not suitable, at least for determining the immunogenicity of the CF components in a nonprimed population. Since initial studies in Swedish volunteers showed a strong correlation between IgA immune responses against the ETEC vaccine in intestinal lavage fluid and the IgA ASC responses in peripheral blood [54], the immunogenicity of the ETEC vaccine has, in most subsequent studies, been determined as circulating ASC responses. This method is clearly superior to the intestinal lavage method in simplicity and sensitivity. However, determination of ASC responses has several disadvantages, such as problems in standardization, difficulties in comparing preimmunization and postimmunization levels on the same day, need for relatively large volumes of peripheral blood and requirements for tissue culturing equipment, etc. Therefore much effort has been made to develop a simple, yet reproducible, approach for assessing mucosal immune responses against the ETEC vaccine. These approaches include determination of immune responses in fecal specimens [54], measurements of specific antibodies in saponin extracts of intestinal biopsies [33], or indirect determination of mucosal immune responses as reflected in serum in immunologically primed populations [55].

C. Phase I/Phase II Trials of the rCTB-CF ETEC Vaccine in Adults

Based on the promising results with the prototype vaccine, a more definitive formulation of the CTB-CF ETEC vaccine

was developed (Table 4). This modified vaccine contained rCTB in combination with five different *E. coli* strains collectively expressing CFA/I and the different subcomponents of CFA/II (CS1, CS2, and CS3) and CFA/IV (CS4 and CS5), respectively. The rCTB-CF ETEC vaccine was first tested extensively in Phase I trials in Sweden and subsequently in the United States and in different ETEC-endemic countries. Such studies in several hundred adult volunteers who received one or two oral doses of the vaccine confirmed that the vaccine was safe and only gave rise to mild gastrointestinal symptoms and borborygmus in a few volunteers [33,54–60].

In initial Phase I trials in Swedish volunteers, the capacity of the rCTB-CF ETEC vaccine to induce ASC responses in peripheral blood was evaluated [56,58]. Two doses of vaccine given 2 weeks apart induced strong increases in CTB-specific IgA ASCs in 95–100% of the vaccinees and significant IgA ASC responses against CFA/I, CFA/II, and CFA/IV, respectively, in 85–95% of the volunteers (Table 5). In some of the volunteers, immune responses in intestinal lavage fluid, fecal extracts, and serum were also evaluated [54]. These analyses showed that ~ 70–90% of the volunteers responded with significant IgA responses to CFA/I, CFA/II, or CFA/IV in intestinal lavages, whereas 45–75% responded in fecal extracts. Responses against CTB were seen in 90–95% of the vaccinees irrespective of whether lavages or fecal specimens were tested [54,56].

Based on the results from these studies, determination of vaccine-specific ASCs in peripheral blood to the rCTB-CF ETEC vaccine has been done in subsequent studies in, e.g., the United States (Taylor et al., unpublished data), Bangladesh [57], Egypt [60], and Israel [59]. Results from studies in adult Bangladeshis and Egyptians show that the frequencies and magnitudes of ASC responses against the different CFs are comparable to those observed in Swedish volunteers (Table 5) [57,60]. Taken together, these trials in different countries indicate that the rCTB-CF ETEC vaccine gives rise to significant mucosal or mucosa-derived (blood ASC) immune responses against the CFs of the vaccine in a majority of the volunteers (70–95%) and against CTB in as many as 90–100% of them. The frequencies and magnitudes of serum antibody responses against the CFs, on the other hand, were considerably lower and were mainly of IgA rather than IgG type, suggesting their intestinal origin (Table 5). Serum antibody responses against CTB were

Table 4 Oral rCTB-CF ETEC Vaccine

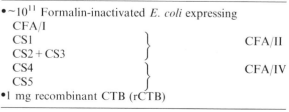

Given as two or three doses 1–2 weeks apart.

Table 5 Antibody-Secreting Cell and Serum IgA Antibody Responses to Oral Immunizations with the rCTB-CF ETEC Vaccine in Adult Volunteers from Different Countries [55,57,58,60]

Residents of	IgA ASC % responders (magnitudes)[a] to			Serum IgA % responders (magnitudes)[b] to		
	CTB	CFA/I	CS2	CTB	CFA/I	CS2
Sweden	95 (724)	95 (79)	90 (28)	95 (50)	65 (2.7)	40 (2.0)
Bangladesh	100 (426)	91 (40)	100 (29)	91 (3.7)	55 (2.1)	n.t.
Egypt	100 (n.d.)	94 (n.d.)	81 (n.d.)	95 (13)	68 (2.1)	31 (1.7)

n.t.—not tested; n.d.—not determined.

[a] Cumulative responses after a first or a second dose given 2 weeks apart; a positive response is a ≥ 2-fold increase between ASC/10^7 MNC between preimmunization and postimmunization values. Magnitudes of responses represent the ratio between baseline and the highest postimmunization level (after one or two doses).

[b] Percent volunteers with significant ≥ 2-fold increase in ELISA titers between preimmunization and postimmunization (after two doses) specimens.

observed in more than 90% of the vaccinees in all different studies. The magnitudes of IgA responses in Swedish volunteers were considerably higher than in vaccinees in ETEC-endemic countries, but this was mainly related to the considerably lower preimmunization levels in the nonprimed Swedes than in adult Bangladeshis or Egyptians.

D. Dose Dependence and Immunological Memory

The rCTB-CF ETEC vaccine has also been tested for reproducibility in production, dose dependence, and capacity to induce an immunological memory in adult Swedish volunteers. Different batches of the vaccine have induced substantial and comparable mucosal immune responses against the different CFs of the vaccine in a majority of the volunteers [58]. Studies have also revealed a clear dose dependence with regard to both mucosal and systemic antibody responses against the CF components of the vaccine, allowing the determination of optimal immunizing doses in different study populations [58]. Compared to adult Swedes given a full dose (see Table 4), those given a one-third dose of the whole cell component exhibited lower frequencies of IgA ASC responses against all the different CFs. The proportion of vaccinees responding with rises in serum IgA antibody titers against the various CFs was also lower after immunization with a reduced dose of ETEC bacteria, and responses in serum were considerably lower than the ASC responses. These findings suggest that measurements of circulating IgA ASCs can be used for quantitative assessment of the immunogenicity of individual fimbrial antigens in various preparations of ETEC vaccine. Based on these results, studies have recently been initiated in Bangladesh to compare a full dose, a half dose, and a quarter dose of ETEC vaccine in children, aged 6–36 months, to determine the lowest dose that can induce strong immune responses also in very young children (Qadri et al., unpublished data).

The immune responses after a single, two, and three doses of vaccine as well as against a booster dose given 1 year later have also been compared in adult Swedish volunteers. These analyses revealed that two doses were optimal in inducing mucosal immune responses in intestinal lavage fluid both against the whole cell component and against

CTB [52,56]. Thus a third dose of vaccine only occasionally resulted in higher anti-CF IgA antibody levels in intestinal lavage than two doses, and, in most instances, there was instead a decrease in IgA level after the third dose [52]. With regard to responses against CTB, on the other hand, equally or, even in a few cases, higher anti-CTB levels were observed after three than two doses. In subsequent studies, it was shown that two doses of vaccine induced considerably higher and more frequent antitoxin IgA levels in intestinal lavage fluid than a single dose. Thus whereas only 37% of 19 vaccinated adult Swedish volunteers responded with a mean 5-fold increase in specific antitoxin/total IgA levels after the first dose, as many as 89% responded with a mean 23-fold rise after the second dose (Åhrén et al., unpublished data). Also, the frequencies of intestinal lavage responses against the different CF components were higher after two than a single dose, although the differences were less marked than observed for the antitoxin immune responses. For example, 42% of the vaccinees responded with significantly elevated IgA anti-CFA/I levels after the first dose and 63% with comparable magnitudes of responses after the second dose (Åhrén et al., unpublished data). Similarly, two doses were more efficient than a single dose in inducing serum IgA antibody responses, i.e., the serum conversion rate was 50% after the first dose vs. 65% after the second dose for CFA/I, 15% vs. 40% for CS2, and 35% vs. 95% for CTB [58]. With regard to IgA ASC responses in peripheral blood, on the other hand, the frequencies and magnitudes of the different anti-CF ASC responses were comparable, or even lower, after the first and the second immunization, whereas the CTB-specific IgA ASC responses were considerably higher ($P < 0.001$) after the second dose [58]. A single booster dose given after 1 year resulted in similar antitoxin responses both in intestinal lavages and as ASC responses in peripheral blood after two initial doses, whereas the CF responses seem to be comparable to those observed after the initial dose (Åhrén et al., unpublished data).

E. Protective Efficacy Studies in Adult Travelers

A number of different studies to evaluate the protective efficacy of the rCTB-CF ETEC vaccine have been initiated in adult travelers going from industrialized areas to different countries in Asia, Africa, and Latin America. In an initial pilot study, the ETEC vaccine was tested for protective efficacy in European travelers going to 20 different countries in Africa, Asia, and Latin America [13]. The protective efficacy of the ETEC vaccine was compared with that of the CTB-WC cholera vaccine and *E. coli* K12 placebo. This study revealed very promising results in that the ETEC vaccine conferred 82% protective efficacy ($P < 0.05$) against ETEC disease, whereas the effect of the cholera vaccine could not be evaluated due to the infrequency of cases associated with LT-positive ETEC. However, the number of cases fulfilling the inclusion criteria overall was low and the findings of this promising pilot study need to be supported in additional studies.

Another trial was initiated several years ago in European travelers going to Kenya. However, due to very few cases fulfilling the inclusion criteria, no conclusions of the protective efficacy of the vaccine could be deduced from this study (Steffen et al., unpublished data).

A large controlled trial was recently completed in American travelers going to Mexico and Guatemala [61]. In that study, 685 adult Americans either received the rCTB-CF ETEC vaccine or *E. coli* K12 placebo in a double-blinded fashion. The vaccine showed a protective efficacy of 77% ($P = 0.039$) against nonmild ETEC diarrheal illness [61], but no significant protection was observed when ETEC diarrheal cases of any severity (also including mild cases) were considered. Another trial is now being completed in the same setting to carefully assess vaccine efficacy against ETEC diarrheal disease where symptoms interfere with the daily activity of the traveler (Bourgeois, personal communication).

F. Pediatric Evaluation of the rCTB-CF ETEC Vaccine

From a public health standpoint, a vaccine against ETEC is most needed for infants and young children in developing countries. Save major improvements in sanitation in these settings, a vaccine is sought that substantially reduces the acute morbidity and mortality of ETEC diarrhea and conceivably stems long-term morbidity such as growth impairment. To investigate suitability of the oral rCTB-CF ETEC vaccine for a pediatric indication, clinical studies have thus far been conducted in Egypt and Bangladesh, two countries where a high incidence of ETEC diarrhea in childhood has been well documented.

Undertaking pediatric clinical trials with an ETEC vaccine presents some special challenges. Ethically, pediatric testing must be confined to children who are at risk from ETEC diarrhea, namely, those living in developing countries. Studies could only be initiated after the accrual of sufficient safety data from adults so as to minimize undue risk to children. In evaluating vaccine immune responses, attention must be paid to the possible effects of preexisting immunity and intercurrent boosting due to natural exposure to ETEC. In evaluating efficacy, the degree and duration of protection are both important considerations since at-risk children are frequently exposed to ETEC throughout childhood and beyond. Delay of onset of ETEC diarrhea rather than disease prevention would be an undesirable consequence of vaccination.

At the outset, a framework for evaluation of the rCTB-CF ETEC vaccine in Egyptian infants and young children was designed that would culminate in the evaluation of vaccine efficacy. As shown in Figure 1, this framework included epidemiological studies to ascertain disease incidence and establish the infrastructure for an efficacy trial and corollary studies to examine feasibility issues, both of which complemented the actual clinical trial pathway. Site selection for vaccine testing in Egypt was made in cooperation with national health authorities based on ETEC incidence data and community interest in the research project. Studies in Bangladesh utilized a longstanding research infrastructure for the evaluation of diarrheal disease interventions. In both locations, safety and immunogenicity studies were completed in native adults before initiating pediatric studies.

In both Egypt and Bangladesh, sequential studies in descending age groups of children have been completed, providing a comprehensive assessment of the safety and immunogenicity of the rCTB-CF ETEC vaccine. All of the trials in Egypt used a randomized, double-blind, placebo-controlled study design. The findings from these trials are summarized in the following sections.

1. rCTB-CF ETEC Vaccine Safety Data in Children

Egyptian children between 2 and 12 years of age given a two-dose (0, 2 weeks) schedule of the oral rCTB-CF ETEC vaccine, coadministered with a graduated dose of antacid, tolerated the vaccine very well. As shown in Table 6, a small proportion of children in this age range experienced gastrointestinal symptoms (i.e., diarrhea and vomiting) in the postdosing interval, with no difference between vaccine and control groups. Safety findings from an uncontrolled study in Bangladeshi children in the same age range were similar [57]. No systemic adverse events were associated with vaccine administration in this age range. Perhaps the most pertinent indicator of safety was the finding that the vast majority of Egyptian children receiving the rCTB-CF ETEC vaccine reported no disturbance in their general well-being after vaccination.

The next study done in Egypt evaluated a three-dose (0, 2, 4 weeks) schedule of the rCTB-CF ETEC vaccine in 6–18 months old children. The vaccine dose was the same as that given to adults and children in earlier trials and was coadministered with 1/10 the adult dose of antacid. Findings confirmed the safety of the vaccine in this age range, although it did raise questions about acceptability of the preparation. Diarrhea and vomiting were the most common adverse events. The proportion of subjects reporting these or other events did not differ significantly between vaccine and control groups, but generally occurred more commonly than in older vaccinated children. Subgroup analyses suggested that the vaccine was associated with an excess of gastrointestinal symptoms in children less than 1 year of age. Due to the mild nature of these symptoms observed in young Egyptian children, this was not regarded as a barrier for

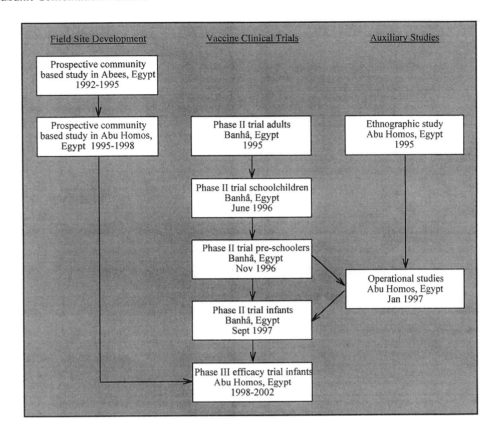

Figure 1   Schematic presentation of research program and interleaved studies undertaken to assess the safety, immunogenicity, and efficacy of the oral rCTB-CF ETEC vaccine in Egypt.

proceeding with an efficacy trial using the same dosing. In a controlled study performed in young Bangladeshi children, children under 18 months of age experienced higher rates of vomiting than older children. This prompted investigators to undertake a dose ranging study to identify a lower dose that resulted in less reactogenicity but undiminished immunogenicity. Preliminary analysis of this study suggests that one quarter of the adult dose of the rCTB-CF ETEC vaccine is well tolerated and immunogenic (Qadri, personal communication).

2.   rCTB-CF ETEC Vaccine Immunogenicity in Children

Following the approach established in adult Phase I clinical trials of the rCTB-CF ETEC vaccine, measurement of circulating B-cell IgA antibody-secreting cell (IgA-ASC) responses to vaccine cellular (CF) antigens was used as the primary determinant of immunogenicity in the initial studies in older (2–12 year age range) Egyptian and Bangladeshi children. Serologic responses were also measured in these

Table 6   Percentage of Egyptian Children with Diarrhea and Vomiting in the 3 days After Each Dose of the rCTB-CF ETEC Vaccine or *E. coli* K12 Control

Age group	Dose	n^a	Diarrhea		Vomiting	
			Vaccine	Control	Vaccine	Control
6–12 years	1	52/55	4	4	0	2
	2	51/54	0	0	4	4
2–5 years	1	54/52	4	4	6	4
	2	49/48	4	6	4	4
6–18 months	1	48/47	19	19	25	17
	2	47/40	17	5	21	15
	3	36/28	3	4	11	14

[a] Number in vaccine group/number in placebo group.

children, permitting an assessment of the correlation between seroconversion and antibody-secreting cell responses. With the exception of two studies in Bangladeshi children [57,62] in which circulating B-cell IgA responses to rCTB were measured, serum anti-rCTB antibody responses served as the endpoint for determining antitoxic immunity in all children. Anti-CF serologic responses were adopted as the primary immune measure in children under 2 years of age due to practical constraints in drawn blood volumes and demonstration that these measures were strongly predictive of IgA-ASC responses in older children as discussed below.

The rCTB vaccine component predictably evoked strong serological responses in the great majority of children [57,62–64]. IgA antitoxin titers increased after each of two doses given to Egyptian children as young as 2 years, whereas a third dose, given to 6- to 18-month Egyptian children only, did not result in a further titer increase (see Figure 2). Dose-to-dose boosting of IgG antitoxin titers was observed in older children given a two-dose vaccine schedule as well as in the 6- to 18-month-old children receiving three doses, as shown in Figure 2. The study in 3- to 9-year-old

Bangladeshi children found a significant correlation between circulating IgA-ASC responses and IgA serological responses to rCTB [57]. These findings extend upon earlier studies of the whole cell cholera B-subunit vaccine in older subjects to show that orally delivered rCTB is a very potent immunogen in children as young as 6 months of age.

Similar to findings in adult vaccinees in Egypt and Bangladesh, a high proportion of children 18 months–12 years of age exhibited circulating IgA antibody-secreting cell (ASC) responses to several of the CF components of the CTB-CF ETEC vaccine [57,62,63] (Table 7). Apparent differences in the timing of maximal CF-specific IgA-ASC responses, which occurred after the first dose in school-aged children in contrast to preschool children who exhibited similar or greater levels after both doses, may reflect the degree of past priming from natural ETEC infection. In Bangladeshi children, the magnitudes of the anti-CF IgA-ASC responses were lower than the corresponding antitoxin IgA-ASC responses [57,62]. These findings show that in children as young as 18 mo of age, the rCTB-CF ETEC vaccine stimulates mucosal immunity to the CF vaccine

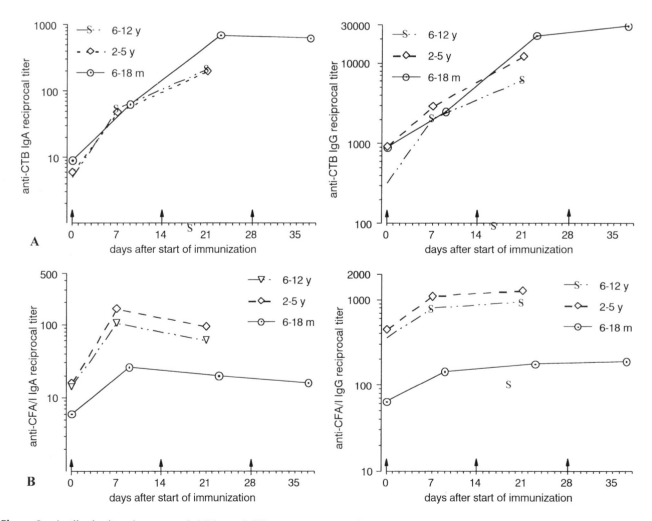

Figure 2 Antibody titers in serum of children of different age groups after 1, 2, and 3 oral doses of rCTB-CF ETEC vaccine. A = antiCTB IgA; B = anti-CTB Igg; C = antiCFA/I IgA; D = antiCFA/I Igg.

Table 7 Percentage of Egyptian Vaccinees Mounting a Mucosal IgA Antibody-Secreting Cell Response, as well as IgA and IgG Seroconversion Against Selected Components of the rCTB-CF ETEC Vaccine

Antigen	Immune measure	Age group		
		6–12 years	2–5 years	6–18 months
CTB	Serum IgA	100[a]	96[a]	97[a]
	Serum IgG	100[a]	94[a]	97[a]
CFA/I	IgA-ASC	100[a]	95[a]	n.t.
	Serum IgA	96[a]	87[a]	61[a]
	Serum IgG	75[a]	70[a]	64[b]
CS2	IgA-ASC	92[a]	83[a]	n.t.
	Serum IgA	78[a]	79[a]	26
	Serum IgG	44[b]	50[b]	53[a]
CS4	IgA-ASC	93[a]	n.t.	n.t.
	Serum IgA	84[a]	70[a]	39[a]
	Serum IgG	44[b]	60[b]	58[a]

n.t.—not tested.

[a] P < 0.001, chi-square test, comparing proportion of responders after any dose to that of the control group.

[b] P < 0.01, chi-square test, comparing proportion of responders after any dose to that of the control group.

components, inasmuch as this is reflected by circulating IgA B cell responses.

The most extensive evaluation of anti-CF serologic responses to the CTB-CF ETEC vaccine in children has thus far been carried out in Egypt. A majority of children aged 6 months to 12 years of age manifest IgG seroconversion (defined as a ≥2-fold increase over baseline titer) to CFA/I, CS2, and CS4 (Table 7), the proportion of seroresponders being comparable across age groups. Over two-thirds of children aged 2–12 years exhibited IgA seroconversion to these same antigens, while a lower proportion of 6- to 18-month-old vaccine recipients exhibited IgA seroconversion to CS2 and CS4. It was also shown that in the age range of 2–45 years, the magnitude of IgA serologic responses was inversely associated with age, even after controlling for baseline titer. This relationship did not, however, hold up with the inclusion of children under 2 years of age, inasmuch

as their fold increases in anti-CF antibody titers were distinctly lower than in 2- to 12-year-old children (see Figure 2).

Since both anti-CF IgA-ASC and plasma IgA and IgG antibody responses were examined in trials of school-aged and preschool Egyptian children, it was possible to assess how well these measures correlated. Considering the IgA-ASC responses as the standard, it was found that a twofold seroconversion of either IgA or IgG antibodies was highly predictive of a positive IgA-ASC response. IgA seroconversion had the advantage of being a more sensitive predictor of IgA-ASC response, whereas IgG seroconversion showed slightly higher specificity. Table 8 depicts these comparisons for CFA/I and CS2 over a range of cutoff points that signify seroconversion. These data suggest the validity of IgA and IgG seroresponses as measures of CTB-ETEC CF vaccine immunogenicity in an endemic population and support the decision of using serologic responses as the primary measure

Table 8 Sensitivity, Specificity, and Positive Predictive Accuracy (Percentages) of IgA and IgG Antibody Seroconversion in Identifying IgA-ASC Responses over the Range of Cutoff Points from ≥2.0- to ≥4.0-fold Increase in Antibody Titer, in Egyptian Children Aged 2–12 Years

Antigen/ titer fold-increase cutoff	IgA isotype			IgG isotype		
	Sensitivity	Specificity	PPA	Sensitivity	Specificity	PPA
CFA/I						
≥2.0[a]	88	91	>99	74	100	100
≥3.0	79	91	>99	47	100	100
≥4.0	68	91	>99	29	100	100
CS2						
≥2.0[a]	81	95	99	56	100	100
≥3.0	74	95	99	33	100	100
≥4.0	67	100	100	22	100	100

[a] Note that the predefined cutoff for defining a positive seroconversion in these studies was ≥2.0 fold-increase over baseline.

of ETEC vaccine immunogenicity in infants and young children. It must be kept in mind that no immune measure has yet to be correlated with protection against ETEC disease, either following natural infection or vaccination. The search for such a protective immune correlate is an important objective to be considered in the design of vaccine efficacy studies as well as studies of naturally occurring ETEC disease and acquisition of immunity.

3. Evaluation of rCTB-CF ETEC Vaccine Efficacy in Children

To date, the only pediatric study to assess efficacy of the rCTB-CF ETEC vaccine has been undertaken in rural Egypt (Savarino et al., unpublished data). Initiated in 1999 and recently completed, this randomized, double-blind, controlled trial was conducted in healthy 6- to 18-month-old children. Two cohorts were entered 1 year apart and randomized to receive a three-dose regimen at 2-week intervals of the rCTB-CF ETEC vaccine or *E. coli* K-12 control. Disease detection was based on active surveillance through semiweekly household visits and culture of fecal specimens from children with diarrhea. The primary disease endpoint is occurrence of a first episode of diarrhea associated with excretion of LTST ETEC or ST ETEC expressing one or more vaccine-shared CFs over the first year of surveillance. The required sample size, based on firm incidence data drawn earlier from the same population, has been achieved and is expected to allow detection of an efficacy of $> 70\%$. Forthcoming results from this trial, currently in the data analysis phase, should be very useful in determining the future course of clinical studies with this and other ETEC vaccines, particularly as it relates to a pediatric indication.

REFERENCES

1. Black RE. The epidemiology of diarrheal disease: Implications for control by vaccines. Vaccine 1993; 11:100–106.
2. Report on Diarrheal Disease Vaccines. Geneva: World Health Organization, 1998.
3. Wennerås C, Erling V. Global distribution of enterotoxigenic *Escherichia coli* (ETEC): Epidemiology and virulence factors. WHO Report. In press.
4. Black RE. Epidemiology of travelers' diarrhea and relative importance of various pathogens. Rev Infect Dis 1990; 12 (Suppl 1):S73–S79.
5. Evans DJ, Evans DG. Determinants of microbial attachment and their genetic control. In: Farthing MJG, Keusch GT, eds. Enteric Infections: Mechanisms, Manifestations and Management. London: Chapman & Hall, 1989:31–40.
6. Qadri F, Das SK, Faruque AS, Fuchs GJ, Albert MJ, Sack RB, Svennerholm AM. Prevalence of toxin types and colonization factors in enterotoxigenic *Escherichia coli* isolated during a 2-year period from diarrheal patients in Bangladesh. J Clin Microbiol 2000; 38:27–31.
7. Black RE, Brown KH, Becker S. Effects of diarrhea associated with specific enteropathogens on the growth of children in rural Bangladesh. Pediatrics 1984; 73:799–805.
8. Lopez-Vidal Y, Calva JJ, Trujillo A, Ponce de Leon A, Ramos A, Svennerholm AM, Ruiz-Palacios GM. Enterotoxins and adhesins of enterotoxigenic *Escherichia coli*: Are they risk factors for acute diarrhea in the community? J Infect Dis 1990; 162:442–447.
9. Cravioto A, Reyes RE, Ortega R, Fernandez G, Hernandez R, Lopez D. Prospective study of diarrhoeal disease in a cohort of rural Mexican children: Incidence and isolated pathogens during the first two years of life. Epidemiol Infect 1988; 101: 123–134.
10. Clemens JD, Sack DA, Harris JR, Chakraborty J, Neogy PK, Stanton B, Huda N, Khan MU, Kay BA, Khan MR, et al. Cross-protection by B subunit-whole cell cholera vaccine against diarrhea associated with heat-labile toxin-producing enterotoxigenic *Escherichia coli*: Results of a large-scale field trial. J Infect Dis 1988; 158:372–377.
11. Peltola H, Siitonen A, Kyronseppa H, Simula I, Mattila L, Oksanen P, Kataja MJ, Cadoz M. Prevention of travellers' diarrhoea by oral B-subunit/whole-cell cholera vaccine. Lancet 1991; 338:1285–1289.
12. Scerpella EG, Sanchez JL, Mathewson IJ, Torres-Cordero JV, Sadoff JC, Svennerholm AM, DuPont HL, Taylor DN, Ericsson CD. Safety, immunogenicity, and protective efficacy of the whole-cell/recombinant B subunit (WC/rBS) oral cholera vaccine against travelers' diarrhea. J Travel Med 1995; 2:22–27.
13. Wiedermann G, Kollaritsch H, Kundi M, Svennerholm AM, Bjare U. Double-blind, randomized, placebo controlled pilot study evaluating efficacy and reactogenicity of an oral ETEC B-subunit-inactivated whole cell vaccine against travelers' diarrhea (preliminary report). J Travel Med 2000; 7:27–29.
14. Gaastra W, Svennerholm AM. Colonization factors of human enterotoxigenic *Escherichia coli* (ETEC). Trends Microbiol 1996; 4:444–452.
15. Peruski LF Jr, Kay BA, El-Yazeed RA, El-Etr SH, Cravioto A, Wierzba TF, Rao M, El-Ghorab N, Shaheen H, Khalil SB, Kamal K, Wasfy MO, Svennerholm AM, Clemens JD, Savarino SJ. Phenotypic diversity of enterotoxigenic *Escherichia coli* strains from a community-based study of pediatric diarrhea in periurban Egypt. J Clin Microbiol 1999; 37: 2974–2978.
16. Holmgren J, Svennerholm AM. Bacterial enteric infections and vaccine development. In: McDermott RP, Elson CO, eds. Mucosal Immunology: Gastroenterology Clinics of North America. Philadelphia: Saunders, 1992:283–302.
17. Wolf MK. Occurrence, distribution, and associations of O and H serogroups, colonization factor antigens, and toxins of enterotoxigenic *Escherichia coli*. Clin Microbiol Rev 1997; 10: 569–584.
18. Takeda Y, Honda T, Sima H, Tsuji T, Miwatani T. Analysis of antigenic determinants in cholera enterotoxin and heat-labile enterotoxins from human and porcine enterotoxigenic *Escherichia coli*. Infect Immun 1983; 41:50–53.
19. Rao MC. Toxins which activate guanylate cyclase: Heat stable enterotoxins. Evered D, Whelan J, eds. Microbial Toxins and Diarrhoeal Disease. Vol. 112. London: Ciba Foundation Symposium, 1985:74–93.
20. Svennerholm AM, Wikstrom M, Lindblad M, Holmgren J. Monoclonal antibodies against *Escherichia coli* heat-stable toxin (STa) and their use in a diagnostic ST ganglioside GM1-enzyme-linked immunosorbent assay. J Clin Microbiol 1986; 24:585–590.
21. Pichel M, Binsztein N, Viboud G. CS22, a novel human enterotoxigenic *Escherichia coli* adhesin, is related to CS15. Infect Immun 2000; 68:3280–3285.
22. Binsztein N, Jouve MJ, Viboud GI, Lopez Moral L, Rivas M, Orskov I, Åhrén C, Svennerholm AM. Colonization factors of enterotoxigenic *Escherichia coli* isolated from children with diarrhea in Argentina. J Clin Microbiol 1991; 29:1893–1898.
23. Wolf MK, Taylor DN, Boedeker EC, Hyams KC, Maneval DR, Levine MM, Tamura K, Wilson RA, Echeverria P. Characterization of enterotoxigenic *Escherichia coli* isolated from US troops deployed to the Middle East. J Clin Microbiol 1993; 31:851–856.

24. Viboud GI, Binsztein N, Svennerholm AM. Characterization of monoclonal antibodies against putative colonization factors of enterotoxigenic *Escherichia coli* and their use in an epidemiological study. J Clin Microbiol 1993; 31:558–564.

25. Paniagua M, Espinoza F, Ringman M, Reizenstein E, Svennerholm AM, Hallander H. Analysis of incidence of infection with enterotoxigenic *Escherichia coli* in a prospective cohort study of infant diarrhea in Nicaragua. J Clin Microbiol 1997; 35:1404–1410.

26. Svennerholm AM, Wenneras C, Holmgren J, McConnell MM, Rowe B. Roles of different coli surface antigens of colonization factor antigen II in colonization by and protective immunogenicity of enterotoxigenic *Escherichia coli* in rabbits. Infect Immun 1990; 58:341–346.

27. Svennerholm AM, McConnell MM, Wiklund G. Roles of different putative colonization factor antigens in colonization of human enterotoxigenic *Escherichia coli* in rabbits. Microb Pathog 1992; 13:381–389.

28. Levine MM, Ristaino P, Marley G, Smyth C, Knutton S, Boedeker E, Black R, Young C, Clements ML, Cheney C, et al. Coli surface antigens 1 and 3 of colonization factor antigen II-positive enterotoxigenic *Escherichia coli*: Morphology, purification, and immune responses in humans. Infect Immun 1984; 44:409–420.

29. Levine MM. Vaccines against enterotoxigenic *Escherichia coli* infections. In: Woodrow GC, Levine MM, eds. New Generation Vaccines. New York: Marcel Dekker Inc., 1990:649–660.

30. Svennerholm AM, Vidal YL, Holmgren J, McConnell MM, Rowe B. Role of PCF8775 antigen and its coli surface subcomponents for colonization, disease, and protective immunogenicity of enterotoxigenic *Escherichia coli* in rabbits. Infect Immun 1988; 56:523–528.

31. Svennerholm AM, Åhren C, Jertborn M. Oral inactivated vaccines against enterotoxigenic *Escherichia coli*. In: Levine MM, Woodrow GC, Kaper JB, Gabon GS, eds. New Generation Vaccines: II ed. New York: Marcel Dekker Inc., 1997:865–874.

32. Stoll BJ, Svennerholm AM, Gothefors L, Barua D, Huda S, Holmgren J. Local and systemic antibody responses to naturally acquired enterotoxigenic *Escherichia coli* diarrhea in an endemic area. J Infect Dis 1986; 153:527–534.

33. Wennerås C, Qadri F, Bardhan PK, Sack RB, Svennerholm AM. Intestinal immune responses in patients infected with enterotoxigenic *Escherichia coli* and in vaccinees. Infect Immun 1999; 67:6234–6241.

34. Evans DG, de la Cabada FJ, Evans DJ Jr. Correlation between intestinal immune response to colonization factor antigen/I and acquired resistance to enterotoxigenic *Escherichia coli* diarrhea in an adult rabbit model. Eur J Clin Microbiol 1982; 1:178–185.

35. Neutra MR, Kraehenbühl JP. Transepithelial Transport and Mucosal Defenced I: The Role of M Cells 1992; Vol. 2. Oxford: Elsevier Science Publishers Ltd, 1992:134–138.

36. Aitken R, Hirst TR. Recombinant enterotoxin as vaccines against *Escherichia coli*-modified diarrhoea. Vaccine 1993; 11: 227–233.

37. Sanchez J, Svennerholm AM, Holmgren J. Genetic fusion of a non-toxic heat-stable enterotoxin-related decapeptide antigen to cholera toxin B-subunit. FEBS Lett 1988; 241:110–114.

38. Clemens JD, Svennerholm AM, Harris JR, Huda S, Rao M, Neogy PK, Khan MR, Ansaruzzaman M, Rahaman S, Ahmed F, et al. Seroepidemiologic evaluation of anti-toxic and anti-colonization factor immunity against infections by LT-producing *Escherichia coli* in rural Bangladesh. J Infect Dis 1990; 162:448–453.

39. Åhren CM, Svennerholm AM. Synergistic protective effect of antibodies against *Escherichia coli* enterotoxin and colonization factor antigens. Infect Immun 1982; 38:74–79.

40. Levine MM, Nalin DR, Hoover DL, Bergquist EJ, Hornick RB, Young CR. Immunity to enterotoxigenic *Escherichia coli*. Infect Immun 1979; 23:729–736.

41. Rudin A, McConnell MM, Svennerholm AM. Monoclonal antibodies against enterotoxigenic *Escherichia coli* colonization factor antigen I (CFA/I) that cross-react immunologically with heterologous CFAs. Infect Immun 1994; 62:4339–4346.

42. Rudin A, Wiklund G, Wenneras C, Qadri F. Infection with colonization factor antigen I-expressing enterotoxigenic *Escherichia coli* boosts antibody responses against heterologous colonization factors in primed subjects. Epidemiol Infect 1997; 119:391–393.

43. Freedman DJ, Tacket CO, Delehanty A, Maneval DR, Nataro J, Crabb JH. Milk immunoglobulin with specific activity against purified colonization factor antigens can protect against oral challenge with enterotoxigenic *Escherichia coli*. J Infect Dis 1998; 177:662–667.

44. Richie E, Punjabi NH, Sidharta YY, Peetosutan KK, Sukandar MM, Wasserman SS, Lesmana MM, Wangsasaputra FF, Pandam SS, Levine MM, O'Hanley PP, Cryz SJ, Simanjuntak CH. Efficacy trial of single-dose live oral cholera vaccine CVD 103-HgR in North Jakarta, Indonesia, a cholera-endemic area. Vaccine 2000; 18:2399–2410.

45. Evans DG, Graham DY, Evans DJ Jr. Administration of purified colonization factor antigens (CFA/I, CFA/II) of enterotoxigenic *Escherichia coli* to volunteers. Response to challenge with virulent enterotoxigenic *Escherichia coli*. Gastroenterology 1984; 87:934–940.

46. Tacket CO, Reid RH, Boedeker EC, Losonsky G, Nataro JP, Bhagat H, Edelman R. Enteral immunization and challenge of volunteers given enterotoxigenic *E. coli* CFA/II encapsulated in biodegradable microspheres. Vaccine 1994; 12:1270–1274.

47. Sanchez J, Holmgren J. Recombinant systems for overexpression of cholera toxin B subunit in *Vibrio cholerae* as a basis for vaccine development. Proc Natl Acad Sci USA 1989; 86: 481–485.

48. Holmgren J, Jertborn M, Svennerholm AM. Oral B subunit killed whole-cell cholera vaccine. In: Levine MM, Woodrow GC, Kaper JB, Gabon GS, eds. New Generation Vaccines. New York: Marcel Dekker Inc., 1997:459–468.

49. Lebens M, Shahabi V, Bäckström M, Houze T, Lindblad N, Holmgren J. Synthesis of hybrid molecules between heat-labile enterotoxin and cholera toxin B subunits: Potential for use in a broad-spectrum vaccine. Infect Immun 1996; 64:2144–2150.

50. Svennerholm AM, Holmgren J, Sack DA. Development of oral vaccines against enterotoxinogenic *Escherichia coli* diarrhea. Vaccine 1989; 7:196–198.

51. Evans DG, Evans DJ Jr, Opekun AR, Graham DY. Nonreplicating oral whole cell vaccine protective against enterotoxigenic *Escherichia coli* (ETEC) diarrhea: Stimulation of anti-CFA (CFA/I) and anti-enterotoxin (anti-LT) intestinal IgA and protection against challenge with ETEC belonging to heterologous serotypes. FEMS Microbiol Immunol 1988; 1: 117–125.

52. Åhren C, Wennerås C, Holmgren J, Svennerholm AM. Intestinal antibody response after oral immunization with a prototype cholera B subunit-colonization factor antigen enterotoxigenic *Escherichia coli* vaccine. Vaccine 1993; 11:929–934.

53. Wennerås C, Svennerholm AM, Åhren C, Czerkinsky C. Antibody-secreting cells in human peripheral blood after oral immunization with an inactivated enterotoxigenic *Escherichia coli* vaccine. Infect Immun 1992; 60:2605–2611.

54. Åhren C, Jertborn M, Svennerholm AM. Intestinal immune responses to an inactivated oral enterotoxigenic *Escherichia coli* vaccine and associated immunoglobulin A responses in blood. Infect Immun 1998; 66:3311–3316.

55. Hall ER, Wierzba TF, Åhren C, Rao MR, Bassily S, Francis W, Girgis FY, Safwat M, Lee YJ, Svennerholm AM, Clemens JD, Savarino SJ. Induction of systemic antifimbria and anti-

toxin antibody responses in Egyptian children and adults by an oral, killed enterotoxigenic *Escherichia coli* plus cholera toxin B subunit vaccine. Infect Immun 2001; 69:2853–2857.

56. Jertborn M, Åhrén C, Holmgren J, Svennerholm AM. Safety and immunogenicity of an oral inactivated enterotoxigenic *Escherichia coli* vaccine. Vaccine 1998; 16:255–260.

57. Qadri F, Wennerås C, Ahmed F, Asaduzzaman M, Saha D, Albert MJ, Sack RB, Svennerholm A. Safety and immunogenicity of an oral, inactivated enterotoxigenic *Escherichia coli* plus cholera toxin B subunit vaccine in Bangladeshi adults and children. Vaccine 2000; 18:2704–2712.

58. Jertborn M, Åhrén C, Svennerholm AM. Dose-dependent circulating immunoglobulin A antibody-secreting cell and serum antibody responses in Swedish volunteers to an oral inactivated enterotoxigenic *Escherichia coli* vaccine. Clin Diagn Lab Immunol 2001; 8:424–428.

59. Cohen D, Orr N, Haim M, Ashkenazi S, Robin G, Green MS, Ephros M, Sela T, Slepon R, Ashkenazi I, Taylor DN, Svennerholm AM, Eldad A, Shemer J. Safety and immunogenicity of two different lots of the oral, killed enterotoxigenic *Escherichia coli*-cholera toxin B subunit vaccine in Israeli young adults. Infect Immun 2000; 68:4492–4497.

60. Savarino SJ, Brown FM, Hall E, Bassily S, Youssef F, Wierzba T, Peruski L, El-Masry NA, Safwat M, Rao M, Jertborn M, Svennerholm AM, Lee YJ, Clemens JD. Safety and immunogenicity of an oral, killed enterotoxigenic *Esche-richia coli*-cholera toxin B subunit vaccine in Egyptian adults. J Infect Dis 1998; 177:796–799.

61. Sack DA, Shimko J, Torres O, Gomes G, Karnell K, Nyquist IBG, Svennerholm AM. Safety and efficacy of a killed oral vaccine for enterotoxigenic *E. coli* diarrhea in adult travelers to Guatemala and Mexico. 42nd Interscience Conference on Antimicrobial Agents and Chemotherapy. San Diego, CA, 2002.

62. Quadri F, et al. Safety and immunogenicity of an oral inactivated enterotoxigenic *Escherichia coli* plus cholera toxin B subunit vaccine in Bangladeshi children 18–36 months of age. Vaccine 2003; 21:2394–2403.

63. Savarino SJ, Hall ER, Bassily S, Brown FM, Youssef F, Wierzba TF, Peruski L, El-Masry NA, Safwat M, Rao M, El Mohamady H, Abu-Elyazeed R, Naficy A, Svennerholm AM, Jertborn M, Lee YJ, Clemens JD. Oral, inactivated, whole cell enterotoxigenic *Escherichia coli* plus cholera toxin B subunit vaccine: Results of the initial evaluation in children. PRIDE Study Group. J Infect Dis 1999; 179:107–114.

64. Savarino SJ, Hall ER, Bassily S, Wierzba TF, Youssef FG, Peruski LF Jr, Abu-Elyazeed R, Rao M, Francis WM, El Mohamady H, Safwat M, Naficy AB, Svennerholm AM, Jertborn M, Lee YJ, Clemens JD. Introductory evaluation of an oral, killed whole cell enterotoxigenic *Escherichia coli* plus cholera toxin B subunit vaccine in Egyptian infants. Pediatr Infect Dis J 2002; 21:322–330.

61

Multivalent *Shigella*/Enterotoxigenic *Escherichia coli* Vaccine

Eileen M. Barry and Myron M. Levine
University of Maryland School of Medicine, Baltimore, Maryland, U.S.A.

I. INTRODUCTION

The disease burdens posed by enterotoxigenic *Escherichia coli* (ETEC) and *Shigella* are described in depth in the chapters by Svennerholm and Savarino and Kotloff et al., respectively. Both pathogens are important causes of diarrheal disease in children in developing countries and are major etiologic agents of traveler's diarrhea.

II. SHIGELLA

A. Strategy to Achieve Broad-Spectrum Protection Against *Shigella*

A globally useful *Shigella* vaccine will have to protect against *Shigella dysenteriae* 1 (cause of severe epidemic disease in the least developed countries), all 15 serotypes of *S. flexneri* (main cause of endemic shigellosis in developing countries), and *S. sonnei* (the serotype most frequently associated with traveler's shigellosis and the most common serotype causing disease in industrialized countries). Infection-derived immunity against *Shigella* is directed towards O antigens. Based on shared O antigens among the 15 *S. flexneri* serotypes, Noriega et al. [1] hypothesized that a vaccine containing *S. flexneri* 2a, *S. flexneri* 3a and *S. flexneri* 6 O antigens could provide broad protection against all 15 *S. flexneri* serotypes. By means of challenge studies in guinea pigs, Noriega et al. [1] generated preclinical evidence supporting this hypothesis. Pursuing this strategy, investigators at the Center for Vaccine Development have concluded that a multivalent *Shigella* vaccine that includes O antigens of five carefully selected serotypes, *S. dysenteriae* 1, *S. flexneri* 2a, *S. flexneri* 3a, *S. flexneri* 6, and *S. sonnei*, could provide broad coverage against the most important *Shigella* serotypes that cause disease worldwide [1–3].

B. Shigella Harboring Mutations in *guaBA* and in the Genes Encoding *Shigella* Enterotoxins 1 and 2

Introduction of a deletion mutation in the *guaBA* operon (which impairs guanine nucleotide biosynthesis) of *S. flexneri* 2a wild-type strain 2457T, renders strain CVD 1204, which is markedly attenuated compared to its wild-type parent [4]. Nevertheless, at high dosage levels in humans, approximately one-half of subjects who ingested CVD 1204 still developed mild diarrhea and full clinical attenuation was not achieved until deletions in the genes encoding *Shigella* enterotoxin 1 (ShET1) (*set*) [5,6] and ShET2 (*sen*) [7] were also introduced, resulting in well-tolerated and immunogenic strain CVD 1208. Based on the favorable experience with *S. flexneri* 2a as a prototype, attenuated *S. dysenteriae* 1, *S. flexneri* 3a, *S. flexneri* 6, and *S. sonnei* strains are also being constructed [1,3] that similarly harbor deletions in *guaBA* and *sen*; in addition, the *S. dysenteriae* 1 strain has a deletion mutation in *stxA* that encodes the A subunit of Shiga toxin. These five carefully selected *Shigella* serotypes should provide broad coverage against the most important serotypes that cause shigellosis worldwide [1].

III. ENTEROTOXIGENIC *ESCHERICHIA COLI*

A. Target Antigens

As a preliminary step in the pathogenesis of diarrhea, ETEC adhere to receptors on enterocytes in the proximal small intestine by means of fimbrial colonization factors, thereby counteracting the peristalsis defense mechanism. Once adherent, they elaborate enterotoxins that cause intestinal secretion, culminating clinically in diarrhea. Considerable evidence, as reviewed in the chapter by Svennerholm and Savarino, indicates that broad-spectrum, relatively long-lived, immunity to ETEC is mediated by intestinal immune responses directed against these fimbrial attachment factors.

B. Antigenic Diversity Among Human ETEC Pathogens

Analysis of the antigenic structure of ETEC strains from endemic areas shows many different O:H serotypes, at least 10 distinct antigenic types of fimbrial colonization factors (of which the most common are CFA/I and CS1–CS6) and three different toxin phenotypes (LT, ST, and LT/ST) [8,9]. CFA/I is a single antigenic moiety. Coli surface antigens 1 (CS1), 2 (CS2) and 3 (CS3) constitute the CFA/II family of antigens. All CFA/II strains express CS3, either alone or in conjunction with CS1 or CS2. CS4, CS5, and CS6 comprise the CFA/IV family of antigens. All CFA/IV strains express CS6, either alone or in conjunction with CS4 or CS5. Other fimbrial colonization factors are much less frequent. Carriage of the genes that encode a particular fimbrial colonization factor is closely correlated with O:H serotype and toxin phenotype. Analysis of ETEC isolates from diverse geographic areas shows that CFA/I and CS1-6 are found on the majority of isolates. Circa 70–90% of isolates that elaborate both heat-labile and heat-stable enterotoxins (LT and ST, respectively) express these CFAs, while they are found on ca. 60% of ST-only strains. Generally, less than 10% of LT-only strains bear these CFAs. Thus, a multivalent ETEC vaccine that contained CFA/I and CS1-6 plus an appropriate antigen (such as B subunit or mutant LT) to elicit neutralizing LT antitoxin might broaden protection to cover ~80–90% of ETEC strains worldwide. Inclusion of less frequent fimbrial antigens in a multivalent vaccine could expand the spectrum of coverage, albeit at the price of even greater complexity.

C. Infection-Derived Immunity to ETEC

Despite the antigenic heterogeneity of ETEC, evidence from both volunteer studies and from epidemiological surveys argues convincingly that prior clinical infection with ETEC confers immunity [10–12]. In endemic areas, multiple infections with strains bearing different fimbrial colonization factors must occur in order for broad-spectrum immunity to be elicited. In less-developed countries, infants and young children experience up to three separate clinical ETEC infections per year during the first three years of life, after which the incidence of ETEC diarrhea plummets [11]. The lower incidence in older persons is due to specific acquired immunity rather than to nonspecific age-related host factors, since adult travelers from industrialized countries who visit less-developed countries where ETEC pediatric diarrhea is endemic suffer high attack rates of ETEC travelers' diarrhea. The fimbrial colonization factor antigenic profile of strains that cause endemic pediatric diarrhea in developing countries and those that cause travelers' diarrhea is the same. Travelers from industrialized countries who remain

in less-developed countries for at least a year and travelers who arrive from other less-developed countries suffer significantly lower incidence rates of ETEC diarrhea than newly arrived travelers from industrialized countries [12]. These data further support the concept of acquired immunity. Data from a prospective epidemiological field study in Mexican infants and young children provide direct evidence that acquired immunity is largely directed at fimbrial colonization factors of ETEC [13].

D. Lessons Learned from Studies with a Prototype Attenuated E. coli Live Oral ETEC Vaccine

Escherichia coli E1392-75-2A is a CFA/II-positive mutant strain derived in the Central Public Health Laboratory, Colindale, UK, wherein the genes encoding LT and ST spontaneously deleted from the CFA/II plasmid. Consequently, E1392-75-2A, which expresses CS1 and CS3 fimbrial antigens, is negative when tested with toxin assays and gene probes for LT and ST. Levine et al. [14–16] utilized strain E1392-75-2A to explore fundamental questions of anticolonization immunity in the absence of antitoxic immunity. All volunteers who were fed 10^{10} CFU of strain E1392-75-2A developed significant rises in intestinal fluid SIgA antibody to CS1 and CS3 fimbriae. The geometric mean titer (GMT) of antifimbrial CS1 and CS3 SIgA antibody in these volunteers was 10-fold higher than the peak postvaccination GMT of volunteers who received enteral immunization with multiple doses of purified CS1 and CS3 fimbriae.

A group of vaccinees who were immunized with a single 5×10^{10} CFU dose of E1392-75-2A with buffer was challenged 1 month later, along with nonimmunized control volunteers. The pathogenic ETEC challenge strain used, E24377A, was of a heterologous serotype O139:H28 but expressed CS1 and CS3 and elaborated LT and ST. The vaccinees were significantly protected ($P < 0.005$, 75% vaccine efficacy) against ETEC diarrhea [14]. By means of bacteriological studies it was shown that anticolonization immunity was responsible for the protection. In the challenge study, all participants, both vaccinees and nonimmunized controls, excreted the ETEC challenge strain and there was no difference between the groups in the mean number of ETEC per gram of stool. In contrast, a striking difference was found in duodenal cultures that monitored colonization of the proximal small intestine, the critical site of ETEC–host interaction. The challenge strain was recovered from duodenal cultures of 5 of 6 controls (mean 7×10^3 CFU per mL) versus only 1 of 12 vaccinees (10^1 CFU per mL) ($P < 0.004$). Levine et al. interpreted these results to mean that SIgA anti-CS1 and anti-CS3 fimbrial antibody in the proximal intestine stimulated by the live oral vaccine prevented challenge ETEC from colonizing the proximal small intestine. Since the immune response was not bactericidal, the ETEC organisms were carried by peristalsis to the large intestine where they could colonize without causing diarrheal illness. Strain E1392-75-2A caused mild diarrhea in approximately 15% of the recipients who ingested it, an unacceptable rate of adverse reactions that made it unworthy of further development. Nevertheless, this strain provided invaluable data on the feasibility of eliciting protection in humans mediated by immune responses directed against fimbrial colonization factors.

IV. MULTIVALENT *SHIGELLA*–ETEC LIVE VECTOR VACCINE

A. Attenuated *Shigella* Strains Expressing ETEC Antigens

Investigators at the Center for Vaccine Development of the University of Maryland have shown that attenuated *Shigella* can be used as live vector vaccines to express ETEC fimbrial antigens and LT toxoids (B subunit or mutant LT) and deliver them to the immune system, resulting in SIgA antifimbrial and anti-LT responses [17–21], as well as *Shigella* anti-O antibody responses in mucosal secretions and serum.

B. The Multivalent Vaccine

The multivalent *Shigella*/ETEC vaccine under development contains five attenuated *Shigella* serotype strains (*S. dysenteriae* 1, *S. flexneri* 2a, *S. flexneri* 3a, *S. flexneri* 6, and *S. sonnei*), each expressing two different ETEC fimbrial antigens and an antigen ("LT toxoid") to stimulate neutralizing LT antitoxin. Both LT B subunit and mutant LT moieties are being evaluated as possible LT toxoids, the former having the attraction of greater potential safety. LT from human ETEC pathogens (LTh), from domestic animals, and cholera toxin, or their respective B subunits, can all elicit antibodies that can neutralize LTh [22]. However, each of these antigens has unique epitopes and the highest antitoxin titers observed are against the homologous antigen [22–24]. Consequently, it is our contention that an antigen based on LTh should be used to stimulate LT antitoxin. Notably, expression of the ETEC fimbriae and LT toxoid does not diminish the capacity of the vector strain to protect against challenge with wild-type *Shigella* in a guinea pig model [17–21].

C. *Shigella* Can Express Combinations of ETEC Fimbria Not Found in Nature

The utility of attenuated *Shigella* as live vectors to coexpress CFA/I and CS3 fimbriae of ETEC, a combination never found in nature, was documented [17]. The immunogenicity of this bivalent *Shigella* live vector strain was evaluated in a guinea pig immunization model in which *Shigella* are administered intranasally following which mucosal SIgA responses are measured in tears. The *Shigella* live vector expressing these two ETEC fimbrial antigens elicited SIgA mucosal antibody responses to both CFA/I and CS3 [17].

D. Genetic Characterization of CS4

In constructing the multivalent *Shigella* live vector ETEC vaccine, one must be able to manipulate the operons encoding biogenesis of each of the fimbrial structures in the vaccine (CFA/I and CS1–CS6). Among these, the CS4 operon

was the last to be elucidated and cloned [20]. Altboum et al. [20] showed that the CS4 (*csa*) operon encodes a 17-kDa major fimbrial subunit (CsaB), a 40-kDa fimbrial tip protein (CsaE), a 27-kDa chaperone (CsaA), and a 97-kDa usher protein (CsaC). Furthermore, they showed that the predicted amino acid sequences of CS4 proteins are highly homologous to CS1, CS2, and CFA/I. With the successful cloning and expression of CS4, it is now possible to express all of the common ETEC fimbrial colonization factors in *Shigella* live vectors.

E. Combinations of *Shigella* Live Vector Strains Expressing Different ETEC Fimbriae

A hurdle faced by a multivalent live vector *Shigella*/ETEC vaccine is to demonstrate convincingly (ultimately in humans) that a mixture of vaccine strains, each expressing different ETEC fimbrial antigens, can elicit strong mucosal responses to all the different antigens in the combination. Towards this goal, initial preclinical studies in the guinea pig model were performed with two bivalent *Shigella* live vector candidates, one expressing CFA/I and CS3 [17] and the other CS2 and CS3 [19]. Each bivalent live vector elicited strong mucosal SIgA responses in tears against both fimbrial antigens; serum antibody responses were also robust. Studies were next undertaken with a pentavalent *Shigella*/ETEC vaccine consisting of attenuated *S. flexneri* 2a expressing either CFA/I, CS2, CS3, CS4 fimbriae or mutant LTh [21]. Following intranasal immunization, SIgA antifimbrial responses were measured in tears of guinea pigs immunized with either one of the monovalent vaccines or the multivalent vaccine (containing the five different live vector strains administered in combination). For each of the ETEC antigens, the combination vaccine, as well as each corresponding monovalent vaccine, stimulated significant rises in antifimbrial or anti-LT antibody. These groups of guinea pigs also exhibited strong *Shigella* anti-O antibody responses and were protected against challenge with wild-type *S. flexneri* 2a [21].

F. Shigella Live Vector Strains Expressing ETEC Fimbriae and LT Toxoids

Plasmids have been constructed that carry both operons for fimbrial biogenesis and for either mutant LTh or LTB subunit expression so that both antifimbrial and antitoxin responses can be stimulated [18,21]. In a related strategy, attenuated *Shigella* strains harboring LT toxoid genes integrated into the chromosome (and under control of a variety of promoters) and carrying plasmids allowing expression of ETEC fimbriae are also being constructed. Preclinical studies with these constructs, individually and in combination, will evaluate these different strategies and will pave the way for proof-of-principle clinical trials.

G. Summary Comment

A multivalent *Shigella*/ETEC vaccine is complex in development and with respect to the control of manufactured lots.

On the other hand, it has a number of distinct potential advantages. A single, albeit complex, vaccine would offer broad-spectrum coverage against two pathogens for which the target populations are the same, travelers and infants in developing countries.

REFERENCES

1. Noriega FR, et al. Strategy for cross-protection among *Shigella flexneri* serotypes. Infect Immun 1999; 67:782–788.

2. Kotloff KL, et al. Global burden of *Shigella* infections: implications for vaccine development and implementation of control strategies. Bull World Health Organ 1999; 77:651–666.

3. Levine MM. Immunization against bacterial diseases of the intestine. J Pediatr Gastroenterol Nutr 2000; 31:336–355.

4. Noriega FR, et al. Engineered Δ*guaB-A*, Δ*virG Shigella flexneri* 2a strain CVD 1205: construction, safety, immunogenicity and potential efficacy as a mucosal vaccine. Infect Immun 1996; 64:3055–3061.

5. Fasano A, et al. *Shigella* enterotoxin 1: an enterotoxin of *Shigella flexneri* 2a active in rabbit small intestine in vivo and in vitro. J Clin Invest 1995; 95:2853–2861.

6. Fasano A, et al. Effect of *Shigella* enterotoxin 1 (ShET1) on rabbit intestine in vitro and in vivo. Gut 1997; 40:505–511.

7. Nataro JP, et al. Identification and cloning of a novel plasmid-encoded enterotoxin of enteroinvasive *Escherichia coli* and *Shigella* strains. Infect Immun 1995; 63:4721–4728.

8. Levine MM, et al. Epidemiologic studies of *Escherichia coli* infections in a low socioeconomic level periurban community in Santiago, Chile. Am J Epidemiol 1993; 138:849–869.

9. Levine MM, et al. Fimbrial vaccines. In: Klemm P, ed. Fimbriae: Adhesion, Biogenics, Genetics and Vaccines. Boca Raton: CRC Press, 1994.

10. Levine MM, et al. Immunity to enterotoxigenic *Escherichia coli*. Infect Immun 1979; 23:729–736.

11. Black RE, et al. Enterotoxigenic *Escherichia coli* diarrhoea: acquired immunity and transmission in an endemic area. Bull World Health Organ 1981; 59:263–268.

12. DuPont HL, et al. Comparative susceptibility of Latin American and United States students to enteric pathogens. N Engl J Med 1976; 285:1520–1521.

13. Cravioto A, et al. Prospective study of diarrhoeal disease in a cohort of rural Mexican children: incidence and isolated pathogens during the first two years of life. Epidemiol Infect 1988; 101:123–134.

14. Levine MM. *Escherichia coli* that cause diarrhea: enterotoxigenic, enteropathogenic, enteroinvasive, enterohemorrhagic, and enteroadherent. J Infect Dis 1987; 155:377–389.

15. Levine MM, et al. Prevention of enterotoxigenic *Escherichia coli* diarrheal infection by vaccines that stimulate antiadhesion (antipili) immunity. In: Boedeker EC, ed. Attachment of organisms to the gut mucosa. Boca Raton: CRC Press, 1984: 223–244.

16. Levine MM. Travellers' diarrhoea: prospects for successful immunoprophylaxis. Scand J Gastroenterol Suppl 1983; 84: 121–134.

17. Noriega FR, et al. Further characterization of Δ*aroA*, Δ*virG Shigella flexneri* 2a strain CVD 1203 as a mucosal *Shigella* vaccine and as a live vector vaccine for delivering antigens of enterotoxigenic *Escherichia coli*. Infect Immun 1996; 64:23–27.

18. Koprowski H II, et al. Attenuated *Shigella flexneri* 2a vaccine strain CVD 1204 expressing colonization factor antigen I and mutant heat-labile enterotoxin of enterotoxigenic *Escherichia coli*. Infect Immun 2000; 68:4884–4892.

19. Altboum Z, et al. Attenuated *Shigella flexneri* 2a Δ*guaBA* strain CVD 1204 expressing enterotoxigenic *Escherichia coli* (ETEC) CS2 and CS3 fimbriae as a live mucosal vaccine against *Shigella* and ETEC infection. Infect Immun 2001; 69: 3150–3158.

20. Altboum Z, et al. Genetic characterization and immunogenicity of coli surface antigen 4 from enterotoxigenic *Escherichia coli* when it is expressed in a *Shigella* live-vector strain. Infect Immun 2003; 71:1352–1360.

21. Barry EM, et al. Immune responses elicited against multiple enterotoxigenic *Escherichia coli* fimbriae and mutant LT expressed in attenuated *Shigella* vaccine strains. Vaccine 2003; 21:333–340.

22. Levine MM, et al. Enzyme-linked immunosorbent assay to measure antibodies to purified heat-labile enterotoxins from human and porcine strains of *Escherichia coli* and to cholera toxin: application in serodiagnosis and seroepidemiology. J Clin Microbiol 1985; 21:174–179.

23. Finkelstein RA, et al. Antigenic determinants of the cholera/coli family of enterotoxins. Rev Infect Dis 1987; 9(suppl 5): S490–S502.

24. Tsuji T, et al. Molecular heterogeneity of heat-labile enterotoxins from human and porcine enterotoxigenic *Escherichia coli*. Infect Immun 1982; 38:444–448.

62

Vaccines Against Gonococcal Infection

Timothy A. Mietzner
University of Pittsburgh School of Medicine, Pittsburgh, Pennsylvania, U.S.A.

Christopher E. Thomas, Marcia M. Hobbs, and Myron S. Cohen
University of North Carolina, Chapel Hill, North Carolina, U.S.A.

I. INTRODUCTION: THE QUEST FOR A GONOCOCCAL VACCINE

Neisseria gonorrhoeae is the causative agent of gonorrhea, a disease of high morbidity responsible for significant global public health consequences. More than 360,000 cases of infection per year are reported in the United States each year, and many millions of cases occur worldwide [1]. There are three important justifications for the development of a gonococcal vaccine. First, sequelae of mucosal infection in women, including pelvic inflammatory disease (PID) and tubo-ovarian abscess, devastate reproductive health and may become life-threatening [2,3]. Second, depending on the infectiousness of the index case and the susceptibility of the sexual partner, gonococcal infections appear to facilitate the transmission of human immunodeficiency virus type 1 (HIV-1) [4,5]. Gonococcal urethritis causes greatly increased shedding of HIV in mucosal secretions and semen [6,7]. Gonococcal infection recruits cells and cytokines capable of enhancing the acquisition of HIV [9], and likely leads to breaks in mucosal integrity, leading to increased virus infectivity [10]. Third, gonococci demonstrate increased resistance to most, if not all, available antibiotic agents [11–15]. Indeed, fluoroquinolone agents can no longer be employed in patients from Asia [16,17].

The National Institute of Allergy and Infectious Diseases initiated a research program in 1971 focusing on the biology of the gonococcus and other sexually transmitted pathogens, with an emphasis on vaccine development. This sustained support led to extensive studies by basic and clinical scientists on gonococcal epidemiology, physiology, ultrastructure, and pathogenesis that allow us to understand the molecular basis for gonococcal infection. Several excellent recent reviews highlight different aspects of gonococcal pathogenesis [18–22]. Animal and human models have provided insights into gonococcal infection, and a unique opportunity to develop and test vaccine candidates. In this chapter, we describe the clinical, bacteriological, and immunological basis for the development of a gonococcal vaccine.

II. PATHOBIOLOGY OF GONOCOCCAL INFECTION

A. Disease

Gonorrhea is caused by the gram-negative diplococcus *N. gonorrhoeae*. At the morphological, phenotypical, and genotypical levels, the gonococcus is closely related to the pathogen *N. meningitidis*, a major cause of bacterial meningitis in infants and adults. However, meningococcal mucosal colonization leads to bacteremia and central nervous system infection, whereas gonococcal infection is primarily localized to the genitourinary tract. Meningococci only rarely colonize the genital mucosa. The success in the development of a meningococcal vaccine (see the chapter by Rappuoli et al.) emphasizes differences in the biology and immunology of these pathogens. However, some important lessons can be learned from the development of a meningococcal vaccine, as discussed below.

Gonococcal infection occurs almost exclusively by horizontal sexual spread, transmitted most efficiently from men to women (90% per episode of intercourse), although both men and women are generally exposed to a large inoculum (10^6 bacteria) during intercourse [8,23]. Because of the differences in the anatomy and physiology of the male urinary and female reproductive tracts, the manifestations of the disease in men and women are significantly different. Within males, gonococcal urethral infection may be asymptomatic [24] or present as painful but ultimately self-limited urethral inflammation. Acute gonococcal urethritis produces an exuberant granulocytic inflammatory discharge. Gonococcal orchitis and epididymitis are infrequent complications of urethral infection. Anal intercourse may lead to gonococcal proctitis, and increasingly antibiotic resistant organisms have been recovered from infected gay men. Gonococcal infection in women can be asymptomatic or can cause endocervical inflammation and upper genital tract disease. Gonococci can cause bacteremia with skin lesions and attendant septic arthritis, with gonococcal arthritis being the most common cause of septic arthritis in young people.

In large part, surface-accessible antigens mediate the efficiency of infection and disease caused by *N. gonorrhoeae*. If vaccination is possible for the prevention of this disease, it is reasonable to suggest that the immunogenic component will be derived from a prominent "Surface-Accessible Gonococcal Antigen."

B. Surface-Accessible Gonococcal Antigens

The gonococcal cell envelope, such as those of other gram-negative bacterial species [25], consists of a cytoplasmic membrane separated from the outer membrane by the periplasmic space. The external leaflet of the outer membrane is strategically arrayed at the interface between the host and the microbe such that molecules associated with this surface (a) implement the host pathology, or (b) represent targets for a host immune response. This external leaflet is comprised of a complex mixture of phospholipids, lipooligosaccharides (LOS), and proteins as diagramed for the gonococcus in Figure 1. However, the gonococcal outer membrane differs from that of *Escherichia coli* in at least two important ways. First, gonococci appear to lack a functional analogue of Braun lipoprotein, which serves to anchor

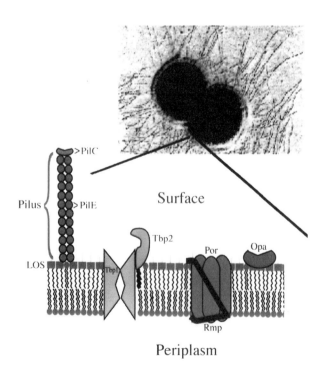

Figure 1 Diagram depicting the most prominent and well-characterized gonococcal surface antigens.

the *E. coli* outer membrane to the relatively rigid middle layer of peptidoglycan [25]. This may explain the spontaneous release of outer membrane fragments or "blebs" from viable gonococci [26]. Because blebs can display surface-associated antigens in their native orientation, they may be capable of binding antibodies to gonococcal outer membrane antigens, thereby serving as antigenic decoys for the organism. In the same regard, blebs may be exploited as vaccines to present novel antigens in their native form, and this has formed the basis for a new class of meningococcal vaccines [27].

Studies of purified gonococcal outer membranes reveal several prominent surface-accessible antigens. The relative molecular masses of these proteins and their quantitative expression depend upon the strain analyzed [28], the extent of in vitro passage [29–32], the growth conditions used for propagation [33–36], and the procedure used to isolate and analyze the outer membrane [33,37]. These surface-accessible gonococcal antigens can be categorized as constitutively expressed, phase variably expressed, or environmentally regulated.

1. Constitutively Expressed Outer Membrane Antigens

Lipooligosaccharide. The most prominent of all surface-accessible gonococcal antigens is LOS. This antigen is the principal component of the gonococcal outer membrane, oriented on the outer leaflet. In this context, it is the "mortar" in which gonococcal protein antigens are presented to the immune system.

Biochemistry of Gonococcal Lipooligosaccharide. Like the rough lipopolysaccharide (LPS) mutants of Enterobacteriaceae [25], gonococcal LOS contains a lipid A molecule attached to two 2-keto-3-deoxy-mannooctulosonic acid (KDO) residues and two heptoses but lacking the *O*-repeating polysaccharide. This basic structure is further modified by the attachment to oligosaccharide chains consisting of two regions: (a) a basal oligosaccharide linked to KDO, and (b) a middle linear segment containing varying numbers of residues that determine the length of the LOS. The nonreducing terminal sugar is similar in monosaccharide content [38] and anomeric linkage [39] to human cell surface glycosphingolipids. Most gonococcal strains produce from one to six LOS species that are antigenically and structurally distinct; this structural heterogeneity can be experimentally appreciated by differences in migration when analyzed by sodium dodecyl sulfate polyacrylamide gel electrophoresis (SDS-PAGE) [40–42]. Like the LOS of *Haemophilus influenzae*, the structural heterogeneity of the LOS oligosaccharide is modulated by the expression of different glycosyltransferases as a result of high-frequency genetic events such as slipped-strand DNA synthesis [43,44]. A demonstration of the genetic basis for LOS variation has been a major contribution to understanding gonococcal pathogenesis.

Variations in gonococcal surface oligosaccharide composition can lead to further modification by host factors. For example, Smith et al. [45] noted that gonococci acquired resistance to killing activity associated with normal human serum after a brief exposure to human blood or secretions, and ascribed this to the sialylation of a 4.2-kDa LOS species that can be identified by binding to a specific monoclonal antibody. The sialylation of gonococci requires a bacterially derived sialyltransferase and the host-derived substrate CMP-NANA, found in saturating concentrations in all human tissues. The sialylation of LOS is enhanced by growth in lactate compared to glucose [45], and lactate is generated by granulocytes that form the gonococcal exudate [46]. Gonococci harvested directly from urethral exudates are sialylated [47].

Contribution of Lipooligosaccharide to Gonococcal Pathogenesis. Antibodies specific for gonococcal LOS can be detected in sera and vaginal fluids of infected patients [48]. In addition, LOS contains a principle antigenic determinant recognized by the "natural" bactericidal antibody of the IgM class that, in combination with serum complement, mediates the killing of serum-sensitive strains. Lipooligosaccharide promotes injury to the mucosa and may be responsible for the loss of ciliary activity and the sloughing of ciliated epithelial cells [49] by inducing the proinflammatory cytokine, TNF-α [50]. This effect is proposed to be an important contributor to gonococcal salpingitis and may mediate postsalpingitis infertility and ectopic pregnancy [50].

Gonococci expressing full-length LOS (containing the lacto-*N*-neotetraose moiety) are serum-sensitive, whereas the sialylation of LOS renders them serum-resistant [51]. The decreased uptake and decreased killing of sialylated gonococci by polymorphonuclear (PMN) cells have been reported [52]. The modulation of LOS may have a significant role in the invasion of cells [53]. Sialylated gonococci are less invasive for a variety of host cells when compared to non-sialylated gonococci [54]. However, other factors also influence this property. For example, the invasiveness of some gonococcal strains depends upon the expression of a terminal glucose [55] or other terminal sugars (e.g., lactosamine) [56].

The structural and antigenic similarity noted above between the terminal oligosaccharides of LOS and human cell surface glycosphingolipids has been examined [39,57]. One terminal LOS trisaccharide was found to resemble a precursor of human blood group antigens, and another was found to be related to the globoseries glycolipids, known to constitute the *E. coli* P-pilus receptor on human uroepithelial surfaces. The "molecular mimicry" of gonococcal LOS with host cells has been proposed to confer three advantages for infection: (a) LOS may resemble "self"-antigens of the host, reducing their immunogenicity; (b) human cell surface lectinlike proteins, which normally recognize specific glycosphingolipids, could bind LOS and thus mediate epithelial cell adherence and invasion by gonococci; and (c) host-derived glycosyltransferases, which normally modify the oligosaccharide moieties of glycosphingolipids, might also modify gonococcal LOS and create neoantigens on the gonococcal surface.

Por and Rmp. Embellishing the analogy of LOS as the mortar of the gonococcal cell surface, two protein antigens, Por and Rmp, act as "bricks" that are prominently displayed on the gonococcal surface. Por and Rmp are unique among other gonococcal surface antigens in that they always associate with the outer membrane in abundant amounts, regardless of how the organism is propagated or how the outer membranes are prepared. Por and Rmp have historically been referred to as Protein I and Protein III, respectively, with Por denoting a well-characterized *por*in function, and Rmp denoting a characteristic *r*eduction *m*odifiable *p*rotein property [28].

Biochemistry of PorB and Rmp. The genomes of the pathogenic *Neisseria* contain two porin genes, *porA* and *porB*. Unlike meningococci, which express both PorA and PorB proteins, gonococci contain mutations in the promoter region and frameshift mutations in the coding region of *porA* that have effectively silenced this locus [56a]. Hence, *N. gonorrhoeae* express a single porin designated as PorB. The deletion of PorB is lethal for *N. gonorrhoeae* propagated in vitro, underscoring its critical presence for gonococcal survival even in the absence of host defenses. By one estimate, PorB comprises ca. 60% by weight of the total repertoire of gonococcal outer membrane proteins [37]. The apparent molecular mass of the gonococcal PorB is between 32 and 39 kDa, depending upon the gonococcal isolate. PorB is organized within the outer membrane as a trimer. In this state, PorB forms an anion-selective channel essential for the diffusion of solutes with molecular masses of less than 1 kDa [58]. PorB forms a trimeric complex in the outer membrane with the monomeric Rmp [59,60].

N. gonorrhoeae isolates from global locations reveal that PorB can be separated into two immunologically distinct classes, referred to as PIA and PIB [61–63]. The differences in antigenicity between PIA and PIB are associated with a substantial variation of surface-exposed loops. More subtle variations within surface loop sequences account for over 40 distinguishable serovars, defined by reactivity with PorB-specific monoclonal antibodies [64]. PorB expression is stable upon passage in vitro; unlike other gonococcal surface antigens, it is not subject to high-frequency phase or antigenic variation within a strain. Nevertheless, gonococcal PorB protein undergoes antigenic variation in vivo over time as evidenced by the diversity of serovars characteristic of the species.

In contrast to PorB, Rmp is a highly conserved, surface-exposed outer membrane protein expressed by all pathogenic *Neisseria*. Its descriptive name derives from its migration properties in SDS-PAGE; Rmp has an apparent molecular mass of approximately 31 kDa under nonreducing conditions, but migrates more slowly in the presence of reducing agents [28]. Gonococcal mutants that do not produce Rmp are viable when cultured in vitro [65], unlike PorB mutants. While surface-exposed, Rmp does not exhibit phase or antigen variation [28]. The precise biochemical function for Rmp is not well understood.

Contribution of Por and Rmp to Gonococcal Pathogenesis. PorB has been implicated in specific responses by host epithelial and phagocytic cells that are relevant to gonococcal pathogenesis [66]. Purified and detergent-solubilized PorB can be incorporated into natural or synthetic lipid bilayers, conferring the property of voltage gating to these bilayers [67]. PorB can translocate from the outer membranes of viable gonococci to the plasma and mitochondrial membranes of eukaryotic cells and to artificial lipid bilayers, where voltage-dependent changes can be detected [68]. The gating properties of certain porins are modulated by nucleotide triphosphates [69]. Purified PorB interferes with degranulation by neutrophils [70], suggesting that PorB may play a role in "managing" the host inflammatory response to gonococcal infection. The addition of purified PorB to human monocytes triggers a Ca^{2+} influx [71]. The significance of this property is that hyperpolarization of plasma membranes activates macrophages and granulocytes [67]. Thus, the disruption of this polarization may limit the ability of host cells to respond to and control gonococcal infection.

The ability of the gonococcus to transcytose through the epithelial cell barrier is recognized as an important property that contributes to infection (Figure 2). The contribution of the gonococcal PorB to transcytosis is suggested by experiments using isogenic gonococcal strains carrying different *por* alleles [72]. This study demonstrated that constructs expressing PorB associated with disseminated gonococcal infection conferred an increased ability to invade epithelial cells. Furthermore, this invasive phenotype was influenced by nucleotide triphosphates or polyphosphates [72]. The current view is that PorB functions to promote invasion in combination with other surface-associated adhesions [18].

The PorB phenotype contributes to complement-mediated killing of gonococci by normal human serum. Nearly all gonococcal strains expressing a PIA PorB are serum-resistant, apparently because serum proteins that downregulate

complement-binding proteins (C4bp and factor H) are bound to loop 5 sequences found in PIA porins, but not in PIBs [73–75]. PIB serum-resistant variants also bind C4bp via a conformational epitope between loops 5 and 7 [74]. Strains sensitive to serum killing fail to bind these factors, but may acquire serum resistance if sialylated LOS binds factor H [75].

Examination of the Rmp sequence reveals an area that is partially homologous with the carboxy-terminal portion of the OmpA proteins of *Shigella dysenteriae*, *E. coli*, and *Enterobacter aerogenes* [76]. It has been proposed that "natural" antibodies to homologous regions of the enterobacterial OmpA proteins cross-react with Rmp and function as "blocking" antibodies [77]. Antibodies to Rmp can be found in the sera and vaginal fluids of patients convalescing from gonorrhea, although in general, Rmp is not as immunogenic as other surface-exposed gonococcal antigens [48]. Binding by these antibodies has a profound blocking effect on the bactericidal activity of sera [78,79]. It is proposed that blocking antibodies to Rmp in these sera may have arisen in response to a previous gonococcal infection, or represent an immune response to enterobacterial OmpA proteins that cross-react with Rmp.

2. Phase-Variable Surface Antigens

Fimbrial Adhesins—PilE and PilC. Fimbriae, also called pili, are long axial appendages (1–4 μm in length, 60

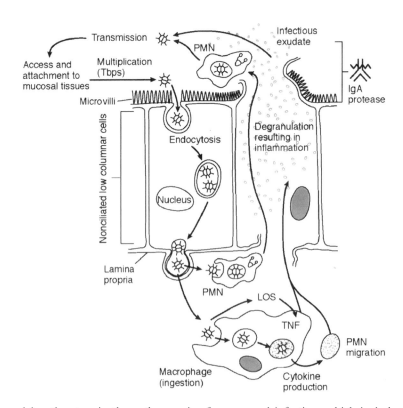

Figure 2 Diagram summarizing the steps in the pathogenesis of gonococcal infection, which include attachment, invasion and transcytosis, multiplication, stimulation of a vigorous immune response, and transmission, as described in the text.

Å in diameter) that extend from the surface of bacteria [80]. Pili participate in a number of different functions including DNA transfer, bacterial attachment to host cells, intrabacterial adhesion, and bacterial movement [81]. As with many bacterial pathogens, gonococcal pili are important for the pathogenesis of infection. First, gonococci undergo natural transformation [82,83], and this property is significantly enhanced by the expression of pili [84]. Second, the attachment properties of gonococcal pili confer tissue tropism as well as the ability to overcome the bacterial–host cell charge repulsion [85]. Finally, gonococcal pili, like other type 4 pili, mediate twitching motility, a mode of migration along liquid–solid or air–liquid interfaces [81]. Twitching motility has been implicated in a wide number of biological processes [18].

Evidence for the involvement of pili in gonococcal pathogenesis came first from the seminal observations by Kellogg et al. [86] in 1963, who reported that clinical materials freshly propagated on solid media gave rise to gonococcal colonies of two morphotypes, termed T_1 and T_2 (now designated as piliated or P^+). Upon nonspecific passage in vitro, two additional colonial forms appeared, termed T_3 and T_4 (now designated as nonpiliated or P^-). P^+ colonial morphotypes were subsequently found to be substantially more infective for male volunteers following intraurethral challenge than types P^- [86]. Later, Jephcott et al. [87] and Swanson et al. [31] described piluslike appendages extending from the surface of organisms comprising P^+ colonies but not P^- colonies. Since this discovery, studies have provided detailed information about the biological properties, molecular structure, immunochemistry, and regulation of expression of gonococcal pili.

Biochemistry of Pili. Among bacteria, several structural classes of pili (e.g., type 1, Gal–Gal, etc.) that have either unique structural or receptor-binding characteristics exist. Gonococci express a type 4 pilus defined by the ordered assembly of a principal repeating polypeptide subunit termed pilin, an 18- to 22-kDa polypeptide encoded by the *pilE* locus [88]. The pilin protein of type 4 fimbriae is synthesized as a precursor protein with a unique secretory signal sequence shared among many type II secretion systems [89]. During processing, the pilin precursor is modified by the PilD prepilin peptidase/transmethylase [90]. The result is a mature pilin subunit with a methylated phenylalanine residue at its N-terminus (*N*-met-Phe). This maturation is coupled with transport and assembly. Recently, a protein identified as PilQ has been described as one of many protein products associated with pilus biogenesis and function [91–93]. This protein was formerly described as a high-molecular-weight common outer membrane antigen and designated as OMP-MC [94]. PilQ is surface-exposed and common to diverse gonococcal isolates. It is thought to function by forming a multimeric channel in the outer membrane through which the assembled pilus fiber is presented. This process results in the aggregation of thousands of pilin molecules in an extended linear structure, which can be readily viewed in negatively stained transmission electron micrographs of gonococci propagated on agar media (Figure 1).

Parge et al. [88] reported the atomic structure of gonococcal pilin. This structural information largely explains much of the serological and biological data described below by demonstrating how packing of the pilus structure is preserved in the context of antigenically variable regions [95]. The pilin monomer contains a C-terminal globular head region and an N-terminal hydrophobic tail that folds into an unusually long α-helix. The helical region packs as a "stalk" presenting an antigenically variable C-terminal "flower." A surprising finding from these studies is the observation that the C-terminal pilin domain can be phosphorylated and glycosylated, further increasing the antigenic diversity of this structure.

Although gonococcal pili were originally thought to exist as a homopolymer, it is now accepted that a 110-kDa protein (PilC) associates with the pilus structure [84,96–98]. The gene for this protein, designated *pilC*, can exist within a single gonococcal strain as two distinct loci (*pilC*1 and *pilC*2) that can undergo phase-variable expression [99,100]. More contentious is whether PilC functions as an adhesin oriented at the pili terminus, distal to the gonococcal cell surface, or whether PilC functions in the assembly, retraction (twitching motility), or genetic competence (transformation) associated with piliated gonococci as reviewed by Merz et al. [18].

Contribution of Pili to Gonococcal Pathogenesis. As originally reported by Kellogg et al. [86] and Cannon et al. [23], all primary clinical isolates are piliated (P^+) upon isolation and nonpiliated (P^-) variants are less infectious in human volunteers challenged intraurethrally. Three properties that likely contribute to these observations are efficiency of infectivity, adherence, and resistance to phagocytosis. More recent work has demonstrated that an engineered *pilE* deletion mutant can cause experimental urethral infection, albeit somewhat different than infection with wild-type gonococcal infection [23]. What is clear from these studies is that the expression of gonococcal pili confers an advantage for the colonization of the male urethral mucosa, presumably mediated by the ability to adhere to this tissue, but not necessarily exclusive of the contribution of the pilus structure to natural competence and twitching motility.

Adherence has been historically recognized as a function of gonococcal pili. When compared to nonpiliated isogenic variants of the same strain, piliated Neisseria are reported to agglutinate human erythrocytes [101], and attach to spermatozoa [102], cultured epithelial cells [103], and explanted fallopian tubes [104]. The eukaryotic antigen CD46 is largely regarded as the pilus receptor; it is widely expressed in epithelial and endothelial cells [21,105,106]. CD46 functions as the receptor for the complement regulatory protein C3b and is associated with the signaling events associated with pilus binding [105]. These observations suggest that pili promote gonococcal adherence to cellular surfaces, thus facilitating the early colonization phase of infection. Proof for this notion is somewhat indirect, however, because electron microscopy studies of infected human tissues seldom reveal convincing piluslike structures [107]. Pilus antigens are nonetheless expressed in some form during the course of infection because pilus antibodies can be readily detected in the sera and vaginal fluids of patients convalescing from gonorrhea [108]. Finally, piliation has historically correlated with the resistance of gonococci to phagocytosis by human neutrophils [109,110].

Antigenic heterogeneity is characteristic of pilin proteins prepared from different gonococcal strains [111]. The antigenic variation of pili expressed by isogenic variants of the same strain also occurs in vivo, where it can be demonstrated using isolates of the same strain from sex partners [112] and from men with experimentally induced gonococcal urethritis [113,114]. Studies clearly demonstrate that (a) pilin variation occurs throughout infection; (b) multiple pilin variants are present at any point during infection; and (c) pilin variants are likely recombinants between previously expressed genes and the silent storage pilin copies, *pilS* [114]. These investigations and others all lead to the same conclusion—during infection, a large repertoire of pilins is produced. As a consequence of this antigenic variation and heterogeneity, gonococci may avoid host immune responses directed at or triggered by pilin proteins.

The genetic basis for gonococcal antigenic variation is beyond the scope of this review and is addressed by several excellent reports [115,116]. In general, most clinical isolates contain a single pilin expression locus [115]. Elsewhere in the gonococcal genome, multiple nontranscribed "silent" pilin (*pilS*) loci exist. Most gonococcal strains have more than a dozen *pilS* loci; each silent locus contains one to several truncated pilin structural genes lacking the 5′ promoter region and the coding sequence for the N-terminal constant region of pilin. The pilin sequences in the silent loci primarily specify the semivariable and hypervariable C-terminal regions of pilin and, consequently, they contain information for the creation of new antigenic determinants that are clearly formed during the process of natural infection [113,114]. It has been proposed that the diversity of pilin variants approaches that of the B-cell repertoire of antigen-combining sites. An equally important property of gonococcal pili is that of "piliation phase syndrome" as first proposed by Brinton et al. [117] in reference to the presence or absence of pili expressed by any given gonococcal isolate. Switching between the P$^+$ or the P$^-$ states occurs at rates as high as one per one thousand cell divisions reversion to the piliated state also occurs, although at slower rates, greater than one per one million cell divisions reversions per generation [82]. Natural recombination events result in the deletion of the pilin expression site, and the upstream promoter sequences lead to a P$^-$ state that is capable of reversion to the P$^+$ state at very low frequencies or not at all. In other cases, pilin is expressed but is undetectable due to rapidly degraded truncated or unassembled pilins, also referred to as soluble pilin [118]. Soluble pilin may provide yet another source of gonococcal protein that antigenically diverts the host immune system during the course of gonococcal infection.

The remarkable structural and antigenic diversity of gonococcal pili deserves a footnote as one of nature's oddities. This property is unique to *N. gonorrhoeae* and its evolution clearly contributes to the efficiency with which this organism causes disease, giving rise to the concept of infection by a "quasi-species" (i.e., a population of multiple clones), reminiscent of HIV-1 infection.

"Afimbrial" Adhesins: Opas. A group of related proteins, historically referred to as Proteins II and now designated as Opas for *op*acity *a*ssociated proteins, are variably expressed on the gonococcal surface. The term Opa is derived from the observation that gonococcal colonies, propagated on clear typing media and viewed through a stereomicroscope using light reflected from a mirror below the stage, exhibit an opacity phenotype ranging from transparent to opaque [119–121]. Colonies appearing transparent by this analysis generally, but not always, lack Opas. These proteins are not presented as part of an extended appendage such as a pilus; rather, they are intimately associated with the gonococcal outer membrane. Whereas pili appear to be crucial for the first contact of gonococci with host cells from rather long-range, Opas are thought to promote more intimate contact with host cells, resulting in subsequent cell signaling.

Biochemistry of Opas. Opas comprise a family of surface-exposed outer membrane proteins with apparent subunit molecular mass between 24 and 30 kDa. As a group, they are basic proteins with isoelectric points above 9.0 [28,122] and are heat-modifiable (i.e., when prepared at 37°C for SDS-PAGE analysis, they migrate with a higher relative mobility than when prepared at 60°C or 100°C). Organisms forming opaque colonies usually express one or more Opas that affect intergonococcal adhesion, giving rise to the opaque appearance of these colonies [120,123–126].

The predicted amino acid sequences corresponding to Opa structural genes contain a relatively conserved "semivariable" region near the N-terminus of the molecule and two hypervariable regions that differ markedly in amino acid sequence and length [127]. Both hypervariable regions appear to contribute to the antigenic and functional properties of individual Opa family members.

Opa expression is variable; different colonies isolated from a single strain may express none, one, or several serologically distinct Opas simultaneously [120]. Fluctuation between different Opa expression patterns in vitro occurs at rates as high as one per 1000 cell divisions [128]. When fully expressed, the Opa content of the outer membrane nearly equals that of PorB. The genetic basis for Opa phase and antigenic variation has been studied in great detail. Within individual strains, Opas are specified by up to 12 independent structural genes that are distributed throughout the gonococcal chromosome [119,127]. Opa protein expression is controlled at the level of translation by the presence of up to 28 identical, tandem pentameric repeats (CTCTT) encoding the signal peptide [129,130]. Intact Opas are produced only when the number of the repeat units places the initiator AUG codon in-frame with the mature protein coding sequence. A change in the number of repeats results from slipped-strand mispairing of the pentameric units during DNA replication and is independent of RecA activity. Translational regulation as described above accounts for the expression of serologically distinct Opas within a single strain. This antigenic diversity is further enhanced through the recombination between *opa* genes within and among gonococcal strains resulting in chimeric *opa* structural genes with different combinations of hypervariable regions [121]. Sequence analysis of gonococcal and meningococcal *opa* genes suggests that horizontal genetic exchange and recombination between *N. gonorrhoeae* and *N. meningitidis* DNA occur in nature [131], as evidenced by the presence of at least one identical *opa* hypervariable locus in isolates of the two species.

Contribution of Opas to Gonococcal Pathogenesis. In addition to promoting interbacterial adhesion, Opa proteins have long been recognized as adhesins that facilitate gonococcal interactions with human epithelial and phagocytic cells [122,132–135]. The expression of certain Opa proteins favors the binding of gonococci to human polymorphonuclear cells but not human epithelial cells [136]. In another study, it was demonstrated that only a subset of Opa proteins could induce oxidative killing by human polymorphonuclear cells, whereas a different subset could induce oxidative killing by human peripheral blood monocytes [133]. Variability in Opa-mediated host cell binding and activation is likely a reflection of variation in host cell receptors and the intracellular pathways stimulated by specific Opa binding to these receptors.

Early studies of naturally infected patients suggest that Opa expression is strongly correlated with the clinical manifestation of gonorrhea. In women, recovery of opaque colonial variants is highly associated with endocervicitis occurring at midcycle. In men, Opa$^+$ gonococci are closely linked with uncomplicated urethritis, pharyngitis, and proctitis. By contrast, recovery of the transparent colonial morphology is associated with disseminated gonococcal infection, pelvic inflammatory disease, and endocervicitis during menstruation [30]. Antibodies to Opa proteins can be detected in the convalescent serum and vaginal fluid of patients treated for gonorrhea, indicating that these proteins are expressed and immunogenic in vivo [112]. In an analysis of 200 variants of a single strain isolated during an outbreak of penicillin-resistant gonorrhea, Schwalbe et al. [137] demonstrated variable Opa expression. Swanson et al. [121,126] demonstrated a transition to the opaque phenotype in vivo in males challenged by urethral inoculation with a transparent colonial variant.

In more recent studies employing the male urethral challenge model, volunteers were challenged with transparent gonococci followed by the characterization of the Opa protein expression of gonococci recovered from the urine, urethra, and semen [138]. The studies confirmed the strong selection for Opa proteins in vivo, which are expressed more rapidly, in greater number, and with more variation than the same strains passaged in vitro. However, no single Opa protein type was preferentially expressed during early infection in the male urethra, and different subjects inoculated with the same bacterial suspension developed infections with gonococci that varied dramatically in the Opas expressed.

Using isogenic gonococci differing only in Opa expression in conjunction with well-defined cell lines, two candidate host receptors have been identified. One receptor appears to be the heparan sulphate proteoglycans (HSPGs)

[132,139,140]. Certain Opa proteins that contain highly cationic surface-exposed loops bind strongly to HSPGs, resulting in invasion of certain epithelial cells such conjunctival cells. This binding is markedly reduced by competition with soluble heparin, heparan sulfate, or HSPGs. In addition, the serum proteins vitronectin and fibronectin, in conjunction with their integrin receptors (and other cell proteins), encourage HSPG-mediated binding [141–143]. Opa-mediated binding to HSPG receptors results in the stimulation of intracellular signaling pathways involving acid sphingomyelinases [144] and cytoskeletal rearrangement [145]. A convincing argument that these events facilitate invasion by gonococci has been made.

A second target for many Opas is the CEACAM (formerly called CD66) family of host cell receptors. These host cell surface antigens are represented by multiple isoforms, each with a different expression pattern on various epithelial and immune cells. This differential expression and subsequent Opa recognition may account for the tissue tropism exhibited by the isogenic gonococcal Opa variants. As in the case of binding to HSPG receptors, binding to CEACAM results in the activation of intracellular signaling cascades, including acid sphingomyelinases [144], protein tyrosine kinases [146], and cytoskeletal rearrangement [145]. Recent studies suggest that Opa$^+$ gonococci binding to CEACAM1 (also called CD66a or BGP) on CD4$^+$ T-cells [146] and to CEACAM3 (CD66d or CGM1a) on B-cells and neutrophils may result in the inhibition of host immune responses.

Opa expression is strongly correlated with the most basic aspects of host–parasite interaction. One interpretation of studies of Opa biology is that this family of proteins and the genetic mechanisms that underlie its phase and antigenic variation are essential to the ecology of the organism, if not for virulence per se. Studies in the male urethral challenge model do not indicate a "programmed" or "selected" Opa, or, for that matter, a pilin expression pattern. Rather, expression of these antigenic and phase-variable surface proteins during infection reflects a certain arbitrariness, placing an apparent premium on antigenic and attachment diversity. Opa expression may also play a role in active immune suppression by gonococci, consistent with the familiar picture of reinfection, even by *N. gonorrhoeae* of the same porin serotype [147].

3. Environmentally Regulated Nutrient Acquisition Proteins

Transferrin-Binding Proteins—TbpA and TbpB. Given the tight regulation of protein expression exhibited by other organisms in response to their growth environment, analysis of the molecular composition of gonococci grown on rich complex medium in a laboratory environment may not accurately reflect the composition of the organism in vivo. The natural environment of the human host is defined by many parameters; notable examples include extremes in temperature, pH [148,149], and growth-essential nutrients. The latter is of particular significance because natural environments are frequently limited in one or more essential nutrients due to depletion by the host and endogenous microbial populations. Hence, nutrient insufficiency may be the most common environmental extreme to which a pathogen is exposed. Investigators have focused on potential gonococcal antigens expressed when this organism is propagated under conditions that simulate those of a less than hospitable host. For example, using continuous culture, Morse et al. [150] were able to modulate the structural and antigenic composition of gonococcal LOS using glucose as a rate-limiting nutrient. Other reports suggest that oxygen tension may influence the synthesis of novel proteins [36,151]. However, the most attention in this area has focused upon the influence of environmental iron concentration on the molecular composition of gonococci [152–154].

Within the human host, there is little free iron, most being complexed to human transferrin in serum and human lactoferrin in secretions [155]. Iron in the form of heme may be available, bound to proteins such as hemoglobin, hapto-globin, or hemopexin [153,156]. These host proteins represent the principal reservoir of growth-essential iron for pathogenic bacteria. In turn, the ability of pathogenic microorganisms to scavenge iron from their host environment and incorporate this element into proteins is a crucial requirement for the production of disease [157]. Many pathogenic bacteria employ soluble low-molecular-weight siderophores that compete for this iron source [158]. The inability to detect the secretion of a soluble siderophore by Norod et al. [159] for the gonococcus, and by Archibald et al. [160] for the meningococcus, was the first indication that these organisms employed a fundamentally different mechanism for iron acquisition from the canonical siderophore-mediated mechanisms of scavenging iron observed in other organisms. Ultimately, this was resolved using a classical experiment by Archibald et al. [160]. These investigators demonstrated that ferri-transferrin, sequestered within a dialysis bag and immersed in iron-limiting media, was able to support the growth of a siderophore-producing strain of *E. coli* but not *N. meningitidis*, leading to the conclusion that transferrin binding was required for meningococci but not for *E. coli*. Almost three decades after these original experiments were performed, the existence of a transferrin receptor-binding complex on the surface of pathogenic *Neisseria* is well accepted [156,161]. For a contemporary review comparing the different mechanisms of iron transport among gram-negative bacteria, the reader is directed to Clarke et al. [162].

All strains of *N. gonorrhoeae* obtained from clinical infections are able to utilize iron from human transferrin [163], whereas only subsets of gonococci are able to utilize iron from human lactoferrin and hemoglobin [164]. The key to this process is the expression of specific receptors that bind human transferrin, human lactoferrin, or hemoglobin at the bacterial surface. One further source of iron is an outer membrane receptor formerly referred to as FrpB [165], but now designated FetA for *f*erric *e*nterobactin *t*ransport [166]. This receptor recognizes phenolate siderophores produced by other microorganisms. A common property of pathogenic *Neisseria* is the exploitation of endogenous host iron sources such as transferrin, lactoferrin, hemoglobin, or phenolate siderophores, without expending metabolic energy to make a scavenging (e.g., siderophore) compound.

The neisserial lactoferrin, hemoglobin, and enterobactin receptors all demonstrate some capacity for phase variation [156,167,168], allowing gonococci expressing these surface proteins to potentially escape immune responses directed at these proteins, and making these poor targets for vaccine development. On the other hand, the transferrin receptor is expressed by all gonococci and does not demonstrate phase variation, making it an attractive target for a vaccine. Thus, subsequent sections of this review on the biochemistry and contributions of iron to gonococcal pathogenesis are focused on the gonococcal transferrin receptor.

Biochemistry of Transferrin-Binding Proteins. The gonococcal transferrin receptor is comprised of a heterodimer transcribed from a bicistronic operon whose promoter is regulated by the iron-dependent transcriptional repressor "Fur" (for *f*erric *u*ptake *r*epressor) [169]. The first gene in this operon encodes a lipoprotein (TbpB) that is tethered to the gonococcal cell surface and imparts binding and recognition properties to the transferrin receptor oligomeric complex [170,171]. The second gene in this operon encodes an integral outer membrane protein (TbpA) that is proposed to function as a gated porin [172]. Sequence analysis of TbpA reveals homology with the TonB-dependent outer membrane siderophore receptors FepA, FecA, IutA, FhuA, and FhuE [162]. By SDS-PAGE, the molecular masses of the gonococcal TbpA and TbpB are estimated to be ~100 and ~85 kDa, respectively [154]. Structural and antigenic diversity is demonstrated for both TbpA [173] and TbpB [174], although the variability appears to be greater for the more surface-accessible TbpB.

The stoichiometry of TbpA to TbpB in the transferrin receptor complex does not appear to be fixed and may vary as a function of the degree of iron starvation of gonococci [172]. Under extreme conditions, there may be as many as 20 copies of TbpB to one copy of TbpA. The specificity of the neisserial TbpA/B receptor complex for transferrin of hominid origin has been well described and may explain why gonococcal infection is confined to humans [156]. The gonococcal transferrin receptor preferentially binds to ferri-transferrin over apo-transferrin [175,176]. TbpA or TbpB can bind human transferrin independently of each other; however, both are required for the efficient transport of growth-essential iron from human transferrin [170,177]. The mechanism by which the gonococcal receptor liberates iron from human transferrin is unclear; the dissociation constant of iron bound to transferrin is 10^{-20} M.

Contribution to Gonococcal Pathogenesis. To accomplish its proposed function, the gonococcal transferrin receptor requires that it be surface-exposed. It has been proposed that human transferrin bound to the gonococcal cell surface may act as a bridging ligand to facilitate the attachment and invasion of organisms [178]. More recent studies using gonococcal invasion of transformed cells propagated in culture report that human epithelial cells infected with *N. gonorrhoeae* have reduced levels of transferrin receptor messenger RNA and cycling of human transferrin receptors, suggesting that infection alters epithelial cell transferrin–iron homeostasis at multiple levels [179]. The expression of a functional transferrin receptor is critical to growth of gonococci in vivo. Cornelissen et al. [180] report that an engineered mutation inactivating the transferrin receptor, in a strain of *N. gonorrhoeae* that naturally lacks the lactoferrin receptor, rendered the bacteria unable to cause experimental urethral infection. These observations underscore the critical relationship between the ability to obtain iron from the host environment and the ability to efficiently cause disease.

4. Other Surface-Exposed Structures

In addition to the well-described gonococcal surface antigens discussed above, recent work from Spence et al. [181] suggests that ribosomal protein, L12, is exposed on the surface of *N. gonorrhoeae* and is involved in the invasion of host cells in the female genital tract bearing the lutropin receptor. This rather surprising observation further emphasizes the complexity and redundancy of mechanisms for the attachment and invasion of host cells in this remarkably versatile pathogen.

C. Experimental Models of Gonococcal Infection

1. Cell Culture Models

Significant progress has been made in recent years with respect to the host cellular receptors and the signal transduction processes involved in neisserial adherence, invasion, and transcytosis. Transformed and well-defined primary cell cultures have provided the most controlled models to analyze gonococcal adherence, invasion, and influence on host cell biology [18,56,135]. These studies have defined CD46 as a receptor for pilus that allows adherence to epithelial and endothelial cells, HSPGs acting in cooperation with vitronectin and fibronectin as receptors for some Opa variants, CEACAMs as the receptors for other Opa variants, and the host cell asialoglycoprotein receptor for gonococcal LOS expressing an appropriate terminal sugar. Binding to these receptors initiates the process of transcytosis through epithelial, endothelial, and phagocytic cells. From these studies, it can be concluded that the surface variation exhibited by gonococci is adaptive, and may modulate tissue tropism, immune evasion and suppression, and survival in the multiple environments (e.g., cervix vs. male urethra) encountered by this organism.

2. Fallopian Tube Culture Model

Explanted cervical, urethral, and fallopian tissues have been used for the purpose of understanding the pathobiology of the gonococcus. McGee et al. [50,182,183] pioneered a fallopian tube model from premenopausal women undergoing oophosalpingohysterectomy. Fallopian tubes obtained from these volunteers can be maintained in tissue culture for several days, exhibiting normal ciliary motion and synthesis of local antibodies and cytokines [184]. Using this model, the temporal sequence of the interaction of the gonococcus with fallopian tube membranes has been defined [183]: Approximately 20 hr after inoculation of the fallopian tube mucosa with piliated gonococci, scanning electron micrographs reveal attachment to nonciliated, low columnar cells. Although few microorganisms interact with the ciliated epithelial cells, many cilia begin to slough from the epithelial cell surface, probably as a result of TNF-α [50]. The attachment of organisms exclusively to the nonciliated columnar cells suggests a highly specific recognition event indicative of a receptor ligand-mediated binding process. Gonococcal adherence to the mucosal surface appears to occur at two levels: Initially, long-range adherence occurs, which is most likely mediated by pili. Subsequently, intimate association between the gonococcal outer membrane and the epithelial cell plasma membrane occurs, which may be mediated by afimbrial adhesins such as Opas and LOS. By 2 hr, invasion of epithelial cells by gonococci is evident. This process appears to begin with the retraction of gonococcal-bound microvilli that, in effect, encompass the organism, leading to its presence in a membrane-bound endocytic vesicle. By 40 hr, the membrane-bound vesicles are found to contain multiple organisms and are located close to the cytoplasmic face of the basal surface of the epithelial cell. Thus, transport of the vesicle from the apical to the basal aspect of the cell has occurred, accompanied by the replication of single organisms within vesicles or the coalescence and fusion of several vesicles leading, in either case, to the existence of larger vesicles containing multiple organisms. Fusion of the basal plasma and vesicular membranes ensues and is followed by exocytosis of gonococci onto the basement membrane and in the lamina propria of the subepithelial space, where they may multiply in a sterile environment devoid of competing commensal organisms. In addition, the gonococcus is positioned in close proximity to local lymphatics and blood.

Although the human fallopian tube culture closely mimics the interaction between host and the insulting gonococcus, it is critical to appreciate the differences between this simulated organ culture model and natural infection. The use of sera of nonhuman origin to sustain fallopian tube viability is not a condition typically encountered by gonococci. Furthermore, many inflammatory and immune processes of gonococcal pathogenesis cannot be studied in the fallopian tube organ model.

3. Murine Models of Gonorrhea

Progressing from cellular models of gonococcal infection to animal models, gonococcal infection has been established in chambers implanted subcutaneously in mice [185]. Corbiel et al. [186] were able to initiate vaginal infection in mice. Two groups extended these early observations using 17-β estradiol to establish the colonization of the vagina with gonococci. Arko et al. [187] investigated the parenteral vaccination of mice with gonococcal antigens and then challenged with live gonococci. Vaginal clearance of gonococci from mice parenterally primed with a gonococcal PIB synthetic peptide and then orally immunized with a γ-irradiated, Rmp-deficient gonococcal strain was significantly more efficient than in corresponding nonimmunized controls. Similarly, Plante et al. [188] used estradiol-treated female mice to study the vaccine potential of outer membranes. Mice receiving nasal immunization with gonococcal outer membranes demonstrated a systemic and vaginal immune response against several outer membrane proteins. Immunized mice cleared gonococci in half the time observed in the control group. These experimental studies suggest that a vaccination approach for the management of gonococcal infection is feasible. Despite its limitations (e.g., inability of gonococci to multiply in mouse serum and the lack of classical symptomology), the mouse model of gonococcal infection is likely to receive increased attention in coming years, especially as results demonstrate predictable results with the human challenge model.

4. Primate Models of Gonorrhea

More relevant animal models are those that have been developed in primates. Some, but not all, primate tissues can be infected with gonococci in vitro [185]. Gonococci bind to chimpanzee epithelial cells. Furthermore, male chimpanzees inoculated with *N. gonorrhoeae* develop purulent urethral infection and transmit the organism to female chimpanzees. However, the cost and ethical issues of working with chimpanzees have limited the extent to which this experimental approach has been and can be used.

5. Human Male Urethral Challenge Model of Gonorrhea

It has long been recognized that gonococci transmitted in urethral pus or grown in vitro can cause urethral infection. Historically, John Hunter first employed the human urethral challenge model experimentally in the now-infamous experiment in 1767 by inoculating himself with a urethral exudate from a patient suffering from gonorrhea. Unfortunately, the exudate was also infected with *Treponema pallidum* and Dr. Hunter tragically acquired the much more serious symptoms of syphilis. In the 1960s, Kellogg et al. [86] employed a human challenge model to detect differences in gonococcal infectivity related to colony morphology (manifested as a result of pilin expression, as described above). In this study, piliated gonococci were 1000-fold more infectious than nonpiliated organisms. In the 1970s, Brinton et al. [80] used the male urethral challenge model to demonstrate protection to homologous challenge using a pilin subunit vaccine.

The male urethral challenge model of gonococcal infection, in its current form, involves the direct inoculation of gonococci 5 cm into the distal urethra through a small-diameter catheter in order to bypass the squamous epithelium (which is believed to be somewhat resistant to gonorrhea relative to the transitional epithelium). Only male subjects have been used in this model because possible complications to females in this model represent an unacceptable risk [189]. Furthermore, treatment of subjects prior to painful symptoms generally limits the model to the very early stages of gonococcal infection. The inoculum required to cause gonococcal infection in men depends on the strain used and the in vitro growth conditions used to prepare this inoculum. Typically, 10^6 organisms are required to attain an infectious dose in 100% of volunteers [189]. However, using organisms recovered from humans with experimental urethritis, infection has been attained with as few as 250 bacteria [190].

Pyogenic urethral discharge (generally asymptomatic) develops 1–3 days after inoculation and is typically preceded by the recovery of gonococcal colonies from the urine and an increased number of white cells in the urine. After infection is established, gonococci can be harvested and quantified within the semen. Experimental subjects excrete 10^3–10^4 organisms per milliliter of semen whereas patients with natural infection excrete 10^6 organisms per milliliter of semen.

The human challenge model can be used for three purposes: (a) to define antigenic variation during infection; (b) to use isogenic mutants to determine gonococcal genes (and structures or enzymes) required to produce mucosal infection in men; and (c) to test a vaccine for efficacy. Using this model, antigenic variation in LOS, pilin, and Opa expression during experimental human infection has been described [113,114,126,128,189–191]. As inferred by the antigenically variable gonococcal surface antigens, recombination (generally facilitated by RecA) would be predicted to be an important property [192,193]. Contrary to this prediction, the inoculation of a RecA-deficient strain was virulent in spite of a single predominant pilin phenotype [193a]. Subjects infected with this strain frequently developed delayed or asymptomatic infection and, in some cases, the urine colony counts began to fall at the time of therapy, thereby suggesting an engagement of host defenses capable of eradicating the organism. From these studies, it is clear that gonococci do not follow a "programmed" order of surface antigen expression. Antigenic variation can be expected to help the organism evade host responses and to provide the organism a better chance to establish infection in the next host. Isogenic pilin, RecA, IgA protease, Opa, and transferrin receptor mutants have been examined [114,126,138,180,189,191, 194,195]. Although some differences were observed when comparing mutant organisms to wild type, the results indicate that the transferrin receptor is absolutely required for infection in organisms that do not use lactoferrin as an iron source [180].

A characteristic of gonorrhea is that repeated infections often occur within an individual and, after clearance, subsequent infections are often caused by the identical organism responsible for the primary infection. This is referred to as gonococcal recidivism and begs the question as to why the infected human host does not mount an effective immune response to prevent subsequent infections as a result of exposure to the primary infection. The human challenge model has been used to determine whether experimental infection limits reinfection. Schmidt et al. [194] used a defined inoculum of Opa⁻ gonococci to infect volunteers, and infection was allowed to progress to a symptomatic state. Two weeks posttreatment, subjects were challenged with a lower number (10%) of the identical gonococcal clone. This challenge infected the same number (ca. 50%) of previously infected subjects as naive controls, indicating that no broadly protective immunity resulted from the initial challenge. However, serological analyses from this small number of rechallenged subjects suggested that the presence of serum IgG antibodies against gonococcal LOS was associated with an increased resistance to reinfection with the lower inoculum. Whether these antibodies resulted from experimental infection or previous community-based encounters could not be discerned.

III. POTENTIAL GONOCOCCAL VACCINE STRATEGIES—PREVIOUS EXPERIENCE, FUTURE DIRECTIONS

A. The Immune Response to Gonococcal Infection

An antibody response that can be amplified by vaccination of the human host forms the basis for most of the bacterial vaccines described in this text. Indeed, the development of capsular vaccines protecting against systemic disease by common strains of meningococcal infection was developed based on landmark work correlating serum bactericidal antibodies with protection [196]. Unlike meningococci, gonococci do not make capsules and previous diseases do not protect from reinfection. Consequently, in the case of gonococcal infection, we are forced to understand a failed immune response rather than to capitalize on the success of the meningococcal vaccine.

The conventional view is that a successful gonococcal vaccine must ultimately induce a mucosal antibody response. Antibodies generated at mucosal surfaces are expected to (a) block bacterial attachment, (b) facilitate granulocyte killing by promoting ingestion, or (c) stimulate complement-mediated lysis. Accordingly, insight into the mucosal response to gonococcal infection is essential. Mucosal and invasive gonococcal infection induces serum antibodies directed against surface-exposed antigens [48,108]. These immune responses, in large part, represent the basis for the selection of existing vaccine candidates. In some studies, serum antibodies directed against some porin types [197] or Opa proteins [198] have been correlated with some levels of protection from infection.

More recently, Hedges et al. conducted quantitative studies of the mucosal immune response in female and male volunteers. In studies with cervical mucus and vaginal wash fluid, these investigators rarely detected the inflammatory cytokines (IL-1, IL-6, and IL-8), except in women with concomitant infections with several pathogens (e.g., gonococci, *Trichomonas*, and *Chlamydia*) [199,200]. Serum cytokines were detected in high levels in some of these subjects. Likewise, the concentration of antibodies detected in the urethral exudate or semen in men with gonorrhea was very low. However, the inflammatory response itself in men was confirmed by an increase in cytokines (IL-1, IL-6, IL-8, and TNF-α) in semen of men with gonococcal urethritis compared to a control group. A similar cytokine profile was detected in the urine of subjects with experimental urethritis [200a]. These findings suggest that antibody formation is not a result of stimulation by interaction between exposed gonococcal antigens and local immune devices.

Studies of blood T-lymphocyte responses to gonococci have been reported. Massari et al. [201] demonstrated that peripheral blood CD4$^+$ and CD8$^+$ T-cells harvested from patients with mucosal gonococcal infection have a demonstrable increased TH$_2$-type response to porin antigens. In addition, increased numbers of CD4$^+$ T-cells have been recovered from the cervicovaginal lavage of women experiencing gonococcal infection. However, the lymphocytic responses to gonococcal infection have not been studied in the context of vaccinologic protection.

Gonococci may exploit the innate metabolic and enzymatic functions of the host to limit the immune response to infection [52]. Examination of outer membrane proteins expressed during natural infection demonstrates that the organism can shift from an aerobic to an anaerobic environment [151,202]. Gonococci are capable of respiration sufficient to limit free radical formation of attacking neutrophils, at least in vitro [203].

Mucosal secretions contain all classes of antibodies, but secretory IgA1 and IgA2 are locally generated, whereas IgG concentration likely reflects transudation from serum. Gonococci (and meningococci) make a protease that can cleave secretory IgA1 (sIgA1) at the hinge region, uncoupling the specificity-determining region (Fab) of sIgA1 from its effector (Fc) region. From this, it is inferred that (a) sIgA is an important local defense, and (b) gonococcal IgA1 protease evolves to support infection [204]. The detection of serum and mucosal antibodies in people with meningococcal infection directed against IgA1 protease proves that this enzyme is generated in vivo [205]. However, it has not been possible to demonstrate a role for this enzyme in gonococcal pathogenesis. sIgA cleavage fragments typical of protease activity are not detected in cervical fluid of women with gonococci. IgA1 protease-deficient gonococcal mutants cause infection in both the fallopian tube model [184] and the urethral challenge model [206], comparable to control organisms. It is possible that the gonococcal IgA1 protease plays an alternative role. More recently, it has been demonstrated that this enzyme can cleave an important phagosomal protein (LAMP-1) and can facilitate intracellular survival and transcytosis [207–210].

B. Vaccine Candidates

Delivery approaches. Experience with both bacterial and viral vaccines suggests several potential approaches that include live attenuated vaccines, killed whole bacterial pathogen vaccines, outer membrane vesicles, purified subunit vaccines, and DNA vaccines. Given the propensity for gonococcal recidivism, a live attenuated vaccine is unlikely to be successful. A killed vaccine consisting of autolyzed gonococci was tested in the 1970s and demonstrated no protective effect [211]. Furthermore, gonococcal LOS limits the use of a live attenuated or killed pathogen. On the other hand, progress has been made in all the other approaches. Subunit vaccines have been tested, or are in clinical development. Outer membrane vesicles have been employed as potential meningococcal group B [27] and gonococcal vaccines [188] using murine models. The use of a gonococcal DNA vaccine using unique vectors has also been reported. Regardless of the delivery system, the key question remains: Can an immune response be directed to any known epitopes that will stimulate a broadly protective immune response against the quasi-species inoculum typified by gonococcal infection? In this regard, three gonococcal subunit vaccines employing pilin, porin, and the transferrin-binding proteins have been focused on and deserve discussion.

1. Pilin Vaccines

Previous Vaccine Experience with Pili. The functional, structural, and serological properties of gonococcal pili described above strongly correlate gonococcal pathogenesis with antibodies to pili that block the attachment of gonococci to human cells and that promote phagocytosis [212, 213]. These antibodies can be found in the sera and genital secretions of individuals convalescing from gonorrhea. Based upon this rationale, a vaccine comprised of pilus filaments was prepared from one gonococcal strain by Brinton et al. [80], Tramont et al. [111,215,216], and McChesney et al. [214] and administered by intramuscular injection to two male volunteers. Approximately 3 months after the primary immunization, the vaccine recipients and three nonimmunized control subjects were challenged by intraurethral inoculation with increasing numbers of the homologous gonococcal strain. In this study, vaccination was associated with a 30-fold increase in resistance to gonococcal infection. One of the immunized volunteers was boosted 15 months later. Upon challenge, a 900-fold increase in resistance, when compared to the nonimmunized control subjects, could be demonstrated. These data led to a larger study of more than 100 subjects, which showed that a higher dose of gonococci was required to cause infection in pilus-vaccinated individuals when compared to a control group [80]. This study established that a parenteral gonococcal pilus vaccine could confer at least partial protection.

Studies of the local and systemic immune response to the same vaccine were performed by Tramont et al. [111,216]. After immunization, antibodies to pili were detected in the serum and genital secretions of 100% and 50% of the vaccine recipients, respectively; the antibodies generated were opsonic and blocked the attachment of gonococci to human buccal cells. The immune sera were assessed for cross-reactivity with pili prepared from several heterologous gonococcal strains and were found to be substantially more broadly reactive than the immune sera elicited by the same vaccine in rabbits and mice. Moreover, the human immune sera contained antibodies that recognized a common pilus epitope; these cross-reacting antibodies seemed to be functionally important, being able to block buccal cell attachment by heterologous strains. Based on this information, the U.S. Army carried out a double-blind, randomized, placebo-controlled field trial with the same vaccine preparation. Gonorrhea occurred in 108 of 1499 (7.2%) men receiving the gonococcal vaccine and in 101 of 1498 (6.7%) men receiving a placebo vaccine. Moreover, no relationship between serum antibody levels to pili and risk of infection could be demonstrated. Four possible reasons for failure of this vaccine include: (a) the number of gonococci encountered in nature may have exceeded the level of protection conferred by the vaccine; (b) the concentration of antibodies to pili in genital secretions may have been too low to provide protection; (c) the antigenic diversity of pili expressed by the heterologous infecting strains may have been too great; and (d) antibodies elicited by the vaccine may have actually been selected for pilus variants unaffected by these antibodies.

Current State of a Pilus-Based Gonococcal Vaccine. The remarkable antigenic diversity of gonococcal pilin subunit has limited enthusiasm for its development as a subunit vaccine candidate. However, demonstrating that the minor pilus-related outer membrane protein, PilC, is a possible adhesin associated with the pilus tip [96,217] represents a significant finding in light of the observation that antibody to similar adhesions from *E. coli* urinary tract isolates significantly reduced infectivity [218]. The finding that PilQ (OMP-MC) is essential for pilus biogenesis and function is interesting because it is surface-accessible and common among diverse gonococcal isolates.

2. Porin Vaccine

Previous Vaccine Experience with Por. Antibodies to PorB are bactericidal [219–223] and opsonic [224]. Furthermore, antibodies are detected in the vaginal fluid and serum of patients convalescing from gonorrhea [48]. Virji et al. [225,226] reported that Por-specific monoclonal antibodies were broadly cross-reactive; two monoclonal antibodies recognized 94% of gonococcal strains tested. These antibodies showed a protective effect when assayed against relevant gonococcal strains by complement activation, opsonic activity, and the ability to protect against challenge to epithelial cells in tissue culture. Elkins et al. [227] presented evidence that bactericidal antibodies could be elicited to peptides derived from Por sequences presumed to be surface-exposed.

Some epidemiological studies have suggested that an immune response to Por could protect against gonococcal infection. Buchanan et al. [228] found that subsequent episodes of salpingitis by gonococci of the same Por serovar were uncommon, indicating that acquired serovar-specific immunity may exist. Rice et al. noted that pelvic inflammatory disease was more common in patients with a reduced ratio of Por/Rmp antibodies [79]. Similarly, a longitudinal study of a cohort of sex workers in Nairobi, Kenya by Plummer et al. [77] found that anti-Rmp antibodies correlated with gonococcal infection. These investigators also reported that particular Por serovars were associated with "specific" but "incomplete" protection against subsequent infection with a homologous serovar [197]. More recent studies in the United States showed no association with Por serovar-specific immunity acquired during the course of natural infection [229].

Blake et al. [211] examined the protection offered from a Por vaccine formulation that likely contained contaminating quantities of Rmp. These investigators noted no protection by the vaccine and more recently have demonstrated that the subjects had a high concentration of antibodies directed against Rmp, suggesting that blocking antibodies could have offset a Por vaccine benefit [79].

Current State of a Por-Based Gonococcal Vaccine. Genetic manipulation allows for the expression of Por in a Rmp-negative gonococcal background [65], or in a genetically altered strain of *E. coli* that does not express OmpA (OmpA is a homologue of Rmp that could elicit blocking antibodies). A purified and renatured Por-based vaccine is currently being evaluated by Wyeth-Lederle in human volunteers for safety.

3. Transferrin-Binding Protein Vaccines

Previous Vaccine Experience with Tbps. By virtue of their surface localization, contribution to gonococcal growth, and high level of expression during the course of natural infection, the transferrin receptor complex is a reasonable target for a candidate vaccine. The phase variation demonstrated by the lactoferrin, hemoglobin, and enterochelin receptors challenges their consideration as a vaccine candidate. A transferrin receptor complex approach is being pursued to produce a protein-based meningococcal vaccine that would be broadly protective across capsular serotypes [174,230,231]. A potential limitation of a Tbp-based vaccine is competition for binding of host transferrin to the receptors; levels of host transferrin exist at micromolar levels, concentrations predicted to saturate the transferrin receptor. Nonetheless, lessons derived from studies of meningococcal Tbp should be very informative for the development of a homologous gonococcal vaccine formulation.

Current State of a Tbp-Based Gonococcal Vaccine. The finding that deleting the transferrin receptor complex from a virulent strain of gonococci renders this organism unable to cause disease [180] is significant and underscores the importance of iron and growth in the host environment. One of the challenges that faces this vaccine approach is the specificity of the gonococcal transferrin receptor complex to human transferrin as a source of iron [156,161]. This limits testing to cell culture models that include human serum in place of sera from animal sources as typically is used, and the use of the human experimental challenge model for testing the efficacy of this vaccine candidate.

C. Other Advances in the Development of a Gonococcal Vaccine

1. Mab2c7 Antiidiotype

Yamasaki et al. [232] demonstrated that a monoclonal antibody, Mab2C7, binds to more than 90% of gonococcal isolates. This antibody is bactericidal (even in the face of sialylation) and opsonic. These investigators have proposed an idiotype/antiidiotype approach to gonococcal vaccine development. This antiidiotype approach allows vaccine development against LOS epitopes without immunization with toxic LOS. However, given the antigenic diversity of LOS and the lack of antiidiotypic vaccines for the prevention of other important infectious disease, this vaccinologic approach should probably be considered more theoretical than practical at this time.

IV. CONCLUSIONS

Regardless of small fluctuations in incidence and prevalence, gonorrhea remains a major global public health problem. Given the challenges for developing a vaccine for the prevention of gonorrhea, in the short term, more aggressive methods of diagnosis and treatment can be employed to decrease the incidence of this disease. One of the major problems in this area is compliance of the infected, typically adolescent, population to undergo STD testing. A significant step toward preserving the privacy of the adolescent would be the implementation of vaginal swabs self-collection used to diagnose *N. gonorrhoeae*. In a study addressing this [233], it was demonstrated that 2% of female students in this age group tested positive for gonorrhea using sensitive polymerase chain reaction (PCR)-based methods. The study also found that self-collection of vaginal swabs was almost uniformly reported as easy to perform and preferable to a gynecological examination. Nearly all of the study participants indicated that they would undergo testing at frequent intervals if self-testing was available. A similar finding regarding the positive merits of self-testing was independently reported by another group of investigators [234]. Clearly one of the most effective ways of controlling gonorrhea is the rapid and private diagnosis of this disease. Self-testing is an option that would empower a high-risk population to detect gonorrhea, and other STDs, that would otherwise remain undetected and untreated. After diagnosis, administration of effective antibiotic treatment will be required, which represents its own challenges given the emergence of antimicrobial resistance by the gonococcus. Furthermore, treating gonococcal infection will not prevent facilitated AIDS transmission and may not prevent reproductive tract sequelae.

The only reasonable conclusion that can be reached is that in the long term, a vaccine for the prevention and management of gonococcal infection remains as important today as when the quest for a gonococcal vaccine began some 30 years previous. Although a vaccine that prevents infection would be ideal, one that reduces transmission from an immunized but still infected host to his/her sexual partner would likely be of equal significance—particularly coupled with effective diagnosis and treatment.

The introductory chapters in this book are devoted to describing the ideal nature of a vaccine for infectious diseases of human significance. In a perfect world, a vaccine for the prevention of gonorrhea could be developed, therefore dispensing with issues of the diagnosis and treatment briefly described above. However, the unique pathobiology of gonococcal infection, which includes surface antigen variation and transient intracellular survival, along with limitations of animal model testing, makes the implementation of a safe and effective gonococcal vaccine very difficult. The development of such a vaccine would represent a "quantum leap" in the management of gonorrhea. In spite of this, we have learned an enormous amount about the biology and immunology of gonococcal infection. These are the data required to develop a rational vaccine. The failure of natural infection to offer protective immunity likely rests in the very poor mucosal response elicited.

Our challenges are clear: (a) we must develop immune strategies that force a vigorous mucosal response, so we can test the hypothesis that such a response can prevent infection; (b) this hypothesis can be explored in a mouse model, imperfect as it is; (c) this hypothesis can be validated rapidly

in the human challenge model, a huge advantage to gonococcal vaccine development; (d) surface-exposed antigens
are attractive vaccine targets, and the fact that gonococci
demonstrate an absolute requirement for iron offers unique
epitopes for focus; and (e) sequencing of the gonococcal
genome offers access to neoantigens that may be important
to the organism and that evoke no response; such conserved
neoantigens may ultimately prove of value. Most importantly, we must not become terminally frustrated or perceive
lack of a vaccine as lack of success. Vaccines against STD
pathogens remain the best way to control their spread [235].
What we learn about one pathogen (whether HIV, HSV, or
gonorrhea) is relevant to the entire STD vaccine effort.
Accordingly, now is the best time for increased effort in the
development of a gonococcal vaccine.

REFERENCES

1. Anonymous. Tracking the Hidden Epidemics: Trends in
   STDs in the United States, 2000. CDC Atlanta, GA.
2. Grodstein F, et al. Relation of tubal infertility to history of
   sexually transmitted diseases. Am J Epidemiol 1993; 137:
   577–584.
3. Ault KA, et al. Pelvic inflammatory disease. Current diagnostic criteria and treatment guidelines. Postgrad Med
   1993; 93:85–86, 89–91.
4. Chakraborty H, et al. Viral burden in genital secretions
   determines male-to-female sexual transmission of HIV-1: a
   probabilistic empiric model. AIDS 2001; 15:621–627.
5. Cohen MS, et al. Sexually transmitted diseases and human
   immunodeficiency virus infection: cause, effect, or both? Int
   J Infect Dis 1998; 3:1–4.
6. Sadiq ST, et al. The effects of antiretroviral therapy on
   HIV-1 RNA loads in seminal plasma in HIV-positive patients with and without urethritis. AIDS 2002; 16:219–225.
7. Cohen MS, et al. Reduction of concentration of HIV-1 in
   semen after treatment of urethritis: implications for
   prevention of sexual transmission of HIV-1. Lancet 1997;
   349:1868–1873.
8. Isbey SF, et al. Characterisation of Neisseria gonorrhoeae in
   semen during urethral infection in men. Genitourin Med
   1997; 73:378–382.
9. Kaul R, et al. Gonococcal cervicitis is associated with reduced systemic $CD8^+$ T cell responses in human immunodeficiency virus type 1-infected and exposed, uninfected sex
   workers. J Infect Dis 2002; 185:1525–1529.
10. Vernazza PL, et al. Sexual transmission of HIV: infectious-
    ness and prevention. AIDS 1999; 13:155–166.
11. Mavroidi A, et al. Multidrug-resistant strains of Neisseria
    gonorrhoeae in Greece. Antimicrob Agents Chemother
    2001; 45:2651–2654.
12. Moodley P, et al. Evolution in the trends of antimicrobial re-
    sistance in Neisseria gonorrhoeae isolated in Durban over a
    5 year period: impact of the introduction of syndromic
    management. J Antimicrob Chemother 2001; 48:853–859.
13. Banwat EB, et al. Antimicrobial susceptibility pattern of
    Neisseria gonorrhoeae isolated at the Jos University
    Teaching Hospital, Jos, Central Nigeria. Niger J Med
    (Natl Assoc Resid Drs Niger) 2001; 10:72–74.
14. Dillon JA, et al. Reduced susceptibility to azithromycin and
    high percentages of penicillin and tetracycline resistance in
    Neisseria gonorrhoeae isolates from Manaus, Brazil, 1998.
    Sex Transm Dis 2001; 28:521–526.
15. Dillon JA, et al. The Caribbean. Antimicrobial susceptibil-
    ity of Neisseria gonorrhoeae isolates from three Caribbean

16. countries: Trinidad, Guyana, St. Vincent. Sex Transm Dis
    2001; 28:508–514.
16. Tanaka M, et al. A remarkable reduction in the suscept-
    ibility of Neisseria gonorrhoeae isolates to cephems and the
    selection of antibiotic regimens for the single-dose treat-
    ment of gonococcal infection in Japan. J Infect Chemother
    2002; 8:81–86.
17. Ye S, et al. Surveillance of antibiotic resistance of Neisseria
    gonorrhoeae isolates in China, 1993–1998. Sex Transm Dis
    2002; 29:242–245.
18. Merz AJ, et al. Interactions of pathogenic Neisseriae with
    epithelial cell membranes. Annu Rev Cell Dev Biol 2000;
    16:423–457.
19. Nassif X, et al. Interactions of pathogenic Neisseria with
    host cells: is it possible to assemble the puzzle? Mol
    Microbiol 1999; 32:1124–1132.
20. Koomey M. Implications of molecular contacts and
    signaling initiated by Neisseria gonorrhoeae. Curr Opin
    Microbiol 2001; 4:53–57.
21. Dehio C, et al. Host cell invasion by pathogenic Neisseriae.
    Sub-cell Biochem 2000; 33:61–96.
22. Naumann M, et al. Host cell interactions and signalling
    with Neisseria gonorrhoeae. Curr Opin Microbiol 1999;
    2:62–70.
23. Cannon J, et al. Infectivity of gonococcal mutants in the
    human challenge model. In: Zollinger W, Frasch C, Deal C,
    eds. Pathogenic Neisseria—Tenth International Pathogenic
    Neisseria Conference, Baltimore, MD, 1996:11–12.
24. Turner CF, et al. Untreated gonococcal and chlamydial
    infection in a probability sample of adults. JAMA 2002;
    287:726–733.
25. Nikaido H, et al. The outer membrane of Gram-negative
    bacteria. Morris AHRaJG ed. Advances in Microbial
    Physiology. Vol. 20. London: Academic Press, 1979:163–
    250.
26. DeVoe IW, et al. Release of endotoxin in the form of cell
    wall blebs during in vitro growth of Neisseria meningitidis. J
    Exp Med 1973; 138:1156–1167.
27. Quakyi EK, et al. Immunization with meningococcal outer-
    membrane protein vesicles containing lipooligosaccharide
    protects mice against lethal experimental group B Neisseria
    meningitidis infection and septic shock. J Infect Dis 1999;
    180:747–754.
28. Blake MS. Functions of the outer membrane proteins of
    Neisseria gonorrhoeae. In: Jackson GG, Thomas H, eds.
    The Pathogenesis of Bacterial Infection, Berlin: Springer,
    1985:51–63.
29. Belland RJ, et al. Expression and phase variation of gono-
    coccal P II genes in Escherichia coli involves ribosomal
    frame shifting and slipped strand mispairing. Mol Micro-
    biol 1989; 3:777–786.
30. James JF, et al. Studies on gonococcus infection: XIII.
    Occurrence of color/opacity colonial variants in clinical
    cultures. Infect Immun 1978; 19:332–340.
31. Swanson JS, et al. Studies on gonococcus infection: I. Pili
    and zones of adhesion and their relation to gonococcal
    growth patterns. J Exp Med 1971; 135:886–906.
32. Swanson JS, et al. Pilus—gonococcal variants. Evidence for
    multiple forms of piliation control. J Exp Med 1985; 162:
    729–744.
33. Mietzner TA, et al. Identification of an iron-regulated
    37,000-dalton protein in the cell envelope of Neisseria gon-
    orrhoeae. Infect Immun 1984; 45:410–416.
34. Norqvist A, et al. The effect of iron-starvation on the outer
    membrane protein composition of Neisseria gonorrhoeae.
    FEMS Microbiol Lett 1978; 4:71–75.
35. Silver LE, et al. Construction of a translational lacZ fusion
    system to study gene regulation in Neisseria gonorrhoeae.
    Gene 1995; 166:101–104.

36. Hoehn GT, et al. Isolation and nucleotide sequence of the gene (aniA) encoding the major anaerobically induced outer membrane protein of *Neisseria gonorrhoeae*. Infect Immun 1992; 60:4695–4703.

37. Johnston KH, et al. Isolation and characterization of the outer membrane of *Neisseria gonorrhoeae*. J Bacteriol 1974; 19:250–257.

38. Arking D, et al. Analysis of lipooligosaccharide biosynthesis in the Neisseriaceae. J Bacteriol 2001; 183:934–941.

39. Mandrell RE, et al. Lipooligosaccharides (LOS) of mucosal pathogens: molecular mimicry and host-modification of LOS. Immunobiology 1993; 187:382–402.

40. Griffiss JM, et al. Lipooligosaccharides: the principal glycolipids of the neisserial outer membrane. Rev Infect Dis 1988; 10:s287.

41. Griffiss JM, et al. The immunochemistry of neisserial LOS. Antonie van Leeuwenhoek 1987; 53:501–507.

42. Griffiss JM, et al. Vaccines against encapsulated bacteria: a global agenda. Rev Infect Dis 1987; 9:176–188.

43. Danaher RJ, et al. Genetic basis of *Neisseria gonorrhoeae* lipooligosaccharide antigenic variation. J Bacteriol 1995; 177:7275–7279.

44. Burch CL, et al. Antigenic variation in *Neisseria gonorrhoeae*: production of multiple lipooligosaccharides. J Bacteriol 1997; 179:982–986.

45. Smith H, et al. The sialylation of gonococcal lipopolysaccharide by host factors: a major impact on pathogenicity. FEMS Microbiol Lett 1992; 79:287–292.

46. Frangipane JV, et al. Anaerobic growth and cytidine 5′-monophospho-*N*-acetylneuraminic acid act synergistically to induce high-level serum resistance in *Neisseria gonorrhoeae*. Infect Immun 1993; 61:1657–1666.

47. Parsons NJ, et al. The serum resistance of gonococci in the majority of urethral exudates is due to sialylated lipopolysaccharide seen as a surface coat. FEMS Microbiol Lett 1992; 69:295–299.

48. Lammel CJ, et al. Antibody–antigen specificity in the immune response to infection with *Neisseria gonorrhoeae*. J Infect Dis 1985; 152:990–1001.

49. Greg CR, et al. Toxic activity of purified lipopolysaccharide of *Neisseria gonorrhoeae* for human fallopian tube mucosa. J Infect Dis 1981; 143:432–439.

50. McGee ZA, et al. Gonococcal infection of human fallopian tube mucosa in organ culture: relationship of mucosal tissue TNF-alpha concentration to sloughing of ciliated cells. Sex Transm Dis 1999; 26:160–165.

51. Gill MJ, et al. Functional characterization of a sialyltransferase-deficient mutant of *Neisseria gonorrhoeae*. Infect Immun 1996; 64:3374–3378.

52. Rest RF, et al. Interaction of pathogenic *Neisseria* with host defenses. What happens in vivo? Ann NY Acad Sci 1994; 730:182–196.

53. van Putten JP, et al. Function of lipopolysaccharide in the invasion of *Neisseria gonorrhoeae* into human mucosal cells. Proc Clin Biol Res 1995; 392:49–58.

54. van Putten JP. Phase variation of lipopolysaccharide directs interconversion of invasive and immuno-resistant phenotypes of *Neisseria gonorrhoeae*. EMBO J 1993; 12:4043–4051.

55. Minor SY, et al. Effect of alpha-oligosaccharide phenotype of *Neisseria gonorrhoeae* strain MS11 on invasion of Chang conjunctival, HEC-1-B endometrial, and ME-180 cervical cells. Infect Immun 2000; 68:6526–6534.

56. Harvey HA, et al. Receptor-mediated endocytosis of *Neisseria gonorrhoeae* into primary human urethral epithelial cells: the role of the asialoglycoprotein receptor. Mol Microbiol 2001; 42:659–672.

56a. Feavers IM, Maiden MC. A gonococcal *porA* pseudogene: implications for understanding the evolution and pathoge-

nicity of *Neisseria* gonorrhoeae. Mol Microbiol 1998; 30: 647–656.

57. Harvey HA, et al. The mimicry of human glycolipids and glycosphingolipids by the lipooligosaccharides of pathogenic *Neisseria* and *Haemophilus*. J Autoimmun 2001; 16: 257–262.

58. Douglas JT, et al. Protein I of *Neisseria gonorrhoeae* outer membrane is a porin. FEMS Microbiol Lett 1981; 12:305–309.

59. Newhall WJ, et al. Cross-linking analysis of the outer membrane proteins of *Neisseria gonorrhoeae*. Infect Immun 1980; 28:785–791.

60. Leith DK, et al. Cross-linking analysis of *Neisseria gonorrhoeae* outer membrane proteins. J Bacteriol 1980; 143:182–187.

61. Carbonetti NH, et al. Molecular cloning and characterization of the structural gene for protein I, the major outer membrane protein of *Neisseria gonorrhoeae*. Proc Natl Acad Sci USA 1987; 84:9084–9088.

62. Gotschlich EC, et al. Genetics of protein I of *Neisseria gonorrhoeae* construction of hybrid porins. Proc Natl Acad Sci USA 1983; 85:6841–6845.

63. Gotschlich EC, et al. Porin protein of *Neisseria gonorrhoeae*: cloning and gene structure. Proc Natl Acad Sci USA 1987; 84:8135–8139.

64. Mee BJ, et al. Structural comparison and epitope analysis of outer-membrane protein PIA from strains of *Neisseria gonorrhoeae* with differing serovar specificities. J Gen Microbiol 1993; 139:2613–2620.

65. Wetzler LM, et al. Gonococcal porin vaccine evaluation: comparison of Por proteosomes, liposomes, and blebs isolated from rmp deletion mutants. J Infect Dis 1992; 166:551–555.

66. Lorenzen DR, et al. *Neisseria gonorrhoeae* porin modifies the oxidative burst of human professional phagocytes. Infect Immun 2000; 68:6215–6222.

67. Young JD, et al. Properties of the major outer membrane protein from *Neisseria gonorrhoeae* incorporated into model lipid membranes. Proc Natl Acad Sci USA 1983; 80:3831–3835.

68. Mauro A, et al. Voltage gating of conductance in lipid bilayers induced by porin from outer membrane of *Neisseria gonorrhoeae*. Proc Natl Acad Sci USA 1988; 85:1071–1075.

69. Rudel TA, et al. Modulation of *Neisseria* porin (PorB) by cytosolic ATP/GTP of target cells: parallels between pathogen accommodation and mitochondrial endosymbiosis. Cell 1996; 85:391–402.

70. Haines KA, et al. Effects of protein I of *Neisseria gonorrhoeae* on neutrophil activation: generation of diacylglycerol from phosphatidylcholine via a specific phospholipase C is associated with exocytosis. J Cell Biol 1991; 114:433–442.

71. Muller A, et al. Neisserial porin (PorB) causes rapid calcium influx in target cells and induces apoptosis by the activation of cysteine proteases. EMBO J 1999; 18:339–352.

72. van Putten JP, et al. Gonococcal invasion of epithelial cells driven by PIA, a bacterial ion channel with GTP binding properties. J Exp Med 1998; 188:941–952.

73. Ram S, et al. C4bp binding to porin mediates stable serum resistance of *Neisseria gonorrhoeae*. Int Immunopharmacol 2001; 1:423–432.

74. Ram S, et al. Binding of C4b-binding protein to porin: a molecular mechanism of serum resistance of *Neisseria gonorrhoeae*. J Exp Med 2001; 193:281–295.

75. Ram S, et al. The contrasting mechanisms of serum resistance of *Neisseria gonorrhoeae* and group B *Neisseria meningitidis*. Mol Immunol 1999; 36:915–928.

76. Gotschlich EC, et al. The DNA sequence of the structural gene of gonococcal protein III and the flanking region containing a repetitive sequence; homology of Protein III with

enterobacterial OmpA proteins. J Exp Med 1987; 165:471–482.

77. Plummer FA, et al. Antibody to Rmp (outer membrane protein 3) increases susceptibility to gonococcal infection. J Clin Invest 1993; 91:339–343.

78. Rice PA, et al. Immunoglobulin G antibodies directed against protein III block killing of serum-resistant *Neisseria gonorrhoeae* by immune serum. J Exp Med 1986; 164:1735–1748.

79. Rice PA, et al. Serum resistance of *Neisseria gonorrhoeae*. Does it thwart the inflammatory response and facilitate the transmission of infection? Ann NY Acad Sci 1994; 730:7–14.

80. Brinton CJ, et al. Uses of pili in gonorrhea control: role of bacterial pili in disease, purification, and properties of gonococcal pili, and progress in the development of a gonococcal pilus vaccine for gonorrhea. In: Brooks GF, Gotschlich EC, Holmes KK, Sawyer WD, Young FE, eds. Immunobiology of *Neisseria gonorrhoeae*. Washington, DC: American Society for Microbiology, 1978:1242–1245.

81. Wall D, et al. Type IV pili and cell motility. Mol Microbiol 1999; 32:1–10.

82. Cannon JG, et al. The genetics of the gonococcus. Annu Rev Microbiol 1984; 38:111–133.

83. Fussenegger M, et al. Transformation competence and type-4 pilus biogenesis in *Neisseria gonorrhoeae*—a review. Gene 1997; 192:125–134.

84. Rudel T, et al. Role of pili and the phase-variable PilC protein in natural competence for transformation of *Neisseria gonorrhoeae*. Proc Natl Acad Sci USA 1995; 92:7986–7990.

85. Long CD, et al. Modulation of gonococcal piliation by regulatable transcription of pilE. J Bacteriol 2001; 183:1600–1609.

86. Kellogg DS Jr, et al. *Neisseria gonorrhoeae*: I. Virulence genetically linked to clonal variation. J Bacteriol 1963; 85:1274–1279.

87. Jephcott AE, et al. *Neisseria gonorrhoeae*: III. Demonstration of presumed appendages to cells from different colony types. Acta Pathol Microbiol Scand 1971; 79:437–439.

88. Parge HE, et al. Structure of the fibre-forming protein pilin at 26 A resolution. Nature 1995; 378:32–38.

89. Sandkvist M, et al. General secretion pathway (*eps*) genes required for toxin secretion and outer membrane biogenesis in *Vibrio cholerae*. J Bacteriol 1997; 179:6994–7003.

90. Lory S, et al. Structure–function relationship of type-IV prepilin peptidase of *Pseudomonas aeruginosa*—a review. Gene 1997; 192:117–121.

91. Collins RF, et al. Analysis of the PilQ secretin from *Neisseria meningitidis* by transmission electron microscopy reveals a dodecameric quaternary structure. J Bacteriol 2001; 183:3825–3832.

92. Tonjum T, et al. Structure and function of repetitive sequence elements associated with a highly polymorphic domain of the *Neisseria meningitidis* PilQ protein. Mol Microbiol 1998; 29:111–124.

93. Tonjum T, et al. The pilus colonization factor of pathogenic neisserial species: organelle biogenesis and structure/function relationships—a review. Gene 1997; 192:155–163.

94. Tsai WM, et al. Cloning and DNA sequence of the *omc* gene encoding the outer membrane protein–macromolecular complex from *Neisseria gonorrhoeae*. Infect Immun 1989; 57:2653–2659.

95. Forest KT, et al. Assembly and antigenicity of the *Neisseria gonorrhoeae* pilus mapped with antibodies. Infect Immun 1996; 64:644–652.

96. Rudel T, et al. *Neisseria* PilC protein identified as type-4 pilus tip-located adhesin. Nature 1995; 373:357–359.

97. Rudel T, et al. Interaction of two variable proteins (PilE and PilC) required for pilus-mediated adherence of *Neisseria gonorrhoeae* to human epithelial cells. Mol Microbiol 1992; 6:3439–3450.

98. Rudel T, et al. Pilus biogenesis and epithelial cell adherence of *Neisseria gonorrhoeae* pilC double knock-out mutants. Mol Microbiol 1995; 17:1057–1071.

99. Jonsson AB, et al. Pilus biogenesis gene, pilC, of *Neisseria gonorrhoeae*: pilC1 and pilC2 are each part of a larger duplication of the gonococcal genome and share upstream and downstream homologous sequences with opa and pil loci. Microbiology 1995; 141:2367–2377.

100. Mellies J, et al. Transcriptional regulation of pilC2 in *Neisseria gonorrhoeae*: response to oxygen availability and evidence for growth-phase regulation in *Escherichia coli*. Mol Gen Genet 1997; 255:285–293.

101. Buchanan TM, et al. Pili as a mediator of the attachment of gonococci to human erythrocytes. Infect Immun 1976; 13:1483–1489.

102. James-Holmquest AN, et al. Differential attachment by piliated and nonpiliated *Neisseria gonorrhoeae* to human sperm. Infect Immun 1974; 9:897–902.

103. Nassif X, et al. Antigenic variation of pilin regulates adhesion of *Neisseria meningitidis* to human epithelial cells. Mol Microbiol 1993; 8:719–723.

104. Gorby GL, et al. Effect of attachment factors (pili plus Opa) on *Neisseria gonorrhoeae* invasion of human fallopian tube tissue in vitro: quantitation by computerized image analysis. Microb Pathog 1992; 13:93–108.

105. Kallstrom H, et al. Attachment of *Neisseria gonorrhoeae* to the cellular pilus receptor CD46: identification of domains important for bacterial adherence. Cell Microbiol 2001; 3:133–143.

106. Fernandez R, et al. Increased adhesiveness and internalization of *Neisseria gonorrhoeae* and changes in the expression of epithelial gonococcal receptors in the Fallopian tube of copper T and Norplant users. Hum Reprod 2001; 16:463–468.

107. Novotney P, et al. An electron microscope study of naturally occurring and cultured cells of *Neisseria gonorrhoeae*. J Med Microbiol 1975; 8:413–427.

108. Lammel CJ, et al. Male and female consorts infected with the same strain of *Neisseria gonorrhoeae* often have different antibody responses to protein IIs and other gonococcal antigens. In: Schoolnik GK, Brooks GF, Falkow S, Frasch CE, Knapp JS, McCutchan JS, Morse SA, eds. The Pathogenic *Neisseria*, Proceedings of the Fourth International Symposium. Washington, DC: American Society for Microbiology, 1985:244–249.

109. Ofek I, et al. Resistance of *Neisseria gonorrhoeae* to phagocytosis: relationship to colonial morphology and surface pili. J Infect Dis 1974; 129:310–316.

110. Cohen MS. Molecular events in the activation of human neutrophils for microbial killing. Clin Infect Dis 1994; 18:s170–179.

111. Tramont E, et al. Gonococcal pilus vaccine: studies of antigenicity and inhibition of attachment. J Clin Invest 1981; 68:881–888.

112. Zak K, et al. Antigenic variation during infection with *Neisseria gonorrhoeae*: detection of antibodies to surface proteins in sera of patients with gonorrhea. J Infect Dis 1984; 149:166–174.

113. Swanson J, et al. Gonococcal pilin variants in experimental gonorrhea. J Exp Med 1987; 165:1344–1357.

114. Seifert H, et al. Multiple gonococcal pilin antigenic variants are produced during experimental human infections. J Clin Invest 1994; 93:2744–2749.

115. Seifert HS. Molecular mechanisms of antigenic variation in *Neisseria gonorrhoeae*. Mol Cell Biol Hum Dis Ser 1992; 1:1–22.

116. Mehr IJ, et al. A homologue of the recombination-dependent growth gene, *rdgC*, is involved in gonococcal pilin antigenic variation. Genetics 2000; 154:523–532.

117. Brinton CC, et al. Electrophoresis and phage susceptibility studies on a filament-producing variant of the *E. coli* B bacterium. Biochim Biophys Acta 1954; 15:533.

118. Koomey JM, et al. Pilin expression and processing in pilus mutants of *Neisseria gonorrhoeae*: critical role of Gly-1 in assembly. Mol Microbiol 1991; 5:279–287.

119. Bhat KS, et al. The opacity proteins of *Neisseria gonorrhoeae* strain MS11 are encoded by a family of 11 complete genes. Mol Microbiol 1992; 6:1073–1076.

120. Swanson J. Studies on gonococcus infection: XIV. Cell wall protein differences among color/opacity colony variants of *Neisseria gonorrhoeae*. Infect Immun 1978; 21:292–302.

121. Swanson J, et al. Neisserial surface variation: how and why? Curr Opin Genet Dev 1992; 2:805–811.

122. Blake MS, et al. Gonococcal opacity: lectin-like interactions between Opa proteins and lipooligosaccharide. Infect Immun 1995; 63:1434–1439.

123. Swanson J. ^{125}I-labeled peptide mapping of some heat-modifiable proteins of the gonococcal outer membrane. Infect Immun 1980; 28:54–64.

124. King GJ, et al. Studies on gonococcus infection: XV. Identification of surface proteins of *Neisseria gonorrhoeae* correlated with leukocyte association. Infect Immun 1978; 21: 575–580.

125. Swanson J, et al. Immunologic characteristics of gonococcal outer membrane protein II assessed by immunoprecipitation, immunoblotting, and coagglutination. J Exp Med 1983; 157:1405–1420.

126. Swanson J, et al. Expression of outer membrane protein II by gonococci in experimental gonorrhea. J Exp Med 1988; 168:2121–2129.

127. Dempsey JA, et al. Physical map of the chromosome of *Neisseria gonorrhoeae* FA1090 with locations of genetic markers, including opa and pil genes. J Bacteriol 1991; 173: 5476–5486.

128. Mayer LW. Rates in vitro changes of gonococcal colony opacity phenotypes. Infect Immun 1982; 37:481–485.

129. Stern A, et al. Opacity determinants of *Neisseria gonorrhoeae*: gene expression and chromosomal linkage to the gonococcal pilus gene. Cell 1984; 37:447–456.

130. Stern A, et al. Opacity genes in *Neisseria gonorrhoeae*: control of phase and antigenic variation. Cell 1986; 47:61–71.

131. Hobbs MM, et al. Microevolution within a clonal population of pathogenic bacteria: recombination, gene duplication and horizontal genetic exchange in the opa gene family of *Neisseria meningitidis*. Mol Microbiol 1994; 12:171–180.

132. Chen T, et al. Adherence of pilus-Opa[+] gonococci to epithelial cells in vitro involves heparan sulfate. J Exp Med 1995; 182:511–517.

133. Belland RJ, et al. Human neutrophil response to recombinant neisserial Opa proteins. Mol Microbiol 1992; 6:1729–1737.

134. Gorby G, et al. *Escherichia coli* that express *Neisseria gonorrhoeae* opacity-associated proteins attach to and invade human fallopian tube epithelium. Ann NY Acad Sci 1994; 730:286–289.

135. Dehio C, et al. The role of neisserial Opa proteins in interactions with host cells. Trends Microbiol 1998; 6:489–495.

136. Kupsch EM, et al. Variable opacity (Opa) outer membrane proteins account for the cell tropisms displayed by *Neisseria gonorrhoeae* for human leukocytes and epithelial cells. EMBO J 1993; 12(2):641–650.

137. Schwalbe RS, et al. Variation of *Neisseria gonorrhoeae* protein II among isolates from an outbreak caused by a single gonococcal strain. Infect Immun 1985; 49:250–252.

138. Jerse AE, et al. Multiple gonococcal opacity proteins are expressed during experimental urethral infection in the male. J Exp Med 1994; 179(3):911–920.

139. Chen T, et al. The CGM1a (CEACAM3/CD66d)-mediated phagocytic pathway of *Neisseria gonorrhoeae* expressing opacity proteins is also the pathway to cell death. J Biol Chem 2001; 276:17413–17419.

140. Grant CC, et al. Proteoglycan receptor binding by *Neisseria gonorrhoeae* MS11 is determined by the HV-1 region of OpaA. Mol Microbiol 1999; 32:233–242.

141. Duensing TD, et al. Vitronectin mediates internalization of *Neisseria gonorrhoeae* by Chinese hamster ovary cells. Infect Immun 1997; 65:964–970.

142. van Putten JP, et al. Entry of OpaA[+] gonococci into HEp-2 cells requires concerted action of glycosaminoglycans, fibronectin and integrin receptors. Mol Microbiol 1998; 29:369–379.

143. Freissler E, et al. Syndecan-1 and syndecan-4 can mediate the invasion of OpaHSPG-expressing *Neisseria gonorrhoeae* into epithelial cells. Cell Microbiol 2000; 2:69–82.

144. Makino S, et al. Phase variation of the opacity outer membrane protein controls the invasion of *Neisseria gonorrhoeae* into human epithelial cells. EMBO J 1991; 10:1307–1315.

145. Grassme HU, et al. Gonococcal opacity protein promotes bacterial entry-associated rearrangements of the epithelial cell actin cytoskeleton. Infect Immun 1996; 64:1621–1630.

146. Boulton IC, et al. Neisserial binding to CEACAM1 arrests the activation and proliferation of CD4[+] T lymphocytes. Nat Immunol 2002; 3:229–236.

147. Hobbs MM. Molecular typing of *Neisseria gonorrhoeae* causing repeated infections: evolution of porin during passage within a community. J Infect Dis 1999; 179:371–381.

148. Pettit RK, et al. Phenotypic modulation of gonococcal lipooligosaccharide in acidic and alkaline culture. Infect Immun 1995; 63:2773–2775.

149. Pettit RK, et al. Alteration of gonococcal protein expression in acidic culture. Infect Immun 1996; 64:1039–1042.

150. Morse SA, et al. Effect of dilution rate on lipopopolysaccharide and serum resistance of *Neisseria gonorrhoeae* grown in continuous culture. Infect Immun 1983; 41:74–82.

151. Lissenden S, et al. Identification of transcription activators that regulate gonococcal adaptation from aerobic to anaerobic or oxygen-limited growth. Mol Microbiol 2000; 37(4): 839–855.

152. Sparling PF. Iron and infection. Clin Infect Dis 1998; 27: 1367–1368.

153. Mietzner TA, et al. Perplasm-to-cytosol free Fe(III) transporters of pathogenic gram-negative bacteria. Curr Top Microbiol Immunol 1998; 225:113–135.

154. Schryvers AB, et al. Comparative analysis of the transferrin and lactoferrin binding proteins in the family Neisseriaceae. Can J Microbiol 1989; 35:409–415.

155. Welch S. Iron metabolism in man. In: Welch S, ed. Transferrin: The Iron Carrier. Boca Raton, FL: CRC Press, 1992: 25–40.

156. Schryvers AB, et al. Iron acquisition systems in the pathogenic *Neisseria*. Mol Microbiol 1999; 32:1117–1123.

157. Weinberg ED. Iron withholding: a defense against infection and neoplasia. Physiol Rev 1984; 64:65–102.

158. Neilands JB, et al. Comparative biochemistry of microbial iron-assimilation. In: Winkelmann G, van der Helm D, Neilands JB, eds. Iron Transport in Microbes, Plants and Animals Weinheim, West Germany: VCH Publishers, 1987: 3–33.

159. Norod P, et al. Growth of *Neisseria gonorrhoeae* in medium deficient in iron without detection of siderophores. Curr Microbiol 1978; 1:281–284.

160. Archibald FS, et al. Removal of iron from human trans-

ferrin by *Neisseria meningitidis*. FEMS Microbiol Lett 1979; 6:159–162.

161. Schryvers AB, et al. Bacterial lactoferrin receptors. Adv Exp Med Biol 1998; 443:123–133.

162. Clarke TE, et al. Structural biology of bacterial iron uptake systems. Curr Top Med Chem 2001; 1:7–30.

163. McKenna WR, et al. Iron uptake from lactoferrin and transferrin by *Neisseria gonorrhoeae*. Infect Immun 1988; 56:785–791.

164. Mickelsen PA, et al. Ability of *Neisseria gonorrhoeae*, *Neisseria meningitidis*, and commensal Neisseria spp. to obtain iron from lactoferrin. Infect Immun 1982; 35:915–920.

165. Beucher M, et al. Cloning, sequencing, and characterization of the gene encoding FrpB, a major iron-regulated, outer membrane protein of *Neisseria gonorrhoeae*. J Bacteriol 1995; 177:2041–2049.

166. Carson SD, et al. Ferric enterobactin binding and utilization by *Neisseria gonorrhoeae*. J Bacteriol 1999; 181(9): 2895–2901.

167. Carson SD, et al. Phase variation of the gonococcal siderophore receptor FetA. Mol Microbiol 2000; 36(3):585–593.

168. Chen CJ, et al. Phase variation of hemoglobin utilization in *Neisseria gonorrhoeae*. Infect Immun 1998; 66:987–993.

169. Ronpirin C, et al. Gonococcal genes encoding transferrin-binding proteins A and B are arranged in a bicistronic operon but are subject to differential expression. Infect Immun 2001; 69:6336–6347.

170. Anderson JE, et al. Gonococcal transferrin-binding protein 2 facilitates but is not essential for transferrin utilization. J Bacteriol 1994; 176:3162–3170.

171. Boulton IC, et al. Purified meningococcal transferrin-binding protein B interacts with a secondary, strain-specific, binding site in the N-terminal lobe of human transferrin. Biochem J 1999; 339:143–149.

172. Masri HP, et al. Specific ligand binding attributable to individual epitopes of gonococcal transferrin binding protein A. Infect Immun 2002; 70:732–740.

173. Cornelissen CN, et al. Antigenic and sequence diversity in gonococcal transferrin-binding protein A. Infect Immun 2000; 68:4725–4735.

174. Rokbi B, et al. Allelic diversity of the two transferrin binding protein B gene isotypes among a collection of *Neisseria meningitidis* strains representative of serogroup B disease: implication for the composition of a recombinant TbpB-based vaccine. Infect Immun 2000; 68:4938–4947.

175. Retzer MD, et al. Discrimination between apo and iron-loaded forms of transferrin by transferrin binding protein B and its N-terminal subfragment. Microb Pathog 1998; 25:175–180.

176. Boulton IC, et al. Transferrin-binding protein B isolated from *Neisseria meningitidis* discriminates between apo and diferric human transferrin. Biochem J 1998; 334:269–273.

177. Cornelissen CN, et al. Expression of gonococcal transferrin-binding protein 1 causes *Escherichia coli* to bind human transferrin. J Bacteriol 1993; 175:2448–2450.

178. Heine RP, Presented at the International Society for STD Research: 9th International Meeting, Banff, Alberta, Canada, 1991.

179. Bonnah RA, et al. Alteration of epithelial cell transferrin-iron homeostasis by *Neisseria meningitidis* and *Neisseria gonorrhoeae*. Cell Microbiol 2000; 2:207–218.

180. Cornelissen CN, et al. The transferrin receptor expressed by gonococcal strain FA1090 is required for the experimental infection of human male volunteers. Mol Microbiol 1998; 27:611–616.

181. Spence JM, et al. Role of ribosomal protein L12 in gonococcal invasion of Hec1B cells. Infect Immun 2000; 68:5002–5010.

182. McGee ZA, et al. Pathogenic mechanisms of *Neisseria gonorrhoeae*: observations on damage to human fallopian tubes in organ culture by gonococci of type 1 and type 4. J Infect Dis 1981; 143:413–422.

183. McGee ZA, et al. Parasite-directed endocytosis. Rev Infect Dis 1988; 10:s311–322.

184. Cooper MD, et al. Attachment to and invasion of human fallopian tube mucosa by an IgA1 protease-deficient mutant of *Neisseria gonorrhoeae* and its wild-type parent. J Infect Dis 1984; 150:737–744.

185. Arko RJ. Animal models for pathogenic *Neisseria* species. Clin Microbiol Rev 1989; 2:s56–59.

186. Corbiel LB, et al. Specific cross-protective antigonococcal immunity in the murine genital tract. Can J Microbiol 1984; 30:482–487.

187. Arko RJ, et al. *Neisseria gonorrhoeae*: vaginal clearance and its correlation with resistance to infection in subcutaneous chambers in orally immunized estradiol-primed mice. Vaccine 1997; 15:1344–1348.

188. Plante M, et al. Intranasal immunization with gonococcal outer membrane preparations reduces the duration of vaginal colonization of mice by *Neisseria gonorrhoeae*. J Infect Dis 2000; 182:848–855.

189. Cohen MS, et al. Human experimentation with *Neisseria gonorrhoeae*: rationale, methods, and implications for the biology of infection and vaccine development. J Infect Dis 1994; 169:532–537.

190. Schneider H, et al. Experimental human gonococcal urethritis: 250 *Neisseria gonorrhoeae* MS11mkC are infective. J Infect Dis 1995; 172:180–185.

191. Cohen MS, et al. Human experimentation with *Neisseria gonorrhoeae*: progress and goals. J Infect Dis 1999; 179: s375–379.

192. Koomey JM, et al. Effects of *rec*A mutations on pilus antigenic variation and phase transition in *Neisseria gonorrhoeae*. Genetics 1987; 117:391–398.

193. Hassett DJ. RecA versus catalase: who's on first? J Clin Invest 1995; 95:924–925.

193a. Cohen MS, et al. In vivo experiments with *Neisseria gonorrhoeae*. In: Evans SE, Yost SE, Maiden MCJ, Feavers IM, eds. Neisseria '94, Proceedings of the Ninth International Pathogenic Neisseria Conference, Winchester, England, 1994:223–224.

194. Schmidt KA, et al. Experimental gonococcal urethritis and reinfection with homologous gonococci in male volunteers. Sex Transm Dis 2001; 28(10):555–564.

195. Schmidt KA, et al. *Neisseria gonorrhoeae* MS11mkC opacity protein expression in vitro and during human volunteer infectivity studies. Sex Transm Dis 2000; 27:278–283.

196. Gotschlich EC. Development of a gonorrhoea vaccine: prospects, strategies and tactics. Bull World Health Organ 1984; 62:671.

197. Plummer FA, et al. Epidemiologic evidence for the development of serovar specific immunity after gonococcal infection. J Clin Invest 1989; 83:1472–1476.

198. Plummer FA, et al. Antibodies to opacity proteins (Opa) correlate with a reduced risk of gonococcal salpingitis. J Clin Invest 1994; 93:1748–1755.

199. Hedges SR, et al. Limited local and systemic antibody responses to *Neisseria gonorrhoeae* during uncomplicated genital infections. Infect Immun 1999; 67:3937–3946.

200. Russell MW, et al. Mucosal immunity in the genital tract: prospects for vaccines against sexually transmitted diseases—a review. Am J Reprod Immunol 1999; 42:58–63.

200a. Ramsey KH, et al. Inflammatory cytokines produced in response to experimental human gonorrhea. J Infect Dis 1995; 172:186–191.

201. Massari P, et al. Cutting edge: immune stimulation by neis-

serial porins is toll-like receptor 2 and MyD88 dependent. J Immunol 2002; 168(4):1533–1537.

202. Hoehn GT, et al. The major anaerobically induced outer membrane protein of *Neisseria gonorrhoeae*, Pan 1, is a lipoprotein. Infect Immun 1992; 60:4704–4708.

203. Alcorn TM, et al. Variation in hydrogen peroxide sensitivity between different strains of *Neisseria gonorrhoeae* is dependent on factors in addition to catalase activity. Infect Immun 1994; 62:2138–2140.

204. Mulks MH, et al. Immunoglobulin A1 protease types of *Neisseria gonorrhoeae*. In: Schoolnik GK, Brooks GF, Falkow S, Frasch CE, Knapp JS, McCutchan JS, Morse SA, eds. The Pathogenic *Neisseria*, Proceedings of the Fourth International Symposium. Washington, DC: American Society for Microbiology, 1985:51–56.

205. Brooks GF, et al. Antibodies against IgA1 protease are stimulated both by clinical disease and asymptomatic carriage of serogroup A *Neisseria meningitidis*. J Infect Dis 1992; 166:1316–1321.

206. Johannsen DB, et al. A *Neisseria gonorrhoeae* immunoglobulin A1 protease mutant is infectious in the human challenge model of urethral infection. Infect Immun 1999; 67:3009–3013.

207. Lin L, et al. The *Neisseria* type 2 IgA1 protease cleaves LAMP1 and promotes survival of bacteria within epithelial cells. Mol Microbiol 1997; 24:1083–1094.

208. Lin L, et al. The IgA1 protease of pathogenic *Neisseriae* increases LAMP1 turnover and promotes survival of bacterial in epithelial cells. In: Zollinger W, Frasch C, Deal C, eds. Pathogenic *Neisseria*: Tenth International Pathogenic *Neisseria* Conference Proceedings, Baltimore, MD, 1996:293–293.

209. Hopper S, et al. Effects of the immunoglobulin A1 protease on *Neisseria gonorrhoeae* trafficking across polarized T84 epithelial monolayers. Infect Immun 2000; 68:906–911.

210. Ayala P, et al. Infection of epithelial cells by pathogenic *Neisseriae* reduces the levels of multiple lysosomal constituents. Infect Immun 1998; 66:5001–5007.

211. Blake MS, et al. Vaccines for gonorrhea: where are we on the curve?. Trends Microbiol 1995; 3:469–474.

212. Heckels JE, et al. Structure and function of pili of pathogenic *Neisseria* species. Clin Microbiol Rev 1989:66–73.

213. Pujol C. Do pathogenic *Neisseriae* need several ways to modify the host cell cytoskeleton? Microbes Infect 2000; 2:821–827.

214. McChesney D, et al. Genital antibody response to a parenteral gonococcal pilus vaccine. Infect Immun 1982; 36:1006–1012.

215. Tramont EC, et al. Antigenic specificity of antibodies in vaginal secretions during infection with *Neisseria gonorrhoeae*. J Infect Dis 1980; 142:23–32.

216. Tramont E, et al. Parenteral gonococcal pilus vaccine. The Pathogenic *Neisseria*: Proceedings of the Fourth International Symposium. Washington, DC: American Society for Microbiology, 1985:316–322.

217. Morand PC, et al. The adhesive property of the type IV pilus-associated component PilC1 of pathogenic *Neisseria* is supported by the conformational structure of the N-terminal part of the molecule. Mol Microbiol 2001; 40:846–856.

218. Langermann S, et al. Prevention of mucosal *Escherichia coli* infection by FimH-adhesin-based systemic vaccination. Science 1997; 276:607–611.

219. Elkins C, et al. Antibodies to N-terminal peptides of gonococcal porin are bactericidal when gonococcal lipopolysaccharide is not sialylated. Mol Microbiol 1992; 6:2617–2628.

220. Nowicki S, et al. Gonococcal infection in a nonhuman host is determined by human complement C1q. Infect Immun 1995; 63:4790–4794.

221. Joiner KA, et al. Monoclonal antibodies directed against gonococcal protein I vary in bactericidal activity. J Immunol 1985; 134:3411–3419.

222. Schoolnik GK, et al. Immunoglobulin class responsible for gonococcal bactericidal activity of normal human sera. J Immunol 1979; 122:1771–1779.

223. Rice PA, et al. Characterization of gonococcal antigens responsible for gonococcal bactericidal antibody in disseminated infection. J Clin Invest 1977; 60:1149–1158.

224. Joiner KA, et al. Gonococcal protein I-specific opsonic IgG in normal human serum. J Infect Dis 1983; 148:1025–1032.

225. Virji M, et al. Monoclonal antibodies to gonococcal outer membrane protein IB: use in the investigation of the potential protective effect of antibodies directed against conserved and type-specific epitopes. J Gen Microbiol 1986; 132:1621–1629.

226. Virji M, et al. The potential protective effect of monoclonal antibodies to gonococcal outer membrane protein IA. J Gen Microbiol 1987; 133:2346–2639.

227. Elkins C, et al. Immunobiology of purified recombinant outer membrane porin protein I of *Neisseria gonorrhoeae*. Mol Microbiol 1994; 14:1059–1075.

228. Buchanan TM, et al. Gonococcal salpingitis is less likely to recur with *Neisseria gonorrhoeae* with the same principal outer membrane protein antigenic type. Am J Obstet Gynecol 1980; 138:978–983.

229. Fox KK, et al. Longitudinal evaluation of serovar-specific immunity to *Neisseria gonorrhoeae*. Am J Epidemiol 1999; 149:353–358.

230. Quentin-Millet MJ, et al. Design and production of meningococcal vaccine based on transferrin binding proteins. In: Zollinger W, Frasch C, Deal C, eds. Pathogenic *Neisseria*—Tenth International Pathogenic *Neisseria* Conference, Baltimore, MD, 1996:131–132.

231. Rokbi B. Identification of two major families of transferrin receptors among *Neisseria meningitidis* strains based on antigenic and genomic features. FEMS Microbiol Lett 1993; 110:51–57.

232. Yamasaki R, et al. Structural and immunochemical characterization of a *Neisseria gonorrhoeae* epitope defined by a monoclonal antibody 2C7; the antibody recognizes a conserved epitope on specific lipo-oligosaccharides in spite of the presence of human carbohydrate epitopes. J Biol Chem 1999; 274:36550–36558.

233. Wiesenfeld HC, et al. Self-collection of vaginal swabs for the detection of chlamydia, gonorrhea, and trichomoniasis: opportunity to encourage sexually transmitted disease testing among adolescents. Sex Transm Dis 2001; 28:321–325.

234. Smith K, et al. Self-obtained vaginal swabs for diagnosis of treatable sexually transmitted diseases in adolescent girls. Arch Pediatr Adolesc Med 2001; 155:676–679.

235. Adimora AA, et al. Vaccines for classic sexually transmitted diseases. Infect Dis Clin North Am 1994; 8:859–876.

63

Vaccines Against *Campylobacter jejuni*

David R. Tribble, Shahida Baqar, and Daniel A. Scott
Naval Medical Research Center, Silver Spring, Maryland, U.S.A.

I. INTRODUCTION

Surveillance data indicate that *Campylobacter jejuni* is the most common bacterial agent associated with diarrhea in the United States and, on a global basis, is an important bacterial cause of both endemic and travelers' diarrhea (TD). Compared to noninvasive causes of diarrhea, *Campylobacter*-associated diarrhea is generally more severe, with a longer duration of symptoms and frequent occurrence of severe cramps, bloody stools, and fever [1–3]. Recognizing the significance of this disease threat to military personnel (particularly when deployed to tropical regions and developing countries) [4–6], the Department of Defense (DOD) has sponsored a *Campylobacter* research program headed by the U.S. Navy that includes vaccine development activities.

II. EPIDEMIOLOGY

Campylobacters are commensals of many wild and domesticated birds and mammals. These animals may become colonized at a very early age, with the organisms establishing themselves as part of their normal bowel flora [7,8]. Humans usually acquire infection by eating contaminated meat or poultry from animals colonized with the bacteria [9]. Diarrhea is by far the most common human illness, and *C. jejuni* is the dominant species associated with disease [2,10,11]. However, *C. jejuni*, as well as other members of the genus, are increasingly being identified as causes of bacteremia and a variety of systemic or localized infections in immuno-compromised hosts [12–17]. *C. jejuni* is identified in association with diarrhea more frequently in developing countries [18–20]. Notable differences exist in the epidemiology of human Campylobacteriosis between developing and industrialized countries (Table 1) in regards to incidence, seasonality, age distribution, identified risk factors, clinical presentation/infection, and the subsequent public health impact.

A. Campylobacter as a Cause of Travelers' Diarrhea

In many studies *Campylobacter* spp. are second only to ETEC as a pathogen isolated in association with TD [19,21–31]. In most industrialized countries with temperate climates *Campylobacter* incidence peaks during summer, whereas in tropical regions no seasonality is observed [18–20]. *Campylobacter*-associated TD appears more severe than TD caused by other enteropathogens [21,31,32].

The high percentage of *Campylobacter* infections associated with diarrhea among U.S. military personnel studied in Southeast Asia does not appear to be related to doxycycline malaria prophylaxis, as it is also seen in troops taking mefloquine [27,33].

Antibiotic resistance to erythromycin, the newer macrolides, and the fluoroquinolones exacerbates the threat of *Campylobacter*-associated diarrhea [34–41]. The trend of increasing fluoroquinolone resistance reinforces the rationale to develop a vaccine against this agent [34,39–41].

B. Campylobacter as a Cause of Endemic Diarrhea

C. jejuni is now believed to be the most common bacterial cause of diarrheal disease in the United States [18,42,43]. Rarely, large community outbreaks occur from consumption of food, particularly raw milk, or contaminated water [10, 44,45]. In contrast, sporadic cases and household epidemics are extremely common, resulting from eating contaminated poultry or other meat. Person-to-person transmission is rare. A Center for Disease Control and Prevention multi-hospital study found that *Campylobacter* sp. were isolated from diarrhea stools twice as frequently as *Salmonella* sp. and over four times as often as *Shigella* sp. [3]. Similar data were obtained in two studies by a Seattle health maintenance organization that found the incidence of laboratory-confirmed *Campylobacter*-associated diarrhea to be 50–71 cases per 100,000 population per year, or about twice as frequent as *Salmonella* and *Shigella* combined [46,47]. Because these

Table 1 *Campylobacter jejuni*-Associated Diarrheal Disease: Lesser Developed Vs. Industrialized Countries

Factors	Lesser developed countries	Industrialized countries	Reference(s)
Incidence	40,000/100,000 annual	14–22/100,000 annual (United States)	[18–20,56]
	0.4–0.6 episodes/child-year (≤3 years old)	50–150/100,000 annual (in other industrialized countries)	
Seasonality	Not evident	Summer peak (in temperate climates)	[18–20]
Age distribution	Typically limited to first 2 years of life (peak at 6–12 months old)	Highest <1 year old (53/100,000 in the United States) Second peak noted in young adulthood (particularly males)	[18–20,56]
Risk factors	Primarily sporadic disease Complex, multiple sources of exposure; identified risks include poor hygienic conditions and presence of animals in household	Primarily sporadic disease Identified risks: poultry consumption, transmission from pets, contaminated drinking water, raw milk consumption, and foreign travel	[18,19,56]
Clinical syndrome	Childhood watery diarrhea Less severe disease observed in developing countries	Spectrum of illness: watery diarrhea to dysentery; frequent fevers and abdominal cramps (less severe in children)	[10,19,20,32]
Infection	Frequent asymptomatic infection in early childhood Duration of excretion ≤1 week	Infrequent asymptomatic infection Duration of excretion 2–3 weeks	[19,20,56,122]
Disease impact	Estimated 400 million cases/year	Estimated 2.4 million cases/year in the United States	[18–20,54,56,74]
	Associated with severe dehydration (13%)	Case fatality rate low (0.08%)	
	Contributor to overall infant morbidity/mortality from diarrheal disease	Significant economic burden	
	Chronic sequelae (not quantified)	Chronic sequelae (Guillain–Barré syndrome— estimated as 1 GBS case/1–3000 *Campylobacter* infections)	

studies included only patients who sought medical attention and had a stool culture done they likely underestimate the true disease incidence. Tauxe has estimated the total incidence of *Campylobacter*-associated illness in the United States by extrapolating from data obtained during investigation of a U.S. waterborne outbreak in which 1 of 18 who became ill consulted a physician [18,48]. Applying the same ratio of ill-to-treated patients to published estimates for the number of laboratory confirmed clinical cases and case-fatality rates, he estimates that the total number of *Campylobacter*-associated diarrhea cases in the United States is as high as 2.4 million per year (1% of the total population), resulting in about 200 to 700 deaths [49].

The major impact of *Campylobacter* diarrheal disease in industrialized countries stems from short-term morbidity and economic burden. Mortality typically is limited to populations at the extremes of age, particularly the elderly, and immunocompromised individuals [50]. Mead et al. estimated

13,000 hospitalizations due to *Campylobacter* spp. occur annually in the United States with approximately 125 deaths [50]. *Campylobacter* is also the leading foodborne pathogen observed in European surveillance systems [18].

In developing countries, where hygiene and sanitation are often suboptimal, the incidence of *Campylobacter* enteritis in children under 5 years of age is as high as 40,000/100,000, or 0.4 episodes per child per year [52,53]. One estimate suggests that as many as 400 million cases of *Campylobacter* diarrhea may occur annually worldwide [54]. Isolation rates of *Campylobacter* in children with diarrheal disease (typically ≤2 years old) range between 5% and 18% [20], but, in contrast to industrialized countries, asymptomatic infections are commonly observed, with prevalence rates as high as 15% [55]. Given the prevalence of this infection in healthy children it is challenging to discriminate the impact of campylobacter on child health in developing countries [56].

III. CLINICAL SPECTRUM OF DISEASE

Campylobacter enteritis can present with a range of symptoms from watery diarrhea to dysentery [32]. Most frequently, there are moderate volumes of watery diarrhea that contain leukocytes and mucus. Frank blood is found in about 20–50% of cases. There is usually an accompanying fever and abdominal cramps which can be severe. Untreated acute infection usually runs its course in 3 to 5 days, followed by shedding of the organism for several days to weeks.

Two strains of *C. jejuni* (81–176 and A2349) fed to healthy adult North American volunteers both caused disease, but strain 81–176 (utilized by our group in a killed whole-cell vaccine) was much more virulent. Clinical illness included diarrhea, fever, dysentery, malaise, and abdominal cramps [1].

Like *Salmonella*, *Shigella*, and *Yersinia*, *Campylobacter* enteritis has been associated with development of a reactive arthritis/arthropathy (RA) [57–64]. Studies of outbreaks [59,63] and case series [60,65] have found an incidence of rheumatic complaints ranging from about 1% to 14% in subjects with evidence of *C. jejuni* infection. However, these studies did not use a consistent definition of reactive arthritis and included patients with joint symptoms that, in some cases, lasted only 3 to 7 days [60]. In the majority of reported cases, symptoms resolved completely. A genetic predisposition to acquiring a seronegative spondyloarthropathy after a bacterial enteric infection (approximate risk gradient: *Yersinia* spp. > *Shigella* spp. (*S. flexneri*) > nontyphoidal *Salmonella* > *C. jejuni*) has been observed in individuals with the human leukocyte antigen HLA-B27 [66]. An overall estimated 18-fold increased risk of reactive arthritis exists for HLA-B27 positive as compared to negative individuals following one of these infections [66].

A more devastating complication of *Campylobacter* infection is Guillain–Barré syndrome (GBS) [9,67–76]. Based on epidemiological studies involving both serology and culture results, approximately 30–40% of patients with GBS have had a *C. jejuni* infection in the preceding 10–21 days [66,70,75]. *C. jejuni*-associated GBS appears to be associated with a more severe clinical presentation [76]. Published data from a large case-control study of *Campylobacter*-associated GBS by Rees and coworkers showed evidence of *C. jejuni* infection in 26% of the 103 GBS and Miller–Fisher syndrome patients, compared to 2% of household controls, and 1% of hospital controls. *Campylobacter*-associated GBS more commonly presented with weakness as a first symptom had less severe sensory deficits at the peak of illness but had significantly greater disability at a 1-year follow-up than non-*Campylobacter*-associated GBS cases [77]. The pathogenesis of *Campylobacter*-associated GBS is unclear but may involve "molecular mimicry" wherein peripheral nerves share epitopes with some *C. jejuni* antigens. Thus an immune response, which is initially mounted against the infection, may be misdirected to the peripheral nerve in some convalescing patients. An association between GBS and infection with *C. jejuni* strains of the heat stable (HS) Penner serotype HS19 has been noted by several groups [67,71,78–81] as well as an association with HS41 serotype, particularly in South Africa [82,83]. The antigenic determinant of the

heat stable serotyping scheme was felt to be lipooligosaccharide (LOS), and structural analyses of *C. jejuni* LOS identified structures that resemble gangliosides (such as GM1, GD1a, and GQ1b) present on human nerves. But the antigenic determinant of the Penner serotyping scheme has recently been shown to be a phase-variable capsule in many strains. Karlyshev et al. found that capsular mutants in five out of six strains had lost the ability to be serotyped in the Penner scheme [84] and Bacon et al. showed that capsule mutants of *C. jejuni* 81–176 lost the HS23 and HS36 serotypes and showed reduced virulence [85]. But a capsule mutant of *C. jejuni* 81–116, which was serotyped as HS6,7, was serotyped as HS6 only, suggesting that the HS serodeterminant in most strains is capsule, but that the situation is complex [84]. The molecular structure of the capsule and any role in the pathogenesis of GBS remain unknown. Genetic predisposition of the host may also play a role [73,86].

IV. ANIMAL MODELS OF CAMPYLOBACTER

Campylobacters naturally colonize numerous domestic and laboratory animal species, but usually without clinical signs of disease. This lack of disease has made the development of an animal model to be used in Campylobacter vaccine development challenging. This has led to the development of models using very young or surgically manipulated models that are cumbersome or not well suited to the study of vaccine efficacy [87–92]. Susceptibility to *C. jejuni*-induced diarrhea decreases rapidly with age, making these models more useful for pathogenesis studies than vaccine development [87,93]. As it has not been established that the mechanism(s) of diarrhea in nonprimate mammalian newborns or manipulated nonprimate animals is the same as that in humans, the relevance for humans of findings made in nonprimate mammals remains unanswered. Campylobacteriosis models investigated include nonhuman primates, piglets, rabbits, ferrets, mice, and chickens.

Experimental infection of very young rhesus monkeys with *C. jejuni* closely mimics human disease and *Campylobacter* enteritis appears to be an important cause of diarrhea in primate colonies [1,87]. After experimental infection, the onset and duration of the disease, infection-associated pathology and development of acquired immunity appear to make nonhuman primates an attractive model for human campylobacteriosis. However, these studies have not been duplicated in older animals. Attempts are underway to develop a Campylobacter disease model using adult rhesus and New World monkeys. Rhesus monkeys have been used to test the safety and immunogenicity of an adjuvanted *Campylobacter* whole-cell vaccine [94].

Gnotobiotic and newborn, colostrum-deprived piglets have both been shown to develop diarrhea when challenged orally with *C. jejuni* [95,96]. The disease affects mainly the colon and is similar histopathologically to that seen in humans. However, the requirement for newborn animals makes this a logistically difficult and expensive model for most laboratories and limits its application to vaccine development.

Overt diarrheal disease can be induced when young (≤1 kg) rabbits are challenged with strains of *Campylobacter*, using the removable intestinal tie adult rabbit diarrhea (RITARD) procedure. In the RITARD surgical model, the cecum is ligated to prevent reabsorption of fluid and a reversible tie is placed below the bacterial inoculum to impede normal bowel motility and improve bacterial attachment and colonization. When young rabbits are challenged in this manner with live motile *C. jejuni*, most animals become bacteremic and develop diarrhea characterized by loose, mucus containing stools [97]. Older rabbits challenged by the RITARD procedure become colonized but fail to develop diarrhea. Therefore it cannot be used to measure protection against disease offered by vaccine candidates. But young rabbits can be orally immunized with either live strains or vaccines and then, approximately 30 days later, challenged via the RITARD procedure with either the same strain or a heterologous organism to measure protection against colonization. Protection against colonization in this model seems to be Lior serotype-specific. Thus immunization with one strain of *Campylobacter* protects against other strains of the same Lior serogroup, but not strains of other Lior serogroups [98,99].

In search of a suitable small animal model, different strains of mice and rats, bacterial isolates and routes of infection have been explored [91–93,100–110]. Mice can be used in a nondiarrheal disease model using oral, intranasal, or intraperitoneal routes of challenge [101,102,109]. An oral/intranasal immunization-intranasal challenge murine model has been adapted from its original use in studies of *Shigella* immunity [102,110]. Naive mice infected intranasally with virulent strains of *Campylobacter* develop pulmonary disease, accompanied by weight loss and other signs of illness including ruffled fur hunched back, dehydration, lethargy, and sometimes death [102]. Following intranasal infection, most strains colonize the intestine and some strains disseminate to the liver, spleen, and other organs. This model of oral/intranasal immunization followed by intranasal challenge appears to be useful in measuring the immune response to candidate vaccine antigens, and protective efficacy as measured by protection against pulmonary disease, intestinal colonization, and disseminated disease.

Young ferrets develop diarrhea when naturally or experimentally infected with *C. jejuni* via the oro-gastric route. Adult ferrets that have been intragastrically inoculated with some strains of live *Campylobacter* (e.g., *C. jejuni* 81–176) develop enteric symptoms lasting up to 3 days and remain colonized for up to 8 days [111]. Ferrets, which have been "immunized" in this manner, do not develop disease when rechallenged with the same strain. However, colonization resistance does not develop until after several additional exposures. This is similar to human volunteers studies where protection against disease develops before colonization resistance. However, difficulty in obtaining *Campylobacter*-free ferrets and the lack of ferret-specific immunologic reagents limit the utility of this model for studying acquired immunity.

An avian model of campylobacteriosis has been employed for studies of pathogenesis and immunity [90,112], and the immunoreactive complication, Guillain–Barré syndrome [113]. Whether results obtained with various animal models can be extrapolated to the human-*C. jejuni* parasitism remains to be seen.

V. IMMUNE RESPONSES TO *CAMPYLOBACTER*

Although infection with *Campylobacter* has been shown to provide protective immunity, relatively little is known about the nature of acquired immunity, correlates of protection, or the mechanism(s) of protection against this infection. Evidence for acquired immunity to *C. jejuni* comes mostly from epidemiological studies of residents of developing countries. Children living in endemic areas have frequent symptomatic infections in the first one to three years of life, but with increasing age and acquired immunity, the frequency of symptomatic disease decreases compared to asymptomatic infection [53,114–122]. Moreover, the number of *C. jejuni* excreted per gram of stool of infected individuals also declines with increasing age [122], as does the duration of excretion of the organism [53].

Direct evidence of acquired immunity to *C. jejuni* in man comes from the study of infection in volunteers. To evaluate the protective immunity induced by prior disease, volunteers who became ill after an initial challenge were rechallenged 28 days later [1]. The rechallenged volunteers were completely protected from illness, and some were protected against colonization after rechallenge with a homologous strain.

During the acute phase of infection IgA or IgM antibodies are elevated followed by induction of IgG in serum [30,123]. In challenge studies, volunteers with the highest prechallenge levels of anti-Campylobacter serum IgA were the least likely to develop disease [1]. In a field study, individuals with higher preexposure levels of *Campylobacter*-specific IgA in circulation were less likely to get *Campylobacter* disease in an endemic area [30]. Naturally acquired *C. jejuni* infection elicits antibodies which recognize *C. jejuni* antigens, and the titers of these antibodies increase with age [114,116,117,120–122]. The antigen preparations used in these studies contain outer membrane and flagellar proteins that appear to be antigenic [124,125]. In a recent *Campylobacter* case report, infecting strain-specific ~ 32 and 34 kDa proteins were detected early in infection (IgA first detected at day 3 after onset) and peaked at 10 (IgA) or 34 (IgG) days. IgA wanes, but IgG persists for at least 4 months [126]. Others have reported similar patterns of *Campylobacter*-specific antibodies of various isotypes [123]. The durability of these antibodies may be dependent on the endemicity of the agent. In endemic areas the level of acquired immunity may be maintained by repeated asymptomatic exposure to the same or cross-reactive *Campylobacter* serotypes. The level of mucosal antibody is probably more important than serum antibody levels in the protection against *Campylobacter* infection. Anti-flagellar IgA has been identified in human breast milk and has been shown to protect children from *C. jejuni* diarrhea [127,128]. A vaccine challenge study conducted at the Naval Medical Research Center also suggests a protective role of *Campylobacter*-specific fecal IgA.

Little information is available on cellular immune responses to *C. jejuni*, and the limited data available are on the role of T cell subset recognition in GBS patients [129,130]. Cellular responses might play important roles as helpers in antibody formation, in the clearance of *C. jejuni* as well as recall of memory response upon reexposure. A vigorous and sustained antigen-specific, IFN-γ-dependent lymphocyte proliferative response was seen in a naturally acquired *C. jejuni* infection [126]. Our unpublished data also support the role of Th-1-type IFN-γ-dependent cell-mediated immune response in protecting volunteers from a homologous rechallenge with *C. jejuni*. Given the complex and highly regulated cytokine network, it is difficult to determine the precise role of a given cytokine in *Campylobacter* infection and immunity. We have recently shown that the high levels of pro-inflammatory cytokines such as IL-1 and IL-8 in stool and, to a lesser magnitude, in serum and CRP in circulation are present during the acute phase of the infection. In contrast, IFN-γ and IL-6 appear in circulation at 4–8 days of onset, suggesting the regulatory roles of these cytokines in immunity [126]. Heretofore, it has not been possible to demonstrate a definitive association between any specific antigen and protection.

VI. PATHOGENESIS/PROTECTIVE EPITOPES

Although *C. jejuni* is a leading cause of diarrheal disease worldwide [4,5,11,18–20,22], little is understood about the mechanisms by which it causes disease. Moreover, compared to other diarrheal agents (e.g., *Shigella* and ETEC), there is a paucity of information available on the development of rational vaccines against *C. jejuni*. Studies aimed at deciphering the virulence mechanisms of *C. jejuni* have been hampered by a number of unique aspects of this pathogen, including limitations in systems of experimental genetics and in nonprimate models of diarrheal disease.

Flagella and motility are clearly virulence determinants in all strains of *C. jejuni* [1,131,132]. Moreover, flagellin is the immunodominant antigen recognized during infection, including human volunteer feeding studies, and has been suggested to be a protective antigen [120]. *C. jejuni* flagellin is a glycoprotein that contains conserved and hypervariable protein domains [133–135]. The carbohydrates are surface exposed in the filament and variations in the structure of the pseudaminic acids found on the filament appear to contribute to the antigenicity of flagellin.

Other putative virulence factors include the PEB proteins and cytolethal distending toxin [136–140]. The PEB proteins may act as adhesins. Cytolethal distending toxin is a multisubunit toxin that causes cell cycle arrest, cytoplasm distention, and, eventually, chromatin fragmentation and cell death [137]. One of the subunits of this toxin, CdtB, was shown to exhibit features of type 1 deoxyribonucleases [141]. The toxin is membrane bound and highly conserved among strains [142].

To better understand *Campylobacter* pathogenesis, the Sanger Institute has sequenced the genome of one strain of *C. jejuni*, NCTC 11168, which was a clinical isolate from the United Kingdom [143]. Analysis of the sequence has revealed a number of interesting features such as the presence of capsule genes [84,85], and hypervariable regions upstream of capsule, LOS, and protein glycosylation genes. Although the sequence provided numerous insights into the ultrastructure, biology, and physiology of *C. jejuni*, it offered few clues into the pathogenesis of the organism. Other than the known cytolethal distending toxin, no cytotoxins or enterotoxins were identified. In addition, there were no genes encoding proteins with homology to known invasins or other known virulence determinants; neither was there evidence of a type III secretion system found in other enteric pathogens.

Current data suggest that comparative genomic studies may yield additional data on pathogenesis that will impact vaccine development efforts. *Campylobacter* infections can present with a variety of symptoms from watery diarrhea to dysentery and there may be multiple mechanisms of pathogenesis, similar to diarrheagenic *E. coli*. There is a range in the ability with which *C. jejuni* can be internalized into intestinal epithelial cells. Strain 81–176, which has been shown to cause disease in volunteer studies, invades at exceptionally high levels (2–5% of the input inoculum) compared to other strains [144–148]. Most other strains invade INT407 cells at levels below that of an *E. coli* K-12 negative control, and this includes NCTC 11168. We have also observed a gradation of symptoms in the ferret model among different strains. In this model the animals are fed different doses of *C. jejuni* and within 24 hr the animals develop diarrhea. Strain 81–176 is the most virulent strain tested in this model and causes a mucus diarrhea, often with occult or frank blood. Mutants of 81–176 defective in invasion show attenuation in the ferret model [85,132,149]. Other, less invasive strains cause a markedly milder diarrhea, and others (e.g., NCTC 11168, as mentioned above) cause no diarrhea [149].

Consistent with the above observations, there are differences in virulence genes among strains of *C. jejuni*. *C. jejuni* 81–176 contains two plasmids not present in NCTC 11168 which encode a number of proteins with significant homology to proteins in type IV secretion systems of other pathogens. Type IV secretion systems are specialized systems of protein transport in bacteria. Additionally, there appear to be differences in the chromosomal genes of different strains of *C. jejuni*. A recent microarray study indicated that as much as 21% of the genome of NCTC 11168 is missing in 11 other strains of *C. jejuni* [150]. This study indicated that 3.9% of the NCTC 11168 genes were missing in 81–176. These data and ongoing comparative studies will be useful in elucidating campylobacter pathogenesis and in identifying widely conserved antigens as vaccine targets.

VII. *CAMPYLOBACTER* VACCINE STRATEGIES

A. Killed Whole Cell Vaccines

Inactivated microorganisms offer several advantages as potential vaccines for mucosal immunization. Physically, they are naturally occurring microparticles, which should enhance interactions between their surface and mucosal lymphoid tissues. As vaccines they are relatively inexpensive to produce and contain multiple antigens that may be important for protection. Presentation of multiple antigens may be particularly important for *Campylobacter*, for which protective antigens are not known. Although not suitable for parenteral administration, whole-cell preparations are safe for mucosal immunization.

Killed whole-cell vaccines have been developed for enterotoxigenic *E. coli* and *V. cholerae* O1, and the cholera vaccine is now marketed in Europe. This vaccine contains heat and formalin-killed *Vibrio cholerae* whole cells (WC), of different biotypes and serotypes, plus the nontoxic B subunit (BS) of cholera toxin. A randomized, double blind, placebo-controlled field trial involving 63,000 individuals in rural Bangladesh established the safety, immunogenicity, and efficacy of an early formulation of the WC/BS cholera vaccine. Three doses of the WC/BS vaccine conferred 85% protection against cholera for the first 6 months in all age groups tested, and 51% overall protection after 3 years [151–154]. No adverse effects attributable to the vaccine were reported. The same WC/rBS vaccine provided 86% protection against ETEC diarrhea in Finnish travelers [158]. More recently, a new formulation of the WC/BS cholera vaccine, containing a recombinant cholera toxin B-subunit (WC/rBS), was also found to be safe and give high levels of protection against symptomatic cholera in Peruvian military recruits [155,156]. Larger-scale studies in civilian populations in Peru have not shown any efficacy for a two-dose regimen but administering a third (booster) dose after 1 year was followed by ~60% protection observed over the ensuing 12 months of follow-up [157]. Although not as immunogenic as live attenuated *V. cholerae* strains [159,160], these vaccines have proven the concept that an orally administered, whole-cell vaccine can be safe and provide reasonable protection against an enteric pathogen.

Because of the success with other killed whole-cell vaccines, the NMRC has studied the hypothesis that a killed whole-cell vaccine against *Campylobacter* could be safe, immunogenic, and protect against disease. But in contrast to *V. cholerae*, campylobacters are invasive, and protection may be more difficult to achieve, so combining the vaccine with a mucosal adjuvant such as *E. coli* heat-labile toxin (LT) or one of its less toxin derivatives was felt to be important [161,162]. Initial studies using *C. coli* VC167 showed that when sonicated cells were combined with 25 μg of LT and given orally to mice, the mucosal immune response was equal to live infection with the same strain [163]. The duration of intestinal colonization after live challenge could also be significantly shortened in mice or rabbits immunized with sonicates plus LT, but not by immunization with sonicates alone. Studies using a mixture of heat and formalin-killed *C. jejuni* 81–176 in mice have shown that LT enhances the mucosal immune response over a wide range of vaccine doses [101]. Mice were orally immunized with three doses of 10^5, 10^7, or 10^9 vaccine particles alone, or in combination with 25 μg of LT. Significant *Campylobacter*-specific IgA and low levels of IgG were detected in intestinal lavage fluid only after immunization with adjuvanted vaccine. In contrast, whole cells with or without LT stimulated similar levels of *Campylobacter*-specific serum antibody levels. The optimal secretory immune response was induced

following vaccination with 10^7 CWC-LT formulation suggesting that the ratio of adjuvant to inactivated cells may be important. When challenged orally with live *C. jejuni* 81–176, mice immunized with any dose of whole cells plus LT showed colonization resistance, whereas only the highest dose of CWC alone (10^9 cells) gave comparable protection. Both vaccine formulations provided similar levels of protection against the systemic spread of challenge organisms [101].

In follow-on experiments, the relative protective efficacy and duration of immunity induced by CWC or CWC-LT vaccines were compared in an oral immunization-intranasal challenge model [102]. Both CWC and CWC-LT formulations provided varying degrees of protection against illness and intestinal colonization for up to 4 months after completing the two-dose primary immunization series (14-day intervals). However, the adjuvanted preparation appeared superior to formalin-inactivated whole cells alone in that immunity in this vaccination group was still evident in mice at 8 months post-immunization (S. Baqar, personal communication). In vitro T-cell proliferative responses to *C. jejuni* antigens were also measurably enhanced by the addition of LT. Two doses of orally administered CWC vaccine with or without LT were well tolerated in rhesus monkeys [101]. Elevated *Campylobacter*-specific IgA and IgG antibody-secreting cells (ASCs) were detected in the peripheral blood of most animals after vaccination, but the IgA ASC response was significantly enhanced by the co-administration of LT in a dose-dependent manner. Heat-labile toxin also significantly enhanced the serum *Campylobacter*-specific IgA and IgG responses. These results suggested that both killed whole-cells alone, and LT-adjuvanted preparations, are promising oral *Campylobacter* vaccine candidates. In various animal models, the addition of LT enhances the mucosal and serum immune response to *Campylobacter* antigens, increases the protective efficacy of the CWC at lower vaccine doses, and prolongs the duration of immunity compared to CWC alone. Given these data, clinical evaluation of a CWC vaccine was undertaken in human volunteers.

Currently, we are studying a monovalent, formalin-inactivated, whole-cell vaccine (CWC) made from *C. jejuni* 81–176 (Penner serotype 23/36; Lior serogroup 5). This strain is invasive in cell culture [148,164] and was originally isolated from the feces of a 9-year-old girl with diarrhea who became ill during a milk-borne outbreak in Minnesota [165]. In 1984, the strain was used in a human volunteer study at the Center for Vaccine Development, University of Maryland, described above [1]. The organism used to make the vaccine was recovered from a challenged volunteer with diarrhea. The vaccine is grown under conditions that maximize motility/flagella expression and ability to invade eukaryotic cells in vitro, and then inactivated using 0.2% formalin. The final preparation was shown to have intact flagella by electron microscopy and to retain its ability to agglutinate in Lior 5 antisera.

Volunteer studies have shown the vaccine to be generally safe and moderately immunogenic. However, when given in a two-dose regimen such as that used for the whole-cell cholera vaccine, the vaccine did not protect in a volunteer challenge study. Nevertheless, there was a trend toward less severe disease in volunteers receiving the vaccine. Recent studies have shown that the immune response to the vaccine can be improved using a four-dose, short-interval vaccination regimen such as that used for live oral typhoid vaccine Ty21a (D. Tribble, unpublished data). Specifically, while a two-dose, 14-day regimen induced no fecal IgA response, the four-dose regimen produced a mean 13-fold rise in fecal IgA. It is not yet known if the enhanced immune responses will be adequate to provide protection against disease.

B. Subunit Vaccines

Another approach is a recombinant protein vaccine based on a conserved surface-exposed antigen that has been shown to induce an immune response after infection. Because such a vaccine would not contain LOS or capsule it would not have any ganglioside mimicry and would therefore, presumably, have no risk of inducing GBS. Several *Campylobacter* antigens have been suggested as subunit vaccine candidates for use either as purified recombinant proteins or expressed in carrier vaccine strains such as live attenuated *Salmonella* or *Shigella*. Purified proteins could be delivered to the mucosa by oral or intranasal administration, or given parenterally.

A general characteristic of *Campylobacter* species is its rapid, darting motility. Sustained motility contributes to pathogenesis of diarrheal disease. Studies have shown that nonmotile mutant *Campylobacter* strains fail to colonize experimental animals or volunteers, nor do they invade epithelial cells in vitro [1,98,131]. A single uni- or bipolar flagellum, composed of a major [1,98,131] flagellin subunit, FlaA, and a minor FlaB subunit, imparts motility. *Campylobacter* flagellin has long been recognized as an immunodominant antigen recognized during infection, and numerous studies have suggested a role in protection [115,120,166,167]. The overall structure of *Campylobacter* flagellins is similar to those of the *Enterobacteriaceae* in that the amino and carboxyl ends, which function in the transport and assembly of the monomers into the filament, are highly conserved among different *Campylobacter* strains, and the central region appears antigenically diverse [134]. Power et al. have studied the antigenicity of *C. coli* VC167 flagellin in detail and have shown that the major immune response seems to reside in the highly conserved amino and carboxy ends of the protein [134].

Epidemiologic studies in children from the developing world provide evidence of protective immunity through investigations of clinical presentation, stool microbiology, and *Campylobacter*-specific immunology. Direct evidence of the importance of flagellin as an immune correlate of clinical outcomes derives from studies of breast-fed Mexican infants (<6 months old) [127]. A lower incidence of *Campylobacter*-associated diarrhea occurred in infants whose mothers had colostral *Campylobacter*-specific secretory IgA antibodies detected in breast milk.

During the last few years, researchers at NMRC have developed a recombinant subunit vaccine composed of truncated FlaA flagellin of *C. coli* VC167 fused to maltose binding protein of *Escherichia coli* [168]. The region of flaA

encoding amino acids 5–337 was chosen because of its high conservation among different strains of *Campylobacter*, and because this region has been demonstrated to be immunogenic [134]. Additionally, native *Campylobacter* flagellin is heavily glycosylated, and the region of the protein between amino acids 5–337 contains only a single glycosylation site [135].

The recombinant truncated flagellin protein (rFla-MBP) has demonstrated cross-species protection in murine models of *C. jejuni* pathogenesis [168]. Intranasal rFla-MBP vaccination induces higher levels of specific intestinal IgA and serum IgA and IgG antibodies than oral administration. In addition, a ferret diarrhea model has been used to study the safety, immunogenicity, and efficacy of the rFla-MBP vaccine. Intranasal immunization with a three-dose regimen of rFla-MBP (100 μg) provided an approximately 60% protective efficacy from diarrheal illness following oral challenge with 1×10^{10} CFU *C. jejuni* strain 81–176.

Another protein which has been suggested as a potential subunit-based vaccine target is PEB1, a highly immunogenic protein conserved among *C. jejuni* strains, which has also been suggested to function as an adhesin to eukaryotic cells [139]. PEB1 has high sequence similarity to the binding component of several amino acid transport systems, an observation that remains to be reconciled with a putative role in virulence. A subunit of cytolethal distending toxin may also be a vaccine candidate. As more is understood about pathogenesis of *Campylobacter* sp., it is likely that additional subunit target proteins will be identified which are conserved among strains sharing the same mechanisms of pathogenesis.

C. Live Attenuated Vaccines

Live attenuated oral vaccines also have the potential to deliver the full complement of protective antigens, even if they have not been identified, and to be effective after only a single dose. Several live attenuated oral vaccines have been shown to effectively stimulate mucosal immunity and provide excellent protection in field or volunteer challenge studies. These include vaccines attenuated by serial passage (oral polio), chemical mutagenesis (the Ty21A vaccine strain of *Salmonella* Typhi), or targeted deletion of genes encoding important virulence factors (e.g., attenuated cholera vaccine strain CVD 103-HgR which has a deletion of the gene encoding cholera toxin A subunit) [169–172]. Using genetic methods to engineer a living attenuated *Campylobacter* vaccine is an attractive approach. This would allow the inclusion of the full complement of antigens, but selecting the appropriate mutations is complicated by the paucity of information on pathogenesis. Recent advances in pathogenesis research and sequencing of the *Campylobacter* genome provide numerous targets, and inclusion of a recA mutation [164] would preclude reversion to wild type by this naturally transformable enteropathogen [173]. On the other hand, the fact that there is currently an incomplete understanding of the mechanisms by which wild-type *Campylobacter* induces Guillain–Barré syndrome argues against pursuing the strategy of developing live attenuated vaccine strains (or at least calls for exercising caution).

REFERENCES

1. Black RE, et al. Experimental *Campylobacter jejuni* infection in humans. J Infect Dis 1988; 157:472–479.
2. Blaser MJ, Reller LB. Campylobacter enteritis. N Engl J Med 1981; 305:1444–1452.
3. Blaser MJ, et al. Campylobacter enteritis in the United States. A multicenter study. Ann Intern Med 1983; 98:360–365.
4. Petruccelli BP, et al. Treatment of traveler's diarrhea with ciprofloxacin and loperamide. J Infect Dis 1992; 165:557–560.
5. Echeverria P, et al. Diarrhea in US troops deployed to Thailand. J Clin Microbiol 1993; 31:3351–3352.
6. Murphy GS, et al. Ciprofloxacin- and azithromycin-resistant Campylobacter causing traveler's diarrhea in US troops deployed to Thailand in 1994. Clin Infect Dis 1996; 22:868–869.
7. Altekruse SF, et al. Food and animal sources of human *Campylobacter jejuni* infection. J Am Vet Med Assoc 1994; 204:57–61.
8. Altekruse SF, et al. *Campylobacter jejuni*—an emerging foodborne pathogen. Emerg Infect Dis 1999; 5:28–35.
9. Allos BM. *Campylobacter jejuni* Infections: update on emerging issues and trends. Clin Infect Dis 2001; 32:1201–1206.
10. Blaser MJ. Epidemiologic and clinical features of *Campylobacter jejuni* infections. J Infect Dis 1997; 176(suppl 2): S103–S105.
11. Blaser MJ, et al. Epidemiology of *Campylobacter jejuni* infections. Epidemiol Rev 1983; 5:157–176.
12. Mishu B, Blaser MJ. *Campylobacter jejuni*, human immunodeficiency virus, and the Guillain–Barre syndrome [letter]. J Infect Dis 1994; 169:1177.
13. Perlman DM, et al. Persistent *Campylobacter jejuni* infections in patients infected with the human immunodeficiency virus (HIV). Ann Intern Med 1988; 108:540–546.
14. Johnson RJ, et al. Persistent *Campylobacter jejuni* infection in an immunocompromised patient. Ann Intern Med 1984; 100:832–834.
15. Pigrau C, et al. Bacteremia due to Campylobacter species: clinical findings and antimicrobial susceptibility patterns. Clin Infect Dis 1997; 25:1414–1420.
16. Tee W, Mijch A. *Campylobacter jejuni* bacteremia in human immunodeficiency virus (HIV)-infected and non-HIV-infected patients: comparison of clinical features and review. Clin Infect Dis 1998; 26:91–96.
17. Snijders F, et al. Prevalence of Campylobacter-associated diarrhea among patients infected with human immunodeficiency virus. Clin Infect Dis 1997; 24:1107–1113.
18. Friedman CR, et al. Epidemiology of *Campylobacter jejuni* infections in the United States and other industrialized nations. In: Nachamkin I, Blaser MJ, eds. Campylobacter. 2d ed. Washington, DC: ASM Press, 2000:121–138.
19. Oberhelman RA, Taylor DN. *Campylobacter* infections in developing countries. In: Nachamkin I, Blaser MJ, eds. *Campylobacter*. 2d ed. Washington, DC: ASM Press, 2000: 139–153.
20. Coker AO, et al. Human campylobacteriosis in developing countries. Emerg Infect Dis 2002; 8:237–244.
21. Mattila L. Clinical features and duration of traveler's diarrhea in relation to its etiology. Clin Infect Dis 1994; 19: 728–734.
22. Mattila L, et al. Seasonal variation in etiology of traveler's diarrhea. Finnish–Moroccan Study Group. J Infect Dis 1992; 165:385–388.
23. Speelman P, et al. Detection of *Campylobacter jejuni* and other potential pathogens in travellers' diarrhoea in Bangladesh. Scand J Gastroenterol Suppl 1983; 84:19–23.
24. Taylor DN, Echeverria P. Etiology and epidemiology of travelers' diarrhea in Asia. Rev Infect Dis 1986; 8(suppl 2): S136–S141.
25. Taylor DN, et al. Polymicrobial aetiology of travellers' diarrhoea. Lancet 1985; 1:381–383.
26. Bourgeois AL, et al. Etiology of acute diarrhea among United States military personnel deployed to South America and west Africa. Am J Trop Med Hyg 1993; 48:243–248.
27. Taylor DN, et al. Campylobacter enteritis during doxycycline prophylaxis for malaria in Thailand. Lancet 1988; 2: 578–579.
28. Kuschner RA, et al. Use of azithromycin for the treatment of Campylobacter enteritis in travelers to Thailand, an area where ciprofloxacin resistance is prevalent. Clin Infect Dis 1995; 21:536–541.
29. Echeverria P, et al. Prophylactic doxycycline for travelers' diarrhea in Thailand. Further supportive evidence of *Aeromonas hydrophila* as an enteric pathogen. Am J Epidemiol 1984; 120:912–921.
30. Walz SE, et al. Pre-exposure anti-*Campylobacter jejuni* immunoglobulin a levels associated with reduced risk of Campylobacter diarrhea in adults traveling to Thailand. Am J Trop Med Hyg 2001; 65:652–656.
31. Sanders JW, et al. An observational clinic-based study of diarrheal illness in deployed US military personnel in Thailand: presentation and outcome of *Campylobacter* infection. Am J Trop Med Hyg, 2002. Accepted for publication.
32. Skirrow MB, Blaser MJ. Clinical aspects of *Campylobacter* infection. In: Nachamkin I, Blaser MJ, eds. *Campylobacter*. 2nd ed. Washington, D.C.: ASM Press, 2000:69–88.
33. Arthur JD, et al. A comparative study of gastrointestinal infections in United States soldiers receiving doxycycline or mefloquine for malaria prophylaxis. Am J Trop Med Hyg 1990; 43:608–613.
34. Engberg J, et al. Quinolone and macrolide resistance in *Campylobacter jejuni* and *C coli*: resistance mechanisms and trends in human isolates. Emerg Infect Dis 2001; 7:24–34.
35. Sack RB, et al. Antimicrobial resistance in organisms causing diarrheal disease. Clin Infect Dis 1997; 24(suppl 1): S102–S105.
36. Adler Mosca H, et al. Development of resistance to quinolones in five patients with campylobacteriosis treated with norfloxacin or ciprofloxacin. Eur J Clin Microbiol Infect Dis 1991; 10:953–957.
37. Hoge CW, et al. Trends in antibiotic resistance among diarrheal pathogens isolated in Thailand over 15 years. Clin Infect Dis 1998; 26:341–345.
38. Rautelin H, et al. Emergence of fluoroquinolone resistance in *Campylobacter jejuni* and *Campylobacter coli* in subjects from Finland. Antimicrob Agents Chemother 1991; 35: 2065–2069.
39. Reina J, et al. Emergence of resistance to erythromycin and fluoroquinolones in thermotolerant Campylobacter strains isolated from feces 1987–1991. Eur J Clin Microbiol Infect Dis 1992; 11:1163–1166.
40. Smith KE, et al. Quinolone-resistant *Campylobacter jejuni* infections in Minnesota, 1992–1998. Investigation Team [see comments]. N Engl J Med 1999; 340:1525–1532.
41. Center for Disease Control and Prevention. National Antimicrobial Resistance Monitoring System. Annual Report. Atlanta, GA: Center for Disease Control and Prevention, 1997.
42. Foodborne Diseases Active Surveillance Network. 1996. MMWR Morb Mortal Wkly Rep 1997; 46:258–261.
43. Preliminary FoodNet data on the incidence of foodborne illnesses-selected sites, United States, 2001. MMWR Morb Mortal Wkly Rep 2002; 51:325–329.
44. Vogt RL, et al. Campylobacter enteritis associated with contaminated water. Ann Intern Med 1982; 96:292–296.

45. Melby K, et al. Clinical and serological manifestations in patients during a waterborne epidemic due to *Campylobacter jejuni*. J Infect 1990; 21:309–316.

46. MacDonald KL, et al. *Escherichia coli* 0157:H7, an emerging gastrointestinal pathogen. Results of a one-year, prospective, population-based study. JAMA 1988; 259:3567–3570.

47. Surveillance of the flow of *Salmonella* and *Campylobacter* in a community. Seattle: Seattle-King County Department of Public Health, 1984.

48. Sacks JJ, et al. Epidemic campylobacteriosis associated with a community water supply. Am J Public Health 1986; 76:424–428.

49. Tauxe RV. Epidemiology of *Campylobacter jejuni* infections in the United States and other industrialized nations. In: Nachamkin I, Blaser MJ, Tompkins LS, eds. *Campylobacter jejuni*: current status and future trends. Washington, DC: American Society for Microbiology, 1992:9–19.

50. Mead PS, et al. Food-related illness and death in the United States. Emerg Infect Dis 1999; 5:607–625.

51. Preliminary FoodNet data on the incidence of foodborne illnesses—selected sites, United States, 2000. MMWR Morb Mortal Wkly Rep 2001; 50:241–246.

52. Calva JJ, et al. Cohort study of intestinal infection with campylobacter in Mexican children. Lancet 1988; 1:503–506.

53. Taylor DN, et al. Influence of strain characteristics and immunity on the epidemiology of Campylobacter infections in Thailand. J Clin Microbiol 1988; 26:863–868.

54. Haberberger RL, Waker RI. Prospects and problems for development of a vaccine against diarrhea caused by *Campylobacter*. Vaccine Res 1994; 3:15–22.

55. Megraud F, et al. Incidence of Campylobacter infection in infants in western Algeria and the possible protective role of breast feeding. Epidemiol Infect 1990; 105:73–78.

56. Rao MR, et al. Pathogenicity and convalescent excretion of Campylobacter in rural Egyptian children. Am J Epidemiol 2001; 154:166–173.

57. Bengtsson A, et al. Reactive arthritis after *Campylobacter jejuni* enteritis. A case report. Scand J Rheumatol 1983; 12:181–182.

58. Ebright JR, Ryan LM. Acute erosive reactive arthritis associated with *Campylobacter jejuni*-induced colitis. Am J Med 1984; 76:321–323.

59. Eastmond CJ, et al. An outbreak of Campylobacter enteritis—a rheumatological follow-up survey. J Rheumatol 1983; 10:107–108.

60. Johnsen K, et al. HLA-B27-negative arthritis related to *Campylobacter jejuni* enteritis in three children and two adults. Acta Med Scand 1983; 214:165–168.

61. Berden JH, et al. Reactive arthritis associated with *Campylobacter jejuni* enteritis. Br Med J 1979; 1:380–381.

62. van de Putte LB, et al. Reactive arthritis after *Campylobacter jejuni* enteritis. J Rheumatol 1980; 7:531–535.

63. Bremell T, et al. Rheumatic symptoms following an outbreak of campylobacter enteritis: a five-year follow up. Ann Rheum Dis 1991; 50:934–938.

64. Leung FY, et al. Reiter's syndrome after *Campylobacter jejuni* enteritis. Arthritis Rheum 1980; 23:948–950.

65. Gumpel JM, et al. Reactive arthritis associated with campylobacter enteritis. Ann Rheum Dis 1981; 40:64–65.

66. Lindsay JA. Chronic sequelae of foodborne disease. Emerg Infect Dis 1997; 3:443–452.

67. Kuroki S, et al. Guillain–Barre syndrome associated with Campylobacter infection. Pediatr Infect Dis J 1991; 10:149–151.

68. Rees JH, et al. *Campylobacter jejuni* and Guillain–Barre syndrome. Q J Med 1993; 86:623–634.

69. Mishu B, Blaser MJ. Role of infection due to *Campylobacter jejuni* in the initiation of Guillain–Barre syndrome. Clin Infect Dis 1993; 17:104–108.

70. Allos BM. Association between Campylobacter infection and Guillain–Barre syndrome. J Infect Dis 1997; 176(suppl 2):S125–S128.

71. Prendergast MM, Moran AP. Lipopolsaccharides in the development of the Guillain–Barre syndrome and Miller Fisher syndrome forms of acute inflammatory peripheral neuropathies. J Endotoxin Res 2000; 6:341–359.

72. Nachamkin I. Campylobacter enteritis and the Guillain–Barre syndrome. Curr Infect Dis Rep 2001; 3:116–122.

73. Nachamkin I. Chronic effects of Campylobacter infection. Microbes Infect 2002; 4:399–403.

74. Nachamkin I, et al. *Campylobacter jejuni* infection and the association with Guillain–Barré syndrome. In: Nachamkin I, Blaser MJ, eds. *Campylobacter*. 2nd ed. Washington, DC: ASM Press, 2000:155–175.

75. Nachamkin I, et al. Campylobacter species and Guillain–Barre syndrome. Clin Microbiol Rev 1998; 11:555–567.

76. Van Der Meche FG. The Guillain–Barre syndrome: pathogenesis and treatment. Rev Neurol Paris 1996; 152:355–358.

77. Rees JH, et al. *Campylobacter jejuni* infection and Guillain–Barre syndrome [see comments]. N Engl J Med 1995; 333:1374–1379.

78. Fujimoto S, et al. Specific serotype of *Campylobacter jejuni* associated with Guillain–Barre syndrome [letter]. J Infect Dis 1992; 165:183.

79. Kuroki S, et al. *Campylobacter jejuni* strains from patients with Guillain–Barre syndrome belong mostly to Penner serogroup 19 and contain beta-N-acetylglucosamine residues. Ann Neurol 1993; 33:243–247.

80. Allos BM, Blaser MJ. *Campylobacter jejuni* infection and the Guillain–Barre syndrome: mechanisms and implications. Int J Med Microbiol Virol Parasitol Infect Dis 1994; 281:544–548.

81. Aspinall GO, et al. Lipopolysaccharides from *Campylobacter jejuni* associated with Guillain–Barre syndrome patients mimic human gangliosides in structure. Infect Immun 1994; 62:2122–2125.

82. Goddard EA, et al. Campylobacter 0:41 isolation in Guillain–Barre syndrome. Arch Dis Child 1997; 76:526–528.

83. Lastovica AJ, et al. Guillain–Barre syndrome in South Africa associated with *Campylobacter jejuni* 0:41 strains. J Infect Dis 1997; 176(suppl 2):S139–S143.

84. Karlyshev AV, et al. Genetic and biochemical evidence of a *Campylobacter jejuni* capsular polysaccharide that accounts for Penner serotype specificity. Mol Microbiol 2000; 35:529–541.

85. Bacon DJ, et al. A phase-variable capsule is involved in virulence of *Campylobacter jejuni* 81–176. Mol Microbiol 2001; 40:769–777.

86. Yuki N, et al. Serotype of *Campylobacter jejuni*, HLA, and the Guillain–Barre syndrome [letter]. Muscle Nerve 1992; 15:968–969.

87. Russell RG, et al. Experimental *Campylobacter jejuni* infection in Macaca nemestrina. Infect Immun 1989; 57:1438–1444.

88. Caldwell MB, et al. Simple adult rabbit model for *Campylobacter jejuni* enteritis. Infect Immun 1983; 42:1176–1182.

89. Saha SK, Sanyal SC. Production and characterisation of *Campylobacter jejuni* enterotoxin in a synthetic medium and its assay in rat ileal loops. FEMS Microbiol Lett 1990; 55:333–338.

90. Sanyal SC, et al. *Campylobacter jejuni* diarrhea model in infant chickens. Infect Immun 1984; 43:931–936.

91. McCardell BA, et al. A mouse model for the measurement of virulence of species of Campylobacter. J Infect Dis 1986; 153:177.

92. Stanfield JT, et al. Campylobacter diarrhea in an adult mouse model. Microb Pathog 1987; 3:155–165.

93. Field LH, et al. Intestinal colonization of neonatal animals by *Campylobacter fetus* subsp. *jejuni*. Infect Immun 1981; 33:884–892.

94. Baqar S, et al. Immunogenicity and protective efficacy of a prototype Campylobacter killed whole-cell vaccine in mice. Infect Immun 1995; 63:3731–3735.

95. Babakhani FK, et al. Newborn piglet model for campylobacteriosis. Infect Immun 1993; 61:3466–3475.

96. Vitovec J, et al. The gnotobiotic piglet as a model for the pathogenesis of *Campylobacter jejuni* infection. Zentralbl Bakteriol 1989; 271:91–103.

97. Walker RI, et al. Studies of Campylobacter infection in the adult rabbit. In: Nachamkin I, Blaser MJ, Tompkins LS, eds. *Campylobacter jejuni*: current status and future trends. Washington, DC: American Society for Microbiology, 1992:139–147.

98. Pavlovskis OR, et al. Significance of flagella in colonization resistance of rabbits immunized with *Campylobacter* spp. Infect Immun 1991; 59:2259–2264.

99. Abimiku AG, Dolby JM. Cross-protection of infant mice against intestinal colonisation by *Campylobacter jejuni*: importance of heat-labile serotyping (Lior) antigens. J Med Microbiol 1988; 26:265–268.

100. Baqar S, et al. Modulation of mucosal immunity against *Campylobacter jejuni* by orally administered cytokines. Antimicrob Agents Chemother 1993; 37:2688–2692.

101. Baqar S, et al. Safety and immunogenicity of a prototype oral whole-cell killed Campylobacter vaccine administered with a mucosal adjuvant in non-human primates. Vaccine 1995; 13:22–28.

102. Baqar S, et al. Murine intranasal challenge model for the study of Campylobacter pathogenesis and immunity. Infect Immun 1996; 64:4933–4939.

103. Newell DG. Animal models of *Campylobacter jejuni* colonization and disease and the lessons to be learned from similar *Helicobacter pylori* models. Symp Ser Soc Appl Microbiol 2001; 57S–67S.

104. Vuckovic D, et al. Primary *Campylobacter jejuni* infection in different mice strains. Microb Pathog 1998; 24:263–268.

105. Yrios JW, Balish E. Colonization and infection of athymic and euthymic germfree mice by *Campylobacter jejuni* and *Campylobacter fetus* subsp. fetus. Infect Immun 1986; 53:378–383.

106. Yrios JW, Balish E. Pathogenesis of *Campylobacter* spp. in athymic and euthymic germfree mice. Infect Immun 1986; 53:384–392.

107. Yrios JW, Balish E. Immune response of athymic and euthymic germfree mice to *Campylobacter* spp. Infect Immun 1986; 54:339–346.

108. O'Sullivan AM, et al. The effect of campylobacter lipopolysaccharide on fetal development in the mouse. J Med Microbiol 1988; 26:101–105.

109. Pancorbo PL, et al. Potential intervention of *Campylobacter jejuni* in the modulation of murine immune response. Curr Microbiol 2001; 43:209–214.

110. Mallett CP, et al. Evaluation of Shigella vaccine safety and efficacy in an intranasally challenged mouse model. Vaccine 1993; 11:190–196.

111. Bell JA, Manning DD. A domestic ferret model of immunity to *Campylobacter jejuni*-induced enteric disease. Infect Immun 1990; 58:1848–1852.

112. Welkos SL. Experimental gastroenteritis in newly-hatched chicks infected with *Campylobacter jejuni*. J Med Microbiol 1984; 18:233–248.

113. Li CY, et al. Experimental *Campylobacter jejuni* infection in the chicken: an animal model of axonal Guillain–Barre

114. Blaser MJ, et al. Serologic study of two clusters of infection due to *Campylobacter jejuni*. J Infect Dis 1983; 147:820–823.

115. Blaser MJ, Duncan DJ. Human serum antibody response to *Campylobacter jejuni* infection as measured in an enzyme-linked immunosorbent assay. Infect Immun 1984; 44:292–298.

116. Blaser MJ, et al. Extraintestinal *Campylobacter jejuni* and *Campylobacter coli* infections: host factors and strain characteristics. J Infect Dis 1986; 153:552–559.

117. Jones DM, et al. Serological response to *Campylobacter jejuni*/coli infection. J Clin Pathol 1980; 33:767–769.

118. Jones DM, et al. Serological studies in two outbreaks of *Campylobacter jejuni* infection. J Hyg (London) 1981; 87:163–170.

119. Kaldor J, et al. Serum antibodies in Campylobacter enteritis. J Clin Microbiol 1983; 18:1–4.

120. Martin PM, et al. Immune response to *Campylobacter jejuni* and *Campylobacter coli* in a cohort of children from birth to 2 years of age. Infect Immun 1989; 57:2542–2546.

121. Svedhem A, et al. Diffusion-in-gel enzyme-linked immunosorbent assay for routine detection of IgG and IgM antibodies to *Campylobacter jejuni*. J Infect Dis 1983; 148:82–92.

122. Taylor DN, et al. Campylobacter immunity and quantitative excretion rates in Thai children. J Infect Dis 1993; 168:754–758.

123. Strid MA, et al. Antibody responses to Campylobacter infections determined by an enzyme-linked immunosorbent assay: 2-year follow-up study of 210 patients. Clin Diagn Lab Immunol 2001; 8:314–319.

124. Blaser MJ, et al. *Campylobacter jejuni* outer membrane proteins are antigenic for humans. Infect Immun 1984; 43:986–993.

125. Mills SD, Bradbury WC. Human antibody response to outer membrane proteins of *Campylobacter jejuni* during infection. Infect Immun 1984; 43:739–743.

126. Baqar S, et al. *Campylobacter jejuni* enteritis. Clin Infect Dis 2001; 33:901–905.

127. Ruiz-Palacios GM, et al. Protection of breast-fed infants against Campylobacter diarrhea by antibodies in human milk. J Pediatr 1990; 116:707–713.

128. Torres O, Cruz JR. Protection against Campylobacter diarrhea: role of milk IgA antibodies against bacterial surface antigens. Acta Paediatr 1993; 82:835–838.

129. Hughes RA, et al. Pathogenesis of Guillain–Barre syndrome. J Neuroimmunol 1999; 100:74–97.

130. Cooper JC, et al. T cell recognition of a non-protein antigen preparation of *Campylobacter jejuni* in patients with Guillain–Barre syndrome. J Neurol Neurosurg Psychiatry 2002; 72:413–414.

131. Wassenaar TM, et al. Inactivation of *Campylobacter jejuni* flagellin genes by homologous recombination demonstrates that flaA but not flaB is required for invasion. EMBO J 1991; 10:2055–2061.

132. Yao R, et al. CheY-mediated modulation of *Campylobacter jejuni* virulence. Mol Microbiol 1997; 23:1021–1031.

133. Doig P, et al. Characterization of a post-translational modification of Campylobacter flagelin: identification of a sero-specific glycosyl moiety. Mol Microbiol 1996; 19:379–387.

134. Power ME, et al. Structural and antigenic characteristics of *Campylobacter coli* FlaA flagelin. J Bacteriol 1994; 176:3303–3313.

135. Thibault P, et al. Identification of the carbohydrate moieties and glycosylation motifs in *Campylobacter jejuni* flagelin. J Biol Chem 2001; 276:34862–34870.

136. Johnson WM, Lior H. A new heat-labile cytolethal distend-

ing toxin (CLDT) produced by *Campylobacter* spp. Microb Pathog 1988; 4:115–126.

137. Whitehouse CA, et al. *Campylobacter jejuni* cytolethal distending toxin causes a G2-phase cell cycle block. Infect Immun 1998; 66:1934–1940.

138. Pickett CL, et al. Prevalence of cytolethal distending toxin production in *Campylobacter jejuni* and relatedness of *Campylobacter* sp. cdtB genes. Infect Immun 1996; 64:2070–2078.

139. Pei Z, Blaser MJ. PEB1, the major cell-binding factor of *Campylobacter jejuni*, is a homolog of the binding component in gram-negative nutrient transport systems. J Biol Chem 1993; 268:18717–18725.

140. Pei Z, et al. Mutation in the peb1A locus of *Campylobacter jejuni* reduces interactions with epithelial cells and intestinal colonization of mice. Infect Immun 1998; 66:938–943.

141. Lara-Tejero M, Galan JE. A bacterial toxin that controls cell cycle progression as a deoxyribonuclease I-like protein. Science 2000; 290:354–357.

142. Hickey TE, et al. *Campylobacter jejuni* cytolethal distending toxin mediates release of interleukin-8 from intestinal epithelial cells. Infect Immun 2000; 68:6535–6541.

143. Parkhill J, et al. The genome sequence of the food-borne pathogen *Campylobacter jejuni* reveals hypervariable sequences. Nature 2000; 403:665–668.

144. Konkel ME, et al. Bacterial secreted proteins are required for the internalization of *Campylobacter jejuni* into cultured mammalian cells. Mol Microbiol 1999; 32:691–701.

145. Konkel ME, et al. Identification of proteins required for the internalization of *Campylobacter jejuni* into cultured mammalian cells. Adv Exp Med Biol 1999; 473:215–224.

146. Konkel ME, et al. Kinetic and antigenic characterization of altered protein synthesis by *Campylobacter jejuni* during cultivation with human epithelial cells. J Infect Dis 1993; 168:948–954.

147. Konkel ME, et al. Translocation of *Campylobacter jejuni* across human polarize epithelial cell monolayer cultures. J Infect Dis 1992; 166:308–315.

148. Oelschlaeger TA, et al. Unusual microtubule-dependent endocytosis mechanisms triggered by *Campylobacter jejuni* and *Citrobacter freundii*. Proc Natl Acad Sci USA 1993; 90: 6884–6888.

149. Bacon DJ, et al. Involvement of a plasmid in virulence of *Campylobacter jejuni* 81–176. Infect Immun 2000; 68:4384–4390.

150. Dorrell N, et al. Whole genome comparison of *Campylobacter jejuni* human isolates using a low-cost microarray reveals extensive genetic diversity. Genome Res 2001; 11: 1706–1715.

151. Clemens JD, et al. Field trial of oral cholera vaccines in Bangladesh. Southeast Asian J Trop Med Public Health 1988; 19:417–422.

152. Clemens JD, et al. Field trial of oral cholera vaccines in Bangladesh: results of one year of follow-up. J Infect Dis 1988; 158:60–69.

153. Clemens JD, et al. Evidence that inactivated oral cholera vaccines both prevent and mitigate Vibrio cholerae O1 infections in a cholera-endemic area. J Infect Dis 1992; 166: 1029–1034.

154. Clemens JD, et al. Field trial of oral cholera vaccines in Bangladesh: results from three-year follow-up [see comments]. Lancet 1990; 335:270–273.

155. Sanchez JL, et al. Safety and immunogenicity of the oral, whole cell/recombinant B subunit cholera vaccine in North American volunteers. J Infect Dis 1993; 167:1446–1449.

156. Sanchez JL, et al. Protective efficacy of oral whole-cell/recombinant-B-subunit cholera vaccine in Peruvian military recruits [see comments]. Lancet 1994; 344:1273–1276.

157. Taylor DN, et al. Two-year study of the protective efficacy of the oral whole cell plus recombinant B subunit cholera vaccine in Peru. J Infect Dis 2000; 181:1667–1673.

158. Peltola H, et al. Prevention of travellers' diarrhoea by oral B-subunit/whole-cell cholera vaccine. Lancet 1991; 338: 1285–1289.

159. Black RE, et al. Protective efficacy in humans of killed whole-vibrio oral cholera vaccine with and without the B subunit of cholera toxin. Infect Immun 1987; 55:1116–1120.

160. Levine MM, Kaper JB. Live oral vaccines against cholera: an update. Vaccine 1993; 11:207–212.

161. Walker RI, Clements JD. Use of the heat labile toxin of enterotoxigenic *Escherichia coli* to facilitate mucosal immunization. Vaccine Res 1993; 2:1–10.

162. Dickinson BL, Clements JD. Dissociation of *Escherichia coli* heat-labile enterotoxin adjuvanticity from ADP-ribosyltransferase activity. Infect Immun 1995; 63:1617–1623.

163. Rollwagen FM, et al. Killed Campylobacter elicits immune response and protection when administered with an oral adjuvant. Vaccine 1993; 11:1316–1320.

164. Yao R, et al. Isolation of motile and non-motile insertional mutants of *Campylobacter jejuni*: the role of motility in adherence and invasion of eukaryotic cells. Mol Microbiol 1994; 14:883–893.

165. Korlath JA, et al. A point-source outbreak of campylobacteriosis associated with consumption of raw milk. J Infect Dis 1985; 152:592–596.

166. Nachamkin I, Hart AM. Western blot analysis of the human antibody response to *Campylobacter jejuni* cellular antigens during gastrointestinal infection. J Clin Microbiol 1985; 21:33–38.

167. Wenman WM, et al. Antigenic analysis of Campylobacter flagellar protein and other proteins. J Clin Microbiol 1985; 21:108–112.

168. Lee LH, et al. Evaluation of a truncated recombinant flagellin subunit vaccine against *Campylobacter jejuni*. Infect Immun 1999; 67:5799–5805.

169. Kaper JB, et al. A recombinant live oral cholera vaccine. Bio/Technology 1984; 2:345–349.

170. Kaper JB, et al. Recombinant nontoxinogenic *Vibrio cholerae* strains as attenuated cholera vaccine candidates. Nature 1984; 308:655–658.

171. Sabin AB. Oral poliovirus vaccine. JAMA 1965; 194:872–876.

172. Black RE, et al. Efficacy of one or two doses of Ty21a *Salmonella typhi* vaccine in enteric-coated capsules in a controlled field trial. Chilean Typhoid Committee. Vaccine 1990; 8:81–84.

173. Taylor DE. Genetics of *Campylobacter* and *Helicobacter*. Annu Rev Microbiol 1992; 46:35–64.

64

Vaccines Against Uropathogenic *Escherichia coli*

Solomon Langermann and W. Ripley Ballou, Jr.
MedImmune, Inc., Gaithersburg, Maryland, U.S.A.

Acute urinary tract infections (UTIs) are among the most common disorders prompting medical evaluation. A recent retrospective analysis demonstrated that 40% of adult women in the United States experience at least one UTI sometime during their lifetime [1], with a per year incidence rate between 0.5% and 0.7% in young adult females [2]. This results in approximately seven million office visits each year with an estimated annual health care cost exceeding $1 billion [3]. *Escherichia coli* are the main causative agents of UTIs [4,5] and account for about 80–85% of cases of acute cystitis and pyelonephritis. *E. coli* also causes 60% of recurrent cystitis cases and at least 35% of recurrent pyelonephritis infections. In children an *E. coli* etiology is still more frequent [6,7]. Childhood pyelonephritis, which is almost exclusively caused by *E. coli*, has been a leading cause of end-stage renal disease [8]. One method of eliminating acute UTIs as well as preventing recurrent UTIs and ascending infections is the use of regular or intermittent antimicrobial prophylaxis [9]. Concern about the emergence of antibiotic-resistant bacterial strains limits the long-term feasibility of this approach. Given the high incidence of both primary and recurrent UTIs, along with the associated morbidity and significant cost of treatment, a prophylactic vaccine to block infection of the urinary tract by *E. coli* would be desirable.

In order for UTIs to occur, *E. coli* that originate in the bowel and ascend into the bladder must first attach to the uroepithelial cells lining the bladder mucosa. Numerous studies have shown that a bacterial ligand or adhesin known as FimH mediates attachment to the bladder epithelium and that the FimH adhesin is critical for cystitis to occur [10,11,12,13,14]. The FimH adhesin protein is located at the distal tip of proteinaceous, filamentous polymeric organelles, known as type 1 pili or fimbriae, expressed on the surface of the bacteria [15]. FimH interacts specifically with mannosylated glycoproteins known as uroplakin 1a and 1b that line the bladder mucosa [16] leading to bacterial colo-

nization and replication. These cellular receptors contain a single N-linked carbohydrate of the high-mannose type [17], common to most glycoproteins recognized by FimH.

Aside from its role in colonization, FimH is also involved in subsequent stages of pathogenesis. FimH-mediated binding to the bladder mucosa induces the expression of proinflammatory cytokines and chemokines by uroepithelial cells, resulting in neutrophil recruitment and the massive inflammatory response characteristic of cystitis. FimH has also been shown to induce exfoliation of uroepithelial cells by an apoptosis-like mechanism upon attachment to the epithelium followed by rapid reconstitution of the urothelium through differentiation of underlying basal and intermediate cells [18]. Furthermore, FimH mediates invasion of *E. coli* into the bladder epithelium, a mechanism that allows for survival and persistence of *E. coli* in the bladder [19].

Given the essential role of type 1 pili and in particular FimH in the initial stages of bladder colonization, antibodies targeting FimH should prevent UTIs. In addition to blocking attachment at the site of entry and colonization of mucosal surfaces at the earliest stage of the disease process, antibodies against FimH might also promote opsonization of bacteria that have invaded beyond the superficial epithelium for clearance by the systemic immune system. Furthermore, antibodies against the FimH adhesin might also be expected to protect against subsequent bacterial invasion or ascending infection into the kidney.

We have developed FimH as a vaccine candidate against UTI and have tested it in various animal models and surrogate in vitro assays. Our efforts have been focused on the development of a recombinant subunit vaccine that contains the FimH adhesin complexed with its cognate chaperone FimC, which is critical for proper folding and stabilization of the full-length adhesin [20]. The FimCH complex (FimC + FimH) forms the basis of a pilus vaccine candidate against *E. coli* UTI. Preclinical data with FimCH indicate that it induces high levels of serum IgG directed against functional domains on the FimH adhesin. Anti-FimH IgG transudates into urogenital secretions and confers protection against colonization of bladder epithelium in several challenge models. The preclinical data suggest that the FimCH vaccine may have utility in preventing UTIs in humans.

I. CHOICE OF THE FIMCH COMPLEX AS A VACCINE VERSUS FIMH SUBUNIT ALONE OR WHOLE PILI

Type 1 pili are composed of single or multiple protein subunits, called pilins or fimbrins, which are typically arranged in a helical fashion. They are expressed peritrichously around individual bacteria and range from a few fractions of a micrometer to greater than 20 µm in length and vary from less than 2 nm up to 11 nm in diameter. The primary function of the type 1 pilus is to act as scaffolding for the presentation of the associated 29.1-kDa FimH adhesin protein. High-resolution electron microscopy of type 1 pili of *E. coli* has revealed that these structures are composite fibers, consisting of a thick pilus rod attached to a thin, short distally located tip fibrillum with the adhesin located at the distal end of the tip fibrillum [15,21,22]. Its location at the distal tip of the pilus allows the FimH adhesin to mediate interactions of bacteria with each other, with inanimate surfaces, and with tissues and cells in susceptible host organisms. Such interactions facilitate the formation of bacterial communities such as biofilms and are often critical to the successful colonization of the host by both commensal and pathogenic bacteria [23].

Early studies using purified whole type 1 pili as immunogens demonstrated that these vaccines induced some protection against *E. coli* infections in animals and man [24,25], although these vaccines were not tested in the context of UTIs. A major disadvantage to pilus-based vaccines has been the fact that the major immunodominant components of pilus fibers are often highly variable antigenically and therefore afford protection against only a limited number of bacterial strains. In contrast, pilus-associated adhesins, such as FimH, are highly conserved proteins among different species and strains of bacteria. However, adhesin-based vaccines have been difficult to develop given the inherent instability of these proteins. Recombinant technology has been used to produce adhesin proteins in pure form but as such are often rapidly proteolytically degraded when the corresponding periplasmic chaperone protein is absent. Adhesins can, however, be readily stabilized by the presence of periplasmic chaperone molecules, which are important in the synthesis of adhesins and assembly of pili, but are not incorporated into the structure.

FimC is the periplasmic chaperone protein that mediates assembly of type 1 pili in bacteria. The FimC chaperone stabilizes the type 1 pilus subunits in the periplasm through formation of distinct periplasmic complexes. FimC binds to and caps interactive surfaces on the pilus subunits, preventing aggregation and allowing for correct folding and assembly. The chaperone–subunit complexes are targeted to a large channel protein in the bacterial outer membrane called the usher where the chaperone is released, exposing interac-

tive surfaces on the subunits that facilitate their assembly into the pilus [26,27]. Each of the pilus subunits are then incorporated into the pilus depending, in part, upon the kinetics with which they are partitioned to the usher in complex with the chaperone [28] (Figure 1).

X-ray diffraction studies of the FimH adhesin in a complex with its chaperone FimC have shed new light on the nature of the chaperone subunit interaction [20]. With regard to the 52.0-kDa FimCH complex, the following was noted. The FimH adhesin has two domains; one interacts with the FimC chaperone (the pilin domain) while the other interacts with mannose (the lectin-binding domain) (Figure 2). The pilin domain that interacts with FimC, as well as FimC itself, has an immunoglobulin-like fold made up of antiparallel β strands. However, the seventh strand is missing from the FimH immunoglobulin fold, exposing a hydrophobic groove on the surface of the pilin domain. This groove would render the FimH unstable were it not for the fact that the FimC chaperone temporarily shares its seventh strand with the FimH subunit without parting with the shared strand, in a process called donor strand complementation. This complementation during formation of the FimCH complex stabilizes the FimH adhesin.

These observations explain in part why initial attempts at developing a subunit adhesin vaccine based on only FimH without its cognate chaperone protein FimC were unsuccessful. The use of hyperexpression systems to produce and purify large amounts of adhesin most likely failed because FimH expressed as an independent moiety, with an exposed hydrophobic groove, enters a nonproductive pathway in the bacterium and is rapidly degraded [29,30]. In contrast, hyperexpression of recombinant FimH in combination with FimC as a FimCH complex allows for high-level expression of the full-length adhesin. Since the FimCH complex is a stable compound, and presents the lectin-binding domain of FimH in the proper conformation, the complex was selected as a vaccine candidate for eliciting functional adhesin-blocking antibodies to type 1 piliated uropathogenic *E. coli*.

II. PRECLINICAL IMMUNOGENICITY AND PROTECTION STUDIES WITH FIMCH

Experiments were conducted in C3H/HeJ mice using purified FimCH complex at doses ranging from 0.3 to 30 µg emulsified in complete Freund's adjuvant (CFA) to test for immunogenicity of FimCH. Booster doses were administered in incomplete Freund's adjuvant (IFA). Antibodies to the FimH adhesin were measured in an enzyme-linked immunosorbent assay (ELISA)-based format using a truncated form of FimH expressed as a histidine-tagged fusion protein (FimH T3) as the capture antigen. FimH T3 is truncated at its carboxy terminus and thus contains the amino-terminal lectin (mannose) binding domain of FimH.

Mice immunized with FimCH developed strong, long-lasting immune responses to FimH T3 and to FimH associated with whole type 1 pilus rods [12]. Serum anti-FimH IgG was detected for more than 30 weeks. An additional dose of FimCH administered after the 30-week time point further boosted responses such that antibodies were detected more

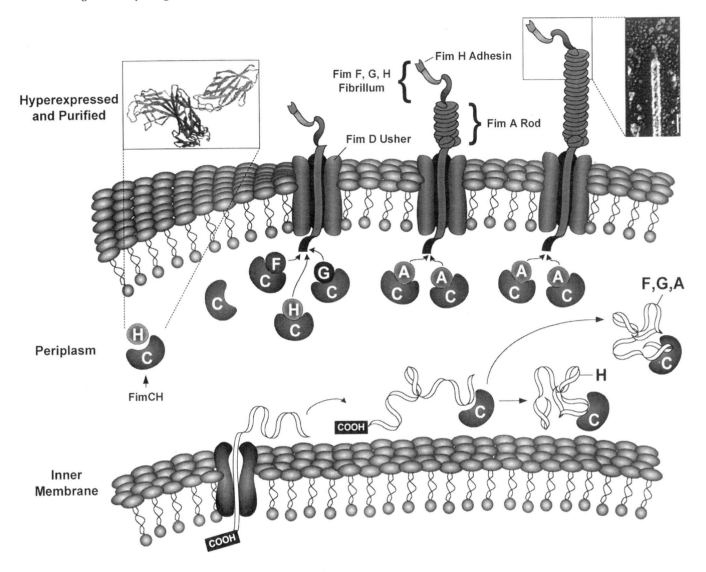

Figure 1 Type 1 pilus biogenesis. Schematic representation of type 1 pilus assembly via the chaperone–usher pathway. FimC chaperone-mediated extraction of subunits from the inner cytoplasmic membrane is coupled to their folding into an assembly-competent state. The G1 β strand of the immunoglobulin-like chaperones, which may serve as a template in the subunit folding pathway, protects nascently folded subunits from premature oligomerization in the periplasmic space by directly capping the newly formed assembled surfaces. These interactive surfaces remain protected until delivery of the preassembly complex to the outer membrane assembly site. Such interactions with the chaperone also prevent the subunit from being proteolytically degraded in the periplasm. In the case of the FimH subunit, its carboxy-terminal domain has an immunoglobulin-like fold in which the seventh strand is missing, leaving part of the hydrophobic core exposed. The chaperone, FimC, donates a strand to complete the pilin domain 20.

than 1 year after immunization. Immunization studies in rabbits demonstrated immunogenicity profiles similar to those seen in mice. FimH-specific IgG was also detected in the urine and vaginal secretions of immunized mice. Antibodies to FimH generated in both mice and rabbits were shown to be biologically active by their ability to block attachment of uropathogenic *E. coli* to bladder cells in vitro; > 94% of primary *E. coli* clinical isolates induced to express type 1 pili were inhibited by FimH sera raised against a single FimH protein. Moreover, in a murine challenge model involving the uropathogenic *E. coli* strain NU14, more than

99% reduction in colonization of the bladder mucosa was observed in vivo. Similarly, immune serum from rabbits was used to passively immunize mice, which then underwent challenge using a panel of 10 diverse uropathogenic *E. coli* strains. Greater than 99% reduction in colonization of the bladder mucosa was observed, and highly significant protection was seen with 9 of 10 uropathogenic strains. Thus, preclinical studies involving active immunization of mice with FimCH in Freund's adjuvant confirmed that the vaccine was immunogenic and able to induce strong, long-lasting, antigen-specific, functional antibody responses that

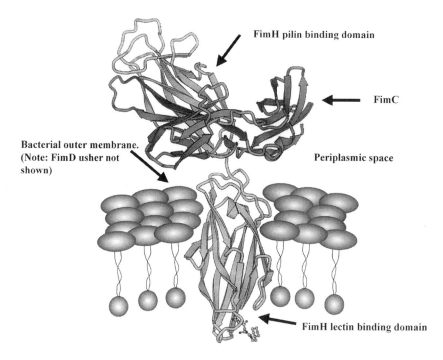

Figure 2 MOLLSCRIPT ribbon diagram of the FimCH complex. The FimH pilin domain and the NH2-terminal domain of FimC form a closed superbarrel with a continuous core made from conserved residues in both proteins. A ball and stick model of a mannoselike compound (C-HEGA) molecule bound to the lectin domain indicates the position of the carbohydrate-binding site at the tip of the domain [20]. This portion of the molecule is also being depicted as it is extruded from the bacterial outer membrane, where it will form the distal tip-associated adhesin on the pilus rod.

were able to block attachment of uropathogenic *E. coli* to bladder cells and protected mice against challenge.

III. DEVELOPING A VACCINE FORMULATION SUITABLE FOR HUMAN STUDIES

The initial preclinical studies involved formulations containing Freund's adjuvant, which is not suitable for use in humans. The data suggested that protection was dependent upon high-titer IgG responses, and therefore a potent formulation suitable for human use would be essential. Additional studies were thus conducted in mice to determine the relative potency of FimCH adsorbed to alum [Al(OH)$_3$], the only adjuvant currently licensed as a component of a vaccine in the United States. As an alternative to alum, FimCH was adjuvanted with MF59C.1, an oil-in-water (squalene) emulsion developed by Chiron that has been extensively tested in humans and that is used in an influenza vaccine that has been licensed in Italy [31,32]. FimCH formulated with alum consistently gave titers to FimH in mice that were 5- to 10-fold lower than those seen with Freund's adjuvant. In contrast, FimCH formulated with MF59C.1 gave titers as high as those seen with Freund's adjuvant. Since there is a relationship between antibody titer to FimH and protection against infection in vivo, subsequent efforts focused on developing FimCH formulated with MF59C.1. At the same time new formulations with alum in combination with different buffers and pH conditions are being investigated in ongoing preclinical studies.

Additional studies were conducted to demonstrate the immunogenicity of different doses of FimCH formulated with MF59C.1. C3H/HeJ mice were immunized with doses ranging from 0.16 to 20 µg per injection. Some groups received two doses at 0 and 18 weeks, while others received three doses at 0, 4, and 18 weeks, either intramuscularly, intraperitoneally, or subcutaneously. The results confirmed the immunogenicity of FimCH formulated with MF59C.1 by all routes at doses as low as 0.8 µg and revealed the superiority of three doses over two. Moreover, IgG antibodies to FimH were detected in urine and vaginal secretions similar to those seen with formulations involving Freund's adjuvant, and active immunization (×3 injections) protected mice against challenge with uropathogenic *E. coli.*

Having identified a highly immunogenic FimCH formulation that was potentially suitable for human use, adult female cynomolgus monkeys (*Macaca fasicularis*) received either 2 or 3 injections of 4, 20, or 100 µg of FimCH mixed 1:1 with MF59C.1. The formulation appeared to be well tolerated and was highly immunogenic, resulting in endpoint titers in excess of 50,000 in monkeys that received 2 doses of vaccine, whereas those that received 3 doses reached endpoint titers in excess of 200,000. Immunized animals underwent challenge studies to determine in vivo efficacy. Vaccination and challenge studies in the primate model corroborated the original murine studies [33]. Monkeys vaccinated with purified recombinant FimCH chaperone–adhesin complex with the MF59 adjuvant developed long-lasting serum IgG antibodies to FimH as well as functional inhibitory titers as measured by the ability of the antibodies to block in vitro binding of type 1-piliated *E. coli* to mannose. The vaccine protected the monkeys from bladder infection by uropathogenic *E. coli* and from an inflammatory response typically associated with cystitis. Three out of four animals were completely protected from colonization by the NU14 *E. coli* strain. Furthermore, although the number of animals was small, there was a direct correlation between the presence of inhibitory antibodies in local (vaginal wash) secretions and protection against colonization and infection [33].

In a second challenge study in monkeys, 2 of 4 monkeys receiving a 100-µg dose of FimCH vaccine (×3 doses) were protected from colonization by a high dose of a highly virulent strain of *E. coli*, DS17 [34]. The two vaccinated monkeys that had *E. coli* in their urine following challenge were nonetheless protected from inflammatory responses and hematuria typically associated with cystitis. In contrast, all four MF59 control monkeys had high levels of *E. coli* in their urine for at least 9 days following challenge, and all had potent inflammatory responses and hematuria. The highly virulent DS17 strain used in the second primate study was originally isolated from a patient with pyelonephritis, and is capable of expressing multiple virulence determinants including P pili in addition to type 1 pili *in vivo*. Thus, these results further point to the potency of the FimCH vaccine and its ability to protect against uropathogenic *E. coli* strains expressing multiple adhesins.

One of the theoretical concerns with development of a FimCH vaccine is the potential to affect the normal *E. coli* flora of the gastrointestinal tract. To address this issue, we collected fecal samples from each monkey over the entire course of this first study to investigate whether vaccination with the FimCH vaccine would affect the normal gut flora. Overall coliform counts per milliliter of fecal suspension were determined at each time point and compared to three preimmune samples taken for each animal. No differences between immunized and control monkeys were observed. To examine whether the vaccine caused a shift in subpopulations within the coliform bacteria, a biochemical profile assay was used for biochemical characterization of the fecal isolates obtained during the immunization period. No differences in the coliform populations were observed. Thus, systemic vaccination with the FimCH adhesin vaccine does not appear to have an effect on the normal gut flora.

In summary, preclinical studies of FimCH formulated in MF59C.1 confirmed its immunogenicity in two animal species, including doses administered to nonhuman primates in the range intended for human studies, and revealed the superiority of three over two doses of vaccine. The vaccine does not appear to have adverse effects on the normal flora of the gastrointestinal tract and should be well tolerated in humans.

IV. CLINICAL EXPERIENCE WITH MEDI-516

A Phase I study of MEDI-516, an *E. coli* FimCH vaccine formulated with MF59C.1 adjuvant, Chiron's proprietary oil (squalene)-in-water adjuvant was conducted as a double-blind, randomized, adjuvant-controlled, dose-escalation study. The study protocol, all amendments to the protocol,

and volunteer informed consent documents were submitted for review to an Institutional Review Board (IRB).Written IRB approvals were obtained prior to implementation. Written informed consent was obtained from each participant prior to conduct of any protocol-specific activity or study entry. The study was conducted in accordance with the Declaration of Helsinki (amended 1989) and with the U.S. Code of Federal Regulations governing the protection of human volunteers (21 CFR 50), Institutional Review Boards (21 CFR 56), and the obligations of clinical investigators (21 CFR 312).

Forty-eight healthy adult women who were seronegative for antibody to FimH as measured by MedImmune's FimH T3 screening ELISA were sequentially randomized to four cohorts (1, 5, 25, or 123 µg FimCH). Within each cohort, nine volunteers were randomized to receive injections of MEDI-516 with MF59C.1 adjuvant and three were randomized to receive adjuvant alone as a control. Injections were administered at 0, 1, and 4 months. Volunteers were followed for the occurrence and intensity of solicited adverse events for the 7-day period following each immunization and unsolicited adverse events for 28 days after each immunization. Volunteers were followed for the occurrence and intensity of serious adverse events occurring during the period starting from the administration of the first dose of vaccine and ending 28 days after administration of the last dose of vaccine. The occurrence of severe solicited and unsolicited adverse events and any serious adverse events after each dose were to be reported immediately and reviewed by the medical monitor.

Dose escalation was by cohort and did not proceed until all of the following had occurred: all volunteers at a given dose level had received an injection of study vaccine; at least 9 of the 12 volunteers had been followed for at least 7 days after immunization; and the Medical Monitor had reviewed the available safety data with the Safety Monitoring Committee (SMC) and the SMC had recommended to continue with dose escalation. Volunteers who received one or more immunizations were asked to provide samples of blood, urine, and cervical secretions for measures of immune responses. Antibody responses were determined by measuring FimH T3-specific immunoglobulin G (IgG) concentrations in serum and the functional activity (binding inhibition) of IgG in serum were measured using methods reported previously [33].

All 48 volunteers were female. The mean ages were similar among treatment groups (range of means: 31–37 years). Most of the volunteers (45, 94%) were White/non-Hispanic; the remaining 3 volunteers were Black (2 in the 25-µg MEDI-516 group and 1 in the 123-mg MEDI-516 group). Of the 48 volunteers who entered the study, 44 completed through study day 364. Four volunteers were lost to follow-up after completing all protocol evaluations on study day 119.

V. SAFETY AND REACTOGENICITY

All volunteers, except 1 in the 5-µg MEDI-516 group, had at least one solicited adverse event. The most common solicited adverse event in all groups was pain at the injection site, reported by 78% to 100% of the volunteers in each group. No redness or swelling at the injection site within 7 days of

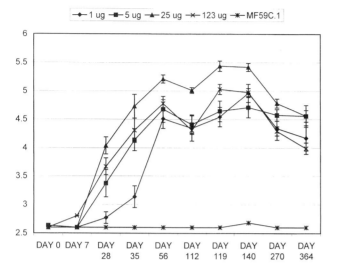

Figure 3 Serum antibody responses to FimH T3 (ELISA titers).

immunization was observed in any volunteer. The most common general reactions among volunteers who received MEDI-516 were headache in 18 (50%), fever in 16 (44%), and fatigue in 13 (36%) volunteers. In the MF59C.1 control group, the most common general reactions were headache in 6 (50%) and fatigue in 3 (25%) volunteers, while fever occurred in only 2 (17%) volunteers. With the exception of fever, each solicited adverse event was reported by similar proportions (≤15 percentage points difference) of MEDI-516 and MF59C.1 volunteers. There were no intensity grade 3 (severe) solicited adverse events and the frequency and intensity grade of solicited adverse events did not increase with increasing vaccine dose or number of injections. Local (site of injection) solicited adverse events were considered to be related to study injections. Systemic adverse events judged to be related to study injections, with the exception of fever, were reported by similar proportions (≤15 percentage points difference) of MEDI-516 and MF59C.1 control volunteers. Fever was more common among MEDI-516 recipients and was reported by 14 (39%) of these volunteers as compared to 1 (8%) in the MF59C.1 control group. Fevers greater than 100.0°F were uncommon. The highest temperature recorded

during the study was 102.0°F (intensity grade 2 fever) on day 3 following the second injection in a volunteer who received 5 μg MEDI-516. Fever in this volunteer was associated with headache, fatigue, and myalgia, and was attributed to the study vaccine. The incidence of unsolicited adverse events was similar between the MEDI-516 and MF59C.1 control groups (29, 81% and 9, 75%, respectively). There were no deaths or other serious adverse events through study day 140. No clinically meaningful changes were noted in vital signs (temperature, pulse, respiration rate, systolic and diastolic blood pressure) in any volunteer in any group from preinjection to 30 min after injection. No volunteers were permanently discontinued from study vaccine due to adverse events. There were no clinically meaningful changes in any of the laboratory parameters followed to assess vaccine safety (complete blood count, liver enzymes, renal function studies, or urinalysis) that were judged to be related to administration of study vaccine.

A. Immunogenicity

All anti-FimH T3 titers were ≤1:800 at baseline (study day 0). All volunteers who received the MF59C.1 control had titers of <1:800 at all time points tested except for one volunteer whose titer was 1:3200 at study day 140. All volunteers who received MEDI-516 seroconverted by study day 56. For each MEDI-516 group, geometric mean antibody titers rose rapidly after the second injection of MEDI-516 was administered, peaked at study day 56, and decreased by approximately 50% of peak values before the administration of the third injection of vaccine. After the third injection, geometric mean antibody titers increased further, exceeding the peak levels achieved after the second injection. For each MEDI-516 group, geometric mean antibody titers decreased between study days 140 and 364. Anti-FimH T3 ELISA data are summarized in Figure 3.

Sera were assayed for the ability to inhibit the in vitro binding of *E. coli* to J82 bladder cells as reported previously [12,33]. The results were reported as IC_{50}, the greatest dilution giving at least 50% reduction in mean channel fluorescence over baseline. For these assays, baseline sera for each group were pooled. Baseline pools were run in the same assay as the test sera, and calculations were made using the results of the baseline pool run on the same day as that assay.

No volunteer had inhibitory serum activity at baseline (Table 1). After three doses of the vaccine (study day 140)

Table 1 Number (%) of Volunteers with Binding Inhibition Activity in Sera (IC_{50} Value ≥50)

| Study day | MEDI-516 | | | | MF59C.1 Adjuvant (N=12) |
	1 μg (N=9)	5 μg (N=9)	25 μg (N=9)	123 μg (N=9)	
0	0 (0%)	0 (0%)	0 (0%)	0 (0%)	0 (0%)
140	6 (67%)	9 (100%)	9 (100%)	8 (89%)	0 (0%)[a]
270	7 (78%)	9 (100%)	8 (100%)[b]	6 (75%)[b]	0 (0%)[a]
364	6 (67%)	7 (78%)	7 (88%)[b]	5 (63%)[b]	0 (0%)[c]

[a] N = 11.
[b] N = 8.
[c] N = 10.

substantial inhibitory activity ($IC_{50} \geq 50$) was seen in 6 (67%), 9 (100%), 9 (100%), and 8 (89%) of the volunteers in the 1-, 5-, 25-, and 123-μg MEDI-516 groups, respectively. In approximately half of these volunteers, significant inhibitory activity was not detectable until after the third injection had been administered.

Urine and cervical secretions were collected at baseline and on study day 140 and IgG responses against FimH T3 were determined by ELISA. Paired urine specimens were available from baseline and study day 140 for all volunteers except 1 in each of the 5-μg MEDI-516 and MF59C.1 control groups. A twofold (or greater) increase over baseline optical density was seen in urine samples from 5 of 9 (56%), 4 of 8 (50%), 9 of 9 (100%), and 3 of 9 (33%) volunteers from the 1-, 5-, 25-, and 123-μg MEDI-516 groups, respectively, and in 1 of 11 (9%) volunteers from the MF59C.1 control group. The highest group mean urine anti-FimH T3 ELISA response was seen in the 25-μg MEDI-516 group. Paired cervical secretion specimens were available from baseline and study day 140 for all volunteers except 1 in the MF59C.1 control group. The optical density readings at baseline varied considerably from volunteer to volunteer. At least a twofold increase over baseline optical density was seen in cervical secretions from 7 of 9 (78%), 8 of 9 (89%), 8 of 9 (89%), and 8 of 9 (89%) volunteers from the 1-, 5-, 25-, and 123-μg MEDI-516 groups, respectively, and in 3 of 11 (27%) volunteers from the MF59C.1 control group. Substantial group mean anti-FimH T3 ELISA response was seen in all MEDI-516 groups.

To confirm the specificity of the antibody responses in urogenital secretions, Western blot analysis was performed using the same specimens that were assayed by ELISA. Western blot analysis using highly purified recombinant FimCH as the antigen and electrophoretic separation of the FimH and FimC proteins permitted assessment of responses to each antigen individually. This analysis confirmed the presence of antibodies reactive with both FimH and FimC in samples from volunteers who had received MEDI-516. In volunteers for whom both urine and cervical samples were analyzed, reactivity against FimH by Western blot was detected in baseline urine and/or cervical secretions in 46% (16/35) of the MEDI-516 group and 55% (6/11) of the MF59C.1 control group, suggesting that these individuals had previous exposure to FimH, presumably through colonization or previous UTIs with bacteria expressing FimH.

In summary, this Phase I study indicated that MEDI-516 appears to be safe and well tolerated. Mild to moderate pain at the injection site was commonly reported following all injections and appeared to be indistinguishable from pain following immunization with MF59C.1 alone. Low-grade fever occurred more frequently after immunization with MEDI-516 than MF59C.1 control. Administration of MEDI-516 resulted in the production of binding-inhibitory antibodies directed against FimH, with optimum results observed at the 25-μg dose. Antibody responses against FimH in urogenital secretions increased significantly after immunization with MEDI-516. On the basis of these results, MedImmune plans to conduct Phase II studies in adult women with and without a history of recurrent UTI to further assess the safety, tolerability and immunogenicity

of the vaccine. These studies will also provide important data on the incidence of *E. coli* UTI in these populations and potentially provide preliminary evidence of vaccine efficacy.

REFERENCES

1. Kunin CM. Urinary tract infections in females. Clin Infect Dis 1994; 18:1–12.
2. Hooton TM, et al. A prospective study of risk factors for symptomatic urinary tract infection in young women. N Engl J Med 1996; 335:468–474.
3. Stamm WE, Hooton TM. Management of urinary tract infections in adults. N Engl J Med 1993; 329:1328–1334.
4. Muhldorfer I, Hacker J. Genetic aspects of *Escherichia coli* virulence. Microb Pathog 1994; 16:171–181.
5. Winberg J, et al. Epidemiology of symptomatic urinary tract infection in childhood. ACTA Paediatr Scand 1974; 63 (Suppl):1–20.
6. Marild S, Jodal U. Incidence rate of first-time symptomatic urinary tract infection in children under 6 years of age. Acta Paediatr 1998; 87:549–552.
7. Winberg J, et al. Epidemiology of symptomatic urinary tract infection in childhood. ACTA Paediatr Scand 1974; 63(Suppl):1–20.
8. Esbjorner E, et al. Epidemiology of chronic renal failure in children: a report from Sweden. Paediatric Nephrol 1997; 11:438–442.
9. Stapleton A, Stamm WE. Prevention of urinary tract infection. Infect Dis Clin North Am 1997; 11:719–733.
10. Keith BR, et al. Receptor-binding function of type 1 pili effects bladder colonization by a clinical isolate of *Escherichia coli*. Infect Immun 1986; 53:693–696.
11. Connell I, et al. Type 1 fimbrial expression enhances *Escherichia coli* virulence for the urinary tract. Proc Natl Acad Sci U S A 1996; 93:9827–9832.
12. Langermann S, et al. Prevention of mucosal *Escherichia coli* infection by FimH-adhesin-based systemic vaccination. Science 1997; 276:607–611.
13. Bahrani-Mougeot FK, et al. Type 1 fimbriae and extracellular polysaccharides are preeminent uropathogenic *Escherichia coli* virulence determinants in the murine urinary tract. Mol Microbiol 2002; 45:1079–1093.
14. Gunther NW IV, et al. Assessment of virulence of uropathogenic *Escherichia coli* type 1 fimbrial mutants in which the invertible element is phase-locked on or off. Infect Immun 2002; 70:3344–3354.
15. Jones CH, et al. FimH adhesin of type 1 pili is assembled into a fibrillar tip structure is the *Enterobacteriaceae*. Proc Natl Acad Sci U S A 1995; 92:2081–2085.
16. Zhou G, et al. Uroplakin Ia is the urothelial receptor for uropathogenic *Escherichia coli*: evidence from in vitro FimH binding. J Cell Sci 2001; 114:4095–4103.
17. Wu XR, et al. In vitro binding of type 1-fimbriated *Escherichia coli* to uroplakins 1a and 1b: relation to urinary tract infections. Proc Natl Acad Sci U S A 1996; 93:9630–9635.
18. Mulvey MA, et al. Induction and evasion of host defenses by type 1-piliated uropathogenic *Escherichia coli*. Science 1998; 282:1494–1497.
19. Martinez JJ, et al. Type 1 pilus-mediated bacterial invasion of bladder epithelial cells. EMBO J 2000; 19:2803–2812.
20. Choudhury D, et al. X-ray structure of the FimC-FimH chaperone–adhesin complex from uropathogenic *Escherichia coli*. Science 1999; 285:1061–1066.
21. Hultgren SJ, et al. Pilus and nonpilus bacterial adhesins: assembly and function in cell recognition. Cell. 1993; 73:887–901.
22. Jacob-Dubuisson F, et al. A novel secretion apparatus for the assembly of adhesive bacterial pili. Trends Microbiol 1993; 1:50–55.

23. Costerton JW, et al. Bacterial biofilms: a common cause of persistent infections. Science 1999; 284:1318–1322.

24. Levine MM, et al. Reactogenicity, immunogenicity and efficacy studies of *Escherichia coli* type 1 somatic pili parenteral vaccine in man. Scand J Infect Dis Suppl 1982; 33:83–95.

25. Guerina NG, et al. Heterologous protection against invasive *Escherichia coli* K1 disease in newborn rats by maternal immunization with purified mannose-sensitive pili. Infect Immun 1989; 57:1568–1572.

26. Dodson K, et al. Outer-membrane PapC molecular usher discriminately recognizes periplasmic chaperone–pilus subunit complexes. Proc Natl Acad Sci USA 1996; 90:3670–3674.

27. Thanassi DG, et al. The PapC usher forms an oligomeric channel: implications for pilus biogenesis across the outer membrane. Proc Natl Acad Sci U S A 1998; 95:3146–3151.

28. Saulino ET, et al. Ramifications of kinetic partitioning on usher-mediated pilus biogenesis. EMBO J 1998; 17:2177–2185.

29. Hultgren SJ, et al. Chaperone-assisted assembly and molecular architecture of adhesive pili. Annu Rev Microbiol 1991; 45:383–415.

30. Kuehn MJ, et al. Immunoglobulin-like PapD chaperone caps and uncaps interactive surfaces of nascently translocated pilus subunits. Proc Natl Acad Sci U S A 1991; 88:10586–10590.

31. Podda A. The adjuvanted influenza vaccines with novel adjuvants: experience with the MF59-adjuvanted vaccine. Vaccine 2001; 21:2673–2680.

32. De Donato S, et al. Safety and immunogenicity of MF59-adjuvanted influenza vaccine in the elderly. Vaccine 1999; 17:3094–3101.

33. Langermann S, et al. Vaccination with FimH adhesin protects *Cynomolgus* monkeys from colonization and infection by uropathogenic *Escherichia coli*. J Infect Dis 2000; 181:774–778.

34. Tullus K, et al. Epidemic outbreaks of acute pyelonephritis caused by nosocomial spread of P fimbriated *Escherichia coli* in children. J Infect Dis 1984; 150:728–736.

65

Vaccine Strategies Against *Helicobacter pylori*

Karen L. Kotloff
University of Maryland School of Medicine, Baltimore, Maryland, U.S.A.

Cynthia K. Lee
Acambis, Inc., Cambridge, Massachusetts, U.S.A.

Giuseppe Del Giudice
Chiron S.r.l., Siena, Italy

I. RATIONALE FOR A *HELICOBACTER PYLORI* VACCINE

Nearly half of the world's population is infected with *H. pylori*, a bacterium that causes chronic gastritis and peptic ulcer and has been strongly incriminated in the etiology of gastric cancer, the second most common fatal malignancy. Although antibiotics can cure infection, multidrug regimens are required which are expensive, have side effects, and may induce resistance. These drugs are not amenable to widespread use for primary prevention, or even for treatment, of infection in some areas of the world. For these reasons, vaccines are being developed.

Because most *H. pylori* infections are acquired during the first years of life, vaccination strategies that target infants are being considered. A series of economic analyses predicted that the cost/benefit ratio of a prophylactic *H. pylori* vaccine for infants would be favorable in the United States [1], even if efficacy were as low as 55% [2]. An infant vaccination campaign lasting only 10 years has the potential to reduce the prevalence of *H. pylori* by 99% by the end of the twenty-first century, and virtually eliminate transmission [3]. A different situation is found in many developing countries, where persistently high rates of transmission would require a continuous vaccination program, a highly efficacious vaccine, and broad population coverage [3]. The large investment of resources needed to implement such a program would be a serious consideration for countries with limited health care budgets.

II. FEASIBILITY OF DEVELOPING A *H. PYLORI* VACCINE

Several factors must be addressed in assessing the feasibility of developing an effective *H. pylori* vaccine. One issue is the remarkable genetic diversity of *H. pylori*. Each patient carries a unique pool of strains [4] and these strains undergo genetic variation over time, presumably as a result of mutation and host-mediated selective pressure [5]. It remains to be determined whether this has implications for the ability to identify shared antigens for inclusion in a vaccine.

There is no clear evidence for infection-derived immunity that could serve as a paradigm for vaccine development. Even in the face of strong humoral and cellular immune responses, *H. pylori* colonization persists for life. The ineffectiveness of the host response to natural infection is further illustrated by studies which demonstrate that reinfection rates in patients who receive successful eradication therapy are similar to those seen in previously uninfected individuals [6]. Nonetheless, reports that transient infections are common in childhood suggest that effective immune surveillance may exist [7,8]. Furthermore, immunomodulation by concurrent enteric helminth infection can ameliorate gastric pathology in *H. pylori*-infected mice despite persistent colonization [9]. Thus even if a *H. pylori* vaccine does not achieve the so-called sterile immunity, it might still protect against adverse clinical outcomes.

It is difficult to rationally select vaccine candidates that appear promising in clinical trial when the desired immune responses are uncertain. In such circumstances, human challenge studies have been used to assess vaccine efficacy. The feasibility of experimentally infecting humans was proven by two investigators, who inoculated themselves with *H. pylori* in an attempt to fulfill Koch's postulates of pathogenicity [10,11]. More recently, investigators have attempted to develop a *H. pylori* challenge model in volunteers using a *cagA*-negative strain [12]. They successfully infected the subjects, and were able to observe clinical symptoms and gastric inflammatory changes. However, the role of volunteer challenge trials in *H. pylori* vaccine development is controversial, and animal studies remain an essential source of information on the mechanisms of vaccine-mediated immunity. These models have illustrated that vaccines can prevent *H. pylori* infection even when infection-derived immunity cannot be demonstrated.

A point of debate is whether the elimination of *H. pylori* infection using prophylactic vaccination would increase the risk of proximal esophageal diseases, such as gastroesophageal reflux, Barrett's esophagus, and esophageal adenocarcinoma [13]. The hypothesis is that *H. pylori* infection inhibits gastric acid secretion and thereby protects the esophagus from injury. Proponents of this theory contend that the natural decline in *H. pylori* infection that has followed industrialization is causally related to the concomitant increase in the incidence of proximal esophageal disease that has been observed in Western countries during the past century. In this scenario, the benefits of preventing peptic ulcer and gastric carcinoma with a *H. pylori* vaccine would have to be weighed against a potential increase in the risk of proximal esophageal disease.

A final consideration is that certain *H. pylori* antigens serologically cross-react with host moieties, such as Lewis b antigens on the surface of gastric epithelial cells, and that this so-called antigenic mimicry could elicit autoimmune sequela. Antibodies recognizing gastric epithelium have been observed in *H. pylori*-infected individuals but are of uncertain clinical significance [14].

III. *H. PYLORI* VIRULENCE FACTORS AND PATHOGENIC MECHANISMS

H. pylori has evolved diverse mechanisms which foster its survival in the harsh environment of the human stomach. Specialized secretory machinery exports macromolecular messengers to subvert the host cell for bacterial needs. The bacterium can endure an acidic milieu, penetrate the viscous mucus layer, and adhere intimately to gastric cells. It effectively eludes the host immune system while silently colonizing the stomach for many years.

Production of a unique urease that is highly active at low pH is thought to be essential for colonization [15]. *H. pylori* urease is encoded by two structural (*ureA* and *ureB*) and seven accessory genes in a single chromosomal cluster. This 550-kDa nickel metalloenzyme catalyzes the hydrolysis of urea to yield ammonia and carbamate, which in turn form ammonium hydroxide and increase the pH of the micorenvironment [16]. Although primarily intracellular [17], after autolysis urease can be found on the bacterial surface by immunogold labeling using monoclonal antibodies [18]. Whether urease has a role in infection-derived immunity is not clear; most chronically infected individuals do not have specific antibodies [19,20] and only a minority of $CD4^+$ T-cell clones from gastric biopsies of infected individuals recognize this antigen [21].

Flagellate-mediated burrowing motility enables this spiral-shaped organism to penetrate the mucus layer and reach the neutral environment of the epithelial surface [22]. Adhesion to gastric cells induces an attaching and effacing epithelial lesion similar to that caused by enteropathogenic *Eschericia coli* [23]. Several outer membrane proteins are candidate adherence factors, including BabA [24], which binds to the Lewis b blood group antigen, and the flagella sheath protein HpaA [25] that binds sialic acid-containing macromolecules.

The dominant virulence factor is a 40-kb DNA sequence within the chromosome, called the *cag* pathogenicity island (PAI). This genetic cassette contains 31 genes, including the gene encoding CagA, a 126- to 145-kDa protein [26]. CagA is one of the most immunogenic proteins of *H. pylori*, stimulating production of both serum antibodies [27] and specific $CD4^+$ T lymphocytes at the level of the gastric mucosa [21]. The PAI genes encode for a type IV secretory machinery that translocates CagA into the host cell cytosol to be tyrosine phosphorylated, leading to actin polymerization with cellular elongation ("hummingbird" phenotype) and formation of adherence pedestals [28–30]. Furthermore, some PAI genes, such as *cagE*, regulate epithelial cell production of the inflammatory mediator IL-8 [31] and activation of nuclear factor (NF)-κβ [32].

Many investigators have tried to correlate human infection with CagA-positive organisms with the occurrence of peptic ulcers and gastric cancer. These studies have yielded discrepant results [33–37], probably because the principal determinant of virulence is a functional PAI. Mutagenesis studies suggest that other PAI genes, such as *cagE*, play a more direct role in the pathogenesis of severe gastric pathology [32]. This organism's genetic metamorphism further complicates the relationship between the PAI and clinical outcome. *H. pylori* infecting the human stomach contain isogenic populations of *cag*-positive and negative strains in which the PAI presumably has been excised [38]. A dynamic state is postulated in which chronically infected patients have periods of *cag*-positive predominance which lead to disease expression [34].

Another protein with an important (albeit incompletely understood) role in gastric injury is the vacuolating cytotoxin A (VacA). *vacA* is a pleomorphic gene present in all *H. pylori* strains and expressed in most strains [39,40]. It encodes VacA, a secreted protein composed of individual ~90-kDa monomers, each formed by two distinct domains (p37 and p58) [41]. When orally administered to mice, VacA induces gastric epithelial erosion similar to that seen in humans with peptic ulcer [42]. It is postulated that after binding to the host cell, VacA becomes internalized via endocytosis [43] and triggers formation of anion-selective channels in the endosomal membrane [44], producing vacuoles [41,45], and ultimately cell death by apoptosis [46]. VacA also enhances permeability of polarized epithelial cells by altering the tight junctions [41,47], a phenomenon that could favor *H. pylori* survival by providing an efflux of nutrients from the gastric submucosa.

The presence of VacA in the late endosomes and the formation of vacuoles alters the capacity of antigen-presenting cells to appropriately process antigens and present them in a Ii-dependent pathway [48]. This may explain the paucity of VacA-specific CD4$^+$ cells in biopsies of infected individuals [21], as well as the reduced ability of *H. pylori*-infected animals to mount CD8$^+$ cell responses specific for a virus concomitantly infecting the mice [49]. However, it remains unclear whether this inhibitory activity of VacA significantly influences in vivo immune responses.

A *H. pylori* protein with chemotactic and proinflammatory properties is the neutrophil-activating protein (NAP) [50], a 170-kDa iron-binding protein [51] that is highly conserved among isolates. After binding to a specific receptor, NAP stimulates leukocytes to produce reactive oxygen intermediates [52] and triggers mast cells to degranulate and release inflammatory mediators such as IL-6 [53]. NAP also enhances the expression of tissue factor and depresses fibrinolysis, thus impeding the physiological mechanisms leading to tissue repair [54].

IV. MECHANISMS OF PROTECTIVE IMMUNITY

The operating assumption when the first successful vaccination studies were performed in mouse models was that vaccine-mediated protection against *Helicobacter* infection was a result of the induction of mucosal antibodies while avoiding proinflammatory, ineffective immune responses associated with active *H. pylori* infection. We have since come to realize that antibodies have little or no role in effector mechanisms that lead to protection, and that vaccine-induced bacterial clearance involves the action of MHC class-II restricted CD4$^+$ T cells. While these mechanisms are not well elucidated, several lines of experimentation have contributed to the current understanding of this rather complex problem.

A role for antibodies in protective immunity was suggested by the finding that passive immunization with *H. pylori*-specific IgA protected mice against *Helicobacter felis* challenge [55]. This notion was further supported by the strong correlation observed between mucosal antibodies and protection in immunized mice [56]. Initial indication that mucosal antibodies were not as important for protection as originally believed was provided by Weltzin and coworkers [57], who showed that a nasal immunization regimen administered without mucosal adjuvants induced high levels of mucosal antibodies against urease but did not protect against challenge. This was defined more clearly in later experiments, in which genetic knock-out agammaglobulinemic mice vaccinated with various regimens were equally protected against *H. pylori* or *H. felis* challenge compared with wild-type mice [58,59]. Furthermore, IgA-deficient humans do not exhibit more severe pathology due to *H. pylori* [60]. Taken together, these findings suggest that antibodies play little or no role in protection against *Helicobacter*. Although mucosal antibody induction is a marker for

successful adjuvant effect of cholera toxin (CT) or *E. coli* heat-labile enterotoxin (LT), protection is mediated by mechanisms coinduced with mucosal antibodies.

A series of experiments in defined knock-out mice attempted to identify the immune mechanisms required for protection. CD8$^+$ T cells were found to play no role in preventing bacterial colonization because MHC Class I-deficient mice were protected from *H. pylori* challenge by using various immunization regimens [58,61]. However, MHC Class II knock-out mice were not able to generate vaccine-related protection [58,61], suggesting that CD4$^+$ T-cell-mediated mechanisms in the gastric mucosa are required. This hypothesis is also supported by studies using adoptive transfer techniques, in which CD4$^+$ T cells from mice immunized by various methods protected syngeneic recipients against challenge with *H. felis* and *H. pylori* [62–64]. To define the effector mechanisms, studies were performed in which cytokine deficient mice were either vaccinated or were used as syngeneic recipients in adoptive transfer experiments. These studies demonstrated that neither IL-4, IL-10 [63], nor IFN-γ [65] are required for protection.

The above studies defined protection microbiologically as lack of colonization with *H. pylori* or *H. felis*; resolution of gastritis, and thus disease, was seldom assessed. Eaton and coworkers [66] further explored the role of IFN-γ and IL-10 in protective immunity by examining their effect on gastric histopathology. When SCID mice were infected with *H. pylori* and then reconstituted with splenocytes from uninfected, immunocompetent syngeneic mice, severe gastritis developed within 2–4 weeks and then gradually resolved [66], accompanied by bacterial clearance. Adoptive transfer of splenocytes from IL-10-deficient mice resulted in more severe gastritis than seen in wild-type mice suggesting that IL-10 modulates gastritis [66]. On the other hand, adoptive transfer of splenocytes from IFN-γ deficient donors resulted in milder gastritis than seen in immunocompetent mice, suggesting that IFN-γ may exacerbate gastric pathology [66]. This last finding was further supported by experiments showing that IFN-γ depletion by specific antibodies inhibited the delayed-type hypersensitivity response in the stomach that occurs with *H. felis* infection or oral immunization with antigen and CT [67].

In sum, vaccine-induced protection against *H. pylori* colonization is not mediated by antibodies or CD8$^+$ T-cell mechanisms but requires CD4$^+$ T cells. IL-4, IL-10, and IFN-γ are not involved in the vaccine-induced protection against colonization. Nevertheless, IL-10 and IFN-γ appear to play a role in disease modulation, and should be considered in the design of vaccines. IL-10 stimulation may be a desirable goal as it ameliorates gastritis, while IFN-γ induction may be undesirable as it exacerbates gastritis.

V. ROUTES, ADJUVANTS, AND DELIVERY SYSTEMS

Most preclinical studies have used mucosal routes of vaccine delivery, usually orogastric. Antigens (either whole-cell lysates, or purified recombinant, or native molecules) have invariably required concomitant mucosal adjuvants for both prophylactic and therapeutic efficacy (reviewed in Ref. [68]). These have included wild-type LT and CT, and various mutants of LT retaining little or no enzymatic activity.

Inspired by successful parenteral vaccination against other mucosal pathogens, such as poliovirus and *Bordetella pertussis*, more recent experiments have utilized the parenteral delivery of *H. pylori* vaccine antigens. Intramuscular immunization with both whole-cell lysate and purified antigens effectively protected animals against *H. pylori* infection prophylactically and therapeutically, although results varied in different models. Adjuvants known to enhance immune responses to parenterally administered antigens were used in these experiments, such as Freund's adjuvant in mice [64] and in gnotobiotic piglets [69], aluminum hydroxide in mice [64], in dogs (G. del Giudice, unpublished), and in gnotobiotic piglets [69], QS21 in mice [70,71], Bay adjuvant in mice [70,71] and in monkeys [72,73], as well as the cationic lipid adjuvant DC Chol in mice [74] and in monkeys [75]. Interestingly, wild-type LT enhanced protective immunity engendered by urease when both were subcutaneously administered [76]. A combined delivery approach in which a mucosal prime is followed by parenteral boosts has been shown to be more efficacious than parenteral immunization alone in a rhesus monkey model [77]. The challenge in human studies involving parenteral immunization will be to understand whether the immune response that no doubt will be vigorous will elicit effector mechanisms leading to protection.

Little work has been reported on the use of DNA vaccines [78,79]. The predilection of DNA vaccination to enhance Th1-type responses may make this an inappropriate method for immunization against *H. pylori*. Th1-type responses may exacerbate *H. pylori* induced inflammation and CD8$^+$ cell responses do not appear to play a major role in vaccine-mediated protection against this organism.

VI. LESSONS FROM ANIMAL MODELS

A. Murine *H. felis* Models

The mouse model provided the first proof-of-principle that a vaccine could be developed to prevent and treat *Helicobacter* infection. Initial studies were performed by inoculating mice with a feline *Helicobacter* isolate designated *H. felis*. Infection caused acute inflammation which progressed to chronic gastritis typified by formation of microabscesses involving neutrophils and lymphocytes [80,81]. Successful mucosal immunization with *H. felis* sonicate antigens [55,82] or purified *H. pylori* antigens conserved between species [56,83–85] required coadministration of CT or LT adjuvant. Therapeutic immunization was often effective in reducing bacterial burden to a nondetectable level [86,87]. However, the agar-swarming nature of *H. felis* prevented the evaluation of bacterial colonization status by culture, and required that histopathology and gastric urease activity be used instead. Initially, urease assays (the least sensitive methods for detecting colonization) suggested that mice protected by vaccination were free of *H. felis* [55,82,85]. This notion was dispelled when gastric histopathology revealed residual bacteria, albeit at levels much lower than those seen in unim-

munized animals [56,84,88]. These residual bacteria were shown to be responsible for a phenomenon termed "postimmunization gastritis," whereby gastric inflammation was observed in immunized mice when they encountered *H. felis* challenge [67]. The inflammation subsides upon antimicrobial treatment to eradicate residual *H. felis* [89].

B. Murine *H. pylori* Models

An early study showing that *H. pylori* can transiently colonize the stomachs of conventional mice [90] led to subsequent studies in which persistent infection was achieved [91]. Marchetti and coworkers inoculated mice with a VacA/CagA-producing *H. pylori* clinical isolate, SPM326, evoking extensive gastric pathology including gastritis and ulcer formation [91]. More fulminate infections with *H. pylori* were achieved when stomach tissues from mice infected with other clinical strains were harvested and used to infect additional mice [92,93]. Initially, a cat *H. pylori* isolate, termed X47-2AL [94], was used [93,95]. Lee and coworkers [92] serially adapted a human isolate, designated as SS1, to colonize mice and offered this strain as a standardized model for vaccination and other studies. SS1 produced chronic gastritis with infiltration of inflammatory cells and mucosal atrophy [92]. Other *H. pylori* strains have been reported to infect mice [65,95], but none achieved the bacterial colonization levels of SS1 and X47-2AL [92,96,97].

The ability to determine colony-forming units (CFU) of *H. pylori* confirmed the histological finding in the *H. felis* model that vaccination does not achieve sterile immunity. Thus the "postimmunization gastritis" phenomenon reported in the *H. felis* model was not observed when mice were infected with *H. pylori*. Using the X47-2AL strain, it was determined that vaccination, at best, resulted in a 100-fold reduction in bacterial burden compared to unimmunized controls [58,98]. Although resolution of gastritis was not apparent in the short-term experiments, it is unknown whether this residual level of bacteria would eventually become an asymptomatic infection.

C. Ferret Models

Ferrets purchased from a commercial vendor were found to be infected with a *Helicobacter* species, *H. mustelae*. Colonization resulted in superficial gastritis consisting of glandular atrophy and a mononuclear leukocytic infiltration [99]. Spontaneous occurrence of adenocarcinoma has also been described in aged infected animals [100]. When naturally infected ferrets were orally immunized with *H. pylori* urease, an antigen that shares a 70% homology with *H. mustelae* urease, plus CT adjuvant, there was eradication or reduction in bacterial colonization in 30% of animals, and gastric inflammation was diminished [101]. This was the first proof-of-principle showing vaccine efficacy in a nonmurine model and one that becomes naturally colonized with a native *Helicobacter* species. The 30% vaccine efficacy was encouraging, considering that a heterologous antigen was used for immunization. This model also suggested that infection does not elicit protective immunity, because the animals whose *H. mustelae* infection was eradicated with antibiotics remained susceptible to reinfection with a homologous strain [102].

D. Feline Models

Cats develop persistent *H. pylori* infections characterized by multifocal gastritis with lymphoid aggregates and occasional neutrophil infiltration [103]. Uninfected cats orally vaccinated with recombinant *H. pylori* urease admixed with LT adjuvant and then challenged with a human isolate of *H. pylori* had a 20-fold lower gastric burden of *H. pylori* and diminished gastric inflammation compared to cats receiving adjuvant alone [104].

E. Primate Models

The rhesus monkey is the only nonhuman primate shown to be useful for evaluating *H. pylori* vaccines [72,73,105]. Rhesus monkeys raised in captivity are ubiquitously infected with *H. pylori* [106]. Infection results in chronic gastritis with intense mononuclear cell infiltrates, but in contrast to humans, neutrophils are rare and gastric ulcers have not been seen [106]. The inability of *H. pylori* infection (that was eradicated with antimicrobials) to confer protection against reinfection with the homologous strain was clearly demonstrated in this model [72]. Nonetheless, prophylactic vaccines have been efficacious. In one study, seronegative juvenile monkeys were orally immunized with *H. pylori* urease admixed with LT and then housed in social groups where they were exposed to *H. pylori* [105]. Ten months later, 93% of unvaccinated monkeys were infected with *H. pylori* compared with only 69% of vaccinated monkeys. In contrast, the same formulation appeared ineffective when administered to specific pathogen-free rhesus monkeys either orally or parenterally [73]. Similarly, therapeutic vaccination of older chronically infected monkeys with oral rUrease plus LT failed to reduce the gastric *H. pylori* burden [72]. However, when the infection was eradicated with antimicrobials and the monkeys rechallenged with *H. pylori*, bacterial colonization was significantly reduced in vaccinated monkeys compared to unvaccinated monkeys [72]. In a follow-up study, antimicrobial-treated monkeys were immunized with different regimens of rUrease. Those primed with oral vaccine and boosted with an intramuscular formulation had a more than 10-fold lower bacterial burden following *H. pylori* challenge compared with placebo recipients [77].

F. Swine Models

The earliest success at developing a *H. pylori* animal model was achieved by Krakowka and coworkers [107,108] using gnotobiotic piglets. Histopathological changes consisted of diffuse and follicular infiltration of mononuclear leukocytes into the gastric mucosa and submucosa with few neutrophils. Infection persisted for at least 90 days even if the piglets were transferred to conventional housing [109]. Two vaccination studies have been performed using this model. Killed bacteria were administered orally with and without LT, or parenterally with incomplete Freund's adjuvant [69,110]. Oral vaccination yielded disappointing results as

LT adjuvant induced diarrhea and the piglets were not protected against challenge [69]. Parenteral immunization provided partial protection but evoked gastritis in both protected and unprotected pigs [69,110].

G. Canine Models

Conventional beagle dogs can be experimentally infected with a *H. pylori* strain previously adapted to the mouse [111]. Infected dogs exhibit inflammatory cell changes in the gastric mucosa that mimic the response in humans. Interestingly, the lymphoid follicles in the gastric mucosa of infected dogs consist of peripheral CD4$^+$ lymphocytes surrounding a germinal center-like structure particularly rich in B (CD21$^+$) lymphocytes [112]. Studies of vaccine efficacy have been carried out in this model (G. Del Giudice, unpublished).

H. Mongolian Gerbils

The mongolian gerbil is not only susceptible to infection with *H. pylori*, but infection results in a high incidence of gastric ulcers (80%) [113] and adenocarcinoma of the stomach (37%) by 62 weeks postinfection [114,115]. The induction of these severe gastric pathologies was strictly associated with presence of the *cag* PAI [32]. This small animal model is useful for testing the efficacy of vaccination in preventing long-term effects of *H. pylori* infection and provides a valuable addition to data gathered in other animal models that mainly focus on bacterial burden.

VII. APPROACHES TO VACCINATION

A. Subunit Vaccines

1. Urease

Recombinant *H. pylori* urease apoenzyme (rUrease) expressed in *E. coli* from the *ureA* and *ureB* structural genes is devoid of enzymatic activity because additional *H. pylori* genes are required for insertion of nickel ion [116]. However, the recombinant protein is fully assembled into the 13-nm diameter, disk-shaped particles that are characteristic of the native protein [56,56,117]. The genes encoding urease are well conserved among *Helicobacter* species and provided an easy antigen to test in the animal models available in the early days of vaccine research.

Subunit vaccines consisting of native *H. pylori* urease [85], recombinant urease subunits expressed as fusion proteins [84,85], or, most commonly, rUrease apoenzyme [56] have been tested in animals. All had comparable efficacy in the *H. felis* challenge model. Subsequent studies in mice [58,98], cats [104], and monkeys [77] used *H. pylori* as the challenge strain. All showed that prophylactic vaccination diminished bacterial colonization (10- to 100-fold), and in many instances ameliorated gastritis and/or other epithelial abnormalities [72,77,104,105]. More recently, mouse studies have shown that parenteral immunization induces levels of protection similar to that achieved with mucosal immunization alone [74], and that mucosal prime followed by parenteral boost may be even more efficacious [58,77].

Promising preclinical data indicating that mucosal immunization with urease induces protective immunity led to a series of clinical trials in which urease was delivered by various mucosal routes. In an initial trial, 12 adults with asymptomatic *H. pylori* infection were randomized to receive either 60 mg rUrease or placebo orally once weekly for 4 weeks. Vaccination was well tolerated but minimally immunogenic, and did not eliminate infection or reduce gastritis [118]. As a next step toward developing a therapeutic vaccine, rUrease was combined with native LT as a mucosal adjuvant. In a double-blind design, 26 volunteers with asymptomatic *H. pylori* infection were randomly assigned to receive four weekly oral doses of either rUrease (20, 60, or 180 mg) plus LT (5–10 μg), LT alone, or placebo [119]. Native LT plus rUrease vaccine induced serum and antibody-secreting cell (ASC) IgA responses, but not local (salivary or gastric) responses to the vaccine antigen [119]. Most subjects (67%) receiving LT developed diarrhea [119]. Although none of the subjects were cured of their *H. pylori* infection, a significant decrease in gastric *H. pylori* density (but not inflammation) was observed in biopsy tissue. It remains to be determined whether sterilizing immunity can be achieved by a *H. pylori* vaccine and, if not, whether suppression alone can prevent the pathological consequences of infection.

Banerjee and coworkers [120] attempted to confirm that LT possesses adjuvanticity for rUrease in humans, and to identify the lowest dose that would be safe and immunogenic. They immunized 42 *H. pylori* uninfected adults with 60 mg rUrease in soluble or encapsulated form, given in four spaced doses (days 1, 8, 29, and 57] with LT at doses ranging from 0 to 2.5 μg. Preliminary results indicate that mild diarrhea (1–4 loose stools) occurred after the first dose in 50% of subjects receiving 2.5 μg LT but not in subjects receiving lower LT doses. A serologic response to urease was seen in 67% of subjects who received 2.5 μg of LT, and in 17–33% of those given lower doses of LT (0.5 and 0.1 μg). These data support the notion that coadministered LT enhances the immune response to oral rUrease vaccine and indicate that at the minimal effective dose of LT (2.5 μg), mild diarrhea occurs.

Rectal delivery of rUrease was evaluated in a clinical trial as a means to achieve an alternative mucosal route of immunization. Eighteen *H. pylori* uninfected volunteers were randomized to receive either 60 mg rUrease alone, or 60 mg rUrease plus native LT (5 or 25 μg). Three doses were given on days 0, 14, and 28. The rectally delivered vaccine was well tolerated. Although most subjects mounted excellent IgG and IgA serum antibody (60–80%) and IgA ASC responses (100%) to LT, few (8–25%) had responses to urease [121]. Interestingly, salivary and fecal antibody responses were not detected.

2. Other *H. pylori* Vaccine Antigens

Although urease has received the most attention for vaccine development, antigens such as VacA, CagA, and NAP, selected because of their contribution to *H. pylori* virulence, have generated promising preclinical results. Both native and recombinant VacA confer prophylactic and therapeutic protection against *H. pylori* infection after oral immuniza-

tion of mice when given with either native LT or with the nontoxic mutant LTK63 [91,122–124]. The full-length molecule was required to achieve high levels of protection, because the mice immunized with recombinant fragments corresponding to the 37- and 58-kDa subunits of VacA did not resist infection [122]. Interestingly, recombinant VacA generates protective immunity although it retains neither its native conformation nor its toxic activity in vitro [123]. The mechanism of immunity is strictly antigen-specific, because VacA does not protect against challenge with an isogenic strain lacking the *vacA* gene [122]. Moreover, therapeutic vaccination with recombinant VacA plus LTK63 prevents reinfection with the same *H. pylori* strain, providing further proof that this regimen induces antigen-specific immunological memory in vivo [124]. Notably, all these studies used the infecting strain to rechallenge, and protection was defined as failure to cultivate *H. pylori* from the excised stomachs of the mice. While the ability of VacA to induce sterilizing immunity is encouraging, it will be important to confirm these findings using heterologous *H. pylori* challenge strains.

Prophylactic and therapeutic protection has also been observed in mice after oral [122,124] and intranasal (G. Del Giudice, unpublished) immunization with CagA plus LTK63. As in the case of VacA, the full-length CagA molecule achieves high levels of protection, whereas neither the A17/12 fragment (known to contain immunodominant epitopes in humans) [122] nor a fusion protein containing a 65-kDa fragment of CagA [95] protects mice against challenge.

Oral immunization of mice with *H. pylori* NAP, along with LTK63 as adjuvant, also provided excellent prophylactic efficacy [52]. It is possible that neutralization of the chemotactic and proinflammatory properties of this protein interferes with the colonization and/or survival of *H. pylori*.

Several other *H. pylori* antigens have been reported as potential vaccine candidates. The bacterial heat shock proteins, for example, were used to immunize mice as recombinant proteins [83,125], as synthetic peptides [126], and as DNA plasmids [78,79]. Other antigens reported as protective in mice following prophylactic immunization are enzymes such as catalase given mucosally [127] or parenterally [74], and a serine protease given parenterally [74], bacterial adhesins such as AlpA and BabB given parenterally [74], heparan sulphate-binding protein covalently linked with the B subunit of the CT given orally [128], outer membrane proteins such as the Lpp20 [129,130], several Hop proteins [131], and a protein of 26 kDa [132], the L7/L12 ribosomal protein [130], and other proteins that are yet to be characterized [130,133].

For some bacterial infections, such as pertussis, optimal protection is achieved by combining multiple antigens in a vaccine formulation [134]. Given the difficulty in identifying protective *H. pylori* antigens in humans, and the likelihood that broader immunity could be achieved by stimulating immune responses against multiple targets, a multivalent approach has been considered for *H. pylori*. Preclinical assessment of this strategy is limited by the fact that optimum protection is often achieved with a single antigen. Nonetheless, improved protection was reported in mice orally immunized with heat shock proteins plus urease B subunit [83] or with VacA plus urease [122], and with combinations of various antigens plus urease given parenterally [74]. More recently, intramuscular immunization of beagles with VacA, CagA, and NAP (formulated together with aluminum hydroxide) was shown to confer significant protection against *H. pylori* challenge (G. Del Giudice, unpublished). This formulation has now been tested in volunteers [135]. A total of 57 *H. pylori*-negative subjects were immunized intramuscularly, with three doses of each antigen ranging from 10 to 25 μg. The vaccine was very well tolerated and induced strong antigen-specific antibody and lymphocyte proliferation responses.

B. Live Vectors

The experience with subunit vaccines illustrates that, although efficacious mucosal immunizations were achieved in animal models, in which the reactogenic doses of CT or LT adjuvants exceeded the level required for successful adjuvant effect, this has not been the case for humans who are exquisitely sensitive to these bacterial toxins [119,120]. Thus the use of live vectors for mucosal delivery was investigated, first in mouse models and then in volunteers.

Attenuated *Salmonella enterica* strains expressing *H. pylori* antigens have shown promise in murine challenge models. Mice immunized with attenuated $\Delta phoP^c$ or $\Delta aroA$ *S. enterica* serovar Typhimurium strains expressing *H. pylori* urease [136,137] or catalase [138] were protected against challenge with *Helicobacter*. These studies formed the basis for several exploratory clinical trials using *S. enterica* vectors. Disappointing results were obtained from a study using a serovar Typhi vector strain deleted for the virulence regulon *phoP/phoQ* (Ty800) and engineered to constitutively express the urease A and B subunit genes from a stabilized multicopy plasmid. Vaccination of eight volunteers with a single oral dose of $\geq 10^{10}$ CFU of this Ty1033 strain was mildly reactogenic and failed to elicit immune responses to urease, although the mucosal and serum antibody to *Salmonella* antigens were detected [139]. Possible reasons for this lack of immunogenicity include the cell-associated presentation of urease or insufficient antigen production by the vector. A similarly meager immune response was observed in nine volunteers orally inoculated with *S. enterica* serovar Typhi Ty21a expressing *H. pylori* rUrease A and B [140].

A more successful outcome was obtained with a similarly constructed $\Delta phoP/phoQ$ serovar Typhimurium strain LH1160 derived from the wild-type mouse virulent strain ATCC 14028 and engineered to express urease [141]. Six subjects received a single oral dose of vaccine containing 5–8×10^7 CFU. Two subjects experienced unacceptable fever and constitutional symptoms, but none had diarrhea. Three subjects mounted urease-specific IgA ASC responses (measured either by ELISPOT or by soluble immunoglobulin release from PBMC grown in tissue culture to high density), and one subject had an increase in serum antiurease IgG antibody. These results suggest that, despite the same attenuating mutation, plasmid expression system, and expressed antigen, even at a 3-log lower dose, serovar Typhimurium appeared to be a superior vector for engendering immune responses to urease compared with serovar Typhi. Enhanced

plasmid stability and more vigorous intestinal colonization were postulated to explain these differences [141]. Nonetheless, issues that must be considered if LH1160 were to be developed further include tolerability, potential transmission to immunodeficient individuals, and the risk for postinfectious reactive arthritis (that may follow wild-type nontyphoidal *Salmonella* infections).

An alternative strategy was studied by McKenzie and coworkers [142], in which two attenuated strains of *S.* Typhi Ty2, CVD 908 ($\Delta aroC$, $\Delta aroD$) [143], and CVD 908-*htrA* ($\Delta aroC$, $\Delta aroD$, $\Delta htrA$) [144], were engineered to express *H. pylori* urease. In an ascending-dose design, volunteers received two oral inoculations 4 weeks apart. Preliminary reports indicate that the less-attenuated strain ($\Delta aroC$, $\Delta aroD$), at doses of 5×10^7 or 2×10^8, caused adverse reactions in several volunteers. The more attenuated $\Delta aroC$, $\Delta aroD$, $\Delta htrA$ strain at doses of 5×10^8 or 5×10^9 was well tolerated. The stool shedding pattern of the two strains was similar but, most interestingly, the more attenuated strain elicited a better immune response to urease. The high dose of the triple mutant stimulated urease-specific IgG ASCs in 10 of the 12 subjects and fecal IgA in 5 subjects. These trials provide encouraging results that mucosal immunization against *H. pylori* can be achieved in humans, but whether or not these immune responses could lead to protection against disease or infection is not known.

C. Inactivated Whole-Cell Vaccines

Administration of inactivated whole cell preparations (as sonicates, lysates, or formalin-treated cells) is an empiric approach to vaccine development that has the potential to elicit immunity to multiple *H. pylori* antigens. Numerous preclinical studies have shown that both mucosal and parenteral vaccination with whole cell preparations of *H. pylori* or *H. felis*, together with appropriate adjuvant confers protection against challenge with the homologous organism [55,56,82,83,91,122]. Similar formulations were also shown to be an effective therapeutic strategy in mice [87,145] and piglets [69] when given mucosally, but not parenterally [69,145].

Formalin-inactivated whole cell *H. pylori* vaccine coadministered with mutant LT_{R192G} adjuvant was evaluated in Phase 1 studies involving subjects with and without *H. pylori* infection [146]. In a double-blind, randomized fashion, 18 *H. pylori*-infected subjects ingested either 2.5×10^{10} vaccine cells or placebo, plus 25 μg LT_{R192G} or placebo. Diarrhea, low-grade fever, and/or vomiting were observed in ~30% of subjects, usually after the first dose. The diarrhea appeared to be related to receipt of mutant LT, but was augmented by increasing doses of vaccine. Whereas serum antibody responses to the whole-cell antigen were marginal and seen only in *H. pylori*-infected subjects, mucosal (fecal and salivary) IgA responses were stronger and occurred among *H. pylori*-infected and uninfected subjects, but only following inoculation with vaccine plus LT_{R192G}. Some *H. pylori*-negative volunteers developed lymphoproliferative and IFN-γ responses. No subjects were cured of their *H. pylori* infection. These results suggest that it is possible to stimulate mucosal and systemic immune responses in humans to *H.*

pylori antigens using a whole-cell vaccine, but more immunogenic, better-tolerated formulations are required.

VIII. FUTURE DIRECTIONS

To date, the design of most *H. pylori* vaccine candidates submitted to preclinical or clinical evaluation has been based on empirical approaches, as in the case of whole cell preparations, outer membrane vesicles, or antigens representing virulence factors. More recently, the genome sequence of *H. pylori* has been explored. Several hundred genes have been cloned and their products tested in the mouse challenge model, some of which elicited protective immunity when given parenterally with adjuvant [74]. However, the lack of immunological correlates of protection against *H. pylori* limits the possibility to exploit the genomics information fully without having to test each antigen empirically. Much interest has thus turned to analyzing the gene products of the bacterium (proteomics) because of considerable progress in protein separation and biochemical analysis. These bacterial extracts can be reacted with a source of specific antibodies, mainly serum samples from infected patients, to select new potential targets for use in vaccines [147–151]. It is likely that the next generation of vaccines will combine multiple *H. pylori* antigens to produce a multivalent vaccine formulation.

We have reached a critical juncture in which animal systems and molecular techniques have identified numerous protective antigens, but available clinical models cannot effectively discern which of these holds promise. Clearly, formulation and delivery systems must be optimized to overcome the meager immunogenicity elicited by most mucosally delivered candidates subjected to clinical trial thus far. Additional data are needed about the requirements for induction of antigen-specific cell populations, homing of these cells to the gastric mucosa, and the mechanisms involved in effector responses that mediate protection against *H. pylori* following immunization. However, even if immunogenic vaccines were constructed, the appropriate clinical endpoints for evaluating these candidates remain undefined. It is unclear whether a therapeutic vaccine should be required to eradicate infection, reduce bacterial burden, or merely ameliorate gastritis. Even if the latter two choices were deemed acceptable, noninvasive means to measure these outcomes are not available for use in larger Phase 2 and 3 trials. Furthermore, gastric injury is patchy, so it is difficult to accurately quantify bacterial load and inflammatory changes. Strategies for selecting promising prophylactic vaccines are also problematic. One approach is to seek vaccines that demonstrate therapeutic efficacy and assume that similar effector mechanisms are operative in prevention. Alternatively, one could develop constructs that appear immunogenic in Phase 1 and 2 trials. Ultimately, prophylactic efficacy must be evaluated, either in an experimental challenge model, which remains controversial, or in field trial. Again, this would require clarification of reasonable endpoints.

In conclusion, remarkable gains have been made in understanding *H. pylori* infection during the two decades since it was discovered. Nonetheless, further progress in *H. pylori* vaccine development will depend on the discovery of innovative approaches to vaccine design, host immunity, and clinical evaluation.

REFERENCES

1. Institute of Medicine. Vaccines for the 21st Century: A Tool for Decision Making. In: Stratton KR, Durch JS, Lawrence RS, eds. Washington, DC: National Academy Press, 2001: 181–188.
2. Rupnow MF, et al. *Helicobacter pylori* vaccine development and use: a cost-effectiveness analysis using the Institute of Medicine Methodology. Helicobacter 1999; 4:272–280.
3. Rupnow MF, et al. Quantifying the population impact of a prophylactic *Helicobacter pylori* vaccine. Vaccine 2001; 20: 879–885.
4. Go MF, et al. Population genetic analysis of *Helicobacter pylori* by multilocus enzyme electrophoresis: extensive allelic diversity and recombinational population structure. J Bacteriol 1996; 178:3934–3938.
5. Blaser MJ, Berg DE. *Helicobacter pylori* genetic diversity and risk of human disease. J Clin Invest 2001; 107:767–773.
6. Ramirez-Ramos A, et al., for the Gastrointestinal Physiology Working Group of the Universidad Peruana Cayetano Heredia and The Johns Hopkins University, Salazar G, et al. Rapid recurrence of *Helicobacter pylori* infection in Peruvian patients after successful eradication. Clin Infect Dis 1997; 25:1027–1031.
7. Malaty HM, et al. Natural history of *Helicobacter pylori* infection in childhood: 12-year follow-up cohort study in a biracial community. Clin Infect Dis 1999; 28:279–282.
8. Kumagai T, et al. Acquisition versus loss of *Helicobacter pylori* infection in Japan: results from an 8-year birth cohort study. J Infect Dis 1998; 178:717–721.
9. Fox JG, et al. Concurrent enteric helminth infection modulates inflammation and gastric immune responses and reduces Helicobacter-induced gastric atrophy. Nat Med 2000; 6:536–542.
10. Marshall BJ, et al. Attempt to fulfil Koch's postulates for pyloric Campylobacter. Med J Aust 1985; 142:436–439.
11. Morris A, Nicholson G. Ingestion of *Campylobacter pyloridis* causes gastritis and raised fasting gastric pH. Am J Gastroenterol 1987; 82:192–199.
12. Graham DY, et al. H. pylori vaccine development in humans: Challenge model. Developments and New Directions in Helicobacter Research: From the Basic Laboratory to the Patient. 26–27 February, 1999. Orlando, Florida, p. 54.
13. Blaser MJ. Hypothesis: the changing relationships of *Helicobacter pylori* and humans: implications for health and disease. J Infect Dis 1999; 179:1523–1530.
14. Negrini R, et al. Autoantibodies to gastric mucosa in *Helicobacter pylori* infection. Helicobacter 1997; 2(Suppl 1):S13–S16.
15. Eaton KA, et al. Essential role of urease in pathogenesis of gastritis induced by *Helicobacter pylori* in gnotobiotic piglets. Infect Immun 1991; 59:2470–2475.
16. Mobley HL, et al. Molecular biology of microbial ureases. Microbiol Rev 1995; 59:451–480.
17. Scott DR, et al. The role of internal urease in acid resistance of *Helicobacter pylori*. Gastroenterology 1998; 114:58–70.
18. Hawtin PR, et al. Investigation of the structure and localization of the urease of *Helicobacter pylori* using monoclonal antibodies. J Gen Microbiol 1990; 136(Pt 10):1995–2000.
19. Leal-Herrera Y, et al. Serologic IgG response to urease in

Helicobacter pylori-infected persons from Mexico. Am J Trop Med Hyg 1999; 60:587–592.

20. Torres J, et al. Specific serum immunoglobulin G response to urease and CagA antigens of *Helicobacter pylori* in infected children and adults in a country with high prevalence of infection. Clin Diagn Lab Immunol 2002; 9:97–100.

21. D'Elios MM, et al. Different cytokine profile and antigen-specificity repertoire in *Helicobacter pylori*-specific T cell clones from the antrum of chronic gastritis patients with or without peptic ulcer. Eur J Immunol 1997; 27:1751–1755.

22. Ottemann KM, Lowenthal AC. *Helicobacter pylori* uses motility for initial colonization and to attain robust infection. Infect Immun 2002; 70:1984–1990.

23. Dytoc M, et al. Comparison of *Helicobacter pylori* and attaching-effacing *Escherichia coli* adhesion to eukaryotic cells. Infect Immun 1993; 61:448–456.

24. Ilver D, et al. *Helicobacter pylori* adhesin binding fucosylated histo-blood group antigens revealed by retagging. Science 1998; 279:373–377.

25. Jones AC, et al. A flagellar sheath protein of *Helicobacter pylori* is identical to HpaA, a putative *N*-acetylneuraminyl-lactose-binding hemagglutinin, but is not an adhesin for AGS cells. J Bacteriol 1997; 179:5643–5647.

26. Censini S, et al. cag, a pathogenicity island of *Helicobacter pylori*, encodes type I-specific and disease-associated virulence factors. Proc Natl Acad Sci USA 1996; 93:14648–14653.

27. Webb PM, et al. Gastric cancer, cytotoxin-associated gene A-positive *Helicobacter pylori*, and serum pepsinogens: an international study. The Eurogst Study Group. Gastroenterology 1999; 116:269–276.

28. Covacci A, Rappuoli R. Tyrosine-phosphorylated bacterial proteins: Trojan horses for the host cell. J Exp Med 2000; 191:587–592.

29. Stein M, et al. c-Src/Lyn kinases activate *Helicobacter pylori* CagA through tyrosine phosphorylation of the EPIYA motifs. Mol Microbiol 2002; 43:971–980.

30. Higashi H, et al. SHP-2 tyrosine phosphatase as an intracellular target of *Helicobacter pylori* CagA protein. Science 2002; 295:683–686.

31. Crabtree JE, et al. Induction of interleukin-8 secretion from gastric epithelial cells by a cagA negative isogenic mutant of *Helicobacter pylori*. J Clin Pathol 1995; 48:967–969.

32. Ogura K, et al. Virulence factors of *Helicobacter pylori* responsible for gastric diseases in Mongolian gerbil. J Exp Med 2000; 192:1601–1610.

33. Parsonnet J, et al. Risk for gastric cancer in people with CagA positive or CagA negative *Helicobacter pylori* infection. Gut 1997; 40:297–301.

34. Hamlet A, et al. Duodenal *Helicobacter pylori* infection differs in cagA genotype between asymptomatic subjects and patients with duodenal ulcers. Gastroenterol 1999; 116:259–268.

35. Crabtree JE, et al. Mucosal IgA recognition of *Helicobacter pylori* 120 kDa protein, peptic ulceration, and gastric pathology. Lancet 1991; 338:332–335.

36. Go MF, Graham DY. Presence of the cagA gene in the majority of *Helicobacter pylori* strains is independent of whether the individual has duodenal ulcer or asymptomatic gastritis. Helicobacter 1996; 1:107–111.

37. Owen RJ, et al. Conservation of the cytotoxin-associated (cagA) gene of *Helicobacter pylori* and investigation of association with vacuolating-cytotoxin activity and gastroduodenal disease. FEMS Immunol Med Microbiol 1994; 9:307–315.

38. van der Ende A, et al. Heterogeneous *Helicobacter pylori* isolates from members of a family with a history of peptic ulcer disease. Gastroenterol 1996; 111:638–647.

39. Xiang Z, et al. Analysis of expression of CagA and VacA virulence factors in 43 strains of *Helicobacter pylori* reveals that clinical isolates can be divided into two major types and that CagA is not necessary for expression of the vacuolating cytotoxin. Infect Immun 1995; 63:94–98.

40. van Doorn LJ, et al. Geographic distribution of vacA allelic types of *Helicobacter pylori*. Gastroenterology 1999; 116:823–830.

41. Reyrat JM, et al. Towards deciphering the *Helicobacter pylori* cytotoxin. Mol Microbiol 1999; 34:197–204.

42. Telford JL, et al. Gene structure of the *Helicobacter pylori* cytotoxin and evidence of its key role in gastric disease. J Exp Med 1994; 179:1653–1658.

43. Sommi P, et al. Significance of ammonia in the genesis of gastric epithelial lesions induced by *Helicobacter pylori*: an in vitro study with different bacterial strains and urea concentrations. Digestion 1996; 57:299–304.

44. Czajkowsky DM, et al. The vacuolating toxin from *Helicobacter pylori* forms hexameric pores in lipid bilayers at low pH. Proc Natl Acad Sci USA 1999; 96:2001–2006.

45. Ricci V, et al. *Helicobacter pylori* vacuolating toxin accumulates within the endosomal–vacuolar compartment of cultured gastric cells and potentiates the vacuolating activity of ammonia. J Pathol 1997; 183:453–459.

46. Galmiche A, et al. The N-terminal 34 kDa fragment of *Helicobacter pylori* vacuolating cytotoxin targets mitochondria and induces cytochrome c release. EMBO J 2000; 19:6361–6370.

47. Papini E, et al. Selective increase of the permeability of polarized epithelial cell monolayers by *Helicobacter pylori* vacuolating toxin. J Clin Invest 1998; 102:813–820.

48. Molinari M, et al. Selective inhibition of Ii-dependent antigen presentation by *Helicobacter pylori* toxin VacA. J Exp Med 1998; 187:135–140.

49. Shirai M, et al. Persistent infection by *Helicobacter pylori* down-modulates virus-specific CD8$^+$ cytotoxic T cell response and prolongs viral infection. J Infect Dis 1998; 177:72–80.

50. Evans DJ Jr, et al. Characterization of a *Helicobacter pylori* neutrophil-activating protein. Infect Immun 1995; 63:2213–2220.

51. Tonello F, et al. The *Helicobacter pylori* neutrophil-activating protein is an iron- binding protein with dodecameric structure. Mol Microbiol 1999; 34:238–246.

52. Satin B, et al. The neutrophil-activating protein (HP-NAP) of *Helicobacter pylori* is a protective antigen and a major virulence factor. J Exp Med 2000; 191:1467–1476.

53. Montemurro P, et al. The neutrophil-activating protein (HP-NAP) of *Helicobacter pylori* is a potent stimulant of mast cells. Eur J Immunol 2002; 32:671–676.

54. Montemurro P, et al. *Helicobacter pylori* neutrophil-activating protein stimulates tissue factor and plasminogen activator inhibitor-2 production by human blood mononuclear cells. J Infect Dis 2001; 183:1055–1062.

55. Czinn SJ, et al. Protection of germ-free mice from infection by *Helicobacter felis* after active oral or passive IgA immunization. Vaccine 1993; 11:637–642.

56. Lee CK, et al. Oral immunization with recombinant *Helicobacter pylori* urease induces secretory IgA antibodies and protects mice from challenge with *Helicobacter felis*. J Infect Dis 1995; 172:161–172.

57. Weltzin R, et al. Novel intranasal immunization techniques for antibody induction and protection of mice against gastric *Helicobacter felis* infection. Vaccine 1997; 15:370–376.

58. Ermak TH, et al. Immunization of mice with urease vaccine affords protection against *Helicobacter pylori* infection in the absence of antibodies and is mediated by MHC class II-restricted responses. J Exp Med 1998; 188:2277–2288.

59. Blanchard TG, et al. Antibody-independent protective mucosal immunity to gastric Helicobacter infection in mice. Cell Immunol 1999; 191:74–80.

60. Bogstedt AK, et al. *Helicobacter pylori* infections in IgA deficiency: lack of role for the secretory immune system. Clin Exp Immunol 1996; 105:202–204.

61. Pappo J, et al. *Helicobacter pylori* infection in immunized mice lacking major histocompatibility complex class I and class II functions. Infect Immun 1999; 67:337–341.

62. Mohammadi M, et al. Murine CD4 T-cell response to Helicobacter infection: TH1 cells enhance gastritis and TH2 cells reduce bacterial load. Gastroenterology 1997; 113:1848–1857.

63. Lucas B, et al. Adoptive transfer of CD4$^+$ T cells specific for subunit A of *Helicobacter pylori* urease reduces *H. pylori* stomach colonization in mice in the absence of interleukin-4 (IL-4)/IL-13 receptor signaling. Infect Immun 2001; 69:1714–1721.

64. Gottwein JM, et al. Protective anti-Helicobacter immunity is induced with aluminum hydroxide or complete Freund's adjuvant by systemic immunization. J Infect Dis 2001; 184:308–331.

65. Sawai N, et al. Role of gamma interferon in *Helicobacter pylori*-induced gastric inflammatory responses in a mouse model. Infect Immun 1999; 67:279–285.

66. Eaton KA, et al. The role of T cell subsets and cytokines in the pathogenesis of *Helicobacter pylori* gastritis in mice. J Immunol 2001; 166:7456–7461.

67. Mohammadi M, et al. Helicobacter-specific cell-mediated immune responses display a predominant Th1 phenotype and promote a delayed-type hypersensitivity response in the stomachs of mice. J Immunol 1996; 156:4729–4738.

68. Del Giudice G, et al. The design of vaccines against *Helicobacter pylori* and their development. Annu Rev Immunol 2001; 19:523–563.

69. Eaton KA, et al. Vaccination of gnotobiotic piglets against *Helicobacter pylori*. J Infect Dis 1998; 178:1399–1405.

70. Guy B, Hessler C, et al. Systemic immunization with urease protects mice against *Helicobacter pylori* infection. Vaccine 1998; 16:850–856.

71. Guy B, Hessler C, et al. Comparison between targeted and untargeted systemic immunizations with adjuvanted urease to cure *Helicobacter pylori* infection in mice. Vaccine 1999; 17: 1130–1135.

72. Lee CK, et al. Immunization with recombinant *Helicobacter pylori* urease decreases colonization levels following experimental infection of rhesus monkeys. Vaccine 1999; 17:1493–1505.

73. Solnick JV, et al. Immunization with recombinant *Helicobacter pylori* urease in specific-pathogen-free rhesus monkeys (*Macaca mulatta*). Infect Immun 2000; 68:2560–2565.

74. Sanchez V, et al. Formulations of single or multiple *H. pylori* antigens with DC Chol adjuvant induce protection by the systemic route in mice. Optimal prophylactic combinations are different from therapeutic ones. FEMS Immunol Med Microbiol 2001; 30:157–165.

75. Guy B, et al. Mucosal, systemic, or combined therapeutic immunization in cynomolgus monkeys naturally infected with *Gastrospirillum hominis*-like organisms. Vaccine Res 1997; 6:141–150.

76. Weltzin R, et al. Parenteral adjuvant activities of *Escherichia coli* heat-labile toxin and its B subunit for immunization of mice against gastric *Helicobacter pylori* infection. Infect Immun 2000; 68:2775–2782.

77. Lee CK, et al. Immunization of rhesus monkeys with a mucosal prime, parenteral boost strategy protects against infection with *Helicobacter pylori*. Vaccine 1999; 17:3072–3082.

78. Todoroki I, et al. Suppressive effects of DNA vaccines encoding heat shock protein on *Helicobacter pylori*-induced gastritis in mice. Biochem Biophys Res Commun 2000; 277:159–163.

79. Miyashita M, et al. Immune responses in mice to intranasal and intracutaneous administration of a DNA vaccine encoding *Helicobacter pylori*-catalase. Vaccine 2002; 20:2336–2342.

80. Lee A, et al. A small animal model of human *Helicobacter pylori* active chronic gastritis. Gastroenterology 1990; 99:1315–1323.

81. Fox JG, et al. Local and systemic immune responses in murine *Helicobacter felis* active chronic gastritis. Infect Immun 1993; 61:2309–2315.

82. Chen M, et al. Immunisation against gastric helicobacter infection in a mouse/*Helicobacter felis* model [letter]. Lancet 1992; 339:1120–1121.

83. Ferrero RL, et al. The GroES homolog of *Helicobacter pylori* confers protective immunity against mucosal infection in mice. Proc Natl Acad Sci USA 1995; 92:6499–6503.

84. Ferrero RL, et al. Recombinant antigens prepared from the urease subunits of *Helicobacter* spp.: evidence of protection in a mouse model of gastric infection. Infect Immun 1994; 62:4981–4989.

85. Michetti P, et al. Immunization of BALB/c mice against *Helicobacter felis* infection with *Helicobacter pylori* urease. Gastroenterology 1994; 107:1002–1011.

86. Corthesy-Theulaz I, et al. Oral immunization with *Helicobacter pylori* urease B subunit as a treatment against Helicobacter infection in mice. Gastroenterology 1995; 109:115–121.

87. Doidge C, et al. Therapeutic immunisation against Helicobacter infection. Lancet 1994; 343:914–915.

88. Saldinger PF, et al. Immunization of BALB/c mice with Helicobacter urease B induces a T helper 2 response absent in Helicobacter infection. Gastroenterology 1998; 115:891–897.

89. Ermak TH, et al. Gastritis in urease-immunized mice after *Helicobacter felis* challenge may be due to residual bacteria. Gastroenterology 1997; 113:1118–1128.

90. Karita M, et al. New small animal model for human gastric *Helicobacter pylori* infection: success in both nude and euthymic mice. Am J Gastroenterol 1991; 86:1596–1603.

91. Marchetti M, et al. Development of a mouse model of *Helicobacter pylori* infection that mimics human disease. Science 1995; 267:1655–1658.

92. Lee A, et al. A standardized mouse model of *Helicobacter pylori* infection: introducing the Sydney strain. Gastroenterology 1997; 112:1386–1397.

93. Kleanthous H, et al. Oral immunization with recombinant *Helicobacter pylori* urease apoenzyme in the treatment of Helicobacter infection. Gut 1995; 37:A94.

94. Handt LK, et al. Evaluation of two commercial serologic tests for the diagnosis of *Helicobacter pylori* infection in the rhesus monkey. Lab Anim Sci 1995; 45, 613–617.

95. Kleanthous H, et al. Sterilizing immunity against experimental *Helicobacter pylori* infection is challenge-strain dependent. Vaccine 2001; 19:4883–4895.

96. van Doorn NE, et al. *Helicobacter pylori*-associated gastritis in mice is host and strain specific. Infect Immun 1999; 67:3040–3046.

97. Ferrero RL, et al. Immune responses of specific-pathogen-free mice to chronic *Helicobacter pylori* (strain SS1) infection. Infect Immun 1998; 66:1349–1355.

98. Kleanthous H, et al. Rectal and intranasal immunizations with recombinant urease induce distinct local and serum immune responses in mice and protect against *Helicobacter pylori* infection. Infect Immun 1998; 66:2879–2886.

99. Fox JG, et al. *Helicobacter mustelae*-associated gastritis in ferrets. An animal model of *Helicobacter pylori* gastritis in humans. Gastroenterology 1990; 99:352–361.

100. Fox JG, et al. *Helicobacter mustelae*-associated gastric adenocarcinoma in ferrets (*Mustela putorius furo*). Vet Pathol 1997; 34:225–229.

101. Cuenca R, et al. Therapeutic immunization against *Helicobacter mustelae* in naturally infected ferrets. Gastroenterology 1996; 110:1770–1775.

102. Batchelder M, et al. Natural and experimental *Helicobacter mustelae* reinfection following successful antimicrobial eradication in ferrets. Helicobacter 1996; 1:34–42.

103. Fox JG, et al. *Helicobacter pylori*-induced gastritis in the domestic cat. Infect Immun 1995; 63:2674–2681.

104. Batchelder M, et al. Oral vaccination with recombinant urease reduces gastric *Helicobacter pylori* colonization in the cat. Meeting of the American Gastroenterology Association, May 19–22, San Francisco, CA, 1996.

105. Dubois A, et al. Immunization against natural *Helicobacter pylori* infection in nonhuman primates. Infect Immun 1998; 66:4340–4346.

106. Baskerville A, Newell DG. Naturally occurring chronic gastritis and *C. pylori* infection in the rhesus monkey: a potential model for gastritis in man. Gut 1988; 29:465–472.

107. Krakowka S, et al. Establishment of gastric *Campylobacter pylori* infection in the neonatal gnotobiotic piglet. Infect Immun 1987; 55:2789–2796.

108. Krakowka S, et al. Manifestations of the local gastric immune response in gnotobiotic piglets infected with *Helicobacter pylori*. Vet Immunol Immunopathol 1996; 52:159–173.

109. Eaton KA, et al. Persistence of *Helicobacter pylori* in conventionalized piglets. J Infect Dis 1990; 161:1299–1301.

110. Eaton KA, Krakowka S. Chronic active gastritis due to *Helicobacter pylori* in immunized gnotobiotic piglets. Gastroenterol 1992; 103:1580–1586.

111. Rossi G, et al. A conventional beagle dog model for acute and chronic infection with *Helicobacter pylori*. Infect Immun 1999; 67:3112–3120.

112. Rossi G, et al. Immunohistochemical study of lymphocyte populations infiltrating the gastric mucosa of beagle dogs experimentally infected with *Helicobacter pylori*. Infect Immun 2000; 68:4769–4772.

113. Honda S, et al. Gastric ulcer, atrophic gastritis, and intestinal metaplasia caused by *Helicobacter pylori* infection in Mongolian gerbils. Scand J Gastroenterol 1998; 33:454–460.

114. Hirayama F, et al. Induction of gastric ulcer and intestinal metaplasia in mongolian gerbils infected with *Helicobacter pylori*. J Gastroenterol 1996; 31:755–757.

115. Watanabe T, et al. *Helicobacter pylori* infection induces gastric cancer in mongolian gerbils. Gastroenterology 1998; 115:642–648.

116. Hu LT, et al. Purification of recombinant *Helicobacter pylori* urease apoenzyme encoded by ureA and ureB. Infect Immun 1992; 60:2657–2666.

117. Austin JW, et al. Macromolecular structure and aggregation states of *Helicobacter pylori* urease. J Bacteriol 1991; 173:5663–5667.

118. Kreiss C, et al. Safety of oral immunisation with recombinant urease in patients with *Helicobacter pylori* infection [letter]. Lancet 1996; 347:1630–1631.

119. Michetti P, et al. Oral immunization with urease and *Escherichia coli* heat-labile enterotoxin is safe and immunogenic in *Helicobacter pylori*-infected adults. Gastroenterology 1999; 116:804–812.

120. Banerjee S, et al. Low dose *E. coli* enterotoxin for urease-based oral immunization against *H. pylori* in healthy volunteers: can it be safe and effective? Gastroenterology 2000; 118:A172.

121. Sougioultzis S, et al. Safety and efficacy of *E. coli* enterotoxin adjuvant for urease-based rectal immunization against *H pylori*. Gastroenterology 2002; 122:A427.

122. Marchetti M, et al. Protection against *Helicobacter pylori* infection in mice by intragastric vaccination with *H pylori*

123. Manetti R, et al. Detoxification of the *Helicobacter pylori* cytotoxin. Infect Immun 1997; 65:4615–4619.

124. Ghiara P, et al. Therapeutic intragastric vaccination against *Helicobacter pylori* in mice eradicates an otherwise chronic infection and confers protection against reinfection. Infect Immun 1997; 65:4996–5002.

125. Ferrero RL, et al. Local immunoglobulin G antibodies in the stomach may contribute to immunity against Helicobacter infection in mice. Gastroenterology 1997; 113:185–194.

126. Yamaguchi H, et al. Immune response against a cross-reactive epitope on the heat shock protein 60 homologue of *Helicobacter pylori*. Infect Immun 2000; 68:3448–3454.

127. Radcliff FJ, et al. Catalase, a novel antigen for *Helicobacter pylori* vaccination. Infect Immun 1997; 65:4668–4674.

128. Ruiz-Bustos E, et al. Protection of BALB/c mice against experimental *Helicobacter pylori* infection by oral immunisation with *H. pylori* heparan sulphate-binding proteins coupled to cholera toxin beta-subunit. J Med Microbiol 2000; 49:535–541.

129. Keenan J, et al. Immune response to an 18-kilodalton outer membrane antigen identifies lipoprotein 20 as a *Helicobacter pylori* vaccine candidate. Infect Immun 2000; 68:3337–3343.

130. Hocking D, et al. Isolation of recombinant protective *Helicobacter pylori* antigens. Infect Immun 1999; 67:4713–4719.

131. Peck B, et al. Characterization of four members of a multigene family encoding outer membrane proteins of *Helicobacter pylori* and their potential for vaccination. Microbes Infect 2001; 3:171–179.

132. Jiang Z, et al. A study of recombinant protective *H pylori* antigens. World J Gastroenterol 2002; 8:308–311.

133. Dunkley ML, et al. Protection against *Helicobacter pylori* infection by intestinal immunisation with a 50/52-kDa subunit protein. FEMS Immunol Med Microbiol 1999; 24:221–225.

134. Rappuoli R. Rational design of vaccines. Nat Med 1997; 3:374–376.

135. Malfertheiner P, et al. Phase I safety and immunogenicity of a three-component *H. pylori* vaccine. Gastroenterology 2002; 122(suppl):A585.

136. Corthesy-Theulaz IE, et al. Mice are protected from *Helicobacter pylori* infection by nasal immunization with attenuated *Salmonella typhimurium* phoPc expressing urease A and B subunits. Infect Immun 1998; 66:581–586.

137. Gomez-Duarte OG, et al. Protection of mice against gastric colonization by *Helicobacter pylori* by single oral dose immunization with attenuated *Salmonella typhimurium* producing urease subunits A and B. Vaccine 1998; 16:460–471.

138. Liao W, et al. Construction of attenuated *Salmonella typhimurium* vaccine strain expressing *Helicobacter pylori* catalase and observation on its protective immunity. Zhonghua Yi Xue Za Zhi 2001; 81:613–616.

139. DiPetrillo MD, et al. Safety and immunogenicity of phoP/phoQ-deleted *Salmonella typhi* expressing *Helicobacter pylori* urease in adult volunteers. Vaccine 1999; 18:449–459.

140. Bumann D, et al. Safety and immunogenicity of live recombinant *Salmonella enterica* serovar Typhi Ty21a expressing urease A and B from *Helicobacter pylori* in human volunteers. Vaccine 2001; 20:845–852.

141. Angelakopoulos H, Hohmann EL. Pilot study of phoP/phoQ-deleted *Salmonella enterica* serovar typhimurium expressing *Helicobacter pylori* urease in adult volunteers. Infect Immun 2000; 68:2135–2141.

142. McKenzie R, et al. A phase I study of the safety and immunogenicity of two attenuated *Salmonella typhi* vectors expressing the urease vaccine antigen of *H pylori*. 102nd Annual Meeting of the American Society of Microbiology, May 19–23, Salt Lake City, Utah, 2002.

antigens is achieved using a non-toxic mutant of *E. coli* heat-labile enterotoxin (LT) as adjuvant. Vaccine 1998;1633–37.

143. Hone DM, et al. Construction of genetically-defined double aro mutants of *Salmonella typhi*. Vaccine 1991; 9:810–816.

144. Galen JE, et al. Optimization of plasmid maintenance in the attenuated live vector vaccine strain *Salmonella typhi* CVD 908-htrA. Infect Immun 1999; 67:6424–6433.

145. Ikewaki J, et al. Therapeutic oral vaccination induces mucosal immune response sufficient to eliminate long-term *Helicobacter pylori* infection. Microbiol Immunol 2000; 44:29–39.

146. Kotloff KL, et al. Safety and immunogenicity of oral inactivated whole-cell *Helicobacter pylori* vaccine with adjuvant among volunteers with or without subclinical infection. Infect Immun 2001; 69:3581–3590.

147. McAtee CP, et al. Identification of potential diagnostic and vaccine candidates of *Helicobacter pylori* by "proteome" technologies. Helicobacter 1998; 3:163–169.

148. McAtee CP, et al. Identification of potential diagnostic and vaccine candidates of *Helicobacter pylori* by two-dimensional gel electrophoresis, sequence analysis, and serum profiling. Clin Diagn Lab Immunol 1998; 5:537–542.

149. Nilsson CL, et al. Identification of protein vaccine candidates from *Helicobacter pylori* using a preparative two-dimensional electrophoretic procedure and mass spectrometry. Anal Chem 2000; 72:2148–2153.

150. Kimmel B, et al. Identification of immunodominant antigens from *Helicobacter pylori* and evaluation of their reactivities with sera from patients with different gastroduodenal pathologies. Infect Immun 2000; 68:915–920.

151. Haas G, et al. Immunoproteomics of *Helicobacter pylori* infection and relation to gastric disease. Proteomics 2002; 2:313–324.

66

Vaccines for *Staphylococcus aureus* Infections

Ali I. Fattom, Gary Horwith, and Robert Naso

W. W. Karakawa Microbial Pathogenesis Laboratory, Nabi Biopharmaceuticals, Rockville, Maryland, U.S.A.

I. INTRODUCTION

Staphylococci are commensal bacteria of the anterior nares, skin, and the gastrointestinal tract of humans that rarely cause systemic infections in otherwise healthy individuals, and therefore are considered opportunistic pathogens. Through various mechanisms, adult humans and animals attain an innate but incomplete natural protection from staphylococcal infections. Partial protection is afforded by mucosal and epidermal barriers, in addition to possible immunological mechanisms that impart resistance. Interruption of these natural barriers as a result of immunosuppressive diseases or therapies, or injuries such as burns, traumas, or surgical procedures involving indwelling medical devices, increases the risk for staphylococcal infections [1,2]. Nasal carriage of *Staphylococcus aureus* is reportedly one of the major risk factors for surgical wound infections after surgery, and for infections of the vascular access site in hemodialysis patients [3–5]. It is estimated that staphylococcal infections account for >50% of all hospital-acquired infections. *S. aureus* alone is responsible for 15–25% of such infections and is surpassed only by *S. epidermidis*, which reportedly accounts for as many as 35% of these infections [6–12]. Staphylococcal infections, especially those caused by *S. aureus*, are associated with high morbidity and mortality [13,14].

II. PATHOGENESIS

S. aureus produces a wide range of extracellular enzymes and toxins that play a significant role in pathogenesis. Enzymes such as hyalurodinase, coagulase, and fibrinolysin, among others, facilitate the establishment of *S. aureus* infections and dissemination of the microorganisms. Toxins produced by *S. aureus* isolates have a wide range of activities that compromise the host's resistance. *S. aureus* include enterotoxins that are responsible for food poisoning; exfoliative exotoxin causes intraepidermal splitting of tissues and necrosis; hemolysins alpha through delta, and toxic shock syndrome toxin-1 cause rash, fever, and, in extreme cases, shock

[15–18]. In addition, *S. aureus* produces extracellular proteins responsible for destroying human polymorphonuclear leukocytes (PMNs), thus, compromising opsonophagocytosis, the mechanism that is believed to play a major role in clearance of staphylococci from infected tissues [19]. *S. aureus* is also a major cause of infections associated with indwelling medical devices such as catheters and orthopedic devices [20]. Multiple surface proteins that play an important role as receptors for plasma proteins, glycoproteins, and tissue matrices, enhance the adherence of *S. aureus* to medical devices and facilitate the initiation of infection [21]. *S. aureus* also produces extracellular and cell-associated enzymes, such as coagulase and clumping factor, that enhance survival of the microorganism and establishment of infection [22]. In addition, *S. aureus* possesses other surface antigens that facilitate its survival in the bloodstream by helping the bacteria evade phagocytic killing by host leukocytes. These surface antigens include cell wall components such as teichoic acid, protein A, and capsular polysaccharides (CPs) [6,7,23–25]. Due in part to the versatility of these bacteria and their ability to produce extracellular products that enhance infectivity and pathogenesis, staphylococcal bacteremia (and its complications such as endocarditis, septic arthritis, and osteomyelitis) continue to be serious and frequently observed nosocomial infections [26,27]. While neutralizing staphylococcal extracellular toxins or blocking adherence of *S. aureus* to medical devices by antibodies may reduce virulence and confer protection against the specific indication [21,28], clearance of the bacteria from the body and elimination of the infectious locus remain the underlining mechanisms of protection against *S. aureus* infections [20,29,30].

The introduction, in the 1940s, of penicillin G temporarily solved the problem of staphylococcal infections. However, by 1948, the prevalence of penicillin-resistant strains had seriously reduced the value of this antibiotic in treating serious staphylococcal infections [31]. By the late 1950s, *S. aureus* clinical isolates had acquired resistance to virtually all the systemic antibiotics then in use, including penicillin, erythromycin, streptomycin, and the tetracyclines. These resistant strains, especially phage type 80/81, caused a global pandemic and were isolated from nosocomial infections in hospitals around the world. The introduction of the semisynthetic penicillins, methicillin and oxacillin, was considered a giant step toward controlling multiresistant *S. aureus* infections, and again temporarily brought *S. aureus* infections back under control [32]. Shortly after the introduction of these semisynthetic agents, however, strains of methicillin-resistant *S. aureus* (MRSA) were isolated in England (in 1961) and, by 1965, these isolates were common in Europe. In 1968, the first outbreak of MRSA in the United States was reported in Boston, MA [33]. Currently, methicillin resistance among staphylococci isolates from nosocomial infections continues to increase in frequency, and resistant *S. aureus* strains continue to cause epidemics in hospitals in spite of developed preventive procedures and extensive research into bacterial epidemiology and antibiotic development [34,35].

While the initial efficiency and efficacy of these antibiotic agents in treating and curing staphylococcal infections has drawn attention away from the development of immunological approaches for dealing with these infections, the emergence of multiple-antibiotic-resistant strains of *S. aureus* has now reduced the options for treatment to virtually one antibiotic, vancomycin. This, in combination with the emergence of vancomycin-resistant enterococci (that in laboratory experiments can transfer vancomycin resistance to *S. aureus*), and of *S. aureus* with reduced sensitivity to vancomycin, has renewed the interest in alternative strategies to prevent and treat *S. aureus* infections [36–39].

III. PREVIOUS EXPERIENCE WITH *S. AUREUS* VIRULENCE AND VACCINES

The late 1950s and early 1960s witnessed vigorous research activities into *S. aureus* virulence, pathogenesis, and the development of vaccines for treatment and prevention of staphylococcal infections. Two experimental vaccines were produced and tested in human trials. The first was comprised of a phage lysate of virulent *S. aureus* isolates belonging to phage groups I and III. This vaccine was evaluated in treatment and cure of severe staphylococcal skin infections in humans. Of 607 patients immunized with this vaccine, 80% reportedly recovered from their infections, which included furunculosis, pustular acne, and eczema, among others [40]. However, this trial was neither randomized nor placebo controlled. A subsequent placebo-controlled study with a similar phage lysate vaccine, comprised of phage group I and Cowan 1 strain *S. aureus*, showed no significant improvement in the number, size, or frequency of furunculosis lesions [41]. Another vaccine containing polyvalent somatic antigens, produced by enzymatic treatment of *S. aureus* clinical isolates representing the four major phage groups, protected immunized animals against intradermal challenge with a variety of clinical *S. aureus* isolates [42,43]. In a clinical trial to treat and prevent impetigo in Native Americans, the vaccine showed a significant curative efficacy for 4 months following two injections of the vaccine [44]. These data appeared to confirm protection results obtained in a previous study with this vaccine [45]. Examination of the

vaccine phage types used in these vaccines as listed by these authors, using data published by Sompolinsky et al. [46] on phage types and the corresponding capsular types, revealed that the polyvalent lysate or the somatic antigens vaccine used in these studies were basically comprised of *S. aureus* strains representative of CP type 5 (phage group III), type 8 (phage group I), and so-called nontypeables (other groups). Observations from these studies testify to a possible role of capsular polysaccharides in the protective activities: (1) the only failed vaccine was that comprised of Group I (CP 8) and the noncapsulated strain Cowan 1 [41], (2) a group-specific protection was observed in the potency test for the release of the polyvalent somatic antigen vaccine, and (3) protection was achieved following one or more rounds of immunization, and was associated with rise of agglutinins in immunized animals [42,43], indicating that the observed protection was mediated by antibodies generated in response to vaccination with these antigens. These preliminary encouraging data were not enough to counter the prevailing opinion among staphylococcal researchers that protective immunity against staphylococcal infections was not a valid approach and led to the conclusion that the immune-based approach to combat staphylococcal infections "has gone as far as it can go" [47].

IV. CAPSULAR POLYSACCHARIDES OF *S. AUREUS* CLINICAL ISOLATES

A renewed interest in staphylococcal immunology was generated by the work of Karakawa and colleagues in the early 1980s, who showed that *S. aureus* isolates associated with bacteremia and other systemic infections possessed CP [48–50]. To date, at least 13 serologically different *S. aureus* capsular types have been found among human and animal infection isolates [51–53]. Surveillance of *S. aureus* infection isolates from the United States and Europe by various laboratories, using Karakawa's serological typing scheme, showed that of the 13 known capsular types, types 5 and 8 comprised >80% of the isolates [50]. Data from several surveillance studies over the last few years have shown that these two types and their variants comprise >90% of all clinical isolates in certain patient populations.

The chemical composition of CP types 5 and 8 is nearly identical. Both are polymers composed of *N*-acetyl-aminouronic acid and *N*-acetyl-fucosamine in a 1:2 ratio but differ in the glycosidic linkages and the site of O-acetylation [23, 54,55]. Despite the similarities, however, no demonstrable immunological cross-reactivity between the two capsular types is found. The subunit structure of these CP molecules is shown below:

Type 5
    →4)-β-D-Man*p*NAcA3Ac-(1→4)-α-L-Fuc*p*NAc
      -(1→3)-β-D-Fuc*p*NAc-(1→

Type 8
    →3)-β-D-Man*p*NAcA4Ac-(1→3)-α-L-Fuc*p*NAc
      -(1→3)-β-D-Fuc*p*NAc-(1→

In vitro studies show that polyclonal and monoclonal antibodies elicited against these CP are biologically active and mediate opsonophagocytic killing of the type-specific bacteria by human PMNs [56]; in this respect, the CP of *S. aureus* are no different from the capsules of other bacterial pathogens [57–60] and, as such, *S. aureus* CP may play a role in protective immunity and serve as vaccine candidates.

V. CONJUGATE VACCINES

A. Rationale and Evaluation in Animals

Bacterial CPs are generally poor immunogens, and their immunogenicity in humans is known to be related to their molecular size and the age of the vaccinee. Infants and toddlers below the age of 2 years, the elderly, and immuno-compromised patients are poor responders to CP vaccines [61,62]. CP vaccines are T-cell independent and they induce humoral antibodies with no boost upon reinjection. Compared to other polysaccharides vaccines used in humans, types 5 and 8 CP are of low molecular size, ~50,000 Da, and as such, they are expected to be poor immunogens in humans, especially in immunocompromised populations with reduced resistance.

Since immunization with a *S. aureus* vaccine would be intended for certain at-risk patients, such as those on chemotherapy, hemodialysis patients, infants, shock-trauma patients, surgical patients, and others with reduced resistance or partially compromised immune systems, we embarked on the development of capsular polysaccharide-conjugate vaccines, a strategy already proven to enhance the immunogenicity of other CP-based vaccines. Conjugation of polysaccharides to protein carriers makes bacterial CP antigens T-cell-dependent immunogens, thus increasing their immunogenicity and potentiating their use in infants and immunocompromised patients [63–67]. The two clinically significant CP types, 5 and 8, were conjugated to a nontoxic, recombinant exoprotein A from *Pseudomonas aeruginosa* (rEPA). The immunogenicity of the two CP and their conjugates was evaluated in mice. While the nonconjugated CP were not immunogenic, the conjugates were highly immunogenic and acquired T-cell-dependent properties such as booster response and carrier priming. CP conjugate vaccines elicited antibodies shown to be biologically active in vitro and mediated the opsonophagocytosis and killing of bacteria of homologous serotype by human PMNs [68,69].

B. Evaluation in Humans

S. aureus type 5 and 8 CP-conjugate vaccines have now been evaluated for their safety and immunogenicity in healthy adult volunteers [70]. In the initial studies, vaccinees received, via intramuscular injection, either type 5 or type 8 CP–rEPA conjugates at a nominal dose of 25 μg CP in 0.5 mL phosphate-buffered saline. A second dose of CP conjugates was administered 6 weeks following the first injection. No serious local or systemic reactions were recorded following the first or second injection. However, most of the volunteers experienced a slight tenderness and erythema after the second injection. These reactions were generally mild and disappeared within 48 hr of the injection. Two volunteers experienced a slight transient elevation in their liver

enzymes for 5 days following the initial injection, but there was no elevation in liver enzymes in any of the volunteers following the second injection.

During the clinical trials described above, it was noted that most volunteers had preimmunization antibodies to type 5 and type 8 CP; their geometric mean IgG antibody titers were in the 5–10 μg/mL range. All volunteers in both groups responded to immunization with greater than fourfold increase in IgG antibody levels. Maximum antibody levels were reached by 6 weeks after the first immunization with a geometric mean rise in antibody titer over preimmunization levels of 35-fold for type 5 and 10-fold for type 8. A significant rise in titer was observed for IgM class antibodies as well. As shown with other conjugate vaccines, the second injection did not stimulate a booster response. This was attributed to the fact that adult humans are already primed to these antigens. Therefore, the immune response following the first immunization is considered a booster [64,71]. The conjugate-induced antibodies were mostly of IgG1 and IgG2 subclasses and the antibodies mediated opsonophagocytic killing of the appropriate CP type *S. aureus* by human PMNs. A decrease in type 5 and type 8 antibody levels was observed in the immunized volunteers by 6 months post-immunization (14–20% and 9%, respectively).

Ultimately, bivalent formulations will be made to simplify immunization. A clinical trial was undertaken to evaluate the immunogenicity of the two monovalent conjugates when injected simultaneously into separate arms of volunteers. Results showed no difference in the anti-CP antibody levels, IgG subclasses, or longevity of the immune response for the two vaccines injected simultaneously compared to data obtained with the monovalent regimen in healthy volunteers [72]. A bivalent CP5–rEPA and CP8–rEPA conjugate was formulated in one vial (StaphVAX™), and evaluated in healthy volunteers. The bivalent formulation containing 25 μg of each CP conjugated to rEPA was well tolerated by the vaccines, with no serious local or systemic reactions being recorded in the vaccine group compared to the placebo control group. IgG antibody levels to type 5 and type 8 CP were comparable to those elicited by the previous monovalent vaccines, 173.4 and 70.8 μg/mL, respectively. Moreover, in a subsequent study, the immunogenicity of the two conjugates in the bivalent formulation was compared to their immunogenicity when administered concurrently as monovalent vaccine in separate arms. The IgG levels to CP5 and CP8 achieved by bivalent formulations were equivalent to those elicited by the double monovalent regimen, 178.2 μg/mL versus 139.3 μg/mL for CP5, and 62.7 μg/mL versus 74.6 μg/mL for CP8, respectively. These results show that the bivalent combination is safe and no immunogenic interference of one component against the other is observed. Furthermore, these data point out to feasibility for combining the two conjugates into one single injection that may simplify the future immunization regimen (unpublished data).

VI. VACCINATION STRATEGIES

S. aureus vaccines are intended for specific populations at heightened risk and not for mass immunization. The target populations for immunization may be divided into two major categories: (1) patients who are able to mount an immune response following active immunization and (2) patients who are unable to respond to a vaccine or who do not have time to respond to active immunization and require the passive administration of antibodies that were previously raised in other hosts.

A. Active Immunization

Active immunization may be a feasible strategy for preventing staphylococcal infections in patients scheduled for cardiac or orthopedic surgery (especially hip replacement) and for patients undergoing implantation of medical devices, including renal failure patients on dialysis. Typically, these target populations are sufficiently immunocompetent to respond to a vaccine and have a sufficient time to mount an immune response.

The safety and immunogenicity of the type 5–rEPA conjugate vaccine was evaluated in hemodialysis patients at Walter Reed Army Medical Center [73]. Seventeen hemodialysis patients were immunized twice, 6 weeks apart, with 25 µg CP type 5–rEPA conjugate vaccine. The vaccine was well tolerated and serious local or systemic reactions were not observed. The type 5 CP specific IgG postimmunization levels were comparable to those achieved in normal volunteers immunized with the same lot of vaccine, 179.5 IgG and 317.8 µg/mL, respectively ($P = 0.11$). A lower percentage of vaccinees responding with greater than fourfold increase in the specific antibody levels compared to preimmunization levels was observed in this hemodialysis patient population compared to the study in normal, healthy volunteers described above, 81% and 100%, respectively [73]. A second immunization at 6 weeks failed to boost immune response beyond levels achieved with the first injection. A significantly larger decrease in antibody levels, 39% versus 14%, respectively, was observed 6 months postimmunization in the hemodialysis patients than was observed in healthy volunteers immunized with the same lot of the conjugate vaccine. These data suggest that active immunization with S. aureus conjugate–polysaccharide vaccine may be feasible even in an immunocompromised target population, although immunogenicity remains an issue. Strategies to improve active vaccination, such as reimmunization when titers fall to low levels, optimizing the dose for each target population, the use of adjuvants, and alternate delivery systems, are under evaluation.

B. Passive Immunization

Populations at high risk for S. aureus infections, where active immunization is unlikely to be helpful, include neonates, especially premature newborns [74]; other more completely immunocompromised individuals (e.g., certain cancer patients on immunosuppressive therapy); and populations where the risk for infection is both high and immediate (e.g., shock-trauma patients). Passive protection may be useful for such high-risk subjects. To accomplish this, vaccines would be used to actively immunize healthy adult plasma donors, whose plasma would then be collected and fraction-

ated to produce specific hyperimmune gamma immunoglobulin (IGIV) for intravenous passive immunization. To this end, plasma donors were immunized with a bivalent type 5 and type 8 CP–rEPA conjugate (StaphVAX, Nabi, Boca Raton, FL) and plasmapheresis was performed. Plasma units collected from this donor stimulation program were pooled and fractionated using licensed fractionation techniques. When compared to the commercially available standard intravenous immunoglobulin (IGIV), the specific hyperimmune IGIV (Altastaph™, aka StaphGAM™, Nabi) contained 30- to 40-fold more S. aureus types 5 and 8 CP-specific IgG. This antibody preparation was opsonic in an in vitro opsonophagocytosis assay and was protective in animal model studies (see below). This vaccine-induced antibody product might have an advantage over screened and or standard IGIV by having a higher specific IgG content. Moreover, preliminary results showed that vaccine-induced IgG had greater than fourfold higher affinity for S. aureus CP than did commercial IgG (unpublished data). Studies are ongoing to optimize the donor vaccination regimen and vaccine dose, and to evaluate the effect of plasmapheresis frequency on the specific antibody levels in plasma donors.

In a study performed in collaboration with the Shock-Trauma Center (STC) at the University of Maryland School of Medicine, Baltimore [75], S. aureus infections in patients admitted to the STC over an 18-month period in 1993–1994 were evaluated. A high S. aureus infection rate was observed (7.54%) with bacteremia and pneumonia as the two major infections; infection rates for bacteremia and pneumonia were 4.9% and 2.64%, respectively. Nearly all of these infections occurred within 2–5 days following the initial day of hospitalization. Since a robust immune response to vaccination with a polysaccharide–conjugate vaccine such as StaphVAX usually takes more than two weeks to develop, the immediate-risk status of shock trauma patients makes active immunization impractical. Studies are therefore planned to passively immunize patients such as these with Altastaph. Based on previous experience with the pharmacokinetics of standard IGIV and other specific polyclonal antibodies, passive immunization is expected to provide protective levels of circulating antibody and possibly protection for at least 3 weeks, more than enough time to protect the shock-trauma patient and potentially emergency surgery patients during the period of highest risk.

It should be noted that for some patients, for example, those receiving prosthetic devices such as hip replacements, it may be necessary to provide both passive and active immunization to protect the individual from infection immediately after surgery and for the longer term. Studies are in progress in animals to evaluate combined passive and active immunization against S. aureus.

VII. IN VIVO AND IN VITRO VIRULENCE AND PROTECTION DATA

A. Early Human and Animal Data

Two clinical trials using a vaccine composed of a whole-cell lysate combined with S. aureus toxoids (Staphypan Berna) were performed in an attempt to prevent *S. aureus* infections in end-stage renal dialysis (ESRD) patients on chronic ambulatory peritoneal dialysis (CAPD). Although conclusions could not be drawn from the results of the first study, the authors expressed optimism about the possible future usefulness of this vaccine in controlling *S. aureus* infections in these patients [76]. This vaccine was subsequently evaluated in a multicenter, placebo controlled, double-blinded trial. Data published from the subsequent trial showed no significant advantage of the vaccine over the placebo [77].

It has been well established since the 1960s that capsules belonging to *S. aureus* strains Smith (capsular type 2) and M (capsular type 1) are virulence factors and protective antigens [78–83]. Subsequent work by Lee et al. [84] showed that mutants that lost their capsules are less virulent than their parent strains and that these capsules, when used as vaccines, induced protective activity against bacterial challenge [85]. In contrast, the role of the clinically significant capsules, types 5 and 8, in virulence and possible protection continues to be controversial. While some authors have reported these capsules to be antiphagocytic (requiring type-specific antibodies to mediate opsonophagocytosis) [48,56,68–70], others have reported that *S. aureus* CP types 5 and 8 are not virulence factors [86]. One study reports that encapsulated isolates are equally phagocytosed in the presence of homologous or heterologous sera as well as sera raised against noncapsulated strains[87]. In fact, it has been reported that capsular polysaccharides actually attenuate the virulence of these clinical strains [88]. In other related studies, immunization of animals with type 5 whole cell vaccine failed to protect against bacterial challenge in rabbit as well as rat endocarditis models [89,90].

B. Current Animal Data

To further evaluate the role of capsule and antibodies to capsular polysaccharides in *S. aureus* infections, we have used a lethal, challenge mouse model to evaluate CP–conjugate vaccines and hyperimmune IGIV. Our data showed that either intraperitoneal or subcutaneous administration of hyperimmune human IGIV (Altastaph, aka StaphGAM) directed to *S. aureus* CP protected mice against lethal intraperitoneal challenge with a clinical *S. aureus* isolate (CP type 5); we observed >90% survival in mice passively immunized with specific polyclonal antibody compared to a 22% survival rate in animals receiving standard IGIV ($P < 0.001$) [91]. Studies in this mouse model have also shown that active immunization with CP–rEPA conjugate vaccine conferred significant protection compared to saline immunized animals. In these studies, survival of immunized animals after challenge with type 5 *S. aureus* was >73% versus <7% survival rate in nonimmunized animals ($P < 0.001$).

Rabbit IgG preparations from animals immunized with a type 5 CP–conjugate vaccine were evaluated in a modified catheter-induced model of staphylococcal endocarditis rat model [92]. Data generated in this model showed that hyperimmune rabbit IgG significantly protected rats against intraperitoneal bacterial challenge of type 5 *S. aureus*. Animals receiving the hyperimmune IgG preparation developed fewer endocarditis episodes compared to those immunized

with nonimmune rabbit IgG (25% and 87.5%, respectively; $P < 0.05$). Furthermore, these animals had reduced bacterial counts in blood, in vegetation on the catheter-damaged heart valve, and in kidneys compared to rats receiving the same amount of nonimmune rabbit IgG ($P < 0.05$ for all three indications) [92].

VIII. STAPHVAX—RECENT CLINICAL RESULTS AND FUTURE PROSPECTIVES

S. aureus is a major cause of infections associated with indwelling medical devices such as catheters and orthopedic devices [93]. Peritonitis, exit-site infections, and bacteremia due to staphylococci are the major cause of morbidity and mortality in patients with ESRD [94–100]. ESRD patients are, therefore, considered to be appropriate targets for evaluation of active vaccination. StaphVAX containing 25 μg of each polysaccharide conjugated to rEPA was evaluated for its safety and immunogenicity in ESRD patients on hemodialysis. Although this dose of vaccine was determined to be safe and immunogenic, specific antibody levels achieved were lower in this population than seen previously in normal, healthy volunteers. In addition, although antibody levels declined over time faster in the ESRD patients than in normal, healthy volunteers, one year after vaccination, CP-specific antibody levels remained significantly elevated over preimmunizaton levels (not shown).

A Phase 2 multicenter, double-blinded efficacy trial of StaphVAX in 237 ESRD patients undergoing chronic ambulatory peritoneal dialysis also demonstrated that a single dose of 25 μg of StaphVAX was safe and well tolerated. However, this dose of vaccine did not decrease the incidence of *S. aureus* peritonitis (unpublished results). Importantly, the results suggested that the vaccine dose selected was suboptimal, since lower antibody levels were achieved than previously observed in normal, healthy volunteers administered that dose.

In an attempt to optimize the performance of Staph-VAX in ESRD patients, a dose-escalating clinical study in ESRD patients on hemodialysis was performed using 50 and 100 μg/mL of each polysaccharide conjugated to rEPA in the bivalent formulation. Data in Table 1 show a dose response to the vaccine in both antibody levels achieved and the percent responders. As shown in Table 1, the antibody levels at 42 days postimmunization at the 100-μg dose in ESRD patients approximated the levels seen in normal healthy volunteers at the 50-μg dose (not shown). However, the antibody levels declined more rapidly in ESRD patients than previously observed in normal, healthy volunteers at all vaccine doses tested (not shown).

In 1998, a single dose of bivalent vaccine containing 100 μg of each polysaccharide conjugated to rEPA was evaluated for safety, immunogenicity, and efficacy in a double-blinded, randomized, placebo-controlled study in ESRD patients (ages 18–91) on hemodialysis [101]. A total of 1804 adult patients at 73 hemodialysis centers received a single intramuscular injection of either vaccine ($n = 894$) or saline ($n = 910$). IgG antibodies to types 5 and 8 CP were measured at intervals for up to 2 years, and episodes of *S. aureus* bac-

Table 1 Dose Response to StaphVAX Immunization in ESRD Patients

Nominal dose (μg)	N	Type 5 IgG antibodies (μg/mL)			Type 8 IgG antibodies (μg/mL)		
		Day 0	Day 42	Responders (%)	Day 0	Day 42	Responders (%)
25/25	15	6	62	80	10	31	47
75/75	16	4	82	75	3	50	75
100/100	17	4	172	88	6	143	88

teremia were recorded. The primary endpoint of the trial was efficacy through 1 year of follow-up postvaccination. Efficacy was estimated by comparing the attack rate of *S. aureus* bacteremia in the vaccine group to that of the controls. Vaccine reactions were generally mild to moderate and most resolved within 2 days. The vaccine elicited a significant CP-specific antibody response in 86% of the patients. Through 54 weeks of follow-up postvaccination, the incidence of *S. aureus* bacteremia was 27/892 in the vaccine group and 37/906 in controls, for a person–time estimate of efficacy of 26%, a value that did not differ significantly from zero (P value = 0.2, 95% confidence interval, 24.5–56.8%). A post hoc analysis of results through 40 weeks postvaccination, however, showed that the incidence of *S. aureus* bacteremia was 11/892 in the vaccine group, and 26/906 in controls for a person–time estimate of efficacy of 57% (nominal P value = 0.02; 95% confidence interval, 10–81%). Analysis of efficacy versus antibody concentrations through 40 weeks postvaccination demonstrated that there was a strong correlation between the falloff of efficacy after approximately 40 weeks postvaccination and the falloff of mean antibody concentrations below 107 μg/mL type 5 antibody (P < 0.0001) and 111 μg/mL type 8 (P < 0.0001) antibody in the vaccinated population. Although this population-based correlation between efficacy and antibody titer appeared evident in this trial, it was clear from the results of the trial that relatively high levels of antibody to CP were insufficient to protect some ESRD patients. The failure to establish a correlation between efficacy and antibody titer in individual ESRD patients may reflect the immunological heterogeneity of the ESRD population and the variable general health of individuals in the population. Factors such as underlying disease, age, variable complement levels and phagocytic competency of leukocytes, and other complicating factors that characterize this population may make it impossible to predict a threshold protective antibody level for any individual ESRD patient.

Another interesting outcome of the ESRD trial with StaphVAX was the results observed in a subset of subjects. It is generally recognized that nasal carriage of *S. aureus* is associated with an increased risk of *S. aureus* bacteremia among hemodialysis patients and other at-risk individuals [96–100]. Although the numbers are small, it appears that nasal carriage put controls but not vaccinees at higher risk of bacteremia (P value = 0.057). This suggests that vaccination may have provided protection against *S. aureus* infection associated with nasal carriage.

Also of note from this large trial was the CP type distribution of *S. aureus* isolates from bacteremic patients. As predicted from earlier typing studies, approximately 80% of clinical isolates of *S. aureus* received for typing were either type 5 or type 8 [46,48–53]. The remainder of isolates were so-called type 336, a new subtype of *S. aureus* characterized by a specific surface polysaccharide (Fattom et al., manuscript in preparation). In this trial, there was also a similar distribution of methicillin resistance among isolates from both the vaccine and placebo groups. These results are consistent with in vitro data showing that both antibiotic-resistant and -sensitive *S. aureus* are killed by vaccine-induced antibody-mediated opsonophagocytosis.

Patients participating in this study, in addition to being on hemodialysis, were elderly (mean age 58.3 + 14.8 years), and many suffer from type 1 or 2 diabetes (51.9%). It is well established that uremia and hyperglycemia have a major debilitating impact on host defense mechanisms, in particular, complement activity and opsonophagocytosis, the two main mechanisms for clearance of gram-positive pathogens [102–105].

In summary, this large, double-blinded, placebo-controlled clinical trial showed that StaphVAX, a bivalent *S. aureus* CP–conjugate vaccine, was able to reduce *S. aureus* bacteremia in an immunocompromised, at-risk, adult patient population. This is the first time that a vaccine against *S. aureus* has shown efficacy in humans in a well-controlled trial. Because of their reduced immune competency, hemodialysis patients are among the patient populations least likely to be protected by immunoprophylaxis. An efficacy of 57% through 10 months postvaccination is a remarkable achievement for StaphVAX in this patient population. It is reasonable to expect that the efficacy of this vaccine might be higher in other more immunocompetent patient populations such as scheduled orthopedic, cardiac, and general surgery patients. Additional clinical trials of StaphVAX are planned in ESRD and other at-risk patient populations.

ACKNOWLEDGMENT

We are grateful to Kimberly L. Taylor and Phyllis Link for reviewing the manuscript.

REFERENCES

1. Weinstein RA. Epidemiology and control of nosocomial infections in adult intensive care units. Am J Med 1991; 91 (suppl 3B):179–184.
2. Musher DM, McKenzie SO. Infections due to *S. aureus*. Medicine 1977; 56:383–409.

3. Kluytmans JA, et al. Nasal carriage of *S. aureus* as major factor for wound infections after cardiac surgery. J Infect Dis 1995; 171:216–219.

4. Kaplowitz LG, et al. Prospective study of microbial colonization of the nose and skin and infection of vascular access site in hemodialysis patients. J Clin Microbiol 1988; 26:1257–1262.

5. Yu VL, et al. *Staphylococcus aureus* nasal carriage and infection in patients on hemodialysis. N Engl J Med 1986; 315:91–96.

6. Nolan CM, Beatty HN. *Staphylococcus aureus* bacteremia. Am J Med 1976; 60:495–500.

7. McGowan JE, et al. Bacteremia at Boston city hospital; occurrence and mortality during selected years (1935–1972), with special reference to hospital-acquired cases. J Infect Dis 1975; 132:316–335.

8. Mylotte JM, et al. Prospective study of 114 consecutive episodes of *Staphylococcus aureus* bacteremia. J Infect Dis 1987; 9:891–907.

9. Tessen I, et al. Incidence and etiology of neonatal septicemia and meningitis in western Sweden 1975–1986. Acta Paediatr Scand 1990; 79:1023–1030.

10. Center For Disease Control. Nosocomial infection surveillance. MMWR Morb Mortal Wkly Rep 1986; 35:17–29.

11. Ford-Jones EL, et al. Epidemiologic study of 4684 hospital-acquired infections in pediatric patients. Pediatr Infect Dis 1989; 8:668–675.

12. Kaiser AB. Surgical wound infections. N Engl J Med 1991; 324:123–124.

13. Cross AS, Steigbigel RT. Infective endocarditis and access site infection in patients on hemodialysis. Ann Intern Med 1978; 88:28–33.

14. Dobkin JF, et al. Septicemia in patients on chronic hemodialysis. Ann Intern Med 1978; 88:28–33.

15. Takiuchi I, et al. Staphylococcal exfoliative toxin induces caseinolytic activity. J Infect Dis 1987; 156:508–509.

16. Kass EH, Parsonnet J. On the pathogenesis of toxic shock syndrome. Rev Infect Dis 1987; 9:S482–S489.

17. Melish ME, Glasgow LA. The staphylococcal scalded-skin syndrome. Development of an experimental model. N Engl J Med 1970; 282:1114–1119.

18. Bergdoll MS, et al. A new staphylococcal enterotoxin, enterotoxin F, associated with toxic-shock-syndrome. Lancet 1981; 1:1017–1027.

19. Suttorp N, Habben E. Effect of staphylococcal alpha-toxin on intracellular Ca^{+2} in polymorphonuclear leukocytes. Infect Immun 1988; 56:2228–2234.

20. Bisno AL, Waldvogel FA. Infections Associated with Indwelling Medical Devices. Washington, DC: ASM Press, 1994.

21. Foster T, McDevitt D. Molecular basis of adherence of staphylococci to biomaterials. In: Bisno AL, Waldvogel FA, eds. Infections Associated with Indwelling Medical Devices. Washington, DC: ASM Press, 1994:31–44.

22. Foster T, McDevitt D. Surface associated protein of *Staphylococcus aureus*: their possible roles in virulence. FEMS Microbiol Lett 1994; 118:199–205.

23. Moreau M, et al. Structure of the type 5 capsular polysaccharide of *Staphylococcus aureus*. Carbohydr Res 1990; 201:285–297.

24. Peterson PK, et al. Influence of capsulation on staphylococcal opsonization and phagocytosis by human polymorphonuclear leukocytes. Infect Immun 1978; 19:943–949.

25. Peterson PK, et al. Dychotomy between opsonization and serum complement activation by encapsulated staphylococci. Infect Immun 1978; 20:770–775.

26. Sheagren JN. *Staphylococcus aureus*: the persistent pathogen. N Engl J Med 1984; 310:1368–1373.

27. Albus A, et al. *Staphylococcus aureus* capsular types and antibody response to lung infection in patients with cystic fibrosis. J Clin Microbiol 1988; 26:2505–2509.

28. Best GK, et al. Protection of rabbits in an infection model of toxic shock syndrome (TSS) by a TSS toxin-1-specific monoclonal antibody. Infect Immun 1988; 56:998–999.

29. Morse S. Staphylococci and other micrococci. In: Dubos RJ, Hirsch J, G., eds. Bacterial and Mycotic Infection of Man. Philadelphia: J.B. Lippincott, 1965:412–439.

30. Quie PG. Bactericidal function of human polymorphonuclear leukocytes. Pediatrics 1972; 50:264–270.

31. Barber M, Rozwadowska-Dawzenko M. Infection by penicillin-resistant staphylococci. Lancet 1948; 2:641–644.

32. Rolinson GN, et al. Bacteriological studies on new penicillin-BRL. Lancet 1960; 2:564–567.

33. Bitar CM, et al. Outbreak due to methicillin and rifampin resistant *Staphylococcus aureus*: epidemiology and eradication of the resistant strain from the hospital. Infect Control 1987; 8:15–23.

34. Cohen SH, et al. A seven-year experience with methicillin-resistant *Staphylococcus aureus*. Am J Med 1991; 91(suppl 3B):233–237.

35. Linnemann CC, et al. Reemergence of epidemic methicillin-resistant *Staphylococcus aureus* in general hospital associated with changing staphylococcal strain. Am J Med 1991; 91(suppl 3B):238–244.

36. Krause RM. Immunity to *Staphylococcus aureus*, a persistent enigma. Emory Univ J Med 1989; 3:77–85.

37. Krause RM. Dynamics of emergence. J Infect Dis 1994; 170:265–271.

38. Foster TJ. Potential for vaccination against infections caused by *Staphylococcus aureus*. Vaccine 1991; 9:221–227.

39. Karakawa WW. The role of capsular antigens in *Staphylococcus aureus* immunity. Zentralbl Bakteriol 1992; 277:415–418.

40. Salmon GG Jr, Symonds M. Staphage lysate therapy in chronic staphyloccocal infections. J Med Assoc NJ 1963; 60:188–193.

41. Bryant RE, et al. Treatment of recurrent furunculosis with staphylococcal bacteriophage-lysed vaccine. JAMA 1965; 194:11–14.

42. Greenberg L, Le Riche WH. Staphylococcal enzyme lysed soluble vaccine. Can J Public Health 1961; 52:479–485.

43. Greenberg L, Cooper MY. Polyvalent somatic antigen for the prevention of staphylococcal infections. Can Med Assoc J 1960; 83:143–147.

44. Dillenberg H, Waldron MPD. A preventive approach to impetigo of treaty Indians using a *Staphylococcus* polyvalent somatic antigen vaccine. Can Med Assoc J 1963; 89:947–949.

45. Dillenberg H. Experience with a polyvalent staphylococcal vaccine with alpha-toxoid. Can J Public Health 1962; 53:248–253.

46. Sompolinsky D, et al. Encapsulation and capsular types in isolates of *Staphylococcus aureus* from different sources and relationship to phage types. Infect Immun 1985; 22:828–834.

47. Rogers DE, Melly MA. Speculation on the immunology of staphylococcal Infection. Ann N Y Acad Sci 1965; 128:274–284.

48. Karakawa WW, Vann WF. Capsular polysaccharides of *Staphylococcus aureus*. In: Weinstein L, Fields BN, eds. Seminars in Infectious Disease. New York: Thieme-Stratton, 1982:285–293.

49. Karakawa WW, et al. Method for the serological typing of the capsular polysaccharides of *Staphylococcus aureus*. J Clin Microbiol 1985; 22:445–447.

50. Arbeit R, et al. Predominance of two newly described capsular polysaccharide types among clinical isolates of *Staphylococcus aureus*. Diagn Microbiol Infect Dis 1984; 2:85–91.

51. Daum RS, et al. Capsular polysaccharides serotypes of co-agulase-positive staphylococci associated with tenosynovo-tis, osteomyelitis, and other invasive infections in chicken and turkeys: evidence for new capsular types. Avian Dis 1994; 38:762–771.

52. Poutrel B, Sutra L. Type 5 and 8 capsular polysaccharides are expressed by *Staphylococcus aureus* isolates from rab-bits, poultry, pigs, and horses. J Clin Microbiol 1993; 31: 467–469.

53. Poutrel B, et al. Prevalence of capsular polysaccharide types 5 and 8 among *Staphylococcus aureus* isolates from cow, goat, and ewe milk. J Clin Microbiol 1988; 26:38–40.

54. Fournier JM, et al. Purification and characterization of *Staphylococcus aureus* type 8 capsular polysaccharide. Infect Immun 1984; 45:87–93.

55. Fournier JM, et al. Isolation of type 5 capsular polysaccha-ride form *Staphylococcus aureus*. Ann Inst Pasteur Micro-biol 1987; 138:561–567.

56. Karakawa WW, et al. Capsular antibodies induce type-specific phagocytosis of capsulated *Staphylococcus aureus* by human polymorphonuclear leukocytes. Infect Immun 1988; 56:1090–1095.

57. Robbins JB, et al. Virulence properties of bacterial capsu-lar polysaccharides: unanswered questions. In: Smith H, Skehel JJ, Turner MJ, eds. The Molecular Basis of Micro-bial Pathogenicity. Weinheim: Verlag Chemie GmbH, 1980: 115–132.

58. Robbins JB, et al. Considerations for formulating the sec-ond generation pneumococcal vaccine with the emphasis of the cross-reactive types within groups. J Infect Dis 1983; 148: 1136–1159.

59. Robbins JB, et al. Prevention of systemic infections caused by group B Streptococcus and *Staphylococcus aureus* by multivalent polysaccharide–protein conjugate vaccines. Ann N Y Acad Sci 1995; 754:68–82.

60. Austrian R. Some observations on the pneumococcal vac-cine and on the current status of pneumococcal disease and its prevention. Rev Infect Dis 1981; 3:S51–S57.

61. Simberkoff MS, et al. Pneumococcal capsular polysacchar-ide vaccination in adult chronic hemodialysis patients. J Lab Clin Med 1980; 96:363–370.

62. Sarnaik S, et al. Studies on pneumococcus vaccine alone or mixed with DTP and on pneumococcus type 6B and *Hae-mophilus influenzae* type B capsular polysaccharide–tetanus toxoid conjugates in two- to five-year-old children with sickle cell anemia. Pediatr Infect Dis 1990; 9:181–186.

63. Schneerson R, et al. Preparation, characterization and im-munogenicity of *Haemophilus influenzae* type B polysaccha-ride–protein conjugates. J Exp Med 1980; 152:361–376.

64. Schneerson R, et al. Quantitative and qualitative analysis of serum antibodies elicited in adults by *Haemophilus influen-zae* type B and pneumococcus type 6A capsular polysac-charide–tetanus toxoid conjugates. Infect Immun 1986; 52: 519–528.

65. Schneerson R, et al. Serum antibody responses of juvenile and infant rhesus monkeys injected with *Haemophilus influ-enzae* type B and pneumococcus type 6A polysaccharide–protein conjugates. Infect Immun 1984; 45:582–591.

66. Robbins JB, Schneerson R. Polysaccharide–protein conju-gates. A new generation of vaccines. J Infect Dis 1990; 161: 821–832.

67. Robbins JB. Vaccines for the prevention of encapsulated bacterial diseases: current status, problems and prospects for the future. Immunochemistry 1978; 15:839–854.

68. Fattom A, et al. Synthesis and immunologic properties in mice of vaccines composed of *Staphylococcus aureus* type 5 and type 8 capsular polysaccharides conjugated to *Pseudo-monas aeruginosa* exotoxin A. Infect Immun 1990; 58:2367–2374.

69. Fattom A, et al. Comparative immunogenicity of conju-gates composed of *Staphylococcus aureus* type 8 capsular polysaccharide bound to carrier proteins by adipic acid dihydrazide or *N*-succinimidyl-3-(2-pyridylthio) propionate. Infect Immun 1992; 60:584–589.

70. Fattom A, et al. Laboratory and clinical evaluation of con-jugate vaccines composed of *Staphylococcus aureus* types 5 and 8 capsular polysaccharides bound to *Pseudomonas aeru-ginosa* recombinant exoprotein A. Infect Immun 1993; 61: 1023–1032.

71. Fattom A, et al. Immune response in adult volunteer elic-ited by injection of *Streptococcus pneumoniae* type 12F polysaccharide alone or conjugated to diphtheria toxoid. Infect Immun 1990; 58:2309–2312.

72. Fattom A, et al. Evaluation in humans of *Staphylococcus aureus* types 5 and 8 capsular polysaccharide conjugate vaccines injected concurrently into separate arms [abstr]. Interscience Conference on Antimicrobial Agents and Che-motherapy, 1994.

73. Welch P, et al. Safety and immunogenicity of *S. aureus* type 5 capsular polysaccharide–*Pseudomonas aeruginosa* recom-binant exoprotein A conjugate vaccine in patients on hemo-dialysis. J Am Soc Nephrol 1996; 7:247–253.

74. Baker CJ, et al. Intravenous immunoglobulin for the pre-vention of nosocomial infection in low-birth-weight neo-nates. N Engl J Med 1992; 327:213–219.

75. Na'was T, et al. Phenotypic and genotypic characterization of nosocomial *S. aureus* isolates from trauma patients. J Clin Microbiol 1998; 36:414–420.

76. Scatizzi A, Strippoli P. Prevention of *Staphylococcus aureus* peritonitis in continuous ambulatory peritoneal dialysis. In: Smeby LC, Jorstad S, Wideroe TE, eds. Immune and Meta-bolic Aspects of Therapeutic Blood Systems. Basel: Karger, 1986:191–196.

77. Atkins R, et al. Vaccination for the prevention of CAPD associated with staphylococcal infections: results of a pro-spective multicenter clinical trial. Clin Nephrol 1991; 35: 198–206.

78. Koening MG, Melly M. The importance of surface antigens in staphylococcal virulence. Ann N Y Acad Sci 1965; 128: 231–250.

79. Koening MG. Factors relating to the virulence of staphylo-cocci: I. Comparative studies of two colonial variants. Yale J Biol Med 1962; 34:537–559.

80. Melly MA, et al. Biological properties of encapsulated *Staphylococcus aureus*. Infect Immun 1974; 10:389–397.

81. Fisher S. Observation on an antistaphylococcal mouse pro-tective antibody in human sera. J Exp Biol 1961; 39:413–422.

82. Fisher MW, et al. A new staphylococcal antigen. Nature 1963; 199:1074–1075.

83. Ekstedt RD. Immune response to surface antigens of *Staph-ylococcus aureus* and their role in resistance to staphylo-coccal disease. Ann N Y Acad Sci 1974; 236:203–220.

84. Lee JC, et al. Virulence studies in mice of transposon-induced mutant of *Staphylococccus aureus* differing in capsular size. J Infect Dis 1987; 156:751–760.

85. Lee CJ, et al. Purified capsular polysaccharide-induced im-munity to *Staphylococcus aureus* infection. J Infect Dis 1988; 157:723–730.

86. Albus AR, et al. Virulence of *Staphylococcus aureus* mutants altered in type 5 capsules production. Infect Immun 1991; 59: 1008–1014.

87. Xu S, et al. Phagocytic killing of encapsulated *Staphylo-coccus aureus* by human polymorphonuclear lymphocytes. Infect Immun 1992; 60:1358–1362.

88. Baddour LM, et al. *Staphylococcus aureus* microcapsule ex-pression attenuates bacterial virulence in rat model of ex-perimental endocarditis. J Infect Dis 1992; 165:749–753.

89. Greenberg DP, et al. Influence of *Staphylococcus aureus* antibody on experimental endocarditis in rabbits. Infect Immun 1987; 55:3030–3034.

90. Nemeth J, Lee CJ. Antibodies to capsular polysaccharides are not protective against experimental *Staphylococcus aureus* endocarditis. Infect Immun 1995; 63:375–380.

91. Fattom AI, et al. *Staphylococcus aureus* capsular polysaccharide (CP) vaccine and CP-specific antibodies protect mice against bacterial challenge. Infect Immun 1996; 64:1659–1665.

92. Lee JC, et al. Protective efficacy of antibodies to the *S. aureus* type 5 capsular polysaccharide in a rat model of endocarditis. Infect Immun 1997; 65:4146–4151.

93. Sheargen JN. Staphylococcus aureus: the persistent pathogen. N Engl J Med 1984; 310:1368–1373.

94. Edmond M, et al. Nosocomial bloodstream infections in United States hospitals: a three-year analysis. Clin Infect Dis 1999; 29:239–244.

95. Rubin RJ, et al. The economic impact of *Staphylococcus aureus* infection in New York City hospitals. Emerg Infect Dis 1999; 5:9–17.

96. Chow JW, Yu V. *Staphylococcus aureus* nasal carriage in hemodialysis patients: its role in infection and approaches to prophylaxis. Arch Intern Med 1989; 149:1258–1262.

97. Kluytmans JA, et al. Elimination of nasal carriage of *Staph-ylococcus aureus* in hemodialysis patients. Infect Control Hosp Epidemiol 1996; 17:793–797.

98. Yu V, et al. *Staphylococcus aureus* nasal carriage and infection in patients on hemodialysis. N Engl J Med 1986; 315:91–96.

99. Dobkin JF, et al. Septicemia in patients on chronic hemodialysis. Ann Intern Med 1978; 88:28–33.

100. Kaplowitz LG, et al. A prospective study of infections in hemodialysis patients: patient hygiene and other risk factors for infection. Infect Control Hosp Epidemiol 1988; 9:534–541.

101. Shinefield H, et al. Use of a *Staphylococcus aureus* types 5 and 8 polysaccharide conjugate vaccine to prevent bacteremia in patients receiving hemodialysis. N Engl J Med 2001; 346:491–496.

102. Minnaganti VR, Cunha BA. Infection associated with uremia and dialysis. Infect Dis Clin North Am 2001; 15:385–406.

103. Haag-Weber M, Hort WH. Uremia and infection: mechanisms of by impaired cellular host defense. Nephron 1993; 63:125–131.

104. Haag-Weber M, et al. Metabolic response of neutrophils to uremia and dialysis. Kidney Int 1989; 36(suppl 27):S293–S298.

105. Bagdade J, et al. Impaired leukocyte function in patients with poorly controlled diabetes. Diabetes 1974; 23:9–15.

67

Moraxella catarrhalis and Nontypable *Haemophilus influenzae* Vaccines to Prevent Otitis Media

Philippe A. Denoel, Fabrice Godfroid, Joelle Thonnard, Cécile Neyt, and Jan T. Poolman
GlaxoSmithKline Biologicals, Rixensart, Belgium

David W. Dyer
Oklahoma University Health Sciences Center, Oklahoma City, Oklahoma, U.S.A.

I. INTRODUCTION

Successful bacterial vaccines are composed of either killed or attenuated whole bacteria, detoxified exotoxins, or polysaccharides (and polysaccharide–protein conjugates). A newer vaccine development approach uses bacterial surface proteins as purified subunits, albeit in combination with a detoxified exotoxin. Acellular pertussis vaccines, the first example of this strategy of exploiting surface protein subunits, may contain, in addition to pertussis toxin (PT), the *Bordetella pertussis* pertactin (PRN), filamentous hemagglutinin (FHA), and fimbriae (FIM). Other nonencapsulated pathogenic bacteria such as nontypable *Haemophilus influenzae* (NTHi) and *Moraxella catarrhalis* (*M. cat*) are potential targets for using surface components other than capsular polysaccharides as vaccine components. However, in terms of immune evasion, there is a major difference between *B. pertussis* and NTHi/*M. cat*. *Bordetella* exhibits rather limited antigenic variability in its various surface components and exotoxins such as PRN, FHA, FIM and pertussis toxin (PT), and adenylate cyclase (AC). *B. pertussis* may evade host immune responses by the immunomodulating effects of PT and AC. Both NTHi and *M. cat* use the antigenic variability of surface and secreted components to evade the human immune response. This hampers the identification of candidate antigens and complicates vaccine development. Although oral immunization with killed NTHi of adults with a history of chronic recurrences of respiratory NTHi infectious diseases has shown an impact on NTHi carriage and subsequent diseases [1–3], the duration of this effect is not known. However, these findings have demonstrated the feasibility of immunization for protecting against NTHi infection. With respect to the potential of immune escape, it can be postulated that a multicomponent vaccine targeting a few components associated with essential biological functions would be needed for successful immunization. Such a multicomponent product can be either killed or live attenuated bacteria, or a multicomponent subunit. In the case of whole bacteria, it would be beneficial to genetically delete highly variable and nonprotective antigens and to up-regulate (minor) conserved, biologically essential, and protective components. Another option could be the use of outer membrane vesicles extracted from such manipulated bacteria.

How can we identify biologically essential, conserved, and protective NTHi/*M. cat* antigens? Various steps in the host–bacterial interaction are being delineated [4,5]. Both NTHi and *M. cat* exploit mechanisms to adhere to or to colonize various host cells [5–16]. Invasion and survival within epithelial cells allow NTHi/*M. cat* to survive/evade immunity [17]. The removal of iron from host proteins such as lactoferrin, transferrin, haptoglobin, and hemoglobin is essential for NTHi/*M. cat* survival within the human host, and various bacterial iron uptake mechanisms have been identified [18–24]. Specific immune evasion processes exist, such as the activity of bacterial immunoglobulin (Ig) A proteases as well as complement binding and degradation or serum resistance [13,25,26]. Animal models that have been developed to study the immunizing potential of various NTHi/*M. cat* components mimic the major clinical infections caused by NTHi/*M. cat* such as otitis media (OM), pneumonia, and other respiratory diseases [27–33].

Although many potential NTHi/*M. cat* candidate antigens have been identified such as adhesins/invasins, iron uptake systems, porins, secretins, etc., many more potentially exist. Nontypable *H. influenzae*/*M. cat* each possesses a single chromosome of ~1.8 and 1.9 Mb, respectively; full sequence information should reveal the identity of new candidates. A similar genomic approach has been applied to the pneumococcus and meningococcus. In the case of the pneumococcus, the genomic approach has identified several new candidate antigens [34]. In the case of the meningococcus, a relatively large number of candidate antigens have been identified via nongenomic approaches, making it more difficult to find new bonafide antigens. New antigens were discovered from the genome sequence of one meningococcal strain, and early studies suggested at least one promising conserved candidate that induces bactericidal antibodies [35]. However, in subsequent studies, this antigen did not prove useful [36]. These examples illustrate that the genomic antigen discovery approach can be valuable, although caveats still exist.

Nontypable *H. influenzae/M. cat* cause clinically important infections such as otitis, pneumonia, and other respiratory diseases. Vaccination, if successful, may allow better control of these diseases. A comprehensive approach that considers previously defined antigens as well as new candidates derived from genomics is needed. Aside from protein antigens, the surface lipopolysaccharides (LPS) must be considered because of their dominance at the bacterial surface, their role in host bacterial interactions, and the greater difficulty of bacteria to vary saccharide structures as compared to protein antigens [14,37–39]. However, NTHi/*M. cat* LPS do show antigenic variability, complicating the identification of conserved epitopes [40–45]. A summary of previously identified antigens and new antigens identified by genomic is presented in this chapter.

II. *M. CAT*

M. cat is a gram-negative bacterium that has long been considered a harmless commensal colonizer of the nasopharynx. Only recently has *Moraxella* been associated as the causative agent of a variety of respiratory tract diseases of which the most important are otitis media in infants and children, and pneumonia in the elderly. *Moraxella* also causes sinusitis, nosocomial infections, and, much less frequently, invasive diseases.

In 1921, Gordon [46] described *M. cat* as a saprophyte of negligible virulence that could be isolated from the throat of healthy adults. This view decreased the scientific interest in *Moraxella* and explained why this bacterium was not well studied until the 1970s. Vaneechoutte et al. [47] critically examined 112 publications stating that *M. cat* is a common commensal and found that no studies provided experimental evidence supporting this view. They concluded that misidentification of *M. cat* and confusion with *Neisseria cinerea*, which is present in 90% of throats, were probably responsible for the original misconception that *M. cat* is only a harmless commensal. Other arguments demonstrating the pathogenic potential of *M. cat* were recently reviewed [48].

The immune response to *M. cat* is poorly characterized. The analysis of strains isolated sequentially from the nasopharynx of babies followed from birth to 2 years of age indicates that they frequently acquire and eliminate new strains. This could indicate that an efficacious immune response against this bacterium is developed by colonized children [49]. The antibody response to outer membrane proteins (OMPs) of *M. cat* in children with otitis media is raised mainly against four dominant targets corresponding to UspA, TbpB, CopB (see below), and a 60-kDa protein [50]. An opsonizing activity has been observed in the sera of children recovering from otitis media. A very low or even undetectable IgG3 antibody response to *M. cat* in children under the age of 4 years having increased otitis media or sinusitis caused by this pathogen has been reported [51,52].

In most adults tested, bactericidal antibodies have been identified [53]. Strains of *M. cat* vary in their capacity to resist serum bactericidal activity; in general, isolates from ill individuals are more resistant than strains isolated from individuals who are simply colonized [25,54]. Serum resistance could therefore be considered as a virulence factor of the bacteria. A recent study indicates that complement-resistant strains represent a separate lineage in the species. The clonal nature of the complement-resistant strains offers an interpretation of the observations made in a previous study, which showed that strains isolated from the upper respiratory tract of healthy children are primarily sensitive to complement-mediated killing. Although several factors have been suggested to be involved in serum resistance (Cop B), no final demonstration has been reported.

M. cat produces outer membrane vesicles (blebs), which have been isolated by different methods [55,56]. The protective capacity of such bleb preparations has been tested in a murine model for pulmonary clearance; active immunization with a bleb vaccine or passive transfer of antibleb antibodies induces significant protection against homologous challenge [57].

Several proteins or bacterial compounds are potential antigens and putative virulence factors of *M. cat*, and can be categorized as factors involved in bacterial attachment to host surfaces, proteins induced by iron limitation, or other antigens.

A. Factors Involved in Bacterial Attachment to Host Surface

1. Pili (Fimbriae)

Type 4 pili on the surface of some *M. cat* strains [58] are expressed during infection. Their length varies between 50 and 80 nm [59]. Pili could be involved in bacterial attachment to bronchial cells. However, nonpiliated strains also adhere to these cells, although in smaller numbers [60]. The host–cell receptor for fimbriae has been identified on pharyngeal cells as ganglioside M2 [16]. It is not known if pili induce a protective immune response.

2. UspA1/2

UspA is a surface protein first recognized by a protective monoclonal antibody. Convalescent-phase sera from patients with *M. cat* pneumonia or otitis media, but not acute-phase sera from these patients, contain anti-UspA antibodies [61,62]. In general, IgG and IgA serum levels are higher in adults than in children [63]. Two UspA genes that encode two distinct proteins bearing conserved epitopes have been identified [64]. UspA1 is involved in bacterial adhesion to human epithelial cells whereas UspA2 is involved in normal human serum resistance [65]. Both proteins have been purified and characterized. Purified UspA2 has an affinity for vitronectin; UspA1 binds Hep-2 cells and fibronectin. Immunization of mice with both proteins induces bactericidal antibodies and protects against pulmonary challenge [66]. Some strains produce a third protein, Uspa2H. Its N-terminal half is similar to the N-terminal half of UspA1, and its C-terminal sequence is nearly identical to the UspA2 C-terminal sequence. UspA2H may be an adhesin [67]. The expression of UspA1 is phase-variable, being affected by the length of a poly(G) tract located upstream of the *uspa1* ORF [68]. UspA1 and UspA2 may belong to the same family of proteins as YadA from *Yersinia* species. These surface proteins form a lollipop-shaped structure resulting in a tripartite organization, with the N-terminal head domain followed by a putative coiled-coil rod, the C-terminal part of the protein being a membrane anchor domain [69]. These proteins are promising vaccine candidates.

3. Omp106

Omp106, which has a molecular weight ranging from about 180 to 230 kDa, displays hemagglutination properties [70]. Antibodies to Omp106 are bactericidal and can block the adhesion of *M. cat* onto epithelial cells. Moreover, immunization with Omp106 enhances bacterial clearance in a pulmonary mouse model (unpublished data). The sequence of the 200-kDa OMP MID, which displays high affinity for IgD [71], is highly similar to Omp106.

B. Proteins Induced by Iron Limitation

M. cat expresses specific iron-repressible proteins in response to iron-limited growth in vitro. Human transferrin and lactoferrin can be used as the sole source of iron in the absence of any detectable siderophore production [18]. *M. cat* was found to express transferrin-binding and lactoferrin-binding proteins. OmpB1 binds human transferrin [19]. OmpB1 and a 74-kDa protein are variants of the same protein, TbpB [72,73]. An 84-kDa OMP and a 95-kDa OMP have been isolated using immobilized human lactoferrin and were proposed to be the LbpA and LbpB proteins, respectively, constituting the lactoferrin receptor [74]. The LbpA and LbpB proteins have been expressed recombinantly and anti-LbpB mouse antibodies are bactericidal [75]. Although some variability between strains has been observed, LbpB remains a potential vaccine candidate. The same observations have been made using recombinant TbpA and TbpB proteins. The conservation of TbpB among strains is lower than that of TbpA. Children infected with *M. cat* show antibodies to OmpB1 in convalescent sera [19]. Recombinant TbpB binds human transferrin (recombinant TbpA does not) and elicits bactericidal antibodies in mice [76]. However, affinity-purified anti-TbpB human antibodies lack bactericidal activity although they react with all isolates tested [73].

1. CopB

CopB, an 81-kDa OMP similar to TonB-dependent OMP, is overexpressed in response to iron limitation. A *copB* mutant is severely impaired in its ability to utilize transferrin and lactoferrin as sole iron sources [77]. The sequence of this OMP is moderately conserved among strains. Most

of the variability is localized within three variable regions of the protein [78]. A monoclonal antibody against CopB-enhanced pulmonary bacterial clearance in an animal model exerts complement-dependent bactericidal activity against *M. cat*. This monoclonal antibody binds a 26-amino acid-oligopeptide corresponding to a surface-exposed region of CopB [79].

C. Other Protein Antigens

1. OmpCD

OmpCD is a 45- to 60-kDa heat-modifiable OMP that is highly conserved among *M. cat* strains. OmpCD might be analogous to OMP P5 of *H. influenzae* (see below) and OmpA from *Escherichia coli*. Moreover, the conservation of the protein sequence has been demonstrated among clinical isolates recovered at a 6-month interval from chronically infected patients [80]. Antibodies to the detergent-extracted and purified OmpCD elicited in mice and guinea pigs were shown to be bactericidal [81]. The protein contains at least two surface-exposed conserved epitopes and one of these epitopes is recognized by human convalescent sera [82]. Recombinant OmpCD induced strong protection in a rat pulmonary challenge model upon mucosal and parenteral immunization. Protection coincided with the presence of anti-OmpCD-specific antibodies in serum and broncho-alveolar lavages [83].

2. OmpE

OmpE is another heat-modifiable OMP. The gene encoding OmpE has been cloned and its sequence is already known. The predicted molecular mass of the matured OMP is 47 kDa. The *ompE* gene is conserved among strains [84]. Sequence analysis of the *ompE* gene from respiratory tract isolates from patients colonized with the same strain for at least 6 months indicated that the OmpE-encoding sequence remains stable during colonization [85]. Adults with chronic bronchitis have IgA antibodies to OmpE in their serum and sputum supernatants [86]. *M. cat* mutant strains lacking the *ompE* gene have been constructed. These mutant strains were more readily killed by human normal serum than the wild-type strains, suggesting that OmpE could be involved in serum resistance [87].

D. Lipopolysaccharide

Lipopolysaccharides may be one of the virulence factors of *M. cat*. Serological typing of *M. cat* using rabbit sera shows that three serotypes account for 95% of the isolates: A (60%), B (30%), and C (5%). However, no correlation between the serotype and the severity of infection has been found [44]. The structural characteristics and antigenic properties of *M. cat* LPS have been reviewed [40]. Lipopolysaccharides and, in particular, an epitope of LPS have been shown to be an important factor in the resistance to normal serum bactericidal activity. Indeed, *galE* mutants have a reduced resistance to serum killing [88].

Detoxified LPS conjugated to tetanus toxoid (TT) or to NTHi high-molecular-weight (HMW) proteins induced a protective immune response in a mouse lung challenge model. This protective immune response correlated with bactericidal antibody titers in the sera of animals [89]. These data suggest that LPS is a potential vaccine candidate.

III. NONTYPABLE *H. INFLUENZAE*

Nontypable *H. influenzae*, a nonmotile fastidious gram-negative rod, is an important cause of localized respiratory tract diseases beginning with the colonization of the upper respiratory mucosa. Otitis media, sinusitis, bronchitis, and community-acquired pneumonia due to NTHi are major causes of morbidity and mortality in both developed and nonindustrialized nations [90,91].

A. Pathogenesis and Variability

Nontypable *H. influenzae* exist as commensals in the human nasopharynx, and 40–80% of healthy children and adults are colonized [92]. Carriage of a given strain may persist for months [93]. Pathogenesis involves a contiguous spread of the bacteria within the respiratory tract, resulting in local disease in the middle ear, sinuses, or lungs. Modifications of the host defenses and the bacterium can transform this natural commensal into an infectious agent. For example, disruption of the mucociliary clearance, mucosal integrity or neutrophil functions by a viral infection, cigarette smoke, or allergies can lead to infection with NTHi. On the other hand, the balance between host defenses and NTHi virulence mechanisms can also be disrupted by a rapid and efficient adaptation of the bacteria. One adaptive mechanism of NTHi is the exchange of genetic information within this naturally transformable population after spread of different subtypes. Another mechanism, called antigenic drift, involves an irreversible substitution of amino acids in immunodominant regions of proteins. Finally, NTHi variability can be enhanced by phase variation that is characterized by reversible loss or gain of a defined structure. This mechanism can occur by *rec*-dependent inversion of DNA fragments but more commonly by slipped-strand mispairing during DNA replication. This leads to variation in the number of nucleotides in a homopolymeric stretch or a number of oligonucleotide repeats in a tandem array within the relevant gene.

By these mechanisms, NTHi has demonstrated the ability to adapt the antigenic character of both proteins and LOS, which constitutes the major component of the outer membrane, in response to a preexisting or developing immune response. Indeed, the proteins P1, P2, and P5 are targets of antibody responses and reveal antigenic drift to avoid the host immune system during persistent infection [94–96]. In the same way, LOS phase variation due to four loci, *lic-1* to *lic-3* and *lgtC*, produce a heterogeneous range of polysaccharides and enhance NTHi-invasive capabilities [43,45,97,98]. Phase variation of protein antigens was also demonstrated with respect to HMW1 and HMW2 as well as hemagglutinating pili [99,100].

Although antibiotic treatment usually eradicates infections caused by NTHi, antimicrobial resistance is increasing worldwide [101]. Thus, there is a demand for NTHi vaccines.

However, the development of NTHi vaccines is hampered by difficulties in identifying protective antigens and the lack of an in vitro correlate of immunity against this pathogen.

B. Killed Whole Cell Vaccines

Oral vaccines containing killed nontypable *H. influenzae* were previously tested in double-blind, randomized, controlled studies for the prevention of acute bronchitis. In the first study on oral immunization with NTHi, Clancy et al. [1] observed a 10-fold reduction in the incidence of acute bronchitis in adults. Nevertheless, without further vaccination, no significant protection was observed during the next winter [1]. In the second trial conducted on adult patients with chronic bronchitis, the incidence rate of acute bronchitis was significantly reduced in the vaccine group as compared with the placebo group. No difference was observed with regards to more severe lower respiratory disease. Protection was maximal at times of peak incidence of acute exacerbation, persisted for the duration of the 12-month follow-up period, and was associated with a reduction in the number of viable *H. influenzae* in sputum samples [2]. A third reported study demonstrated protection against the occurrence of acute infection in elderly subjects with chronic bronchitis. This protection correlated with transient reduction in the level of colonization by *H. influenzae* and allowed a reduced use of antibiotics [3]. Despite promising results, follow-up studies have not been reported.

C. Subunit Vaccines

Recombinant DNA technology offers the possibility of developing subunit vaccines, a strategy that uses only part of the pathogen to raise a protective immune response. Several antigenic components have been identified for nontypable *H. influenzae*.

D. Potential Protein Vaccine Antigens

1. Lipoprotein D

Lipoprotein D (LPD), encoded by the *hpd* gene, is a 42-kDa membrane-associated IgD-binding protein [102,103]. Lipoprotein D consists mainly of hydrophilic amino acids and contains a typical bacterial lipoprotein consensus sequence at its N-terminal region. The classification of LPD as a lipoprotein was further confirmed by the presence of covalently attached ester-linked and amine-linked fatty acids to the N-terminal cysteine residue [104]. Lipoprotein D is homologous to the periplasmic glycerophosphodiesterase GlpQ of *E. coli* and catalyzes the reaction of glycerophosphodiester to glycerol-3-phosphate [105]. Lipoprotein D is antigenically conserved and has been implicated in NTHi adhesion and invasion into host cells [105–107]. Akkoyunlu et al. [108] have demonstrated that in human donors, the levels of IgG antibodies to LPD start to increase after 1 year of age, and IgA after 2 years of age, whereas IgM levels start to increase as early as 6 months of age.

In rats, LPD was highly immunogenic and induced bactericidal antibodies [109]. Although immunization with LPD failed to protect rats from developing otitis media, it might affect the course of otitis media by promoting faster recovery [109]. In a chinchilla model of otitis media, bacteria were cleared more rapidly from the middle ear fluids of LPD-immunized animals [110]. The same authors also demonstrated that the delivery of anti-LPD serum by passive transfer reduced the incidence of middle ear effusion [110]. In a rat model [111], immunization with LPD tended to clear NTHi from the middle ear and induced a significant reduction of bacterial counts in the lungs.

2. P5 (LB1)

The P5 protein is a heat-modifiable, antigenically variable, major outer membrane protein that has been shown to bind to nasopharyngeal mucin [112] or to RSV-infected respiratory epithelial cells [8]. Recently, P5 was described as a ligand for the carcinoembryonic antigen family of cell adhesion molecules (CEACAMs) [7,113]. Anti-P5-specific antibodies had no protective capacity in an infant rat bacteremic model [114]. However, it has been shown that purified mouse anti-P5 antibodies were bactericidal for the homologous NTHi strain and a few heterologous strains. P5 is predicted to adopt an eight-stranded β-barrel structure with four extracellular loop regions [115–117].

One synthetic peptide, called LB1 and corresponding to the sequence of the third loop in P5 fused to a T-cell epitope, was designed by Bakaletz et al. [27]. Based on sequence variability of this region, NTHi strains were clustered in three groups (LB1-1, LB1-2, and LB1-3) [115,118]. The LB1 peptide was able to inhibit the adherence of NTHi to chinchilla ciliated tracheal mucosal epithelium (65% reduction in adhering bacteria). In a chinchilla NTHi nasopharyngeal colonization model, significantly earlier clearance was observed in animals immunized with this peptide. In two other experiments, chinchillas immunized with P5 or LB1 with either Freund's adjuvant or alum had lower nasopharyngeal and middle ear NTHi colonization than control animals [110]. A passive transfer of anti-LB1 antibodies or antibodies generated against a fusion of LPD and three LB1 variant peptide sequences designated LPD-LB1(f)$_{2,1,3}$ to chinchillas prior to intranasal challenge with NTHi significantly reduced the severity of signs and incidence of otitis media development [110]. In recent passive transfer experiments, antisera directed against LB1 or LPD-LB1(f)$_{2,1,3}$ were found to be highly protective against the induction of otitis media following intranasal challenge with heterologous NTHi strains [119].

3. OMP26

The OMP26 protein was originally purified from NTHi by preparative electrophoresis (sodium dodecyl sulfate polyacrylamide gel electrophoresis, SDS-PAGE) of an outer membrane preparation. It contains 174 amino acids, has a molecular mass of 26 kDa, and displays no heat-modifiable characteristics. Analysis of the deduced sequence shows that this protein bears a cleavable signal sequence of 23 amino acids. The deduced amino acid sequence of OMP26 is 56% identical to that of the *Pasteurella multocida* Skp protein. In the Enterobacteriaceae, the highly conserved Skp protein is a periplasmic protein (chaperone) that might be involved in

the translocation of LPS or OMPs to the outer membrane [120]. Nevertheless, the role of OMP26 in NTHi strains has yet to be determined. Southern blot analysis of the genomic DNA of NTHi strains with an *OMP26* gene probe demonstrated the high conservation of OMP26 among NTHi strains.

Rats immunized with OMP26 purified from NTHi displayed a significantly enhanced bacterial lung clearance following intranasal challenge with NTHi. An experiment with a heterologous NTHi strain resulted in a similarly enhanced clearance. Lymphocytes from animals immunized with OMP26 proliferated in vitro upon restimulation with OMP26 or OMP extracts from NTHi strains. Like immunization with killed bacteria [121], immunization with OMP26 resulted in protection that correlated with a greater number of phagocytic cells in the lungs [120].

In further studies, two recombinant forms of OMP26, a full length 28-kDa protein and a 26-kDa protein lacking the 23-amino-acid leader peptide, were evaluated. The protein that included the leader peptide was described as more effective in enhancing pulmonary clearance, and it induced better cell-mediated responses and higher titers of systemic and mucosal antibody [122].

4. HMW1/HMW2

High-molecular-weight surface-exposed proteins of NTHi that are major targets of human serum antibody during NTHi infection were shown to be implicated in bacterial adherence to human epithelial cells [9,123]. The two high-molecular-weight proteins of prototypic strain 12 were characterized. The HMW1 protein is 125 kDa in size and is encoded by a 4.6-kb open reading frame (ORF). The HMW2 protein has an apparent molecular mass of 120 kDa and is encoded by a 4.4-kb open reading frame. Despite their overall sequence similarity of 80%, HMW1 and HMW2 proteins display distinct cellular specificities, suggesting the recognition of distinct receptors. Both proteins are antigenically related to filamentous hemagglutinin, a known adhesin and colonization factor of *B. pertussis*. Although absent from encapsulated strains of *H. influenzae*, approximately 75% of NTHi clinical isolates expressed proteins immunologically and antigenically related to HMW1 and HMW2 produced by *H. influenzae* strain 12 [124]. By Southern blot analysis, the presence of HMW1 and HMW2 structural genes (referred to as hmw1A and hmw2A, respectively) was identified in 80% of strains tested [125]. Both *hmw1A* and *hmw2A* are flanked downstream by two additional genes, designated B and C, respectively [126]. HMW1B/HMW1C and HMW2B/HMW2C proteins are interchangeable and required for the normal processing and secretion of HMW1 and HMW2 [127]. By generating complementary chimeric proteins, the binding domains of HMW1 and HMW2 were recently localized to an approximately 360-amino-acid region near the N-terminus of the mature protein [128].

In the chinchilla model of otitis media, immunization with a purified protein preparation containing primarily HMW1 or HMW2 provided partial protection against intra-bullar challenge with NTHi strain 12 [129]. Interestingly, among animals immunized with either HMW1 or HMW2 that developed otitis media, isolates from the middle ear uniformly expressed reduced amount of HMW1 or HMW2, respectively. This suggested a downmodulation of the expression of those proteins. More recently, it has been demonstrated that the expression of both HMW1 and HMW2 is subject to phase variation and varies based on the number of 7-bp tandem repeats in the *hmw1A* and *hmw2A* promoters [99].

5. Hia/Hsf

Hia (*H. influenzae* adhesin) is a high-molecular-weight adhesion protein that is highly immunogenic. Expression of the *hia* gene in nonadherent *E. coli* strains was associated with adherence to cultured Chang conjunctival cells [6]. Hia is an autotransporter protein that undergoes no processing between the internal and C-terminal domains, and thus remains full-length and completely cell-associated, allowing maximal adhesive activity [130]. This protein is expressed by only a subset of NTHi strains (20–25%) and is absent in HMW1-expressing and HMW2-expressing strains [6]. As 95% of NTHi strains contain either *hmw* or *hia* genes [125], several authors envisioned that a combination of those two major nonpilus adhesins could be an effective vaccine formulation.

6. Hemagglutinating Pili

Hemagglutinating pili are helical structures of approximately 5 nm in diameter and up to 450 nm in length that promote agglutination of human erythrocytes and attachment to some, but not all, cells derived from human respiratory tissues and to human mucins [10,12,131]. *H. influenzae* pili show strain-to-strain immunological diversity, and 14 different pilus serotypes have been described [132]. Pili are present on both typable and NTHi strains, but pili expression is phase-variable [133]. Phase variation could be required during the course of infection because pili are important for the initial colonization of the human nasopharynx, but their expression may hinder subsequent steps in infection [10,134–136]. Antibodies directed against *H. influenzae* type B pili were bactericidal for the homologous strains but not for strains expressing heterologous pili [137]. In the same way, immunization with purified pili from a NTHi strain induced protection against homologous, but not heterologous, strains in an NTHi chinchilla model of otitis media [138]. It is interesting to note that a gene cluster containing five genes (*hifA–hifE*) is required for pilus assembly and function [133,139]. HifA is the major pilin subunit, HifB is a periplasmic chaperone, HifC is an outer membrane usher, and HifD and HifE are minor tip proteins, localized at the end of the pili. HifE antiserum completely blocks pilus-mediated hemagglutination, suggesting that HifE contains the pilus-binding domain and mediates pilus adherence [140,141]. Recent data demonstrated that anti-HifA antibodies inhibited the adhesion of type B and NTHi strains on mucins [12].

The expression of pili and the carriage of the *hic* gene (no function identified yet) are mutually exclusive in NTHi strains [142]. Irreversible loss of *hif* genes may represent an adaptative mechanism that profoundly influences the interactions of NTHi with its human host. This mechanism could be related to the reversible shutting off of *hif* genes by phase variation observed during Hib-persistent infection. An average of 18% of nonencapsulated *Haemophilus* strains has a fimbria gene cluster consisting of *hifA* to *hifE*, but differences in the frequency of fimbria cluster-positive strains were observed, depending on the source of isolates [143].

7. P1

This heat-modifiable surface-exposed protein accounts for ~ 10% of *H. influenzae* OMP content. Significant variability in the primary protein sequence and its ability to be heat-modified allowed it to be used as a form of subtyping for *H. influenzae* type B strains [94,144]. P1 has eight potentially surface-exposed loops [145]. Several distinct surface-exposed epitopes were identified in the antigenic domain of P1 but do not induce protective antibodies against a Hib infection in an animal challenge model [145,146]. Nevertheless, P1 extracted from NTHi enhanced homologous bacterial clearance from the lungs of rats after mucosal immunization [147]. More recently, chinchillas actively immunized with recombinant P1 protein were protected against otitis media due to homologous, but not heterologous, NTHi strains [148]. Strain-specific protective responses suggest that P1-based strategy will require the development of a polyvalent vaccine reflecting the P1 variability.

8. P2

This is the most prominent outer membrane protein. It self-associates as a homotrimer and acts as a porin, allowing the passage of molecules of 1.4 kDa or less through the outer membrane [149]. P2 protein is a target for bactericidal antibodies elicited during the antibody response against NTHi in humans [150]. Immunization with P2 protein induced enhanced pulmonary clearance of a homologous strain of NTHi in a rat model of infection [151]. Among the eight potential surface-exposed regions, loops 5, 6, and 8 were further studied [152–154]. For instance, antibodies directed against loop 6 of P2 induced complement-mediated bactericidal killing of several heterologous NTHi strains [155]. A potential drawback of using the P2 protein or a more conserved region thereof as vaccine molecules is that P2 porin exhibits marked diversity among strains of NTHi. Moreover, the horizontal transfer of P2 genes was demonstrated in four aboriginal infants persistently colonized with multiple strains of NTHi. The horizontal transfer of P2 genes encoding P2 with a highly heterogeneous surface-exposed region would function as a mechanism to evade a protective immune response [156].

9. P4

This 28-kDa surface-exposed lipoprotein is ubiquitous and conserved among *H. influenzae* strains [157]. P4 has a phosphomonoesterase activity and is involved in heme transport [23,158,159]. Despite some controversies, P4 appeared to induce bactericidal antibodies in mice and rabbits [157]. No bactericidal antibody production nor protection from infection was observed in chinchillas immunized with a mixture of P4, P6 (see below), and PCP (see below), but effusion and inflammation were significantly reduced [160]. Further evaluation of the P4 vaccine potential remains to be done.

10. P6

P6 is a 16-kDa peptidoglycan-associated lipoprotein (PAL), which is present in the outer membrane of all strains of NTHi and shows a high degree of sequence conservation [161–163]. P6 has been demonstrated as being immunogenic and able to induce bactericidal antibodies in rabbits, rats, and mice [30,160,162,164–166]. Moreover, clearance was observed after mucosal immunization with P6 in rat and mouse respiratory models as well as in an otitis media model [30,167,168]. In chinchillas, contradictory results were obtained probably because of differences in methods used. Green et al. [160] raised P6 antisera in chinchillas, but neither bactericidal activity nor protection against NTHi challenge was obtained. In subsequent studies, bactericidal antibodies and/or protection against otitis media in chinchillas were observed [169,170]. In humans, bactericidal antibodies directed against P6 were described [171]. In otitis-prone children, failure to recognize P6 as a specific immunogen may account for recurrent infections [172]. Moreover, antibodies directed against P6 in breast milk and nasopharyngeal secretions are associated with a decreased incidence of colonization with NTHi [173,174].

11. D15

This ~ 80-kDa OMP is conserved in both typable and NTHi strains [175,176]. Antibodies directed against D15 were found in eight of nine convalescent-phase sera from children with invasive Hib infection, suggesting that it might be an important immunogen. Affinity-purified D15-specific antibodies induced protection against the development of bacteremia in a rat pup model [175]. Also, anti-rD15 antibodies protected infant rats from bacteremia caused by *H. influenzae* type B or type A [176]. In a recent study, rabbit antisera directed against a 20-kDa N-terminal fragment protected infant rats against Hia or Hib bacteremia, indicating that immunodominant protective B-cell epitopes are located within this D15 fragment [177].

12. OapA

The opacity-associated protein A is a cell envelope protein responsible for the transparent colony phenotype of *H. influenzae* and required for efficient colonization of the nasopharynx in an infant rat model of *H. influenzae* carriage [178]. Further studies demonstrated that OapA contributes to binding to Chang epithelial cells and that its sequence appeared highly conserved among both encapsulated and nontypable *H. influenzae* strains [179].

13. Hap

This *H. influenzae* surface protein is associated with the capacity for intimate interactions with cultured epithelial cells and formation of microcolonies [11,13]. This nonpilus adhesin is an autotransporter protein composed of three domains: an N-terminal leader sequence, a serine protease domain (Hap_s), and a C-terminal outer membrane domain (Hap_s). The Hap_s domain is extracellularly released by autoproteolysis. Interestingly, the inhibition of Hap autoproteolysis resulted in augmented Hap-mediated adherence to respiratory epithelial cells and bacterial aggregation [11,180]. Recently, the Hap autoproteolysis mechanism was more fully characterized [181].

14. HtrA

This moiety (also called Hin 47) is a stress response protein of 46 kDa that functions as a serine protease and is highly conserved among encapsulated and NTHi strains [182]. Although predicted to be a periplasmic protein, surface expression under stress conditions may occur. The protective capacities of recombinant HtrA protein and two site-directed mutants (H91A and S197A) lacking the serine protease activity were evaluated. The three proteins were immunogenic and equally protective in a passive infant rat model of bacteremia. In a chinchilla model of otitis media, only the rHtrA and the H91A mutant induced protection [182]. Absence of protection with the S197A mutant may come from an improper folding observed by circular dichroism spectroscopy [183].

15. PCP

This 16-kDa outer membrane lipoprotein is conserved in all *H. influenzae* tested, and antiserum directed against this protein showed high complement-mediated bactericidal activity [184]. When combined with P4 and P6 proteins, PCP did not induce protection in a chinchilla model of otitis media, but effusion and inflammation measured by tympanometry were significantly reduced [160].

E. Iron and Heme Acquisition Proteins

Iron acquisition by *H. influenzae* occurs by a complex process involving several outer membrane or secreted proteins binding to hemoglobin or hemoglobin–haptoglobin (HhuA, HgpA, HgbA, HgbB, and HgbC) [185–187], hemopexin (HxuA and HxuC) [188,189], transferrin (Tbp1 and Tbp2) [20,190,191], and lactoferrin [191]. Sera from healthy adults recognized Tbp1 and Tbp2, suggesting that both proteins are expressed in vivo [21]. More recently, the expression of *tbpA*, *tbpB*, and *hgpA* genes by *H. influenzae* during acute otitis media was confirmed by reverse transcription polymerase chain reaction (RT-PCR) [24]. Outer membrane localization and expression in in vivo conditions suggest a potential role for these iron transport proteins as vaccine immunogens.

F. Lipopolysaccharide

The LPS of gram-negative bacteria is a complex amphipathic molecule composed of lipids and sugars that represents the main component of the outer leaflet of the bacterial outer membrane. In contrast to the Enterobacteriaceae, the *H. influenzae* LPS lacks the O-antigen (repeating side chain) and

Table 1   List of In Silico Discovered *M. cat* Potential Vaccine Candidates

GSK number	Homology	Type	Tested
1	Adhesin component	Adhesin	Yes
2	Adhesin component	Adhesin	Yes
3	Hsf	Adhesin/autotransporter	Yes
4	UspA1	Adhesin/autotransporter	
5	UspA2	Adhesin/autotransporter	
6	Ail adhesin	Adhesin/porin	Yes
7	OmpA	Adhesin/porin	
8	Opacity protein	Adhesin/porin	
9	Outer membrane esterase	Enzyme/autotransporter	
10	Phospholipase	Enzyme/porin	Yes
11	OmpCD	Outer membrane	
12	OmpE	Outer membrane	
13	Outer membrane	Outer membrane	
14	YtfN	Outer membrane	Yes
15	—	Outer membrane	
16	TolC/CyaE	Efflux	
17	TolC/MtrE	Efflux	Yes
18	D15/Omp85	Porin	Yes
19	YtfM/D15	Porin	
20	FHAC/HecB	Porin	
21	PorB	Porin	
22	Porin	Porin	
23	Porin	Porin	
24	PilQ (type IV pili)	Porin/secretin	Yes
25	CopB	Porin/tonB-dependent	
26	HasR	Porin/tonB-dependent	
27	Hemoglobin binding	Porin/tonB-dependent	
28	TonB-dependent receptor	Porin/tonB-dependent	
29	TonB-dependent receptor	Porin/tonB-dependent	
30	TbpB	Porin/tonB-dependent	
31	TbpA	Porin/tonB-dependent	
32	LbpB	Lipoprotein OM	
33	TbpB	Lipoprotein OM	
34	Pal	Lipoprotein OM	Yes
35	PliP	Lipoprotein OM	
36	NlpE	Lipoprotein OM	Yes
37	Pna1	Lipoprotein OM	Yes
38	Pal	Lipoprotein OM	Yes
39	PlpA	Lipoprotein OM	Yes
40	NlpD	Lipoprotein OM	Yes
41	Putative outer membrane lipoprotein	Lipoprotein OM	Yes
42	OmlA	Lipoprotein	Yes
43	Putative hemolysin	Lipoprotein	Yes
44	Putative fimbrial biogenesis	Lipoprotein	Yes
45	Putative lipoprotein	Lipoprotein	Yes
46	No	Lipoprotein	
47	No	Lipoprotein	Yes
48	No	Lipoprotein	Yes
49	No	Lipoprotein	
50	No	Lipoprotein	
51	No	Lipoprotein	
52	No	Lipoprotein	Yes
53	No	Lipoprotein	Yes
54	MtrC	Lipoprotein	
55	Substrate binding	Lipoprotein	
56	Solute binding	Lipoprotein	
57	Solute binding	Lipoprotein	
58	BRO β-lactamase	Lipoprotein	

Table 1 Continued

GSK number	Homology	Type	Tested
59	Hypothetical	Lipoprotein	
60	Hypothetical	Lipoprotein	
61	No	Lipoprotein	
62	No	Lipoprotein	
63	No	Lipoprotein	
64	No	Lipoprotein	
65	No	Lipoprotein	
66	HtrA	Periplasmic	Yes
67	Macrophage infectivity potentiator	Periplasmic	Yes
68	Pal	Periplasmic	
69	HlyA hemolysin *Serratia*	Protease	
70	TlyC hemolysin	Protease	Yes
71	Collagenase	Protease	

is therefore often called lipooligosaccharide (LOS). The LOS of NTHi is antigenically heterogenous. This is mainly due to NTHi outer core region variability, the lipid A and inner core region being more conserved. Nontypable *H. influenzae* LOS is a major surface antigen that may be implicated in virulence and is described as a potential protective antigen. Human antibodies and mouse monoclonal antibodies directed against LOS are bactericidal for NTHi [123,192]. A mouse monoclonal antibody directed against NTHi LOS was opsonic and enhanced clearance in a murine pulmonary challenge model [193].

Using anhydrous hydrazine-detoxified NTHi strain 9274 LOS (type III) lacking the terminal lacto-*N*-neotetraose, Gu et al. [194,195] prepared two conjugates using tetanus toxoid or high-molecular-weight proteins HMW as carriers. Both conjugates were immunogenic in mice and rabbits. Conjugate-induced LOS antibodies elicited complement-mediated bactericidal activity against homologous and heterologous NTHi strains [194,195]. Moreover, vaccination with the two conjugates resulted in significant protection against experimental otitis media in chinchillas. This protection correlated with high anti-LOS titers in the chinchilla sera and middle ear fluids. Biological activities in the sera of the protected chinchillas sera were measured and 46% of the serum samples induced inhibition of NTHi adherence onto epithelial cells, 49% induced bactericidal activity, and 49% showed opsonophagocytic activity [196].

G. In Silico Antigen Discovery

Whole genome sequencing opens the possibility of identifying "in silico" new surface-exposed or secreted proteins that can be tested as new potential vaccine candidates. We have followed such a strategy to identify new *M. cat* and NTHi vaccine candidates.

1. *M. cat*

The genome from *M. cat* strain ATCC43617 was used for screening while the sequencing was still in progress. The genome was sequenced by Incyte Genomics, Palo Alto, CA. The last version of the genome screened was split into 41 DNA fragments (Patent WO0078968, Genbank accession nos. AX067426–AX06766) of a total length of 1.91 Mb, where 1513 open reading frames were predicted.

To identify surface-exposed proteins, such as porins, fimbrial and nonfimbrial adhesins, lipoproteins, other outer membrane proteins, and periplasmic and secreted proteins, the strategy was based on screening by homology. Surface-exposed or antigenic proteins previously described in other bacteria were used as query for performing Blast searches. To increase the sensitivity, hidden Markov models (HMMs) derived from multiple alignments of protein domains were used to screen the ORFs [197,198]. Specific identification of porins or porinlike proteins and lipoproteins was used as second strategy. Porin detection was based on the identification of signal sequence within ORF, prediction of β-strand predominance, and presence of a C-terminal aromatic amino acid. Lipoprotein detection was based on identification of a type II secretion signal. The ORFs selected were annotated by homology and analyzed for detection of signal sequence, transmembrane regions, and specific features from Prosite, Pfam, Blocks, and Prints [199–204].

Among the *M. cat*-predicted ORFs, 71 ORFs were selected for further evaluation; 61 previously unknown ORFs included 6 predicted adhesins, 2 outer membrane enzymes, 3 proteins of unknown function, 2 outer membrane proteins involved in a type I secretion system, 6 porins, 4 additional porins involved in heme acquisition, 1 porinlike protein component of type IV pili, 31 lipoproteins of which eight were predicted to be anchored in the outer membrane, 3 periplasmic proteins, 2 potential hemolysins, and 1 potential collagenase (Table 1).

The protective potential of 27 proteins was assessed in vitro by anti-adhesion and bactericidal tests and in vivo in a mouse lung infection model. The 27 genes were cloned and expressed in *E. coli*; recombinant proteins were then purified and injected in rabbit and mice. The antiadhesion activity of induced antibodies was tested by measuring the inhibition of adhesion of *M. cat* onto epithelial cells in the presence of immune sera. The bactericidal activity of the antibodies was tested by measuring the complement-mediated cytotoxic activity of immune sera. The mouse lung infection model was based on the analysis of lung invasion by *M. cat* following a standard intranasal challenge to vaccinated mice. Nine proteins yielded positive results with the mouse infection model; four of them were also positive in the bactericidal assay and one was positive in the antiadhesion assay. Furthermore, one protein was positive in the anti-adhesion assay only, and one in the bactericidal assay only (data not shown).

2. Nontypable *H. influenzae*

The genome of nontypable *H. influenzae* strain 3224A was sequenced to 4× coverage by the University of Oklahoma. The shotgun sequence data were assembled into 535 DNA fragments for a total length of 1.67 Mb, covering 90% of the genome, and around 1800 ORFs were identified. The comparison of the NTHi genome with the HiRd genome [205] showed that the DNA sequences are very similar (around 95% identity) but that both genomes contained specific regions. NTHi-specific regions are, together, longer than 0.1 Mb and comprise more than 100 ORFs.

The strategy for identifying NTHi surface-exposed proteins was similar to that used to screen the *M. cat* genome. Because many NTHi ORFs were not complete, the ORFs of HiRd have been used as reference [205]. The corresponding sequence in NTHi was subsequently determined by sequencing. Furthermore, each ORF located within the NTHi-specific regions has been examined.

With respect to known antigens, 14 have been found, with Hmw1, Hmw2, and Hap being located in the NTHi-specific regions. Additional selected proteins comprise three adhesins VirG, YadA, and YadA-c, but none was in-frame (confirmed by sequencing). We also selected 16 lipoproteins of which 14 are potentially anchored in the outer membrane, 1 protein is involved in a type I secretion system, 8 porins are involved in iron acquisition, 5 porins or porinlike proteins, 5 other outer membranes, 2 periplasmic proteins, and 2 secreted proteins (Table 2). Furthermore, in an NTHi-specific region, there were four neighboring ORFs similar to one another (around 80% identity). They were predicted to have a signal sequence and were homologous to potentially antigenic surface exposed proteins.

In another NTHi-specific region, a set of genes similar to bacteriophage P1 was found. At the end of this phagelike genome, six hypothetical genes were predicted. They might encode proteins playing a role in virulence. Indeed, phage-associated virulence genes have been observed in other bacterial genomes such as *Streptococcus pyogenes* and *N. meningitidis*. Some of them encode proteins able to induce bactericidal antibodies against the organism from which they were derived [206,207]. Those six hypothetical proteins could thus be protein vaccine candidates.

The protective potential of five proteins has been assessed in vivo in a mouse infection lung model similar to the one used for *M. cat* proteins. Of those, three proteins yielded positive results. These proteins are well conserved among NTHi strains.

IV. FUTURE CHALLENGES

Nontypable *H. influenzae* and *M. cat* cause a number of respiratory infectious diseases, particularly in the very young and very old. Immune prophylaxis by way of active or passive immunization represents an important tool toward improved control of these diseases. It is very likely that such control programs will eventually result in improved public health and are to be welcomed, in addition to similar programs aimed to prevent infectious diseases due to influenza, pneumococci, and RSV, among others. A further clarification of the relative importance of each of these infectious agents in diseases such as otitis media warrants careful epidemiological studies. Pediatric pneumonia in developing countries has, to some extent, been investigated [208–210]. Further information from various regions of the world is needed. Pediatric otitis has been studied extensively. It appears that a wide variety of viral agents (RSV influenza, parainfluenza, adenoviruses, and rhinoviruses) and a limited number of bacteria (pneumococci, NTHi/*M. cat*) are the predominant causes. Quite often, it seems that a mild viral infection precedes a bacterial otitis [211]. It is remarkable that group A streptococci have gradually disappeared as a major otitis-causing agent as compared to 50–100 years ago [212]. Adult (particularly in the very old)-sustaining pneumonia, bronchitis, and chronic obstructive pulmonary disease (COPD) also are infections where population-based immunization programs are likely to become important tools to improve public health. Influenza and pneumococcal vaccines already play an important role in the elderly and the public acceptance is still growing. Further epidemiological data on the relative importance of infections agents causing adult pneumonia are highly needed to allow rational vaccine development and societal implementation to become a reality.

The identification of protective antigens from NTHi and *M. cat* is difficult. These bacteria are noncapsulated, the surface proteins and lipopolysaccharides demonstrate a high variability, and no major exotoxins have been identified. This suggests that the successful principles used in developing many bacterial vaccines such as targeting capsular polysaccharides (preferentially conjugated to protein), detoxified exotoxins, or single surface proteins cannot be applied.

On the other hand, some success has been achieved with oral killed whole cell NTHi, implying that a combination of a number of protective surface antigens can lead to effective vaccines. Over the years, a number of surface antigens that represent candidate antigens, such as the adhesins (HMW proteins, Hia, pili, Hap, P5), the iron uptake systems (Tbps, Lbps, hemoglobin/hemopexin uptake systems), and other candidates as described in this review have been identified. Similar candidates have been identified for *M. cat* (Omp106, UspAs, pili, Tbps, Lbps, etc.). Aside from surface proteins, the lipopolysaccharides of NTHi and *M. cat* represent attractive antigens because these are major surface components and these molecules play an important role in the pathogenesis of NTHi/*M. cat* infectious diseases. Unfortunately, LPS also reveals extensive antigenic and phase variability [40–45]. Nowadays, the unraveling of the sequence of a bacterial genome has become standard practice, although the first genome available in 1995 for *H. influenzae* strain Rd was a major scientific breakthrough [205]. However, strain Rd is not representative for the major NTHi clonal lineages responsible for infectious diseases [213].

Table 2 List of In Silico Discovered NTHi Potential Vaccine Candidates

GSK	Homology	Type	NTHi-specific	Comment	Lung infection
1	YadA	Adhesin		No start	
2	VirG	Adhesin	Yes	No start	
3	Hap	Adhesin	Yes		
4	YadA-c	Adhesin	Yes	No start	
5	Hmw1	Adhesin	Yes		
6	Hmw2	Adhesin	Yes		
7	Hap	Adhesin/autotransporter	Yes		
8	P5	Adhesin/porin			
20	LPD	Lipoprotein OM			
21	P4	Lipoprotein OM			
22	P6	Lipoprotein OM			
23	PCP	Lipoprotein OM			
34	TbpB	Lipoprotein OM			
35	LbpB	Lipoprotein OM			
24	HlpA	Lipoprotein OM			−
31	MltA	Lipoprotein OM			
28	NlpB	Lipoprotein OM			
30	NlpC1	Lipoprotein OM			
27	NlpC2	Lipoprotein OM			+
25	NlpD	Lipoprotein OM			
29	NlpD2	Lipoprotein OM			
26	Slp	Lipoprotein OM			+
32	Lipo930	Lipoprotein			
33	Lipo162	Lipoprotein			
9	MtrE	Efflux			
43	comE	Porin			
44	P1/FadL	Porin			
45	P2	Porin			
46	D15	Porin			
47	D15b	Porin			−
50	TbpA	TonB/porin			
51	LbpA	TonB/porin			
52	HasR	TonB/porin			
53	Fe receptor	TonB/porin			
54	Fe receptor	TonB/porin			
55	Fe receptor	TonB/porin			
56	Fe receptor	TonB/porin			
57	Fe receptor	TonB/porin			
36	OstA	OMP			
37	YtfN	OMP			
38	—	OMP			
39	—	OMP			+
40	—	OMP			
41	Omp26	Peri			
42	Htra	Peri			
48	IgA protease	Protease/secreted/autotransporter			
49	OapA	Secreted			
10	Antigenic ORF	Periplasmic or secreted	Yes		
11	Antigenic ORF	Periplasmic or secreted	Yes		
12	Antigenic ORF	Periplasmic or secreted	Yes		
13	Antigenic ORF	Periplasmic or secreted	Yes		
14	—	Phage-associated	Yes		
15	—	Phage-associated	Yes		
16	—	Phage-associated	Yes		
17	—	Phage-associated	Yes		
18	—	Phage-associated	Yes		
19	—	Phage-associated	Yes		

We decided to sequence strain 3224A and discovered that approximately 100 additional open reading frames (absent in Rd) are present. In silico antigen discovery is a powerful tool that enables one to screen the genome systematically for homologues of known protective antigens from other bacterial species. It is also possible to look for specific sequence features associated with families of proteins such as porins, lipoproteins, proteins containing signal peptides, etc. In silico mining has been successful in finding conserved protective surface proteins in case of the pneumococcus [214]. A similar approach has been used for the meningococcus, but conserved candidates remain to be found from genome sequence, as opposed to antigens described previously. The availability of full genome sequences will likely disclose further possible candidates within many bacterial species.

The consolidation of an antigen as a robust vaccine candidate requires multiple preclinical evaluations using stringently validated animal models and other tests. An example of such a model is the pertussis mouse lung clearance assay that accurately mimics the clinical effectiveness of the different acellular pertussis vaccines, being composed of pertussis toxin filamentous hemagglutinin, pertactin, and/or fimbriae in various combinations [215]. It is hoped that similar lung clearance/pneumonia models are equally predictive for protection induced by candidate antigens in case of *Streptococcus pneumoniae*, NTHi, and *M. cat*. Aside from preclinical models, one can evaluate antigens by using human nasopharyngeal colonization as readout after challenge. Preclinical otitis models have been developed to be able to evaluate vaccine candidates from the pneumococcus and NTHi [27,216].

Carefully designed preclinical and human nasopharyngeal challenge studies are needed to investigate a number of preselected candidates before clinical studies in the target populations (infants and elderly). The preselection process is a critical step and depends upon high-throughput but still robust preclinical models. Finally, formulation, adjuvantation, and route of administration represent critical parameters for immunization efforts against NTHi and *M. cat* respiratory infectious diseases for which mucosal immunity likely plays an important role.

REFERENCES

1. Clancy R, et al. Oral immunisation with killed *Haemophilus influenzae* for protection against acute bronchitis in chronic obstructive lung disease. Lancet 1985; 2:1395–1397.
2. Lehmann D, et al. Reduction in the incidence of acute bronchitis by an oral *Haemophilus influenzae* vaccine in patients with chronic bronchitis in the highlands of Papua New Guinea. Am Rev Respir Dis 1991; 144:324–330.
3. Tandon MK, Gebski V. A controlled trial of a killed *Haemophilus influenzae* vaccine for prevention of acute exacerbations of chronic bronchitis. Aust NZ J Med 1991; 21:427–432.
4. Foxwell AR, et al. Nontypeable *Haemophilus influenzae*: pathogenesis and prevention. Microbiol Mol Biol Rev 1998; 62:294–308.
5. Rao VK, et al. Molecular determinants of the pathogenesis of disease due to non-typable *Haemophilus influenzae*. FEMS Microbiol Rev 1999; 23:99–129.
6. Barenkamp SJ, St Geme JWI. Identification of a second family of high-molecular-weight adhesion proteins expressed by non-typable *Haemophilus influenzae*. Mol Microbiol 1996; 19:1215–1223.
7. Hill DJ, et al. The variable P5 proteins of typeable and nontypeable *Haemophilus influenzae* target human CEACAM1. Mol Microbiol 2001; 39:850–862.
8. Jiang Z, et al. Fimbria-mediated enhanced attachment of nontypeable *Haemophilus influenzae* to respiratory syncytial virus-infected respiratory epithelial cells. Infect Immun 1999; 67:187–192.
9. St Geme JWI, et al. High-molecular-weight proteins of nontypable *Haemophilus influenzae* mediate attachment to human epithelial cells. Proc Natl Acad Sci USA 1993; 90: 2875–2879.
10. Gilsdorf JR, et al. Role of pili in *Haemophilus influenzae* adherence to, and internalization by, respiratory cells. Pediatr Res 1996; 39:343–348.
11. Hendrixson DR, St Geme JWI. The *Haemophilus influenzae* Hap serine protease promotes adherence and microcolony formation, potentiated by a soluble host protein. Mol Cell 1998; 2:841–850.
12. Kubiet M, et al. Pilus-mediated adherence of *Haemophilus influenzae* to human respiratory mucins. Infect Immun 2000; 68:3362–3367.
13. StGeme JWI, et al. A *Haemophilus influenzae* IgA protease-like protein promotes intimate interaction with human epithelial cells. Mol Microbiol 1994; 14:217–233.
14. Swords WE, et al. Non-typeable *Haemophilus influenzae* adhere to and invade human bronchial epithelial cells via an interaction of lipooligosaccharide with the PAF receptor. Mol Microbiol 2000; 37:13–27.
15. Lafontaine ER, et al. The UspA1 protein and a second type of UspA2 protein mediate adherence of *Moraxella catarrhalis* to human epithelial cells in vitro. J Bacteriol 2000; 182:1364–1373.
16. Ahmed K, et al. Attachment of *Moraxella catarrhalis* to pharyngeal epithelial cells is mediated by a glycosphingolipid receptor. FEMS Microbiol Lett 1996; 135:305–309.
17. van Schilfgaarde M, et al. *Haemophilus influenzae* localized in epithelial cell layers is shielded from antibiotics and antibody-mediated bactericidal activity. Microb Pathog 1999; 26:249–262.
18. Campagnari AA, et al. Growth of *Moraxella catarrhalis* with human transferrin and lactoferrin: expression of iron-repressible proteins without siderophore production. Infect Immun 1994; 62:4909–4914.
19. Campagnari AA, et al. Outer membrane protein B1, an iron-repressible protein conserved in the outer membrane of *Moraxella (Branhamella) catarrhalis*, binds human transferrin. Infect Immun 1996; 64:3920–3924.
20. Gray-Owen SD, et al. Identification and characterization of genes encoding the human transferrin-binding proteins from *Haemophilus influenzae*. Infect Immun 1995; 63:1201–1210.
21. Holland J, et al. Evidence for in vivo expression of transferrin-binding proteins in *Haemophilus influenzae* type b. Infect Immun 1992; 60:2986–2991.
22. Luke NR, Campagnari AA. Construction and characterization of *Moraxella catarrhalis* mutants defective in expression of transferrin receptors. Infect Immun 1999; 67:5815–5819.
23. Reidl J, Mekalanos JJ, et al. Lipoprotein e(P4) is essential for hemin uptake by *Haemophilus influenzae*. J Exp Med 1996; 183:621–629.
24. Whitby PW, et al. Transcription of genes encoding iron and heme acquisition proteins of *Haemophilus influenzae* during acute otitis media. Infect Immun 1997; 65:4696–4700.
25. Hol C, et al. Complement resistance in *Branhamella (Moraxella) catarrhalis*. Lancet 1993; 341:1281.

26. Williams BJ, et al. Serum resistance in an invasive, non-typeable *Haemophilus influenzae* strain. Infect Immun 2001; 69:695–705.

27. Bakaletz LO, et al. Relative immunogenicity and efficacy of two synthetic chimeric peptides of fimbrin as vaccinogens against nasopharyngeal colonization by nontypeable *Haemophilus influenzae* in the chinchilla. Vaccine 1997; 15:955–961.

28. Fulghum RS, et al. Longitudinal studies of experimental otitis media with *Haemophilus influenzae* in the gerbil. Int J Pediatr Otorhinolaryngol 1985; 9:101–114.

29. Kyd J, et al. Investigation of mucosal immunisation in pulmonary clearance of *Moraxella* (*Branhamella*) *catarrhalis*. Vaccine 1999; 18:398–406.

30. Kyd JM, et al. Enhanced respiratory clearance of nontypeable *Haemophilus influenzae* following mucosal immunization with P6 in a rat model. Infect Immun 1995; 63:2931–2940.

31. Melhus A, et al. Nontypeable and encapsulated *Haemophilus influenzae* yield different clinical courses of experimental otitis media. Acta Otolaryngol 1994; 114:289–294.

32. Soriano F, et al. Role of *Streptococcus pneumoniae* and *Haemophilus influenzae* in the development of acute otitis media and otitis media with effusion in a gerbil model. J Infect Dis 2000; 181:646–652.

33. Westman E, et al. *Moraxella catarrhalis*-induced purulent otitis media in the rat middle ear. Structure, protection, and serum antibodies. APMIS 1999; 107:737–746.

34. Wizemann TM, et al. Use of a whole genome approach to identify vaccine molecules affording protection against *Streptococcus pneumoniae* infection. Infect Immun 2001; 69: 1593–1598.

35. Pizza M, et al. Identification of vaccine candidates against serogroup B meningococcus by whole-genome sequencing. Science 2000; 287:1816–1820.

36. Granoff DM, et al. A novel mimetic antigen eliciting protective antibody to *Neisseria meningitidis*. J Immunol 2001; 167:6487–6496.

37. Jacques M. Role of lipo-oligosaccharides and lipopolysaccharides in bacterial adherence. Trends Microbiol 1996; 4:408–409.

38. Moxon ER, et al. Bacterial lipopolysaccharides: candidate vaccines to prevent *Neisseria meningitidis* and *Haemophilus influenzae* infections. Adv Exp Med Biol 1998; 435:237–243.

39. Swords WE, et al. Binding of the non-typeable *Haemophilus influenzae* lipooligosaccharide to the PAF receptor initiates host cell signalling. Cell Microbiol 2001; 3:525–536.

40. Holme T, et al. The lipopolysaccharide of *Moraxella catarrhalis* structural relationships and antigenic properties. Eur J Biochem 1999; 265:524–529.

41. Inzana TJ. Electrophoretic heterogeneity and interstrain variation of the lipopolysaccharide of *Haemophilus influenzae*. J Infect Dis 1983; 148:492–499.

42. Maskell DJ, et al. Molecular biology of phase-variable lipopolysaccharide biosynthesis by *Haemophilus influenzae*. J Infect Dis 1992; 165(suppl 1):S90–S92.

43. Tong HH, et al. Evaluation of phase variation of nontypeable *Haemophilus influenzae* lipooligosaccharide during nasopharyngeal colonization and development of otitis media in the chinchilla model. Infect Immun 2000; 68: 4593–4597.

44. Vaneechoutte M, et al. Serological typing of *Branhamella catarrhalis* strains on the basis of lipopolysaccharide antigens. J Clin Microbiol 1990; 28:182–187.

45. Weiser JN, Pan N. Adaptation of *Haemophilus influenzae* to acquired and innate humoral immunity based on phase variation of lipopolysaccharide. Mol Microbiol 1998; 30: 767–775.

46. Gordon JE. The gram-negative cocci in colds and influenza. Influenza studies VII. J Infect Dis 1921; 29:462–494.

47. Vaneechoutte M, et al. Respiratory tract carrier rates of *Moraxella* (*Branhamella*) *catarrhalis* in adults and children and interpretation of the isolation of *M. catarrhalis* from sputum. J Clin Microbiol 1990; 28:2674–2680.

48. Sethi S, Murphy TF. Bacterial infection in chronic obstructive pulmonary disease in 2000: a state-of-the-art review. Clin Microbiol Rev 2001; 14:336–363.

49. Faden H, et al. Epidemiology of *Moraxella catarrhalis* in children during the first 2 years of life: relationship to otitis media. J Infect Dis 1994; 169:1312–1317.

50. Mathers K, et al. Antibody response to outer membrane proteins of *Moraxella catarrhalis* in children with otitis media. Pediatr Infect Dis J 1999; 18:982–988.

51. Goldblatt D, et al. Association of Gm allotypes with the antibody response to the outer membrane proteins of a common upper respiratory tract organism, *Moraxella catarrhalis*. J Immunol 1994; 153:5316–5320.

52. Goldblatt D, et al. *Branhamella catarrhalis*: antigenic determinants and the development of the IgG subclass response in childhood. J Infect Dis 1990; 162:1128–1135.

53. Chapman AJ Jr, et al. Development of bactericidal antibody during *Branhamella catarrhalis* infection. J Infect Dis 1985; 151:878–882.

54. Jordan KL, et al. A comparison of serum bactericidal activity and phenotypic characteristics of bacteremic, pneumonia-causing strains, and colonizing strains of *Branhamella catarrhalis*. Am J Med 1990; 88:28S–32S.

55. Murphy TF, Loeb MR. Isolation of the outer membrane of *Branhamella catarrhalis*. Microb Pathog 1989; 6:159–174.

56. Unhanand M, et al. Pulmonary clearance of *Moraxella catarrhalis* in an animal model. J Infect Dis 1992; 165:644–650.

57. Maciver I, et al. Effect of immunization of pulmonary clearance of *Moraxella catarrhalis* in an animal model. J Infect Dis 1993; 168:469–472.

58. Marrs CF, Weir S. Pili (fimbriae) of *Branhamella* species. Am J Med 1990; 88:36S–40S.

59. Ahmed K, et al. Expression of fimbriae and host response in *Branhamella catarrhalis* respiratory infections. Microbiol Immunol 1994; 38:767–771.

60. Rikitomi N, et al. *Moraxella* (*Branhamella*) *catarrhalis* adherence to human bronchial and oropharyngeal cells: the role of adherence in lower respiratory tract infections. Microbiol Immunol 1997; 41:487–494.

61. Helminen ME, et al. A large, antigenically conserved protein on the surface of *Moraxella catarrhalis* is a target for protective antibodies. J Infect Dis 1994; 170:867–872.

62. Samukawa T, et al. Immune response to surface protein A of *Streptococcus pneumoniae* and to high-molecular-weight outer membrane protein A of *Moraxella catarrhalis* in children with acute otitis media. J Infect Dis 2000; 181:1842–1845.

63. Chen D, et al. The levels and bactericidal capacity of antibodies directed against the UspA1 and UspA2 outer membrane proteins of *Moraxella* (*Branhamella*) *catarrhalis* in adults and children. Infect Immun 1999; 67:1310–1316.

64. Aebi C, et al. A protective epitope of *Moraxella catarrhalis* is encoded by two different genes. Infect Immun 1997; 65:4367–4377.

65. Aebi C, et al. Phenotypic effect of isogenic uspA1 and uspA2 mutations on *Moraxella catarrhalis* 035E. Infect Immun 1998; 66:3113–3119.

66. McMichael JC, et al. Isolation and characterization of two proteins from *Moraxella catarrhalis* that bear a common epitope. Infect Immun 1998; 66:4374–4381.

67. Lafontaine ER, et al. The UspA1 protein and a second type of UspA2 protein mediate adherence of *Moraxella catarrhalis* to human epithelial cells in vitro. J Bacteriol 2000; 182:1364–1373.

68. Lafontaine ER, et al. Expression of the *Moraxella*

catarrhalis UspA1 protein undergoes phase variation and is regulated at the transcriptional level. J Bacteriol 2001; 183:1540–1551.

69. Hoiczyk E, et al. Structure and sequence analysis of *Yersinia* YadA and *Moraxella* UspAs reveal a novel class of adhesins. EMBO J 2000; 19:5989–5999.

70. Tucker K, et al. *Moraxella catarrhalis* outer membrane protein-106 polypeptide, gene sequence and uses thereof. US Patent US6214981 B1. Antex Biologics Inc., Application No. 08/968685, 2001, filed November 12, 1997.

71. Forsgren A, et al. Isolation and characterization of a novel IgD-binding protein from *Moraxella catarrhalis*. J Immunol 2001; 167:2112–2120.

72. Mathers KE, et al. Characterisation of an outer membrane protein of *Moraxella catarrhalis*. FEMS Immunol Med Microbiol 1997; 19:231–236.

73. Chen D, et al. Evaluation of a 74-kDa transferrin-binding protein from *Moraxella (Branhamella) catarrhalis* as a vaccine candidate. Vaccine 1999; 18:109–118.

74. Bonnah RA, et al. Biochemical and immunological properties of lactoferrin binding proteins from *Moraxella (Brannhamella) catarrhalis*. Microb Pathog 1998; 24:89–100.

75. Du RP, et al. Cloning and expression of the *Moraxella catarrhalis* lactoferrin receptor genes. Infect Immun 1998; 66:3656–3665.

76. Myers LE, et al. The transferrin binding protein B of *Moraxella catarrhalis* elicits bactericidal antibodies and is a potential vaccine antigen. Infect Immun 1998; 66:4183–4192.

77. Aebi C, et al. Expression of the CopB outer membrane protein by *Moraxella catarrhalis* is regulated by iron and affects iron acquisition from transferrin and lactoferrin. Infect Immun 1996; 64:2024–2030.

78. Sethi S, et al. Antigenic heterogeneity and molecular analysis of CopB of *Moraxella (Branhamella) catarrhalis*. Infect Immun 1997; 65:3666–3671.

79. Aebi C, et al. Mapping of a protective epitope of the CopB outer membrane protein of *Moraxella catarrhalis*. Infect Immun 1998; 66:540–548.

80. Hsiao CB, et al. Outer membrane protein CD of *Branhamella catarrhalis*: sequence conservation in strains recovered from the human respiratory tract. Microb Pathog 1995; 19:215–225.

81. Yang YP, et al. The major outer membrane protein, CD, extracted from *Moraxella (Branhamella) catarrhalis* is a potential vaccine antigen that induces bactericidal antibodies. FEMS Immunol Med Microbiol 1997; 17:187–199.

82. Murphy TF, et al. Analysis of antigenic structure and human immune response to outer membrane protein CD of *Moraxella catarrhalis*. Infect Immun 1999; 67:4578–4585.

83. Murphy TF, et al. Enhancement of pulmonary clearance of *Moraxella (Branhamella) catarrhalis* following immunization with outer membrane protein CD in a mouse model. J Infect Dis 1998; 178:1667–1675.

84. Bhushan R, et al. Molecular cloning and characterization of outer membrane protein E of *Moraxella (Branhamella) catarrhalis*. J Bacteriol 1994; 176:6636–6643.

85. Murphy TF, et al. Conservation of outer membrane protein E among strains of *Moraxella catarrhalis*. Infect Immun 2001; 69:3576–3580.

86. Bhushan R, et al. Antigenic characterization and analysis of the human immune response to outer membrane protein E of *Branhamella catarrhalis*. Infect Immun 1997; 65:2668–2675.

87. Murphy TF, et al. Antigenic structure of outer membrane protein E of *Moraxella catarrhalis* and construction and characterization of mutants. Infect Immun 2000; 68:6250–6256.

88. Zaleski A, et al. Lipooligosaccharide P(k) (Galalpha1–

4Galbeta1–4Glc) epitope of *Moraxella catarrhalis* is a factor in resistance to bactericidal activity mediated by normal human serum. Infect Immun 2000; 68:5261–5268.

89. Hu WG, et al. Enhancement of clearance of bacteria from murine lungs by immunization with detoxified lipooligo-saccharide from *Moraxella catarrhalis* conjugated to proteins. Infect Immun 2000; 68:4980–4985.

90. Cuthill SL, et al. Nontypable *Haemophilus influenzae* meningitis. Pediatr Infect Dis J 1999; 18:660–662.

91. Klein JO. Role of nontypeable *Haemophilus influenzae* in pediatric respiratory tract infections. Pediatr Infect Dis J 1997; 16:S5–S8.

92. St Geme JWI. Nontypeable *Haemophilus influenzae* disease: epidemiology, pathogenesis, and prospects for prevention. Infect Agents Dis 1993; 2:1–16.

93. Faden H, et al. Epidemiology of nasopharyngeal colonization with nontypeable *Haemophilus influenzae* in the first 2 years of life, Part 1. J Infect Dis 1995; 172:132–135.

94. Barenkamp SJ, et al. Subtyping isolates of *Haemophilus influenzae* type b by outer-membrane protein profiles. J Infect Dis 1981; 143:668–676.

95. Groeneveld K, et al. Antigenic drift of *Haemophilus influenzae* in patients with chronic obstructive pulmonary disease. Infect Immun 1989; 57:3038–3044.

96. Moller LV, et al. Multiple *Haemophilus influenzae* strains and strain variants coexist in the respiratory tract of patients with cystic fibrosis. J Infect Dis 1995; 172:1388–1392.

97. High NJ, et al. The role of a repetitive DNA motif (5′-CAAT-3′) in the variable expression of the *Haemophilus influenzae* lipopolysaccharide epitope alpha Gal(1–4)beta Gal. Mol Microbiol 1993; 9:1275–1282.

98. Hood DW, et al. Identification of a lipopolysaccharide alpha-2,3-sialyltransferase from *Haemophilus influenzae*. Mol Microbiol 2001; 39:341–350.

99. Dawid S, et al. Variation in expression of the *Haemophilus influenzae* HMW adhesins: a prokaryotic system reminiscent of eukaryotes. Proc Natl Acad Sci U S A 1999; 96:1077–1082.

100. van Ham SM, et al. Phase variation of *H. influenzae* fimbriae: transcriptional control of two divergent genes through a variable combined promoter region. Cell 1993; 73:1187–1196.

101. Felmingham D, Gruneberg RN. The Alexander Project 1996–1997: latest susceptibility data from this international study of bacterial pathogens from community-acquired lower respiratory tract infections. J Antimicrob Chemother 2000; 45:191–203.

102. Janson H, et al. Protein D, an immunoglobulin D-binding protein of *Haemophilus influenzae*: cloning, nucleotide sequence, and expression in *Escherichia coli*. Infect Immun 1991; 59:119–125.

103. Ruan MR, et al. Protein D of *Haemophilus influenzae*. A novel bacterial surface protein with affinity for human IgD. J Immunol 1990; 145:3379–3384.

104. Janson H, et al. Protein D, the immunoglobulin D-binding protein of *Haemophilus influenzae*, is a lipoprotein. Infect Immun 1992; 60:1336–1342.

105. Janson H, et al. Protein D, the glycerophosphodiester phosphodiesterase from *Haemophilus influenzae* with affinity for human immunoglobulin D, influences virulence in a rat otitis model. Infect Immun 1994; 62:4848–4854.

106. Janson H, et al. Effects on the ciliated epithelium of protein D-producing and -nonproducing nontypeable *Haemophilus influenzae* in nasopharyngeal tissue cultures. J Infect Dis 1999; 180:737–746.

107. Duim B, et al. Sequence variation in the *hpd* gene of non-encapsulated *Haemophilus influenzae* isolated from patients with chronic bronchitis. Gene 1997; 191:57–60.

108. Akkoyunlu M, et al. Biological activity of serum antibodies to a nonacylated form of lipoprotein D of *Haemophilus influenzae*. Infect Immun 1996; 64:4586–4592.

109. Akkoyunlu M, et al. The acylated form of protein D of *Haemophilus influenzae* is more immunogenic than the nonacylated form and elicits an adjuvant effect when it is used as a carrier conjugated to polyribosyl ribitol phosphate. Infect Immun 1997; 65:5010–5016.

110. Bakaletz LO, et al. Protection against development of otitis media induced by nontypeable *Haemophilus influenzae* by both active and passive immunization in a chinchilla model of virus–bacterium superinfection. Infect Immun 1999; 67:2746–2762.

111. Poolman JT, et al. Developing a nontypeable *Haemophilus influenzae* (NTHi) vaccine. Vaccine 2000; 19(suppl 1):S108–S115.

112. Reddy MS, et al. Binding between outer membrane proteins of nontypeable *Haemophilus influenzae* and human nasopharyngeal mucin. Infect Immun 1996; 64:1477–1479.

113. Virji M, et al. Carcinoembryonic antigens are targeted by diverse strains of typable and non-typable *Haemophilus influenzae*. Mol Microbiol 2000; 36:784–795.

114. Munson RS Jr, Granoff DM. Purification and partial characterization of outer membrane proteins P5 and P6 from *Haemophilus influenzae* type b. Infect Immun 1985; 49:544–549.

115. Webb DC, Cripps AW. Secondary structure and molecular analysis of interstrain variability in the P5 outer-membrane protein of non-typable *Haemophilus influenzae* isolated from diverse anatomical sites. J Med Microbiol 1998; 47:1059–1067.

116. Webb DC, Cripps AW. A method for the purification and refolding of a recombinant form of the nontypeable *Haemophilus influenzae* P5 outer membrane protein fused to polyhistidine. Protein Expr Purif 1999; 15:1–7.

117. Munson RS Jr, et al. Molecular cloning and sequence of the gene for outer membrane protein P5 of *Haemophilus influenzae*. Infect Immun 1993; 61:4017–4020.

118. Duim B, et al. Molecular variation in the major outer membrane protein P5 gene of nonencapsulated *Haemophilus influenzae* during chronic infections. Infect Immun 1997; 65:1351–1356.

119. Bakaletz LO. Peptide and recombinant antigens for protection against bacterial middle ear infection. Vaccine 2001; 19:2323–2328.

120. Kyd JM, Cripps AW. Potential of a novel protein, OMP26, from nontypeable *Haemophilus influenzae* to enhance pulmonary clearance in a rat model. Infect Immun 1998; 66:2272–2278.

121. Foxwell AR, et al. Kinetics of inflammatory cytokines in the clearance of non-typeable *Haemophilus influenzae* from the lung. Immunol Cell Biol 1998; 76:556–559.

122. El Adhami W, et al. Characterization of the gene encoding a 26-kilodalton protein (OMP26) from nontypeable *Haemophilus influenzae* and immune responses to the recombinant protein. Infect Immun 1999; 67:1935–1942.

123. Barenkamp SJ, Bodor FF. Development of serum bactericidal activity following nontypeable *Haemophilus influenzae* acute otitis media. Pediatr Infect Dis J 1990; 9:333–339.

124. Barenkamp SJ, Leininger E. Cloning, expression, and DNA sequence analysis of genes encoding nontypeable *Haemophilus influenzae* high-molecular-weight surface-exposed proteins related to filamentous hemagglutinin of *Bordetella pertussis*. Infect Immun 1992; 60:1302–1313.

125. St Geme JWI, et al. Prevalence and distribution of the hmw and hia genes and the HMW and Hia adhesins among genetically diverse strains of nontypeable *Haemophilus influenzae*. Infect Immun 1998; 66:364–368.

126. Barenkamp SJ, St Geme JWI. Genes encoding high-molec-

127. St Geme JWI, Grass S. Secretion of the *Haemophilus influenzae* HMW1 and HMW2 adhesins involves a periplasmic intermediate and requires the HMWB and HMWC proteins. Mol Microbiol 1998; 27:617–630.

128. Dawid S, et al. Mapping of binding domains of nontypeable *Haemophilus influenzae* HMW1 and HMW2 adhesins. Infect Immun 2001; 69:307–314.

129. Barenkamp SJ. Immunization with high-molecular-weight adhesion proteins of nontypeable *Haemophilus influenzae* modifies experimental otitis media in chinchillas. Infect Immun 1996; 64:1246–1251.

130. St Geme JWI, Cutter D. The *Haemophilus influenzae* Hia adhesin is an autotransporter protein that remains uncleaved at the C terminus and fully cell associated. J Bacteriol 2000; 182:6005–6013.

131. Gilsdorf JR, et al. Comparison of hemagglutinating pili of *Haemophilus influenzae* type b with similar structures of nontypeable *H. influenzae*. Infect Immun 1992; 60:374–379.

132. Brinton CC Jr, et al. Design and development of pilus vaccines for *Haemophilus influenzae* diseases. Pediatr Infect Dis J 1989; 8:S54–S61.

133. Farley MM, et al. Pilus- and non-pilus-mediated interactions of *Haemophilus influenzae* type b with human erythrocytes and human nasopharyngeal mucosa. J Infect Dis 1990; 161:274–280.

134. Weber A, et al. Inability to express fimbriae results in impaired ability of *Haemophilus influenzae* b to colonize the nasopharynx. Infect Immun 1991; 59:4724–4728.

135. Pichichero ME, et al. Do pili play a role in pathogenicity of *Haemophilus influenzae* type B? Lancet 1982; 2:960–962.

136. Gilsdorf JR, et al. Role of pili in *Haemophilus influenzae* adherence and colonization. Infect Immun 1997; 65:2997–3002.

137. LiPuma JJ, Gilsdorf JR. Structural and serological relatedness of *Haemophilus influenzae* type b pili. Infect Immun 1988; 56:1051–1056.

138. Karasic RB, et al. Evaluation of pilus vaccines for prevention of experimental otitis media caused by nontypable *Haemophilus influenzae*. Pediatr Infect Dis J 1989; 8:S62–S65.

139. van Ham SM, et al. The fimbrial gene cluster of *Haemophilus influenzae* type b. Mol Microbiol 1994; 13:673–684.

140. McCrea KW, et al. Identification of two minor subunits in the pilus of *Haemophilus influenzae*. J Bacteriol 1997; 179:4227–4231.

141. McCrea KW, et al. Immunologic and structural relationships of the minor pilus subunits among *Haemophilus influenzae* isolates. Infect Immun 1998; 66:4788–4796.

142. Mhlanga-Mutangadura T, et al. Evolution of the major pilus gene cluster of *Haemophilus influenzae*. J Bacteriol 1998; 180:4693–4703.

143. Geluk F, et al. The fimbria gene cluster of nonencapsulated *Haemophilus influenzae*. Infect Immun 1998; 66:406–417.

144. Munson R Jr, et al. Comparative analysis of the structures of the outer membrane protein P1 genes from major clones of *Haemophilus influenzae* type b. Infect Immun 1989; 57:3300–3305.

145. Chong P, et al. Immunogenicity of synthetic peptides of *Haemophilus influenzae* type b outer membrane protein P1. Infect Immun 1995; 63:3751–3758.

146. Proulx C, et al. Epitope analysis of an immunodominant domain on the P1 protein of *Haemophilus influenzae* type b using synthetic peptides and anti-idiotypic antibodies. Microb Pathog 1992; 12:433–442.

147. Cripps AW, et al. Respiratory immunity stimulated by

intestinal immunization with purified nontypeable *Haemophilus influenzae* antigens. J Infect Dis 1992; 165(suppl 1): S199–S201.

148. Bolduc GR, et al. Variability of outer membrane protein P1 and its evaluation as a vaccine candidate against experimental otitis media due to nontypeable *Haemophilus influenzae*: an unambiguous, multifaceted approach. Infect Immun 2000; 68:4505–4517.

149. Vachon V, et al. Transmembrane permeability channels across the outer membrane of *Haemophilus influenzae* type b. J Bacteriol 1985; 162:918–924.

150. Murphy TF, Bartos LC. Human bactericidal antibody response to outer membrane protein P2 of nontypeable *Haemophilus influenzae*. Infect Immun 1988; 56:2673–2679.

151. Kyd JM, Cripps AW. Modulation of antigen-specific T and B cell responses influence bacterial clearance of nontypeable *Haemophilus influenzae* from the lung in a rat model. Vaccine 1996; 14:1471–1478.

152. Yi K, Murphy TF. Importance of an immunodominant surface-exposed loop on outer membrane protein P2 of nontypeable *Haemophilus influenzae*. Infect Immun 1997; 65: 150–155.

153. Duim B, et al. Antigenic drift of non-encapsulated *Haemophilus influenzae* major outer membrane protein P2 in patients with chronic bronchitis is caused by point mutations. Mol Microbiol 1994; 11:1181–1189.

154. Haase EM, et al. Mapping of bactericidal epitopes on the P2 porin protein of nontypeable *Haemophilus influenzae*. Infect Immun 1994; 62:3712–3722.

155. Neary JM, et al. Antibodies to loop 6 of the P2 porin protein of nontypeable *Haemophilus influenzae* are bactericidal against multiple strains. Infect Immun 2001; 69:773–778.

156. Smith-Vaughan HC, et al. Nonencapsulated *Haemophilus influenzae* in aboriginal infants with otitis media: prolonged carriage of P2 porin variants and evidence for horizontal P2 gene transfer. Infect Immun 1997; 65:1468–1474.

157. Green BA, et al. The e (P4) outer membrane protein of *Haemophilus influenzae*: biologic activity of anti-e serum and cloning and sequencing of the structural gene. Infect Immun 1991; 59:3191–3198.

158. Reilly TJ, et al. Outer membrane lipoprotein e (P4) of *Haemophilus influenzae* is a novel phosphomonoesterase. J Bacteriol 1999; 181:6797–6805.

159. Reilly TJ, et al. Contribution of the DDDD motif of *H. influenzae* (P4) to phosphomonoesterase activity and heme transport. FEBS Lett 2001; 494:19–23.

160. Green BA, et al. Evaluation of mixtures of purified *Haemophilus influenzae* outer membrane proteins in protection against challenge with nontypeable *H. influenzae* in the chinchilla otitis media model. Infect Immun 1993; 61:1950–1957.

161. Murphy TF, et al. Identification of a specific epitope of *Haemophilus influenzae* on a 16,600-dalton outer membrane protein. J Infect Dis 1985; 152:1300–1307.

162. Deich RA, et al. Cloning of genes encoding a 15,000-dalton peptidoglycan-associated outer membrane lipoprotein and an antigenically related 15,000-dalton protein from *Haemophilus influenzae*. J Bacteriol 1988; 170:489–498.

163. Nelson MB, et al. Molecular conservation of the P6 outer membrane protein among strains of *Haemophilus influenzae*: analysis of antigenic determinants, gene sequences, and restriction fragment length polymorphisms. Infect Immun 1991; 59:2658–2663.

164. Green BA, et al. A recombinant non-fatty acylated form of the Hi-PAL (P6) protein of *Haemophilus influenzae* elicits biologically active antibody against both nontypeable and type b *H. influenzae*. Infect Immun 1990; 58:3272–3278.

165. Badr WH, et al. Immunization of mice with P6 of nontypeable *Haemophilus influenzae*: kinetics of the antibody response and IgG subclasses. Vaccine 1999; 18:29–37.

166. Yang YP, et al. Effect of lipid modification on the physicochemical, structural, antigenic and immunoprotective properties of *Haemophilus influenzae* outer membrane protein P6. Vaccine 1997; 15:976–987.

167. Hotomi M, et al. Specific mucosal immunity and enhanced nasopharyngeal clearance of nontypeable *Haemophilus influenzae* after intranasal immunization with outer membrane protein P6 and cholera toxin. Vaccine 1998; 16:1950–1956.

168. Sabirov A, et al. Intranasal immunization enhances clearance of nontypeable *Haemophilus influenzae* and reduces stimulation of tumor necrosis factor alpha production in the murine model of otitis media. Infect Immun 2001; 69:2964–2971.

169. DeMaria TF, et al. Immunization with outer membrane protein P6 from nontypeable *Haemophilus influenzae* induces bactericidal antibody and affords protection in the chinchilla model of otitis media. Infect Immun 1996; 64:5187–5192.

170. Yang YP, et al. Nasopharyngeal colonization with nontypeable *Haemophilus influenzae* in chinchillas. Infect Immun 1998; 66:1973–1980.

171. Murphy TF, et al. Identification of a 16,600-dalton outer membrane protein on nontypeable *Haemophilus influenzae* as a target for human serum bactericidal antibody. J Clin Invest 1986; 78:1020–1127.

172. Yamanaka N, Faden H. Antibody response to outer membrane protein of nontypeable *Haemophilus influenzae* in otitis-prone children. J Pediatr 1993; 122:212–218.

173. Harabuchi Y, et al. Human milk secretory IgA antibody to nontypeable *Haemophilus influenzae*: possible protective effects against nasopharyngeal colonization. J Pediatr 1994; 124:193–198.

174. Harabuchi Y, et al. Nasopharyngeal colonization with nontypeable *Haemophilus influenzae* and recurrent otitis media. Tonawanda/Williamsville Pediatrics. J Infect Dis 1994; 170:862–866.

175. Thomas WR, et al. Expression in *Escherichia coli* of a high-molecular-weight protective surface antigen found in nontypeable and type b *Haemophilus influenzae*. Infect Immun 1990; 58:1909–1913.

176. Loosmore SM, et al. Outer membrane protein D15 is conserved among *Haemophilus influenzae* species and may represent a universal protective antigen against invasive disease. Infect Immun 1997; 65:3701–3707.

177. Yang Y, et al. A 20-kilodalton N-terminal fragment of the D15 protein contains a protective epitope(s) against *Haemophilus influenzae* type a and type b. Infect Immun 1998; 66:3349–3354.

178. Weiser JN, et al. Identification and characterization of a cell envelope protein of *Haemophilus influenzae* contributing to phase variation in colony opacity and nasopharyngeal colonization. Mol Microbiol 1995; 17:555–564.

179. Prasadarao NV, et al. Opacity-associated protein A contributes to the binding of *Haemophilus influenzae* to Chang epithelial cells. Infect Immun 1999; 67:4153–4160.

180. Hendrixson DR, et al. Structural determinants of processing and secretion of the *Haemophilus influenzae* hap protein. Mol Microbiol 1997; 26:505–518.

181. Fink DL, et al. The *Hemophilus influenzae* Hap autotransporter is a chymotrypsin clan serine protease and undergoes autoproteolysis via an intermolecular mechanism. J Biol Chem 2001; 276:39492–39500.

182. Loosmore SM, et al. The *Haemophilus influenzae* HtrA protein is a protective antigen. Infect Immun 1998; 66:899–906.

183. Cates GA, et al. Properties of recombinant HtrA: an otitis media vaccine candidate antigen from non-typeable *Haemophilus influenzae*. Dev Biol (Basel) 2000; 103:201–204.

184. Deich RA, et al. Antigenic conservation of the 15,000-dalton outer membrane lipoprotein PCP of *Haemophilus influenzae* and biologic activity of anti-PCP antisera. Infect Immun 1990; 58:3388–3393.

185. Cope LD, et al. Detection of phase variation in expression of proteins involved in hemoglobin and hemoglobin–haptoglobin binding by nontypeable *Haemophilus influenzae*. Infect Immun 2000; 68:4092–4101.

186. Maciver I, et al. Identification of an outer membrane protein involved in utilization of hemoglobin–haptoglobin complexes by nontypeable *Haemophilus influenzae*. Infect Immun 1996; 64:3703–3712.

187. Jin H, et al. Cloning of a DNA fragment encoding a heme-repressible hemoglobin-binding outer membrane protein from *Haemophilus influenzae*. Infect Immun 1996; 64:3134–3141.

188. Cope LD, et al. The 100 kDa haem:haemopexin-binding protein of *Haemophilus influenzae*: structure and localization. Mol Microbiol 1994; 13:863–873.

189. Cope LD. Involvement of HxuC outer membrane protein in utilization of hemoglobin by *Haemophilus influenzae*. Infect Immun 2001; 69:2353–2363.

190. Morton DJ, Williams P. Siderophore-independent acquisition of transferrin-bound iron by *Haemophilus influenzae* type b. J Gen Microbiol 1990; 136(Part 5):927–933.

191. Schryvers AB. Identification of the transferrin- and lactoferrin-binding proteins in *Haemophilus influenzae*. J Med Microbiol 1989; 29:121–130.

192. Ueyama T. Identification of common lipooligosaccharide types in isolates from patients with otitis media by monoclonal antibodies against nontypeable *Haemophilus influenzae* 9274. Clin Diagn Lab Immunol 1999; 6:96–100.

193. McGehee JL, et al. Effect of primary immunization on pulmonary clearance of nontypable *Haemophilus influenzae*. Am J Respir Cell Mol Biol 1989; 1:201–210.

194. Gu XX, et al. Synthesis, characterization, and immunologic properties of detoxified lipooligosaccharide from nontypeable *Haemophilus influenzae* conjugated to proteins. Infect Immun 1996; 64:4047–4053.

195. Gu XX, et al. Detoxified lipooligosaccharide from nontypeable *Haemophilus influenzae* conjugated to proteins confers protection against otitis media in chinchillas. Infect Immun 1997; 65:4488–4493.

196. Sun J, et al. Biological activities of antibodies elicited by lipooligosaccharide based-conjugate vaccines of nontypeable *Haemophilus influenzae* in an otitis media model. Vaccine 2000; 18:1264–1272.

197. Corpet F, et al. ProDom and ProDom-CG: tools for protein domain analysis and whole genome comparisons. Nucleic Acids Res 2000; 28:267–269.

198. Eddy SR. Profile hidden Markov models. Bioinformatics 1998; 14:755–763.

199. Bateman A, et al. The Pfam protein families database. Nucleic Acids Res 2002; 30:276–280.

200. Falquet L, et al. The PROSITE database, its status in 2002. Nucleic Acids Res 2002; 30:235–238.

201. Henikoff JG, et al. Blocks-based methods for detecting protein homology. Electrophoresis 2000; 21:1700–1706.

202. King RD, et al. DSC: public domain protein secondary structure predication. Comput Appl Biosci 1997; 13:473–474.

203. Nielsen H, et al. Identification of prokaryotic and eukaryotic signal peptides and prediction of their cleavage sites. Protein Eng 1997; 10:1–6.

204. Sonnhammer EL, et al. A hidden Markov model for predicting transmembrane helices in protein sequences. Proc Int Conf Intell Syst Mol Biol 1998; 6:175–182.

205. Fleischmann RD, et al. Whole-genome random sequencing and assembly of *Haemophilus influenzae* Rd. Science 1995; 269:496–512.

206. Ferretti JJ, et al. Complete genome sequence of an M1 strain of *Streptococcus pyogenes*. Proc Natl Acad Sci USA 2001; 98:4658–4663.

207. Masignani V, et al. Mu-like Prophage in serogroup B *Neisseria meningitidis* coding for surface-exposed antigens. Infect Immun 2001; 69:2580–2588.

208. Heffelfinger JD, et al. Evaluation of children with recurrent pneumonia diagnosed by World Health Organization criteria. Pediatr Infect Dis J 2002; 21:108–112.

209. Sniadack DH, et al. Potential interventions for the prevention of childhood pneumonia: geographic and temporal differences in serotype and serogroup distribution of sterile site pneumococcal isolates from children—implications for vaccine strategies. Pediatr Infect Dis J 1995; 14:503–510.

210. McIntosh K. Community-acquired pneumonia in children. N Engl J Med 2002; 346:429–437.

211. Heikkinen T. The role of respiratory viruses in otitis media. Vaccine 2000; 19(suppl 1):S51–S55.

212. Faden H. The microbiologic and immunologic basis for recurrent otitis media in children 2. Eur J Pediatr 2001; 160:407–413.

213. van Alphen L, Caugant DA, Duim B, O'Rourke M, Bowler LD. Differences in genetic diversity of nonencapsulated *Haemophilus influenzae* from various diseases. Microbiology 1997; 143(Part 4):1423–1431.

214. Adamou JE, et al. Identification and characterization of a novel family of pneumococcal proteins that are protective against sepsis. Infect Immun 2001; 69:949–958.

215. Guiso N, et al. Intranasal murine model of *Bordetella pertussis* infection: I. Prediction of protection in human infants by acellular vaccines. Vaccine 1999; 17:2366–2376.

216. Giebink GS. Otitis media: the chinchilla model. Microb Drug Resist 1999; 5:57–72.

68

Vaccines for *Chlamydia trachomatis* and *Chlamydia pneumoniae*

Andrew D. Murdin
Aventis Pasteur, Toronto, Ontario, Canada

Robert C. Brunham
University of British Columbia, Vancouver, British Columbia, Canada

The history of chlamydia vaccine research is characterized both by empirical approaches using whole inactivated organism and, more recently, by rational molecular vaccine design. Unfortunately, human trials with inactivated vaccines ended in the late 1960s, and no rational design approach has been successful enough to move to clinical testing. Although several chlamydia vaccines are at various stages of development by several vaccine manufacturers there is little information on these in the scientific literature. To provide an overview of the current status of chlamydia vaccine development this chapter focuses on *Chlamydia pneumoniae* and *Chlamydia trachomatis*, which are the two main chlamydial pathogens of humans, on our understanding of protective and pathologic immune responses to these pathogens, and on past and present attempts to develop human vaccines against these organisms. For another recent perspective on this subject, see Igietseme et al. [1]. It should be noted that although there are veterinary vaccines available or under development that may inform vaccine strategies for humans, veterinary vaccine development is beyond the scope of this chapter.

I. THE PATHOGENS

C. pneumoniae and *C. trachomatis* are obligate intracellular parasites, which share a unique intracellular developmental cycle [2]. The extracellular stage or elementary body (EB) is infectious but metabolically inert, whereas the intracellular stage or reticulate body (RB) is noninfectious but metabolically active. Intracellullar replication occurs within a membrane-bound inclusion, the development of which appears to be mediated by the multiple chlamydial proteins associated with the inclusion membrane. There is evidence for a cryptic or latent intracellular stage associated with persis-

tent infection, but this stage is not well characterized. Persistent infection may be an important cause of much of the long-term tissue damage secondary to chlamydial infection [3,4].

C. pneumoniae has been associated with a broad spectrum of diseases, including sinusitis, bronchitis, community-acquired pneumonia, chronic obstructive pulmonary disease, asthma, cardiovascular disease, multiple sclerosis, and Alzheimer's disease. The association with cardiovascular disease, which is of particular recent interest, is strong but not yet proven to be causal [5,6]. *C. trachomatis* infection is associated with trachoma, lymphogranuloma venereum, and sexually transmitted infections of the genital tract. It is the most common sexually transmitted disease in the United States with an estimated three million cases occurring in 1999 [7]. Up to 70% of infected women are asymptomatic, making the infection difficult to diagnose despite the availability of effective and accurate diagnostic tests. Serious sequelae of infection in women include endometritis and/or salpingitis, pelvic inflammatory disease, infertility, ectopic pregnancy, and possibly cervical cancer [8,9].

The genome sequences of several chlamydia isolates have been determined [10–13,13a]. These reveal organisms well adapted to their intracellular lifestyle, auxotrophic for many amino acids, ribonucleotides, and cofactors, and dependant on the host for energy. With respect to vaccine development, the available *C. pneumoniae* genome sequences reveal a highly clonal organism, which arguably occurs as a single strain with global distribution [10–13,13a]. There is the possibility that members of a family of 21 putative membrane proteins (pmps) may carry antigenic determinants that vary to some extent among isolates, and that expression of these proteins may vary from cell to cell in a process analogous to phase variation [14], but this is not yet clear. The pathogen possesses an array of virulence determinants including an apparently functional type III secretion system, three Hsp60 homologs, and an array of proteases, kinases, and other enzymes with homologies to known bacterial virulence factors [2]. The *C. trachomatis* genome sequences show both strong similarities to and important differences from *C. pneumoniae* [11,12]. In particular, both sequence and serological data reveal an organism with much greater antigenic variation than *C. pneumoniae*. There are 15 well-established serovars of *C. trachomatis*, with several more proposed [15,16]. Surprisingly, the genetic basis for specific disease association found among chlamydiae remains unknown even with genomic information in hand.

Both *C. pneumoniae* and *C. trachomatis* appear well adapted to evade the host immune response, possessing a sophisticated multilayered repertoire of immune evasion strategies. First, replication of the bacterium within a membrane-bound inclusion limits exposure of bacterial antigens to the host–cell antigen presentation machinery. Second, the bacterium is in any case able to moderate the effectiveness of host–cell antigen presentation by downregulating the expression of MHC I and MHC II by infected cells [17,18]. Third, the pathogen elaborates at least one protein able to inhibit host–cell apoptosis, rendering infected cells resistant to fas-mediated killing [19]. The organism's biphasic developmental cycle can also be viewed as an immune evasion mechanism, in that the extracellular EBs are susceptible only to antibody-mediated immunity, and the intracellular RBs are susceptible only to cell-mediated immunity. One of the developmental stages might be able to persist in the face of a relatively weak cellular or humoral response, and it is speculated that when the overall host response has declined active infection may recur.

II. IMMUNITY TO CHLAMYDIAL INFECTIONS

Despite the ability of the pathogen to circumvent the host response, both innate and adaptive immune responses can confer protection. Innate immunity falls outside the scope of this chapter, but see Brunham [3] for a discussion of the protective effects of innate immune responses against chlamydial infection. Evidence that adaptive immune responses can be protective against infection and disease is provided by early human challenge studies and vaccine trials, by epidemiological studies, and by studies of animal models of infection. Numerous observations of chlamydial persistence in various tissues raise the possibility that complete elimination of an infection does not occur in many individuals, and that a common effect of a protective immune response is to hold the pathogen in a quiescent state in certain preferred sites within the body rather than to clear it completely. This leads to important questions about host–pathogen interaction, in particular regarding the nature of the interactions that occur among chlamydial antigens, antigen-presenting molecules, and antigen-specific lymphocytes that determine the heterogeneity in the clearance rate of chlamydial infection. We will briefly review what is known of immunity to *C. pneumoniae* and *C. trachomatis*, and highlight areas where differences are known to occur.

A. Observations in Humans

Jawetz et al. [20] first demonstrated strain-specific immunity to ocular *C. trachomatis* infection in challenge studies using human subjects, and these observations were subsequently replicated in immunization and challenge studies in both humans and primates (see, e.g., Refs. 21,22). Epidemiological studies in human populations show similar evidence for the development of protective immune responses following infection [23,24]. In aggregate, the human data are strongly supportive of the notion that *C. trachomatis* infection or immunization induces strain-specific, but possibly short-lived, resistance to reinfection.

Several immunoepidemiological studies of host resistance and susceptibility to human ocular and genital *C. trachomatis* infection have demonstrated the importance of cell-mediated responses in protective immunity. Individuals spontaneously clearing an ocular chlamydial infection exhibited enhanced lymphoproliferative responses to chlamydia compared to individuals with persistent ocular disease, whereas individuals with conjunctival scarring in the advanced stages of trachoma had markedly depressed lymphoproliferative responses to chlamydia in comparison to controls without scarring [25]. Other studies have indicated that enhanced Th2 and depressed Th1 responses may be associated with the development of scarring trachoma [26,27]. Most data suggest that class II-restricted $\alpha\beta$ CD4$^+$ T cells are essential for immunity to chlamydial infection (e.g., Refs. 24,28). A protective role for CD8$^+$ T cells is less clearly defined, and may differ between *C. trachomatis* and *C. pneumoniae*. Several studies have demonstrated CD8$^+$ cytotoxic T-lymphocyte (CTL) responses specific for *C. trachomatis* major outer membrane protein (MOMP) and Hsp60 in the peripheral blood of infected individuals [29,30] and demonstrated their cytolytic function through specific lysis of *C. trachomatis*-infected epithelial cells in vitro [30]. Based on these findings, it seems probable that MHC I-restricted CD8$^+$ T-cell responses to *Chlamydia* antigens can contribute to effective immunity against these pathogens.

B. Observations in Mice

Cell-mediated responses play a key protective role in mice as well as in humans. In the case of *C. trachomatis*, in vivo depletion studies [31], studies using mice defective in CD8$^+$ T-cell function [31], and adoptive transfer studies [32] all indicate a dominant protective role for CD4$^+$ T cells and a lesser role for CD8$^+$ T cells in host defense against primary *C. trachomatis* infection. The bulk of the animal data regarding protective immunity to *C. pneumoniae* infection suggest that the CD8$^+$ T-cell subset plays a more prominent, although not exclusive, role in defense. In vivo depletion of CD8$^+$ T cells resulted in an increase in the chlamydial burden in the lungs of infected animals and an extended duration of secondary infection [33]. Furthermore, various knockout mice lacking functional CD8$^+$ T cells are all more susceptible to *C. pneumoniae* infection than normal mice [34,35].

The mechanisms through which both the CD4$^+$ T-cell and the CD8$^+$ T-cell populations contribute to protection include the release of IFNγ, a key cytokine in the resolution of both *C. pneumoniae* and *C. trachomatis* infections [34–40]. Studies of other cytokines and their receptors have demonstrated an important role for both IL-12 and IL-10 in antichlamydia responses. IL-12 is known to be a differentiating cytokine for IFNγ-production by sensitized Th1 cells, and can clearly drive antichlamydial responses toward that pathway [38,41,42]. By contrast, IL-10 has been shown to have a negative regulatory role, and can attenuate the Th1 type response [43–45]. In addition to the important role of these two molecules, TNF-α, IL-1β, and IL-8, have all been shown to be released from chlamydia-infected cells [46], and presumably serve to activate specific leukocytes and recruit them to sites of infection.

Although B cells appear not to be required for protection from chlamydial infection [47], recent evidence obtained from in vivo T-cell depletion studies in normal and B-cell-deficient mice indicate that B cells can play a key role during the resolution of secondary, but not primary, *C. trachomatis* vaginal infections [48,49]. Depletion of either CD4$^+$ T cells or CD8$^+$ T cells, or both, in previously infected wild-type C57BL/6 mice had a limited effect on resistance to reinfection, whereas depletion of CD4$^+$ T cells, but not CD8$^+$ T cells, in previously infected B-cell-deficient mice resulted in a chronic infection which did not resolve until anti-CD4 treatment was halted. That is, either CD4$^+$ T cells or B cells were sufficient to resolve a secondary chlamydial infection, indicating a previously unrecognized but significant role for B cells in resistance to chlamydial reinfection. The mechanism by which B cells contribute to immunity to *C. trachomatis* infections and how B cells and CD4$^+$ T cells interact during an intact immune response are unknown, but represent important goals for future research. It will also be important to determine whether B cells make a similar contribution to immunity to *C. pneumoniae* infections.

C. Role of Antibody in Humans

In contrast with the clear role for T cells in immunity to *Chlamydia*, the evidence for a direct protective role of antibodies is less convincing. In many instances, high serum antibody responses often correlate with complications of chlamydial disease. Elevated anti-*C. pneumoniae* serum IgG titers in patients with atherosclerosis were the first indication of the association between *C. pneumoniae* and cardiovascular disease (CVD) [50]. Serum antibodies against *C. trachomatis* are produced at surprisingly high titers among women with acute salpingitis [51], the Fitz–Hugh–Curtis syndrome [52], and postsalpingitis tubal infertility [53]. As such, it appears that high-serum antibodies do not protect against the complications of chlamydial infection except, perhaps, in some special circumstances [54]. In contrast to serum antibodies, secretory immunoglobulin A (IgA) antibodies may play a more important role in protection, from both ocular [55,56] and genital infection [57,58]. Furthermore, the possibility that synergistic interactions between cellular and humoral immune responses are required for optimal protec-

tion from chlamydial infection should not be overlooked (see, e.g., *Francisella* [59]).

D. Immunopathology

Many immunological findings seen with chlamydial disease are highly reminiscent of immune correlates in other infectious diseases that exhibit a spectrum of host immunological responses, such as leishmaniasis and leprosy [60]. In aggregate, the results suggest that MOMP-specific Th1-like CD4$^+$ T cells are important in immunity to and clearance of *C. trachomatis* infection and disease and that Hsp60-specific Th2-like CD4$^+$ T cells are associated with the pathological sequelae of persistent *C. trachomatis* infection. Similar responses may govern the outcome of *C. pneumoniae* infection, although the target antigens in this case are less easy to identify. Persistent infection is a common correlate of the more severe manifestations of chlamydial disease. Some hosts fail to clear chlamydial infection and remain persistently infected or susceptible to frequent reinfection [61–67]. These individuals appear to be at increased risk of developing the long-term sequelae of chlamydial disease [68], which arise as a result of inflammation and fibrosis. Cytokine synthesis by chronically infected cells together with persistent antigen synthesis in the face of an ineffective or partially effective immune response is thought to contribute to chronic inflammation, tissue damage, and immunopathology [69]. For a complete discussion of chlamydia-induced immunopathology, see Ward [9].

Much remains to be learned regarding the identity of the chlamydial antigens contributing to the development of immunopathology. Several antigens, including Hsp60, lipopolysaccharide (LPS), OmcB, and Cpn0483, have been implicated as potential virulence factors playing a role in these processes [70–72], but the inability to generate chlamydial mutants has inhibited more extensive studies of chlamydial virulence and pathogenesis. The availability of multiple chlamydial genome sequences offers new potential for defining chlamydial virulence factors and their role in the disease process, and it will be critical to take advantage of this information to ensure that chlamydia vaccines do not inadvertently elicit immunopathological responses in vaccinees.

III. VACCINES FOR CHLAMYDIAL INFECTIONS

A. Vaccine Antigens

Early efforts at developing a chlamydial vaccine were based on parenteral immunization with various partially purified preparations of live or inactivated chlamydial elementary bodies. A good overview of this early body of work is provided by Collier [73]. Although this approach met with some success in human trials, protection was short-lived and serovar-specific [74–79]. More significantly, these whole-organism vaccines sometimes exacerbated the incidence and/or severity of disease during subsequent infection episodes, possibly because of pathological reactions to certain chlamydial antigens [77–79]. Exacerbation was not seen in all cases, and tended to be more obvious in monkeys than in humans [80, 81, 82; Grayston, personal communication cited in 83]. On reading these accounts one is left with a suspicion that the choice of adjuvant may have been a significant influence on this effect, but it is impossible to be sure because the various vaccine preparations were so diverse. Regardless, the potential for the induction of immunopathogenesis has deterred more recent investigators from considering live or inactivated whole organisms as vaccine candidates.

However, because chlamydial infection confers partial protection against reinfection, it has been suggested that an avirulent, nonimmunopathological strain of *Chlamydia* might have potential as a vaccine. A significant practical restriction in pursuing this idea has been the lack of a system for the genetic manipulation of *Chlamydia*; nevertheless, the idea of an attenuated vaccine still receives attention. In a study to evaluate the potential efficacy of a live attenuated vaccine, the effect of an attenuated chlamydia strain was simulated by treating mice with a subchlamydiacidal concentration of oxytetracycline following vaginal infection [84]. Antibiotic-treated mice generated levels of *Chlamydia*-specific antibody and cell-mediated immunity equivalent to those of infected but untreated control mice and were as immune as control mice when rechallenged vaginally. In particular, these mice produced a minimal inflammatory response in urogenital tissue and did not experience infection-related sequelae, suggesting that protective and immunopathological immune responses can be separated. This result is interesting, but further research into the molecular basis of chlamydial virulence and immunopathology will be required before an attenuated vaccine candidate can confidently be expected to be safe.

An alternative to the killed whole-organism approach has been described by Pal et al. [85] who investigated a subunit vaccine consisting of *C. trachomatis* outer membrane complexes (COMCs). Mice immunized with COMCs were challenged by inoculation of the mouse pneumonitis (MoPn) strain of *C. trachomatis* into the ovarian bursa, then assessed for vaginal shedding of chlamydia and for fertility. The mice developed significant humoral and lymphoproliferative immune responses, including vaginal IgA chlamydia-specific antibodies. COMC-immunized mice exhibited a significant decrease in the intensity and duration of vaginal shedding post challenge and were as fertile as normal control mice. This is a promising result, particularly in view of the relatively severe intrabursal challenge, but the potential of COMCs to induce immunopathology requires additional study. The reason for the enhanced immunogenicity of the COMCs also remains to be determined, because it is unclear which of the multiple antigens in the COMC are the targets for protective responses, or how these antigens are processed by the immune system.

Many recent attempts at *C. trachomatis* vaccine development have focused on MOMP, which is the dominant surface antigen and comprises over 60% of the total membrane protein [86]. It is recognized by sera from infected humans and is a principal target of neutralizing antibodies [87]. The extensive antigenic variation observed in *C. trachomatis* MOMP means that a cocktail of several MOMPs would be required to produce a vaccine. Candidate vaccines have typically been based on a subunit design using whole MOMP protein, or fragments or peptides. These vaccines have had mixed success, perhaps because the immunogens do not reliably induce protective cellular and humoral immune responses recalled by native epitopes on the organism [88–93]. Some success was reported with whole recombinant MOMP in a mouse model of genital tract infection [94], but the result was heavily dependent on the route of immunization and challenge.

The most effective MOMP protein vaccines have been based on the intact native protein extracted from chlamydial EBs, although the results obtained have been dependent on the method of extraction and the adjuvant used. MOMP extracted using SDS is largely denatured and no more effective as an antigen than synthetic peptides, whereas MOMP extracted with the nonionic detergent n-octyl-beta-D-glucopyranoside has been found to elicit partial protection in mouse and primate models [91,95,96]. This is possibly because MOMP extracted in this way remains as multimers [96,97], which may retain at least some elements of the native conformation, but the mechanism of protection in these studies is unclear. In one study, OGP-extracted MOMP formulated into immune stimulating complexes (ISCOMs) [98] raised a protective cell-mediated response in mice that could be adoptively transferred to naïve recipient animals [95]. It is not obvious that MOMP conformation would be important to raising this kind of cellular immune response, but recent data suggest that it may be. MOMP extracted with the detergent Zwittergent 3-14, and estimated to be >99% pure, was refolded by dialysis against glutathione–PBS [96]. Refolded MOMP was obtained as multimers, as shown by nonreducing SDS-PAGE, but could be converted to monomers by sonication. Refolded MOMP in complete Freund's adjuvant elicited strong humoral and lymphoproliferative responses in mice, and conferred partial protection from vaginal shedding and infertility following an intrabursal chlamydia challenge. In contrast, refolded and sonicated MOMP elicited only a humoral response, conferred only minimal protection from vaginal shedding, and had no effect on infertility following chlamydial challenge. The authors speculate that conformational differences between monomeric and multimeric MOMP influence the development of CD4$^+$ T-cell responses, citing the precedent of the *Leishmania major* surface antigen PSA-2 [99]. It will be important to determine the extent to which MOMP conformation actually influences the induction of cellular responses because despite the data for refolded MOMP, the successful use of DNA vaccines encoding MOMP [100–102] argues that the correct conformation is not an absolute requirement for eliciting a protective response.

Until recently few chlamydial antigens other than MOMP had been seriously evaluated as vaccine candidates. The most noteworthy of these is the secreted glycolipid GLXA, a soluble genus-specific glycolipid that is secreted into the extracellular environment during the chlamydial developmental cycle [103–105]. A guinea pig anti-idiotypic antibody (anti-id) mimicking the immunogenicity of GLXA of *C. trachomatis* was reported to elicit antibodies in rabbits that could neutralize heterologous chlamydiae in vitro and in vivo [106]. Furthermore, mice immunized with a murine monoclonal anti-id encapsulated in polylactide micro-spheres were significantly protected against ocular and genital challenge with human strains of *C. trachomatis* [107,108]. In contrast to the studies with MOMP, but consistent with the use of the anti-id as an immunogen, protection was apparently associated with induction of anti-GLXA antibody and antichlamydial neutralizing antibody. However, significant questions remain regarding the induction of a protective immune response to GLXA. For example, is neutralizing antibody the sole or dominant protective effector mechanism, or does the anti-id somehow elicit a protective cell-mediated response to a nonprotein antigen? It will be important to achieve a better understanding of the immunobiology of GLXA to properly interpret these findings.

Chlamydial LPS was found to be ineffective as a protective antigen against *C. trachomatis* ocular disease when administered orally to monkeys as a recombinant antigen expressed by an *E. coli* vector [109]. DNA vaccines encoding *C. pneumoniae* Hsp60 have been found to be protective in mice, with efficacy comparable to a similar vaccine encoding *C. pneumoniae* MOMP [35,102]. However, the extensive homology between human and chlamydial Hsp60s may prevent the use of chlamydial Hsp60 in a vaccine for human use. The *C. pneumoniae* cysteine-rich outer membrane protein 2 (Omp2) has been reported by one group to be nonprotective when administered via DNA immunization [102], whereas another group has found the antigen to be at least as protective as the MOMP using similar methods of immunization and animal models [110]. The reasons for this discrepancy are unclear.

The recent determination of several chlamydial genome sequences [10–13,13a] has greatly expanded opportunities for chlamydial antigen discovery and vaccine development in the last few years [111,112]. Strategies for the postgenomic discovery of protective antigens fall into two broad categories. In sequence-based strategies, antigens selected from the genome sequence according to predefined criteria are screened for protective efficacy in an animal model of infection [14,101,113,114], whereas in biology-based strategies antigens of demonstrated biological relevance are identified with the help of the genome sequence and then cloned and evaluated for protective efficacy [115]. An example of a sequence-based strategy might be to test all predicted membrane proteins [116], whereas an example of a biology-based strategy might be to sequence MHC-bound peptides by mass spectrometry [117], identify the parent protein from the genome data, then clone and test that protein.

The screening approach has been used with relatively broad selection criteria to test over 200 *C. pneumoniae* ORFs for protective efficacy in a mouse model of *C. pneumoniae* lung infection, resulting in the identification of multiple protective antigens including MOMP, OMP2, an ATP/ADP translocase and a homolog of the 76-kDa antigen [101,110, 118]. Interestingly, the *C. pneumoniae* ATP/ADP translocase is highly conserved with *C. trachomatis* and preliminary results show that it elicits protection against *C. trachomatis* in addition to *C. pneumoniae* (Murdin, Lu, and Brunham, unpublished data). Screening approaches utilizing a greater degree of genome analysis to focus on specific antigens, thus limiting the amount of animal testing required, have also

been successful at identifying other candidate protective antigens, including a serine–threonine kinase gene selected because of its potential role as an effector protein secreted by the chlamydial type III secretion system. Whether the protein is actually a type III secretion-associated effector is unknown, but DNA immunization with the ORF encoding the protein elicited partial protection from a *C. trachomatis* MoPn lung challenge in a mouse model [113]. The genome sequence has also played a primary role in identifying and characterizing other potentially protective antigens such as PorB, a novel chlamydial porin [114], and in characterizing the full extent of the family of pmps [14].

The alternative approach to antigen discovery, the identification and characterization of antigens of known biological relevance, has been used by Fling et al. [115] to identify the protein recognized by a protective *C. trachomatis*-specific CD8$^+$ T-cell line. Clones of P815 cells transduced with fragments of a *C. trachomatis* expression library were screened for their ability to stimulate the protective T-cell line, and one stimulating clone was identified. The chlamydial DNA fragment from this clone was sequenced and mapped to a predicted *C. trachomatis* ORF, CT529, encoding a 31-kDa inclusion membrane-associated protein, Cap1. The CD8$^+$ T-cell line and CTLs derived from *C. trachomatis*-infected mice were able to lyse P815 targets pulsed with a nine amino acid peptide derived from Cap1, confirming the immunological relevance of the protein. Fling et al. were then able to complete the final step of the antigen discovery process by demonstrating that mice immunized with a recombinant vaccinia virus expressing a 70 amino acid fragment of Cap1 were weakly but significantly protected from an intravenous challenge with *C. trachomatis* serovar L2.

B. Adjuvants and Delivery Systems

Based on our current understanding of protective immunity, adjuvants eliciting a Th1-biased response are likely to be most effective at eliciting protection against chlamydial infection. Several adjuvants and delivery systems have been evaluated for their utility in chlamydia vaccines. However, these studies have used different antigens, immunization routes, immunization schedules, challenge protocols, and animal models, so a direct comparison of the efficacy of the various adjuvants or delivery systems used is not possible.

Early *C. trachomatis* vaccine trials in humans made use of mineral oil or alum adjuvants, with mixed results [74,75], but of these adjuvants only alum would be acceptable for human use today, and this elicits a Th2-biased response. All recent studies have focused on animal, usually murine, models of infection, and the evaluation of a particular adjuvant has often not been a central theme of these studies. A number of adjuvants have been used with MOMP or MOMP peptides, again with mixed success. The use of cholera toxin [88] and liposomes containing monophosphoryl lipid A [119] elicited modest serum antibody responses to MOMP, but not protection. In contrast, purified MOMP formulated into ISCOMs did elicit an immune response protective against vaginal challenge with *C. trachomatis* serovar D [95]. Adoptive transfer of peripheral blood lymphocytes from immunized mice to naïve recipients was able to confer protection upon the recipients, indicating that MOMP-ISCOMs were able to elicit systemic cell-mediated responses and that such responses could make an important contribution to local immunity at genital mucosal surfaces.

An analogous approach to the use of synthetic lipophilic particles such as ISCOMs and liposomes is the use of bacterial cell walls and outer membranes, or ghosts, to deliver vaccine antigens. In addition to providing a particulate delivery vehicle, ghosts utilize the intrinsic adjuvant properties of many bacterial wall and membrane components and are effective at eliciting cell-mediated and local immune responses [120,121]. As noted above, the use of chlamydial outer membrane complexes has been successful at eliciting quite strong protective responses [85] but potentially risks eliciting immunopathological responses in addition to protective responses. The use of recombinant bacterial ghosts expressing selected chlamydial antigens should allow the antichlamydial response to be focused on selected protective antigens [1]. Preliminary studies of *Vibrio cholerae* ghosts expressing *C. trachomatis* MOMP indicates that this approach has the potential to elicit protective immune responses in a mouse model of *C. trachomatis* genital tract infection (J. Igietseme, personal communication, 2001).

Several live bacterial and viral delivery systems have also been used to deliver chlamydial antigens, although the use of live vectors for chlamydial antigens is lagging behind the use of other adjuvants and delivery systems. The bacterial vectors used include *Salmonella*, which failed to elicit strong immune responses when a Salmonella construct expressing *C. trachomatis* MOMP epitopes was tested in mice [122], and *Lactobacillus*, which could express *C. psittaci* MOMP but was not tested for immunogenicity [123]. The use of viral vectors has been more encouraging, but much remains to be done in this area also. MOMP epitopes have been expressed on a filamentous phage vector [124] and upon poliovirus [125–127]. Both approaches were successful at raising antibodies against chlamydia EBs, but only the poliovirus construct has been tested for protective efficacy in an animal model, where it was unable to elicit a protective response against an ocular challenge in monkeys (Caldwell and Murdin, unpublished data). Poxvirus vectors have so far received relatively little attention in the context of *Chlamydia*, although their ability to elicit both humoral and cell-mediated immune responses suggest that they should be effective vectors for chlamydial antigens. Preliminary studies suggest that they may be an effective delivery system for chlamydial antigens, including Cap1 [115] and MOMP (Murdin, Raudonikiene, Millar, and Dunn, unpublished data).

Unlike protein or peptide-based subunit vaccines, DNA vaccination provides protective immunity following endogenous expression of foreign proteins by host T cells, thus allowing the presentation of antigen to the immune system in a manner that may be closer to that which occurs during natural infection with viruses or other intracellular pathogens. In the context of chlamydial infection, the potential advantages of DNA vaccination include the induction of a broad spectrum of immune responses including Th1-like CD4 responses and mucosal immunity. DNA immunization with several chlamydial antigens including the homologous

MOMP gene produces significant protective immunity to lung challenge infection with *C. trachomatis* MoPn [100,113] or *C. pneumoniae* [35,101,102], and elicited cellular and humoral immune responses consistent with a predominantly Th1-mediated response [35,128]. It should be noted that although DNA immunization appears to be able to reliably protect against a lung chlamydial challenge in several different models, it failed to protect mice from a genital chlamydial challenge in the one published account using such a model [129]. Mice immunized with MOMP DNA mounted weak humoral and cell-mediated immune responses but were not protected from vaginal shedding of *Chlamydia* following a vaginal challenge, or from infection-associated infertility. The reason for this failure is unclear, but may indicate that the genital tract is a more difficult site to protect than the lung when using a systemic DNA immunization strategy.

Subsequent studies showed that a MOMP-DNA prime followed by a MOMP-ISCOM boost was highly effective at inducing immunity to pulmonary *C. trachomatis* challenge, eliciting protection comparable to that conferred by a prior infection [130]. This is a significant result because most immunization strategies elicit partial protection significantly weaker than that elicited by a previous infection. The result is consistent with the observation that prime-boost strategies are often superior to single-adjuvant or single-vector strategies for several intracellular pathogens [131], and such strategies probably deserve to receive more attention in the context of *Chlamydia*. It is also worth noting in this context that prime-boost strategies employing a mucosal route of immunization may elicit different responses from similar strategies using a systemic route of immunization [132].

C. The Importance of Dendritic Cells in Anti-*Chlamydia* Immunization

Perhaps the most interesting studies in the recent *Chlamydia* vaccine literature are those which have used dendritic cells (DCs) for antigen delivery, or have sought to recruit DCs during immunization. This approach seems to hold considerable promise for establishing firm correlates of antichlamydial immunity and for identifying truly effective antichlamydial immunization strategies. The first of these studies, by Su et al. [133], established that DCs pulsed ex vivo with killed *Chlamydiae* could efficiently phagocytose, process, and present chlamydial antigens, accompanied by the secretion of IL-12. Intravenous immunization of mice with chlamydial-pulsed DCs elicited protective immunity against vaginal challenge equal to that obtained after infection with live organisms, and protection was correlated with a *Chlamydia*-specific Th1-biased response similar to that elicited by chlamydial infection. Similar results were subsequently obtained in a mouse lung infection model by Lu and Zhong [42], who showed that *Chlamydia*-pulsed DCs, but not macrophages, could elicit strong protection which correlated with Th1-biased immune responses. In an important additional finding, Lu and Zhong [42] demonstrated the importance of IL-12 secretion by the antigen-pulsed DCs in directing Th1 response. DCs from mice deficient in the IL-12 p40 gene failed to produce IL-12 following an ex vivo

Chlamydia pulse, and immunization with these DCs failed to induce either a Th1-biased response or protection against chlamydial infection. Conversely, as might be expected, downregulation of endogenous IL-10 expression of *Chlamydia*-pulsed DCs also enhances Th1 responses and protection [44]. Mice genetically engineered to be IL-10$^{-/-}$ were highly resistant to chlamydial genital infection, and induced a greater frequency of *Chlamydia*-specific Th1 responses following *C. trachomatis* infection. The negative effect of IL-10 in the development of a protective response acts at the level of the antigen-presenting DC itself, since immunization with DCs from IL-10$^{-/-}$ mice or with IL-10 antisense-treated DCs from wild-type mice was able to elicit strong protective responses in IL-10$^{+/+}$ C57BL/6 mice against vaginal challenge with *C. trachomatis* serovar D. These observations suggest that the ability of DCs to efficiently process and present chlamydial antigens to naive T-cells *in vivo* and to direct a Th1 immune response by the secretion of high levels of IL-12 in comparison to IL-10 are important components in eliciting effective antichlamydial immunity.

Recognizing that immunization with live *Chlamydia* elicits stronger protective immunity than does immunization with the inactivated organism, Zhang et al. [41] studied immune responses in mice immunized with viable or UV-killed chlamydia. Immunization with viable chlamydiae induced a Th1-biased response, including high levels of antigen-specific delayed-type hypersensitivity, IFNγ, and local IgA, GM-CSF, and IL-12 production, whereas immunization with killed chlamydia induced Th2-biased responses including IL-10 production and IgG1. Interestingly, mice immunized with viable organisms exhibited a recruitment of a DC-like cell population to the site of immunization, consistent with the important role of DCs indicated by the DC immunization studies described above. Developing the hypothesis that early induction of proinflammatory cytokines and the activation and differentiation of DCs may be key to the induction of protective responses by viable organisms, the same group studied the use of an adenovirus vector expressing GM-CSF (Ad-GM-CSF) to recruit DCs to the site of immunization [134]. Mice were inoculated with the Ad-GM-CSF 7 days prior to immunization with UV-inactivated chlamydia. Both routes of immunization recruited DCs to the site of immunization and elicited significant levels of systemic Th1 immune responses, but the intranasal immunization also elicited antichlamydial IgA in the lung. Intranasal, but not intraperitoneal, immunization elicited strong protection against a pulmonary chlamydial challenge, comparable to that elicited by live chlamydiae. Immunization with UV-inactivated chlamydia in the absence of Ad-GM-CSF was not protective. This result provides further support for the importance of DCs in eliciting a protective Th1 immune response and indicates the contribution of local IgA responses to immunity from chlamydial infection. It is not clear that protection was due solely to local IgA in this study; effector T-cells arising from intraperitoneal immunization may not have been recruited to the lung as quickly or efficiently as those arising from intranasal immunization, for example. Nevertheless, the result is a reminder that local antibody responses may have a role to play in protection from chlamydial infection.

Overall, these studies indicate the central importance of DCs in the induction of protective immunity to chlamydial infection. Vaccination strategies based on the use of antigen-pulsed DCs as the immunizing agent are not realistic for mass use, at least with current technology, but vaccination strategies intended to recruit DCs to the site of immunization and to target antigen to those DCs appear to be well worth exploring. Recruitment of DCs might be achieved, for example, by the expression of not only GM-CSF but also other molecules such as IL-1β, TNF-α, MIP-1α, MIP-1β, MIP-3α, and RANTES. Achieving a better understanding of the factors influencing the expression of effective immunity at mucosal sites distant from the site of immunization will also be an important goal of studies in this area.

D. Routes of Immunization

Route of immunization is a critical variable determining the success of immunization, but the data for chlamydia is fragmented and sometimes contradictory. Several routes have been evaluated in several different models, including conjunctival [88,91], intranasal [95,100,101,108], oral [88,94,107–109,122], vaginal [84], intravenous [122], subcutaneous [85,94,96,108], intramuscular [94–96,100–102], intraperitoneal [94], and presacral [94]. The results from this considerable body of work are often hard to interpret, and it may seem that all that can be concluded is that under some circumstances some routes are effective for inducing antichlamydial immunity. For example, MOMP DNA given intranasally may be more effective than DNA given intramuscularly, at least at protecting the lung [100]. MOMP DNA given intramuscularly will protect the lung [100] but may not protect the genital tract [129], whereas purified MOMP formulated with ISCOMs given intramuscularly will protect the genital tract [95]. Orally administered anti-id to GLXA encapsulated in polylactide microspheres elicits protection versus ocular and vaginal challenge [107,108], whereas orally administered MOMP and LPS elicited little or no protection [88,94,109].

However, at the risk of stating the obvious, some tentative guidelines can be proposed. Firstly, intranasal immunization appears to be one of the more effective routes of immunization at eliciting protective responses in both the lungs and the genital tract, a finding that matches experience with other mucosal pathogens [135,136]. In light of these findings and because of the clear importance of eliciting effective mucosal antichlamydial responses it would make sense to include this route in future evaluations of candidate vaccines. Second, the systemic route of immunization should not be ignored. Intramuscular delivery of both protein and DNA can elicit protective immunity against lung and genital tract challenges [see, e.g., Refs. 95, 96, and 100], and should continue to be evaluated if for no other reason than that it is acceptable and easy to use in humans. It may prove useful to vary the site of intramuscular immunization to target selected (or multiple) draining lymph nodes. Third, given the important role of DCs in eliciting protective immune responses, routes targeting DC-rich sites such as the skin [137] may repay further study, although the experience of Lu et al. [134] indicates that the site at which DCs are targeted can influence the effectiveness of the subsequent immune response. Finally, the use of multiple routes of inoculation in a single immunization schedule should be investigated. Combined intramuscular and intranasal immunizations have been effective for DNA immunization against *C. pneumoniae* lung infection, for example [101], and in the absence of a thorough understanding of the induction of effective antichlamydial protective immunity in different organs approaches targeting multiple inductive sites may be more effective at inducing widespread distribution of appropriate immune effectors.

E. Animal Models for Vaccine Testing

The outcome and interpretation of vaccination studies depend not only upon the vaccine but also upon the species, strain, and age of the vaccinated animal and upon the strain of the pathogen used for challenge. The models most commonly used for recent vaccine studies are mouse models of *C. trachomatis* genital or lung infection [138–140], and mouse models of *C. pneumoniae* lung infection [141], although some important studies have used mouse models of *C. trachomatis* ocular infection [107]. The lung infection model using *C. trachomatis* MoPn is convenient and easy to use, but it should be recognized that MoPn is a murine isolate of *C. trachomatis* [142] that is antigenically distinct from human isolates and more virulent than those in the mouse. Furthermore, human *C. trachomatis* infection targets the eyes or genital tract. *C. pneumoniae* lung infection models have the advantage of targeting a clinically relevant organ. They produce consistent results in different laboratories, although the strain of mouse and the strain of chlamydia used will affect the outcome [141].

With respect to the genital infection models, there are several variations in protocol that can influence the outcome of an experiment and need to be taken into account when designing and interpreting studies. Intrabursal and intrauterine challenge inoculations [138,139] ensure infection of the upper genital tract and are usually used when fertility or salpingitis is an endpoint. However, the route of inoculation is clearly unnatural and bypasses vaginal barriers to infection, both innate and adaptive, which may be significant in vaccination studies. Intravaginal inoculation is more realistic, but older mice in particular may be resistant to chlamydial infection by this route, and infection may not ascend past the cervix, unless the mice are treated with progesterone [139]. This may be acceptable for studies of chlamydial biology and pathogenesis, but because progesterone has strong immunomodulatory properties [143] its use should be avoided when testing vaccines. The use of human *C. trachomatis* isolates for genital tract challenge overcomes the objection that *C. trachomatis* MoPn is not a human pathogen, but many human strains are relatively avirulent in mice, possibly because of increased sensitivity to IFNγ [144,145] or differential expression of virulence determinants [146].

When considering testing a *C. pneumoniae* vaccine for cardiovascular disease, several mouse [147–149] and rabbit [150,151] models are available. The murine models are in $LDLR^{-/-}$ or $ApoE^{-/-}$ mice, which will develop atherosclerosis independently of *C. pneumoniae* infection. In these models *C. pneumoniae* strain AR39 [147–149], but apparently not the Kajaani strain [152,153], is an exacerbating factor in the development of atherosclerosis. However, it should be recognized that the underlying genetic lesion dominates the atherosclerotic process and may influence the outcome of immunization studies.

IV. SUMMARY AND FUTURE DIRECTIONS

L. H. Collier, writing in 1966 on the then current status of *C. trachomatis* vaccine development, concluded "that, although some vaccines now being tested are partially effective, much remains to be learned about immunity to trachoma and methods of inducing it artificially" [73]. Thirty-five years later, skeptics might argue that nothing much has changed. Candidate *C. trachomatis* and *C. pneumoniae* vaccines are at best partially effective in animals and have not been tested in humans, the nature of protective immune responses is only partially defined, and methods of eliciting effective protection in animals models are arrived at empirically following strategies that may not be acceptable or effective for human use. This criticism is, of course, too harsh, but does highlight the often frustrating lack of progress caused by the unusually difficult challenges inherent to chlamydia vaccine development [83]. In reality, real and significant progress has been made in our understanding of the chlamydiae and their interaction with their host and specifically with their host's immune system.

The single most important advance in the last few years has been the sequencing of several chlamydial genomes. For an organism such as chlamydia that is not susceptible to genetic manipulation, the ability to analyze and compare the genome sequences has provided an insight into chlamydia biology that was simply not available before. In the context of vaccine development this has allowed the identification of novel protective antigens, in some cases has provided an insight into the biological significance of these antigens, and has generally propelled the field beyond the MOMP-based vaccine studies that characterized the pregenome literature. The recent studies of the role of DCs in immunity to chlamydial infection hold the promise of defining the requirements for the induction of strong, enduring and properly localized protective immune responses. Parallel advances in developing novel adjuvants and delivery systems offer tools with which to present selected antigens to the immune system in such a way that these requirements for the induction of protectivity immunity can be fulfilled safely and effectively.

In conclusion, it does not seem overly optimistic to paraphrase Collier [73] as follows: most vaccines now being tested are only partially effective, but recent advances in our understanding of the biology and immunology of chlamydial infection should allow the rapid development of effective methods of inducing protective immunity.

ACKNOWLEDGMENTS

The authors gratefully acknowledge the help and advice of Dr. Joseph Igietseme, Dr. Luis de la Maza, Dr. Pamela

Dunn, Dr. Hang Lu, and the staff of the Aventis Pasteur library in Toronto, Canada.

REFERENCES

1. Igietseme JU, et al. Chlamydial vaccines: strategies and status. BioDrugs 2002; 16:19–35.
2. Stephens RS. *Chlamydia*: Intracellular Biology, Pathogenesis and Immunity. Washington, DC: American Society for Microbiology, 1999.
3. Brunham RC. Human immunity to chlamydiae. In: Stephens RS, ed. *Chlamydia*: Intracellular Biology, Pathogenesis and Immunity. Washington, DC: American Society for Microbiology, 1999:211–238.
4. Beatty WL, et al. Persistent chlamydiae: from cell culture to a paradigm for chlamydial pathogenesis. Microbiol Rev 1994; 58:686–699.
5. Grayston JT. Background and current knowledge of *Chlamydia pneumoniae* and atherosclerosis. J Infect Dis 2000; 181 (suppl 3):S402–S410.
6. Rutherford JD. *Chlamydia pneumoniae* and atherosclerosis. Curr Atheroscler Rep 2000; 2:218–225.
7. Centers for Disease Control and Prevention. Sexually Transmitted Disease Surveillance, 2000. Atlanta, GA: U.S. Department of Health and Human Services, Centers for Disease Control and Prevention, September 2001.
8. Anttila T, et al. Serotypes of *Chlamydia trachomatis* and risk for development of cervical squamous cell carcinoma. JAMA 2001; 285:47–51.
9. Ward ME. Mechanisms of *Chlamydia*-induced disease. In: Stephens RS, ed. *Chlamydia*: Intracellular Biology, Pathogenesis and Immunity. Washington, DC: American Society for Microbiology, 1999:171–210.
10. Stephens RS, et al. Genome sequence of an obligate intracellular pathogen of humans: *Chlamydia trachomatis*. Science 1998; 282:754–759.
11. Kalman S, et al. Comparative genomes of *Chlamydia pneumoniae* and *C. trachomatis*. Nat Genet 1999; 21:385–389.
12. Read TD, et al. Genome sequences of *Chlamydia trachomatis* MoPn and *Chlamydia pneumoniae* AR39. Nucleic Acids Res 2000; 28:1397–1406.
13. Shirai M, et al. Comparison of whole genome sequences of *Chlamydia pneumoniae* J138 from Japan and CWL029 from USA. Nucleic Acids Res 2000; 28:2311–2314.
13a. Griffais R. *Chlamydia pneumoniae* genome sequence. International Patent Application WO 99/27105.
14. Christiansen G, et al. Potential relevance of *Chlamydia pneumoniae* surface proteins to an effective vaccine. J Infect Dis 2000; 181(suppl 3):S528–S537.
15. Newhall WJ 5th, et al. Serovar determination of *Chlamydia trachomatis* isolates by using type-specific monoclonal antibodies. J Clin Microbiol 1986; 23:333–338.
16. Wang SP, et al. Three new serovars of *Chlamydia trachomatis*: Da, Ia, and L2a. J Infect Dis 1991; 163:403–405.
17. Zhong G, et al. *Chlamydia* inhibits interferon γ-inducible major histocompatibility complex class II expression by degradation of upstream stimulatory factor 1. J Exp Med 1999; 189:1931–1938.
18. Zhong G, et al. Degradation of transcription factor RFX5 during the inhibition of both constitutive and interferon γ-inducible major histocompatibility complex class I expression in *Chlamydia*-infected cells. J Exp Med 2000; 191:1525–1534.
19. Fan T, et al. Inhibition of apoptosis in *Chlamydia*-infected cells: blockade of mitochondrial cytochrome *c* release and caspase activation. J Exp Med 1998; 187:487–496.
20. Jawetz E, et al. Experimental inclusion conjunctivitis in man. JAMA 1965; 194:150–162.
21. Grayston JT, et al. The potential for vaccine against infection of the genital tract with *Chlamydia trachomatis*. Sex Transm Dis 1978; 5:73–77.
22. Taylor HR. Development of immunity to ocular chlamydial infection. Am J Trop Med Hyg 1990; 42:358–364.
23. Katz BP, et al. Effect of prior sexually transmitted disease on the isolation of *Chlamydia trachomatis*. Sex Transm Dis 1987; 14:160–164.
24. Brunham RC, et al. The epidemiology of *Chlamydia trachomatis* within a sexually transmitted diseases core group. J Infect Dis 1996; 173:950–956.
25. Mabey D, et al. Immunity to *Chlamydia trachomatis*: lessons from a Gambian village. J Med Microbiol 1996; 45:1–2.
26. Holland MJ, et al. T helper type-1 (Th1)-Th2 profiles of peripheral blood mononuclear cells (PBMC); responses to antigens of *Chlamydia trachomatis* in subjects with severe trachomatous scarring. Clin Exp Immunol 1996; 105:429–435.
27. Bobo LD, et al. Severe disease in children with trachoma is associated with persistent *Chlamydia trachomatis* infection. J Infect Dis 1997; 176:1524–1530.
28. Kimani J, et al. Risk factors for *Chlamydia trachomatis* pelvic inflammatory disease among sex workers in Nairobi, Kenya. J Infect Dis 1996; 173:1437–1444.
29. Holland MJ, et al. Synthetic peptides based on *Chlamydia trachomatis* antigens identify cytotoxic T lymphocyte responses in subjects from a trachoma-endemic population. Clin Exp Immunol 1997; 107:44–49.
30. Kim SK, et al. Direct detection and magnetic isolation of *Chlamydia trachomatis* major outer membrane protein-specific CD8$^+$ CTLs with HLA class I tetramers. J Immunol 2000; 165:7285–7299.
31. Magee DM, et al. Role of CD8 T cells in primary *Chlamydia* infection. Infect Immun 1995; 63:516–521.
32. Su H, et al. CD4$^+$ T cells play a significant role in adoptive immunity to *Chlamydia trachomatis* infection of the mouse genital tract. Infect Immun 1995; 63:3302–3308.
33. Penttila JM, et al. Depletion of CD8$^+$ cells abolishes memory in acquired immunity against *Chlamydia pneumoniae* in BALB/c mice. Immunology 1999; 97:490–496.
34. Rottenberg ME, et al. Role of innate and adaptive immunity in the outcome of primary infection with *Chlamydia pneumoniae*, as analyzed in genetically modified mice. J Immunol 1999; 162:2829–2836.
35. Svanholm C, et al. Protective DNA immunization against *Chlamydia pneumoniae*. Scand J Immunol 2000; 51:345–353.
36. Lampe MF, et al. Gamma interferon production by cytotoxic T lymphocytes is required for resolution of *Chlamydia trachomatis* infection. Infect Immun 1998; 66:5457–5461.
37. Vuola JM, et al. Acquired immunity to *Chlamydia pneumoniae* is dependent on gamma interferon in two mouse strains that initially differ in this respect after primary challenge. Infect Immun 2000; 68:960–964.
38. Geng Y, et al. Roles of interleukin-12 and gamma interferon in murine *Chlamydia pneumoniae* infection. Infect Immun 2000; 68:2245–2253.
39. Wang S, et al. IFN-gamma knockout mice show Th2-associated delayed-type hypersensitivity and the inflammatory cells fail to localize and control chlamydial infection. Eur J Immunol 1999; 29:3782–3792.
40. Johansson M, et al. Studies in knockout mice reveal that antichlamydial protection requires Th1 cells producing IFN-gamma: is this true for humans? Scand J Immunol 1997; 46:546–552.
41. Zhang D, et al. Immunity to *Chlamydia trachomatis* mouse pneumonitis induced by vaccination with live organisms correlates with early granulocyte–macrophage colony-stimulating factor and interleukin-12 production and with dendritic cell-like maturation. Infect Immun 1999; 67:1606–1613.

42. Lu H, Zhong G. Interleukin-12 production is required for chlamydial antigen-pulsed dendritic cells to induce protection against live *Chlamydia trachomatis* infection. Infect Immun 1999; 67:1763–1769.

43. Yang X, et al. IL-10 gene knockout mice show enhanced Th-1-like protective immunity and absent granuloma formation following *Chlamydia trachomatis* lung infection. J Immunol 1999; 162:1010–1017.

44. Igietseme JU, et al. Suppression of endogenous IL-10 gene expression in dendritic cells enhances antigen presentation for specific Th1 induction: potential for cellular vaccine development. J Immunol 2000; 164:4212–4219.

45. Caspar-Bauguil S, et al. *Chlamydia pneumoniae* induces interleukin-10 production that down-regulates major histocompatibility complex class I expression. J Infect Dis 2000; 182:1394–1401.

46. Redecke V, et al. Interaction of *Chlamydia pneumoniae* and human alveolar macrophages: infection and inflammatory response. Am J Respir Cell Mol Biol 1998; 19:721–727.

47. Johansson M, et al. Immunological memory in B-cell-deficient mice conveys long-lasting protection against genital tract infection with *Chlamydia trachomatis* by rapid recruitment of T cells. Immunology 2001; 102:199–208.

48. Morrison SG, et al. Immunity to murine *Chlamydia trachomatis* genital tract reinfection involves B cells and CD4(+) T cells but not CD8(+) T cells. Infect Immun 2000; 68:6979–6987.

49. Morrison SG, et al. Resolution of secondary *Chlamydia trachomatis* genital tract infection in immune mice with depletion of both CD4$^+$ and CD8$^+$ T cells. Infect Immun 2001; 69: 2643–2649.

50. Saikku P, et al. Serological evidence of an association of a novel *Chlamydia*, TWAR, with chronic coronary heart disease and acute myocardial infarction. Lancet 1988; ii:983–985.

51. Treharne JD, et al. Antibodies to *Chlamydia trachomatis* in acute salpingitis. Br J Vener Dis 1979; 55:26–29.

52. Wang S-P, et al. *Chlamydia trachomatis* infection in Fitz–Hugh–Curtis syndrome. Am J Obstet Gynecol 1980; 138: 1034–1038.

53. Punnonen R, et al. Chlamydial serology in infertile women by immunofluorescence. Fertil Steril 1979; 31:656–659.

54. Osser S, et al. Postabortal pelvic infection associated with *Chlamydia trachomatis* and the influence of humoral immunity. Am J Obstet Gynecol 1984; 150:699–703.

55. Bailey RL, et al. The influence of local antichlamydial antibody on the acquisition and persistence of human ocular chlamydial infection: IgG antibodies are not protective. Epidemiol Infect 1993; 111:315–324.

56. Ghaem-Maghami S, et al. Characterization of B-cell responses to *Chlamydia trachomatis* antigens in humans with trachoma. Infect Immun 1997; 65:4958–4964.

57. Brunham RC, et al. Correlation of host immune response with quantitative recovery of *Chlamydia trachomatis* from the human endocervix. Infect Immun 1983; 39:1491–1494.

58. Puolakkainen M, et al. Persistence of chlamydial antibodies after pelvic inflammatory disease. J Clin Microbiol 1986; 23: 924–928.

59. Rhinehart-Jones TR, et al. Transfer of immunity against lethal murine Francisella infection by specific antibody depends on host gamma interferon and T cells. Infect Immun 1994; 62:3129–3137.

60. Abbas AK, et al. Functional diversity of helper T lymphocytes. Nature 1996; 383:787–793.

61. Campbell LA, et al. Detection of *Chlamydia trachomatis* deoxyribonucleic acid in women with tubal infertility. Fertil Steril 1993; 59:45–50.

62. Patton DL, et al. Detection of *Chlamydia trachomatis* in fallopian tube tissue in women with postinfectious tubal infertility. Am J Obstet Gynecol 1994; 171:95–101.

63. Taylor-Robinson D, et al. Detection of *Chlamydia trachomatis* DNA in joints of reactive arthritis patients by polymerase chain reaction. Lancet 1992; 340:81–82.

64. Bas S, et al. Amplification of plasmid and chromosome *Chlamydia* DNA in synovial fluid of patients with reactive arthritis and undifferentiated seronegative oligoarthropathies. Arthritis Rheum 1995; 38:1005–1013.

65. Campbell LA, et al. *Chlamydia pneumoniae* and cardiovascular disease. Emerg Infect Dis 1998; 4:571–579.

66. Maass M, et al. Endovascular presence of viable *Chlamydia pneumoniae* is a common phenomenon in coronary artery disease. J Am Coll Cardiol 1998; 31:827–832.

67. Ramirez JA. Isolation of *Chlamydia pneumoniae* from the coronary artery of a patient with coronary atherosclerosis. The *Chlamydia pneumoniae*/Atherosclerosis Study Group. Ann Intern Med 1996; 125:979–982.

68. Hillis SD, et al. Recurrent chlamydial infections increase the risks of hospitalization for ectopic pregnancy and pelvic inflammatory disease. Am J Obstet Gynecol 1997; 176:103–107.

69. Beatty WL, et al. Persistent chlamydiae: from cell culture to a paradigm for chlamydial pathogenesis. Microbiol Rev 1994; 58:686–699.

70. Kalayoglu MV, et al. Chlamydial virulence determinants in atherogenesis: the role of chlamydial lipopolysaccharide and heat shock protein 60 in macrophage–lipoprotein interactions. J Infect Dis 2000; 181(suppl 3):S483–S489.

71. Lenz DC, et al. A *Chlamydia pneumoniae*-specific peptide induces experimental autoimmune encephalomyelitis in rats. J Immunol 2001; 167:1803–1808.

72. Bachmaier K, et al. *Chlamydia* infections and heart disease linked through antigenic mimicry. Science 1999; 283:1335–1339.

73. Collier LH. The present status of trachoma vaccination studies. Bull Wld Hlth Org 1966; 34:233–241.

74. Grayston JT, et al. Prevention of trachoma with vaccine. Arch Environ Health 1964; 8:518–526.

75. Grayston JT, et al. Field studies of protection from infection by experimental trachoma virus vaccine in preschool-aged children on Taiwan. Proc Soc Exp Biol Med 1963; 112:589–595.

76. Sampaio AA, et al. Studies on tachoma. IV. Investigations in Portugal on formalin-killed trachoma vaccines with special reference to serologic response. Am J Trop Med Hyg 1963; 12:909–915.

77. Sowa S, et al. Trachoma vaccine field trials in The Gambia. J Hyg Camb 1969; 67:699–717.

78. Woolridge RL, et al. Field trial of a monovalent and of a bivalent mineral oil adjuvant trachoma vaccine in Taiwan school children. Am J Ophthalmol 1967; 63(suppl):1645–1650.

79. Woolridge RL, et al. Long-term follow-up of the initial (1959–1960) trachoma vaccine field trial on Taiwan. Am J Ophthalmol 1967; 63(suppl):1650–1655.

80. Wang S-P, et al. Trachoma vaccine studies in monkeys. Am J Ophthalmol 1967; 63(suppl):1615–1630.

81. Grayston JT, et al. The effect of trachoma virus vaccine on the course of experimental trachoma infection in blind human volunteers. J Exp Med 1962; 115:1009–1024.

82. Collier LH, et al. Immunogenicity of experimental trachoma vaccines in baboons. II. Experiments with adjuvants, and tests of cross-protection. J Hyg (Lond) 1966; 64:529–544.

83. Murdin AD, et al. Collaborative multidisciplinary workshop report: progress toward a *Chlamydia pneumoniae* vaccine. J Infect Dis 2000; 181(suppl 3):S552–S557.

84. Su H, et al. Subclinical chlamydial infection of the female mouse genital tract generates a potent protective immune

response: implications for development of live attenuated chlamydial vaccine strains. Infect Immun 2000; 68:192–196.

85. Pal S, et al. Immunization with an acellular vaccine consisting of the outer membrane complex of *Chlamydia trachomatis* induces protection against a genital challenge. Infect Immun 1997; 65:3361–3369.

86. Caldwell HD, et al. Structural analysis of chlamydial major outer membrane proteins. Infect Immun 1982; 38:960–968.

87. Brunham RC, et al. *Chlamydia trachomatis* antigens: role in immunity and pathogenesis. Infect Agents Dis 1994; 5:218–233.

88. Taylor HR, et al. Oral immunization with chlamydial major outer membrane protein (MOMP). Invest Ophthalmol Vis Sci 1988; 29:1847–1853.

89. Tan T-W, et al. Protection of sheep against *Chlamydia psittaci* infection with a subcellular vaccine containing the major outer membrane protein. Infect Immun 1990; 58:3101–3108.

90. Batteiger BE, et al. Partial protection against genital reinfection by immunization of guinea-pigs with isolated outer-membrane proteins of the chlamydial agent of guinea-pig inclusion conjunctivitis. J Gen Microbiol 1993; 139: 2965–2972.

91. Campos M, et al. A chlamydial major outer membrane protein extract as a trachoma vaccine candidate. Invest Ophthalmol Vis Sci 1995; 36:1477–1491.

92. Su H, et al. Protective efficacy of a parenterally administered MOMP-derived synthetic oligopeptide vaccine in a murine model of *Chlamydia trachomatis* genital tract infection: serum neutralizing IgG antibodies do not protect against chlamydial genital tract infection. Vaccine 1995; 13:1023–1032.

93. Zhong G, et al. Immunogenicity evaluation of lipidic amino acid-based synthetic peptide vaccine for *Chlamydia trachomatis*. J Immunol 1993; 151:3728–3736.

94. Tuffrey M, et al. Heterotypic protection of mice against chlamydial salpingitis and colonization of the lower genital tract with a human serovar F isolate of *Chlamydia trachomatis* by prior immunization with recombinant serovar LI major outer-membrane protein. J Gen Microbiol 1992; 138:1707–1715.

95. Igietseme JU, et al. Induction of protective immunity against *Chlamydia trachomatis* genital infection by a vaccine based on major outer membrane protein-lipophilic immune response-stimulating complexes. Infect Immun 2000; 68:6798–6806.

96. Pal S, et al. Immunization with the *Chlamydia trachomatis* mouse pneumonitis major outer membrane protein can elicit a protective immune response against a genital challenge. Infect Immun 2001; 69:6240–6247.

97. Mccafferty MC, et al. Electrophoretic analysis of the major outer membrane protein of *Chlamydia psittaci* reveals multimers which are recognized by protective monoclonal antibodies. Infect Immun 1995; 63:2387–2389.

98. Morein B, et al. Iscom, a delivery system for parenteral and mucosal vaccination. Dev Biol Stand 1998; 92:33–39.

99. Sjolander A, et al. Vaccination with recombinant parasite surface antigen 2 from *Leishmania major* induces a Th1 type of immune response but does not protect against infection. Vaccine 1998; 16:2077–2084.

100. Zhang D-J, et al. DNA vaccination with the major outer-membrane protein gene induces acquired immunity to *Chlamydia trachomatis* (mouse pneumonitis) infection. J Infect Dis 1997; 176:1035–1040.

101. Murdin AD, et al. Use of a mouse lung challenge model to identify antigens protective against *Chlamydia pneumoniae* lung infection. J Infect Dis 2000; 181(suppl 3):S544–S551.

102. Penttilä T, et al. Immunity to *Chlamydia pneumoniae* induced by vaccination with DNA vectors expressing a cytoplasmic protein (Hsp60) or outer membrane proteins (MOMP and Omp2). Vaccine 2000; 19:1256–1265.

103. Stuart ES, et al. Characterization of an antigen secreted by *Chlamydia*-infected cell culture. Immunology 1987; 61:527–533.

104. Stuart ES, et al. Some characteristics of a secreted chlamydial antigen recognized by IgG from *C. trachomatis* patient sera. Immunology 1989; 68:469–473.

105. Stuart ES, et al. Examination of chlamydial glycolipid with monoclonal antibodies: cellular distribution and epitope binding. Immunology 1991; 74:740–747.

106. An L-L, et al. Biochemical and functional antigenic mimicry by a polyclonal anti-idiotypic antibody for chlamydial exoglycolipid antigen. Pathobiology 1997; 65:229–240.

107. Whittum-Hudson JA, et al. Oral immunization with an anti-idiotypic antibody to the exoglycolipid antigen protects against experimental *Chlamydia trachomatis* infection. Nat Med 1996; 2:1116–1121.

108. Whittum-Hudson JA, et al. The anti-idiotypic antibody to *Chlamydial glycolipid* exoantigen (GLXA) protects mice against genital infection with a human biovar of *Chlamydia trachomatis*. Vaccine 2001; 19:4061–4071.

109. Taylor HR, et al. Attempted oral immunization with chlamydial lipopylsaccharide subunit vaccine. Invest Ophthalmol Vis Sci 1987; 28:1722–1726.

110. Murdin AD, et al. *Chlamydia* antigens and corresponding DNA fragments and uses thereof. International Patent Application WO 00/55326.

111. Stephens RS, et al. *Chlamydia* outer membrane protein discovery using genomics. Curr Opin Microbiol 2001; 4:16–20.

112. Stephens RS. Chlamydial genomics and vaccine antigen discovery. J Infect Dis 2000; 181(suppl 3):S521–S523.

113. Brunham RC, et al. The potential for vaccine development against chlamydial infection and disease. J Infect Dis 2000; 181(suppl 3):S538–S543.

114. Kubo A, et al. Characterization and functional analysis of PorB, a chlamydia porin and neutralizing target. Mol Microbiol 2000; 38:772–780.

115. Fling SP, et al. CD8$^+$ T cells recognize an inclusion associated protein from the pathogen *Chlamydia trachomatis*. Proc Natl Acad Sci U S A 2001; 98:1160–1165.

116. Pizza M, et al. Identification of vaccine candidates against serogroup B meningococcus by whole-genome sequencing. Science 2000; 287:1816–1820.

117. Chicz RM, et al. Analysis of MHC-presented peptides: applications in autoimmunity and vaccine development. Immunol Today 1994; 15:155–159.

118. Murdin AD, et al. *Chlamydia* antigens and corresponding DNA fragments and uses thereof. International Patent Application WO 00/66739.

119. Motin VL, et al. Immunization with a peptide corresponding to chlamydial heat shock protein 60 increases the humoral immune response in C3H mice to a peptide representing variable domain 4 of the major outer membrane protein of *Chlamydia trachomatis*. Clin Diagn Lab Immunol 1999; 6:356–363.

120. Lubitz W, et al. Extended recombinant bacterial ghost system. J Biotechnol 1999; 73:261–273.

121. Szostak MP, et al. Bacterial ghosts: non-living candidate vaccines. J Biotechnol 1996; 44:161–170.

122. Hayes LJ, et al. *Clamydia trachomatis* major outer membrane protein epitopes expressed as fusions with LamB in an attenuated aroA strain of *Salmonella typhimurium*: their application as potential immunogens. J Gen Microbiol 1991; 137:1557–1564.

123. Turner MS, et al. Expression of *Chlamydia psittaci*- and human immunodeficiency virus-derived antigens on the cell surface of *Lactobacillus fermentum* BR11 as fusions to BspA. Infect Immun 1999; 67:5486–5489.

124. Zhong G, et al. Conformational mimicry of a chlamydial neutralization epitope on filamentous phage. J Biol Chem 1994; 269:24183–24188.

125. Murdin AD, et al. A poliovirus hybrid expressing a neutralization epitope from the major outer membrane protein of *Chlamydia trachomatis* is highly immunogenic. Infect Immun 1993; 61:4406–4414.

126. Murdin AD, et al. Poliovirus hybrids expressing neutralization epitopes from variable domains I and IV of the major outer membrane protein of *Chlamydia trachomatis* elicit broadly cross-reactive *C. trachomatis*-neutralizing antibodies. Infect Immun 1995; 63:1116–1121.

127. Burke KL, et al. A cassette vector for the construction of antigen chimaeras of poliovirus. J Gen Virol 1989; 70:2475–2479.

128. Zhang DJ, et al. Characterization of immune responses following intramuscular DNA immunization with the MOMP gene of *Chlamydia trachomatis* mouse pneumonitis strain. Immunology 1999; 96:314–321.

129. Pal S, et al. Vaccination of mice with DNA plasmids coding for the *Chlamydia trachomatis* major outer membrane protein elicits an immune response but fails to protect against a genital challenge. Vaccine 1999; 17:459–465.

130. Dong-Ji Z, et al. Priming with *Chlamydia trachomatis* major outer membrane protein (MOMP) DNA followed by MOMP ISCOM boosting enhances protection and is associated with increased immunoglobulin A and Th1 cellular immune responses. Infect Immun 2000; 68:3074–3078.

131. Ramshaw IA, et al. The prime-boost strategy: exciting prospects for improved vaccination. Immunol Today 2000; 21:163–165.

132. Eo SK, et al. Prime-boost immunization with DNA vaccine: mucosal route of administration changes the rules. J Immunol 2001; 166:5473–5479.

133. Su H, et al. Vaccination against chlamydial genital tract infection after immunization with dendritic cells pulsed ex vivo with nonviable Chlamydiae. J Exp Med 1998; 188:809–818.

134. Lu H, et al. GM-CSF transgene-based adjuvant allows the establishment of protective mucosal immunity following vaccination with inactivated *Chlamydia trachomatis*. J Immunol 2002; 169:6324–6331.

135. Rosenthal KL, et al. Challenges for vaccination against sexually-transmitted diseases: induction and long-term maintenance of mucosal immune responses in the female genital tract. Semin Immunol 1997; 9:303–314.

136. Staats HF, et al. Intranasal immunization is superior to vaginal, gastric, or rectal immunization for the induction of systemic and mucosal anti-HIV antibody responses. AIDS Res Hum Retroviruses 1997; 13:945–952.

137. Knight SC, et al. A peptide of *Chlamydia trachomatis* shown to be a primary T-cell epitope in vitro induces cell-mediated immunity *in vivo*. Immunology 1995; 85:8–15.

138. Barron AL, et al. A new animal model for the study of *Chlamydia trachomatis* genital infections: infection of mice with the agent of mouse pneumonitis. J Infect Dis 1981; 143:63–66.

139. Tuffrey M, et al. Progesterone as a key factor in the development of a mouse model for genital-tract infection with *Chlamydia trachomatis*. FEMS Microbiol Lett 1981; 12:111–115.

140. Kuo C, et al. A mouse model of *Chlamydia trachomatis* pneumonitis. J Infect Dis 1980; 141:198–202.

141. Saikku P, et al. Animal models for *Chlamydia pneumoniae* infection. Atherosclerosis 1998; 140(suppl 1):S17–S19.

142. Nigg C. An unidentified virus which causes pneumonia and systemic infection in mice. Science 1942; 95:49–50.

143. Szekeres-Bartho J, et al. Progesterone as an immunomodulatory molecule. Int Immunopharmacol 2001; 1:1037–1048.

144. Perry LL, et al. Differential sensitivity of distinct *Chlamydia trachomatis* isolates to IFN-gamma-mediated inhibition. J Immunol 1999; 162:3541–3548.

145. Morrison RP. Differential sensitivities of *Chlamydia trachomatis* strains to inhibitory effects of gamma interferon. Infect Immun 2000; 68:6038–6040.

146. Belland RJ, et al. *Chlamydia trachomatis* cytotoxicity associated with complete and partial cytotoxin genes. Proc Natl Acad Sci USA 2001; 98:13984–13989.

147. Moazed TC, et al. *Chlamydia pneumoniae* infection accelerates the progression of atherosclerosis in apolipoprotein E-deficient mice. J Infect Dis 1999; 180:238–241.

148. Hu H, et al. The atherogenic effects of chlamydia are dependent on serum cholesterol and specific to *Chlamydia pneumoniae*. J Clin Invest 1999; 103:747–753.

149. Liu L, et al. *Chlamydia pneumoniae* infection significantly exacerbates aortic atherosclerosis in an LDLR −/− mouse model within six months. Mol Cell Biochem 2000; 215:123–128.

150. Fong IW, et al. De novo induction of atherosclerosis by *Chlamydia pneumoniae* in a rabbit model. Infect Immun 1999; 67:6048–6055.

151. Muhlestein JB, et al. Infection with *Chlamydia pneumoniae* accelerates the development of atherosclerosis and treatment with azithromycin prevents it in a rabbit model. Circulation 1998; 97:633–636.

152. Caligiuri G, et al. *Chlamydia pneumoniae* infection does not induce or modify atherosclerosis in mice. Circulation 2001; 103:2834–2838.

153. Aalto-Setälä K, et al. *Chlamydia pneumoniae* does not increase atherosclerosis in the aortic root of apolipoprotein E-deficient mice. Arterioscler Thromb Vasc Biol 2001; 21:578–584.

69

Overview of Vaccine Strategies for Malaria

Michael F. Good and David Kemp
The Queensland Institute of Medical Research, Brisbane, Queensland, Australia

Malaria remains one of the leading causes of morbidity and mortality in the world. Of the approximately 50 million deaths worldwide each year, about 2 million are attributed to malaria. Throughout the last century there were many exciting developments with the promise to eradicate or at least control malaria. These included the discovery of chloroquine and other drugs, and insecticides to kill the mosquito vector. While it was very natural to think of vaccine development as a way to prevent malaria infection, classical approaches such as attenuation and the use of killed organisms were not useful for malaria principally because the parasites require red cells for their growth and it is not practical to culture and administer parasites cultivated in such a manner. Safety considerations would also be of paramount concern. It was thus a time of great excitement when malaria genes were first cloned [1,2], opening the possibility for the development of a subunit vaccine. Chapters 70–73 outline the different approaches in some detail, but the purpose of this chapter is to discuss the overall strategies for malaria vaccine development.

The ultimate goal of a vaccine is to prevent disease. In the case of malaria this can theoretically be achieved by interrupting the life cycle at various stages or possibly by inducing a state of "tolerance" to parasites. Interrupting the life cycle and reducing parasite densities and the prevalence of parasitemia will also reduce parasite transmission between individuals. The life cycle thus provides the strategic framework to vaccine development (Figure 1). The major vaccine programs aim to induce immunity that will kill parasites in different locations either within the body or indeed in the mosquito.

Infection commences with the bite of an anopheline mosquito that injects sporozoites into the circulation. It is difficult to calculate how many sporozoites are inoculated but it is likely that under conditions of natural exposure, very few sporozoites ($\approx$10) enter the circulation. The pioneering work of Fairley and colleagues [3] demonstrated using blood transfer between volunteers that sporozoites remain in the circulation for up to 30 min. They can be cleared by various tissues but those that enter hepatocytes are capable of continuing the life cycle. If sporozoites are killed or removed from the circulation prior to entering hepatocytes, the life cycle will be interrupted and disease will not eventuate. Antibodies targeting sporozoite surface proteins are capable of neutralizing sporozoites [4,5].

When the sporozoite enters the hepatocyte there is hepatic schizogony over a period of about 1 week after which merozoites are liberated into the circulation. If infected hepatocytes are destroyed, the life cycle will not continue. T cells (CD8$^+$ and CD4$^+$) [6,7] are able to kill infected hepatocytes. When merozoite forms of the parasite emerge from hepatocytes they enter normal red blood cells (RBCs). Here they undergo exponential growth. The two major species of human parasites, *Plasmodium falciparum* and *P. vivax*, have a 48-hr lifecycle in RBCs. During this time they develop from ring stages to schizonts that rupture the red cell to release more merozoites (approximately 16) to invade fresh cells. Antibodies directed at merozoite surface proteins can prevent merozoites from entering fresh red cells and so antigens on the surface of merozoites represent one class of potential vaccine candidates. With the sequencing of the malaria genome in recent years, the number of known merozoite surface proteins has increased substantially and at least seven have been described so far. Another class of merozoite proteins that are potential vaccine candidates are proteins of merozoite organelles (rhoptries), which are involved in the invasion of the red cell.

The parasite modifies the red cell significantly both in terms of structure and expression of parasite-encoded proteins on the red cell membrane. An important class of antigens are the variant surface antigens of which PfEMP1 is the best studied [8,9,10]. There are approximately 50 variant copies of PfEMP1 represented in each parasite genome but typically only one is expressed at any time. Determinants

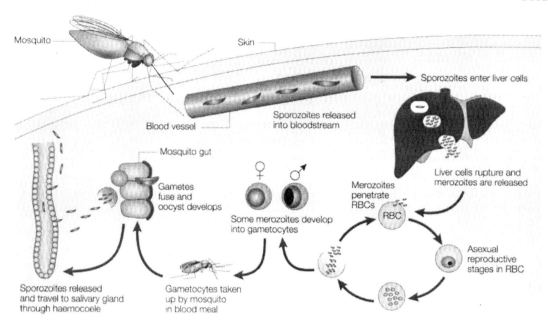

Figure 1 Life cycle of the malaria parasite. The lifecycle in the mammalian host commences with the inoculation of sporozoites by an infected anopheline mosquito which travel by the circulation to the liver. After about 1 week (depending on the species of malaria) parasites have multiplied intracellularly and merozoites rupture from infected hepatocytes to invade red blood cells (RBCs). For *Plasmodium falciparum* and *P. vivax* there is a 48-hr period inside the RBCs during which merozoites multiply and approximately 16 fresh merozoites are released from ruptured red cells to invade fresh cells. Sexual forms (gametocytes) develop within RBCs and are taken up by the mosquito. These emerge in the gut of the mosquito as gametes, which fuse to form an oocyst, and sporozoites develop. Sporozoites are released and travel to the salivary gland of the mosquito. (From *Good, Nature Review Immunology*, 1:117–125, 2001.)

within PfEMP1 are responsible for adhesion of infected RBCs to host receptors on vascular endothelium and placenta and antibodies that are capable of agglutinating infected RBCs and which likely target PfEMP1 are associated with strain-specific immunity [11]. Although the protein is variant, it is an important candidate for a vaccine against the blood stage of the parasite because certain regions of the protein are conserved and monoclonal antibodies that can agglutinate multiple strains have been described [12]. Other molecules have been implicated in adhesion [13] but their vaccine candidacy has not been established.

Although red cells do not express MHC molecules and would not be directly recognized by either CD4$^+$ or CD8$^+$ T cells, there is evidence from animal and human systems that CD4$^+$ T cells can inhibit parasite growth both in vitro and in vivo [14]. It is likely that antigens from infected red cells are processed by antigen presenting cells and presented to T cells in association with MHC. Activated T cells are thought to inhibit parasite growth via nonspecific effector molecules, such as NO and oxygen radicals [15,16]. Identifying the target antigens of antibody-independent cell mediated immunity represents an additional strategy for vaccine development to the blood stage of the parasite.

The sexual forms of malaria parasites are "gametocytes" and these develop within red blood cells. Once taken up by mosquitoes the gametocytes emerge from the red cell and become "gametes," which fertilize to give rise to zygotes and then ookinetes which lodge in the wall of the mosquito's

midgut as oocysts. Immature sporozoites develop within the cysts and then travel to the salivary gland. Antibodies directed to gamete surface antigens are able to either block gamete fertilization or block zygote development. These antibodies do not have an effect within the human host because gametocytes are located within RBCs and are not accessible to antibodies. Gamete surface antigens have been identified and cloned and have been tested in immunogenicity trials in volunteers.

Despite the fact that a number of molecules representing the life-cycle stages and cellular locations described are known and have been cloned and recombinant proteins prepared, hurdles to the development of a malaria vaccine remain. Whatever combination of antigens will be most effective for a human vaccine is not only unknown but difficult to establish. The latter is true because while the parasites can be grown with limitations in a few species of monkeys, human malaria parasites are adapted specifically to humans and trials in human volunteers are time consuming and costly because of the important safety issues that must be addressed. Furthermore, it is not clear which route of administration of a vaccine will be most appropriate. While the concept of DNA vaccines is attractive because of the reduced need for a "cold chain" in tropical areas where a vaccine is most needed, there is as yet no clear evidence for efficacy. Choice between the alternatives of recombinant proteins or peptides and identification of the best adjuvant for use with these, or of live viral vectors, are other outstanding issues. The combinatorial nature of such problems presents a substantial challenge indeed.

REFERENCES

1. Kemp DJ, Coppel RL, Cowman AF, Saint RB, Brown GV, Anders RF. Expression of Plasmodium falciparum blood-stage antigens in *Escherichia coli*: detection with antibodies from immune humans. Proc Natl Acad Sci USA 1983; 80(12): 3787–3791.

2. Ellis J, Ozaki LS, Gwadz RW, Cochrane AH, Nussenzweig V, Nussenzweig RS, Godson GN. Cloning and expression in *E coli* of the malarial sporozoite surface antigen gene from *Plasmodium knowlesi*. Nature 1983; 302(5908):536–538.

3. Fairley NH, et al. Sidelights on malaria in man obtained by subinoculation experiments. Trans R Soc Trop Med Hyg 1947; 40:621–676.

4. Nussenzweig V, Nussenzweig RS. Rationale for the development of an engineered sporozoite malaria vaccine Adv Immunol 1989; 45:283–334.

5. Hoffman SL, Franke ED, Hollingdale MR, Druilhe P. Attacking the infected hepatocyte. In: Hoffman SL, ed. Malaria Vaccine Development: a multi-immune response approach. Washington, DC: American Society for Microbiology Press, 1996:35–76.

6. Good MF, Doolan DL. Immune effector mechanisms in malaria. Curr Opin Immunol 1999; 11(4):412–419.

7. Renia L, Grillot D, Marussig M, Corradin G, Miltgen F, Lambert PH, Mazier D, Del Giudice G. Effector functions of circumsporozoite peptide-primed CD4$^+$ T cell clones against *Plasmodium yoelii* liver stages. J Immunol 1993; 150(4):1471–1478.

8. Baruch DI, Pasloske BL, Singh HB, Bi X, Ma XC, Feldman M, Taraschi TF, Howard RJ. Cloning the *P falciparum* gene encoding PfEMP1, a malarial variant antigen and adherence receptor on the surface of parasitized human erythrocytes. Cell 1995; 82:77–87.

9. Su XZ, Heatwole VM, Wertheimer SP, Guinet F, Herrfeldt JA, Peterson DS, Ravetch JA, Wellems TE. The large diverse gene family var encodes proteins involved in cytoadherence and antigenic variation of *Plasmodium falciparum*-infected erythrocytes. Cell 1995; 82:89–100.

10. Smith JD, Chitnis CE, Craig AG, Roberts DJ, Hudson-Taylor DE, Peterson DS, Pinches R, Newbold CI, Miller LH. Switches in expression of *Plasmodium falciparum var* genes correlate with changes in antigenic and cytoadherent phenotypes of infected erythrocytes. Cell 1995; 82:101–110.

11. Marsh K, Howard RJ. Antigens induced on erythrocytes by *P falciparum*: expression of diverse and conserved determinants. Science 1986; 231:150–153.

12. Gamain B, Miller LH, Baruch DI. The surface variant antigens of *Plasmodium falciparum* contain cross-reactive epitopes. Proc Natl Acad Sci USA 2001; 98:2664–2669.

13. Trenholme KR, Gardiner DL, Thomas EA, Holt DC, Kemp DJ, Cowman AF. Malaria: a new gene family (clag) involved in adhesion—reply. Parasitol Today 2000; 16(9):405.

14. Good MF. Towards a blood stage vaccine for malaria: Are we following all the leads? Nat Rev Immunol 2001; 1:117–125.

15. Stevenson MM, Tam MF, Wolf SF, Sher A. IL-12-induced protection against blood-stage *Plasmodium chabaudi* AS requires IFN.- and TNF.- and occurs via a nitric oxide-dependent mechanism. J Immunol 1995; 155:2545–2556.

16. Su Z, Stevenson MM. Central role of endogenous gamma interferon in protective immunity against blood-stage *Plasmodium chabaudi* AS infection. Infect Immun 2000; 68:4399–4406.

70

Adjuvanted RTS,S and Other Protein-Based Pre-Erythrocytic Stage Malaria Vaccines

D. Gray Heppner, Jr., James F. Cummings, Christian F. Ockenhouse, and Kent E. Kester
Walter Reed Army Institute of Research, Silver Spring, Maryland, U.S.A.

Joe D. Cohen and W. Ripley Ballou, Jr.
GlaxoSmithKline Biologicals, Rixensart, Belgium

I. INTRODUCTION

A. Imperative for a Pre-Erythrocytic Malaria Vaccine

The march of drug-resistant parasite strains [1], the spread of insecticide-resistant mosquito vectors [2], and the recognition that global morbidity and mortality due to malaria equals that of HIV/AIDS [3] have made malaria vaccine development a global imperative [4]. In broad terms, there are three possible goals for a malaria vaccine. Each goal requires a specific vaccine development strategy targeted against specific parasite stages. A malaria vaccine intended to confer sterile immunity would target pre-erythrocytic stages of the malaria parasite, i.e., the sporozoite, liver stages, or hepatic merozoites prior to initial red cell invasion. A vaccine designed to prevent severe disease or death, but not necessarily preventing parasitemia, should aim immune responses against asexual blood stages or toxins. Lastly, a vaccine designed to prevent transmission of malaria from host to vector to host would direct immune responses against sexual stage antigens present in either the host or the mosquito vector. A long-term goal of researchers in this field has been to develop and license a multistage, multiantigen vaccine against *Plasmodium falciparum* that protects malaria-naïve children and adults against infection, limits morbidity in those who develop infection, and is effective for at least 12 months. This goal may require the inclusion of multiple parasite antigens including antigens from more than one stage of the parasite's life cycle. Since the mid 1980s, our efforts have focused upon the development of a safe, well-tolerated, and effective pre-erythrocytic vaccine. This chapter emphasizes recent progress in our co-development with GlaxoSmithKline Biologicals of the sporozoite-based RTS,S/AS02A vaccine and reviews other protein-based pre-erythrocytic malaria vaccines currently in clinical development.

B. Feasibility of a Pre-Erythrocytic Vaccine

As is the case for most parasitic infections, sterile immunity to malaria parasites rarely, if ever, occurs naturally, even under the most intense exposure conditions [5]. However, there is circumstantial evidence that naturally acquired cellular immunity against pre-erythrocytic antigens may reduce disease severity [6,7], and that specific MHC alleles governing T-cell responses to pre-erythrocytic antigens have been positively selected for endemic populations [8,9]. The theoretical feasibility of developing an effective pre-erythrocytic vaccine was established more than 30 years ago by experimental immunization of human subjects with large numbers of radiation-attenuated sporozoites [10,11]. This impractical but effective process rendered immunized subjects completely protected from sporozoite challenge with homologous or heterologous parasites of the same species. However, subjects immunized with radiation-attenuated sporozoites remained susceptible to other plasmodial species and to blood stage infection, thus demonstrating the species and stage specificity of this approach. An ideal pre-erythrocytic vaccine would therefore elicit the same immune responses, capable of eliminating sporozoites from the circulation, or killing all infected hepatocytes, or preventing all hepatic merozoites from invading erythrocytes, thereby conferring "sterile immunity."

C. Uses of a Pre-Erythrocytic Vaccine

An effective pre-erythrocytic vaccine would be of great benefit to the nonimmune traveler or deploying member of the military. It would be especially important that a pre-erythrocytic vaccine be highly effective in nonimmune subjects as these individuals would have no effective immunity against blood-stage parasites. Vaccine efficacy for the nonimmune traveler should exceed the protection afforded by available chemoprophylactic drugs, although the vaccine might be used in conjunction with chemoprophylaxis in areas where multidrug resistance is high or other plasmodial species, such as *Plasmodium vivax*, are transmitted. Cost, extended duration of efficacy, and boostability by natural infection would be lesser considerations for nonimmune travelers than for endemic populations. A moderately effective pre-erythrocytic vaccine, even of short-term duration, could be of potential benefit to populations for whom short-term chemoprophylaxis has been beneficial. Such indications would include infants [12] and pregnant women, especially primagravidae [13,14]. Broader public health indications for a pre-erythrocytic vaccine in endemic populations might also include reduction in malaria intensity in a manner analogous to the use of bed nets [15], and as an adjunct to malaria eradication efforts. Ultimately, an ideal pre-erythrocytic vaccine would also include blood stage antigens able to reduce disease severity, and sexual stage antigens able to limit transmission of vaccine-resistant parasites.

D. Obstacles to Pre-Erythrocytic Vaccine Development

There is not a licensed vaccine for malaria or any other parasitic affliction of mankind. The obstacles are formidable, chief of which is the inadequate knowledge of the requirements for immunity. Classical vaccine approaches such as immunization with atttenuated or killed whole organisms are impractical. Hence development is based upon a subunit approach that seeks to include one or more protective antigens and may lead to a multicomponent formulation. Positive selection factors for antigen development in order of decreasing importance include 1) demonstration that antigen-specific immune responses correlate with those associated with protection in volunteers immunized by exposure to radiation-attenuated sporozoites or in previous pre-erythrocytic stage subunit vaccine trials; 2) accessibility of the host immune system to the targeted plasmodial antigen; 3) demonstration that immunization with the homologous antigen confers protection against sporozoite-transmitted infection in analogous animal models; and, potentially, 4) correlation of antigen-specific immune responses with protection against severe disease in epidemiological studies.

Antigen selection is further complicated by the existence of allelic polymorphisms that have presumably arisen as means of evading protective immunity and may ultimately require the inclusion of more than one allele of the same antigen. Another consideration is the role of host genetic restriction of immune responses to protective epitopes, an additional argument in favor of including more antigens in a vaccine intended for use in genetically diverse populations.

E. Design Considerations for a Malaria Vaccine

The design of candidate malaria vaccines involves the selection of antigens that target the parasite at vulnerable portions of its life cycle. Malaria species that have been adapted to robust rodent models, such as *Plasmodium berghei* and

Plasmodium yoelii, have been powerful tools for identifying both candidate antigens and immunization strategies. Sporozoites transmitted by the bite of female *Anopheles* mosquitoes can be targeted by antibodies directed against their surface antigens as they travel through the bloodstream [16]. These antibodies block the ability of sporozoites to invade liver cells. A variety of cell-mediated responses, including lymphokines and cellular cytotoxicity, are able to kill infected liver schizonts and thus prevent the maturation and release of mature *P. falciparum* exo-erythrocytic forms into the bloodstream [17,18]. To date, most vaccine candidates tested in humans have been based on a small number of sporozoite surface antigens that have been extensively investigated using these rodent systems.

F. Decision Criteria and the Human Sporozoite Challenge Model

Adherence to the critical path for malaria vaccine development requires that definitive decisions be made for each potential improvement to the current vaccine candidate. The human sporozoite challenge model using laboratory-reared *Anopheles* mosquitoes that become infected by feeding on in vitro cultured *P. falciparum* was developed at WRAIR to assess the efficacy of candidate sporozoite vaccines and new antimalarial drugs [19]. The model has proven to be safe, standardized, and highly reliable for the experimental inoculation of infectivity controls in Phase 2 trials. Since 1992, we have conducted over 400 experimental infections of malaria-naïve malaria vaccine recipients and concomitant unimmunized infectivity controls. The endpoint for efficacy is the appearance of blood stage infection as detected by light microscopy. Typical pre-patent periods are 9–12 days in the infectivity controls. Comparing vaccine efficacy [20] and the duration of efficacy [21] in malaria-naïve vaccinees to that observed in malaria-experienced vaccinees in the field [22] suggests this model has strong negative and positive predictive value. Thus we have incorporated proof of efficacy in the human sporozoite challenge model as the Go/NoGo decision criteria for incorporation of potential new antigens/adjuvants into a multicomponent pre-erythrocytic malaria vaccine.

II. CIRCUMSPOROZOITE PROTEIN (CSP) AS THE BASIS OF A PRE-ERYTHROCYTIC VACCINE

A. First CSP-Based Vaccines

One of the first malaria genes to be identified through this model was the circumsporozoite (CS) protein [23]. The CS proteins of all malaria species contain a central segment of species-specific amino acid repeat sequences flanked by non-repeat regions. In the case of *P. falciparum*, the central portion contains approximately 40 repeats of the amino acid sequence asparagine–alanine–asparagine proline (NANP) and several asparagine–valine–aspartic acid–proline (NVDP) repeats [24]. The central repeating unit is immunodominant relative to the flanking regions and is the portion of the molecule to which protective antibody responses are principally directed [25]. Two alum-adjuvanted candidate vaccines based on the CS repeat sequences were developed in the mid-1980s, tested in humans, and found to be safe, but both suffered from generally poor immunogenicity [26,27]. In most of the volunteers, repeated immunization induced relatively low titers of antibodies against the repeat region of the CS protein. Nevertheless, a small number of volunteers who did respond well were protected against homologous experimental sporozoite challenge. These pivotal challenge data confirmed that sterile immunity against malaria could be induced in humans by immunization with a synthetic pre-erythrocytic stage subunit vaccine. Because, in these studies involving a limited number of volunteers, protection seemed to be associated with high antibody levels, it was felt that the development of more immunogenic versions of these vaccines would lead to better efficacy.

Subsequent sporozoite vaccines, also based on the NANP repeat, contained modifications conducive to the enhancement of immune responses, such as conjugation of recombinant CS repeat protein with *Pseudomonas aeruginosa* exotoxin A (R32ToxA) [28], and formulation of a similar antigen (R32NS1) in liposomes containing monophosphoryl lipid A (MPL) [29] or an emulsion of MPL, mycobacterial cell wall skeleton, and squalene (Detox®, Ribi Immunochem) [30,31]. Each of these strategies resulted in generally higher antibody levels but surprisingly did not significantly enhance efficacy.

While these clinical studies were in progress, the role of protective T-cell responses directed against the liver-stage form of the parasite was elucidated in greater detail. Studies in rodents and humans immunized with irradiated sporozoites revealed that not only antibodies but also $CD4^+$, $CD8^+$, and cytotoxic T-cell (CTL) responses and cytokines such as interferon-gamma were important components of the protective immune responses against the pre-erythrocytic stage of *P. falciparum* [32,33]. Target epitopes for these T cells have been localized to the C-terminal region of the CS protein [34–39]. Region II, a charged highly conserved sequence that lies in this portion of the molecule, was implicated in the binding of sporozoites to hepatocytes [40]. The recognition that peptide sequences lying outside the CS repeat were important for induction of humoral and cellular responses against the hepatic stage led to the inclusion of nonrepeat portions of the molecule in the next generation of CS-based vaccines. One such candidate (NS1RLF) was constructed so as to be completely devoid of repeat epitopes and contained both N-terminal and C-terminal flanking regions. This vaccine was formulated as a recombinant protein encapsulated in liposomes and adjuvanted with MPL. The vaccine was found to stimulate a potent CTL response in mice and induced a brisk immune response in humans that included antibodies that recognized sporozoites [41]. Unfortunately, no protection from experimental sporozoite challenge was observed and this vaccine has been abandoned.

B. Initial Development of Candidate Malaria Vaccine "RTS,S"

In collaboration with then GlaxoSmithKline Biologicals (GSK Bio) our group at the Walter Reed Army Institute of Research turned to what has become a more promising approach. This strategy was based upon GSK Bio's development of an expression system in which the CS repeats as well as the C-terminal region were incorporated into highly immunogenic HBsAg particles. The components of this new vaccine are two polypeptides (RTS and S) that are synthesized simultaneously in genetically engineered *Saccharomyces cerevisiae* yeast cells. During purification they spontaneously form composite particulate structures (RTS,S) that constitute the vaccine antigen. RTS is a single polypeptide chain corresponding to amino acids 207–395 of the CS protein gene in the 7G8 strain of *P. falciparum* fused to the amino terminus of the hepatitis B surface antigen (HBsAg; adw serotype). S is a polypeptide of 226 amino acids that corresponds to HBsAg. RTS includes 19 copies of the tetrapeptide repeat motif (NANP) plus the C-terminal region of the protein devoid of the hydrophobic anchor sequence. Several formulations of the vaccine were developed and manufactured at GSK Bio and preclinical studies included a series of increasingly potent adjuvants. The initial clinical studies involved one formulation in which RTS,S was adsorbed to alum, and a second in which it was adsorbed to alum to which was added the immunostimulant 3-deacyl-MPL (MPL, see Table 1). This second adjuvant formulation is designated AS04 (formerly SBAS4). Although antibody responses were modest, most volunteers developed proliferative cellular responses against the CS protein. More importantly, following sporozoite challenge, two of eight volunteers in the RTS,S/AS04 group were protected whereas all six volunteers that received the alum formulation developed malaria [42]. Encouraged by these results that suggested that greater immunogenicity would be associated with greater efficacy, two additional formulations were studied in a Phase 1/2a trial [20]. In this and in all subsequent trials, RTS was re-engineered to represent the NF54 strain (3D7 clone) of *P. falciparum*. In that study, the AS04 formulation was tested along with two additional formulations developed by GSK Bio: AS03 (formerly SBAS3) containing a proprietary oil-in-water emulsion, and AS02A (formerly SBAS2) containing the same emulsion plus the immunostimulants MPL and QS21. These new adjuvant systems were chosen on the basis of preclinical studies in rhesus monkeys that demonstrated their safety and immunogenicity. The primate data showed that AS03 promoted strong antibody responses while AS02A induced both humoral and cellular responses (Heppner DG, unpublished data). Human volunteers immunized with either RTS,S/AS03 or RTS,S/AS02A developed some of the highest anti-repeat antibody responses induced by any sporozoite-based vaccine, but both the AS04 and AS03 formulations were only marginally protective following laboratory-based sporozoite challenge. In contrast, an unprecedented six of seven volunteers who received the AS02A formulation were protected. Type 1 cellular responses, especially the production of IFN-gamma upon stimulation with CS peptides, were promoted by the AS02A formulation of RTS,S and were presumed to be an important component of the protective immune responses. Subsequently, expanded safety and immunogenicity trials of RTS,S/AS02A in over 400 malaria-naïve and malaria-immune subjects have revealed the vaccine to be safe and highly

Table 1 Synopsis of Phase 2 Trials of RTS,S 1996–2003

	Adjuvants (Adjuvant System) formerly SBAS	Additional antigens	Antigen formulation	Antibody	CMI	Phase 2a efficacy	Phase 2b efficacy
RTS,S	Alum	–	Liquid	+	–	–	Nd
RTS,S	AS04 = MPL® + alum	–	Liquid	+ +	+	+	Nd
RTS,S	AS03 = O-i-W	–	Liquid	+ + +	+	+	Nd
RTS,S	AS02A = O-i-W, MPL, QS21	–	Liquid	+ + +	+ +	+ +	Nd
RTS,S	AS02A	–	Lyophilized	+ + +	+ +	+ +	+ +
RTS,S	AS02A	TRAP / 3D7	Lyophilized	+ + +	+ +	+	Nd
RTS,S	AS02A	MSP-1 / 3D7	Lyophilized	+ + +	+ +	+ +	2004
RTS,S	AS01B = liposome, MPL®, QS21	–	Lyophilized	2003	2003	2003	???

Relative scale: – absent; + slight; + + moderate, + + + substantial; Nd = not done; TRAP = thrombospondin-related anonymous protein; MSP-1 = merozoites surface protein 1; O-i-W = oil in water emulsion.

immunogenic, and recent experimental challenge studies involving more than 50 volunteers indicate that the vaccine consistently induces significant protection when given on two- or three-dose schedules [43].

C. Initial Field Trials of RTS,S/AS02A Candidate Malaria Vaccine

These encouraging preliminary results were followed up recently with GSK Bio-sponsored clinical trials involving malaria-immune adult male residents of The Gambia, West Africa. A Phase I safety and immunogenicity study was conducted by investigators at the Medical Research Council (MRC) laboratories in Banjul, at a study site where there was minimal ongoing malaria transmission. This study indicated that the vaccine was safe, mildly reactogenic, and immunogenic in otherwise healthy malaria semi-immune adults [44]. A follow-up Phase 2b pilot efficacy study was conducted at a separate site characterized by high and seasonal transmission rates in malaria semi-immune adult Gambian men who were immunized during a period of low transmission and followed for the occurrence of new malaria infections during a period of active malaria transmission [45]. In this study, conducted at the MRC Field Station in Basse, Upper River Division, The Gambia, 360 men were randomized to receive three doses of either RTS,S/AS02A or human diploid rabies vaccine, given intramuscularly at 0, 1, and 6 months. The vaccination schedule was timed to coincide with the dry season during which transmission of *P. falciparum* was low. The final dose was administered approximately 1 month before the expected onset of the rainy season. Volunteers were treated with sulfadoxine/pyrimethamine to clear asexual-stage parasites 1 month before the beginning of the 15-week efficacy follow-up period. The vaccine was again found to be safe, mildly reactogenic, and immunogenic in this semi-immune population. Two hundred and fifty of the volunteers enrolled in this study received all three doses of the vaccine and had adequate follow-up data. Vaccine efficacy was estimated to be 71% (95% CI 46–85%) during the first 2 months of follow-up but decreased to 0% during the last 6 weeks of the follow-up period. The reasons for the short

duration of efficacy are likely to be multiple. Subset analysis revealed that younger, less malaria-experienced men became infected in the control group earlier than did the older, more highly immune members of their cohort. As vaccine efficacy waned, the incidence in the RTS,S/AS02A group was being compared to the control group from which the most susceptible subjects had been removed. Antibody responses also declined during the period of follow-up such that the mean levels at the end of the follow-up period were equivalent to those after a single dose of vaccine. As has been seen in other studies of sporozoite vaccines, no boosting of antibody responses was seen following sporozoite exposure. Finally, it is likely that the entomologic inoculation rate was typical of that previously described for this region and was higher at the end of the transmission season than it was at the beginning. Importantly, a fourth booster dose was administered to 158 volunteers a year later and prior to the next peak of malaria transmission. Antibody responses were significantly boosted and, during a 9 week follow-up, efficacy was 47% (95% CI:4–71%; P = 0.037). This important field study extended encouraging data previously obtained in studies of malaria-naïve volunteers immunized with RTS,S/AS02A and exposed to sporozoites using the WRAIR standard sporozoite challenge model. First, it confirmed the predictive value of the model—efficacy in the field was similar in magnitude and duration to that observed with the same vaccine in the laboratory-based clinical trial [21]. Second, there was no evidence of strain-specific immunity, as polymerase chain reaction analysis of CS genes from isolates collected from subjects who became infected during the study revealed that the frequency of polymorphic sequence variants at the Th2R and Th3R regions characteristic of the NF54 clone (from which the vaccine was derived) was similar for the RTS,S/AS02A and rabies vaccine groups [46]. Third, it demonstrated that natural boosting through exposure to sporozoites was unlikely to enhance or sustain vaccine-induced immunity. Finally, the data again suggest the importance of high levels of antibodies against CS repeat epitopes as a potential correlate of immunity, although a specific protective cutoff value could not be identified. The results obtained with RTS,S/AS02A in The Gambia must be viewed cautiously. However, clearly they mark an important milestone—the first time that vaccine-induced protection from infection with *P. falciparum* has ever been observed in a field setting, and the capacity building and experience gained with African co-investigators were invaluable.

D. Additional Development of RTS,S

In 2003, RTS,S adjuvanted with AS02A, now renamed AS02, is the only malaria vaccine in clinical development that has been demonstrated to prevent *Plasmodium falciparum* infection. However, further improvements in the magnitude and duration of efficacy are clearly desirable. Parallel efforts are underway to define the benefit of RTS,S/AS02A in pediatric population at greatest risk of malaria and to improve the efficacy of RTS,S through the addition of new vaccination schedules, adjuvants, antigens, and platform technologies.

1. Pediatric Trials of RTS,S/AS02

In January 2000, GSK Bio and the Malaria Vaccine Initiative (MVI) at PATH (Program for Appropriate Technology in Health) entered into a private/public partnership that initiated the clinical pediatric development of RTS,S/AS02. Two sequential Phase 1 studies in children were conducted by the MRC in The Gambia: a study in older children (6–11 years), followed by a second study in younger children (1–5 years). In each study, a double-blind, randomized, controlled, staggered dose-escalation design was used to evaluate 1/5, 1/2, and a full dose. The RTS,S/AS02A vaccine had a good safety profile and there were no serious adverse events related to vaccination. All doses were highly immunogenic for anti-CS and anti-HBs antibodies. Subsequent pediatric development of RTS,S/AS02A is now underway in Mozambique [4].

2. New Schedules and Doses of RTS,S/AS02A Administration

Initial trials of RTS,S/AS02A administered this vaccine on a 0-, 1-, and 6–9-month schedule. Subsequent trials at WRAIR demonstrated no apparent change in efficacy when given as a half (25 µg RTS,S/0.25 ml of AS02A) or full (50 µg RTS,S/0.50 ml of AS02A) dose [43]. A recent Phase 2 trial of RTS,S/AS02A compared the safety, immunogenicity, and efficacy of two accelerated regimens of RTS,S/AS02A. Forty malaria-naïve volunteers were randomized to receive full dose RTS,S/AS02A on either a 0-, 1-, and 3-month or 0-, 7-, and 28-day schedule. Both immunization schedules were well tolerated and comparably immunogenic. Following standard sporozoite challenge, 45% and 38% volunteers were completely protected against parasitemia. The study supported the safety of short-course immunization and underscored the need to improve vaccine efficacy for use in travelers (Kester KE, unpublished data).

3. New Adjuvants

As reviewed earlier, initial formulations of RTS,S with alum, alum and MPL, or oil-in-water emulsions had conferred marginal protection. In contrast, formulation of RTS,S with AS02A, a proprietary formulation containing MPL®, QS21 and an oil-in-water emulsion, elicited strong antibody and a Th1 cellular immune response (Krzych U, unpublished data) [47] and unprecedented efficacy. Working closely with GSK Bio, we have systematically compared RTS,S/AS02A to RTS,S formulated with additional new adjuvants using the standardized rhesus monkey safety and immunogenicity vaccine model. One alternative adjuvant, designated AS01B, induced a sustained and improved RTS,S-specific IFN-gamma ELISPOT response and an equivalent antibody response to that seen with the AS02A (Stewart A, unpublished data). A Phase 2a trial in malaria-naïve adults of RTS,S/AS01B versus RTS,S/AS02A to be initiated in late 2003 at WRAIR will compare the magnitude and duration of protection against malaria challenge at 2 weeks and 6 months after the last immunization.

4. RTS,S in Combination with a Second Antigen

Thrombospondin-Related Anonymous Protein. *P. falciparum* thrombospondin-related anonymous protein [48] (Pf-TRAP) is a candidate vaccine antigen found in a patchy distribution on the surface and within the micronemes of the sporozoite [49]. Thrombospondin-related anonymous protein is required for the gliding motility and infectivity of sporozoites [50]. *P. falciparum* thrombospondin-related anonymous protein was recombinantly expressed in SF9 insect cells, lyophilized, and bottled as single-dose vials. One formulation contained 20 µg of TRAP per human dose; a second formulation contained 20 µg of TRAP and a standard 50-µg dose of RTS,S. Preclinical safety and immunogenicity testing of these two formulations with the AS02 adjuvant in a standardized rhesus malaria vaccine model demonstrated a good safety and local reactogenicity profile. Serologic analysis as determined by ELISA showed no interference by TRAP in the antibody response to RTS,S; and there was an increase in the IFA titers to RTS,S/TRAP/AS02A as compared to that seen with either antigen alone (Heppner DG, unpublished data). A subsequent Phase 1/2 trial of TRAP/AS02A and RTS,S/TRAP/AS02 given on a 0- and 1-month schedule confirmed the preclinical safety and immunogenicity of these formulations (Kester KE, unpublished data). In the efficacy phase of this study, none (0 of 4) of the TRAP/AS02 vaccinees and only 1 of 12 of the RTS,S/TRAP/AS02A vaccinees was protected. This cautionary result suggests that vaccine development efforts should first determine the marginal utility of additional antigens prior to their incorporation into a multicomponent vaccine, and that attention should be paid to the possibility of immunological interference between the antigens in the combination.

Merozoite Surface Protein-1. Merozoite surface protein-1 (MSP-1), the first antigen discovered on the surface of the erythrocytic stage merozoites, is also expressed in merozoites released at the end of hepatic schizogony [51]. Merozoite Surface Protein-1 is the target of protective immunity, particularly the C-terminal portion, against severe disease as suggested by epidemiological studies [52], and as demonstrated by immunization studies of Aotus monkeys with purified native merozoite surface protein [53]. Recently, J. Lyon and E. Angov at WRAIR expressed and produced a

42-kDa C-terminal MSP-1 protein based on the *P. falciparum* 3D7 clone in *E. coli*. In preclinical [54] and Phase 1 clinical trials (Ockenhouse CF, unpublished data), a full dose of 50 µg of MSP-1 formulated with 0.5 ml of AS02A was shown to be safe and well tolerated. Seroconversion to MSP-1/AS02A occurred in volunteers who received a single immunization with a 1/5 (*N* = 5), 1/2 (*N* = 5), or full dose (*N* = 5), and serum antibody from each volunteer recognized native protein as determined by a merozoite immunflourescence assay. Encouraged by these results, a Phase 2A trial in 2001 evaluated the combination of RTS,S and MSP-1, adjuvanted with AS02A (Cummings JF, unpublished data). The trial demonstrated that the extemporaneous combination of MSP-1/AS02 and RTS,S/AS02A caused no interference in the protective efficacy of RTS,S/AS02A against sporozoite challenge. Accordingly, the MSP-1/AS02A formulation is now in field efficacy trials in Kenya. If successful in reducing clinical disease, the two antigens will be co-formulated and field tested.

5. RTS,S and New Platform Technologies

Improved B- and T-cell responses have been achieved in numerous nonmalaria preclinical trials that combine heterologous platform vaccine technologies. This approach, referred to as "prime-boost," yields results dependent not only upon the vaccines but upon the sequence, interval, and number of immunizations administered. Preclinical proof of concept for enhanced immunologic responses to plasmodial antigens has been demonstrated for immunizations with protein vaccines in combination with either DNA [55], vaccinia [56], or adenovirus [57] vaccine carriers. Recently, a Phase I clinical trial of a CSP–DNA plasmid vaccine expressing the full-length CS protein was conducted [58,59]. Cytotoxic T-cell responses were observed, but no antibody responses were detected, even at very high doses. Volunteers from this trial were subsequently enrolled into a Phase 1 prime-boost pilot study to evaluate the safety and immunogenicity of boosting these volunteers previously immunized with three doses of a CSP–DNA plasmid given by various routes with two full doses of RTS,S/AS02A at 0 and 1 month. Despite an unfavorable dosing interval, DNA immunization did appear to prime for improved cellular responses to RTS,S (Wang R, and Epstein J, unpublished data).

A second prime-boost approach involves a current Phase 2 trial of RTS,S/AS02 and a modified vaccinia Ankara (MVA) expressing the *P. falciparum* CS gene now underway at the University of Oxford. Detailed immunogenicity assessment and efficacy data will be available in 2003. However, the excellent safety profile, potency, and vectorial capacity of vaccinia are offset by the current prospect of widespread immunization with vaccinia against smallpox that might interfere with subsequent use of vaccinia-based malaria vaccines.

E. Other CSP-Based Protein Subunit Vaccines

As the only antigen to reproducibly confer protection when used as a subunit vaccine, CSP is a logical target for proof of concept studies for new vaccine platform technologies.

1. Multiple Antigen Peptides

Although initial CSP tetrapeptide-based malaria vaccines were poorly immunogenic and gave scant protection, correlations were made between anti-CSP repeat antibody titer and protective efficacy against sporozoite challenge [26,27]. These vaccines were recognized to have potential design deficiencies [60], such as a low malaria epitope density, the potential for carrier epitope suppression when conjugated with tetanus toxoid [61], and the absence of parasite-specific T-cell helper epitopes needed to elicit memory responses upon natural exposure to sporozoites. A second generation of synthetic, well-defined CSP-based vaccines known as "multiple antigen peptides" or "MAPs" were developed that contained the B-epitope (NANP)₃ and a T-helper cell epitope from the CSP repeat region found in all *P. falciparum* isolates known as "T1" [62]. This construct, described as (T1B4)₄MAP, elicited high titer antibodies in a subset of volunteers whose class II DR or DQ molecules were known to more avidly bind the T1 epitope [63]. Encouragingly, these antibodies recognized native sporozoites in both an IFA assay and in a CS precipitin reaction. No sporozoite challenge was conducted to assess the efficacy of this vaccine. The occurrence of hypersensitivity reactions to this vaccine led to the abandonment of this construct.

In an effort to broaden the immune response, a third generation malaria peptide vaccine was designed that added a second universal T-cell helper epitope found in the C-terminal portion of the CS protein to the T1 epitope and the (NANP)₃ CS repeats [64]. This tri-epitope vaccine incorporated a lipopeptide adjuvant and was constructed by joining epitope modules to a branched lysine core via oxime bonds, hence the short-hand term, "polyoxime." A Phase 1 trial elicited antibodies in vaccinees of diverse class II haplotypes that recognized native sporozoites in both an IFA assay and in a CS precipitin reaction. Again, no sporozoite challenge to assess for protective efficacy was conducted and the future of this vaccine construct remains uncertain [65].

2. Modified Hepatitis B Core Particle as a Carrier

Modified hepatitis B core particles are an immunologically potent carrier of heterologous epitopes [66]. Proof of concept of this platform technology for malaria was first achieved in a *P. berghei* mouse malaria model at WRAIR in the early 1990s [67] and again demonstrated by protection against sporozoite challenge in a *P. yoellii* model [70]. To design a vaccine for human use, a preliminary series of modified recombinant HBc particles containing *P. falciparum* CS protein T- and B-cell epitopes were assayed for immunogenicity in rodents [69,70]. The optimal *P. falciparum* HBc vaccine candidate, termed ICC-1132, contains T- and B-cell epitopes from the CS protein repeat region and a universal T-cell epitope from the C terminus of the CS protein [65]. Preclinical studies in rhesus and cynomolgus monkeys have demonstrated that ICC-1132, formulated in Seppic ISA-720, is a potent B-cell immunogen (Birkett A, personal communication). In mice, a single injection of ICC-1132 elicited strong anamnestic antibody responses following priming with *P. falciparum* sporozoites. Human CD4⁺ T-cell clones specific for the CS-derived universal T-cell epitope proliferated and produced cytokines following in vitro stimulation with ICC-1132. These findings suggest that the candidate vaccine, in addition to inducing strong cellular and humoral immunity in naïve individuals, may have particular utility in enhancing the sporozoite-primed immune responses of individuals living in malaria-endemic areas. ICC-1132, which was developed by Apovia Inc., San Diego, CA, in collaboration with scientists at New York University, entered Phase 1 clinical trials at the University of Tuebingen in November 2002.

3. Long Synthetic Peptides as Vaccines

Long synthetic peptides (LSP) are a maturing technology that enable the effective presentation of defined CS protein B- and T-cell epitopes to the immune system. Proof of concept of this approach was first achieved in primates by Roggero et al. who used a 102-amino acid LSP representing the CSP to elicit CD4$^+$ and CD8$^+$ T cells and antibodies [71]. A subsequent Phase 1 study in 16 malaria naïve adults evaluated four separate formulations containing either 100 or 300 μg of the LSP adjuvanted with aluminum hydroxide or Montanide ISA-720 [72]. Antigen-specific CD4$^+$ and CD8$^+$ T cells were elicited with both formulations; however, only the Montanide ISA-720 formulation induced positive IFA results. The utility of this approach awaits proof of efficacy in experimental Phase 2 trials and definition of manufacturing costs for large-scale synthesis.

III. CLINICAL TRIALS OF NON-CSP PRE-ERYTHROCYTIC PROTEIN VACCINES

At present, there are no trials of non-CSP pre-erythrocytic vaccines in progress.

However, recent advances in recombinant protein expression and in peptide synthesis suggest such Phase 1/2 trials will occur in the next two years of two antigens, liver stage antigen 1 (LSA-1) and liver stage antigen 3 (LSA-3).

A. Liver Stage Antigen 1

Since the discovery of *Plasmodium falciparum* LSA-1 [73], mounting evidence supports its development as a vaccine [71]. In studies in endemic populations, protection against malarial disease has been associated with LSA-1-specific cellular and humoral immune responses. Likewise, in studies of irradiated sporozoite-immunized volunteers challenged with infectious sporozoites, cellular responses to LSA-1 were higher in protected than in unprotected volunteers [75]. A recombinant *E. coli–P. falciparum* LSA-1 protein is scheduled for Phase 1/2 trials at WRAIR in 2004.

B. Liver Stage Antigen 3

Liver stage antigen 3 is a 205-kDa protein found in both sporozoite and liver stages. Recent testing of LSA-3 LSP constructs in vitro reveals multiple B- and T-cell epitopes recognized by malaria-immune individuals in Africa [78]. Subsequent studies of either LSA3-LSP formulated in AS02A or LSA3-lipopeptides in chimpanzees demonstrated induction of antibody and T-helper and T-cytotoxic responses and apparent protection of two chimpanzees against sporozoite challenge [77]. The initial Phase 1 trials of GMP LSA-3 LSP are scheduled for 2003 in Europe.

IV. CONCLUSIONS

"There must be a beginning of any great matter, but the continuing unto the end until it be thoroughly finished yields the true glory"—Sir Frances Drake

Of all the pre-erythrocytic antigens, none has been exhaustively evaluated, and only CSP has been systematically tested in clinical development. New antigens, adjuvants, and technologies offer great hope. Ultimate success, the development of an effective malaria vaccine, demands bold leadership, undeterred by myriad failures, able to marshal scarce resources against this formidable foe.

ACKNOWLEDGMENTS

We thank Carter Diggs, Jeff Lyon, Urszula Krzych, Evelina Angov, Ashley Birkett, Ann Stewart, Ruobing Wang, and Judy Epstein for sharing unpublished results.

REFERENCES

1. Wongsrichanalai C, et al. Epidemiology of drug-resistant malaria. Lancet Infect Dis 2002; 2:209–218.
2. Chandre, et al. Status of pyrethroid resistance in Anopheles sensu lato. Bull World Health Org 1999; 77:230–234.
3. Sachs J, Malany P. The economic and social burden of malaria. Nature 2002; 415:670–672.
4. http://www.MalariaVaccine.org
5. Trape JF, et al. The Dielmo project: a longitudinal study of natural malaria infection and the mechanisms of protective immunity in a community living in a holoendemic area of Senegal. Am J Trop Med Hyg 1994; 51:123–137.
6. Kun JF, et al. Nitric oxide synthase2 (Lambarene) (G-954C), increased nitric oxide production, and protection against malaria. J Infect Dis 2001; 84:330–336.
7. Kurtis JD, et al. Pre-erythrocytic immunity to *Plasmodium falciparum*: the case for an LSA-1 vaccine. Trends Parasitol 2001; 17:219–223.
8. Hill AVS, et al. Common west African HLA antigens are associated with protection from severe malaria. Nature 1991; 352:595–600.
9. Hill AVS, et al. Molecular analysis of the association of HLA-B53 and resistance to severe malaria. Nature 1992; 360:434–439.
10. Clyde DF. Immunization of man against *falciparum* and vivax malaria by use of attenuated sporozoites. Am J Trop Med Hyg 1975; 24:397–401.
11. Clyde DF, et al. Specificity of protection of man immunized against sporozoite-induced *falciparum* malaria. Am J Med Sci 1973; 266:398–403.
12. Schellenberg D. Intermittent treatment for malaria and anemia control at time of routine vaccinations in Tanzanian infants; a randomised, placebo-controlled trial. Lancet 2001; 357:1471–1477.
13. Schultz LJ, et al. The effect of antimalaria regimens containing sulfadoxine-pyrimethamine and/or chloroquine in

preventing peripheral and placental *Plasmodium falciparum* infection among pregnant women in Malawi. Am J Trop Med Hyg 1994; 51:515–522.

14. Schulman CE, et al. Intermittent sulfadoxine-pyrimethamine to prevent severe anaemia secondary to malaria in pregnancy: a randomised placebo-controlled trial. Lancet 1999; 353:632–636.

15. D'Alessandro U, et al. Mortality and morbidity from malaria in Gambian children after introduction of an impregnated bednet programme. Lancet 1995; 345:479–483.

16. Potocnjak P, et al. Monovalent fragments (Fab) of monoclonal antibodies to a sporozoite surface antigen (Pb44) protect mice against malarial infection. J Exp Med 1980; 151:1504–1513.

17. Weiss WR, et al. CD8+ T cells (cytotoxic/suppressors) are required for protection in mice immunized with malaria sporozoites. Proc Natl Acad Sci USA 1988; 85:573–576.

18. Krzych U, et al. The role of intrahepatic lymphocytes in mediating protective immunity induced by attenuated Plasmodium berghei sporozoites. Immunol Rev 2000; 174:123–134.

19. Chulay JD, et al. Malaria transmitted to humans by mosquitoes infected from cultured *Plasmodium falciparum*. Am J Trop Med Hyg 1986; 35:66–88.

20. Stoute JA, et al. A preliminary evaluation of a recombinant circumsporozoite protein vaccine against *Plasmodium falciparum* malaria. N Engl J Med 1997; 336:86–91.

21. Stoute JA, et al. Long-term efficacy and immune responses following immunization with the RTS,S.malaria vaccine. J Infect Dis 1998; 178:1139–1144.

22. Bojang KA, et al. Efficacy of RTS,S/AS02 malaria vaccine against *Plasmodium falciparum* infection in semi-immune adult men in The Gambia: a randomised trial. Lancet 2001; 358:1927–1934.

23. Dame JB, et al. Structure of the gene encoding the immunodominant surface antigen on the sporozoite of the human malaria parasite *Plasmodium falciparum*. Science 1984; 225:593–599.

24. Enea V, et al. DNA cloning of *Plasmodium falciparum* circumsporozoite gene: amino acid sequence of repetitive epitope. Science 1984; 225:628–630.

25. Burkot TR, et al. Fine specificities of monoclonal antibodies against the *Plasmodium falciparum* circumsporozoite protein: recognition of both repetitive and non-repetitive regions. Parasite Immunol 1991; 13:161–170.

26. Ballou WR, et al. Safety and efficacy of a recombinant DNA *Plasmodium falciparum* sporozoite vaccine. Lancet 1987: 1227–1281.

27. Herrington DA, et al. Safety and immunogenicity in man of a synthetic peptide malaria vaccine against *Plasmodiumialciparum* sporozoites. Nature 1987; 328:257–259.

28. Fries LF, et al. Safety, immunogenicity, and efficacy of a *Plasmodium falciparum* vaccine comprising a circumsporozoite protein repeat region peptide conjugated to *Pseudomonas aeruginosa* toxin A. Infect Immun 1992; 60:1834–1839.

29. Fries LF, et al. Liposomal malaria vaccine in humans: a safe and potent adjuvant strategy. Proc Natl Acad Sci USA 1992; 89:358–362.

30. Ribi E, et al. Biological activities of monophosphoryl lipid A. In: Levine L, Bonventre PF, Morello IA, et al. eds. Microbiology. Washington: American Society for Microbiology, 1986.

31. Hoffman SL, et al. Safety, immunogenicity, and efficacy of a malaria sporozoite vaccine administered with monophosphoryl lipid A, cell wall skeleton of mycobacteria, and squalene as adjuvant. Am J Trop Med Hyg 1994; 51:603–612.

32. Schofield L, et al. Interferon-gamma, CD8+ T cells and antibodies required for immunity to malaria sporozoites. Nature 1987; 330:664–666.

33. Hoffman SL, et al. Protection of humans against malaria by immunization with radiation-attenuated *Plasmodium falciparum* sporozoites. J Infect Dis 2002; 185:1155–1164.

34. Good MF, et al. Human T-cell recognition of the circumsporozoite protein of *Plasmodium falciparum*: immunodominant T-cell domains map to the polymorphic regions of the molecule. Proc Natl Acad Sci USA 1998; 85:199–203.

35. Kumar S, et al. Cytotoxic T cells specific for the circumsporozoite protein of *Plasmodium falciparum*. Nature 1988; 334:258–260.

36. Sinigaglia F, et al. A malaria T-cell epitope recognized in association with most mouse and human MHC class II molecules. Nature 1988; 336:778–780.

37. Sinigaglia F, et al. *Plasmodium falciparum* specific human T cell clones: evidence for helper and cytotoxic activities. Eur J Immunol 1987; 17:187–192.

38. Malik A, et al. Human cytotoxic T lymphocytes against the *Plasmodium falciparum* circumsporozoite protein. Proc Natl Acad Sci USA 1991; 88:3300–3304.

39. Moreno A, et al. CD4+ T cell clones obtained from *Plasmodium falciparum* sporozoite-immunized volunteers recognize polymorphic sequences of the circumsporozoite protein. J Immunol 1993; 151:489–499.

40. Cerami C, et al. The basolateral domain of the hepatocyte plasma membrane bears receptors for the circumsporozoite protein of *Plasmodium falciparum* sporozoites. Cell 1992; 70:1021–1033.

41. Heppner DG, et al. Safety, immunogenicity, and efficacy of *Plasmodium falciparum* repeatless circumsporozoite protein vaccine encapsulated in liposomes. J Infect Dis 1996; 174:361–366.

42. Gordon DM, et al. Safety, immunogenicity, and efficacy of a recombinantly produced *Plasmodium falciparum* circumsporozoite protein-hepatitis B surface antigen subunit vaccine. J Infect Dis 1995; 171:1576–1585.

43. Kester KE, et al. Efficacy of recombinant circumsporozoite protein vaccine regimens against experimental *Plasmodium falciparum* malaria. J Infect Dis 2001; 183:640–647.

44. Doherty JF, et al. Phase I safety and immunogenicity trial with the candidate malaria vaccine RTS,S/SBAS2 in semi-immune adults in The Gambia. Am J Trop Med Hyg 1999; 61:865–868.

45. Bojang KA, et al. Efficacy of RTS,S/AS02 malaria vaccine against *Plasmodium falciparum* infection in semi-immune adult men in The Gambia: a randomised trial. Lancet 2001; 358:1927–1934.

46. Alloueche A, et al. Protective efficacy of the R2S,S/AS02A *Plasmodium falciparum* malaria vaccine is not stain specific. Am J Trop Med Hyg 2003; 68:97–101.

47. Lalvani A, et al. Potent induction focused Th1-type cellular and humoral immune responses by RTS,S/SBAS2, a recombinant *Plasmodium falciparum* malaria vaccine. J Infect Dis 1999; 180:1656–1664.

48. Robson KJ, et al. A highly conserved amino-acid sequence in thrombospondin, properdin, and in proteins from sporozoites and blood stages of a human malaria parasite. Nature 1988; 335:79–82.

49. Rogers WO, et al. Characterization of *Plasmodium falciparum* sporozoite surface protein 2. Proc Natl Acad Sci USA 1992; 89:9176–9180.

50. Sultan AA, et al. TRAP is necessary for gliding motility and infectivity of *Plasmodium* sporozoites. Cell 1996; 84:933–939.

51. Szarfman A, et al. Mature liver stages of cloned *Plasmodium falciparum* share epitopes with proteins from sporozoites and asexual blood stages. Parasite Immunol 1988; 10:339–351.

52. Egan AF, et al. Clinical immunity to *Plasmodium falciparum* is associated with serum antibodies to the19 kDa C terminal fragment of the merozoite surface antigen, PfMSP1. J Infect Dis 1996; 173:765–769.

53. Siddiqui WA, et al. Merozoite surface coat precursor protein completely protects Aotus monkeys against *Plasmodium falciparum* malaria. Proc Natl Acad Sci USA 1987; 84: 3014–3018.

54. Pichyangkul S, et al. Pre-clinical evaluation of vaccine candidate *P. falciparum* MSP-1(42) formulated with novel adjuvants in comparison with clinically approved alum. Manuscript in preparation.

55. Jones TR, et al. Protection of Aotus monkeys by *Plasmodium falciparum* EBA-175 region II DNA prime-protein boost mmunization regimen. J Infect Dis 2001; 183:303–312.

56. Plebanski M, et al. Protection from *Plasmodium* berghei infection by priming and boosting T cells to a single class I-restricted epitope with recombinant carriers suitable for human use. Eur J mmunol 1998; 28:4345–4355.

57. Gilbert SC, et al. Enhanced CD8 T cell immunogenicity and protective efficacy in a mouse malaria model using a recombinant adenoviral vaccine in heterologous prime-boos immunisation regimes. Vaccine 2002; 20:1039–1045.

58. Le TP, et al. Safety, tolerability and humoral immune responses after intramuscular administration of a malaria DNA vaccine to healthy adult volunteers. Vaccine 2000; 18:1893–1901.

59. Wang R, et al. Induction of antigen-specific cytotoxic T lymphocytes in humans by a malaria DNA vaccine. Science 1998; 282:476–480.

60. Reed RC, et al. Re-investigation of the circumsporozoite protein-based induction of sterile immunity against *Plasmodium* berghei infection. Vaccine 1996; 14:828–836.

61. Di John D, et al. Effect of priming with carrier on response to conjugate vaccine. Lancet 1989; 2:1415–1418.

62. Nardin EH, et al. Synthetic peptide malaria vaccine elicits high levels of antibodies in vaccinees of defined HLA genotypes. J Infect Dis 2000; 182:1486–1496.

63. Calvo-Calle JM, et al. Binding of malaria T cell epitopes to DR and DQ molecules in vitro correlates immunogenicity in vivo: identification of a universal T cell epitope in the *Plasmodum falciparum* circumsporozoite protein. J Immunol 1997; 159:1362–1373.

64. Nardin EH, et al. *Plasmodium falciparum* polyoximes: highly immunogenic synthetic vaccines constructed by chemoselective ligation of repeat B-cell epitopes and a universal T-cell epitope of CS protein. Vaccine 1998; 16:590–600.

65. Nardin EH, et al. A totally synthetic polyoxime malaria vaccine containing *Plasmodium falciparum* B cell and uni-

versal T cell epitopes elicits immune responses in volunteers of diverse HLA types. J Immunol 2001; 166:481–499.

66. Ulrich R, et al. Core particles of hepatitis B virus as carrier for foreign epitopes. Adv Virus Res 1998; 50:141–182.

67. Schodel F, et al. Immunity to malaria elicited by hybrid hepatitis B virus core particles carrying circumsporozoite protein epitopes. J Exp Med 1994; 180:1037–1046.

68. Schodel F, et al. Immunization with hybrid hepatitis B virus core particles carrying circumsporozoite antigen epitopes protects mice against *Plasmodium* yoelii challenge. Behring-Inst Mitt 1997; 98:114–119.

69. Birkett A, et al. Hepatitis core antigen particles containing minimal T and B cell epitopes of *P. falciparum* CS protein elicit high levels of malaria specific immune responses in mice and non-human primates. American Society for Tropical Medicine and Hygiene, November 11–15, 2001, Atlanta, GA.

70. Milich DR, et al. Conversion of poorly immunogenic malaria repeat sequences into a highly immunogenic vaccine candidate. Vaccine 2001; 20:771–788.

71. Roggero MA, et al. *Plasmodium falciparum* CS C-terminal fragment: preclinical evaluation and Phase 1 clinical studies. Parassitologia 1999; 41:421–424.

72. Lopez JA, et al. A synthetic malaria vaccine elicits a potent CD8+ and CD4+ T lymphocyte immune response in humans. Implications for vaccination strategies. Eur J Immunol 2001; 31:1989–1998.

73. Guerin-Marchand C, et al. A liver stage-specific antigen of *Plasmodium falciparum* characterized by gene cloning. Nature 1987; 329:164–167.

74. Kurtis JD, et al. Pre-erythrocytic immunity to *Plasmodium falciparum*: the case for an LSA-1 vaccine. Trends Parasitol 2001; 17:219–223.

75. Krzych U, et al. T lymphocytes from volunteers immunized with irradiated *Plasmodium falciparum* sporozoites recognize liver and blood stage malaria antigens. J Immunol 1995; 155:4072–4077.

76. Perllaza BL, et al. Long synthetic peptides encompassing the *Plasmodium falciparum* LSA3 are the target of human B and T cells and are potent inducers of B helper, T helper and cytolytic responses in mice. Eur J Immunol 2001; 31:2200–2209.

77. Daubersies P, et al. Protection against *Plasmodium falciparum* malaria in chimpanzees by immunization with the conserved pre-erythrocytic liver-stage antigen 3. Nat Med 2000; 6:1258–1263.

71

Malaria: A Complex Disease that May Require a Complex Vaccine

Stephen L. Hoffman
Sanaria Inc., Gaithersburg, Maryland, U.S.A.

Denise L. Doolan and Thomas L. Richie
Naval Medical Research Center, Silver Spring, Maryland, U.S.A.

I. THE NEED FOR A MALARIA VACCINE

Malaria, caused by *Plasmodium falciparum*, *Plasmodium vivax*, *Plasmodium malariae*, or *Plasmodium ovale*, is a major health problem in most countries in the tropics. For years, it has been estimated that more than 2 billion people live in countries where malaria is transmitted, that there may be 300–500 million new infections and 1–3 million deaths annually caused by malaria, and that the majority of cases and more than 90% of the deaths occur in sub-Saharan Africa, where malaria is, in many places, the leading cause of death among children less than 5 years of age. Recent analyses suggest that the medical impact of malaria may actually have been significantly underestimated [1], and that the enormous economic impact of malaria has never been adequately considered [2]. It has been estimated that malaria reduces annual gross domestic product (GDP) in affected countries in sub-Saharan Africa by more than 1.3% [2]. As we begin the twenty-first century, it is troubling that a treatable infectious disease has such an "intolerable" impact. Yet, the increasing resistance of the *Plasmodium* sp. parasite to chemoprophylactic and chemotherapeutic agents, the resistance of the *Anopheles* sp. mosquito vector to insecticides, including the pyrethroids used in insecticide-impregnated bed-nets, and the inability of the most affected countries to mobilize and sustain the resources required for malaria control, as evidenced by the resurgence of malaria in areas formerly free of the disease, highlight the urgency for developing an effective malaria vaccine. A vaccine would dramatically improve the chances of optimally controlling, and eventually eradicating, malaria.

Additionally, malaria remains a major public health threat to nonimmune visitors to areas where malaria is transmitted. Of the nearly 700 million international tourist arrivals recorded worldwide in 2000, approximately 9 million were bound for West, Central, or East Africa, 37 million were to Southeast Asia, 6 million to South Asia, and 10 million to Oceania [3]. Although it is not possible to ascertain what proportion of these travelers visited malaria-endemic areas, an estimate of 30% would yield 18 million international travelers to areas potentially exposed to malaria transmission. This estimate can be supplemented by arrivals to malarious areas of the Middle East, the Caribbean, and South America, and by nontourist travel, such as deployment of military personnel. Serological studies of various traveling populations suggest that from 2% to 21% (but as high as 80%) of travelers are actually inoculated with *Plasmodium* spp. sporozoites during their stay in the tropics [4]. In addition to international travelers, a growing number of people residing in malaria-free regions of malaria-endemic countries travel locally to areas where malaria is transmitted [5]. Whether the purpose is tourism, family visits, business, government service, military deployment, religious service, emigration or escaping civil strife or persecution, malaria is one of the most significant health risks faced by travelers today. Factors associated with use of chemoprophylaxis, such as availability, costs, contraindications, side effects, inconvenience, and compliance, along with the many cases of malaria in returning travelers, and the threat of increasing drug resistance, form the rationale for a traveler's vaccine for the prevention of malaria. In order to be used as a substitute for chemoprophylaxis, such a vaccine would have to provide greater than 85–90% protective efficacy for a sustained period, perhaps at least 6 months.

There are four chapters on malaria vaccine development in this book. In this chapter, we summarize our perspective on the current efforts to develop malaria vaccines. We emphasize the work we performed to utilize a sequential immunization approach (DNA prime and recombinant virus or protein boost) to maximize the antibody and T-cell responses against the sporozoite, liver, and asexual erythrocytic stages of the parasite life cycle, and introduce recent work to develop an attenuated whole sporozoite *P. falciparum* vaccine.

II. THE POTENTIAL FOR DIFFERENT MALARIA VACCINES FOR DIFFERENT TARGET POPULATIONS

Many malariologists believe that different types of malaria vaccines may be necessary for different populations. The primary requirement is to reduce the incidence of severe malaria and malaria-associated mortality in infants and children with heavy exposure to *P. falciparum*, such as those living in sub-Saharan Africa (Type 1 vaccine). At the other extreme is the requirement to prevent all clinical manifestations of malaria in individuals from areas with no exposure, who travel to regions where malaria is endemic, primarily malaria caused by *P. falciparum* and *P. vivax* (Type 2 vaccine). This "extremes" approach to malaria vaccine development does not take into account specific populations affected by malaria which fall between these extremes, such as individuals in endemic regions at high risk of *P. vivax* infections [6]. In fact, as Type 1 and Type 2 vaccines are developed, they will need to be assessed in many different populations.

For the Type 1 vaccine designed to reduce mortality among children in sub-Saharan Africa, the problem is complicated by the varied epidemiology of the disease. In areas with extremely intense transmission, such as northern Ghana, it is primarily infants who die of malaria, with severe anemia as a major cause of death. In areas with less intense transmission, such as The Gambia, 2- to 5-year-olds appear to face the greatest risk of dying, with cerebral malaria as the major cause of death [7]. It is even possible that different vaccines or vaccination strategies, tailored to the predominant pathophysiology of a particular region or targeting the age groups at greatest risk, may be the most effective response to this heterogeneous epidemiology.

For the Type 2 vaccine designed to prevent all clinical manifestations of malaria in nonimmune travelers to malaria-endemic areas, the target populations are also varied. One generally thinks that the major recipients of such a vaccine would be travelers from North America, Europe, Japan, Australia, and other highly developed malaria-free areas of the world. However, there are hundreds of millions of people living in nonmalarious areas of malaria-endemic countries who travel to malarious areas of their own country. For example, it is not infrequent for someone born in western Kenya, where transmission is high, to attend a university in Nairobi, where there is no malaria transmission, and then settle in Nairobi. The children of these Nairobi residents are nonimmune to malaria, and the parents themselves may lose their immunity if sufficient time passes. When they, their children, or other Kenyans born in Nairobi visit western Kenya on holidays, they are at high risk of contracting malaria and rapidly developing

severe disease. There is little mention in the malaria literature of the increasing numbers of nonimmunes living in countries with endemic malaria who must receive short-term protection against malaria by a vaccine. Because of their susceptibility to rapidly developing severe disease and because of their brief exposure to transmission, we think that these in-country travelers, including their children, would require a vaccine with the same protective profile as a vaccine for travelers from North America or Europe.

There is a third type of vaccine being developed, a transmission-blocking vaccine. This vaccine is designed to protect the entire community rather than the immunized individual, by reducing transmission intensity. The target populations for such a vaccine are not yet clearly defined. Such a vaccine could eventually be combined with the Type-1 and -2 vaccines described above. Such a vaccine would unquestionably be of great value, perhaps even on its own, in islands with malaria or in areas with only modest transmission. It might also be useful during prolonged epidemics. It is not clear how useful such a vaccine will be in areas such as sub-Saharan Africa, where transmission is intense. However, a recent article has suggested that such a vaccine could be quite useful, particularly when combined with vaccines targeting other parasite stages, for preventing a selective process favoring the emergence of fast-growing, and therefore, virulent parasites [8]. Even if not able to impact overall transmission levels, a transmission-blocking component included in a Type 1 or Type 2 vaccine could block the escape of resistant mutants, thus preserving vaccine efficacy in the community and preventing the emergence of virulent parasite strains.

III. THE FEASIBILITY OF A MALARIA VACCINE IS SUPPORTED BY HUMAN MODELS

Functional human models demonstrate that both pre-erythrocytic stage and erythrocytic stage vaccines are feasible. In humans, pre-erythrocytic stage immunity can be induced by exposure to irradiated sporozoites [9], and a clinically important degree of erythrocytic stage immunity can be induced by exposure to repeated blood stage infection [10,11].

The first model, immunization with radiation-attenuated sporozoites, is for the design of a vaccine to prevent all clinical manifestations of malaria. In 1967, it was demonstrated that mice immunized with *Plasmodium* sporozoites attenuated by radiation, such that they could invade the host hepatocyte and undergo limited development but could not mature into blood-stage parasites, were protected against challenge with live sporozoites [12]. In late 1973 and early 1974, two groups independently reported that human volunteers could likewise be protected against infectious sporozoite challenge by immunization with radiation-attenuated *P. falciparum* sporozoites [13–15]. The attenuated sporozoite vaccine is administered by exposing vaccinees to at least 1000 bites of irradiated, infected mosquitoes over the course of several months. These attenuated parasites undergo partial development in the liver but do not progress to the blood-stage. They stimulate an immune response that is sporozoite- and liver-stage-specific and, provided the number of immunizations is sufficient, are able to sterilize subsequent challenge with intact sporozoites for up to 42 weeks [9]. This cumbersome procedure presents a technical barrier to large-scale immunization that has not yet been overcome. Nonetheless, the induction of sterile immunity by attenuated sporozoites provides proof-of-principle regarding the feasibility of making a sporozoite/liver-stage malaria vaccine that prevents blood-stage infection and clinical disease entirely.

The second model of immunity to malaria in humans is for a vaccine to prevent death and severe disease without preventing erythrocytic-stage infection, and the model is naturally acquired immunity [11]. In areas where malaria is transmitted, individuals that survive past a certain age will become reinfected and may become clinically ill, but will not develop severe disease or die. In areas with stable transmission, there is little to no severe disease or malaria-associated deaths after the age of 7–10 years; in areas with very intense transmission, this transition may occur as early as the second or third year of life. The decrease in the incidence of *P. falciparum* infections, the prevalence and density of parasitemia, and the morbidity and mortality associated with *Plasmodium* spp. infection with natural exposure is consistent with acquisition of antimalarial immunity in humans [7,16]. The existence of naturally acquired immunity provides a strong rationale for including blood-stage antigens designed to induce antibody responses as the second "tier" of a "two-tiered" vaccine: pre-erythrocytic components to destroy the majority of developing parasites during the 5-day window of liver stage development, and erythrocytic components to protect against severe disease and death in individuals who experience breakthrough blood-stage infections.

In the case of naturally acquired immunity, the genetics of the human host, the transmission dynamics of the parasite, and probably even the age of the host, contribute to the complexity of the immune response to infection and therefore may add to the difficulty of developing a vaccine. Although it is clear that sickle-cell trait protects against severe disease, and that other genetic traits may influence outcome, our understanding of the relationship between host genetics and the response to infection is limited. The elucidation of the sequence of the human genome and the development of scientific tools to use these data should lead to a better understanding of the role of host factors in determining the severity of disease associated with infection.

IV. APPROACHES TO MALARIA VACCINE DEVELOPMENT

Vaccines have eliminated the natural transmission of smallpox from the world, nearly eliminated polio, and eliminated *Hemophilus influenza* as a cause of severe disease in industrialized countries. We know that it is possible for the immune system to control malaria, yet despite much effort, there is currently no commercially available malaria vaccine. It is not possible to consider immunizing people by

exposure to live infectious parasites, which is what occurs in naturally acquired immunity, because the individuals would become clinically ill. It has not been considered practical to immunize by the bite of irradiated, infected mosquitoes, or by intravenous injection of live radiation-attenuated sporozoites, to duplicate the immunity elicited by the irradiated sporozoite vaccine.

During the past 20 years, therefore, there has been considerable work performed to develop subunit vaccines that provide protective immunity comparable to that of the human models of radiation-attenuated sporozoite immunization and naturally acquired immunity. However, no vaccine has yet provided comparable protection. There are numerous potential explanations for the lack of current success. One is that exposure to the whole parasite elicits a more potent, protective immune response than the subunit vaccines tested thus far. However, in the case of people protected by the irradiated sporozoite vaccine or by naturally acquired immunity, T-cell and antibody responses against current candidate antigens or against whole parasites (in the case of antibody responses) are generally modest at best and often lower than those achieved by subunit vaccination. A more likely explanation is that immunization with only one or a few parasite proteins cannot duplicate the immunity elicited by exposure to a parasite that has thousands of proteins.

The disappointments in the initial clinical trials considered in the context of the two human models have resulted in a reappraisal of malaria vaccine development strategies. The general approach has been to attempt to delineate the immune responses responsible for the protective immunity seen in models, determine the antigens against which these protective immune responses are directed, package these antigens or their critical epitopes in a vaccine formulation that is immunogenic and suitable for manufacture and administration, and develop a vaccine delivery system that would induce the required responses against the identified targets. During the past decade, significant progress has been made in each of these areas. Three general approaches to malaria vaccine development have been delineated. A fourth approach has been added in the past 6 months.

The most work has been done and progress achieved on an approach focused on maximizing the magnitude and quality of immune responses to a single or a few key antigens, such as the circumsporozoite protein (CSP) and the merozoite surface protein-1 (MSP1), by immunizing with synthetic peptides or recombinant proteins in an adjuvant. These vaccines are being designed to primarily induce antibody [17] and CD4$^+$ T-cell responses [18], but there is also interest in eliciting CD8$^+$ T-cell responses. Researchers focusing on this approach consider that the subset of parasite antigens currently identified as potential vaccine targets is adequate, and that the major obstacle to fielding an effective vaccine lies with optimizing the induction of the desired immune response by vaccination. Some success with this approach has been shown with the demonstration that a vaccine composed of partial-length *P. falciparum* circumsporozoite protein (PfCSP) fused to hepatitis B surface antigen and expressed together with unfused HbsAg (called

RTS,S) formulated in adjuvant provided short-term protection of malaria-naïve volunteers against experimental challenge [19,20], and of semi-immune adults resident in The Gambia against naturally transmitted malaria [21]. These results support the potential for RTS,S as a core component for a vaccine. However, the transient nature of the RTS,S-induced protection and the inability of the vaccine to induce the class I restricted responses considered important for pre-erythrocytic stage protection, despite the induction of class II-restricted anti-PfCSP IFN-γ responses and antibody responses, establish that the vaccine is not yet optimal as currently formulated. These data clearly indicate that this vaccine will not be adequate for preventing all clinical manifestations of malaria in travelers and military personnel, but do not preclude the possibility that this vaccine, on its own, could reduce severe morbidity and mortality in children in Africa. For this reason, it is now being tested in field trials in children in Africa.

The second approach to malaria vaccine development is to induce good or optimal immune responses against each of approximately 5–15 identified potential target antigens, by immunizing with DNA vaccines or recombinant viruses, and boosting with either DNA, recombinant viruses or bacteria, or recombinant proteins in adjuvant, or replicons. The goal here is to elicit CD8$^+$ and CD4$^+$ T-cell as well as antibody responses. To date, the primary target antigens at the pre-erythrocytic stage, those antigens expressed by *P. falciparum*-irradiated sporozoites within infected hepatocytes, include CSP, SSP2, LSA1, and Exp1 [22]. Recently, LSA3 has been proposed as an additional candidate [23]. Researchers focusing on this multivalent, multi-immune response approach are skeptical regarding the ability of a vaccine based on a single antigen to protect against a parasite as complex as *Plasmodium*, considering the problems posed by the severe genetic restriction of the host immune response and parasite variation of target epitopes. Efforts to date on the development of a multivalent and multi-immune response malaria vaccine have primarily focused on the technology of DNA-based vaccines, with both whole-gene and multiepitope vaccines being evaluated in the clinic [24,25] (AVS Hill, unpublished results; TL Richie, unpublished results). In the case of the whole gene, the *P. falciparum* circumsporozoite protein (PfCSP) has been used to provide the foundation and establish the proof-of-principle for safety, tolerability, and immunogenicity of DNA-based vaccines in normal healthy humans. Initial Phase I studies have established that DNA vaccines are safe and well tolerated [26,27], and that antigen-specific and genetically restricted CD8$^+$ T-cell responses can be induced by vaccination with plasmid DNA [28,29] (Figures 1 and 2). However, these first-generation DNA vaccines are suboptimal, as indicated by the frequency and magnitude of induced immune responses in humans, and by the demonstrations in multiple animal models of the potential of a number of immune enhancement strategies. In particular, prime-boost approaches involving priming with DNA and boosting with poxvirus or recombinant protein in adjuvant offer an excellent means of inducing protective antibody and T-cell responses of significantly greater magnitude than DNA vaccine approaches on their own [30].

The third approach is to develop a subunit vaccine that duplicates the whole-organism immunity induced by immunization with radiation-attenuated sporozoites or by natural exposure to malaria. Success in this area will be dependent on utilizing data from the malaria genome projects [31,32] and developing methods for exploiting this genomic sequence data. It remains to be established how such multiantigen vaccines will be constructed, but it is likely that DNA-based vaccines will be the core technology used for this approach.

The fourth approach is to develop a practical nonreplicating, metabolically active (attenuated) *P. falciparum* sporozoite vaccine that provides the sustained greater-than-90% protection in humans that has been achieved by exposing volunteers to the bites of irradiated mosquitoes carrying *P. falciparum* sporozoites in their salivary glands [9]. Success of this approach will require development methods of practically producing sterile sporozoites, and demonstrating that administration in the skin, subcutaneous tissue, or muscle of the sporozoites by needle and syringe, or some other practical method provides protection.

V. RATIONAL DESIGN OF SUBUNIT VACCINES

Although many approaches have been adopted by various laboratories for vaccine development, there is a rough consensus regarding certain principles for rational subunit malaria vaccine design.

A. Consider Evolutionary Selection Pressures

Because of *P. falciparum*'s history of circumventing interventions through evolutionary change, designing vaccines which are minimally susceptible to the development of resistance should be a priority. Review of the history of malaria control reveals that despite the deployment of highly effective drugs (e.g., chloroquine, which enjoyed many years of 100% efficacy against all species of human malaria parasites in most tropical regions) and insecticides (e.g., DDT, which has had the greatest impact on malaria transmission to date of any specific intervention), malaria remains deeply entrenched in most tropical countries. This is because the basic reproduction rate (i.e., the number of individuals who will become infected if one infected individual enters an area with *Anopheles* mosquitoes) often far exceeds the minimum rate required to maintain the parasite's life cycle, thereby making it very difficult to interrupt transmission through control measures. This "excess" transmission also results in the potential for evolutionary change in the parasite and vector populations when selection pressures are applied through the application of drugs or insecticides. In other words, both parasite and vector populations can be dramatically reduced in numbers, yet still maintain transmission, allowing the emergence of resistant genotypes. For example, chloroquine resistance by *P. falciparum*, which probably originated independently at least four times [33], is now widespread and increasing, and is also expanding to *P. vivax* [34,35] and to *P. malariae* [36]. Studies of the *P. falciparum* genome highlight the genetic complexity of the organism and its potential for evolutionary

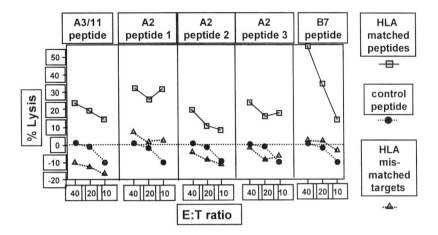

Figure 1 DNA-induced CTL responses against the PfCSP are restricted by multiple HLA alleles. Fresh peripheral blood mononuclear cells (PBMCs) from a volunteer immunized with 500 μg PfCSP DNA, who expressed the alleles HLA-A2, -A3, and -B7, were assayed for antigen-specific, genetically restricted CTLs against PfCSP-derived peptides. The assay was repeated with coded frozen PBMCs that were collected before and after vaccination; the results confirmed that the peptide-specific (the same five peptides), genetically restricted CTLs were induced by vaccination with plasmid DNA. (From Ref. 29.)

change [37]. It is imperative that vaccine developers consider the parasite's potential for evolutionarily "escaping" susceptibility to the immune responses induced by a vaccine, leading to lost efficacy of hard-won vaccine antigens. Vaccines targeting travelers may not exert significant selection pressures, because infections in this population would, in most cases, have little impact on within-country malaria transmission, and therefore would not contribute to the evolution of resistance to the vaccine by the parasite. However, widespread use of an effective vaccine in endemic areas favors the transmission of resistant genotypes.

B. Define the Immune Responses to Be Induced by Vaccination

1. For irradiated sporozoite-induced immunity, protection is thought to be primarily mediated by T cells directed against peptide epitopes from parasite proteins expressed in infected hepatocytes (function-independent killing via elimination of infected host cells) (Figure 3). More specifically, CD8[+] T cells specific for parasite-derived peptide/class I MHC molecule complexes on the surface of infected hepatocytes [38] are considered the primary immune effectors, where elimination of the infected hepatocytes is mediated by interferon-gamma (IFN-γ) released by CD8[+] T cells (as well as other cells) and not by direct cytolysis of the infected hepatocyte by parasite-specific CD8[+] T cells [39,40]. Humans immunized with radiation-attenuated sporozoites [41–43] (Doolan, submitted) or naturally exposed to malaria [44–48] have been shown to have CD8[+] cytotoxic T lymphocytes and CD8[+] IFN-γ responses against pre-erythrocytic stage proteins. However, data regarding the importance of T cells in the immunity elicited by radiation-attenuated sporozoites come entirely from rodent experiments [39,40,49–53], in which T-

cell subsets were depleted or adoptively transferred. In rodent models, protection is absolutely dependent on CD8[+] T cells and IFN-γ, and often dependent on IL-12 and nitric oxide [39,40] (Fig. 3). Also, CD8[+] T cells eliminate *Plasmodium berghei*- or *Plasmodium yoelii*-infected mouse hepatocytes from in vitro culture in an MHC-restricted and antigen-restricted manner [38,54]. Nonetheless, CD4[+] T cells that recognize parasite-derived peptide/class II MHC molecule complexes on hepatocytes are also thought to play a role in sporozoite-induced protection, because the adoptive transfer of antigen-specific CD4[+] T cells can protect against sporozoite challenge [55,56], and depletion of CD4[+] T cells can eliminate protection in some strains of genetically inbred mice [40]. Finally, antibodies against sporozoite surface proteins, such as CSP, that neutralize the infectivity of sporozoites for hepatocytes (function-inhibiting activity) may also be involved [22,57,58]. Sporozoite-induced protective immunity is complex with a number of different cell types, cytokines, or chemokines potentially playing roles in a multifaceted and integrated fashion. Attempts to dissect this immunity using molecular immunology are underway. Other areas of uncertainty regarding sporozoite-induced protective immunity include the site of immune induction, the infected hepatocyte as the target of protective CD8[+] T cells, the infected hepatocyte as the antigen presenting cell (APC), the role of dendritic cells, macrophages, and other professional APCs, the mechanism of antigen processing and presentation, the mechanism for and factors influencing induction of long-term protective immunity, the requirement for persistence of antigen for induction of long-term protective immunity, and identification of appropriate in vitro correlate(s) of protective immunity.

In general, the immune responses induced by immunization with irradiated sporozoites are not as robust as those

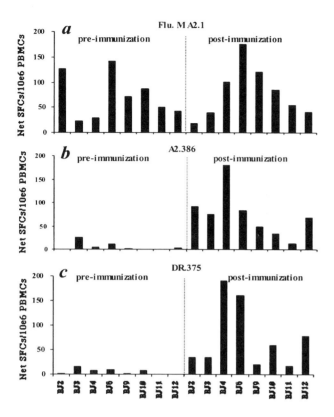

Figure 2 Antigen-specific IFN-γ responses against the PfCSP induced by DNA vaccination. IFN-γ responses against: (a) HLA-A2.1-restricted positive control peptide from influenza matrix protein (Flu. A2.1); (b) HLA-A2.1-restricted peptide from PfCSP (A2.386); or (c) HLA-DR-restricted peptide from PfCSP (DR.375) with coded and double-blinded frozen PBMCs collected from eight volunteers pre- and postimmunization with PfCSP DNA administered by Biojector® intramuscularly (BJ2, -33, and -4), by Biojector® intramuscularly and intradermally (BJ6, -9, and -10), and by needle intramuscularly (BJ11 and -1). (From Ref. 28.)

induced by subunit vaccination. We favor the hypothesis that irradiated sporozoite-induced protective immunity reflects the sum of many immune responses of low magnitude against multiple targets, where the low magnitude of response results from density of epitope presentation. However, there may be other explanations; a single or few "key" antigens could be responsible for the protection and are as yet unidentified.

2. With regard to naturally acquired immunity, passive transfer experiments in humans indicate that antidisease/antiparasite immunity is mediated, at least in part, by antibodies against parasite proteins expressed on the surface of infected erythrocytes and merozoites and in merozoite apical organelles. Passive transfer of immunoglobulin derived from adults with naturally acquired immunity following lifelong exposure to endemic malaria rapidly reduced parasitemia and led to resolution of symptoms in parasitemic recipients [59–62]. Antibodies directed against parasite proteins ex-

pressed on the surface of erythrocytes that prevent sequestration in the microcirculation (function-inhibiting) [63], antibodies directed against parasite proteins expressed on the surface of merozoites that prevent invasion of erythrocytes (function-inhibiting) [64], and antibodies expressed against either type of parasite protein that are capable of mediating antibody-dependent cellular inhibition (ADCI) [65], whereby biologically active molecules, including cytokines, nitric oxide, and free oxygen intermediates are released from reticuloendothelial or other cells after activation through the Fc component of the bound antibody molecule (function-independent killing), are implicated. One such protein is *P. falciparum* erythrocyte membrane protein 1 (PfEMP1), which mediates cytoadherence and sequestration. Cytoadherence of infected erythrocytes to endothelial cells in the microcirculation during maturation of the parasite, thereby preventing removal of the infected erythrocyte in the spleen, is thought to be responsible for the microcirculatory obstruction important to the pathogenesis of severe disease. Biologically active molecules released from CD4[+] T cells after an antigen-specific interaction also probably contribute to naturally acquired immunity. Furthermore, pathogenesis of the clinical disease [66–68] may be mediated by these same host-derived biologically active molecules, or by toxins released from the infected erythrocytes [68–70], and neutralization of these toxins via antibodies may contribute to naturally acquired immunity.

Finally, antibody responses against sporozoites as well as T-cell responses against parasite proteins expressed within infected hepatocytes also probably contribute to naturally acquired disease modulating immunity. By reducing the number of *Plasmodium* spp. parasites maturing within the host hepatocyte, these pre-erythrocytic stage protective immune responses would be expected to reduce the initial blood-stage parasite burden and consequently the magnitude of the subsequent asexual stage amplification. In both hospitalized populations and semi-immune populations, most investigators have demonstrated a direct correlation between *P. falciparum* parasite density and morbidity and mortality associated with *P. falciparum* infection [71–75].

C. Identify the Antigenic Targets of Protective Immune Responses

The parasites causing malaria are more complex than the viruses and bacteria that heretofore have been controlled by vaccination, this complexity being reflected in their genetic make-up and their multistage life cycle. When *P. falciparum* sporozoites are inoculated into humans by *Anopheles* mosquitoes, they circulate extracellularly in the bloodstream for less than 30 min before entering the liver. Within the hepatocyte, a uninucleate sporozoite develops into a schizont with an estimated 10,000–40,000 uninucleate merozoites. These merozoites rupture from the hepatocyte and each can invade an erythrocyte, initiating the cycle of intraerythrocytic-stage development, rupture, and reinvasion that leads to a 10- to 20-fold increase in the number of parasites in the bloodstream every 48 hr. The asexual erythrocytic stage parasites are responsible for the clinical manifestations and pathology of malaria. Sexual erythrocytic stage parasites

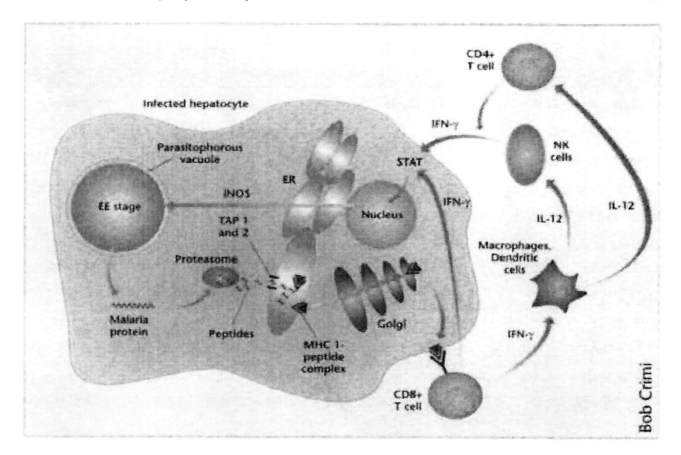

Figure 3 Proposed mechanism of protective immunity directed against the *Plasmodium*-infected hepatocyte. Protective immunity directed against pre-erythrocytic stage (EE stage) malaria is primarily mediated by antigen-specific CD8[+] T cells which recognize parasite-derived peptides presented in association with class 1 MHC molecules on the surface of infected hepatocytes. Short peptides are derived from the cytoplasmic malaria protein by the proteolytic action of proteosomes. The peptides are imported into the endoplasmic reticulum (ER) via the transporters associated with antigen processing, TAP1 and TAP2. In the ER, the peptides associated with the MHC class 1 molecule, and the peptide/MHC complex pass through the Golgi apparatus to the cell surface where they can be recognized by the T-cell receptor on the surface of CD8[+] T cells. IFN-γ is produced as a direct consequence of the CD8[+] T-cell activation, and subsequent production of IFN-γ may be upregulated by a positive feedback loop involving IL-12 (produced by dendritic cells, macrophages, or other cells), NK cells and/or CD4[+] T cells, depending on the host. IFN-γ, via signal transducers associated with transcription (STAT), activates nitric oxide synthase (iNOS) and induces the L-arginine-dependent NO pathway to eliminate the infected hepatocyte or the intrahepatic schizonts. (From Hoffman SL, Doolan DL. Malaria vaccines-targeting infected hepatocytes. Nat Med 2000;6:1218–1219.)

(gametocytes) are ingested by mosquitoes and develop over a period of 14–21 days to sporozoites.

Elucidation of the genomic sequence of the *P. falciparum* parasite [31] and its proteome [76] reveals that *P. falciparum* has approximately 5400 genes [31]. In general, proteins expressed at each of the stages in the parasite life cycle are antigenically distinct. Thus, if a vaccine elicits protective antisporozoite antibodies, those antibodies will often fail to recognize asexual erythrocytic stage parasites. Furthermore, for many of the genes/proteins characterized to date, allelic or antigenic variation has been demonstrated, and a single individual can be infected simultaneously with at least eight different strains [77] that may vary at critical T- and B-cell epitopes. This allelic heterogeneity is expanded by extensive antigenic variation present within a single isolate. PfEMP1 is

encoded by 59 different genes in the sequenced 3D7 isolate of *P. falciparum*, each with some variation in its sequence [31]. The parasite likely expresses only one at a time, each new variant escaping from antibodies induced by the previous variant and therefore capable of generating a new wave of parasitemia.

In summary, the large number of parasite proteins, stage-specific expression of proteins, the presence of multiple antigenically distinct strains in nature, and within-strain antigenic variation are critical to the parasite's survival; these factors are also unfavorable for the host and greatly complicate the challenge for vaccine developers. Nonetheless, the malaria genome project [31] and the single nucleotide polymorphism (SNP) projects currently nearing completion may provide knowledge of all potential targets and their variability at the epitope level, thereby laying the foundation for duplicating whole-organism immunity with subunit vaccines.

D. Select the Antigenic Target(s)

Antigens meeting the following criteria are likely to be good candidates for inclusion in a vaccine.

1. Accessibility to the immune system due to expression on the surface of free parasites or on the surface of infected host cells, with characteristics thought to be critical for induction of protective immunity (e.g., T-cell epitopes for vaccines to induce cellular immunity, secondary structures, and transmembrane domains for antibody vaccines). There is no algorithm that can be used to identify the targets of protective antibody or T-cell responses from genomic sequence data. In the case of antibody responses, one approach has been to focus on predicted surface or secreted molecules presumably accessible to antibody. In the case of T-cell responses, the subcellular location and function of the target protein are important as well as the presence of appropriate MHC binding epitopes in the sequence. Therefore, in order to select appropriate vaccine target candidates, one approach is to identify stage-specific expression of proteins encoded by all open reading frames (ORFs) from the genomic sequence and to determine subcellular localization of the proteins at least to the level of distinguishing between cytoplasmic, surface, and secreted organellar proteins.

2. Conserved antigenic structure among diverse strains (reduced chance of evolutionary "escape").

3. Mediation of critical biological functions. The assumption is that as long as the role played by a target antigen in the functioning of a critical molecular pathway, such as host cell invasion [78], depends on the molecular structure of the target antigen, and as long as that structure constrains the variability permissible in the peptide sequence (in the case of T-cell responses) or the epitope specificity (in the case of antibodies) of the target antigen, the parasite will be evolutionarily restricted. In other words, mutations that allow escape from the immune response via alterations in amino acid sequence would also necessarily negate biological function, selecting against such escape mutants. Antigens derived from "low complexity regions," such as the tandem repeats present in many parasite molecules, might be poor choices in that these rapidly evolving nonglobular domains are thought to be nonessential for protein function [79]. There must be cognizance that critical biological functions may possess redundant pathways (e.g., nine distinct receptors on endothelial surfaces and four on uninfected erythrocytes mediate binding of *Pf*-parasitized erythrocytes [80]), and that each pathway must be simultaneously blocked to achieve the desired vaccine effect.

4. Elicitation of protective responses in animal models. It is a reasonable assumption that the *P. falciparum* orthologs of murine or simian malarial antigens shown to be protective in animal models will be good candidates for a human vaccine.

5. Antigens containing promiscuous epitopes recognized by superfamilies of HLA alleles. Such antigens provide broader population coverage for eliciting genetically restricted T-cell responses [81].

6. Compatibility with other antigens in the mixture. This question—compatibility of antigens combined into a cocktail—is potentially a major issue in vaccine design (see E(6) below).

E. Determine the Number of Antigenic Components to Include in a Vaccine

Neither of the two human models described above, the irradiated sporozoite vaccine nor natural exposure to malaria, elicit immune responses of great magnitude, suggesting that immune responses against many parasite proteins are responsible for protection. Modest immune response against multiple parasite proteins may be additive or synergistic. Preliminary data (Doolan et al., submitted) support this contention. It is likely that a multiantigen vaccine will be required to produce comparable protective immunity.

The most advanced candidate malaria vaccine, RTS,S, consists of a recombinant fusion protein of a portion of the *P. falciparum* circumsporozoite protein (CSP) with the surface protein of hepatitis B. This vaccine consistently protects 40–50% of volunteers against experimental challenge for a period of at least 2–3 weeks after last immunization [19,20] and protected 70% of adult, lifelong residents of endemic areas from parasitemia for a period of up to 2 months [21]. If the magnitude and duration of protection could be increased, the simplicity of a single protein vaccine would make this any extremely attractive vaccine. However, there are significant potential limitations associated with a univalent vaccine.

1. Improved efficacy: Combining antigens, each with a partially protective effect, should synergize to improve overall vaccine efficacy [82], provided that they do not interfere with each other. However, few systematic experiments have been conducted to determine whether more antigens are better than a few. In the *P. yoelii*-rodent model, combining two antigens given as DNA vaccines (PyCSP and PyHep17) [82] and combining two antigens (PyCSP and PySSP2) given as recombinant tumor cells conferred additive protection [83]. In the *P. knowlesi*-rhesus model, protection has been demonstrated by immunization with four antigens (two pre-erythrocytic and two erythrocytic) in heterologous DNA prime/virus boost vaccination regimens [84,85], but the protection of the tetravalent vaccine has not been dissected to determine the relative role of the individual components. It will not be easy to determine in humans if adding antigens improves protection.

2. Genetic restriction of the host immune response: Cell-mediated immune responses directed against T-cell epitopes are genetically restricted; the genetic background (MHC haplotype) of the vaccine recipient determines which epitopes can bind to MHC molecules, interact with the T-cell receptor, and be recognized by vaccine-induced T cells. Immune responses directed against a single epitope will generally be insufficient to protect hosts with different MHC types, and sufficient numbers of T-cell epitopes derived from one or more antigens and recognized in the context of multiple

genetic restrictions must be included in a vaccine to protect individuals of all genetic backgrounds. Using DNA vaccines, it has been shown that epitopes from multiple antigens are required to elicit a high degree of protective immunity against *P. yoelii* parasite challenge in genetically distinct inbred mice [82]. Multivalent vaccines can circumvent the problem of genetic restriction by increasing the likelihood of "offering something for everyone" [86,87].

3. Parasite heterogeneity: Many *P. falciparum* genes exhibit antigenic heterogeneity; a malaria vaccine may require several forms of these proteins to protect against all *P. falciparum* strains. This may stem from allelic heterogeneity at a single locus (e.g., there are two major antigenic families of the leading blood-stage antigen merozoite surface protein-1, MSP1 [88]), or from the presence of multiple copies of a single gene. The best example of the latter is the *var* (variable) gene family [63], which encodes PfEMP1, a molecule expressed on the surface of infected erythrocytes that mediates their adhesion to endothelial cells. Fifty-nine [31] members of this family are present in the 3D7 *P. falciparum* genome, each encoding an antigenically variant molecule. Variant forms are expressed sequentially on the surface of infected erythrocytes, with each newly expressed variant allowing escape from immune responses generated against the previously expressed variant, resulting in recurring waves of parasitemia. For immune responses PfEMP1 is a natural target, but a vaccine would have to include all members of the family or else employ conserved domains of the molecule. With regard to the pre-erythrocytic stage, it has been demonstrated that CSP polymorphism primarily maps to identified $CD8^+$ and $CD4^+$ T-cell epitopes [89], and cytotoxic T-lymphocyte (CTL) responses to some variants do not cross-react [90–92], suggesting that polymorphism has been evolutionarily selected to allow parasite evasion of host immunity [93]. In African children with malaria, the CTL epitope variants present may be influenced by the presence of an HLA type that restricts the immune response to the epitope [86]. In the same individuals, these variants can lead to the inhibition or impairment of CTL responses by altered peptide ligand antagonism. Variant epitopes may narrow the CTL repertoire by interfering with T-cell priming [92].

4. Stage-specific antigen expression: Stage-specific expression of many malaria parasite antigens indicates that to protect against both pre-erythrocytic and erythrocytic stages of the parasite, vaccines must include antigens which are expressed at each of these stages. Moreover, as also discussed above, it is likely that even within one stage of the life cycle, many antigens will be needed to confer protection.

5. Evolution of resistance: If the protection afforded by each antigen in a vaccine is independent of that afforded by others, a multivalent vaccine provides insurance against the evolution of resistance by the parasite. The likelihood that spontaneous mutations would simultaneously circumvent *multiple* immune responses is low (the product of the individual likelihoods if protective effects are truly independent).

6. Downsides to multiantigen formulations include interference among antigens, as well as issues associated with dose reduction for each component relative to single-antigen formulations. Current formulations of DNA vaccines

are limited to approximately 4 mg/mL of solution, resulting in a several fold dose reduction for each component of a multiplasmid cocktail as compared with the concentration achievable if each component were formulated separately. Furthermore, interference and dose reduction significantly reduce immunogenicity of vaccine components, potentially negating the advantages of a multicomponent vaccine. To avoid this, careful selection of antigens is needed. This can be accomplished by "subtraction experiments," in which a full cocktail is tested for immunogenicity against the same cocktail minus one of its components. If all combinations are assessed, it may be possible to identify suppressive antigens that can be removed, partially or completely restoring the immunogenicity of the remaining antigens (Sedegah, submitted). However, because these mixing studies can be only performed in mice or other small animal models (requirement for large numbers) and immunogenicity but not protection can be assessed (because of the unnatural host–parasite combination), it is uncertain as to whether these studies actually predict compatible antigen mixtures for humans.

F. Select Vaccine Delivery Systems that Induce Required Immune Response(s) Against Identified Target(s)

A major challenge is how to induce the appropriate responses against each antigen included in a vaccine. A range of subunit vaccines based on whole gene/protein (all epitopes) and partial gene/protein (defined epitopes; multiple epitopes) have been considered, including recombinant proteins, linear synthetic peptides, multiple antigen peptides, recombinant or attenuated viruses/bacteria, plasmid DNA, and replicons. Exposed parasite targets, such as proteins on the surface of extracellular sporozoites, merozoites, gametes, and ookinetes, and on the surface of infected erythrocytes are amenable to neutralization by antibodies, as demonstrated by antibody-mediated in vitro assays, and by the effectiveness of IgG infusions in humans for resolving the symptoms of blood-stage infection and for reducing parasitemia. Destruction of intracellular parasites such as those in infected hepatocytes and infected erythrocytes relies primarily on cell-mediated responses. Certain adjuvants may direct the response appropriately, but the challenge of how to direct immune responses toward antibody production for some antigens and T-cell responses for others, when the antigens are mixed together in a cocktail, has not been solved. Approaches include splitting the vaccine into liver-stage and blood-stage formulas that are injected into separate sites, or trying to induce both cellular and antibody responses to all antigens in the cocktail. Other considerations include route of immunization, dose, and kinetics of response. The choice and validity of animal models in preclinical studies (mice, rhesus monkeys, *Aotus* monkeys, cynomolgi monkeys, etc.) also warrant attention. A major obstacle to adopting the "right kind" of immune response is that as yet, there is no established specific immunological correlate of immunity. Finally, for a vaccine to be optimally effective it must elicit protective immune responses that are sustained over time, either due to vaccine administration or boosting by exposure to parasites. Progress has been made, but no delivery system has been shown to be optimal or adequate for delivering the multiple antigens likely required to induce immune responses comparable to those elicited by natural exposure to parasites or by the irradiated sporozoite vaccine.

VI. WHOLE, ATTENUATED PARASITE VACCINE DEVELOPMENT

The only proof thus far of significant, sustained protection against malaria in humans comes from immunization of humans with the whole parasite, irradiated sporozoite vaccine, and naturally acquired immunity. Nonetheless, there has been little to no effort expended on developing an attenuated parasite vaccine during the past 20 years. It was deemed impractical (or impossible) to develop such a vaccine, and with the advent of monoclonal antibodies and molecular biology, it was generally considered not necessary. However, given the difficulty in producing effective subunit vaccines, and the general consensus in the field of how long it will take to launch such vaccines [94], we are now focusing efforts on developing an attenuated (nonreplicating, metabolically active) *P. falciparum* sporozoite vaccine that is expected to completely prevent all manifestations of infections in nonimmune travelers and military personnel, and reduce severe morbidity and mortality in infants and children in Africa.

VII. THE CHALLENGE OF DESIGNING AND EXECUTING FIELD TRIALS OF MALARIA VACCINES

It will be critical to consider which outcome variables to measure in field trials of malaria vaccines, and which population groups to study. For vaccines designed to prevent asexual erythrocytic stage infections and thereby prevent all clinical manifestations of malaria, clinical trials are quite straightforward to design. However, for vaccines not expected to prevent infection in all recipients, but expected to prevent severe disease and mortality, trials will be more difficult and much larger. There is a potential problem that a vaccine may be discarded as a result of initial studies because the proper outcome variables were not measured. It will be difficult to use severe disease and death as the primary outcome variables in initial studies, because of the very large sample sizes required. It is important to identify groups at highest risk so that sample sizes can be reduced. Current investigations seek to identify surrogates of severe disease and death: parasitological, hematological, biochemical, or clinical manifestations that are predictive of severe outcome.

Several other areas of field research could provide data to help vaccine development. The most important area is the identification of target groups for vaccines in different areas (see above) and the exclusion of groups, like those with sickle-cell trait, who are at decreased risk and do not need to be immunized. It is important to determine if there are measurable outcome variables that have a high predictive value for severe disease- and malaria-associated mortality. The impact of bed-nets and other interventions on epidemiology and the age-specific attributable reduction in mortality must be assessed. More data are needed on the effects of radical cure (elimination of all parasites from the body) on host protective and clinical immunity so as to design trials better. Better assays are needed for predicting protective immunity, involving more detailed characterization of the proteins and epitopes on these proteins involved in protective immunity.

VIII. FUTURE PROSPECTS REGARDING MALARIA VACCINE DEVELOPMENT

The human models (attenuated sporozoite and naturally acquired immunity) indicate that the development of a malaria vaccine is feasible. An intense effort at making the attenuated sporozoite vaccine practical may prove to be the most direct route to a licensed, deployed malaria vaccine, but several years of studies will be required to prove the principle that this approach is feasible. However, genomics, proteomics, molecular biology, molecular immunology, vaccinology, population genetics, population biology, and quantitative epidemiology have created great expectations for the development, licensing, and deployment of effective malaria vaccines. It will be a formidable task to determine which antigens/epitopes from specific stages of the life cycle are required for sustainable protection, how to measure immune responses that predict protection, which vaccine delivery systems are optimal, who and when in life to immunize, and how to establish surveillance systems able to assess the true impact of a malaria vaccine on public health. At a recent scientific meeting [94], scientists, many of whom have devoted their careers to malaria vaccine development, were polled as to when they thought a vaccine might be launched. Responses ranged from 7 to 25 years. We believe that the next 7–25 years will bear witness to the development of effective malaria vaccines, and that these will be used to control the effects of the disease worldwide and, when combined with other interventions, will be able to eradicate malaria from many areas.

The importance, difficulty, and cost of this task must not be underestimated. We are still far from controlling the enormous suffering and loss of life caused by malaria. Everyday, 2500–8000 children die of malaria, and no research finding during the past 25 years in molecular biology, cell biology, genomics, immunology, vaccinology, or protein chemistry has resulted in the saving of a single life from malaria. We believe that the development of malaria vaccines will be crucial to the successful, widespread control of malaria.

ACKNOWLEDGMENT

This work was supported in part by funds from the Naval Medical Research Center work units 61102A.S13.F.A0009, 62787A.870.F.A0010, and 60000.000.000.A0062. The assertions here are private ones by the authors and are not to be construed as official or to reflect the views of the U.S. Navy or the Naval service.

REFERENCES

1. Breman JG. Ears of the hippopotamus: manifestations, determinants, and estimates of the malaria burden. Am J Trop Med Hyg 2001; 64:1–11.
2. Gallup JL, et al. The economic burden of malaria. Am J Trop Med Hyg 2001; 64:85–96.
3. World Tourism Organization. International tourist arrivals by (sub)region. June 2002; http://www.world-tourism.org/market_research/facts&figures/latest_data/tita01_07-02.pdf.
4. Jelinek T, et al. Imported *Falciparum malaria* in Europe: sentinel surveillance data from the European network on surveillance of imported infectious diseases. Clin Infect Dis 2002; 34:572–576.
5. Martens P, et al. Malaria on the move: human population movement and malaria transmission. Emerg Infect Dis 2000; 6:103–109.
6. Mendis K, et al. The neglected burden of *Plasmodium vivax* malaria. Am J Trop Med Hyg 2001; 64:97–106.
7. Snow RW, et al. Relation between severe malaria morbidity in children and level of *Plasmodium falciparum* transmission in Africa. Lancet 1997; 349:1650–1654.
8. Gandon S, et al. Imperfect vaccines and the evolution of pathogen virulence. Nature 2001; 414:751–756.
9. Hoffman SL, et al. Protection of humans against malaria by immunization with radiation-attenuated *Plasmodium falciparum* sporozoites. J Infect Dis 2002; 185:1155–1164.
10. Jeffery GM. Epidemiological significance of repeated infections with homologous and heterologous strains and species of *Plasmodium*. Bull WHO 1966; 35:873–882.
11. Baird JK. Host age as a determinant of naturally acquired immunity to *Plasmodium falciparum*. Parasitol Today 1995; 11:105–111.
12. Nussenzweig RS, et al. Protective immunity produced by the injection of X-irradiated sporozoites of *Plasmodium berghei*. Nature 1967; 216:160–162.
13. Clyde DF, et al. Specificity of protection of man immunized against sporozoite-induced falciparum malaria. Am J Med Sci 1973; 266:398–401.
14. Clyde DF, et al. Immunization of man against sporozoite-induced falciparum malaria. Am J Med Sci 1973; 266:169–177.
15. Rieckmann KH, et al. Sporozoite induced immunity in man against an Ethiopian strain of *Plasmodium falciparum*. Trans R Soc Trop Med Hyg 1974; 68:258–259.
16. Baird JK. Age-dependent characteristics of protection v. susceptibility to *Plasmodium falciparum*. Ann Trop Med Parasitol 1998; 92:367–390.
17. Nardin E, et al. Pre-erythrocytic malaria vaccine: mechanisms of protective immunity and human vaccine trials. Parassitologia 1999; 41:397–402.
18. Lalvani A, et al. Potent induction of focused Th1-type cellular and humoral immune responses by RTS,S/SBAS2, a recombinant *Plasmodium falciparum malaria* vaccine. J Infect Dis 1999; 180:1656–1664.
19. Stoute JA, et al. A preliminary evaluation of a recombinant circumsporozoite protein vaccine against *Plasmodium falciparum* malaria. N Engl J Med 1997; 336:86–91.
20. Stoute JA, et al. Long-term efficacy and immune responses following immunization with the RTS,S malaria vaccine. J Infect Dis 1998; 178:1139–1144.
21. Bojang KA, et al. Efficacy of RTS,S/AS02 malaria vaccine against *Plasmodium falciparum* infection in semi-immune adult men in The Gambia: a randomised trial. Lancet 2001; 358:1927–1934.
22. Hoffman SL, et al. Attacking the infected hepatocyte. In: Hoffman SL, ed. Malaria Vaccine Development: A Multi-Immune Response Approach. Washington, DC: ASM Press, 1996:35–75.
23. Daubersies P, et al. Protection against *Plasmodium falciparum malaria* in chimpanzees by immunization with the conserved pre-erythrocytic liver-stage antigen 3. Nat Med 2000; 6:1258–1263.
24. Doolan DL, et al. DNA-based vaccines against malaria: status and promise of the Multi-Stage Malaria DNA Vaccine Operation. Int J Parasitol 2001; 31:753–762.
25. Kumar S, et al. A multilateral effort to develop DNA vaccines against *Falciparum malaria*. Trends Parasitol 2002; 18:129–135.
26. Le TP, et al. Safety, tolerability and humoral immune responses after intramuscular administration of a malaria DNA vaccine to healthy adult volunteers. Vaccine 2000; 18:1893–1901.
27. Epstein JE, et al. Safety, tolerability, and lack of antibody responses after administration of a PfCSP DNA malaria vaccine via needle or needle-free jet injection, and comparison of intramuscular and combination intramuscular/intradermal routes. Hum Gene Ther 2002; 13:1551–1560.
28. Wang R, et al. Induction of CD4(+) T cell-dependent CD8(+) type 1 responses in humans by a malaria DNA vaccine. Proc Natl Acad Sci USA 2001; 98:10817–10822.
29. Wang R, et al. Induction of antigen-specific cytotoxic T lymphocytes in humans by a malaria DNA vaccine. Science 1998; 282:476–480.
30. Schneider J, et al. Induction of CD8$^+$ T cells using heterologous prime-boost immunisation strategies. Immunol Rev 1999; 170:29–38.
31. Gardner MJ, et al. Genome sequence of the human malaria parasite *Plasmodium falciparum*. Nature 2002; 419:498–511.
32. Carlton JM, et al. Genome sequence and comparative analysis of the model rodent malaria parasite *Plasmodium yoelii yoelii*. Nature 2002; 419:512–519.
33. Wootton JC, et al. Genetic diversity and chloroquine selective sweeps in *Plasmodium falciparum*. Nature 2002; 418:320–323.
34. Whitby M. Drug resistant *Plasmodium vivax* malaria. J Antimicrob Chemother 1997; 40:749–752.
35. Murphy GS, et al. Vivax malaria resistant to treatment and prophylaxis with chloroquine. Lancet 1993; 341:96–100.
36. Maguire JD, et al. Chloroquine-resistant *Plasmodium malariae* in south Sumatra, Indonesia. Lancet 2002; 360:58–60.
37. Mu J, et al. Chromosome-wide SNPs reveal an ancient origin for *Plasmodium falciparum*. Nature 2002; 418:323–326.
38. Hoffman SL, et al. Sporozoite vaccine induces genetically restricted T cell elimination of malaria from hepatocytes. Science 1989; 244:1078–1081.
39. Doolan DL, et al. IL-12 and NK cells are required for antigen-specific adaptive immunity against malaria initiated by CD8$^+$ T cells in the *Plasmodium yoelii* model. J Immunol 1999; 163:884–892.
40. Doolan DL, et al. The complexity of protective immunity against liver-stage malaria. J Immunol 2000; 165:1453–1462.
41. Malik A, et al. Human cytotoxic T lymphocytes against the *Plasmodium falciparum* circumsporozoite protein. Proc Natl Acad Sci USA 1991; 88:3300–3304.
42. Wizel B, et al. HLA-A2-restricted cytotoxic T lymphocyte responses to multiple *Plasmodium falciparum* sporozoite surface protein 2 epitopes in sporozoite-immunized volunteers. J Immunol 1995; 155:766–775.
43. Wizel B, et al. Irradiated sporozoite vaccine induces HLA-B8-restricted cytotoxic T lymphocyte responses against two overlapping epitopes of the *Plasmodium falciparum* surface sporozoite protein 2. J Exp Med 1995; 182:1435–1445.
44. Sedegah M, et al. Naturally acquired CD8$^+$ cytotoxic T

lymphocytes against the *Plasmodium falciparum* circumsporozoite protein. J Immunol 1992; 149:966–971.

45. Aidoo M, et al. Identification of conserved antigenic components for a cytotoxic T lymphocyte-inducing vaccine against malaria. Lancet 1995; 345:1003–1007.

46. Lalvani A, et al. Cytotoxic T lymphocytes to *Plasmodium falciparum* epitopes in an area of intense and perennial transmission in Tanzania. Eur J Immunol 1996; 26:773–779.

47. Doolan DL, et al. Degenerate cytotoxic T cell epitopes from *P. falciparum* restricted by HLA-A and HLA-B supertypes alleles. Immunity 1997; 7:97–112.

48. Flanagan KL, et al. Unique T cell effector functions elicited by *Plasmodium falciparum* epitopes in malaria-exposed Africans tested by three T cell assays. J Immunol 2001; 167:4729–4737.

49. Schofield L, et al. Gamma-interferon, CD8$^+$ T cells and antibodies required for immunity to malaria sporozoites. Nature 1987; 330:664–666.

50. Weiss WR, et al. CD8$^+$ T cells (cytotoxic/suppressors) are required for protection in mice immunized with malaria sporozoites. Proc Natl Acad Sci USA 1988; 85:573–576.

51. Romero P, et al. Cloned cytotoxic T cells recognize an epitope in the circumsporozoite protein and protect against malaria. Nature 1989; 341:323–325.

52. Weiss WR, et al. A T cell clone directed at the circumsporozoite protein which protects mice against both *Plasmodium yoelii* and *Plasmodium berghei*. J Immunol 1992; 149:2103–2109.

53. Khusmith S, et al. Complete protection against *Plasmodium yoelii* by adoptive transfer of a CD8$^+$ cytotoxic T cell clone recognizing sporozoite surface protein 2. Infect Immun 1994; 62:2979–2983.

54. Weiss WR, et al. Cytotoxic T cells recognize a peptide from the circumsporozoite protein on malaria-infected hepatocytes. J Exp Med 1990; 171:763–773.

55. Renia L, et al. In vitro activity of CD4$^+$ and CD8$^+$ T lymphocytes from mice immunized with a synthetic malaria peptide. Proc Natl Acad Sci USA 1991; 88:7963–7967.

56. Renia L, et al. Effector functions of circumsporozoite peptide-primed CD4$^+$ T cell clones against *Plasmodium yoelii* liver stages. J Immunol 1993; 150:1471–1478.

57. Potocnjak P, et al. Monovalent fragments (Fab) of monoclonal antibodies to a sporozoite surface antigen (Pb44) protect mice against malaria infection. J Exp Med 1980; 151:1504–1513.

58. Sinnis P, et al. Preventing sporozoite invasion of hepatocytes. In: Hoffman SL, ed. Malaria Vaccine Development: A Multi-Immune Response Approach. Washington, DC: ASM Press, 1996:15–33.

59. Cohen S, et al. Gamma-globulin and acquired immunity to human malaria. Nature 1961; 192:733–737.

60. Edozien JC, et al. Adult and cord-blood gamma-globulin and immunity to malaria in Nigerians. Lancet 1962; ii:951–955.

61. McGregor A, et al. Treatment of East African *P. Falciparum* malaria with West African human gamma-globulin. Trans R Soc Trop Med Hyg 1963; 57-3:170–175.

62. Sabchareon A, et al. Parasitologic and clinical human response to immunoglobulin administration in falciparum malaria. Am J Trop Med Hyg 1991; 45:297–308.

63. Duffy PE, et al. Variant proteins on the surface of malaria-infected erythrocytes-developing vaccines. Trends Parasitol 2001; 17:354–356.

64. Sim BK, et al. Induction of biologically active antibodies in mice, rabbits, and monkeys by *Plasmodium falciparum* EBA-175 region II DNA vaccine. Mol Med 2001; 7:247–254.

65. Bouharoun Tayoun H, et al. Mechanisms underlying the monocyte-mediated antibody-dependent killing of *Plasmodium falciparum* asexual blood stages. J Exp Med 1995; 182:409–418.

66. Miller LH, et al. Malaria pathogenesis. Science 1994; 264:1878–1883.

67. Marsh K, et al. The pathogenesis of severe malaria in African children. Ann Trop Med Parasitol 1996; 90:395–402.

68. Clark IA, et al. Pathogenesis of malaria. Parasitol Today 2000; 16:451–454.

69. Playfair JHL. An antitoxic vaccine for malaria? In: Hoffman SL, ed. Malaria Vaccine Development: A Multi-Immune Response Approach. Washington, DC: ASM Press, 1996:167–180.

70. Schofield L, et al. Synthetic GPI as a candidate anti-toxic vaccine in a model of malaria. Nature 2002; 418:785–789.

71. Mbogo CN, et al. Relationships between *Plasmodium falciparum* transmission by vector populations and the incidence of severe disease at nine sites on the Kenyan coast. Am J Trop Med Hyg 1995; 52:201–206.

72. McElroy PD, et al. Predicting outcome in malaria: correlation between rate of exposure to infected mosquitoes and level of *Plasmodium falciparum* parasitemia. Am J Trop Med Hyg 1994; 51:523–532.

73. Beadle C, et al. Impact of transmission intensity and age on *Plasmodium falciparum* density and associated fever: Implications for malaria vaccine design. J Infect Dis 1995; 172:1047–1054.

74. McElroy PD, et al. Dose- and time-dependent relations between infective *Anopheles* inoculation and outcomes of *Plasmodium falciparum* parasitemia among children in western Kenya. Am J Epidemiol 1997; 145:945–956.

75. Vounatsou P, et al. Apparent tolerance of *Plasmodium falciparum* in infants in a highly endemic area. Parasitology 2000; 120:1–9.

76. Florens L, et al. A proteomic view of the *Plasmodium falciparum* life cycle. Nature 2002; 419:520–526.

77. Felger I, et al. Genotypes of merozoite surface protein 2 of *Plasmodium falciparum* in Tanzania. Trans R Soc Trop Med Hyg 1999; 93:3–9.

78. Berzins K. Merozoite antigens involved in invasion. Chem Immunol 2002; 80:125–143.

79. Pizzi E, et al. Low-complexity regions in *Plasmodium falciparum* proteins. Genome Res 2001; 11:218–229.

80. Craig A, et al. Molecules on the surface of the *Plasmodium falciparum* infected erythrocyte and their role in malaria pathogenesis and immune evasion. Mol Biochem Parasitol 2001; 115:129–143.

81. Sette A, et al. Nine major HLA class I supertypes account for the vast preponderance of HLA-A and -B polymorphism. Immunogenetics 1999; 50:201–212.

82. Doolan DL, et al. Circumventing genetic restriction of protection against malaria with multi-gene DNA immunization: CD8$^+$ T cell, interferon-gamma, and nitric oxide dependent immunity. J Exp Med 1996; 183:1739–1746.

83. Khusmith S, et al. Protection against malaria by vaccination with sporozoite surface protein 2 plus CS protein. Science 1991; 252:715–718.

84. Rogers WO, et al. Multistage multiantigen heterologous prime boost vaccine for *Plasmodium knowlesi* malaria provides partial protection in rhesus macaques. Infect Immun 2001; 69:5565–5572.

85. Rogers WO, et al. Protection of rhesus macaques against lethal *Plasmodium knowlesi* malaria by a heterologous DNA priming and poxvirus boosting immunization regimen. Infect Immun 2002; 70:4329–4335.

86. Gilbert SC, et al. Association of malaria parasite population structure, HLA, and immunological antagonism. Science 1998; 279:1173–1177.

87. Sette A, et al. Epitope identification and vaccine design for cancer immunotherapy. Curr Opin Invest Drugs 2002; 3:132–139.

88. Miller LH, et al. Analysis of sequence diversity in the *Plasmodium falciparum* merozoite surface protein-1 (MSP-1). Mol Biochem Parasitol 1993; 59:1–14.

89. Doolan DL, et al. Cytotoxic T lymphocyte (CTL) low-responsiveness to the *Plasmodium falciparum* circumsporozoite protein in naturally-exposed endemic populations: analysis of human CTL response to most known variants. Int Immunol 1993; 5:37–46.

90. Hill AVS, et al. Molecular analysis of the association of HLA-B53 and resistance to severe malaria. Nature 1992; 360:434–439.

91. Udhayakumar V, et al. Antigenic diversity in the circumsporozoite protein of *Plasmodium falciparum* abrogates cytotoxic T-cell recognition. Infect Immun 1994; 62:1410–1413.

92. Plebanski M, et al. Altered peptide ligands narrow the repertoire of cellular immune responses by interfering with T-cell priming. Nat Med 1999; 5:565–571.

93. Hughes AL, et al. Extensive polymorphism and ancient origin of *Plasmodium falciparum*. Trends Parasitol 2002; 18:348–351.

94. Long CA, et al. Parasitology. Malaria—from infants to genomics to vaccines. Science 2002; 297:345–347.

72

Plasmodium falciparum Asexual Blood Stage Vaccine Candidates: Current Status

Danielle I. Stanisic, Laura B. Martin*, and Michael F. Good
The Queensland Institute of Medical Research, Brisbane, Queensland, Australia

Robin F. Anders
LaTrobe University and the Australian Co-operative Centre for Vaccine Technology, Bundoora, Victoria, Australia

I. INTRODUCTION AND LIFE CYCLE OF *PLASMODIUM*

Humans are the definitive host of four plasmodial species that cause malaria: *Plasmodium falciparum, P. vivax, P. malariae,* and *P. ovale.* The four species exhibit differences in their periodicity of paroxysms (chills, fever) because of differences in replication time in the red blood cell, preferences for different aged erythrocytes, and different geographical distributions. *P. falciparum* infection is the most dangerous as it can cause life-endangering complications such as cerebral malaria and severe anemia.

Infection begins when a female mosquito of the genus *Anopheles* takes a blood meal from a host (e.g., a human). When a mosquito feeds, she injects an anticoagulant from her salivary glands into the subcutaneous tissue and less frequently the blood stream; this is normally accompanied by injection of the sporozoite stage of the parasite if the mosquito is infected. The sporozoites then invade the liver and form the nonpathogenic pre- or exo-erythrocytic schizont stage. During this time (5–15 days), the parasite grows and multiplies, resulting in the lysis of the infected hepatocyte and the release of thousands of merozoites. One exoerythrocytic schizont may contain 10,000–30,000 merozoites [1a]. During the next stage of development, the merozoites target the red blood cells (RBC) for invasion, and once inside become an erythrocytic trophozoite, which ingests and digests hemoglobin and asexually multiplies to become an

erythrocytic schizont. Two to three days after entry into the RBC (depending on the species of *Plasmodium*), 6–24 new merozoites are released upon rupture of the cell and rapidly invade new blood cells. This asexual reproductive cycle is repeated several times. It is this repeated cycle of multiplication that causes the symptoms of malaria including the periodic fever initiated by the release of pyrogens when infected red blood cells burst.

The red blood cell stage is the phase of exponential growth of the parasite within the host. As the life cycle starts with so few parasites and the number of red cells is so large, it takes several days of parasite multiplication (the prepatent period) before parasites can be detected by microscopy. More sensitive detection methods (e.g., polymerase chain reaction, PCR) can detect parasites in the blood before they can be microscopically detected [1].

Some asexual parasites differentiate into gametocytes, the sexual form of the parasite, which mature to extracellular gametes in the midgut of another female mosquito. This is followed by fertilization of the gametes, producing a zygote, which becomes a motile ookinete that burrows into the midgut wall, encysts on the outer surface, and becomes an oocyst. Within the oocyst, the sporozoites develop and are shed into the insect's hemocele and migrate to the salivary glands.

All malaria parasites have a similar life cycle (Figure 1), with some exceptions. The prepatent period for malaria varies from species to species; it can be as short as 9 days, but typically 12 (*P. falciparum*) to 30 days (*P. malariae*) from the time of initial infection. *P. vivax* and *P. ovale* differ from *P. falciparum* in their ability to cause true relapses as the sporozoites are able to lay dormant in liver stages (such resting stages are known as hypnozoites), and become active

---

*Current affiliation: National Institutes of Health, Rockville, Maryland, U.S.A.

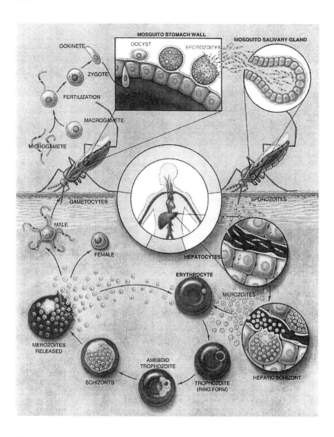

Figure 1 The life cycle of the malaria parasite. (From Ref. 141.)

at a later stage, releasing merozoites months after the initial infection. This is in comparison with *P. malariae*, which can remain dormant in the blood for years, without causing any sign of disease, but may suddenly cause clinical symptoms. This reappearance of parasite is known as a recrudescence.

Four species of parasites that can infect rodents, *P. yoelii*, *P. berghei*, *P. chabaudi*, and *P. vinckei*, are frequently used to model human disease. Although they are not exact replicas of the human situation, the rodent parasite models allow examination of the interactions between the hosts' immune system and the different stages of the parasite. They are used in concert with different rodent strains, with the combinations resulting in different disease patterns [2]. The rodent malaria parasite spends only 24 hr within each red blood cell. This may in part explain the higher parasite densities observed in the blood of rodents compared with those in humans [3].

II. VACCINE APPROACHES AND DESIGN

There have been numerous vaccine success stories with smallpox eradication and the virtual elimination of polio being the best examples. However, the development of a malaria vaccine is a major challenge. The parasite's complex biology contributes to this, with the parasite existing in different forms in different tissues and in the mosquito (Figure 1). Different stages of the parasite express different

antigens (stage-specific antigens) and many of these exhibit degrees of antigenic polymorphism. For each stage, different vaccine strategies must be employed. An alternative approach is the multicomponent vaccine, which involves either combining antigens from the various life cycle stages (multistage vaccine) or combining multiple antigens from a single life cycle stage (multivalent vaccines). Other hurdles to overcome include immunological nonresponsiveness to vaccine antigens (especially low molecular weight antigens), heterogeneity of the human immune response as determined by HLA type, the technological hurdles encountered in folding recombinant antigens, and the lack of potent adjuvants for use in humans.

Although the possibility of developing live-attenuated vaccines for malaria has been discussed, logistical problems have focused malaria vaccine development on the subunit approach. This review will discuss different strategies being taken to develop a blood stage malaria vaccine. However, it is critical to properly understand the nature of malaria immunity before considering vaccine strategies. Immune mechanisms are the least understood for the blood stage of malaria, responsible for all the symptoms and pathology, and present the greatest challenge.

Because the parasite density in blood is generally proportional to disease severity, a vaccine must limit parasite density. It may not be necessary to induce sterile immunity (complete eradication of parasites) but this may be possible and would be advantageous as it would prevent parasite transmission from infected humans to mosquitoes. However, it is worth considering the immune state of adults living in malaria endemic regions. They have nonsterile clinical immunity characterized by low-density parasitemia and absence of clinical symptoms. This type of immunity may ultimately be a more realistic and achievable goal.

III. THE ACQUIRED SPECIFIC IMMUNE RESPONSE AGAINST MALARIA

Specific immune responses induced by infections with *Plasmodium* spp. provide protection against the consequences of subsequent infections. Naturally acquired immunity to the malaria parasite requires years of exposure in an endemic region, presumably as this allows the development of antibodies to multiple parasite strains and continual boosting of existing immune mechanisms. Although highly effective immunity is slow to develop and not sterilizing, recent studies in Kenya have shown that some protection against severe disease is provided by a single *P. falciparum* infection [4]. Two separate types of antimalarial immunity can be distinguished: immunity that limits parasite development (antiparasite immunity); and immunity to disease-causing parasite "toxins" (antitoxic immunity) [5,6].

A. Antiparasite Immunity

1. Antibodies

Although parasite density is not a precise predictor of the clinical consequences of infection, the acquisition of immunity in children living in endemic areas is associated with a very significant reduction in mean densities of asexual blood-stage parasitemias. Thus the mean density of parasitemias in 5–9 year olds living in the Wosera region of Papua New Guinea is <20% of the mean density of 1–4 year olds in the same communities and the older group of children suffer little malaria morbidity [7]. Much information has accumulated about the nature of immune effector mechanisms that inhibit parasite development, either in vitro or in human and animal hosts, but there is no consensus concerning the nature or the specificity of the immune effector mechanisms responsible for limiting the development of asexual blood-stage parasites in semi-immune individuals living in endemic areas.

Antibodies clearly have a role in antiasexual blood-stage immunity in humans and the transfer of immunoglobulins from immune adults to infected children results in a significant decrease in the density of parasitemias in the recipients. Such antibodies may directly act, either by preventing merozoite invasion of host erythrocytes or by blocking cytoadherence of infected erythrocytes to vascular endothelium, and thereby increasing the likelihood of clearance by phagocytic cells in the spleen. Alternatively, antibodies may indirectly act as mediators of cellular effector mechanisms. Druilhe and colleagues have provided extensive evidence that a process of antibody-dependent cellular inhibition (ADCI), where antibodies to merozoite antigens activate monocytes to kill intra-erythrocytic parasites, is a major effector mechanism regulating the density of asexual blood-stage parasitemias [8,9]. Although studies with *P. falciparum* in vitro have shown that human antibodies can inhibit parasite development in the absence of effector cells the unusual bias towards cytophilic IgG isotypes in the human antibody response to a number of merozoite surface antigens is consistent with the operation of antibody-dependent cellular effectors [10]. Studies in animal models, particularly using rodent parasites and in-bred strains of mice, have provided much evidence that both antibody and non-antibody effector mechanisms limit the development of asexual blood-stage parasites.

2. Cell-Mediated Immunity

Cell-mediated immunity (CMI) generally refers to $CD4^+$ T cells acting in the absence of antibody to limit parasite growth. A number of studies elegantly showed that CMI can be effective in controlling parasite growth [11–13]. $CD4^+$ T cell lines and clones can limit or eradicate parasites following adoptive transfer [14–16].

$CD4^+$ T cells are thought to exert their antiparasite effect in the spleen following processing of parasites by antigen-presenting cells and ending with the death of parasites following phagocytosis and via inflammatory molecules such as oxygen and nitric oxide radicals [15,17,18]. Cell-mediated immunity is regulated by interleukin 12 (IL-12) and involves interferon-γ (IFN-γ) and tumor necrosis factor-α (TNF-α) [17–19]. Although most data has been generated in the mouse, it has recently been shown that humans can be immunized by exposure to ultralow doses of parasites and that in this situation immunity is apparently entirely mediated by CMI (involving IFN-γ and upregulation of nitric oxide synthase) and the complete lack of any detectable antibodies [20].

$\gamma\delta$ T cells (expressing $\gamma\delta$ receptors) may also play a role in immunity and may act independently of $CD4^+$ T cells and antibody [21,22]. Although protective CMI can be induced in both mice and humans, the role of CMI in natural immunity to malaria is much less clear. A number of studies have examined the impact of human immunodeficiency virus (HIV) on malaria severity and prevalence as a means to ascertain the role of naturally occurring CMI. The greatest impact of HIV is on pregnancy-associated malaria (PAM). The human immunodeficiency virus delays the development of immunity to PAM. The evidence that HIV affects CMI to malaria is less convincing. This has recently been summarized and discussed [23].

B. Antitoxic Immunity

Exposure to infection induces immunity to the toxic effects of asexual blood-stage parasitemias more rapidly than to the parasite itself so that after some exposure children in endemic areas will remain asymptomatic despite having parasitemias that would cause severe disease in malaria-naïve individuals. Tumor necrosis factor-α plays a central role in the pathogenesis of severe malaria [24–26] and there is considerable evidence that the glycosylphosphatidylinositol (GPI) anchor released from merozoite surface proteins, such as MSP1 and MSP2, induces the release of TNF-α from monocytes [27]. This GPI structure is conserved across more than 20 geographically distinct isolates of *P. falciparum* examined so far [28]. Monoclonal antibodies specific for malarial GPI can neutralize the production of TNF-α and nitric oxide in response to whole parasite extracts [29] and a synthetic vaccine based on the GPI of *P. falciparum* successfully immunized mice against *P. berghei* ANKA infection [6] and prevented cerebral malaria and respiratory distress syndrome. An antidisease vaccine such as the synthetic GPI vaccine trialed in mice, which induces immune responses that neutralize the TNF-α-inducing activity of these GPI moieties, could be highly effective at reducing the incidence of severe morbidity. However, a vaccine that does not limit parasite development will be difficult to evaluate and test in preclinical and clinical human vaccine trials.

IV. VACCINE CANDIDATES ON THE MEROZOITE

There are essentially three groups of antigens associated with the merozoite, and all have been identified as potential vaccine candidates (Figure 2). The first group is found on the merozoite surface, including merozoite surface proteins. To date, eight different *P. falciparum* MSPs designated MSP1–MSP8 have been described [10,30–36]. The second group includes soluble proteins including the serine repeat antigen (SERA). The third group consists of proteins in the apical organelles and includes apical membrane antigen 1 (AMA-1) and the rhoptry associated proteins, RAP1–RAP3.

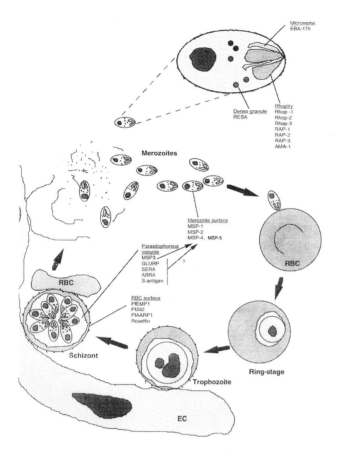

Figure 2 Subcellular localization of *P. falciparum* erythrocytic stage vaccine antigens. (Modified from Ref. 142.)

A. MSP1

Merozoite surface protein 1 (MSP1) is a 185–220 kDa glycoprotein (depending on the parasite species) found on the surface of the free merozoite and is synthesized during schizogony. The function of MSP1 is still unclear, but it is thought that the intact unprocessed protein may be involved in the initial recognition of the erythrocyte and attachment to receptors on the red cell surface [37,38]. As these proteins are found on the surface of the parasite, their exposure to the hosts' immune system makes them a target of the immune response.

Upon merozoite release from the rupturing erythrocyte, the high molecular weight precursor is proteolytically cleaved into four smaller fragments ($MSP1_{83}$, $MSP1_{30}$, $MSP1_{38}$, and $MSP1_{42}$) that form a noncovalently associated complex held together by the 42-kDa fragment on the surface of the merozoite [30]. Just prior to invasion of a new RBC, a secondary proteolytic processing step, which is critical for invasion, occurs with the 42-kDa carboxyl terminal fragment cleaved into a 19-kDa fragment ($MSP1_{19}$) and a 33-kDa fragment ($MSP1_{33}$) [39,40]. $MSP1_{33}$ is shed with the other fragments forming the complex [41], while $MSP1_{19}$ remains on the surface of the merozoite and is the only part of MSP1 carried into the RBC [42].

Antibodies raised against MSP1 could work in a number of ways: neutralization by agglutination or opsonization of merozoites, prevention of invasion of the red blood cell, or inhibition of the growth of the parasite within the red blood cell. Parasite-specific antibodies may act by binding to a portion of MSP1 ($MSP1_{19}$) on the surface of the merozoite thereby blocking invasion of the RBC [42]. Alternatively, they may prevent a crucial processing step of the protein. For example, the secondary processing step of MSP1 to $MSP1_{19}$, thought to be critical for initiation of the invasion process [43], can be inhibited by specific antibodies. Recently, a class of blocking antibodies have been identified that act in the parasite's favor. Anti-MSP1 monoclonal antibodies have been identified that compete with the binding of processing-inhibiting antibodies to their epitopes [44,45]. Additionally, it was shown that naturally acquired antibodies in humans specific for a region within the N-terminus of MSP1 could block the ability of an anti-MSP1 monoclonal antibody to inhibit the processing step [42,44,46]. The potential for these blocking antibodies to interfere or even abolish protection induced by immunization or infection cannot be underestimated. To this end, mutant forms of recombinant $MSP1_{19}$ have been designed that are no longer recognized by known blocking antibodies but retain the structure necessary for immune recognition [45].

MSP1 shows much promise as a vaccine candidate. Studies involving MSP1 purified from *P. falciparum* showed partial or complete protection following challenge in primates [47,48]. Additional studies using recombinant proteins produced similar results [47,49].

The structure of MSP1 is critical for the protein's antigenicity and immunogenicity. Various expression systems for the production of recombinant protein have been utilized in an effort to maintain correct conformation. Recombinant MSP1 has been produced using bacterial [50], mammalian [51], baculovirus [52,53], and yeast systems [54,55].

It is the C-terminus of this molecule, from which $MSP1_{19}$ is derived, that has been the focus of most attempts to elucidate the immune response to this molecule. $MSP1_{19}$ is cysteine-rich and contains two epidermal growth factor (EGF)-like domains [56]. The native conformation is dependent on the correct formation of multiple disulfide bonds within each domain. Reduction and alkylation of these disulfide bonds in recombinant MSP1 or $MSP1_{19}$ abolishes or greatly reduces the recognition by polyclonal and monoclonal antibodies [57–59]. Most of the antibody-binding sites in $MSP1_{19}$ appear to be conformation dependent requiring both EGF-like motifs for the formation of the dominant epitopes [60].

Studies using the rodent model of malaria have shown that protection induced by $MSP1_{19}$ immunization is MHC restricted, correlating with genes present in the H-2 loci [61]. T cells from C57BL/6 ($H-2^b$) and BALB/c ($H-2^d$) mice immunized with $MSP1_{19}$ proliferate in response to different regions within $MSP1_{19}$, indicating they recognize different T cell epitopes [62]. In addition, C57BL/10 ($H-2^b$) and BALB/c ($H-2^d$) mice are protected when immunized with GST–$MSP1_{19}$ expressed by *Escherichia coli* while B10.BR ($H-2^k$)

mice are not [61]. This appears to reflect the level and type of antibody present at the time of challenge.

High-titer MSP1$_{19}$-specific antibodies present in the serum of the mice are required at the time of challenge for protection [61,63–65]. These specific antibodies do not function via Fc-mediated interactions as evidenced by the ability of passively transferred antibodies to reduce parasite burden in Fc-receptor-deficient mice [66,67]. It was further found that vaccination of B cell deficient mice with MSP1$_{19}$ did not result in protection [65] nor could adoptively transferred CD4+ T cells, specific for defined MSP1$_{19}$ T helper epitopes, protect normal mice [62]. This not only emphasizes the vital role for MSP1$_{19}$-specific antibodies but it also suggests that the antibody-mediated parasite clearance is not reliant on antibody-dependent cell-mediated cytotoxicity and Fc-mediated phagocytosis.

Although it has been shown that antibodies are required at the time of challenge to reduce parasite density, high titer passively transferred MSP1$_{19}$ antibody is unable to completely eradicate parasites from mice lacking a functional immune system [68]. It is apparent that even in the presence of high-titer antibody, a complete immune response including B cells and CD4+ T cells is required for protection in mice. The high-titer MSP1$_{19}$ antibodies most likely act to reduce the parasite burden, providing the recipient time to mount a protective immune response independent of the vaccine [23]. Whether this reflects the situation in humans following vaccination with MSP1$_{19}$ is yet to be determined.

The relevance of MSP1 to human malaria has been shown by longitudinal studies, which demonstrate that reduced susceptibility to clinical malaria is associated with elevated antibody levels and T-cell proliferative and cytokine responses to the C-terminal region of MSP1 [60,69,70]. T cell epitopes have been identified in both the conserved [71,72] and variant regions [73] of MSP1$_{19}$.

MSP1 has been included in a number of combination antigen human vaccine trials [74,75,77] with varying degrees of success. Yet, MSP1 remains one of the leading malaria vaccine candidates with varied forms of the antigen being developed for further Phase I clinical trials.

B. MSP2

Merozoite surface protein 2 (MSP2) is a 43–56 kDa polypeptide attached to the surface of the merozoite [32,78]. The primary structure consists of three domains: highly conserved N- and C-terminal regions flanking a central dimorphic variable region. Based on the variable region, MSP2 genes can be grouped into two main families [79].

Initially, the importance of MSP2 was identified when specific monoclonal antibodies resulted in the inhibition of *P. falciparum* growth in vitro [78,80]. Further studies found that the acquired antibody response in humans is primarily directed against the polymorphic central region [81,82], although antibodies to conserved regions may develop in an age-dependent manner following extensive malaria exposure [81]. Recent epidemiological studies have associated the presence of antibodies against the conserved region of MSP2 with the reduced frequency of clinical malaria [81]. In a malaria endemic region, a Phase I/IIb trial of a vaccine containing RESA, MSP1, and MSP2 showed a vaccine-induced selective pressure exerted on the reinfecting parasites. This resulted in a skewing of the parasite population towards the alternate dimorphic form of MSP2 not included in the vaccine [76]. This argues for the inclusion of all important allelic types of a parasite antigen to be included in a vaccine; in the instance of MSP2, both allelic families should be included. An alternative approach to a vaccine based on MSP2 might be to include just the conserved regions.

Polyclonal antibodies to MSP2 have been identified that enhance the invasion of RBC by merozoites resulting in an increased proportion of RBC containing more than one ring-stage parasite [83]. It has been proposed that multiple invasion may reflect the ability of merozoites cross-linked by the antibody to reorientate so that their apical surfaces can contact the RBC surface. Alternatively, it is possible that the separation of previously cross-linked parasites attracted to the same RBC enables them to invade the same cell individually [83,84]. The identification of deleterious antibodies emphasizes the need to identify minimal epitopes capable of inducing protective antibodies for inclusion in malaria vaccines.

C. MSP3

MSP3 has an N-terminal secretion signal but no structural features characteristic of an integral membrane protein or signal for a GPI anchor. It is now assumed to associate with the merozoite surface as a peripheral membrane protein after being secreted into the parasitophorous vacuole of schizonts [85]. The major form of MSP3 on the merozoite surface is derived by proteolysis from full-length MSP3, but the site of cleavage is unknown.

A striking feature of the MSP3 primary structure is three blocks of heptad repeats in the N-terminal half of the polypeptide. Such sequences are highly predictive of a coiled-coil structure and a model of how the three blocks of heptads could form an intramolecular three-stranded coiled-coil has been proposed [86]. The C-terminal half of MSP3 is highly charged with aspartate, glutamate, and lysine residues comprising ~50% of the 164 residues C-terminal to the third block of heptads. A central 51-residue segment of this region of MSP3 is particularly acidic containing 36 glutamate or aspartate residues. Diversity in MSP3 appears to be restricted to the N-terminal heptad-containing half of the polypeptide and again much of the diversity reflects an underlying dimorphism [87,88]. Additional mutational events have added to the diversity in MSP3 and one of the sequenced alleles (D10) appears to have been generated by intragenic recombination between alleles representative of each dimorphic family [88]. The bias towards nonsynonymous substitutions seen in the genes of many malarial antigens is also seen in *msp3* genes, consistent with diversifying selection of protective immune responses directed against MSP3.

MSP3 was originally detected as a target of cytophilic human antibodies that induce monocytes to inhibit the development of asexual blood-stage parasites in a process known as antibody-dependent cellular inhibition (ADCI) [10]. Druilhe and colleagues have extensively documented the activity of MSP3 antibodies in ADCI using *P. falciparum* cultured in vitro [9]. Additional evidence implicating anti-MSP3 antibodies in ADCI has been obtained using *P. falciparum*-infected BXN mice that were reconstituted with human erythrocytes [89]. The anti-MSP3 antibodies used in these ADCI studies were affinity purified on a 64-residue recombinant fragment of MSP3 or on MSP3b, a 27-residue synthetic peptide derived from the 64-residue fragment of MSP3. Despite the extensive documentation of the ADCI phenomenon, it seems improbable that the dominant specificity of antibodies acting to limit the development of *P. falciparum* asexual blood stages is restricted to such a short, linear sequence of one merozoite antigen.

D. MSP4 and MSP5

MSP4 and MSP5 are both 40-kDa proteins attached to the surface of the merozoite by a GPI anchor and contain a single EGF-like domain in the C-terminal region [31,33]. In *P. falciparum*, the genes that encode MSP4 and MSP5 are closely linked on chromosome 2, next to the gene encoding MSP2 [33]. Homologs of the *P. falciparum* proteins have been identified in *P. berghei*, *P. chabaudi*, and *P. yoelii*, and are represented by a single gene in the rodent *Plasmodium* strains [90,91]. A recombinant *P. yoelii* MSP4/5 protein was used in murine immunization studies and was effective at protecting mice from lethal challenge [92]. A significant correlation between prechallenge antibody titers and peak parasitemia was observed. Antibodies in sera from individuals living in malaria endemic areas recognized at least four different epitopes within MSP4 and were mainly of the IgG1 and IgG3 isotypes [93,94]. Disruption of the disulfide bonds in the C-terminus of the protein abrogated the binding of antibodies to epitopes both within and removed from the EGF-like domain, indicating the recognition of conformation-dependent epitopes.

E. SERA (SERP)

The serine repeat antigen (SERA) or serine-rich protein (SERP) is a 126-kDa protein found within the parasitophorous vacuole in late-stage parasites [95]. Following schizogony, the protein is cleaved into 73- and 50-kDa fragments. It is a conserved protein, rich in serine (as the name suggests), and very similar in structure to cysteine proteases [96]. It was demonstrated that monoclonal antibodies specific for SERA act to block entry of *P. falciparum* merozoites into red blood cells [97,98]. Immunization of nonhuman primates with SERA purified from parasites [99] or recombinant protein [100,101] could induce varying degrees of protection.

F. AMA-1

Apical membrane antigen-1 (AMA-1) is an 80-kDa integral membrane protein and is probably found in micronemes. At the time of merozoite release, the 83-kDa molecule is at the apical pole while a 66-kDa N-terminally processed form is distributed on the merozoite surface [102,103].

Immunization of monkeys and rodents with native [104] or recombinant [105–108] forms of the protein resulted in protection from homologous challenge. Passive immunization of mice with AMA-1-specific antibodies protected them from lethal challenge with *P. chabaudi* [107]. This indicated an important role for anti-AMA-1 antibodies in mediating protection from malaria. Maintenance of the conformation is critical for recognition of epitopes by the antibodies as reduction and alkylation of AMA-1 abrogates the protection seen in previously protected mice [107].

Additional studies have also suggested a role for T cells. Depletion of CD4 + T cells in mice immunized with AMA-1 partially affects their ability to control parasitemia, despite the presence of anti-AMA-1 antibodies, indicating a role for antibody-independent T-cell-mediated immunity [109]. This was consistent with an earlier study showing protection following the adoptive transfer of CD4 + T cells specific for a cryptic epitope on AMA-1 into T-cell-deficient mice [106]. Therefore both AMA-1-specific antibodies and CMI contribute to protection against malaria.

Early human clinical trials have commenced with *P. falciparum* AMA-1, and the immunogenicity and safety assessed in an escalating dose–response Phase 1 trial. In this study, immune responses were poor, and further analysis has been hindered by vaccine formulation problems [110]. The development of AMA-1 for use in human Phase 1 clinical trials continues, with protein from various recombinant expression systems being explored.

G. RAP1, RAP2, and RAP3

A number of proteins located within the rhoptries of *P. falciparum* have been identified ranging in size from 37 to 86 kDa, which form the low molecular mass rhoptry complex. Rhoptry-associated proteins 1 and 2 (RAP1 and RAP2) form a tightly associated complex in the rhoptries [111]. Recently, it has been shown that RAP3 can also complex with RAP1 [112]. The RAP2 and RAP3 proteins are closely related and are highly conserved across *Plasmodium* species. RAP1 appears to act as a chaperone protein facilitating the intracellular trafficking of RAP2 and presumably RAP3 to the rhoptries [113]. However, the precise function of the RAP complex is unknown. It has been suggested that RAP2 and RAP3 play a role in merozoite invasion [112].

The proteins of the RAP complex have long been considered candidate vaccine antigens and the antigenic diversity that presents a major difficulty for other antigens is less problematic for the RAP complex proteins. Antibodies to RAP1 can inhibit parasite invasion and immunization with purified native RAP complex has protected against *P. falciparum* challenge in *Saimiri* monkeys [114,115]. Recombinant forms of RAP1 and RAP2 were found to be immunogenic in mice and rabbits [116,117]. Studies in nonhuman primates using recombinant and parasite-derived protein established a significant correlation between antibody titers to RAP2 and the degree of protection [118]. Additionally, naturally occurring antibodies to RAP1 and RAP2 have been measured in humans residing in malaria endemic areas; recognition was found to correlate with age [119]. These serum antibodies are also capable of recognizing epitopes present in the recombinant protein. Presently, only RAP2 is currently undergoing development for human vaccine trials.

V. VACCINE CANDIDATES ON THE INFECTED RED BLOOD CELL

A. PfEMP1

P. falciparum erythrocyte membrane protein-1 (PfEMP1) is a variant protein found expressed on the surface of infected erythrocytes [120]. It is involved in the cytoadherence of the infected RBC to vascular endothelium [121], and is thought to play a role in the pathogenesis of cerebral malaria. It may also serve as a ligand for rosetting [122]. A multigene family, containing between 50 and 150 *var* genes, occurring on multiple parasite chromosomes [123] encodes this protein [124,125]. The differential expression of these genes is thought to be responsible for the different binding properties to adhesion molecules during sequestration exhibited by different strains of the parasite [126,127]. It also forms the basis for the extensive antigenic variation associated with the parasite. During infection, switching of the *var* genes results in expression of different PfEMP1 variants on the surface of the infected RBC [126–128]. This process allows the parasite to multiply in the presence of antibodies that were directed at PfEMP1 variants previously expressed.

The extraordinary antigenic variation means that the development of a vaccine using this molecule will need to focus on conserved yet functional domains. The regions of this protein that mediate the binding of the merozoites to the RBC, or infected RBC to endothelium, are potential candidates. A recent study immunized monkeys with a minimal fragment derived from PfEMP1, known to function in the binding of CD36 [129]. The immunized animals experienced lower parasite densities than control animals and this protection occurred despite the expression of different *var* genes during waves of recurrent parasitemia.

B. RESA (Pf155)

Ring-infected erythrocyte surface antigen (RESA) is found in the dense granules of the apical organelles in merozoites [130]. Following invasion, it is released from the merozoite when it translocates to the cytoplasmic side of the erythrocyte membrane [131]. This protein contains two regions of tandem repeats [132] containing both B and T cell epitopes [133,134]. The antigen appears not to be expressed on the surface of the parasitized RBC [135], although a portion of it is accessible to the immune system [136]. Epidemiological studies in malaria endemic regions have presented conflicting results with some studies demonstrating a correlation between repeat region-specific antibody levels and reduced parasitemias and clinical episodes. Additional studies have been unable to establish a correlation [137–139]. It is thought that this may reflect differences in human genetics and patterns of endemicity [139,140]. Ring-infected erythrocyte surface antigen has been included in a number of combination antigen vaccines for human trials [75,76].

VI. THE FUTURE

The prospects of developing a subunit malaria vaccine are good. We now understand to a significant degree the nature of protective immune responses and have defined a number of subunit vaccine candidates that are targets of antiparasite antibodies and antitoxin antibodies. We are also in the process of defining target antigens for CMI. However, most importantly, we are now aware of many of the great difficulties involved in developing an effective malaria vaccine.

While it would be ideal, but unlikely, that a single antigen were to be a successful blood-stage subunit vaccine, it is more likely that success will come from combining multiple antigens that each stimulate different types of protective immune responses. In parallel, it is hoped that there will be success in developing vaccines that target the parasite at the pre-erythrocytic stage and in the mosquito. Success in one or more of these three major strategies will have an enormous impact on world health.

ACKNOWLEDGMENT

We gratefully acknowledge the input of Dr Louis Miller who kindly reviewed the manuscript.

REFERENCES

1. Cheng Q, et al. Measurement of *Plasmodium falciparum* growth rates in vivo: a test of malaria vaccines. Am J Trop Med Hyg 1997; 57(4):495–500.
1a. Fujioka H, Aikawa M. The malaria parasite and its lifecycle. In: Wahlgren M, Perlmann P, eds. Malaria: Molecular and Clinical Aspects. Amsterdam: Harwood Academic Publishers, 1999: 19–55.
2. Li C, et al. Rodent malarias: the mouse as a model for understanding immune responses and pathology induced by the erythrocytic stages of the parasite. Med Microbiol Immunol (Berl) 2001; 189:115–126.
3. Good MF, et al. Pathways and strategies for developing a malaria blood-stage vaccine. Annu Rev Immunol 1998; 16:57–87.
4. Gupta S, et al. Immunity to non-cerebral severe malaria is acquired after one or two infections. Nat Med 1999; 5:340–343.
5. Clark IA, Schofield L. Pathogenesis of malaria. Parasitol Today 2000; 16:451–454.
6. Schofield L, et al. Synthetic GPI as a candidate anti-toxic vaccine in a model of malaria. Nature 2002; 418:785–789.
7. Genton B, et al. The epidemiology of malaria in the Wosera area, East Sepik Province, Papua New Guinea, in preparation for vaccine trials. I. Malariometric indices and immunity. Ann Trop Med Parasitol 1995; 89:359–376.
8. Bouharoun-Tayoun H, et al. Antibodies that protect humans against *Plasmodium falciparum* blood stages do not on their own inhibit parasite growth and invasion in vitro, but act in cooperation with monocytes. J Exp Med 1990; 172:1633–1641.
9. Bouharoun-Tayoun H, et al. Mechanisms underlying the monocyte-mediated antibody-dependent killing of *Plasmodium falciparum* asexual blood stages. J Exp Med 1995; 182:409–418.
10. Oeuvray C, et al. Merozoite surface protein-3: a malaria protein inducing antibodies that promote *Plasmodium fal-*

ciparum killing by cooperation with blood monocytes. Blood 1994; 84:1594–1602.

11. Grun JL, Weidanz WP. Antibody-independent immunity to reinfection malaria in B-cell-deficient mice. Infect Immun 1983; 41:1197–1204.

12. van der Heyde HC, et al. The resolution of acute malaria in a definitive model of B cell deficiency, the JHD mouse. J Immunol 1994; 152:4557–4562.

13. von der Weid T, et al. Gene-targeted mice lacking B cells are unable to eliminate a blood stage malaria infection. J Immunol 1996; 156:2510–2516.

14. Brake DA, et al. Adoptive protection against *Plasmodium chabaudi adami* malaria in athymic nude mice by a cloned T cell line. J Immunol 1988; 140:1989–1993.

15. Taylor-Robinson AW, et al. The role of TH1 and TH2 cells in a rodent malaria infection. Science 1993; 260:1931–1934.

16. Amante F, Good M. Prolonged Th1-like response generated by a *Plasmodium yoelii*-specific T cell clone allows complete clearance of infection in reconstituted mice. Parasite Immunol 1997; 19:111–126.

17. Stevenson MM, et al. IL-12-induced protection against blood-stage *Plasmodium chabaudi* AS requires IFN-gamma and TNF-alpha and occurs via a nitric oxide-dependent mechanism. J Immunol 1995; 155:2545–2556.

18. Favila-Castillo L, et al. Protection of rats against malaria by a transplanted immune spleen. Parasite Immunol 1996; 18:325–331.

19. Su Z, Stevenson MM. Central role of endogenous gamma interferon in protective immunity against blood-stage *Plasmodium chabaudi* AS infection. Infect Immun 2000; 68:4399–4406.

20. Pombo D, et al. Immunity to malaria after administration of ultra-low doses of red cells infected with *Plasmodium falciparum*. Lancet 2002; 360:610.

21. van der Heyde HC, et al. Gamma delta T cells function in cell-mediated immunity to acute blood-stage *Plasmodium chabaudi adami* malaria. J Immunol 1995; 154:3985–3990.

22. Seixas EM, Langhorne J. Gammadelta T cells contribute to control of chronic parasitemia in *Plasmodium chabaudi* infections in mice. J Immunol 1999; 162:2837–2841.

23. Good MF. Towards a blood-stage vaccine for malaria: are we following all the leads. Nat Rev Immunol 2001; 1:117–125.

24. Clark IA, et al. Possible importance of macrophage-derived mediators in acute malaria. Infect Immun 1981; 32:1058–1066.

25. Bate CA, et al. Malarial parasites induce TNF production by macrophages. Immunology 1988; 64:227–231.

26. Bate CA, et al. Soluble malarial antigens are toxic and induce the production of tumour necrosis factor in vivo. Immunology 1989; 66:600–605.

27. Schofield L, Hackett F. Signal transduction in host cells by a glycosylphosphatidylinositol toxin of malaria parasites. J Exp Med 1993; 177:145–153.

28. Berhe S, et al. Conservation of structure among glycosylphosphatidylinositol toxins from different geographic isolates of *Plasmodium falciparum*. Mol Biochem Parasitol 1999; 103:273–278.

29. Schofield L, et al. Neutralizing monoclonal antibodies to glycosylphosphatidylinositol, the dominant TNF-alpha-inducing toxin of *Plasmodium falciparum*: prospects for the immunotherapy of severe malaria. Ann Trop Med Parasitol 1993; 87:617–626.

30. McBride JS, Heidrich HG. Fragments of the polymorphic Mr 185,000 glycoprotein from the surface of isolated *Plasmodium falciparum* merozoites form an antigenic complex. Mol Biochem Parasitol 1987; 23:71–84.

31. Marshall VM, et al. A second merozoite surface protein (MSP-4) of *Plasmodium falciparum* that contains an epidermal growth factor-like domain. Infect Immun 1997; 65:4460–4467.

32. Miettinen-Baumann A, et al. A 46,000 dalton *Plasmodium falciparum* merozoite surface glycoprotein not related to the 185,000–195,000 dalton schizont precursor molecule: isolation and characterization. Parasitol Res 1988; 74:317–323.

33. Marshall VM, et al. Close linkage of three merozoite surface protein genes on chromosome 2 of *Plasmodium falciparum*. Mol Biochem Parasitol 1998; 94:13–25.

34. Trucco C, et al. The merozoite surface protein 6 gene codes for a 36 kDa protein associated with the *Plasmodium falciparum* merozoite surface protein-1 complex. Mol Biochem Parasitol 2001; 112:91–101.

35. Pachebat JA, et al. The 22 kDa component of the protein complex on the surface of *Plasmodium falciparum* merozoites is derived from a larger precursor, merozoite surface protein 7. Mol Biochem Parasitol 2001; 117:83–89.

36. Black CG, et al. Merozoite surface protein 8 of *Plasmodium falciparum* contains two epidermal growth factor-like domains. Mol Biochem Parasitol 2001; 114:217–226.

37. Perkins ME, Rocco LJ. Sialic acid-dependent binding of *Plasmodium falciparum* merozoite surface antigen. Pf200, to human erythrocytes. J Immunol 1988; 141:3190–3196.

38. Herrera S, et al. A conserved region of the MSP-1 surface protein of *Plasmodium falciparum* contains a recognition sequence for erythrocyte spectrin. EMBO J 1993; 12:1607–1614.

39. Blackman MJ, et al. A conserved parasite serine protease processes the *Plasmodium falciparum* merozoite surface protein-1. Mol Biochem Parasitol 1993; 62:103–114.

40. Blackman MJ, et al. Processing of the *Plasmodium falciparum* major merozoite surface protein-1: identification of a 33-kilodalton secondary processing product which is shed prior to erythrocyte invasion. Mol Biochem Parasitol 1991; 49:35–44.

41. Blackman MJ, Holder AA. Secondary processing of the *Plasmodium falciparum* merozoite surface protein-1 (MSP1) by a calcium-dependent membrane-bound serine protease: shedding of MSP133 as a noncovalently associated complex with other fragments of the MSP1. Mol Biochem Parasitol 1992; 50:307–315.

42. Blackman MJ, et al. A single fragment of a malaria merozoite surface protein remains on the parasite during red cell invasion and is the target of invasion-inhibiting antibodies. J Exp Med 1990; 172:379–382.

43. Blackman MJ, et al. Antibodies inhibit the protease-mediated processing of a malaria merozoite surface protein. J Exp Med 1994; 180:389–393.

44. Guevara Patino JA, et al. Antibodies that inhibit malaria merozoite surface protein-1 processing and erythrocyte invasion are blocked by naturally acquired human antibodies. J Exp Med 1997; 186:1689–1699.

45. Uthaipibull C, et al. Inhibitory and blocking monoclonal antibody epitopes on merozoite surface protein 1 of the malaria parasite *Plasmodium falciparum*. J Mol Biol 2001; 307:1381–1394.

46. Nwuba RI, et al. The human immune response to *Plasmodium falciparum* includes both antibodies that inhibit merozoite surface protein 1 secondary processing and blocking antibodies. Infect Immun 2002; 70:5328–5331.

47. Etlinger HM, et al. Ability of recombinant or native proteins to protect monkeys against heterologous challenge with *Plasmodium falciparum*. Infect Immun 1991; 59:3498–3503.

48. Siddiqui WA, et al. Merozoite surface coat precursor protein completely protects *Aotus* monkeys against *Plasmodium falciparum* malaria. Proc Natl Acad Sci USA 1987; 84:3014–3018.

49. Herrera S, et al. Immunization of *Aotus* monkeys with *Plas-*

modium falciparum blood-stage recombinant proteins. Proc Natl Acad Sci USA 1990; 87:4017–4021.

50. Daly TM, Long CA. A recombinant 15-kilodalton carboxyl-terminal fragment of *Plasmodium yoelii yoelii* 17XL merozoite surface protein 1 induces a protective immune response in mice. Infect Immun 1993; 61:2462–2467.

51. Pan W, et al. Vaccine candidate MSP-1 from *Plasmodium falciparum*: a redesigned 4917 bp polynucleotide enables synthesis and isolation of full-length protein from *Escherichia coli* and mammalian cells. Nucleic Acids Res 1999; 27:1094–1103.

52. Chang SP, et al. A recombinant baculovirus 42-kilodalton C-terminal fragment of *Plasmodium falciparum* merozoite surface protein 1 protects *Aotus* monkeys against malaria. Infect Immun 1996; 64:253–261.

53. Perera KL, et al. Baculovirus merozoite surface protein 1 C-terminal recombinant antigens are highly protective in a natural primate model for human *Plasmodium vivax* malaria. Infect Immun 1998; 66:1500–1506.

54. Hui GS, et al. Immunogenicity of the C-terminal 19-kDa fragment of the *Plasmodium falciparum* merozoite surface protein 1 (MSP1), yMSP1(19) expressed in *S. cerevisiae*. J Immunol 1994; 153:2544–2553.

55. Morgan WD, et al. Expression of deuterium-isotope-labelled protein in the yeast *Pichia pastoris* for NMR studies. J Biomol NMR 2000; 17:337–347.

56. Blackman MJ, et al. Proteolytic processing of the *Plasmodium falciparum* merozoite surface protein-1 produces a membrane-bound fragment containing two epidermal growth factor-like domains. Mol Biochem Parasitol 1991; 49:29–33.

57. Ling IT, et al. The combined epidermal growth factor-like modules of *Plasmodium yoelii* Merozoite Surface Protein-1 are required for a protective immune response to the parasite. Parasite Immunol 1995; 17:425–433.

58. Burghaus PA, Holder AA. Expression of the 19-kilodalton carboxy-terminal fragment of the *Plasmodium falciparum* merozoite surface protein-1 in *Escherichia coli* as a correctly folded protein. Mol Biochem Parasitol 1994; 64:165–169.

59. Chappel JA, Holder AA. Monoclonal antibodies that inhibit *Plasmodium falciparum* invasion in vitro recognize the first growth factor-like domain of merozoite surface protein-1. Mol Biochem Parasitol 1993; 60:303–311.

60. Egan AF, et al. Serum antibodies from malaria-exposed people recognize conserved epitopes formed by the two epidermal growth factor motifs of MSP1(19), the carboxy-terminal fragment of the major merozoite surface protein of *Plasmodium falciparum*. Infect Immun 1995; 63:456–466.

61. Tian JH, et al. Genetic regulation of protective immune response in congenic strains of mice vaccinated with a subunit malaria vaccine. J Immunol 1996; 157:1176–1183.

62. Tian JH, et al. Definition of T cell epitopes within the 19 kDa carboxylterminal fragment of *Plasmodium yoelii* merozoite surface protein 1 (MSP1(19)) and their role in immunity to malaria. Parasite Immunol 1998; 20:263–278.

63. Daly TM, Long CA. Humoral response to a carboxyl-terminal region of the merozoite surface protein-1 plays a predominant role in controlling blood-stage infection in rodent malaria. J Immunol 1995; 155:236–243.

64. Hirunpetcharat C, et al. Intranasal immunization with yeast-expressed 19 kD carboxyl-terminal fragment of *Plasmodium yoelii* merozoite surface protein-1 (yMSP119) induces protective immunity to blood stage malaria infection in mice. Parasite Immunol 1998; 20:413–420.

65. Hirunpetcharat C, et al. Complete protective immunity induced in mice by immunization with the 19-kilodalton carboxyl-terminal fragment of the merozoite surface protein-1 (MSP1[19]) of *Plasmodium yoelii* expressed in *Saccharomyces cerevisiae*: correlation of protection with an-

tigen-specific antibody titer, but not with effector CD4+ T cells. J Immunol 1997; 159:3400–3411.

66. Rotman HL, et al. Fc receptors are not required for antibody-mediated protection against lethal malaria challenge in a mouse model. J Immunol 1998; 161:1908–1912.

67. Vukovic P, et al. Immunoglobulin G3 antibodies specific for the 19-kilodalton carboxyl-terminal fragment of *Plasmodium yoelii* merozoite surface protein 1 transfer protection to mice deficient in Fc-gammaRI receptors. Infect Immun 2000; 68:3019–3022.

68. Hirunpetcharat C, et al. Absolute requirement for an active immune response involving B cells and Th cells in immunity to *Plasmodium yoelii* passively acquired with antibodies to the 19-kDa carboxyl-terminal fragment of merozoite surface protein-1. J Immunol 1999; 162:7309–7314.

69. Riley EM, et al. Naturally acquired cellular and humoral immune responses to the major merozoite surface antigen (PfMSP1) of *Plasmodium falciparum* are associated with reduced malaria morbidity. Parasite Immunol 1992; 14:321–337.

70. Riley EM, et al. A longitudinal study of naturally acquired cellular and humoral immune responses to a merozoite surface protein (MSP1) of *Plasmodium falciparum* in an area of seasonal malaria transmission. Parasite Immunol 1993; 15:513–524.

71. Crisanti A, et al. Epitopes recognized by human T cells map within the conserved part of the GP190 of *P. falciparum*. Science 1988; 240:1324–1326.

72. Sinigaglia F, et al. Nonpolymorphic regions of p190, a protein of the *Plasmodium falciparum* erythrocytic stage, contain both T and B cell epitopes. J Immunol 1988; 140:3568–3572.

73. Udhayakumar V, et al. Identification of T and B cell epitopes recognized by humans in the C-terminal 42-kDa domain of the *Plasmodium falciparum* merozoite surface protein (MSP)-1. J Immunol 1995; 154:6022–6030.

74. Lawrence GW, et al. Phase I trial in humans of an oil-based adjuvant SEPPIC MONTANIDE ISA 720. Vaccine 1997; 15:176–178.

75. Saul A, et al. Human phase I vaccine trials of 3 recombinant asexual stage malaria antigens with Montanide ISA720 adjuvant. Vaccine 1999; 17(23–24):3145–3159.

76. Genton B, et al. A recombinant blood-stage malaria vaccine reduces *Plasmodium falciparum* density and exerts selective pressure on parasite populations in a phase 1-2b trial in Papua New Guinea. J Infect Dis 2002; 185:820–827.

77. Keitel WA, et al. Phase I trial of two recombinant vaccines containing the 19 kd carboxy terminal fragment of *Plasmodium falciparum* merozoite surface protein 1 (MSP-1(19)) and T helper epitopes of tetanus toxoid. Vaccine 1999; 18(5–6):531–539.

78. Clark JT, et al. 46–53 kilodalton glycoprotein from the surface of *Plasmodium falciparum* merozoites. Mol Biochem Parasitol 1989; 32:15–24.

79. Smythe J, et al. Structural diversity in the *Plasmodium falciparum* merozoite surface antigen 2. Proc Natl Acad Sci USA 1991; 88:1751–1755.

80. Epping RJ, et al. An epitope recognised by inhibitory monoclonal antibodies that react with a 51 kilodalton merozoite surface antigen in *Plasmodium falciparum*. Mol Biochem Parasitol 1988; 28:1–10.

81. al-Yaman F, et al. Relationship between humoral response to *Plasmodium falciparum* merozoite surface antigen-2 and malaria morbidity in a highly endemic area of Papua New Guinea. Am J Trop Med Hyg 1994; 51:593–602.

82. Taylor RR, et al. Human antibody response to *Plasmodium falciparum* merozoite surface protein 2 is serogroup specific and predominantly of the immunoglobulin G3 subclass. Infect Immun 1995; 63:4382–4388.

83. Ramasamy R, et al. Antibodies to a merozoite surface protein promote multiple invasion of red blood cells by malaria parasites. Parasite Immunol 1999; 21:397–407.

84. Ramasamy R, et al. Antibodies and *Plasmodium falciparum* merozoites. Trends Parasitol 2001; 17:194–197.

85. McColl DJ, et al. Molecular variation in a novel polymorphic antigen associated with *Plasmodium falciparum* merozoites. Mol Biochem Parasitol 1994; 68:53–67.

86. Mulhern TD, et al. Solution structure of a polypeptide containing four heptad repeat units from a merozoite surface antigen of *Plasmodium falciparum*. Biochemistry 1995; 34:3479–3491.

87. McColl DJ, Anders RF. Conservation of structural motifs and antigenic diversity in the *Plasmodium falciparum* merozoite surface protein-3 (MSP-3). Mol Biochem Parasitol 1997; 90:21–31.

88. Huber W, et al. Limited sequence polymorphism in the *Plasmodium falciparum* merozoite surface protein 3. Mol Biochem Parasitol 1997; 87:231–234.

89. Badell E, et al. Human malaria in immunocompromised mice: an in vivo model to study defense mechanisms against *Plasmodium falciparum*. J Exp Med 2000; 192:1653–1660.

90. Black CG, et al. Identification of the *Plasmodium chabaudi* homologue of merozoite surface proteins 4 and 5 of *Plasmodium falciparum*. Infect Immun 1999; 67:2075–2081.

91. Kedzierski L, et al. Characterization of the merozoite surface protein 4/5 gene of *Plasmodium berghei* and *Plasmodium yoelii*. Mol Biochem Parasitol 2000; 105:137–147.

92. Kedzierski L, et al. Immunization with recombinant *Plasmodium yoelii* merozoite surface protein 4/5 protects mice against lethal challenge. Infect Immun 2000; 68:6034–6037.

93. Wang L, et al. Structural and antigenic properties of merozoite surface protein 4 of *Plasmodium falciparum*. Infect Immun 1999; 67:2193–2200.

94. Wang L, et al. Naturally acquired antibody responses to *Plasmodium falciparum* merozoite surface protein 4 in a population living in an area of endemicity in Vietnam. Infect Immun 2001; 69:4390–4397.

95. Delplace P, et al. Localization, biosynthesis, processing and isolation of a major 126 kDa antigen of the parasitophorous vacuole of *Plasmodium falciparum*. Mol Biochem Parasitol 1987; 23:193–201.

96. Higgins DG, et al. Malarial proteinase? Nature 1989; 340:604.

97. Perrin LH, et al. Inhibition of *P. falciparum* growth in human erythrocytes by monoclonal antibodies. Nature 1981; 289:301–303.

98. Banyal HS, Inselburg J. Isolation and characterization of parasite-inhibitory *Plasmodium falciparum* monoclonal antibodies. Am J Trop Med Hyg 1985; 34:1055–1064.

99. Perrin LH, et al. Antimalarial immunity in *Saimiri* monkeys. Immunization with surface components of asexual blood stages. J Exp Med 1984; 160:441–451.

100. Inselburg J, et al. Protective immunity induced in *Aotus* monkeys by recombinant SERA proteins of *Plasmodium falciparum*. Infect Immun 1991; 59:1247–1250.

101. Inselburg J, et al. Protective immunity induced in *Aotus* monkeys by a recombinant SERA protein of *Plasmodium falciparum*: further studies using SERA 1 and MF75.2 adjuvant. Infect Immun 1993; 61:2048–2052.

102. Narum DL, Thomas AW. Differential localization of full-length and processed forms of PF83/AMA-1 an apical membrane antigen of *Plasmodium falciparum* merozoites. Mol Biochem Parasitol 1994; 67:59–68.

103. Peterson MG, et al. Integral membrane protein located in the apical complex of *Plasmodium falciparum*. Mol Cell Biol 1989; 9:3151–3154.

104. Deans JA, et al. Vaccination trials in rhesus monkeys with a minor, invariant, *Plasmodium knowlesi* 66 kD merozoite antigen. Parasite Immunol 1988; 10:535–552.

105. Crewther P, et al. Protective immune responses to apical membrane antigen 1 of *Plasmodium chabaudi* involve recognition of strain-specific epitopes. Infect Immun 1996; 68:3310–3317.

106. Amante FH, et al. A cryptic T cell epitope on the apical membrane antigen 1 of *Plasmodium chabaudi adami* can prime for an anamnestic antibody response: implications for malaria vaccine design. J Immunol 1997; 159:5535–5544.

107. Anders RF, et al. Immunisation with recombinant AMA-1 protects mice against infection with *Plasmodium chabaudi*. Vaccine 1998; 16:240–247.

108. Collins WE, et al. Protective immunity induced in squirrel monkeys with recombinant apical membrane antigen-1 of *Plasmodium fragile*. Am J Trop Med Hyg 1994; 51:711–719.

109. Xu H, et al. CD4 + T cells acting independently of antibody contribute to protective immunity to *Plasmodium chabaudi* infection after apical membrane antigen 1 immunization. J Immunol 2000; 165:389–396.

110. Anders RF, Saul A. Malaria vaccines. Parasitol Today 2000; 16:444–447.

111. Bushell GR, et al. An antigenic complex in the rhoptries of *Plasmodium falciparum*. Mol Biochem Parasitol 1988; 28:105–112.

112. Baldi DL, et al. Identification and disruption of the gene encoding the third member of the low-molecular-mass rhoptry complex in *Plasmodium falciparum*. Infect Immun 2002; 70:5236–5245.

113. Baldi DL, et al. RAP1 controls rhoptry targeting of RAP2 in the malaria parasite *Plasmodium falciparum*. EMBO J 2000; 19:2435–2443.

114. Perrin LH, et al. Immunization with a *Plasmodium falciparum* merozoite surface antigen induces a partial immunity in monkeys. J Clin Invest 1985; 75:1718–1721.

115. Ridley RG, et al. A rhoptry antigen of *Plasmodium falciparum* is protective in *Saimiri* monkeys. Parasitology 1990; 101:187–192.

116. Stowers A, et al. Immunogenicity of recombinant *Plasmodium falciparum* rhoptry associated proteins 1 and 2. Parasite Immunol 1995; 17:631–642.

117. Stowers AW, et al. A peptide derived from a B cell epitope of *Plasmodium falciparum* rhoptry associated protein 2 specifically raises antibodies to rhoptry associated protein 1. Mol Biochem Parasitol 1996; 82:167–180.

118. Collins WE, et al. Efficacy of vaccines containing rhoptry-associated proteins RAP1 and RAP2 of *Plasmodium falciparum* in *Saimiri boliviensis* monkeys. Am J Trop Med Hyg 2000; 62:466–479.

119. Stowers A, et al. Assessment of the humoral immune response against *Plasmodium falciparum* rhoptry-associated proteins 1 and 2. Infect Immun 1997; 65:2329–2338.

120. Leech JH, et al. Identification of a strain-specific malarial antigen exposed on the surface of *Plasmodium falciparum*-infected erythrocytes. J Exp Med 1984; 159:1567–1575.

121. Baruch DI, et al. *Plasmodium falciparum* erythrocyte membrane protein 1 is a parasitized erythrocyte receptor for adherence to CD36, thrombospondin, and intercellular adhesion molecule 1. Proc Natl Acad Sci USA 1996; 93: 3497–3502.

122. Chen Q, et al. Identification of *Plasmodium falciparum* erythrocyte membrane protein 1 (PfEMP1) as the rosetting ligand of the malaria parasite *P. falciparum*. J Exp Med 1998; 187:15–23.

123. Rubio JP, et al. The *var* genes of *Plasmodium falciparum* are located in the subtelomeric region of most chromosomes. EMBO J 1996; 15:4069–4077.

124. Baruch DI, et al. Cloning the *P. falciparum* gene encoding PfEMP1, a malarial variant antigen and adherence receptor on the surface of parasitized human erythrocytes. Cell 1995; 82:77–87.

125. Su XZ, et al. The large diverse gene family *var* encodes proteins involved in cytoadherence and antigenic variation of *Plasmodium falciparum*-infected erythrocytes. Cell 1995; 82:89–100.

126. Roberts DJ, et al. Rapid switching to multiple antigenic and adhesive phenotypes in malaria. Nature 1992; 357:689–692.

127. Smith JD, et al. Switches in expression of *Plasmodium falciparum* var genes correlate with changes in antigenic and cytoadherent phenotypes of infected erythrocytes. Cell 1995; 82:101–110.

128. Peters J, et al. High diversity and rapid changeover of expressed *var* genes during the acute phase of *Plasmodium falciparum* infections in human volunteers. Proc Natl Acad Sci USA 2002; 99:10689–10694.

129. Baruch D, et al. Immunization of Aotus monkeys with a functional domain of the *Plasmodium falciparum* variant antigen induces protection against a lethal parasite line. Proc Natl Acad Sci USA 2002; 99:3860–3865.

130. Aikawa M, et al. Pf155/RESA antigen is localized in dense granules of *Plasmodium falciparum* merozoites. Exp Parasitol 1990; 71:326–329.

131. Culvenor JG, et al. *Plasmodium falciparum* ring-infected erythrocyte surface antigen is released from merozoite dense granules after erythrocyte invasion. Infect Immun 1991; 59:1183–1187.

132. Favaloro JM, et al. Structure of the RESA gene of *Plasmodium falciparum*. Nucleic Acids Res 1986; 14:8265–8277.

133. Kabilan L, et al. T-cell epitopes in Pf155/RESA, a major candidate for a *Plasmodium falciparum* malaria vaccine. Proc Natl Acad Sci USA 1988; 85:5659–5663.

134. Perlmann H, et al. Dissection of the human antibody response to the malaria antigen Pf155/RESA into epitope specific components. Immunol Rev 1989; 112:115–132.

135. Berzins K. Pf155/RESA is not a surface antigen of *Plasmodium falciparum* infected erythrocytes. Parasitol Today 1991; 7:193–194.

136. Saul A, et al. A portion of the Pf155/RESA antigen of *Plasmodium falciparum* is accessible on the surface of infected erythrocytes. Immunol Cell Biol 1988; 66(Pt 4): 269–276.

137. al-Yaman F, et al. Assessment of the role of the humoral response to *Plasmodium falciparum* MSP2 compared to RESA and SPf66 in protecting Papua New Guinean children from clinical malaria. Parasite Immunol 1995; 17: 493–501.

138. Riley EM, et al. Association between immune recognition of the malaria vaccine candidate antigen Pf155/RESA and resistance to clinical disease: a prospective study in a malaria-endemic region of west Africa. Trans R Soc Trop Med Hyg 1991; 85:436–443.

139. Modiano D, et al. Humoral response to *Plasmodium falciparum* Pf155/ring-infected erythrocyte surface antigen and Pf332 in three sympatric ethnic groups of Burkina Faso. Am J Trop Med Hyg 1998; 58:220–224.

140. Riley EM, et al. MHC and malaria: the relationship between HLA class II alleles and immune responses to *Plasmodium falciparum*. Int Immunol 1992; 4:1055–1063.

141. Strickland G, Hoffman S. Strategies for the control of malaria. Sci Am 1994, July/August, 24–33.

142. Berzins K, Anders R. The malaria antigens. In: Wahlgren M, Perlmann P, eds. Malaria: Molecular and Clinical Aspects. Amsterdam: Harwood Academic Publishers, 1999:181–216.

73

Malaria Transmission-Blocking Vaccines

Allan Saul
Malaria Vaccine Development Unit, National Institutes of Health, Rockville, Maryland, U.S.A.

I. INTRODUCTION

By any criterion, malaria is a disease of major global significance. The World Health Organization (WHO) estimates that approximately 1 million people die each year from malaria, primarily children in Africa. However, this is just the "ears of the hippopotamus." The number of clinical cases is estimated at perhaps 500 million per year and 1.5 billion people at risk [1]. Besides the disease, malaria is a major economic problem, directly through the cost of health care and the cost of maintaining control programs that prevent the spread of malaria, and indirectly through the loss of productivity [2]. Vector control and the detection and drug treatment of human cases remain the only weapons available. Although innovative ways of using existing technologies are being developed by programs such as Roll Back Malaria [3], these programs face technical difficulties with the spread of insecticide resistance in mosquitoes and the spread of drug resistance in the parasite [4]. Drug resistance and insecticide resistance are not the only impediments—malaria is overwhelmingly a disease of poverty. This leads to logistical difficulties in establishing and maintaining the infrastructure to continuously deliver vector-based control and human treatment and prophylaxis in areas with very limited health resources. For all these reasons, malaria vaccines have been promoted as having the potential to make a quantum difference. A long-lived vaccine may provide a cost-effective prophylaxis against the disease without requiring a major investment in infrastructure.

Malaria is caused by four species of *Plasmodium* parasites, *Plasmodium falciparum*, *P. vivax*, *P. malariae*, and *P. ovale*. Of the four, *P. falciparum* and *P. vivax* are responsible for most of the diseases, and *P. falciparum* is responsible for most of the deaths. These four species are sufficiently different that a vaccine directed against one species will probably not protect against the others. Although common in some localities, *P. malariae* and *P. ovale* are not responsible for enough diseases to currently attract vaccine development. Because of its importance in causing death and because it is the only human malaria parasite that can be cultured, most vaccine developments are aimed at producing a vaccine for *P. falciparum* alone. However, the development of transmission-blocking vaccines (TBVs) for both *P. falciparum* and *P. vivax* is proceeding in parallel. In the low to medium endemic areas that are the prime targets of transmission-blocking vaccines, diseases caused by *P. vivax* and *P. falciparum* are both of considerable importance, and both components will be required as part of integrated control programs.

Several types of antimalaria vaccines are being developed (see other chapters). Vaccines are commonly described by the stage of parasite they target. These include the following:

Preerythrocytic vaccines that target the form of the parasite, the sporozoite injected by the mosquito, or the resulting liver stage parasites. These stages of the parasite cause no disease, but an effective vaccine would stop the infection from developing into the next stage, the erythrocytic stage, which does cause diseases. Preerythrocytic vaccines are likely to be of particular importance for travelers.

Erythrocytic stage vaccines that target the forms of the parasite that replicate in the bloodstream. This is the stage of the parasite that causes disease. Vaccines directed against this stage are seen as particularly important in endemic areas, where, in conjunction with natural immunity, they may protect against severe disease and death even if they do not provide sterile immunity.

Mosquito stage vaccines, commonly called "transmission-blocking vaccines" that target the sexual and subsequent stages of the parasite as it develops in the mosquito. These vaccines are designed for people living in endemic areas and are aimed at preventing new infections. Although they provide no immediate direct benefit for the person immunized, malaria transmission is highly localized, so a successful transmission-blocking vaccine would result in considerable indirect benefits to the individual vaccinated (e.g., through decreased malaria infection rates in other family members and neighbors).

Vaccines against all stages of malaria potentially block transmission. Preerythrocytic stage vaccines are designed to prevent the transmission of malaria from mosquitoes to people. Erythrocytic stage vaccines, either by decreasing the probability of becoming infected or by decreasing the time that a person remains infectious, would decrease the reservoir of infection in a community, thereby decreasing transmission. In fact, computer models of malaria transmission in areas of low endemic malaria or seasonal malaria predict that preerythrocytic, erythrocytic stage, and mosquito stage vaccines could all have similar effects on malaria transmission [5]. However, this review will only discuss vaccines aimed at directly blocking transmission from people to mosquitoes (Figure 1).

Within this definition, the current design of malaria transmission-blocking vaccines involves several unusual concepts:

Malaria TBVs are designed to work outside the person or animal vaccinated. This both simplifies and con-

strains the vaccine design. These vaccines appear to work primarily through antibody-mediated effects [6]. Therefore, TBVs aim to obtain high-level and persistent antibodies. Ideally, protective antibody would last for several years. However, for areas of seasonal or epidemic malaria, protection that lasted a minimum of one transmission season (typically 4 months) would be useful in the context of integrated control programs. Fortunately, mosquito stage antigens are exposed for many hours, so transmission-blocking immunity (TBI) is unlikely to require the very high antibody levels required to block merozoite invasion [7].

Some target antigens (e.g., Pfs48/45 and Pfs230) are expressed in gametocytes. Naturally occurring antibodies against these proteins can be detected in exposed human populations. However, other targets (e.g., Pfs25) are only expressed in the mosquito midgut [8]. It is unlikely that these proteins have ever been under significant immune pressure. Consistent with this idea, these antigens have minimal sequence diversity. Transmission-blocking vaccines based on these may avoid some of the complica-

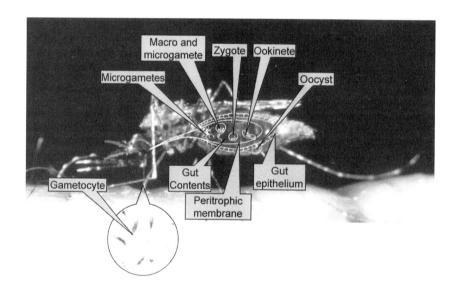

Figure 1 Targets of transmission-blocking immunity. Parasite and mosquito targets for transmission-blocking immunity are shown diagrammatically superimposed on a feeding *A. gambiae*, one of the most dangerous mosquito vectors. Gametocytes in the blood meal are ingested with uninfected blood cells. In the mosquito, each gametocyte rapidly transforms, escaping from its host red cell to produce approximately eight microgametes (♂) or a single macrogamete (♀). These fuse to form a zygote that transforms into a motile ookinete. This penetrates the peritrophic membrane, an acellular membrane secreted by the mosquito to surround the blood meal, and then crosses the mosquito gut wall to form an oocyst. Approximately 10 days after taking a blood meal, the oocyst ruptures to release thousands of sporozoites (not shown) that travel to the salivary glands. When injected with a subsequent blood meal, the sporozoites may infect another person.
Potential vaccine targets (listed in the text) on these stages are:

Gametocyte	Gametes	Zygote	Ookinete	Oocyst	Gut contents	Gut epithelium
Pfs48/45	Pfs48/45	Pfs230	Pfs25	Pfs25	Trypsin	Surface macromolecules
Pfs230	Pfs230	Pfs25	Pfs28	Pfs28	Other proteases	
			Chitinase			
			CTRP			

tions that vaccines aimed at other stages face with antigenic diversity but cannot be boosted by natural infection.

- In addition to protecting the vaccinated individual, most vaccines aimed at infectious diseases have a major herd immunity effect, protecting people not immunized by reducing the human reservoir of infection. However, TBVs are only designed to protect communities though a herd immunity effect and will not immediately protect the person vaccinated against the disease.

Four distinct uses for transmission-blocking vaccines are anticipated [8,9].

(1) *As a component of integrated control programs to eliminate endemic malaria in low to mesoendemic areas.* To eliminate malaria, a control program needs to reduce the potential number of new cases of malaria resulting from each existing case to less than one (i.e., in epidemiological terms, to reduce the $R_0 < 1$). We anticipate that a TBV alone could realistically achieve a threefold reduction in R_0 (e.g., a vaccine inducing high levels of antibody in vaccinees, with a 70% compliance). This would be sufficient in some areas but, coupled with other measures such as the use of insecticide-treated bed nets (ITNs) and better early case detection and treatment, could eliminate malaria from much of the world at risk from low to mesoendemic malaria. This includes almost all areas of *P. vivax* transmission and most of the world population at risk outside of Africa. Approximately 1.4 billion people are at risk outside Africa, with 50 million cases of *P. falciparum* malaria and 65 million cases of *P. vivax*

malaria annually [10]. Within Africa, the pattern is more complex, with a significant proportion of the 550 million people at risk from malaria living in areas of such high transmission that these measures would not interrupt transmission. However, even in sub-Saharan Africa, the epidemiology of malaria is not uniform. A recent study [11] of endemicity in West Africa, excluding Niger, found that of the 219 million at some risk of malaria in this region, 50 million live in low endemic areas (areas with a malaria prevalence in 2- to 10-year-old children <30%) where transmission-blocking vaccines could form part of an elimination program (Table 1). People in such sites are bitten by very few [1,2] infectious mosquitoes each year [12]. There are a further 153 million in areas of moderate endemicity (30–70% prevalence in 2- to 10-year-old children), where TBVs alone will not be effective but may be a component of an effective integrated control program. Only 16 million lived in high endemic areas (>70% prevalence in 2- to 10-year-old children) where elimination is not feasible in the foreseeable future [11].

(2) *To protect populations against epidemics of malaria in low endemic areas.* Epidemics of malaria usually occur as a result of unseasonable weather conditions, or accompany natural or man-made disasters in tropical areas. Although a high proportion of the population can be infected in an epidemic, the biology of the parasite limits the rate at which such epidemics can build up. For example, following the bite of an infectious mosquito, for *P. falciparum*, it takes 6 days before parasites are released into the blood, a further 6 days before the parasite density is high enough to generate significant numbers of gametocytes, another 10 days before these are mature enough to infect mosquitoes, and another

Table 1 Malaria Prevalence in West Africa

Country[a]	Percentage of total population in each risk category[b]			
	Predicted prevalence of <10%	Predicted prevalence of 10–30%	Predicted prevalence of 30–70%	Predicted prevalence of >70%
Benin	0	5	43.4	12
Burkino Faso	0	17	76	0
Cameroon	1	16	58	2
Côte d'Ivoire	0	4	75	0
Gambia	0	8	44	0
Ghana	1	15	46	17
Guinea	1	12	57	3
Guinea Bissau	2	30	13	0
Liberia	0	1	81	2
Mali	3	28	66	1
Mauritania	20	30	6	1
Nigeria	0	8	48	8
Senegal	1	22	41	2
Sierra Leone	0	0	79	2
Togo	0	0	39	38
Entire region	2.4	14.8	52.7	5.4
Total population at risk	7,006,869	42,941,669	152,779,264	15,698,929

[a] Excludes Niger for which statistics were not available.

[b] Percentages do not add up to 100% as urban populations have been excluded and parts of some countries lie outside of the area for which statistics were available.

Source: From Ref. 11.

10 days before a mosquito feeding on an infectious person will become infectious—a minimum of 32 days for one person receiving an infectious bite before that could result in a secondary infectious mosquito bite. *P. vivax* has a faster life cycle, but even for this parasite, the minimum generation time is about 4 weeks. In low to mesoendemic areas, it takes, on average, several days or weeks before a vector mosquito feeds on a potentially infectious person, happens to get infected, happens to survive long enough to transmit to another person, and happens to successfully transmit parasites. In practice, mean generation times from one person becoming infected to the next infection will be substantially longer than these minimum times. Computer modeling shows that relatively modest reductions (3×) in the transmission rate, which could be achieved by transmission-blocking vaccines alone, could have a major impact on the total number of cases of malaria that will occur before seasonal or other factors change to limit an epidemic [5]. Furthermore, the long malaria generation time allows adequate time to instigate a vaccination program at the first sign of an epidemic, provided rapid immunity can be achieved after vaccination. In areas prone to epidemics, one could envisage a strategy to combine TBV and the childhood Expanded Program on Immunization (EPI) program so that a rapid response could be achieved from a single booster vaccination when required.

(3) *To decrease disease in high endemic areas.* Two types of studies show that the incidence of disease caused by malaria in medium to high endemic areas correlates with the transmission intensity.

(a) Although initial studies suggested that morbidity from malaria is independent of transmission rates in Africa [13], a more recent and more comprehensive study has shown a highly significant correlation between transmission and death in infants [14]. In this study, a 10-fold reduction in transmission in the high endemic regions would be expected to result in a decrease of about 20 deaths per 1000 infants per year.

(b) Insecticide-treated bed nets in areas of relatively high transmission rates, where they reduce but not prevent transmission, have still resulted in significant reductions in mortality and morbidity due to malaria [15] with a measured reduction in mortality of six children per 1000 protected. Insecticide-treated bed nets work in two ways: by protecting individuals against infectious mosquito bites and by preventing uninfected mosquitoes from biting infectious people. Transmission-blocking vaccines will have an action similar to the latter. However, unlike bed nets that only work while a person is using the bed net, vaccination will give 24-hr protection and, after vaccination, requires no further active participation. The relative merits of ITN and TBV (and preferably both) will depend on the exact epidemiology and human behavior in a particular environment. However, the experience with ITNs strongly suggests that TBV will lead to a substantial reduction of malaria deaths in high endemic areas.

(4) *To slow the spread of drug-resistant or vaccine-resistant mutant parasites in all endemic areas.* A tragedy of malaria control has been the loss of safe, inexpensive, and effective antimalarial drugs through the development and spread of drug resistance. In the case of chloroquine, molecular typing of the chloroquine resistance locus and linked microsatellite markers suggests that chloroquine resistance present in *P. falciparum* has probably arisen from just four mutated parasites followed by its spread throughout the world over a period of 10–20 years [16]. Chloroquine-resistant *P. vivax* has now emerged in Papua New Guinea and adjacent areas in Indonesia, and may similarly spread [17]. Even in areas where a transmission-blocking vaccine may not decrease parasite prevalence, it would slow the spread of resistance mutants. Unfortunately, we anticipate that the problems observed with the spread of drug-resistant malaria will be mimicked by the spread of vaccine-resistant parasites as effective preerythrocytic or blood stage vaccines are developed. The incorporation of a transmission-blocking vaccine with vaccines targeting these stages may be an important strategy to preserve their effective life.

Three different types of TBV may be required:

1. A *P. vivax*-only vaccine. From WHO country profiles, there are approximately 130 million people living in regions where *P. vivax* is the only—or overwhelmingly dominant—parasite with a reported 700,000 cases. The actual number of cases will be much larger. For example, the Roll Back Malaria [18] program estimates that the number of cases of *P. vivax* malaria in Afghanistan alone was approximately 2–3 million in 2000.

2. A *P. vivax*/*P. falciparum* combination vaccine. The majority of the world's population at risk from malaria live in areas affected by both species. Mendis et al. [10] estimate that approximately 1.4 billion people outside of Africa live in malaria risk areas, experience approximately 116 million cases of malaria, with *P. vivax* accounting for 60% of these. Even in Africa where *P. falciparum* dominates, some areas (e.g., Sudan, Ethiopia, and other East African countries) have significant rates of *P. vivax* [10].

3. A *P. falciparum*-only vaccine. This vaccine would be required for most of Africa and countries where the population is primarily of West African origin (e.g., Haiti). About 500 million people are at risk in these areas, resulting in 200–300 million cases of malaria and approximately 1 million deaths annually [10,19].

The concept of a malaria TBV was demonstrated by vaccination of chickens with formalin-treated or X-irradiated blood drawn from birds infected with *P. gallinaceum* [20], or with partially purified preparations of extracellular gametes of *P. gallinaceum* [21]. These birds were not immune to the blood stage infection, but were markedly less infectious to *Aedes aegypti*, one of the mosquitoes that can transmit *P. gallinaceum*. With multiple immunizations with extracellular gametes, 99.99% suppression of infectivity was achieved

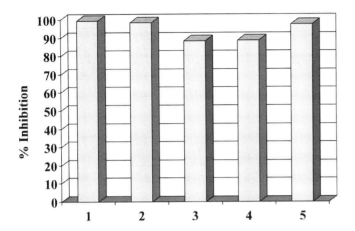

Figure 2 Membrane feeding assay of transmission-blocking immunity. Blood containing mature gametocytes is mixed with a test antiserum and placed in a small glass chamber whose base is sealed with a thin membrane. A glass jacket through which warm water circulates surrounds the chamber. Mosquitoes attracted to the warm blood feed through the membrane. Mosquitoes are then held in an insectory until oocysts have developed, the gut has been removed and stained, and the number of oocysts has been counted. (From Refs. 31,32,34,135.)

Transmission-blocking activity is measured by either (a) the decrease in the average number of oocysts on mosquitoes fed test antisera compared with mosquitoes fed control sera (i.e., a decrease in the intensity of infection), or (b) the decrease in the proportion of mosquitoes that have at least one oocyst (i.e., a decrease in the frequency of infection).

A decrease in the average number of oocysts is used in our laboratory to assess experimental vaccines because the mosquitoes and source of parasites have been chosen to give reproducibly high infection rates to maximize the statistical significance of the assay. In part, this is achieved by using relatively high gametocyte densities that tend to produce high oocyst numbers. Under these conditions, antisera that gave even a 90% blockage of oocyst development may have a minimal impact on the proportion of mosquitoes infected.

In the field, the efficacy of a vaccine is likely to be proportional to the number of mosquitoes that fail to become infected at all (i.e., have zero oocysts). In predicting the impact of a TBV, it will be critical to know the distribution of oocysts in naturally infected mosquitoes. The data available from wild caught feeds and laboratory simulations show that this distribution is highly skewed, with most mosquitoes infected with very few (often only one or two) oocysts but a small number of mosquitoes infected with large numbers. (From Refs. 164–168.) Under these conditions, predictions of vaccine efficacy based on reduction in oocyst numbers in the laboratory will overestimate field efficacy because the vaccine will probably fail to prevent the infection of a small proportion of mosquitoes that would have been infected with a large number of oocytes. However, provided that most natural infections result in few oocysts per gut, then this error will not be large. On the other hand, because of the very great differences in the average numbers of oocysts per gut in laboratory infections compared with field data, predictions of efficacy based on the proportion of mosquitoes failing to be infected in the laboratory are likely to grossly underestimate field efficacy.

[22]. Panels of monoclonal antibodies (mAbs) that inhibited transmission [23] and immunoprecipitated proteins of 240,000, 56,000, and 54,000 kDa [24] on the surface of male and female gametes were developed. As detailed below, homologs of these proteins and other targets of transmission-blocking immunity have been identified on *P. falciparum*, *P. vivax*, other primate malarias, and rodent malarias. Many studies with monoclonal antibodies used in vitro or by passive transfer of polyclonal antibody raised against parasite-derived and recombinant gamete, zygote, or ookinete proteins have demonstrated that blocking transmission through vaccination is feasible (see later sections for specific references).

Antibodies to the *P. falciparum* homologs, Pfs230 and Pfs48/45, can be demonstrated in populations living in highly endemic areas who have a high prevalence of infection with gametocytes [25–30]. As assayed by the ability of sera to block the infection of mosquitoes when mixed either with parasites ex vivo or laboratory-derived parasites and fed to mosquitoes via an artificial membrane (Figure 2) [31,32], naturally occurring TBI can be demonstrated [25,33–41]. Correlations have been found with the level of TBI for both anti-Pfs230 [25,42] and anti-Pfs48/45 antibody [38,39].

II. TARGETS OF TRANSMISSION-BLOCKING VACCINE

The potential components of TBV can be conveniently grouped in four categories:

The six-cys motif gamete and zygote surface antigens
The epidermal growth factor (EGF) domain ookinete surface antigens
Other malaria proteins
Mosquito proteins.

A. The Six-Cys Motif Gamete and Zygote Surface Proteins

Early studies of gamete surface proteins identified three proteins that are synthesized in both male and female gametocytes. Following the release of the gametes from their red cells, these proteins are found on the surface of gametes. They coprecipitated with polyclonal and monoclonal antibodies that blocked transmission. These three proteins from *P. falciparum* had apparent sizes of 230, 48, and 45 kDa on reducing sodium dodecyl sulfate (SDS) polyacrylamide electrophoresis [43,44]. The 230-kDa protein can be separated from the 48- and 45-kDa proteins by phase separation using Triton X-114 [45]. Subsequently, it was shown the 48- and 45-kDa proteins are different forms of a single protein [46] (although the reasons for the two forms are still not understood) and so these gamete proteins were described as Pfs230 and Pfs48/45. When the genes encoding these proteins were cloned, it became clear that both belong to the same superfamily of genes, characterized by domains with up to six cysteines [47]. Genes encoding at least seven proteins in this family are now known in the *P. falciparum* genome [48]. The repeating motif in these proteins has not been found outside the genus *Plasmodium*. The predicted proteins all have signal peptides and some have a C-terminal hydrophobic peptide that probably is recognized as a GPI anchor signal by the parasite.

1. Pfs48/45 and Orthologs

The genes coding for the Pfs48/45 orthologs (P48/45 proteins) have been cloned from *P. falciparum* [46], *P. reichenowi* [49], *P. vivax*, and *P. berghei* [50]. The four orthologs show considerable similarity: the *P. berghei* and *P. vivax* proteins share 54% and 55% amino acids, respectively, with the *P. falciparum* sequence. Pfs48/45 is 448 amino acids long, starts with a signal peptide, contains three copies of the six-cys motif, and terminates with a putative GPI anchor. Consistent with the presence of a GPI anchor, Pfs48/45 can be labeled with [^{3}H]glucosamine or [^{3}H]mannose [44,51]. In *P. falciparum*, *P. vivax*, and *P. berghei* genomes, the gene encoding P48/45 is adjacent to a similar gene encoding P47, another member of the six-cys domain family. Presumably, this arrangement has arisen by gene duplication [50].

Four epitopes were defined on Pfs48/45 by monoclonal antibodies [44,52,53] and human recombinant antibodies [54]. Epitopes I, II, and III are reduction-sensitive. Monoclonal antibodies directed against epitope I are efficient at blocking transmission either as the intact antibody or as a Fab fragment [52,55]. At least one mAb (1A3-B8) directed against epitope II has transmission-blocking activity that increases in the presence of a complement. Another mAb (IIC5-B10) directed against region III has weak transmission-blocking activity, although no transmission-blocking activity of other rat and mouse antiepitope II and III mAbs has been observed [55]. However, marked synergistic blocking (>98% inhibition of transmission) was found when mosquitoes were fed a mixture of epitope II and epitope III mAbs 1A3-B8 and IIC5-B10 [52,56].

Based on reactivity with different parasites, mAbs directed against region II can be divided into two groups: the panspecific IIb and the polymorphic allelic forms IIa/IIc. Binding to the latter correlates with two adjacent amino acid substitutions in the second six-cys motif [47,57]. A further three amino acids have been observed to be polymorphic in the third motif [57], but as yet, these have not been associated with antigenic diversity. The geographical distribution of these polymorphisms is highly biased [58–60].

Gene knockout experiments confirm the essential role of Pfs48/45 and its *P. berghei* ortholog, Pbs48/45, in fertilization. Knockout mutants form gametocytes and gametes but have greatly reduced zygote formation. Although P48/45 is on both male and female gametes, surprisingly, the gene knockout only affected the male gametes. Female knockout gametes were efficiently fertilized by wild-type male gametes, but not vice versa [50].

So far, the expression of Pfs48/45 for use as a vaccine has not been achieved. In *Escherichia coli*, the full-length protein (including signal peptide and C-terminal transmembrane domain) was toxic to the host cells. A truncated protein missing the last two cysteines of the third six-cys motif was expressed at a high level as an insoluble inclusion body, as the free protein, or as a GST fusion protein. When solubilized and used to immunize mice and rabbits, the GST fusion protein gave high-titer antibody, but this did not recognize gametes or block transmission [61]. Expression in eukaryotes is complicated by the presence of seven potential glycosylation sites that are not used in *P. falciparum*. Attempts to express the protein in eukaryotic systems with a variety of constructs—with and without the glycosylation sites removed, or with optimized codon use in *Saccharomyces*, Pichia [62], or in a vaccinia system [63]—have not yielded materials suitable for human vaccines.

2. Pfs230

When the gene coding Pfs230 was cloned and sequenced [64], the full-length protein was much larger than the apparent size of 230 kDa observed in immunoprecipitates of surface-labeled gametes. The gene encodes a 360-kDa protein, consisting of a signal peptide, a relatively unremarkable 260-amino-acid N-terminal domain, a stretch of 25 consecutive glutamic acids, 16 copies of a tetrapeptide repeat (EEGV), and 14 copies of the six-cys motif. These 14 motifs are arranged in seven pairs, with the odd-numbered motifs containing only one or two of the consensus three consensus disulfides [47]. Other than the signal peptide, Pfs230 has no transmembrane domain and the mature protein is presumably anchored to the gamete surface through its interaction with Pfs48/45 [45].

The protein is present in gametocytes as the 360-kDa form predicted from the gene sequence. On transformation to gametes, Pfs230 is cleaved to give proteins of 300 and 307 kDa on the gamete surface. Cleavages occur between amino acids 477–487 and 523–555, respectively [65], resulting in a mature protein that lacks the poly-glutamic acid region and the EEGV repeats. It has been speculated that the N-terminal region may act as an immune evasion mechanism to divert an immune system response to this N-terminal region shed on the emergence of the gametes in the mosquito [66]. Consistent with this hypothesis, EEGV repeat was the region recognized most frequently by sera from adults living in a highly endemic region of The Gambia [67], although this study may not have detected antibodies directed against conformational epitopes. It is also consistent with the early observation in the *P. gallinaceum* model that gametes were much more effective in inducing transmission-blocking antibodies than gametocytes [22].

Full-length sequences are available from four isolates [68] (GenBank locus AF269242; Z. X. Shan et al., unpublished) and partial sequences from two other isolates [60]. By comparison with asexual stage surface proteins, Pfs230 is highly conserved. In the ~300-kDa gamete form, only 18 of 2650 amino acids are polymorphic. In addition, there is a short, low-complexity region (amino acids 2413–2420 in the 3D7 sequence) in which there is some variation in an EEQQ repeat. Consistent with this lack of sequence diversity, 17 mAbs out of a panel 18 of mAbs, known to recognize at least nine different epitopes, bound to gametocytes from all isolates tested [53,69].

At least 15 anti-Pfs230 mAbs, which block the transmission of parasites to mosquitoes, have been identified [69–

72]. With one exception (a mAb that recognizes a linear epitope present on at least three gamete proteins [73] and whose transmission-blocking target is therefore not clear), all recognize reduction-sensitive epitopes, all are of complement-fixing IgG2a or IgG2b subclasses, and all require the presence of active complements to kill parasites. As judged by competition experiments, these mAbs recognize at least five different epitopes. In fact, all known anti-Pfs230 IgG2a and IgG2b mAbs are able to block transmission in a complement-dependent manner [69,70,72]. Transmission-blocking activity in the mosquito correlates with the lysis of female gametes and zygotes in vitro [69,70]. The dependence for complement fixation was dramatically illustrated by the subclass switching of a nonblocking IgG1 mAb to transmission-blocking, complement-dependent IgG2a and IgG2b subclass mAbs [71].

The size, the number of cysteines, and the apparent requirement for correct folding make the expression of full-length Pfs230 suitable for use as a vaccine, a daunting task. Williamson et al. [74] and Bustamante et al. [75] have approached vaccine development by expressing domains of the protein in *E. coli*. One region covering the first pair of six-cys motifs and expressed as a maltose-binding protein chimeria (r230/MBP.C) elicited significant transmission blocking, although this was substantially lower than the transmission-blocking activity of monoclonal antibodies. None of the domains gave a strong signal on Western blotting with 19 anti-Pfs230 mAbs, suggesting that *E. coli*-expressed proteins are not correctly folded [67].

As for P48/45, the development of a transmission-blocking vaccine based on Pfs230 remains an attractive goal, but will require the development of ways of efficiently expressing correctly folded six-cys motifs.

B. The P25 and P28 EGF Domain Zygote, Ookinete, and Oocyst Antigens

Two proteins with sizes of 26 and 28 kDa on reducing SDS gels were identified by surface labeling of *P. gallinaceum* zygotes and ookinetes. These proteins were present on ookinetes but not earlier stages [43,76–78]. The 26-kDa protein appeared about 2 hr postfertilization and the 28-kDa protein appeared 3–5 hr postfertilization [43]. Both could be labeled with glucosamine and palmitic acid [51]. Monoclonal antibodies directed against these proteins blocked the development of parasites in mosquitoes, identifying them as potential targets of transmission-blocking antibodies [76, 78].

A similar 25-kDa protein was identified on the surface of *P. falciparum* ookinetes as the target of transmission-blocking antibody [79,80]. When the gene coding the *P. falciparum* 25-kDa protein was cloned and sequenced, it was found that the protein consisted of four-tandem EGF-like domains [81]. As expected for a surface protein, the sequence encoded a typical signal peptide. The translated protein sequence ended with a hydrophobic domain and, consistent with earlier observations that the protein could be labeled with glucosamine and palmitic acid [44], this sequence probably is replaced by a GPI anchor in the mature protein.

Subsequently, the genes encoding the 26-kDa *P. gallinaceum* protein [82] and the ortholog from *P. reichenowi* [83] were cloned. As expected from their close evolutionary relationship, the *P. falciparum* and *P. reichenowi* genes are closely related. Surprisingly, a striking similarity was also found between the genes from the more distantly related *P. falciparum* and *P. gallinaceum* parasites [82]. Subsequently, the Pfs25 orthologs (P25 family) have been cloned from *P. berghei* [84], *P. yoelii* [85], *P. vivax* [86], and *P. ovale* [87].

The cloning of the 28-kDa surface protein from *P. gallinaceum* (Pgs28) showed that this protein had a structure similar to those Pfs25 and Pgs25, with a signal peptide, four EGF domains, and a C-terminal anchor sequence [88], but differed in the last EGF domain, which was truncated and ended with a short repeat region.

A 21-kDa protein, Pbs21, had also been identified on the surface of zygotes and ookinetes of the rodent malaria, *P. berghei*, as the target of monoclonal antibodies that blocked transmission [89,90]. Affinity-purified Pbs21 was able to induce transmission-blocking immunity in mice [91]. When the corresponding gene was cloned and sequenced, it was found that this protein was also a member of this four-EGF domain surface antigen family, the ortholog of Pgs28 [92]. Pgs28 orthologs (P28 family) have been cloned from *P. falciparum* [93], *P. yoelii* [85], *P. chabaudi* [94], *P. vinckei* [94], *P. vivax* [86], and *P. ovale* [87]. Unlike all other species so far examined, *P. ovale* has three members of the EGF surface protein family: Pos25, Pos28-1, and Pos28-2.

The expression of P25 and P28 family members has been studied in *P. gallinaceum*, *P. berghei*, *P. falciparum*, and *P. vivax*. Kumar and Carter [51] showed that in *P. gallinaceum*, Pgs25 is synthesized from approximately 2 hr postgametogenesis and continues to be synthesized for about another 8–10 hr. The expression of Pgs28 starts later, 3–5 hr postfertilization, but this continues until at least 22 hr postfertilization.

The low-level synthesis of Pfs25 was detected in immature *P. falciparum* gametocytes, but production dramatically increased following gametogenesis and fertilization [44]. In contrast, Fries et al. [95] only detected synthesis postinduction of gametes. Pfs28 is synthesized later. By immunofluorescence, Pfs28 is first observed on retort stages, the transitional stage between a zygote and an ookinete [93]. Similar results have been obtained with the P25 and P28 proteins from *P. vivax*. Anti-Pvs25 antibodies stained parasites ranging from zygotes to mature ookinetes, whereas anti-Pvs28 antibodies mainly stained retort and mature ookinete stage parasites [96]. In *P. berghei*, the protein expression of both the P25 (Pbs25) and P28 (Pbs21) proteins commenced in the macrogamete, with Pbs25 detectable 30 min following gametocyte activation and Pbs21 detectable after 2 hr [97]. The expression of Pbs21 reached the peak level approximately 10 hr postfertilization [98]. Surprisingly, the transcription of the *Pbs25* and *Pbs21* genes occurs in gametocytes prior to the release of gametes; thus, the translation of protein is subject to some unknown posttranscriptional controls [92,97]. Pbs21 is shed during the invasion of mosquito epithelial cells [99], but presumably, further synthesis results in the presence of antigens for at least 6 days [99,100]. Similarly, Pfs25 is also present in *P. falciparum* oocysts until rupture [101], and anti-

Pfs25 antibody has been used to improve the detection of early-stage oocysts in mosquito midguts [102].

Pfs25 and Pfs28 are closely linked to chromosome 10 [88]. Preliminary data available from both the *P. falciparum* and *P. yoelii* genome projects show in both species that the *P25* and *P28* genes are located approximately 1.5 kb apart. The close proximity of the genes and their related structure suggests that these proteins have arisen through gene duplication that preceded the speciation of the present-day *Plasmodium*.

Studies of the P25 and P28 proteins suggest that they are functionally redundant. In *P. berghei*, knockout of either the *P25* or the *P28* gene had little impact on the viability of ookinetes or the ability to invade the mosquito gut wall to form oocysts, but in the double knockout, the formation of ookinetes was significantly inhibited and the double knockout ookinetes had a much reduced capacity to transform into oocyts [103]. A variety of roles have been proposed for the P25 and P28 proteins. These include a surface coat to protect the parasite against lethal factors in the mosquito gut [103–106], and as specific receptors for endothelium and basal membrane proteins. The *P. berghei* P25 protein has been shown to interact with laminin [107], whereas the *P. gallinaceum* P28 has been shown to interact with both laminin and collagen IV [108].

Many studies show that antibodies against these two proteins can disrupt several stages in the development of parasites, including killing of zygotes/ookinetes and the prevention of the interaction of the ookinete with the mosquito midgut epithelium [8,78,88–91,93,96,97,109–126]. In mosquito feeds, intact monoclonal antibody, FAb fragments, or recombinant single-chain antibody targeting the P28 protein in *P. berghei* (Pbs21) were approximately equally efficacious at blocking transmission, suggesting that complement activation or interaction with cells via Fc receptors is not required in vivo [121,124,126]. These studies contrast with results obtained in culture, where intact antibodies and the presence of peripheral blood leukocytes were critical [125]. A mAb directed against Pgs25 in *P. gallinaceum* failed to affect the development of ookinetes in vitro. When taken up with gametocytes in a blood meal, it did not slow the development of ookinetes, but prevented oocyst formation [127]. That study concluded that antibodies bound on the ookinete prevented ookinetes from crossing the peritrophic membrane, rather than preventing the invasion of the gut epithelium. The peritrophic membrane separates the blood meal from the endothelial cells of the midgut, and must be crossed by malaria ookinetes before they can invade the actual gut wall.

In vivo, the available mechanisms for killing parasites will be further limited by the life of antibodies in the mosquito blood meal [128]. Although not conclusive, the available data suggest that both monoclonal and polyclonal antibodies against the P25 proteins are more efficient at preventing transmission than antibodies against the P28 proteins. This has been observed with monoclonal antibodies recognizing the Pgs25 and Pgs28 proteins of *P. gallinaceum* [78], monoclonal antibodies recognizing the Py25 and Pys28 of *P. yoelii* [118], and polyclonal antibodies directed against Pvs25 and Pvs28 of *P. vivax* [129].

Early results suggested that antibodies to a fusion protein of Pfs25 and Pfs28 were much more potent in transmission blocking than antibodies to Pfs25 alone [112]. However, subsequent studies with more highly characterized antigens failed to confirm these results. Antibodies to Pfs25 gave better transmission blocking than antibodies to the chimeric Pfs25–Pfs28 [110]. The trend that anti-P25 antibodies are more potent than anti-P28 antibodies is consistent with the earlier expression of the P25 proteins, suggesting that early events in the killing of parasites are important in transmission-blocking immunity.

Two studies have shown that the P25 and P28 proteins persist in the oocyst wall for up to 8 days, and that these remain accessible to antibodies. Mosquitoes typically feed every 2–4 days; thus, oocysts would be potentially susceptible to antibodies directed against P25 and P28 proteins taken up with feeds several days after becoming infected. Mouse polyclonal anti-Pfs25 taken up on days 3 and 6 following a feed containing *P. falciparum* gametocytes reduced the number of resulting sporozoites [101]. Monoclonal antibodies recognizing the P28 protein in *P. berghei* (Pbs21) reduced the number of oocysts present and the subsequent number of sporozoites when added to a second mosquito blood feed. The effect was greatest with a second feed 2 days after the primary feed [124]. These experiments have an important implication for transmission-blocking vaccines used in endemic regions where mosquitoes are highly anthropophagic: vaccines may be more effective than expected at less than 100% coverage because there will be several chances for transmission to be blocked following a feed by a mosquito on an infectious person.

1. Antigenic Diversity and Natural Immunity

As the P25 and P28 proteins are not expressed at significant levels in the vertebrate host, there is probably no immune selection driving antigenic diversity. Indeed, serological surveys failed to find antibodies directed against Pfs25 in human sera from highly endemic areas [130,131]. Some antigenic diversity has been reported from one study of field isolates. Foo et al. used a panel of monoclonal antibodies that recognized two epitopic regions of Pfs25. Two mAbs recognizing the "epitope II" recognized all 45 Malaysian isolates tested by an immunofluorescence assay (IFA) [53]. Three epitope I mAbs tested on the same parasite panel showed some variation in the IFA positivity. Several isolates gave no or weak fluorescence with one or more mAb. However, it is not clear if these weak IFA results represent true antigenic diversity because sequence data are not available to confirm these observations. The limited polymorphism seen in this study contrasts with the ability of an anti-Pfs25 mAb to block transmission in 13 of 13 field isolates from Cameroon [119] and the very limited diversity found by direct sequencing of the genes. For Pfs25, two amino acids have been found to be polymorphic from isolates tested from eight laboratory lines, 14 isolates from Brazil and 20 from Papua New Guinea [132,133]. Both of these substitutions were highly conservative: an alanine/glycine substitution at amino acid 131 and an alanine/valine substitution at amino acid amino acid 142.

The antigenic diversity of Pfs28 has not been studied. Very limited sequence polymorphism has been observed with a single arginine/lysine substitution observed in seven laboratory lines and 32 field isolates from the Philippines [134]. Greater sequence variation has been seen in Pvs25 and Pvs28 with three amino acid substitutions in Pvs25 and seven point substitutions in Pvs28, and with variation in the number of C-terminal repeats from four isolates [86]. One of the substitutions in the Pvs28 was nonconservative (a lysine/threonine polymorphism substitution at amino acid 65). The remainder conserved amino acid properties.

The low substitution frequencies, the conservative nature of the substitutions, and the likelihood that these have not been selected as a result of immune pressure [94,135] suggest that antigenic diversity will not be a major issue for P25- and P28-based vaccines.

2. P25/P28 Vaccine Development

Two major issues face the production of an effective P25- or P28-based vaccine: the production of the antigen in immunologically active form and the development of a formulation that generates a high-level, long-lasting antibody response.

Not surprising in view of the 10 or 11 disulfides present in the mature proteins, initial studies with Pfs25 and Pbs21 showed that antigens produced in E. coli were effective at eliciting antibodies, but these had poor transmission-blocking activities [114,136]. Three approaches have been taken to circumvent this obstacle:

Search for linear epitopes that induce transmission-blocking immunity
Use of live viral vectors and DNA vaccines to generate folded antigen in situ
Use of eukaryotic expression systems to produce correctly folded antigen.

Although most mAbs that recognize the P25/P28 proteins are sensitive to reduction of the protein, at least two monoclonal antibodies, 32F81 [137] and 4B7 [116], both block transmission and recognize linear or at least denatured proteins [138]. Based on this observation, Quakyi et al. [139] constructed a series of overlapping peptides spanning the sequence of Pfs25 and tested their ability to elicit transmission-blocking antibodies in mice. Peptides that gave consistent transmission-blocking activity were found, but the levels were low compared to the transmission-blocking activity induced by recombinant proteins, vaccinia constructs, or DNA vaccines (see below).

Although common in extracellular proteins of higher animals, EGF domains have not been found in any lower eukaryotes other than malaria parasites. Consistent with this phylogeny, they are not efficiently synthesized and correctly folded in prokaryotic or lower eukaryotic expression systems [140]. Therefore, vaccination by in situ expression of P25 and P28 family proteins in the vertebrate host is attractive because correct secretion and folding are likely to occur. Vaccinia constructs containing Pfs25 used to immunize mice gave potent transmission-blocking activity at relatively low antibody titers [117]. Pfs25 expression on the surface of

HeLa cells infected with Pfs25 containing vaccinia was readily detected and rhesus monkeys immunized with these constructs made fair titers of anti-Pfs25 antibodies that were able to react with Pfs25 on the surface of zygotes [141]. Thirty-six of 39 human volunteers vaccinated with NYVAC-Pf7, a vaccinia expressing seven P. falciparum antigens, had detectable antibodies against Pfs25. However, none of the sera had detectable transmission-blocking activity when mixed with infected blood and fed to mosquitoes in a membrane feeding apparatus [142], although several volunteers generated significant TBI when boosted with a recombinant Pfs25 adsorbed to alum [169].

The DNA vaccines expressing Pfs25 have been tested in mice [109,143]. High antibody levels were obtained with a vector containing a tissue plasminogen activator secretion signal, but not when the Pfs25 was expressed in the absence of a secretion signal [109]. Antibodies induced by this construct gave 95% transmission blocking when assayed in a membrane feeding experiment.

Three approaches have been taken to the expression of correctly folded antigen: expression in baculovirus [120,122, 123] and expression in Saccharomyces cerivisiae [96,110–116, 129,140,144].

The baculovirus system has been used to investigate vaccine production and immunization strategies using Pbs21, the P. berghei P28 protein. Expression of the full-length Pbs21 resulted in a GPI-anchored, hydrophobic protein that was difficult to purify [145]. Nevertheless, the immunization of mice with crude homogenates of insect cells expressing recPbs21 elicited similar anti-Pbs21 antibody titers as the native protein, and both were comparable at blocking transmission [123]. The removal of the C-terminal hydrophobic sequence resulted in a soluble secreted protein [120,145]. On nonreduced Western blots, this protein lacking the GPI anchor was strongly recognized by a mAb reacting with a linear epitope, but compared to the GPI-anchored recombinant protein, it was weakly recognized by a conformationally dependent anti-Pbs21 mAb. After two immunizations, either intramuscularly or subcutaneously with no adjuvant, native Pbs21 elicited higher antibody levels than the GPI-anchored recombinant Pbs21 and much higher levels that the secreted recPbs21 when assayed on native protein. After a third immunization, the secreted Pbs21 was able to generate high-level antibody and all three gave substantial transmission-blocking activity [120]. It is not clear if the difference in immunogenicity is due to structural differences of the antigen, adjuvant activity in the GPI anchor, or a combination of these. If baculovirus-produced P28 requires a membrane anchor for optimal immunogenicity and structure (as determined by the binding of mAbs recognizing conformational epitopes), then this makes it less attractive for vaccine manufacture.

Initial results of the expression of a recPfs25 (TBV25B) in S. cerevisae were encouraging. The secreted recombinant protein induced transmission-blocking antibodies in mice and monkeys when immunized with Freund's adjuvant or MF59 adjuvant containing muramyl tripeptide, even though a truncation in the construct must have resulted in an incompletely formed fourth EGF domain [116]. This protein reacted with several conformationally dependent mAbs but not as well as native proteins, suggesting that its conformation was not optimal. Subsequently, it was shown that in mice and Aotus monkeys, the protein was poorly immunogenic without adjuvants, but that alum was significantly more potent as an adjuvant than the MTP/MF59 combination [114,115]. A second-generation construct, TBV25H, which had a complete fourth EGF domain, was prepared, and production conditions were developed for producing materials suitable for Phase I human trials. With alum, TBV25H was more immunogenic that the earlier TBV25B but still showed some heterogeneity on nonreducing SDS electrophoresis [113]. TBV25H bound to alhydrogel has been used in a Phase I trial [169]. This trial was stopped when one of the volunteers experienced an atypical hypersensitivity reaction.

Although a similar *Saccharomyces* system has been used to express a number of P25 and P28 proteins for experimental use, close examination shows that a substantial proportion of EGF domains in malarial proteins expressed by *Saccharomyces* are incorrectly folded [140]. Detailed examination showed that only about 10% of Pfs25 or Pvs25 expressed in this system has all four EGF domains correctly folded. These observations led to a third-generation experimental vaccine based on Pfs25 and Pvs25 that relies on very high expression levels and an efficient purification system to prepare homogeneous, correctly folded antigen. Clinical-grade Pfs25 and Pvs25 have been produced. A Phase I clinical trial with Pvs25 is underway and a trial of Pfs25 will commence in the near future. In preclinical studies, Pvs25 and Pfs25 are able to elicit antibodies that efficiently block the transmission of malaria to mosquito using adjuvants that are, in principle, suitable for human vaccines. For example, when mixed with chimpanzee blood infected with *P. vivax* and fed to mosquitoes in a membrane feeding apparatus,

sera from rhesus monkeys immunized with Pvs25 emulsified in Montanide ISA720 adjuvant gave near-total transmission blockage (Figure 3).

At least for Phase I/II trials, a satisfactory method of producing antigen appears to have been achieved. The next challenge that can only be addressed in human trials will be to find a formulation that is well tolerated and elicits long-lasting and potent antibodies.

C. Other Malaria Proteins

Besides the six-cys motif and the EGF domain proteins, parasite-encoded chitinase and the circumsporozoite protein and thrombospondin-related protein (TRAP)-related protein (CTRP) [146] have been identified as having potential as transmission-blocking vaccine components.

Mosquitoes secrete an acellular chitin-containing membrane, the peritrophic membrane, that separates the blood meal from the endothelial cells of the midgut, which malaria ookinetes must cross before they can invade the actual gut wall. Ookinetes secrete a prochitinase, activated by endogenous mosquito proteases, that facilitates the passage of the ookinete through the peritrophic membrane [147,148]. Ingestion of allosamidin, a chitinase inhibitor, with the blood meal prevented oocyst formation. Two distinct chitinases secreted by *P. gallinaceum* ookinetes were separated by high-performance liquid chromatography [149] and the gene (*PgCHT1*) encoding one of these has been cloned [149]. An ortholog of this gene, PbCHT1, has been identified in *P. berghei* [150] and a gene *PfCHT1* encoding a chitinase in *P. falciparum* [151]. From the structure of the genes and the corresponding proteins, PbCHT1 is probably the ortholog of PgCHT1, whereas the *P. falciparum* PfCHT1 is likely to be a paralog of the PbCHT1 and PgCHT1 and an ortholog

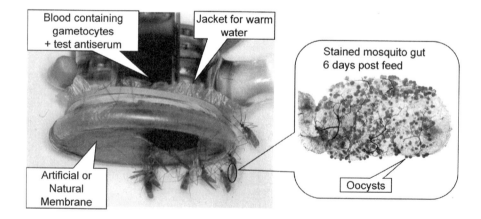

Figure 3 Transmission blockage of *P. vivax* to mosquitoes by anti-Pvs25 sera from immunized rhesus monkeys. Five rhesus monkeys were immunized with two injections at a 4-week interval with 25 μg of Pvs25H emulsified in Montanide ISA720. Sera were collected 2 weeks after the boost immunization and a 1:2 dilution was mixed with chimpanzee cells infected with *P. vivax* and fed to *A. stephensi* mosquitoes. Control mosquitoes received infected cells mixed with a 1:2 dilution of preimmunization serum from each monkey. Mosquitoes were dissected after 10 days and the number of oocysts present in the mosquitoes fed on the prevaccinated and postvaccinated sera was counted. Percent inhibition was calculated as the $100 \times [1-($Number of oocysts in postvaccination feeds$)/$ (Number of oocyts in prevaccination feeds$)]$. Mosquitoes fed prevaccination sera plus infected red cells had an average of 80 oocysts per mosquito (unpublished data).

of the as yet uncloned gene coding for the second chitinase in *P. gallinaceum* [152]. The two groups of chitinases differ in several aspects. PfCHT1 lacks a putative chitin-binding domain found in PgCHT1 and PbCHT1. It also lacks the proenzyme domain and is fully active when expressed in *E. coli* [151]. Interestingly, an ortholog of PbCHT1 cannot be identified in *P. falciparum* genome, nor can an ortholog of PfCHT1 be identified in the *P. yoelii* genome project, although the PbCHT1 ortholog is present in this database. Therefore, it is likely that *P. falciparum* and the rodent malarias have only one chitinase, whereas *P. gallinaceum* has two genes: one of each type. For both *P. falciparum* [153] and *P. berghei* [150], knockout of the identified chitinase gene reduces the infectivity of ookinetes. Recombinant parasite chitinases will now make it possible to test if this enzyme has potential as a vaccine candidate [8,154].

The CTRP is found in the microneme organelle at the apical end of mature ookinetes [155]. This protein has six copies of an integrin I adhesion domain (also found in extracellular vertebrate proteins such as von Willebrand factor) followed by seven copies of another binding domain, the thrombospondin type I domain [146]. Integrin I and TSP I domains are also found in another *Plasmodium* protein, TRAP, and a TSP I domain is found in the circumsporozoite protein. Similar genes encoding CRTP have been identified in *P. falciparum* [146] and *P. berghei* [156]. Knockout of the *CTRP* gene from *P. berghei* [155,157] or *P. falciparum* [158] interferes with the motility of the ookinete, invasion of the mosquito midgut, and transformation to oocysts.

Both chitinase and CRTP appear to play critical roles in the development of the mosquito stage parasites. However, both are expressed relatively late in the development cycle of the parasite in the mosquito midgut. It is not clear if sufficient antibodies against these proteins would survive the digestion of blood meal by mosquito proteolytic enzymes long enough to impact on parasite development to make them useful vaccine targets.

D. Antimosquito Approaches

The development of a commercial veterinary vaccine for protecting cattle against infestation with cattle ticks [159,160], and for preventing tick-borne disease such as babesiosis demonstrated the feasibility of producing transmission-blocking vaccines by attacking the concealed antigens in the vector. Several target antigens that may form the basis of a TBV have now been identified in mosquitoes.

A trypsinlike protease is secreted by the mosquito gut following a blood meal. Antitrypsin antibodies are able to block the activity of this enzyme and prevent parasite development [161]. Interestingly, these antibodies appear to have no detrimental effect on the mosquito survival or fecundity, and appear to work, not by preventing the digestion of the blood meal, but by preventing the activation of the prochitinase secreted by the ookinete. Because this is required for the parasite to cross the peritrophic membrane, blocking trypsin effectively prevents the escape of the ookinete out of the blood meal bolus.

Polyclonal antibodies raised against midgut proteins of *Anopheles gambiae* block the transition of *P. falciparum* and *P. vivax* ookinetes to oocysts [162]. Three monoclonal antibodies derived from mice immunized with midgut preparations blocked parasite development, gave a small decrease in mosquito survival, and decreased fecundity. Periodate treatment of extracted gut proteins prevented the binding of two of the mAbs, suggesting that their targets are oligosaccharides.

Unexpectedly, monoclonal antibodies directed against 29- and 100-kDa proteins in the salivary gland, when present in the blood meal, are able to attain a high-enough concentration in the mosquito hemolymph to partially block the invasion of sporozoites into the salivary gland [163]. The mechanism by which antibodies can cross the gut wall and appear in the hemolymph is not known, although there are several reports to show that this is not limited to these particular antibodies.

III. HUMAN TRIALS AND VACCINE DEVELOPMENT PLANS

With two vaccine candidates Pvs25 and Pfs25 entering Phase I human trials in 2002, issues of how to test and develop TBV are now assuming greater importance.

On one hand, transmission-blocking vaccines have a number of features that simplify their development. These include:

A well-defined mechanism of action (i.e., neutralization of parasites by antibody)

A powerful in vitro test, the membrane feed (Fig. 3), that is believed to provide a useful prediction of protection

Target groups in which the presence or absence of naturally occurring immunity is not likely to be a major modulator of the efficacy of the vaccine.

As a result, it should be feasible to experiment with different formulations, dose, etc., to give optimal transmission blocking in a series of relatively small Phase I vaccine trials. Importantly, from a vaccine development perspective, these tools should provide a solid basis for a decision not to proceed to field trials if the level of transmission-blocking activity elicited in a Phase I trial has been insufficient. Effectively, much of the information (i.e., a demonstration of a biological effect on parasites) that would require Phase II trials of other vaccines will be obtained as part of a Phase I study with transmission-blocking vaccines.

Provided the encouraging results obtained so far with Pvs25 and Pfs25 in preclinical studies translate to human trials, progress through Phase I studies is likely to be relatively rapid. On the other hand, Phase III and preregistration trials of transmission-blocking vaccines, where the aim is to document the level of village-wide reduction in malaria transmission, will require considerable resources. Because these vaccines are unlikely to attract substantial commercial investment, the development of appropriate partnerships between the public and private sectors for the development, manufacture, and deployment of transmission-blocking vaccines will be as important as the underlying biotechnology. An important step toward this goal has been the creation of a collaborative network of researchers interested in developing and testing transmission-blocking vaccines [8] under the umbrella of the Malaria Vaccine Initiative at the Program for Appropriate Technology in Health (PATH) through a grant from the Bill and Melinda Gates Foundation [8].

ACKNOWLEDGMENTS

I thank my colleagues at the Malaria Vaccine Development Unit and the MVI Transmission-Blocking Vaccine Consortium, Dr. John Beier, Professor Robert Sinden, and Professor Richard Carter for review of the manuscript and their suggestions. Thanks to Dr. Robert Gwadz for the photographs.

REFERENCES

1. Breman JG. The ears of the hippopotamus: manifestations, determinants, and estimates of the malaria burden. Am J Trop Med Hyg 2001; 64:1–11.
2. Gallup JL, Sachs JD. The economic burden of malaria. Am J Trop Med Hyg 2001; 64:85–96.
3. Remme JHE, et al. Toward a framework and indicators for monitoring Roll Back Malaria. Am J Trop Med Hyg 2001; 64:76–84.
4. Trape JF. The public health impact of chloroquine resistance in Africa. Am J Trop Med Hyg 2001; 64:12–17.
5. Saul AJ. Vaccine strategies for malaria: applicability in areas of seasonal or epidemic malaria. Southeast Asian J Trop Med Public Health 1992; 23(suppl 4):89–92.
6. Healer J, et al. Phagocytosis does not play a major role in naturally acquired transmission-blocking immunity to Plasmodium falciparum malaria. Infect Immun 1999; 67:2334–2339.
7. Saul A. Kinetic constraints on the development of a malaria vaccine. Parasite Immunol 1987; 9:1–9.
8. Carter R. Transmission blocking malaria vaccines. Vaccine 2001; 19:2309–2314.
9. Carter R, et al. Malaria transmission-blocking vaccines—how can their development be supported? Nat Med 2000; 6:241–244.
10. Mendis K, et al. The neglected burden of Plasmodium vivax malaria. Am J Trop Med Hyg 2001; 64:97–106.
11. Kleinschmidt I, et al. An empirical malaria distribution map for West Africa. Trop Med Int Health 2001; 6:779–786.
12. Beier JC, et al. Short report: entomologic inoculation rates and Plasmodium falciparum malaria prevalence in Africa. Am J Trop Med Hyg 1999; 61:109–113.
13. Snow RW, Marsh K. Will reducing Plasmodium falciparum transmission alter malaria mortality among African children? Parasitol Today 1995; 11:188–190.
14. Smith TA, et al. Child mortality and malaria transmission intensity in Africa. Trends Parasitol 2001; 17:145–149.
15. Lengeler C. Insecticide-treated bed nets and curtains for preventing malaria. Cochrane Libr 2001.
16. Wootton JC, et al. Genome-wide haplotypes, linkage disequilibrium, and chloroquine selection sweeps in the falciparum parasite. Nature 2002; 418:320–323.
17. Schuurkamp GJ, et al. Chloroquine-resistant Plasmodium vivax in Papua New Guinea. Trans R Soc Trop Med Hyg 1992; 86:121–122.
18. Roll Back Malaria. Country Profiles. http://mosquito.who.int/cgi-bin/rbm/countryprofile.jsp 2001.
19. Breman JG, et al. The intolerable burden of malaria: a new look at the numbers. Am J Trop Med Hyg 2001; 64:iv–vii.
20. Gwadz RW. Successful immunization against the sexual stages of Plasmodium gallinaceum. Science 1976; 193:1150–1151.
21. Carter R, Chen DH. Malaria transmission blocked by immunisation with gametes of the malaria parasite. Nature 1976; 263:57–60.
22. Carter R, et al. Plasmodium gallinaceum: transmission-blocking immunity in chickens I. Comparative immunogenicity of gametocyte- and gamete-containing preparations. Exp Parasitol 1979; 47:185–193.
23. Rener J, et al. Anti-gamete monoclonal antibodies synergistically block transmission of malaria by preventing fertilization in the mosquito. Proc Natl Acad Sci USA 1980; 77:6797–6799.
24. Kaushal DC, et al. Monoclonal antibodies against surface determinants on gametes of Plasmodium gallinaceum block transmission of malaria parasites to mosquitoes. J Immunol 1983; 131:2557–2562.
25. Graves PM, et al. Antibodies to Plasmodium falciparum gamete surface antigens in Papua New Guinea sera. Parasite Immunol 1988; 10:209–218.
26. Graves PM, et al. Naturally occurring antibodies to an epitope on Plasmodium falciparum gametes detected by monoclonal antibody-based competitive enzyme-linked immunosorbent assay. Infect Immun 1988; 56:2818–2821.
27. Graves PM, et al. Association between HLA type and antibody response to malaria sporozoite and gametocyte epitopes is not evident in immune Papua New Guineans. Clin Exp Immunol 1989; 78:418–423.
28. Graves PM, et al. High frequency of antibody response to Plasmodium falciparum gametocyte antigens during acute malaria infections in Papua New Guinea highlanders. Am J Trop Med Hyg 1990; 42:515–520.
29. Ong CS, et al. The primary antibody response of malaria patients to Plasmodium falciparum sexual stage antigens which are potential transmission-blocking vaccine candidates. Parasite Immunol 1990; 12:447–456.
30. Riley EM, et al. Human antibody responses to Pfs 230, a sexual stage-specific surface antigen of Plasmodium falciparum: non-responsiveness is a stable phenotype but does not appear to be genetically regulated. Parasite Immunol 1994; 16:55–62.
31. Graves PM. Studies on the use of a membrane feeding technique for infecting Anopheles gambiae with Plasmodium falciparum. Trans R Soc Trop Med Hyg 1980; 74:738–742.
32. Ponnudurai T, et al. Infectivity of cultured Plasmodium falciparum gametocytes to mosquitoes. Parasitology 1989; 98 (Part 2):165–173.
33. Drakeley CJ, et al. Transmission-blocking effects of sera from malaria-exposed individuals on Plasmodium falciparum isolates from gametocyte carriers. Parasitology 1998; 116:417–423.
34. Lensen A, et al. Measurement by membrane feeding of reduction in Plasmodium falciparum transmission induced by endemic sera. Trans R Soc Trop Med Hyg 1996; 90:20–22.
35. Lensen A, et al. Mechanisms that reduce transmission of Plasmodium falciparum malaria in semiimmune and nonimmune persons. J Infect Dis 1998; 177:1358–1363.
36. Mulder B, et al. Plasmodium falciparum: membrane feeding assays and competition ELISAs for the measurement of transmission reduction in sera from Cameroon. Exp Parasitol 1999; 92:81–86.
37. Roeffen W, et al. A comparison of transmission-blocking activity with reactivity in a Plasmodium falciparum 48/45-kD molecule-specific competition enzyme-linked immunosorbent assay. Am J Trop Med Hyg 1995; 52:60–65.

38. Roeffen W, et al. Association between anti-Pfs48/45 reactivity and *P. falciparum* transmission-blocking activity in sera from Cameroon. Parasite Immunol 1996; 18:103–109.

39. Graves PM, et al. Human antibody responses to epitopes on the *Plasmodium falciparum* gametocyte antigen PFS 48/45 and their relationship to infectivity of gametocyte carriers. Am J Trop Med Hyg 1992; 46:711–719.

40. Ranawaka MB, et al. Boosting of transmission-blocking immunity during natural *Plasmodium vivax* infections in humans depends upon frequent reinfection. Infect Immun 1988; 56:1820–1824.

41. Mendis C, et al. Characteristics of malaria transmission in Kataragama, Sri Lanka: a focus for immuno-epidemiological studies. Am J Trop Med Hyg 1990; 42:298–308.

42. Healer J, et al. Complement-mediated lysis of *Plasmodium falciparum* gametes by malaria-immune human sera is associated with antibodies to the gamete surface antigen Pfs230. Infect Immun 1997; 65:3017–3023.

43. Kumar N, Carter R. Biosynthesis of the target antigens of antibodies blocking transmission of *Plasmodium falciparum*. Mol Biochem Parasitol 1984; 13:333–342.

44. Vermeulen AN, et al. Characterization of *Plasmodium falciparum* sexual stage antigens and their biosynthesis in synchronised gametocyte cultures. Mol Biochem Parasitol 1986; 20:155–163.

45. Kumar N. Phase separation in Triton X-114 of antigens of transmission-blocking immunity in *Plasmodium gallinaceum*. Mol Biochem Parasitol 1985; 17:343–358.

46. Kocken CH, et al. Cloning and expression of the gene coding for the transmission blocking target antigen Pfs48/45 of *Plasmodium falciparum*. Mol Biochem Parasitol 1993; 61:59–68.

47. Carter R, et al. Predicted disulfide-bonded structures for three uniquely related proteins of *Plasmodium falciparum*, Pfs230, Pfs48/45 and Pf12. Mol Biochem Parasitol 1995; 71:203–210.

48. Templeton TJ, Kaslow DC. Identification of additional members define a *Plasmodium falciparum* gene superfamily which includes Pfs48/45 and Pfs230. Mol Biochem Parasitol 1999; 101:223–227.

49. Milek RL, et al. *Plasmodium reichenowi*: deduced amino acid sequence of sexual stage-specific surface antigen Prs48/45 and comparison with its homologue in *Plasmodium falciparum*. Exp Parasitol 1997; 87:150–152.

50. van Dijk MR, et al. A central role for P48/45 in malaria parasite male gamete fertility. Cell 2001; 104:153–164.

51. Kumar N, Carter R. Biosynthesis of two stage-specific membrane proteins during transformation of *Plasmodium gallinaceum* zygotes into ookinetes. Mol Biochem Parasitol 1985; 14:127–139.

52. Carter R, et al. Properties of epitopes of Pfs 48/45, a target of transmission blocking monoclonal antibodies, on gametes of different isolates of *Plasmodium falciparum*. Parasite Immunol 1990; 12:587–603.

53. Foo A, et al. Conserved and variant epitopes of target antigens of transmission-blocking antibodies among isolates of *Plasmodium falciparum* from Malaysia. Am J Trop Med Hyg 1991; 44:623–631.

54. Roeffen WF, et al. Recombinant human antibodies specific for the Pfs48/45 protein of the malaria parasite *Plasmodium falciparum*. J Biol Chem 2001; 276:19807–19811.

55. Roeffen W, et al. *Plasmodium falciparum*: production and characterization of rat monoclonal antibodies specific for the sexual-stage Pfs48/45 antigen. Exp Parasitol 2001; 97, 45–49.

56. Graves PM, et al. Effects of transmission-blocking monoclonal antibodies on different isolates of *Plasmodium falciparum*. Infect Immun 1985; 48:611–616.

57. Kocken CH, et al. Variation in the transmission-blocking vaccine candidate Pfs48/45 of the human malaria parasite *Plasmodium falciparum*. Mol Biochem Parasitol 1995; 69: 115–118.

58. Drakeley CJ, et al. Geographical distribution of a variant epitope of Pfs48/45, a *Plasmodium falciparum* transmission-blocking vaccine candidate. Mol Biochem Parasitol 1996; 81:253–257.

59. Conway DJ, et al. Extreme geographical fixation of variation in the *Plasmodium falciparum* gamete surface protein gene Pfs48/45 compared with microsatellite loci. Mol Biochem Parasitol 2001; 115:145–156.

60. Niederwieser I, et al. Limited polymorphism in *Plasmodium falciparum* sexual-stage antigens. Am J Trop Med Hyg 2001; 64:9–11.

61. Milek RL, et al. Immunological properties of recombinant proteins of the transmission-blocking vaccine candidate, Pfs48/45, of the human malaria parasite *Plasmodium falciparum* produced in *Escherichia coli*. Parasite Immunol 1998; 20:377–385.

62. Milek RL, et al. Assembly and expression of a synthetic gene encoding the antigen Pfs48/45 of the human malaria parasite *Plasmodium falciparum* in yeast. Vaccine 2000; 18:1402–1411.

63. Milek RL, et al. *Plasmodium falciparum*: heterologous synthesis of the transmission-blocking vaccine candidate Pfs48/45 in recombinant vaccinia virus-infected cells. Exp Parasitol 1998; 90:165–174.

64. Williamson KC, et al. Cloning and expression of the gene for *Plasmodium falciparum* transmission-blocking target antigen, Pfs230. Mol Biochem Parasitol 1993; 58:355–358.

65. Brooks SR, Williamson KC. Proteolysis of *Plasmodium falciparum* surface antigen, Pfs230, during gametogenesis. Mol Biochem Parasitol 2000; 106:77–82.

66. Williamson KC, et al. Stage-specific processing of Pfs230, a *Plasmodium falciparum* transmission-blocking vaccine candidate. Mol Biochem Parasitol 1996; 78:161–169.

67. Riley EM, et al. Human immune recognition of recombinant proteins representing discrete domains of the *Plasmodium falciparum* gamete surface protein, Pfs230. Parasite Immunol 1995; 17:11–19.

68. Williamson KC, Kaslow DC. Strain polymorphism of *Plasmodium falciparum* transmission-blocking target antigen Pfs230. Mol Biochem Parasitol 1993; 62:125–127.

69. Read D, et al. Transmission-blocking antibodies against multiple, non-variant target epitopes of the *Plasmodium falciparum* gamete surface antigen Pfs230 are all complement-fixing. Parasite Immunol 1994; 16:511–519.

70. Quakyi IA, et al. The 230-kDa gamete surface protein of *Plasmodium falciparum* is also a target for transmission-blocking antibodies. J Immunol 1987; 139:4213–4217.

71. Roeffen W, et al. Transmission blockade of *Plasmodium falciparum* malaria by anti-Pfs230-specific antibodies is isotype dependent. Infect Immun 1995; 63:467–471.

72. Roeffen W, et al. *Plasmodium falciparum*: a comparison of the activity of Pfs230-specific antibodies in an assay of transmission-blocking immunity and specific competition ELISAs. Exp Parasitol 1995; 80:15–26.

73. Wizel B, Kumar N. Identification of a continuous and cross-reacting epitope for *Plasmodium falciparum* transmission-blocking immunity. Proc Natl Acad Sci USA 1991; 88:9533–9537.

74. Williamson KC, et al. Recombinant Pfs230, a *Plasmodium falciparum* gametocyte protein, induces antisera that reduce the infectivity of *Plasmodium falciparum* to mosquitoes. Mol Biochem Parasitol 1995; 75:33–42.

75. Bustamante PJ, et al. Differential ability of specific regions of *Plasmodium falciparum* sexual-stage antigen, pfs230, to induce malaria transmission-blocking immunity. Parasite Immunol 2000; 22:373–380.

76. Carter R, et al. Target antigens in malaria transmission-blocking immunity. Philos Trans R Soc Lond B Biol Sci 1984; 307:201–213.

77. Carter R, Kaushal DC. Characterization of antigens on mosquito midgut stages of *Plasmodium gallinaceum*. III. Changes in zygote surface proteins during transformation to mature ookinete. Mol Biochem Parasitol 1984; 13:235–241.

78. Grotendorst CA, et al. A surface protein expressed during the transformation of zygotes of *Plasmodium gallinaceum* is a target of transmission-blocking antibodies. Infect Immun 1984; 45:775–777.

79. Vermeulen AN, et al. Sequential expression of antigens on sexual stages of *Plasmodium falciparum* accessible to transmission-blocking antibodies in the mosquito. J Exp Med 1985; 162:1460–1476.

80. Vermeulen AN, et al. *Plasmodium falciparum* transmission blocking monoclonal antibodies recognize monovalently expressed epitopes. Dev Biol Stand 1985; 62:91–97.

81. Kaslow DC, et al. A vaccine candidate from the sexual stage of human malaria that contains EGF-like domains. Nature 1988; 333:74–76.

82. Kaslow DC, et al. Comparison of the primary structure of the 25 kDa ookinete surface antigens of *Plasmodium falciparum* and *Plasmodium gallinaceum* reveal six conserved regions. Mol Biochem Parasitol 1989; 33:283–287.

83. Lal AA, et al. Primary structure of the 25-kilodalton ookinete antigen from *Plasmodium reichenowi*. Mol Biochem Parasitol 1990; 43:143–145.

84. Tsuboi T, et al. Primary structure of a novel ookinete surface protein from *Plasmodium berghei*. Mol Biochem Parasitol 1997; 85:131–134.

85. Tsuboi T, et al. Comparison of *Plasmodium yoelii* ookinete surface antigens with human and avian malaria parasite homologues reveals two highly conserved regions. Mol Biochem Parasitol 1997; 87:107–111.

86. Tsuboi T, et al. Sequence polymorphism in two novel *Plasmodium vivax* ookinete surface proteins, Pvs25 and Pvs28, that are malaria transmission-blocking vaccine candidates. Mol Med 1998; 4:772–782.

87. Tachibana M, et al. Presence of three distinct ookinete surface protein genes, Pos25, Pos28-1, and Pos28-2, in *Plasmodium ovale*. Mol Biochem Parasitol 2001; 113:341–344.

88. Duffy PE, et al. Pgs28 belongs to a family of epidermal growth factor-like antigens that are targets of malaria transmission-blocking antibodies. J Exp Med 1993; 177:505–510.

89. Winger LA, et al. Ookinete antigens of *Plasmodium berghei*. Appearance on the zygote surface of an M_r 21 kD determinant identified by transmission-blocking monoclonal antibodies. Parasite Immunol 1988; 10:193–207.

90. Tirawanchai N, Sinden RE. Three non-repeated transmission blocking epitopes recognized in the 21 kD surface antigen of zygotes–ookinetes of *Plasmodium berghei*. Parasite Immunol 1990; 12:435–446.

91. Tirawanchai N, et al. Analysis of immunity induced by the affinity-purified 21-kilodalton zygote–ookinete surface antigen of *Plasmodium berghei*. Infect Immun 1991; 59:36–44.

92. Paton MG, et al. Structure and expression of a post-transcriptionally regulated malaria gene encoding a surface protein from the sexual stages of *Plasmodium berghei*. Mol Biochem Parasitol 1993; 59:263–275.

93. Duffy PE, Kaslow DC. A novel malaria protein, Pfs28, and Pfs25 are genetically linked and synergistic as *falciparum* malaria transmission-blocking vaccines. Infect Immun 1997; 65:1109–1113.

94. Taylor D, et al. Sequence diversity in rodent malaria of the Pfs28 ookinete surface antigen homologs. Mol Biochem Parasitol 2000; 110:429–434.

95. Fries HC, et al. Biosynthesis of the 25-kDa protein in the macrogametes/zygotes of *Plasmodium falciparum*. Exp Parasitol 1990; 71:229–235.

96. Hisaeda H, et al. Antibodies to malaria vaccine candidates Pvs25 and Pvs28 completely block the ability of *Plasmodium vivax* to infect mosquitoes. Infect Immun 2000; 68:6618–6623.

97. del Carmen R, et al. Characterisation and expression of pbs25, a sexual and sporogonic stage specific protein of *Plasmodium berghei*. Mol Biochem Parasitol 2000; 110:147–159.

98. Sinden RE, et al. Ookinete antigens of *Plasmodium berghei*: a light and electron-microscope immunogold study of expression of the 21 kDa determinant recognized by a transmission-blocking antibody. Proc R Soc Lond B Biol Sci 1987; 230:443–458.

99. Han YS, et al. Molecular interactions between *Anopheles stephensi* midgut cells and *Plasmodium berghei*: the time bomb theory of ookinete invasion of mosquitoes. EMBO J 2000; 19:6030–6040.

100. Simonetti AB, et al. Kinetics of expression of two major *Plasmodium berghei* antigens in the mosquito vector, *Anopheles stephensi*. J Eukaryot Microbiol 1993; 40:569–576.

101. Lensen AH, et al. Transmission blocking antibody of the *Plasmodium falciparum* zygote/ookinete surface protein Pfs25 also influence sporozoite development. Parasite Immunol 1992; 14:471–479.

102. Gouagna LC, et al. The use of anti-Pfs 25 monoclonal antibody for early determination of *Plasmodium falciparum* oocyst infections in *Anopheles gambiae*: comparison with the current technique of direct microscopic diagnosis. Exp Parasitol 1999; 92:209–214.

103. Tomas AM, et al. P25 and P28 proteins of the malaria ookinete surface have multiple and partially redundant functions. EMBO J 2001; 20:3975–3983.

104. Yeates RA, Steiger S. Ultrastructural damage of in vitro cultured ookinetes of *Plasmodium gallinaceum* (Brumpt) by purified proteinases of susceptible *Aedes aegypti* (L.). Z Parasitenkd 1981; 66:93–97.

105. Grotendorst CA, et al. Complement effects on the infectivity of *Plasmodium gallinaceum* to *Aedes aegypti* mosquitoes. I. Resistance of zygotes to the alternative pathway of complement. J Immunol 1986; 136:4270–4274.

106. Grotendorst CA, Carter R. Complement effects of the infectivity of *Plasmodium gallinaceum* to *Aedes aegypti* mosquitoes. II. Changes in sensitivity to complement-like factors during zygote development. J Parasitol 1987; 73:980–984.

107. Vlachou D, et al. *Anopheles gambiae* laminin interacts with the P25 surface protein of *Plasmodium berghei* ookinetes. Mol Biochem Parasitol 2001; 112:229–237.

108. Adini A, Warburg A. Interaction of *Plasmodium gallinaceum* ookinetes and oocysts with extracellular matrix proteins. Parasitology 1999; 119(Part 4):331–336.

109. Lobo CA, et al. Immunization of mice with DNA-based Pfs25 elicits potent malaria transmission-blocking antibodies. Infect Immun 1999; 67:1688–1693.

110. Gozar MM, et al. *Plasmodium falciparum*: immunogenicity of alum-adsorbed clinical-grade TBV25-28, a yeast-secreted malaria transmission-blocking vaccine candidate. Exp Parasitol 2001; 97:61–69.

111. Stowers AW, et al. A region of *Plasmodium falciparum* antigen pfs25 that is the target of highly potent transmission-blocking antibodies. Infect Immun 2000; 68:5530–5538.

112. Gozar MM, et al. *Saccharomyces cerevisiae*-secreted fusion proteins Pfs25 and Pfs28 elicit potent *Plasmodium falciparum* transmission-blocking antibodies in mice. Infect Immun 1998; 66:59–64.

113. Kaslow DC, Shiloach J. Production, purification and immunogenicity of a malaria transmission-blocking vaccine

candidate: TBV25H expressed in yeast and purified using nickel-NTA agarose. Biotechnology (New York) 1994; 12: 494–499.

114. Kaslow DC, et al. *Saccharomyces cerevisiae* recombinant Pfs25 adsorbed to alum elicits antibodies that block transmission of *Plasmodium falciparum*. Infect Immun 1994; 62: 5576–5580.

115. Kaslow DC, et al. Induction of *Plasmodium falciparum* transmission-blocking antibodies by recombinant Pfs25. Mem Inst Oswaldo Cruz 1992; 87(suppl 3):175–177.

116. Barr PJ, et al. Recombinant Pfs25 protein of *Plasmodium falciparum* elicits malaria transmission-blocking immunity in experimental animals. J Exp Med 1991; 174:1203–1208.

117. Kaslow DC, et al. Induction of *Plasmodium falciparum* transmission-blocking antibodies by recombinant vaccinia virus. Science 1991; 252:1310–1313.

118. Tsuboi T, et al. Two antigens on zygotes and ookinetes of *Plasmodium yoelii* and *Plasmodium berghei* that are distinct targets of transmission-blocking immunity. Infect Immun 1997; 65:2260–2264.

119. Mulder B, et al. Anti-Pfs25 monoclonal antibody 32F81 blocks transmission from *Plasmodium falciparum* gametocyte carriers in Cameroon. Trans R Soc Trop Med Hyg 1996; 90:195.

120. Martinez AP, et al. The roles of the glycosylphosphatidylinositol anchor on the production and immunogenicity of recombinant ookinete surface antigen Pbs21 of *Plasmodium berghei* when prepared in a baculovirus expression system. Parasite Immunol 2000; 22, 493–500.

121. Yoshida S, et al. A single-chain antibody fragment specific for the *Plasmodium berghei* ookinete protein Pbs21 confers transmission blockade in the mosquito midgut. Mol Biochem Parasitol 1999; 104:195–204.

122. Matsuoka H, et al. Induction of anti-malarial transmission-blocking immunity with a recombinant ookinete surface antigen of *Plasmodium berghei* produced in silkworm larvae using the baculovirus expression vector system. Vaccine 1996; 14:120–126.

123. Margos G, et al. Expression of the *Plasmodium berghei* ookinete protein Pbs21 in a baculovirus-insect cell system produces an efficient transmission blocking immunogen. Parasite Immunol 1995; 17:167–176.

124. Ranawaka G, et al. The effect of transmission-blocking antibody ingested in primary and secondary bloodfeeds, upon the development of *Plasmodium berghei* in the mosquito vector. Parasitology 1993; 107:225–231.

125. Ranawaka GR, et al. Characterization of the effector mechanisms of a transmission-blocking antibody upon differentiation of *Plasmodium berghei* gametocytes into ookinetes in vitro. Parasitology 1994; 109:11–17.

126. Ranawaka GR, et al. Characterization of the modes of action of anti-Pbs21 malaria transmission-blocking immunity: ookinete to oocyst differentiation in vivo. Parasitology 1994; 109:403–411.

127. Sieber KP, et al. The peritrophic membrane as a barrier: its penetration by *Plasmodium gallinaceum* and the effect of a monoclonal antibody to ookinetes. Exp Parasitol 1991; 72: 145–156.

128. Beier JC, et al. Bloodmeal identification by direct enzyme-linked immunosorbent assay (ELISA), tested on *Anopheles* (Diptera: Culicidae) in Kenya. J Med Entomol 1988; 25:9–16.

129. Hisaeda H, et al. Antibodies to *Plasmodium vivax* transmission-blocking vaccine candidate antigens Pvs25 and Pvs28 do not show synergism. Vaccine 2001; 20:763–770.

130. Carter R, et al. Restricted or absent immune responses in human populations to *Plasmodium falciparum* gamete antigens that are targets of malaria transmission-blocking antibodies. J Exp Med 1989; 169:135–147.

131. Quakyi IA, et al. Differential non-responsiveness in humans of candidate *Plasmodium falciparum* vaccine antigens. Am J Trop Med Hyg 1989; 41:125–134.

132. Kaslow DC, et al. Minimal variation in a vaccine candidate from the sexual stage of *Plasmodium falciparum*. Mol Biochem Parasitol 1989; 32:101–103.

133. Shi YP, et al. Single amino acid variation in the ookinete vaccine antigen from field isolates of *Plasmodium falciparum*. Mol Biochem Parasitol 1992; 50:179–180.

134. Hafalla JC, et al. Minimal variation in the Pfs28 ookinete antigen from Philippine field isolates of *Plasmodium falciparum*. Mol Biochem Parasitol 1997; 87:97–99.

135. Tsuboi T, et al. Transmission-blocking vaccine of *Plasmodium vivax* malaria. Parasitol Int 2003; 52:1–11.

136. Matsuoka H, et al. Studies on the immunogenicity of a recombinant ookinete surface antigen Pbs21 from *Plasmodium berghei* expressed in *Escherichia coli*. Parasite Immunol 1994; 16:27–34.

137. van-Amerongen A, et al. Identification of a peptide sequence of the 25 kD surface protein of *Plasmodium falciparum* recognized by transmission-blocking monoclonal antibodies: implications for synthetic vaccine development. Parasite Immunol 1989; 11:425–428.

138. van-Amerongen A, et al. Peptides reactive with a transmission-blocking monoclonal antibody against *Plasmodium falciparum* Pfs25: 2000-fold affinity increase by. Pept Res 1992; 5:269–274.

139. Quakyi IA, et al. Synthetic peptides from *P. falciparum* sexual stage 25-kDa protein induce antibodies that react with the native protein: the role of IL-2 and conformational structure on immunogenicity of Pfs25. Pept Res 1995; 8:335–344.

140. Stowers AW, et al. Structural conformers produced during malaria vaccine production in yeast. Yeast 2001; 18:137–150.

141. Tine JA, et al. NYVAC-Pf7: a poxvirus-vectored, multiantigen, multistage vaccine candidate for *Plasmodium falciparum* malaria. Infect Immun 1996; 64:3833–3844.

142. Ockenhouse CF, et al. Phase I/IIa safety, immunogenicity, and efficacy trial of NYVAC-Pf7, a pox-vectored, multiantigen, multistage vaccine candidate for *Plasmodium falciparum* malaria. J Infect Dis 1998; 177:1664–1673.

143. Grifantini R, et al. Multi-plasmid DNA vaccination avoids antigenic competition and enhances immunogenicity of a poorly immunogenic plasmid. Eur J Immunol 1998; 28:1225–1232.

144. Wang MY, et al. Production of a malaria transmission-blocking protein from recombinant yeast. Ann NY Acad Sci 1996; 782:123–132.

145. Blanco AR, et al. The biosynthesis and post-translational modification of Pbs21 an ookinete-surface protein of *Plasmodium berghei*. Mol Biochem Parasitol 1999; 98:163–173.

146. Trottein F, Triglia T, Cowman AF. Molecular cloning of a gene from *Plasmodium falciparum* that codes for a protein sharing motifs found in adhesive molecules from mammals and plasmodia. Mol Biochem Parasitol 1995; 74:129–141.

147. Huber M, et al. Malaria parasite chitinase and penetration of the mosquito peritrophic membrane. Proc Natl Acad Sci USA 1991; 88:2807–2810.

148. Shahabuddin M, et al. Transmission-blocking activity of a chitinase inhibitor and activation of malarial parasite chitinase by mosquito protease. Proc Natl Acad Sci USA 1993; 90:4266–4270.

149. Vinetz JM, et al. Chitinases of the avian malaria parasite *Plasmodium gallinaceum*, a class of enzymes necessary for parasite invasion of the mosquito midgut. J Biol Chem 2000; 275:10331–10341.

150. Dessens JT, et al. Knockout of the rodent malaria parasite

chitinase pbcht1 reduces infectivity to mosquitoes. Infect Immun 2001; 69:4041–4047.

151. Vinetz JM, et al. The chitinase PfCHT1 from the human malaria parasite *Plasmodium falciparum* lacks proenzyme and chitin-binding domains and displays unique substrate preferences. Proc Natl Acad Sci USA 1999; 96:14061–14066.

152. Langer RC, Vinetz JM. *Plasmodium* ookinete-secreted chitinase and parasite penetration of the mosquito peritrophic matrix. Trends Parasitol 2001; 17:269–272.

153. Tsai YL, et al. Disruption of *Plasmodium falciparum* chitinase markedly impairs parasite invasion of mosquito midgut. Infect Immun 2001; 69:4048–4054.

154. Kaslow DC. Transmission-blocking vaccines: uses and current status of development. Int J Parasitol 1997; 27:183–189.

155. Dessens JT, et al. CTRP is essential for mosquito infection by malaria ookinetes. EMBO J 1999; 18:6221–6227.

156. Yuda M, et al. Structure and expression of an adhesive protein-like molecule of mosquito invasive-stage malarial parasite. J Exp Med 1999; 189:1947–1952.

157. Yuda M, et al. Targeted disruption of the *Plasmodium berghei* CTRP gene reveals its essential role in malaria infection of the vector mosquito. J Exp Med 1999; 190:1711–1716.

158. Templeton TJ, et al. Development arrest of the human malaria parasite *Plasmodium falciparum* within the mosquito midgut via CTRP gene disruption. Mol Microbiol 2000; 36:1–9.

159. Willadsen P, Jongejan F. Immunology of the tick–host interaction and the control of ticks and tick-borne diseases. Parasitol Today 1999; 15:258–262.

160. De La FJ, et al. Immunological control of ticks through vaccination with Boophilus microplus gut antigens. Ann NY Acad Sci 2000; 916:617–621.

161. Shahabuddin M, et al. Antibody-mediated inhibition of *Aedes aegypti* midgut trypsins blocks sporogonic development of *Plasmodium gallinaceum*. Infect Immun 1996; 64: 739–743.

162. Lal AA, et al. Anti-mosquito midgut antibodies block development of *Plasmodium falciparum* and *Plasmodium vivax* in multiple species of *Anopheles* mosquitoes and reduce vector fecundity and survivorship. Proc Natl Acad Sci USA 2001; 98:5228–5233.

163. Brennan JD, et al. *Anopheles gambiae* salivary gland proteins as putative targets for blocking transmission of malaria parasites. Proc Natl Acad Sci USA 2000; 97:13859–13864.

164. Carter R, Graves PM. Gametocytes. In: Wernsdorfer W, McGregor I, eds. Malaria. Edinburgh: Churchill Livingstone, 1988:235–305.

165. Graves PM, et al. Measurement of malarial infectivity of human populations to mosquitoes in the Madang area, Papua, New Guinea. Parasitology 1988; 96:251–263.

166. Sattabongkot J, et al. *Plasmodium vivax*: gametocyte infectivity of naturally infected Thai adults. Parasitology 1991(Part 1); 102:27–31.

167. Medley GF, et al. Heterogeneity in patterns of malarial oocyst infections in the mosquito vector. Parasitology 1993; 106:441–449.

168. Toure YT, et al. Gametocyte infectivity by direct mosquito feeds in an area of seasonal malaria transmission: implications for Bancoumana, Mali as a transmission-blocking vaccine site. Am J Trop Med Hyg 1998; 59:481–486.

169. Kalsow DC. Transmission-blocking vaccines. Chem Immunol 2002; 80:287–307.

74

Vaccines Against *Leishmania*

Farrokh Modabber and Antonio Campos-Neto*
Infectious Disease Research Institute, Seattle, Washington, U.S.A.

Steven G. Reed
Corixa Corporation and Infectious Disease Research Institute, Seattle, Washington, U.S.A.

I. INTRODUCTION

More than a dozen identified and characterized species of the genus *Leishmania* cause diseases, ranging from simple self-healing cutaneous lesions to debilitating and lethal (if untreated) visceral leishmaniasis (VL) known as kala-azar (Table 1). Other less frequent forms are mucosal leishmaniasis (ML), a highly disfiguring disease of oral and nasal cavities, and diffuse cutaneous leishmaniasis (DCL), with hundreds of nodular lesions spread over the body. Self-limiting visceral infections with some *Leishmania* species (*Leishmania infantum* [1], *L. donovani* [2], and, possibly *L. tropica* [3]) may also occur. These asymptomatic individuals as well as cured cases would later develop disease if their immune responses are depressed by drugs or human immunodeficiency virus (HIV) infection, indicating nonsterile immunity following cure [4]. The persistence of parasites in resistant mouse strains long after the recovery of the initial lesion has been documented [5,6], and leishmaniasis recidivans (reappearance of new satellite lesions) around the original healed lesion is occasionally seen with *L. tropica* infection. In this respect, leishmaniasis is considered as an opportunistic infection [7]. All forms of leishmaniasis are naturally transmitted by the bites of female sandflies either from infected humans (anthroponotic leishmaniasis) or from infected animals (zoonotic). Generally, there is a good association between the organism and the type of disease it produces in humans (Table 1). However, *L. tropica*, usually the causative agent of anthroponotic cutaneous leishmaniasis (ACL), may cause VL as was seen in U.S. soldiers returning from the Desert Storm operation [3], and *L.*

infantum, the causative agent of zoonotic VL, can cause CL [8]. Approximately 350 million people are believed to be at risk of infection and the annual incidence of new cases is about 2 million, mostly in children and young adults (1.5 million CL and the rest VL). The current estimated prevalence is 12 million, distributed in 88 countries [9]. These figures do not include epidemics, which can claim the lives of tens of thousands of individuals, eliminate communities, and cause massive migration [10].

With resistance to first-line drugs (antimonials) up to 60%, in certain parts of India, the mortality rate from VL is very high [11]. The pattern of disease has changed dramatically in the past decade in southwestern Europe where HIV infection has shifted from what was a pediatric disease to one of adults. In different countries of Southern Europe, between 25% and 75% of all cases of VL emerge from people infected with the HIV. Moreover, 1.5–9.5% of all patients with acquired immunodeficiency syndrome (AIDS) suffer from newly acquired or reactivated VL (http://www.who.int/inf-fs/en) in different countries of Europe.

Leishmaniasis is present in all continents except in Oceania, but is restricted to temperate and tropical climates (45° north to 35° south) perhaps due to the survival and activity period of the vectors. More than two dozen sandfly species are vectors of leishmaniasis (*Lutzomya* in the Americas and *Phlebotomus* in the rest of the world). Transmission by contaminated needles in drug abusers has been documented [12]. Leishmaniasis has diverse epidemiological characteristics, and transmission occurs intradomiciliary or paradomiciliary, or in the wild, with forests, deserts, and mountains making reservoir or vector control difficult or impossible. The first-line drugs (antimonials) developed almost a century ago require repeated injections (4 weeks of daily injections for VL), are costly, are often associated with side effects, and are becoming ineffective in many endemic foci. Therefore, an effective, safe, and affordable

---

Current affiliation: The Forsyth Institute, Boston, Massachusetts, U.S.A.

Table 1 Most Common Etiological Agents of Human
Leishmaniasis

Disease	Old world	New world
Cutaneous leishmaniasis	*L. tropica*	*L. mexicana*
	L. major	*L. amazonensis*
	L. aetiopica	*L. brasiliensis*
	L. infantum	*L. panamensis*
		L. guynensis
		L. peruviana
		Others
Mucosal leishmaniasis	*L. aetiopica*	*L. brasiliensis*
		L. guynensis
		L. panamensis
Visceral leishmaniasis	*L. donovani*	*L. chagasi*[a]
	L. infantum	
	L. archibaldi?	
Diffuse cutaneous	*L. aetiopica*	*L. amazonensis*
leishmaniasis		*L. pifanoi*

[a] May be the same as *L. infantum*.

vaccine is regarded as the best control means for all forms of leishmaniasis.

Antigenic cross-reactivity among *Leishmania* is so high that sera of patients cannot be used to identify the causative species; hence, it is hoped that with a single vaccine, it might be possible to protect against different *Leishmania* species. Some experimental and epidemiological data support this notion [13,14], but exception is also seen in experimental leishmaniasis [15]. Several reviews have been published on experimental vaccines against leishmaniasis [16–20]. Here we emphasize those in development and in clinical trials.

II. IMMUNOLOGY OF LEISHMANIASIS

Acquired resistance to leishmaniasis is mediated by T cells. T-cell-deficient mice rapidly succumb after infection with most species of *Leishmania*, and adoptive transfer of normal T cells confers resistance to the animals. Moreover, as mentioned before, patients with AIDS are highly susceptible to leishmaniasis either as a result of concurrent infection, or as a reactivation of older subclinical infection [4]. Among the T cells, CD4$^+$ are crucial for resistance whereas CD8$^+$ T cells seem to participate more in the memory events of the immune response than as effector cells involved in parasite elimination. These conclusions were reached from a series of experiments using mice genetically engineered to lack either the class I or class II major histocompatibility complex (MHC) molecules, or in mice lacking CD4 or CD8 cells. In addition, the spectrum of susceptibility of different strains of mice to *L. major* infection has been extremely helpful for the understanding of the genetic control of the disease and the mechanism of protection or susceptibility mediated by different subsets of CD4$^+$ T cells [21–24]. Hence, the outcome of *L. major* infection in mice is under a multigene control system. Most of these genes do not map in the MHC systems of either humans or mice [25–27]. Resistant strains such as

C3H C57BL/6, CBA/J, or B10D2 normally develop a small lesion, which heals spontaneously within 4–6 weeks, whereas the BALB/c strain is so exquisitely susceptible that even a few metacyclic parasites will cause a full-blown lethal disease that cannot be treated with first-line drugs (antimonials). The BALB/c mice develop a progressive local lesion and a systemic, visceralized disease [28] with a pathology somewhat similar to human VL, including weight loss, hepatosplenomegaly, lymphadenopathy, hyperglobulinemia, anemia, leucopenia and thrombocytopenia, and, finally, death. In addition, this outcome is directly related to the typical Th2 response observed in these animals [29]. Mice of the resistant phenotype clearly develop a dominant Th1 phenotype of immune response to the parasite's antigens and interference with this response will make them susceptible [30,31].

In contrast to T cells, B cells are apparently important only during the early events involving the development of parasite-specific immune response. However, B cells themselves and the specific antibodies they produce are not involved in the host effector mechanisms against the parasites. When B-cell-deficient mice of the resistant phenotype were infected with either *L. mexicana* or *L. donovani*, they did not develop the disease [32–34].

In humans, circumstantial observations that show a direct correlation between Th1 response and resistance are primarily applicable to CL. A predominance of IFN-γ producing cells has generally been found in healing cutaneous lesions whereas in chronic cutaneous or mucosal lesions, a mixture of type 1 and type 2 cytokines with a striking abundance of IL-4 mRNA has been consistently found [35,36]. In VL, however, no association with increased IL-4 and active disease could be found. Both splenic IFN-γ mRNA and IL-4 mRNA are elevated during active disease, and decline significantly after cure. This same pattern of cytokine profile production occurs after antigenic stimulation of peripheral blood mononuclear cells (PBMCs) of patients with active disease and after cure [37]. However, a direct correlation between IL-10 production and active disease was reported in VL patients [38,39]. In conclusion, human studies similar to the murine observations point to a preferential association of Th1 cytokines with resistance against cutaneous leishmaniasis. Therefore, the design of a vaccine against CL should involve immunization protocols that generate primarily IFN-γ and little or no IL-4 responses to the leishmanial vaccine components.

III. ANIMAL MODELS FOR VACCINE STUDIES

Many *Leishmania* species infect mice, hamsters, and nonhuman primates. In addition, the natural hosts of some parasites [i.e., *Psammomys* (the wild rodent for *L. major*) and dogs (for *L. infantum*)] have been used as laboratory animals. These models have been very important in studying the parasite biology, natural history, and, particularly, the immunology of leishmaniasis as mentioned above. However, none of these animal models has been validated for vaccine studies for human diseases. Although a few investigators have used the resistant strains, the BALB/c and *L. major* infection have been most extensively used for vaccine studies. It is thought that if a vaccine can protect BALB/c mice, then it should also protect humans. Laboratory animals are usually challenged by cultured promastigotes without the components of sandflies, which have a profound impact on the fate of the infection [40]. Sometimes amastigotes are injected intravenously when promastigote injection intradermally does not produce rapid or uniform infection (i.e., in dogs), or infection with *L. donovani* in mice and hamsters. Skin-associated immune responses are crucial for protection against all forms of leishmaniasis as the port of entry is skin. Hence, a vaccine may protect against an intravenous injection of amastigotes but has no impact against natural disease [41]. To promote infection, promastigotes isolated from infected sandflies just prior to injection of dogs [42], or exudates of salivary glands of sandflies mixed with culture promastigotes have been used in mice [40] and monkeys [43]. Belkaid et al. [44] have developed a model by which infected sandflies deliver the parasite to the ears of mice. This is the most natural mode of delivering the challenge organism; however, it is not easily quantifiable.

IV. TARGET ANTIGENS FOR VACCINE DEVELOPMENT

The life cycle of the parasite is relatively simple. *Leishmania* exists in two principal forms: promastigote, the flagellated form in the invertebrate host that can be grown in cell-free tissue culture media, and amastigote, the round intracellular form in the vertebrate's macrophages. There is some differential antigen expression in these two forms and most vaccine candidates are selected to be present at least in the amastigotes, although their presence in promastigotes as well is an added advantage. The promastigotes also undergo antigenic changes in the process of maturation from procyclical (noninfective attached to the wall of the midgut of sandflies) to infective metacyclical form (released to the foregut for delivery during blood meal). This maturation also occurs in culture for most *Leishmania*. These antigens, essentially lipophosphoglycans of the promastigote surface, are considered as possible antigens for transmission-blocking vaccines as are components of sandfly guts [45–49]. Specific antibodies to these antigens transferred to the sandfly during the blood meal could, in principle, prevent the normal maturation of the parasite within the vector.

Another intriguing target for vaccine development against leishmaniasis is the sandfly saliva. Recent observations in mouse models point to a protective effect of the phlebotomine's saliva components against challenge with *L. major*. The mechanism of this protection has not yet been completely elucidated. However, it has been suggested that the immunization of mice with the saliva of *Phlebotomus papatasi* induces a strong delayed-type hypersensitivity (DTH) to the saliva components. When parasites are delivered with salivary gland excretions during a blood meal, a local delayed-type hypersensitivity reaction, which could mediate parasites killing, is induced [50,51]. That a DTH to unrelated antigens at the site of infection could enhance healing was shown long ago [52]. The inclusion of sandfly

components that may induce hypersensitivity in a vaccine given to normal individuals who are exposed to bites of sandflies (mostly uninfected) may not be without risks. Further studies are needed to validate this approach.

V. VACCINES IN USE

There is no current prophylactic vaccine available for general use against leishmaniasis. "Leishmanization,"an ancient preventive practice, is still used in high-risk populations in Uzbekistan. This consists of inoculating live virulent *L. major* to produce a self-healing lesion at a covered part of the body. This lesion will induce a protective response against natural infection, with multiple lesions on the face and other exposed parts of the body. Resistance to reinfection following recovery from CL was known to be very high when the natural history of the disease was described more than 500 years ago [53]. In its initial practice, pus from an active lesion was used for inoculation. Later, when the parasite was grown in vitro, axenically grown *L. major* was used for inoculation [54,55].

Presently, in Uzbekistan, a mixture of dead and live *L. major* is given, which usually produces a lesion of 1–2 cm in diameter that lasts 3–4 months and heals spontaneously. The Israeli group also used leishmanization in the 1960s and 1970s on over 5000 high-risk individuals [56]. It was noted that the "take" rate of the vaccine dropped precipitously (from 85% to 15%) over the years using the same organism, which was repeatedly subcultured [57]. To overcome this, Greenblatt et al. [58] developed a simple method to produce stabilates by freezing the parasite, which preserved its virulence for long periods. Nevertheless, the program was discontinued due to unwanted side effects, including allergic response in preexposed individuals, long duration of active lesion, and lack of immunity in the "nontake" individuals [59]. Leishmanization was practiced in large scale primarily in soldiers as the last resort in Iran during the Iran–Iraq war in the 1980s [60], following a trial in civilians [59] that showed over 98% efficacy. The leishmanization program was stopped after the war mainly due to the prolonged duration of lesions and the appearance of a few nonhealing cases, which were very difficult to treat. At present, stabilates have been prepared under the guidelines of good manufacturing practices (GMP) and leishmanization is being used in hyperendemic foci following vaccination with killed *Leishmania* vaccines as a live challenge for the evaluation of the efficacy of the killed vaccines (Khamesipour et al., personal communication).

Although antigen selection studies have led to the identification of several candidate molecules and most (but not all) have been produced as recombinant proteins (see "Second-Generation Vaccines"below), none has been taken into clinical development yet. This is primarily because the market for a leishmaniasis vaccine is conceived to be very limited and only of local importance within the endemic regions. Most laboratories do not have the resources required for preclinical and clinical development and the large pharmaceutical industries are not interested because of small markets. The best solution is to promote a vaccine-producing facility in a developing country (where leishmaniasis is of public health importance) to good manufacturing practices standards and to seek local governments' support for purchasing and distribution. Philanthropic support for the transfer of technology and production under GMP conditions is needed as most donor agencies for medical research are not interested in development. Hence, the generous grant of the Bill and Melinda Gates Foundation has allowed one such candidate vaccine (a trifusion of leishmanial antigens with a novel adjuvant) to enter clinical development with the view of transferring the production to an endemic country to assure low cost and sustainability, should the vaccine prove to be efficacious.

VI. FIRST-GENERATION VACCINES (KILLED LEISHMANIA WITH OR WITHOUT ADJUVANTS)

Whole killed parasites, if given by appropriate route, and adjuvants can protect many experimental animals and hence have been used as a gold standard to evaluate different vaccine candidates. Because most *Leishmania* species can easily be grown in cell-free cultures, killed parasites have been tried as a vaccine much in the same way as early bacterial vaccines. The history of vaccine trials using killed *Leishmania* goes back to the 1920s and 1930s first for immunotherapy and then in the 1940s for prophylaxis (reviewed by Genaro et al. [61]). More recently, Mayrink et al. in Brazil, following the earlier studies of Pessoa [62] and Convit et al. using bacille Calmette–Guérin (BCG) as an adjuvant in Venezuela, initiated vaccine trials with killed *Leishmania* in prophylactic trials as well as therapeutical trials (see below).

VII. NEW WORLD (MULTIPLE STRAINS)

The initial vaccine of Mayrink et al. [63,64] consisted of five different *Leishmania*, and several trials were conducted [65].Three injections were given intramuscularly 1 week apart to volunteers with a negative leishmania skin test (LST) (also called a Montenegro skin test). The antigen is a low-concentration (5–10 μg) phenol-killed parasite. Vaccination induced LST conversion (> 5 mm induration after 48–72 hr) in 35–70% of volunteers in different trials ranging from 480 to 2500 volunteers in each trial. The vaccine was well tolerated, acute adverse reactions were rare (mild pain), and long-time follow-up showed no untoward responses, including the presence of autoantibodies. Collectively, the trials showed the safety of this approach and revealed that skin test conversion is a powerful tool in field studies to monitor the responsiveness of the population. Antunes et al. [65] demonstrated that LST converters have a lower incidence of disease, which has been repeatedly seen in subsequent trials (ALM trial, see Sec.IX). A three-species autoclave-killed vaccine was produced in the laboratory of Armijos et al. [66] and the safety, immunogenicity, and efficacy of two injections against cutaneous leishmaniasis were tested in rural Ecuadorian children in a randomized, BCG-controlled, double-blinded study. Live BCG was used

as adjuvant. Within the 1-year follow-up, the incidence of CL was significantly reduced in the vaccine group compared with the control group (2.1% vs. 7.6%, *P* < 0.003). The protective efficacy of the vaccine was 72.9% (95% confidence interval = 36.1–88.5%). This is the only trial in which a significant difference was observed between killed *Leishmania* + BCG vs. BCG alone.

VIII. NEW WORLD (SINGLE STRAIN)

A. Brazil

A single-strain *L. amazonensis* vaccine was produced by Biobras after a careful comparison of different strains [61]. This vaccine was tested in a dose-escalating trial for safety and skin test conversion [67], and further trials were conducted to analyze the immune responses [68–71]. The vaccine induced primarily a Th1-type response with demonstrable IFN-γ but mostly from CD8$^+$ cells—a pattern associated with the healing process in mice [72] and humans [73]. This vaccine was shown to be effective (96% cure) as an adjunct to low-dose treatment with antimonials (15% cure) and is the first human antiparasitic vaccine (therapeutic) to be registered. It is of interest, although so far only for a single case, that this vaccine was effective against mucocutaneous leishmaniasis in a patient concomitantly suffering from AIDS [74].

B. Colombia

Mayrink et al.'s vaccine was formulated by Biobras at higher concentrations for use in combination with BCG, which is given intradermally. This formulation was compared for safety and immunogenicity with the intramuscular formulation in a double-blind, randomized, placebo-controlled trial in Medellin, Colombia [75]. Because of the side effects of BCG (active lesion for about 3 weeks), volunteers refused to receive the third injection; hence, a comparative study could not be completed. Nevertheless, the three injections of Mayrink et al.'s vaccine were shown to be well accepted with minor side effects. There were 86% and 90% LST conversion on day 80 postvaccination and a year later, respectively; there was no antibody production to the vaccine antigens; and the cytokine pattern was that of a Th1 response. Based on this, an efficacy trial has been started in a high-risk population and the results are expected in 2004.

C. Venezuela

Convit et al. were the first to use BCG as an adjuvant and autoclaved *Leishmania* as the immunogen for immunoprophylaxis as well as immunotherapy [76,77]. Without the addition of antimonials, three injections of the vaccine (autoclaved *L. mexicana* + BCG) given a month apart can cure about 90% of CL patients (slightly below drug treatment), but at a much lower cost and with no serious side effects. In contrast, drug treatment (60 injections) produced 18% serious (cardiopathy and renal toxicity) and 16% moderate adverse reactions. Although drug treatment reached over 90% cure in a shorter time, immunotherapy (three injections) is far more applicable and cost-effective than drug treatment. The BCG treatment alone cured about 40% during the same period. Historical controls without treatment usually take much longer to heal. This treatment is now being given initially, and if patients do not respond to three injections, they will be treated with chemotherapy [78].

IX. OLD WORLD (KILLED L. MAJOR + BACILLE CALMETTE–GUÉRIN)

Following the establishment of a seed bank from the *L. major*, which was used in the mass leishmanization program (see above), the Razi Institute in Iran produced different formulations of killed parasites, which were tested in randomized, double-blind, and controlled (RDBC) trials with single and multiple injections for safety, dose finding, and immunogenicity [79]. Finally, autoclaved *L. major* (ALM) produced similarly to Convit's method was chosen for efficacy trials at a dose of 1 mg per injection. This preparation has been used for all further trials of ALM + BCG in single or multiple injections against homologous or heterologous parasites [80–82]. All studies were double-blind and randomized, and BCG was used as control. Bacille Calmette–Guérin, rather than a placebo, was used to assure blindness even though BCG clearly converts some individuals (5–15%) from LST^- to LST^+ (>5 mm), has a nonspecific immunopotentiation, and has antigenic cross-reactivity with *Leishmania*. The results of three efficacy trials of ALM + BCG are shown in Table 2. These consist of a single injection against zoonotic CL [80], a single injection against (heterologous) ACL [81], and two injections against VL [82]. In contrast to the trial of Armijos et al. [66], in none of these trials with ALM + BCG vs. BCG was there a significant difference between the two groups. However, individually

and collectively, these trials produced interesting findings as indicated below:

(1) In all the trials, the vaccine produced more skin test conversion than BCG alone as expected, but BCG alone also produced LST conversion in 3.2–7.9% of individuals when tested 40–80 days postinjection and as high as 35% after a year.

(2) In all the trials, the LST-converted individuals had a reduced incidence of disease. This was significant for the homologous trial and the trial with two injections against VL, but although the same trend was seen, the difference was not significant ($P < 0.6$). These findings confirm the earlier studies with the vaccine of Antunes et al. [65].

(3) The rate of skin test conversion in the volunteers living in the nonendemic regions was significantly higher than that in the endemic regions. This indicates that immunogenicity studies must be conducted in the endemic foci prior to deciding on the dose for formulation in efficacy trials. The reason for this is not clear; however, the LST-negative individuals living in an endemic focus may be genetically "nonresponders," whereas those in the nonendemic focus would be mixed.

(4) Bacille Calmette–Guérin alone induces LST conversion and may protect a small proportion of volunteers for a short period of time. Bacille Calmette–Guérin is known to have cross-reactive antigens with *Leishmania* and to stimulate the cellular immune response nonspecifically for a limited period of time. Hence, the use of BCG as control in these trials may have obliterated the true protective value of the vaccine.

(5) The vaccine is not sufficiently immunogenic as presented and stronger adjuvants should be used to enhance its immunogenicity.

Table 2 Summary of Three Field Efficacy Trials with ALM + BCG

Trial	Vaccine	Disease	Groups	% LST	Incidence per 2 years	Other outcomes
1	ALM + BCG	ZCL[a]	BCG	7.9 (80)	18.5	35% ↓ incidence in LST[a] ($P < 0.05$)
	Single injection	2453[b]	ALM + BCG	36.2 (80)	18.0	↓ severity in vaccinated children ($P < 0.04$)
2	ALM + BCG	ACL[c]	BCG	3.2 (80)	3.3	Boys protected greater than girls ($P < 0.01$)
	Single injection	3637[b]	ALM + BCG	16.5 (80)	2.8	
3	ALM + BCG	VL[d]	BCG	7 (42)	12.7	43% ↓ incidence in LST conversion ($P < 0.003$)
	Double injection	2306[b]	ALM + BCG	30 (42)	7.2	

Numbers in parentheses represent time (in days after vaccination) when the LST was performed.
[a] *L. major*.
[b] Number of volunteers.
[c] *L. tropica*.
[d] *L. donovani*.

X. NEW FORMULATION OF AUTOCLAVED L. MAJOR+BACILLE CALMETTE–GUÉRIN

To increase immunogenicity, the Razi Serum and Vaccine Research Institute, Iran, added alum to the vaccine. Single injections of Alum–ALM plus IL-12 or BCG were shown to protect against CL (caused by *L. amazonensis* [83]) and against VL (after a lethal dose of *L. donovani*) in nonhuman primates [84]. Preliminary safety and immunogenicity human trials with this vaccine are ongoing in Sudan and Iran (Khalil et al., in preparation; Khamesipour et al., personal communication).

XI. ANTI-LEISHMANIA SUBUNIT VACCINE COMPOSED OF RECOMBINANT PROTEINS

Several investigators, including us, have, over the past decade, searched for gene-encoding leishmanial proteins that could induce protection against cutaneous and visceral leishmaniasis in several experimental models of the disease. Table 3 contains many of the recombinant proteins that have been described and obtained using a variety of lucidly planned cloning strategies [85–99]. However, soon after the great success in producing these recombinant molecules, it became evident that a critical step to successfully deliver them to induce the right type of immune response against leishmaniasis was missing (i.e., the induction of a strong

antigen-specific Th1 response in the absence of a Th2 response). Most of the adjuvants used in these initial experiments, including adjuvants licensed for human use such as alum, and adjuvants used in animal experimentation were not selective, or they stimulated primarily a Th2-type of response. Several different strategies, including IL-12, live vectors, naked DNA, oligonucleotides (CpG sequences), etc., have been tested, aiming to circumvent this impasse. These alternative means of antigen delivery are discussed in detail in Chapters 20–34.

IL-12 injected subcutaneously with leishmanial soluble antigens (SLAs) induces a strong anti-SLA Th1 response and no detectable Th2 response to this antigen. Importantly, this protocol of immunization confers excellent protection in BALB/c mice challenged with *L. major* [100]. Therefore, the presence of IL-12 in the milieu of the antigen stimulation of the T cells by the antigen-presenting cells (APCs) provides the necessary signal that causes the responding antigen-specific T cells to differentiate to a Th1 phenotype [101]. IL-12 has been successfully used as a Th1 adjuvant for a variety of antigens in both the murine and in the nonhuman primate models of several infectious diseases including leishmaniasis [83,98,100,102,103]. One of the drawbacks of IL-12 is the fact that its adjuvant effect is essentially restricted to the modulation of the immune response to the Th1 phenotype (i.e., there is no depot effect and, consequently, the amplitude of the immune response is not augmented as it is for conventional adjuvants). Moreover, in contrast with

Table 3 Leishmanial Recombinant Proteins Tested as Vaccine Candidates

| Antigen | Homology | Parasite species | Adjuvant | Species specific protection | | | Ref. |
				Mice	Hamster	Monkey	
Gp63	Zn binding-metalloproteases	*L. major*	*C. parvum* BCG, IL-12, MPL, QS21	Partial/No		Partial	[85–88]
GP46/M2		*L. amazonensis*	rVaccinia virus *C. Parvum*	Partial			[89]
LeIF	Eukaryotic ribosomal protein eIF4A	*L. brasiliensis*	None	Partial[a]			[90]
LACK	Receptors for Activated C Kinase	*L. major*	IL-12	Partial	No[b]		[91,92]
PSA-2	GP46/M2	*L. major*	*C. parvum*	Good/No			[93]
ORFF and BT1	??? Biopterin transporter	*L. donovani*	?	Partial			[94]
HASPB1	Hydrophilic acylated surface protein	*L. donovani*	None	Partial			[95]
CPB	Cathepsin	*L. major*	DNA	Partial			[96]
TSA	Thiol anti-oxidant	*L. major*	IL-12 MPL-SE	Partial	Partial[c]	Good[d]	[97,98]
LmSTI1	Stress Inducible Protein	*L. major*	IL-12 MPL-SE	Good	Partial[c]	Good[d]	[98]
A2	S antigen of *Plasmodium falciparum*	*L. donovani*	None ?	Partial			[99]

[a] Effect seen in an immunotherapeutic protocol.
[b] Challenge with *L. donovani*.
[c] Protection against challenge with *L. chagasi* (combination of TSA + LmSTI1, ACN, unpublished).
[d] Combination of TSA + LmSTI1.

conventional adjuvants and with DNA immunization, it seems that the immunological memory to the immunizing antigen is not stimulated appropriately when IL-12 is used as adjuvant. Thus, vaccination of BALB/c mice with the leishmanial antigen LACK mixed with IL-12 as an adjuvant resulted in short-term protection against challenge with *L. major*. In contrast, vaccination with LACK–DNA induced long-term protection. In addition, these studies suggested that the short-term nature of protection could not be overcome by creating a depot condition after immunization with LACK plus IL-12. Thus, mice immunized with a mixture of LACK + IL-12 + alum (added as a component of the vaccine to create the depot effect) developed a strong Th1 response to LACK, but short-term protection could not be overcome by the generation of depot [104,105]. These results question the utility of IL-12 for general use in vaccine development. Moreover, at the present time, the manufacture of IL-12 in large scale is difficult and expensive, imposing serious logistical restrictions to its use in mass vaccination of humans.

Although DNA vaccines are still in relatively early stages of development, they have been shown experimentally to induce excellent protection against several intracellular pathogens including *Leishmania*. Recent studies have demonstrated that DNA encoding the leishmanial proteins LACK, LmSTI1, and thiol-specific antioxidant (TSA) could effectively immunize susceptible BALB/c mice against *L. major* by inducing CD4$^+$ and CTL responses [104–106]. DNA immunization may provide an effective way to deliver leishmanial vaccines. However, DNA vectors currently available are less effective in stimulating appropriate human immune responses and still require validation and safety studies.

CpG ODN alone has been shown to induce a state of partial resistance in BALB/c mice up to 5 weeks against challenge with *L. major* [107]. If the CpG ODN is injected in conjunction with leishmanial soluble antigen, significant protection is obtained in these animals, which is maintained for as long as 6 months. In these experiments, the immunostimulatory properties of the CpG ODN were associated with the production of IL-12 and the emergence of strong Th1 response to SLA [108,109]. However, further studies are required to optimize CpG ODN as an adjuvant for humans.

XII. VACCINE DEVELOPMENT WITH THE RECOMBINANT ANTIGENS TSA, LMSTI1, AND LEIF

Based on protection seen in mice and nonhuman primates [98], we have selected three leishmanial antigens to be included as a single protein in a recombinant vaccine. The vaccine will be developed both for prophylaxis as well as therapy for different forms of leishmaniasis.

A. Thiol-Specific Antioxidant

A novel protein of *L. major* with sequence homology to eukaryotic thiol-specific antioxidant was discovered in experiments performed to characterize the immune responses elicited by *L. major* promastigote culture filtrate

proteins (CFPs). To identify the immunogenic components of the promastigote CFP, serum samples from CFP-vaccinated BALB/c mice, prior to challenge with *L. major*, were used to screen an *L. major* cDNA expression library. Southern blot hybridization analyses indicate that there are multiple copies of the *TSA* gene in all species of *Leishmania* that were analyzed (*L. tropica*, *L. donovani*, *L. infantum*, *L. chagasi*, *L. amazonensis*, *L. braziliensis*, and *L. guyanensis*). Northern blot analyses indicated that the *TSA* gene is constitutively expressed in *L. major* promastigotes and amastigotes. Immunization of BALB/c mice with recombinant TSA protein resulted in the development of strong cellular immune responses and conferred protective immune responses against infection with *L. major* when the protein was combined with IL-12 [97,98].

B. LmSTI1

The screening of an *L. major* amastigote cDNA library with sera from *L. major*-infected BALB/c mice identified one clone with strong homology with eukaryotic Stress-Inducible Protein-1, designated as LmSTI1. LmSTI1 contains six copies of the tetratricopeptide consensus motif that is common to stress-inducible proteins. Recombinant LmSTI1 protein plus IL-12 elicited a mixed cellular response that was skewed toward a Th1 phenotype and protected susceptible BALB/c mice [98,110].

C. Leishmania Elongation and Initiation Factor

Leishmania elongation and initiation factor (LeIF) was identified by expression cloning using sera from a patient with mucosal leishmaniasis to screen a *L. braziliensis* genomic library. Immunoreactive antigens were purified and analyzed in patient T-cell assays for the ability to stimulate proliferative responses and preferential Th1 cytokine production. Several cDNAs were identified, one of which was LeIF, a *L. braziliensis* homologue of the eukaryotic initiation factor 4A, selected because this unique molecule has two important properties: (a) it is a powerful stimulator of the innate immune system for the production of IL-12, IL-18, and IFN-γ, and therefore a Th1 inducer; and (b) because of its immunotherapeutical properties in mice infected with *L. major* [90,111,112].

Subsequent to the studies in which we showed that these individual antigens are protective against experimental leishmaniasis in both mice and monkeys, the three proteins LmSTI1, TSA, and LeIF were engineered as a single polyprotein (trifusion or Leish-111f) in tandem. The expression construct for Leish-111f protein was engineered in a multistep process as shown in Figure 1. First, each gene was cloned into the pCDNA vector: TSA and LmSTI1 were amplified by polymerase chain reaction (PCR) from *L. major* Friedlin strain VI genomic DNA and cloned into the *Bam*HI/*Eco*RI sites of the pCDNA vector. The gene for LeIF was amplified by PCR of an excised vector from a ZAP-cDNA library constructed with poly-A$^+$ RNA from *L. major* and cloned into the pCDNA vector. In the next phase, the fusion was built by first amplifying the individual genes off the pCDNA constructs and subcloning the *TSA* gene into

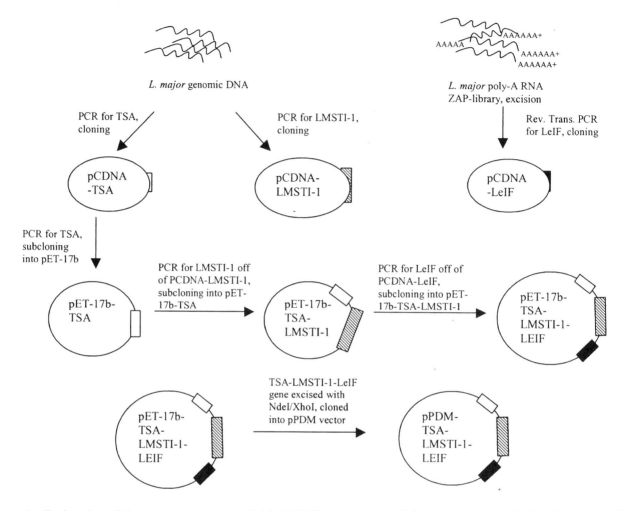

Figure 1 Engineering of the expression construct Leish-111f. The engineering of the construct proceeded in three steps: (1) A cloning phase in which each of the coding sequences were cloned from *Leishmania major* Friedlin nucleic acids into pCDNA vectors; (2) a building phase in which the pCDNA vectors were used as templates for PCR to build the fusion construct in pET-17b; and (3) a subcloning step in which the final manufacturing construct (pPDM-TSA-LmSTI1-LeIF) was made.

pET-17b. Next, the gene for LmSTI1 was fused to TSA in pET-17b via a *Bam*HI linker. Finally, the amplified gene for LeIF was fused to this construct with an *Eco*RI linker. For manufacturing, a variant of pET-28, pPDM, was created by inserting a polylinker sequence from pET-17b into pET-28, resulting in an expression vector with an *Nde*I site in the polylinker and a kanamycin resistance marker. The coding sequence for the TSA–LmSTI1–LeIF fusion from pET-17b was excised by *Nde*I/*Xho*I restriction digestion and cloned into the pPDM vector. This DNA was then transformed into the HMS174 pLysS strain of *Escherichia coli* and used for testing, cell banking, and manufacture. The final construct is shown in Figure 1. This polyprotein (Leish-111f) was then tested in protection experiments in mice challenged with *L. major*. In addition, the adjuvant MPL-SE® was employed instead of IL-12. This adjuvant, a monophosphoryl lipid A derived from *Salmonella minessota* plus the emulsifier Squalene, has been proven to be an excellent modulator of Th1 responses [113]. More importantly, this adjuvant is suitable

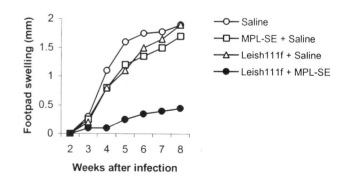

Figure 2 Vaccination of BALB/c mice against *L. major* with Leish111f. Mice (five per group) were immunized s.c., in the left footpad, twice (3 weeks apart) with 10μg of Leish111 plus the adjuvant MPL-SE. Three weeks after the last immunization the mice were infected in the right footpad with 10^5 promastigote forms (metacyclics) of *L. major* and footpad swelling was measured weekly thereafter.

for human use. BALB/c mice immunized with Leish111f plus MPL-SE mounted a strong Th1 response to epitopes of the three individual proteins and, more importantly, they were totally protected against challenge with a high dose of virulent *L. major* (10^6 metacyclical forms) (Figure 2). These highly promising results were the basis for selecting this construct for clinical development. Hence, Leish-111f has now been produced under conditions of GMP at large scale and an IND application has been submitted for conducting Phase 1 studies in the United States. Following safety evaluation and the identification of the optimal dose, clinical trials in endemic foci will commence. The transfer of technology and local production in a leishmaniasis endemic country will follow as soon as safety and protective efficacy are confirmed in clinical trials.

XIII. CONCLUSION

During the past 4–5 years, several well-designed, double-blind, randomized trials have been conducted using various preparations of killed *Leishmania* (whole parasite) with or without BCG as adjuvant. With the exception of one report from Ecuador (72% protection), little or no efficacy was seen. A lower incidence of disease was seen in those who responded by converting from negative to positive DTH reaction (ranging from 15% to 35% in different trials with different doses). Alum has been added to increase immunogenicity and this formulation has been shown in preliminary trials to induce skin conversion in all recipients. It remains to be seen if the new formulation can induce significant protection against leishmaniasis. It should be noted, however, that the first-generation vaccines are crude antigens and it is difficult, if not impossible, to standardize them. The BCG used as adjuvant, although the most widely utilized vaccine in the world, is not standardized and various strains have different activities. Hence, even if the first-generation vaccines show efficacy, there will still be a need to develop a well-defined, safe, efficacious, and standardized vaccine.

The alternative, developing a second-generation subunit vaccine composed of recombinant antigens, is now moving from the laboratory bench to clinical trials. Over the past 5 years, several *Leishmania* recombinant proteins have been tested as vaccine candidates in mice and more recently in rhesus monkeys. A mixture of three leishmanial antigens, TSA, LmSTI1, and LeIF, engineered in tandem as a polyprotein named Leish111f and mixed with the adjuvant MPL-SE (Corixa Corporation, Seattle, WA), consistently induced protection in animals challenged with several *Leishmania* species. In view of these promising results, the first second-generation vaccine (Leish-111f plus MPL-SE) is being formulated under GMP for clinical development. This has become possible because of a generous grant from the Bill and Melinda Gates Foundation to the Infectious Disease Research Institute and the collaboration with Corixa Corporation. The vaccine will be tested both for its prophylactic efficacy as well as therapeutic efficacy. One condition of the grant is an assurance of the affordability of the vaccine, should it be shown to be efficacious. To this end, every effort is being made to transfer the technology of GMP production

to suitable vaccine manufacturing facilities in one of the leishmaniasis-afflicted countries to seek local government support for the reduction of cost.

Of the major human infectious diseases for which vaccines do not currently exist, leishmaniasis represents an opportunity for success. The induction of protective immunity appears to be exclusively T-cell-mediated, with a strong dependence on type 1 cytokines. Intensive work during the last two decades, made possible by molecular techniques, has completely changed the prospects for the development of a safe and effective vaccine for leishmaniasis. Of equal importance is the recent development of potent T-cell adjuvants, which have been shown to be safe and effective in both animal models and in clinical studies. The employment of such adjuvants will expedite the development of a range of new vaccines not possible a decade ago. Furthermore, the demonstration that both whole parasite and defined antigen vaccines can be used to treat incurable drug-resistant leishmaniasis not only provides strong support for the concept of a leishmaniasis vaccine, but indicates that the demonstration of therapeutical efficacy may speed up the development of candidate vaccines. Finally, leishmaniasis vaccine efforts are providing important insights into approaches for the development of safe and effective T-cell vaccines for a range of human diseases.

REFERENCES

1. Badaro R. New perspectives on a subclinical form of visceral leishmaniasis. J Infect Dis 1986; 154:1003–1011.
2. Sharma MC, et al. *Leishmania donovani* in blood smears of asymptomatic persons. Acta Trop 2000; 76:195–196.
3. Magill AJ, et al. Visceral infection due to *Leishmania tropica* in a veteran of Operation Desert Storm who presented 2 years after leaving Saudi Arabia. Clin Infect Dis 1994; 19:805–806.
4. Montalban C, et al. Visceral leishmaniasis (kala-azar) as an opportunistic infection in patients infected with the human immunodeficiency virus in Spain. Rev Infect Dis 1989; 11: 655–660.
5. Leclerc C, et al. Systemic infection of *Leishmania tropica* (major) in various strains of mice. Trans R Soc Trop Med Hyg 1981; 75:851–854.
6. Aebischer T, et al. Persistence of virulent *Leishmania major* in murine cutaneous leishmaniasis: a possible hazard for the host. Infect Immun 1993; 61:220–226.
7. Medrano FJ, et al. Visceral leishmaniasis in HIV-1-infected individuals: a common opportunistic infection in Spain? AIDS 1992; 6:1499–1503.
8. Belazzoug S. Leishmaniasis in Mediterranean countries. Vet Parasitol 1992; 44:15–19.
9. Desjeux P. Leishmaniasis. Public health aspects and control. Clin Dermatol 1996; 14:417–423.
10. Seaman J, et al. The epidemic of visceral leishmaniasis in western Upper Nile, southern Sudan: course and impact from 1984 to 1994. Int J Epidemiol 1996; 25:862–871.
11. Sundar S. Drug resistance in Indian visceral leishmaniasis. Trop Med Int Health 2001; 6:849–854.
12. Alvar J, et al. AIDS and *Leishmania infantum*. New approaches for a new epidemiological problem. Clin Dermatol 1996; 14:541–546.
13. Gicheru MM, et al. Heterologous protection by *Leishmania donovani* for *Leishmania major* infections in the vervet monkey model of the disease. Exp Parasitol 1997; 85:109–116.

14. Zijlstra EE, et al. Endemic kala-azar in eastern Sudan: a longitudinal study on the incidence of clinical and subclinical infection and post-kala-azar dermal leishmaniasis. Am J Trop Med Hyg 1994; 51:826–836.

15. Alexander J. A radioattenuated *Leishmania major* vaccine markedly increases the resistance of CBA mice to subsequent infection with *Leishmania mexicana mexicana*. Trans R Soc Trop Med Hyg 1982; 76:646–649.

16. Modabber F. Vaccines against leishmaniasis. Ann Trop Med Parasitol 1995; 89(suppl 1):83–88.

17. Cox FE. Designer vaccines for parasitic diseases. Int J Parasitol 1997; 27:1147–1157.

18. Hommel M, et al. Experimental models for leishmaniasis and for testing anti-leishmanial vaccines. Ann Trop Med Parasitol 1995; 89(suppl 1):55–73.

19. Modabber F. First generation leishmaniasis vaccines in clinical development: moving, but what next? Curr Opin Anti-Infect Invest Drugs 2000; 2:35–39.

20. Melby PC. Vaccination against cutaneous leishmaniasis: current status. Am J Clin Dermatol 2002; 3:557–570.

21. Locksley RM, et al. Induction of Th1 and Th2 CD4$^+$ subsets during murine *Leishmania major* infection. Res Immunol 1991; 142:28–32.

22. Reiner SL, Locksley RM. The regulation of immunity to *Leishmania major*. Annu Rev Immunol 1995; 13:151–177.

23. Muller I, et al. T-cell responses and immunity to experimental infection with *Leishmania major*. Annu Rev Immunol 1989; 7:561–578.

24. Solbach W, Laskay T. The host response to *Leishmania* infection. Adv Immunol 2000; 74:275–317.

25. Blackwell JM. Genetic susceptibility to leishmanial infections: studies in mice and man. Parasitology 1996; 112(suppl): S67–S74.

26. Mock B, et al. Genetic control of *Leishmania major* infection in congenic, recombinant inbred and F2 populations of mice. Eur J Immunogenet 1993; 20:335–348.

27. Blackwell JM, et al. Genetic regulation of macrophage priming/activation: the *Lsh* gene story. Immunol Lett 1991; 30:241–248.

28. Scott PA, Farrell JP. Experimental cutaneous leishmaniasis: disseminated leishmaniasis in genetically susceptible and resistant mice. Am J Trop Med Hyg 1982; 31:230–238.

29. Scott P, et al. Immunoregulation of cutaneous leishmaniasis. T cell lines that transfer protective immunity or exacerbation belong to different T helper subsets and respond to distinct parasite antigens. J Exp Med 1988; 168:1675–1684.

30. Locksley RM, et al. Murine cutaneous leishmaniasis: susceptibility correlates with differential expansion of helper T-cell subsets. Ann Inst Pasteur Immunol 1987; 138:744–749.

31. Heinzel FP, et al. Reciprocal expression of interferon gamma or interleukin 4 during the resolution or progression of murine leishmaniasis. Evidence for expansion of distinct helper T cell subsets. J Exp Med 1989; 169:59–72.

32. Kima PE, et al. Internalization of *Leishmania mexicana* complex amastigotes via the Fc receptor is required to sustain infection in murine cutaneous leishmaniasis. J Exp Med 2000; 191:1063–1068.

33. Smelt SC, et al. B cell-deficient mice are highly resistant to *Leishmania donovani* infection, but develop neutrophil-mediated tissue pathology. J Immunol 2000; 164:3681–3688.

34. Babai B, et al. Depletion of peritoneal CD5$^+$ B cells has no effect on the course of *Leishmania major* infection in susceptible and resistant mice. Clin Exp Immunol 1999; 117: 123–129.

35. Pirmez C, et al. Cytokine patterns in the pathogenesis of human leishmaniasis. J Clin Invest 1993; 91:1390–1395.

36. Caceres-Dittmar G, et al. Determination of the cytokine profile in American cutaneous leishmaniasis using the polymerase chain reaction. Clin Exp Immunol 1993; 91: 500–505.

37. Kenney RT, et al. Splenic cytokine responses in Indian kala-azar before and after treatment. J Infect Dis 1998; 177: 815–818.

38. Ghalib HW, et al. Interleukin 10 production correlates with pathology in human *Leishmania donovani* infections. J Clin Invest 1993; 92:324–329.

39. Karp CL, et al. In vivo cytokine profiles in patients with kala-azar. Marked elevation of both interleukin-10 and interferon-gamma. J Clin Invest 1993; 91:1644–1648.

40. Titus RG, Ribeiro JM. Salivary gland lysates from the sand fly *Lutzomyia longipalpis* enhance *Leishmania* infectivity. Science 1988; 239:1306–1308.

41. Mayrink W, et al. Vaccination of dogs against *Leishmania* (Viannia) *braziliensis*. Rev Inst Med Trop Sao Paulo 1990; 32:67–69.

42. Killick-Kendrick R, et al. A laboratory model of canine leishmaniasis: the inoculation of dogs with *Leishmania infantum* promastigotes from midguts of experimentally infected phlebotomine sandflies. Parasite 1994; 1:311–318.

43. Gicheru MM, et al. Vervet monkeys vaccinated with killed *Leishmania major* parasites and interleukin-12 develop a type 1 immune response but are not protected against challenge infection. Infect Immun 2001; 69:245–251.

44. Belkaid Y, et al. Development of a natural model of cutaneous leishmaniasis: powerful effects of vector saliva and saliva preexposure on the long-term outcome of *Leishmania major* infection in the mouse ear dermis. J Exp Med 1998; 188:1941–1953.

45. Saraiva EM, et al. Changes in lipophosphoglycan and gene expression associated with the development of *Leishmania major* in *Phlebotomus papatasi*. Parasitology 1995; 111:275–287.

46. Sacks DL, et al. Stage-specific binding of *Leishmania donovani* to the sand fly vector midgut is regulated by conformational changes in the abundant surface lipophosphoglycan. J Exp Med 1995; 181:685–697.

47. Volf P, et al. Sandfly midgut lectin: effect of galactosamine on *Leishmania major* infections. Med Vet Entomol 1998; 12:151–154.

48. Palanova L, Volf P. Carbohydrate-binding specificities and physico-chemical properties of lectins in various tissue of phlebotominae sandflies. Folia Parasitol (Praha) 1997; 44: 71–76.

49. Sacks DL, et al. Stage-specific binding of *Leishmania donovani* to the sand fly vector midgut is regulated by conformational changes in the abundant surface lipophosphoglycan. J Exp Med 1995; 181:685–697.

50. Valenzuela JG, et al. Toward a defined anti-*Leishmania* vaccine targeting vector antigens: characterization of a protective salivary protein. J Exp Med 2001; 194:331–342.

51. Belkaid Y, et al. Delayed-type hypersensitivity to *Phlebotomus papatasi* sand fly bite: an adaptive response induced by the fly? Proc Natl Acad Sci USA 2000; 97: 6704–6709.

52. Behin R, et al. Mechanisms of protective immunity in experimental cutaneous leishmaniasis of the guinea-pig: III. Inhibition of leishmanial lesion in the guinea-pig by delayed hypersensitivity reaction to unrelated antigens. Clin Exp Immunol 1977; 29:320–325.

53. Bray BS, Modabber F. History of leishmaniasis. In: Gills HM, ed. Protozoal Diseases. London: Arnold, 1999:413–421.

54. Senekji HA, Beattie CP. Artificial infection and immunization of man with cultures of *L. tropica*. Trans R Soc Trop Med Hyg 1941; 34:415–419.

55. Marzinowsky EI, Schurenkova A. Oriental sore and immunity against it. Trans R Soc Trop Med Hyg 1924; 18:67–69.

56. Greenblatt CL. The present and future of vaccination for cutaneous leishmaniasis. Prog Clin Biol Res 1980; 47:259–285.

57. Gunders AE, et al. Follow-up study of a vaccination programme against cutaneous leishmaniasis: I. Vaccination with

a 5 year-old human strain of *L. tropica* from the Negev. Trans R Soc Trop Med Hyg 1972; 66:235–238.

58. Greenblatt CL, et al. An improved protocol for the preparation of a frozen promastigote vaccine for cutaneous leishmaniasis. J Biol Stand 1980; 8:227–232.

59. Nadim A, et al. Effectiveness of leishmanization in the control of cutaneous leishmaniasis. Bull Soc Pathol Exot 1983; 76:377–383.

60. Nadim A, Javadian E. Leishmanization in the Islamic Republic of Iran. In: Walton B, Wijeyarertne PM, Modabber F, eds. Research on Strategies for the Control of Leishmaniasis. Ottawa: International Development Research Center, 1988:336–339.

61. Genaro O, et al. Vaccine for prophylaxis and immunotherapy, Brazil. Clin Dermatol 1996; 14:503–512.

62. Pessoa SB. Profilaxia da leishmaniose tegumentar no Estado de Sao Paulo. Folia Med 1941; 22:157–161.

63. Mayrink W, et al. Further trials of a vaccine against American cutaneous leishmaniasis. Trans R Soc Trop Med Hyg 1986; 80:1001.

64. Mayrink W, et al. An experimental vaccine against American dermal leishmaniasis: experience in the State of Espirito Santo, Brazil. Ann Trop Med Parasitol 1985; 79: 259–269.

65. Antunes CM, et al. Controlled field trials of a vaccine against New World cutaneous leishmaniasis. Int J Epidemiol 1986; 15:572–580.

66. Armijos RX, et al. Field trial of a vaccine against New World cutaneous leishmaniasis in an at-risk child population: safety, immunogenicity, and efficacy during the first 12 months of follow-up. J Infect Dis 1998; 177:1352–1357.

67. Marzochi KB, et al. Phase 1 study of an inactivated vaccine against American tegumentary leishmaniasis in normal volunteers in Brazil. Mem Inst Oswaldo Cruz 1998; 93: 205–212.

68. Mendonca SC, et al. Characterization of human T lymphocyte-mediated immune responses induced by a vaccine against American tegumentary leishmaniasis. Am J Trop Med Hyg 1995; 53:195–201.

69. Mayrink W, et al. Short report: evaluation of the potency and stability of a candidate vaccine against American cutaneous leishmaniasis. Am J Trop Med Hyg 1999; 61:294–295.

70. De Luca PM, et al. Evaluation of the stability and immunogenicity of autoclaved and nonautoclaved preparations of a vaccine against American tegumentary leishmaniasis. Vaccine 1999; 17:1179–1185.

71. De Luca PM, et al. A randomized double-blind placebo-controlled trial to evaluate the immunogenicity of a candidate vaccine against American tegumentary leishmaniasis. Acta Trop 2001; 80:251–260.

72. Muller I, et al. Expansion of gamma interferon-producing $CD8^+$ T cells following secondary infection of mice immune to *Leishmania major*. Infect Immun 1994; 62: 2575–2581.

73. Coutinho SG, et al. T-cell responsiveness of American cutaneous leishmaniasis patients to purified *Leishmania pifanoi* amastigote antigens and *Leishmania braziliensis* promastigote antigens: immunologic patterns associated with cure. Exp Parasitol 1996; 84:144–155.

74. Da Cruz AM, et al. Atypical mucocutaneous leishmaniasis caused by *Leishmania braziliensis* in an acquired immunodeficiency syndrome patient: T-cell responses and remission of lesions associated with antigen immunotherapy. Mem Inst Oswaldo Cruz 1999; 94:537–542.

75. Velez ID, et al. Safety and immunogenicity of a killed *Leishmania* (L.) *amazonensis* vaccine against cutaneous leishmaniasis in Colombia: a randomized controlled trial. Trans R Soc Trop Med Hyg 2000; 94:698–703.

76. Convit J, et al. Immunotherapy versus chemotherapy in localised cutaneous leishmaniasis. Lancet 1987; 1:401–405.

77. Convit J, et al. Immunotherapy of localized, intermediate,

and diffuse forms of American cutaneous leishmaniasis. J Infect Dis 1989; 160:104–115.

78. Convit J. Leishmaniasis: immunological and clinical aspects and vaccines in Venezuela. Clin Dermatol 1996; 14:479–487.

79. Bahar K, et al. Comparative safety and immunogenicity trial of two killed *Leishmania major* vaccines with or without BCG in human volunteers. Clin Dermatol 1996; 14:489–495.

80. Momeni AZ, et al. A randomised, double-blind, controlled trial of a killed *L. major* vaccine plus BCG against zoonotic cutaneous leishmaniasis in Iran. Vaccine 1999; 17:466–472.

81. Sharifi I, et al. Randomised vaccine trial of single dose of killed *Leishmania major* plus BCG against anthroponotic cutaneous leishmaniasis in Bam, Iran. Lancet 1998; 351: 1540–1543.

82. Khalil EA, et al. Autoclaved *Leishmania major* vaccine for prevention of visceral leishmaniasis: a randomised, double-blind. BCG-controlled trial in Sudan. Lancet 2000; 356:1565–1569.

83. Kenney RT, et al. Protective immunity using recombinant human IL-12 and alum as adjuvants in a primate model of cutaneous leishmaniasis. J Immunol 1999; 163:4481–4488.

84. Dube A, et al. Vaccination of langur monkeys (*Presbytis entellus*) against *Leishmania donovani* with autoclaved *L. major* plus BCG. Parasitology 1998; 116:219–221.

85. Connell ND, et al. Effective immunization against cutaneous leishmaniasis with recombinant bacille Calmette–Guerin expressing the *Leishmania* surface proteinase gp63. Proc Natl Acad Sci USA 1993; 90:11473–11477.

86. Rivier D, et al. Vaccination against *Leishmania major* in a CBA mouse model of infection: role of adjuvants and mechanism of protection. Parasite Immunol 1999; 21:461–473.

87. Olobo JO, et al. Vaccination of vervet monkeys against cutaneous leishmaniasis using recombinant *Leishmania* "major surface glycoprotein" (gp63). Vet Parasitol 1995; 60: 199–212.

88. Aebischer T, et al. Subunit vaccination of mice against new world cutaneous leishmaniasis: comparison of three proteins expressed in amastigotes and six adjuvants. Infect Immun 2000; 68:1328–1336.

89. McMahon-Pratt D, et al. Recombinant vaccinia viruses expressing GP46/M-2 protect against *Leishmania* infection. Infect Immun 1993; 61:3351–3359.

90. Skeiky YA, et al. LeIF: a recombinant *Leishmania* protein that induces an IL-12-mediated Th1 cytokine profile. J Immunol 1998; 161:6171–6179.

91. Mougneau E, et al. Expression cloning of a protective *Leishmania* antigen. Science 1995; 268:563–566.

92. Melby PC, et al. *Leishmania donovani* p36(LACK) DNA vaccine is highly immunogenic but not protective against experimental visceral leishmaniasis. Infect Immun 2001; 69: 4719–4725.

93. Handman E, et al. Protective vaccination with promastigote surface antigen 2 from *Leishmania major* is mediated by a TH1 type of immune response. Infect Immun 1995; 63: 4261–4267.

94. Dole VS, et al. Immunization with recombinant LD1 antigens protects against experimental leishmaniasis. Vaccine 2000; 19:423–430.

95. Stager S, et al. Immunization with a recombinant stage-regulated surface protein from *Leishmania donovani* induces protection against visceral leishmaniasis. J Immunol 2000; 165:7064–7071.

96. Rafati S, et al. Identification of *Leishmania major* cysteine proteinases as targets of the immune response in humans. Mol Biochem Parasitol 2001; 113:35–43.

97. Webb JR, et al. Human and murine immune responses to a novel *Leishmania major* recombinant protein encoded by

members of a multicopy gene family. Infect Immun 1998; 66:3279–3289.

98. Campos-Neto A, et al. Protection against cutaneous leishmaniasis induced by recombinant antigens in murine and nonhuman primate models of the human disease. Infect Immun 2001; 69:4103–4108.

99. Ghosh A, et al. Immunization with A2 protein results in a mixed Th1/Th2 and a humoral response which protects mice against *Leishmania donovani* infections. Vaccine 2001; 20:59–66.

100. Afonso LC, et al. The adjuvant effect of interleukin-12 in a vaccine against *Leishmania major*. Science 1994; 263:235–237.

101. Mosmann TR, Sad S. The expanding universe of T-cell subsets: Th1, Th2 and more. Immunol Today 1996; 17:138–146.

102. Biron CA, Gazzinelli RT. Effects of IL-12 on immune responses to microbial infections: a key mediator in regulating disease outcome. Curr Opin Immunol 1995; 7:485–496.

103. Trinchieri G. Function and clinical use of interleukin-12. Curr Opin Hematol 1997; 4:59–66.

104. Gurunathan S, et al. Vaccination with DNA encoding the immunodominant LACK parasite antigen confers protective immunity to mice infected with *Leishmania major*. J Exp Med 1997; 186:1137–1147.

105. Gurunathan S, et al. DNA vaccines: a key for inducing long-term cellular immunity. Curr Opin Immunol 2000; 12:442–447.

106. Campos-Neto A, et al. Vaccination with plasmid DNA encoding TSA/LmSTI1 leishmanial fusion proteins confers protection against *Leishmania major* infection in susceptible BALB/c mice, 2002; 70:4215–4225.

107. Zimmermann S, et al. CpG oligodeoxynucleotides trigger protective and curative Th1 responses in lethal murine leishmaniasis. J Immunol 1998; 160:3627–3630.

108. Stacey KJ, Blackwell JM. Immunostimulatory DNA as an adjuvant in vaccination against *Leishmania major*. Infect Immun 1999; 67:3719–3726.

109. Walker PS, et al. Immunostimulatory oligodeoxynucleotides promote protective immunity and provide systemic therapy for leishmaniasis via IL-12- and IFN-gamma-dependent mechanisms. Proc Natl Acad Sci USA 1999; 96: 6970–6975.

110. Webb JR, et al. Molecular cloning of a novel protein antigen of *Leishmania major* that elicits a potent immune response in experimental murine leishmaniasis. J Immunol 1996; 157:5034–5041.

111. Skeiky YA, et al. A recombinant *Leishmania* antigen that stimulates human peripheral blood mononuclear cells to express a Th1-type cytokine profile and to produce interleukin 12. J Exp Med 1995; 181:1527–1537.

112. Borges MM, et al. Potent stimulation of the innate immune system by a *Leishmania brasiliensis* recombinant protein. Infect Immun 2001; 69:5270–5277.

113. Ulrich JT, Myers KR. Monophosphoryl lypid A as an adjuvant. In: Powell MF, Newman MJ, eds. Vaccine Design: The Subunit Adjuvant Approach. New York: Plenum Press, 1995:495–524.

75
Vaccines Against Schistosomiasis

André Capron and Gilles J. Riveau
Institut Pasteur de Lille, Lille, France

Paul B. Bartley and Donald P. McManus
Queensland Institute of Medical Research, Brisbane, Queensland, Australia

I. INTRODUCTION

Schistosomiasis is a major helminth infection that, even at the beginning of the twenty-first century, still represents an important public health problem in many developing countries. As the second major parasitic disease in the world after malaria, schistosomiasis affects 200 million people, with 800 million at risk of infection. It is estimated that 20 million individuals suffer from severe consequences of this chronic and debilitating disease responsible for at least 500,000 deaths per year.

Infection is characterized by the presence of adult worms in the portal and mesenteric veins of humans and various mammalian species, as part of a complex migratory cycle initiated by cutaneous penetration of infective larvae (cercariae) shed by infected freshwater snails. The infective larvae transform into schistosomula in the skin of appropriate hosts and, over several weeks, develop into sexually mature, egg-laying worms. The adult worms can survive for up to 15 years in the definitive host. Female worm fecundity is characterized by the deposition in mucosae and tissues (in particular liver) of millions of eggs that are responsible for the pathology and disease associated with schistosomiasis.

In spite of undeniable chemotherapeutic progress and the existence of active molecules such as praziquantel (PZQ), there is a considerable spreading of schistosomiasis, particularly in West Africa. The construction of dams and the development of important irrigation schemes are often followed by impressive epidemic outbreaks, as for instance observed in the region of St Louis in Senegal. The massive Three Gorges Dam across the Yangtze River in Southern China, soon to be completed, is expected to significantly increase schistosomiasis transmission and introduce the disease into areas currently unaffected [1]. After some 20 years' experience, it is generally agreed that chemotherapy, although the mainstay of current control programs, does have significant limitations. In particular, mass treatment does not prevent reinfection. This rapidly occurs in exposed populations in most endemic areas so that within a period of 6–8 months following chemotherapy, the prevalence returns to its baseline level. Efficient drug delivery requires a substantial infrastructure to regularly cover all parts of an endemic area. This makes chemotherapy an expensive and often impractical approach [2]. Although there is still no clear-cut evidence for the existence of PZQ-resistant schistosome strains, decreased susceptibility to the drug has been observed in several countries [3–5]. As a result, vaccine strategies represent an essential component for the future control of schistosomiasis.

Vaccination can be either targeted toward the prevention of infection or to the reduction of parasite fecundity. A reduction in worm numbers is the "gold standard" for antischistosome vaccine development but, as schistosome eggs are responsible for both pathology and transmission, a vaccine targeted on parasite fecundity and egg viability also appears entirely relevant. This review considers aspects of antischistosome protective immunity that are important in the context of vaccine development. The current status in the development of vaccines against the African (*Schistosoma mansoni* and *Schistosoma haematobium*) and Asian (*Schistosoma japonicum*) schistosomes is then discussed, as are new approaches that may improve on the efficacy of available vaccines and aid in the identification of new targets for immune attack. Earlier comprehensive reviews of the area are available [6–8].

II. EFFECTOR MECHANISMS AND CLINICAL EXPRESSION OF IMMUNITY

Research developed on *S. mansoni* and *S. japonicum* for over 20 years has led to the identification of in vitro mechanisms of protective immunity against infection or reinfection in animal models and in humans. The most significant contributions of these studies have been the demonstration in vivo of the protective role of IgE [9] and eosinophils [10]. In humans, epidemiological correlations supporting these experimental observations and arising from several different studies in various parts of the world strongly suggest that IgE may be one of the key components of protective immunity [11,12].

Together with IgE, high levels of IgG4 are produced during helminthic infection. Preliminary evidence was first reported of a significant correlation between susceptibility to reinfection of *S. mansoni* in humans and increased production of IgG4 to defined schistosome antigens [13]. In fact, in subsequent studies, elevated production of IgG4 and IgG2 antibodies was consistently associated with increased susceptibility to reinfection [14]. From these studies, it was concluded that immunity to reinfection was more closely related to the IgE/IgG4 balance than to the absolute level of each isotype. Similar findings have been obtained with *S. haematobium* and *S. japonicum* infections [8,12].

Contrasting effects of IgE and IgG4 could not be dissociated in the analysis indicating that these isotypes were probably antagonizing each other in terms of protection. Although both IgE and IgG4 responses initially depend on IL4 and IL13 production, it has recently been shown that the production of IgG4 antibodies is regulated in an antigen-specific context by IL10 and IFN-γ produced by Th0 cells [15]. This supports the view that IgE and IgG4 can be dissociated in spite of their reported dependence on IL4. The putative role of IL10 in the preferential induction of an IgG4 response should be placed in the broader perspective of the general properties of this cytokine. Indeed, it is now well established that IL10 prevents antigen presenting cell (APC)-dependent IgE synthesis and IgE-dependent cytokine

release from host cells causes activation of eosinophils as well as IL5 release [16].

The evidence that IL10 has an inhibitory function toward several essential effector arms of the immune response should prompt further studies on its production profile and biological activity in human schistosomiasis. The clinical expression of immunity to schistosome infection is obviously not simply determined by the mere balance between IgE and IgG4 antibodies. It cannot exclude the participation of additional mechanisms observed in experimental models. The evidence for additional protective mechanisms operating in man has been provided by the recently observed relationship between IgA responses to the protective antigen Sm28GST and acquired resistance. Initial studies in the rat first indicated a potential protective role for IgA antibodies produced after vaccination with Sm28GST, as well as the synergistic association of IgA and IgE antibodies in rat eosinophil-dependent cytotoxicity [17]. A significant association between IgA antibodies to Sm28GST and the age-dependent decrease in egg excretion in infected humans was demonstrated [18]. The potential protective role of IgA antibodies in human schistosomiasis has now been supported by a series of convergent correlation studies in several parts of the word including *S. haematobium* and *S. japonicum* infection (see below). Within the limits of our current knowledge, the effector function of IgA antibodies appears to be associated with a decrease in female worm fecundity and egg viability [19].

Confirming initial observations made in Kenyan populations [17], recent studies in Senegal have shown a significant association between the IgA response to Sm28GST and a decrease in egg excretion, whereas neutralization of glutathione *S*-transferase (GST) enzymatic activity by antibodies

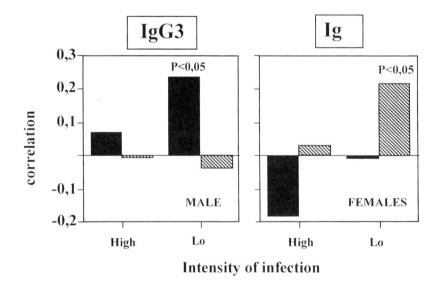

Figure 1 Association of specific isotype response in males and females with Sm28GST enzymatic inhibition. Kendall's test was used to evaluate individual correlation of the presence of specific IgG3 and IgA in male (*n* = 76) and female (*n* = 79) volunteers with the neutralizing activity of the serum. Each population was divided into two levels of infection intensity (high and low) according to the geometric mean for both sexes and the WHO Technical Report Series, no. 830. The value of correlation coefficient *r* and the significance are indicated. (From Ref. 22.)

appeared closely related with inhibition of female worm fecundity [20]. Again, IgA does not appear to be the only isotype with such neutralizing properties, considering that IgG antibodies have also demonstrated this activity in cattle (*S. mattheei*), primates (*S. haematobium*) [21], and humans [20]. In the latter case, IgG3 to Sh28GST, especially in male populations, seemed to be correlated with the age-dependent decrease in egg output in *S. haematobium* infection [22]. Indeed, before any treatment, specific IgG3 response was predominant in the male population with low intensity of infection, and was associated with maximal glutathione *S*-transferase (GST) inhibition (Figure 1). In contrast, the neutralizing activity of serum samples from women with a low intensity of infection was correlated with high specific IgA response especially directed toward a peptide constitutive to the GST enzyme site (see Figure 2).

The potential role of IgA in immunity to schistosomes and, in particular, its antifecundity effect has led, over the past 3 years, to the development of novel strategies of mucosal immunization. Multiple vectors (synthetic or recombinant live vectors) have been used in the mouse model and have now established for the first time the feasibility of inducing a protective response associated with IgA production against a systemic parasitic disease [23,24]. This will probably lead to second-generation vaccines as soon as the optimal delivery conditions have been defined. Another question arising from these observations concerns the regulation of the IgA response in the general framework of antischistosome immunity. Although our current knowledge of the regulation of the IgA response (notably secretory IgA production) in man remains fragmentary, there are convincing pieces of evidence suggesting that both Th1 and Th2 cytokines are involved. There is also evidence that IL10 and TGF-β positively regulate IgA production. It has been

postulated that Th3 cells which produce high amounts of TGF-β significantly participate in IgA regulation [22]. This suggests that the overall cytokine pattern expressed in the context of human schistosomiasis might result from a complexity ranging from a simple (Th1/Th2) to a more sophisticated (Th0/Th3) model. Indeed, a continuously changing cytokine profile according to the different developmental stages, together with a continuum of different combinatory of cytokines, is the most likely scenario.

Although the existence of highly complex networks of regulation does not allow any attempt at oversimplification, by and large, it is still the case that clinical expression of protective immunity to schistosomes in human is largely associated with a Th2 profile of immune response, among which distinct mechanisms (either IgE- or IgA-dependent) might be implicated in the control of infection or of egg-induced pathology.

III. FROM CONCEPTS TO VACCINE DEVELOPMENT—*S. MANSONI*

Based on these immunological studies, the identification and the molecular cloning [25] in the laboratory in Lille of a target antigen (Sm28GST) of the effector response has made it possible in the last 10 years to develop numerous approaches regarding its vaccine potential. At present, of six *S. mansoni* vaccine candidates (Table 1) that have been selected by the World Health Organization (WHO) for further development [6], the 28-kDa glutathione *S*-transferase (Sm28GST) is unquestionably the best-characterized and most promising molecule, and it has already entered into Phase II Clinical trials [6].

Identified as an enzyme, this molecule, initially cloned from a cDNA library from *S. mansoni* [25], has been crystallized [26], making the elucidation of its three-dimensional structure possible (Figure 2). The gene encoding for Sm28GST has been fully sequenced, leading to a series of studies concerning the control of protein expression [27]. Vaccination experiments performed with the recombinant protein [expressed in *Saccharomyces cerevisiae*, in various experimental models (rodents, primates, and cattle)] have demonstrated not only a partial but significant protective effect of the molecule against schistosome infection (reduction of 40–60% of the worm burden); they also provide evidence for a very significant inhibitory effect on female worm fecundity and egg viability [6]. It has been further shown that the inhibition of fecundity and of egg viability is associated with the inhibition of the enzymatic activity of the GST expressed in the N (24–43)- and C (190–211)-terminal regions of the molecule [28]. Research undertaken to identify the immune mechanisms induced by vaccination and implied in the inhibition of parasite fecundity led to the original demonstration of the potential role played by IgA antibodies in animal models [28]. In infected human populations, schistosome antifecundity immunity is associated with IgA and IgG3 responses together with neutralizing antibodies [20].

The extension of these observations to various animal models and to several schistosome species was made possible thanks to the molecular cloning in the laboratory in Lille of

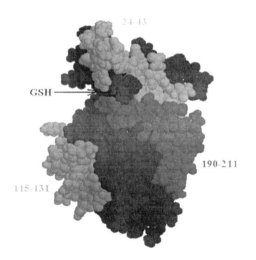

Figure 2 3-D structure of the *Schistosoma mansoni* 28-kDa gluthatione *S*-transferase. The enzymatic site of the GST implicates the N (24–43)- and C (190–211)-terminal regions of the protein. Specific antibody response against these regions inhibits the enzymatic activity and induces a significant inhibitory effect on the female worm fecundity and egg viability. (From Ref. 28. Image kindly provided by M. Hervé.)

Table 1 *Schistosoma mansoni* Vaccine Candidates

Antigen and reference	Short form	Size (kDa)	Stage expressed	Particular property	Claimed protection[a] (%)			Legal status	Place of antigen development
					Mouse	Rat	Other		
Glutathione S-transferase 28	GST 28	18	All stages	Enzyme	30–60	40–60	40 (baboon)	Patented	Institut Pasteur de Lille, France
Paramyosin	Sm97	97	Somula Adult	Muscle Protein	30			Public domain	Cornell/CWRU/NIAID, USA
Irrad. vaccine antigen no. five	IrV-5	62	All stages	Muscle protein	50–70	95	25 (baboon)	Patented	J. Hopkins School of Med., Baltimore, USA
Triose phosphate isomerase (TPI)	MAP-4	28	All stages	Synthetic peptide	30–40			Public domain	Harvard School of Public Health, Boston, USA
Membrane antigen Sm23	MAP-3	23	All stages	Synthetic peptide	40–50			Public domain	J. Hopkins/Harvard
Fatty-acid-binding protein	Sm14	14	Somula Adult	Membrane antigen	65		90–100 (rabbit)	Patented	Oswaldo Cruz Found., Rio de Janeiro, Brazil

[a] Reduction in worm burdens.

the genes encoding 28 GST from the other schistosome species *S. haematobium, S. japonicum,* and *Schistosoma bovis* [29]. It is noteworthy that the C-terminal regions of the various schistosome GSTs, apart from that of *S. japonicum,* exhibit a remarkable degree of conservation and they are very closely homologous.

Preclinical studies performed in primates by homologous and heterologous immunization [30], as well as in cattle, have confirmed the remarkable antiparasite fecundity or anti-egg effect achieved by vaccination—reaching 75–85% in primates and 94% in young calves [31]. Although no cross-protection against challenge could be induced by heterologous immunization (*S. mansoni* vs. *S. haematobium*), a dramatic reduction in egg production and viability has been achieved, entirely consistent with the predictive comparison of the molecular structure of the various GSTs. This effect correlated in all cases with the induction of antibodies capable of neutralizing GST after vaccination, leading to the concept of a cross-species-specific antifecundity vaccine [6].

It is particularly noteworthy that a significant antiworm fecundity effect has now been observed in experiments performed with GSTs of all schistosome species (including *S. japonicum,* see below) by homologous immunization, leading to a wider view of the function of these molecules in schistosomes. In this context, the recent demonstration in the laboratory in Lille that schistosomes release significant amounts of prostaglandin D2 (PGD2), which regulates various stages of the immune response, and the demonstration that PGD2 synthase is an entire homolog of 28 GST [32] reinforces our views regarding the key role played by this enzyme in schistosome biology [33] and its relevance as a vaccine target.

IV. FROM CONCEPTS TO CLINICAL TRIALS

All these results have encouraged the initiation of Phase I human trials to evaluate the safety and immunogenicity of the schistosome GST vaccine. Although most of the research of the team in Lille has been primarily based on the model of *S. mansoni* infection, we have decided to concentrate in this initial project on *S. haematobium* GST (Sh28GST), the rationale being based on the following considerations.

1. It has been established that resistance to *S. haematobium* is strongly associated with immune mediated inhibition of parasite fecundity.
2. The methods of quantitative evaluation of eggs in urine through filtration procedures are reliable and easier to handle than stool examinations.
3. Urinary schistosomiasis provides a unique opportunity to follow by noninvasive methods (bladder and urinary tract ultrasound tomography) the evolution of inflammatory lesions associated with infection.
4. It is now well established from various surveys that in adolescents there is a rapid normalization of these indicators following chemotherapy and a rapid reappearance following reinfection. In addition, the existence of a demonstrated synergy between the

immune response and praziquantel treatment provides a unique opportunity to evaluate, under strict ethical conditions, the efficacy of the vaccine in association with chemotherapy compared with chemotherapy alone.

It should also be emphasized that preclinical studies in primates have clearly shown that vaccination performed either with Sm28 or Sh28GST leads to an identical decrease in egg excretion and egg viability after *S. haematobium* challenge.

Sh28GST has been produced under GMP conditions by our industrial partner (Pharos, Eurogentec, Belgium) and named *BILHVAX*. Phase I clinical trials were initiated in September 1998 and performed in Lille at the Center for Clinical Investigation. The main objective of this study, which involved 24 healthy volunteers (Caucasian males), was the evaluation of the safety of Sh28GST immunization and as a secondary objective the evaluation of its immunogenicity.

Consistent with toxicity testing performed in rats, rabbits, and dogs, where no systemic or local toxicity was observed and no cross-reactivity with rat and human GST was detected, no adverse reactions either local or systemic were observed in human volunteers. No cross-reactivity with the human GST(Pi), was detected in spite of high titers of specific antibody produced. The evaluation of immunogenicity led to noteworthy results. Following three injections of 100 μg of Bilhvax in alum hydroxide, a strong immune response was elicited in all immunized individuals. Specific IgG response was significantly induced after the first administration in 6 out of 8 vaccinated adults, the mean IgG titer strongly increased after the second infection, and all vaccinated adults showed positive responses.

Analysis of isotypic profiles indicated that the IgG1 response was predominant; low IgG2 and IgA responses were observed whereas, strikingly, the IgG3 response was high in 7 out of 8 adults. During the Phase Ib trial performed in Saint Louis, Senegal, specific antibody responses observed in healthy children after vaccination (two injections of 100 μg of Bilhvax) showed a similar profile compared to vaccinated adults and a high specific IgG3 response was observed in 10 out of 12 vaccinated children. The most striking feature of the antibody response was the production of high titers of neutralizing antibodies. In the Phase Ia study, all vaccinated adults demonstrated significant titers of neutralizing antibodies, which were strongly boosted after the third injection, reaching a concentration of 100-fold over the IC_{50} usually observed in infected patients. It was evident that these antibodies were able to neutralize not only the recombinant, but also the native GST enzymatic activity. During Phase Ib, as observed in adults, two injections of Sh28GST induced a high titer of neutralizing antibodies in all vaccinated children.

As anticipated, no production of Th1 cytokines was observed in Phase Ia or Phase Ib. In contrast, there was a prominent production of IL-5 and IL13, again strongly boosted after the third injection in all vaccinated individuals. Identical cytokine profiles were observed in vaccinated children during Phase Ib, but the production of IL-5 and IL13 was higher, and a significant production of IL2 and IL10 was observed. The follow-up of vaccinated individuals, during the 4-month period after the first shot, indicated that Bilhvax induced a high and lasting specific immune response associated with a Th2-type profile generally regarded as associated with protective immunity in human schistosomiasis [34].

It is also particularly noteworthy that the major features of the immune response induced by vaccination in humans are perfectly consistent with the concepts that our Lille group had derived from our studies of experimental models. In particular, if the close association between neutralizing antibodies and the inhibition of parasite fecundity already observed in experimental models and in human infected populations can be regarded, based on these results, as a surrogate marker of vaccine efficacy, then we have undoubtedly moved a significant step toward the feasibility of a clinical vaccine against one of the major human parasitic disease [35].

V. VACCINES AGAINST *S. JAPONICUM*— BASIC CONSIDERATIONS

Schistosomiasis japonica is endemic in Southern China and the Philippines [36]. As stressed earlier, the control of schistosomiasis requires an integrated approach involving large-scale population-based chemotherapy in addition to environmental and behavioral modification [37]. Further, population movements [1] and the construction of dams already referred to, have contributed to the spread of schistosomiasis into new areas. As with the African schistosomes, there is therefore an important role for a vaccine to provide long-term prevention against Asian schistosomiasis. Unlike *S. mansoni* or *S. haematobium*, mammals other than humans (such as dogs, bovines, and pigs) can act as definitive hosts for *S. japonicum*. Zoonotic transmission adds to the complexity of control programs, but may provide opportunities for novel approaches in vaccine development to prevent human disease. When available for wide-scale use, it is envisaged that the vaccine would be applied in the first instance, at least in China, in water buffalo reservoir hosts (to impact on human transmission), and then, perhaps, if required, clinically (to prevent or reduce disease).

Recent progress has provided the basic framework for the development of an effective vaccine against this complex parasite. Schistosomulum lifecycle stage antigens are likely to be major vaccine candidate targets of protective immune responses. As with the *S. mansoni* mouse model, vaccination with radiation-attenuated cercariae induces significant levels of resistance to *S. japonicum* challenge in mice, rats, rabbits, sheep, and bovines [8]. Worm burden reduction ranges from 40% to >85%—with less protection evident in mice than rabbits or larger animals. Like *S. mansoni*, the initial protection is conferred by Th1 cellular immunity with lymphoid proliferation in regional and mediastinal lymph nodes. Subsequent vaccination (at least in mice) did not appear to confer additional protection. Appropriately timed passive transfer of sera from vaccinated mice can also confer protection. This protection is antibody-mediated, with predominantly IgG (less so by IgM) antibodies acting on the lung schistosomula stage. IgE depletion did not influence protection in these studies. Some later studies suggest that both Th1 and Th2 responses may contribute to protection [8].

Human immunity to *S. japonicum* has been predominantly assessed by reinfection and immune-correlative studies. As in *S. mansoni* and *S. haematobium*, acquired immunity to *S. japonicum* develops with age [8,12]. Like the African schistosomes, a high IgG4/IgE ratio to adult worm antigen (AWA) and soluble egg antigen (SEA) correlates susceptibility to reinfection, whereas IgE excess correlates with resistance to reinfection [38]. Further, peripheral blood mononuclear cells taken from resistant individuals in China produce significantly greater amounts of IL-10 in response to parasite extracts and recombinant antigens in vitro [39]. Preliminary field studies from the Philippines suggest that IgE antibodies to a 22.6-kDa tegument-associated antigen (Sj22.6) are associated with resistance to reinfection [8]. It should be stressed that, whereas much of our understanding of the effector mechanisms and clinical expression of immunity against *S. japonicum* has been extrapolated from the extensive studies on *S. mansoni* and *S. haematobium*, this may prove not to be the case, so different are the African and Asian schistosomes.

VI. VACCINES AGAINST *S. JAPONICUM*— CURRENT STRATEGIES

While offering, in some cases, high levels of protection, the irradiated cercarial vaccine is impractical, cumbersome, and impossible to standardize. Additionally, the protection conferred is species- and often strain-specific. Therefore considerable efforts have been made aimed at the identification of relevant schistosome antigens that may be involved in inducing protective immune responses, with a view to developing either a recombinant protein, synthetic peptide, or DNA vaccine [8]. As emphasized earlier, coordinated laboratory and field research have identified a set of well-defined *S. mansoni* molecules with protective potential with the *S. mansoni* and *S. haematobium* 28-kDa GSTs being the best characterized and most studied of the candidate vaccine antigens. Several of these molecules are also recognized as major vaccine targets against *S. japonicum* (Table 2). One leading candidate is paramyosin.

Paramyosin is a 97-kDa myofibrillar protein with a coiled-coil structure and is exclusively found in invertebrates. It is expressed on the surface tegument of lung-stage schistosomula and may function as a receptor for Fc [40]. Native and recombinant paramyosin confer significant protection (approximately 35% decreased worm burden and 45% decreased liver egg burden) against *S. japonicum* in mice and buffaloes [41]. There is greater than 95% homology between the paramyosin genes of *S. japonicum* (Chinese and Philippine strains), *S. haematobium*, and *S. mansoni* [41]. This may facilitate development of a "consensus" molecule as a vaccine against all three human pathogens should efficacy be improved. Currently, mathematical modeling of the likely benefits of rec-Sj-97 at its current level of efficacy as an antifecundity vaccine suggest it would prove a useful adjunct to existing control programs [1,42].

A calcium-activated neutral proteinase (calpain) may be another "consensus molecule" vaccine. It has been identified in *S. mansoni* and *S. japonicum*, and has been localized to the

Table 2 *Schistosoma Japonicum* Vaccine Candidates

Antigen[a]	Short form	Size (kDa)	Stage expressed	Biological function(s)	Claimed protection[b] (%)	
					Mouse	Other
Paramyosin (native)	Sj97	97	Somula Adult	Contractile protein + others	27–86	31–48 (sheep/cattle)
Paramyosin (recombinant)	recSj97	97	Somula Adult	Contractile protein + others	20–60	7–60 (buffalo/pigs/sheep)
Triose phosphate Isomerase (native)	TPI	28	All stages	Enzyme	21–24	
Integral membrane protein (recombinant)	Sj23	23	Adult	Membrane protein		32–59 (buffalo/cattle/sheep)
Aspartic protease (recombinant)	SjASP	46	All stages	Digestion of hemoglobin	21–40	
Calpain large subunit (recombinant)	r-calpain	80	Adult	Protease	40	
Glutathione *S*-transferase (recombinant)	Sj28-GST	28	All stages	Enzyme	0–35	33–69 (buffalo/sheep)
Glutathione *S*-transferase (recombinant)	Sj26-GST	26	All stages	Enzyme	24–30	25–62 (buffalo/pigs/sheep)

[a] All in public domain.

[b] Reduction in worm burdens. Significant egg reduction also recorded with the majority of candidates. (See Refs. 8,41 and 45.)

extracellular domain [43]. The protein is recognized by sera from infected patients. Vaccination results in approximately 40% reduction in worm and egg burdens in mouse models of *S. mansoni* and *S. japonicum* infection. The *S. mansoni* and *S. japonicum* 22.6-kDa (Sm22.6 and Sj22.6) tegument-associated antigens may also be useful vaccine targets. While the function of this family of proteins remains unknown, they are expressed near the surface of lung-stage schistosomula [44], and specific IgE and IgA antibodies appear associated with resistance to reinfection in human studies [8]. Mouse studies of bacterially expressed and purified recombinant Sj22.6 have demonstrated specific IgG and IgE production but no protection [44]. Also, vaccination with *Escherichia coli* and baculovirus-expressed recombinant *S. japonicum* aspartic protease—cathepsin D—generated high levels of specific antibodies but only a limited level of protection [45].

More encouraging results have been obtained with recombinant 26-kDa GST of *S. japonicum*, which induces a pronounced antifecundity effect, as well as a low but significant level of protection in terms of reduced worm burden. The molecule is capable of stimulating antifecundity immunity in mice (up to 59% decrease in liver eggs) [46] and pigs (53.5% decrease in liver eggs) [47], following challenge infection with *S. japonicum*. Similar vaccination experiments have been carried out on water buffaloes (*Bos buffelus*), the major reservoir for transmission of schistosomiasis japonica in China, using purified reSjc26GST in order to investigate its vaccine potential [48]. Anti-Sjc26GST antibodies were produced in the immunized buffaloes and, following challenge with *S. japonicum* cercariae, a small but significant reduction in worm numbers was evident in vaccinated subjects when compared with control animals. The typical antifecundity effect was manifest, characterized by a significant decrease in fecal egg output and eggs deposited in host tissues with those in the liver and intestine being reduced by

about 50%. In addition to the antifecundity effect, reSjc26GST reduced by nearly 40% the egg-hatching capacity of *S. japonicum* eggs into viable miracidia.

In summary, all of the proteins mentioned above have shown some promise as candidate vaccines although they generally produce modest reductions in worm and egg burdens. It is important, therefore, to explore alternative vaccination strategies to improve vaccine efficacy, and to identify new target antigens.

VII. VACCINATION AGAINST SCHISTOSOMES—DNA VACCINES

DNA vaccination offers many potential advantages including cost-effective production, thermal stability and the ability to induce a wide variety of immune responses—including induction of cytotoxic T-lymphocytes (CTLs) [49,50]. In addition to schistosomiasis, DNA vaccination is being explored for a wide variety of parasite, including helminthic infections [49,51]. Large reductions in parasite burdens have been demonstrated in animal models of some of these infections namely: *Taenia crassiceps* [52], *Fasciola hepatica* [53], and *Onchocerca volvulus* [54]. A prime-boost strategy of DNA vaccination followed by recombinant modified vaccinia virus Ankara (MVA) encoding pre-erythrocytic stage antigens has induced sterilizing immunity to malaria [55,56]. Similar prime-boost strategies have conferred protection against influenza [55] and swine fever [57]. A DNA prime-protein boost strategy using the *Plasmodium falciparum* 175-kDa erythrocyte binding protein induces a significant reduction in parasitaemia in *Aotus* monkeys [58]. Prime-boost vaccination along similar lines may prove valuable against schistosomiasis.

Table 3 Some DNA Vaccines Tested in Mice Against *Schistosoma* spp.

Organism	Vector	cDNA	Method	Specific immune response	Worm burden reduction (%)	Egg burden reduction (%)
S. japonicum	VR1020 (Vical Inc., USA)	22-kDa Tegument antigen	Gene gun	Yes	Nil	Nil
S japonicum	VR1020 (Vical Inc., USA)	Paramyosin	IMI—Quadriceps	Yes	Nil	Nil
S. japonicum	PcDNA1/Amp	Paramyosin	IMI—*Tibialis anterior*	Yes	35–40	50–80
S. mansoni	pNI	28 kDa GST	IMI—IL-18 plasmid adjuvant	Yes	23	28
S. mansoni	pcDNA1.1	Sm23 surface protein	IMI—IL-12 or IL-4 plasmid adjuvant	Yes	20–44	Not evaluated
S. japonicum	VR1020 (Vical Inc., USA)	Sj62, Sj28, Sj23 and Sj14-3-3	IMI—Cocktail vaccination ± IL-12 plasmid adjuvant	Yes	40	Not evaluated
S. japonicum	VR1020 (Vical Inc., USA)	62 kDa myosin	IMI—Naked DNA or liposomal	Yes	Nil	Nil

Indeed, there has already been considerable interest in the development of a DNA-based vaccine against schistosomiasis (Table 3). The modulation of immune responses possible with DNA vaccination renders this as an attractive prospect, given what is known about human and animal immunity to schistosomes. DNA vaccines tested to date have included plasmid DNA of *S. japonicum* paramyosin [59,60] and 62-kDa myosin [61], *S. japonicum* 22-kDa [62] and 23-kDa [63] tegument-associated antigens, *S. japonicum* 28-kDa GST [64], *S. mansoni* 28-kDa GST [65–68], *S. mansoni* 23-kDa integral membrane protein (Sm23) [69], and *S. mansoni* calpain [70].

Unlike vaccination with native or recombinant protein [41,71], DNA vaccination with paramyosin has yielded conflicting results. Early studies demonstrated specific antibody production without protection [59]. However, another group [60] recently demonstrated a 35–40% reduction in worm burden and 50–80% reduction in visceral egg burdens following intramuscular DNA vaccination into the *tibialis anterior* muscle of a different inbred mouse strain. The authors concluded that the differences in mouse strain and site of injection could account for the contrasting results. It is well described that intramuscular immunization (IMI) of DNA vaccines into the tibialis anterior induces significantly greater immune responses than IMI into the quadriceps muscle in mice [50]. DNA prime-protein boost with paramyosin is an attractive prospect.

DNA vaccination with either the 22- or 23-kDa *S. japonicum* tegument-associated antigens [62,63] has induced high titers of specific murine antibodies without protection. This is despite manipulation of the route of administration and fusion of the antigen cDNA to an Ig κ-chain secretory leader sequence [62]. Equally, DNA vaccination with a 62-kDa fragment of *S. japonicum* myosin did not induce protection in several strains of mice despite cationic lipid adjuvant and additional CpG motifs [61].

DNA vaccine plasmids encoding Sm28GST have also been the subject of much interest [65–68]. These vaccines induce specific antibody responses which are boosted by challenge infection [66]. These antibody responses can mediate antibody-dependent cytotoxity against schistosomulae [66] and also assist in immune-mediated killing of injured adult worms [68]. When coadministered with an IL-18-encoding plasmid, profound Th1 stimulation occurred with a 28% reduction in worm burden [67]. In general, however, Sm28GST DNA vaccines appear to evoke less protection than the recombinant protein.

DNA vaccines containing cDNAs from two other *S. mansoni* surface-associated proteins (calpain and Sm23) have undergone initial protection trials with promising results [69,70]. The Sm23pcDNA vaccine elicited a 21–44% reduction in worm burden in mice [69]. Protection was not enhanced by the addition of plasmids encoding either IL-12 or IL-4 to influence the immune response toward Th1 or Th2, respectively. A DNA plasmid encoding the large calpain subunit (p80) conferred a 60% reduction in worm burden [70]. Interestingly, the 5′UTR of p80 needed to be included in the DNA vaccine for this protection to be achieved. Vaccination of mice with "cocktail" DNA vaccines is another potentially promising avenue. A recent report demonstrated modest reduction of worm and egg burdens with a cocktail of DNA plasmids encoding four *S. japonicum* tegument-associated peptide antigens [72]. The recent assembly of multiple defined and different epitopes of *S. mansoni* into a variety of covalent structures, including a DNA plasmid vaccine encoding different epitopes in tandem, failed to protect mice from subsequent challenge infection [73].

VIII. VACCINATION AGAINST SCHISTOSOMES—NEW ANTIGEN DISCOVERY

Secreted or transmembrane proteins are likely to encounter the host immune system and are, therefore, potential vaccine candidates. This portion of the schistosome proteome is poorly characterized. Only 30 of the ~15,000 schistosome DNA expressed sequence tags (EST) in public databases, are known to possess coding sequence for signal peptides. Signal peptides are positioned at the N-terminus of secreted protein precursors. They initiate export of the precursor proteins across the endoplasmic reticulum. The ratio of known proteins with predicted signal peptides to ESTs is far greater in other parasites (e.g., *Brugia malayi*). It is therefore rational to identify additional schistosome cDNAs that encode proteins with functional signal peptides and assess their efficacy as vaccine candidates—in addition to determining their biological function. This approach is very much in its infancy. An alkaline-phosphatase signal sequence trap method [74] has been used to isolate sequences encoding secreted and transmembrane proteins from *S. mansoni* adult worm cDNA [75]. Among the 18 clones identified and sequenced to date, two encode novel tetraspanin-like proteins, five sequences have no known homologs, and several others are homologous to known *S. mansoni* ESTs. There is a likelihood of discovering a group of important secreted and surface schistosome proteins, potentially involved in central roles in the schistosome host–mammal relationship. In addition to the determination of their biological functions and interactions, some proteins may also be interesting vaccine candidates.

B-cell antigenic determinants appear to be dependent on the conformational integrity of the molecule in question. Conformational epitopes may be important in generating protective immunity against parasites. One example is the recent determination that the protection conferred against experimental cystic hydatid disease by the EG95 vaccine, a recombinant oncospheral protein, relies on conformational integrity rather than linear epitopes [76]. Indeed, the absence of tertiary structure and therefore conformational epitopes in the recombinant Sj22.6 vaccine is one possible explanation for the apparent lack of protection associated with this molecule [44]. Clearly, further evaluation of synthetic protein vaccines may need to take conformational epitopes into consideration. Likewise, improved efficacy of antischistosome vaccines may require more powerful adjuvants than those currently available for clinical use. In this respect, the recent demonstration that Lewis-type carbohydrate Lacto-*N*-fucopentose III (LNFPIII) found on *S. mansoni* egg antigens is a potent inducer of a Th2-type response and can also act as an adjuvant by inducing antibody against coupled protein antigen (human serum albumin) [77] suggests this molecule might prove useful for future development as an adjuvant for application with schistosome vaccines.

IX. CONCLUDING COMMENTS

Taking the breadth of consolidated, international efforts to generate antischistosome vaccines, there is considerable optimism that these endeavors will prove successful [8,78]. Indeed, the promising preclinical trials with the Sh28GST vaccine followed by very encouraging Phase 1a and 1b human trials auger well for Phase II and Phase III efficacy trials underway or planned for the future. In addition, re-

markable recent progress in schistosome gene discovery [79,80] may lead to the identification of additional vaccine candidate molecules. When developed and employed, antischistosome vaccines will not be a panacea. They need to be regarded as one component, albeit a very important one, of integrated schistosomiasis control programs that complement existing strategies including chemotherapy and health education.

REFERENCES

1. Ross AGP, et al. Schistosomiasis in the People's Republic of China: prospects and challenges for the 21st century. Clin Microbiol Rev 2001; 14:270–295.
2. Bergquist RN, Colley DG. Schistosomiasis vaccines: research to development. Parasitol Today 1998; 14:99–104.
3. Fallon PG, et al. Short report: diminished susceptibility to praziquantel in a Senegal isolate of *Schistosoma mansoni*. Am J Trop Med Hyg 1995; 53:61–62.
4. Stelma FF, et al. Efficacy and side effects of praziquantel in an endemic focus of *Schistosoma mansoni*. Am J Trop Med Hyg 1995; 53:167–170.
5. Ismail M, et al. Characterization of isolates of *Schistosoma mansoni* from Egyptian villagers that tolerate high dose of praziquantel. Am J Trop Med Hyg 1996; 55:214–218.
6. Riveau GJ, Capron A. Vaccination against schistosomiasis: concepts and strategies. In: Kaufmann SHE, ed. Concepts in Vaccine Design. Berlin, New York: Walter de Gruyter, 1996: 509–532.
7. Riveau GJ, Capron A. Vaccines against schistosomiasis. In: Levine MM, ed. New Generation Vaccines. 2d ed. New York: Marcel Dekker, 1997:1081–1093.
8. McManus DP. The search for a vaccine against schistosomiasis—a difficult path but an achievable goal. Immunol Rev 1999; 171:149–161.
9. Capron A, et al. Specific IgE antibodies in immune adherence of normal macrophages to *Schistosoma mansoni* schistosomules. Nature 1975; 253:474–475.
10. Capron M, et al. Evidence for IgE-dependent cytotoxicity by rat eosinophils. J Immunol 1981; 126:1764–1768.
11. Capron M, Capron A. Rats, mice and men. Models for immune effector mechanisms against schistosomiasis. Parasitol Today 1986; 2:69–75.
12. Ross AGP, et al. Is there immunity to *Schistosoma japonicum*? Parasitol Today 2000; 16:159–164.
13. Hagan P, et al. Human IgE, IgG4 and resistance to reinfection with *Schistosoma haematobium*. Nature 1991; 349:243–245.
14. Demeure CE, et al. Resistance to *S. mansoni* in humans: influence of IgE/IgG4 balance and IgG2 in immunity to reinfection after chemotherapy. J Infect Dis 1993; 168:1000–1008.
15. Gascan H, et al. Anti-CD40 monoclonal antibodies or CD4+ T cell clones and IL-4 induce IgG4 and IgE switching in purified human B cells via different signalling pathways. J Immunol 1991; 147:8–13.
16. Akdis CA, et al. Role of IL-10 in specific immunotherapy. J Clin Invest 1998; 102:98–106.
17. Grezel D, et al. Protective immunity induced in rat Schistosomiasis by a single dose of the Sm28GST recombinant antigen: effector mechanisms involving IgE and IgA antibodies. Eur J Immunol 1993; 23:455–460.
18. Grzych JM, et al. IgA antibodies to a protective antigen in human schistosomiasis mansoni. J Immunol 1993; 150:527–635.
19. Grzych JM, et al. Relationship of impairment of Schistosome 28-kilodalton glutathione *S*-transferase (GST) activity

to expression of immunity to *Schistosoma mattheei* in calves vaccinated with recombinant *Schistosoma bovis* 28-kilodalton GST. Infect Immun 1998; 66:1142–1148.

20. Remoué F, et al. Sex-dependent neutralizing humoral response to *S. mansoni* 28GST antigen in infected human population. J Infect Dis 2000; 181:1855–1859.

21. Boulanger D, et al. Immunization of mice and baboons with the recombinant Sm28GST affects both worm viability and fecundity after experimental infection with *Schistosoma mansoni*. Parasite Immunol 1991; 13:473–490.

22. Remoué F, et al. Gender-dependent specific immune response during chronic human schistosomiasis haematobia. Clin Exp Immunol 2001; 124:62–68.

23. Ivanoff N, et al. Mucosal vaccination against schistosomiasis using liposome-associated Sm28kDa glutathione *S*-transferase. Vaccine 1996; 14:1123–1131.

24. Mielcarek N, et al. Homologous and heterologous protection after single intranasal administration of live attenuated recombinant *Bordetella pertussis*. Nat Biotechnol 1998; 16:454–457.

25. Balloul JM, et al. Molecular cloning of a protective antigen of schistosomes. Nature 1987; 326:149–153.

26. Trottein F, et al. Crystallisation and preliminary X-ray diffraction studies of a protective cloned 28kDa GST from *S. mansoni*. J Mol Biol 1992; 224:515–518.

27. McNair AT, et al. Cloning and characterisation of the gene encoding the 28kDa GST of *S. mansoni*. Gene 1993; 124:245–249.

28. Xu CB, et al. *Schistosoma mansoni* 28-kDa glutathione *S*-transferase and immunity against parasite fecundity and egg viability. Role of the amino- and carboxyl-terminal domains. J Immunol 1993; 150:940–949.

29. Trottein F, et al. Interspecies variation of schistosome 28 kDa glutathione *S*-transferase. Mol Biochem Parasitol 1992; 54:63–72.

30. Boulanger D, et al. Vaccination of patas monkeys experimentally infected with *Schistosoma haematobium* using a recombinant glutathione *S*-transferase clone from *S. mansoni*. Parasite Immunol 1995; 17:361–369.

31. De Bont J, et al. Potential of a recombinant *Schistosoma bovis*-derived glutahione *S*-transferase to protect cattles against experimental and natural *S mattheei* infection. I. Parasitological results. Parasitology 1997; 115:249–255.

32. Angeli V, et al. Role of the parasite-derived prostaglandin D2 in the inhibition of epidermal Langerhans cell migration during schistosomiasis infection. J Exp Med 2001; 193:1135–1147.

33. Capron A. Schistosomiasis: forty years' war on the worm. Parasitol Today 1998; 14:379–384.

34. Dunne DW, et al. Prospects for immunological control of schistosomiasis. Lancet 1995; 345:1488–1492.

35. Capron A, et al. Vaccine strategies against schistosomiasis: from concepts to clinical trials. Int Arch Allergy Immunol 2001; 124:9–15.

36. Chitsulo L, et al. The global status of schistosomiasis and its control. Acta Trop 2000; 77:41–51.

37. Morel C. Reaching maturity—25 years of the TDR. Parasitol Today 2000; 16:522–529.

38. Li Y, et al. Human susceptibility to *Schistosoma japonicum* in China correlates with antibody isotypes to native antigens. Trans R Soc Trop Med Hyg 2001; 95:441–448.

39. McManus DP, et al. Production of interleukin-10 by peripheral blood mononuclear cells from residents of a marshland area in China endemic for *Schistosoma japonicum*. Parasitol Int 1999; 48:169–177.

40. Loukas A, et al. Receptor for Fc on the surfaces of schistosomes. Infect Immun 2001; 69:3646–3651.

41. McManus DP, et al. Recombinant paramyosin (rec-Sj-97) tested for immunogenicity and vaccine efficacy against *Schistosoma japonicum* in mice and water buffaloes. Vaccine 2002; 20:870–878.

42. Williams G, et al. Mathematical modelling of *Schistosoma japonicum*: comparison of control strategies in the People's Republic of China. Acta Trop. 2002; 82:253–262

43. Zhang R, et al. Vaccination with calpain induces a Th1-biased protective immune response against *Schistosoma japonicum*. Infect Immun 2001; 69:386–391.

44. Li Y, et al. Immunogenicity and immunolocalization of the 22.6kDa antigen of *Schistosoma japonicum*. Parasite Immunol 2000; 22:415–424.

45. Verity C, et al. Vaccine efficacy of recombinant cathepsin D aspartic protease from *Schistosoma japonicum*. Parasite Immunol 2001; 23:153–162.

46. Liu S, et al. Immunization of mice with recombinant Sjc26GST induces a pronounced anti-fecundity effect after experimental infection with Chinese *Schistosoma japonicum*. Vaccine 1995; 13:603–607.

47. Liu SX, et al. Anti-fecundity immunity induced in pigs vaccinated with recombinant *Schistosoma japonicum* 26kDa glutathione-*S*-transferase. Parasite Immunol 1995; 17:340–355.

48. Liu SX, et al. Anti-fecundity immunity to *Schistosoma japonicum* induced in Chinese water buffaloes (*Bos bufelus*) after vaccination with recombinant 26kDa glutathione-*S*-transferase (reSjc26GST). Vet Parasitol 1997; 69:39–47.

49. Alarcon J, et al. DNA vaccines: technology and application as anti-parasite and anti-microbial agents. Adv Parasitol 1999; 42:343–410.

50. Gurunathan S, et al. DNA vaccines: immunology, application, and optimization. Annu Rev Immunol 2000; 18:927–974.

51. Kofta W, Wedrychowicz H. c-DNA vaccination against parasitic infections: advantages and disadvantages. Vet Parasitol 2001; 100:3–12.

52. Mantoucharian K, et al. Protection against murine cysticercosis using cDNA expression library immunization. Immunol Lett 1998; 62:131–136.

53. Kofta W, et al. Successful DNA vaccination of rats against fasciolosis. Vaccine 2000; 18:2985–2990.

54. Harrison R, et al. DNA immunization with *Onchocerca volvulus* chitinase induces partial protection against challenge infection with L3 larvae in mice. Vaccine 1999; 18:647–655.

55. Degano P, et al. Gene gun intradermal DNA immunization followed by boosting with modified vaccinia virus Ankara: enhanced CD8$^+$ T cell immunogenicity and protective efficacy in the influenza and malaria models. Vaccine 1999; 18:623–632.

56. Gilbert SC, et al. Enhanced CD8 T cell immunogenicity and protective efficacy in a mouse malaria model using a recombinant adenoviral vaccine in heterologous prime-boost immunisation regimes. Vaccine 2002; 20:1039–1045.

57. Hammond J, et al. A prime-boost vaccination strategy using naked DNA followed by recombinant porcine adenovirus protects pigs from classical swine fever. Vet Microbiol 2001; 80:101–119.

58. Jones T, et al. Protection of *Aotus* monkeys by *Plasmodium falciparum* EBA-175 region II DNA prime-protein boost immunization regimen. J Infect Dis 2001; 183:303–312.

59. Waine G, et al. DNA-based vaccination using *Schistosoma japonicum* (Asian blood-fluke) genes. Vaccine 1997; 15:846–848.

60. Zhou S, et al. Protective immunity induced by the full-length cDNA encoding paramyosin of Chinese *Schistosoma japonicum*. Vaccine 2000; 18:3196–3204.

61. Zhang Y, et al. Immunogenicity of plasmid DNA encoding the 62 kDa fragment of *Schistosoma japonicum* myosin. Vaccine 2000; 18:2102–2109.

62. Waine G, et al. DNA immunization by intramuscular injection or gene gun induces specific IgG antibodies against a *Schistosoma japonicum* 22kDa antigen, Sj22, when fused to

the murine Ig K-chain secretory leader sequence. Parasite Immunol 1999; 21:53–56.

63. Waine G, et al. Genetic immunization of mice with DNA encoding the 23 kDa transmembrane surface protein of *Schistosoma japonicum* (Sj23) induces antigen-specific immunoglobulin G antibodies. Parasite Immunol 1999; 21:377–381.

64. Shi F, et al. Laboratory and field evaluation of *Schistosoma japonicum* DNA vaccines in sheep and water buffalo in China. Vaccine 2001; 20:462–467.

65. Kayes S, et al. Overproduction of SM28GST in a baculovirus expression vector and its use to evaluate the in vivo immune responses of mice vaccinated against *Schistosoma mansoni* with naked DNA encoding the SM28GST gene. J Parasitol 1998; 84:764–770.

66. Dupre L, et al. Intradermal immunization of rats with plasmid DNA encoding *Schistosoma mansoni* 28 kDa glutathione S-transferase. Parasite Immunol 1997; 19:505–513.

67. Dupre L, et al. Immunostimulatory effect of IL-18-encoding plasmid in DNA vaccination against murine *Schistosoma mansoni* infection. Vaccine 2001; 19:1373–1380.

68. Dupre L, et al. Control of schistosomiasis pathology by combination of Sm28GST DNA immunization and praziquantel treatment. J Infect Dis 1999; 180:454–463.

69. Da'dara A, et al. Immunization with plasmid DNA encoding the integral membrane protein, Sm23, elicits a protective immune response against schistosome infection in mice. Vaccine 2001; 20:359–369.

70. Hota-Mitchell S, et al. Recombinant vaccinia virus and gene gun vectors expressing the large subunit of *Schistosoma mansoni* calpain used in a murine immunization-challenge model. Vaccine 1999; 17:1338–1354.

71. Flanigan T, et al. Induction of resistance to *Schistosoma mansoni* infection in mice by purified parasite paramyosin. J Clin Invest 1989; 83:1010–1014.

72. Zhang Y, et al. Vaccination of mice with a cocktail DNA vaccine induces a Th1-type immune response and partial protection against *Schistosoma japonicum* infection. Vaccine 2001; 20:724–730.

73. Yang W, et al. Multi-epitope schistosome vaccine candidates tested for protective immunogenicity in mice. Vaccine 2000; 19:103–113.

74. Chen H, Leder P. A new signal sequence trap using alkaline phosphatase as a reporter. Nucleic Acids Res 1999; 27:1219–1222.

75. Smyth DJ, et al. Isolation of cDNAs encoding secreted and transmembrane proteins from *Schistosoma mansoni* using signal sequence trap. Inf Immun 2003; 71:2548–2554.

76. Woollard D, et al. Protection against hydatid disease induced with the EG95 vaccine is associated with conformational epitopes. Vaccine 2000; 19:498–507.

77. Okano M, et al. Lacto-*N*-fucopentaose III found on *Schistosoma mansoni* egg antigens functions as adjuvant for proteins by inducing Th2-type response. J Immunol 2001; 167:442–450.

78. Hagan P, et al. Schistosomiasis vaccines: a response to a Devil's Advocate view. Parasitol Today 2000; 16:322–323.

79. Hu W, et al. Evolutionary and biomedical implications of a *Schistosoma japonicum* complementary DNA resource. Nature Genetics 2003; 35:139–147.

80. Verjovski-Almeida, et al. Transcriptome analysis of the acoelomate human parasite *Schistosoma mansoni*. Nature Genet 2003; 35:148–157.

76

Vaccines Against *Entamoeba histolytica*

Christopher D. Huston* and William A. Petri, Jr.
University of Virginia School of Medicine, Charlottesville, Virginia, U.S.A.

I. INTRODUCTION

Amebic colitis and liver abscess are due to infection with the enteric protozoan parasite, *Entamoeba histolytica*. This parasite has recently been separated using modern diagnostic techniques from the nonpathogenic parasite *E. dispar*, which is more common and identical in appearance to *E. histolytica* [2]. The World Health Organization (WHO) estimates that approximately 50 million people worldwide suffer from invasive amebic infection each year, with a resultant 40,000–100,000 deaths annually [1]. Infection with *E. histolytica* occurs worldwide, but people living in Central and South America, Africa, and India suffer from the bulk of the morbidity and mortality [2,3]. Carefully conducted serological studies in Mexico, where amebiasis is endemic, demonstrated antibody to *E. histolytica* in 8.4% of the population [4]. In the urban slum of Fortaleza, Brazil, 25% of the people tested carried antibody to *E. histolytica*; the prevalence of antiamebic antibodies in children aged 6–14 years was 40% [5]. A prospective study of preschool children in a slum of Dhaka Bangladesh demonstrated new *E. histolytica* infection in 39% of children over a 1-year period of observation, with 10% of the children having an *E. histolytica* infection associated with diarrhea and 3% with dysentery [6].

Recent advances include not only the reclassification of *E. histolytica* from *E. dispar* but also the identification of several amebic proteins associated with virulence, which are potential vaccine candidates [7–10]. More is also becoming known about the human immune response to amebic infection, and about the feasibility of a vaccine. This chapter summarizes the current knowledge of how *E. histolytica* causes invasive disease, the role of the host innate and acquired immune responses to limiting amebic infection, and recent progress in the development of a vaccine for amebiasis.

II. PATHOGENESIS

It is generally accepted that *E. histolytica* invades tissues and causes clinical disease through a well-defined sequence of events that starts with the ingestion of the infectious cyst form of the parasite from fecally contaminated food or water [11–14]. Excystation of the amebic trophozoites occurs in the intestinal lumen. The trophozoites adhere to the colonic mucus and epithelial cells through the binding of a parasite galactose and *N*-acetyl-D-galactosamine (Gal/GalNac)-inhibitable lectin with host Gal/GalNac-containing glycoconjugates [7,15]. Secretion of proteolytic enzymes by the parasite may aid the disruption of the intestinal mucus and epithelial barrier, and may facilitate tissue penetration [8]. The trophozoite kills host epithelial and immune cells at points of invasion, causing the characteristic flask-shaped colonic ulcers for which it is known. Finally, *E. histolytica* resists the host's immune response and survives to cause prolonged extraintestinal infection such as amebic liver abscesses.

III. ADHERENCE

The adherence of *E. histolytica* trophozoites in vivo to the colonic mucosal surface occurs prior to tissue penetration or cytotoxicity [12–14]. The adherence of the parasite to the host is mediated by a parasite lectin that binds to *N*-acetyl-D-galactosamine and D-galactose (Gal/GalNAc) (reviewed in Ref. 7) [15,16]. The blockade of amebic Gal/GalNAc lectin activity with millimolar concentrations of Gal or GalNAc prevents the contact-dependent cytotoxicity for which the organism is named [16]. Additionally, Chinese hamster ovary (CHO) cell glycosylation-deficient mutants lacking terminal Gal/GalNAc residues on *N*-linked and *O*-linked sugars are nearly totally resistant to amebic adherence and cytolytic activity [17,18]. Importantly, the Gal/GalNac lectin also mediates adherence to human neutrophils, colonic mucins, and epithelial cells—the in vivo targets of *E. histolytica* [7,19]. The disruption of the lectin (via inducible expression in the parasite of a dominant-negative mutant of

---
* *Current affiliation*: University of Vermont College of Medicine, Burlington, Vermont, U.S.A.

the lectin) inhibits amebic abscess formation in an animal model [20].

The Gal/GalNAc lectin is composed of a 260-kDa heterodimer of disulfide-linked heavy (170 kDa) and light (35/31 kDa) subunits, which is noncovalently associated with an intermediate subunit of 150 kDa (Figure 1) [15,20–26]. The 170-kDa subunit contains a carboxyl-terminal cytoplasmic and transmembrane domain adjacent to a cysteine-rich extracellular domain [23,24]. Five distinct genes (termed *hgl1–hgl5*) encoding the lectin's heavy subunit have been identified and at least partially sequenced in strain HM1: IMSS, and simultaneous expression of three different heavy subunit genes has been demonstrated in cultures of trophozoites [25]. At least 89% sequence homology exists within this gene family, and the number and location of every cysteine residue are conserved [22,23,25]. The carbohydrate recognition domain (CRD) is located within the cysteine-rich domain of the heavy subunit [26,27]. A peptide encompassing cysteine-rich region amino acids 895–998 expressed in *Escherichi coli* has been shown to bind to Gal/GalNAc in vitro [26].

The function of the light and intermediate subunits of the Gal/GalNAc lectin remains unclear. Six to seven gene loci and at least three unique genes coding for the light subunit exist and are simultaneously expressed [25]. Interference with the overall production of light subunit via antisense production results in a reduction in heterodimeric lectin and a decrease in cytotoxicity [28]. The intermediate subunit is encoded by two genes, which share 81% amino acid sequence

identity and are in turn members of a much larger family of amebic genes containing CXXC and CXC motifs [22].

IV. INVASION

In most human infections, the host remains asymptomatic [6,30,31]; alternatively, the trophozoite may penetrate the colonic mucus and epithelial barrier in a first step toward invasive disease. Penetration of the lamina propria can occur in the absence of local inflammation [12,13]. A discussion of parasite mechanisms of invasion can logically be divided into the roles of amebic proteinases and contact-dependent cytotoxicity [32].

Two classes of amebic proteinases believed to play a role in pathogenesis have been isolated: thiol (cysteine) proteinases, which are secreted as well as located on the amebic cell surface, and a surface-bound metallocollagenase (reviewed in Ref. 8). Several investigators have independently purified amebic cysteine proteinases and have confirmed their ability to degrade relevant tissue proteins in vitro including type I collagen and the anchoring proteins fibronectin and laminin [33–35]. The cysteine proteinases also degrade IgA, IgG, and the complement anaphylatoxins C3a and C5a [36–39].

A total of six distinct *E. histolytica* genes (termed *EhCP1–EhCP6*) encoding typical precursors of cysteine proteinases have been identified and partially sequenced [40]. Cysteine proteinase activity in lysates from various *E. histolytica* isolates can be almost completely attributed to the expression of three of these genes: *EhCP1*, *EhCP2*, and *EhCP5*. *E. dispar* carries genes homologous to four of the six genes carried by *E. histolytica* (termed *EdCP2*, *EdCP3*, *EdCP4*, and *EdCP6*), but appears to lack genes similar to *EhCP1* and *EhCP5* [40]. In *E. dispar*, the most abundant RNA encoding a cysteine proteinase corresponds to the *EdCP3* gene, which contributes very little to *E. histolytica*'s proteinase activity [41]. Differences in the genes encoding cysteine proteinases and in their expression could partially explain the differences in pathogenicity between *E. histolytica* and *E. dispar*.

The release of the cysteine proteinases by *E. histolytica* is spontaneous [42], and the in vitro ability of trophozoites to degrade collagen correlates with virulence [43,44]. Amebic cysteine proteinases with the ability to activate interleukin-1β have also been implicated in intestinal inflammation [45]. The inhibition of cysteine proteinases of *E. histolytica* by the use of irreversible chemical inhibitors or antisense RNA results in a reduction or elimination of the ability of the amebae to form liver abscesses in animal models following intrahepatic injection of virulent trophozoites, supporting the role of cysteine proteinases in pathogenicity [46,47].

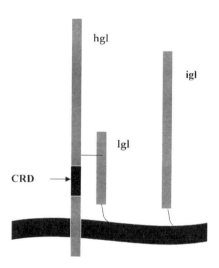

Figure 1 Gal/GalNAc adherence lectin of *E. histolytica*. The Gal/GalNAc lectin mediates parasite adherence to and killing of host cells. It is present on the plasma membrane of the ameba and is composed of three subunits. The integral membrane heavy subunit (hgl) has a short cytoplasmic tail implicated in intracellular signaling. The CRD is located within hgl. Hgl is disulfide-bonded to a lipid-anchored light subunit (lgl). Finally, the lipid-anchored intermediate subunit (igl) is noncovalently associated with the hgl–lgl heterodimer. The functions of lgl and igl in adherence and killing are unknown.

V. CYTOLYTIC ACTIVITY

The cause of the remarkable cytolytic activity for which *E. histolytica* is named has been the subject of intense investigation (Figure 2). Moments after the trophozoite contacts the host via the Gal/GalNAc lectin, host cells undergo membrane blebbing and loss of cytoplasmic granules and membrane integrity followed by cell death within 5–15 min

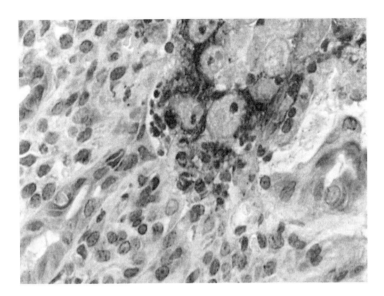

Figure 2 Parasite-induced apoptosis of host cells at the site of colonic invasion. C3H/HeJ mice were infected intracecally with *E. histolytica* trophozoites. Twenty-four days after infection, cecal tissues were examined for apoptosis with the terminal deoxynucleotidyl transferase-mediated dUTP-biotin nick-end labeling (TUNEL) stain. Apoptotic cells labeled brown by the TUNEL stain can be seen in contact with and within amebic trophozoites (arrows) (b, original magnification ×600). (Reprinted from Ref. 54.)

[16]. The parasite's ability to form abscesses is impaired in amebae rendered defective in cytotoxicity, either by inducible expression of a dominant negative mutant of the Gal/GalNAc lectin, or by expression of antisense RNA to the Gal/GalNAc lectin [20,28]. Therefore, *E. histolytica* cytotoxicity appears crucial to the ability of the parasite to cause disease.

Studies using cinemicrography show that blebbing and cell death of CHO cell monolayers occur only upon direct contact between amebae and their target cell [32]. The calcium channel blockers, verapamil and bepridil, significantly inhibit amebic cytotoxicity, as do the calcium chelator, ethylenediaminetetraacetate (EDTA), and the putative blocker of intracellular calcium flux, 8-(*N,N*-diethylamino)octyl-3,4,5-trimethoxybenzoate (TMB-8) [48,49]. As determined by studies utilizing the fluorescent calcium probe Fura-2 AM, the target cell's intracellular calcium concentration rises irreversibly and approximately 300-fold within 30 sec of contact with a trophozoite. The addition of D-galactose completely blocks both this calcium flux [50] and cytolysis [16,32]. Because abutment of trophozoites and target cells via centrifugation in the presence of galactose was not adequate to promote killing, the Gal/GalNac lectin appears to participate actively in the cytolytic process rather than simply bringing host cells and amebae together [16]. Upon the incubation of CHO cells with purified Gal/GalNac lectin at sublethal concentrations, a reversible rise in intracellular calcium concentration of magnitude and speed comparable to that observed with whole amebae occurs [51]. Minimal chromium release from CHO cells incubated with affinity-purified lectin, however, suggests that the lectin alone is not sufficient to induce cytotoxicity [51].

The ultimate cause of target cell lysis induced by *E. histolytica* may involve both programmed cell death and necrosis. Compaction of nuclear chromatin, cytoplasmic condensation, and membrane blebbing, as well as DNA fragmentation characteristic of apoptotic cell death have been observed in a murine myeloid cell line killed by *E. histolytica* [52]. In contrast, other investigators have observed changes consistent with necrosis, including cytoplasmic swelling, and compromised membrane integrity [53]. The killing of the Jurkat human T lymphocyte cell line occurred via apoptosis, as judged by DNA fragmentation and caspase 3 activation. This killing was inhibited by galactose. Classical upstream caspases seemed not to be involved, as caspase 8-deficient cells, resistant to killing by FasL, were readily killed by *E. histolytica* [54]. Caspase 8-deficient cells treated with a caspase 9 inhibitor (Ac-LEHD-fmk) (at a level sufficient to inhibit apoptosis via etoposide) were readily killed as well. In contrast, the caspase 3 inhibitor, Ac-DEVD-CHO, at 100 μM (sufficient to block killing via actinomycin D) blocked *E. histolytica* killing, as measured both by DNA fragmentation and ^{51}Cr release, indicating that it was necessary both for the apoptotic death phenotype and for necrosis to occur [54]. The blockade of caspases has been shown to block amebic liver abscess formation in mice [55]. The mechanism by which the parasite activates caspase 3 to initiate cell death is unknown [54].

Several laboratories have reported the isolation of amebic pore-forming proteins similar in function to the pore-forming proteins of the immune system [56–60]. A 5-kDa polypeptide with pore-forming activity in liposomes, which may be a major effector molecule mediating *E. histolytica*'s ability to kill endocytosed bacteria, has been described [58]. The amoebapore (reviewed in Ref. 9) is a 77-amino-acid polypeptide. Computer-aided analysis of secondary structure predicts four adjacent α-helices with tertiary structure maintained by three disulfide bonds [60]. Synthetic peptides based on the amino acid sequence of the amoebapore possess cytolytic activity against bacteria and eukaryotic cells, and antisense RNA inhibition of amoebapore synthesis decreases amebic cytotoxicity [61,62].

VI. SERUM RESISTANCE

Invasion of the colon and hematogenous spread to the liver result in the continuous exposure of the extracellular trophozoite to the human complement system. The complement system is one of the first barriers to infection in nonimmune individuals; circumvention of this defense is central to the pathogenesis of amebiasis. Trophozoites activate the classical and alternative complement pathways in the absence of antiamebic antibodies. The incubation of trophozoites in normal human sera results in the depletion of human complement, as measured by CH50 and C5b-9 hemolytic assays and C3 and C4 depletion [63]. The amebic 56-kDa cysteine proteinase cleaves C3 at a site one amino acid distal to that of the human C3 convertase, and may be the route by which the complement is activated [64,65]. Depletion of complement in hamsters by cobra venom factor treatment increases both the frequency and the severity of amebic liver abscess, providing evidence of the protective role of the complement system in amebiasis [66].

E. histolytica freshly isolated from patients with invasive amebiasis and laboratory strains passed through animals activate the alternative complement pathway but are resistant to C5b-9 complexes deposited on the membrane surface [63–65]. On the other hand, amebae cultured from the stool of asymptomatically infected individuals or virulent amebae attenuated by axenic (in the absence of associated bacteria) culture activate the alternative complement pathway and are killed by C5b-9 [63–65].

The killing of amebae is mediated by the terminal complement components. and the direct lysis of sensitive, but not resistant, *E. histolytica* has been demonstrated with purified complement components C5b-9 [65]. Resistance to terminal complement attack in *E. histolytica* could be due to an amebic cell surface protein with C5b-9-inhibitory activity, or to endocytosis or shedding of the C5b-9 complex. Rapid membrane repair via shedding or endocytosis of the membrane-inserted C5b-9 complex has been postulated to confer C5b-9 resistance to several different cells, including nucleated mammalian cells and the metacyclical (infective promastigote) stage of *Leishmania major*. However, the shedding or release of C9 from the membrane does not appear to be the explanation for C5b-9 resistance in *E. histolytica*, as C9 binding is higher in resistant than sensitive amebae.

Braga et al. produced monoclonal antibodies against serum-resistant amebae and identified an antibody that increased *E. histolytica* lysis by human sera and by purified human complement components C5b-9. It was a surprise that the antigen recognized by the antibody was the 170-kDa lectin subunit [67]. The inhibition of complement resistance by the anti-170 kDa mAb was shown to be specific to mAb-recognizing epitopes 6 and 7. An examination of the sequence of the 170-kDa subunit showed limited identity with CD59, a human inhibitor of C5b-9 assembly, and the purified lectin was recognized by anti-CD59 anti-

bodies. The lectin bound to purified human C8 and C9, and blocked assembly in the amebic membrane of the complement membrane attack complex at the steps of C8 and C9 insertion.

The lectin gene family therefore appears to participate not only in adherence and host cell killing, but also in the evasion of the complement system of defense via a remarkable mimicry of human CD59. Gal/GalNAc inhibition of lectin activity had only a minor effect on C5b-9 resistance of trophozoites, suggesting that the lectin and complement regulatory domains of the lectin are distinct.

VII. THE INNATE AND ACQUIRED IMMUNE RESPONSE TO AMEBIASIS

Although the precise roles and importance of humoral and cellular responses in immunity remain to determined, protective immunity is likely to involve elements of both. Immunization of animals with several *E. histolytica* antigens provides protection from an intrahepatic challenge with *E. histolytica* [68]. These antigens include serine-rich and cysteine-rich proteins and the Gal/GalNAc adherence lectin.

Antibodies appear to play a role in immunization-mediated protection, as evidenced from studies using a severe combined immunodeficient (SCID) mouse model of amebic liver abscess. The passive transfer to SCID mice of antibodies against whole *E. histolytica* proteins, serine-rich proteins, or cysteine-rich domains of the galactose lectin resulted in a faster resolution of amebic liver abscess [26, 69–71].

Proinflammatory cytokines also appear to be important for protective immunity. Lymphocytes from patients recovered from invasive amebic disease proliferate in response to amebic antigens, have amebicidal activity, and produce interleukin-2 and interferon gamma (IFN-γ) [72,73]. Macrophages and neutrophils activated by IFN-γ and tumor necrosis factor alpha (TNF-α) are endowed with the capability of killing *E. histolytica* trophozoites, whereas in the absence of activation, these immune effector cells were killed by the amebae [72,73]. Proinflammatory cytokine production in response to *E. histolytica* infection may, in part, be an innate immune response: the purified Gal/GalNAc lectin promotes the production of IL-12 and TNF-α production by macrophages [74,75]. In murine macrophages, TNF-α was shown to play a central role in activating macrophages for nitric oxide-dependent cytotoxicity against *E. histolytica* [76]. Mice with targeted disruption ("knockout") of either IFN-γ or inducible nitric oxide synthase had more severe amebiasis, providing in vivo evidence of the importance of proinflammatory cytokines in protection [76].

VIII. ACQUIRED IMMUNITY IN HUMANS

Until recently, little was known about the existence or nature of acquired immunity. The development of invasive amebiasis in some *E. histolytica*-colonized individuals and documented second infections led many to conclude that acquired immunity was nonexistent or, at best, incomplete [77–80]. There was little in the way of clinical research to contradict

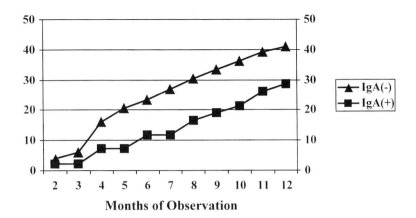

Figure 3 Cumulative percentage of *E. histolytica* infection in children with or without mucosal lectin-specific IgA at the time of enrollment. The two groups are statistically significantly different at 5 months ($P = 0.03$) and 7 months ($P = 0.04$). (Reprinted from Ref. 6.)

this conclusion. Confounding the problem was the fact that most researchers failed to distinguish the invasive parasite *E. histolytica* from the noninvasive but identical in appearance parasite *E. dispar*, making their work difficult to interpret.

The existence of acquired immunity to amebiasis was discovered in a prospective observational study of amebiasis in preschool children in Dhaka, Bangladesh. Immunity was linked to a mucosal antiadherence lectin IgA response. The association of mucosal antilectin IgA with protection was demonstrated three ways. First, in a cross-sectional analysis, *E. histolytica* colonization was absent in all 64 children with stool antilectin IgA. Second, children with stool antilectin IgA acquired fewer new *E. histolytica* infections over a prospective period of observation [3/42 IgA (+) vs. 47/227 IgA (−); $P = 0.03$] (Figure 3). Finally, the appearance of a stool IgA antilectin response coincided with the resolution of infection. Mucosal antilectin IgA is therefore an indicator of

immune protection and may prove effective as a surrogate marker of vaccine efficacy [6].

IX. VACCINE CANDIDATES

Although whole *E. histolytica* proteins elicit a protective immune response indicating that an effective antiamebic vaccine is possible, vaccines using native antigens are expensive and impractical to produce. This has driven an aggressive search for antigens that might form the basis of a cheap, recombinant vaccine (reviewed in Refs. 10 and 68). Candidate proteins (see Table 1) that have been developed have mostly been cell surface or secreted. Among these are amebic proteins implicated in pathogenesis, including the Gal/Gal-Nac lectin, the cysteine proteinases, and the amoebapore. The use of cDNA libraries has resulted in the isolation of two

Table 1 Known Characteristics of Current Antiamebic Vaccine Candidates

Amebic protein	Putative function	Surface expression?	Conserved?	Immunogenic?	Protective in animal models?
Amoebapore	Cytolytic activity	Yes, secreted	Yes	Unknown	Unknown
Cysteine proteinase	Tissue penetration/ degrades IgA, IgG, C3a, and C5a	Yes, secreted	Yes	Yes	Unknown
Gal/GalNac lectin	Adherence/ complement resistance	Yes	Yes	Yes	Yes
SREHP	Possible role in adherence	Yes	No	Yes	Yes
29-kDa cysteine-rich antigen	Thiol-dependent peroxidase	Controversial, probably yes	Yes	In liver abscess only	Yes

Source: Ref. 68.

additional candidates: the serine-rich *E. histolytica* protein (SREHP) and the 29-kDa cysteine-rich *E. histolytica* antigen [81,82].

X. PARENTERAL VACCINES

The Gal/GalNac lectin plays an essential role in adherence and cytotoxicity, as well as in resistance to serum complement. In addition, the lectin's cysteine-rich extracellular domain is highly conserved [83,84]. The 170-kDa heavy subunit is the predominant amebic protein recognized by immune sera of individuals cured of invasive amebiasis from geographically diverse areas including the United States, Mexico, Africa, India, and Jordan [83,84]. More than 90% of sera from individuals with amebic liver abscess or asymptomatic colonization with *E. histolytica* contain antilectin antibodies [83–85]. Furthermore, as mentioned above, acquired immunity in humans is associated with the production of mucosal IgA against the lectin.

In one study, 100% of gerbils immunized with purified native Gal/GalNac lectin in complete Freund's adjuvant developed high-titer serum antibodies to the heavy subunit. Immune sera completely blocked amebic adherence to CHO cells at 1/10 dilutions, and 67% of gerbils were completely protected from liver abscess following intrahepatic injection of trophozoites. Surprisingly, the remaining animals developed larger abscesses [86]. Antibodies to different epitopes on the lectin's 170-kDa heavy subunit variably enhance or inhibit amebic adherence to CHO cells and to human colonic mucin, but no differences in the development of antilectin antibodies or their adherence-inhibitory properties were observed in the immunized gerbils [86].

Parenteral immunization with two different recombinant peptides based on the cysteine-rich extracellular portion of the lectin's heavy subunit has been protective in the gerbil model of amebic liver abscess. In one study, immunization of gerbils with the recombinant LC3 region and Titermax adjuvant elicited a high-titer serum IgG response capable of inhibiting amebic adherence to CHO cells. There was a 71% reduction in the number of animals with liver abscesses following intrahepatic challenge and, in contrast to abscesses following immunization with the native lectin, abscesses in the immunized gerbils that developed them were no larger than in controls [87]. Similarly, Lotter et al. immunized gerbils with several recombinant peptides based on the carboxyl-terminal portion of the lectin's cysteine-rich extracellular domain. Immunization with a 115-amino-acid peptide (termed 170CR2) completely prevented abscess development in 62.5% of animals, and the remaining animals in this study developed significantly smaller abscesses than unimmunized controls. Antibody production to a 25-amino-acid sequence within 170CR2 correlated strongly with the development of protective immunity. Successful passive immunization of SCID mice with rabbit serum raised against the peptide reconfirmed the importance of humoral immunity in the prevention of amebic liver abscess [88].

Stanley et al. [81] identified the SREHP by screening cDNA libraries. This protein contains multiple-tandem dodecapeptide repeats reminiscent of the repetitive circum-

sporozoite antigens of malarial species. Indirect immunofluorescent staining localizes the native SREHP to the cell surface and to focal areas within the cytoplasm [89]. Different *E. histolytica* isolates have different numbers of dodecapeptide repeats encoded within their SREHP genes [90]. Western blots for the presence of anti-SREHP antibodies in patients from diverse geographical regions with acute invasive amebiasis were positive in 82%. Seropositivity ranged from 65% in Durban, South Africa to 91% in Mexico City [91]. Differences in the observed rates of anti-SREHP antibody production may have been due to differences in the timing of serum sampling during the course of acute illness. They also raise the possibility that local populations have differing abilities to produce anti-SREHP antibodies, or that differences in the number of SREHP repeats in different *E. histolytica* isolates affect immunogenicity [91].

Zhang et al. tested the ability of recombinant SREHP to elicit a protective immune response against amebic liver abscess in gerbils. Gerbils were immunized either subcutaneously in a single shot, or intraperitoneally in a series of three shots with a recombinant SREHP/maltose-binding protein (MBP) fusion protein combined with complete Freund's adjuvant. Immunization completely prevented amebic liver abscess following intrahepatic challenge in 64% of gerbils immunized intraperitoneally and 100% of gerbils immunized with a single subcutaneous shot. All of the immunized animals developed delayed-type hypersensitivity reactions [92]. African green monkeys immunized with three doses of the SREHP/MBP fusion protein developed serum antiamebic antibodies 10 days after the first booster. Unfortunately, the control monkeys in this trial did not develop liver abscesses following intrahepatic challenge, so vaccine efficacy could not be assessed [93].

Screening of cDNA libraries also identified the 29-kDa cysteine-rich *E. histolytica* antigen, another immunogenic protein that may be suitable for inclusion in a vaccine [82]. The 29-kDa antigen appears to be a thiol-dependent peroxidase because it possesses hydrogen peroxide-removing capacity in the presence of reducing agents such as thioredoxin [97,98]. It may, therefore, protect *E. histolytica* from oxidative attack by activated neutrophils and macrophages. The location of the 29-kDa antigen within the ameba remains controversial. Immunofluorescent staining of formalin-fixed cells with monoclonal antibodies shows the protein within both the nucleus and the cytoplasm [97,98]. An enzyme-linked immunosorbent assay (ELISA) using purified native and recombinant 29-kDa proteins demonstrated the presence of anti-29-kDa antibodies in 79% of people with amebic liver abscess, but failed to show significant antibody production in patients suffering from amebic colitis and in asymptomatic carriers [98]. Intraperitoneal immunization of gerbils with a recombinant fusion protein based on the 29-kDa protein and Titermax adjuvant elicited production of antigen-specific IgG and was partially protective (54% vaccine efficacy) against amebic liver abscess following intrahepatic challenge with virulent trophozoites [99].

The cysteine proteinases and the amoebapore are additional amebic proteins associated with virulence that must be considered. Each has yet to be evaluated as a potential vaccine component. Numerous studies document the central role of amebic cysteine proteinases in the penetration of host tissues and in the evasion of host defenses via the degradation of IgA, IgG, C3a, and C5a. Patients with amebic liver abscess, moreover, develop antibodies to histolysain (*EhCP2*), and the use of protease inhibitors in SCID mice reduces the size of liver abscesses following intrahepatic injection of trophozoites. The recombinant amoebapore's cytotoxicity toward eukaryotic cells prohibits its use in a vaccine. The identification of antigenic regions within this peptide, however, should yield other possible vaccinogens.

XI. ORAL VACCINES

Two major oral vaccine strategies have been used: the incorporation of amebic antigens into attenuated bacterial strains, and the creation of fusion proteins composed of amebic antigens and cholera toxin or its subunits. An effective oral vaccine against *E. histolytica* could have several advantages over parenteral preparations. A direct stimulation of the gut-associated lymphoid tissue (GALT) might stimulate the production of secretory IgA more effectively than parenteral immunization, and prevent both colonization and invasive disease. By establishing a limited invasive infection in the host, moreover, an oral vaccine carried by an attenuated bacterial strain might provide more prolonged immunity than parenteral vaccines based on the same antigens. Combination vaccines providing protection against multiple organisms may also be possible. For example, immunization with attenuated *Salmonella typhi* strains engineered to express amebic antigens might protect against both amebiasis and typhoid fever. Finally, the lower cost and ease of administering an oral vaccine would increase acceptance in developing nations.

An oral attenuated vaccine for typhoid fever is currently in use in humans. Foreign antigens expressed in attenuated *Salmonella* species can effectively stimulate both cell-mediated immunity and production of secretory IgA. Oral immunization of mice and gerbils with an attenuated strain of *S. typhimurium* that expresses the SREHP/MBP fusion protein at high levels resulted in the production of secretory IgA and serum IgG. Anti-lipopolysaccharide (LPS) antibodies also developed in both sham-immunized and immunized animals, suggesting that the amebic antigen did not impair the immune response to the *Salmonella* infection. A vaccine protective against both, therefore, might be possible. Following intrahepatic injection with amebic trophozoites, 100% of control gerbils and only 22% of immunized gerbils developed abscesses in this study [100]. In another study, oral immunization of gerbils with *S. dublin* expressing a fragment of the Gal/GalNac lectin resulted in significant reduction in mean abscess weight, but no significant difference in the number of animals developing abscesses. No serum antiamebic antibody production was observed in this study, suggesting that the observed protection may have been cell-mediated [101]. The plasmid carrying the lectin fragment, however, was somewhat unstable in vitro; higher or more prolonged expression of the antigen may have resulted in antibody production and in greater vaccine efficacy [101].

Cholera toxin has two subunits, a 28-kDa A subunit with ADP-ribosylating activity and an 11.5-kDa B or binding subunit. The A subunit contains A1, the active toxin domain, and A2, which noncovalently links subunit A to five B subunits. A pentamer of B subunits binds the intestinal epithelium. Whole cholera toxin stimulates the production of serum IgG and secretory IgA when orally administered, and also stimulates immunity to coadministered antigens [102]. In humans, the B subunit retains some of whole cholera toxin's oral adjuvant properties. Parenteral immunization of rats with native Gal/GalNac lectin in complete Freund's adjuvant followed by intra-Peyer's patch injection of lectin with cholera toxin's B subunit stimulates the production of antilectin secretory IgA [103]. Oral immunization of mice with the recombinant LC3 portion of the lectin and whole cholera toxin induced the production of secretory IgA capable of inhibiting the adherence of amebic trophozoites to CHO cells. Interestingly, there was a negative correlation between intestinal IgA production, and serum IgA and IgG titers in this study [104]. High-dose oral immunization with streptococcal antigens by other investigators has resulted similarly in a strong mucosal immune response with no systemic antibody production, whereas lower doses led both to mucosal and systemic antibody production [105].

A potential limitation of strategies combining recombinant peptides with cholera toxin's B subunit is that large, attached molecules might prevent the pentamerization of the B subunit and reduce its adjuvant properties by changing its ability to bind to intestinal epithelium. The coupling of antigens to the B subunit via A2 to create holotoxin-like molecules could potentially increase their immunogenicity as well as facilitate the use of larger recombinant antigens. A holotoxin-like molecule containing the SREHP fused to the A2 domain of cholera toxin (SREHP-H) has been created. Oral immunization of mice with SREHP-H coexpressed with the cholera toxin B subunit in *E. coli* resulted in the production of mucosal IgA and serum IgG antiamebic antibodies [106].

XII. CONCLUSIONS AND AREAS FOR FURTHER INVESTIGATION

The identification of acquired immunity to amebiasis in humans lends tremendous credence to the development of a vaccine against *E. histolytica*. Many obstacles to the production of a vaccine have fallen by the wayside in the last decade. Effective immunity in humans is now known to be associated with a mucosal IgA response against the Gal/GalNAc lectin, one of several well-characterized virulence factors of the parasite. A mouse model of amebic colitis has been developed and allows for the first-time identification of protective immune responses at the mucosal surface where infection occurs. Well-characterized cohorts of children with *E. histolytica* infection have been described. The extremely high rates of new *E. histolytica* infection in these children should enable the testing of vaccine efficacy using small numbers of patients. Although much progress has been made, the burden of disease due to amebiasis throughout the tropical and subtropical world makes vaccine development an urgent task.

ACKNOWLEDGMENTS

Work from the authors' laboratory was supported by NIH grant AI26649. W. A. P. is a Burroughs Wellcome Scholar in Molecular Parasitology and C. D. H. is a recipient of a Howard Hughes Medical Institute Postdoctoral Fellowship for Physicians.

REFERENCES

1. WHO. Amoebiasis. WHO Wkly Epidemiol Rec 1997; 72(14): 97–100.
2. Diamond LS, Clark CG. A redescription of *Entamoeba histolytica* Schaudinn 1903 (emended Walker 1911) separating it from *Entamoeba dispar* (Brumpt 1925). J Eukaryot Microbiol 1993; 40(3):340–344.
3. Petri WA. Recent advances in amebiasis. Crit Rev Clin Lab Sci 1996; 33(1):1–37.
4. Caballero-Salcedo A, et al. Seroepidemiology of amebiasis in Mexico. Am J Trop Med Hyg 1994; 50(4):412–419.
5. Braga LL, et al. Seroepidemiology of *Entamoeba histolytica* in a slum in Northeastern Brazil. Am J Trop Med Hyg 1996; 55(6):693–697.
6. Haque R, et al. Amebiasis and mucosal IgA antibody against the *Entamoeba histolytica* adherence lectin in Bangladeshi children. J Infect Dis 2001; 183:1787–1793.
7. Petri WA Jr, et al. The bittersweet interface of parasite and host: lectin–carbohydrate interaction during human invasion by the parasite *Entamoeba histolytica*. Annu Rev Microbiol 2002; 56:39–64.
8. McKerrow JH, et al. The protease and pathogenicity of parasitic protozoa. Annu Rev Microbiol 1993; 47:821–853.
9. Leippe M, Muller-Eberhard HJ. The pore-forming peptide of *Entamoeba histolytica*, the protozoan parasite causing human amebiasis. Toxicology 1994; 87(1–3):5–18.
10. Stanley SL. Progress towards development of a vaccine for amebiasis. Clin Microbiol Rev 1997; 10(4):637–649.
11. Ravdin JI. Amebiasis now. Am J Trop Med Hyg 1989; 41(3):40–48.
12. Takeuchi A, Phillips BP. Electron microscope studies of experimental *Entamoeba histolytica* infection in the guinea pig. Am J Trop Med Hyg 1975; 24(1):34–48.
13. Beaver PC, et al. Invasive amebiasis in naturally infected new world and old world monkeys with and without clinical disease. Am J Trop Med Hyg 1988; 39(4):343–352.
14. Chadee K, Meerovitch E. *Entamoeba histolytica*: early progressive pathology in the cecum of the gerbil (*Meriones unguiculatus*). Am J Trop Med Hyg 1985; 34(2):283–291.
15. Petri WA, et al. Isolation of the galactose-binding lectin which mediates the in vitro adherence of *Entamoeba histolytica*. J Clin Invest 1987; 80(5):1238–1244.
16. Ravdin JI, Guerrant RL. Role of adherence in cytopathogenic mechanisms of *Entamoeba histolytica*. Study with mammalian tissue culture cells and human erythrocytes. J Clin Invest 1981; 68(5):1305–1313.
17. Li E, et al. Chinese hamster ovary cells deficient in *N*-acetylglucosaminyltransferase I activity are resistant to *Entamoeba histolytica*-mediated cytotoxicity. Infect Immun 1989; 57:8–12.
18. Ravdin JI, et al. Characterization of cell surface carbohydrate receptors for *Entamoeba histolytica* adherence lectin. Infect Immun 1989; 57:2179–2186.
19. Chadee K, et al. Rat and human colonic mucins bind to and inhibit adherence lectin of *Entamoeba histolytica*. J Clin Invest 1987; 80(5):1245–1254.
20. Vines RR, et al. Regulation of adherence and virulence by the *Entamoeba histolytica* lectin cytoplasmic domain, which contains an β2 integrin motif. Mol Biol Cell 1998; 9:2069–2079.
21. Petri WA, et al. Subunit structure of the galactose and *N*-acetyl-D-galactosamine inhibitable adherence lectin of *Entamoeba histolytica*. J Biol Chem 1989; 264(5):3007–3012.
22. Cheng X-J, et al. The 150 kDa Gal/GalNac lectin co-receptor of *Entamoeba histolytica* is a member of a gene family containing multiple CXXC sequence motifs. Infect Immun 2001; 69:5892–5898.
23. Tannich E, et al. Primary structure of the 170-kDa surface lectin of pathogenic *Entamoeba histolytica*. Proc Natl Acad Sci USA 1991; 88:1849–1853.
24. Mann BJ, et al. Sequence of the cysteine-rich heavy subunit of the galactose lectin in *Entamoeba histolytica*. Proc Natl Acad Sci USA 1991; 88(8):3248–3252.
25. Ramakrishnan G, et al. Physical mapping and expression of gene families encoding the *N*-acetyl-D-galactosamine adherence lectin of *Entamoeba histolytica*. Mol Microbiol 1996; 19(1):91–100.
26. Dodson JM, et al. Role of the *Entamoeba histolytica* adhesin carbohydrate recognition domain in infection and immunity. J Infect Dis 1999; 179:460–466.
27. Pillai DR, et al. The cysteine-rich region of the *Entamoeba histolytica* adherence lectin (170-kilodalton subunit) is sufficient for high affinity Gal/GalNAc-specific binding in vitro. Infect Immun 1999; 67:3836–3841.
28. Ankri S, et al. Antisense inhibition of expression of the light subunit (35 kDa) of the Gal/GalNac lectin complex inhibits *Entamoeba histolytica* virulence. Mol Microbiol 1999; 33:327–337.
29. Petri WA, et al. Monoclonal antibodies directed against the galactose-binding lectin of *Entamoeba histolytica* enhance adherence. J Immunol 1990; 144(12):4803–4809.
30. Gathiram V, Jackson TFHG. Frequency distribution of *Entamoeba histolytica* zymodemes in a rural South African population. Lancet 1985; 1(8431):719–721.
31. Meza I, et al. Isoenzyme patterns of *Entamoeba histolytica* isolates from asymptomatic carriers: use of gradient acrylamide gels. Am J Trop Med Hyg 1986; 35(6):1134–1139.
32. Ravdin JI, et al. Cytopathogenic mechanisms of *Entamoeba histolytica*. J Exp Med 1980; 152(2):377–390.
33. Keene WE, et al. The major neutral proteinase of *Entamoeba histolytica*. J Exp Med 1986; 163(3):536–549.
34. Luaces AL, Barrett AJ. Affinity purification and biochemical characterization of histolysin, the major cysteine proteinase of *Entamoeba histolytica*. Biochem J 1988; 250(3): 903–909.
35. Lushbaugh WB, et al. *Entamoeba histolytica*: purification of cathepsin B. Exp Parasitol 1985; 59(3):328–336.
36. Kelsall BL, Ravdin JI. Degradation of human IgA by *Entamoeba histolytica*. J Infect Dis 1993; 168(5):1319–1322.
37. Thran VQ, et al. The neutral cysteine proteinase of *Entamoeba histolytica* degrades IgG and prevents its binding. J Infect Dis 1998; 177(2):508–511.
38. Herdman DS, et al. Cleavage of IgG by the neutral cysteine proteinase of *Entamoeba histolytica*. Arch Med Res 1997; 28:178–179.
39. Reed SL, et al. The extracellular neutral cysteine proteinase of *Entamoeba histolytica* degrades anaphylatoxins C3a and C5a. J Immunol 1995; 155(1):266–274.
40. Bruchhaus I, et al. *Entamoeba histolytica* and *Entamoeba dispar*: differences in numbers and expression of cysteine proteinase genes. Mol Microbiol 1996; 22(2):255–263.
41. Bruchhaus I, Tannich E. A gene highly homologous to ACPI encoding cysteine proteinase 3 in *Entamoeba histolytica* is present and expressed in *Entamoeba dispar*. Parasitol Res 1996; 82(2):189–192.

42. Leippe M, et al. Spontaneous release of cysteine proteinases but not of pore-forming peptides by viable *Entamoeba histolytica*. Parasitology 1995; 111(5):569–574.

43. Gadasi H, Kessler E. Correlation of virulence and collagenolytic activity in *Entamoeba histolytica*. Infect Immun 1983; 39(2):528–531.

44. Reed SL, et al. Thiol proteinase expression and pathogenicity of *Entamoeba histolytica*. J Clin Microbiol 1989; 27(12):2772–2777.

45. Zhang Z, et al. *Entamoeba histolytica* cysteine proteinases with interleukin-1 beta converting enzyme (ICE) activity cause intestinal inflammation and tissue damage in amoebiasis. Mol Microbiol 2000; 37:542–548.

46. Stanley SL, et al. Role of the *Entamoeba histolytica* cysteine proteinase in amebic liver abscess formation in severe combined immunodeficient (SCID) mice. Infect Immun 1995; 63(4):1587–1590.

47. Ankri S, et al. Antisense inhibition of expression of cysteine proteinases affects *Entamoeba histolytica*-induced formation of liver abscess in hamsters. Infect Immun 1999; 67:421–422.

48. Ravdin JI, et al. Effect of ion channel inhibitors on the cytopathogenicity of *Entamoeba histolytica*. J Infect Dis 1982; 146(3):335–340.

49. Ravdin JI, et al. Effect of calcium and phospholipase A on the cytopathogenicity of *Entamoeba histolytica*. J Infect Dis 1985; 152(3):542–549.

50. Ravdin JI, et al. Relationship of free intracellular calcium to the cytolytic activity of *Entamoeba histolytica*. Infect Immun 1988; 56(6):1505–1512.

51. Saffer LD, Petri WA. Role of the galactose lectin of *Entamoeba histolytica* in adherence-dependent killing of mammalian cells. Infect Immun 1991; 59(12):4681–4683.

52. Ragland BD, et al. *Entamoeba histolytica*: target cells killed by trophozoites undergo DNA fragmentation which is not blocked by Bcl-2. Exp Parasitol 1994; 79(3):460–467.

53. Berninghausen O, Leippe M. Necrosis vs. apoptosis as the mechanism of target cell death induced by *Entamoeba histolytica*. Infect Immun 1997; 65(9):3615–3621.

54. Huston CD, et al. Caspase 3 dependent killing of human cells by the parasite *Entamoeba histolytica*. Cell Microbiol 2000; 2:617–625.

55. Le Yan L, Stanley SL Jr. Blockade of caspases inhibits amebic liver abscess formation in a mouse model of disease. Infect Immun 2001; 69:7911–7914.

56. Young JD, et al. Characterization of a membrane pore-forming protein from *Entamoeba histolytica*. J Exp Med 1982; 156(6):1677–1690.

57. Lynch EC, et al. An ion-channel forming protein produced by *Entamoeba histolytica*. EMBO J 1982; 1(7):801–804.

58. Leippe M, et al. Pore-forming peptide of pathogenic *Entamoeba histolytica*. Proc Natl Acad Sci USA 1991; 88(17): 7659–7663.

59. Leippe M. Ancient weapons: NK-lysin is a mammalian homolog to pore-forming peptides of a protozoan parasite. Cell 1995; 83(1):17–18.

60. Leippe M, et al. Primary and secondary structure of the pore-forming peptide of pathogenic *Entamoeba histolytica*. EMBO J 1992; 11(10):3501–3506.

61. Leippe M, et al. Cytolytic and antibacterial activity of synthetic peptides derived from amoebapore, the pore-forming peptide of *Entamoeba histolytica*. Proc Natl Acad Sci USA 1994; 91(7):2602–2606.

62. Bracha R, et al. Antisense inhibition of amoebapore expression in *Entamoeba histolytica* causes a decrease in amoebic virulence. Mol Microbiol 1999; 34:463–472.

63. Reed SL, et al. Activation of complement by pathogenic and nonpathogenic *Entamoeba histolytica*. J Immunol 1986; 136:2265–2270.

64. Reed SL, et al. Cleavage of C3 by a neutral cysteine proteinase of *Entamoeba histolytica*. J Immunol 1989; 143:189–195.

65. Reed SL, Gigli I. Lysis of complement-sensitive *Entamoeba histolytica* by activated terminal complement components. J Clin Invest 1990; 86:1815–1822.

66. Capin R, et al. Effect of complement depletion on the induction of amebic liver abscess in the hamster. Arch Invest Med (Mexico) 1980; 11(suppl 1):173–180.

67. Braga LL, et al. Inhibition of the complement membrane attack complex by the galactose-specific adhesin of *Entamoeba histolytica*. J Clin Invest 1992; 90(3):1131–1137.

68. Huston CD, Petri WA Jr. Host–pathogen interaction in amebiasis and progress in vaccine development. Eur J Clin Microbiol Infect Dis 1998; 17:601–614.

69. Cieslak PR, et al. A severe combined immunodeficient (SCID) mouse model for infection with *Entamoeba histolytica*. J Exp Med 1992; 176:1605–1609.

70. Zhang T, Stanley SL Jr. Protection of gerbils from amebic liver abscess by immunization with a recombinant protein derived from the 170-kilodalton surface adhesin of *Entamoeba histolytica*. Infect Immun 1994; 62:2605–2608.

71. Lotter H, et al. Identification of an epitope on the *Entamoeba histolytica* 170 kD lectin conferring antibody-mediated protection against invasive amebiasis. J Exp Med 1997; 185: 1793–1801.

72. Salata RA, et al. Interaction of human leukocytes with *Entamoeba histolytica*: killing of virulent amebae by the activated macrophage. J Clin Invest 1985; 76:491–499.

73. Lin JY, et al. Tumor necrosis factor alpha augments nitric oxide-dependent macrophage cytotoxicity against *Entamoeba histolytica* by enhanced expression of the nitric oxide synthase gene. Infect Immun 1994; 62:1534–1541.

74. Campbell D, et al. A subunit vaccine candidate region of the *Entamoeba histolytica* galactose-adherence lectin promotes interleukin 12 gene transcription and protein production in human macrophages. Eur J Immunol 2000; 30:423–430.

75. Seguin R, et al. The tumor necrosis factor alpha-stimulating region of galactose-inhibitable lectin of *Entamoeba histolytica* activates gamma interferon-primed macrophages for amebicidal activity mediated by nitric oxide. Infect Immun 1997; 65:2522–2527.

76. Seydel KB, et al. Innate immunity to amebic liver abscess is dependent on gamma interferon and nitric oxide in a murine model of disease. Infect Immun 2000; 68:400–402.

77. Bray RS, Harris WG. The epidemiology of infection with *Entamoeba histolytica* in the Gambia, West Africa. Trans R Soc Trop Med Hyg 1977; 71:401–407.

78. Choudhari G, et al. Protective immunity to *Entamoeba histolytica* infection in subjects with amtiamoebic antibodies residing in a hyperendemic zone. Scand J Infect Dis 1991; 23:771–776.

79. Gathiram V, Jackson TFHG. Frequency distribution of *Entamoeba histolytica* zymodeme in a rural South Africa population. Lancet 1985; 1:719–721.

80. Wanke C, et al. Epidemiologic and clinical features of invasive amebiasis in Bangladesh: a case-control comparison with other diarrheal diseases and postmortem findings. Am J Trop Med Hyg 1988; 38:335–341.

81. Stanley SL, et al. Cloning and expression of a membrane antigen of *Entamoeba histolytica* possessing multiple tandem repeats. Proc Natl Acad Sci USA 1990; 87(13):4976–4980.

82. Torian BE, et al. cDNA sequence analysis of a 29-kDa cysteine-rich surface antigen of pathogenic *Entamoeba histolytica*. Proc Natl Acad Sci USA 1990; 87(16):6358–6362.

83. Petri WA, et al. Antigenic stability and immunodominance of the Gal/GalNac adherence lectin of *Entamoeba histolytica*. Am J Med Sci 1989; 297(3):163–165.

84. Ravdin JI, et al. Association of serum antibodies to adherence lectin with invasive amebiasis and asymptomatic in-

fection with pathogenic *Entamoeba histolytica*. J Infect Dis 1990; 162(3):768–772.

85. Petri WA, et al. Recognition of the galactose- or *N*-acetyl-galactosamine-binding lectin of *Entamoeba histolytica* by human immune sera. Infect Immun 1987; 55(10):2327–2331.

86. Petri WA, Ravdin JI. Protection of gerbils from amebic liver abscess by immunization with the galactose-specific adherence lectin of *Entamoeba histolytica*. Infect Immun 1991; 59(1):97–101.

87. Soong CJG, et al. A recombinant cysteine-rich section of the *Entamoeba histolytica* galactose-inhibitable lectin is efficacious as a subunit vaccine in the gerbil model of amebic liver abscess. J Infect Dis 1995; 171(3):645–651.

88. Lotter H, et al. Identification of an epitope on the *Entamoeba histolytica* 170-kDa lectin conferring antibody-mediated protection against invasive amebiasis. J Exp Med 1997; 185 (10):1793–1801.

89. Stanley SL, et al. The serine-rich *Entamoeba histolytica* protein is a phosphorylated membrane protein containing *O*-linked terminal *N*-acetylglucosamine residues. J Biol Chem 1995; 270(8):4121–4126.

90. Clark CG, Diamond LS. *Entamoeba histolytica*: a method for isolate identification. Exp Parasitol 1993; 77(4):450–455.

91. Stanley SL, et al. Serodiagnosis of invasive amebiasis using a recombinant *Entamoeba histolytica* protein. JAMA 1991; 266(14):1984–1986.

92. Zhang T, et al. Protection of gerbils from amebic liver abscess by immunization with a recombinant *Entamoeba histolytica* antigen. Infect Immun 1994; 62(4):1166–1170.

93. Stanley SL, et al. Immunogenicity of the recombinant serine rich *Entamoeba histolytica* protein (SREHP) in African green monkeys. Vaccine 1995; 13(10):947–951.

94. Poole LB, et al. Peroxidase activity of a TSA-like antioxidant protein from a pathogenic amoeba. Free Radic Biol Med 1997; 23(6):955–959.

95. Bruchhaus I, et al. Removal of hydrogen peroxide by the 29 kDa protein of *Entamoeba histolytica*. Biochem J 1997; 326 (3):758–759.

96. Tachibana H, et al. Identification of a pathogenic isolate-specific 30,000-M_r antigen of *Entamoeba histolytica* by using a monoclonal antibody. Infect Immun 1990; 58(4):955–960.

97. Reed SL, et al. Molecular and cellular characterization of the 29-kilodalton peripheral membrane protein of *Entamoeba histolytica*: differentiation between pathogenic and non-pathogenic isolates. Infect Immun 1992; 60(2):L542–L549.

98. Flores BM, et al. Serologic reactivity to purified recombinant and native 29-kilodalton peripheral membrane protein of pathogenic *Entamoeba histolytica*. J Clin Microbiol 1993; 31(6):1403–1407.

99. Soong CG, et al. Protection of gerbils from amebic liver abscess by immunization with recombinant *Entamoeba histolytica* 29-kilodalton antigen. Infect Immun 1995; 63(2):472–477.

100. Zhang T, Stanley SL. Oral immunization with an attenuated vaccine strain of *Salmonella typhimurium* expressing the serine-rich *Entamoeba histolytica* protein induces an anti-amebic immune response and protects gerbils from amebic liver abscess. Infect Immun 1996; 64(5):1526–1531.

101. Mann BJ, et al. Protection in a gerbil model of amebiasis by oral immunization with *Salmonella* expressing the galactose/ *N*-acetyl-D-galactosamine inhibitable lectin of *Entamoeba histolytica*. Vaccine 1997; 15(6–7):659–663.

102. Elson CO. Cholera toxin and its subunits as potential oral adjuvants. Curr Top Microbiol Immunol 1989; 146:29–33.

103. Kelsall BL, Ravdin JI. Immunization of rats with the 260-kilodalton *Entamoeba histolytica* galactose-inhibitable lectin elicits an intestinal secretory immunoglobulin A response that has in vitro adherence-inhibitory activity. Infect Immun 1995; 63(2):686–689.

104. Beving DE, et al. Oral immunization with a recombinant cysteine-rich section of the *Entamoeba histolytica* galactose-inhibitible lectin elicits an intestinal secretory immunoglobulin A response that has in vitro adherence inhibition activity. Infect Immun 1996; 64(4):1473–1476.

105. Holmgren J, et al. Strategies for the induction of immune responses at mucosal surfaces making use of cholera toxin B subunit as immunogen, carrier, and adjuvant. Am J Trop Med Hyg 1994; 50(suppl):42–54.

106. Zhang TE, et al. Oral immunization with the dodecapeptide repeat of the serine-rich *Entamoeba histolytica* protein (SREHP) fused to cholera toxin B subunit induces a mucosal and systemic anti-SREHP antibody response. Infect Immun 1995; 63(4):1349–1355.

77

Vaccines Against Human Hookworm Disease

Peter J. Hotez, Zhan Bin, Alex Loukas, Jeff M. Bethony, James Ashcom, Kashinath Ghosh, John M. Hawdon, Walter Brandt, and Philip K. Russell
The Sabin Vaccine Institute and George Washington University, Washington, D.C., U.S.A.

I. INTRODUCTION

Human hookworm infection is a soil-transmitted intestinal helminthiasis caused by either *Necator americanus* or *Ancylostoma duodenale* [1]. In a few focal areas, intestinal infections with the canine hookworms *Ancylostoma ceylanicum* and *Ancylostoma caninum* occur as a consequence of zoonotic transmission [2]. Hookworms are one of the most ubiquitous infectious agents of humankind; some estimates suggest that as many 1.2 billion people are infected worldwide [3]. The infection is found wherever rural poverty intersects with a tropical or subtropical climate and adequate moisture. In the Western Hemisphere, hookworm is common in the rural areas of Central America and the tropical regions of South America, including Brazil and Venezuela. In Asia, hookworm is highly endemic in China, Southeast Asia, and the Indian subcontinent. Hookworm is common throughout sub-Saharan Africa and Egypt. *N. americanus* is the predominant species worldwide, except in some northerly latitudes of China and India, Argentina and Paraguay, and in Egypt, where *A. duodenale* is focally endemic [1]. Mixed infections with both major hookworm species are common. Human infections with *A. ceylanicum* and *A. caninum* have been sporadically reported from Asia and Australia, respectively.

Hookworms injure their human host by causing intestinal blood loss, leading to iron deficiency and protein malnutrition [1,4,5]. As these processes are typically insidious and chronic and do not usually result in death, until recently hookworms were often overlooked as significant causes of morbidity. For instance, hookworms were not placed on the World Health Organization's (WHO) priority list for its Tropical Disease Research (TDR) program during the 1980s. Instead, hookworm was recognized for its devastating effects by its victims living in the rural tropics or by small numbers of biomedical researchers and public health practitioners, such as Norman Stoll of the Rockefeller Foundation and Institute, who labeled hookworm "the great infection of mankind" [6]. Public health interest in hookworm was renewed in the 1990s when new quantitative estimates of disease burden based on disability adjusted life years (DALYs) revealed its global impact [7]. As shown in Table 1, soil-transmitted helminthiases, which include hookworm, ascariasis, and trichuriasis, are the most significant parasitic infections of humans with the exception of malaria. The disease burden caused by hookworm alone exceeds three tropical infectious diseases under investigation in the WHO-TDR program, namely African trypanosomiasis, Chagas disease, and leprosy. Hookworm outranks dengue fever. However, even these DALY measurements probably underestimate the true disease burden impact of hookworm. Iron-deficiency anemia is one of the leading causes of morbidity in the developing world, possibly exceeding the impact of HIV/AIDS (Table 1). New data on the epidemiology of iron deficiency anemia in East Africa and elsewhere points to the important contribution of hookworms to this condition [4,5,8].

Some of the most accurate data on the prevalence and intensity of hookworm comes from China, where the Ministry of Health conducted fecal examinations on almost 1.5 million people as part of their nationwide survey of intestinal parasites between 1988 and 1992 [9]. An estimated 194 million cases of hookworm occur in a belt across South China that extends from the eastern coast to the western provinces of Sichuan and Yunnan (Table 2a). Subsequent data obtained after 1997 reveal that hookworm remains highly endemic wherever rural poverty occurs [10–16] (Table 2b). In addition to its health impact, hookworm may also affect regional economic development in China [16].

II. RATIONALE FOR VACCINATION

Hookworm remains highly endemic in the developing countries of the tropics and subtropics despite the widespread availability for almost two decades of relatively safe and inexpensive benzimidazole anthleminthic drugs, such as mebendazole or albendazole. The failure to control hookworm with benzimidazoles is largely a reflection of the high rates of

Table 1 Causes of Selected Infectious Disease-Related DALYs (Specific Etiology), 1990[a]

Rank	Disease	DALYs (Thousands)	% of Total
7	Tuberculosis	38,426	2.8
8	Measles	36,520	2.7
11	Malaria	31,706	2.3
14	**Iron-deficiency anemia**	**24,613**	**1.8**
28	HIV/AIDS	11,172	0.8
43	Meningitis/Meningococcemia	6242	0.5
49	**Soil-transmitted helminthes**	**5022**	**0.4**
55	Lymphatic filariasis	3997	0.3
69	Leishmaniasis	2092	0.2
78	Schistosomiasis	1514	0.1
79	**Hookworm**	**1484**	**0.1**
80	Trypanosomiasis	1467	0.1
87	Trachoma	1024	0.1
89	Dengue	750	0.1
92	Chagas Disease	641	0.1
94	Leprosy	384	0.0

[a] From Ref. 7, Table 5.2, pp. 262–265.

reinfection following treatment. Studies sponsored by WHO in a highly endemic region of East Africa, for instance, revealed that hookworm returns to its original pretreatment level within 4–12 months following deworming with mebendazole [17]. Similar results have been reported from Papua New Guinea [18]. The high rates of reinfection are indicative of inadequate host natural immunity to hookworm, which leads to the observation that experience with the infection does not confer resistance [19], except in selected individuals who somehow acquire parasite-specific IgE responses [20,21]. The absence of natural immunity has been confirmed in volunteer infections with *N. americanus* [22].

The inability to mount natural immunity to hookworm means that effective control with benzimidazoles in a given population would require frequent deworming treatments on, at least, a semiannual basis. The ability to provide the infrastructure required for regular deworming for the rural poor is often not sustainable. One solution under investigation is to implement a practice of providing regular benzimidazole anthelminthic treatments in the schools [23]. School-based deworming programs were rationalized based on the observation that *Ascaris* and *Trichuris* infections exhibit their highest prevalence and intensity among school-age children between the ages of 5 and 14 years [23]. However, this is unlikely to be a feasible control strategy for hookworm. In many areas, hookworm infections exhibit epidemiologic patterns that are distinct from infections with *Ascaris* and *Trichuris* [24]. Although hookworm has an important impact on childhood growth and cognitive development [25,26], in much of the developing world, the highest prevalence and intensity of hookworm infections occur among young and middle aged adults [27–29]. This accounts for the observation that an estimated 44 million pregnant women are infected with hookworm [29]. Hookworm during pregnancy is a major contributor to iron deficiency anemia

Table 2a China's Helminth Infections Based on the Nationwide Parasite Survey[a]

Helminth infection	Estimated number of cases
Ascariasis (large roundworm infection)	531 million
Trichuriasis (whipworm infection)	212 million
Hookworm infection (Necatoriasis and Ancylostomiasis)	194 million
Clonorchiasis (oriental liver fluke infection)	4 million
Fasciolopsiasis (intestinal fluke infection)	2 million
Taeniasis (pork and beef tapeworm infection)	1 million
Schistosomiasis (blood fluke infection)	1 million

[a] Numbers derived from data obtained during China's nationwide parasite survey of 1,477,742 individuals between 1988 and 1992 [9]. Modified from Ref. 16.

Table 2b Prevalence of Human Hookworm Infection in Selected Provinces 1997–1998

Province No.	Patients	Prevalence	Age Group (yr) Highest prevalence	Reference
Anhui	488	33%	41–50	[12]
Hainan	631	60%	>40	[14]
Jiangsu	876	12%	>50.	[10]
Sichuan	520	67%	>65	[11]
Yunnan	766	37%	>60	[13]

Table 2c Causes of Infectious Disease-Related DALYs in China (Specific Etiology) Among Females Aged 14–44 (1990)[a]

Rank	Infectious disease	DALYs (thousands)
1	Tuberculosis	753
2	Bacterial meningitis	170
3	Hepatitis (B and C)	72
4	Chlamydia	61
5	Trachoma	57
6	**Hookworm**	**36**
7	Lymphatic filariasis	28
8	Japanese encephalitis	18
8	Gonorrhea	18
9	Malaria	13
10	Tetanus	11

[a] From Ref. 7, Annex Table 9.d, p. 553.

of pregnancy [8,29], and is associated with a number of adverse fetal outcomes. As shown in Table 2c, hookworm is a major cause of disease burden in women of child-bearing age in China, where it exceeds Japanese encephalitis, malaria, and tetanus as significant causes of infectious disease morbidity. Further epidemiologic investigations of hookworm in China and Southeast Asia have also identified the elderly as an important population that suffers from heavy hookworm infections [14–16,30]. In rural Hainan, where the overall hookworm prevalence exceeds 50%, age alone accounts for 27% of the variance attributed to hookworm [15]. Hookworm is now emerging as an important geriatric infection among a rapidly expanding population of elderly in the developing world [16].

In addition to the inability of school-based deworming programs to control hookworm, there are also new concerns about the emergence of anthelminthic drug resistance. Outright failure of mebendazole has been reported from Mali [31], with other anecdotal reports of failure from China. Benzimidazole resistance occurs as a consequence of point mutations in nematode tubulin genes, which can lead to widespread resistance among parasite populations. Among the nematode parasites of livestock, for instance, high rates of benzimidazole drug resistance now occur in South Africa, Australia, New Zealand, and South America [32]. These concerns have led to the need to consider alternative or complementary approaches to control that rely on vaccination [33].

III. VACCINE PERFORMANCE CHARACTERISTICS

Because no human vaccine against a parasitic helminth vaccine currently exists, the desired attributes and efficacy of an effective antihookworm vaccine are difficult to define and predict. Hookworms, like most other human parasitic helminths, do not replicate in their host. For that reason, there is frequently a disparity between hookworm infection and hookworm disease. Clinical disease resulting from hookworms usually only occurs with moderate and heavy infections. The degree of iron deficiency and protein malnu-

trition resulting from hookworms depends on the following: (1) numbers of hookworms, (2) hookworm species (*A. duodenale* causes greater blood loss than *N. americanus*), and (3) dietary iron and protein intake and host reserves.

From experience with live larval vaccines (see below), it is almost certain that sterilizing immunity that provides 100% hookworm burden reductions will not be achieved by vaccination. Fortunately, sterile immunity is not a prerequisite for a nematode vaccine and, in fact, may prove detrimental in the long term [34]. Computer modeling of veterinary antinematode vaccines for sheep and cattle based on population dynamics demonstrate that adequate control can be achieved with vaccine efficacy well below 100%, and possibly, as low as 60% worm burden reduction [35]. However, these models are heavily biased to limit helminth egg deposition on modest-sized grazing pastures, which would then lead to the interruption of nematode transmission [34]. For that reason, reductions in parasite egg fecundity are considered as important, or even more important for domestic animal veterinary vaccines than worm burden reductions. This situation would not be applicable to human helminthiases. Instead, the goals of successful antihookworm vaccination include targets aimed at reducing intestinal blood loss and hookworm disease. This could either be accomplished by reducing the number of third-stage infective larvae that reach the intestine or by impairing the ability of surviving adult hookworms to feed at the attachment site in the intestinal mucosa and submucosa.

A two-tiered strategy that attempts to target both third-stage infective larvae (L3) as well as adult hookworms is analogous to some antimalarial vaccine strategies that target both sporozoites and asexual blood stages of *Plasmodium* spp. It is likely that an optimal antihookworm vaccine will therefore include a cocktail of antigens derived from both L3 and adult worms. As will be detailed below, an effective vaccination strategy will likely become one that elicits a strong T-helper type 2 (Th2) response with high levels of parasite antigen-specific IgE.

In summary, the optimal hookworm vaccine will be one that blocks the establishment, development, fecundity, and survival of the adult parasites in the human intestine [36]. The major parasitological parameters are outlined below.

Reduced worm burden. As noted above, reduced worm burden is a critical component of successful vaccinations. Decreased numbers of hookworms in the human intestine could either result from diminished numbers of larval hookworms that enter the intestine (decreased establishment), or from increased mortality of adult hookworms at the site of their intestinal attachment [37]. The former might be achieved by employing larval-specific antigens as immunogens, while the latter might result from selecting adult-specific antigens. In the case of *A. duodenale* infections, acquired immunity could also reduce worm burden by forcing the infective larval stages to arrest their development in the musculature or other tissues.

Worm size. Parasite stunting has been ascribed to the effects of an anthelminthic immune response. A reduced length might be attributable to inhibited growth, a selective expulsion of large worms, or shrinkage of worms during infection [37]. It is anticipated that vaccinations conducted with adult worm-derived secreted proteins might have this effect, as well as cross-reacting antigens shared between L3 and adult hookworms [38].

Altered worm morphology. Reduced size of the nematode vulval flap has been described from nematodes recovered from vaccinated ruminants. This effect has not yet been described for hookworm vaccinations [37].

Altered habitat selection. Recently, vaccinations with *Escherichia coli* expressed recombinant proteins that encode adult hookworm-specific proteinase inhibitors and enzymes were found to alter the habitat selection of adult hookworms in the canine small intestine [39]. Dogs with high levels of antihookworm antibodies were shown to exit their classical habitat in the small intestine and migrate past the ileocecal valve into the colon. It is uncertain whether adult hookworms have the ability to survive for long periods in the colon, or whether this observation reflects a transition-phase of the adult hookworms before they are expelled per rectum [39].

Fecal egg counts. This is the only parasitological parameter that can be regularly obtained from the same animal during infection [37]. Reduced fecal egg count in immune animals can either be the result of reduced numbers of female worms or reduced egg production per female worms. Fecal egg counts do not strictly reflect the fecundity of the parasite population, although there is typically a good correlation between fecal egg counts and number of eggs in utero [37].

Hematologic parameters. For reasons outlined below, it is likely that successful vaccination will require induction of Th2 responses, including the induction of prominent antigen-specific IgE responses and eosinophilia. This is discussed under the section on "Mechanism of Protection." An important hematologic parameter will be the reductions in intestinal blood loss as manifested by host circulating hemoglobin concentration, hematocrit, and ferritin concentration.

IV. FEASIBILITY OF ANTIHOOKWORM VACCINATIONS

No human clinical trials with an antinematode vaccine have ever been conducted. Instead, proof-of-concept that it is possible to vaccinate against hookworms is based on over 70 years of experience with laboratory animal models of infection [33,40]. The two major lines of evidence for the feasibility of an antihookworm vaccine are: (1) the success of vaccinating against canine infections with the dog hookworm *A. caninum*, using either trickle doses of living L3 or L3 attenuated by ionizing radiation, and (2) the success of vaccinating ruminants with chemically defined antigens against the blood-feeding nematode *Haemonchus contortus.*

A. Protection with Live Nematode Larval Vaccines

It is possible to immunize laboratory animals against infection by using killed L3. However, achieving this goal requires heroic efforts with large numbers of larvae and multiple injections. For instance, rats were successfully vaccinated against *Strongyloides ratti* by administering a total 16,000 killed L3 in 13 subcutaneous injections at intervals of 3 days

[34,41]. The vaccination series can be completed in a more efficient and timely manner by substituting living larvae. This was best shown by using vaccinated and challenged with *A. caninum* L3. Studies conducted at the Johns Hopkins School of Hygiene and Public Health during the 1930s and 1940s revealed that protective immunity could be obtained by administration of repeated doses of live *A. caninum* L3 over a period of several weeks [42–47]. These studies were recently reviewed and summarized [40]. Vaccine immunity could be stimulated by either subcutaneous or oral injections of L3. Specific immunity was not absolute but instead was demonstrable by diminished intensity of infection. Resistance induced by graded doses of larvae was manifested by reduction in worm burden, delayed development of worms, reduced size of the worms developing and lower fecundity [40]. These observations led to the development of a commercial canine hookworm vaccine that relied on *A. caninum* L3 attenuated by exposure to x-rays and other forms of ionizing radiation [38,48,49]. The advantage of using irradiated larvae was that larger numbers of L3 could be administered over a much shorter period of time. This practice allowed L3 to be manufactured into a product of potential commercial utility. Single and double vaccination schedules with x-irradiated larvae protected vaccinated pups against the establishment of potentially severe challenge infections by reducing worm burdens 37% and 90%, respectively [38,48]. The vaccine was marketed in Florida in 1973 and then the eastern United States in 1974 [48]. Ultimately, the vaccine failed as a commercial product because of high production costs (to harvest L3 from canine feces), some respiratory side effects (some irradiated L3 still migrated into the lung and even reached the intestine), short shelf life (dead and dying L3 were not effective immunogens), and an absence of sterilizing immunity, which sometimes resulted in the appearance of hookworm eggs in the feces. This last observation led both pet owner and veterinarian to erroneously conclude that the vaccine had failed [48].

Despite the commercial failure of live L3 vaccines, these early experiments led to the important observation that the protective antigens might not present in sufficient quantity in extracts of dead parasites but might be actively secreted by the living parasites [50]. The first experiments pointing to the importance of larval secreted products were conducted at the University of Chicago during the 1930s by Sarles and Taliaferro [51,52], who found that when L3 of the rodent nematode *Nippostrongylus brasiliensis* are maintained in serum from immunized rats, precipitates form at the L3 amphid, oral opening, and excretory pore; similar precipitates were detected histologically around the orifices of L3 in the skin and lungs of immune rats. These precipitates did not appear to damage the worm directly, but may have blocked a secretion, such as an enzyme required for survival in the host [34]. Subsequently, it was shown that sera from children with low hookworm burdens, despite repeated endemic *N. americanus* L3 exposure, also forms immune precipitates around hookworm L3 [53,54]. Because rats and guinea pigs could be successfully protected by vaccination with L3 secreted products [55,56], it was anticipated that humans could also be protected by *N. americanus* L3 secreted proteins. This situation is analogous to the development of antimalaria vaccines in which irradiated sporozoites and their corresponding circumsporozoite antigens elicit high levels of protection [57].

The absence of sufficient quantities of available hookworm L3 secreted proteins blocked progress in developing hookworm vaccines. For that reason, the major hookworm L3 secreted antigens were produced in bacteria by genetic engineering [58–60]. Mice immunized with recombinant L3 hookworm antigens acquired parasite-specific antibody and Th2-dependent immunity that blocked larval migration and entry into the lungs [61–63]. A homolog of the major secreted hookworm L3 antigens were subsequently shown to protect guinea pigs against challenge with L3 of the sheep stomach-worm *H. contortus* [56].

B. Protection with Purified Nematode Antigens

Because animal and human hookworms are not usually available in sufficient quantities for antigen purification, there are very few reported vaccine trials with isolated hookworm proteins. Instead, most antinematode vaccine development programs are focused on trichostrongyle nematodes, which parasitize the alimentary tract and lungs of ruminants. Cattle and sheep infections with *Trichostrongylus colubriformis* and *H. contortus* are major veterinary problems in subtropical and temperate climates, particularly South Africa, South America, Australia, New Zealand, and the Southeastern United States. High rates of benzimidazole drug resistance have encouraged some veterinary pharmaceutical companies to embark on vaccine development programs [32]. A major advantage of selecting *T. colubriformis* and *H. contortus* is the relatively abundant quantities of parasite material available for purifying antigens. In some cases, millions of L3 and thousands of adult worms can be recovered from a single ruminant infection.

For comparison with hookworm, vaccine trials against infections with *H. contortus*, the "stomach worm" or "wireworm" from the abomasums of sheep, goats, and cattle, are particularly instructive. The hookworms and *H. contortus* each belong to different families within the order Strongylida of the phylum Nematoda [64] (Table 3). Like hookworm disease, the principal clinical feature of haemonchiasis is anemia, which occurs when the adult and fourth-stage larvae ingest blood and leave mucosal wounds that hemorrhage [64]. The average blood loss has been calculated at 0.05 ml blood per parasite per day and blood first appears in the feces 6–12 days postinfection.

Two major classes of antigens from trichostrongyles offer promise as vaccine targets: (1) secreted molecules that are essential for parasite survival, and (2) biochemically extracted molecules from the parasite alimentary canal and other parasite organs [34].

Secreted parasite molecules. This category includes molecules released by the parasite during in vitro culture; in the parasite literature, fluids containing these molecules are typically referred to as excretory–secretory (ES) products. ES products may be derived from the parasite surface, from specialized secretory glands, or as byproducts of parasite digestion [34]. Almost 70 years ago, Asa Chandler [65,66] first theorized that antibody directed against critical parasite

Table 3 Phylogenetic Relationship Between Hookworms and Trichostrongyles

Phylum Nematoda	
Order or family	Representative species
Order Ascaridida	*Ascaris lumbricoides*
Order Rhabditida	*Strongyloides stercoralis*
	Caenorhabditis elegans
Order Strongylida	
Family Trichostrongylidae	*Haemonchus contortus*
	Trichostrongylus colubriformis
Family Ancylostomatidae	*Ancylostoma caninum*
	Ancylostoma ceylanicum
	Ancylostoma duodenale
	Necator americanus
Order Spirurida	*Wuchereria bancrofti*
Order Enoplida	*Trichuris trichiura*

From Ref. 64.

secreted enzymes mediates a successful anthelminthic immune response. These antibodies may "prevent the worms from digesting and assimilating host proteins," thereby creating an unfavorable environment for helminths living in the small intestine [39,65,66]. Thorson [67] subsequently provided proof of principle of the anti-ES enzyme hypothesis when he observed that serum obtained from dogs immunized against *A. caninum* contained antiprotease properties that could neutralize proteolytic enzyme activity from hookworm esophageal extracts. Abundant quantities of ES antigens are available from trichostrongyles. For instance, it was estimated that 25,000 *T. colubriformis* adults produce 1 mg protein/day [34,37].

To date, promising results were obtained by using purified or enriched preparations of a secreted cysteinyl protease from *H. contortus* [34] and an acetylcholinesterase (ACH) and superoxide dismutase from the trichostrongyle lungworm *Dictyocaulus viviparous* [68–70]. The corresponding enzymes have been identified from *Ancylostoma* and *Necator*. However, the most promising ES antigens belong to a family of adult and L3 cysteine-rich secretory proteins with homology to the *Ancylostoma* secreted proteins (ASPs) [58,59,71]. These include Hc24 and Hc15 isolated from *H. contortus* adult worm ES products and Hc40 from *H. contortus* L3 ES products (Table 4). Hc24 and Hc15 were discovered and selected based on their reactivity to serum obtained from sheep that were partly immune to primary and secondary infections [72]. Vaccination of sheep with Hc24 and Hc15 results in substantial reductions in fecal egg output and final worm burdens of 77% and 85%, respectively [73,74]. Similarly biochemical fractionation of *H. contortus* L3 ES products resulted in the isolation of Hc40 [56]. Vaccination of guinea pigs with either naturally purified Hc40 or Hc40 expressed in baculovirus provides a high level of protection (worm burden reduction) against *H. contortus* challenge of >80% and 45%, respectively [56].

Biochemical fractionation of worms. Another approach for isolating trichostrongyle natural products that effectively

Table 4 The Ancylostoma-Secreted Proteins (ASPs) and Their Homology to Hc24 and Hc40

	Size	Source	N-CHO	Hc24 homology[a]	Hc40 homology[b]
Single domain					
ASP-2	245	L3	1	50%	None
ASP-3	200	Adult	1	25%	None
ASP-5	ND	Adult	ND	32%	None
NIF	257	Adult	7	23%	None
PI	181	Adult	0	28%	None
Double Domain					
ASP-1	424	L3	0	NTD 26%	NTD 27%
				CTD 43%	CTD 23%
ASP-4	508	Adult	2	NTD 0%	None
				CTD 30%	
ASP-6	444	Adult	2	NTD 25%	NTD 28%
				CTD 26%	CTD 26%

ND = Full sequence not yet determined.

[a] From Refs. [73–74].

[b] From Ref. [56]. More than a single "Hc40" exists. The larval Hc40 is different from an adult derived Hc40 that is reported in GenBank.

function as vaccines is to progressively fractionate parasite extracts. The fractionation procedure is followed by vaccine testing of each fraction. Although extremely labor-intensive, at least two vaccine molecules have been successfully purified by this approach, including an ASP from *H. contortus* adults [75], and a tropomyosin homolog from *T. colubriformis* L3 [76].

To expedite biochemical fractionation, successful attempts have been made to narrow the search by isolating specific antigens from defined parasite organs that can serve as targets for antibody or immune effector cells. The trichostrongyle target organ most successfully exploited for purposes of antigen discovery has been the nematode gut. This approach is based partly on proof-of-principle obtained in developing vaccines against gut antigens derived from the tick *Boophilus microplus*. The Bm86 antigen, an 89-kDa glycoprotein with an extracellular location on the digestive cells of the tick gut, has been shown to be function as an effective antitick vaccine for cattle. Bm86 is not ordinarily recognized by the host bovine immune system during tick infestation. However, forcing an immune response against Bm86 through vaccination results in the appearance of specific antibodies that can be ingested by the tick as it takes up a bloodmeal. In doing so, the antibody acts as a "Trojan horse" by targeting the tick gut and interfering with the tick's ability to digest blood [77]. Although the *E. coli*-expressed recombinant protein is not as effective as the native Bm86 [78], recent success with Bm86 expressed in the methanol utilizing yeast *Pichia pastoris*, suggests that yeast-derived recombinant proteins might successfully reproduce the conformational epitopes of the Bm86 glycoprotein [79].

Based on this success, efforts in several laboratories have attempted to isolate antigens or enzymes that line the alimentary canal of trichostrongyle nematodes. Lambs have been successfully immunized with several different antigens extracted from the gut of adult *H. contortus*, including contortin, a helical polymeric structure [80]; H11, an integral membrane 110-kDa glycoprotein aminopeptidase [81–83]; H-gal-GP, a lectin-binding galactose-containing complex,

which is composed of galectin [84], cystatin [85,86], thrombospondin [87], a pepsinogen-like aspartic protease [88], and a metalloprotease (MTP) [34,89]; thiol sepharose binding proteins (TSBP) comprised of cathepsin B-like cysteinyl proteases [90] and GA1, a carbohydrate containing complex of two proteins of 46 and 52 kDa [91]. These gut-derived complexes of proteins have produced high levels of protection. To date, however, no protection has been obtained when these proteins are expressed in *E. coli* and tested as recombinant vaccines [92]. Presumably, *E. coli* expression vectors do not accurately reproduce the conformational epitopes of the native protein. The conformational dependence of these proteins is illustrated by studies in which protection with H11 is reduced when it is progressively denatured with SDS and dithiothreitol [81], suggesting that conformational epitopes are required for the full expression of protective immunity [34,92].

V. CANDIDATE ADULT HOOKWORM ANTIGENS

A. Adult Hookworm Secretory Antigens

Studies are in progress to isolate the major adult *A. caninum* secreted proteins. A partial listing of the predominant gene products are listed in Table 5.

1. Single-Domain *Ancylostoma* Secreted Proteins (ASP-3, ASP-5, Platelet Inhibitor)

The ASPs are a family of cysteine-rich secretory proteins from adult and larval hookworms (Table 4). Ac-ASP-1 and Ac-ASP-2 from *A. caninum* are the two most abundant proteins released from infective third-stage larvae (L3) of *A. caninum* upon host stimulation, and were the first two members of the family that were cloned and expressed (see below). It was noted that the ASPs share consensus sequences in their C-termini with antigen 5, a major venom allergen from stinging insects of the order Hymenoptera, and its

Table 5 Major Recombinant Hookworm Antigens Undergoing Preclinical Testing

Antigen	Description	M_W [kDa]	Ref.
Adult hookworm ES antigens			
ASP-3	Single-domain Ancylostoma secreted protein	24	Unpublished
ASP-4	Double-domain Ancylostoma secreted protein	50	Unpublished
ASP-5	Single-domain Ancylostoma secreted protein	24	Unpublished
ASP-6	Double-domain Ancylostoma secreted protein	45	Unpublished
NIF	Neutrophil inhibitory factor	45	[95]
CP-1	Cysteinyl protease	35	[103]
TMP	Tissue inhibitor of metalloproteases	16	[96]
AP	Factor Xa anticoagulant peptide	8	[98]
Adult hookworm gut-associated antigens			
APR-1	Aspartic protease	45	[113]
APR-2	Pepsinogen	45	Unpublished
MEP	Metalloendopeptidase	99	[110]
L3 ES antigens			
ASP-1	Double-domain Ancylostoma secreted protein	45	[58]
ASP-2	Single-domain Ancylostoma secreted protein	24	[59]
MTP	Astacin-like metalloprotease	62	[123]
ACH	Acetylcholinesterase	60	Unpublished
TTR	Transthyreitin-like retinol binding protein	16	Unpublished
L3 surface antigens			
103	Surface antigen with homology to Ov7		Unpublished

mammalian evolutionary counterpart, a sperm-derived protein known as testes-specific protein [58,59]. No functions have yet been ascribed to the ASPs, antigen 5, or testes-specific protein. There are two classes of ASPs. Single-domain ASPs are monomeric structures that contain between 200 and 245 amino acids, and double-domain ASPs are heterodimorphic repeats of monomeric-like sequences. The major adult single-domain ASPs are composed of ASP-3, ASP-5, and a protein that was isolated as an inhibitor of platelet aggregation. The single-domain ASPs share conserved KLGCAV sequences.

Rationale for vaccine selection. The adult hookworm-derived, single-domain ASPs have significant amino-acid sequence homology to Hc24, the 24-kDa protective antigen secreted from adult *H. contortus* [73,74] (Table 4). Some homology is also apparent between Hc15 and the ASPs. As noted above, a cocktail vaccine comprised of Hc24 and Hc15 is highly protective in sheep [73,74,93]. The two adult *A. caninum* secreted single-domain ASPs, ASP-3 and ASP-5, exhibit 25% and 32% homology to Hc24, respectively. ASP-3 is the most abundant single-domain ASP isolated from adult *A. caninum* secretory products. Vaccine trials with ASP-2, which has 50% homology with Hc24, are in progress.

2. Double-Domain ASPs (ASP-4, ASP-6)

Double-domain ASPs are heterodimorphic repeats of the monomeric single-domain structures [33], and are composed of anywhere between 424 and 508 amino acids. Adult *A. caninum* hookworms secrete two different double-domain ASPs, Ac-ASP-4 and Ac-ASP-6.

Rationale for vaccine selection. In *H. contortus* vaccinations, adult parasite-derived double-domain ASPs were shown to be highly protective. Successive column fractionation of adult *H. contortus* worms resulted in a consistent

peak of protein that associated with vaccine protection in a guinea pig model [75]. Final purification resulted in the isolation of a single 45-kDa glycoprotein corresponding to a double-domain ASP.

3. Neutrophil Inhibitor Factor (NIF)

Ac-NIF from *A. caninum* is a 41-kDa glycoprotein that potently inhibits CD11/CD18 in vitro [94]. It blocks the adhesion of activated neutrophils to vascular endothelial cells. The mature protein is composed of 257 amino acids (with a 17-amino-acid secretory leader peptide), and has 10 cysteines and 7 potential N-linked glycosylation sites. Ac-NIF from *A. caninum* exhibits 43% amino acid sequence homology to Ac-ASP-3.

Rationale for vaccine selection. In hamsters, *Pichia*-expressed recombinant *A. ceylanicum* NIF reduces parasite fecundity when used as a vaccine (85.8% by day 21 postinfection) [95]. However, it does not reduce host worm burdens or hematocrit values. No comparable vaccine protection experiments have been conducted with *A. caninum*.

4. Tissue Inhibitor of Metalloproteinase (TMP)

Ac-TMP is the most abundant protein secreted by adult *A. caninum* hookworms [96]. A cDNA encoding a putative TMP was cloned from an *A. caninum* adult hookworm cDNA library by immunoscreening with antihookworm ES antiserum. Ac-TMP is encoded by a 480-bp mRNA with a predicted open reading frame (ORF) of 140 amino acids ($M_W = 16,100$) that contains one potential N-linked glycosylation site, and an N-terminal C–X–C consensus sequence. The ORF is 33% identical and 50% similar to the N-terminal domain of human TIMP-2. Reverse transcription-polymerase chain reaction (RT-PCR) analysis indicates that transcription is restricted to the adult stage. Ac-TMP can be successfully expressed in *E. coli* as a soluble product and purified.

Rationale for vaccine selection. In a canine model, vaccination with *E. coli* expressed recombinant Ac-TMP (precipitated with alum) resulted in 11% reduction in the number of adult hookworms recovered from the small intestine relative to alum-injected dogs [39]. There was a 500% increase noted in the number of adult hookworms recovered from the colon. No effects on hookworm fecal egg counts were observed.

5. Anticoagulant Peptide (AP)

Ac-AP is an 8-kDa factor Xa inhibitor released from the amphidial (cephalic) glands of adult *A. caninum* [97–100]. It belongs to a family of nematode anticoagulant peptides (NAPs), which also includes a factor VIIa/tissue factor inhibitor [100]. Ac-AP can be expressed as a soluble product in *E. coli* [98].

Rationale for vaccine selection. Ac-AP precipitates with calcium phosphate but not with alum [39]. Vaccination of dogs with a combination of alum and calcium phosphate-precipitated Ac-AP does not result in consistent host antigen-specific antibody responses [39]. However, in a single dog that exhibited prominent antibody responses, adult hookworms were found to significantly alter their habitat selection by migrating out of the small intestine (35% reduction of small intestinal hookworms) and into the colon (1083% increase).

6. Cysteinyl Proteases (CP-1)

Adult *A. caninum* hookworm secrete cathepsin-B-like proteases [101,102]. These might function as hemoglobinases. Modeling of one of these enzymes, Ac-CP-1 indicates that it preferentially cleaves Phe–Arg over Arg–Arg, thereby providing an explanation of why the enzyme contains cathepsin-L-like substrate specificity, although structurally it more closely resembles cathepsin B [103]. Ac-CP-1 exhibits 51% homology to the *H. contortus* cysteinyl protease HMCP4.

Rationale for vaccine selection. A cysteine protease enriched fraction from *H. contortus* that binds to thiol-sepharose elicits 47% reduced worm burdens and 77% reduced egg excretion [92,104]. In *H. contortus*, the predominant CP appears to localize to the gut membrane [92], whereas it is a secreted amphidial antigen in hookworms. Cysteinyl proteases were also shown to function as effective antigens for some laboratory animal trematode infections.

7. Other Secreted Adult Antigens

Among the other secreted proteins described from hookworms are a broad spectrum Kunitz-type serine protease inhibitor from *A. ceylanicum* [105], glutathione *S*-transferases [106], a Cu/Zn superoxide dismutase [107,108], and a calreticulin-like molecule from *N. americanus* [109]. *Necator* calreticulin interacts with C1q and the cytoplasmic signaling domains of some integrins [109]. Of these, the superoxide dismutase (SOD) might hold the most promise as a vaccine antigen, based on reports of worm burden reduction with the

Haemonchus enzyme (David Knox, personal communication).

B. Adult Hookworm Gut-Associated Antigens

As noted above, the gut-associated antigens of *H. contortus* are a potent vaccine that elicits high levels of protection. In particular, the H-gal-GP complex, composed of a metalloprotease(s), aspartic protease, cysteinyl protease, cystatin, thrombospondin, and galectin, results in 72% reduction in worm burdens and 93% reduction in fecal egg counts. However, the cDNAs encoding most of the components of H-gal-GP have been expressed in *E. coli* and, to date, none of these recombinant proteins have been reported to be protective [92]. For that reason, efforts are underway to express both the hookworm and *Haemonchus* components in *Pichia* (yeast) and insect cells.

1. Metalloendopeptidase (MEP)

Ac-MEP is encoded by a 2.8-kb mRNA with a predicted ORF of 870 amino acids ($M_W = 99$ kDa) that contains four potential *N*-linked glycosylation sites and predicted zinc-binding domains (HexxH and EnxADxGG) [110]. These domains represent signature sequences of the neprilysin family of enzymes. RT-PCR indicates that the transcription of Ac-MEP occurs only in the adult stage. Experiments in which adult worms are probed with Ac-MEP-specific antiserum localize this enzyme to the microvilli of the worm gastrointestinal tract. The function of Ac-MEP is unknown, although by its localization, it may be involved in the digestion of a blood meal. Culley et al. [111] recently showed that host eotaxin, a potent eosinophil chemoattractant that acts selectively through CCR2 expressed on eosinophils, basophils, mast cells, and Th2-type T cells is specifically cleaved by hookworm metalloproteases. Eotaxin also elicits rapid vesicular transport mediated release of preformed IL-4 from human eosiniphils [112]. Therefore, Ac-MEP may have an important immunoregulatory function for the parasite.

Rationale for vaccine selection. In addition to its possible importance in modulating host Th-2 type effector immunity, Ac-MEP also exhibits strong amino acid sequence homology to Hc-MEP-1 and MEP-3 from *H. contortus*. The Hc-MEPs are prominent components of the H-gal-GP protective antigen complex against haemonchiasis. Hc-MEP-3, in particular appears to be an important component for protection (David Knox, personal communication).

2. Aspartic Proteases (APRs)

Two gut membrane-bound aspartic proteases have been cloned from *A. caninum*. Ac-APR-1 (also known as Ac-ASP in some literature) is a 422-cathepsin-D-like aspartic protease that exhibits 48.5% homology to human cathepsin D [113]. APR-1 also localizes to the microvillar brush border of the adult hookworm gastrointestinal tract (A. Williamson and A. Loukas, unpublished observation). A second, related aspartic protease (APR-2) with homology to pepsinogen from *H. contortus* [88] has also been cloned from adult *A. caninum* and *N. americanus* (A. Williamson and A. Loukas, unpublished observation).

Rationale for vaccine selection. Aspartic proteases from hookworms are key enzymes required for blood feeding [114,115]. Vaccination of dogs with alum-precipitated APR-1 followed by *A. caninum* larval challenge resulted in an 18% reduction in the number of hookworms in the small intestine relative to alum-injected dogs [39]. The APR-1 homolog of *H. contortus* is not considered to be a prominent component of the H-gal-GP complex (David Knox, personal communication). Instead, the major aspartic protease component of the complex is probably pepsinogen [92].

3. Other H-gal-GP Components

Homologs of the other predominant H-gal-GP components, namely cystatin [85], thrombospondin [87], and galectin [84], have not yet been cloned from hookworms, although expressed sequence tags (ESTs), encoding at least two distinct *A. caninum* cystatins, have been recovered from an EST database. If cloned, hookworm cystatin may be a particularly attractive component based on the observations that nematode cystatins inhibit host class II MHC-restricted antigen processing [116,117], and a cystatin homolog from the infective larval stages of *Onchocerca volvulus* (Ov7) elicits high levels of protection when formulated with alum and used as a vaccine in a mouse model [86]. Whereas the cysteinyl protease of *H. contortus* is a gut membrane-bound antigen, Ac-CP-1, the predominant hookworm cysteinyl protease, is secreted from amphidial glands, suggesting a potentially distinct role in the parasite's pathobiology.

VI. CANDIDATE INFECTIVE LARVAL (L3) HOOKWORM ANTIGENS

A. Larval Secretory Antigens

Secreted larval antigens are attractive hookworm vaccine candidates because they may provide the basis by which irradiated larval vaccines elicit protection. The *A. caninum* and *H. contortus* homologs of larval ASPs elicit high levels of protection in laboratory animal models [56,61–63]. Further rationale for targeting L3-secreted antigens is based on early studies with antibody from animals vaccinated with living L3, which resulted in immune precipitates at the openings of glandular ducts near the anterior end of the parasite. There are at least two major sites of secretion by infective hookworm larvae: amphidial glands and esophageal glands. Amphids are nematode organs of chemosensation; in parasitic L3, the amphids are modified to have elaborate glandular structures. The amphids are one of the only exposed organs in the environmental life history of the parasite prior to host entry. In contrast, the mouth and pharynx of L3 are sealed with an electron-dense plug while the L3 is in the soil. Therefore L3 are nonfeeding stages and believed to be developmentally arrested [118,119]. Upon host entry, the electron-dense plug is either dissolved or dislodged. This stimulates the L3 to resume feeding. Resumption of larval feeding is coupled to the resumption of development and associated with the transition to parasitism [119]. The observation that host antibody in animals rendered resistant by larval vaccination localizes to either the amphids or the oral

pore connected to the parasite esophagus, suggests that secretions originating from either of these two sources might be a rich source of protective antigens. Knox [34] has theorized that immune responses to these openings may block release of these molecules that are critical for parasite survival.

1. ASP-1 and ASP-2

Ac-ASP-1 and Ac-ASP-2 are the most abundant proteins released in vitro by *A. caninum* hookworm L3 activated under host-stimulatory conditions and represent, double-domain (heterdimorphic repeat) and single-domain (monomeric form) ASPs, respectively [33,58,59]. *Ac-asp-1* cDNA encodes a 424-amino acid protein ($M_W = 45,735$), including an 18-amino-acid secretory signal sequence. ASP-1 is released from the L3 amphidial glands. Similar to other ASPs, ASP-1 exhibits homology with a family of antigenic molecules from hymenoptera venoms, such as antigen 5 from the yellow jacket *Vespula squamosa*, and antigen 3 from the red imported fire ant, *Solenopsis invicta*. ASP-1 is released within 30 min after host-stimulated activation of the parasite, with the majority released by 4 hr. Complementary DNAs homologous to *Ac-asp-1* cDNA were cloned from the human hookworms *A. duodenale* and *N. americanus* [71]. Each of the predicted proteins exhibits characteristic heterodimorphic repeat structure. *Ad-asp-1* from *A. duodenale* L3 encodes a 424-amino-acid protein with a 19-amino-acid hydrophobic signal sequence. There are three potential *N*-linked glycosylation sites, none of which are present in Ac-ASP-1. The *Na-asp-1* cDNA from *N. americanus* also encodes a 424-amino-acid protein, but like Ac-ASP-1, it contains no potential *N*-linked glycosylation site. Surprisingly, the Na-ASP-1 sequence from *N. americanus* is more similar to the Ac-ASP-1 sequence than the sequence from the congeneric species *A. duodenale* (97% vs. 88% amino acid homology) [33,71]. Ac-ASP-2 is the second most abundant molecule released by activated *A. caninum*. The Ac-asp-2 cDNA encodes a single-domain ASP of 219 amino acids ($M_W = 23,954$), which also has homology to the hymenoptera venom antigens [59]. Of the ASP cDNAs cloned from *A. caninum*, it is of interest to note that the ORF encoded by *Ac-asp-1* most closely resembles Hc40 from *H. contortus* L3, while *Ac-asp-2* cDNA most closely resembles Hc24 from *H. contortus* adults (Table 4). ASP-1 is most likely derived from L3 amphids whereas ASP-2 is released through the oral opening from L3 esophageal/pharyngeal glands.

Rationale for vaccine selection. The rationale for targeting L3 amphidial or esophageal gland secretory products is outlined above. In addition, vaccine studies conducted with recombinant Ac-ASP-1 expressed in *E. coli*, indicate that this will function as a protective antigen in laboratory mice challenged with *A. caninum* L3 [61–63]. Because L3 do not develop to adult hookworms in mice [44,61], vaccine protection was measured by counting the number of L3 that enter the lungs after either oral or subcutaneous inoculation. These studies also confirmed that vaccine protection is antibody mediated and IgE-dependent [62]. Bm-VAL-1, an ASP from the filarial parasite *Brugia malayi* protects jirds against challenge infection [120]. Similarly, Hc40, an ASP homolog from *H contortus* L3 elicits high levels of protection in guinea pigs, either as the natural product (>80% protection) or as a baculovirus expressed recombinant protein (45% protection) after *H. contortus* challenge [56].

2. Astacin-Like Metalloprotease (MTP)

In addition to the ASPs, *A. caninum* L3 also release a zinc metalloprotease upon in vitro stimulation with host serum ultrafiltrate [121–123]. A cDNA encoding Ac-MTP was isolated by screening an *A. caninum* L3 cDNA expression library with serum from human patients that are putatively resistant to hookworm infection [123]. The protease is a member of the astacin family of metalloproteases, and is characterized by a conserved zinc binding region, HExx-HxxGFxHExxRxDRDm, and a "Met turn," SxMHY. The domains of Ac-MTP-1 are typical of astacin family members, and include a signal peptide, a prosequence that is cleaved during protease activation, a highly conserved catalytic domain, and C-terminal EGF-like and CUB domains. RT-PCR from life cycle stages indicated the presence of *Ac-mtp* mRNA in both L3 and adult stages, but not in the egg, or L1/L2 stages. Western blots using a polyclonal antiserum against recombinant MTP-1 indicate that only infective larvae stimulated in vitro with host serum components secrete the metalloprotease.

Rationale for vaccine selection. The stage specificity and secretion of Ac-MTP during L3 activation suggests a critical function in the infective process. Possibly, the enzyme is used either in tissue invasion or molting. For that reason, together with its apparent immunoreactivity to patient serum [123], Ac-MTP is an attractive vaccine antigen candidate.

3. Acetylcholinesterase (ACH)

A 1851 cDNA encoding an ORF of 594 with predicted homology to nematode acetylcholinesterase has been cloned from *N. americanus*. By western blots using anti-Na-ACH-specific antiserum, ACH was secreted by both L3 and adult stages of *A. caninum*.

Rationale for vaccine selection. The observation that *Dictyocaulus* and *Trichostrongylus* protective immunity can be stimulated with purified ACH [68–70] suggests that this antigen is worth pursuing for vaccine development. *Necator* ACH is also immunogenic in humans [124]. The function of nematode ACH is unknown. However, an older body of literature also points to the importance of nematode ACH for parasite survival [125], while newer data indicates that ACH and related enzymes affect host immunity [126–128].

4. Transthyreitin (TTR)

Both larval and adult stages secrete proteins with homologies to *Caenorhabditis elegans* retinol binding proteins. The larval retinol binding protein is a 144-amino-acid polypeptide with homology to a protein known as transthyreitin. Its predicted M_W is 15,934 (with signal peptide). Its function is unknown, although it may serve to scavenge host retinol. A protein with partial homology to TTR from *O. volvulus* (Ov20) was shown to elicit partial protection.

B. Larval Surface Proteins

Two cDNAs encoding *A. caninum* larval surface proteins have been cloned and expressed. Ac-103 is a homolog of Ov-103, a protective antigen from *O. volvulus*. A second protein was obtained by immunoscreening using antiserum from a rabbit immunized with live *A. caninum* L3. The protein has regions of predicted homology to von Willebrand factor.

VII. MECHANISMS OF VACCINE PROTECTION

There are very few studies on the mechanisms by which recombinant nematode antigens protect against challenge infections. However, increasing evidence points to the importance of host IgE responses and Th2-type immunity for a successful vaccine outcome. Kooyman et al. [93] found that vaccine protection with the adult *H. contortus* secretory proteins Hc24 and Hc15 depends on the age of the cohort and that this correlates with the magnitude of host IgE responses. Vaccinated sheep, 9, 6, or 3 months of age, were protected for 83%, 77%, and −34%, respectively. The difference between these vaccinated groups significantly correlated with antigen-specific IgE responses. Increased eosinophilia and mucosal mast cells were also noted [93]. Mice vaccinated with Ac-ASP-1 elicit Th2 responses marked by high antigen-specific IgG1 and IgE [62]. This vaccine protection is abrogated when mice receive injections of antimouse IgE, or if vaccinations are conducted in mice deficient in host IL-4. In contrast, vaccine protection is unaffected in mice receiving antimouse IgG or if the vaccinations are conducted in mice deficient in gamma interferon (K. Ghosh, unpublished observations). Mice vaccinated with recombinant antigens derived from *O. volvulus* exhibit increased protection when the antigens are first formulated with alum (a Th2-inducing adjuvant) instead of Freund's complete adjuvant [86]. Human correlates of immunity to hookworm antigens have not been extensively investigated. However, in two preliminary unpublished studies, human IgE antibody to recombinant Ac-ASP-1 [129] and Ac-MEP was associated with lower fecal egg counts (J. Bethony, unpublished communication).

The importance of IgE in mediating antigen-specific vaccine protection may also partly explain why purified proteins elicit worm burden reductions and lowered fecundity when the corresponding recombinant *E. coli* proteins fail. Most investigators interpret this finding on the basis of conformational epitopes that are not preserved in the *E. coli* expressed product. Indeed, baculovirus-expressed Hc40 protects, whereas the *E. coli*-expressed Hc40 fails [56]. However, as an alternative explanation, Holland et al. [130] found that proteins secreted by parasitic nematodes act as natural adjuvants for Th2 responses, whereas comparable Th2 stimulating adjuvants are possibly missing in *E. coli* expressed proteins.

The mechanisms by which IgE results in worm burden reductions are unknown. IgE may promote eosinophil attachment to parasite surfaces and result in antibody-dependent cell mediated toxicity (ADCC). In the case of amphidial-derived proteins, cellular attachment at the amphidial opening could interfere with parasite-secretory mechanisms or chemosensation. Alternatively, generation of relatively high levels of specific IgE may be important in mast cell mediated effector responses [37]. The observation that eosinophils released cytokines [112] has led to the suggestion that eosinophils may function as antigen presenting cells, particularly after IgE binding to Fc receptors. In this case, the appearance of IgE might possibly break tolerance to masked parasite antigens.

In contrast to vaccinations with single antigens, vaccinations using living L3 appear to operate by redundant pathways. For instance, anti-IgE has no effect on protective immunity against *S. stercoralis* L3 in mice [131], and IL-4 deficient mice vaccinated with *A. caninum* L3 are still protected against challenge infections. Vigorous cellular inflammatory responses to challenge L3 are seen after live L3 vaccinations [132–138], but cellular inflammation is typically absent during single antigen vaccinations.

VIII. PRECLINICAL TESTING

Successful preclinical testing of recombinant hookworm antigens requires their appropriate soluble expression in a prokaryotic or eukaryotic vector and isolation by chromatographic methods, selection of an appropriate laboratory animal for vaccine testing, appropriate adjuvant formulation to elicit high levels of antigen-specific IgE, and selection of an optimal challenge route of infection.

A. Protein Expression

Experience with recombinant *Haemonchus* antigens suggests that *E. coli*-expressed proteins will not be suitable for hookworm vaccinations. To date, no *E. coli*-expressed recombinant protein has been reported to offer protection against *H. contortus* challenge infection. The reason for this has been largely explained on the need to preserve conformational epitopes, which are not typically preserved in many *E. coli*-expressed antigens. Recently, baculovirus-expressed Hc40 (ASP homolog) was shown to exhibit significant protection [56], whereas baculovirus-expressed H11 did not [92]. There are no reports of vaccine studies with *Pichia*-expressed *Haemonchus* proteins, although *Pichia*-expressed NIF from *A. ceylanicum* was reported to elicit reduced fecundity among female *A. ceylanicum* hookworms in hamsters [95]. A distinct advantage of *Pichia* expression over insect cell expression are the lower costs and higher yields associated with the former, and therefore the possibility of developing Pichia recombinant proteins as low-cost, public sector vaccines. Recently, Na-ASP-1 from *N. americanus* was expressed in *Pichia*, and Ac-APR-1 from *A. caninum* was expressed in baculovirus. A number of platform technologies also offer potential promise for hookworm vaccine development.

B. Laboratory Animals

N. americanus infections have been successfully established in nonhuman primates, such as the chimpanzee and patas monkey [139]. However, the expense and support required for maintaining nonhuman primates and conducting preclinical trials precludes their use for routine vaccination studies. Although the dog, rabbit, and hamster have demonstrated some degree of susceptibility to infection with *N. americanus* [140–143], they do not yield reproducible and consistent numbers of adult hookworms in the small intestine and therefore are not considered reliable models for preclinical vaccine testing. *A. duodenale* has been successfully adapted to dogs [144], but steroids are usually required in order to ensure that large numbers of L3 successfully mature into adult hookworms. Mice can be employed to model L3 tissue migrations of a number of hookworm species [44, 61,62], but L3 seldom if ever mature to adult hookworms in mice.

Currently, the two laboratory animal systems that have been successfully used for vaccine development are: (1) hamster infections with *A. ceylanicum* [95,145] and (2) canine infections with *A. caninum* [146]. Of the two, only canine infections with *A. caninum* model a natural host–parasite relationship. For that reason, *A. caninum* infections in dogs most closely resemble *A. duodenale* human hookworm infections. Like *A. duodenale*, *A. caninum* L3 are both orally and percutaneously infective. The L3 of both species have the capacity to undergo developmental arrest and possibly undergo lactogenic transmission. Among the differences between canine and human hookworm infections is the observation that an age-related innate resistance develops in the former. This feature shortens the window period when a vaccine can be successfully studied. For vaccine studies, purpose-bred beagles are usually vaccinated with hookworm antigens formulated with adjuvant beginning at 8–10 weeks of age. Up to 2 months are often required in order to complete the immunizations series, followed by challenge infections. In nonvaccinated dogs, challenge doses of 400 L3 result in the establishment of 100–150 adult *A. caninum* hookworms in the gastrointestinal tract [146].

C. Adjuvant Selection

The importance of antigen-specific IgE in mediating antigen-specific vaccine protection may require specific augmentation of host Th2 immune responses through new adjuvants. To date, alum and aluminum hydroxide (Alhydrogel™) have been the most reliable adjuvant for promoting this type of responses [61–63,86]. Although the Glaxo Smith Kline adjuvant SBAS2 promotes high levels of antibody, it does not elicit vigorous IgE responses (unpublished observations). The Lewis-type carbohydrate lacto-*N*-fucopentaose III (LNFPIII) found on *Schistosoma mansoni* egg antigens was recently found to promote Th2-type immunity [147], and may become useful for parasite vaccinations. LNFPIII may also find a role in DNA vaccinations, which have not yet successfully stimulated protective immunity against gastrointestinal helminths.

D. Route of Immunization and Challenge

Both subcutaneous and intramuscular injections of antigens have elicited high levels of antihookworm immunoglobulin in mice, hamsters, and dogs [61–63,145,146]. In mice, intraperitoneal injections are also effective in eliciting high titers of Th2 antibody [62]. Both oral and subcutaneous challenge doses of hookworm L3 have been used successfully in laboratory animals. Subcutaneous challenge is used commonly to substitute for skin penetration. The advantage of subcutaneous challenge in dogs is that high percentages of L3 successfully migrate into the lungs and gastrointestinal tract. Therefore it is possible to standardize the challenge dose with relative ease. This is in contrast to percutaneous challenges in which only a small percentage of the L3 successfully penetrate skin even in nonvaccinated controls [49]. Concerns have been raised, however, that subcutaneous challenge bypasses the skin, which is an important organ of immunity against hookworm [49]. Intradermal inoculation may therefore be a more preferable route of challenge.

IX. HUMAN CLINICAL TRIALS

No human clinical trials have been conducted with recombinant hookworm vaccines. Successful preclinical testing will warrant the good manufacturing practices (GMP) manufacture of hookworm antigens suitable for immunogenicity testing in nonhuman primates followed by Phase 1 safety testing in the United States. Possible toxicities include the requirement to elicit IgE responses that could potentially cross-react to other antigens, including autoantigens in human tissue. For instance, the ASPs exhibit a small region of homology with testes-specific protein found in mammalian sperm [58,59]. These issues will require resolution prior to safety testing.

Because of the public-sector nature of a hookworm vaccine, it is not likely that GMP manufacture will be carried out by one of the traditional large pharmaceutical companies. Instead, its manufacturing may occur offshore, presumably in a country with a proven track record for producing high-quality vaccines, and presumably in a country with endemic hookworm. This list might include Brazil, Mexico, India, or China. Target age populations and appropriate dosing schedules for the vaccine may depend on the in-country epidemiology of hookworm. Studies in China and elsewhere suggest that women of child-bearing age might represent one such target population. To date, there is no evidence of significant geographic antigenic variation of the major hookworm-vaccine candidates under investigation [148].

The development of a hookworm vaccine has the potential to enormously impact on the health, education, and economic underdevelopment for the rural poor living in the tropics and subtropics. It would diminish the reliance on benzimidazole anthelminthics and, at the same time, lower hookworm burdens among at-risk populations including children, pregnant women, and the elderly.

ACKNOWLEDGMENTS

These studies were supported by the Human Hookworm Vaccine Initiative of the Sabin Vaccine Institute and The Bill and Melinda Gates Foundation, as well as grants from the NIAID, NIH (AI-32726 and AI-39461).

REFERENCES

1. Hotez PJ, Pritchard DI. Hookworm infection. Sci Am 1995; 272:68–74.
2. Prociv P, Croese J. Human enteric infection with *Ancylostoma caninum*: hookworms reappraised in the light of a "new" zoonosis. Acta Trop 1996; 62:23–44.
3. Chan MS, et al. The evaluation of potential global morbidity attributable to intestinal nematode infections. Parasitology 1994; 109:373–387.
4. Stoltzfus RJ, et al. Epidemiology of iron deficiency anemia in Zanzibari schoolchildren: the importance of hookworms. Am J Clin Nutr 1997; 65:153–159.
5. Stoltzfus RJ, et al. Hookworm control as a strategy to prevent iron deficiency. Nutr Rev 1997; 55:223–232.
6. Stoll NR. On endemic hookworm, where do we stand today? Exp Parasitol 1962; 12:241–248.
7. Murray CJL, Lopez AD, eds. The Global Burden of Disease, Global Burden of Disease and Injury Series. Geneva: World Health Organization, 1996.
8. Dreyfuss ML, et al. Hookworms, malaria and vitamin A deficiency contribute to anemia and iron deficiency among pregnant women in the plains of Nepal. J Nutr 2000; 130: 2527–2536.
9. Hotez PJ, et al. Emerging and reemerging helminthiases and the public health of China. Emerg Infect Dis 1997; 3: 303–310.
10. Sun FH, et al. Epidemiology of human intestinal nematode infections in Wujiang and Pizhou Counties, Jiangsu Province, China. Southeast Asian J Trop Med Publ Health 1998; 29:605–610.
11. Liu CG, et al. Epidemiology of human hookworm infections among adult rural villagers in Heijiang and Santai Counties, Sichuan Province, China. Acta Trop 1999; 73:255–265.
12. Wang Y, et al. Epidemiology of human ancylostomiasis in Nanlin County (Zhongzhou Village), Anhui Province China: 1. Prevalence, intensity and hookworm species identification. Acta Trop 1999; 30(4):692–697.
13. Zhan LL, et al. Epidemiology of human geohelminth infections (ascariasis, trichuriasis, and necatoriasis) in Lushui and Puer Counties, Yunnan Province, China. Southeast Asian J Trop Med Publ Health 2000; 31(3):448–453.
14. Gandhi NS, et al. Epidemiology of *Necator americanus* hookworm infections in Xiulongkan Village, Hainan Province, China: high prevalence and intensity among middle-aged and elderly residents. J Parasitol 2001; 87:739–743.
15. Bethony J, et al. Emerging patterns of hookworm infection: influence of aging on the intensity of *Necator* infection in Hainan Province, People's Republic of China. Clin Infect Dis 2002; 35:1336–1344.
16. Hotez PJ. China's hookworms. China Q 2002; 172:1029–1041.
17. Albonico M, et al. Rate of reinfection with intestinal nematodes after treatment of children with mebendazole or albendazole in a highly endemic area. Trans R Soc Trop Med Hyg 1995; 89:538–541.
18. Quinnell RJ, et al. Reinfection with hookworm after chemotherapy in Papua New Guinea. Parasitology 1993; 106: 379–385.
19. Pritchard DI, et al. Epidemiology and immunology of *Necator americanus* infection in a community in Papua New Guinea: humoral responses to excretory secretory and cuticular collagen antigens. Parasitology 1990; 100:317–326.

20. Pritchard DI, Walsh EA. The specificity of the human IgE response to *Necator americanus*. Parasite Immunol 1995; 17: 605–607.

21. Pritchard DI, et al. Immunity in humans to *Necator americanus*: IgE, parasite weight and fecundity. Parasite Immunol 1995; 17:71–75.

22. Maxwell C, et al. The clinical and immunologic responses of normal human volunteers to low dose hookworm (*Necator americanus*) infection. Am J Trop Med Hyg 1987; 37:126–134.

23. Albonico M, et al. Control strategies for human intestinal nematode infections. Adv Parasitol 1999; 42:277–341.

24. Bundy DAP. Is the hookworm just another geohelminth? In: Schad GA, Warren KS, eds. Hookworm Disease, Current Status and New Directions. London: Taylor & Francis, 1990:147–164.

25. Hotez PJ. Hookworm disease in children. Pediatr Infect Dis J 1989; 8:516–520.

26. Sakti H, et al. Evidence for an association between hookworm infection and cognitive function in Indonesian school children. Trop Med Int Health 1999; 4:322–334.

27. Chan MS, et al. Transmission patterns and the epidemiology of hookworm infection. Int J Epidemiol 1997; 26:1392–1400.

28. Behnke JM, et al. The epidemiology of human hookworm infections in the southern region of Mali. Trop Med Int Health 2000; 5:343–354.

29. Bundy DA, et al. Hookworm infection in pregnancy. Trans R Soc Trop Med Hyg 1995; 89:521–522.

30. Humphries DL, et al. The use of human faeces for fertilizer is associated with increased intensity of hookworm infection in Vietnamese women. Trans R Soc Trop Med Hyg 1997; 91:518–520.

31. De Clercq D, et al. Failure of mebendazole in treatment of human hookworm infections in the southern region of Mali. Am J Trop Med Hyg 1997; 57:25–30.

32. Conder GA, Campbell WC. Chemotherapy of nematode infections of veterinary importance, with special reference to drug resistance. Adv Parasitol 1995; 35:1–84.

33. Hotez P, et al. Experimental approaches to the development of a recombinant hookworm vaccine. Immunol Rev 1999; 171:163–171.

34. Knox DP. Development of vaccines against gastrointestinal nematodes. Parasitology 2000; 120:S43–S61.

35. Barnes EH, et al. Worm control and anthelmintic resistance: adventures with a model. Parasitol Today 1995; 11:56–63.

36. Quinnell RJ, Keymer AE. Acquired immunity and epidemiology. In: Behnke JM, ed. Parasites: Immunity and Pathology. The Consequences of Parasitic Infection in Mammals. London: Taylor & Francis, 1990:317–343.

37. Claerebout E, Vercruysse J. The immune response and the evaluation of acquired immunity against gastrointestinal nematodes in cattle: a review. Parasitology 2000; 120:S25–S42.

38. Miller TA. Vaccination against the canine hookworm diseases. Adv Parasitol 1971; 9:153–183.

39. Hotez PJ, et al. Effect of vaccinations with recombinant fusion proteins on *Ancylostoma caninum* habitat selection in the canine intestine. J Parasitol 2002; 88:684–690.

40. Hotez PJ, et al. Molecular approaches to hookworm vaccines. Pediatr Res 1996; 40:515–521.

41. Sheldon AJ. Studies on active acquired resistance, natural and artificial, in the rat to infection with *Strongyloides ratti*. Am J Hyg 1937; 25:53–65.

42. McCoy OR. Immunity reactions of the dog against hookworm (*Ancylostoma caninum*) under conditions of repeated infection. Am J Hyg 1931; 14:268–303.

43. Foster AO. The immunity of dogs to *Ancylostoma caninum*. Am J Hyg 1935; 22:65–105.

44. Kerr KB. Studies on acquired immunity to the dog *Ancylostoma caninum*. Am J Hyg 1936; 23:381–406.

45. Otto GF, Kerr KB. The immunization of dogs against hookworm *Ancylostoma caninum*, by subcutaneous injection of graded doses of larvae. Am J Hyg 1939; 29(D):25–45.

46. Otto GF. A serum antibody in dogs actively immunized against the hookworm *Ancylostoma caninum*. Am J Hyg 1940; 31(D):23–27.

47. Otto GF. Further observations on the immunity induced in dogs by repeated infection with the hookworm *Ancylostoma caninum*. Am J Hyg 1941; 33(D):39–57.

48. Miller TA. Industrial development and field use of the canine hookworm vaccine. Adv Parasitol 1978; 16:333–342.

49. Miller TA. In: Soulsby EJL, ed. Immune Responses in Parasitic Infections: Immunology, Immunopathology and Immunoprophylaxis. Vol. I. Nematodes. Boca Raton, FL: CRC Press, 1987.

50. Clegg JA, Smith MA. Dead vaccines against helminthes. Adv Parasitol 1978; 16:165–218.

51. Sarles MP. The in vitro action of immune serum on the nematode *Nippostrongylus muris*. J Infect Dis 1938; 62:337–348.

52. Taliaferro WH, Sarles MP. The cellular reactions in the skin, lungs and intestine of normal and immune rats after infection with *Nippostrongylus muris*. J Infect Dis 1939; 64:157–192.

53. Sheldon AJ, Groover ME Jr. An experimental approach to the problem of acquired immunity in human hookworm (*Necator americanus*) infections. Am J Hyg 1942; 36:183–186.

54. Morisita T. Immunity to hookworm infections. In: Komiya Y, Yasuraoka Y, eds. Progress in Medical Parasitology in Japan. Meguro Japan: Meguro Parasitology Museum, 1966:371–383.

55. Thorson RE. Studies on the mechanisms of immunity in rats to the nematode *Nippostrongylus muris*. Am J Hyg 1953; 58:1–15.

56. Sharp PJ, Wagland BM. Nematode vaccine. United States Patent Number 5,734,035, March 31, 1998.

57. Hotez PJ. Parasitic disease vaccines (chapter 40). Vaccines. third edition. Philadelphia: WB Saunders, 1999:983–987.

58. Hawdon JM, et al. Cloning and expression of *Ancylostoma* secreted protein: a polypeptide associated with the transition to parasitism by infective hookworm larvae. J Biol Chem 1996; 271:6672–6678.

59. Hawdon JM, et al. *Ancylostoma* secreted protein 2 (ASP-2): cloning and characterization of a second member of a novel family of nematode secreted proteins from *Ancylostoma caninum*. Mol Biochem Parasitol 1999; 99:149–165.

60. Hotez PJ, et al. Progress in the development of a recombinant vaccine for human hookworm disease: the human hookworm vaccine initiative. Int J Parasitol 2003. In press.

61. Ghosh K, et al. Vaccination with alum-precipitated ASP-1 protects mice against challenge infections with infective hookworm (*Ancylostoma caninum*) larvae. J Infect Dis 1996; 174:1380–1383.

62. Ghosh K, Hotez PJ. Antibody-dependent reductions in mouse hookworm burden after vaccination with *Ancylostoma caninum* secreted protein 1 (Ac-ASP-1). J Infect Dis 1999; 180:1674–1681.

63. Liu S, et al. Hookworm burden reductions in BALB/c mice vaccinated with *Ancylostoma* secreted protein 1 (ASP-1) from *Ancylostoma duodenale*, *A. caninum* and *Necator americanus*. Vaccine 2000; 18:1096–1102.

64. Soulsby EJL. Helminths, Arthropods and Protozoa of Domesticated Animals. 7th Edition. Philadelphia: Lea & Febiger, 1982:141–142.

65. Chandler AC. Susceptibility and resistance to helminthic infections. J Parasitol 1932; 3:135–152.

66. Chandler AC. Studies on the nature of immunity to intestinal helminths III. Renewal of growth and egg production in *Nippostrongylus* after transfer from immune to non-immune rats. Am J Hyg 1936; 23:36–54.

67. Thorson RE. The stimulation of acquired immunity in dogs by the injection of extracts of the oesophagus of adult hookworms. J Parasitol 1956a; 42:501–504.

68. McKeand JB. Vaccine development and diagnostics of *Dictyocaulus viviparous*. Parasitology 2000; 120:S17–S23.

69. McKeand JB, et al. Immunisation of guinea pigs against *Dictyocaulus viviparous* using adult ES products enriched for acetylcholinesterases. Int J Parasitol 1995; 25:829–837.

70. Griffiths G, Pritchard DI. Vaccination against gastrointestinal nematodes of sheep using purified secretory acetylcholinesterase from *Trichostrongylus colubriformis*—an initial pilot study. Parasite Immunol 1994; 16:507–510.

71. Zhan B, et al. *Ancylostoma* secreted protein-1 (ASP-1) homologues from human hookworms. Mol Biochem Parasitol 1999; 98:143–149.

72. Schallig HDFH, et al. Immune responses of sheep to excretory/secretory products of adult *Haemonchus contortus*. Parasitology 1994; 108:351–357.

73. Schallig HDFH, et al. Protective immunity induced by vaccination with two *Haemonchus contortus* excretory secretory proteins in sheep. Parasite Immunol 1997a; 19:447–453.

74. Schallig HDFH, et al. Molecular characterization and expression of two putative protective excretory secretory proteins of *Haemonchus controtus*. Mol Biochem Parasitol 1997b; 88:203–213.

75. Sharp PJ, et al. Nematode vaccine. International patent application number PCT/AU92/00041, International Publication Number WO92/13889 and 13890, 1992.

76. Cobon GS, et al. Vaccines against animal parasites. World patent application No. WO 89/00163, 1989.

77. Willadsen P. Commercialisation of a recombinant vaccine against *Boophilus microplus*. Parasitology 1995; 110:S43–S50.

78. Rand KN, et al. Cloning and expression of a protective antigen from the cattle tick *Boophilus microplus*. Proc Natl Acad Sci USA 1989; 86:9657–9661.

79. Rodriquez M, et al. High level expression of the *B. microplus* Bm86 antigen in the yeast *Pichia pastoris* forming highly immunogenic particles for cattle. J Biotechnol 1994; 33:135–146.

80. Munn EA, Greenwood CA. The occurrence of the submicrovillar endotube (modified terminal web) and associated cytoskeletal structure in the intestinal epithelia of nematodes. Philos Trans R Soc 1984; 306:1–18.

81. Munn EA, et al. Vaccination against *Haemonchus contortus* with denatured forms of the protective antigen H11. Parasite Immunol 1997; 19:243–248.

82. Smith TS, et al. Purification and evaluation of the integral membrane protein H11 as a protective antigen against *Haemonchus contortus*. Int J Parasitol 1993; 23:271–277.

83. Smith TS, et al. Cloning and characterization of a microsomal aminopeptidase from the intestine of the nematode *Haemonchus contortus*. Biochim Biophys Acta 1997; 1338:295–306.

84. Greenhalgh CJ, et al. A family of galectins from *Haemonchus contortus*. Mol Biochem Parasitol 2000; 107:117–121.

85. Newlands GF, et al. Cloning and expression of cystatin, a potent cysteine protease inhibitor from the gut of *Haemonchus contortus*. Parasitology 2001; 122:371–378.

86. Abraham D, et al. Development of a recombinant antigen vaccine against infection with the filarial worm *Onchocerca volvulus*. Infect Immun 2001; 69:262–270.

87. Skuce PJ, et al. Cloning and characterization of thrombospondin, a novel multidomain glycoprotein found in association with a host protective gut extract from *Haemonchus contortus*. Mol Biochem Parasitol 2001; 117:241–244.

88. Redmond DL, et al. Expression of *Haemonchus contortus* pepsinogen in *Caenorhabditis elegans*. Mol Biochem Parasitol 2001; 112:125–131.

89. Redmond DL, et al. Molecular cloning and characterisation of a developmentally regulated putative metallopeptidase present in a host protective extract of *Haemonchus contortus*. Mol Biochem Parasitol 1997; 85:77–87.

90. Knox DP, et al. Thiol binding proteins, patent application no. PCT/GB95/00665, 1995.

91. Rehman A, Jasmer JP. A tissue-specific approach for analysis of membrane and secreted protein antigens from *Haemonchus contortus* gut and its application to diverse nematode species. Mol Biochem Parasitol 1998; 97:55–68.

92. Knox DP, Smith WD. Vaccination against gastrointestinal nematode parasites of ruminants using gut-expressed antigens. Vet Parasitol 2001; 100:21–32.

93. Kooyman FNJ, et al. Protection in lambs vaccinated with *Haemonchus contortus* antigens is age related, and correlates with IgE rather than IgG1 antibody. Parasite Immunol 2000; 22:13–20.

94. Moyle M, et al. A hookworm glycoprotein that inhibits neutrophil function is a ligand of the integrin CD11b/CD18. J Biol Chem 1994; 269:10008–10015.

95. Ali F, et al. Vaccination with neutrophil inhibitory factor reduces the fecundity of the hookworm *Ancylostoma ceylanicum*. Parasite Immunol 2001; 23:237–249.

96. Zhan B, et al. Molecular cloning and purification of AcTMP a developmentally regulated putative tissue inhibitor of metalloprotease released in relative abundance by adult *Ancylostoma* hookworms. Am J Trop Med Hyg 2002; 66:238–244.

97. Cappello M, et al. *Ancylostoma caninum* anticoagulant peptide (AcAP): a novel hookworm derived inhibitor of human coagulation factor Xa. Proc Natl Acad Sci USA 1995; 92:6152–6156.

98. Cappello M, et al. Cloning and expression of *Ancylostoma caninum* anticoagulant peptide (AcAP). Mol Biochem Parasitol 1996; 80:113–117.

99. Harrison LM, et al. *Ancylostoma caninum* anticoagulant peptide-5: immunolocalization and in vitro neutralization of a major hookworm anti-thrombotic. Mol Biochem Parasitol 2001; 115:101–107.

100. Stanssens P, et al. Anticoagulant repertoire of the hookworm *Ancylostoma caninum*. Proc Natl Acad Sci USA 1996; 93:2149–2154.

101. Harrop SA, et al. Characterization and localization of cathepsin B proteinases expressed by adult *Ancylostoma caninum* hookworms. Mol Biochem Parasitol 1995; 71:163–171.

102. Loukas A, et al. Purification of a diagnostic, secreted cysteine protease-like protein from the hookworm *Ancylostoma caninum*. Parasitol Int 2000; 49:327–333.

103. Harrop SA, et al. Amplification and characterization of cysteine proteinase genes from nematodes. Trop Med Parasitol 1995; 46:119–122.

104. Knox DP, et al. Immunization with an affinity purified protein extract from the adult parasite protects lambs against *Haemonchus contortus*. Parasite Immunol 1999; 21:201–210.

105. Milstone AM, et al. A broad spectrum Kunitz type serine protease inhibitor secreted by the hookworm *Ancylostoma ceylanicum*. J Biol Chem 2000; 275:29391–29399.

106. Brophy PM, et al. Glutathione S-transferase (GST) expression in the human hookworm *Necator americanus*: potential roles for excretory–secretory forms of GST. Acta Trop 1995; 59:259–263.

107. Taiwo FA, et al. Cu/Zn superoxide dismutase in excretory–secretory products of the human hookworm *Necator americanus*. An electron spectrometry study. Eur J Biochem 1999; 264:434–438.

108. Pritchard DI. Do hematophagous parasites secrete SOD and promote blood flow? Int J Parasitol 1996; 26:1339–1340.

109. Kasper G, et al. A calreticulin-like molecule from the human hookworm *Necator americanus* interacts with C1q and the cytoplasmic signaling domains of some integrins. Parasite Immunol 2001; 23:141–152.

110. Jones BF, Hotez PJ. Molecular cloning and characterization of Ac-MEP-1 a developmentally regulated gut luminal metalloendopeptidase from adult *Ancylostoma caninum* hookworm. Mol Biochem Parasitol 2001; 119:107–116.

111. Culley FJ, et al. Eotaxin is specifically cleaved by hookworm metalloproteases preventing its action in vitro and in vivo. J Immunol 2000; 165:6447–6453.

112. Bandeira-Melo C, et al. Cutting edge: eotaxin elicits rapid vesicular transport-mediated release of preformed IL-4 from human eosinophils. J Immunol 2001; 166:4813–4817.

113. Harrop SA, et al. Acasp, a gene encoding a cathepsin D-like aspartic protease from the hookworm *Ancylostoma caninum*. Biochem Biophys Res Commun 1996; 227:294–302.

114. Brinkworth RI, et al. Host specificity in blood feeding parasites: a defining contribution by haemoglobin-degrading enzymes? Int J Parasitol 2000; 30:785–790.

115. Brinkworth RI, et al. Hemoglobin-degrading aspartic proteases of blood-feeding parasites: substrate specificity revealed by homology models. J Biol Chem 2001; 276:38844–38851.

116. Manoury B, et al. Bm-CPI-2, a cystatin homolog secreted by the filarial parasite *Brugia malayi*, inhibits class II MHC-restricted antigen processing. Curr Biol 2001; 11:447–451.

117. Dainichi T, et al. Nippocystatin, a cystein protease inhibitor from *Nippostrongylus brasiliensis*, inhibits antigen processing and modulates antigen-specific immune responses. Infect Immun 2001; 69:7380–7386.

118. Hotez PJ, et al. Hookworm larval infectivity, arrest and amphiparatenesis: the *Caenorhabditis elegans* Daf-c paradigm. Parasitol Today 1993; 9:23–26.

119. Hawdon JM, Hotez PJ. Hookworm: developmental biology of the infectious process. Curr Opin Genet Dev 1996; 6:618–623.

120. Murray J, et al. Expression and immune recognition of *Brugia malayi* VAL-1, a homologue of vespid venom allergens and *Ancylostoma* secreted proteins. Mol Biochem Parasitol 2001; 118:89–96.

121. Hotez PJ, et al. Infective *Ancylostoma* hookworm larval metalloproteases and their possible functions in tissue invasion and ecdysis. Infect Immun 1990; 58:3883–3892.

122. Hawdon JM, et al. *Ancylostoma caninum*: resumption of hookworm larval feeding coincides with metalloprotease release. Exp Parasitol 1995; 80:205–211.

123. Zhan B, et al. A developmentally regulated metalloprotease secreted by host-stimulated *Ancylostoma caninum* third-stage infective larvae is a member of the astacin family of proteases. Mol Biochem Parasitol 2002; 120:291–296.

124. Brown A, Pritchard DI. The immunogenicity of hookworm (*Necator americanus*) acetylcholinesterase (AchE) in man. Parasite Immunol 1993; 15:195–203.

125. Ogilve BM, et al. Acetylcholinesterase secretion by parasitic nematodes. I. Evidence for the secretion of the enzyme by a number of species. Int J Parasitol 1973; 3:589–597.

126. Ziaie Z, Kefalides NA. Inhibition of polymorphonuclear leukocyte activation by acetylcholinesterase. Mol Cell Biol Res Commun 1999; 2(1):11–14.

127. Kawashima K, Fujii T. Extraneuronal cholinergic system in lymphocytes. Pharmacol Ther 2000; 86:29–48.

128. Selkirk ME, et al. Acetylcholinesterase secretion by nematodes. In: Kennedy MW, Harnett W, eds. Parasitic Nematodes. Oxon, UK: CABI International, 2001:211–228.

129. Bethony JM. Epidemiology and immunology of *Necator americanus* infection in rural Thailand: the role of acquired immunity in determining infection intensity. Master of Science Thesis, State University of New York at Buffalo, 1998.

130. Holland MJ, et al. Proteins secreted by the parasitic nematode *Nippostrongylus brasiliensis* act as adjuvants for Th2 responses. Eur J Immunol 2000; 30:1977–1987.

131. Abraham D, et al. *Strongyloides stercoralis*: protective immunity to third-stage larvae in BALB/cByJ mice. Exp Parasitol 1995; 80:297–307.

132. Xiao SH, et al. Protective immunity in mice elicited by living infective third-stage hookworm larvae (Shanghai strain of *Ancylostoma caninum*). Chin Med J 1998a; 111: 43–48.

133. Xiao SH, et al. Electron microscopy of peritoneal cellular immune responses in mice vaccinated and challenged with third-stage infective hookworm (*Ancylostoma caninum*) larvae. Acta Trop 1998b; 71:155–167.

134. Xiao SH, et al. Length of protection afforded by murine vaccination with living infective third-stage hookworm larvae (Shanghai strain of *Ancylostoma caninum*). Chin Med J 1999; 112:1129–1132.

135. Xiao SH, et al. Electron and light microscopy of neutrophil responses in mice vaccinated and challenged with third-stage infective hookworm (*Ancylostoma caninum*) larvae. Parasitol Int 2001; 50:241–248.

136. Yang YQ, et al. Cutaneous and subcutaneous granulomata formation in mice immunized and challenged with third-stage infective hookworm (*Ancylostoma caninum*) larvae. Acta Trop 1998; 69:229–238.

137. Yang YQ, et al. Cutaneous and subcutaneous mast cell and eosinophil responses in mice vaccinated with living infective third-stage hookworm larvae (Shanghai strain of *Ancylostoma caninum*). Chin Med J 1999; 112:1020–1023.

138. Yang YQ, et al. Histochemical alterations of infective third-stage hookworm larvae (L3) in vaccinated mice. Southeast Asian J Trop Med Pub Health 1999; 30:356–364.

139. Orihel TC. *Necator americanus* infection in primates. J Parasitol 1971; 57:117–121.

140. Yoshida YK, et al. Studies on the development of *Necator americanus* in young dogs. Jpn J Parasitol 1960; 9:735–743.

141. Yoshida YK, Fukutome S. Experimental infection of rabbits with the human hookworm, *Necator americanus*. J Parasitol 1967; 53:1067–1073.

142. Sen HG. *Necator americanus*: behavior in hamsters. Exp Parasitol 1972; 32:26–32.

143. Sen HG, Seth D. Complete development of the human hookworm, *Necator americanus*, in golden hamsters, *Mesocricetus auratus*. Nature 1967; 214:609–610.

144. Schad GA. *Ancylostoma duodenale*: maintenance through six generations in helminth-naïve pups. Exp Parasitol 1979; 47:246–252.

145. Bungiro RD, et al. Mitigation of hookworm disease by immunization with soluble extracts of *Ancylostoma ceylanicum*. J Infect Dis 2001; 183:1380–1387.

146. Hotez PJ, et al. Natural history of primary canine hookworm infections following three different oral doses of third-stage infective larvae of *Ancylostoma caninum*. Comp Parasitol 2002; 69:72–80.

147. Okano M, et al. Lacto-*N*-fucopentaose III found on *Schistosoma mansoni* egg antigens functions as adjuvant for proteins by inducing Th2-type response. J Immunol 2001; 167: 442–450.

148. Shan Q, et al. Variation between ASP-1 molecules from *Ancylostoma caninum* in China and the U.S. J Parasitol 2000; 86:181–185.

78

Principles of Therapeutic Vaccination for Viral and Nonviral Malignancies

Drew M. Pardoll
Johns Hopkins University School of Medicine, Baltimore, Maryland, U.S.A.

I. INTRODUCTION

In contrast to the success of many prophylactic vaccines, therapeutic vaccination for established chronic infections as well as cancer has yet to achieve widespread acceptance. To date, no therapeutic vaccine has been approved for general use in the United States, despite there being a number that have recently been tested in Phase III registration trials. The striking differences in success between immunoprophylaxis and immunotherapy are based on the fact that, in order to become successfully established within the host, either pathogens or cancer cells have developed mechanisms to avoid recognition and elimination by the immune system (Table 1). Potential mechanisms for immune invasion are best understood for tumors and viruses, which often use common strategies. Downmodulation of components of the antigen processing and presentation system to T cells represents one of the best defined mechanisms for both viruses and tumors [1–31]. Production of cytokines that inhibit or divert productive effector responses [32–35] as well as induction of antigen-specific tolerance through normal pathways of self-tolerance generation [36–46] represents additional mechanisms by which tumors and some viruses can avoid recognition by the immune system. However, these mechanisms of immune resistance do not represent absolute barriers. Most chronic viral infections involve expression of at least one viral gene which provides a target for immunotherapy. Although they are derived from "self," all tumors express antigens recognizable by the immune system, either as unique antigens (the result of genetic alterations), tissue-specific antigens or upregulated self-antigens (Table 2) [47,48]. While most successful prophylactic vaccines protect through the induction of long-lived neutralizing antibody responses, successful immunotherapy of established cancer or pathogenic infections will likely depend to a larger extent upon diverse effector pathways regulated by both CD4 and CD8 T cells [49].

Despite the barriers to immunotherapy of chronic viral infection and cancer, the fundamental knowledge about the molecular and cellular basis for immune regulation, particularly at the level of T-cell responses, provides a new arsenal of approaches to enhance antigen-specific responses in both these settings. In the case of cancer, immune responses to antigens can be induced through both engineering of the tumor cells themselves or by engineering responses against specific tumor antigens.

II. THE LINK BETWEEN CHRONIC VIRAL INFECTION AND CANCER

Many of the strategies for development of immunotherapy are applicable to both cancer and chronic viral infections. The immunobiology of these two diseases has indeed intersected for a number of reasons. First, chronic viral infections are carried in the form of integrated or episomal proviruses within viable cells. Recognition and elimination of these virally infected cells appears to involve similar mechanisms to the recognition and elimination of tumor cells. In the case of viral infections, viral antigens expressed during the chronic carrier state represent ideal targets for antigen-specific immunotherapy. While the delineation of immunodominant antigens in tumors is a much more complex endeavor, chronic viral infection offers defined antigens to target with immunotherapy. The most significant link between immunotherapy efforts for viruses and cancer comes from the fact that some of the most common human cancers in immunocompetent individuals are induced by chronic viral infection and actually harbor proviral elements.

The most clear-cut link between viruses and human cancer is represented by human papillomavirus (HPV) infection, whose prooncogenic properties depend on the expression of the E6 and E7 antigens [50–53]. E6 binds and induces the degradation of the tumor suppressor gene p53 whereas E7 binds and induces the inactivation of the tumor suppressor gene, Rb. These events are not transforming but enhance the probability of transformation significantly by

Table 1 Contrasting Features of Prophylactic Vaccines and Therapeutic Vaccines Indicate Significant Differences Between the Two

Prophylactic vaccines	Therapeutic vaccines
• Typically infectious dz • Antibody mediated • Immune system is naive to vaccinating antigen—no tolerance or immune evasion • Antigens are known	• Typically cancer • T-cell responses key • Immune system has been exposed to vaccinating antigen—tolerance and/or immune evasion operative • Relevant antigens may not be known

reducing genome integrity, thereby facilitating the accumulation of additional transforming mutations. Essentially all cervical cancer as well as anal cancer and a proportion of head and neck cancer arises from HPV-infected cells in the cervix, anus, and oral/laryngeal epithelium, respectively. Of the over 100 HPV types, only 8–10 predispose to cancer, with HPV-16 and HPV-18 being the most common. One of the most compelling arguments for the development of a therapeutic vaccine for premalignant HPV infection is that a majority of HPV infections are naturally eliminated by the immune system in immunocompetent individuals. Even late-stage premalignant HPV lesions (so-called CIN II or CIN III) resolve spontaneously in a significant proportion of women. The dramatic increase in HPV persistence in immunodeficient individuals confirms the central role of the immune system in viral elimination in immunocompetent women. It is thus possible that a relatively modest enhancement of the right type of immune response directed at E6 and/or E7 might tip the balance toward immune elimination of infected cells.

Hepatocellular carcinoma, a leading cancer killer worldwide, is associated with chronic hepatitis B or hepatitis C chronic virus infection in the majority of cases [54–57]. Chronic hepatitis is a precursor to cancer with both viruses. The etiologic link between these viruses and cancer is less clear than with HPV. Both viruses elicit potent immune responses during acute infection. While the acute hepatitis accompanying hepatitis B infection is relatively strong and results in viral clearance >90% of the time, the acute response to hepatitis C infection is generally mild (and asymptomatic) and clears the virus only about 20% of the time. While gene products of both viruses have been implicated in carcinogenesis, it is believed that the nonsterilizing inflammatory responses during the chronic phase of both these viruses may be the major contributor to cancer formation.

While Epstein–Barr virus is best known for its role in lymphomagenesis in immunodeficient patients, it also causes cancers such as Burkitts lymphoma, nasopharyngeal carcinoma, and Hodgkins disease in immunocompetent individuals [58–60]. Almost everybody is infected with EBV, whose transition from latency (generally in B cells) is rapidly perceived by the immune system such that EBV transformed cells are rapidly eliminated by a T-cell-dependent response. This is the classic example of successful immune surveillance. It is still unclear how EBV evades immune surveillance in cases of EBV-associated cancers in immunocompetent individuals, as they all express a subset of EBV antigens capable of recognition by T cells. The finding that the EBNA-1 antigen contains sequences that prevent its processing via the proteasome provides a hint at mechanisms of immune evasion [61], although other antigens such as LMP-2 appear to be perfectly recognizable. In any case, all of the chronic viral infections associated with premalignant states are good candidates for therapeutic vaccination.

III. PRINCIPLES IN THE CANCER–IMMUNE SYSTEM INTERACTION UNDERLYING CANCER VACCINE STATEGIES

Successful immunotherapy of cancer will ultimately require understanding the natural relationship between the immune system and tumors as they transform, invade, and metastasize. There is evidence that immune responses against tumor antigens bear both similarities and differences to immune responses against "self" tissue antigens. That immunity to tumors would resemble immunity to normal tissues is not surprising as tumors are, of course, transformations of normal cells in which growth control has become disregulated. However, dissection of the molecular events of tumori-

Table 2 Categories of Tumor Antigen[a]

1) Produces of mutations (or rearrangements): ras-12V, cdk-4, caspase-8, bcr-abl
2) Tissue specific antigens: tyrosinase, gp100, MART-1/melan A
3) Antigens selectively expressed in tumor ≫ normal tissue: MAGE1-3, BAGE, GAGE ("cancer-testes ag"), HER-2/neu
4) Viral antigens in virus associated malignancies: HPV (E6 and E7), EBV (EBNA-1, LMP-1, and 2), HBV, HCV

[a] The list of candidate tumor rejection antigens continues to grow. The most specific tumor antigens arise from mutations, however, these are usually unique to individual tumors. The other three categories (tissue specific antigens, tumor selective antigens, and viral antigens) are shared among many tumors.

ginesis together with the pathophysiology of cancer progression teaches us that there are significant features that distinguish cancer cells from their normal counterparts. Some of these differences significantly impact the nature of their interaction with the immune system. It is these distinctive features that may well represent the immunologic Achilles heel of cancer, capable of being exploited therapeutically.

Specifically, tumors differ fundamentally from their normal cell counterparts in antigenic composition and biologic behavior. The molecular hallmark of carcinogenesis is genetic instability [62]. Genetic instability in cancers is a consequence of deletion and/or mutational inactivation of genome guardians, such as p53 [63]. Indeed, many of the genetically defined familial cancer syndromes, such as hereditary nonpoliposis colon cancer and familiar breast cancer, are due to mutation in genes that mediate responses to DNA damage [64–69]. The genetic instability of cancer cells means that new antigens are constantly being generated in tumors as they develop and progress. This does not occur in normal, nontransformed tissues, which maintain a very stable antigenic profile. In addition to the thousands of mutational events that occur during tumoriginesis, hundreds of genes that are either inactive in the normal tissue of origin or expressed at relatively low levels are activated dramatically in cancers. While these epigenetic changes do not formally create tumor-specific neoantigens, they raise the concentration of encoded proteins many orders of magnitude, thereby dramatically affecting antigenicity.

While uncontrolled growth is certainly a common biological feature of all tumors, the major pathophysiologic characteristics of malignant cancer responsible for morbidity and mortality are the ability to invade across natural tissue barriers and to metastasize. Both of these characteristics, which are never seen with normal tissues or benign tumors, are associated with dramatic disruption of tissue architecture. One of the important consequences of tissue disruption, even when caused by noninfectious mechanisms, is the elaboration of pro-inflammatory signals. These signals, generally in the form of cytokines and chemokines, are central initiators of both innate and adaptive immune responses. Thus, unlike normal tissues, cancers are constantly confronted with inflammatory responses as they invade tissues and metastasize through the body. How they handle and modulate these responses dictates the interplay with the host immune system [70].

Despite a continuing interest in the concept of natural immune surveillance of cancer, there is an ample wealth of evidence that the normal immune response to tumor antigens is tolerance induction, rather than activation. In considering the concept of tolerance induction by tumors, it is critical to distinguish between induction of unresponsiveness through mechanism such as anergy or deletion vs. resistance mechanisms to recognition and killing of tumor cells by activated immunologic effectors. In contrast to tolerance induction, which implies a failure of immune surveillance, the presence of resistance mechanisms that cloak the tumor from recognition by T cells or inhibit the function of immune effectors implies that the tumor was either selected or has adapted to survive an environment in which immune surveillance is operative.

While there is a huge body of literature on tumor resistance mechanisms, virtually all of the evidence is circumstantial and does not prove that the observed alterations in antigen processing machinery or expression of immune inhibitory molecules is a response on the part of the tumor to activate antitumor immunity. Downregulation of the antigen processing machinery—particularly the MHC class I pathway—has been documented extensively in a large variety of tumors. In the human, downregulation of the MHC class I molecules has been observed in a diversity of tumor types, particularly breast cancer, prostate cancer, and lung cancer [1–18]. Downmodulation of MHC class I genes can result from multiple mechanisms affecting transcription [13,23,71]. Downregulation of TAP genes as well as components of the immunoproteosome such as LMP-2 and LMP-7 has likewise been documented in a number of tumor types [25–30]. In the majority of cases where the MHC class I processing machinery is downmodulated, it is usually rapidly upregulated by IFN-γ, suggesting that the diminished expression is epigenetic in origin and reversible.

The other major mechanism for putative immune resistance by tumors is the expression of secreted or cell surface molecules that either kill or inhibit cellular components of the effector immune response. The most clear-cut example is TGF-β, which is produced by many different tumors particularly of epithelial origin [32–35]. Relatively little evidence exists that expression of TGF-β by tumors protects them from recognition and killing by effector components of the immune response once they have been successfully activated. It is in fact more likely that TGF-β inhibits the generation of pro-inflammatory responses during tumor invasion and therefore inhibits the induction of immune responses at the outset. It is thus a more likely agent to participate in the induction of true immune tolerance (see below) rather than immune resistance. A more controversial effector of immune tolerance is FasL. After an initial spate of reports that many tumors express FasL and that FasL expression provides immunologic resistance with consequent enhanced in vivo tumor growth [72–77], subsequent reports have called these conclusions into serious question [78–80]. Difficulties in assessing the true levels of cell surface FasL expression by monoclonal antibodies have been a major technical problem. Thus expression of FasL by tumors is unlikely an important mechanism in resistance to recognition by effector components of the immune system.

In contrast to persistent uncertainties regarding tumor resistance mechanisms, experiments employing TCR transgenic mice have provided strong evidence for the capacity of tumor cells to induce tolerance to their antigens [36–45]. Tolerance appears to be operative predominately at the level of T cells; B-cell tolerance to tumors is less certain as there is ample evidence for the induction of antibody responses in animals bearing tumors as well as human patients with tumors. With the exception of antibodies against members of the epidermal growth factor receptor family, there is little evidence that the humoral response to tumors provides significant or relevant antitumor immunity. In contrast, numerous adoptive transfer studies have demonstrated the potent capacity of T cells to kill growing tumors, either directly through CTL activity or indirectly through multiple

CD4-dependent effector mechanisms [81,82]. It is thus likely that from the tumor's standpoint, induction of antigen-specific tolerance among T cells is of paramount importance for survival. Likewise, breaking tolerance to tumor antigens is absolutely critical if therapeutic vaccines are to have a significant clinical impact against cancer.

IV. CENTRAL ROLE OF THE DENDRITIC CELL AS A TARGET FOR THERAPEUTIC VACCINES

The most common theme among active immunotherapy strategies is enhancement or modulation of APC function. Indeed, presentation of antigen by APCs is the critical initial step in the initiation of adaptive immunity. The quantitative and qualitative characteristics of T-cell responses to antigen depend upon the signals they receive from the APC. Elucidation of the molecular events of APC proliferation, differentiation, and activation, together with the molecular definition of signals communicated between APCs to T cells, is transforming the design of therapeutic vaccines. Among the major bone marrow-derived APC subtypes (B cells, macrophages, and dendritic cells), the dendritic cell (DC) has emerged as the most potent APC type responsible for initiating immune responses (Figure 1). As virtually all phases of DC differentiation and function can be modulated by engineered vaccines, it is important to understand the molecular signals that regulate their role in the activation of T-cell-dependent immunity [83,84].

At sites of infection and inflammation, bone marrow-derived progenitor cells (either circulating or resident in the tissue) respond to both proliferative and differentiative signals in order to develop into mature DCs. The cytokine GM-CSF is the most potent known mitogenic factor for DCs at both immature and mature stages. Other cytokines such as FLT-3L, IL-3, and IL-4 can also serve as mitogenic or comitogenic factors for DCs, particularly in conjunction with GM-CSF [85–89]. Initially, immature DCs pass through a stage of differentiation that is specialized for antigen uptake and processing but not for presentation to T cells. Antigen uptake occurs through both micropinocytosis ("drinking of fluid-phase antigens") and receptor-mediated endocytosis, dependent upon lectin-like membrane molecules such as CD36 and DEC-205 [90,91]. Once in endosomal compartments, antigens are digested into peptide, peptidoglycan, and glycolipid fragments which are shunted to lysosome-like compartments where they associate with MHC class II as well as class Ib molecules [92]. In addition to processing within vesicular compartments, antigens are also transferred out of endosomes and into the cytosol where they can undergo proteosome-dependent processing and TAP-dependent transport into the ER for association with MHC class I molecules [93].

Once they have ingested antigens at inflammatory sites in the tissue, immature DCs differentiate in response to a number of distinct "maturation" signals. While many diverse molecules induce DC maturation, most appear to signal DCs via binding to two classes of receptor—the toll-like receptors (TLR) and the TNF receptor (TNFR) family. Toll-like receptors are "pattern recognition receptors" (PRR) which bind common chemical moieties expressed by pathogens termed pathogen-associated molecular patterns (PAMPs) [94]. Lipopolysaccharide (LPS) is the prototypical PAMP and activates the maturation of DCs through binding

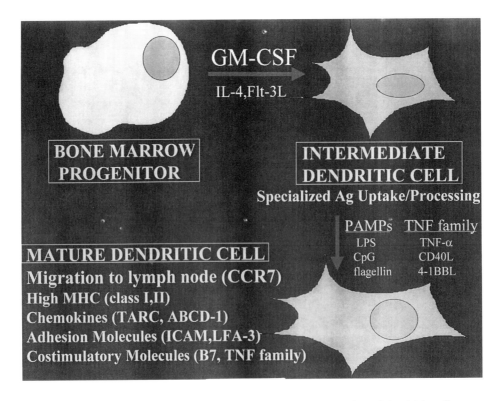

Figure 1 Signals involved in the differentiation and maturation of dendritic cells.

to a TLR-4-containing complex. Other examples include zymosan which binds to TLR-2 and unmethylated CpG DNA sequences which bind to TLR-9. The TNFR family members deliver maturation signals in response to endogenously produced ligands. The two best characterized endogenous DC maturation factors are TNF-α itself and CD40L [95–97]. It is as yet unclear whether these different DC maturation signals result in distinct phenotypes of activated DCs. They all appear to have at least one signaling pathway in common, which is activation of NF-κB.

One of the first consequences of DC maturation is the expression of chemokine receptors such as CCR7 which cause migration from the peripheral tissues to the draining lymph nodes via afferent lymphatics [98]. Once in the draining lymph node, full maturation transforms DC function from antigen uptake and processing into antigen-presentation to T cells. This maturation phase involves the traffic of MHC class II molecules from MHC loading compartments onto the cell surface where they present peptides derived from antigens ingested during the immature tissue phase [99,100]. Presentation of MHC class II-restricted antigens to CD4 cells in the paracortical regions of the lymph node sets up a cross talk in which CD4 cells further activate DCs through CD40 as well as CD40-independent pathways [101–104]. These activated DCs are particularly potent in presenting antigens to and activating CD8 cells. Mature DCs also produce chemokines that selectively attract immature T cells to their surface. This function together with expression of high levels of adhesion molecules such as ICAM-1 can be dramatically observed through clustering of as many as 100 T cells onto the surface of a single dendritic cell [105].

In addition to provision of high densities of peptide-MHC complexes for T-cell stimulation (termed signal 1), DCs regulate T-cell activation and differentiation through provision of costimulatory signals in the form of soluble and membrane-bound ligands (collectively termed signal 2). The best characterized soluble signal delivered to T cells by DCs is the cytokine IL-12, which induces IFN-γ production and promotes Th1 differentiation via a STAT-4-dependent pathway. The best characterized membrane-bound costimulatory ligands are represented by the B7 family. Activation of naïve T cells is critically dependent upon the engagement of the CD28 receptor by B7.1 and B7.2, the first two B7 family members to be discovered [106–109]. While essentially all APC types express B7.1 and B7.2 to varying degrees upon activation, mature DCs express higher levels of B7.2 than any other APC [96,110]. At least three other more recently discovered B7 family members—B7H1/PDL1, B7-DC/PDL2, and B7H3—are also expressed by DCs [111–115]. These B7 family members fail to bind CD28 (or its counter-regulatory partner CTLA-1), indicating that a complex family of costimulatory ligand-receptor pairs participate in the delivery of signals to naive T cells. These distinct B7 family members appear to induce different patterns of cytokine production by T cells.

In addition to the B7 family members, other TNF family members expressed by DCs costimulate T cells. 4-1BBL and OX40-L represent examples of this category of costimulatory signals [116–118]. The ever-expanding panoply of costimulatory signals utilized by DCs to instruct T cells as to their pathway of differentiation and effector function defines

a high degree of complexity to the communications that occur between APC and T cell. Each of the molecular events involved in proliferation, antigen presentation, and costimulation represents potential targets that are being exploited in the design of immunotherapy approaches.

V. GENETICALLY MODIFIED CELL-BASED TUMOR VACCINES THAT ENHANCE DENDRITIC CELL FUNCTION

The elucidation of specific molecules that induce DC proliferation and maturation has provided an important tool kit for the engineering of vaccines with enhanced therapeutic potency. The prototypical example has been the incorporation of GM-CSF into cell-based tumor vaccines (Figure 2). Prior to the discovery of GM-CSF transduced tumors as potent vaccines a large number of genetically modified tumor vaccines had been evaluated. Genes introduced into tumor cells included MHC genes, genes encoding foreign antigens (so-called xenogenization) [119–121], costimulatory genes [122–124], and cytokine genes [125–134]. A detailed comparison of the potency of tumor cell vaccines transduced with different cytokine and immunoregulatory genes demonstrated that GM-CSF-transduced cell vaccines produce the most potent systemic immunity against challenge with wild-type tumor. GM-CSF-transduced vaccines were further shown to cure animals of established micrometastatic tumors [135,136]. Biopsy analysis of the local vaccine sites of GM-CSF-transduced tumor vaccines demonstrates a strong infiltrate of mononuclear cells expressing markers characteristic of the DC lineage. Within a few days of vaccination, one can find increased numbers of mature DCs in the draining lymph node together with active T-cell proliferation in the paracortical regions. As GM-CSF is strictly a DC proliferation factor, it is unclear what stimuli induce DC maturation. The most likely maturation stimulus in GM-CSF-transduced vaccines comes from endogenous factors released by dying cells, such as heat shock proteins. Indeed, a recent report demonstrated that transduction of tumor cells with the hsp-70 gene, thereby significantly increasing the concentration of intracellular hsp-70, enhanced tumor cell immunogenicity [137]. In fact, co-transduction of tumor cells with the GM-CSF gene as well as certain hsp genes or simple heat shocking of GM-CSF-transduced tumor cell vaccines prior to vaccination results in enhancement of vaccine potency relative to the GM-CSF vaccines alone [138]. Another example of vaccine engineering using a combination of DC proliferative and maturation stimuli was provided by Colombo and colleagues. They found that vaccination with tumor cells co-transduced with GM-CSF and CD40L genes generated a dramatic increase in activated DCs at the vaccine site as well as enhanced vaccine potency [139].

The adjuvant effects of paracrine GM-CSF either in the form of transduced cells or incorporated into recombinant nucleic acid vaccines (see below) results in enhancement of diverse effector functions characterized by mixtures of both TH1 and TH2 components. In addition to CTL generation, documented TH1 effector pathways induced by paracrine GM-CSF vaccines include macrophage activation resulting in the production of both superoxides and nitric oxide as

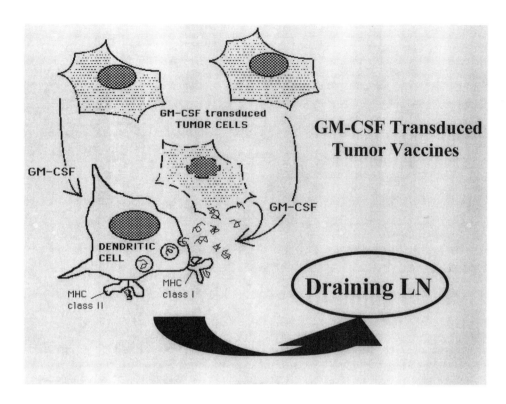

Figure 2   GM-CSF-transduced tumor vaccines.

tumorocidal effectors. TH2 effector pathways involve the activation of eosinophils at the site of tumor metastases. These mixed effector responses have been documented in clinical trials using GM-CSF-transduced vaccines in renal cell cancer, melanoma, and pancreatic cancer [81,140].

A number of early stage clinical trials using both autologous [141,142] and allogeneic [143] GM-CSF gene-transduced cell-based vaccines have demonstrated both immunization and occasional clinical responses in diverse cancer types, including renal cancer, prostate cancer, melanoma, and pancreatic cancer. While these results are promising, they must be viewed with caution, particularly because earlier generations of BCG-based cancer vaccines that showed promise in initial reports failed to demonstrate significant clinical benefit in larger multicenter randomized clinical trials [144–146]. Two principles form the basis for application of allogeneic genetically modified vaccines. First, tumor antigen discovery studies in human cancer—particularly melanoma—have demonstrated a significant proportion of recognized antigens to be shared [47,48]. Second, a number of murine studies have demonstrated that the critical pathway for processing of tumor antigens is crosspresentation by bone marrow-derived APCs [39,46,147,148]. Thus it is not necessary to match HLA alleles between patient and allogeneic vaccine lines. Indeed, a recent analysis of immune responses generated after vaccination with an allogeneic GM-CSF-transduced pancreatic vaccine definitively demonstrated the crosspriming pathway [143,149].

One of the major challenges in the development of autologous GM-CSF-transduced vaccines clinically is the difficulty in achieving reproducibly high transduction and subsequent GM-CSF production with each individual tumor harvest.

Additionally, it is difficult to obtain or culture large numbers of tumor cells from many cancers. In cases where large numbers of tumor cells can be easily obtained (i.e., leukemias, lymphomas, multiple myeloma, and solid tumors where a large mass of relatively pure tumor can be obtained), Borrello et al. have developed a bystander cell approach that obviates the need for individualized transduction. They have demonstrated that simply admixing a GM-CSF-producing bystander cell with unmodified tumor cells produces a vaccine effect equivalent to direct tumor cell transduction [150]. Clinical trials using a human GM-CSF-expressing bystander cell are currently in progress in multiple myeloma, acute myelocytic leukemia, and colon cancer.

VI.   EX VIVO LOADED DENDRITIC CELL VACCINES

The ability to culture DCs ex vivo has led to a plethora of studies of ex vivo antigen-loaded DCs as tumor vaccines. Initially, it was demonstrated that loading of ex vivo cultured DCs with either MHC class I-restricted peptides or whole proteins followed by administration back into the animal led to the generation of immune responses against the loaded antigen [151,152]. Subsequently, significant antitumor responses were demonstrated after injection of DCs loaded with either tumor-derived peptides or tumor lysates

[153,154]. More recently, the advent of more efficient gene transfer vectors has led to approaches in which ex vivo cultured DCs are transduced with genes encoding relevant viral or tumor antigens [155–157]. A number of recombinant replication defective viruses have been used to transduce DCs. In addition, Gilboa and colleagues have demonstrated that purified RNA can be used to effectively transduce DCs with resultant presentation of encoded antigens [158]. This strategy offers the interesting possibility that DCs could be transduced with the entire amplified transcriptome of a tumor cell, even when only tiny amounts of tumor tissue are available.

Another approach aimed at providing DCs with a full complement of tumor antigens has been DC-tumor fusion vaccines [159]. The concept behind this approach is to fuse autologous tumor cells with dendritic cells, thereby allowing for the coexpression of all relevant tumor antigens together with all relevant DC molecules within the same cell. One of the major limitations to clinically translating an approach of this type is the efficiency with which fusion can be achieved between DCs and tumor cells in the absence of selection.

Elucidation of proliferative and maturation signals for DCs has led recently to approaches in which DCs are not only loaded with antigen but are transduced with genes encoding proliferation and maturation signals. This would result in autocrine DC stimulation in vivo after reinjection. In one study, DCs loaded with antigen were transduced with genes encoding GM-CSF and CD40L. These genetically modified DCs resulted in much more potent stimulation of antitumor immunity than immunization with DCs only loaded with antigen [160].

A major issue with regard to ex vivo loaded DC vaccines is the degree of maturation that is induced in vitro and its relevance to homing and function of loaded DCs after reinjection. Concern has been raised that full-blown maturation/activation of DCs ex vivo to a stage normally achieved once they are within paracortical regions of the lymph node will impair their ability to home to lymph nodes after reinjection. This has led to the suggestion that DCs should be loaded and reinjected in an immature state and allowed to mature in vivo. Such an approach has potential negative consequences as Steinman, Bardwaj, and colleagues have demonstrated that immunization of patients with antigen-loaded immature DCs can actually result in tolerance/suppression of antigen-specific responses as compared with activation induced by immunization with antigen-loaded DCs matured in vitro prior to injection [161,162].

There are currently active clinical development of ex vivo loaded DC vaccines so the therapeutic value of various DC manipulations will hopefully be sorted out. At present, the paucity of direct comparative studies leaves open the question of which method of loading DCs ex vivo will be the most effective.

VII. ANTIGEN-SPECIFIC VACCINES—TARGETING ANTIGEN TO MHC PROCESSING PATHWAYS OF DENDRITIC CELLS

A major advantage of cell-based vaccines is the diversity of expressed tumor antigens and the lack of necessity to know the immunorelevant tumor antigens for a given patient's cancer (Table 3). However, the continuing elucidation of specific immunodominant antigens at the molecular level (Table 2) allows for new generations of antigen-specific vaccines that previously were only possible in infectious diseases vaccines. The elucidation of specific receptors on DCs that are responsible for receptor-mediated endocytosis provides a strategy to modify antigens so that they can be more efficiently bound to these DC uptake receptors. Indeed, the antigen-GM-CSF fusion proteins represent a potential example of DC targeting as the GM-CSF component of the antigen not only stimulates DC proliferation but also may act to target the antigen into endosomal compartments once it binds the GM-CSF receptor. Linkage of GM-CSF to antigen in the form of recombinant protein, nucleic acid, and viral vaccines has been shown to significantly enhance immunization. In the case of protein vaccines, both preclinical and clinical trials have been done with idiotype vaccination for B-cell lymphomas. Levy and colleagues demonstrated that fusion proteins of idiotype with GM-CSF-enhanced vaccine potency to the greatest extent relative to fusion of idiotype proteins to other cytokines such as IL-2 [163]. In these fusion vaccines, GM-CSF may also enhance targeting of antigen to endosomal antigen processing compartments after binding to its receptor on DC progenitors. GM-CSF protein has also been mixed with idiotype vaccines in an attempt to recapitulate the paracrine physiology of cytokines. While simple mixture is simple and can add some immunization potency, the effect is not nearly as great as when GM-CSF is genetically or physically linked to the vaccinating antigen.

More direct antigen-targeting approaches have utilized fusion genes between antigen and immunoglobulin Fc regions to enhance Fc receptor-mediated antigen uptake by APCs [164,165]. Such an approach is likely to be more effective in targeting antigens to macrophages which have

Table 3 Cell-Based vs. Antigen-Based Cancer Vaccines[a]

Cell-based	Antigen-based
• Do not need to know relevant antigens	• Must know the relevant antigens
• Highly polyvalent	• Mono/oligovalent
• Full of "irrelevant" and self antigens	• Ability to completely define vaccinating ag
• Limitations in ability to manipulate antigen for maximal stimulation	• Tremendous potential versatility for antigen manipulation

[a] The two major categories of tumor vaccines are cell-based and antigen-specific. Cell-based vaccines use either autologous or allogeneic tumor cells as the source of antigen.

higher levels of FcR than do DCs. Approaches that modify antigens so that they can be selectively targeted to DC receptors such as CD36 and DEC-205 may ultimately provide more effective priming [166]. A recent study demonstrated that conjugation of antigens to anti-DEC-205 antibodies dramatically enhanced the targeting of antigen to DEC-205$^+$ DCs. Importantly, this maneuver alone failed to produce sustained antigen-specific immunity, owing to the failure to activate DCs in vivo. Addition of an activating anti-CD40 antibody to the DEC-205-antigen conjugate did produce sustained immunity, demonstrating the importance of combining MHC targeting and APC activation strategies.

Another interesting category of proteins that may target antigen effectively to DCs and furthermore into MHC processing pathways are the heat shock proteins. It is now well established that complexing of peptide antigens to certain heat shock proteins such as gp96, hsp-70, calreticulin, and hsp-110 enhances their immunogenicity significantly [167–169]. Heat shock proteins were first utilized as tumor vaccines by purifying them from tumor cells followed by immunization. Heat shock proteins isolated from tumors are naturally complexed with a whole array of tumor-associated peptides. Other approaches to link antigen to heat shock protein have included the production of recombinant fusion proteins in which antigenic peptides are linked to the heat shock protein as well as nucleic acid-based vaccines in which fusion genes between antigen and heat shock protein gene are incorporated [170,171]. In one direct comparative study using the HPV-E7 antigen as a model, it was demonstrated that nucleic acid vaccines encoding an E7-hsp70 fusion gene

were 30-fold more effective than the wild-type E7 gene in generating CD8 responses [171]. Immunogenic hsps complexed with antigenic peptides have been shown to efficiently load the MHC class I processing pathway [172]. Although the intracellular pathway by which heat shock proteins effectively load MHC class I molecules with their associated peptides has not yet been elucidated, Srivastava and colleagues have identified CD91, the α2 macroglobulin receptor, as an important receptor for multiple types of heat shock protein (gp96, hsp-70, hsp-90) [173]. Blockade of CD91 on antigen-presenting cells resulted in inhibition of hsp-mediated in vitro crosspresentation into MHC on MHC class I molecules. Ultimately, the immunogenicity of heat shock proteins has been proposed to result from their ability to activate APCs in addition to targeting antigens to MHC processing pathways. One report has suggested that hsp-70 can activate macrophages via CD14/TLR-4 (LPS receptor)-dependent and -independent pathways [174]. Heat shock proteins have also been reported to activate DCs although the receptors that mediate these putative activation functions have yet to be elucidated [175].

Another approach to enhance peptide-MHC ligand density on DCs is to enhance the targeting of antigens into the MHC processing pathways. Two approaches have been utilized to accomplish this goal. One approach has utilized the linkage of targeting signals onto the antigen that will more effectively target them into MHC processing compartments and pathways. Strategies for antigen targeting to the MHC class II processing pathway have utilized the invariant chain targeting signal and the endosomal/lysosomal target-

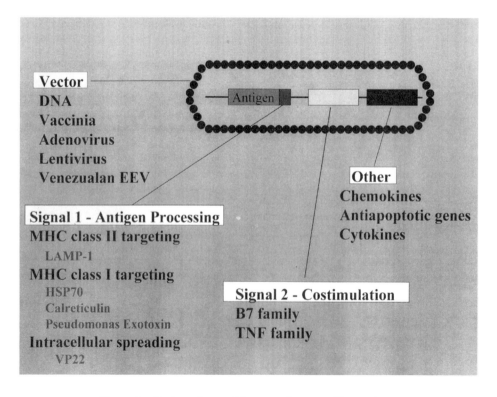

Figure 3 Design of recombinant antigen-specific vaccines.

ing signal in the cytoplasmic tail of the LAMP-1 protein. In the case of the LAMP-1 sorting signal, fusion genes of the E7 antigen linked to the LAMP-1 sorting signal resulted in increased targeting E7 into the MHC class II processing pathway and resultant enhancement of presentation to E7-specific MHC class II-restricted CD4 T cells [176–178]. Incorporation of the LAMP targeting signal onto the E7 gene enhanced CD4 responses and ultimate antitumor potency of both recombinant vaccinia and recombinant nucleic acid vaccines.

A number of MHC class I targeting approaches have also resulted in enhanced immunization potency [179–181]. The antigen-hsp70 fusion genes described above represent such an example, selectively enhancing antigen-specific CD8 responses. Other validated targeting signals that enhance CD8 priming include calreticulin, VP22, and Pseudomonas exotoxin B. Another strategy for enhanced MHC class I processing has been the construction of "epitopes on a string." This approach separates out individual epitopes from a given antigen and strings them together separated by linkers that encode basic amino acids that are good substrates for proteosome cleavage [182]. As a number of these strategies likely function via distinct mechanisms, maximal loading of MHC on APCs will likely be achieved through combining different targeting signals (Figure 3).

VIII. EPITOPE MODIFICATION TO ENHANCE THE T-CELL RECEPTOR SIGNAL

Just as with APC development and activation, the tremendous explosion in knowledge about T-cell development, antigen recognition and activation provides opportunities to engineer immunotherapies that directly modify T-cell responses. Because virtually all of the signals to T cells begin at the cell membrane, vaccines and other immunotherapies can be enhanced by inclusion of ligands that bind these cell membrane receptors. As will be discussed, the enhanced versatility of new vector systems allows for combinatorial construction of immunotherapies containing multiple elements that target multiple points in the pathway of T-cell activation.

In considering the immunogenicity of various antigenic formulations, it is commonly assumed that alterations in the immune response will depend strictly on the set of costimulatory signals (Signal-2) provided to T cells at the time of antigen recognition. However, it is now clear that both qualitative and quantitative characteristics of the peptide MHC interaction with TCR (Signal-1) are equally important in determining the outcome of T-cell responses. The two most well-defined parameters of TCR engagement are ligand density and TCR affinity. Multiple studies with altered peptide ligands have indicated that there is a relatively narrow range of TCR affinities that will produce optimal T-cell stimulation [183]. Lower affinity ligands result in partial agonist properties and ultimately in antagonist properties—under certain circumstances resulting in anergy induction. The favored model to explain these findings is a kinetic proofreading model which suggests that the TCR must be engaged by the peptide MHC complex for a long

enough time period to initiate the complete set of intracellular biochemical signaling events for T-cell activation. Engagement of the T-cell receptor for time periods less than that requisite for complete activation of signaling cascades results in incomplete activation. Suboptimal TCR engagement may ultimately deplete substrates or activate negative feedback pathways resulting in abortive T-cell stimulation and leading to a state of unresponsiveness. Even for high affinity ligands, it has been demonstrated that exposure of T cells to ligand densities below activation threshold can also result in induction of T-cell unresponsiveness. Evidence in favor of the kinetic proofreading model comes from the finding that exposure of T cells to altered peptide ligands with lower affinity for TCR results in partial phosphorylation of the zeta chain as well as other incomplete signaling events. A fundamental corollary of the hypothesis that tumors arising endogenously are capable of inducing tolerance among T cells specific for neoantigens is that the residual repertoire of tumor antigen-specific T cells will either be low affinity or specific for epitopes presented at low density. Similar mechanisms may be operative when viruses evade immune elimination and set up a chronic carrier state.

Analysis of T-cell responses specific for defined tumor antigens has indeed provided experimental evidence for this notion. The human tumor for which immunodominant antigens have been best characterized is melanoma. The majority of melanoma-specific T cells that have been grown in culture appear to recognize melanocyte-specific differentiation antigens such as MART-1/melan-A, GP100, and tyrosinase. As specific MHC class I and class II-restricted epitopes have been identified, a surprisingly large number appear to have extremely low affinities for their presenting MHC molecule, resulting in low-density peptide MHC complexes both on the tumor and on APCs loaded with the antigen. This low MHC affinity is generally associated with undesirable residues at critical anchor positions. In other cases, tumor peptides bind well to MHC molecules but available T cells display low affinities for the peptide–MHC complex [48]. T-cell responses to the immunodominant antigen of the murine CT26 colon tumor represent an example of this latter case [184]. This antigen, derived from an endogenous retroviral gp70 gene, is the target for roughly 90% of the total CD8 response in animals vaccinated with this tumor. The particular immunodominant epitope was shown to display a high affinity for its restricting MHC class I molecule. However, when the peptide–MHC affinity of the T-cell receptor expressed by T cells grown from vaccinated animals was measured, it was significantly lower than affinities measured for T cells specific for standard foreign antigens.

As tumor antigens continue to be identified, there will be important opportunities to modify epitopes so that they are presented to T cells in a fashion that provides the most effective transmission of signal 1 (Figure 4). For antigens that have poor MHC binding affinity, a number of groups have demonstrated that alteration of MHC anchor residues to more favorable amino acids can result in dramatic enhancement of MHC binding while nonetheless retaining the capacity for enhanced activation of T cells specific for the

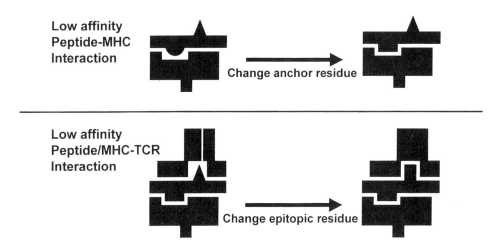

Figure 4 Peptide-MHC binding vs. peptide/MHC-TCR binding in immunogenicity of tumor antigens.

original wild-type epitope [185,186]. This results in a hetero-clitic response in which vaccines containing the anchor-modified epitope can produce greater immune responses against the wild-type peptide in vivo as well as enhanced antitumor immunity. Epitope engineering can also generate enhanced immunity at the level of TCR affinity for peptide-MHC. Thus in the case of the low affinity response to the GP70-derived peptide described above, a single amino acid alteration was identified which did not affect MHC binding but increased the affinity of peptide-MHC for the T-cell receptor by threefold. Immunization with DCs loaded with this altered peptide resulted in a dramatic enhancement in the expansion of T cells in vivo specific for the original wild-type peptide and enhancement of systemic antitumor immunity [184].

The effect of T-cell affinity is not only manifest at the level of T-cell priming but also at the level of T-cell effector function. This concept was most effectively demonstrated by Greenberg and colleagues who were able to separate tyrosinase-specific T cells cloned from melanoma patients into high and low affinity populations based on their level of staining with peptide-MHC tetramers. Higher affinity T cells bind greater amounts of tyrosinase peptide-A2 tetramer at equilibrium than low affinity T cells. When analyzed on peptide-loaded targets (which express artificially high ligand densities) both high and low affinity T-cell clones lysed targets with relatively equivalent efficacy. However, only the high affinity T-cell clones were capable of lysing the original tumor cells in vitro. These findings have led to clinical trials in which T-cell clones are first selected based on levels of tetramer binding prior to expansion and reinfusion [187].

IX. ENHANCEMENT OF COSTIMULATION IN THERAPEUTIC VACCINE DESIGN

As mentioned above, qualitative and quantitative elements of T-cell activation and differentiation are determined in large part by signals delivered by costimulatory molecules.

As the number of costimulatory molecules increase, a picture is emerging in which T-cell activation requires integration of a large number of different signals. The best characterized costimulatory signals fall into three families: the B7 family, the TNF family, and cytokines. Among these three categories of costimulatory molecules, the B7 family appears to be the only one with a unidirectional vector of signaling, namely, from APC to T cell. In contrast, different members of the TNF family and cytokine families provide multidirectional signaling, i.e., from APC to T cell, from T cell to APC, and T cell to T cell. Tremendous effort has been placed in engineering costimulatory molecules into vaccines and other immunotherapies in an attempt to enhance their activity. In the case of the B7 family members, virtually all of the focus thus far has been on B7.1 and B7.2. It will be interesting to see how the new B7 family members B7H1/PDL1, B7-DC/PDL2, and B7H3 [111–115] will fit into the armamentarium as they bind distinct receptors from B7.1 and B7.2 and have only partially overlapping biological activity.

There are three primary approaches that have been used to build B7.1/B7.2 into immunotherapeutic approaches. One involves the transduction of tumor cells with B7 genes in order to enhance their immunogenicity as vaccines [122–124]. The original concept behind introducing B7 genes into tumors came from the idea that tumors fail to stimulate immune responses against them under normal circumstances because they did not express costimulatory molecules. Therefore presentation of signal 1 (peptide/MHC) in the absence of costimulatory signals would result in either failure to effectively activate tumor-specific T cells or tolerance induction. Transduction of tumor cells with the genes encoding either B7.1 or B7.2 would reconstitute costimulation and therefore might activate antitumor immune responses through direct presentation. Indeed, multiple studies have confirmed that B7-transduced tumor cells are effectively rejected when high enough B7 levels are achieved. However, when the transduced tumor is poorly immunogenic (as is presumably the case in human tumors) transduction with B7 fails to induce systemic protective immunity although the B7-transduced cells themselves are rejected. As described above, more detailed analysis of the mechanisms of both rejection and immune priming by B7-transduced tumors supports the emerging view that direct presentation by tumor cells to the immune system is a relatively minor pathway as compared with the indirect presentation pathway via bone marrow-derived APCs (crosspriming). Rejection of B7-transduced tumor cells involves a major NK-mediated component. Indeed, NK cells appear to recognize B7 as a target for activation and lysis. Bone marrow chimera studies demonstrated that after initial vaccination with B7-transduced tumors, the majority of T-cell priming came from bone marrow-derived APCs rather than from the B7-transduced tumor cells themselves. Once a primed population of T cells had been induced, then B7-transduced tumor cells could amplify those responses through direct presentation [188].

A more promising application of the B7 molecules to vaccine design has been the inclusion of B7 genes into recombinant nucleic acid and viral vaccine vectors for antigen-specific vaccination [189,190]. The basis for the inclusion of B7 genes into recombinant nucleic acid or viral vaccines comes from the idea that one of the methods by which these vaccines immunize is through direct transduction or infection of APCs. Theoretically, although professional APCs (i.e., dendritic cells) naturally express B7 molecules, the increased expression provided by B7 genes engineered into recombinant vaccines as well as altered patterns or ratios of expression of the different B7 family members could significantly modify the ultimate outcome of T-cell priming in vivo. A number of studies have demonstrated that incorporation of either B7.1 or B7.2 into DNA vaccines as well as recombinant vaccinia vaccines enhances the generation of CTL responses and in some cases antibody responses against the specific antigen expressed by the recombinant vaccine. Interestingly, while these studies have failed to corroborate early suggestions that B7.1 predominantly costimulated TH1 responses and B7.2 predominantly costimulated TH2 responses in vivo, they have in some cases demonstrated differential activity between B7.1 and B7.2. One common theme has been that the B7.2 gene appears to be superior to the B7.1 gene in the generation of CTL responses in vivo.

Another approach that has been utilized to enhance immunization with the B7 costimulatory molecules has been the infusion of B7-Ig dimers either systemically or mixed with vaccine formulations [191]. Chimeric immunoglobulin-B7 fusion molecules, which display B7 as a dimer, are extremely potent costimulators for T cells in vitro and have been shown to enhance the potency of tumor vaccines in vivo. No toxicity has been observed with systemic administration of B7-Ig dimers, presumably because CD28 engagement in the absence of TCR engagement has little or no effect on T cells. One might imagine that this approach could have detrimental effects on tolerance to self-antigens if administered chronically. However, it is unlikely that administration of these molecules over short periods of time together with a vaccine or adoptively transferred T cells would have major effects on the maintenance of self-tolerance.

The list of potential TNF receptor family molecules expressed by T cells that may participate in modifying T-cell responses (either upward or downward) continues to grow. Two very interesting candidate costimulatory receptors of the TNFR family are 4-1BB and OX40. Administration of putatively agonist anti-4-1BB and anti-OX40 antibodies has been shown to induce antitumor immunity when administered either alone or in the context of a vaccine [116–118]. Using a TCR transgenic model for tolerance induction, Parker and colleagues derived evidence that activation through OX40 might even be able to break anergic tolerance. 4-1BB ligand and OX40 ligand are expressed on antigen-presenting cells and these ligand-receptor pairs therefore represent candidate costimulatory signals from APC to T cell. CD27 and CD30 represent two additional TNF receptor family members on T cells that may represent interesting targets either for activation or inhibition of antigen-specific responses [192,193].

X. APPLICATION OF CYTOKINES IN CANCER IMMUNOTHERAPY

Cytokines represent by far and away the largest category of immunoregulatory molecules and have been utilized as systemic agents, as local agents and as components of both genetically modified cell-based and recombinant antigen-specific vaccines. Rather than discussing the detailed application of cytokines to immunotherapy, a topic covered in numerous reviews, some general principles and a few selected examples of cytokine application to immunotherapy will be covered here. The major clinical application of cytokines has been in the form of systemic administration of the recombinant cytokine protein. In general, systemic administration of cytokines as single agents in cancer immunotherapy has been quite disappointing. Of all the many cytokines tested, interleukin-2 (IL-2) has an established track record in patients with metastatic renal cancer and melanoma and has been demonstrated to induce durable complete responses in these two cancers in between 3% and 10% of individuals [194]. Unfortunately, the toxicity of systemically administered cytokines (including IL-2) is quite high and significantly limits their widespread application. The therapeutic effects of IL-2 in murine tumor systems as well as in human melanoma and renal cancer are immunologically mediated, as IL-2 has no direct effect on the tumor cells themselves. However, it is unclear whether systemically administered IL-2, particularly at higher doses, enhances antigen-specific antitumor immunity when administered as a single systemic agent. Indeed, the serum concentrations achieved with "high-dose IL-2" are high enough to bind to the intermediate affinity IL-2 receptor expressed on NK cells (IL-2Rβ). Likewise, the antitumor effects of high-dose IL-12 in mice are at least partially mediated by NK and NKT cells without clear evidence that antigen-specific T-cell immunity is enhanced. Application of systemic IL-2 in conjunction with vaccination may potentially be a more effective way to utilize IL-2 to enhance systemic antigen-specific T-cell immunity. When T cells are initially activated by their cognate antigen, they express a high affinity IL-2 receptor consisting of the IL-2Rα and IL-2Rβ subunits (together with the non-IL-2 binding IL-2Rγ signaling subunit). Thus antigen-specific T cells activated in response to a vaccine will transiently respond to much lower doses of IL-2 based on their expression of the high affinity IL-2 receptor. Indeed, preliminary studies combining vaccination with lower doses of IL-2 have demonstrated evidence of synergy between these two agents.

One of the disappointing surprises in systemic cytokine administration has been the vast differences in tolerability of systemic cytokines between mice and humans. Thus cytokines, such as IL-2, TNF-α, and IL-12, which induce regressions of established tumors in mice at high systemic doses, are lethal to humans at doses that achieve therapeutic serum concentrations in mice. For example, the LD50 for systemic IL-2 in mice is estimated roughly 50-fold higher than in humans whereas the LD50 for TNF-α is roughly 300-fold higher in mice than in humans. Toxicity determinations for IL-12 are more complicated as lower doses of IL-12 can "tolerize" individuals to higher doses of IL-12. Nonetheless, the maximal tolerable doses of IL-12 in humans are significantly below the doses that achieve significant antitumor responses in mice.

As virtually all cytokines behave physiologically as autocrine or paracrine factors, it is not surprising that applying them as systemic agents results in unacceptable toxicities and side effects owing to the loss of geographical specificity that is so critical to normal cytokine physiology. Indeed, the primary motivation for building cytokines into tumor cell vaccines as well as recombinant nucleic acid or viral vectors is to maximize the expression of the cytokine at the site of antigen delivery. In the case of cytokine gene-transduced tumor vaccines, introduction of genes encoding cytokines targeted at the T cell has been less successful in priming immune responses than transduction of cytokines aimed at APCs, particularly dendritic cells. Considering that the vaccines are typically administered intradermally or in the subcutaneous space, whereas T-cell priming generally occurs in the draining lymph node, it is not surprising that tumor cell vaccines engineered to produce dendritic cell-targeted cytokines would ultimately be more effective. One important approach to cytokine-based therapeutics is the targeting of cytokines to areas of tumor metastasis where T cells originally activated in the draining lymph nodes would subsequently traffic and discharge their effector function. The function of these effector T cells would be significantly enhanced by the presence of cytokines at the sites of metastatic tumor in the periphery. Proof of principle for the efficacy of such an approach has come from studies by Reisfeld and colleagues who have linked cytokines such as IL-2 to the Fc regions of antitumor antibodies [195]. While the antitumor antibodies themselves demonstrate limited efficacy, owing to limited penetration into solid tumors by most monoclonal antibodies infused systemically, there is enough concentration in the tumors to increase the local concentration of IL-2, thereby enhancing antitumor immune responses in a T-cell-dependent fashion. It will be of great interest in the future to evaluate combination approaches between vaccination that would generate an increased population of tumor-specific T cells expressing high affinity IL-2 receptors together with IL-2-linked antitumor antibodies.

Engineering approaches to maximize the efficacy of cytokine signaling during the effector phase of antitumor

immunity have also been applied to adoptive T cell transfer approaches. Ridell and Greenberg have demonstrated that adoptively transferred tumor-specific CD8 T-cell clones home to tumors and can exert transient effector function but, in the absence of adequate T-cell help, are rapidly lost from both the circulation and sites of tumor. The requirement that CD8 effector cells have for T-cell help comes from the fact that they are very inefficient at providing their own helper cytokines such as IL-2. Provision of systemic IL-2 after adoptive transfer of CD8 cells can enhance their longevity and activity [196,197], but this approach is ultimately limited by the toxicities of systemic IL-2 as described above. In order to circumvent this problem, tumor-specific CD8 cells were transduced with chimeric receptors expressing the extracellular domains for cytokines normally secreted by CD8 cells, e.g., GM-CSF, linked to the cytoplasmic signaling domain of the IL-2 receptors. Specifically, the GM-CSFRα extracellular domain was linked to the IL-2Rβ domain and the GM-CSFRβ extracellular domain was linked to the IL-2Rγ intracellular signaling domain. T cells transduced with these chimeric receptors transmitted IL-2-dependent signals in response to GM-CSF, thus converting GM-CSF into an autocrine growth factor for CD8 cells [198]. These engineered CD8 cells become relatively helper cell-independent and generate enhanced numbers of effectors as well as memory cells upon encounter of antigen in vivo.

Possibly the most promising application of T-cell costimulatory or proliferative cytokines is their incorporation as genes into recombinant nucleic acid and viral vaccines (Figure 3). Multiple studies have demonstrated that incorporation of cytokine genes to recombinant vaccines of this sort cannot only quantitatively enhance T-cell responses but can also alter the differentiation pattern of antigen-specific T cells. Again, this approach is based on the notion that both nucleic acid and viral vaccines act in part through direct infection of antigen-presenting cells thereby maximizing the paracrine effect of the cytokine on T cells to which the infected or transduced APC is presenting antigen. For example, Bersofsky and colleagues performed a detailed analysis of the type of immune responses generated by nucleic acid vaccines in which multiple different cytokine genes were incorporated. As described above, they found that GM-CSF, which acts on APCs, generated the greatest level of T-cell immunity, although the characteristics of the responses were mixed TH1 and TH2. When interleukin-12 was incorporated into the nucleic acid vaccine, antigen-specific responses were predominantly TH1 in character whereas when IL-4 or IL-10 was incorporated into the vaccine, TH1 responses were quenched and the predominant response was TH2 in character [199].

XI. RECOMBINANT VIRAL VACCINE VECTORS FOR ANTIGEN-SPECIFIC IMMUNOTHERAPY OF CANCER

For all of the added value that recombinant DNA technology provides in engineering elements into vaccine constructs that enhance their potency, nature itself provides a virtually limitless array of delivery systems in the form of diverse microbes with potent intrinsic immunologic properties. Of the three major microbial classes: virus, bacterium, and fungi, viruses and bacteria have been the most intensively investigated. A recent report of engineered yeast vaccines emphasizes the potential immunologic utility of the third microbial class.

Viruses are the most diverse and efficient gene transfer agents whose natural cell tropism and biologic features can significantly enhance the immunogenicity of antigens carried within them. Using standard recombination approaches, Moss and Paoletti were the first to generate recombinant viruses as vaccine vectors [200–202]. They utilized vaccinia virus because this virus had been administered to hundreds of millions of individuals in the smallpox eradication campaign. Vaccinia is a highly immunogenic virus related to smallpox; its reduced virulence is in part due to its high immunogenicity. In most cases, a single immunization with recombinant vaccinia carrying a gene expressing an antigen will generate significantly greater immune responses against that antigen than the corresponding protein or peptide epitopes mixed with standard adjuvants. This is particularly true for CTL generation. To date, many viruses have been explored as recombinant vaccine vectors, including attenuated replication-deficient poxviruses such as modified vaccinia ancara, fowl pox, and canary pox [203,204]. Adenovirus, herpesviruses, and venezuelan equine encephalitis virus represent additional promising viruses that have been engineered to express specific tumor and other antigens [205,206]. Each of these viruses has various advantages and disadvantages and no clear "winner" has emerged as the absolute vector of choice. However, a number of principles are emerging. Features of viruses that can enhance their potency as vaccine vectors include their ability to replicate, thereby increasing the antigen load, to induce immunologic "danger" signals at sites of infection, and to directly infect antigen-presenting cells, thereby leading to efficient processing and presentation of encoded epitopes, particularly in the MHC class I pathway. Elements of viruses that can diminish their potency as vaccine vectors include the presence of virally encoded inhibitors of immunity [207]. These include molecules that block processing and presentation in the MHC class I pathway (such as TAP inhibitors and inhibitors of MHC class I traffic out of the endoplasmic reticulum) and cytokine decoys, to mention a few. Thus deleting immunologic inhibitory genes from recombinant viruses may enhance their vaccine potency while attenuating their virulence.

Another major limitation of virus-based vaccination comes from the presence of neutralizing antibodies in pre-exposed individuals that inhibit the initial round of infection and replication, thereby quenching their ability to immunize. The presence of neutralizing antibodies has been a major factor limiting the efficacy of recombinant adenoviral vaccines and recombinant vaccinia vaccines in previously exposed (adenovirus) or vaccinated (vaccinia) individuals. Even in individuals who have never been exposed to the vaccinating virus previously or who have very low titers at the time of initial vaccination will tend to generate very high titers of neutralizing antibody after the first vaccination,

thereby precluding subsequent vaccination with the same vector. This finding has led to the concept of cycling different viral vectors in "prime-boost" formats [208,209]. Dramatic enhancement of immunization potency has been observed in prime-boost formats between both different viruses such as fowl pox followed by vaccinia as well as between nucleic acid vaccines and recombinant viral vaccines. DNA-virus prime-boost regimens look particularly promising because, while DNA-based vaccines tend to be of relatively low potency, they are not subject to the limitations of neutralizing humoral immunity for multiple vaccinations. Furthermore, even when ineffective on their own, DNA vaccines appear to prime populations of antigen-specific T cells that respond particularly vigorously to boosting with a recombinant viral vaccine. One hypothesis for this synergy is that nucleic acid vaccines generate a population of memory T cells specific for the encoded antigen that compete more effectively with virus-specific T cells upon boosting with recombinant virus.

XII. RECOMBINANT BACTERIAL VACCINES

The diverse set of bacteria whose immunopathogenesis is becoming elucidated has led to a number of interesting and promising recombinant bacterial vaccines. Genetic engineering of intracellular bacteria has produced enhanced immune responses in the case of BCG, Salmonella, Shigella, and Listeria [210–214]. The basic principle behind recombinant bacterial vaccines is that bacteria that enter antigen-presenting cells may represent a good vehicle for delivery of recombinant antigens. In certain cases, such as Listeria, the bacteria exhibit complex life cycles that involve both phagolysosomal and cytoplasmic stages. Thus recombinant Listeria monocytogenese engineered to secrete antigens will load the MHC class II processing pathway during the phagolysosomal phase and the MHC class I pathway during the cytosolic phase of the life cycle. In addition, a number of recombinant bacteria actively induce infected APCs to secrete proinflammatory cytokines such as IL-12 (Figure 5). These proinflammatory cytokines can have very potent effects on adaptive immunity.

More recently, recombinant bacteria have been appreciated to be an interesting new vector for delivery of nucleic acid vaccines [215,216]. Thus engineering plasmids with eukaryotic promoter and enhancer elements driving the antigen gene results in more potent immunity induction than when the plasmids utilize prokaryotic promoters. These results indicate that the bacteria can directly transfer plasmids into eukaryotic transcriptional compartments within infected APCs.

XIII. AMPLIFICATION OF IMMUNITY THROUGH BLOCKADE OF INHIBITORY PATHWAYS AND REGULATORY T CELLS

As engineered immunotherapeutics continue to improve, a potency ceiling will be reached owing to the presence of hardwired inhibitory pathways that negatively regulate lymphocyte responses—so-called immunologic checkpoints. It is now clear that the quantitative response to antigen is

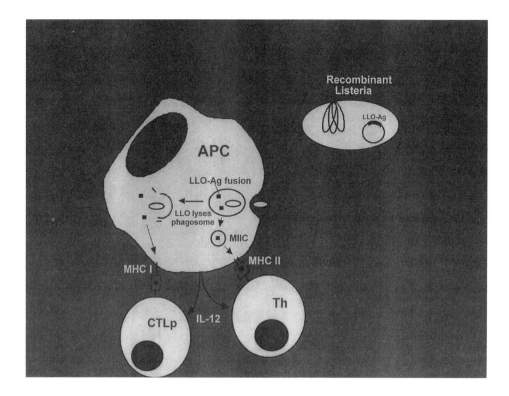

Figure 5 Listeria monocytogenes vaccine.

balanced by both positive (costimulatory) and negative (checkpoint) signaling pathways. In the case of T-cell responses, a number of these pathways appear to have components that are either exclusively or at least selectively expressed by T cells. As they become elucidated, the signaling molecules of immunologic checkpoints will represent a major target for pharmacologic intervention. Past efforts in the development of pharmacologic agents that target the immune system have exclusively identified drugs that either inhibit or activate immune responses in a nonspecific, antigen-independent fashion. The discovery of specific negative regulatory signaling pathways that check immune responses by dampening TCR or costimulatory signaling pathways provides a wonderful opportunity for antigen-specific immunopharmacology by applying drugs (or antibodies) that block these pathways utilized together with antigen-specific activation stimuli.

Among the best studied of these counter-regulatory pathways is the one initiated by engagement of CTLA-4. Naive T cells express the costimulatory B7 receptor CD28, whose engagement amplifies TCR-dependent responses in a number of ways including increased cytokine gene transcription rates, increased cytokine mRNA stability, and inhibition of activation-induced cell death. Subsequent to T-cell activation, a second B7 receptor, CTLA-4, becomes expressed. CTLA-4 has a much higher affinity for B7.1 and B7.2 than does CD28. CTLA-4 delivers inhibitory signals to T cells that oppose the costimulatory signals delivered by CD28 [217]. CTLA-4 knockout mice die at a relatively young age of "hyperimmune" infiltrates into multiple organs, indicating that CTLA-4 is a critical negative regulator of

T-cell activity (Figure 6). Allison and colleagues have demonstrated that transient in vivo blockade of CTLA-4 with a blocking antibody administered at the time of tumor vaccination can enhance vaccine potency and subsequent antitumor immunity [218–220]. The immune-enhancing effect of anti-CTLA-4 blocking antibodies was demonstrated in the context of a number of different cell-based vaccines including B7-transduced and GM-CSF-transduced tumor cell vaccines. Results with combinations of GM-CSF-transduced prostate cancer and melanoma vaccines together with CTLA-4 blockade illustrated two important points. First, the combination of an activating stimulus (vaccine) together with blockade of an immunologic checkpoint (anti-CTLA-4) was able to induce elimination of macroscopic established and spontaneously arising tumors whereas either vaccine alone or CTLA-4 blockade alone failed to achieve these results. Second, while the combination approach induced autoimmune disease, the autoimmunity was confined to the tissue from which the tumor vaccine was derived. Thus treatment of mice with B16 melanoma-GM-CSF + anti-CTLA-4 exclusively resulted in vitiligo—an autoimmune response restricted to melanocytes. Mice receiving the prostate cancer-GM-CSF vaccine + anti-CTLA-4 developed prostatitis but no other signs of autoimmunity. These findings demonstrate that there is a hierarchy of tolerance induction in which tolerance to tissue-specific antigens may be maintained less stringently than tolerance to more ubiquitous self-antigens. This hierarchy thus provides a therapeutic window for cancers derived from dispensable tissues in which tissue-specific antigens shared by the cancer represent viable immunologic targets.

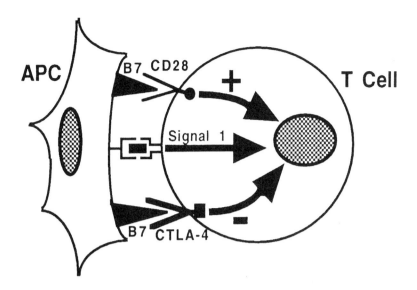

Figure 6 The CTLA-4 checkpoint in T-cell activation.

Dissection of signaling pathways in T cells has revealed a number of additional potential targets for inhibitors of immunologic checkpoints. PD-1, a membrane molecule induced subsequent to T-cell activation, is a CTLA-4-like inhibitory molecule that decreases cytokine responses in T cells and may enhance activation-induced cell death of T cells. PD-1 is now appreciated to be a receptor for two of the newer B7 family members, B7-H1/PDL-1 and B7-DC/PDL-2. Given that both B7-H1 and B7-DC can costimulate enhanced cytokine production by naive T cells, it is likely that PD-1 represents a counter-regulatory inhibitory receptor matched against an as yet unidentified costimulatory receptor on naive T cells. PD-1 knockout mice do not develop the broad hyperimmune organ infiltrates that CTLA-4 knockout mice develop but rather display a more focal autoimmunity. PD-1 therefore represents an interesting potential target for blockade in the context of immunization analogous to CTLA-4 blockade.

A number of intracellular inhibitory signaling pathways in T cells represent promising targets for pharmacologic intervention. Some of the best candidates include Cbl-b, Cabin, certain protein tyrosine phosphatases (PTPs) as well as the tyrosine kinase Csk. Among the phosphatases, SHiP-1, SHP-1, and SHP-2 have all been implicated in down-modulating signaling pathways activated by TCR engagement [221]. More recently, the CD45 PTP has been demonstrated to negatively regulate immune responses by inhibiting JAK-1 and 2 activation, thereby downmodulating responses to certain cytokines [222]. Downstream of the JAK kinases, activation of the STAT transcription factors is inhibited by the CIS/SOCS family [223]. Csk has been well demonstrated to inhibit or downmodulate TCR signaling through phosphorylation of regulatory tyrosines on the src family tyrosine kinases, which are critical for T-cell activation [224]. Cbl-b is an adaptor protein that appears to negatively regulate T-cell activation by antagonizing CD28-mediated costimulatory pathways. Thus T cells from

Cbl-b knockout mice are hypersensitive to low doses of T-cell stimulatory ligands and are furthermore relatively CD28-independent in their activation [225,226]. Cabin is a molecule that appears to have multiple functions, including as a scaffold for coordinating transcription factors. Cabin was originally identified as a molecule that binds to and inhibits calcineurin, a critical serine phosphatase that mediates TCR-dependent cytokine activation through dephosphorylation of NFAT-c, a critical step in nuclear translocation [227]. The calceneurin-inhibiting portion of Cabin has been localized and thus represents an interesting target for pharmacologic intervention.

In light of the resurrection of suppressor T cells under the new alias of T-regulatory (Treg) cells [228,229], a discussion of tumor tolerance would be incomplete without considering the potential role of this important subset. There is relatively little specific information on the role of Treg cells in inducing or maintaining tumor tolerance under normal circumstances; however, two studies strongly support the notion that they significantly limit the efficacy of vaccine-induced antitumor immune responses and their inhibition or elimination could significantly enhance tumor immunotherapy. In one study, a combination of a GM-CSF-transduced tumor vaccine plus anti-CTLA4 was much more effective at eliminating established tumors when animals were treated with anti-IL2 receptor α antibodies prior to vaccination/ anti-CTLA4 treatment [230]. The notion of eliminating Treg cells came from the surprising finding that while CD4 depletion of animals significantly diminished the ability of GM-CSF vaccine/anti-CTLA4 to protect animals from subsequent tumor challenge (with B16 melanoma), the opposite effect was observed for therapy of established B16 tumors [231]. These results suggested the idea that CD4 cells predominately played an enhancing helper role when vaccine/anti-CTLA4 treatment was done prior to tumor inoculation, but once tumors were established they induced a dominant population of CD4$^+$ T regulatory cells. As T regulatory cells typically express IL2 receptor, it was reasoned that depletion of IL2 receptor positive cells prior to vaccination/anti-CTLA4 would eliminate these Treg cells.

In a second set of studies, Jaffee and colleagues demonstrated that treatment of mice with low-dose cytoxan prior to vaccination enhanced the ability of HER-2/neu/GM-CSF vaccines to protect HER-2/neu transgenic mice from challenge with HER-2/neu-expressing tumors [232]. As the cytoxan and vaccine treatments were performed prior to the tumor challenge, the enhanced effect of cytoxan could not be explained by a direct antitumor effect. Indeed, low-dose cytoxan treatment has long been touted to inhibit or kill suppressor cells, although this effect had been more recently attributed to the creation of lymphoid "space." However, adoptive transfer experiments with $CD4^+IL2R^+$ cells from noncytoxan-treated HER-2/neu transgenic mice proved that the cytoxan effect was indeed due to inhibition of Treg cells. It is likely that the next few years will see many additional demonstrations for an important role of Treg cells in blunting or blocking antitumor immunity, likely because they are a natural consequence of tolerance induction. They represent a very tempting target for inhibition as part of combination immunotherapy strategies.

XIV. TUMOR VACCINATION IN THE CONTEXT OF BONE MARROW TRANSPLANTATION

The curative effects of bone marrow transplantation stand as the major example of the ability of the immune system to cure cancer in humans. A paradigm shift in the bone marrow transplant field has been the appreciation that bone marrow transplantation represents a potent approach to modify host immunity and generate significant antitumor immune responses. It is now quite clear that the major antitumor effects of allogeneic bone marrow transplantation have an immunologic basis. Specifically, antitumor immunity is generated by contaminating mature donor T cells in the marrow infusion. Under some circumstances, donor-derived T cells selectively recognize tumor cells (graft-vs.-tumor effect) that express higher levels of minor histocompatibility antigens than host tissues. Graft-vs.-tumor effect is of course balanced by the significant toxicity of graft-vs.-host disease [233–235].

Ironically, the original mechanism on which allogeneic bone marrow transplantation is based—namely, the ability to deliver higher doses of radio-chemotherapy followed by rescue with tumor-free donor bone marrow—plays relatively little role in the antitumor effects of allogeneic bone marrow transplantation. While less well documented, it is likely that autologous bone marrow transplantation exerts some of its antitumor effects through immunologic means. It is now clear that autologous BMT, even with documented tumor-contaminated marrow, can result in long-term tumor-free survival and cancer cure.

Given the documented immunologically based antitumor effects of bone marrow transplantation, but also the severe toxicity of this procedure, it was logical to combine bone marrow transplantation and vaccination in an attempt to more selectively focus immune responses on tumor-specific antigens. Initially, Borrello et al. demonstrated that vaccination with a GM-CSF-transduced cell-based vaccine generated more potent antitumor effects when delivered in a window of time post autologous bone marrow transplantation [236]. They demonstrated that vaccination in this setting resulted in a greater expansion of antigen-specific T cells. This effect was attributed to two potential mechanisms—general systemic enhancement of APC activation in the bone marrow transplant setting and increased "lymphoid space" created by the initial induction regimen prior to bone marrow transplantation. Indeed, evidence exists for both mechanisms. The radiation and chemotherapy regimens used for induction prior to bone marrow transplantation cause subclinical gut damage, which results in the release of bacterial products such as LPS systemically. These ultimately serve to globally activate antigen-presenting cells that are critical to the activity of virtually all vaccines, as described above. It is also well documented that lympoablation results in the upregulation of cytokines, such as IL7 and IL15, which not only participate in "homeostatic" T-cell expansion but also enhance the generation and persistence of memory T cells subsequent to immunization [237,238].

Synergistic effects between allogeneic bone marrow transplantation and vaccination with both antigen-based vaccines and cell-based vaccines have likewise been documented in a number of animal models [239,240]. Because the basis for the antitumor effect of allogeneic transplantation comes from donor mature T cells, it would be expected that these donor lymphocytes would not have been rendered tolerant to tumor antigens as they come from a tumor-free individual. Indeed, vaccination of donors prior to BMT plus DLI can result in dramatic enhancements of antitumor immunity; however, concomitant increase in graft-vs.-host disease is also observed [241,242].

A very different mechanism of antitumor immunity has been observed when vaccination is applied in the context of nonmyeloblative allogeneic BMT. Originally, nonmyeloblative allogeneic BMT was developed in order to produce diminished graft-vs.-host disease, allowing one to titrate in doses of donor lymphocytes to skirt the balance between graft-vs.-tumor effect and graft-vs.-host disease [243–245]. Despite initially encouraging reports, the value of this approach remains to be validated. Standard conditioning regimens for nonmyeloblative bone marrow transplant ultimately inhibit the host immune system to the extent that full donor reconstitution ultimately ensues. However, Luznik and Fuchs have developed modified conditioning regimens that can result in stable mixed chimerism in which host and donor immune systems coexist [246]. Under such a circumstance, tumor vaccination exhibits much greater potency without any significant graft-vs.-host disease [247]. The enhanced antitumor effect surprisingly comes predominantly from activation of host tumor-specific T cells but nonetheless requires both CD4 and CD8 cells in the donor lymphocyte infusion. Experiments in CD40 knockout mice suggest a mechanism in which host DLI recognize minor histocompatibility antigens on host APCs, thereby enhancing their activation state and ability to present tumor antigens from the vaccine to residual host T cells. These findings point out both the promise and complexity of generating antitumor immune response in the bone marrow transplant setting.

XV. FUTURE PROSPECTS FOR SUCCESSFUL IMMUNOTHERAPY

The weight of evidence that established cancers induce immune tolerance to their antigens defines the major challenge to successful immunotherapy. While the mechanisms by which chronic viral infections avoid immune elimination are still largely unknown, it is likely that common mechanisms as well as distinct mechanisms relative to non-virus-associated cancers will be operative. The barriers of immunologic tolerance, together with the failure of cancer vaccines as single agents to achieve sufficient success in randomized Phase III trials in patients with advanced cancer, have raised a significant degree of skepticism about immunotherapy of cancer in general. However, the most promising vaccination strategies—indeed, most of those described in this chapter—have only just begun to enter early stage clinical trials. It is therefore premature to conclude that the cryptic repertoire of tumor-specific (and virus-specific) T cells known to exist in patients with cancer and chronic viral disease cannot be mobilized with therapeutic success.

A major theme to have emerged from the growing preclinical animal model immunotherapy investigations is the importance of combination approaches that target different regulatory points in the immune response from priming to amplification to effector function. The most clear-cut benefits of combination approaches are demonstrated by the synergy observed with vaccination and CTLA-4 blockade as well as vaccination after elimination or inhibition of T regulatory cells. In addition, vaccination in the context of bone marrow transplantation shows great promise due to the effects of BMT on multiple elements of T-cell-dependent immune responses. Innovative combinatorial immunotherapies are becoming a major focus of translational efforts in many different cancer types.

Finally, as with all cancer therapies, the selection of appropriate patient populations is as critical as the therapy itself. A number of potentially promising cancer vaccine approaches have been tested in patients with advanced bulky metastatic disease. In fact, multiple lines of evidence suggest that immunotherapies may be most effective in the minimal residual disease state. An analogous circumstance with chronic viral diseases has been the shift in emphasis on the application of therapeutic HPV vaccines to women with premalignant cervical lesions rather than established cervical cancer. Given the relative lack of toxicity of most immunotherapies—particularly vaccines—their application in earlier stages of disease seems quite reasonable. Rapid advances in early detection as well as prognostication have resulted in detection of many cancers at a much earlier stage. These advances should lay the groundwork for development of the most promising immunotherapies in the most effective possible fashion.

REFERENCES

1. Esteban F, et al. Lack of MHC class I antigens and tumour aggressiveness of the squamous cell carcinoma of the larynx. Br J Cancer 1990; 62:1047–1051.
2. Esteban F, et al. Histocompatibility antigens in primary and metastatic squamous cell carcinoma of the larynx. Int J Cancer 1989; 43:436–442.
3. Esteban F, et al. MHC class I antigens and tumour-infiltrating leucocytes in laryngeal cancer: long-term follow-up. Br J Cancer 1996; 74:1801–1804.
4. Ferrone S, Maricola F. Loss of HLA class I antigens by melanoma cells: molecular mechanisms, functional significance and clinical relevance. Immunol Today 1995; 16:487–497.
5. Natali PG, et al. Distribution of human Class I (HLA-A,B,C) histocompatibility antigens in normal and malignant tissues of nonlymphoid origin. Cancer Res 1984; 44:4679–4687.
6. Natali P, et al. Heterogeneous expression of melanoma-associated antigens and HLA antigens by primary and multiple metastatic lesions removed from patients with melanoma. Cancer Res 1985; 45:2883–2889.
7. Natali PG, et al. Antigenic heterogeneity of surgically removed primary and autologous metastatic human melanoma lesions. J Immunol 1983; 130:1462–1466.
8. Natali PG, et al. Selective changes in expression of HLA class I polymorphic determinants in solid tumors. Proc Natl Acad Sci USA 1989; 86:6719–6723.
9. Perez E, et al. Heterogeneity of the expression of class I and I HLA antigens in human breast carcinoma. J Immunogenet 1986; 13:247–253.
10. Whitwell HL, et al. Expression of major histocompatibility antigens and leucocyte infiltration in benign and malignant human breast disease. Br J Cancer 1984; 49:161–172.
11. Zuk JA, Walker RA. Immunohistochemical analysis of HLA antigens and mononuclear infiltrates of benign and malignant breast. J Pathol 1987; 152:275–285.
12. Ruiz-Cabello F, et al. Phenotypic expression of histocompatibility antigens in human primary tumours and metastases. Clin Exp Metastasis 1989; 7:213–226.
13. Ruiz-Cabello F, et al. Molecular analysis of MHC-class-I alterations in human tumor cell lines. Int J Cancer Suppl 1991; 6:123–130.
14. Cabrero T, et al. High frequency of altered HLA class I phenotypes in invasive breast cell lines. Hum Immunol 1996; 50:127–134.
15. Cabrero T, et al. High frequency of altered HLA class I phenotypes in invasive colorectal carcinomas. Tissue Antigens 1998; 52:114–123.
16. van den Ingh HF, et al. HLA antigens in colorectal tumours—low expression of HLA class I antigens in mucinous colorectal carcinomas. Br J Cancer 1987; 55:125–130.
17. van Driel WJ, et al. Association of allele-specific HLA expression and histopathologic progression of cervical carcinoma. Gynecol Oncol 1996; 62:33–41.
18. Marincola F, et al. Escape of human solid tumors from T-cell recognition: molecular mechanisms and functional significance. Adv Immunol 2000; 74:181–273.
19. D'Urso CM, et al. Lack of HLA class I antigen expression by cultured melanoma cells FO-1 due to defect in B2m gene expression. J Clin Invest 1991; 87:284–292.
20. Wang Z, et al. Lack of HLA class I antigen expression by melanoma cells SK-MEL-33 caused by a reading frameshift in beta 2-microglobulin messenger RNA. J Clin Invest 1993; 91:684–692.
21. Bicknell DC, et al. Beta 2-microglobulin gene mutations: a study of established colorectal cell lines and fresh tumors. Proc Natl Acad Sci USA 1994; 91:4751–4756.

22. Benitez R, et al. Mutations of the beta2-microblobuline gen result in a lack of HLA class I molecules on melanoma cells of two patients immunized with MAGE peptides. Tissue Antigens 1998; 52:520–529.

23. Blanchet O, et al. Altered binding of regulatory factors to HLA class I enhancer sequence in human tumor cell lines lacking class I antigen expression. Proc Natl Acad Sci USA 1992; 89:3488–3492.

24. Doyle A, et al. Markedly decreased expression of class I histocompatibility antigens, protein, and mRNA in human small-cell lung cancer. J Exp Med 1985; 161:1135–1151.

25. Restifo NP, et al. Loss of functional beta 2-microglobulin in metastatic melanoms from five patients receiving immunotherapy. J Natl Cancer Inst 1996; 88:100–108.

26. Rowe M, et al. Restoration of endogenous antigen processing in Burkitt's lymphoma cells by Epstein–Barr virus laten membrane protein-1: coordinate up-regulation of peptide transporters and HLA-class I antigen expression. Eur J Immunol 1995; 25:1374–1384.

27. Sanda MG, et al. Molecular characterization of defective antigen processing in human prostate cancer. J Natl Cancer Inst 1995; 87:280–285.

28. Alpan RS, et al. Cell cycle-dependent expression of TAP1, TAP2, and HLA-B27 messenger RNAs in a human breast cancer cell line. Cancer Res 1996; 56:4358–4361.

29. Seliger B, et al. Reduced membrane major histocompatibility complex class I density and stability in a subset of human renal cell carcinoms with low TAP and LMP expression. Clin Cancer Res 1996, 1427–1433.

30. Hilders CG, et al. The expression of histocompatibility-related leukocyte antigens in the pathway to cervical carcinoma. Am J Clin Pathol 1994; 101:5–12.

31. Koopman L, et al. Multiple genetic alterations cause frequent and heterogeneous human histocompatibility leukocyte antigen class I loss in cervical cancer. J Exp Med 2000; 191:961–976.

32. Schmid P, et al. In situ analysis of transforming growth factor-beta s (TGF-beta 1, TGF-beta 2, TGF-beta 3), and TGF-beta type II receptor expression in malignant melanoma. Carcompgemesos 1995; 16:1499–1503.

33. Moretti S, et al. In situ expression of transforming growth factor beta is associated with melanoma progression and correlates with Ki67, HLA-DR and beta 3 integrin expression. Melanoma Res 1997; 7:313–321.

34. Van Belle P, et al. Melanoma-associated expression of transforming growth factor-beta isoforms. Am J Pathol 1996; 148:1887–1894.

35. Wojtowicz-Praga S, et al. Modulation of b16 melanoma growth and metastasis by anti-transforming growth factor beta antibody and interleukin-2. Immunotherapy 1996; 19:169–175.

36. Bogen B, et al. Naive CD4+ T cells confer idiotype-specific tumor resistance in the absence of antibodies. Eur J Immunol 1995; 25:3079–3086.

37. Bogen B. Peripheral T cell tolerance as a tumor escape mechanism: deletion of CD4+ T cells specific for a monoclonal immunoglobulin idiotype secreted by a plasmacytoma. Eur J Immunol 1996; 26:2671–2679.

38. Staveley-O'Carroll K, et al. Induction of antigen-specific T cell anergy: an early event in the course of tumor progression [In Process Citation]. Proc Natl Acad Sci USA 1998; 95:1178–1183.

39. Sotomayor EM, et al. Cross-presentation of tumor antigens by bone marrow-derived antigen-presenting cells is the dominant mechanism in the induction of T-cell tolerance during B-cell lymphoma progression. Blood 2001; 98:1070–1077.

40. Wick M, et al. Antigenic cancer cells grow progressively in immune hosts without evidence for T cell exhaustion or systemic anergy. J Exp Med 1997; 186:229–238.

41. Speiser DE, et al. Self antigens expressed by solid tumors Do not efficiently stimulate naive or activated T cells: implications for immunotherapy. J Exp Med 1997; 186:645–653.

42. Doan T, et al. Peripheral tolerance to human papillomavirus E7 oncoprotein occurs by cross-tolerization, is largely Th-2-independent, and is broken by dendritic cell immunization. Cancer Res 2000; 60:2810–2815.

43. den Boer AT, et al. Longevity of antigen presentation and activation status of APC are decisive factors in the balance between CTL immunity versus tolerance. J Immunol 2001; 167:2522–2528.

44. Shrikant P, et al. CTLA-4 blockade reverses CD8+ T cell tolerance to tumor by a CD4+ T cell-and IL-2-dependent mechanism. Immunity 1999; 11:483–493.

45. Schell TC, et al. Sequential loss of cytotoxic T lymphocyte responses to simian virus 40 large T antigen epitopes in T antigen transgenic mice developing osteosarcomas. Cancer Res 2000; 60:3002–3012.

46. Robinson BW, et al. Lack of ignorance to tumor antigens: evaluation using nominal antigen transfection and T-cell receptor transgenic lymphocytes in Lyons–Parish analysis—implications for tumor tolerance. Clin Cancer Res 2001; 7:811s–817s.

47. Boon T, OL. Cancer tumor antigens. Curr Opin Immunol 1997; 9:681–683.

48. Robbins PF, Kawakami Y. Human tumor antigens recognized by T cells. Curr Opin Immunol 1996; 8:628–636.

49. Pardoll DM. Cancer vaccines. Nat Med 1998; 4:525–531.

50. Scheffner M, et al. The E6 oncoprotein encoded by human papillomavirus types 16 and 18 promotes the degradation of p53. Cell 1990; 63:1129–1136.

51. Munger K, et al. Complex formation of human papillomavirus E7 proteins with the retinoblastoma tumor suppressor gene product. EMBO 1989; 8:4099–4105.

52. Galloway DA, Jenison SA. Characterization of the humoral immune response to genital papillomaviruses. Mol Biol Med 1990; 7:59–72.

53. Howley PM. In: Fields BN, Knipe DM, eds. Fundamental Virology. New York: Raven Press, 1991:743–763.

54. Beasley RP, et al. Hepatocellular carcinoma and hepatitis B virus. A prospective study of 22 707 men in Taiwan. Lancet 1981; 2:1129–1133.

55. Brechot C. What is the role of hepatitis B virus in the appearance of hepatocellular carcinomas in patients with alcoholic cirrhosis? Gastroenterol Clin Biol 1982; 6:727–730.

56. Szmuness W. Hepatocellular carcinoma and the hepatitis B virus: evidence for a casual association. Prog Med Virol 1987; 24:40–46.

57. Shafritz DA, et al. Integration of hepatitis B virus DNA into the genome of liver cells in chronic liver disease and hepatocellular carcinoma. Studies in percutaneous liver biopsies and post-mortem tissue specimens. N Engl J Med 1981; 305:1067–1073.

58. zur Hausen H, et al. EBV DNA in biopsies of Burkitt tumors and anaplastic carcinomas of the nasopharynx. Nature 1970; 228:1056–1059.

59. Weiss LM, et al. Detection of Epstein–Barr viral genomes in Reed–Sternberg cells of Hodgkin's disease. N Engl J Med 1989; 320:502–506.

60. Wu TC, et al. Detection of EBV gene expression in Reed–Sternberg cells of Hodgkin's disease. Int J Cancer 1990; 46:801–804.

61. Levitskaya J, et al. Inhibition of ubiquitin/proteasome-dependent protein degradation by the Gly–Ala repeat domain of the Epstein–Barr virus nuclear antigen 1. Proc Natl Acad Sci USA 1997; 94:12616–12621.

62. Fearon ER, Vogelstein B. A genetic model for colorectal tumorigenesis. Cell 1990; 61:759–767.

63. Lu X, Lane DP. Differential induction of transcriptionally

active p53 following UV or ionizing radiation: defects in chromosome instability syndromes? Cell 1993; 75:765–778.

64. Gowen L, et al. BRCA1 required for transcription-coupled repair of oxidative DNA damage. Science 1998; 281:1009–1012.

65. Sharan SK, et al. Embryonic lethality and radiation hypersensitivity mediated by Rad51 in mice lacking Brca2. Nature 1997; 386:804–810.

66. Fishel R, et al. The human mutator gene homolog MSH2 and its association with hereditary nonpolyposis colon cancer. Cell 1993; 75:1027–1038.

67. Leach FS, et al. Mutations of a mutS homolog in hereditary nonployposis colorectal cancer. Cell 1993; 75:1215–1225.

68. Bronner CE, et al. Mutation in the DNA mismatch repair gene homologue hMLH1 is associated with hereditary nonployposis colon cancer. Nature 1994; 368:258–261.

69. Papadopoulos N, et al. Mutation of a mutL homolog in hereditary colon cancer. Science 1994; 263:1625–1629.

70. Pardoll D. T cells and tumours. Nature 2001; 411:1010–1012.

71. Doyle A, et al. Markedly decreased expression of class I histocompatibility antigens, protein, and mRNA in human small-cell lung cancer. J Exp Med 1985; 161:1135–1151.

72. Hahne M, et al. Melanoma cell expression of Fas (Apo-1/CD95) ligand: implications for tumor immune escape. Science 1996; 274:1363–1366.

73. Gratas C, et al. Fas ligand expression in glioblastoma cell lines and primary astrocytic brain tumors. Brain Pathol 1997; 7:863–869.

74. Bennett MW, et al. The fas counterattack in vivo: apoptotic depletion of tumor-infiltrating lymphocytes associated with Fas ligand expression by human esophageal carcinoma. J Immunol 1998; 160:5669–5675.

75. Niehans, et al. Human lung carcinomas express Fas ligand. Cancer Res 1997; 57:1007–1012.

76. O'Connell J, et al. The Fas counterattack: Fas-mediated T cell killing by colon cancer cells expressing Fas ligand. J Exp Med 1996; 184:1075–1082.

77. Shiraki K, et al. Expression of Fas ligand in liver metastases of human colonic adenocarcinomas. Proc Natl Acad Sci USA 1997; 94:6420–6425.

78. Chappel DB, et al. Human melanoma cells do not express Fas (Apo-1/CD95) ligand. Cancer Res 1999; 59:59–62.

79. Seino K, et al. Antitumor effect of locally produced CD95 ligand. Nat Med 1997; 3:165–170.

80. Arai H, et al. Gene transfer of Fas ligand induces tumor regression in vivo. Proc Natl Acad Sci USA 1997; 94:13862–13867.

81. Hung K, et al. The central role of CD4+ T cells in the antitumor immune response. J Exp Med 1998; 188:2357–2368.

82. Qin Z, et al. B cells inhibit induction of T cell-dependent tumor immunity. Nat Med 1998; 4:627–630.

83. Steinman RM, et al. The dendritic cell system and its role in immunogenicity. Annu Rev Immunol 1991; 9:271–296.

84. Bancherau J, Steinman RM. Dendritic cells and the control of immunity. Nature 1998; 392:245–252.

85. Inaba K, et al. Identification of proliferating dendritic cell precursors in mouse blood. J Exp Med 1992; 175:1157–1167.

86. Caux C, et al. GM-CSF and TNF-alpha cooperate in the generation of dendritic Langerhans cells. Nature 1992; 360:258–261.

87. Kiertscher SM, RM. Human CD14+ leukocytes acquire the phenotype and function of antigen-presenting dendritic cells when cultured in GM-CSF and IL-4. J Leukoc Biol 1996; 59:208–218.

88. Romani N, RD, et al. Generation of mature dendritic cells from human blood. An improved method with special regard to clinical applicability. J Immunol Methods 1996; 196:137–151.

89. Maraskovsky E, et al. Dramatic increase in the numbers of functionally mature dendritic cells in Flt3 ligand-treated mice: multiple dendritic cell subpopulations identified. J Exp Med 1996; 184:1953–1962.

90. Ren Y, et al. CD36 gene transfer confers capacity for phagocytosis of cells undergoing apoptosis. J Exp Med 1995; 181:1857–1862.

91. Nussenzweig M, et al. A monoclonal antibody specific for mouse dendritic cells. Proc Natl Acad Sci USA 1982; 79:161–165.

92. Mellman I, Steinman R. Dendritic cells: specialized and regulated antigen processing machines. Cell 2001; 106:255–258.

93. Yewdell J, et al. Mechanisms of exogenous antigen presentation by MHC class I molecules in vitro and in vivo: implications for generating CD8+ T cell responses to infectious agents, tumors, transplants and vaccines. Adv Immunol 1999; 73:1–77.

94. Akira, S TK, Kaisho T. Toll-like receptors: critical proteins linking innate and acquired immunity. Nat Immunol 2001; 2:675–680.

95. Sallusto F, Lanzavecchia A. Efficient presentation of soluble antigen by cultured human dendritic cells is maintained by granulocyte/macrophage colony-stimulating factor plus interleukin 4 and downregulated by tumor necrosis factor alpha. J Exp Med 1994; 179:1109–1118.

96. Caux C, et al. Activation of human dendritic cells through CD40 cross-linking. J Exp Med 1994; 180:1263–1272.

97. Cella M, et al. Ligation of CD40 on dendritic cells triggers production of high levels of interleukin-12 and enhances T cell stimulatory capacity: T-T help via APC activation. J Exp Med 1996; 184:747–752.

98. Saeki H, et al. Cutting edge: secondary lymphoid-tissue chemokine (SLC) and CC chemokine receptor 7 (CCR7) participate in the emigration pathway of mature dendritic cells from the skin to regional lymph nodes. J Immunol 1999; 162:2472–2475.

99. Cella M, et al. Inflammatory stimuli induce accumulation of MHC class II complexes on dendritic cells. Nature 1997; 388:782–787.

100. Pierre P, et al. Developmental regulation of MHC class II transport in mouse dendritic cells. Nature 1997; 388:787–792.

101. Schoenberger SP, et al. T help for CTL is mediated by CD40–CD40L interactions. Nature 1998; 393:480–483.

102. Bennett SR, et al. Help for cytotoxic-T-cell responses is mediated by CD40 signalling. Nature 1998; 393:478–480.

103. Ridge JP, et al. A conditioned dendritic cell can be a temporal bridge between a CD4+ T-helper and a T-killer cell. Nature 1998; 393:474–478.

104. Lu Z, et al. CD40-independent pathways of T cell help for priming of CD8(+) cytotoxic T lymphocytes. J Exp Med 2000; 191:541–550.

105. Chang C, et al. Selective regulation of ICAM-1 and major histocompatibility complex class I and II molecular expression on epidermal Langerhans cells by some of the cytokines released by keratinocytes and T cells. Eur J Immunol 1994; 24:2889–2895.

106. Linsley PS, et al. Binding of the B cell activation antigen B7 to CD28 costimulates T cell proliferation and interleukin 2 mRNA accumulation. J Exp Med 1991; 173:721–730.

107. Schwartz RH. Costimulation of T lymphocytes: the role of CD28, CTLA-4, and B7/BB1 in interleukin-2 production and immunotherapy. Cell 1992; 71:1065–1068.

108. Shahinian A, et al. Differential T cell costimulatory requirements in DC28-deficient mice. Science 1993; 261:609–612.

109. Borriello F, et al. B7-1 and B7-2 have overlapping, critical roles in immunoglobulin class switching and germinal center formation. Immunity 1997; 6:303–313.

110. Caux C, et al. B70/B7-2 is identical to CD86 and is the major functional ligand for CD28 expressed on human dendritic cells. J Exp Med 1994; 180:1841–1847.

111. Dong H, et al. B7-H1, a third member of the B7 family, co-stimulates T-cell proliferation and interleukin-10 secretion [see comments]. Nat Med 1999; 5:1365–1369.

112. Freeman GJ, et al. Engagement of the PD-1 immunoinhibitory receptor by a novel B7 family member leads to negative regulation of lymphocyte activation [In Process Citation]. J Exp Med 2000; 192:1027–1034.

113. Tseng S-Y, et al. B7-DC, a new dendritic cell molecule with unique costimulatory properties for T cells. J Exp Med 2001; 193:839–846.

114. Latchman Y, et al. PD-L2 is a second ligand for PD-I and inhibits T cell activation. Nat Immunol 2001; 2:261–268.

115. Chapoval A, et al. B7-H3: a costimulatory molecule for T cell activation and IFN-gamma production. Nat Immunol 2001; 2:269–274.

116. Melero I, et al. Monoclonal antibodies against the 4-1BB T-cell activation molecule eradicate established tumors. Nat Med 1997; 3:682–685.

117. Weinberg AD, et al. Engagement of the OX-40 receptor in vivo enhances antitumor immunity. J Immunol 2000; 164: 2160–2169.

118. Bansal-Pakala P, et al. Signaling through OX40 (CD134) breaks peripheral T-cell tolerance. Nat Med 2001; 7:907–912.

119. Fearon ER, et al. Induction in a murine tumor of immunogenic tumor variants by transfection with a foreign gene. Cancer Res 1988; 48:2975–2980.

120. Itaya T, et al. Xenogenization of a mouse lung carcinoma (3LL) by transfection with an allogeneic class I major histocompatibility complex gene (H-2Ld). Cancer Res 1987; 47:3136–3140.

121. Plautz GE, et al. Immunotherapy of malignancy by in vivo gene transfer into tumors [see comments]. Proc Natl Acad Sci USA 1993; 90:4645–4649.

122. Townsend SE, Allison JP. Tumor rejection after direct costimulation of CD8 + T cells by B7-transfected melanoma cells [see comments]. Science 1993; 259:368–370.

123. Chen L, et al. Costimulation of antitumor immunity by the B7 counterreceptor for the T lymphocyte molecules CD28 and CTLA-4. Cell 1992; 71:1093–1102.

124. Baskar S, et al. Constitutive expression of B7 restores immunogenicity of tumor cells expressing truncated major histocompatibility complex class II molecules. Proc Natl Acad Sci USA 1993; 90:5687–5690.

125. Golumbek PT, et al. Treatment of established renal cancer by tumor cells engineered to secrete interleukin-4. Science 1991; 254:713–716.

126. Restifo NP, et al. A nonimmunogenic sarcoma transduced with the cDNA for interferon gamma elicits $CD8^+$ T cells against the wild-type tumor: correlation with antigen presentation capability. J Exp Med 1992; 175:1423–1431.

127. Asher M, et al. Murine tumor cells transduced with the gene for tumor necrosis factor-a. J Immunol 1991; 146:3227–3229.

128. Bannerji R, et al. The role of IL-2 secreted from genetically modified tumor cells in the establishment of antitumor immunity. J Immunol 1994; 152:2324–2332.

129. Gansbacher B, et al. Retroviral vector-mediated gamma-interferon gene transfer into tumor cells generates potent and long lasting antitumor immunity. Cancer Res 1990; 50:7820–7826.

130. Li WQ, et al. Lack of tumorigenicity of interleukin 4 autocrine growing cells seems related to the anti-tumor function of interleukin 4. Mol Immunol 1990; 27:1331–1337.

131. Hock H, et al. Interleukin 7 induces $CD4^+$ T cell-dependent tumor rejection. J Exp Med 1991; 174:1291–1298.

132. Colombo MP, et al. Granulocyte colony-stimulating factor gene transfer suppresses tumorigenicity of a murine adenocarcinoma in vivo. J Exp Med 1991; 173:889–897.

133. Porgador A, et al. Interleukin 6 gene transfection into Lewis lung carcinoma tumor cells suppresses the malignant phenotype and confers immunotherapeutic competence against parental metastatic cells. Cancer Res 1992; 52:3679–3686.

134. Blankenstein T, et al. Tumor suppression after tumor cell-targeted tumor necrosis factor via gene transfer. J Exp Med 1991; 173:1047–1052.

135. Dranoff G, et al. Vaccination with irradiated tumor cells engineered to secrete murine granulocyte–macrophage colony-stimulating factor stimulates potent, specific, and long-lasting anti-tumor immunity. Proc Natl Acad Sci USA 1993; 90:3539–3543.

136. Pardoll D, Jaffee E. Principles and Practice of Biologic Therapy of Cancer. Charlottesville: Silverchair, 1999.

137. Okamoto M, et al. The combined effect against colon-26 cells of heat treatment and immunization with heat treated colon-26 tumour cell extract. Int J Hyperther 2000; 16:263–273.

138. Wang X, et al. Hsp110 overexpression increases the immunogenicity of the murine CT26 colon tumor. Cancer Immunol Immunother 2002; 51:311–319.

139. Chiodoni C, et al. Dendritic cells infiltrating tumors cotransduced with granulocyte–macrophage colony-stimulating (GMCSF) and CD40 ligand genes take up and present endogenous tumor-associated antigens, and prime naive mice for a cytotoxic T-lymphocyte response. J Exp Med 1999; 190: 125–133.

140. Tendler DS, et al. Intersection of interferon and hypoxia signal transduction pathways in nitric oxide-induced tumor apoptosis. Cancer Res 2001; 61:3682–3688.

141. Simons JW, et al. Bioactivity of autologous irradiated renal cell carcinoma vaccines generated by ex vivo granulocyte–macrophage colony-stimulating factor gene transfer. Cancer Res 1997; 57:1537–1546.

142. Soiffer R, et al. Vaccination with irradiated autologous melanoma cells engineered to secrete human granulocyte–macrophage colony-stimulating factor generates potent antitumor immunity in patients with metastatic melanoma. Proc Natl Acad Sci USA 1998; 95:13141–13146.

143. Jaffee EM, et al. Novel allogeneic granulocyte–macrophage colony-stimulating factor-secreting tumor vaccine for pancreatic cancer: a phase i trial of safety and immune activation. J Clin Oncol 2001; 19:145–156.

144. Wittes R. Bacille Calmette–Guerin vaccine. Clin Infect Dis 2000; (suppl 3):S115–S121.

145. Foon K. Immunotherapy for colorectal cancer. Curr Oncol Rep 2001; 3:116–126.

146. Zeh H, et al. Vaccines for colorectal cancer. Trends Mol Med 2001; 7:307–313.

147. Huang AY, et al. Role of bone marrow-derived cells in presenting MHC class I-restricted tumor antigens. Science 1994; 264:961–965.

148. Nguyen LT, et al. Tumor growth enhances cross-presentation leading to limited T cell activation with out tolerance. J Exp Med 2002; 195:423–435.

149. Morck A, et al. Functional genomics identifies mesothelin as an immunodominant pancreatic cancer antigen, 2002. Submitted.

150. Borrello I, et al. A universal GM-CSF producing bystander cell line for use in the formulation of autologous tumor cell-based vaccines. Human Gene Therapy 1999; 10:1983–1991.

151. Porgador A, Gilboa E. Bone marrow-generated dendritic cells pulsed with a class I-restricted peptide are potent inducers of cytotoxic T lymphocytes. J Exp Med 1995; 182: 255–260.

152. Mayordomo JI, et al. Bone marrow-derived dendritic cells pulsed with synthetic tumour peptides elicit protective and therapeutic antitumour immunity. Nat Med 1995; 1:1297–1302.

153. Lambert LA, et al. Equipotent generation of protective antitumor immunity by various methods of dendritic cell

loading with whole cell tumor antigens. J Immunother 2001; 24:232–236.

154. Shimizu K, et al. Enhancement of tumor lysate- and peptide-pulsed dendritic cell-based vaccines by the addition of foreign helper protein. Cancer Res 2001; 61:2618–2624.

155. Song W, et al. Dendritic cells genetically modified with an adenovirus vector encoding the cDNA for a model tumor antigen induce protective and therapeutic antitumor immunity. J Exp Med 1997; 186:1247–1256.

156. Specht JM, et al. Dendritic cells retrovirally transduced with a model tumor antigen gene are therapeutically effective against established pulmonary metastases. J Exp Med 1997; 186:1213–1221.

157. Dyall J, et al. Lentivirus-transduced human monocyte-derived dendritic cells efficiently stimulate antigen-specific cytotoxic T lymphocytes. Blood 2001; 97:114–121.

158. Boczkowski D, et al. Dendritic cells pulsed with RNA are potent antigen-presenting cells in vitro and in vivo. J Exp Med 1996; 184:465–472.

159. Gong J, et al. Induction of antitumor activity immunization with fusion of dendritic and carcinoma cells. Nat Med 1997; 3:558–561.

160. Klein C, et al. Comparative analysis of genetically modified dendritic cells and tumor cells as therapeutic cancer vaccines. J Exp Med 2000; 191:1699–1708.

161. Reddy A, et al. A monocyte conditioned medium is more effective than defined cytokines in mediating the terminal maturation of human dendritic cells. Blood 1997; 90:3640–3646.

162. Bender A, et al. Improved methods for the generation of dendritic cells from nonproliferating progenitors in human blood. J Immunol Methods 1996; 196:121–135.

163. Tao MH, Levy R. Idiotype/granulocyte–macrophage colony-stimulating factor fusion protein as a vaccine for B-cell lymphoma. Nature 1993; 362:755–758.

164. Boyle JS, et al. Enhanced responses to a DNA vaccine encoding a fusion antigen that is directed to sites of immune induction. Nature 1998; 392:408–411.

165. You Z, et al. Targeting dendritic cells to enhance DNA vaccine potency. Cancer Res 2001; 61:3704–3711.

166. Mahnke K, et al. The dendritic cell receptor for endocytosis, DEC-205, can recycle and enhance antigen presentation via major histocompatibility complex class II-positive lysosomal compartments. J Cell Biol 2000; 151:673–684.

167. Srivastava PK. Roles of heat-shock proteins in innate and adaptive immunity. Nat Rev Immunol 2002; 2:185–194.

168. Udono H, Srivastava PK. Comparison of tumor-specific immunogenicities of stress-induced proteins gp96, hsp90, and hsp70. J Immunol 1994; 152:5398–5403.

169. Wang XY, et al. Characterization of heat shock protein 110 and glucose-regulated protein 170 as cancer vaccines and the effect of fever-range hyperthermia on vaccine activity. J Immunol 2001; 166:490–497.

170. Castellino F, et al. Receptor-mediated uptake of antigen/heat shock protein complexes results in major histocompatibility complex class I antigen presentation via two distinct processing pathways. J Exp Med 2000; 191:1957–1964.

171. Chen C-H, WT-L, et al. Enhancement of DNA vaccine potency by linkage of antigen gene to an HSP70 gene. Cancer Res 2000; 60:1035–1042.

172. Suto R, Srivastava PK. A mechanism for the specific immunogenicity of heat shock protein-chaperoned peptides. Science 1995; 269:1585–1588.

173. Basu S, et al. CD91 is a common receptor for heat shock proteins gp96, hsp90, hsp70, and calreticulin. Immunity 2001; 14:303–313.

174. Asea A, et al. HSP70 stimulates cytokine production through a CD14-dependant pathway, demonstrating its dual role as a chaperone and cytokine. Nat Med 2000; 6:435–442.

175. Kuppner MC, et al. The role of heat shock protein (hsp70) in dendritic cell maturation: hsp70 induces the maturation of immature dendritic cells but reduces DC differentiation from monocyte precursors. Eur J Immunol 2001; 31:1602–1609.

176. Wu TC, et al. Engineering an intracellular pathway for major histocompatibility complex class II presentation of antigens. Proc Natl Acad Sci USA 1995; 92:11671–11675.

177. Lin KY, et al. Treatment of established tumors with a novel vaccine that enhances major histocompatibility class II presentation of tumor antigen. Cancer Res 1996; 56:21–26.

178. Ji H, et al. Targeting human papillomavirus type 16 E7 to the endosomal/lysosomal compartment enhances the antitumor immunity of DNA vaccines against murine human papillomavirus type 16 E7-expressing tumors. Hum Gene Ther 1999; 10:2727–2740.

179. Chen CH, et al. Enhancement of DNA vaccine potency by linkage of antigen gene to an HSP70 gene. Cancer Res 2000; 60:1035–1042.

180. Hung CF, et al. Improving vaccine potency through intercellular spreading and enhanced MHC class I presentation of antigen. J Immunol 2001; 166:5733–5740.

181. Hung CF, et al. Cancer immunotherapy using a DNA vaccine encoding the translocation domain of a bacterial toxin linked to a tumor antigen. Cancer Res 2001; 61:3698–3703.

182. Livingston BD, et al. Optimization of epitope processing enhances immunogenicity of multiepitope DNA vaccines. Vaccine 2001; 19:4652–4660.

183. Boniface JJ, Davis MM. T-cell recognition of antigen. A process controlled by transient intermolecular interactions. Ann N Y Acad Sci 1995; 766:62–69.

184. Slansky JE, et al. Enhanced antigen-specific antitumor immunity with altered peptide ligands that stabilize the MHC–peptide–TCR complex. Immunity 2000; 13:529–538.

185. Parkhurst MR, et al. Improved induction of melanoma-reactive CTL with peptides from the melanoma antigen gp100 modified at HLA-A*0201-binding residues. J Immunol 1996; 157:2539–2548.

186. Dyall R, et al. Heteroclitic immunization induces tumor immunity. J Exp Med 1998; 188:1553–1561.

187. Yee C. Adoptively transferred antigen-specific CD8[+] T cell clones persist in vivo, migrate to tumor sites and mediate antigen-specific immune response in patients with metastatic melanoma. Proc Natl Acad Sci 2002; 99:16168–16173.

188. Huang AY, et al. Does B7-1 expression confer antigen-presenting cell capacity to tumors in vivo? J Exp Med 1996; 183:769–776.

189. Kim JJ, et al. Engineering of in vivo immune responses to DNA immunization via codelivery of costimulatory molecule genes. Nat Biotechnol 1997; 15:641–646.

190. Agadjanyan MG, et al. CD86 (B7-2) can function to drive MHC-restricted antigen-specific CTL responses in vivo. J Immunol 1999; 162:3417–3427.

191. Sturmhoefel K, et al. Potent activity of soluble B7-IgG fusion proteins in therapy of established tumors and as vaccine adjuvant. Cancer Res 1999; 58:4964–4972.

192. Schmitter D, et al. Involvement of the CD27–CD70 co-stimulatory pathway in allogeneic T-cell response to follicular lymphoma cells. Br J Haematol 1999; 106:64–70.

193. Watts T, DeBenedette M. T cell co-stimulatory molecules other than CD28. Curr Opin Immunol 1999; 11:286–293.

194. Atkins MB, et al. High-dose recombinant interleukin 2 therapy for patients with metastatic melanoma: analysis of 270 patients treated between 1985 and 1993. J Clin Oncol 1999; 17:2105–2116.

195. Lode HN, et al. Immunocytokines: a promising approach to cancer immunotherapy. Pharmacol Ther 1998; 80:277–292.

196. Cheever M, et al. Interleukin 2(IL 2) administered in vivo: influence of IL 2 route and timing on T cell growth. J Immunol 1985; 134:3895–3900.

197. Kern D, et al. Requirements for the generation of a Lyt-2$^+$ T cell proliferative response to a syngeneic tumor in the absence of L3T4$^+$ T cells. Cancer Res 1990; 50:6256–6263.

198. Evans L, et al. Expression of chimeric granulocyte–macrophage colony-stimulating factor/interleukin2 receptors in human cytotoxic T lymphocyte clones results in granulocyte–macrophage colony-stimulating factor-dependent growth. Hum Gene Ther 1999; 10:1941–1951.

199. Ahlers JD, et al. Cytokine-in-adjuvant steering of the immune response phenotype to HIV-1 vaccine constructs: granulocyte–macrophage colony-stimulating factor and TNF-alpha synergize with IL-12 to enhance induction of cytotoxic T lymphocytes. J Immunol 1997; 158:3947–3958.

200. Smith GL, et al. Construction and characterization of an infectious vaccinia virus recombinant that expresses the influenza hemagglutinin gene and induces resistance to influenza virus infection in hamsters. Proc Natl Acad Sci USA 1983; 80:7155–7159.

201. Panicali D, et al. Construction of live vaccines by using genetically engineered poxviruses: biological activity of recombinant vaccinia virus expressing influenza virus hemagglutinin. Proc Natl Acad Sci USA 1983; 80:5364–5368.

202. Moss B. Genetically engineered poxviruses for recombinant gene expression, vaccination, and safety. Proc Natl Acad Sci USA 1996; 93:11341–11348.

203. Carroll MW, et al. Highly attenuated modified vaccinia virus Ankara (MVA) as an effective recombinant vector: a murine tumor model. Vaccine 1997; 15:387–394.

204. Paoletti E, et al. Highly attenuated poxvirus vectors: NYVAC, ALVAC and TROVAC. Dev Biol Stand 1995; 84:159–163.

205. Velders MP, et al. Eradication of established tumors by vaccination with venezuelan equine encephalitis virus replicon particles delivering human papillomavirus 16 e7 RNA. Cancer Res 2001; 61:7861–7867.

206. Elzey BD, et al. Immunization with type 5 adenovirus recombinant for a tumor antigen in combination with recombinant canarypox virus (alvac) cytokine gene delivery induces destruction of established prostate tumors. Int J Cancer 2001; 94:842–849.

207. Gewurz BE, et al. Virus subversion of immunity: a structural perspective. Curr Opin Immunol 2001; 13:442–450.

208. Irvine KR, et al. Enhancing efficacy of recombinant anticancer vaccines with prime/boost regimens that use two different vectors. J Natl Cancer Inst 1997; 89:1595–1601.

209. Ramshaw IA, Ramsay AJ. The prime-boost strategy: exciting prospects for improved vaccination. Immunol Today 2000; 21:163–165.

210. Pan ZK, et al. A recombinant Listeria monocytogenes vaccine expressing a model tumour antigen protects mice against lethal tumour cell challenge and causes regression of established tumours. Nat Med 1995; 1:471–477.

211. Thole JE, et al. Live bacterial delivery systems for development of mucosal vaccines. Curr Opin Mol Ther 2000; 2:94–99.

212. Killeen K, et al. Bacterial mucosal vaccines: vibrio cholerae as a live attenuated vaccine/vector paradigm. Curr Top Microbiol Immunol 1999; 236:237–254.

213. Ohara N, Yamada T. Recombinant BCG vaccines. Vaccine 2001; 19:4089–4098.

214. Shata MT, et al. Recent advances with recombinant bacterial vaccine vectors. Mol Med Today 2000; 6:66–71.

215. Sizemore DR, et al. Attenuated Shigella as a DNA delivery vehicle for DNA-mediated immunization. Science 1995; 270:299–302.

216. Darji A, et al. Oral somatic transgene vaccination using attenuated S. typhimurium. Cell 1997; 91:765–775.

217. Chambers CA, et al. CTLA-4-mediated inhibition in regulation of T cell responses: mechanisms and manipulation in tumor immunotherapy. Annu Rev Immunol 2001; 19: 565–594.

218. van Elsas A, et al. Combination immunotherapy of B16 melanoma using anti-CTLA-4 and GM-CSF producing vaccines induces rejection of subcutaneous and metastatic tumors accompanied by autoimmune depigmentation. J Exp Med 1999; 190:355–366.

219. Hurwitz AA, et al. CTLA-4 blockade synergizes with tumor-derived granulocyte–macrophage colony-stimulating factor for treatment of an experimental mammary carcinoma. Proc Natl Acad Sci USA 1998; 95:10067–10071.

220. Hurwitz AA, et al. Combination immunotherapy of primary prostate cancer in a transgenic mouse model using CTLA-4 blockade. Cancer Res 2000; 60:2444–2448.

221. Ibarra-Sanchez MJ, et al. The T-cell protein tyrosine phosphatase. Semin Immunol 2000; 12:379–386.

222. Irie-Sasaki J, et al. CD45 is a JAK phosphatase and negatively regulates cytokine receptor signalling. Nature 2001; 409:349–354.

223. Greenhalgh CJ, Hilton DJ. Negative regulation of cytokine signaling. J Leukoc Biol 2001; 70:348–356.

224. Vang T, et al. Activation of the COOH-terminal Src kinase (Csk) by cAMP-dependent protein kinase inhibits signaling through the T cell receptor. J Exp Med 2001; 193:497–507.

225. Chiang YJ, et al. Cbl-b regulates the CD28 dependence of T-cell activation. Nature 2000; 403:216–220.

226. Bachmaier K, et al. Negative regulation of lymphocyte activation and autoimmunity by the molecular adaptor Cbl-b. Nature 2000; 403:211–216.

227. Sun L, et al. Cabin 1, a negative regulator for calcineurin signaling in T lymphocytes. Immunity 1998; 8:703–711.

228. Sakaguchi S, et al. Immunologic tolerance maintained by CD35$^+$CD4$^+$ regulatory cells: their common role in controlling autoimmunity, tumor immunity, and transplantation tolerance. Immunol Rev 2001; 182:18–32.

229. Shevach E. CD4$^+$CD25$^+$ suppressor T cells: more questions than answers. Nat Rev Immunol 2002; 2:389–400.

230. Sutmuller R, et al. Synergism of cytotoxic T lymphocyte-associated antigen 4 blockade and depletion of CD24$^+$ regulatory cells in antitumor therapy reveals alternative pathways for suppression of autoreactive cytoxic T lymphocyte responses. J Exp Med 2001; 194:823–832.

231. van Elsas A, et al. Elucidating the autoimmune and antitumor effector mechanisms of a treatment based on cytotoxic T lymphocyte antigen-4 blockade in combination with a B16 melanoma vaccine: comparison of prophylaxis and therapy. J Exp Med 2001; 194:481–489.

232. Ercolini A, et al. Identification and characterization of the immunodominant rat HER-2/neu MHC class I epitope presented by spontaneous mammary tumors from HER-2/neu-transgenic mice. J Immunol 2003; 170:4273–4280.

233. Pardoll D. Taming the sinister side of BMT: Dr. Jekyll and Mr. Hyde. Nat Med 1997; 3:833–834.

234. van den Brink M, Burakoff S. Cytolytic pathways in haematopoietic stem-cell transplantation. Nat Rev Immunol 2002; 2:273–281.

235. Levitsky H. Augmentation of host immune responses to cancer: overcoming the barrier of tumor antigen-specific T-cell tolerance. Cancer J 2000; 6(suppl):S281–S290.

236. Borrello I, et al. Sustaining the graft-versus-tumor effect through posttransplant immunization with granulocyte–macrophage colony-stimulating factor (GM-CSF)-producing tumor vaccines. Blood 2000; 95:3011–3019.

237. Tan J, et al. Interleukin (IL)-15 and IL-7 jointly regulate homeostatic proliferation of memory phenotype CD8$^+$ cells but are not required for memory phenotype CD4$^+$ cells. J Exp Med 2002; 195:1523–1532.

238. Goldrath A, et al. Cytokine requirements for acute and Basal

homeostatic proliferation of naive and memory CD8[+] T cells. J Exp Med 2002; 195:1515–1522.

239. Anderson LJ, et al. Immunization of allogeneic bone marrow transplant recipients with tumor cell vaccines enhances graft-versus-tumor activity without exacerbating graft-versus-host disease. Blood 2000; 95:2426–2433.

240. Teshima T, et al. Donor leukocyte infusion from immunized donors increases tumor vaccine efficacy after allogeneic bone marrow transplantation. Cancer Res 2002; 62:796–800.

241. Anderson L, et al. Enhancement of graf-versus-tumor activity and graft-versus-host disease by pretransplant immunization of allogeneic bone marrow donors with a recipient. Cancer Res 1999; 59.

242. Morecki S, et al. Cell therapy with preimmunized effector cells mismatched for minor histocompatible antigens in the treatment of a murine mammary carcinoma. J Immunother 2001; 24, 114–121.

243. Childs R, et al. Engraftment kinetics after nonmyeloablative allogeneic peripheral blood stem cell transplantation: full donor T cell chimerism precedes alloimmune responses. Blood 1999; 1999:3390–3400.

244. Georges G, et al. Adoptive immunotherapy in canine mixed chimeras after nonmyeloablative hematopoietic cell transplantation. Blood 2000; 95:3262–3269.

245. Progozhina T, et al. Nonmyeloablative allogeneic bone marrow transplantation as immunotherapy for hematologic malignancies and metastatic solid tumors in preclinical models. Exp Hematol 2002; 30:89–96.

246. Luznik L, et al. Posttransplantation cyclophosphamide facilitates engraftment of major histocompatibility complex-identical allogeneic marrow in mice conditioned with low-dose total body irradiation. Biol Blood Marrow Transplant 2002; 8:131–138.

247. Luznik L, et al. Successful therapy of metastatic cancer using tumor vaccines in mixed allogeneic bone marrow chimeras. Blood 2003; 101:1645–1652.

79

Vaccines Against Human Papillomavirus Infection

John Boslego
Merck Research Laboratories, West Point, Pennsylvania, U.S.A.

Xiaosong Liu and Ian H. Frazer
The University of Queensland, Brisbane, Queensland, Australia

ABSTRACT

Cervical cancer is one of the commonest causes of cancer death among women worldwide, and is initiated by infection with a limited subset of human papillomaviruses (PV). Prophylactic vaccines, based on recombinant virus particles, are designed to produce virus neutralizing antibody. They are now in late-phase clinical trials, and, if these trials demonstrate efficacy, it is anticipated that vaccines might be available for routine clinical use within the next 5 years. Therapeutic vaccines, based on viral nonstructural proteins, are in early-phase clinical trials. There is little information on the nature of the immune response that will be required for a therapeutic effect. This article reviews the current knowledge base on human papillomavirus vaccines, discusses some areas of uncertainty concerning vaccine development and deployment, and highlights where the field may progress over the next few years.

I. NATURAL IMMUNITY TO PAPILLOMAVIRUS CAPSIDS

Papillomaviruses (PV) infect the superficial epithelium of many vertebrate species. As nonlytic viruses whose non-structural proteins alter the growth and differentiation of epithelial cells, this family of viruses produces lesions ranging from macroscopically undetectable disturbances of epithelial architecture to floridly protuberant warts. There are estimated to be in excess of 200 human papillomavirus (HPV) genotypes [1], and these can be divided into several major phenotypic groups (Table 1).

The World Health Organization recognizes several papillomaviruses as antecedents of cervical cancer, and current data [2] suggest that 99.8% of cervical cancer is caused by infection with human papillomavirus. Since the first recog-

nition in the 1980s of an association between cervical cancer and papillomavirus infection [3], development of a vaccine has been mooted. Productive infection with genital and skin genotypes of papillomavirus is generally self-limiting, and resolution of infection, which occurs over months to years, requires an immunocompetent host. Immune responses to PV infection are generally slow to appear, and less robust in comparison with those seen with lytic or systemic virus infections [4]. Deficits in cell-mediated immunity reduce the clearance of existing infections, and increase the risk of progression of infection to malignancy [5,6]. The extent to which prior infection protects against subsequent exposure to the same or other genotypes of HPV is moot. However, infection with cutaneous papillomaviruses is universal in early childhood, and is rare among adults, including those involved with the care of young children. Similarly, infection of the genital tract is commonest among those recently sexually active [7,8], and is not common among older sexually active individuals, including sex workers at high risk through exposure [9]. Thus while there is some epidemiological data for HPV16 to suggest that prior infection may convey only partial protection on subsequent exposure, a broad conclusion can be entertained that infection with papillomaviruses protects against subsequent exposure in immunocompetent subjects, giving reasonable grounds for believing that a prophylactic vaccine is possible.

II. CROSS PROTECTION BETWEEN PAPILLOMAVIRUS GENOTYPES

More than 80 sequenced papillomaviruses infect man, and several hundred genotypes are postulated to exist based on partial sequence data. While over 80% of cervical cancers are associated with one of the five common genital genotypes of PV [10], even these have minor sequence variations within

Table 1 Broad Classification of Papillomaviruses

Papillomavirus group	Typical member	Clinical manifestations	Natural history	Precursor of malignancy
Epithelial	HPV1,2	Flat or verrucous warts on squamous epithelium	Self-limiting over months to years in immunocompetent subjects	No
EV associated	HPV5,8	Minimal lesions in healthy individuals Warts in patients with epidermodysplasia verruciformis	Persistent infection without lesions in immunocompetent subjects?	Uncertain in healthy individuals Definite in patients with EV or chronic immunosuppression
Genital warts	HPV6, 11	Protuberant warts on anogenital mucosal epithelium and in aerodigestive mucosa	Self-limiting over months to years in immunocompetent subjects	Rarely in aerodigestive tract
Genital cancer associated	HPV16, 18, 33, 35	Minimal dysplastic epithelial changes of anogenital epithelium	Generally self-limiting over months to years in immunocompetent subjects: 2% persistence rate	Up to 10% lifetime risk of cancer, particularly of transition zones between squamous and glandular epithelium, if infection persists

their capsid proteins. Therefore it becomes of considerable importance to understand the extent to which genotypes are immunotypes, and whether there is cross-protection between closely sequence related PV types, or even more distantly related types. Clinical data suggest that infection with one PV genotype conveys little or no protection against subsequent infection with another type [11], despite relative conservation of the sequence of the L1 protein between different PV genotypes. The solution of the crystal structure of a $t = 1$ structure comprising 12 HPV 16 L1 pentamers [12] allowed recognition as to which regions of the L1 protein are external to the virion, and therefore likely to be susceptible to the effects of neutralizing antibody. Perhaps unsurprisingly, in view of previous data on genotype specificity of neutralizing antibody, the majority of intraspecies genotypic variation in the generally highly conserved L1 protein was found among amino acid residues that were exposed to solvent on the external face of the virus. Thus it seems unlikely that antibody raised to one PV genotype will provide protection against challenge with others, and to the extent that animals reflect humans, this observation seems to be valid for data generated using vaccines designed to prevent infection with animal PVs [13]. The relative conservation of PV L1 sequence across genotypes might nevertheless allow for development of T helper responses active across a range of PV genotypes, which might result in some partial cross protection against persistent or severe disease. T helper cell cross reactivity has been observed in man following immunization with HPV 11 viruslike particles (VLPs) [14], and in experimental models following immunization with a HPV6b polynucleotide vaccine [15], although the biological significance of such cross reactivity remains to be established.

III. PRODUCTION AND QUALITY ASSURANCE OF PAPILLOMAVIRUS CAPSIDS FOR VACCINES

Papillomaviruses are icosahedral viruses comprising 360 copies of the major L1 capsid protein, assembled from 72 pentameric rings [16,17]. Although they were among the first demonstrably infectious filterable agents [18], a major problem with developing a vaccine to prevent papillomavirus-associated disease has been production of sufficient virus material to be the basis of a vaccine. Papillomaviruses cannot easily be grown in tissue culture, and therefore recombinant DNA technology has been required to produce papillomavirus capsids that, by analogy with effective virus vaccines, might be used to induce neutralizing antibody and thus prevent papillomavirus infection. Recognition that the capsid proteins of papillomavirus self-assemble into viruslike particles, if expressed in eukaryotic expression systems [19], has facilitated development of particle-based prophylactic vaccines [20]. Although early studies on expression of the L1 and L2 capsid proteins of papillomavirus using recombinant DNA technology demonstrated production of capsid protein in prokaryotic and eukaryotic expression systems [21–24], attempts to isolate virus particles were unsuccessful, although self-assembly of capsid proteins in cell culture had been shown for other viruses [25]. Observation that the L1 protein of HPV16, if expressed from the second methionine initiation codon, could assemble into virus-like particles in Cos 1 cells [19] stimulated further work on production of VLPs in a range of expression systems [26–31]. Papillomavirus L1 proteins of a range of genotypes produced VLPs in greater yield than was initially observed for HPV16, and production of HPV16 VLPs was improved following recognition that the prototype HPV16 L1 clone had a nonconservative mutation [32], not seen in subsequent clinical isolates, that impaired assembly of VLPs from L1 protein. Production of VLPs on a larger scale was facilitated by expression of L1 protein in insect cells using recombinant baculovirus, and in yeasts. These observations paved the way for early vaccine studies in a range of animals using species-specific papillomaviruses [31,33].

The desire for efficient production of VLPs for vaccine use has prompted more thorough examination of the minimal requirements for assembly of capsid proteins into quaternary structures sufficiently resembling the virus to invoke host protective immunity. Expression of PV capsid protein in *E. coli* produces small amounts of VLPs [34] as determined by density gradient purification and electron microscopy analysis—following denaturation and renaturation from amorphous inclusion bodies, significant amounts of L1 protein assemble into L1 pentamer capsomers, which are immunogenic [35] and retain at least some of the structures necessary to induce virus neutralizing antibody. When L1 is expressed in *S. typhimurium*, VLP particles are also observed [36], although the practical utility of a particle or capsomer production system based on prokaryotic systems remains uncertain.

Stability of virus particles once assembled is critical for the development of a successful vaccine. While it is clear that the current generation of vaccines is stable for sufficient time to allow their use in clinical trials, there is little published literature on PV stability [37,38]. One strategy to avoid issues of VLP stability and the requirement for a cold chain for vaccine deployment might be to use polynucleotide vaccines to express the L1 capsid protein, as the stability of polynucleotide vaccines is well defined. Efficient expression of the L1 protein in mammalian cells can be achieved by codon modification of the primary gene sequence to avoid codon biases, which prevent efficient expression of the PV protein [39,40]. A polynucleotide vaccine expressing a codon-modified L1 protein invokes expression of L1 protein that assembles into capsid structures, as the induced antibody recognizes virus-like particles rather better than denatured L1 [41].

IV. PAPILLOMAVIRUS CAPSIDS AS PROPHYLACTIC VACCINES

Demonstration that papillomavirus vaccines induce antibody, and protection against virus challenge, in a range of natural PV infections in animals including the Cottontail rabbit [31], the cow [42], and the beagle dog [43], paved the way for early-phase clinical trials in man. These studies, in subjects with and without HPV infection, have confirmed the safety and immunogenicity of VLP-based vaccines of HPV types 6, 11, and 16, given intramuscularly with or without adjuvant (Table 2). Three administrations of VLPs with adjuvant induce peak antibody levels at least 10 times those seen in subjects naturally infected with HPV, and levels of antibody above those produced by natural infection are sustained for at least 18 months post vaccination. In experimental animals, small doses of VLPs (<1 µg) are immuno-

genic [33]. In the clinical trials published to date, and in others reported at international meetings but not yet published [44], a dose of 10–50 µg, given on three occasions, gives optimal antibody titers. Antibodies are neutralizing in a range of in vitro and in vivo assays [45–48], including the neutralization of PV virions mixed with foreskin epithelial cells and transplanted under the renal capsule of a nude mouse, and the prevention of infection of susceptible cell lines by papillomavirus pseudovirions.

The primary aim of prophylactic vaccination with HPV vaccines is to prevent cervical cancer, and pre–cervical cancer lesions (e.g., CIN 2/3), which require evaluation and treatment. Secondary aims of vaccination are to prevent less severe cervical lesions (e.g., CIN 1), genital warts, and persistent infection/transmission of HPV. A large Phase II study to evaluate the efficacy of an HPV 16 L1 VLP vaccine against incident persistent HPV infection has recently been completed [49]. Two thousand, three hundred and ninety-two (2392) young women (aged 16–23 years) were enrolled in a randomized, double-blind, multicenter study. Subjects received three doses of either 40 µg of HPV 16 L1 VLP vaccine or placebo over a 6 months vaccination regimen. Subjects were evaluated for HPV 16 infection and disease at baseline and every 6 months by collection of cervicovaginal samples for HPV 16 DNA testing and Pap smear. Colposcopy and biopsy were performed as indicated based upon Pap smear findings. Subjects with polymerase chain reaction (PCR) or serologic evidence of HPV 16 infection at baseline or PCR evidence of HPV infection prior to completion of the vaccination regimen were excluded from the primary analysis. With a median duration of 17.4 months of follow-up after completion of the vaccination regimen, the combined incidence of persistent HPV 16 infection or HPV16-related CIN was 3.8/100 subject–years at risk (SYR) in the placebo group and 0.0/100 SYR in the vaccine group for an estimated vaccine efficacy of 100% (95% CI = 90–100%). Of the 41 cases in the placebo group, 31 had persistent HPV 16 infection without CIN, 5 had HPV 16-related CIN 1, 4 had HPV 16-related CIN 2, and 1 had a single HPV 16 PCR+ finding at her last visit prior to being lost to follow-up. These results suggest that intramuscular administration of an HPV L1 VLP vaccine induces a systemic immune response that is sufficient to prevent vaccine-type HPV infection and HPV-related CIN in a high majority of young women. Furthermore, the anti-HPV 16 titers persisted at levels at least fivefold to tenfold higher than those seen after natural HPV 16 infection during the course of follow-up.

VLPs have also been delivered to humans without adjuvant [50]. Delivery without adjuvant is more likely to induce Th1-type responses and CTL, perhaps because of the ability of VLPs to be efficiently taken up by dendritic cells via both the endogenous and exogenous antigen presentation pathways,* and to directly activate immature dendritic cells [51,52] to produce a more mature phenotype. However, delivery with alum adjuvant may give a more sustained immune response, perhaps because adjuvanting proteins with alum can increase their stability in vivo.

---

*Gao et al, submitted.

Table 2 Published Studies of Papillomavirus VLP Vaccines in Man

Recruitment strategy	Dose and delivery schedule	Population size	Outcome measures	Conclusions	Ref.
19–45 years, healthy, not at risk for STD	Baculovirus HPV11 VLPs 3, 9, 30 or 100 μg im with alum 3:1 active: placebo 0, 4, 16 weeks	24 m, 41 f	Antibody to VLPs T cell proliferation Cytokine release (7-day in vitro stimulation	Safe (pain in most, rash in 6, hives in 1) Immunogenic at all doses—no real dose–response curve Antibody non-cross-reactive Proliferation/cytokines cross-reactive between types	[14]
18–29 years, healthy, not at risk for STD	Baculovirus HPV16 VLPs 10, 50 μg im with nil, alum, or MF59 5: 1 active to placebo 0, 4, 16 weeks	14 m, 58 f	Antibody	Safe (pain in most) Antibody, more with higher dose antigen, more with no adjuvant or MF59 than alum	[50]
18–56 years, warts, no other active STD	Baculovirus HPV6 VLPs 1,5,10 μg im with nil no placebo 0, 4 ,8 (12, 16, 20) weeks	6 m, 27 f	Antibody, DTH	Safe Antibody, more with 5 and 10 than 1 μg DTH, most subjects Wart resolution, 25 of 33 subjects	[99]

Papillomaviruses naturally infect mucosal surfaces and there is therefore a case for utilizing a vaccine designed to induce neutralizing antibody specifically through the mucosal immune system. A number of studies have shown that VLPs delivered to mucosal surfaces [53–56] or, perhaps surprisingly, systemically can induce significant titers of antibody at mucosal surfaces. However, administration of VLPs to dogs intranasally, while producing reasonable titers of mucosal antibody, did not protect against challenge with canine oral papillomavirus (COPV) whereas systemic administration was protective [57]. These data, together with the somewhat erratic immune responses to mucosally administered vaccines, cast some doubt on the viability of a vaccine program based on mucosally administered VLPs.

V. FURTHER DEVELOPMENT AND USE OF PROPHYLACTIC HUMAN PAPILLOMAVIRUS VACCINES

The encouraging Phase II results described above have lead to initiation of Phase III testing. Although the primary aim of vaccination is to prevent cervical cancer, and pre–cervical cancer lesions, Phase III study endpoints were primarily based on pre–cervical cancer lesions because such lesions serve as a suitable surrogate marker for cancer as they are treated and removed when discovered in clinical practice. Recent data from epidemiologic and clinical studies suggest that high-grade cytologic abnormalities (HSIL or CIN 2/3) may develop relatively early (within months to several years) after incident HPV infection with high-risk HPV types. Thus Phase III studies utilizing high-grade cytologic abnormali-

ties as endpoints are feasible and ongoing, albeit large (10,000–15,000 subjects) and logistically challenging.

To bolster the benefits of a prophylactic HPV vaccine, efficacy against low-grade cytologic abnormalities (e.g., CIN 1), genital warts, and persistent HPV infection is also highly desirable and the subject of Phase III evaluations. Although most CIN 1 lesions spontaneously resolve, they often result in patient anxiety, increased health care costs because of follow-up evaluations, and potentially unnecessary diagnostic and ablative procedures. Genital warts cause discomfort and psychosocial problems, and are often prolonged and difficult to eradicate. Persistent HPV infection allows for HPV transmission (and subsequent HPV disease) to sexual partners and throughout the sexually active community.

When prophylactic HPV vaccines become available for routine use, predictions of their role and impact on public health strategies for reduction of HPV disease await findings from large-scale clinical trials. If HPV vaccines are shown to be effective for preventing pre–cervical cancer lesions, administration to all young teenage girls before the onset of sexual intercourse should be considered to increase the proportion of young women who will benefit from the intervention. If HPV vaccines are also demonstrated to be effective for preventing genital warts, and for preventing persistent HPV infection/carriage in men, their routine use in young boys might be warranted as well.

The impact of vaccination on HPV disease will also be a function of the number of high-risk HPV types included in the vaccine and will vary according to the health care practices in regions where they are used. In populations without cervical cancer screening programs, the impact of vaccination should be greater than in populations with active screening programs. But even in populations with active screening programs, a highly effective prophylactic HPV vaccine should further reduce cervical cancer rates, particularly in young women, beyond what has been gained from cervical cancer screening programs and may allow a recommendation for an increase in the age for first Pap smear testing and a longer interval between routine Pap smear testings.

Although results from early clinical trials offer promise for an effective prophylactic HPV vaccine, such a vaccine would not be expected to have an immediate and profound impact on HPV disease worldwide. The absence of obvious clinical disease in the majority of those infected with the virus, long periods of infectivity following virus acquisition, difficulties in achieving high rates of vaccine uptake in adolescent populations, and problems with cost and distribution of vaccine to developing world populations combine to suggest that HPV disease would continue as a public health problem for decades to come.

VI. VIRUS-LIKE PARTICLES INCORPORATING ADDITIONAL ANTIGENS

The observed natural immunogenicity of VLPs from a range of viruses in animals and man has provoked studies of their use as delivery systems for antigens other than the major viral capsid proteins [58,59], and papillomavirus VLPs have also been tested in this manner [60–62]. In general, PV VLPs seem to behave like other particulate antigens of viral size, which are good inducers of immunity and can carry nonviral epitopes to the immune system to induce potent humoral and cellular immune responses. The particular ability of PV virus-like particles to activate dendritic cells [52] is not essential for their immunogenicity, as particles coated with additional protein that do not in consequence invoke DC activation (J. Schiller, personal communication), are nevertheless potent inducers of a humoral immune response to the incorporated epitopes [63].

Three alternative methods have been used to incorporate antigen into PV VLPs. Firstly, there is a region at the C′ terminal of the L1 protein of most tested PV genotypes that is relatively permissive for deletion and replacement with incorporation of novel amino acid sequences of up to about 60 amino acids [60]. Secondly, the incorporation of the L2 minor capsid protein into VLPs allows substitution of portions of this protein with novel epitopes [61] that may be displayed on the virus surface. The advantage of incorporating novel epitopes into L2 is that this protein can harbor longer amino acid sequences, although the copy number is lower than that incorporated to L1, and the natural immune response to L2 is not as striking as that to L1. Thirdly, additional proteins can be physically or chemically conjugated to the VLPs using a range of technologies [63]. Each of these methods has the potential to impair to greater or lesser extent the stability of the virus particle structure—particles may appear larger and may degrade faster, to produce the characteristic ~40 kDa cleavage product of L1 protein. It has been recently shown that pentameric L1 capsomers can induce protective immunity against COPV challenge [35]. Therefore chimeric pentamers expressed in bacteria might be

the basis of a more stable chimeric VLP-like vaccine, although the relative immunogenicity of pentamers and VLPs has yet to be established in man.

In experimental animals, robust immune responses can be obtained to epitopes incorporated into VLPs from a range of proteins, including the nonstructural proteins of papillomavirus, and the L2 capsid protein [64]. There is particular interest in VLPs incorporating nonstructural proteins because of their potential to invoke cell-mediated immunity that might be host protective against PV infection, or alternatively therapeutic for early preclinical infection, as has been shown in the rabbit [65,66] and the beagle dog. In a range of models, both humoral and cellular immune responses have been invoked using chimeric particles that can be variously therapeutic for transplanted tumors [61,62], or neutralizing of soluble autoantigen cytokines [63]. Responses to incorporated epitopes can be similarly invoked using polynucleotide vaccines, although it is necessary to encode a ubiquitin sequence at the N′ terminal of the protein to allow efficient degradation of the chimeric protein, and induction of good CTL responses to the incorporated epitope [67]. A vaccine combining a ubiquitinated and non-ubiquitinated sequence can invoke both host protective neutralizing antibody against PV virions and cell-mediated immune responses against PV early proteins, allowing one approach to a combined prophylactic/therapeutic vaccine for PV infection for the developing world.

The concept of using chimeric VLPs as a delivery system for antigens of interest raises the issue of the effects of prior immunity to the carrier protein on the immune response mounted to the novel epitope. Established immunity to the carrier PV genotype enhances the response to the carrier VLP, following administration as a vaccine, but specifically blocks induction of at least some cellular immune responses to a novel incorporated epitope. High titers of VLP-specific antibody can passively transfer inhibition [68]. Inhibition, which can be overcome by choosing a carrier VLPs of a type not immunologically cross reactive with the existing VLP-specific response, does not appear to be a consequence of CTL epitope dominance [15].

VII. THERAPEUTIC VACCINES FOR CERVICAL CANCER AND PRECANCER

Papillomavirus capsid vaccines using conventional adjuvants are likely to be available within the foreseeable future, as discussed in the preceding section. These vaccines induce high titers of virus neutralizing antibody and will likely prevent new viral infections, but antibody is unlikely to have a therapeutic effect against existing infection. It can be estimated that 5 million women worldwide will die with cervical cancer over the next 20 years, and the majority of these women are already infected with the papillomavirus that will initiate their cancer. A prophylactic HPV vaccine will not offer protection against tumor development to already infected women; therefore papillomavirus-specific immunotherapy is a much-needed adjunct to a prophylactic HPV vaccine program. As therapeutic vaccines are currently not available for any infection, successful development of

PV-specific immunotherapy will require new understanding about how immune responses might eliminate virally infected cells in the absence of local inflammation, and about how such responses might be induced in man.

Direct and indirect evidence allows the conclusion that virus-specific immune responses occur following natural infection with PV, and may cause resolution of infection. Greater than 50% of HPV infections resolve without intervention [69], and resolution is significantly impaired in subjects immunocompromised by immunosuppressive therapy [6] or by HIV infection [70]. Further, the relative risk of cervical cancer is significantly increased in subjects immunosuppressed in relation to renal transplantation, and the median time from onset of immunosuppression to development of cancer is about 4 years [71], suggesting that the role of the protective immune response is predominantly to prevent persistence or progression of HPV associated premalignancy, rather than to prevent initial infection. More direct evidence comes from a study demonstrating that resolution of CIN is significantly associated with cutaneous delayed type hypersensitivity to peptides derived from two transforming proteins (E6 and E7) of human papillomavirus [72]. It is noteworthy that while cell-mediated immune responses are described to PV nonstructural proteins in a number of studies of patients with CIN, there is little evidence of humoral immune responses to these proteins [73], prior to the onset of invasive cervical cancer [74], suggesting that the common immune response to PV nonstructural protein is predominantly Th1 type.

VIII. THE NATURE OF THE IMMUNE RESPONSE REQUIRED TO ELIMINATE INFECTED EPITHELIUM

The immune effector mechanisms that might result in elimination in vivo of epithelial cells expressing a non-self–non-MHC antigen in somatic cells are not completely understood. In different systems, either CD4 or CD8 restricted antigen-specific T cell responses can be necessary and sufficient for elimination of skin grafts expressing such antigen [75–77]: In these models, antigen is also expressed in professional antigen-presenting cells. Elimination can be specific for cells expressing antigen [78], or alternatively can also eliminate neighboring cells not expressing the relevant antigen [79]. Indeed, immune responses recognizing antigen (cross) presented only by professional APC in skin can eliminate the surrounding epithelial cells [80]. Thus it seems likely that a range of T cell delivered effector mechanism may be able to eliminate infected epithelium, including direct lytic mechanisms such as perforin and granzymes, or fas–fasL interactions, which would be expected only to eliminate cells expressing the relevant antigen, and indirect cytokine-mediated mechanisms including IFN γ or TNF α, which might induce more general epithelial damage. The extent of local activation of the effector mechanisms of a primed antigen-specific effector T cell will likely depend not only on the level of expression of the relevant MHC/peptide on the target epithelial or antigen-presenting cell, but also on the local pro- or anti-inflammatory cytokine environment in the epithelium, and on the levels of costimulatory molecules expressed by the target [81]. A key question for HPV immunotherapy will be to establish which mechanism is the most effective for eliminating PV-infected epithelium. No particular immune effector mechanism response has proven sufficient for effective elimination of E7 + epithelium in vivo in an animal model involving grafted skin expressing HPV16 E7 [82], although such elimination can be induced by coadministration of E7 expressing skin and nonspecific immune stimuli [83], and CD4 + and CD8 + T cells are each necessary and sufficient for graft rejection in this model (unpublished data) as for other grafting models in which antigen other than MHC is expressed in skin. In vitro, CD8-restricted, E7-specific CTL clones are unable to kill E7 transgenic keratinocytes in a 4-hr cytotoxicity assays [83a], although epithelial cell killing could be observed following IFN γ treatment, which we deduced increased the processing of E7 protein for presentation. However, using a keratinocyte colony formation assay, the same CTL clone over a longer period was able to specifically inhibit formation of epithelial colonies from E7 transgenic epithelial precursors, and the inhibition of colony formation could also be achieved with perforin −/− CTL clones (Harris, unpublished observation) suggesting that slower, cytokine-mediated inhibition of growth may be important for eradication of HPV-infected epithelium.

IX. THE VIRAL ANTIGENS TO TARGET

Expression of papillomavirus proteins in epithelium following HPV infection is spatially and temporally controlled [84]. Episomal PV DNA replicates in the most basal cells, requiring E1 and E2 protein [85]. Expression of PV E6 and E7 protein is observed in the basal and suprabasal epithelium [86]. These proteins direct amplification of the pool of PV-infected cells by disturbing the progress of epithelial cells toward a differentiated phenotype. E4 nonstructural protein, and the viral capsid proteins (L1 and L2), are regarded as late genes, which are abundantly expressed in cells already terminally differentiated, although mRNA encoding these proteins can be detected earlier in the process of cell development. E6 and E7 papillomavirus proteins have been demonstrated to be targets for immunotherapy when overexpressed in transplantable tumors in murine models [87,88]. However, it is not clear from these data whether sufficient protein is expressed, or, if expressed, processed and presented by the relevant epithelial cells, such that an immune response could eliminate the infected epithelium. Thus it is necessary to establish in natural infection what PV antigens can be effectively targeted, as well as to determine what sort of immune response is required for immune-mediated elimination of infected epithelium.

X. IMMUNOTHERAPY OF NATURAL HUMAN PAPILLOMAVIRUS INFECTION IN ANIMAL MODELS

Defining an effective therapeutic immune response for PV-infected skin is hard using transplantable tumors, in part because the tumors used can grow faster than the immune response following immunization, and in part because the transplanted tumors are not epithelial. However, for at least one model transplantable tumor expressing PV antigens, TC-1, therapeutic responses can be shown in primary and metastatic models [89,90]. In this system, many antigen delivery systems have proven effective, although a hierarchy of efficacy becomes apparent under limiting conditions of initial tumor burden.

Three well-characterized animal papillomavirus infections might be used to examine for immunotherapeutic effects. Bovine papillomavirus (BPV) produces skin lesions following viral challenge, which spontaneously regress over weeks to months. Canine oral papillomavirus (COPV) produces mucosal warts that spontaneously regress over weeks. Cottontail rabbit papillomavirus(CRPV) produces nonregressing skin warts, which in some rabbit strain can progress to invasive cancer. The natural course of established CRPV infection, which at least to some extent mimics nonregressing PV infection in man, can be modified by immunization with a cocktail of PV E1, E2, E6, or E7 proteins; significant inhibition of the progression of infection to malignancy is seen, and some regression of existing lesions is reported. Immunization can be delivered as recombinant protein [65,91], or as a polynucleotide vaccine [65], and immunization with single proteins have some efficacy, although the efficacy seems greater if more are used. The natural regression of BPV-associated warts can be accelerated by immunization with E7 [92]; similar studies have been initiated with COPV, although the rapid natural regression of these diseases makes interpretation of therapeutic efficacy difficult.

XI. HUMAN TRIALS OF IMMUNOTHERAPY OF HUMAN PAPILLOMAVIRUS INFECTION AND TUMORS

Trials of immunotherapy of PV-associated cancer or precancer with papillomavirus proteins have been undertaken in man [93–96]. Published studies have utilized the E6 and E7 nonstructural proteins of HPV16, as these proteins are expressed in invasive cancer cells, and HPV16 is the PV genotype most commonly associated with cervical cancer. These early-phase studies have used peptides [97] or whole protein [95] delivered with proprietary adjuvants, or recombinant vaccinia virus encoding E6 and E7 proteins modified to ablate the transforming functions of the proteins [96]. They have generally been conducted in patients with late-stage cervical cancer, although more recent unpublished studies have also been undertaken in patients with precancerous lesions of the cervix or the anus. Early-phase therapeutic studies have also been undertaken in subjects with genital warts [98]. Each of these studies have established that immunotherapy appears safe in the short term, and that immune responses can be induced to the relevant viral proteins in at least some immunized patients. A recent study has examined the safety and efficacy of specific immunotherapy for high-risk HPV. Patients with CIN (n = 31) were recruited to a placebo-controlled dose ranging study of

immunotherapy with CerVax™16 vaccine, a mixture of HPV 16 E6E7 fusion protein formulated with the ISCOM ® adjuvant. Immunotherapy was well tolerated, and immunized subjects mounted HPV16 E6E7 specific humoral and cellular immune responses. Of 14 subjects presenting with CIN associated with HPV16 infection, 7 had no measurable HPV16 after immunotherapy, and HPV copy number in cervical tissue was significantly reduced in the other 7. Thus CerVax™16 vaccine was shown to be safe and immunogenic, and immunotherapy may facilitate clearance of HPV16 infection from cervical epithelium, which should reduce the risk of progression of HPV infection to cervical cancer.

Until a papillomavirus therapeutic vaccine has been demonstrated efficacious, no immunological marker can be held to be a surrogate for an effective immune response. To date, antibody, cutaneous DTH, T helper, and cytotoxic T cell responses have all been reported in some percentage of immunized subjects, and, as many have significant tumor burdens and have had chemotherapy and or radiotherapy, these results must be regarded as encouraging. Studies have not been designed to look for clinical efficacy, and the clinical outcomes reported to date, while encouraging in some patients, are anecdotal.

XII. THE FUTURE

Many studies over a number of years have demonstrated problems with the antigen-presenting machinery in a wide range of epithelial tumors including cervical cancers. These variously result in reversible or nonreversible downregulation of MHC class I expression on tumor cells. These observations, together with those on the requirement for CD4-mediated immune responses for elimination of epithelial grafts in vivo, and the capacity of CD4 cells to mediate bystander killing, suggest that immunotherapy for HPV infection may be more focused on generating an appropriate CD4 response than on producing CD8-restricted cytotoxic T cells specific for papillomavirus antigen. It remains to be established whether any particular papillomavirus antigens are sufficiently cross-presented by the professional APCs in infected lesions to allow immune elimination by this mechanisms. If such is the case, it will then be necessary to determine how to induce and target such immune responses in man.

ACKNOWLEDGMENTS

The authors thank Dr. John Schiller for helpful comments on this manuscript.

REFERENCES

1. Galloway DA. Navigating the descent into papillomavirus hell. J Infect Dis 1994; 170:1075–1076.
2. Bosch FX, et al. Papillomavirus research update: highlights of the Barcelona HPV 2000 international papillomavirus conference. J Clin Pathol 2001; 54(3):163–175.
3. Durst M, et al. A papillomavirus DNA from a cervical car-

cinoma and its prevalence in cancer biopsy samples from different geographic regions. Proc Natl Acad Sci USA 1983; 80: 3812–3815.

4. Carter JJ, et al. Comparison of human papillomavirus types 16, 18, and 6 capsid antibody responses following incident infection. J Infect Dis 2000; 181(6):1911–1919.

5. Frisch M, et al. Human papillomavirus-associated cancers in patients with human immunodeficiency virus infection and acquired immunodeficiency syndrome. JNCI 2000; 92(18): 1500–1510.

6. Bouwes BJ, Berkhout RJ. HPV infections and immunosuppression. Clin Dermatol 1997; 15(3):427–437.

7. Franco EL, et al. Cervical cancer: epidemiology, prevention and the role of human papillomavirus infection. Can Med Assoc J 2001; 164(7):1017–1025.

8. Tyring SK. Human papillomavirus infections: epidemiology, pathogenesis, and host immune response. J Am Acad Dermatol 2000; 43(1):S18–S26.

9. Kjaer SK, et al. Human papillomavirus infection in Danish female sex workers—Decreasing prevalence with age despite continuously high sexual activity. Sex Transm Dis 2000; 27(8): 438–445.

10. Munoz N. Human papillomavirus and cancer: the epidemiological evidence. J Clin Virol 2000; 19(1–2):1–5.

11. Thomas KK, et al. Concurrent and sequential acquisition of different genital human papillomavirus types. J Infect Dis 2000; 182(4):1097–1102.

12. Chen XJS, et al. Structure of small virus-like particles assembled from the L1 protein of human papillomavirus 16. Mol Cell 2000; 5(3):557–567.

13. Breitburd F, et al. Immunization with virus-like particles from cottontail rabbit papillomavirus (CRPV) can protect against experimental CRPV infection. J Virol 1995; 69(6): 3959–3963.

14. Evans TG, et al. A phase 1 study of a recombinant virus-like particle vaccine against human papillomavirus type 11 in healthy adult volunteers. J Infect Dis 2001; 183(10):1485–1493.

15. Liu XS. Mucosal Immune Responses to Chimeric Papillomavirus Like Particles in Mice. Ph.D. thesis, The University of Queensland, 2002.

16. Baker TS, et al. Structures of bovine and human papillomaviruses. Analysis by cryoelectron microscopy and three-dimensional image reconstruction. Biophys J 1991; 60:1445–1456.

17. Hagensee ME, et al. Three-dimensional structure of vaccinia virus-produced human papillomavirus type 1 capsids. J Virol 1994; 68(7):4503–4505.

18. McFadyean J, Hobday F. Notes on the experimental transmission of warts in the dog. J Comp Pathol Ther 1898; 11: 341–342.

19. Zhou J, et al. Expression of vaccinia recombinant HPV 16 L1 and L2 ORF proteins in epithelial cells is sufficient for assembly of HPV virion-like particles. Virology 1991; 185(1): 251–257.

20. Schiller JT, Hidesheim A. Developing HPV virus-like particle vaccines to prevent cervical cancer: a progress report. J Clin Virol 2000; 19(1–2):67–74.

21. Thompson H, Roman A. Expression of human papillomavirus type 6 E1, E2, L1 and L2 open reading frames in *Escherichia coli*. Gene 1987; 56:289–295.

22. Tomita Y, et al. Expression of human papillomavirus types 6b and 16 L1 open reading frames in *Escherichia coli*: detection of a 56,000-dalton polypeptide containing genus-specific (common) antigens. J Virol 1987; 61:2389–2394.

23. Browne HM, et al. Analysis of the L1 gene product of human papillomavirus type 16 by expression in a vaccinia virus recombinant. J Gen Virol 1988; 69:1263–1273.

24. Xi S-Z, Banks LM. Baculovirus expression of the human papillomavirus type 16 capsid proteins: detection of L1–L2 protein complexes. J Gen Virol 1991; 72:2981–2988.

25. French TJ, et al. Assembly of double-shelled, virus-like particles of bluetongue virus by the simultaneous expression of four structural proteins. J Virol 1990; 64,12:5695–5700.

26. Kirnbauer R, et al. Papillomavirus L1 major capsid protein self-assembles into virus-like particles that are highly immunogenic. Proc Natl Acad Sci USA 1992; 89:12180–12184.

27. Hagensee ME, et al. Self-assembly of human papillomavirus type 1 capsids by expression of the L1 protein alone or by coexpression of the L1 and L2 capsid proteins. J Virol 1993; 67:315–322.

28. Park DS, et al. Human papillomavirus type 16 E6, E7 and L1 and type 18 E7 proteins produced by recombinant baculoviruses. J Virol Methods 1993; 45(3):303–318.

29. Rose RC, et al. Expression of human papillomavirus type 11 L1 protein in insect cells: in vivo and in vitro assembly of virus-like particles. J Virol 1993; 67:1936–1944.

30. Heino P, et al. Human papillomavirus type 16 capsid proteins produced from recombinant Semliki forest virus assemble into virus-like particles. Virology 1995; 214(2):349–359.

31. Jansen KU, et al. Vaccination with yeast-expressed cotton-tail rabbit papillomavirus (CRPV) virus-like particles protects rabbits from CRPV-induced papilloma formation. Vaccine 1995; 13(16):1509–1514.

32. Kirnbauer R, et al. Efficient self-assembly of human papillomavirus type 16 L1 and L1–L2 into virus-like particles. J Virol 1993; 67:6929–6936.

33. Suzich JA, et al. Systemic immunization with papillomavirus L1 protein completely prevents the development of viral mucosal papillomas. Proc Natl Acad Sci USA 1995; 92(25): 11553–11557.

34. Zhang W, et al. Expression of human papillomavirus type 16 L1 protein in *Escherichia coli*: denaturation, renaturation, and self-assembly of virus-like particles in vitro. Virology 1998; 243(2):423–431.

35. Yuan H, et al. Immunization with a pentameric L1 fusion protein protects against papillomavirus infection. J Virol 2001; 75(17):7848–7853.

36. Nardelli-Haefliger D, et al. Human papillomavirus type 16 virus-like particles expressed in attenuated *Salmonella typhimurium* elicit mucosal and systemic neutralizing antibodies in mice. Infect Immun 1997; 65(8):3328–3336.

37. Ishizu KI, et al. Roles of disulfide linkage and calcium ion-mediated interactions in assembly and disassembly of virus-like particles composed of simian virus 40 VP1 capsid protein. J Virol 2001; 75(1):61–72.

38. Caparros-Wanderley W, et al. Intratype sequence variation among clinical isolates of the human papillomavirus type 6 L1 ORF: clustering of mutations and identification of a frequent amino acid sequence variant. J Gen Virol 1999; 80(Pt 4):1025–1033.

39. Zhou J, et al. Papillomavirus capsid protein expression level depends on the match between codon usage and tRNA availability. J Virol 1999; 73(6):4972–4982.

40. Leder C, et al. Enhancement of capsid gene expression: preparing the human papillomavirus type 16 major structural gene L1 for DNA vaccination purposes. J Virol 2001; 75(19): 9201–9209.

41. Liu WJ, et al. Polynucleotide viral vaccines: codon optimisation and ubiquitin conjugation enhances prophylactic and therapeutic efficacy. Vaccine 2001; 20(5–6):862–869.

42. Jarrett WFH, et al. Studies on vaccination against papillomaviruses: the immunity after infection and vaccination with bovine papillomaviruses of different types. Vet Rec 1990; 126:473–475.

43. Bell JA, et al. A formalin-inactivated vaccine protects against mucosal papillomavirus infection: a canine model. Pathobiology 1994; 62:194–198.

44. Bosch FX, et al. Papillomavirus research update: highlights of the Barcelona HPV 2000 international papillomavirus conference. J Clin Pathol 2001; 54(3):163–175.

45. Christensen ND, et al. Monoclonal antibody-mediated neutralization of infectious human papillomavirus type 11. J Virol 1990; 64:5678–5681.

46. Roden RB, et al. Assessment of the serological relatedness of genital human papillomaviruses by hemagglutination inhibition. J Virol 1996; 70(5):3298–3301.

47. Bryan JT, et al. Human papillomavirus type 11 neutralization in the athymic mouse xenograft system: correlation with virus-like particle IgG concentration. J Med Virol 1997; 53(3):185–188.

48. Peng SW, et al. Capture ELISA and in vitro cell binding assay for the detection of antibodies to human papillonavirus type 6b virus-like particles in anogenital warts patients. Pathology 2000; 31:418–422.

49. Koutsky LA, et al. A controlled trial of human papilomavirus type 16 vaccine. N Engl J Med 2002; 347:1645–1651.

50. Harro CD, et al. Safety and immunogenicity trial in adult volunteers of a human papillomavirus 16 L1 virus-like particle vaccine. JNCI 2001; 93(4):284–292.

51. Rudolf MP, et al. Human dendritic cells are activated by chimeric human papillomavirus type-16 virus-like particles and induce epitope-specific human T cell responses in vitro. J Immunol 2001; 166(10):5917–5924.

52. Lenz P, et al. Papillomavirus-like particles induce acute activation of dendritic cells. J Immunol 2001; 166(9):5346–5355.

53. Lowe RS, et al. Human papillomavirus type II (HPV-11) neutralizing antibodies in the serum and genital mucosal secretions of African green monkeys immunized with HPV-11 virus-like particles expressed in yeast. J Infect Dis 1997; 176 (5):1141–1145.

54. Balmelli C, et al. Nasal immunization of mice with human papillomavirus type 16 virus-like particles elicits neutralizing antibodies in mucosal secretions. J Virol 1998; 72(10):8220–8229.

55. Liu XS, et al. Mucosal immunisation with papillomavirus virus-like particles elicits systemic and mucosal immunity in mice. Virology 1998; 252(1):39–45.

56. Gerber S, et al. Human papillomavirus virus-like particles are efficient oral immunogens when coadministered with *Escherichia coli* heat-labile enterotoxin mutant R192G or CpG DNA. J Virol 2001; 75(10):4752–4760.

57. Bosch FX, et al. Papillomavirus research update: highlights of the Barcelona HPV 2000 international papillomavirus conference. J Clin Pathol 2001; 54(3):163–175.

58. Burns NR, et al. Production and purification of hybrid Ty-VLPs. Mol Biotechnol 1994; 1(2):137–145.

59. Pumpens P. Grens E. HBV core particles as a carrier for B cell/T cell epitopes. Intervirology 2001; 44(2–3):98–114.

60. Müller M, et al. Chimeric papillomavirus-like particles. Virology 1997; 234(1):93–111.

61. Greenstone HL, et al. Chimeric papillomavirus virus-like particles elicit antitumor immunity against the E7 oncoprotein in an HPV16 tumor model. Proc Natl Acad Sci USA 1998; 95(4):1800–1805.

62. Peng SW, et al. Papillomavirus virus-like particles can deliver defined CTL epitopes to the MHC class I pathway. Virology 1998; 240(1):147–157.

63. Chackerian B, et al. Conjugation of a self-antigen to papillomavirus-like particles allows for efficient induction of protective autoantibodies. J Clin Invest 2001; 108(3):415–423.

64. Campo MS, et al. A peptide encoding a B-cell epitope from the N-terminus of the capsid protein L2 of bovine papillomavirus-4 prevents disease. Virology 1997; 234(2):261–266.

65. Han R, et al. DNA vaccination prevents and/or delays carcinoma development of papillomavirus-induced skin papillomas on rabbits. J Virol 2000; 74(20):9712–9716.

66. Han R, et al. Immunization of rabbits with cottontail rabbit papillomavirus E1 and E2 genes: protective immunity induced by gene gun-mediated intracutaneous delivery but not by intramuscular injection. Vaccine 2000; 18(26):2937–2944.

67. Liu WJ, et al. Codon modified human papillomavirus type 16 E7 DNA vaccine enhances cytotoxic T-lymphocyte induction and anti-tumour activity. Virology. In press.

68. Da Silva DM, et al. Effect of preexisting neutralizing antibodies on the anti-tumor immune response induced by chimeric human papillomavirus virus-like particle vaccines. Virology 2001; 290(2):350–360.

69. Franco EL, et al. Epidemiology of acquisition and clearance of cervical human papillomavirus infection in women from a high-risk area for cervical cancer. J Infect Dis 1999; 180(5): 1415–1423.

70. Ahdieh L, et al. Prevalence, incidence, and type-specific persistence of human papillomavirus in human immunodeficiency virus (HIV)-positive and HIV-negative women. J Infect Dis 2001; 184(6):682–690.

71. Shiel AGR. Cancer Report. In: Disney APS, ed. ANZDATA report 1991. Adelaide, South Australia: Australia and New Zealand Dialysis and Transplant Registry, 1991:100–108.

72. Höpfl R, et al. Spontaneous regression of CIN and delayed-type hypersensitivity to HPV-16 oncoprotein E7. Lancet 2000; 356(9246):1985–1986.

73. Malcolm K, et al. Multiple conformational epitopes are recognized by natural and induced immunity to the E7 protein of human papilloma virus type 16 in man. Intervirology 2000; 43(3):165–173.

74. Jochmus-Kudielka I, et al. Antibodies against the human papillomavirus type 16 early proteins in human sera: correlation of anti-E7 reactivity with cervical cancer. JNCI 1989; 81:1698–1704.

75. Oukka M, et al. Major histocompatibility complex class I presentation of exogenously acquired minor alloantigens initiates skin allograft rejection. Eur J Immunol 1997; 27(12): 3499–3506.

76. Watarai Y, et al. Intraallograft chemokine RNA and protein during rejection of MHC-matched/multiple minor histocompatibility-disparate skin grafts. J Immunol 2000; 164(11): 6027–6033.

77. Zelenika D, et al. Rejection of H-Y disparate skin grafts by monospecific CD4+ Th1 and Th2 cells: no requirement for CD8+ T cells or B cells. J Immunol 1998; 161(4):1868–1874.

78. Rosenberg AS, Singer A. Evidence that the effector mechanism of skin allograft rejection is antigen-specific. Proc Natl Acad Sci USA 1988; 85(20):7739–7742.

79. Doody DP, et al. Immunologically nonspecific mechanisms of tissue destruction in the rejection of skin grafts. J Exp Med 1994; 179:1645–1652.

80. Braun MY, et al. Acute rejection in the absence of cognate recognition of allograft by T cells. J Immunol 2001; 166(8): 4879–4883.

81. Nickoloff BJ, et al. Direct and indirect control of T-cell activation by keratinocytes. J Invest Dermatol 1995; 105(1):25S–29S.

82. Frazer IH, et al. Potential strategies utilised by papillomavirus to evade host immunity. Immunol Rev 1999; 168(2):131–142.

83. Frazer IH, et al. Tolerance or immunity to a tumor antigen expressed in somatic cells can be determined by systemic proinflammatory signals at the time of first antigen exposure. J Immunol 2001; 167(11):6180–6187.

83a. Leggatt GR, et al. Interferon-gamma enhances cytotoxic T lymphocyte recognition of endogenous peptide in Keratinocytes without lowering the requirement for surface peptide. Immunol Cell Biol 2002; 80:415–424.

84. Higgins GD, et al. Transcription patterns of human papillomavirus type 16 in genital intraepithelial neoplasia: evidence for promoter usage within the E7 open reading frame during epithelial differentiation. J Gen Virol 1992; 73:2047–2057.

85. Mohr IJ, et al. Targeting the E1 replication protein to the papillomavirus origin of replication by complex formation with the E2 transactivator. Science 1990; 250:1694–1699.

86. Zur Hausen H, De Villiers E-M. Human papillomaviruses. Annu Rev Microbiol 1994; 48:427–447.

87. Meneguzzi G, et al. Immunization against human papillomavirus type 16 tumor cells with recombinant vaccinia viruses expressing E6 and E7. Virology 1991; 181:62–69.

88. Chen L, et al. Induction of cytotoxic T lymphocytes specific for a syngeneic tumor expressing the E6 oncoprotein of human papillomavirus type 16. J Immunol 1992; 148:2617–2621.

89. Ji HX, et al. Antigen-specific immunotherapy for murine lung metastatic tumors expressing human papillomavirus type 16 E7 oncoprotein. Int J Cancer 1998; 78(1):41–45.

90. Lamikanra A, et al. Regression of established human papillomavirus type 16 (HPV-16) immortalized tumors in vivo by vaccinia viruses expressing different forms of HPV-16 E7 correlates with enhanced CD8$^+$ T-cell responses that home to the tumor site. J Virol 2001; 75(20):9654–9664.

91. Selvakumar R, et al. Immunization with nonstructural proteins E1 and E2 of cottontail rabbit papillomavirus stimulates regression of virus-induced papillomas. J Virol 1995; 69:602–605.

92. McGarvie GM, et al. T cell responses to BPV-4 E7 during infection and mapping of T cell epitopes. Virology 1995; 206: 504–510.

93. Adams M, et al. Clinical studies of human papilloma vaccines in pre-invasive and invasive cancer. Vaccine 2001; 19(17–19): 2549–2556.

94. Van der Burg SH, et al. Pre-clinical safety and efficacy of TA-CIN, a recombinant HPV16 L2E6E7 fusion protein vaccine, in homologous and heterologous prime-boost regimens. Vaccine 2001; 19(27):3652–3660.

95. Frazer IH, et al. Safety and immunogenicity of HPV16 E7/Algammulin immunotherapy for cervical cancer. In: Tindle RW, ed. Vaccines for Human Papillomavirus Infection and Anogenital Disease. Austin, Texas: Landes Bioscience, 1999: 91–104.

96. Borysiewicz LK, et al. A recombinant vaccinia virus encoding human papillomavirus types 16 and 18, E6 and E7 proteins as immunotherapy for cervical cancer. Lancet 1996; 347(9014): 1523–1527.

97. Van Driel WJ, et al. Vaccination with HPV16 peptides of patients with advanced cervical carcinoma: clinical evaluation of a phase I–II trial. Eur J Cancer [A] 1999; 35(6):946–952.

98. Lacey CJN, et al. Phase IIa safety and immunogenicity of a therapeutic vaccine, TA-GW, in persons with genital warts. J Infect Dis 1999; 179(3):612–618.

99. Zhang LF, et al. HPV6b virus like particles are potent immunogens without adjuvant in man. Vaccine 2000; 18(11–12):1051–1058.

80

Active Immunization with Dendritic Cells Bearing Melanoma Antigens

Ralph M. Steinman
The Rockefeller University, New York, New York, U.S.A.

Karolina Palucka and Jacques Banchereau
Baylor Institute for Immunology Research, Dallas, Texas, U.S.A.

Beatrice Schuler-Thurner and Gerold Schuler
University of Erlangen-Nuremberg, Erlangen, Germany

I. INTRODUCTION

This chapter considers an approach to vaccination that is being tested in the setting of malignant melanoma. The method constitutes actively immunizing cancer patients with a sample of their own dendritic cells (DCs) charged with melanoma antigens (MelAgs). The latter can range from previously defined melanoma peptides to a broad group of MelAgs delivered with melanoma cells or RNA derived from there. This active immunization approach is very different from standard approaches of injecting vaccine antigens intramuscularly or intracutaneously, and, clearly, cell therapy is useful only in select contexts. Nevertheless, research on DCs in cancer therapy could be broadly instructive. First, the approach provides a means to load DCs with many tumor antigens, which may be vital in eliciting protective immunity to human cancers. Second, the use of ex vivo-derived, antigen-loaded DCs provides an opportunity to monitor and to manipulate several aspects of DC physiology that are pertinent to the control of immune responses. Third, DC therapy represents a nontoxic means to study the immune response to human cancers in patients who often do not have alternative therapies, as in stage IV melanoma. At this stage, it is not established if active immune cells, once generated by active immunization with DCs, will bring about tumor regression and prolong survival in patients, but some preliminary Phase I studies are encouraging, as summarized briefly below.

Our plan is to outline some of the roles of the distinct lineage of DCs in the control of immunity, and then to consider a few points from studies of DC vaccination to date.

The field is just in its infancy, with many variables to be worked out. In spite of the demands of human research, the methods and rationale are improving continually.

II. FUNCTIONS OF DENDRITIC CELLS IN THE CONTROL OF IMMUNITY

A. Adjuvants—Enhancing Adaptive Immunity

After it became apparent that DCs were specialized and potent stimulators of T-cell-mediated immunity in tissue culture, it was decided to use these cells as adjuvants in vivo in rodents. Some of the first examples of this transition from in vitro to in vivo experiments are described below. Dendritic cells were found to be powerful stimulators of the mixed leukocyte reaction in tissue culture. Lechler and Batchelor [1] were able to show that DCs were major stimulators of graft rejection in vivo and at small doses. Likewise, hapten-modified DCs were noted to be potent stimulators of hapten-specific CD8 T-cell responses in culture. Macatonia et al. [2] tested hapten-modified DCs in vivo, and the cells induced contact sensitivity. Dendritic cells also primed antigen-specific helper T cells in culture. Inaba et al. [3] pulsed DCs ex vivo with protein antigens, reinfused the cells, and found that the animals could be primed specifically to the protein antigen captured by the DCs. In the latter experiments, the proteins first had to be given to the DCs in their immature or antigen-capturing state (which is the state of most DCs in vivo), and then the maturing DCs were injected.

Investigators then considered more challenging antigenic targets. Again the DCs served as adjuvants for strong T-cell priming. Dendritic cells pulsed with tumor antigenic peptides, or with viral vectors recombinant for tumor antigens, were able to elicit protective immunity to tumor challenge, and in some instances caused existing tumors to undergo some regression [4,5]. Dendritic cells pulsed with microbial antigens could also induce protective immunity to infection [6,7], whereas DCs bearing autoantigens could trigger autoimmunity [8,9]. Because it is well known that proteins and preprocessed antigenic peptides are poor immunogens unless they are administered together with adjuvants, DCs seemed to be functioning as "nature's adjuvants" [3].

B. Sentinels—Innate Immunity

Dendritic cells are specialized to respond quickly to the entry of a pathogen and set the stage for an adaptive immune response (above). For example, DCs can mobilize other innate effector cells, such as NK cells and NKT cells. Another example of an innate response is the capacity of DCs to make large amounts of certain cytokines, usually upon stimulation of Toll-like receptors (TLRs) by microbial ligands. The curious finding is that different subsets of DCs can express different TLRs and, upon signaling, make different cytokines [10]. The plasmacytoid DC expresses TLR9 and, upon stimulation with CpG deoxyoligonucleotides, produces large amounts of IFNα (also IFNβ and IFNψ). In contrast, certain monocyte-derived DCs express TLR4 and make abundant IL-12 and tumor necrosis factor-α (TNFα) upon stimulation with lipopolysaccharide. When a TLR receptor is shared, as is the case of TLR7, stimulation with the ligand imiquimod leads to IFNα production by plasmacytoid DCs, and IL-12 and TNFα from monocyte-derived DCs [11]. Therefore the type of DC subset that will be used in immune therapy can influence the type of cytokine that can be produced, and perhaps other features. More details are provided below.

C. Gatekeepers—Immune Tolerance

It is becoming increasingly apparent that DCs have important roles in immune tolerance. It is accepted that DCs in the thymic medulla contribute to negative selection, efficiently capturing self antigens and deleting newly formed self-reactive T cells. In addition, peripheral tolerance mechanisms are available for the immune system to avoid reactivity to antigens that escape negative selection, or environmental proteins to which reactivity must not be induced. The need for peripheral tolerance is dramatized by the fact that when DCs are eliciting immunity to microbial antigens, they are also capturing self-antigens in the form of dying infected cells, as well as harmless environmental proteins in the environment. Therefore it has been proposed that DCs function in the steady state, prior to infection or inflammation, to capture dying self-cells and environmental proteins and to induce peripheral tolerance [12].

When proteins or dead cells are targeted to DCs in vivo in the steady state, the antigens are processed with high efficiency and tolerance is induced [13–15]. The tolerance can occur through the deletion of reactive T cells, or, alternatively, DCs might induce regulatory T cells that suppress the function of other T cells. Therefore in terms of immunotherapy, it is important that the correct DC be used to avoid the tolerizing roles of DCs. In addition, it is possible that autoreactivity will not be a major obstacle to immunotherapy because DCs will have controlled this problem prior to the exposure to antigens from tumor cells.

III. SOME MECHANISMS OF DENDRITIC CELL FUNCTION

A. Dendritic Cells as Antigen Processing Machines—Antigen Uptake and Formation of Major Histocompatibility Complex–Peptide Complexes

Dendritic cells have a very large number of receptors for adsorptive uptake. Through the use of antigens incorporated into antireceptor antibodies, it is evident that these endocytic receptors enhance presentation on major histocompatibility complex (MHC) class II. In some cases, such as DEC-205 and FcγR, endocytosed antigens are also delivered to MHC class I, the so-called "exogenous" pathway to MHC class I. Once taken into the DCs, the conversion of antigen into MHC–peptide complexes seems to be efficient, although more quantitative work needs to be done. To illustrate, when DCs process a membrane protein from dead B cells, the formation of MHC class II peptide complexes is >1000 times more efficient than if the DCs are exposed to preprocessed peptides [16]. Therefore DCs are efficient at processing complex antigens, including whole cells, and present antigenic fragments on both MHC class I and class II products to CD8$^+$ and CD4$^+$ T cells, respectively.

B. Dendritic Cells as Costimulatory Cells—T-Cell Binding and Activation

Even when antigens do not require processing (such as superantigens, allogeneic MHC–peptide complexes, and anti-CD3 antibodies), DCs are much more potent stimulators of T-cell responses than other antigen-presenting cells. Two potentially relevant mechanistic features are the expression of DC-SIGN, a C-type lectin that allows DCs to bind resting T cells via ICAM-3 [17], and high levels of CD86 [18,19], a T-cell costimulator that clusters with MHC–peptide complexes on DCs [20]. Dendritic cells express several other families of molecules. These include molecules for T-cell adhesion (such as CD54/ICAM-1 and CD58/LFA-3), TNF receptors (CD40 and CD95/fas), TNF family members (CD27, 4-1BBL, and OX40L), and several B7 family members (CD80, CD86, ICOS-L, and PD-L2). In addition to these many cell surface molecules for productive T-cell interactions, DCs can produce cytokines such as IL-2 [21] and IL-12 [22,23], and additional growth factors such as cysteine and thioredoxins. These products help to explain the potent effects of DCs on the magnitude and quality of the T-cell response.

C. Dendritic Cell Properties In Vivo—Positioning for Antigen Capture and Migration to the T-Cell Areas

Dendritic cells are designed to navigate peripheral tissues, where they can pick up antigens, enter the afferent lymphatics, and then home to the T-cell areas (reviewed in Refs. 24 and 25). During DC-based immunotherapy, these homing properties should allow the antigen-bearing DCs to find those T cells that are capable of producing an immune response. To execute these migratory functions, DCs control their expression of chemokine receptors in a sequential manner. CCR6 (responding to MIP-3α or CCL20) may target DCs to epithelial surfaces. During inflammation, additional DCs bearing CCR5 (responding to MIP-1α and MIP-1β) or CXCR3 (responding to IP-10, Mig, ITAC, and CCL9-11) may be recruited from the blood. With maturation, CCR7 (responding to CCL19 and CCL21) is upregulated, enhancing entry into lymphatics and homing to the T-cell areas. An important intermediary in the function of chemokine receptors are the cysteinyl leukotrienes LTC and LTD, which are pumped out of DCs through multidrug resistance family proteins and then act on the DCs to influence chemokine responsiveness. In summary, DCs are specialized to capture and handle antigens, to migrate into tissues and then to lymphoid organs in vivo, and to stimulate and control the quality of the immune response.

IV. INTERFACING DENDRITIC CELL PHYSIOLOGY WITH IMMUNOTHERAPY

A. Method of Antigen Loading into Dendritic Cells

From the above considerations, DC-based immunotherapy has considerable demands but potential as well. One example is the capacity to load DCs ex vivo with a large spectrum of tumor antigens, which in turn can be presented on both MHC class I and class II to elicit a combined immune response by CD4$^+$ helper and CD8$^+$ cytotoxic T lymphocytes (CTLs). This ex vivo step may bypass a fundamental defect in the patient's natural immune response, which is that in spite of their many potential antigens, tumor cells are ineffective in presenting their antigens to T cells, or the tumor cells may not be captured by DCs in vivo. The status of the patient's immune system in progressive cancer was recently assessed directly in multiple myeloma [26]. In this tumor, it is possible to take T cells from the tumor environment (the bone marrow) and to assess their capacity to develop immunity to authentic myeloma tumor cells as targets. No immunity was detected ex vivo, but strong immunity could be generated when DCs were loaded with myeloma cells (coated with antisyndecan antibody) and used to expand bone marrow T cells to form strong myeloma-specific CTL responses. The optimal method for tumor antigen loading is far from established for DC-based active immunization. The approaches under consideration for delivering a large spectrum of tumor antigens are antibody-coated tumor cells, apoptotic and necrotic tumor cells, exosomes, mixtures of MHC class I and class II binding peptides, and tumor-derived RNA. Some of these approaches provide an opportunity for tailoring the immunotherapy to those tumor antigens that are being expressed in a patient-specific manner.

B. Monocyte-Derived Dendritic Cells

Beyond the methods for antigen delivery, the subset of DCs could prove critical. Much of the current research is being carried out with monocyte-derived DCs [27–29], which are potent and homogenous stimulators of immunity. Monocyte-derived DCs can be reproducibly generated within a few days in large numbers (300–500 million mature DCs per apheresis) from precursors in blood without any need for pretreating the patients with cytokines such as granulocyte–macrophage colony-stimulating factor (GM-CSF) or Flt3-L [27–29]. It is possible to obtain populations of immature DCs by exposing monocytes to GM-CSF$^+$ IL-4, and these can then be differentiated into mature DCs by various stimuli such as TLR ligands (e.g., microbial products such as LPS or poly I:C), inflammatory cytokines such as those in monocyte-conditioned medium (IL-1β, TNFα, IL-6, and PGE$_2$), or CD40L. The use of DCs that have received a maturation stimulus is likely to be important to induce strong immunity, as it has become clear that antigen delivered on immature or incompletely matured DCs can even induce tolerance (above). However, the type and the duration of the maturation stimulus remain to be determined and may influence efficacy. For example, the use of PGE$_2$ as part of the maturation stimulus allows one to obtain CCR7-expressing Mo-DC that migrates in response to CCL19 and CCL21 and should help guide DCs into lymphoid organs [30,31]. At this time, the monocyte-derived DC populations are the most accessible and homogenous preparations of DCs.

C. Two Dendritic Cell Subsets with Distinct Biological Functions Emerge from Cultures of Cord Blood CD34$^+$ Hematopoietic Progenitor Cells

Early studies with CD34$^+$ hematopoietic progenitor cells (HPCs) used cord blood to produce DCs, including distinct subsets of DCs. Differentiation was induced by culture with GM-CSF/TNF or IL-3/TNF [32,33]. In these culture conditions, the cooperation between TNFα and GM-CSF/IL-3 was critical for the development of DCs from CD34$^+$ HPC. Indeed, although prior work had suggested TNF as an inhibitor of hematopoiesis, TNF was then observed to stimulate the proliferation of CD34-HPC together with either IL-3 or GM-CSF [34]. Limiting dilution analysis indicated that TNF increased both the frequency of IL-3 responding cells and the average size of the IL-3-dependent clones [34]. After 12 days of liquid culture, CD34-HPC cultured with GM-CSF and TNF generated both adherent and nonadherent cells with a dendritic morphology. For optimal generation of DC, TNF was mainly required during the first days of the culture, where it upregulated the expression of the common γ-chain subunit of the GM-CSF/IL-3/IL-5 receptor. Another important site of action of TNF in the CD34-HPC cultures was the inhibition of granulopoietic differentiation and proliferation [35]. In particular, TNF reversibly blocked granulocytic differentiation at the level of uncommitted $CD13^-$ $CD15^-$ blast cells that accumulated in TNF-enriched cultures. Furthermore, the growth of committed granulocytic progenitors ($CD15^+$) was inhibited through an arrest of cell cycle in G_0/G_1. Tumor necrosis factor also blocked erythropoiesis in these cultures [36]. These effects of TNF on growing CD34-HPC were mediated through the p55 TNF receptor [37].

Two precursor subpopulations emerged under these culture conditions: $CD1a^+$ and $CD14^+$ [38,39]. Both precursor subsets matured at days 12–14 into DCs with typical morphology, phenotype (CD80, CD83, CD86, CD58, and high HLA class II), and function. $CD1a^+$ precursors gave rise to cells with the characteristics of epidermal Langerhans cells (Birbeck granules, Lag antigen, and E-cadherin). In contrast, the $CD14^+$ precursors matured into $CD1a^-$ DCs lacking Birbeck granules, E-cadherin, and Lag antigen, but expressing CD2, CD9, CD68, and the coagulation factor XIIIa described for dermal or interstitial DCs. Interestingly, the $CD14^+$ precursors, but not the $CD1a^+$ precursors, represented bipotent cells that could be induced to differentiate, in response to M-CSF, into macrophage-like cells, lacking accessory function for T cells. These DC subsets differed with regard to: (a) antigen capture—interstitial DCs were more efficient in Dextran uptake and in binding immune complexes than LC; (b) lysosomal activity—interstitial DCs expressed higher levels of enzymatic activity; (c) capacity to induce naive B cell differentiation—interstitial DCs were uniquely able to prime naïve B cells, including differentiation into IgM-secreting plasma cells through the secretion of IL-12 [40,41]; and (d) whereas both subsets expressed IL-12 upon CD40 ligation, only interstitial DCs expressed IL-10. Unique functions of LCs remain to be established, but there are some reports suggesting that CD34-DCs with an LC component are more efficient in CD8 T-cell priming than monocyte-derived DCs [42,43]. In circumstances such as the induction of tumor-specific CTLs, CD34-DCs could thus be advantageous.

Granulocyte colony-stimulating factor (G-CSF)-mobilized $CD34^+$ HPCs from adult blood also yielded two DC subsets, including peripheral blood mobilized by G-CSF in patients with advanced melanoma. As in cord blood cultures, two populations could be identified at day 9 (i.e., $CD1a^+$ $CD14^-$ LCs and $CD1a^-$ $CD14^+$ interstitial DCs). About 50% of cells in these cultures remained at a precursor stage and only gave rise to DCs upon further culture. Thus, these cultures are asynchronic, a parameter that needs to be taken into consideration when using these DC preparations for vaccination.

D. The Efficiency with Which Dendritic Cells Home and Survive In Vivo

This critical area needs to be assessed further and more likely controlled better in human studies to improve the efficacy of DC therapy. It is of concern that, currently, DCs are being injected into skin sites in large numbers, possibly more than the lymphatics can handle, especially when the lymphatics

may not be expressing sufficient chemokines needed for proper DC entry and migration. In addition, once DCs reach the T-cell area, they can die within hours to 1–2 days and be processed by other DCs. The death may limit function, and the reprocessing by recipient DCs in the steady state could lead to tolerance. At this time, the vast majority of DCs that are being injected during immunotherapy studies may not gain access to their proper site of action in the lymphoid organs.

V. RESULTS FROM VACCINATION OF HEALTHY VOLUNTEERS

When methods became available to generate large numbers of DCs from monocytes, using culture methods that required only human products (recombinant cytokines and human plasma), it became feasible to assess if autologous DCs could act as immune adjuvants in healthy volunteers. It was evident that humans could be stimulated with their own DCs pulsed with KLH or with an influenza virus peptide, in the absence of any other adjuvant. The antigens by themselves were not detectably immunogenic. Interestingly, the $CD4^+$ T-cell response to KLH was decidedly Th1 in nature [44], whereas the memory $CD8^+$ T-cell response to flu matrix peptide seemed to select for higher-affinity T cells (i.e., T cells responsive to low doses of peptide) [45]. Importantly, when the DCs were of an immature type, antigen-specific IL-10-producing T cells were generated and the cells suppressed the responses of IFNγ-producing T cells [46]. These initial proof-of-concept studies suggest that DCs have the potential to enhance or to dampen the human immune response in patients.

VI. ADVANCED MELANOMA PATIENTS IMMUNIZED WITH CD34-DERIVED DENDRITIC CELLS PULSED WITH MELANOMA PEPTIDES

Banchereau et al. [47] vaccinated 18 HLA $A*0201^+$ patients in stage IV melanoma with CD34-HPC-derived DCs pulsed with six antigens: influenza matrix peptide (Flu-MP), KLH, and peptides derived from the four MelAgs: MART-1/Melan A, gp100, tyrosinase and MAGE-3. The DCs were loaded with KLH, Flu matrix peptide and HLA-A2 binding peptides derived from four MelAgs, MAGE-3, MART-1/MELAN A, GP-100, and tyrosinase, and administered biweekly over 6 weeks (four subcutaneous injections). Vaccination of patients with advanced melanoma with antigen-pulsed CD34-DCs has proven to be well tolerated and results in enhanced immunity to both "nonself" (viral peptide and KLH protein) and "self" (melanoma peptides) antigens [47]. It was observed that the level of immune responses in the blood correlated with early outcome at the tumor sites. Indeed, antigen-pulsed $CD34^+$ HPC-derived DCs induced primary and recall immune responses detectable directly in the blood. An immune response to control antigens (KLH and Flu-MP) was observed in 16 of 18 patients. An enhanced immune response to one or more MelAgs was seen in these same 16 patients, including 10 patients who responded to > 2 MelAg. The MelAg-specific T cells elicited after DC vaccine are functional and detectable in effector T-cell assays without the need for prior ex vivo expansion. They are also capable of proliferation and effector function after short-term (1 week) coculture with antigen-bearing DCs, without the need for exogenous cytokines or multiple restimulations with antigen. The two patients failing to respond to both control and tumor antigens experienced rapid tumor progression. Of 17 patients with evaluable disease, six of seven patients with immunity to two or less MelAg had progressive disease at 10 weeks after study entry, in contrast to tumor progression in only 1 of 10 patients with immunity to more than two MelAg. Regression of more than one tumor metastases was observed in seven of these patients. The overall immunity to MelAgs following DC vaccination was associated with clinical outcome ($P = 0.015$). This initial study suggests that the measurement of immune responses in the blood helps evaluate vaccine efficacy.

The analysis of blood immune responses demonstrated that antigen-pulsed CD34-DCs could lead to rapid induction of CD4$^+$ and CD8$^+$ T-cell immunity. Indeed, a single DC vaccination was sufficient for the induction of KLH-specific responses in six patients and Flu-MP-specific responses in eight patients. A single DC vaccine was sufficient to induce tumor specific effectors to ≥1 MelAg in five patients. None of these five patients showed early disease progression. Only one of six patients with rapid KLH response experienced early disease progression. Rapid and slow Flu-MP responders did not differ with regard to disease progression. Thus, a patient's ability to rapidly respond to CD4 epitopes and MelAgs could be an early indicator of clinical outcome after DC-based vaccination. In other studies in which the induction of immunity was demonstrated [48,49], such correlation was less strict. This might be due, in part, to the fact that more advanced stage IV patients with a larger number of metastases were included. Such a situation clearly enhances the chances of tumor escape, for example, by loss of MHC class I molecules and/or tumor antigens, which occurs in about half of melanoma metastases. The number of metastases will have to be considered in comparing clinical outcome.

VII. ACTIVE IMMUNIZATION WITH MONOCYTE-DERIVED DENDRITIC CELLS

Monocyte-derived DCs were the first DCs to be used for the treatment of melanoma patients, and several pilot studies have been published (see Table 1). Most used defined antigens in the form of peptides, but in some studies, tumor lysates or autologous DC tumor hybrids were also employed. The first trial published in 1998 by Nestle et al. [50] aroused great interest given an overall response rate of 30% in stage IV patients (i.e., distant metastases) including complete responses. The DCs were delivered directly into the inguinal nodes under ultrasonographical guidance, to circumvent the need for the active migration of the DCs from the skin into the nodes, but this rationale remains to be substantiated. The first study also used fetal calf serum (FCS) during DC gener-

ation, and this might have contributed to the observed effects by providing unspecific helper epitopes and by promoting the maturation of DCs. Jonuleit et al. [51] directly compared within each of eight patients the immunogenicity of immature DCs (generated according to Nestle et al. in FCS containing media using GM-CSF and IL-4) versus mature DCs [generated in the absence of FCS and matured by a cocktail consisting of TNFα, IL-1β, IL-6, and PGE$_2$ (these mimic the composition of monocyte-conditioned medium)] upon intranodal administration into opposite inguinal lymph nodes. FCS-free mature DCs induced stronger T-cell responses, both to the two recall antigens used (tetanus toxoid and PPD/tuberculin) and to tumor peptides. Interestingly, however, both immature as well as mature DCs showed an expansion of peptide-specific T cells by tetramer staining, yet only mature DCs induced IFNγ-producing and lytic CD8$^+$ T cells. These findings indicate the interesting possibility that the immature DCs might have induced regulatory T cells, rather than effector T cells, as observed in volunteers [44,46].

Thurner et al. used monocyte-derived DCs matured by monocyte-conditioned medium and cultured in the absence of FCS. The cells were pulsed with MAGE-3 peptide and tetanus toxoid, and injected into HLA-A1$^+$ melanoma patients who suffered from advanced stage IV disease [48]. In contrast to the study by Nestle et al., the patients in this study had all been treated by chemotherapy or chemoimmunotherapy and were nevertheless progressive. For three biweekly vaccinations, 3 million DCs were administered intradermally and 3 million were administerd subcutaneously followed, after 2 weeks, by 6 million and, finally, 12 million intravenously. Immune monitoring involved a simplified form of a limiting dilution assay. Significant expansions of MAGE-3A1-specific CD8$^+$ CTL responses were observed in 8 of 11 patients. This was an encouraging finding given the advanced disease status and the fact that CTL responses (by the methodology used) had not been observed previously in less advanced melanoma patients vaccinated with MAGE-3 A1 peptide itself [52]. Regression of individual metastases was observed in 6 of 11 patients. A complete response did not occur upon short-term follow up, but upon prolonged vaccinations (including also other tumor peptides), disease proved stable in several patients and resolved completely in one.

In a follow-up study, Schuler-Thurner et al. [53] immunized terminal HLA-A2.1$^+$ stage IV melanoma patients. They found that three to five biweekly vaccinations of mature, monocyte-derived DC (three vaccinations of 6 million subcutaneously followed by two intravenous doses of 6 and 12 million, respectively) pulsed with MAGE-3A2.1 tumor and influenza matrix A2.1-positive control peptides as well as the recall antigen tetanus toxoid (in three of eight patients) generated in all eight patients antigen-specific, IFNγ-producing effector CD8$^+$ T cells that were detectable in blood directly ex vivo [53]. The lack of significant clinical responses (only one disease stabilization was observed) despite the induction of antitumor immunity may be due to the properties of the MAGE-3A2 epitope, which is now known to be presented suboptimally by most melanomas.

Recently, Schuler-Thurner et al. reported that mature, monocyte-derived DCs loaded with multiple (five HLA-1-

Table 1

Authors	DC	Antigen (s)	Number of cells / vaccinations (vacc) / interval	Application	Journal	Date	Number of patients / AJCC stag syst. 6th ed.	Pretreatment[b]	Clinical response	Adverse events
Nestle et al.	imMo	Peptide(n = 12): HLA-A1: MAGE-1+3, HLA-A2.1: Gp 100, MelA, Tyr. Lysate(n=4): all KLH	1×10^6 4 vacc weekly, 5th after 2 wk. up to 10 vacc 4wkly	in	Nat Med	1998	16 stage IV (4 M1a, 3 M1b, 9 M1c)	4 Ch 5 lt	2CR, 1MR, 2SD	I[c]
Thurner et al.	mMo	Peptide: HLA-A1: MAGE-3, TT	6 vacc bi weekly: vacc $1-36 \times 10^6$ id + sc, vacc 46×10^6 iv, vacc 512×10^6 iv	id + sc then iv (vacc 4–5)	J Exp Med	1999	11 stage IV (3 M1b, 8 M1c)	11 Ch 6 lt	6MxR	I-II[d]
Mackensen et al.	CD34	Peptide: HLA-A1: MAGE-1 + 3, HLA A2.1: MelA, gp100, Tyr	$5 \times 10^5 - 5 \times 10^7$ ≥4 vacc bi-weekly	iv	Int J Cancer	2000	14 stage III and IV (1 III, 2 M1a, 4 M1b, 7 M1c)	n.d.[a]	1MR, 7SD	I-II[c] vitiligo in 1 patient
Sculer-Thurner et al.	mMo	Peptide: HLA-A2.1: MAGE-3, Flu Matrix; TT (except n = 3)	6 vacc bi weekly: vacc $1-36 \times 10^6$ id + sc, vacc 46×10^6 iv, vacc 512×10^6 iv	sc, then lv (vacc 4–5)	J Immunol	2000	8 stage IV (8 M1c)	8 Ch 8 lt	1SD	I-II[d]
Panelli et al.	ImMo	Peptides: HLA-A2.1: MelA, gp100–209M	$6 \times 10^7 / 2 \times 10^8 (+/ \text{ IL 2})$ 4 vacc at 3 week intervals	iv	J Immunother	2000	10 stage IV (4 M1b, 6 M1c)	8 Ch 7 lt 2 Pt	1PR	I-II[d]
Banchereau et al.	CD34	Peptides: gp100, MelA. Mage-3, Tyr, Flu; KLH	$1-10 \times 10^5$ 4 vacc bi weekly	sc	Cancer Res	2001	18 stage IV (6 M1a, 3 M1b, 11 M1c)	4 Ch 5 l	3CR, 1PR, 3SD, 3MR	I[d] vitiligo in 2 patients
Toungouz et al.	imMo	Peptides: HLA-A1: Mage-1,–3; HLA-A2.1: Mage-3: HLA-B44: Mage-3 (+/ − KLH)	$6 - 60 \times 10^6$ 3 vvacc at 3 week intervals, vacc 4 after 6 weeks	lv + sc	J Leucocyte Biology	2001	16 stage III and IV (9 III, 2 M1b, 5 M1c)	4 Ch 7 lt 3 DC 1 Pt	1CR, PR, 2SD (4)	I
Lau et al.	imMo	Peptides: HLA-A2.1: MelA, Tyr, gp100	$10^7, 3 \times 10^7, 10^8$ 2 vacc biweekly	iv	J Immunother	2001	16 stage IV (5 M1a, 3 M1b, 8 M1c)	7 Ch 8 lt	1CR, 2SD, 2MR.	I-II, patients III (fever)
Andersen et al.	mMo	Peptides: HLA-A2.1: Mage-3, MelA, gp100: Lysate	$20-30 \times 10^6 + \text{IL-2}$ bi-weekly	sc	Int J Cancer	2001	2 stage IV (2 M1c)	2 Ch 1 lt	2SD	n.d.[a]
Jonuleit et al.	Im/m Mo	Peptides: HLA-A2.1: Mage-1, MelA, gp100; II, PPD	8×10^6 (vacc 1–3) 12×10^6 (vacc 4–6) 6 vacc bi-weekly	in	Int J Cancer	2001	8 stage IV (1 M1a, 7 M1c)	7 CH 7 lt	3MR, 1MxR. 1SD	I-II[d]
Chang et al.	imMo	DC + tumor Lysate plus DC + KLH (1:1 mixture)	$10^6, 10^7, 10^8$ 3 vacc bi-weekly	id	Clinical Cancer Res	2002	11 stage IV (4 M1a, 1 Mia, 6 M1c)	4 lt 7 Untreated	1MR, 3SD (4)	I-II[d]
Schuler-Thurner et al.	mMo	Peptides: Mage-3/1/4/10, Mela, gp100, Tyr, GnTV; I + II	$4 \times 10^6/$ MHC class I peptide 5 vacc bi-weekly vacc 6 after 4 weeks	sc	J Exp Med	2002	16 stage III and IV (4 III, 1 M1a, 1 M1b, 10 M1c)	9 Ch 13 lt	1CR, 8SD	I-II[d]

[a] n.d. = not defined in the manuscript.

[b] Partially overlapping.

[c] WHO grading.

[d] National Cancer Institute Common Toxicity Scale.

Abbreviations: KLH = keyhole limpet hemocyanine; TT = tetanus toxoid; PPD = protein purified derivative/tuberculin; im = immature; m = mature; in = intranodal; id = intradermal; sc = subcutaneous; iv = intravenous; vacc = vaccination(s); Ch = systematic chemotherapy; it = systematic immunotherapy; DC = dendritic cell therapy; Pt = peptide therapy; CR = complete remission; MxR = mixed response; MR = minor response; PR = partial response; SD = stable disease.

restricted, eight HLA-A2.1-restricted, and three HLA-A3-restricted) MHC class I peptides (each peptide pulsed onto a separate batch of 4 million DCs to avoid competition at the level of a given MHC molecule) and MHC class II peptides (again loaded in a noncompeting fashion) rapidly induced MAGE-3.DR13 and MAGE-3.DP4-restricted, IFN-γ-producing Th1-type, tumor-specific T cells. The T cells were detectable directly ex vivo [49]. The basic characteristics of several other studies employing monocyte-derived DCs are listed in Table 1 and compared to those employing CD34$^+$ HPC-derived ones [47,54–59].

It is of note that many trials employing monocyte-derived DCs have not used maturing DCs. Mature DCs, when reinjected following ex vivo loading with tumor peptides, express demonstrable migration to lymph nodes, induction of tumor-specific cytotoxic and helper T cells, and movement of tumor antigen-specific T cells into regressing metastases. Recently, newer approaches to charge DC with antigens have been developed, such as the capacity of DCs to express antigens introduced through RNA electroporation [60]. This now allows one to administer to DCs both defined antigens, including universal ones such as telomerase or survivin as well as the total antigenic repertoire of a given tumor (as total tumor or polymerase chain reaction-amplified RNA). The use of dying tumor cells, notably antibody-coated ones, is an alternative [26]. Other preclinical research works have shown that the delivery of defined antigens as antigen–antibody complexes to DC enhances cross-presentation and allows for the potent induction of both CD4$^+$ and CD8$^+$ T-cell responses [61–63]. Therefore it is rational and timely to optimize the use of DCs as vectors for the delivery of antigens to vaccinate against cancer, although Phase III studies with current methods are underway.

In summary, vaccination with monocyte-derived DCs loaded with tumor antigens in the form of peptides has been shown to induce: (a) tumor-specific killer and helper T cells ("proof of concept"), and (b) occasional regression of metastases even in far-advanced cancer patients, including rare complete responses with (c) absence of significant toxicity. The final safety profile is, however, clearly not yet defined as the number of patients is still small, and it is not yet established what happens if, upon optimization of the strategy, stronger immune responses result and prolonged vaccinations are performed. At this point, the various trials are difficult to compare as the maturational status of DC, and many other variables such as DC dose, interval, and route are also very much different.

VIII. DISCUSSION

The field of active immunization with autologous DCs charged with tumor antigens is underway. A small sample of published studies has been discussed here to illustrate that it is feasible to energize a patient's endogenous immune response to tumor antigens. There are many additional questions to be studied: the optimization of Th1 and CTL responses to tumors, the induction of immunity to large numbers of tumor antigens, and the capacity of DCs and T cells to infiltrate and function within tumors. From a re-

search perspective, DC therapy additionally provides an opportunity to assess the incidence of tumor-specific tolerance. Fortunately, answers to these questions are going to be facilitated by the improved capacity to monitor the human immune response in tandem with the measurement of clinical endpoints including survival.

This discussion emphasizes active immunotherapy based on DC priming of tumor-specific T cells. Dendritic cells also provide an opportunity to control the function of other types of lymphocytes—NK, NKT, and B cells—and not just T cells. Many of the current studies emphasize patients with advanced cancer, but vaccination in the setting of minimal residual disease could show enhanced value. Long-term vaccination studies also remain to be described.

REFERENCES

1. Lechler RI, Batchelor JR. Restoration of immunogenicity to passenger cell-depleted kidney allografts by the addition of donor strain dendritic cells. J Exp Med 1982; 155:31–41.
2. Macatonia SE, et al. Dendritic cells and the initiation of contact sensitivity to fluorescein isothiocyanate. Immunology 1986; 59:509–514.
3. Inaba K, et al. Dendritic cells pulsed with protein antigens in vitro can prime antigen-specific, MHC-restricted T cells in situ. J Exp Med 1990; 172:631–640.
4. Mayordomo JI, et al. Bone marrow-derived dendritic cells pulsed with synthetic tumour peptides elicit protective and therapeutic antitumour immunity. Nat Med 1995; 1:1297–1302.
5. Zitvogel L, et al. Therapy of murine tumors with tumor peptide pulsed dendritic cells: dependence on T-cells, B7 costimulation, and Th1-associated cytokines. J Exp Med 1996; 183:87–97.
6. Ludewig B, et al. Dendritic cells efficiently induce protective antiviral immunity. J Virol 1998; 272:3812–3818.
7. Su H, et al. Vaccination against chlamydial genital tract infection following immunization with dendritic cells pulsed ex vivo with non-viable chlamydiae. J Exp Med 1998; 188:809–818.
8. Ludewig B, et al. Dendritic cells induce autoimmune diabetes and maintain disease via de novo formation of local lymphoid tissue. J Exp Med 1998; 188:1493–1501.
9. Dittel BN, et al. Presentation of the self antigen myelin basic protein by dendritic cells leads to experimental autoimmune encephalomyelitis. J Immunol 1999; 163:32–39.
10. Kadowaki N, et al. Subsets of human dendritic cell precursors express different Toll-like receptors and respond to different microbial antigens. J Exp Med 2001; 194:863–870.
11. Ito T, et al. Interferon-α and interleukin-12 are induced differentially by Toll-like receptor 7 ligands in human blood dendritic cell subsets. J Exp Med 2002; 195:1507–1512.
12. Steinman RM, Nussenzweig MC. Avoiding horror autotoxicus: the importance of dendritic cells in peripheral T cell tolerance. Proc Natl Acad Sci USA 2002; 99:351–358.
13. Hawiger D, et al. Dendritic cells induce peripheral T cell unresponsiveness under steady state conditions in vivo. J Exp Med 2001; 194:769–780.
14. Liu K, et al. Immune tolerance after delivery of dying cells to dendritic cells in situ. J Exp Med 2002; 196:1091–1097.
15. Bonifaz L, et al. Efficient targeting of protein antigen to the dendritic cell receptor DEC-205 leads in the steady state to antigen presentation on MHC class I and peripheral CD8$^+$ T cell tolerance. J Exp Med 2002; 196: 1627–1638.

16. Inaba K, et al. Efficient presentation of phagocytosed cellular fragments on the MHC class II products of dendritic cells. J Exp Med 1998; 188:2163–2173.

17. Geijtenbeek TBH, et al. Identification of DC-SIGN, a novel dendritic cell-specific ICAM-3 receptor that supports primary immune responses. Cell 2000; 100:575–585.

18. Inaba K, et al. The tissue distribution of the B7-2 costimulator in mice: abundant expression on dendritic cells in situ and during maturation in vitro. J Exp Med 1994; 180:1849–1860.

19. Caux C, et al. B70/B7-2 is identical to CD86 and is the major functional ligand for CD28 expressed on human dendritic cells. J Exp Med 1994; 180:1841–1847.

20. Turley SJ, et al. Transport of peptide–MHC class II complexes in developing dendritic cells. Science 2000; 288:522–527.

21. Granucci F, et al. Inducible IL-2 production by dendritic cells revealed by global gene expression analysis. Nat Immunol 2001; 2:882–888.

22. Koch F, et al. High level IL-12 production by murine dendritic cells: upregulation via MHC class II and CD40 molecules and downregulation by IL-4 and IL-10. J Exp Med 1996; 184:741–746.

23. Cella M, et al. Ligation of CD40 on dendritic cells triggers production of high levels of interleukin-12 and enhances T cell stimulatory capacity: T–T help via APC activation. J Exp Med 1996; 184:747–752.

24. Sallusto F, Lanzavecchia A. Mobilizing dendritic cells for tolerance, priming, and chronic inflammation. J Exp Med 1999; 189:611–614.

25. Randolph GJ. Is maturation required for Langerhans cell migration? J Exp Med 2002; 196:413–416.

26. Dhodapkar MV, et al. T cells from the tumor microenvironment of patients with progressive myeloma can generate strong, tumor-specific cytolytic responses to autologous, tumor-loaded dendritic cells. Proc Natl Acad Sci USA 2002; 99: 13009–13013.

27. Berger T, et al. Large-scale generation of mature monocyte-derived dendritic cells for clinical application in cell factories. J Immunol Methods 2002; 268:131.

28. Thurner B, et al. Generation of large numbers of fully mature and stable dendritic cells from leukapheresis products for clinical application. J Immunol Methods 1999; 223:1–15.

29. Feuerstein B, et al. A method for the production of cryopreserved aliquots of antigen-preloaded, mature dendritic cells ready for clinical use. J Immunol Methods 2000; 245:15–29.

30. Luft T, et al. Functionally distinct dendritic cell (DC) populations induced by physiologic stimuli: prostaglandin E(2) regulates the migratory capacity of specific DC subsets. Blood 2002; 100:1362–1372.

31. Scandella E, et al. Prostaglandin E2 is a key factor for CCR7 surface expression and migration of monocyte-derived dendritic cells. Blood 2002; 100:1354–1361.

32. Caux C, et al. GM-CSF and TNF-α cooperate in the generation of dendritic Langerhans cells. Nature 1992; 360:258–261.

33. Caux C, et al. Tumor necrosis factor α cooperates with interleukin 3 in the recruitment of a primitive subset of human CD34+ progenitors. J Exp Med 1993; 177:1815–1820.

34. Caux C, et al. Tumor necrosis factor-alpha strongly potentiates interleukin-3 and granulocyte–macrophage colony-stimulating factor-induced proliferation of human CD34+ hematopoietic progenitor cells. Blood 1990; 75:2292–2298.

35. Caux C, et al. Potentiation of early hematopoiesis by tumor necrosis factor-α is followed by inhibition of granulopoietic differentiation and proliferation. Blood 1991; 78:635–644.

36. Jacobsen SEW, et al. Tumor necrosis factor α directly and indirectly regulates hematopoietic progenitor cell proliferation: role of colony-stimulating factor receptor modulation. J Exp Med 1992; 175:1759–1772.

37. Rusten LS, et al. Bifunctional effects of tumor necrosis factor alpha (TNF alpha) on the growth of mature and primitive human hematopoietic progenitor cells: involvement of p55 and p75 TNF receptors. Blood 1994; 83:3152–3159.

38. Caux C, et al. CD34+ hematopoietic progenitors from human cord blood differentiate along two independent dendritic cell pathways in response to GM-CSF + TNF α. J Exp Med 1996; 184:695–706.

39. Caux C, et al. CD34+ hematopoietic progenitors from human cord blood differentiate along two independent dendritic cell pathways in response to granulocyte–macrophage colony-stimulating factor plus tumor necrosis factor α. Blood 1997; 90:1458–1470.

40. Dubois B, et al. Dendritic cells enhance growth and differentiation of CD40-activated B lymphocytes. J Exp Med 1997; 185:941–951.

41. Dubois B, et al. Critical role of IL-12 in dendritic cell-induced differentiation of naive B lymphocytes. J Immunol 1998; 161:2223–2231.

42. Mortarini R, et al. Autologous dendritic cells derived from CD34+ progenitors and from monocytes are not functionally equivalent antigen-presenting cells in the induction of Melan-A/Mart-1 27–35-specific CTLs from peripheral blood lymphocytes of melanoma patients with low frequency of CTL precursors. Cancer Res 1997; 57:5534–5541.

43. Ferlazzo G, et al. Dendritic cells generated from CD34+ progenitor cells with flt3 ligand, c-kit ligand, GM-CSF, IL-4, and TNF-alpha are functional antigen-presenting cells resembling mature monocyte-derived dendritic cells. J Immunother 2000; 23:48–58.

44. Dhodapkar MV, et al. Antigen specific inhibition of effector T cell function in humans after injection of immature dendritic cells. J Exp Med 2001; 193:233–238.

45. Dhodapkar MV, et al. Mature dendritic cells boost functionally superior T cells in humans without foreign helper epitopes. J Clin Invest 2000; 105:R9–R14.

46. Dhodapkar MV, Steinman RM. Antigen-bearing, immature dendritic cells induce peptide-specific, CD8+ regulatory T cells in vivo in humans. Blood 2002; 100:174–177.

47. Banchereau J, et al. Immune and clinical responses in patients with metastatic melanoma to CD34(+) progenitor-derived dendritic cell vaccine. Cancer Res 2001; 61:6451–6458.

48. Thurner B, et al. Vaccination with MAGE-3A1 peptide-pulsed mature, monocyte-derived dendritic cells expands specific cytotoxic T cells and induces regression of some metastases in advanced stage IV melanoma. J Exp Med 1999; 190:1669–1678.

49. Schuler-Thurner B, et al. Rapid induction of tumor-specific type 1 T helper cells in metastatic melanoma patients by vaccination with mature, cryopreserved, peptide-loaded monocyte-derived dendritic cells. J Exp Med 2002; 195:1279–1288.

50. Nestle FO, et al. Vaccination of melanoma patients with peptide- or tumor lysate-pulsed dendritic cells. Nat Med 1998; 4:328–332.

51. Jonuleit H, et al. A comparison of two types of dendritic cells as adjuvants for the induction of melanoma-specific T cell responses in humans following intranodal injection. Int J Cancer 2001; 93:243–251.

52. Marchand M, et al. Tumor regressions observed in patients with metastatic melanoma treated with an antigenic peptide encoded by gene MAGE-3 and presented by HLA-A1. Int J Cancer 1999; 80:219–230.

53. Schuler-Thurner B, et al. MAGE-3 and influenza-matrix peptide-specific cytotoxic T cells are inducible in terminal stage HLA-A2.1+ melanoma patients by mature monocyte-derived dendritic cells. J Immunol 2000; 165:3492–3496.

54. Panelli MC, et al. Phase 1 study in patients with metastatic melanoma of immunization with dendritic cells presenting

epitopes derived from the melanoma-associated antigens MART-1 and gp100. J Immunother 2000; 23:487–498.

55. Toungouz M, et al. Transient expansion of peptide-specific lymphocytes producing IFN-gamma after vaccination with dendritic cells pulsed with MAGE peptides in patients with MAGE-A1/A3-positive tumors. J Leukoc Biol 2001; 69:937–943.

56. Lau R, et al. Phase I trial of intravenous peptide-pulsed dendritic cells in patients with metastatic melanoma. J Immunother 2001; 24:66–78.

57. Andersen MH, et al. Induction of systemic CTL responses in melanoma patients by dendritic cell vaccination: cessation of CTL responses is associated with disease progression. Int J Cancer 2001; 94:820–824.

58. Chang AE, et al. A phase I trial of tumor lysate-pulsed dendritic cells in the treatment of advanced cancer. Clin Cancer Res 2002; 8:1021–1032.

59. Mackensen A, et al. Phase I study in melanoma patients of a vaccine with peptide-pulsed dendritic cells generated in vitro from CD34$^+$ hematopoietic progenitor cells. Int J Cancer 2000; 86:385–392.

60. Van Tendeloo VF, et al. Highly efficient gene delivery by mRNA electroporation in human hematopoietic cells: superiority to lipofection and passive pulsing of mRNA and to electroporation of plasmid cDNA for tumor antigen loading of dendritic cells. Blood 2001; 98:49–56.

61. Kalergis AM, Ravetch JV. Inducing tumor immunity through the selective engagement of activating Fcγ receptors on dendritic cells. J Exp Med 2002; 195:1653–1659.

62. Rafiq K, et al. Immune complex-mediated antigen presentation induces tumor immunity. J Clin Invest 2002; 110:71–79.

63. Ferlazzo G, et al. Human dendritic cells activate resting NK cells and are recognized via the NKp30 receptor by activated NK cells. J Exp Med 2002; 195:343–351.

81
Vaccines Against Alzheimer's Disease

Roy M. Robins-Browne, Richard A. Strugnell, and Colin L. Masters
University of Melbourne, Parkville, Victoria, Australia

I. INTRODUCTION

Alzheimer's disease (AD) is a progressive neurological disorder that imposes an enormous burden on society [1]. Unlike some other progressive neurological diseases, such as subacute sclerosing panencephalitis, progressive multifocal leukoencephalopathy, and Creutzfeldt–Jakob disease, there is no evidence to suggest that AD is the result of an infection. Hence it is all the more remarkable that AD may be the first of the chronic degenerative neurological diseases to be amenable to specific intervention through therapeutic and preventative immunization.

In common with other degenerative diseases of the nervous systems, AD is characterized by gradually evolving progressive neuronal degeneration, which leads to global impairment of memory and other cognitive functions in a way that interferes with normal social or occupational performance (dementia) [2]. As the disease progresses, behavioral changes occur including passivity and withdrawal, accompanied by impairment of attention, judgment, recognition, insight, and language. Later, agitation, suspiciousness, wandering, and hallucinations may occur. In the final stages, patients may enter a vegetative state and be mute and uncomprehending.

The condition was formally described in 1907 by Alois Alzheimer who reported the clinical and pathological findings of a disease in a 51-year-old woman with progressive dementia [3]. Although senile dementia (dementia occurring in older people) was well known at that time, this patient was unusual because of her young age and because an autopsy revealed large numbers of "amyloid plaques" and "neurofibrillary tangles" in her brain. This unique combination of clinical and pathological features came to be known as AD, a term which was originally limited to "presenile" dementia, i.e., dementia occurring below the age of 65, but now is applied to all patients with these clinicopathological features regardless of age.

Although AD may affect people in younger age groups, most patients are aged over 65 with the prevalence increasing with advancing age, such that up to 10% of the population over 65 and 50% over 80 may be affected [2]. The duration of the disease from the time of diagnosis to death may exceed 20 years, although the average length is from 8 to 10 years. In 1993, Rice et al. [4] estimated the cost of AD in the United States to be $63.3 billion, made up from direct financial outlays, such as nursing care, and indirect costs, including loss of productivity of the patients themselves and the family members who care for them. As people born in the population boom which followed World War II reach their 60s and 70s, these costs are poised to escalate considerably unless something is done to reduce the incidence of AD.

II. PATHOLOGY

The hallmark pathological lesions of AD are the extracellular neuritic or amyloid plaques and the intracellular neurofibrillary tangles originally described by Alzheimer. The characteristic plaques are distributed throughout the cerebral cortex at a high density and are made up mainly of degenerated neuronal processes (neurites) and deposits of beta-amyloid (Aβ) protein, which also occurs within the walls of cerebral blood vessels. Neurofibrillary tangles are intraneuronal structures that appear as paired helical filaments when viewed by electron microscopy. They are particularly evident in medial temporal lobe structures, including the hippocampus, a region of the brain that is important for memory [2]. Neurons which contain these tangles have a tendency to lose their synaptic connections and eventually die leaving "ghost tangles." Although the accumulation of amyloid plaques and neurofibrillary tangles may occur in the brain of nondemented persons, both types of lesion occur at a far higher density in the brain of patients with AD [2].

III. PATHOGENESIS

An overwhelming body of evidence points to the fact that the Aβ protein plays a central role in the pathogenesis of AD. Aβ is derived from amyloid precursor protein (APP), a type I transmembrane protein encoded by the *APP* gene on chromosome 21 [5]. Amyloid precursor protein is expressed in a variety of tissues, including neurons and glia, and contains a large extracellular domain, a single transmembrane domain, and a small cytoplasmic tail (Figure 1). There are three main isoforms of APP derived by alternative splicing of the single APP gene. The two larger forms known as APP_{751} and APP_{770} contain a 56-amino acid domain with homology to serine protease inhibitors [6]. APP_{695} is the shortest form because it lacks this domain and is the most common form in neurons. The function of APP_{695} is not known, but in neurons it occurs mainly in synapses and seems likely to influence neuronal communication. Over-expression of APP suggests that it may have an antiadhesion function. Mice lacking APP show only minor defects in neural function, perhaps due to compensation by an APP-like protein. Amyloid precursor protein is subject to extensive posttranslational modification in the endoplasmic reticulum, the Golgi apparatus, and the trans-Golgi network before being exported to the cell surface [5]. It is then further modified by proteolytic cleavage by a series of enzymes collectively termed secretases. Most APP is processed by cleavage with α-secretase releasing a soluble ectodomain $APPs_{\alpha}$, into the extracellular space with retention of an intracellular C-terminal fragment (CTF_{α}). Processing via this pathway prevents the formation of full-length Aβ (Figure 1). By contrast, β-secretase (also known as β-APP cleaving enzyme or BACE-1) cleaves APP at a site immediately N-terminal to the Aβ sequence, approximately 16 amino acids closer to the extracellular N-terminus of APP [7] (Figure 1). In the nervous system, β-secretase activity is more prominent than in other tissues, thus favoring the production of Aβ. Another key enzyme in the production of Aβ is γ-secretase which cleaves APP within the transmembrane region at the C-terminus of Aβ in a manner that releases soluble Aβ from the cell [8]. The exact cleavage site of γ-secretase may vary slightly giving

rise to peptides 40 to 43 amino acids in length. The most common species is $A\beta_{40}$ which is typically found in non-neuronal cells and tends to be more soluble than $A\beta_{42}$ and $A\beta_{43}$ [8]. However, neuronal cells have a greater propensity to produce $A\beta_{42}$ which is a major protein species at the center of senile plaques. Even in the brain, however, 90% of Aβ is $A\beta_{40}$, with the remainder being the less soluble and more fibrillogenic $A\beta_{42/43}$ [5]. If the rate of production of $A\beta_{42}$ exceeds its rate of clearance, it may accumulate in the brain to cause neuronal toxicity.

The basis of the toxic action of Aβ is unknown, but there is a suggestion that secreted oligomers of Aβ can inhibit hippocampal long-term potentiation, thus interfering the development of memory [9]. In addition, the accumulation of Aβ fibrils on the cell surface may encourage the formation of free radicals that damage cell membranes and lead to neuronal death [10].

The neurofibrillary tangles, which are the other hallmark histopathological lesion of AD, are made up mainly from the microtubule-associated protein *tau*, the normal function of which appears to be to stabilize microtubules. This function is regulated in the cell by the reversible phosphorylation and dephosphorylation of *tau*. The observation that *tau* in neurofibrillary tangles is excessively phosphorylated suggests that in affected neurons, the balance between the action of kinases and phosphatases is disturbed [1]. In neurons, microtubules are involved in the axonal transport of proteins. The accumulation of abnormally phosphorylated *tau* may lead to destabilization of the cytoskeleton, neuronal dysfunction, and eventually to neuronal death. One possible underlying cause of the abnormal phosphorylation of *tau* in AD may be the presence of Aβ itself. Interestingly, mutations in the *tau* gene lead to accumulation of aggregated *tau* [11]. Patients with this type of disordered *tau* present with dementia which unlike AD is characterized by frontal lobe atrophy and prominent behavioral abnormalities.

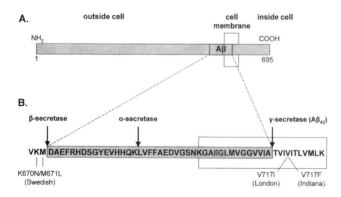

Figure 1 A. Diagrammatic representation of amyloid precursor protein (APP_{695}). B. An enlarged view of amyloid β-protein (Aβ). The α-, β-, and γ-secretase cleavage sites are indicated by arrows, and selected familial Alzheimer disease mutations are shown below. Transgenic mice with the Swedish, London, and Indiana mutations and variations thereof have been used in some immunization studies.

IV. GENETICS OF ALZHEIMER'S DISEASE

Apart from age, the most significant risk factor for the development of AD is genetic. Familial AD, which accounts for fewer than 10% of all cases, is inherited in an autosomal dominant fashion. Apart from the fact that it generally occurs at a younger age, often less than 60, familial AD is indistinguishable, clinically and pathologically, from the sporadic form of the disease. Importantly, unraveling the genetic basis of familial AD has provided key insights into the molecular pathogenesis of AD in general, including strong support for the idea that Aβ plays a central role in its pathogenesis.

Early evidence for the role of chromosome 21 in the development of AD came from the observation that individuals with Down's syndrome (trisomy 21) show identical pathological changes in the brain to those found in AD and often develop this condition while still in their 30s [12]. Intensive study of chromosome 21 revealed that some individuals with familial AD carry a point mutation within the APP gene [5,13]. One of these mutations is the so-called

"Swedish" mutation, a two-point mutation at amino acids 670 and 671 from Lys-Met to Asp-Leu. This change is upstream of the β-cleavage site (Figure 1) and results in a fivefold to eightfold increase in the formation of both $A\beta_{40}$ and $A\beta_{42}$. A second mutation at amino acid 717, the "London" mutation, Val→Ile, is adjacent to the γ-cleavage site and specifically increases the production of $A\beta_{42}$. Although cases with these mutations account for less than 3% of all patients with early onset familial AD, the discovery of these mutations was vital in showing the clear link between abnormal APP processing and AD. Presumably, the association of Down's syndrome with AD is due to the overproduction of APP and consequently Aβ [12].

The largest proportion of patients with familial AD carries mutations in the presenilin gene (*PS1*) on chromosome 14 [5]. The product of this gene is a large transmembrane protein that is likely to be an integral component of γ-secretase [14]. *PS1* shares homology with a gene on chromosome 1 known as *PS2* [15]. One consequence of *PS1* mutations is enhanced production of $A\beta_{42}$, suggesting that these mutations influence the activity of γ-secretase. Thus, collectively, most early onset familial forms of AD are explained by excessive production of $A\beta_{42}$ either as a result of missense mutations in APP at or near the cleavage site of β- or γ-secretase or by abnormal γ-secretase activity per se.

Despite the persuasive evidence incriminating Aβ metabolism as the key abnormality in familial forms of AD, the molecular pathogenesis of sporadic, late onset of AD is poorly understood. The risk of late onset AD is linked with the inheritance of particular isoforms of apolipoprotein E (ApoE) [16]. Apolipoprotein E is a major serum protein involved in cholesterol metabolism transport and storage. The gene for ApoE is located on chromosome 19 and occurs as three common allelic variants termed ApoE2, ApoE3, and ApoE4, the products of which differ by only 1 amino acid. Individuals with the ApoE4 allele are significantly more likely to develop AD than those without it, with ApoE4 homozygous individuals at greatest risk [16]. Although there is no evidence to suggest that ApoE4 is directly responsible for the development of AD, it may modify the expression of the disease by involvement in Aβ deposition or clearance.

V. ANIMAL MODELS

Because much of the research which led to the serendipitous possibility of prophylactic and therapeutic immunization for AD has come from animal models of this disease, it is useful to consider some of these models. Before the identification of the genetic mutations associated with familial AD, animal models were mainly developed to reproduce the nonspecific neuropathology of AD, such as neuronal damage. The discovery of the genetic basis of familial AD, however, permitted the generation of transgenic mice which display various features of AD [5,13,17].

Early attempts to develop transgenic AD mice involved transfection with the normal human APP gene either in its entirety or as a C-terminal fragment. However, these animals failed to develop plaques presumably because they produced APP at approximately endogenous concentrations. Subsequent work showed that a key factor in plaque development is an elevated concentration of $A\beta_{42}$. This can be achieved through the use of promoters, such as platelet-derived growth factor (PDGF), prion protein, or Thy-1, to drive higher levels of protein expression [5]. High concentrations of Aβ are also obtained when APP with the Indiana, London, or Swedish mutations are used for transfection instead of the wild-type gene.

The first successful mouse model of AD was reported in 1995 by Games et al. and termed PDAPP[18]. This model is based on a complex genetic construct consisting of the promoter for the β-chain of PDGF and a mini-gene containing cDNA of portions of APP introns 6–8 bearing a V717F mutation in APP. PDAPP mice contain approximately 40 copies of the transgene and produce human APP mRNA at levels significantly greater than endogenous App transcripts and levels of APP approximately 10 times greater than endogenous mouse APP. At 8 months of age, these animals develop deposits of Aβ in the hippocampus, corpus callosum, and cerebral cortex. Although they suffer no significant loss of neurons, they do show impaired ability to perform novel "spatial" memory tasks in an age-dependent manner that correlates with the accumulation of Aβ deposits [19].

In 1996, a second mouse model, termed Tg2576, was developed. These animals express the 695 amino acid form of human APP carrying the Swedish mutation (K670N/M671L) under the transcriptional control of the hamster prion gene promoter, PrP [20]. The levels of APP produced by these mice are approximately 5 to 6 times higher than endogenous App, and they develop Aβ deposits at 9 to 11 months of age. Tg2576 mice also show disordered behavior and memory in tasks involving different types of mazes. Another cDNA transgenic model that has been used in vaccine studies is termed TgCRND8 [21]. These mice carry full-length APP695 cDNA with both the K670N/M671L and V717F mutations under the control of hamster PrP. In these animals, the APP transgene is expressed at levels 5 times greater than endogenous App, and Aβ deposits occur as early as 3 months of age. The development of these and several other varieties of transgenic mice, which express abnormal APP, has established the relationship between APP, Aβ production, and disorders of memory. Interestingly, however, although some of these transgenic mice show modest loss of neurons and nerve synapses, none of these animals develops full-blown neurofibrillary tangles or shows the pronounced neurodegeneration that is found in patients with AD [5]. These observations suggest that the production of Aβ is not directly related to the development of tangles in mice, although it is possible that mice do not live long enough to develop this pathological change.

VI. IMMUNIZATION

The first indication that AD may be amenable to prevention or even treatment by immunization came in 1999 from a report by Schenk et al. [22] of Elan Pharmaceuticals. In this study, PDAPP transgenic mice were immunized 11 times with 100 μg of a synthetic peptide preparation of human Aβ42 together with Freund's adjuvant. Control mice received either serum amyloid peptide (SAP), phosphate-buffered saline (PBS), or were left untreated. Mice given Aβ42 developed and maintained high titers of serum antibody to this peptide. These antibodies cross-reacted with mouse Aβ without causing obvious tissue damage. One group of mice in this study was immunized over a period of 11 months starting at 6 weeks of age, i.e., before the development of amyloid plaques. These mice were killed at age 13 months, and their brains were compared to those of the three control groups. The results showed that mice immunized with Aβ42 had significantly less ($P \leq 0.001$) Aβ burden (0%, as measured by quantitative image analysis) compared with the groups which received PBS (2.2%), SAP (5.7%), or no treatment (2.7%). In addition, the presence of dystrophic neurites was reduced from 0.3% in controls to 0% in immunized animals, and immunoreactivity for glial fibrillary acidic protein, which is a marker of Aβ plaque-associated gliosis, was reduced from 6% in control mice to 1.6% in those given Aβ42. This study indicates that immunization with Aβ42 can prevent the development of AD-like neuropathological lesions in PDAPP mice. However, it was unclear if immunization could influence the course of the disease if plaques were present when immunization was started. To address this important issue, Schenk et al. [22] immunized some PDAPP mice that were 11 months old, an age when numerous Aβ plaques are already present. Half the mice were killed after 4 months of treatment, and the rest were killed 3 months later. The results were that immunized mice showed a 96% reduction in plaques after 4 months treatment, and greater than 99% reduction after 7 months, compared with controls ($P < 0.001$). Moreover, the Aβ burden in the 7-month treatment group was 0.01% compared with 4.9% in control animals given PBS. Similar findings have been reported by other workers using DgCRND8 and Tg2576 mice [21,23].

Despite these encouraging results, it was not known if the reduction in pathological changes due to the immunization would result in improvements in cognitive function. This question was addressed by Morgan et al. [23] who used a combination of a swim maze and radial arm maze to evaluate cognitive defects in Tg2576 and PS1N146L double transgenic mice. These mice show high levels of Aβ production and plaque development by 12 weeks of age that increases nearly 200-fold by 1 year. The memory task used by Morgan et al. [23] requires mice to learn the spatial location of a submerged escape platform on the basis of visual clues and to navigate the platform from different starting points. Transgenic and control mice were immunized with either Aβ42 or a placebo protein, the keyhole limpet hemocyanin (KLH). Normal mice showed no change in cognitive function after immunization with either protein, demonstrating that immunization with Aβ42 has no overt deleterious effect on these animals. As expected, transgenic mice immunized with KLH at 11.5 months of age showed virtually no learning ability 4 months later, but the Aβ-immunized transgenic mice showed cognitive performance similar to that of nontransgenic animals. Aβ-immunized mice also demonstrated a partial reduction in amyloid burden at the

end of the study. Similar findings were obtained by Janus et al. [21] in TgCRND8 mice (APP695K670N/M671L and V717F), which normally develop increased soluble Aβ, amyloid plaques, and deficits in spatial learning at 3 months of age. In this study, age- and sex-matched transgenic mice and nontransgenic littermates were immunized at 6, 8, 12, 16, and 20 weeks of age with either Aβ42 or a control protein, islet-associated polypeptide, as β-pleated sheets. Through the use of the more conventional water maze than that used by Morgan et al. [23], these investigators showed that repeated vaccination of TgCRND8 mice with Aβ42 reduced cognitive dysfunction concurrently with reduced cerebral fibrillar Aβ compared with control mice, although total levels of Aβ in the brain were not affected. Based on these somewhat unexpected results, Janus et al. concluded that either an approximately 50% reduction in dense-core Aβ plaques is sufficient to improve cognition or that immunization may modulate the activity or abundance of a small subpopulation of especially toxic Aβ species [21].

Analysis of the immune response of *PS1* transgenic mice to immunization with Aβ42 in complete Freund's adjuvant revealed that specific antibodies are detectable only after the third boost [24], with highest antibody responses directed against the N-terminus of Aβ. After the sixth dose, antibody titers tend to plateau and thereafter are maintained above the half-maximal titer for at least 5 months without further boosting. Assays of specific immunoglobulin isotypes in mice immunized with Aβ have demonstrated a preponderance of specific IgG$_1$ and IgG$_{2B}$, indicating a Th2-type immune response [24].

The key role of specific antibodies in mediating the amyloid depleting effects of Aβ immunization has been shown in a series of studies involving passive immunization with anti-Aβ antibodies. Bard et al. [25] treated 8- to 12-month-old PDAPP mice for 5 months with weekly injections of murine monoclonal or polyclonal antibodies directed against Aβ and reduced plaque burden by more than 80% with a corresponding reduction in cortical levels of Aβ42. The key role of antibodies was confirmed by the finding that T cells from passively immunized mice showed no proliferative response when stimulated with Aβ, indicating that plaque clearance does not require T-cell immunity. An important finding in this study was that, contrary to expectations, antibodies that had been administered peripherally entered the central nervous system and bound to amyloid plaques [25]. An ex vivo assay with sections of brain tissue from PDAPP mice or patients with AD showed that antibodies to Aβ could trigger microglial cells to clear plaque through Fc receptor-mediated phagocytosis with subsequent peptide disaggregation. A separate study showed that the direct application of anti-Aβ antibodies to the surface of the brain of living PDAPP mice can reduce Aβ deposits in the immediate vicinity of the application [26]. The unexpected finding that peripherally administered antibodies can traverse the blood–brain barrier may be explained by the fact that Aβ itself is transported across this barrier by a receptor-mediated pathway, and that antibodies bound to Aβ may be able to utilize the same pathway [27]. For passive immunization to succeed in humans, therefore, there needs to be a critical concentration of circulating Aβ, which generally is far lower than in transgenic mice [28]. Another potential problem with passive immunization of humans against AD is that Aβ peptides within the plaques of transgenic mice are physically and chemically distinct from those found in AD, with the latter often displaying a degraded N-terminus, extensive posttranslational modifications, and a reduced tendency towards disaggregation [29]. On the other hand, some studies suggest that the major targets of anti-Aβ antibodies are not plaques per se, but soluble toxic oligomers of Aβ [9,30]. This observation provides an explanation for the finding that the cognitive function of TgCRND8 mice immunized with Aβ showed significant improvements without a major reduction in plaque burden [21].

An alternative view of how peripherally administered antibodies may be beneficial in mouse models of AD has been provided by DeMattos et al. [31] who administered an anti-Aβ monoclonal antibody intravenously to PDAPP mice and showed that this leads to a 1000-fold increase in plasma levels of Aβ. Because levels of Aβ in plasma of untreated animals are low, DeMattos et al. proposed that antibodies in the plasma act as a "peripheral sink" which promotes the efflux of Aβ from the brain to the plasma. These authors went on to show that long-term administration of antibody significantly reduced Aβ burden in the brain without the antibody crossing the blood–brain barrier or binding to intracerebral Aβ. The reasons for the differences between the findings of Bard et al. [25] and DeMattos et al. [31] regarding the transport of anti-Aβ antibodies across the blood–brain barrier are not clear, but there is no doubt that peripherally administered antibodies can deplete Aβ in the brain of transgenic mice. Whether such treatment will be effective in humans with AD is unknown. If the principal target of anti-Aβ is soluble Aβ, active or passive immunization of patients with established AD may be less effective than vaccinating individuals with early disease. Accordingly, effective implementation of a vaccine for AD would necessitate large-scale screening of the general population to identify at-risk individuals who could benefit from immunization.

Because there are no established animal models of AD other than transgenic mice, further studies of Aβ vaccine efficacy would need to be undertaken in humans. In preparation for this, several investigators have examined modes of vaccine delivery that do not require Freund's adjuvant, which is not licensed for use in humans. Some of the alternative approaches to vaccine delivery, which have been successfully trialed in animal models, include mucosal (intranasal) immunization with Aβ40 [32] and parenteral administration of Aβ42 in biodegradable poly(lactide-co-glycolide) microspheres [33].

In an attempt to reduce the potential toxicity of Aβ42, which can cross the blood–brain barrier to form toxic fibrils and possibly seed new fibril formation, Sigurdsson et al. [34] used nontoxic–nonamyloidogenic Aβ homologous peptide $(K6A\beta_{1-30}-NH_2)$ to immunize Tg2576 mice. This peptide retains the two major immunogenic sites of intact Aβ, which are contained within residues 1–11 and 22–28 of Aβ42. This study showed that administration of this compound for 7 months reduced cortical and hippocampal brain amyloid

burden by between 80% and 90% and reduced brain levels of soluble Aβ42 by 57% [34]. An even more reductionist approach to immunization was taken by Frenkel et al. [35] who immunized guinea pigs with a genetically engineered filamentous phage displaying the epitope, EFRH, which correspond to amino acids 3–6 within Aβ (Figure 1). As this region of Aβ controls the formation and the disaggregation of Aβ fibrils, binding of antibodies to this epitope prevents self-aggregation of Aβ as well as enabling the resolubilization of preformed aggregates [36]. Apart from lower toxicity, the phage delivery system also has the advantage of being highly immunogenic, thus obviating the need for separate adjuvants. The use of a phage delivery system may also overcome the immune hyporesponsiveness to Aβ found in certain strains of transgenic mice, which could of itself contribute to the pathogenesis of AD while simultaneously reducing the potential efficacy of future immunization strategies based on Aβ [37].

VII. IMMUNIZATION OF HUMANS

The encouraging results obtained with Aβ immunization of transgenic mice were followed by safety data in monkeys and led to fast tracking of human trials of Aβ immunization [38]. A Phase I/II trial to examine the safety of a synthetic Aβ42 vaccine, known as AN-1792, administered as a single dose to patients with moderate AD was commenced in December 1999 and showed the vaccine to be well tolerated. In early 2002, however, reports emerged of a severe reaction resembling experimental allergic encephalitis in 15 of 400 recipients of AN-1792 [39]. As a result, all clinical trials with this material have been suspended [40]. Whether other modalities of Aβ immunization would produce similar reactions is not known, but clearly, this early setback will necessitate improved understanding of vaccine action and toxicity. Possible explanations for the toxicity of AN-1792 include harm directly attributable to the peripheral administration of Aβ42 per se or the development of immunity to APP and Aβ peptides which are normal constituents of brain tissue. In this regard, the success of Aβ immunization in transgenic mice may rely on the fact that immunity is directed against a protein of human origin and that endogenous mouse proteins are less well recognized or affected by antihuman Aβ antibodies. For this reason, it would be important to know the effects of hyperimmunizing mice with murine Aβ.

The setback experienced in early human trials of AD vaccines does not necessarily spell the end of immunization against this disease. One major consequence of the experience with AN-1792, however, will be an increased need to address the safety of future vaccine candidates. Strategies to avoid vaccine-induced encephalitis could include the construction of vaccines lacking the T-cell epitopes which trigger adverse reactions or vaccines that target novel epitopes on abnormal forms of Aβ. The design of such second-generation vaccines would be facilitated by an improved understanding of the pathogenesis of AD, including the physiological roles of APP and Aβ and the consequences of artificially induced anti-Aβ immunity. The increasing prevalence of AD, its potentially enormous costs, and the promise of its prevention or arrest through immunological interventions ensure that the search for an effective AD vaccine will continue.

REFERENCES

1. Gilman S. Alzheimer's disease. Perspect Biol Med 1997; 40: 230–245.
2. Bennett DA, Evans DA. Alzheimer's disease. Dis-Mon 1992; 38:1–64.
3. Alzheimer A, et al. An English translation of Alzheimer's 1907 paper, "Über eine eigenartige Erkankung der Hirnrinde". Clin Anat 1995; 8:429–431.
4. Rice DP, et al. The economic burden of Alzheimer's disease care. Health Aff (Millwood, Va) 1993; 12:164–176.
5. Chapman PF, et al. Genes, models and Alzheimer's disease. Trends Genet 2001; 17:254–261.
6. Sinha S, Lieberburg I. Cellular mechanisms of β-amyloid production and secretion. Proc Natl Acad Sci USA 1999; 96: 11049–11053.
7. Vassar R, et al. β-secretase cleavage of Alzheimer's amyloid precursor protein by the transmembrane aspartic protease BACE. Science 1999; 286:735–741.
8. Hardy J. Amyloid, the presenilins and Alzheimer's disease. Trends Neurosci 1997; 20:154–159.
9. Walsh DM, et al. Naturally secreted oligomers of amyloid β protein potently inhibit hippocampal long-term potentiation in vivo. Nature 2002; 416:535–539.
10. Sano M, et al. A controlled trial of selegiline, alpha-tocopherol, or both as treatment for Alzheimer's disease. The Alzheimer's Disease Cooperative Study. N Engl J Med 1997; 336: 1216–1222.
11. Wilhelmsen KC. The tangled biology of tau. Proc Natl Acad Sci USA 1999; 96:7120–7121.
12. Beyreuther K, et al. Regulation and expression of the Alzheimer's β/A4 amyloid protein precursor in health, disease, and Down's syndrome. Ann NY Acad Sci 1993; 695:91–102.
13. Hock BJ Jr, Lamb BT. Transgenic mouse models of Alzheimer's disease. Trends Genet 2001; 17:S7–S12.
14. Selkoe DJ. Presenilin, Notch, and the genesis and treatment of Alzheimer's disease. Proc Natl Acad Sci USA 2001; 98: 11039–11041.
15. Rogaev EI, et al. Familial Alzheimer's disease in kindreds with missense mutations in a gene on chromosome 1 related to the Alzheimer's disease type 3 gene. Nature 1995; 376:775–778.
16. Strittmatter WJ, Roses AD. Apolipoprotein E and Alzheimer disease. Proc Natl Acad Sci USA 1995; 92:4725–4727.
17. Duff K, Rao MV. Progress in the modeling of neurodegenerative diseases in transgenic mice. Curr Opin Neurol 2001; 14:441–447.
18. Games D, et al. Alzheimer-type neuropathology in transgenic mice overexpressing V717F β-amyloid precursor protein. Nature 1995; 373:523–527.
19. Dodart JC, et al. Behavioral disturbances in transgenic mice overexpressing the V717F β-amyloid precursor protein. Behav Neurosci 1999; 113:982–990.
20. Hsiao K, et al. Correlative memory deficits, Aβ elevation, and amyloid plaques in transgenic mice. Science 1996; 274: 99–102.
21. Janus C, et al. Aβ peptide immunization reduces behavioural impairment and plaques in a model of Alzheimer's disease. Nature 2000; 408:979–982.
22. Schenk D, et al. Immunization with amyloid-β attenuates Alzheimer-disease-like pathology in the PDAPP mouse. Nature 1999; 400:173–177.
23. Morgan D, et al. A β peptide vaccination prevents memory loss in an animal model of Alzheimer's disease. Nature 2000; 408:982–985.
24. Dickey CA, et al. Duration and specificity of humoral immune responses in mice vaccinated with the Alzheimer's disease-associated β-amyloid peptide. DNA Cell Biol 2001; 20:723–729.
25. Bard F, et al. Peripherally administered antibodies against amyloid β-peptide enter the central nervous system and reduce pathology in a mouse model of Alzheimer disease. Nat Med 2000; 6:916–919.
26. Bacskai BJ, et al. Imaging of amyloid-β deposits in brains of living mice permits direct observation of clearance of plaques with immunotherapy. Nat Med 2001; 7:369–372.
27. Poduslo JF, Curran GL. Amyloid β peptide as a vaccine for Alzheimer's disease involves receptor-mediated transport at the blood-brain barrier. NeuroReport 2001; 12:3197–3200.
28. Scheuner D, et al. Secreted amyloid β-protein similar to that in the senile plaques of Alzheimer's disease is increased in vivo by the presenilin 1 and 2 and APP mutations linked to familial Alzheimer's disease. Nat Med 1996; 2:864–870.
29. Kalback W, et al. APP transgenic mice Tg2576 accumulate Aβ peptides that are distinct from the chemically modified and insoluble peptides deposited in Alzheimer's disease senile plaques. Biochemistry 2002; 41:922–928.
30. McLean CA, et al. Soluble pool of Aβ amyloid as a determinant of severity of neurodegeneration in Alzheimer's disease. Ann Neurol 1999; 46:860–866.
31. DeMattos RB, et al. Peripheral anti-Aβ antibody alters CNS and plasma Aβ clearance and decreases brain Aβ burden in a mouse model of Alzheimer's disease. Proc Natl Acad Sci USA 2001; 98:8850–8855.
32. Lemere CA, et al. Nasal vaccination with β-amyloid peptide for the treatment of Alzheimer's disease. DNA Cell Biol 2001; 20:705–711.
33. Brayden DJ, et al. Encapsulation in biodegradable microparticles enhances serum antibody response to parenterally-delivered β-amyloid in mice. Vaccine 2001; 19:4185–4193.
34. Sigurdsson EM, et al. Immunization with a nontoxic/nonfibrillar amyloid-β homologous peptide reduces Alzheimer's disease-associated pathology in transgenic mice. Am J Pathol 2001; 159:439–447.
35. Frenkel D, et al. Immunization against Alzheimer's β-amyloid plaques via EFRH phage administration. Proc Natl Acad Sci USA 2000; 97:11455–11459.
36. Solomon B, et al. Disaggregation of Alzheimer β-amyloid by site-directed mAb. Proc Natl Acad Sci USA 1997; 94:4109–4112.
37. Monsonego A, et al. Immune hyporesponsiveness to amyloid β-peptide in amyloid precursor protein transgenic mice: implications for the pathogenesis and treatment of Alzheimer's disease. Proc Natl Acad Sci USA 2001; 98:10273–10278.
38. Thatte U. AN-1792 (Elan). Curr Opin Investig Drugs 2001; 2:663–667.
39. Check E. Nerve inflammation halts trial for Alzheimer's drug. Nature 2002; 415:462462.
40. Munch G, Robinson SR. Alzheimer's vaccine: a cure as dangerous as the disease? J Neural Transm 2002; 109:537–539.

82

Vaccines Against Atherosclerosis

Carl R. Alving
Walter Reed Army Institute of Research, Silver Spring, Maryland, U.S.A.

I. SUMMARY

The possibility of creating vaccines against atherosclerosis has evolved from epidemiological analyses based on statistical correlations that suggest that certain metabolic states, or even infections, might play a role in the initiation of the atherosclerotic process. Although many theories exist, it is well known that alterations in lipoprotein metabolism, including elevations in low-density lipoprotein (LDL) cholesterol or decreased levels of high-density lipoprotein (HDL) cholesterol, are associated with increased risk of atherosclerosis. Low-density lipoprotein cholesterol may be deposited in vessel walls, leading to buildup of plaque, and HDL serves as a scavenger for removal of circulating cholesterol. The atherosclerotic plaque lesions are associated with chronic inflammatory reactions affecting the endothelial layer of vessel walls.

In recent years, atherosclerotic lesions or adverse events due to atherosclerosis have also been associated with a variety of infectious agents, particularly bacteria (*Chlamydia pneumoniae* and *Helicobacter pylori*), viruses (cytomegalovirus, herpes simplex viruses, and hepatitis A virus), and even periodontal infections, or combinations of the above. Although a vaccine against a single organism (such as *C. pneumoniae*) might have utility, such a vaccine might not serve as a generic antiatherosclerosis vaccine. This is because the adverse effect caused by the total pathogen burden of multiple infections appears to be a much greater risk factor than that associated with any single organism. Among the mechanisms associated with infections, the process of inflammation, as detected by elevation of serum C-reactive protein (CRP), may be an important factor that correlates with atherosclerosis.

Other atherosclerosis vaccine strategies that have been proposed, besides those directed at infectious organisms, include metabolic vaccines that directly target cholesterol or influence lipoprotein distribution patterns. Cholesterol is a strong antigen when combined with the proper adjuvant, and antibodies to cholesterol react with LDL but not HDL. Immunization with cholesterol results in a lowering of serum LDL levels and partial protection against cholesterol-induced atherosclerosis in rabbits. An alternative metabolic vaccine consists of therapeutic immunization against endogenous cholesteryl ester transfer protein (CETP), a key intermediary in the distribution of cholesterol between HDL and LDL. Antibody-mediated inhibition of CETP causes substantial elevation of HDL relative to LDL in rabbits. If this result is also observed in the Phase 2 studies that are currently ongoing in humans, it may be an important observation because elevations of HDL are not easily achieved by current drug therapy strategies. Metabolic vaccines may serve as an alternative to, or may be complementary to, current dietary or therapeutic methods for control of LDL cholesterol levels.

II. INTRODUCTION

Although deaths due to atherosclerosis in the United States declined approximately 20% between 1978 and 1998, cardiovascular disease still contributes 80% as much total mortality as all other diseases combined, and 71% of the total cardiovascular disease is due to atherosclerosis-related diseases [1,2]. This is all the more remarkable because mortality due to atherosclerotic coronary heart disease, one of the biggest killers, decreased by about 60% between 1963 and 1998 [2]. More than 400,000 coronary artery bypass graft (CABG) surgeries are performed each year [3]. If each CABG were to cost an average between $50,000 and $75,000, this alone would amount to an annual economic outlay of $20–$30 billion. The annual bill for pharmaceuticals or nutriceuticals for lowering cholesterol levels also amounts to tens of billions of dollars. These staggering statistics make a strong case that development of a vaccine strategy for controlling atherosclerosis would have immense public health benefits for reducing pain and suffering, and such a strategy would also have extremely important economic benefits.

The purpose of this chapter is to introduce two general types of vaccine strategies that have been proposed for prophylaxis or treatment of atherosclerosis. First, a brief overview of recent data is presented that suggests that certain infectious diseases that might be controlled with vaccines may be associated with atherosclerosis. Second, it is well known that high levels of LDL and low levels of HDL are classic and important risk factors for atherosclerosis. Unique vaccines, which I refer to as metabolic vaccines, are described that may serve to improve the profile of circulating lipoproteins and thereby decrease the risk of atherosclerosis.

A. What Is Atherosclerosis?

Amazing as it may seem, the answer to the above question has not yet been completely worked out. There are multiple conflicting theories. The most popular viewpoint among those who specialize in this field is that atherosclerosis is an ongoing process. The atherosclerotic process may be viewed as either a local inflammatory reaction involving endothelial linings and smooth muscles of arterial vessels, or a local immune reaction leading to destructive inflammatory effects [4,5]. The popular term for atherosclerosis, hardening of the arteries, is a reflection of the gradual buildup of inflammatory atherosclerotic plaque below the endothelial surface that becomes hardened due to accumulation of inflammatory cells and deposition of fibrous material containing cholesterol, lipoproteins, calcium, and other molecules, a process known as atherogenesis. In the advanced stages of this process the enlarging plaque may either directly interfere with the flow of blood, or may rupture, often with the resultant formation of a thrombus in the vasculature that prevents the delivery of oxygen to tissues and causes the diseases known as myocardial or cerebral infarction, gangrene of extremities, or other diseases or syndromes that are commonly associated with oxygen deprivation.

The histological evidence for a pathological local inflammatory reaction in arterial walls seems clear enough, but what causes the process to begin, and why does it continue? Definitive answers to these important questions would yield significant benefits for continued scientific development of rational preventive or therapeutic measures that could help to control atherosclerosis and its sequelae. Many etiological theories have been floated, among which are the so-called "insult" hypothesis; the metabolic dysfunction hypothesis; the processes of pathological innate or adaptive immune reactions; and various theories about the colonization of arterial walls by infectious agents.

According to the insult hypothesis, "The lesions result from an excessive inflammatory-fibroproliferative response to various forms of insult to the endothelium and smooth muscle of the artery wall" [4]. One view of the metabolic dysfunction hypothesis is that "Atherosclerosis is an inflammatory disease induced by a lipid metabolic disturbance at sites of hemodynamic strain in the vasculature." [5]. According to the innate or adaptive immunity hypothesis, "The inflammatory response is controlled by the immune system, components of which are abundant in the atherosclerotic plaque" [5].

Atherosclerosis is obviously a multifactorial process that probably does not have a single cause. Epidemiological studies have identified numerous risk factors that have led to a variety of recommendations by the National Cholesterol Education Program for prevention of coronary heart diseases (CHDs) [6]. Primary among these risk factors are high LDL cholesterol, low HDL cholesterol, cigarette smoking, hypertension, family history of premature CHD, and increased age [6]. Numerous other risk factors have also been cited, including abdominal obesity, and secondary dyslipidemia due to diabetes, hypothyroidism, obstructive liver diseases, chronic renal failure, and certain drugs, such as progestins, anabolic steroids, and corticosteroids, that increase LDL cholesterol and decrease HDL cholesterol [6]. If the cardiovascular system were viewed as a kind of river, the identification of risk factors for atherosclerosis at any given point would provide epidemiological evidence of upstream factors unrelated to atherosclerosis that may or may not encourage the downstream development of localized atherosclerotic lesions in vessel walls in a given individual. Just as the deposition of silt occurs at the outlet of a river, or accumulation of pollution occurs at a downstream location, atherosclerosis in an artery is an adverse local effect that may be caused or initiated by upstream forces that may be quite distant or unrelated to the local environment of the damaged area. Research on risk factors for atherosclerosis has led to the pinpointing of effective public health measures and therapeutic strategies for lowering the incidence of cardiovascular diseases.

III. INFECTIOUS DISEASE HYPOTHESIS

A. Chlamydia pneumoniae as an Etiological Agent for Atherosclerosis

The infectious disease hypothesis of initiation of atherosclerosis is an idea proposed many decades ago (reviewed in Ref. 7). The hypothesis was given renewed impetus by the rediscovery, in Finland, of an epidemiological association of a serological reaction to lipopolysaccharide from *Chlamydia* species, a gram-negative bacterial venereal infection associated with lymphogranuloma venereum, with acute myocardial infarction [8–10]. *C. pneumoniae* probably existed for many decades, or longer, but the organism was first isolated in 1965 [11]. It causes mild episodes of chronic pneumonia [12], and has been estimated to be the cause of perhaps 10% of community-acquired pneumonia, and 5% of bronchitis and sinusitis [11]. Infection with *C. pneumoniae* is thought to occur in virtually all individuals in their lifetimes, and it can have a detectable antibody prevalence of 80% in certain populations [11]. *C. pneumoniae* has been directly suggested as a factor in the initiation or exacerbation of atherosclerosis-associated diseases and in precipitation of acute thrombotic events [13–18].

The case for *C. pneumoniae* as an etiological agent has been further strengthened by direct observation of the organism in lesions, both by electron microscopy and by a variety of other microscopic and analytic techniques, and by culture of the organism from atherosclerotic lesions [19,20].

Interestingly, it has also been reported that peptides isolated from outer membrane proteins of several *Chlamydia* species exhibit sequence homology to murine heart muscle-specific alpha myosin heavy chain [21]. When *Chlamydia* DNA was used as an adjuvant, the peptides also induced autoantibodies and inflammatory heart disease in mice [21].

It has been estimated that "since 1988 more than 30 worldwide, epidemiological studies indicated correlations between *C. pneumoniae*-associated serological markers ... and atherosclerotic vascular disease" [22]. However, the conclusion that *C. pneumoniae* is a risk factor has caused considerable controversy, and other serological studies have failed to identify *C. pneumoniae* as a risk factor for atherosclerosis [23,24]. Therefore, despite the large amount of interesting data that suggests that *C. pneumoniae* may be a risk factor, the precise role, if any, of the organism in initiation of atherosclerosis is an important question that is still unresolved. Nonetheless, the hypothesis, and the considerable evidence, that *C. pneumoniae* might play a role, has started a growing interest in the possible effects of infectious agents in atherosclerosis.

B. Role of Other Infectious Agents

Numerous other infections have also been implicated in the pathogenesis of atherosclerosis including, most prominently *H. pylori*, cytomegalovirus, herpes simplex virus. Epstein–Barr virus, measles virus, hepatitis A virus, and even markers of chronic dental infection, such as severe periodontal disease and missing teeth [24–26]. Although the infectious disease risk hypothesis for atherosclerosis was initially associated mainly with *C. pneumoniae*, other studies have found independent risks associated with other infections, but not for *C. pneumoniae* [24]. In evaluating the role that infection may play in atherosclerosis, it is not clear why some individuals who have been exposed to an organism associated with atherosclerosis develop severe disease, while others similarly exposed, who have equivalent levels of additional risk factors, are disease free.

Regardless of the specific role of any single infectious entity, the exciting possibility has been introduced from the above studies that atherosclerosis and its associated diseases might be prevented with one or more vaccines. To date, the major vaccine focus has been associated with *C. pneumoniae* [27]. Numerous studies on the effects of antibiotics on development of atherosclerosis have also been undertaken [28–34], but definitive results have not yet been reported that could lead to a recommendation for preventive or therapeutic interventions.

C. Role of Total Burden of Infectious Pathogens

As indicated above, the evidence is abundant and strong for including various infections as risk factors for atherosclerosis. Many of the pathogens that have been studied "were selected because each was either an obligate intracellular pathogen known to establish a persistent lifelong infection and/or elicited a persistent lifelong immune response (as manifested by increased antibody levels)" [35]. However, the remarkable number of organisms that have been implicated

has also generated a complicated and confusing picture. Likewise, it is not clear why some cross-sectional or prospective epidemiological studies seem to implicate certain organisms and other studies implicate entirely different organisms. The overall evidence does not unequivocally point to a single organism that could be a sole target for a generic vaccine against atherosclerosis.

Because of the above issues, the concept was introduced by Zhu et al. that "total pathogen burden" is more important as a risk factor than infection with any individual pathogen [36]. Although each pathogen may or may not be independently associated with increased risk for adverse atherosclerotic events or death, the accumulated risks of multiple infections may be additive [36–38]. Figure 1 illustrates a study of 233 patients in the United States in which the association between exposure to different numbers of pathogens, as determined by seropositivity, was correlated with the prevalence of, and odds ratio for, coronary artery disease [36]. As a further example of some of the considerable

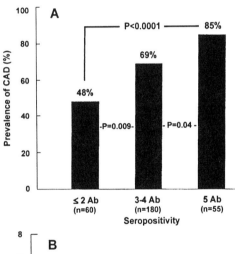

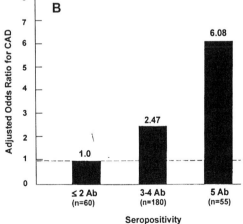

Figure 1 (A) Association between numbers of pathogens to which individuals were exposed (as reflected by seropositivity) and the prevalence of coronary artery disease. Overall linear trend achieves significance ($P = 0.001$). (B) Adjusted odds ratios for coronary artery disease. Overall linear trend achieves significance ($P = 0.001$). Ab = antibody. (From Ref. 36.)

evidence that has recently been accumulated for this concept, it was estimated that after a follow-up of 3.2 years of 572 patients studied in Germany, "cardiovascular mortality was 7.0% in patients with advanced atherosclerosis and seropositive for 0 to 3 pathogens compared with 20% in those seropositive for 6 to 8 pathogens" [39].

D. Multiple Mechanisms by Which Infections May Induce or Exacerbate Atherosclerosis

When the focus shifts from a single organism to multiple organisms, the question naturally arises whether infection per se is the underlying mechanism or whether other factors are more important and whether infection might even be an epiphenomenon rather than an etiological agent. For example, increased infections are also associated with poor socio-economic status, decreased access to vaccination, and lessened access to health care in general. This has been partly considered by studying relatively homogeneous populations [24], but the point is well taken. Of course, other risk factors, such as smoking, could have a confounding effect on determining the etiology of atherosclerosis in the presence of chronic infections [37].

The existence of inflammations, often associated with chronic infections, may sometimes be detected by elevation of serum CRP levels, and correlations between CRP levels and atherosclerotic risk have been reported. However, CRP elevation is a nonspecific indicator, the exact significance of which is ill-defined. Moreover, it is likely that the increased risk for coronary artery disease and increased CRP levels are both related to the primary variable of infectious burden [35,36].

The focus of understanding the possible role of infections has shifted in some laboratories to efforts to understand multiple possible direct and indirect effects that could link infection, particularly the effects of increased pathogen burden and atherosclerosis [25,35] (Figure 2). Where does this leave the question of whether vaccines can be developed for targeting atherosclerotic disease? There is no clear answer to this. Numerous infections do constitute risk factors for atherosclerosis, but recent data suggest that the risk posed by the burden of many infections is greater than the risk associated with any particular single infection. For this reason, a vaccine against a single organism, such as *C. pneumoniae*, probably could not serve as a generic vaccine against infection-associated atherosclerosis, but would reduce the atherosclerotic risk associated with this particular infection.

IV. METABOLIC VACCINES

Two metabolic vaccines have been proposed for inducing beneficial autoimmunity that changes distribution patterns of plasma lipoprotein cholesterol, with the aim of preventing cholesterol buildup in atherosclerotic plaques. Vaccines that have been proposed, or are being developed, have targeted either cholesterol itself [mainly in the form of LDL cholesterol or very low density lipoprotein (VLDL) cholesterol], or cholesteryl ester transfer protein, as an antigen. The latter protein is an important factor that regulates cholesterol

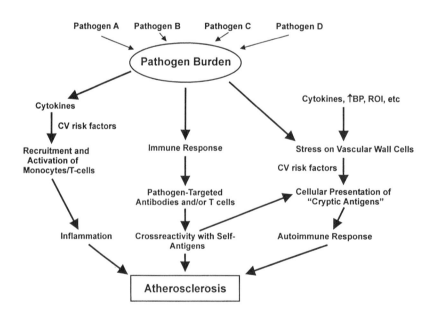

Figure 2   Multiple mechanisms by which infection may contribute to atherosclerosis development and course. The model depicted illustrates the role that infections by multiple pathogens, contributing to pathogen burden, has on the development of atherosclerosis. The mechanisms include factors leading to inflammation, and to immune and autoimmune responses, as well as their complex interactions. These mechanisms play out on a background of cardiovascular risk factors, which importantly influence any effect infection has on atherosclerosis development and progression. CV indicates cardiovascular; ROI, reactive oxygen intermediates. (From Ref. 35.)

transfer and distribution of cholesteryl esters among lipoproteins. In each case, the purpose of a metabolic vaccine is to increase the ratio of HDL/LDL, either by lowering LDL or by raising HDL.

A. Anticholesterol Vaccine

The question of the immunogenicity of cholesterol, whether as a hapten or as an antigen, indeed even the issue of the possible existence of antibodies to cholesterol, has had a long and interesting history that goes back as far as 1925 (reviewed in Ref. 40). Antibodies that apparently could bind to cholesterol or phospholipids were produced in rabbits by intravenous injection of cholesterol or phospholipid mixed together with heterologous serum (pig serum). Numerous studies with cholesterol-haptenated compounds subsequently suggested that antibodies that could bind to cholesterol could be produced [40]. The immunogenicity of cholesterol, and the existence of antibodies to cholesterol, were definitively demonstrated by immunization with a protein-free cholesterol-loaded liposome/lipid A formulation that was used for the production of murine monoclonal antibodies that reacted directly with highly purified cholesterol [41].

The goal of preventing atherosclerosis by creating a vaccine that induces antibodies against cholesterol is based on the intriguing idea that antibodies might be induced that could differentially bind to, and reduce the levels of, LDL, VLDL, and intermediate-density (IDL) lipoprotein cholesterol, without reducing HDL cholesterol [42–45]. Murine monoclonal and polyclonal antibodies induced by injection of cholesterol-loaded liposomes containing lipid A do indeed bind to LDL but not to HDL cholesterol [44]. The antibodies recognize the 3-hydroxy group of cholesterol, and this group is apparently sterically blocked from binding to anticholesterol antibodies by the greater amount of overlying apoprotein that is present in HDL compared to LDL.

Studies with heterologous beta-LDL [46,47] and with a cholesteryl–albumin conjugate [48,49] suggested that immunization with a formulation containing a heterologous protein could partially protect rabbits against diet-induced hypercholesterolemia and aortic atherosclerosis. Subsequent work with the rabbit model demonstrated that a protein-free formulation of liposomes heavily loaded with cholesterol, and containing lipid A as an adjuvant, could induce antibodies that reacted with purified cholesterol and with LDL cholesterol, IDL cholesterol, and VLDL cholesterol, and that also partially blocked diet-induced hypercholesterolemia and aortic atherosclerosis [43]. Protection against diet-induced hypercholesterolemia and atherosclerosis was confirmed after intravenous immunization with cholesterol-loaded liposomes lacking lipid A [50]. Immunization against cholesterol was performed intravenously rather than intramuscularly in the latter study, and complete blockade of cholesterol-induced atherosclerosis was observed.

It would be reasonable to worry whether a vaccine that induces antibodies against such a fundamental compound as cholesterol might be detrimental to health. Cholesterol plays a central role in the dynamics of cell membranes and it is a precursor in the synthesis of all of the steroid hormones. Nonetheless, immunization of rabbits and mice against cholesterol does not appear to induce any detectable toxicity in the animals. However, perhaps the most convincing evidence that antibodies to cholesterol are not deleterious is provided by the discovery that antibodies to cholesterol, both IgG and IgM, occur naturally in virtually all normal humans [45,51] (Figure 3). Based partly on this observation, it has been proposed that naturally occurring antibodies to cholesterol might play a beneficial role in helping to regulate the normal levels of LDL cholesterol [45]. A secondary consequence of this latter hypothesis, of course, is that many of the circulating anticholesterol antibodies in plasma might be hidden in the form of immune complexes with LDL. This would be analogous to the circulation of hidden antiphospholipid antibodies in normal human plasma, in which the antibodies are bound as immune complexes with phospholipids [52].

In view of the ubiquitous existence of varying levels of naturally occurring antibodies to cholesterol, it would seem reasonable to conclude that induction of higher levels of antibodies to cholesterol as part of a vaccine strategy would not be expected to have any adverse consequences. Of course, if subsequent research were to indicate that complement activation by naturally occurring antibodies to cholesterol also play some role in acute pathogenesis of atherosclerosis, for example, a role in accelerated atherosclerosis or acute reactions due to interaction of antibodies with cholesterol derived from a ruptured plaque, as suggested elsewhere [53–55], then the antibodies induced by the vaccine might also contribute to this hypothetical situation [40].

The summation of the anticholesterol vaccine approach is that it appears to be effective for preventing diet-induced hypercholesterolemia and atherosclerosis in animal models. There are experimental data, both in animal models and in the detection of naturally occurring antibodies to cholesterol in humans, that suggest that, although the immunization induces autoantibodies to an important body constituent (i.e., cholesterol), it may be expected to be safe for application as a human vaccine. The safety issue would have to be resolved through clinical trials in humans. It is possible that such a vaccine could be effective as an adjunct to other dietary and drug treatment strategies for lowering serum LDL levels in humans.

B. Anticholesteryl Ester Transfer Protein

Levels of plasma HDL and LDL are strongly and continuously influenced by remodeling of lipoproteins caused by the activity of CETP [56,57]. CETP serves as a transfer protein, one function of which involves facilitating donation of cholesteryl esters from HDL to LDL. It is a hydrophobic glycoprotein that is secreted by the liver, and it circulates mainly bound to HDL. Most of the circulating cholesteryl esters originate from HDL, where they are initially deposited by the catalytic action of lecithin:cholesterol acyl transferase. Triglycerides, originally derived from chylomicrons and VLDL, are also transferred to HDL and LDL. The CETP then changes the different lipoproteins by promoting an equilibrium of various lipids between lipoprotein classes. A

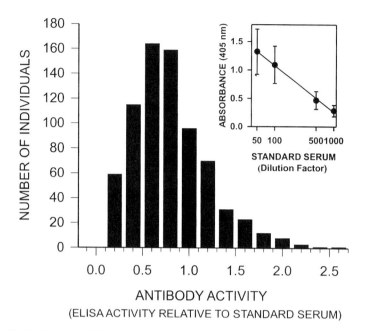

Figure 3 Anticholesterol antibodies in normal human sera. Dilutions (1:50) of each of 742 human sera were tested in triplicate by ELISA with purified nonoxidized cholesterol as antigen and mixed-affinity purified anti-human IgG, IgM, and IgA (H and L chains). Titrations of a standard serum used for comparison was performed with each group of ~15 volunteers (inset shows mean ±SD of 52 assays of the standard serum). Binding was not observed when cholesterol was omitted. (From Ref. 45.)

net effect of this activity is a pattern of chemical and physical changes in the HDL particles that results in a remodeling of, and reduction in the amount of, cholesterol-rich HDL particles.

High-density lipoprotein is generally viewed as an anti-atherogenic fraction, and the action of CETP may therefore have atherogenic effects through the reduction of HDL cholesterol. As noted earlier, reduced HDL has been cited as a risk factor for atherosclerosis [6]. In contrast to the numerous therapeutic agents that are available for reduction of LDL, therapeutic interventions for elevation of plasma HDL levels are inefficient and limited in their potency [6,58,59].

Through the induction of autoantibodies to CETP, an ongoing active immunotherapeutic vaccine program seeks to promote elevated HDL and lowered LDL levels in humans [60–62]. Preliminary experiments in rabbits have suggested that significant increases of HDL can be achieved by inhibition of CETP with a monoclonal antibody to CETP [63], or by immunization with a vaccine that induces antibodies to CETP [60]. The vaccine consists of a 31 amino acid synthetic chimeric peptide that contains 16 residues of human CETP that contain a B-cell epitope, an additional 14 residues containing a T-cell epitope from tetanus toxin, and a linker peptide [60]. The vaccine, known as CETi-1, has successfully completed Phase 1 safety studies in humans, and "measurable antibody titers" were observed in all groups in a pattern that suggested a dose–response relationship [62]. The sponsoring company (Avant Immunotherapeutics, Inc.) initiated a Phase 2 placebo-controlled efficacy trial in patients with low levels of HDL cholesterol in August 2001 [61,62].

Clearly, the net effect of CETP is proatherogenic in rabbits, and inhibition of CETP has a beneficial effect for

reduction of diet-induced atherosclerosis in that species. However, because of uncertainty regarding the role of CETP in transferring cholesteryl esters between lipoproteins in different species, it is not yet certain whether the enhancement of plasma HDL by active immunization that was observed in rabbits will carry over to humans. Nonetheless, there is a strong likelihood that the same result will occur in humans in view of the very high levels of HDL that characterize individuals who are genetically deficient in CETP (reviewed in Ref. 60).

Despite this latter theoretical prediction of a favorable outcome, and despite the promising safety results of the Phase 1 trials, it is still not clear whether the fundamental role and net effect of CETP is universally proatherogenic or antiatherogenic in humans, or whether CETP might have one effect in certain populations and another effect in others (reviewed and discussed in Refs. 57 and 60). CETP plays a very complicated role in lipoprotein distribution patterns, and it does have certain functions that are viewed as antiatherogenic. For example, by virtue of its ability to transport cholesterol from peripheral tissues to the liver for excretion in bile, a process known as reverse cholesterol transport (RCT), CETP can promote the elimination of cholesterol from tissues. Inhibition of CETP therefore might have proatherogenic effects in certain individuals [57,60]. One example that has been cited as circumstantial evidence of a proatherogenic effect associated with deficiency of CETP is an epidemiological study that found that a subset of Japanese-American men having a genetic deficiency of CETP and only modest elevations of HDL had an increased tendency to coronary heart disease [64]. In the same study, deficient individuals with higher HDL did not have higher atherosclerotic risk, and it was concluded that although CETP deficiency is an independent risk factor for coronary heart disease under certain circumstances, the dynamics of RCT and the HDL concentration both play a role in the epidemiological determination of risk. In contrast to this, a much larger epidemiological study of men and women in Japan concluded that increased HDL was associated with a low prevalence of coronary heart disease, including among those with genetic CETP deficiency [65]. Because of various remaining uncertainties, although a vaccine against CETP is interesting, and potentially exciting, the jury is still out as to whether autoantibodies to CETP will be beneficial (antiatherogenic), or perhaps even detrimental (proatherogenic), in some or all humans who might require therapeutic alterations of lipoprotein metabolism [57,60]. Further judgement on the efficacy and safety of this approach must await additional data from ongoing human trials.

REFERENCES

1. Oberman A. Epidemiology and prevention of cardiovascular disease. In: Kelley WN, ed. Textbook of Internal Medicine. 3d ed. Philadelphia: Lippincott-Raven, 1997:158–163.
2. National Heart, Lung, and Blood Institute FY 2000 Fact BookBethesda: NHLBI, NIH, 2001.
3. Gheorghiade M, Bonow RO. Coronary artery disease. In: Kelley WN, ed. Textbook of Internal Medicine. 3d ed. Philadelphia: Lippincott-Raven, 1997:371–385.
4. Ross R. The pathogenesis of atherosclerosis: a perspective for the 1990s. Nature 1993; 362:801–809.
5. Hansson GK, et al. The role of adaptive immunity in atherosclerosis. Ann NY Acad Sci 2000; 902:53–64.
6. Expert Panel on Detection, Evaluation, and Treatment of High Blood Cholesterol in Adults. Executive summary of the third report of the National Cholesterol Education Program (NCEP) Expert Panel on Detection, Evaluation, and Treatment of High Blood Cholesterol in Adults (Adult Treatment Panel III). J Am Med Assoc 2001; 285:2486–2497 (Also available as National Institutes of Health Publication No. 01-3670, May 2001).
7. Nieto FJ. Infections and atherosclerosis: new clues from an old hypothesis. Am J Epidemiol 1998; 148:937–948.
8. Saikku P, et al. Serological evidence of an association of a novel *Chlamydia*, TWAR, with chronic coronary heart disease and acute myocardial infarction. Lancet, 1988; Oct 29:983–986.
9. Mattila KJ. Viral and bacterial infections in patients with acute myocardial infarction. J Intern Med 1989; 225:293–296.
10. Saikku P. Epidemiologic association of *Chlamydia pneumoniae* and atherosclerosis: the initial serologic observation and more. J Inf Dis 2000; 181(suppl 3):S411–S413.
11. Grayston JT. Background and current knowledge of *Chlamydia pneumoniae* and atherosclerosis. J Infect Dis 2000; 181(suppl 3):S402–S410.
12. Saikku P, et al. An epidemic of mild pneumonia due to an unusual strain of *Chlamydia psittaci*. J Infect Dis 1985; 151:832–839.
13. Leinonen M, et al. Circulating immune complexes containing chlamydial lipopolysaccharide in acute myocardial infarction. Microb Pathog 1990; 9:67–73.
14. Linnanmäki E, et al. *Chlamydia pneumoniae*-specific circulating immune complexes in patients with coronary heart disease. Circulation 1993; 87:1130–1134.
15. Maass M, et al. Endovascular presence of viable *Chlamydia*

pneumoniae is a common phenomenon in coronary artery disease. J Am Coll Cardiol 1998; 31:827–832.
16. Mattila KJ, et al. Role of infection as a risk factor for atherosclerosis, myocardial infarction, and stroke. Clin Infect Dis 1998; 26:719–734.
17. Campbell LA, et al. *Chlamydia pneumoniae* and cardiovascular disease. Emerg Infect Dis 1998; 4:571–579.
18. O'Connor S. Fulfillment of Koch's postulates and the causes of atherosclerosis. Am Heart J 1999; 138:S550–S551.
19. Shor A, et al. Detection of *Chlamydia pneumoniae* in coronary arterial fatty streaks and atheromatous plaques. S Afr Med J 1992; 82:158–161.
20. Shor A, Phillips JI. *Chlamydia pneumoniae* and atherosclerosis. J Am Med Assoc 1999; 282:2071–2073.
21. Bachmaier K, et al. *Chlamydia* infections and heart disease linked through antigenic mimicry. Science 1999; 283:1335–1339.
22. Ngeh J, Gupta S. *C. pneumoniae* and atherosclerosis: causal or coincidental link? ASM News 2000; 66(12):732–737.
23. Danesh J, et al. *Chlamydia pneumoniae* IgG titres and coronary heart disease: prospective study and meta-analysis. Br Med J 2000; 321(7255):208–213.
24. Zhu J, et al. Prospective study of pathogen burden and risk of myocardial infarction or death. Circulation 2001; 103:45–51.
25. Danesh J, et al. Chronic infections and coronary heart disease: is there a link? Lancet 1997; 350:430–436.
26. Morré SA, et al. Microorganisms in the aetiology of atherosclerosis. J Clin Pathol 2000; 53:647–654.
27. Murdin AD, et al. Collaborative multidisciplinary workshop report: progress toward a *Chlamydia pneumoniae* vaccine. J Infect Dis 2000; 181(suppl 3):S552–S557.
28. Lip GYH, Beevers DG. Can we treat coronary artery disease with antibiotics? Lancet 1997; 350:378–379.
29. Gurfinkel E, et al. for the ROXIS study group. Randomised trial of roxithromycin in non-Q-wave coronary syndromes: ROXIS pilot study. Lancet 1997; 350:404–407.
30. Fong IW. Antibiotics effects in a rabbit model of *Chlamydia pneumoniae*-induced atherosclerosis. J Infect Dis 2000; 181(suppl 3):S514–S518.
31. Muhlestein JB. *Chlamydia pneumoniae*-induced atherosclerosis in a rabbit model. J Infect Dis 2000; 181(suppl 3):S505–S507.
32. Meier CR. Antibiotics in the prevention and treatment of coronary heart disease. J Infect Dis 2000; 181(suppl 3):S558–S562.
33. Dunne MW. Rationale and design of a secondary prevention trial of antibiotic use in patients after myocardial infarction: The WIZARD (Weekly Intervention with Zithromax [azithromycin] for Atherosclerosis and Its Related Disorders) trial. J Infect Dis 2000; 181(suppl 3):S5572–S5578.
34. Anderson JL, Muhlestein JB. The ACADEMIC study in perspective (Azithromycin in Coronary Artery Disease: Elimination of Myocardial Infection with *Chlamydia*). J Infect Dis 2000; 181(suppl 3):S569–S571.
35. Epstein SE. The multiple mechanisms by which infection may contribute to atherosclerosis development and course. Circ Res 2002; 90:2–4.
36. Zhu J, et al. Effects of total pathogen burden on coronary artery disease risk and C-reactive protein levels. Am J Cardiol 2000; 85:140–146.
37. Roivainen M, et al. Infections, inflammation, and the risk of coronary heart disease. Circulation 2000; 101:252–257.
38. Rupprecht HJ, et al. For the AtheroGene Investigators. Impact of viral and bacterial infectious burden on long-term prognosis in patients with coronary artery disease. Circulation 2001; 104:25–31.
39. Espinola-Klein C, et al. For the AtheroGene Investigators. Circulation 2002; 105:15–21.

40. Alving CR, Swartz GM Jr. Antibodies to cholesterol, cholesterol conjugates, and liposomes: implications for atherosclerosis and autoimmunity. Crit Rev Immunol 1991; 10:441–453.

41. Swartz GM Jr, et al. Antibodies to cholesterol. Proc Natl Acad Sci USA 1988; 85:1902–1906.

42. Alving CR, et al. Prospects for an anticholesterol vaccine. Clin Immunother 1995; 3:409–414.

43. Alving CR, et al. Immunization with cholesterol-rich liposomes induces anti-cholesterol antibodies and reduces diet-induced hypercholesterolemia and plaque formation. J Lab Clin Med 1996; 127(1):40–49.

44. Dijkstra J, et al. Interactions of anti-cholesterol antibodies with human lipoproteins. J Immunol 1996; 157:2006–2013.

45. Alving CR, Wassef NM. Naturally-occurring antibodies to cholesterol: a new theory of LDL cholesterol metabolism. Immunol Today 1999; 20:362–366.

46. Gero S, et al. Inhibition of cholesterol atherosclerosis by immunisation with beta-lipoprotein. Lancet, 1959; 4 July: 6–7.

47. Gerö S, et al. Inhibition of cholesterol atherosclerosis by immunisation with beta-lipoprotein. Lancet, 1961; 20 May: 1119.

48. Bailey JM, et al. Immunization with a synthetic cholesterol–ester antigen and induced atherosclerosis in rabbits. Nature 1964; 201:407–408.

49. Bailey JM, Butler J. Synthetic cholesterol–ester antigens in experimental atherosclerosis. In: Di Luzio NR, Paoletti R, eds. The Reticuloendothelial System and Atherosclerosis-New York: Plenum Press, 1967:433–441.

50. Istvan H, et al. Influence of cholesterol liposome immunisation and immunostimulation on rabbits atherosclerosis induced by a high cholesterol diet. Med Sci Monit 1998; 4(3):403–407.

51. Alving CR, et al. Naturally-occurring autoantibodies to cholesterol in humans. Biochem Soc Trans 1989; 17:637–639.

52. Cabiedes J, et al. Hidden anti-phospholipid antibodies in normal human sera circulate as immune complexes whose antigen can be removed by heat, acid, hypermolar buffers or phospholipase treatments. Eur J Immunol 1998; 28:2108–2114.

53. Alving CR, et al. Cholesterol-dependent human complement activation resulting in damage to liposomal model membranes. J Immunol 1977; 118:342–347.

54. Hammerschmidt DE, et al. Cholesterol and atheroma lipids activate complement and stimulate granulocytes. A possible mechanism for amplification of ischemic injury in atherosclerotic states. J Lab Clin Med 1981; 98:68–77.

55. Niculescu F, et al. Localization of the terminal C5b-9 complement complex in the human aortic atherosclerotic wall. Immunol Lett 1985; 10:109–114.

56. Tall AR. Plasma cholesteryl ester transfer protein. J Lipid Res 1993; 34:1255–1274.

57. Barter P. CETP and atherosclerosis. Arterioscler Thromb Vasc Biol 2000; 20:2029–2031.

58. Havel RJ, Rapaport E. Management of primary hyperlipidemia. N Engl J Med 1995; 332:1491–1498. [Correction appears in N Engl J Med 1996; 333:467].

59. Gotto AM Jr. Cholesterol management in theory and practice. Circulation 1997; 96:4424–4430.

60. Rittershaus CW, et al. Vaccine-induced antibodies inhibit CETP activity in vivo and reduce aortic lesions in a rabbit model of atherosclerosis. Arterioscler Thromb Vasc Biol 2000; 20:2106–2112.

61. Maeder T. Down with the bad, up with the good. A biotech firm develops a vaccine to raise good cholesterol levels. Sci Am 2002; 286(2):32–33.

62. Avant Immunotherapeutics Inc web site: http://www.avant-immune.com.

63. Whitlock ME, et al. Monoclonal antibody inhibition of cholesteryl ester transfer protein activity in the rabbit. Effects on lipoprotein composition and high density lipoprotein cholesteryl ester metabolism. J Clin Invest 1989; 84:129–137.

64. Zhong S, et al. Increased coronary heart disease in Japanese-American men with mutation in the cholesteryl ester transfer protein gene despite increased HDL levels. J Clin Invest 1996; 97:2917–2923.

65. Moriyama Y, et al. A low prevalence of coronary heart disease among subjects with increased high-density lipoprotein cholesterol levels, including those with plasma cholesteryl ester transfer protein deficiency. Prev Med 1998; 27:659–667.

83
Vaccine Therapy

Donald S. Burke
Johns Hopkins Bloomberg School of Public Health, Baltimore, Maryland, U.S.A.

I. INTRODUCTION

The word *vaccine* is usually restricted to describe an immunogen administered to healthy subjects at risk prior to their becoming exposed to a microbial pathogen. This word is also often used when the immunogen is administered early after exposure but before the onset of disease manifestations; in such circumstances the qualifying prefix "postexposure" is employed. Given the conventional use of the word vaccine, the term vaccine therapy might seem to be an oxymoron. However, historical precedent suggests that the term *vaccine therapy* should be used to describe administration of a microbe-specific antigen for therapeutic purposes (after the onset of established disease) [1]. Indeed, "vaccine therapy" and "vaccinotherapy" have been used continuously for this purpose as medical subject headings in the *Index Medicus* since 1911. While alternative terms have been proposed (immunoregulation, immunotherapy, immunostimulation), they are overly general and fail to convey the meaning that the immunity sought in vaccine therapy is both active and directed against microbe-specific antigens. Thus vaccine usage can be categorized relative to the time of microbial exposure: (1) true prevention or prophylaxis, (2) postexposure prophylaxis, and (3) therapy or reduction of recurrences.

Modern biotechnology has led to a renewed interest in vaccine therapy [2–5]. This chapter reviews the usage of vaccines after the moment of exposure (infection), emphasizing the therapeutic use of vaccines; however, postexposure vaccination is also reviewed for the purpose of comparison.

II. HISTORY OF VACCINE THERAPY

Edward Jenner, in his epochal 1798–1800 papers on the use of vaccinia in preventing smallpox, briefly commented on the apparent success of postexposure vaccination (see below) to prevent clinical smallpox [6]. However, he never proposed treatment of established smallpox with vaccinia. The French syphilologist Joseph-Alexandre Auzias-Turenne saw paral-

lels between the benign and fatal pox disease variants and the benign and fatal variants of genital chancres and proposed that matter from benign chancres be used for protection against or even treatment of syphilis. He championed syphilization—an intentional contraction of the terms syphilis and vaccination—as a public health tool [7,8]. For therapy he proposed that matter from a benign lesion could be inoculated serially, up to dozens of times, into the skin of a patient with established syphilis in an effort to achieve a cure. "Syphilization" was a major topic of debate at the 1st International Medical Congress in Paris in 1867. Of course, the clinical efficacy of his approach was never proved or even fully accepted, because he clearly confused syphilis with chancroid and genital herpes.

As Louis Pasteur was beginning his studies of vaccines in the late 1870s, he chanced to receive a copy of Auzias-Turenne's collected works. Pasteur's nephew and laboratory assistant, Adrian Loir, contends that Pasteur read this book avidly and that he was greatly influenced by Auzias' ideas [9]. Loir reports that Pasteur repeated some of Auzias' experiments of pre- and postexposure immunization, particularly with bovine pleuropneumonia [10]. Pasteur also almost certainly read Auzias' speculative paper (written in 1864) on possible uses of material from rabies-infected tissues for purposes of therapeutic vaccination [7,11].

Pasteur's legendary success with postexposure prophylaxis in the case of 9-year-old Joseph Meister led to widespread acceptance of postexposure vaccination for rabies [12,13]. Less widely known is the fact that Pasteur had already used a rabbit brain rabies vaccine in attempts to treat two cases of clinically apparent rabies [14]. These two cases are probably the first true trials of antigen-specific "vaccine therapy." One patient died less than a day after receiving the therapy but the other apparently survived. Pasteur never published or otherwise publicly reported on these cases (Geison discovered the cases in Pasteur's laboratory notebooks [14]).

Robert Koch reported in 1890 that he had discovered a cure for tuberculosis, leading tuberculosis patients from around the world to flock to Berlin to receive the treatment

[15–19]. The "cure" was a solution or suspension of glycerin and extracts from tubercle bacillus cultures, a composition similar to "tuberculin." Like Pasteur, Koch had reported that microbe-derived antigens could stimulate immunity in patients who were already infected. However, reports from colleagues using the material were less than enthusiastic [20]. Cures and remissions were infrequent, and severe reactions, including several deaths, were commonplace. While tuberculin was a failure as a vaccine therapy, these trials led to its use as a diagnostic reagent and opened the field of delayed-type hypersensitivity.

Impressed by Koch's experiments, Almroth Wright in England developed vaccine therapies for other microbes that could be cultivated in vitro [21,22]. He reported the use of heat-killed cultures of *Staphylococcus aureus* as a vaccine therapy [23]. Using an assay developed by William Boog Leishman, he measured the ability of sera to facilitate the ingestion of bacteria by leukocytes. He coined the term opsonization for this activity and correlated changes in the serum opsonic index with outcome in his vaccine therapy patients [24]. Almroth Wright became a zealous champion of vaccine therapy [25].

Based on his discussions with Wright, George Bernard Shaw wrote *The Doctor's Dilemma*, a play whose plot revolved around the selection of patients for slots in a tuberculosis vaccine therapy trial [26]. One memorable line from this play—a vaccine therapist's credo—reads: "There is at bottom only one genuinely scientific treatment for all diseases, and that is to stimulate the phagocytes. Stimulate the phagocytes. Drugs are a delusion." Of course, not everyone was persuaded by Sir Almorth Wright's data. One wag dubbed him "Sir Almost Wright."

Vaccine therapy flourished during the first decades of the 20th century. Even Alexander Fleming wrote an effusive testimonial about its virtues [27]. A *Journal of Vaccine Therapy* appeared, and textbooks with guidelines on vaccine therapy for general practitioners were published. Pharmaceutical companies advertised concoctions of heat-inactivated organisms, typically 10 to 100 million per inoculation, for use as therapeutic vaccines [28,29]. Different mixtures were to be used for different disease syndromes such as pneumonia, urinary tract infections, or skin infections; U.S. practitioners commonly used vaccine therapy in their practice, most often for furunculosis or tuberculosis [30].

Despite their widespread use, bacterial therapeutic vaccines were never proved to have clinical efficacy. The early literature on vaccine therapy is difficult to interpret due to the total lack of appropriately controlled trials. Clinicians who used tuberculin vaccine therapy frequently reported increased inflammation at the sites of clinical tuberculosis, especially at readily visible sites on the skin [31]. Similarly, Wright and coworkers show reproducible increases in the serum opsonic index in *Staphylococcus* trials [32,33]. Some experimental studies in animal models also suggested immunogenicity (but none showed proof of efficacy) [34]. Enthusiasm for vaccine therapy plummeted when potent antibiotics such as streptomycin, chloramphenicol, and penicillin became available. In the 1950s and 1960s there continued to be sporadic efforts to develop and test therapeutic vaccines but none showed much promise [35–42]. By the

1970s, antibiotic treatment completely eclipsed antigen-specific treatment, and vaccine therapy became a forgotten art.

III. EFFICACY OF VACCINATION FOR POSTEXPOSURE PROPHYLAXIS

The observation that vaccination *after exposure* to an infectious agent can afford protection against clinical disease carries obvious implications for a general understanding about how vaccines work: complete or "sterilizing" immunity, with total suppression of the very first rounds of microbe replication, is not necessary for a vaccine to be effective. This suggests that in some circumstances vaccines might be useful even later in the course of an infection, for therapy of overt disease.

There is reasonable evidence for the efficacy of postexposure vaccination in at least four human infectious diseases. All four are viral infections where an exact time of exposure can be determined with relative ease, the incubation period is at least 2 weeks, and an effective vaccine is available. Because these reports on postexposure vaccination are the only evidence that vaccines can be effective after, rather than before, infection, they are presented here in some detail, in historical order.

A. Smallpox

In 1800, Edward Jenner presented the first anecdotal evidence for the efficacy of postexposure vaccination [6]: "Some striking instances of the power of the cow-pox in suspending the progress of the smallpox after the patients had been several days casually exposed to the infection have been laid before me…" The largest and most detailed study of postexposure vaccination against smallpox was conducted by Dr. William Hanna, Medical Office of the Port of Liverpool, who collected 75 cases [43]. Most were travelers from Boston who landed incubating smallpox during the severe outbreak in that city in 1902–1903. All were promptly vaccinated regardless of the time since exposure and then confined to the Port Isolation Hospital. Among those who were previously vaccinia-naive and vaccinated within 6 days of exposure, all 10 of 10 developed only mild or moderate disease; of those vaccinated within 7–14 days of exposure but before rash, 7 developed mild moderate and 6 severe disease (1 death); of those vaccinated only after the rash had begun, 3 developed moderate and 4 severe disease (2 deaths).

Among those who had previously been vaccinated and then revaccinated within 6 days of exposure, 10 developed mild disease, 2 moderate, and 1 severe disease; of those revaccinated within 7–14 days of exposure but before rash, 14 developed mild disease and 1 moderate disease; and of those revaccinated only after the rash had begun, 7 developed mild disease and 10 moderate disease.

Evidence of a successful vaccine "take"—local vesiculation—during the incubation period also correlated strongly with protection against severe disease in the vaccinia-naive cases [43]. Among those not previously vaccinated, a successful take during the incubation period led to severe disease in only 2 of 19, whereas an unsuccessful vaccination (which occurred typically in those cases vaccinated later after exposure, often where symptoms had already begun) led to severe disease in 8 of 11.

Dixon reported on the efficacy of post-exposure vaccination in Tripoli in 1946 and compared the spectrum of disease severity among persons who had never been vaccinated to that among those who were successfully vaccinated postexposure [44]. His findings were remarkably similar to those of Hanna: among 21 cases successfully vaccinated with 5 days of exposure, all developed only mild illness. But when successful vaccination was not performed until the 6th to the 10th day after contact ($n = 36$ cases), the spectrum of disease severity was not different from that among unvaccinated persons.

For obvious ethical reasons, there are no prospective controlled trials of administration of vaccinia at different intervals after exposure, so precise data are impossible to obtain. The two retrospective series presented here identified cases for inclusion by the appearance of at least some smallpox papules. Persons with no evidence at all of smallpox would have been excluded. Indeed, the data in these two series may present a conservative estimate of the efficacy of postexposure vaccination against smallpox, because some individuals that were completely protected would not have been counted.

Fenner pointed out that the clinical course of infection following intradermal vaccinia inoculation (fever in 6–7 days) is much more rapid than the clinical course of typical variola major in an unvaccinated subject (fever in 14 days) or even that of intradermal inoculation smallpox in a naive subject (10–12 days) [45]. He speculates that this alacrity of vaccinia might be an important factor in the success of postexposure vaccination against smallpox.

B. Rabies

Surprisingly, active vaccination for postexposure prophylaxis of rabies, widely considered to be the classic example of postexposure prophylaxis, is of uncertain clinical benefit. The first attempts at rabies postexposure prophylaxis in humans were conducted by Pasteur in mid-1885. By this time he had already tried vaccine therapy of clinically apparent rabies in two patients, with inconclusive results [46]. He first used postexposure rabies vaccine on July 6 on Joseph Meister, who had been bitten 2 days earlier. The boy apparently did well. On October 20, Pasteur began vaccination of his second case, teenager Jean-Baptiste Jupille, who had been severely bitten while defending a group of younger children from an apparently rabid dog. Six days later Pasteur announced his new method to the Academy of Science in Paris. One eminent colleague took the floor to proclaim that date of October 26, 1885, would live "forever memorable in the history of medicine and forever glorious for French science." Pasteur had presented only two clinical cases, with follow-up periods of 4 months and 1 week, respectively. During the next year, over 2000 rabies-exposed patients from throughout Europe flocked to Paris to receive the postexposure vaccination. No controlled clinical studies were done.

Geison has recently shown that there are serious reasons to doubt the efficacy of Pasteur's original postexposure vaccine [47]. The first were "scientific" concerns. For treatment of Meister and Jupille, Pasteur employed a 14-day series of injections of ground-up rabid spinal cords taken from rabbits intracranially inoculated with a "fixed" (rabbit brain-adapted) rabies virus. For the human cases, he began with 14-day dried rabbit cord and progressively each day inoculated a 1-day fresher cord until, on the last day, he inoculated fresh rabbit brains. Although never clearly expounded, his theory was that he was inoculating successively "less attenuated" virus each day. Modern authorities have established that rabbit brain-fixed virus can be virulent for humans. Most of Pasteur's colleagues assumed that his animal experimental work had laid a careful foundation for postexposure rabies vaccination of bitten humans. However, at the time he treated Joseph Meister, Pasteur had not tested the efficacy of the regimen used on him in animals but instead only a variety of other exploratory vaccines and regimens. Furthermore, Gieson has also raised legitimate questions about the statistical significance of Pasteur's animal experiments [47].

Serious concerns (and lawsuits stemming from those concerns) were promptly raised about rabies cases in humans that occurred despite (or perhaps because of?) the first-generation Pasteur vaccine. Within a few years, the Pasteur Institute switched to a carbolic acid-inactivated vaccine. Nonetheless, the bulk of uncontrolled clinical data on postexposure rabies vaccination suggested that the method was reasonably safe and (arguably) effective.

Webster reviewed the world's literature on experimental rabies postexposure vaccination in animal models [48,49] and concluded "it appears that Pasteur's tests on the immunization of dogs by vaccination following bite have not been confirmed. Nine workers over a period of 50 years have stressed the relatively unsatisfactory results obtained in a series of over ninety experiments." McKendrick, after reviewing results of the first 1 million rabies postexposure vaccinations at Pasteur institutes throughout the world [50], concluded that there were no differences in rabies mortality with respect to the type of vaccine employed (killed, live, heated, or other), regardless of the probability of the presence of rabies in the biting animal, location, or severity of the bite. Furthermore, delay in commencing vaccine treatment, even beyond 14 days, failed to show increases in rabies mortality. Other studies also failed to demonstrate any significant efficacy of postexposure rabies vaccination in humans [51].

Although passive postexposure immunization with antirabies immune serum was used sporadically as early as the 1890s, it was not until the 1950s that the efficacy of antirabies serum was studied in controlled field trials in humans [52,53]. Wolf-bite victims were solidly protected by postexposure vaccine plus serum but not by vaccine alone. Subsequent experimental studies of rabies in dogs and in mice have shown that passive immunity with serum and active immunity with vaccine is synergistic when given in the right doses [54,55]. There have been no controlled trials, or even uncontrolled trials, of the newer, safer "third-generation" cell culture-grown rabies vaccines alone (without passive antibodies) for postexposure vaccination. Current recommendations for rabies postexposure prophylaxis call for simultaneous administration of rabies immune globulin, regardless of the type (human diploid cell, Vero cell, rhesus diploid cell), route (intramuscular or intradermal), or dose of vaccine. Early experience with vaccinia and canarypox-vectored rabies proteins suggests that these genetically engineered vaccines might have advantages [56,57].

C. Hepatitis B Virus

By comparison to rabies, the history of hepatitis B virus (HBV) postexposure vaccination is straightforward; evidence for postexposure efficacy was found in the first prevention vaccine trials. In 1978–1980, a randomized, placebo-controlled, double-blind study of plasma-derived vaccine was conducted among 1083 homosexual men in New York who were known to be at risk for HBV infection [58]. The overall reduction in incident infections was 92%. Hepatitis B events occurring in the first 75 days after the first vaccine injection were analyzed as a subset, as these were thought to be HBV infections that were incubating at the time of vaccination. Although the total *incidence* of new infections in the first 75 days was not reduced by vaccination, disease *severity* was substantially less in vaccine recipients than placebo recipients.

The same postexposure protective effect was found among early infections in another study of the plasma-derived vaccine conducted among 1402 homosexual men in five American cities in 1980–1981 [59]. After the plasma-derived vaccine was proved efficacious, it became difficult to prove the efficacy of the newer genetically engineered HBV vaccines in placebo-controlled trials. Data from a placebo-controlled trial and a comparative trial (compared to plasma-derived vaccine) in China have shown that yeast-expressed recombinant HBV vaccine alone (without HB immune globulin) was highly efficacious in postexposure prophylaxis to prevent chronic perinatal HBV infection [60,61].

D. Varicella

Evidence for the efficacy of postexposure vaccination against varicella has also been directly demonstrated in several studies. In one early study where vaccine was administered within 3 days of exposure, protective efficacy against disease was essentially 100% [62]. Subsequent studies have shown that protective efficacy against disease is directly related to how soon after exposure the vaccine is administered and how much vaccine virus is administered [63]. When a dose of vaccine greater than 1000 PFU is administered within 3 days of exposure, postexposure protection is excellent. Although postexposure vaccination against varicella is an efficacious strategy, preexposure vaccination is recommended for persons at risk as a more reliable approach.

E. Vaccine Therapy for Infections that Are Preventable or Modifiable by Postexposure Vaccination

There is no evidence that the vaccination of patients with *clinically overt* smallpox, rabies, or varicella has any favorable impact on disease course. Similarly, studies of chronic

HBV infection have not recorded any beneficial effect of immunization (see below).

IV. CONTEMPORARY VACCINE THERAPY EFFORTS

New findings in immunology and molecular biology have prompted a modest resurgence of interest in vaccine therapy for chronic infectious diseases. Today there are ongoing efforts to develop and test therapeutic vaccines for several problems of public health significance; dozens of clinical trials have been reported just within the past few years. However, because there is no solid proof of efficacy for any of the therapeutic vaccines in these studies, they are reviewed here in outline form only.

A. Human Immunodeficiency Virus

When acquired immunodeficiency syndrome (AIDS) was discovered to be caused by human immunodeficiency virus type 1 (HIV-1) and it became understood that symptomatic illness was the end stage of a slow but inexorable progressive viral infection, several groups began vaccine therapy trials. The vaccines tested thus far have spanned the full gamut of conceivable approaches from crude unpurified preparations to genetically engineered replicating vectors.

Some of the earliest attempts were made to treat HIV with crude infusions of infected whole blood or materials derived from blood [64–66]. One approach has been to autovaccinate patients with autologous-inactivated HIV obtained by cytapheresis of the patient's blood, in an effort to stimulate immunity against the patient's own viral quasi-species. Another approach has been to infuse infected blood taken directly from patients with stable asymptomatic infections into patients with advanced disease, in the hope that the newly introduced virus would be more immunogenic and provoke an effective immune response. There is little evidence that these attempts at therapeutic vaccinations with blood products had any favorable impact. More promising early results were obtained by vaccine therapy with inactivated antigens or subunit proteins. Zagury and colleagues immunized patients with paraformaldehyde-fixed autologous lymphocytes that expressed genetically cloned vaccinia-expressed HIV antigens [67–70], but this approach had some inherent safety problems for use in persons with compromised immune systems [71].

Within the past 5 years there have been at least 20 published reports on clinical vaccine therapy trials of 11 different HIV vaccine approaches (see Table 1).

Salk and colleagues inoculated patients with cell culture-grown whole inactivated virions [72–76]. The vaccine test product, "Remune," was studied in a large multicenter, double-blind, placebo-controlled, randomized trial conducted at 77 centers among HIV-infected adults with early-to mid-stage disease progression (at least 300 CD4 cells per cubic mm) [77]. A total of 2527 patients were randomized to receive the vaccine or adjuvant only. Fifty-three subjects clinically progressed in each treatment group, and there were 19 and 23 deaths in the placebo and immunogen groups.

Table 1 Recent Vaccine Therapy Trials for HIV-Associated Diseases

Vaccine	Disease	Country	N patients	Placebo	Year	Author	Reference
Whole inactivated virions	Early stage	United States	2527	yes	2000	Kahn	77
Whole inactivated virions	Early stage	United States	252	yes	2001	Turner	78
Whole inactivated virions	Early stage	Thailand	297	yes	2001	Churdboonchart	80
Envelope protein gp 160 (baculovirus)	Early stage	Italy	99	yes	1998	Pontesilli	84
Envelope protein gp 160 (baculovirus)	Early stage	Canada	278	yes	1998	Tsoukas	85
Envelope protein gp 160 (baculovirus)	Early stage	Sweden	835	yes	1999	Sandstrom	86
Envelope protein gp 160 (baculovirus)	Early stage	Sweden	40	no	1999	Bratt	87
Envelope protein gp 160 (baculovirus)	Early stage	United States	608	yes	2000	Birx	88
Envelope protein gp 160 (baculovirus)	Late stage	United States	142	no	2000	DeMaria	89
Envelope protein gp 160 (mammalian cell)	Early stage	Germany	208	yes	1999	Goebel	90
Envelope protein gp 160 (mammalian cell)	Early stage	United States	22	yes	2001	Kundu	91
Envelope protein gp120 (mammalian cell)	Early stage	United States	573	yes	1996	Eron	92
Envelope protein gp120 (mammalian cell) or gp 120 (yeast)	Early stage and late stage	United States	128 and 164	yes	2000	Schooley	93
gag/pol/env/nef canarypox	Primary infection	United Kingdom	148	yes	2001	Goh	94
Core protein p17–p24 viruslike particles	Early stage	United Kingdom	74	yes	2002	Lindenberg	95
Core protein p24 viruslike particles	Early stage	Australia	24	yes	1999	Benson	96
Envelope peptides	Early stage	United States	8	no	1999	Pinto	97
tat toxoid	Early stage	Italy	14	no	1998	Gringeri	98
nef or rev or tat DNA	Early stage	Sweden	4	no	1999	Calarota	99
gp160 DNA	Early stage	Switzerland	4	no	2001	Weber	100

These results were taken as evidence by the principal investigator and his colleagues that Remune failed to demonstrate an increase in HIV progression-free survival. In a separate publication, measurements of HIV viral load, CD4 cells, and HIV-1-specific immunity all in a predefined subset of 252 subjects were reported to show beneficial effects from vaccination [78]. In an unprecedented step, the parent company, the Immune Response Corporation, brought legal action against the principal investigator of the clinical trial for refusing to include what they referred to as these more "meaningful and detailed" data in the full report on clinical outcomes [79]. Another adjuvant-controlled double-blind trial of Remune was conducted among 297 asymptomatic patients in Thailand [80]. Over a relatively short 40 weeks of follow-up, the vaccine group was reported to show a better preservation of CD4 cell levels. No effect on disease progression or mortality was reported from this study.

Other early pioneers of HIV-specific vaccine therapy were Redfield and Birx who studied vaccine therapy with a genetically engineered HIV surface envelope protein (gp160) that had been expressed from recombinant baculoviruses in

insect cells; they demonstrated that the approach was safe and immunogenic [81–83]. Results of six large and/or long-term clinical trials, carried out in several countries, have been reported in the last few years. In Italy, 99 early-stage patients were treated with gp160 for a 2-year period, but the treatment was inferior to zidovudine monotherapy [84]. In Canada, 278 early-stage patients were treated for 3 years, but no differences were observed in CD4 cells, time to initiation of therapy, plasma viral loads, or death [85]. In Sweden, 835 early-stage patients received gp160 every 3 months for 3 years [86]. HIV-1 T-cell immunoreactivity was induced in vaccine recipients, but the treatment did not lead to clinical benefit. In another study in Sweden, repeated immunizations for 5 years among 40 asymptomatic patients were safe and may have resulted in a transient improvement in CD4 cell count, but the study was too small to measure clinical impact [87]. In the United States, a large long-term (5-year) carefully conducted study among 608 HIV-infected asymptomatic patients found no evidence for efficacy as measured by the change in CD4 cell count or Walter Reed stage [88]. As in the Swedish study, a transient improvement in CD4 cell count was observed, but this did not translate into improved clinical outcome. Only one study has been reported of vaccine therapy with gp160 among patients with advanced HIV infection [89]. As in early-stage patients, the treatment was safe, and new and augmented immune responses were observed, but there were no evident clinical benefits.

The third major class of candidate therapeutic HIV vaccines to be tested in clinical trials is envelope protein subunits expressed in mammalian cells. Two trials of gp160 (expressed by vaccinia in Vero cells) were recently reported. In Germany, 208 patients were immunized repeatedly over 2 years [90]. Despite the induction of new lymphoproliferative responses, there was no clinical benefit. A smaller study in the United States showed similar findings [91]. Several trials of gp120 expressed from Chinese hamster ovary cells have recently been reported from the United States. In one study, 573 early-stage patients were randomized in a placebo-controlled double-blind study; more vaccine-treated patients than placebo recipients showed a 50% decrease in CD4 cell count, but the result was not statistically significant [92]. Schooley and colleagues studied four different gp120 candidate vaccine preparations [93]: 164 late-stage patients were immunized with CHO expressed gp120 (MN strain) and alum adjuvant, while 128 early-stage patients were randomized to receive either that vaccine, CHO expressed gp120 (III B strain), CHO expressed gp120 (SF-2 strain) in MF-59 adjuvant, or a nongycosylated gp120 (SF-2 strain) produced in yeast. New lymphoproliferative responses developed in only 30% of patients, more commonly among patients who had an undetectable level of HIV-1 RNA at baseline. Proliferative responses were usually HIV-1 strain restricted.

A fourth HIV-1 therapeutic vaccine approach reported to have been carefully studied is a canarypox engineered to express gag, pol, env, and nef gene products (ALVAC vCP1452) [94]. This study was unusual in that only patients with primary HIV infection were studied. All 148 patients were treated with highly active antiretroviral treatment (HAART), and those with sustained ablation of viremia were continued on HAART and randomized to receive ALVAC, ALVAC plus Remune, or no vaccine. The study is ongoing.

The long-term effects of p17/p24 viruslike particles as therapeutic vaccines have also been studied. In HIV-infected early-stage patients, the vaccine is well tolerated but does not induce new anti-p24 antibodies nor consistently induce cellular responses. Fifty-six patients were followed long-term, but no effect on disease progression was observed [95,96].

Other HIV-1 therapeutic vaccine approaches that have been reported recently are envelope peptides, tat toxoid, and DNA vaccines [97–100]. These approaches appear safe and moderately immunogenic, and clinical studies continue. Studies to determine the clinical efficacy of these approaches have not yet been done.

B. DNA Containing Viruses: Herpesviruses, Papillomaviruses, and Hepadnaviruses

DNA viruses that can cause chronic or recurrent clinical disease, including herpes simplex viruses, varicella-zoster vi-

ruses, papillomaviruses, and hepadnaviruses, are logical targets for vaccine therapy (Table 2).

1. Herpes Simplex Viruses

Because recurrent herpes infections are thought to occur as a consequence of a decline in antiherpes immunity, this disease has been a particularly attractive target for vaccine therapy. Numerous therapeutic herpes vaccines produced by inactivation of cell culture-grown virus have been tested in humans [101]. Most early trials were inadequately controlled, and in those few clinical therapeutic herpes vaccine trials done where controls were adequate, results were inconsistent [102–105]. Nonetheless, there continues to be reports in the medical literature of uncontrolled series of thousands of patients treated with therapeutic herpes simplex vaccines [106].

Recent scientific efforts have focused on the development and testing of herpes subunit protein vaccines. HSV-2 envelope protein gD2 with an alum adjuvant was used to prevent the recurrence of genital herpes in a double-blind placebo-controlled trial among 98 patients with frequent recurrences [107]. Vaccine recipients reported fewer recurrences and had fewer virologically confirmed recurrences. The authors of this study concluded that "these results inspire optimism about the potential use of vaccine for the treatment of chronic, recurring viral diseases." The same research group then studied what was thought to be an improved vaccine that included envelope proteins gD2 and gB2 in MF59, and oil-in-water adjuvant. Although glycoprotein-specific and neutralizing antibodies were boosted by vaccination, and the duration and severity of the first study outbreak was reduced significantly, overall the rate of recurrences was not significantly improved [108]. The investigators were unsure why the gD2/gB2/MF59 vaccine failed to show efficacy whereas the gD2/alum vaccine did in the preliminary study. One possible reason is that a lower dose of envelope protein antigens (10 µg each of gD2 and gB2) was used in the second study, compared to (100 µg of gD2) the first study.

2. Varicella Zoster Viruses

The varicella zoster virus (VZV) has also been thought to be a good candidate for vaccine therapy, but for prevention of zoster, not treatment of acute disease. After primary infection VZV remains latent in dorsal root ganglia cells and can reactivate to cause pain and skin lesions. Reactivation is thought to be the result of an age-related decline in VZV-specific T-cell immunity. At least four studies have been reported on the use of live attenuated varicella vaccine to boost immunity to VZV in the elderly [109–116]. Doses ranging from 3000 to 42,000 PFU have been tested. Collectively, local reactions are present in less than one-third of patients and are usually mild. Increased immunity to VZV has been documented by skin testing, lymphocyte proliferation assays, and responder cell frequency assays. Levin summarized studies to date by concluding that "there is anecdotal information from approximately 1200 patient years of follow-up that the incidence of zoster will not be reduced" but that in these preliminary studies "a clinical impression was that all of the events were unusually mild and pain was rarely

Table 2 Recent Vaccine Therapy Trials for Chronic DNA Viruses

Vaccine	Disease	Country	N patients	Placebo	Year	Author	Reference
gD2 HSV-2 (alum)	Recurrent genital herpes	United States	98	yes	1994	Straus	107
gD2 and gB2 HSV-2 (MF-59)	Recurrent genital herpes	United States	202	yes	1997	Straus	108
Live Oka strain (3000 to 42,000)	None (elderly)	United States	200	no	1998, 2000	Berger, Tranoy	109 110
Live Oka strain (4000)	None (elderly)	United States	167	no	1994. 1994, 2000	Hayward, Levin, Levine	111 112 113
Live Oka strain (3000 to 12,000)	None (elderly)	United States	202	no	1998, 2001	Levin, Levin	114 115
Live Oka strain (30,000)	None (elderly)	Japan	30	no	2001	Takahashi	116
E6 and E7 HPV 16 and 18 Vaccinia	Cervical cancer	United Kingdom	8	no	1996	Borysiewicz	121
E7 HPV 16 lipopeptides	Cervical and vulvar cancer	United States	12 (HLA A2)	no	1998	Steller	122
E7 HPV 16 E. coli	Cervical cancer	Australia	5	no	2000	Malcolm	123
E7 HPV 16 peptides	Cervical cancer	Europe	19 (HLA A2)	no	1999, 2000	vanDriel, Ressing	124 125
E7 HPV 16	Cervical and vulvar cancer	United States	18 (HLA A2)	no	2000	Muderspach	126
E6 and E7 HPV 16 and 18 Vaccinia	Advanced, early, and in situ cervical cancer	United Kingdom	44	no	2001	Adams	127
L2 and E7 HPV 6 E. coli	Genital warts	United Kingdom	27	no	1999	Lacey	128
L1 HPV 6b Viruslike particles	Genital warts	Republic of China	32	no	2000	Zhang	129
preS2/S or S	Chronic hepatitis	France	80	yes	2001, 2001	Pol, Soussan	130 131
preS2	Chronic hepatitis	France	27	no	1998, 1999	Pol, Covillin	133 132
S	Chronic hepatitis	Germany	18	no	2001	Heintges	134

significant and never persistent" [115]. The impression is that the "breakthrough zoster" is converted into a minor illness analogous to the "breakthrough varicella" seen in vaccinated children. A large 38,000-patient study—the Shingles Prevention Study—is now underway in the United States in an effort to collect reliable efficacy information.

3. Papillomaviruses

Vaccine therapy for cutaneous warts in cattle has been a common veterinary practice for decades [117]. Infections with bovine papillomavirus typically result in benign lesions that regress spontaneously. Occasionally warts can persist and give rise to squamous cell carcinomas. Commercial therapeutic wart vaccines were widely used but had questionable efficacy. Autogenous vaccines (made from glycerol-saline suspensions of lesions) were reported to have excellent efficacy and were recommended by experts [118,119]. Remarkably, in some locales autogenous vaccines continue to be used as experimental therapy in humans [120]. One recent report proposed that excision followed by autogenous tissue

vaccine is the most effective treatment for perianal condyloma acuminata [120].

There is now solid proof that human papillomavirus infection is causally associated with cervical cancer, most often HPV type 16. Recent research has shown that the E6 and E7 early gene products are nucleoproteins that can malignantly transform human cells, and there is evidence that continued expression of these proteins occurs in cancer cells. At least six small studies have been reported on the use of HPV16 E7 (with or without E6) to treat patients with cervical cancer [121–127]. In some of these trials only patients with the common HLA haplotype A2 were studied, so as to assure optimal HLA class I antigen presentation and epitope-specific recognition. All of the vaccine approaches thus far tested have been safe, and varying degrees of immunogenicity have been detected. In one careful study, vaccine therapy with short E7 peptides provoked and increased dendritic cell infiltrate in cervical biopsies, with clearing of HPV from cervical scrapings but not HPV RNA from biopsy samples [126]. None of the studies thus far conducted has been blinded or controlled, then there has been no compelling evidence of clinical efficacy. Larger clinical trials are ongoing.

Genital warts are benign neoplastic tumors in humans most often caused by HPV types 6 and 11. At least two studies have been reported on using HPV structural proteins (L1 or L2) as a therapeutic vaccine. In one uncontrolled open label study, a fusion protein consisting of HPV 6 L2 and E7 was given to 27 subjects [128]. Of these, 19 made antigen-specific T-cell proliferative responses to L2/E7, and 5 patients completely cleared their warts. A report from China describes a study in which patients with genital warts were immunized with an HPV 6b L1 viruslike particle vaccine [129]. Remarkably, complete regression of genital warts was observed in 25 of 33 evaluable subjects. Although increased anti-L1 antibodies were found, no studies of cellular immunity were reported.

4. Hepatitis B Virus

Hepatitis B virus infection can lead to chronic infection with a high risk for chronic hepatitis and/or hepatocellular carcinoma. Two European groups have recently reported on their studies of HBV envelope proteins as therapeutic vaccines. In France, a pilot open study and a randomized controlled study have been done on patients with chronic HBsAg carriage, detectable serum HBV DNA, and chronic hepatitis [130–133]. Antigen-specific lymphocyte proliferative responses were detected, but in only a minority of patients. Disappearance of serum HBsAg was not observed in any of the patients, but there was a transient decline in serum HBV DNA in the vaccinated groups. Because of a concern that escape mutants might emerge, amino acid sequences of the "a" antigenic determinants were determined for nonresponder and responder patients. No common escape mutations were detected. In Germany, a combination of immunotherapy with alpha-interferon and vaccine therapy with HBsAg was tested in 18 patients who were unresponsive to alpha-interferon alone [134]. HBV DNA became undetectable and liver enzyme profiles became normal in half of the patients.

C. Mycobacteria: Tuberculosis and Leprosy

1. Mycobacterium Tuberculosis

Vaccine therapy for tuberculosis, championed by Koch and widely employed for decades, is undergoing yet another revival (Table 3). Intradermal injections of *Mycobacterium vaccae* have been used to boost immunity to *Mycobacterium tuberculosis* in symptomatic patients [135–137]. The method has been aggressively pursued as cost-effective for developing countries [138,139]. Also, vaccine therapy is seen as perhaps the only alternative for patients infected with multidrug-resistant bacilli [140]. At least five intermediate size trials of the vaccine therapy using heat-killed *M. vaccae* have been reported from countries throughout the world in the last several years. In Romania, the *M. vaccae* vaccine was used as an adjunct to a chemotherapeutic regimen in newly diagnosed cases [141]. Although there were no differences in final outcome, those receiving vaccine therapy showed modestly more rapid improvement. Vaccine therapy was also studied in patients with chemotherapeutic treatment failures [142]. Patients were randomized to receive either *M. vaccae* or saline injections. After 22 months, only 13 of 56 patients receiving vaccine therapy had an unfavorable outcome compared to 26 of 46 patients in the control group. Vaccinated patients were also reported to have better success as measured by chest x-ray and bacteriological cultures. However, there was no significant difference in the number of patients who died in this trial. Two small trials in Argentina,

Table 3 Recent Vaccine Therapy Trials for Mycobacteria

Vaccine	Disease	Country	N patients	Placebo	Year	Author	Reference
Heat-killed *M. vaccae*	Pulmonary, newly diagnosed	Romania	206	yes	1997	Corlan	141
Heat-killed *M. vaccae*	Pulmonary, treatment failure	Romania	102	yes	1997	Corlan	142
Heat-killed *M. vaccae*	Pulmonary, newly diagnosed (HIV-)	Argentina	40	yes	1999	Dlugovitzky	143
Heat-killed *M. vaccae*	Pulmonary, newly diagnosed	Uganda	120	yes	2000	Johnson	144
Heat-killed *M. vaccae*	Pulmonary, multidrug resistant	Several countries	337	no	2001	Stanford	145
Killed *Mycobacterium* "w"	Multibacillary	India	156	yes	1999, 2000	Talwar, Sharma	164 165
BCG + killed *M. leprae*	Advanced lepromatous	India	50	no	1996	Majumder	166
BCG + killed *M. leprae* or BCG or killed *M. leprae*	Borderline, lempromin negative	India	100	no	1997	Chadhury	167
BCG + killed *M. leprae*	Paucibacillary, single lesion	India	60	no	2000	Majumder	168
Killed *Mycobacterium habana*	Lepromatous	India	31	no	2001	Wakhlu	169

involving a total of 40 newly diagnosed HIV negative pulmonary tuberculosis patients, were reported to show that vaccine therapy provided added clinical benefit to chemotherapy alone [143]. In this trial, serum levels of IL-4, IL-10, and TNF-alpha fell and levels of INF-gamma rose in vaccine therapy patients compared to placebo-controlled recipients. In Uganda, adjunctive vaccine therapy with heat-killed *M. vaccae* was studied in a placebo-controlled trial among 120 newly diagnosed HIV negative pulmonary tuberculosis patients [144]. Sputum culture conversion to negative and radiographic improvement were more rapid in the vaccinated patients. A larger open label multinational study of adjunctive vaccine therapy with *M. vaccae* was carried out among 337 patients with multidrug-resistant *M. tuberculosis* in Estonia, Iran, Kuwait, New Zealand, Romania, Vietnam, and the United Kingdom [145]. Although there were no placebo-controlled inoculated patients in this study, the authors concluded that the vaccine therapy improved the rate of cure of multidrug-resistant tuberculosis, most effectively in patients with short histories of disease.

2. Leprosy

In studies of the immunology of tuberculoid and lepromatous leprosy, Convit in Venezuela observed that patients with lepromatous leprosy did not clear heat-inactivated *Mycobacterium leprae* organisms that were experimentally inoculated intradermally [146,147]. However, these patients did clear inoculated live attenuated bacille Calmette-Guerin (BCG). When heat-killed *M. leprae* organisms were mixed with the live BCG, the *M. leprae* organisms were also cleared. Other studies suggested that *M. leprae* was directly suppressive of a delayed-type hypersensitivity response [148–154]. These experimental observations led to clinical trials of vaccine therapy of leprosy in which mixtures of *M. leprae* and BCG were inoculated into hundreds of patients [155,156]. Although treated patients showed improvements in a number of measures of antileprosy immunity (such as increased antibody titers, increased skin-test reactivity, and increased specific lymphocyte proliferation), clinical benefits were not clear-cut. Combined chemotherapy and vaccine therapy is reported to lead to shorter duration of treatment and faster hospital release [157–159].

Injections of 5 units of purified protein derivative of tuberculin also lead to clearing of *M. leprae* at the site of inoculation, as do injections of other mycobacterial antigen preparations [160–162]. It has been speculated that the widespread use of BCG has been a significant factor in the decline in incidence of leprosy in many countries [163].

Results of at least five clinical studies, all in India, have been reported in the last few years. One product has received authorization from the Drugs Controller of India for industrial manufacture, based on the killed *Mycobacterium* "w." This product has been used as an adjunct to drug therapy in 156 multibacillary leprosy patients [164,165]. Control patients received a placebo injection. Ninety percent of vaccinated patients converted from lepromin skin test negative to positive, compared to only 38% in the placebo group. Clinical scores and bacteriological indices improved more rapidly among the vaccinated patients for the first 3 years. Three

trials have been reported using the "Convit" vaccine consisting of live BCG plus killed *M. leprae*, in various stages of leprosy [166–168]. In all three there is a trend toward favorable results, but in the setting of chemotherapy it is difficult to assess these nonrandomized and not completely controlled studies. One Phase I safety and immunogenicity study was reported in which a vaccine consisting of irradiated *Mycobacterium habana* was used to treat 31 patients with lepromatous leprosy [169]. Vaccination induced lepromin conversion in 100% of the vaccines. However, the vaccine produced small cutaneous ulcerations at the injection site in all patients.

D. Leishmaniasis

Convit noted the similarities between the clinical and histopathological features of leprosy and cutaneous leishmaniasis and hypothesized that the pathogenesis of the two diseases was similar. Given the apparent success of treatment of leprosy with BCG, Convit and colleagues conducted clinical trials of vaccine therapy for leishmaniasis with inoculations of BCG mixed with killed *Leishmania* promastigotes [170–173]. Although in vitro markers of antileishmanial immunity have not shown marked changes, clinical efficacy in one study was reported to be excellent [174,175]. Other studies with soluble leishmanial antigens have suggested clinical efficacy [176]. Two vaccine therapy clinical studies of cutaneous leishmaniasis have recently been reported. In Venezuela, 43 patients were studied in an effort to find the immunologic correlates of efficacy [177]. The authors detected enhanced antigen-specific IFN-gamma responses to both components of the vaccine, *M. bovis* BCG and *L. amazonensis*. In Brazil, a vaccine composed of killed promasitgotes was used as an adjunctive therapy to standard chemotherapy with antimonium salts [178]. Fifty-three patients were randomized to receive the adjunctive vaccine therapy or antimonium salts only. Vaccinated patients showed increased lymphoproliferative responses, but there was no difference in the time for complete healing of the lesions between the two groups.

V. SUMMARY AND CONCLUSIONS

Vaccine therapy has been an alluring concept since the dawn of microbiology as a laboratory science and Pasteur, Koch, and Wright were all drawn to the idea that it should be possible to manipulate and direct the immune response in ways favorable to the patient. Will vaccine therapy ever live up to its conceptual promise? If effective therapeutic vaccines are to be developed, this will require a more complete understanding of the mechanisms that microbes use to establish and maintain chronic steady-state infections. Thoughtful new vaccine designs may be necessary to counter suppression, reinforce subverted costimulatory signals, or escort antigens in correct conformations to responsive cells. Vaccine therapy may not only be a goal in itself but, following the precedent set by Pasteur, Koch, and Wright, may also be a valuable tool to dissect the host–pathogen relationship so as to understand its crucial facets.

REFERENCES

1. Burke DS. Vaccine therapy for HIV: a historical review of the treatment of infectious diseases by active specific immunization with microbe-derived antigens. Vaccine 1993; 11:883–891.

2. Sereti I, Lane HC. Immunopathogenesis of human immunodeficiency virus: implications for immune-based therapies. Clin Infect Dis 2002; 32:1738–1755.

3. Raeder CK, Hayney MS. Immunology of varicella immunization in the elderly. Ann Pharmacother 2000; 34:228–234.

4. Gissmann L, et al. Therapeutic vaccines for human papillomaviruses. Intervirology 2001; 44:167–175.

5. Michel ML, Loirat D. DNA Vaccines for prophylactic or therapeutic immunization against hepatitis B. Intervirology 2001; 44:78–87.

6. Jenner E. A continuation of facts and observations relative to the variole vaccinae, or cow-pox, 1800. In: Eliot CW, ed. The Harvard Classics, Scientific Papers 1910. Vol. 38. New York: Collier, 1910.

7. Burke DS. Joseph-Alexander Auzias-Turenne, Louis Pasteur, and early concepts of virulence, attenuation, and vaccines. Perspect Biol Med 1996; 39:171–186.

8. Auzias-Turenne JA. La Syphilisation. Publication d l'Oeuvre du Docteur Auzias-Turenne: Faite par les Soins de ses Amis. (Syphilization, The collected works of Dr. Auzias-Turenne: Compiled through the efforts of his friends). Paris: Librairie Germer Bailliere, 1878:3–5.

9. Loir A. A l' ombre de Pasteur, la documentation medicale de Pasteur. (In the shadow of Pasteur: Pasteur's Medical Sources.) Mouve Sanit 1937; 14:387–392.

10. Loir A. Recherches sur le charbon et sur la peripneumonie bovine. Arch Med Exp 1892; 4:813–826.

11. Auzias-Turenne JA. La Syphilisation. Publication d l' Oeuvre du Docteur Auzias-Terenne: Faite par les Soins de ses Amis. (Syphilization, The collected works of Dr. Auzias-Turenne: Compiled through the efforts of his friends). Paris: Librairie Germer Bailliere, 1878:751–753.

12. Vallery-Radot R. La Vie de Pasteur. Paris: Librairie Hachette, 1924:619–621.

13. Dubos RJ. Louis Pasteur, Free Lance of Science. Boston: Little, Brown, 1951:326.

14. Geison G. The Private Science of Louis Pasteur. Princeton, NI: Princeton University Press, 1995:177–205.

15. Burke DS. Of postulates and peccadilloes: Robert Koch and vaccine (tuberculin) therapy for tuberculosis. Vaccine 1993; 11:795–804.

16. Koch R. Uber bakteriologische Forschung. (On bacterial research.) English translation of address delivered to the Tenth International Medical Congress, Berlin, August 1890. In: Carter KC, ed. Essays of Robert Koch. Westport, CT: Greenwood Press, 1987:179–186.

17. Minard EJC. The tenth international congress at Berlin, as I saw it. JAMA 1891; 16:589–591.

18. Koch R. Fortsetzung der Mittheilungen uber das Tuberkulin. (Continuation of the announcement concerning a cure for tuberculosis.) Dtsch Med Wochenschr, January 1891; 15:101–102.

19. Koch R. Weitere Mitteilung uber das Tuberkulin. (Additional information about tuberculin.) Dtsch Med Wochenschr, October 1891; 22:1189–1192.

20. Anonymous. Official report on the results of Koch's treatment in Prussia. JAMA Apr 1891; 11:526–529.

21. Wright AE. Vaccine therapy: its administration, value, and limitations. Proc R Soc Med 1910; 3:1–38.

22. Colebrook L. Almroth Wright: Provocative Doctor and Thinker. London: Heinemann, 1954:47–61.

23. Wright AE. Notes on the treatment of furunculosis, sycosis,

24. Keating P. Vaccine therapy and the problem of opsonins. J Hist Med Allied Sci 1988; 43:275–296.

25. Cope Z. Almroth Wright: Founder of Modern Vaccine-Therapy. London: Thomas Nelson, 1966:43–45.

26. Shaw B. "The Doctor's Dilemma" with a Preface on Doctors. In: Shaw B, ed. Complete Plays with Prefaces 1906. Vol. I. New York: Dodd, Mead, 1962.

27. Fleming A. Vaccine therapy in regard to general practice. Br Med J February 1921; 19:255–259.

28. Sherman GH. The Bacterial Therapist: A Journal of Vaccine Therapy. Vol. I. Detroit: Sherman, 1912:255–259.

29. Sherman GH. Vaccine News. Vols. 1 and 2. Detroit: Sherman, 1931.

30. Hektoen L, Irons EE. Vaccine therapy: result of a questionnaire to American physicians. JAMA 1929; 92:864–869.

31. Lister J. Lecture on Koch's treatment of tuberculosis. Lancet 1890; 68:1257–1259.

32. Wright AE. Vaccine therapy: its administration, value, and limitations. Proc R Soc Med 1910; 3:1–38.

33. Colebrook L. Almroth Wright: Provocative Doctor and Thinker. London: Heinemann, 1954.

34. Trudeau EL. The treatment of experimental tuberculosis by Koch's Tuberculin. Hunter's modifications and other products of the tubercle bacillus. Trans Assoc Am Phys, 1892:87–101.

35. Lazar MP. Vaccination for recurrent herpes simplex infection. Arch Dermatol 1956; 73:70–71.

36. Ooldman L. Reactions of autoinoculation for re-current herpes simplex. Arch Dermatol 1961; 84:1025–1026.

37. Kern AB, Schiff BL. Vaccine therapy in recurrent herpes simplex. Arch Dermatol 1964; 89:844–845.

38. Miller RI. Treatment of equine phycomycosis by immunotherapy and surgery. Aust Vet J 1981; 57:377–382.

39. Beemer AM, et al. Vaccine and mycostatin in treatment of cryptococcosis of the respiratory tract. Sabouraudia 1976; 14:171–179.

40. Jesiotr M, Beemer AM. Vaccine and antimicrobial therapy in pulmonary nocardiosis. Scand J Respir Dis 1969; 50:54–60.

41. Beemer AM, et al. Treatment with antifungal vaccines. Contrib Microb Immunol 1977; 4:136–146.

42. Bryant RE, et al. Treatment of recurrent furunculosis with staphylococcal bacteriophage-lysed vaccine. JAMA 1965; 164:123–126.

43. Hanna W. Studies of Smallpox and Vaccination. New York: William Wood, 1913.

44. Dixon CW. Smallpox in Tripolitania: an epidemiological and clinical study of 500 cases, including trials of penicillin treatment. J Hyg 1948; 46:351–377.

45. Fenner F, et al. Smallpox and Its Eradication. Geneva: World Health Organization, 1988:65.

46. Geison G. The Private Science of Louis Pasteur. Princeton, NJ: Princeton University Press, 1995:177–205.

47. Geison G. The Private Science of Louis Pasteur. Princeton, NJ: Princeton University Press, 1995:234–253.

48. Webster LT. The immunizing potency of antirabies vaccines: a critical review. Am J Hyg 1939; 30(Sec B):113–134.

49. Webster LT. Rabies. New York: Macmillan, 1942.

50. McKendrick AG. A ninth analytical review of reports from Pasteur Institutes on the results of anti-rabies treatment. Bull Health Org League Nations 1940; 9:31–78.

51. Baltazard M, Ghodssi M. Prevention de la rage humaine. Rev Immunol 1953; 17:366–375.

52. Habel K, Koprowski H. Laboratory data supporting the

clinical trial of antirabies serum in persons bitten by a rabid wolf. Bull WHO 1955; 13:773–779.

53. Baltazard M, Bahmanyar M. Essai pratique du serum antirabique chez les mordus par loups enrages. Bull WHO 1955; 13:747–772.

54. Cho HC, Lawson KF. Protection of dogs against death from experimental rabies by postexposure administration of rabies vaccine and hyperimmune globulin (human). Can J Vet Res 1989; 52:434–437.

55. Baer GM, Cleary WF. A model in mice for the pathogenesis and treatment of rabies. J Infect Dis 1972; 125:520–527.

56. Taylor J, et al. Biological and immunogenic properties of a canarypox-rabies recombinant. ALVAC-RG (vCP 65) in non-avian species. Vaccine 1995; 13:539–549.

57. Fujii H, et al. Protective efficacy in mice of post-exposure vaccination with vaccinia virus recombinant expressing either rabies virus glycoprotein or nucleoprotein. J Gen Virol 1994; 75:1339–1344.

58. Szmuness W, et al. Hepatitis B vaccine: demonstration of efficacy in a controlled clinical trial in a high-risk population in the United States. N Engl J Med 1980; 303:833–841.

59. Francis DP, et al. The prevention of hepatitis B with vaccine: report of the Centers for Disease Control Multicenter efficacy trial among homosexual men. Ann Intern Med 1982; 97:362–366.

60. Xu ZY, et al. Long-term efficacy of active postexposure immunization of infants for prevention of hepatitis B virus infection. J Infect Dis 1995; 171:54–60.

61. Zhu QR, et al. Long term immunogenicity and efficacy of recombinant yeast derived hepatitis B vaccine for interruption of mother–infant transmission of hepatitis B virus. Chin Med J 1994; 107:915–918.

62. Asano Y, et al. Protection against varicella in family contacts by immediate inoculation with live varicella vaccine. Pediatrics 1977; 59:1–8.

63. Asano Y, et al. Protective effect of immediate inoculation of a live varicella vaccine in household contacts in relation to the viral dose and interval between exposure and vaccination. Biken J 1982; 25:43–45124.

64. Bruster H, et al. Autovaccination in ARC and AIDS patients: a clinical report and a statistical analysis of nearly 7 years therapy. Int Conf AIDS 1992; 8(3):6060.

65. Scolaro M, et al. Potential molecular competitor for HIV. Lancet 1991; 1:731–732.

66. Mathisen GE, et al. Self-mononuclear cell vaccine as a therapy for HIV disease. Natl Conf Hum Retrovir Relat Infect, 1993.

67. Zagury D, et al. Immunization against AIDS in humans (letter). Nature 1987; 326:249–250.

68. Zagury D, et al. A group specific anamnestic immune reaction against HIV-1 induced by a candidate vaccine against Ams. Nature 1988; 332:728–731.

69. Zagury D. Anti-HIV cellular immunotherapy in AIDS (letter). Lancet 1991; 338:694–695.

70. Zagury D, et al. One-year follow-up of vaccine therapy in HIV-infected immune-deficient individuals: a new strategy. J AIDS 1992; 5:676–681.

71. Picard O, et al. Complication of intramuscular/subcutaneous immune therapy in severely immune-compromised individuals. J AIDS 1991; 4:641–643.

72. Salk J. Prospects for the control of AIDS by immunizing seropositive individuals. Nature 1987; 327:473–476.

73. Gibbs CJ Jr, et al. Observations after human immunodeficiency virus immunization and challenge of human immunodeficiency virus seropositive and seronegative chimpanzees. Proc Natl Acad Sci USA 1991; 88:3345–3352.33.

74. Moss RB, et al. Inactivated HIV-1 immunogen: impact on markers of disease progression. J AIDS 1994; 7(suppl 1): S21–S27.

75. Levine AM, et al. Initial studies on active immunization of HIV-infected subjects. J AIDS Hum Retrovir 1996; 11:351–364.

76. Ferre F, et al. Viral load in peripheral blood mononuclear cells as surrogate for clinical progression. J AIDS Hum Retrovir 1995; 10(suppl 2):S51–S56.

77. Kahn J, et al. Evaluation of HIV-1 immunogen, and immunologic modifier, administered to patients infected with HIV having 300 to 549 × 10(6)/L CD4 cell counts: a randomized controlled trial. JAMA 2000; 284(17):2193–2202.

78. Turner J, et al. The effect of HIV-1 immunogen (Remune) on viral load, CD4 cell counts and HIV-specific immunity in a double-blind, randomized, adjuvant-controlled subset study in HIV infected subjects regardless of concomitant antiviral drugs. HIV Med 2001; 2(2):68–77.

79. Torassa U. Drug firm battles UCSP on research results: test showed AIDS medicine no help. San Francisco Examiner. 11-1-2000.

80. Churdboonchart V, et al. A double-blind adjuvant-controlled trial on human immunodeficiency virus type 1 (HIV-1) immunogen (Remune) monotherapy in asymptomatic HIV-1 infected Thai subject with CD4-cell counts of >300. Clin Diagn Lab Immunol 2000; 7(5):728–733.

81. Redfield RR, et al. Phase I evaluation of the safety and immunogenicity of vaccination with recombinant gp160 in patients with early human immunodeficiency virus infection. N Engl J Med 1991; 324:1678–1684.

82. Redfield RR, Birx DL. HIV-specific vaccine therapy: concepts, status, and future directions. AIDS Res Hum Retrovir 1992; 8:1051–1058.

83. Vahey M, et al. Assessment of gag DNA and genomic RNA in peripheral blood mononuclear cells in HIV-infected patients receiving intervention with a recombinant gp160 subunit vaccine in a phase I study. AIDS Res Hum Retrovir 1994; 10:649–654.

84. Pontesilli O, et al. Phase II controlled trial of post-exposure immunization with recombinant gp 160 versus antiretroviral therapy in asymptomatic HIV-1 infected adults. VaxSyn Protocol Team. AIDS 1998; 12:473–480.

85. Tsoukas C, et al. Active immunization of patients with HIV infection: a study of the effect of VaxSyn, a recombinant HIV envelope subunit vaccine, on progression of immunodeficiency. AIDS Res Hum Retrovir 1998; 14:483–490.

86. Sandstrom E, Wahren B. Therapeutic immunization with recombinant gp160 in HIV-1 infection: a randomised double-blind placebo-controlled trial. Lancet 1999; 353:1735–1742.

87. Bratt G, et al. Long-term immunotherapy in HIV infection, combined with short-term antiretroviral treatment. Int J STD AIDS 1999; 10:514–521.

88. Birx D, et al. Efficacy testing of recombinant human immunodeficiency virus (HIV) gp160 as a therapeutic vaccine in early-stage HIV-1-infected volunteers. rgp160 Phase II Vaccine Investigators. J Infect Dis 2000; 181:881–889.

89. DeMaria AJ, et al. Immune responses to a recombinant human immunodeficiency virus type 1 (HIV-1) gp160 vaccine among adults with advanced HIV infection. Massachusetts gp160 Working Group. J Hum Virol 2000; 3: 182–192.

90. Goebal F, et al. Recombinant gp160 as a therapeutic vaccine for HIV-infection: results of a large randomized, controlled trial. European Multinational IMMUNO AIDS Vaccine Study Group. AIDS 1999; 13:1461–1468.

91. Kundu-Raychaudhuri S, et al. Effect of therapeutic immunization with HIV type 1 recombinant glycoprotein 160 ImmunoAG vaccine in HIV-infected individuals with CD4$^+$ T cell counts of > or = 500 and 200–400/m^3 (AIDS

Clinical Trials Group Study 246/946). AIDS Res Hum Retrovir 2001; 17:1371–1378.

92. Eron JJ, et al. Randomized trial of MNrgpl120 HIV-1 vaccine in symptonless HIV-1 infection. Lancet 1996; 348: 1547–1551.

93. Schooley R, et al. Two double-blinded, randomized, comparative trials of 4 human immunodeficiency virus across a spectrum of disease severity: AIDS Clinical Trials Groups 209–214. J Infect Dis 2000; 182:1357–1364.

94. Goh LE, et al. Study protocol for the evaluation of the potential durable viral suppression after quadruple HAART with or without HIV vaccination: the QUEST study. HIV Clin Trials 2001; 2:438–444.

95. Lindenburg CEA, et al. Long-term follow-up: no effect of therapeutic vaccination with HIV-1 p17/p24:Ty virus-like particles on HIV-1 disease progression. Vaccine 2002; 20:2343–2347.

96. Benson E, et al. Therapeutic vaccination with p24-VLP and zidovudine augments HIV-specific cytotoxic T lymphocyte activity in asymptomatic HIV-infected individuals. AIDS Res Hum Retrovir 1999; 15:105–113.

97. Pinto L, et al. HIV-specific immunity following immunization with HIV synthetic envelope peptides in asymptomatic HIV-infected patients. AIDS 1999; 13:2003–2012.

98. Gringeri A, et al. Safety and immunogenicity of HIV-1 Tat toxoid in immunocompromised HIV-1 infected patients. J Hum Virol 1998; 1:293–298.

99. Calarota S, et al. Immune responses in asymptomatic HIV-1 infected patients after HIV-DNA immunization followed by highly active antiretroviral treatment. J Immunol 1999; 163:2330–2338.

100. Weber R, et al. Phase I clinical trial with HIV-1 gp160 plasmid vaccine in HIV-1 infected asymptomatic subjects. Eur J Clin Microbiol Infect Dis 2001; 20:800–803.

101. Meigner B. Vaccination against herpes simplex virus infections. In: Roizman B, Lopez C, eds. The Herpesviruses: Immunobiology and Prophylaxis of Human Herpes virus Infection. New York: Plenum Press, 1985:265–296.

102. Anderson SO, et al. An attempt to vaccinate against herpes simplex. Aust J Exp Biol Med Sci 1950; 28:579–584.

103. Hall MI, Katrak K. The quest for a herpes simplex virus vaccine: background and recent developments. Vaccine 1986; 4:138–150.

104. Kern AB, Schiff BL. Vaccine therapy in recurrent herpes simplex. Arch Dermatol 1964; 89:844–845.

105. Weitgasser H. Controlled clinical study of herpes antigens Lupidon-H and Lupidon-G. Z Hautkr 1977; 52:625–628.

106. Dundarov S, Andonov P. Seventeen years of application of herpes vaccine in Bulgaria. Acta Virol 1994; 38:205–208.

107. Straus S, et al. Placebo-controlled trial of vaccination with recombinant glycoprotein D of herpes simplex virus type 2 for immunotherapy of genital herpes. Lancet 1994; 343: 1460–1463.

108. Straus S, et al. Immunotherapy of recurrent genital herpes with recombinant herpes simplex virus 2 glycoproteins D and B: results of a placebo-controlled vaccine trial. J Infect Dis 1997; 176:1129–1134.

109. Berger R, et al. A dose–response study of a live attenuated varicella-zoster virus (Oka strain) vaccine administered to adults 55 years of age and older. J Infect Dis 1998; 178:99–103.

110. Trannoy E, et al. Vaccination of immunocompetent elderly subjects with a live attenuated Oka strain of varicella zoster virus: a randomized, controlled, dose–response trial. Vaccine 2000; 18:1700–1706.

111. Hayward A, et al. Immune response to secondary immunization with live or inactivated VZV vaccine in elderly adults. Viral Immunol 1994; 7:31–36.

112. Levin MJ, et al. Immune responses of elderly persons 4

113. Levine MJ, et al. Comparison of live attenuated and an inactivated varicella vaccine to boost the varicella-specific immune response in seropositive people 55 years of age and older. Vaccine 2000; 18:2915–2920.

114. Levin MJ, et al. Use of live attenuated varicella vaccine to boost varicella-specific immune responses in seropositive people 55 years of age or older: duration of booster effect. J Infect Dis 1998; 178:109–112.

115. Levin MJ. Use of varicella vaccines to prevent herpes zoster in older individuals. Arch Virol Suppl, 2001:151–160.

116. Takahashi M, et al. Immunization of elderly to boost immunity against varicella-zoster virus (VZV) as assesses by VZV skin test reaction. Arch Virol Suppl 2001; 17:161–172.

117. Olson C, Skidmore LV. Therapy of experimentally produced bovine cutaneous papillomatosis with vaccines and excision. J Am Vet Med Assoc 1959; 135:339–343.

118. Pearson JKL, et al. Tissue vaccines in the treatment of bovine papillomas. Vet Record 1958; 79:971–973.

119. Anonymous. Treatment of warts in cattle. Mod Vet Pract September 1978:651–652.

120. Wiltz OH, et al. Autogenous vaccine: the best therapy for perianal condyloma acuminata? Dis Colon Rectum 1995; 38:838–841.

121. Borysiewicz LK, et al. A recombinant vaccinia virus encoding human papillomavirus types 16 and 18, E6 and E7 proteins as immunotherapy for cervical cancer. Lancet 1996; 347:1523–1527.

122. Steller MA, et al. Cell-mediated immunological responses in cervical and vaginal cancer patients immunized with a lipidated epitope of human papillomavirus type 16 E7. Clin Cancer Res 1998; 4:2103–2109.

123. Malcom K, et al. Multiple conformational epitopes are recognized by natural and induced immunity to the E7 protein of human papilloma virus type 16 in man. Intervirology 2000; 43:165–173.

124. van Driel WJ, et al. Vaccination with HPV16 peptides of patients with advanced cervical carcinoma: clinical evaluation of a phase I–II trial. Eur J Cancer 1999; 35:946–952.

125. Ressing M, et al. Detection of T helper responses, but not of human papillomavirus-specific cytotoxic T lymphocyte responses, after peptide vaccination of patients with cervical carcinoma. J Immunother 2000; 23:255–266.

126. Muderspach L, et al. A phase I trial of a human papillomavirus (HPV) peptide vaccine for women with high-grade cervical and vulvar intraepithelial neoplasia who are HPV 16 positive. Clin Cancer Res 2000; 6:3406–3416.

127. Adams M, et al. Clinical studies of human papilloma vaccines in pre-invasive and invasive cancer. Vaccine 2001; 19: 2549–2556.

128. Lacey CJ, et al. Phase IIa safety and immunogenicity of a therapeutic vaccine, TA-GW, in persons with genital warts. J Infect Dis 1999; 179:612–618.

129. Zhang L, et al. HPV6b viruslike particles are potent immunogens without adjuvant in man. Vaccine 2000; 18:1051–1058.

130. Pol S, et al. Efficacy and limitations of a specific immunotherapy in chronic hepatitis B. J Hepatol 2001; 34:917–921.

131. Soussan P, et al. Vaccination of chronic hepatitis B virus carriers with preS2/S envelope protein is not associated with the emergence of envelope escape mutants. J Gen Virol 2001; 82:367–371.

132. Couillin I, et al. Specific vaccine therapy in chronic hepatitis B: induction of T cell proliferative responses specific for envelope antigens. J Infect Dis 1999; 180:15–26.

133. Pol S, et al. Immunotherapy of chronic hepatitis B by anti HBV vaccine. Acta Gastroenterol Belg 1998; 61:228–233.

134. Heintges T, et al. Combination therapy of active HBsAg vaccination and interferon-alpha in interferon-alpha non-responders with chronic hepatitis B. Dig Dis Sci 2001; 46: 901–906.

135. Stanford JL, et al. Immunotherapy with *Mycobacterium vaccae* as an adjunct to chemotherapy in the treatment of pulmonary tuberculosis. Tubercle 1990; 71:87–93.

136. Bahr GM, et al. Improved immunotherapy for pulmonary tuberculosis with *Mycobacterium vaccae*. Tubercle 1990; 71: 259–266.

137. Stanford JL, Stanford CA. Immunotherapy of tuberculosis with *Mycobacterium vaccae* NCTC 11659. Immunobiology 1994; 191:555–563.

138. Standford JL, et al. Is Africa Lost? Lancet 1991; 338:557–558.

139. Onyebujoh PC. Immunotherapy with *Mycobacterium vaccae* as an addition to chemotherapy for the treatment of pulmonary tuberculosis under difficult conditions in Africa. Respir Med 1995; 89:199–207.

140. Prior JG, et al. Immunotherapy with *Mycobacterium vaccae* combined with second line chemotherapy in drug-resistant abdominal tuberculosis. J Infect 1995; 31:59–61.

141. Corlan E, et al. Immunotherapy with *Mycobacterium vaccae* in the treatment of tuberculosis in Romania: 1. Newly-diagnosed pulmonary disease. Respir Med 1997; 91:13–19.

142. Corlan E, et al. Immunotherapy with *Mycobacterium vaccae* in the treatment of tuberculosis in Romania: 2. Chronic or relapsed disease. Respir Med 1997; 91:21–29.

143. Dlugovitzky D, et al. Clinical and serological studies of tuberculosis patients in Argentina receiving immunotherapy with *Mycobacterium vaccae* (SRL 172). Respir Med 1999; 93:557–562.

144. Johnson JL, et al. Randomized controlled trial of *Mycobacterium vaccae* immunotherapy in non-human immuno-deficiency virus-infected Ugandan adults with newly diagnosed pulmonary tuberculosis. The Uganda-Case Western Reserve University Research Collaboration. J Infect Dis 2000; 181:1304–1312.

145. Stanford JL, et al. Does immunotherapy with heat-killed *Mycobacterium vaccae* offer hope for the treatment of multi-drug-resistant pulmonary tuberculosis? Respir Med 2001; 95:444–447.

146. Convit J, et al. Immunological changes observed in indeterminate and lepromatous leprosy patients and Mitsuda-negative contacts after the inoculation of a mixture of *Mycobacterium leprae* and BCG. Clin Exp Immunol 1979; 36:214–220.

147. Rada EM, et al. Immunosuppression and cellular immunity reactions in leprosy patients treated with a mixture of *Mycobacterium leprae* and BCG. Int J Lepr 1987; 55:646–650.

148. Kaplan G, et al. Influence of *Mycobacterium leprae* and its soluble products on the cutaneous responsiveness of leprosy patients to antigen and recombinant interleukin 2. Proc Natl Acad Sci USA 1989; 86:6269–6273.

149. Modlin RL, et al. Genetically restricted suppressor T-cell clones derived from lepromatous leprosy lesions. Nature 1986; 322:459–461.

150. Kaplan G, et al. *Mycobacterium leprae* antigen-induced suppression of T cell proliferation in vivo. J Immunol 1987; 138:3028–3034.

151. Gelber RH, et al. Vaccination with pure *Mycobacterium leprae* proteins inhibits *M. leprae* multiplication in mouse footpads. Infect Immun 1994; 62:4250–4255.

152. Modlin RL. Th1–Th2 paradigm: insights from leprosy. J Invest Dermatol 1994; 102:828–832.

153. Sieling PA, et al. Immunosuppressive roles for IL-10 and IL-4 in human infection: in vitro modulation of T cell responses in leprosy. J Immunol 1993; 150:5501–5510.

154. Kaplan G. Cytokine regulation of disease progression in leprosy and tuberculosis. Immunobiology 1994; 191:564–568.

155. Convit J, et al. Immunotherapy with a mixture of *Mycobacterium leprae* and BCG in different forms of leprosy and in Mitsuda-negative contacts. Int J Lepr 1982; 50:415–424.

156. Convit J, et al. Immunotherapy and immunoprophylaxis of leprosy. Lepr Rev 1983; special issue:47S–60S.

157. Rada E, et al. A longitudinal study of immunologic reactivity in leprosy patients treated with immunotherapy. Int J Lepr Mycobact Dis 1994; 64:552–558.

158. Kar HK, et al. Reversal reaction in multibacillary leprosy patients following MDT with and without immunotherapy with a candidate for an antileprosy vaccine. *Mycobacterium* w. Lepr Rev 1993; 64:219–226.

159. Walia R, et al. Field trials on the use of *Mycobacterium* w vaccine in conjunction with multidrug therapy in leprosy patients for immunotherapeutic and immunoprophylactic purposes. Lepr Rev 1993; 64:302–311.

160. Kaplan G, et al. Efficacy of a cell-mediated reaction to the purified protein derivative of tuberculin in the disposal of *Mycobacterium leprae* from human skin. Proc Natl Acad Sci USA 1988; 85:5210–5214.

161. Zaheer SA, et al. Immunotherapy with *Mycobacterium* w vaccine decreases the incidence and severity of type 2 (ENL) reactions. Lepr Rev 1993; 64:7–14.

162. Zaheer SA, et al. Addition of immunotherapy with *Mycobacterium* w vaccine to multi-drug therapy benefits multibacillary leprosy patients. Vaccine 1995; 13:1102–1110.

163. Fine PEM, Smith PG. Efficacy of leprosy vaccine. Lancet 1992; 360:406.

164. Talwar GP. An immunotherapeutic vaccine for multibacillary leprosy. Int Rev Immunol 1999; 18:229–249.

165. Sharma P, et al. Induction of lepromin positivity and immunoprophylaxis in household contacts of multibacillary leprosy patients: a pilot study with a candidate vaccine, *Mycobacterium* w. Int J Lepr Other Mycobact Dis 2000; 68: 136–142.

166. Majumder V, et al. Immunotherapy of far-advanced lepromatous leprosy patients with low-dose convit vaccine along with multidrug therapy (Calcutta trial). Int J Lepr Other Mycobact Dis 1996; 64:26–36.

167. Chaudhury S, et al. Immunotherapy of lepromin-negative borderline leprosy patients with low-dose Convit vaccine as an adjunct to multidrug therapy; a six-year follow-up study in Calcutta. Int J Lepr Other Mycobact Dis 1997; 65:56–62.

168. Majumder V, et al. Efficacy of single-dose ROM therapy plus low-dose convit vaccine as an adjuvant for treatment of paucibacillary leprosy patients with a single skin lesion. Int J Lepr Other Mycobact Dis 2000; 68:283–290.

169. Wakhlu A, et al. Response of *Mycobacterium habana* vaccine in patients with lepromatous leprosy and their household contacts. A pilot clinical study. Lepr Rev 2001; 72:179–191.

170. Convit J. The Kellersberger Memorial Lecture. Leprosy and leishmaniasis: similar clinical–immunological pathology. Ethiop Med I 1974; 12:187–195.

171. Convit J, et al. Immunotherapy versus chemotherapy in localized cutaneous leishmaniasis. Lancet 1987; 1:401–405.

172. Convit J, Ulrich M. Antigen-specific immunodeficiency and its relation to the spectrum of American cutaneous leishmaniasis. Biol Res 1993; 26:159–166.

173. Modlin RL, et al. Learning from lesions: patterns of tissue inflammation in leprosy. Proc Natl Acad Sci USA 1988; 85:1213–1217.

174. Convit J, et al. Immunotherapy of localized, intermediate, and diffuse forms of American cutaneous leishmaniasis. J Infect Dis 1989; 160:104–115.

175. Castes M, et al. Cell mediated immunity in localized cuta-
     neous leishmaniasis patients before and after treatment with
     immunotherapy of chemotherapy. Parasite Immunol 1989;
     11:211–222.
176. Monjour L, et al. Immunotherapy as treatment of
     cutaneous leishmaniasis. J Infect Dis 1991; 164:1244–1245.
177. Cabrera M, et al. Immunotherapy with live BCG plus heat

     killed Leishmania induces a T helper 1-like response in
     American cutaneous leishmaniasis patients. Parasite Im-
     munol 2000; 22:73–79.
178. Toledo VP, et al. Immunochemotherapy in American
     cutaneous leishmaniasis: immunological aspects before
     and after treatment. Mem Inst Oswaldo Cruz 2001; 96:
     89–98.

84

Vaccination-Based Therapies in Multiple Sclerosis

Jacqueline Shukaliak-Quandt and Roland Martin
National Institutes of Health, Bethesda, Maryland, U.S.A.

I. INTRODUCTION

Multiple sclerosis (MS) is a chronic inflammatory disease of the central nervous system (CNS) characterized by extensive leukocytic infiltration and associated demyelination. The end result is invariably damage to myelin and also to oligodendrocytes, with varying degrees of axonal destruction resulting in neurologic impairment [1–3]. While the exact cause of MS is unknown, an immunological component has been suggested based on the examination of lesions showing scattered inflammatory infiltrates (particularly mononuclear cells) [4,5], the positive therapeutic results after immune modulation or immunosuppression [6,7], and the genetic association of disease to the major histocompatibility complex (MHC) or human leukocyte antigen (HLA) in humans, which presents antigen to T cells [8–10]. Also convincing are the striking similarities between disease in humans and an animal model of MS, experimental autoimmune encephalomyelitis (EAE) [11,12], which is generated in several species following immunization with myelin proteins. The T-cell-mediated response that ensues and that can be passively transferred to naive individuals strongly implicates the involvement of these autoantigen-specific T cells in autoimmune disease.

A. The Schema of Central Nervous System Autoimmunity: Targets for Therapy

Advances in understanding the immunopathogenesis of MS have given rise to several immunomodulatory therapies. Potential therapies for MS under experimental or practical application to date have focused on several steps of disease pathogenesis (Figure 1). While the precise triggering event that activates autoreactive T cells is unknown, studies using the animal model EAE have shed light on the events following T cell activation. Initial activation likely occurs outside the CNS, as myelin-reactive CD4 + T cells encounter an antigen (bacterial, viral, or otherwise) presented in the context of an antigen-presenting cell (APC) with sufficient costimulation to induce full T cell activation. Activated cells are able to cross the blood–brain barrier (BBB) through complex interactions involving adhesion molecules, chemokines, and metalloproteinases, and enter the CNS where they encounter the cross-reactive antigen [13]. Both reactivation and subsequent clonal expansion with inflammatory cytokine and chemokine production within the CNS are requirements for disease development in animal models [13,14], and serve to recruit a multitude of immunocompetent cells. Extensive damage and increased permeability at the BBB also allows for the passage of soluble factors including serum proteins, complement, and antibodies that can contribute to the process of demyelination. The recruitment or presence of macrophages/microglia at this stage is the cornerstone of the effector phase of the disease [15] as these cells perpetuate immune-mediated demyelination via phagocytosis with concomitant release of several cytokines, proteases, and toxic nitrogen and oxygen intermediates [16].

The drugs in widest clinical use include immunomodulatory therapies such as the β-interferons and glatiramer acetate (GA). While their mechanism is far from completely characterized, they can inhibit T cell activation, alter levels of various cytokines, or reduce the trafficking of leukocytes across and reduce BBB permeability. However, they are only moderately effective, and at therapeutic doses can cause organ toxicity and complications that can be difficult to manage. They may also impair the activities of all immune cells, including those with regulatory properties. Newer immunomodulatory strategies are continuously being explored in animal models of MS (Table 1) and include the administration of antibodies to inflammatory mediators, systemic administration/gene therapy to deliver suppressive factors, and most recently the application of vaccine-like strategies.

B. Vaccines to Combat Autoimmune Disease

The traditional concept of a vaccine is the prophylactic administration of an antigen or attenuated infectious agents in preparedness for subsequent exposure. Typically, the goal is to mount a more rapid and potent humoral and cellular

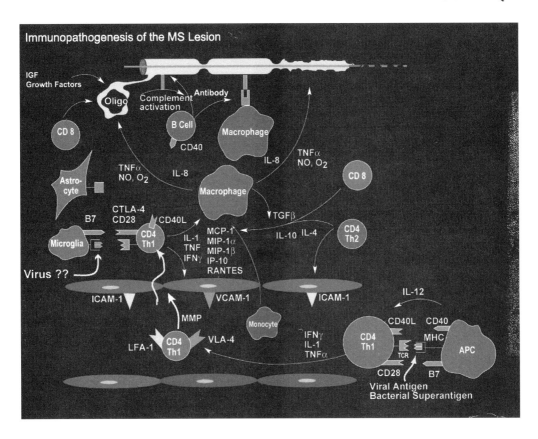

Figure 1 Immunopathogenesis of MS. While the precise triggering event activating autoreactive T cells is unknown, studies using the animal model EAE have shed light on the likeliest mechanisms of disease initiation. Most probably, the initial activation occurs outside the CNS, as myelin-reactive CD4+ T cells encounter an antigen presented in the context of an antigen-presenting cell (APC) with sufficient costimulation to induce full T cell activation. Activation may result from the sharing of epitopes between microbes and CNS antigens (molecular mimicry), superantigen-driven nonspecific T cell activation [172], or cytokine-mediated bystander activation. Upon activation, these cells acquire the ability to cross the blood–brain barrier (BBB) localized to the tight, nonfenestrated endothelial cells lining the microvasculature of the brain [173,174]. Through complex interactions involving adhesion molecules, chemokines, and metalloproteinases, T cells enter the CNS where they encounter the specific autoantigen (presumably a neuroantigen). T cell reactivation and subsequent clonal expansion with inflammatory cytokine and chemokine production within the CNS is a requirement for disease development in animal models [13,14], and serve to recruit several immunocompetent cells. Extensive damage and increased permeability at the BBB also allows for the passage of soluble factors including serum proteins and antibodies that can contribute to the process of demyelination. The recruitment or presence of macrophages/microglia at this stage is the cornerstone of the effector phase of the disease [15] as the cells that perpetuate immune-mediated demyelination via phagocytosis with concomitant release of several cytokines, proteases, and toxic oxygen and nitrogen intermediates [16,175]. (Courtesy of H.F. McFarland, NINDS, NIH, Bethesda, Maryland.)

immune response to microbial pathogens. Recently, vaccines have also been explored in the treatment of cancers where they drive a cellular, antigen-specific response. To be effective in autoimmunity, vaccines could be (1) globally modulatory or suppressive, and by eliminating proinflammatory mediators thus reduce some (and possibly all) immune responses for at least a short time, or (2) antigen-specific, and target only antigen-specific T cells thought to mediate disease. Thus the goal of the vaccination in autoimmune diseases is very different from that to combat viral infection or cancer.

The majority of vaccines applied in EAE for immunomodulatory purposes consist of naked DNA encoding cytokines found at high levels in autoimmune disorders and thus

implicated in disease development. Vaccination with cytokine genes induces a breakdown in tolerance and generates self-specific immunity against that gene product in the form of a high affinity, highly specific antibody response at higher levels than natural antibodies. Ideally, these antibodies can then block the accumulation/activity of an overproduced cytokine, thus inhibiting pathogenic effects. Following naked DNA vaccination, EAE was prevented by limiting in vivo responses to MIP-1α and MCP-1, two chemokines critical in disease progression [17]. Similar protective effects were observed with DNA for TNF-α [18]. While not yet pursued in patients, data suggests that cytokine DNA vaccination could effectively induce anti-self-protective immunity to restrain harmful reactivity. However, the limits of

Table 1 Antigen-Irrelevant Immunotherapies in EAE and MS

Approach	EAE	MS
Cytokine-based		
IFN-β	Suppressive	Approved therapy
IFN-γ	Protective	Worsens
Anti-TNF-α	Conflicting	Worsens/failed
TNF-α DNA vaccination	Suppressive	ND
IL-10	Conflicting	Stopped
Retroviral delivery to brain	Suppressive	ND
IL-4	Suppressive	ND
Retroviral delivery to brain	Suppressive	ND
TGF-β2	Suppressive	Negative side effects
Trafficking of Leukocytes		
MIP-1α DNA vaccination	Protective	ND
MCP-1 DNA vaccination	Protective	ND
Anti-ICAM-1	Suppressive/conflicting	ND
Anti-LFA-1	Suppressive	ND
Anti-α4	Suppressive/cures	Phase II promising, Phase III planned
Chemokine receptor antagonists	Protective	Phase I in progress
Matrix metalloproteinase inhibitors	Suppressive	ND/planning
Altering costimulation		
Anti-B7-1	Protective	ND
Anti-CD40L (CD154)	Suppressive	Side effects with one antibody; another ongoing
Anti-CTLA-4	Worsens	ND
CTLA-4 Ig	Conflicting	ND (promising in psoriasis)
Immunosuppressive		
Mitoxantrone	Suppressive	Successful, approved
Azathioprine	Suppressive	Suppressive
Cyclophosphamide	Suppressive	Suppressive, side effects
Cyclosporin	Suppressive	Moderately suppressive, side effects

such therapy are clear: Long-term reactivity to inflammatory mediators may not be beneficial, especially when difficulties in directing therapies to the target organ may lend to global administration and subsequent systemic suppression of cytokine responses or reduced leukocyte extravasation. Thus a major goal is developing therapies whose modalities specifically target the activity of pathogenic autoreactive T cells, leaving the remainder of the immune system relatively intact.

C. Vaccines as Antigen-Specific Therapies

The purpose of this review is to define the goals of and potential for vaccine usage in MS with a focus on antigen-specific therapies (Table 2). Compared to the development of microbial-oriented vaccines, two great challenges exist in developing an antigen-specific vaccine effective in autoimmune diseases. The first of these is determining the precise identity and specificity of the autoantigen in question, and subsequently characterizing the phenotype and role of the autoantigen-specific T cell in mediating disease. While one may consider targeting the autoreactive pathogenic T cells as the

most specific means of treating T-cell-mediated autoimmune diseases, it is important to consider that autoreactive T cells are not uncommon, and give rise to disease only in a minority of individuals. The incredible degeneracy in T cell recognition begs that in any given T cell repertoire, at least some autoreactive T cells escape negative selection during lymphoid development in the thymus. Selection occurs in the thymus as T cells encounter antigen. T cells recognizing self-antigen with high affinity are deleted, yet those with low affinity can escape this negative selection. Antigens from the brain and other "immunoprivileged" organs were originally thought to be sequestered; thus T cells reactive to proteins from these areas could not be selected against, neither in the thymus nor in the periphery, as they had no access to antigen. However, studies have shown that several myelin antigens are indeed expressed in the thymus and that T cells with high affinity for these antigens are indeed negatively selected. While it is postulated that autoreactive cells become activated via "molecular mimicry," the evidence for its involvement in MS or autoimmune diseases in general is very limited. It has rather been suggested that autoreactive T cells encountering antigen may contribute to T cell survival, mainte-

Table 2 Antigen-Specific Immunotherapies in EAE and MS

Type of vaccine	Mode of action
DNA Vaccines Delivering	
Autoantigen (protein/peptides) MBP, PLP, MOG	Depletion, anergy of autoreactive T cells
T cell receptor peptides	Depletion of autoreactive T cells, immune deviation
Protein/Peptide Vaccines	
Autoantigens (proteins/peptides) MBP, PLP, MOG	Systemic administration→deletion, anergy Mucosal administration→bystander suppression
Altered peptide ligands (APL)	Bystander suppression
Glatiramer acetate	Bystander suppression
Cellular Vaccines	
Autoreactive T cells	Idiotypic depletion of autoreactive T cells, Bystander suppression
Spleen cells coupled to autoantigen	Depletion/anergy of autoreactive T cells
Dendritic cells coupled to autoantigen	Depletion/anergy of autoreactive T cells

nance, and possibly also the homeostasis of the immune system, and rarely cause disease [19].

Secondly, the presence of self-reactive cells in healthy individuals suggests that regulatory mechanisms are physiological, and that in affected individuals this balance of "self-tolerance" has gone awry either at the level of regulation or by particularly strong activation. The objective becomes determining what mechanisms have allowed for this break in tolerance that otherwise keep autoreactive T cells at bay, and how to reestablish a balance. Tolerance can arise in the thymus early in life during T cell development (deemed central tolerance), or occur throughout life in the periphery (peripheral tolerance). Given that MS is not diagnosed until typically the third decade of life, the more common therapeutic approaches currently being explored involve attempts to induce peripheral tolerance in patients, i.e., at a time when the central tolerance-generating organ, the thymus, has already undergone its physiological involution. To this end, studies to date have focused on generating antigen-specific peripheral tolerance via one of the following mechanisms:

1. Anergy and T cell receptor (TCR) downmodulation: Eliminating the responsiveness of antigen-specific T cells to antigen.
2. Deletion: Targeting antigen-specific cells for death by attack from the host's immune system or inducing death/apoptosis pathways within the cell itself.
3. Immune deviation: Altering the profile of autoreactive T cells from proinflammatory to nonpathogenic by shifting cytokine patterns.
4. Bystander suppression: Generating cells with specific regulatory properties and the potential to regulate or suppress autoreactive T cells in a shared environment.

D. Antigen Specificity and Phenotype of Autoreactive T Cells in Multiple Sclerosis and Experimental Autoimmune Encephalomyelitis—Are They the Same?

The extension of therapies from experimental models to humans is based on similarities in factors including antigens, pathogenic mechanisms, and disease phenotypes between MS and EAE. EAE can be actively induced by immunization with brain or spinal cord homogenate, myelin protein, or peptide in complete Freund's adjuvant (CFA), or passively following the transfer of myelin-reactive CD4+ T cells [20]. Several models exist that vary in species, strain, and the initiating autoantigen. Depending on these factors, the inflammatory response and subsequent demyelination can manifest as an acute, chronic, or relapsing course of paralysis. These models are considered effective tools for studying the immunology of MS as they share a gender bias, genetic associations with MHC class II genes, histopathological correlations, and disease patterns. Although EAE shows clinical similarities to MS, controversy exists over the extrapolation of therapies to the latter, partially because the autoantigen/s in MS has/have not been confirmed. Differences also exist in the incidence of disease: MS spontaneously occurs, whereas EAE must be induced either by active immunization or the transfer of activated autoreactive T cells. As such, EAE models may each only represent certain aspects of the heterogeneous course of MS.

In the search to identify candidate autoantigens in MS, proteins within myelin are popular because myelin sheath degradation is a central event in MS pathogenesis, and many proteins are shared between humans and animal models. Myelin basic protein (MBP) is by far the most characterized and investigated autoantigen in MS and EAE: Classical studies have focused on the human T cell response to MBP using T cell lines and clones to characterize their phenotype, reactivity (epitope specificity), effector functions, and T cell receptor identity. Immunodominant regions include MBP 83–99 (described in more detail below), MBP 111–129, MBP 145–170, and a few others in both MS patients and healthy controls [21–28]. T cells specific for these are restricted by those HLA-DR molecules most often associated with disease in different ethnic backgrounds (alleles of the DR15, DR4, DR3, and DR6 haplotypes). Interestingly, similar MBP peptides from the middle region [29,30] (MBP 89–101 in SJL mice and Lewis rats; MBP 111–129 in guinea pigs) or C terminus regions (in marmosets or rhesus monkeys) are capable of inducing EAE in several species with a similar association to MHC class II molecules. These studies show strong yet indirect evidence that similarities in peptide binding affinities or as yet unidentified characteristics exist between HLA-DR and MHC class II molecules in humans and mice that allows for sharing of these disease-associated peptides (review Ref. 31).

T cells specific for another myelin antigen, proteolipid protein (PLP), are encephalitogenic in different EAE models, i.e., in SJL mice: PLP 139–151 (immunodominant), PLP 178–191, 56–70, 104–117 (subdominant); Lewis rats: PLP 217–233; Biozzi mice: PLP 56–70. Similar peptides are immunodominant in both healthy control subjects and in MS patients [32–34]. Myelin oligodendroglia glycoprotein (MOG) is another attractive candidate autoantigen, with a unique location at the outer surface of the myelin sheath accessible to antibodies. It exhibits several encephalitogenic T cell epitopes in different rodent strains and primates [35–37], MOG 1–30, 35–55, 94–116. MOG 1–22, 34–56, and 63–87 are immunodominant in humans [38,39], and interestingly MOG 97–108 was recently reported as immunodominant in humanized transgenic mice expressing the HLA-DR4 allele, suggesting that immunodominance can be linked to the same MHC in two different species [40]. In this regard, further studies characterizing encephalitogenic epitopes in transgenic humanized HLA-DR mice could be an effective tool for identifying relevant pathogenic epitopes in humans. Several other myelin and nonmyelin proteins have also been described as target autoantigens, including myelin-associated oligodendrocytic basic protein (MOBP) [41], S100 protein [42], and 2′,3′-cyclic nucleotide 3′phosphodiesterase (CNPase) [43], where MOBP and another protein, alpha-B crystallin [44], were found to be both encephalitogenic and immunogenic in humans. Once better characterized, these antigens may also be desirable prospects for antigen-specific therapy.

While these studies have focused on the prevalence of single antigens in disease, one must be aware of studies describing the process of determinant- or epitope "spreading," with the introduction of new autoantigens subsequent to myelin breakdown and damage in the CNS following the initial insult. EAE induced by PLP 139–151 in SJL mice remits and later relapses with a preponderance of T cells reactive to a new epitope, PLP 178–191; a third relapse in turn shows highest reactivity to MBP 84–104 [45]. Given the numerous reactivities to myelin components documented in MS patients and their variance on different MHC backgrounds, and studies describing the existence of epitope spreading [46], the potential challenges of targeting multiple antigens in a specific manner are obvious.

Cell analysis in EAE has shown that encephalitogenic T cells are typically major histocompatibility (MHC) class-II-restricted CD4+ T helper cells that produce the inflammatory cytokines IFN-γ, TNF-β, and IL-2. Over the past decade, immunologists have defined the effector functions of T helper cells and grouped them according to their cytokine profile. T-helper 1 or Th1 cells are proinflammatory cells producing IFN-γ, TNF-α, or IL-1β and associated with a delayed-type hypersensitivity response. In contrast, Th2 cells produce the immunosuppressive cytokines IL-4, IL-5, IL-13 [47], or IL-10, and are thought to play a greater role in disease suppression. In EAE, MBP- and PLP-specific Th1 clones could induce disease, whereas Th2 clones with the same specificity did not. In fact, mucosally derived MBP-specific Th2 clones were able to suppress MBP- or PLP-induced EAE [48]. In MS, this was paralleled in a study of cytokine secretion by myelin-reactive T cells at defined points throughout the disease course that suggested the profile of these cells changes with disease status. Relapsing–remitting patients tested for PLP reactivity displayed a Th1 profile loosely correlating with an acute attack that was shifted to a mixture of Th0, Th1, and Th2 cytokine expressing clones during disease remission [49]. Such studies suggest that not only the antigenic specificity but also the phenotype and effector function of these cells may be critical in influencing their pathogenic potential. While this Th1/Th2 paradigm has been interesting for studying immune regulation in several models, one must be aware that this distinction is likely oversimplified. For example, T cells producing both Th1 and Th2 cytokines exist in abundance (termed Th0), and it is clear that T cell clones are capable of producing a myriad of these cytokines, often simply in differing proportions depending on the activation stimulus and environment [47].

E. Activation of Encephalitogenic T Cells

Lymphocytes cannot recognize antigen in a soluble form, rather it must be "presented" to the T cell as a complex with the MHC on the surface of antigen-presenting cells (APC). The specific interactions at this trimolecular complex (Figure 2) [antigen complexed to the MHC and the T cell receptor (TCR)] (primary signals) as well as those between costimulatory molecules located on the T cell and the APC (secondary signals) influence the outcome of T cell antigen recognition. Full activation requires formation of an immunological synapse [50] comprised of the TCR, antigen:MHC, and costimulatory molecules in very close proximity to allow for sustained TCR engagement and subsequent activation. Naive cells that have not previously encountered antigen in the periphery call for a stronger stimulus to become activated, and typically require the primary signal as well as secondary signals to undergo full activation. Cells that have previously encountered antigen in the periphery (memory cells) need a less potent signal to undergo activation. In differentiated memory T cells, a theory of hierarchy exists in the activation of cellular functions, each occurring as the strength of the TCR stimulus increases [51,52]. While cytotoxicity and cytokine secretion appear to be less complex cell

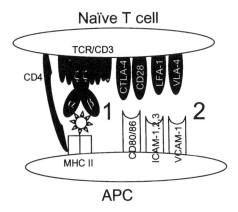

Figure 2 Formation of the immunological synapse. Two signals are required for the full activation of naive T cells. The first (1) is the a signal through the formation of the trimolecular complex that consists of the TCR, Ag:MHC complex. Naive cells also require a costimulatory signal (2) delivered through CD28 and its ligands CD80 (B7.1) or CD86 (B7.2) in addition to adhesion molecules expressed on the T cell and the APC. In contrast, previously activated T cells are less dependent on CD28 signaling and costimulation in subsequent rounds of restimulation. Once activated, cells express CLTA-4 that acts as a negative regulator of activation upon B7 ligation.

functions and thus require a less potent stimulus, proliferation in turn requires "full" activation. Above and beyond these cellular functions, the differential expression of cell surface molecules including cell adhesion molecules and chemokine receptors resulting from partial to full activation also influence the effector function, particularly the trafficking abilities, of these cells [53].

1. The Affinity of the T Cell Receptor for Antigen–Major Histocompatibility Complex

A single TCR has been found able to bind thousands of different peptides [54] based on studies using alanine substitutions in TCR ligands [55,56] and more recently using combinatorial peptide library predictions [52]. So what makes one antigen better than the next? Crystallography studies reveal pockets in the surface of the TCR and MHC that vary both in size and electrostatic charge, into which amino acids of potential ligands may fit in a linear conformation. Those ligands that can best align each of their residues both energetically and structurally to both the TCR and MHC, bringing them into the closest possible proximity, would seem biochemically ideal. Structural and MHC binding data based on these electrostatic predictions have supported this theory [57,58]. By sustaining the formation of the trimolecular complex for the longest possible duration, the "ideal" peptide has the greatest potential for full immunological synapse formation, whereas all other peptides can sustain this formation for less time [59]. A distinct correlation exists between the TCR affinity for the peptide:MHC and their related dissociation rate with biological outcome: "Agonists" are ligands that bind with relatively high affinity and

lower dissociation rates and, while an agonist can induce the full range of T cell effector functions described above for "full activation," partial agonists with substitutions in one or more of the key TCR or MHC contacts are likely to only induce a subset of these T cell functions. "Antagonist" ligands have a high enough binding affinity to compete with agonists for the TCR, but typically cannot induce effector functions, and the binding affinity of null compounds is so low that they simply cannot engage the TCR. Thus the sequence of the antigen and how it influences binding to the TCR is a key component in influencing the extent of T cell activation.

2. Anergy Induction

T cell receptor stimuli can also result in T cell unresponsiveness or even cell death depending on the stage of preactivation. Anergy can describe several forms of unresponsiveness, each induced by different means [60]. For a short time after T cell activation, T cells exhibit a state of hyporesponsiveness with decreased Ca^{2+} mobilization, reduced IL-2 production, and a diminished response to subsequent antigen exposure. This refractory state is most often associated with downregulation of the TCR, and accounts for "blindness" or "partial sightedness" of the T cell to antigen. A more favorable definition of anergy would be "a state of long-lasting, partial or total unresponsiveness induced by partial T cell activation." The most extensively investigated type of anergy is induced in mouse or human T cell clones upon TCR ligation in the absence of full costimulation (i.e., typically the absence of B7 molecules) [60]. Most commonly, it refers to an inability of T cells to produce or respond to proliferative signals [61], and is characterized by an inability to secrete IL-2 by cells otherwise capable of producing IL-2. Importantly, anergy can be partial, as cytotoxic T cells capable of producing IL-2 once rendered anergic no longer produce IL-2, but maintain their cytotoxic potential [62]. Ligation of TCR in the presence of IL-10 also induces IL-2 irreversible unresponsiveness or anergy in T cells [63], giving rise to a unique phenotype. These T cells secrete high levels of IL-10 and are subject to intense investigation for their associated regulatory properties [64]. Importantly, IL-2 can reverse anergy, thus suggesting a potential problem for antigen-specific therapies aimed to anergize autoreactive cells. Infection or any immune response generating IL-2 could reactivate these cells and thus restore their pathogenic potential.

3. Activation-Induced Cell Death

Cell death can be the result of activation at the wrong time, i.e., activation-induced cell death (AICD), or stem from cell-mediated immunity, i.e., the lysis of cells targeted with antibodies. AICD is a form of programmed cell death following TCR engagement/T cell activation and physiologically plays a key role in shaping the T cell repertoire during T cell development. Model systems initially studied responses in thymocytes activated with antibodies to CD3, and were recently extended with antibodies against CD3/TCR to mature T lymphocytes in the periphery. Resting T cells are generally resistant to AICD and in vitro require several days of stimulation before these freshly isolated mature peripheral T cells acquire sensitivity toward AICD. Activated T cells are highly susceptible [65]; thus AICD is thought to a be a key means of "turning off" immune responses by limiting the reactivation of T cells. The death receptors Fas/Fas ligand (CD95/CD95L) are key mediators of AICD. A common scenario describes that following stimulation of an activated T cell via the CD3/TCR complex, CD95L mRNA and cell surface expression are rapidly induced. CD95L then binds to CD95 on activated T cells. A complex signaling cascade is initiated, ultimately resulting in apoptosis. The Fas receptor (CD95) is a key initiator of apoptotic death in several cell types but CD4+ T cells are unique in their ability to undergo autocrine (self) and paracrine (fratricide) death induction by stimulating their own Fas receptors or those on neighboring cells with their secreted or membrane-bound Fas upon activation [66–68]. Thus reexposure to antigen too rapidly after previous encounter is a pathway to death and seems an intriguing means to controlling autoimmunity by the selective induction of apoptosis in autoreactive peripheral T cells.

4. Immune Deviation

Several other factors including the type of antigen, dose, frequency, portal of entry, the involvement of the innate immune system, and the genetic makeup of the host can influence the cytokine repertoire and consequently the phenotype of the activated T cell. For example, nasally or orally introduced allergens at low doses in an environment with high levels of the anti-inflammatory cytokines IL-4 or IL-13 generate Th2 effector cells. Alternatively, naive T cells encountering virus at high doses through the skin in the presence of the proinflammatory mediators IFN-γ and IL-12 become Th1 effector cells. The local cytokine environment is a key factor in CD4+ T helper response to antigen: IL-12 is the major immunomodulatory cytokine associated with Th1-polarized responses vs. IL-4 for inducing Th2 responses. IL-10, an important immunomodulatory cytokine implicated in tolerance via anergy induction [63], decreases proliferation and Th1 cytokine production with effects on MHC class II dependent antigen presentation [69–72]. Activation status and costimulatory molecule expression also play a role. Engagement of leukocyte-associated antigen (LFA-1) by different plate-bound costimulatory intracellular adhesion molecules (ICAMs) alters the T helper profile: ICAM-1 induced high IL-10 production compared to ICAM-2 or -3, which induced higher TNF-α production [73]. Blocking ICAM-1 or -2 with neutralizing antibodies during T cell/APC interactions resulted in a Th2 phenotype [74]. Initial studies suggested that CD28 engagement by CD80/B7.1 or CD86/B7.2 can induce Th1 vs. Th2 responses respectively, but more likely reflected differences in the expression course of these molecules and relative binding affinities [75,76]. More definitively, CD28/B7 costimulation overall regulates the Th1/Th2 balance. While Th2 differentiation of naive CD4+ T cells is strictly dependent on CD28/B7 costimulation, blockade of this pathway has only minor effects on in vitro IFN-γ production (Th1 differentiation) [74,77–79]. The inducible costimulatory molecule (ICOS) is a

member of the CD28 family that provides a unique costimulatory signal with its ligand B7RP-1 or LICOS. Previously activated memory T cells appear to require ICOS costimulation (ICOS is not expressed on naive T cells), and ICOS stimulation appears to be required for significant IFN-γ and IL-10 production, also suggesting a role in T helper cell differentiation [80].

While environment and stimulus can allow for "immune deviation" by alternating potential profiles of naive T cells, similar attempts with differentiated cells have been relatively unsuccessful and are probably prevented by changes in the DNA methylation of cytokine gene loci [81]. Because it is as yet unclear whether terminally differentiated cells can undergo such a shift in their immune profile (i.e., Th1 to Th2 or vice versa), immune deviation may be ineffective at targeting effector or memory cells in autoimmunity.

5. Bystander Suppression and Regulatory T Cells

While anergy, deletion, or ignorance can account for the maintenance of peripheral tolerance, numerous studies in experimental models of organ-specific autoimmune disease convincingly show that specialized T cells exist that are capable of controlling autoimmunity and are an integral part of the T cell repertoire in normal animals. In spontaneous diabetes models [82,83] and in an EAE model of mice transgenic for an MBP-specific TCR [84,85], CD4+ T cells from normal animals inhibit the spontaneous development of disease. Historically, CD8+ T cells were termed cytotoxic/ suppressor cells, but were eventually replaced by the Th2 cells described above. Recently, the whole field has rapidly evolved and identified several regulatory T cell types distinct from Th2 cells involved in the suppression/regulation of autoreactive T cells. T regulatory cells (Treg) have been extensively characterized in rodents and more recently in humans as professional regulatory/suppressor cells that actively and dominantly prevent the activation and effector functions of other T cells [86]. One type are named CD4+ CD25+ for their expression of the IL-2 receptor α chain in mice, (one component of the T cell marker CD25 transiently expressed on activated T cells). These cells are rather homogeneous [87], derive from the thymus [88], and are naturally anergic (nonproliferative) to TCR stimulation. However, TCR stimulation of this cell type is required to inhibit the proliferation of CD4+ or CD8+ T cells through antigennonspecific, largely cytokine-independent/contact-dependent mechanisms [89–91]. Murine CD4+CD25+ Treg cells can inhibit autoimmune diabetes in mice [92] and rats [93], induce tolerance to alloantigens [94–96], impede antitumor immunity [97], and regulate the expansion of other peripheral CD4+ T cells (a mechanism that is IL-10 dependent) [98]. The mechanisms of suppression are ill defined, but thus far suggest the inhibition of responder cell IL-2 production [99] and the downregulation of costimulatory molecules on APC [100]. Notably, CD4+CD25+ Treg cells represent 5–15% of human and murine CD4+ T cells in the periphery of healthy individuals [86,101,102], and their equivalent frequency in the thymus of humans, rats, and mice [103] suggests an evolutionary conservation of their function.

Studies are continuously attributing new functions to these cells, which seem to vary in their reliance upon cytokine production vs. cell–cell contact.

To date, several reports have described different types of regulatory T cells. Repeated stimulation of naive cord blood cells with immature dendritic cells (DC) was found to generate another type of regulatory cell but with more profound production of the regulatory cytokine IL-10 [104]. In mice and humans, another type of regulatory Tr1 cell arose from continuous antigenic stimulation of naive T cells in the presence of IL-10; these cells showed a low proliferative capacity, but upon stimulation released remarkably high levels of IL-10 that inhibited the expansion of other cells [64], rendering them anergic. Additionally, the mucosal administration of antigen gives rise to Th3 cells, a unique T helper profile characterized by TGF-β-associated immunomodulation and associated regulatory properties. Whether or not the above "natural" regulatory cells exist or others can be "induced" in MS patients has yet to be determined, and is an important focus for future studies. For vaccination purposes, the transfer of these cells into mice has shown promise, but the concept of generating these cells for transfer into humans seems not only cumbersome, but challenging because of the large numbers that would be required. Therefore the ability to induce or expand Treg cells in vivo as well as in vitro could have important implications in autoimmunity. Those Treg cells that exert bystander suppression in a nonantigen-specific manner need not necessarily recognize the target antigen(s) that are the subject of immune attack. Identification of the sites of action of these cells will be paramount in regulatory T cell therapies. Thus the notion of administering a regulatory T cell that upon activation within the target organ would produce a wealth of modulatory cytokines and "dim" the activity of autoreactive T cells at the lesion site is very attractive. As such, regulatory cells, even beyond the Th2 profile, remain a hopeful, "undiscovered country" of therapeutic vaccine potential in MS.

II. ANTIGEN-SPECIFIC VACCINES

A. Administration of Autoantigen

In several models of autoimmunity, systemic administration of antigen has been an effective means of establishing antigen-specific T cell tolerance. The creation of mice expressing a transgenic TCR of a single specificity has allowed a unique opportunity to study responses by an otherwise rare population of antigen-specific T cells. Intraperitoneal (i.p.), subcutaneous (s.c.), or intravenous (i.v.) administration of soluble proteins or peptides in high doses were all found to have some effect in inducing tolerance in autoimmune models [105]. Experimental evidence has shown that systemic injection of antigen induces tolerance in several ways. Concurrent with the observation that T cells undergo apoptosis in vitro and in vivo following exposure to high or repeat-dose antigen, repeated i.v. administration of high-dose soluble MBP deleted peripheral autoreactive T cells and improved the course of EAE [106]. Notably, apoptosis is achieved only if T cells are preactivated and have entered the

S phase of the cell cycle [107], complicating the use of such a therapy in humans where the in vivo state of activation of autoreactive cells is not known.

An alternate approach to systemic antigen delivery has been oral or nasal administration of myelin antigens. Mucosal antigen uptake results in a state of unresponsiveness to EAE induction [108]. Success and mechanisms of protection are largely determined by both the antigen administered and the amount/dose, but generally depend on uptake by the gastric mucosa and subsequent processing. Several groups report that oral administration of MBP to mice or rats before disease induction suppresses acute EAE [109–111]. Suppression was shown to be highly specific for the fed antigen [112], and notably myelin administration was ineffective compared to whole MBP [113]. Administration before induction or at the onset of clinical symptoms could suppress chronic relapsing EAE, but multiple doses were required once relapsing disease had been established. At least five mechanisms have been proposed for oral antigen-induced tolerance: immune deviation, deletion, alternate trafficking patterns, active suppression, and anergy. Higher doses favor anergy or deletion of autoantigen-specific cells, whereas lower doses induce regulatory CD4+ T cells that mediate bystander suppression by producing the immuno-modulatory cytokines IL-4, IL-10, and TGF-β [48]. A recent report describes tolerance induction as a dynamic process, and each mechanism may contribute to tolerance albeit at different times: After a rapid removal of antigen-specific cells from the periphery as soon as 1 hr after oral antigen treatment, cells gradually return for about 1 week, followed by a final depletion that results in the protection of mice from severe EAE [114]. Th2 cytokines (IL-10 in particular) increased but only transiently, and is significant in light of work by Groux et al. [63] describing a role for IL-10 in the generation of peripheral unresponsiveness. Recently, others describe the in vivo activation and enrichment of CD4+CD25+ regulatory T cells following oral and i.v. antigen administration, with suppressor function in vitro at least partially dependent on IL-10 and TGF-β [115,116].

While generally effective in mice, several issues need to be addressed before administration of self-antigen becomes an acceptable approach to prevent/treat MS. The precise role of CD4+ T cells, CD8 T cells, and B cells in mediating MS will have to be clarified better to optimize the therapeutic effect and to avoid unwanted side effects. An obvious danger exists in that cells require activation prior to their deletion via activation-induced cell death [117], activation, which may, if only transiently, worsen disease [118,119]. Antigen administration heavily relies on meeting the challenges of defining pathogenic autoantigens, the spread of the response to different antigens, and sparing regulatory T cell populations that assist in reducing the immune response. Notably, i.p. injection of MOG following active induction of EAE with MOG in marmosets was found to block T cell proliferation to MOG and clinical signs during the treatment period, but upon treatment cessation resulted in a hyperacute form of the disease mediated by autoantibodies and associated with increased anti-MOG antibody levels [120]. Of special concern was demyelination induced in marmosets by priming with MBP and PLP that was associated with spreading of the response to MOG determinants that generated anti-MOG serum antibodies and subsequent immunoglobulin deposition in CNS white matter lesions [121].

Thus far, only oral administration of MBP has been extended to humans. In a 1-year, double-blind, placebo-controlled study of relapsing–remitting MS patients receiving a daily mixture of bovine MBP and PLP, few side effects or toxicities were observed. Patients generated more MBP- or PLP-specific T cells secreting TGF-β1 compared to placebo-treated controls, without increasing the proportion of Th1/IFN-γ-secreting myelin specific cells [122,123], supporting the EAE studies. The results of the trial, although not statistically significant, showed a positive trend with improvement in terms of EDSS and attacks, particularly among males [124]. After a longer period of study, results seemed immunologically desirable and showed a trend for betterment, but positive clinical effects in the placebo-controlled group in a small cohort made for statistical insignificance and the trial was deemed unsuccessful [125]. Lastly, the subsequent failure of a Phase III multicenter placebo-controlled study using oral bovine myelin suggests that oral tolerance in humans is thus far not as successful as in mice.

1. Vaccination with DNA Encoding Autoantigenic Peptide

As an alternative to antigen delivered as protein, DNA vaccination has been effective in both infectious disease and experimental cancer vaccines through the delivery of prolonged expression of antigen in ways similar to the systemic administration of antigen. Advantages include the ease of handling, stability, the potential for tissue targeting, and sustained delivery/expression. DNA delivery of auto-antigens to treat EAE has met with conflicting results. DNA vaccination with PLP 139–151 in SJL mice [126], MBP 68–85 in Lewis rats [127], and others suppressed disease. However, protection induced by i.m. DNA specific for MBP 68–85 was lost following a single amino acid exchange in position 79. Here protection was unlikely via bystander effects because protection was highly specific for MBP 68–85 and not for a second encephalitogenic sequence, MBP 89–101 [128]. However, difficulties were again observed in the administration of MOG DNA: Mice developed an exacerbated form of EAE when challenged with either MOG or an unrelated encephalitogen, PLP [129]. Further studies are required to determine whether problems relevant to MOG antigen-specific therapies result from induction of T cell without B cell tolerance, knowing that B cells and antibodies are a definitive and possibly unique element of MOG-induced autoimmunity.

2. Cellular Delivery of Peptide: Trojan Horses

The delivery of antigens already fixed to antigen-presenting cells has also shown particular promise in several models, and allows for management not only of the antigen delivered but also accompanying costimulatory signals. Antigen-specific tolerance could be induced in established, relapsing–remitting EAE by the transfer of PLP 139–151 coupled to chemically fixed splenocytes [130]. Animals were pro-

tected from further relapse associated with epitope spreading to different myelin antigens. Even tolerance induction prior to disease induction with relapse-associated antigens remarkably reduced relapse rates, albeit after a typical primary attack [131]. Thus tolerance induced via antigen-coupled splenocytes does not result in immune deviation or TGF-β-mediated bystander suppression as in other tolerance protocols. In a model of autoimmune myocarditis [132], a similar protocol effected peripheral tolerance in both T and B cells, suggesting even stronger potential for this approach in autoimmunity mediated by both B and T cells. The method of fixing the APCs and thus protecting against in vivo stimuli that may alter the nature of their activating potential (i.e., tolerization changing to full activation and subsequent T cell effector function) enhances its promise for immunotherapy. While cancer vaccine strategies have focused on dendritic cells with their potent stimulating properties (nondesirable properties in combating autoimmunity), the tolerogenic properties of immature or IL-10 cultured DC show promise for their use in tolerization protocols in autoimmunity. Dendritic cells loaded with MBP 68–86 conferred resistance to subsequent EAE induction [133]. Interestingly, transfer of DC isolated from MBP 68–86-induced EAE rats (without antigen loading) also afforded protection in naive rats prior to MBP 68–86 immunization [134]. By negating the need for antigen loading, these DCs are also promising for antigen-specific tolerization.

B. Altered Peptide Ligands

The strength of the signal for T cell activation can determine either full T cell activation (with induction of a Th1 inflammatory response), partial activation (and induction of a Th2 type response), or unresponsiveness/anergy. Thus altering the peptide acts to influence the strength of this signal and thereby also the final effector profile of the T cell. In several animal models, altered peptide ligands (APLs) were created by changing TCR contact residues in immunodominant self-epitopes to impair the strength of the TCR signal. By design, therapeutic mechanisms of APL were postulated to involve MHC blockade [135], TCR antagonism [136], or anergy induction [137] via "imposter" interactions with autoreactive cells at the trimolecular complex. Administration of APL was originally speculated to result in immune deviation of the pathogenic cells in vivo, a difficult task in vitro. When administered with the wild-type peptide to SJL mice, an APL with two amino acid substitutions at key TCR binding sites of the encephalitogen PLP 139-151 induced PLP-specific Th2 cells that secreted IL-4, IL-10, and protected from disease. While immunization also protected against subsequent disease induction with PLP 178-191, MOG 92-106, or mouse MBP, APL immunization did not prevent the generation of PLP 139–151 specific T cells [138]. EAE protection after the adoptive transfer of Th2/Th0 cytokine producing APL-specific T cell clones suggested instead that the main mechanism of action resides in the delivery of suppressor cytokines [139], where protection was abolished with combinations of neutralizing antibodies to IL-4, IL-10, IL-13, and TGF-β [140]. Thus APLs are most likely to afford their greatest protection in vivo through the generation of regulatory cells with effector cytokine production and bystander suppression rather than antagonism or other mechanisms.

As with other TCR- or antigen-targeted therapies, APL therapy heavily relies on the identification of autoreactive T cell specificities if one is truly interested in targeting the autoreactive cells. In developing potential APLs, one must consider numerous interactions at the tri-molecular complex in light of MHC structural variance and the incredible diversity of TCR recognition. As an example, in vitro studies identified immunodominant epitopes of MBP in the amino acid region of 80–100 [21]. While MBP 83–99 is the immunodominant region of MBP in humans and is also encephalitogenic in two animal models (PL/JxSJL/J F1 mice and Lewis rats), different amino acids are important in each system for MHC and TCR recognition. For example, a proline to alanine substitution in MBP 87–99 (96P→A) APL could treat disease in mice, but not rats. Conversely, MBP 87–99 (91K→A) treated the disease in rats, but not in mice [136].

Studies within the past 2 years have strengthened the pathological relevance of T cells specific for MBP 83-99 and thus described an epitope with considerable promise for APL therapy. The in vivo immunolocalization of MBP 85-99 bound to HLA DR2, the HLA molecule highly associated with MS, to the brain tissue of MS patients indicates that MBP 85–99 in the context of HLA-DR2 is present in MS lesions [141]. Transgenic mice carrying a human TCR specific for MBP 83–99 and the human HLA-DR2 allele further revealed the pathogenic potential of these T cells with the spontaneous development of demyelinating disease [142]. In humans, the binding motifs of MBP 83–99 to the HLA-DRB1*0501 and -DRB5*0101 alleles of the MS-associated DR2 haplotype were identified (represented in Figure 3), and extensive in vitro studies using MS-derived MBP 83–99 specific T cell clones revealed critical TCR contact points

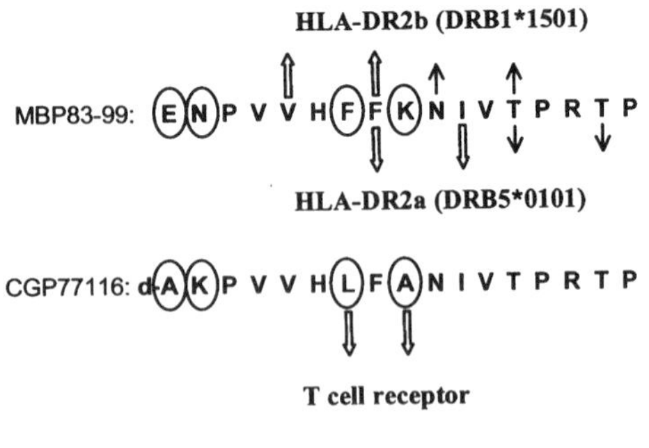

[56,143,144]. In human autoreactive clones from a DR2 MS patient, a TCR-APL (MBP 83-99K→A) was able to induce MBP 85–99 reactive T cells to secrete IL-4 in the absence of IFN-γ [145]; yet this cross-reactivity is not predictable and probably specific for individual repertoires [146].

Based on these observations, an APL of human MBP 83–99 in the context of HLA DR2 was developed. The APL CGP77116 was designed with changes at the N-terminus to extend in vivo half life and alterations in the presumed TCR contacts F89 and K91 to prevent activation of encephalitogenic T cells. Phase I testing showed good tolerability with a significant expansion of APL-reactive T cells, but a concern of poor immunogenicity suggested a higher dosage might be more beneficial [143]. Two Phase II trials were initiated: one smaller baseline-to-treatment cross-over, open label Phase II study [147] and a larger multicenter, double-blind, placebo-controlled study [148]. Both were terminated before the completion of enrollment and/or dosing: The first as a result of atypical MS exacerbations and the second due to the occurrence of APL-induced systemic hypersensitivity. It was concluded that APL treatment activated autoreactive MBP-specific T cells and caused a flare-up of disease in some patients. A review by Bielekova et al. [147] provides insight into the mechanisms of failures of these two studies, and proposes modifications to dosing, but more importantly to the APL design itself, to reduce the potential for pathogenic T cell activation.

C. Glatiramer Acetate

Glatiramer acetate (GA or Copolymer 1, Cop 1) is the active ingredient of Copaxone, which was approved by the FDA in 1996 for the treatment of relapsing remitting MS. Initially designed with high homology to MBP and to experimentally induce EAE, the acetate salt of a synthetic copolymer of L-glutamic acid, L-lysine, L-alanine, and L-tyrosine did the opposite. Suppression of EAE was demonstrated in all species studied [149], although different encephalitogenic determinants of MBP are implicated in disease induction in the different species. Although the different mechanisms of action are still being defined, they appear to rely heavily on immunological cross-reactivity with myelin basic protein both at the antibody [150] and the T cell level. In vitro, GA can competitively inhibit the immune response to MBP of several MBP-specific murine and human T cell lines and clones different in both MHC restriction and epitope specificity [151,152]. GA demonstrates high binding to different MHC class II haplotypes. Therefore it was suggested that it competes for binding with MBP and other myelin-associated proteins including PLP and MOG, which it can efficiently displace from the MHC binding site [153]. While several reports describe a competition-based or antagonistic mode of action, such competition in vivo is unlikely as it would require access to the CNS and substantially larger doses. Perhaps the greatest effect of GA is its ability to generate GA-specific suppressor cells in the peripheral immune system. These IL-4, IL-10, and TGF-β secreting (Th2/Th3) cells that are induced both in humans and mice upon GA administration most likely act via "bystander suppression" to inhibit MBP-specific effector lines and thus EAE in vivo

HLA-DR2b (DRB1*1501)

MBP83-99: (E)(N) P V V H (F)(K) N I V T P R T P

HLA-DR2a (DRB5*0101)

CGP77116: d(A)(K) P V V H (L)(A) N I V T P R T P

T cell receptor

Figure 3 Schema of MBP 83–99 with HLA-DR2 binding motifs compared to an APL CGP77116. Positions 89F and 91K were identified as important TCR contact sites for the majority of autoreactive MBP 83–99-specific T cell clones in vitro; these were modified in the APL along with N terminus regions to increase half life (alterations are highlighted). MHC class II binding motifs of MBP 83–99 to DRB1*1501 and DRB5*0101 alleles (coexpressed in the MS-associated HLA-DR2 haplotype) are shown with large arrows (major MHC contacts) and small arrows (minor MHC contacts). (Courtesy of B. Bielekova, NINDS, NIH, Bethesda, Maryland.)

[154]. In addition, cross-reactivity to myelin results in suppressor cytokine release upon exposure to MBP, suggesting a very potent role in mediating/suppressing pathogenic MBP-specific T cell responses in vivo at the site of myelin breakdown. Such action is supported by observations that GA-specific T lines are capable of crossing the blood–brain barrier and accumulating in the CNS [155]. Recently, oral administration of GA has been found more effective than oral MBP in suppressing EAE in rats, mice, and in primates [156,157], and has led to further human clinical trials.

GA is very well tolerated. Because of its intrinsic heterogeneity, neutralizing antibodies are not observed, so loss of efficacy attributed to depletion is not a concern. Via mechanisms largely attributable to the induction of suppressor/regulatory cells, GA reduced disease exacerbations by about 30% or delayed disease progression or onset in large Phase III trials [158], and has become one of the treatments for MS today. However, it has little effect in preventing disability accumulation once patients have entered a secondary progressive phase of illness. Like the interferons, the success of GA is thus far limited to patients early in disease, and cannot significantly slow progressive MS. However, the converging observations of increased efficacy following oral administration in mice with an increased incidence of regulatory T cells may increase the therapeutic potential of GA.

D. T Cell- or T Cell Receptor Vaccination

Immunologists have long been attracted by the idea that the specificity of cellular and/or humoral immune reactions can be exploited for targeted elimination of antigen-specific T cells, e.g., autoreactive cells. This approach would simulate idiotypic network interactions that are well studied for B cell responses, but clearly less for the cellular immune system. A wealth of evidence suggests that mechanisms act in the peripheral organs to regulate autoantigen-specific T cell responses. Initial studies theorized that pathogenic autoreactive T cells (the "pathogens" in MS) attenuated by irradiation or chemical treatment could be used as vaccines to prevent disease based on the possibility of an idiotype anti-idiotypic T cell response to TCR-related structures on autoreactive T cells [159,160]. In EAE models, vaccination of naive animals with attenuated autoreactive (and otherwise pathogenic) T cells afforded protection from disease induction, and also induced remission of established T-cell-mediated EAE [159–161]. Protection was specific, long lasting, and attributed to direct killing of the target cells or other inhibitory mechanisms such as cytokine secretion.

The antigen–MHC binding region of the TCR is a heterodimer composed of α and β glycoprotein chains with variable (V) regions. One of the striking features of experimental autoimmunity is the tendency of autoreactive T cells to possess a limited V gene repertoire in forming functional TCRs specific for defined autoantigens [162]. In many murine autoimmune disease models and in the Lewis rat, autoreactive T cells utilizing the TCR Vβ8.2 gene segment are instrumental in disease induction [163–165]; thus experiments focused on targeting these cells by vaccination with peptides homologous to regions of their variable chains.

Following vaccination, the induction and expansion of regulatory CD4+ T cells recognizing a portion of the Vβ8.2 chain was operative in spontaneous recovery from EAE in B10.PL mice [166] and immune deviation from a Th1 to a Th2 profile [167]. Each approach modulated disease when administered before EAE induction, with lesser effects upon later administration.

In other strains of mice, as well as in humans, T cell responses to myelin appear more complex and the TCR usage is not as strict. As a result, studies are divided into those targeting specific TCR peptides and those targeting the myelin-reactive T cell population as a whole. One approach in humans was the induction of clonotypic regulatory networks by immunization with bulk preparations of irradiated MBP-specific T cells [168]; here CD8+ regulatory T cells subsequently depleted myelin-reactive T cells. This pilot clinical trial suggested an excellent safety profile with a moderate clinical improvement in some relapsing–remitting MS patients with a reduced exacerbation rate and EDSS stabilization. However, treatment efficacy must be fully evaluated in controlled studies in the future, and such a study is currently being conducted. In a small cohort of MS patients, a detailed determinant analysis of the human anti-T-cell response was reported and showed circulating T cells specific for human Vβ5.2 and Vβ6.1 [169,170].

Protection due to T cell vaccination is likely a result of (1) anti-idiotypic antibody responses, (2) anti-idiotypic T cell regulation by CD8+ T cells [163], or (3) immune deviation through the generation of CD4+ Th2 cell regulatory responses. Following administration of TCR peptides, regulatory cells are generated that produce cytokines or directly kill to suppress/eliminate autoreactive T cells. While promising in animals, caveats do exist. The major disadvantages center on the heterogeneous repertoires of autoreactive T cells possible not only between patients, but also within one patient over time. With the possibility of clonal shift or epitope spreading, the TCR of the target cells could be forever changing, and might preclude the ineffectiveness of this therapy in some murine models. However, the ability of this technique to generate regulatory cells producing anti-inflammatory cytokines such as IL-10 that suppress activation and expansion of MBP-reactive T cells [171] may compensate for shortcomings associated with epitope spreading by limiting disease at earlier stages.

The major concerns with T cell or TCR peptide vaccination approaches are theoretical at this point. The existence of a regulatory, truly idiotypic network of T cells is not well grounded experimentally at this time. Further, the number of individual T cells in our organism, i.e., in the order of $1 \times 10^{11} - 1 \times 10^{12}$ in humans, and even more the number of individual TCR, which is much lower, are far outnumbered by the possible antigens. In this context, it appears teleologically highly wasteful to afford a system of regulation that would produce an equal diversity of regulatory TCR to keep in check those that respond to foreign or self-antigen. In addition, it is now evident that T cells are not as specific as previously thought. Because of these considerations, we deem it unlikely both that a true idiotypic network exists and consequently also that it could be employed for specific immune intervention approaches.

III. CONCLUSIONS AND FUTURE DIRECTIONS

Our increasing understanding of the pathogenesis of MS will be our most powerful tool in generating novel or increasing the effectiveness of existing MS therapies. The heterogeneity of detectable responses against autoantigens, the potential spread of antigen reactivity, diverse genetic backgrounds, and the diversity of the T cell repertoire have made antigen-specific therapy design challenging at best. Treatment involving the administration of peptides or proteins with any significant homology to myelin antigens appears to require at least some degree of autoantigen-specific T cell activation, whether it be on a pathway to death, anergy, regulatory, or encephalitogenic function. However, if the stimulus with which the autoantigen is delivered can be controlled, such therapies retain their promise. Perhaps the most promising alternative to specific pathogenic T cell targeting looks instead to the generation of a mutually exclusive set of cells with a specificity that allows their activation in a setting of demyelination but with a beneficial effector profile. To this end, mucosal administration of antigens has shown some promise, as have observations using Copaxone and the generation of nonpathogenic T cells mediating strong bystander suppression. Some of the future approaches will be testable in appropriate experimental murine or primate models of MS; however, there will be instances in which the full complexity of the immunotherapy will need to be evaluated in MS patients. This assessment should include a pathogenetically well-based rationale and be performed with an optimal trial design. While driving to eliminate or suppress autoreactive T cells, one must also be reminded of the underlying mechanisms that have allowed for this fundamental break in tolerance. If regulatory responses are truly lacking in MS patients as a means of quieting significant immune responses, therapies aimed at boosting these responses may be less effective. Likewise, what underlying factors have prevented natural regulatory T cells, presumably present in MS patients at least before the onset of disease, from mediating recovery from disease?

The next few years will undoubtedly see an increasing number of trials aimed at both the old and the new. They will include extensions of the existing therapies either by reducing the complexity of antigens, or simply altering their route of administration. Novel vaccination strategies employing genetically modified T cells or other immune populations that can be coupled to delivery of autoantigens or other therapeutic factors are on the horizon. While several approaches to vaccination in MS thus far have not shown remarkable clinical efficacy, a lack of deleterious outcome can be built upon. However, the underlying theme must rely on using vaccines in MS to aim to maximize tolerance, while decreasing the potential for pathogenic immunity.

REFERENCES

1. Martin R, et al. Immunological aspects of demyelinating diseases. Annu Rev Immunol 1992; 10:153–187.
2. McFarlin DE, McFarland HF. Multiple sclerosis (second of two parts). N Engl J Med 1982; 307:1246–1251.
3. McFarlin DE, McFarland HF. Multiple sclerosis (first of two parts). N Engl J Med 1982; 307:1183–1188.
4. Raine CS. Multiple sclerosis: immune system molecule expression in the central nervous system. J Neuropathol Exp Neurol 1994; 53:328–337.
5. Lassmann H, et al. Inflammation in the nervous system. Basic mechanisms and immunological concepts. Rev Neurol (Paris) 1991; 147:763–781.
6. Hohlfeld R. Biotechnological agents for the immunotherapy of multiple sclerosis. Principles, problems and perspectives. Brain 1997; 120(Pt 5):865–916.
7. Bashir K, Whitaker JN. Current immunotherapy in multiple sclerosis. Immunol Cell Biol 1998; 76:55–64.
8. Ebers GC, et al. A full genome search in multiple sclerosis. Nat Genet 1996; 13:472–476.
9. Haines JL, et al. A complete genomic screen for multiple sclerosis underscores a role for the major histocompatability complex. The Multiple Sclerosis Genetics Group. Nat Genet 1996; 13:469–471.
10. Sawcer S, et al. A genome screen in multiple sclerosis reveals susceptibility loci on chromosome 6p21 and 17q22. Nat Genet 1996; 13:464–468.
11. Zamvil SS, Steinman L. The T lymphocyte in experimental allergic encephalomyelitis. Annu Rev Immunol 1990; 8:579–621.
12. Wekerle H, et al. Ann Neurol 1994; 36 Suppl:S47–S53.
13. Flugel A, et al. Migratory activity and functional changes of green fluorescent effector cells before and during experimental autoimmune encephalomyelitis. Immunity 2001; 14: 547–560.
14. Jee Y, Matsumoto Y. Two-step activation of T cells, clonal expansion and subsequent Th1 cytokine production, is essential for the development of clinical autoimmune encephalomyelitis. Eur J Immunol 2001; 31:1800–1812.
15. Benveniste EN. Role of macrophages/microglia in multiple sclerosis and experimental allergic encephalomyelitis. J Mol Med 1997; 75:165–173.
16. Bo L, et al. Detection of MHC class II-antigens on macrophages and microglia, but not on astrocytes and endothelia in active multiple sclerosis lesions. J Neuroimmunol 1994; 51: 135–146.
17. Youssef S, et al. Long-lasting protective immunity to experimental autoimmune encephalomyelitis following vaccination with naked DNA encoding C–C chemokines. J Immunol 1998; 161:3870–3879.
18. Wildbaum G, Karin N. Augmentation of natural immunity to a pro-inflammatory cytokine (TNF-alpha) by targeted DNA vaccine confers long-lasting resistance to experimental autoimmune encephalomyelitis. Gene Ther 1999; 6:1128–1138.
19. Hemmer B, et al. Probing degeneracy in T-cell recognition using peptide combinatorial libraries. Immunol Today 1998; 19:163–168.
20. Tabira T. Cellular and molecular aspects of the pathomechanism and therapy of murine experimental allergic encephalomyelitis. Crit Rev Neurobiol 1989; 5:113–142.
21. Ota K, et al. T-cell recognition of an immunodominant myelin basic protein epitope in multiple sclerosis. Nature 1990; 346: 183–187.
22. Martin R, et al. Fine specificity and HLA restriction of myelin basic protein-specific cytotoxic T cell lines from multiple sclerosis patients and healthy individuals. J Immunol 1990; 145: 540–548.
23. Pette M, et al. Myelin basic protein-specific T lymphocyte lines from MS patients and healthy individuals. Neurology 1990; 40:1770–1776.
24. Pette M, et al. Myelin autoreactivity in multiple sclerosis: recognition of myelin basic protein in the context of HLA-DR2 products by T lymphocytes of multiple-sclerosis

patients and healthy donors. Proc Natl Acad Sci USA 1990; 87:7968–7972.

25. Meinl E, et al. Myelin basic protein-specific T lymphocyte repertoire in multiple sclerosis. Complexity of the response and dominance of nested epitopes due to recruitment of multiple T cell clones. J Clin Invest 1993; 92:2633–2643.

26. Valli A, et al. Binding of myelin basic protein peptides to human histocompatibility leukocyte antigen class II molecules and their recognition by T cells from multiple sclerosis patients. J Clin Invest 1993; 91:616–628.

27. Richert JR, et al. Evidence for multiple human T cell recognition sites on myelin basic protein. J Neuroimmunol 1989; 23:55–66.

28. Muraro PA, et al. Immunodominance of a low-affinity major histocompatibility complex-binding myelin basic protein epitope (residues 111–129) in HLA-DR4 (B1*0401) subjects is associated with a restricted T cell receptor repertoire. J Clin Invest 1997; 100:339–349.

29. Offner H, et al. T cell determinants of myelin basic protein include a unique encephalitogenic I–E-restricted epitope for Lewis rats. J Exp Med 1989; 170:355–367.

30. Sakai K, et al. Characterization of a major encephalitogenic T cell epitope in SJL/J mice with synthetic oligopeptides of myelin basic protein. J Neuroimmunol 1988; 19:21–32.

31. Martin R, McFarland HF. Immunological aspects of experimental allergic encephalomyelitis and multiple sclerosis. Crit Rev Clin Lab Sci 1995; 32:121–182.

32. Markovic-Plese S, et al. T cell recognition of immunodominant and cryptic proteolipid protein epitopes in humans. J Immunol 1995; 155:982–992.

33. Pelfrey CM, et al. Identification of a second T cell epitope of human proteolipid protein (residues 89–106) recognized by proliferative and cytolytic CD4+ T cells from multiple sclerosis patients. J Neuroimmunol 1994; 53:153–161.

34. Pelfrey CM, et al. Identification of a novel T cell epitope of human proteolipid protein (residues 40–60) recognized by proliferative and cytolytic CD4+ T cells from multiple sclerosis patients. J Neuroimmunol 1993; 46:33–42.

35. Kerlero de Rosbo N, et al. Rhesus monkeys are highly susceptible to experimental autoimmune encephalomyelitis induced by myelin oligodendrocyte glycoprotein: characterisation of immunodominant T- and B-cell epitopes. J Neuroimmunol 2000; 110:83–96.

36. Linington C, et al. T cells specific for the myelin oligodendrocyte glycoprotein mediate an unusual autoimmune inflammatory response in the central nervous system. Eur J Immunol 1993; 23:1364–1372.

37. Lindert RB, et al. Multiple sclerosis: B- and T-cell responses to the extracellular domain of the myelin oligodendrocyte glycoprotein. Brain 1999; 122(Pt 11):2089–2100.

38. Wallstrom E, et al. Increased reactivity to myelin oligodendrocyte glycoprotein peptides and epitope mapping in HLA DR2(15)+ multiple sclerosis. Eur J Immunol 1998; 28:3329–3335.

39. Kerlero de Rosbo N, et al. Predominance of the autoimmune response to myelin oligodendrocyte glycoprotein (MOG) in multiple sclerosis: reactivity to the extracellular domain of MOG is directed against three main regions. Eur J Immunol 1997; 27:3059–3069.

40. Forsthuber TG, et al. T cell epitopes of human myelin oligodendrocyte glycoprotein identified in HLA-DR4 (DRB1* 0401) transgenic mice are encephalitogenic and are presented by human B cells. J Immunol 2001; 167:7119–7125.

41. Holz A, et al. Myelin-associated oligodendrocytic basic protein: identification of an encephalitogenic epitope and association with multiple sclerosis. J Immunol 2000; 164:1103–1109.

42. Kojima K, et al. Experimental autoimmune panencephalitis and uveoretinitis transferred to the Lewis rat by T

lymphocytes specific for the S100 beta molecule, a calcium binding protein of astroglia. J Exp Med 1994; 180:817–829.

43. Rosener M, et al. 2′,3′-Cyclic nucleotide 3′-phosphodiesterase: a novel candidate autoantigen in demyelinating diseases. J Neuroimmunol 1997; 75:28–34.

44. Thoua NM, et al. Encephalitogenic and immunogenic potential of the stress protein alphaB-crystallin in Biozzi ABH (H-2A(g7)) mice. J Neuroimmunol 2000; 104:47–57.

45. Miller SD, Eagar TN. Functional role of epitope spreading in the chronic pathogenesis of autoimmune and virus-induced demyelinating diseases. Adv Exp Med Biol 2001; 490:99–107.

46. Tuohy VK, et al. Diversity and plasticity of self recognition during the development of multiple sclerosis. J Clin Invest 1997; 99:1682–1690.

47. Dong C, et al. Th1 and Th2 cells. Curr Opin Hematol 2001; 8:47–51.

48. Chen Y, et al. Regulatory T cell clones induced by oral tolerance: suppression of autoimmune encephalomyelitis. Science 1994; 265:1237–1240.

49. Correale J, et al. Patterns of cytokine secretion by autoreactive proteolipid protein-specific T cell clones during the course of multiple sclerosis. J Immunol 1995; 154:2959–2968.

50. Bromley SK, et al. The immunological synapse. Annu Rev Immunol 2001; 19:375–396.

51. Hemmer B, et al. Contribution of individual amino acids within MHC molecule or antigenic peptide to TCR ligand potency. J Immunol 2000; 164:861–871.

52. Hemmer B, et al. Predictable TCR antigen recognition based on peptide scans leads to the identification of agonist ligands with no sequence homology. J Immunol 1998; 160:3631–3636.

53. Gonzalez-Amaro R, Sanchez-Madrid F. Cell adhesion molecules: selectins and integrins. Crit Rev Immunol 1999; 19:389–429.

54. Hemmer B, et al. Identification of candidate T-cell epitopes and molecular mimics in chronic Lyme disease. Nat Med 1999; 5:1375–1382.

55. Hemmer B, et al. Identification of high potency microbial and self ligands for a human autoreactive class II-restricted T cell clone. J Exp Med 1997; 185:1651–1659.

56. Hemmer B, et al. Human T-cell response to myelin basic protein peptide (83–99): extensive heterogeneity in antigen recognition, function, and phenotype. Neurology 1997; 49:1116–1126.

57. Baker BM, et al. Conversion of a T cell antagonist into an agonist by repairing a defect in the TCR/peptide/MHC interface: Implications for TCR signaling. Immunity 2000; 13:475–484.

58. Ding YH, et al. Four A6-TCR/peptide/HLA-A2 structures that generate very different T cell signals are nearly identical. Immunity 1999; 11:45–56.

59. Davis MM, et al. Ligand recognition by alpha beta T cell receptors. Annu Rev Immunol 1998; 16:523–544.

60. Schwartz RH. Models of T cell anergy: is there a common molecular mechanism? J Exp Med 1996; 184:1–8.

61. Lechler R, et al. The contributions of T-cell anergy to peripheral T-cell tolerance. Immunology 2001; 103:262–269.

62. Otten GR, Germain RN. Split anergy in a CD8+ T cell: receptor-dependent cytolysis in the absence of interleukin-2 production. Science 1991; 251:1228–1231.

63. Groux H, et al. Interleukin-10 induces a long-term antigen-specific anergic state in human CD4+ T cells. J Exp Med 1996; 184:19–29.

64. Groux H, et al. A CD4+ T-cell subset inhibits antigen-specific T-cell responses and prevents colitis. Nature 1997; 389:737–742.

65. Klas C, et al. Activation interferes with the APO-1 pathway in mature human T cells. Int Immunol 1993; 5:625–630.

66. Brunner T, et al. Cell-autonomous Fas (CD95)/Fas-ligand interaction mediates activation-induced apoptosis in T-cell hybridomas. Nature 1995; 373:441–444.

67. Dhein J, et al. Autocrine T-cell suicide mediated by APO-1/(Fas/CD95). Nature 1995; 373:438–441.

68. Ju ST, et al. Fas(CD95)/FasL interactions required for programmed cell death after T-cell activation. Nature 1995; 373:444–448.

69. de Waal Malefyt R, et al. Direct effects of IL-10 on subsets of human CD4+ T cell clones and resting T cells. Specific inhibition of IL-2 production and proliferation. J Immunol 1993; 150:4754–4765.

70. de Waal Malefyt R, et al. Interleukin 10(IL-10) inhibits cytokine synthesis by human monocytes: an autoregulatory role of IL-10 produced by monocytes. J Exp Med 1991; 174:1209–1220.

71. de Waal Malefyt R, et al. Interleukin 10 (IL-10) and viral IL-10 strongly reduce antigen-specific human T cell proliferation by diminishing the antigen-presenting capacity of monocytes via downregulation of class II major histocompatibility complex expression. J Exp Med 1991; 174:915–924.

72. Koppelman B, et al. Interleukin-10 down-regulates MHC class II alphabeta peptide complexes at the plasma membrane of monocytes by affecting arrival and recycling. Immunity 1997; 7:861–871.

73. Bleijs DA, et al. Co-stimulation of T cells results in distinct IL-10 and TNF-alpha cytokine profiles dependent on binding to ICAM-1, ICAM-2 or ICAM-3. Eur J Immunol 1999; 29: 2248–2258.

74. Salomon B, Bluestone JA. LFA-1 interaction with ICAM-1 and ICAM-2 regulates Th2 cytokine production. J Immunol 1998; 161:5138–5142.

75. Kuchroo VK, et al. B7-1 and B7-2 costimulatory molecules activate differentially the Th1/Th2 developmental pathways: application to autoimmune disease therapy. Cell 1995; 80: 707–718.

76. Hathcock KS, et al. Comparative analysis of B7-1 and B7-2 costimulatory ligands: expression and function. J Exp Med 1994; 180:631–640.

77. Schweitzer AN, Sharpe AH. Studies using antigen-presenting cells lacking expression of both B7-1 (CD80) and B7-2 (CD86) show distinct requirements for B7 molecules during priming versus restimulation of Th2 but not Th1 cytokine production. J Immunol 1998; 161:2762–2771.

78. Rulifson IC, et al. CD28 costimulation promotes the production of Th2 cytokines. J Immunol 1997; 158:658–665.

79. Rogers PR, Croft M. CD28, Ox-40, LFA-1, and CD4 modulation of Th1/Th2 differentiation is directly dependent on the dose of antigen. J Immunol 2000; 164:2955–2963.

80. Sporici RA, Perrin PJ. Costimulation of memory T-cells by ICOS: a potential therapeutic target for autoimmunity? Clin Immunol 2001; 100:263–269.

81. Rao A, Avni O. Molecular aspects of T-cell differentiation. Br Med Bull 2000; 56:969–984.

82. Fowell D, Mason D. Evidence that the T cell repertoire of normal rats contains cells with the potential to cause diabetes. Characterization of the CD4+ T cell subset that inhibits this autoimmune potential. J Exp Med 1993; 177:627–636.

83. Roncarolo MG, Levings MK. The role of different subsets of T regulatory cells in controlling autoimmunity. Curr Opin Immunol 2000; 12:676–683.

84. Olivares-Villagomez D, et al. Regulatory CD4(+) T cells expressing endogenous T cell receptor chains protect myelin basic protein-specific transgenic mice from spontaneous autoimmune encephalomyelitis. J Exp Med 1998; 188:1883–1894.

85. Van de Keere F, Tonegawa S. CD4(+) T cells prevent spontaneous experimental autoimmune encephalomyelitis in anti-myelin basic protein T cell receptor transgenic mice. J Exp Med 1998; 188:1875–1882.

86. Dieckmann D, et al. Ex vivo isolation and characterization of CD4(+)CD25(+) T cells with regulatory properties from human blood. J Exp Med 2001; 193:1303–1310.

87. Shevach EM. Regulatory T cells in autoimmunity*. Annu Rev Immunol 2000; 18:423–449.

88. Itoh M, et al. Thymus and autoimmunity: production of CD25+CD4+ naturally anergic and suppressive T cells as a key function of the thymus in maintaining immunologic self-tolerance. J Immunol 1999; 162:5317–5326.

89. Thornton AM, Shevach EM. Suppressor effector function of CD4+CD25+ immunoregulatory T cells is antigen non-specific. J Immunol 2000; 164:183–190.

90. Shevach EM, et al. Control of autoimmunity by regulatory T cells. Adv Exp Med Biol 2001; 490:21–32.

91. Shevach EM. Certified professionals: CD4(+)CD25(+) suppressor T cells. J Exp Med 2001; 193:F41–46.

92. Salomon B, et al. B7/CD28 costimulation is essential for the homeostasis of the CD4+CD25+ immunoregulatory T cells that control autoimmune diabetes. Immunity 2000; 12:431–440.

93. Stephens LA, Mason D. CD25 is a marker for CD4+ thymocytes that prevent autoimmune diabetes in rats, but peripheral T cells with this function are found in both CD25+ and CD25-subpopulations. J Immunol 2000; 165:3105–3110.

94. Hara M, et al. IL-10 is required for regulatory T cells to mediate tolerance to alloantigens in vivo. J Immunol 2001; 166:3789–3796.

95. Gao Q, et al. CD4+CD25+ cells regulate CD8 cell anergy in neonatal tolerant mice. Transplantation 1999; 68:1891–1897.

96. Taylor PA, et al. CD4(+)CD25(+) immune regulatory cells are required for induction of tolerance to alloantigen via costimulatory blockade. J Exp Med 2001; 193:1311–1318.

97. Shimizu J, et al. Induction of tumor immunity by removing CD25+CD4+ T cells: a common basis between tumor immunity and autoimmunity. J Immunol 1999; 163:5211–5218.

98. Annacker O, et al. CD25+ CD4+ T cells regulate the expansion of peripheral CD4 T cells through the production of IL-10. J Immunol 2001; 166:3008–3018.

99. Thornton AM, Shevach EM. CD4+CD25+ immunoregulatory T cells suppress polyclonal T cell activation in vitro by inhibiting interleukin 2 production. J Exp Med 1998; 188:287–296.

100. Cederbom L, et al. CD4+CD25+ regulatory T cells down-regulate co-stimulatory molecules on antigen-presenting cells. Eur J Immunol 2000; 30:1538–1543.

101. Jonuleit H, et al. Identification and functional characterization of human CD4(+)CD25(+) T cells with regulatory properties isolated from peripheral blood. J Exp Med 2001; 193:1285–1294.

102. Levings MK, et al. Human cd25(+)cd4(+) t regulatory cells suppress naive and memory T cell proliferation and can be expanded in vitro without loss of function. J Exp Med 2001; 193:1295–1302.

103. Stephens LA, et al. Human CD4(+)CD25(+) thymocytes and peripheral T cells have immune suppressive activity in vitro. Eur J Immunol 2001; 31:1247–1254.

104. Jonuleit H, et al. Induction of interleukin 10-producing, nonproliferating CD4(+) T cells with regulatory properties by repetitive stimulation with allogeneic immature human dendritic cells. J Exp Med 2000; 192:1213–1222.

105. Liblau R, et al. Systemic antigen in the treatment of T-cell-mediated autoimmune diseases. Immunol Today 1997; 18: 599–604.

106. Critchfield JM, et al. T cell deletion in high antigen dose therapy of autoimmune encephalomyelitis. Science 1994; 263:1139–1143.

107. Schmied M, et al. Apoptosis of T lymphocytes in exper-

imental autoimmune encephalomyelitis. Evidence for pro-grammed cell death as a mechanism to control inflammation in the brain. Am J Pathol 1993; 143:446–452.

108. Chen Y, et al. Oral tolerance in myelin basic protein T-cell receptor transgenic mice: suppression of autoimmune encephalomyelitis and dose-dependent induction of regulatory cells. Proc Natl Acad Sci USA 1996; 93:388–391.

109. Meyer AL, et al. Suppression of murine chronic relapsing experimental autoimmune encephalomyelitis by the oral administration of myelin basic protein. J Immunol 1996; 157:4230–4238.

110. Bitar DM, Whitacre CC. Suppression of experimental autoimmune encephalomyelitis by the oral administration of myelin basic protein. Cell Immunol 1988; 112:364–370.

111. Higgins PJ, Weiner HL. Suppression of experimental autoimmune encephalomyelitis by oral administration of myelin basic protein and its fragments. J Immunol 1988; 140:440–445.

112. Javed NH, et al. Exquisite peptide specificity of oral tolerance in experimental autoimmune encephalomyelitis. J Immunol 1995; 155:1599–1605.

113. Benson JM, et al. Oral administration of myelin basic protein is superior to myelin in suppressing established relapsing experimental autoimmune encephalomyelitis. J Immunol 1999; 162:6247–6254.

114. Meyer AL, et al. Rapid depletion of peripheral antigen-specific T cells in TCR-transgenic mice after oral administration of myelin basic protein. J Immunol 2001; 166:5773–5781.

115. Zhang X, et al. Activation of cd25(+)cd4(+) regulatory t cells by oral antigen administration. J Immunol 2001; 167:4245–4253.

116. Thorstenson KM, Khoruts A. Generation of anergic and potentially immunoregulatory CD25+CD4 T cells in vivo after induction of peripheral tolerance with intravenous or oral antigen. J Immunol 2001; 167:188–195.

117. Benson JM, et al. T-cell activation and receptor down-modulation precede deletion induced by mucosally administered antigen. J Clin Invest 2000; 106:1031–1038.

118. Blanas E, et al. Induction of autoimmune diabetes by oral administration of autoantigen. Science 1996; 274:1707–1709.

119. Blanas E, Heath WR. Oral administration of antigen can lead to the onset of autoimmune disease. Int Rev Immunol 1999; 18:217–228.

120. Genain CP, et al. Late complications of immune deviation therapy in a nonhuman primate. Science 1996; 274:2054–2057.

121. McFarland HI, et al. Determinant spreading associated with demyelination in a nonhuman primate model of multiple sclerosis. J Immunol 1999; 162:2384–2390.

122. Fukaura H, et al. Antigen-specific TGF-beta 1 secretion with bovine myelin oral tolerization in multiple sclerosis. Ann N Y Acad Sci 1996; 778:251–257.

123. Fukaura H, et al. Induction of circulating myelin basic protein and proteolipid protein-specific transforming growth factor-beta1-screting Th3 T cells by oral administration of myelin in multiple sclerosis patients. J Clin Invest 1996; 98:70–77.

124. Weiner HL, et al. Double-blind pilot trial of oral tolerization with myelin antigens in multiple sclerosis. Science 1993; 259:1321–1324.

125. Hohol MJ, et al. Three-year open protocol continuation study of oral tolerization with myelin antigens in multiple sclerosis and design of a phase III pivotal trial. Ann N Y Acad Sci 1996; 778:243–250.

126. Ruiz PJ, et al. Suppressive immunization with DNA encoding a self-peptide prevents autoimmune disease: modulation of T cell costimulation. J Immunol 1999; 162:3336–3341.

127. Lobell A, et al. Vaccination with DNA encoding an immunodominant myelin basic protein peptide targeted to Fc of immunoglobulin G suppresses experimental autoimmune encephalomyelitis. J Exp Med 1998; 187:1543–1548.

128. Weissert R, et al. Protective DNA vaccination against organ-specific autoimmunity is highly specific and discriminates between single amino acid substitutions in the peptide auto-antigen. Proc Natl Acad Sci USA 2000; 97:1689–1694.

129. Bourquin C, et al. Myelin oligodendrocyte glycoprotein–DNA vaccination induces antibody-mediated autoaggression in experimental autoimmune encephalomyelitis. Eur J Immunol 2000; 30:3663–3671.

130. Kennedy KJ, et al. Induction of antigen-specific tolerance for the treatment of ongoing, relapsing autoimmune encephalomyelitis: a comparison between oral and peripheral tolerance. J Immunol 1997; 159:1036–1044.

131. Vanderlugt CL, et al. Pathologic role and temporal appearance of newly emerging autoepitopes in relapsing experimental autoimmune encephalomyelitis. J Immunol 2000; 164:670–678.

132. Godsel LM, et al. Prevention of autoimmune myocarditis through the induction of antigen-specific peripheral immune tolerance. Circulation 2001; 103:1709–1714.

133. Huang YM, et al. Autoantigen-pulsed dendritic cells induce tolerance to experimental allergic encephalomyelitis (EAE) in Lewis rats. Clin Exp Immunol 2000; 122:437–444.

134. Xiao BG, et al. Bone marrow-derived dendritic cells from experimental allergic encephalomyelitis induce immune tolerance to EAE in Lewis rats. Clin Exp Immunol 2001; 125:300–309.

135. Samson MF, Smilek DE. Reversal of acute experimental autoimmune encephalomyelitis and prevention of relapses by treatment with a myelin basic protein peptide analogue modified to form long-lived peptide–MHC complexes. J Immunol 1995; 155:2737–2746.

136. Karin N, et al. Reversal of experimental autoimmune encephalomyelitis by a soluble peptide variant of a myelin basic protein epitope: T cell receptor antagonism and reduction of interferon gamma and tumor necrosis factor alpha production. J Exp Med 1994; 180:2227–2237.

137. Gaur A, et al. Amelioration of relapsing experimental autoimmune encephalomyelitis with altered myelin basic protein peptides involves different cellular mechanisms. J Neuroimmunol 1997; 74:149–158.

138. Nicholson LB, et al. An altered peptide ligand mediates immune deviation and prevents autoimmune encephalomyelitis. Immunity 1995; 3:397–405.

139. Nicholson LB, et al. A T cell receptor antagonist peptide induces T cells that mediate bystander suppression and prevent autoimmune encephalomyelitis induced with multiple myelin antigens. Proc Natl Acad Sci USA 1997; 94:9279–9284.

140. Young DA, et al. IL-4, IL-10, IL-13, and TGF-beta from an altered peptide ligand-specific Th2 cell clone down-regulate adoptive transfer of experimental autoimmune encephalomyelitis. J Immunol 2000; 164:3563–3572.

141. Krogsgaard M, et al. Visualization of myelin basic protein (MBP) T cell epitopes in multiple sclerosis lesions using a monoclonal antibody specific for the human histocompatibility leukocyte antigen (HLA)-DR2-MBP 85–99 complex. J Exp Med 2000; 191:1395–1412.

142. Madsen LS, et al. A humanized model for multiple sclerosis using HLA-DR2 and a human T-cell receptor. Nat Genet 1999; 23:343–347.

143. Vergelli M, et al. Differential activation of human autoreactive T cell clones by altered peptide ligands derived from myelin basic protein peptide (87–99). Eur J Immunol 1996; 26:2624–2634.

144. Kozovska M, et al. T cell recognition motifs of an immuno-

dominant peptide of myelin basic protein in patients with multiple sclerosis: structural requirements and clinical implications. Eur J Immunol 1998; 28:1894–1901.

145. Ausubel LJ, et al. Changes in cytokine secretion induced by altered peptide ligands of myelin basic protein peptide 85–99. J Immunol 1997; 159:2502–2512.

146. Ausubel LJ, et al. Cross-reactivity of T-cell clones specific for altered peptide ligands of myelin basic protein. Cell Immunol 1999; 193:99–107.

147. Bielekova B, et al. Encephalitogenic potential of the myelin basic protein peptide (amino acids 83–99) in multiple sclerosis: results of a phase II clinical trial with an altered peptide ligand. Nat Med 2000; 6:1167–1175.

148. Kappos L, et al. Induction of a non-encephalitogenic type 2 T helper-cell autoimmune response in multiple sclerosis after administration of an altered peptide ligand in a placebo-controlled, randomized phase II trial. The Altered Peptide Ligand in Relapsing MS Study Group. Nat Med 2000; 6:1176–1182.

149. Sela M, Teitelbaum D. Glatiramer acetate in the treatment of multiple sclerosis. Expert Opin Pharmacother 2001; 2:1149–1165.

150. Teitelbaum D, et al. Cross-reactions and specificities of monoclonal antibodies against myelin basic protein and against the synthetic copolymer 1. Proc Natl Acad Sci USA 1991; 88:9528–9532.

151. Teitelbaum D, et al. Specific inhibition of the T-cell response to myelin basic protein by the synthetic copolymer Cop 1. Proc Natl Acad Sci USA 1988; 85:9724–9728.

152. Racke MK, et al. Copolymer-1-induced inhibition of antigen-specific T cell activation: interference with antigen presentation. J Neuroimmunol 1992; 37:75–84.

153. Fridkis-Hareli M, et al. Binding motifs of copolymer 1 to multiple sclerosis- and rheumatoid arthritis-associated HLA-DR molecules. J Immunol, 1999, 4697–4704.

154. Aharoni R, et al. Copolymer 1 induces T cells of the T helper type 2 that crossreact with myelin basic protein and suppress experimental autoimmune encephalomyelitis. Proc Natl Acad Sci USA 1997; 94:10821–10826.

155. Aharoni R, et al. Specific Th2 cells accumulate in the central nervous system of mice protected against experimental autoimmune encephalomyelitis by copolymer 1. Proc Natl Acad Sci USA 2000; 97:11472–11477.

156. Teitelbaum D, et al. Immunomodulation of experimental autoimmune encephalomyelitis by oral administration of copolymer 1. Proc Natl Acad Sci USA 1999; 96:3842–3847.

157. Weiner HL. Oral tolerance with copolymer 1 for the treatment of multiple sclerosis. Proc Natl Acad Sci USA 1999; 96:3333–3335.

158. Johnson KP, et al. Copolymer 1 reduces relapse rate and improves disability in relapsing–remitting multiple sclerosis: results of a phase III multicenter, double-blind placebo-controlled trial. The Copolymer 1 Multiple Sclerosis Study Group. Neurology 1995; 45:1268–1276.

159. Lider O, et al. Vaccination against experimental autoimmune encephalomyelitis using a subencephalitogenic dose of auto-immune effector T cells. (2). Induction of a protective anti-idiotypic response. J Autoimmun 1989; 2:87–99.

160. Lider O, et al. Suppression of experimental autoimmune encephalomyelitis by oral administration of myelin basic protein. II. Suppression of disease and in vitro immune responses is mediated by antigen-specific CD8 + T lymphocytes. J Immunol 1989; 142:748–752.

161. Ben-Nun A, et al. Vaccination against autoimmune encephalomyelitis with T-lymphocyte line cells reactive against myelin basic protein. Nature 1981; 292:60–61.

162. Heber-Katz E, Acha-Orbea H. The V-region disease hypothesis: evidence from autoimmune encephalomyelitis. Immunol Today 1989; 10:164–169.

163. Gaur A, et al. Requirement for CD8 + cells in T cell receptor peptide-induced clonal unresponsiveness. Science 1993; 259:91–94.

164. Kumar V, Sercarz E. T cell regulatory circuitry: antigen-specific and TCR-idiopeptide-specific T cell interactions in EAE. Int Rev Immunol 1993; 9:287–297.

165. Vandenbark AA, et al. Immunization with a synthetic T-cell receptor V-region peptide protects against experimental autoimmune encephalomyelitis. Nature 1989; 341:541–544.

166. Kumar V, Sercarz EE. The involvement of T cell receptor peptide-specific regulatory CD4 + T cells in recovery from antigen-induced autoimmune disease. J Exp Med 1993; 178:909–916.

167. Kumar V, et al. Induction of a type 1 regulatory CD4 T cell response following V beta 8.2 DNA vaccination results in immune deviation and protection from experimental autoimmune encephalomyelitis. Int Immunol 2001; 13:835–841.

168. Zhang J, Raus J. Clonal depletion of human myelin basic protein-reactive T-cells by T-cell vaccination. Ann N Y Acad Sci 1995; 756:323–326.

169. Vandenbark AA, et al. Treatment of multiple sclerosis with T-cell receptor peptides: results of a double-blind pilot trial. Nat Med 1996; 2:1109–1115.

170. Chou YK, et al. Immunity to TCR peptides in multiple sclerosis. II. T cell recognition of V beta 5.2 and V beta 6.1 CDR2 peptides. J Immunol 1994; 152:2520–2529.

171. Zang YC, et al. The immune regulation induced by T cell vaccination in patients with multiple sclerosis. Eur J Immunol 2000; 30:908–913.

172. Brocke S, et al. Induction of relapsing paralysis in experimental autoimmune encephalomyelitis by bacterial superantigen. Nature 1993; 365:642–644.

173. Brightman MW, Reese TS. Junctions between intimately apposed cell membranes in the vertebrate brain. J Cell Biol 1969; 40:648–677.

174. Reese TS, Karnovsky MJ. Fine structural localization of a blood–brain barrier to exogenous peroxidase. J Cell Biol 1967; 34:207–217.

175. Santambrogio L, et al. Antigen presenting capacity of brain microvasculature in altered peptide ligand modulation of experimental allergic encephalomyelitis. J Neuroimmunol 1999; 93:81–91.

85

Vaccine Therapy for Autoimmune Diabetes

Irun R. Cohen

The Weizmann Institute of Science, Rehovot, Israel

I. TYPE I DIABETES MELLITUS

Type I diabetes is caused by an autoimmune attack, apparently by the combined forces of CD4$^+$ and CD8$^+$ T cells, directed to the insulin-producing β cells of the pancreatic islets [1]. Destruction of the β cells can proceed very quickly (within weeks to months) in some patients (mostly children) or very slowly (over years) in others (mostly adults); the reasons for this variable rate of progression are not really known, but variable degrees of autoimmune regulation probably affect the rate of destruction. Type I diabetes was once called "juvenile" diabetes because most cases occurred in young people; but now the incidence is rising and the disease is seen to develop in older persons. Indeed, about 10–15% of persons originally diagnosed as suffering from type II diabetes may actually be undergoing a slowly progressive autoimmune process called latent autoimmune diabetes of the adult (LADA) [2]. Type I diabetes is thus among the most prevalent of autoimmune diseases; a specific therapy would help many people.

The factors that initiate the onset of the autoimmune process are unknown, but susceptibility to type I diabetes is associated with certain HLA class II alleles [1]. Like other prevalent autoimmune diseases, type I diabetes is marked by T-cell reactivity to a collective of self-antigens, and not by autoimmunity to only one self-antigen [3]. Unlike most other autoimmune diseases, autoimmune destruction of β cells produces no symptoms; so type I diabetes is usually diagnosed clinically only by the collapse of glucose homeostasis after the destruction of a critical number of β cells, thought to be about 85% of the normal β-cell mass [1].

II. PRECLINICAL BACKGROUND

Mice of the NOD strain, particularly the females, spontaneously develop a form of type I diabetes similar in many ways to that seen in humans [4]. My colleagues and I reported the serendipitous observation that the 60-kDa heat shock protein (HSP60) was among the collective of antigens targeted by the autoimmune reaction responsible for β-cell destruction in NOD mice [5]. HSP60 is hyperexpressed in all stressed cells and not just in β cells [6], so it did not seem likely at the time that autoimmunity to HSP60 could play an exclusive role in the destruction of β cells. Nevertheless, the immunology of HSP60 was intriguing and we wondered whether the molecule might give us a handle on the disease process. We proceeded to identify a target epitope for T cells in the HSP60 molecule composed of amino acids 337–360, which we called peptide p277 (277 was the identification number used by the peptide synthesis unit). We found that β-cell destruction could be stopped in NOD mice by the subcutaneous administration of 100 μg of peptide p277 in incomplete Freund's adjuvant (IFA) [7]. However, it was known that diabetes could be prevented by a variety of treatments administered to young NOD mice early in the course of the autoimmune process, including "nonspecific" immune stimulation [8]; hence we tested whether p277 vaccination late in the autoimmune process could still halt β-cell destruction. Indeed, we found that p277 peptide treatment was effective even after the mice were clinically diabetic [9]; residual β cells could indeed be saved by p277 vaccination.

Successful treatment with p277 was associated with a temporary shift of the spontaneous autoimmune response to HSP60 from a destructive Th1 reaction to an anti-inflammatory Th2 reaction [10]. This Th2 shift was accompanied by downregulation of spontaneous autoimmune reactivity to other antigens in the diabetes collective such as insulin and glutamic acid decarboxylase. Immune reactivity to bacterial antigens remained in the Th1 mode in the treated mice; vaccination with p277 did not debilitate the immune system indiscriminately. After some weeks, the Th2 autoimmunity induced by vaccination spontaneously resolved, and the mice appeared to return to a preautoimmune state; the Th1 autoimmunity did not recur. Moreover, animals treated with p277 showed no toxic reactions or immunological deviations from normal. At this point, we felt that therapeutic vaccination with p277 might be of use in human diabetes, and we sought the human connection. We found that peptide p277 fit the MHC class II binding groove of the HLA susceptibility allele of humans as well as the H2-IA susceptibility allele of NOD mice [11]. Moreover, a significant number of humans, like NOD mice, manifested T-cell autoimmunity to p277 during the development of type I diabetes [12]. It now appeared reasonable to test p277 vaccination in human disease.

There remained two technical problems to solve: IFA could not be used in humans and peptide p277 was chemically unstable. We surveyed several potential vehicles for p277 and discovered that a metabolizable vegetable oil approved for human injection could be used in place of IFA. After experimenting with various amino acid substitutions, we discovered that the p277 peptide could be made stable by substituting the two cysteine residues of the native sequence with valines [9]. The amino acids serine, alanine, or alpha-amino-butyric acid were not effective in substituting for the problematic cysteines (not published). The valine modification was completely cross-reactive with the native p277 peptide; valine-modified p277 does not function as an altered peptide ligand (see below). The valine-modified p277 in vegetable oil is presently called DiaPep277.

We can summarize the background for human trials as follows:

1. Peptide 277 is a target for spontaneous autoimmune T cells in type I diabetes in both NOD mice and human diabetes patients.
2. Therapeutic vaccination using p277 can arrest the progression of β-cell destruction in NOD mice.
3. Preservation of β cells induced by p277 vaccination is associated with temporary activation of a Th2 response to p277 and by lasting downregulation of the Th1 autoimmune reactions associated with type I diabetes.
4. Vaccination with p277 safely leaves intact immune reactions to other antigens not involved in the autoimmune diabetes process.

The question now was whether humans developing type I diabetes would, like NOD mice, respond to p277 vaccination by stopping their β-cell destruction.

III. PHASE I TRIALS FOR THERAPEUTIC VACCINES

Phase I clinical trials are designed to test safety, and not effectiveness. For this reason, Phase I trials traditionally recruit healthy volunteers: persons who would not be expected to benefit from the test treatment, but who still could manifest any adverse effects of the treatment. Consider, however, that exposing a person to a vaccine will leave a mark on the person's immune system. The immune system, like the central nervous system, learns from experience [13]. Both systems continuously organize their repertoires in response to the ongoing interactions of the individual with the individual's internal and external environments. Any immune experience, like any cognitive experience, is formative. Indeed, this cognitive capability of the immune system is what makes vaccination possible; the immune system is

educable [13]. This means that the effects of a vaccine, unlike those of classical pharmaceutical agents, will outlive the catabolism or excretion of the active substance. Hence, any Phase I trial of vaccination will intrude enduringly, if not permanently, in the internal structure of the immune systems of the trial subjects. This consideration led us to disqualify healthy volunteers for a Phase I trial of p277 vaccination.

In place of healthy volunteers, we opened the trial to persons who were already ill with type I diabetes and who had no residual β cells to be saved. We recruited adult male volunteers who had been diagnosed as suffering from type I diabetes for at least 5 years and in whom β-cell function was undetectable: they failed to produce endogenous insulin despite stimulation with intravenous glucagon. We excluded females so as not to expose yet-to-be-born children to the unknown effects of any maternal anti-p277 antibodies transported across the placenta. No adverse reactions to Dia-Pep277 were noted. The stage was set for a Phase II trial of vaccination.

IV. PHASE II TRIALS

Phase II clinical trials are designed to test effectiveness, as well as toxicity. The proof of clinical effectiveness for a therapeutic vaccine for type I diabetes would have to be the arrest of β-cell destruction. Likewise, aggravation of β-cell destruction would indicate a negative clinical effect. Our studies in NOD mice indicated that the immunological effectiveness of the DiaPep277 vaccine would be manifest in the induction of a specific Th2 response to HSP60 and the p277 epitope. Thus, the end points for the Phase II trial focused on detecting endogenous insulin production as a measure of β-cell survival and on assaying the cytokine profile of T-cell autoimmunity to HSP60 and p277.

Thirty-five consecutive male patients, aged 16–55 years, presenting at the Endocrine Clinic of the Hadassah University Hospital, Jerusalem, with type I diabetes of less then 6 months' duration, who manifested basal C-peptide [14] levels of greater that 0.1 nM, were randomized into two groups. The test group was treated by subcutaneous injections of 1 mg of p277 in the vegetable oil vehicle (DiaPep277) at entry and at 1 and 6 months later, a total of three injections. The control group was treated with three placebo injections of the vegetable oil vehicle without p277. The effect of vaccination on β-cell function was detected by glucagon-stimulated C-peptide production; the amount of C-peptide is the standard indicator of the amount of endogenous insulin produced by a subject [14]. We also measured exogenous insulin requirements. T-cell autoimmunity to HSP60 and to p277 was assayed by cytokine secretion. Thirty-one subjects completed the follow-up period of 10 months and were included in the final analysis [15].

During the 10 months, the placebo-treated control subjects manifested a continuous decline in their stimulated C-peptide levels and a persistent rise in their need for exogenous insulin. In contrast, the subjects treated with DiaPep277 maintained their C-peptide response and manifested a reduced need for exogenous insulin ($P = 0.04$ for both measurements compared to the control group). Immunologically, the T-cell reactivity to HSP60 and to p277 of the DiaPep277-treated group showed a significantly enhanced Th2 cytokine phenotype. The T-cell responses to bacterial antigens were not modified by the treatment, and no adverse affects were noted [15]. Thus, therapeutic vaccination of new-onset type I diabetes patients with DiaPep277 preserved endogenous insulin production, as forecast by the experimental mouse model [9]. Without unblinding the trial, test and control subjects were treated with a fourth injection at 12 months. The differences between the two groups were even more significant statistically at 12 and 18 months (unpublished).

So much for the clinical results. We shall now consider why therapeutic vaccination should work at all and how we might proceed from there.

V.   ORGANIZED AUTOIMMUNITY

The results of our trials are promising for the future of DiaPep277, but, clearly, much remains to be learned about the optimal way to use this particular therapeutic vaccine. Nevertheless, the present findings by themselves constitute a proof-of-concept: a destructively progressive autoimmune process can still be halted, even at its peak activity, by a few injections of a relatively small amount of a single peptide in a vegetable oil vehicle. The apparent simplicity of this therapeutic vaccination is remarkable: how can a collective of different autoimmune T-cell clones [3] be shifted into a Th2 mode and the disease arrested by such a humble stimulus? Even if it would turn out that repeated vaccine boosts were needed to maintain the benefits of peptide treatment, the obedience of a complex autoimmune process to a simple peptide signal remains a fact.

Note that the effectiveness of therapeutic peptide vaccination contradicts the "forbidden clone" concept of autoimmune disease as taught by the clonal selection theory of the immune system [16]. Indeed, the forbidden clone concept explains neither the standard collectives of autoreactivities that characterize many autoimmune diseases nor the ability of vaccination with a self-peptide to abort the process. Clearly, an autoimmune disease is not the work of a renegade clone, but the expression of the internal organization of the immune system. What is this internal organization and how does it empower the p277 epitope of HSP60 to shut off the autoimmune disease process?

We shall discuss an attribute of HSP60 immunology that might explain the effectiveness of therapeutic vaccination: HSP60 is a dominant self-antigen within the immunological homunculus [13,17,18]. The scope of this chapter does not accommodate a detailed exposition of the immunological homunculus, and our discussion will mention only the essential concepts.

VI.   HSP60 AND THE IMMUNOLOGICAL HOMUNCULUS

The term immunological homunculus encompasses two elements: a set of observations and a theory proposed to explain these observations.

Empirically, it is clear that a healthy immune system is biased toward responding to a particular group of self-antigens; HSP60 is paradigmatic. The cord blood of new-born human babies is populated with a high frequency of T cells responsive to an HSP60 variant [19]; about a third of healthy adults express spontaneous anti-HSP60 T-cell activity [12] and anti-HSP60 antibodies; and microbial variants of HSP60 are among the most dominant of immunogens, despite the close similarity of these variants to host self-HSP60 [20]. In short, the healthy immune system is not purged of immune reactivity to the HSP60 self-antigen; on the contrary, the adaptive arm of the system is primed from birth to respond and does respond to self-HSP60. Other dominant self-antigens that are the targets of autoimmunity in healthy subjects include myelin basic protein [21], thyroglobulin [22], insulin [23], p53 [24], and the acetylcholine receptor [25]. The immunological homunculus refers to the totality of this natural autoimmunity.

Other observations, thus far only in animal models, show that existing autoimmunity to HSP60 is controlled by several regulatory mechanisms; one of them appears to be an anti-idiotypic T-cell network directed to a T-cell receptor (TCR) relevant to the particular self-antigen. In NOD mice, for example, the onset of autoimmune inflammation in the islets is accompanied by the activation of these anti-idiotypic regulatory T cells; these T cells recognize the TCR (the idiotype) of a particular clone of anti-p277 T cells [26]. The anti-p277 T-cell receptor idiotype of this clone is expressed in the TCR repertoires of different NOD mice. In other words, this anti-p277 idiotype is a shared idiotype [27]. Unfortunately for the mice, the anti-idiotypic response decays spontaneously, and β-cell destruction progresses [26]. The important point is that anti-idiotypic regulation can be rescued; therapeutic vaccination with a TCR peptide or adoptive transfer of lines of anti-idiotypic T cells can arrest the progression of β-cell destruction in most NOD mice [26]. The idiotype-vaccinated mice make anti-idiotypic T cells that shut off the disease process. Additional regulatory mechanisms controlling autoimmune T cells include anti-ergotypic T cells [28], CD25$^+$ T cells [29] and Th2/3 regulatory T cells [30]. These natural regulatory mechanisms are within the immunological homunculus concept. They account for the effectiveness of therapeutic vaccination.

Note that the diabetiogenic autoimmunity developing in NOD mice can be halted by administering either of two peptide vaccines: the p277 peptide from the HSP60 molecule or an idiotypic peptide from a TCR clone that recognizes p277. The two vaccines are composed of different peptides, but they may both activate similar regulatory mechanisms. It turns out that the TCR peptide vaccine, which triggers anti-idiotypic T cells, also activates a Th2 shift in autoimmunity to peptide p277 [26]. In other words, arrest of the disease process by either vaccine is marked by a similar Th2 response to the p277 peptide of HSP60. Likewise, vaccination of NOD mice with the p277 peptide sustains the anti-idiotypic T cells as it halts the disease process [26].

Theoretically, therefore, the regulation of autoimmunity to HSP60 seems to be built into the NOD immune system, and that regulation can be strengthened by therapeutic vaccination. This is the rationale for active vaccination as a means to induce the arrest of autoimmune disease.

It would not be surprising if DiaPep277 treatment strengthens anti-idiotypic T cells as it induces the Th2 shift in human subjects. Humans, of course, are not inbred and homozygous, as are NOD mice. Therefore, it is likely that the T cells in each individual human respond to peptide p277 with unique T-cell receptors; humans, unlike inbred mice, do not express commonly shared T-cell receptor idiotypes. Therefore, we cannot expect to be able to effectively vaccinate different humans with a single T-cell receptor peptide. Each person has his or her own private regulatory networks. Nevertheless, the result of the clinical trial reviewed here does demonstrate that different individuals will respond effectively to vaccination with the *same target peptide vaccine.* There seems to be a uniformity of target antigens among different individuals. Truly, the organization of autoimmunity around HSP60 provides a working definition of the immunological homunculus. The immunological homunculus is not a "little man" inside the immune system; the immunological homunculus is the organization of the natural autoimmune repertoire [13,17].

I borrowed the term *homunculus* from neurology. Neurons in the sensory and motor areas of the brain form a localized anatomical representation of the various organs they innervate; the central nervous system operates on the body using a built-in representation of the body. As can be seen in any neurology textbook, the brain's image of the body is bizarre when traced out on the cerebral cortex because the area of cortex devoted to each organ reflects the function of the organ and not its relative size in the body. For example, the thumb occupies more cortical area than does the whole body truck. By analogy to the central nervous system, the autoimmune clonal repertoire of the immune system creates a functional image of the self [13]. The immune image is a molecular image; the immunological homunculus refers to the sets of naturally autoimmune T cells and B-cells whose antigen receptors form a kind of mirror image of the self-antigens they bind. The immunological image formed by the homunculus, like the image of the neurological homunculus, is bizarre; only some relatively few self-antigens are represented. HSP60 is prominent among them. The function of the immunological homunculus in health is only beginning to be studied, but it seems that some of the autoimmune clones may serve to supply the healthy inflammation needed to maintain the body [31].

VII. AUTOIMMUNE DISEASE

Homunculus theory proposes that pathogenic autoimmune diseases emerge from natural autoimmunity gone awry [13]. A failure of the natural regulatory mechanisms, such as that seen in NOD mice, unleashes the pathogenic potential of the natural autoimmunity present in the immunological homunculus. True, we do not know how homuncular regulation fails or is weakened, but the immunological homunculus concept does explain the observed order of autoimmune

disease unexplainable by classical clonal selection: the autoantigen collectives involved in various diseases, the relatively few diseases and their similar immunological expression in different individuals and in different species, and, most importantly, the ability of a simple vaccination to shut off the disease process. Homunculus theory, in short, proposes that both the disease and its regulation are built into the system of each subject.

Obviously, much remains to be discovered about the homunculus. How do the clones responsive to homuncular self-antigens avoid negative selection? What makes self-antigens such as HSP60 so immunogenic? It was recently discovered that the self-HSP60 molecule can act as a "cytokine" to activate antigen-presenting cells through an innate receptor, toll-like receptor (TLR)-4 [32]. Study of the effects of self-molecules on the innate arm of the immune system may provide new insights into both the immunogenicity of some self-antigens and the mechanisms that regulate natural autoimmunity. Indeed, activation of TLR-9 by vaccination with oligonucleotides bearing the CpG bacterial motif can inhibit the development of NOD diabetes [33]. CpG treatment was associated with a shift of HSP60 autoimmunity into a Th2 mode. Thus, the phenotype of autoimmunity is influenced by innate interactions with signal molecules of infectious agents. The self-organization of the immunological homunculus is molded by the totality of the individual's immune experience [13].

VIII. THE LOGIC OF THERAPEUTIC VACCINATION

Theory leads to practice. Different immunological theories provide rationales for different clinical trial protocols. The forbidden clone theory of autoimmune disease implies its own strategy for therapy; kill or inactivate the forbidden clone and the autoimmune disease will vanish [16]. The homunculus theory of autoimmune disease does not support the strategy of clonal inactivation; on the contrary, the homunculus suggests that once we reactivate natural regulation, the immune system itself will control the autoimmune collective and shut down the disease [13,34]. The two theories recommend opposite approaches: inactivation versus activation. Inactivation of autoimmune T cells by blocking peptides or by toxin conjugates were proposed early on as the solution to autoimmune disease, but the proponents of these approaches are now less assertive. Altered peptide ligands are the latest approach to inactivation therapy, as we shall discuss below.

The apparent success of therapeutic peptide vaccination reviewed here suits well the idea of homuncular activation. In this light, vaccination with a suitable self-antigen or self-peptide would appear to be a natural choice. Each autoimmune disease will need its own particular vaccine, and the challenge will be to find the most effective vaccine for each disease. Multiple sclerosis, for example, might respond to vaccination with a peptide of a myelin antigen [21], myasthenia gravis to a peptide of the acetylcholine receptor [25], lupus to a peptide of p53 [24], and so on. Dose of vaccine and schedule of treatments will be critical factors.

IX. COMPARATIVE IMMUNOMODULATION

Peptide vaccination is only one of several modalities in clinical trials for autoimmune disease therapy. T-cell vaccination refers to a procedure in which a therapeutic vaccine is prepared using cultures of autoimmune T cells obtained from the individual patient [35]. T-cell vaccination was first discovered to be effective in regulating experimental autoimmune diseases in animal models [26,36]. The rationale for T-cell vaccination, as we discussed above, is to activate natural anti-idiotypic and anti-ergotypic networks using the patient's own autoimmune T-cell clones, suitably attenuated [36]. Several hundreds of multiple sclerosis patients have been treated in various open trials, with encouraging results. However, randomized, placebo-controlled studies are just now being undertaken, and proof of effectiveness awaits the results of these trials [35].

Oral, or mucosal, tolerization is another form of immune therapy that could be viewed as a kind of vaccination. Foodstuffs along with other antigens that enter the body through mucosal surfaces have been shown to induce anti-inflammatory Th2/3 cytokine immune reactions [37]. The idea behind oral tolerance is to exploit this natural property of the mucosae and induce resistance to autoimmune attack by administering target self-antigens via this "immunomodulatory" portal [38]. Despite the success of oral tolerance in animal models, this form of treatment has failed to demonstrate effectiveness in clinical trials [39]. Perhaps the development of suitable monitoring assays will make it possible to adjust the dose and dose schedule of oral immunomodulation to the needs of the individual patient's gut absorption and immune state. Until then, protocols for oral tolerization will continue to suffer from uncertainty.

Altered peptide ligand (APL) therapy is yet another type of specific immunomodulation [40]. APL peptides are modifications of natural self-ligands engineered so that they will interact with specific clones of autoimmune T cells through low-affinity binding. Such interactions have been shown to inactivate or "anergize" the specific T cells [40]. Note, however, that the APL approach is quite the opposite of vaccination. The APL concept fits the classical clonal selection theory that attributes autoimmune diseases to the emergence of forbidden clones of autoimmune lymphocytes. The rational way to treat autoimmune disease, according to that idea, is to rid the body of the renegade lymphocytes, and the APL "anergizer" is the latest version of clonal therapy. To insure that all the "forbidden" T cells are inactivated, APL therapy involves relatively high doses of peptide and frequent and prolonged administration. Vaccination therapies, as we have discussed here, aim to reactivate natural immune regulation [17] using limited vaccination protocols [15]. Natural regulation mechanisms are tuned to natural self-epitopes, and not to APLs. Altered peptide ligands, therefore, are likely to be recognized as independent antigens by additional clones of lymphocytes. Indeed, a trial of APL therapy in multiple sclerosis had to be stopped because of the appearance of allergic reactions [41] and aggravated disease [42]. It is conceivable that APL therapy could be safer and more effective when administered in small amounts, infrequently and with adjuvants.

But then, the APL would no longer be an anergizer, but a true vaccine.

ACKNOWLEDGMENTS

I am the incumbent of the Mauerberger Chair in Immunology and Director of the Robert Koch Minerva Center for Research in Autoimmune Disease, at the Weizmann Institute of Science, Director of the Center for the Study of Emerging Diseases, Jerusalem, and a consultant for Peptor, LTD, Rehovot, Israel.

REFERENCES

1. Bach JF. Insulin-dependent diabetes mellitus as an autoimmune disease. Endocr Rev 1994; 15:516–542.
2. Pozzilli P, Di Mario U. Autoimmune diabetes not requiring insulin at diagnosis (latent autoimmune diabetes of the adult): definition, characterization, and potential prevention. Diabetes Care 2001; 24:1460–1467.
3. Roep BO. T-cell responses to autoantigens in IDDM. The search for the Holy Grail. Diabetes 1996; 45:1147–1156.
4. Makino S, et al. Breeding of a non-obese, diabetic strain of mice. Exp Anim 1980; 29:1–13.
5. Elias D, et al. Induction and therapy of autoimmune diabetes in the non-obese diabetic (NOD/LT) mouse by a 65-kDa heat shock protein. Proc Natl Acad Sci USA 1990; 87:1576–1580.
6. Cohen IR. Autoimmunity to chaperonins in the pathogenesis of arthritis and diabetes. Annu Rev Immunol 1991; 9:567–589.
7. Elias D, et al. Vaccination against autoimmune mouse diabetes with a T-cell epitope of the human 65 kDa heat shock protein. Proc Natl Acad Sci USA 1991; 88:3088–3091.
8. Bowman MA, et al. Prevention of diabetes in the NOD mouse: implications for therapeutic intervention in human disease. Immunol Today 1994; 15:115–120.
9. Elias D, Cohen IR. Peptide therapy for diabetes in NOD mice. Lancet 1994; 343:704–706.
10. Elias D, et al. Hsp60 peptide therapy of NOD mouse diabetes induces a Th2 cytokine burst and down-regulates autoimmunity to various beta-cell antigens. Diabetes 1997; 46:758–764.
11. Reizis B, et al. The peptide-binding strategy of the MHC class II I-A molecules. Immunol Today 1998; 19:212–216.
12. Abulafia-Lapid R, et al. T-cell responses of type I diabetes patients and healthy individuals to human hsp60 and its peptides. J Autoimmun 1999; 12:121–129.
13. Cohen IR. Tending Adam's Garden: Evolving the Cognitive Immune SelfLondon: Academic Press, 2000.
14. Berger B, et al. Random C-peptide in the classification of diabetes. Scand J Clin Lab Invest 2000; 60:687–693.
15. Raz I, et al. β-Cell function in new-onset type 1 diabetes and immunomodulation with a heat-shock protein peptide (DiaPep277): a randomized, double-blind, phase II trial. The Lancet 2001; 358:1749–1753.
16. Burnet FM. Self and Not-Self. Cambridge: Cambridge University Press, 1969.
17. Cohen IR. The cognitive paradigm and the immunological homunculus. Immunol Today 1992; 13:490–494.
18. Cohen IR. Discrimination and dialogue in the immune system. Semin Immunol 2000; 12:215–219, 269–271; 321–323.
19. Fischer HP, et al. High frequency of cord blood lymphocytes

against mycobacterial 65-kDa heat-shock protein. Eur J Immunol 1992; 22:1667–1669.

20. Cohen IR, Young DB. Autoimmunity, microbial immunity and the immunological homunculus. Immunol Today 1991; 12:105–110.

21. Burns J, et al. Isolation of myelin basic protein-reactive T-cell lines from normal human blood. Cell Immunol 1983; 81:435–440.

22. Ruf J, et al. Various expressions of a unique anti-human thyroglobulin antibody repertoire in normal state and autoimmune disease. Eur J Immunol 1985; 15:268–272.

23. Petersen KG, et al. Insulin as a target antigen in autoimmune diabetes: a natural repertoire as the source of antibody response. Acta Diabetol 1994; 31:66–72.

24. Herkel J, et al. Systemic lupus erythematosus in mice, spontaneous and induced, is associated with autoimmunity to the C-terminal domain of p53 that recognizes damaged DNA. Eur J Immunol 2000; 30:977–984.

25. Vassilev T, et al. Normal human immunoglobulin suppresses experimental myasthenia gravis in SCID mice. Eur J Immunol 1999; 29:2436–2442.

26. Elias D, et al. Regulation of NOD mouse autoimmune diabetes by T cells that recognize a T-cell receptor CDR3 peptide. Int Immunol 1999; 11:957–966.

27. Tikochinski Y, et al. A shared VDJ beta sequence associated with T cells in mouse autoimmune diabetes. Int Immunol 1999; 11:951–956.

28. Lohse AW, et al. Control of experimental autoimmune encephalomyelitis by T cells responding to activated T cells. Science 1989; 244:820–822.

29. Sakaguchi S, et al. Immunologic tolerance maintained by CD25+ CD4+ regulatory T cells: their common role in controlling autoimmunity, tumor immunity, and transplantation tolerance. Immunol Rev 2001; 182:18–32.

30. Weiner HL. Induction and mechanism of action of transforming growth factor-beta-secreting Th3 regulatory cells. Immunol Rev 2001; 182:207–214.

31. Schwartz M, Cohen IR. Autoimmunity can benefit self-maintenance. Immunol Today 2000; 21:265–268.

32. Ohashi K, et al. Heat shock protein 60 is a putative endogenous ligand of the toll-like receptor-4 complex. J Immunol 2000; 164:558–561.

33. Quintana FJ, et al. Vaccination with empty plasmid DNA or CpG oligonucleotide inhibits diabetes in NOD mice: modulation of spontaneous HSP60 autoimmunity. J Immunol 2000; 165(11):6148–6155.

34. Cohen IR. Treatment of autoimmune disease: to activate or to deactivate? Chem Immunol 1995; 60:150–160.

35. Kumar V, et al. T-cell vaccination: from basics to the clinic. Trends Immunol 2001; 22:539.

36. Cohen IR. T-cell vaccination for autoimmune disease: a panorama. Vaccine 2001; 20(5–6):706–710.

37. Maron R, et al. Oral administration of insulin to neonates suppresses spontaneous and cyclophosphamide induced diabetes in the NOD mouse. J Autoimmun 2001; 16:21–28.

38. Weiner HL, et al. Oral tolerance: immunologic mechanisms and treatment of animal and human organ-specific autoimmune diseases by oral administration of autoantigens. Annu Rev Immunol 1994; 12:809–837.

39. Chaillous L, et al. Oral insulin administration and residual β-cell function in recent-onset type 1 diabetes: a multicentre randomized controlled trial. Lancet 2000; 356:545–549.

40. Bielekova B. Martin R Antigen-specific immunomodulation via altered peptide ligands. J Mol Med 2001; 79:552–565.

41. Kappos L, et al. Induction of a non-encephalitogenic type 2 T helper-cell autoimmune response in multiple sclerosis after administration of an altered peptide ligand in a placebo-controlled, randomized phase II trial. The Altered Peptide Ligand in Relapsing MS Study Group. Nat Med 2000; 6:1176–1182.

42. Bielekova B, et al. Encephalitogenic potential of the myelin basic protein peptide (amino acids 83–99) in multiple sclerosis: results of a phase II clinical trial with an altered peptide ligand. Nat Med 2000; 6:1167–1175.

86

Vaccines for the Treatment of Autoimmune Diseases

David C. Wraith
University of Bristol, Bristol, England

I. BACKGROUND

A. Definition of a Vaccine

The term vaccine is defined as follows: "A vaccine is a material originating from a microorganism or other parasite that induces an immunologically mediated resistance to disease" [1]. It is now clear, however, that vaccines can be created for treatment of disorders other than infectious diseases including cancer, allergy, and autoimmune disease. The Mims definition may therefore be simplified to "A vaccine is a material that induces an immunologically mediated resistance to disease."

It is quite straightforward to extrapolate from infectious disease vaccines to cancer vaccines. Many tumors express tumor-specific antigens, and the hope is that these may be used, just as the specific antigens of many infectious agents have been in the past, as the basis for effective vaccines. A paradox arises, however, when we consider vaccines for allergy and autoimmune disease. The aim, in the case of infectious diseases and cancer, is to induce as strong an immune response to the vaccine antigen as possible. In allergy and autoimmune disease, however, the pathology is caused by the immune response itself. Hence, the aim has to be quite the opposite of the conventional infectious disease or cancer vaccine. Here we must aim to dampen down or suppress the disease by desensitizing the individual.

B. The Inadequacy of Current Treatments for Autoimmune Diseases

Current therapies for autoimmune diseases are based on treatments that nonspecifically suppress the patient's immune system. These therapies can be quite potent and their use is associated with a range of complications.

1. Continuous suppression of the immune system can allow infectious organisms to colonize the individual. Drastic immune suppression may also disturb the normal immune surveillance that prevents tumor growth.
2. Chronic autoimmune disease requires long-term immune suppression. Compliance with treatment is difficult to ensure especially when the treatment is associated with obvious side effects.
3. Nonspecific immune suppression can disturb natural immune regulatory processes. Recent evidence demonstrates that drugs such as cyclosporine can interfere with tolerance mechanisms including apoptosis and anergy induction [2,3].
4. Long-term treatment is expensive.

C. The Case for Antigen-Specific Immunotherapy of Autoimmune Disease

Autoimmune diseases arise as a consequence of autoimmunity, i.e., an immune response to a self-antigen. Autoimmunity is a common feature of the immune system [4] and can be identified in all individuals whether or not they have disease. Disease is prevented by various central and peripheral mechanisms that lead to the deletion or regulation of autoreactive lymphocytes [5]. Autoimmune disease can therefore be seen as a "breakdown in self-tolerance." The Holy Grail for treatment of autoimmune diseases must be to discover how to reinstate self-tolerance, preferably by making such treatments as specific for the disease as possible.

Autoimmune diseases may be defined either as systemic or organ specific. Among organ-specific diseases, there may be a single antigenic target, such as the acetylcholine receptor in myasthenia gravis [6], or a variety of antigenic targets, as is likely to be the case in multiple sclerosis (MS) [7]. The ideal situation would be to induce antigen-specific tolerance to avoid global immune suppression and hence maintain the immune response to infectious agents. Where several different antigens are involved it will be necessary to induce a bystander mechanism that would direct suppression to the appropriate anatomic site and the range of antigens expressed at that site. The systemic autoimmune diseases may be more complex to treat by this approach because the pathology is widespread. Nevertheless, recent studies in mice raise the hope that peptide vaccination could suppress autoantibody generation and hence prolong survival in systemic lupus [8].

D. Vaccines for Autoimmune Disease: A Paradox

The idea that one can vaccinate to suppress an immune response would appear, at face value, to be a contradiction in terms. Yet, we have known for more than a century that it is possible to suppress immunity by encounter with antigen. It was a French physician, Dakin, who noted that the hypersensitivity reaction to poison ivy could be avoided by eating the forbidden leaves [9]. This early description of "mucosal tolerance" was placed on a more scientific footing by Alexandre Besredka who noted that guinea pigs fed milk became resistant to the anaphylactic reaction induced by intracerebral injection of milk proteins [10]. Subsequently, Merrill Chase demonstrated that antigen feeding had an antigen-specific suppressive effect on subsequent immune challenge [11].

There is an attractive logic inherent in the concept of mucosal tolerance. We accept that the immune system generally tolerates encounter with noninfectious antigens. Think of the bulk of antigens that we must eat and inhale each day. Normally we tolerate this material unless, that is, we suffer from allergy to food or an airborne particle such as pollen or dust mite feces. The question is whether mucosal delivery of a self-antigen would enhance the state of tolerance to that antigen. Here I will introduce some recent advances in our understanding of self-tolerance and discuss

how this is guiding our approach to the design of effective vaccines for the treatment of autoimmune disease.

II. THE CONCEPT OF IMMUNE REGULATION

Immunological tolerance toward self-antigens is provided by central and peripheral mechanism. These apply to both B and T lymphocytes, although it appears that the mechanisms relating to T cells are especially important. This is because B cells have evolved to continuously mutate their antigen receptor through the process of affinity maturation. B cells are dependent on T cells for both isotype switching and affinity maturation, and it is therefore logical that tolerance to self-antigens should depend largely on T cells. Tolerance is induced in immature T cells as they mature in the thymus by an avidity-dependent process [12,13]. There is clear evidence that central tolerance is incomplete despite the fact that many self-antigens are expressed in the thymus [14]. Thus, T cells specific for antigens such as myelin basic protein (MBP) are commonly found in the peripheral lymphoid tissues of man [15] as well as rodents [16]. It is increasingly clear that such self-reactive cells are under the tight control of various regulatory mechanisms acting on mature lymphocytes [17]. These include homeostatic [18] as well as regulatory mechanisms [19] (Figure 1).

It is now evident that various types of regulatory cells serve to suppress autoimmunity in healthy individuals. One subset of regulatory cells (Treg) develops naturally in the thymus [20]. These cells constitutively express CD25, proliferate poorly in response to antigen, and regulate the growth of neighboring T cells through cell–cell contact. It is now apparent, however, that distinct CD4 positive Treg cells can be induced with antigen. Antigen-induced Treg cells fall into

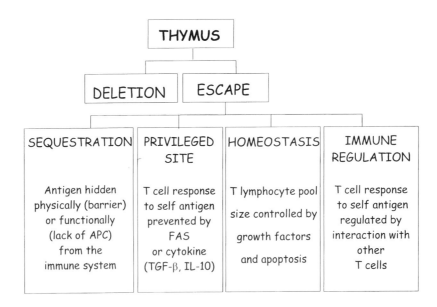

Figure 1 Mechanisms of peripheral tolerance among T lymphocytes. Many self-reactive T cells are deleted as they develop in the thymus. Some self-reactive T cells escape deletion in the thymus and appear in peripheral tissues. Autoimmune disease is prevented by a variety of mechanisms ranging from the sequestration of antigen to immune regulation.

Table 1 The Nature of Induced Regulatory T Lymphocytes

	Th3	Tr1	Tr1/Th10
How raised	Oral antigen	L-10 in vitro	Systemic sol. antigen in vivo
Mechanism	TGF-β	IL-10	Cell–cell contact, IL-10
Reference	[21]	[29]	[23, 25]

Th3 cells are induced by oral administration of intact antigen and regulate autoimmune disease through the production of TGF-β. Tr1 cells may be generated in vitro by repeated stimulation with antigen in the presence of IL-10. IL-10-secreting cells may also be induced in vivo by repeated administration of superantigens or soluble, preferably peptide, antigens.

two categories (Table 1), those induced by oral administration of intact antigen [21] and those induced by repeated administration of either peptide antigens [22] or superantigens [23]. The cells induced by oral administration of intact antigenic proteins include T helper (Th) type 3 (Th3) cells, the helper cells for IgA production, as well as more conventional Th2 cells. Th3 cells produce transforming growth factor beta (TGF-β), the isotype switch factor for IgA. Cells induced by oral administration of antigen suppress autoimmune disease in animal models [24] indicating that TGF-β has a direct anti-inflammatory effect on organ-specific autoimmunity. Cells generated by oral or intranasal peptide antigen administration have, on the other hand, been shown to produce interleukin 10 (IL-10) [25,26] rather than TGF-β and to resemble cells generated by culture in the presence of this cytokine [27]. The cells generated in culture have been termed T regulatory type 1 (Tr1) cells and have been shown to inhibit both Th1 and Th2 responses and to prevent expansion of naïve T cells [28,29]. The fact that Treg cells can be induced by mucosal administration of intact or protein antigen raises the exciting possibility that they could be specifically induced by vaccines to suppress the inflammation associated with autoimmune disease.

III. WHAT FORM SHOULD THE ANTIGEN TAKE?

A. HLA Association

Many autoimmune diseases are associated with a predisposing genotype (Table 2). Among the predisposing genes, the MHC-associated immune response genes (HLA in man) often show the strongest association. This is not, however, direct and most HLA-associated diseases do not follow a simple Mendelian mode of inheritance, frequently involving several different HLA alleles in addition to non-HLA loci. Nevertheless, association with HLA certainly demonstrates the strongest genetic linkage in diseases such as MS, rheumatoid arthritis, and type I diabetes [30–33]. This raises the hope that specific peptide or protein vaccines could be designed to fit a specific, disease-associated HLA allele.

B. The Case for Intact Antigens

Protein antigens are made up of a series of linked epitopes that may be antigenic for T cells from individuals expressing different HLA genes. As mentioned above, HLA association with autoimmune disease is rarely absolute. It is then not likely that a single peptide epitope would be sufficient to induce tolerance in the heterogeneous human population. It was hoped, therefore, that systemic or mucosal administration of whole proteins would effectively induce tolerance and could thus be used for treatment of autoimmune conditions. Even then, there was evidence from experimental animal models of autoimmune disease that more than a single protein would be required. In the experimental model of MS, experimental autoimmune encephalomyelitis (EAE), there was evidence that protein x would be encephalitogenic in one mouse strain whereas protein y would cause disease in another mouse strain [34]. There was therefore no reason to believe that a single protein entity would be responsible for

Table 2 HLA Disease Association in Autoimmune Disease

Disease	HLA allele	Sex ratio (F:M)	Relative risk
Ankylosing spondylitis	B27	0.3	87.4
Type I diabetes	DR3/4 heterozygote	~1	~25
Goodpasture's disease	DR2	~1	15.9
Pemphigus vulgaris	DR4	~1	14.4
Systemic lupus erythematosus	DR3	10–20	5.8
Multiple sclerosis	DR2	10	4.8
Rheumatoid arthritis	DR4	3	4.2
Graves' disease	DR3	4–5	3.7
Hashimoto's thyroiditis	DR5	4–5	3.2
Myasthenia gravis	DR3	4–5	3.7

Many autoimmune diseases display an association with particular HLA genes. Among these associations with class II MHC (HLA DR) molecules are more common.

disease in every single patient suffering from MS. Indeed, there is evidence for T-cell reactivity against a variety of T-cell antigens in MS [7] and further evidence of fluctuation in the nature of the response between antigens during the course of disease [35]. A logical step was therefore to develop tolerance strategies based on the use of mixtures of antigens.

Trials of oral tolerance have involved extracts of myelin in MS, retinal extract for autoimmune uveitis, bovine collagen in rheumatoid arthritis, and insulin in type I diabetes [36]. Unfortunately, none of these treatments provided a dramatic improvement in clinical symptoms. In fact, the uveitis trial indicated that mucosal administration of complex antigens could exacerbate disease. In this trial, patients were treated with either the purified S-antigen or a combination of this antigen with a crude retinal extract [37]. The group receiving the purified S antigen alone appeared to "taper off" their immunosuppressive medication more successfully compared with patients given placebo, whereas all other groups appeared to do worse than did those receiving placebo. This would indicate that the use of complex combinations of antigens should be treated with caution.

Why have clinical trials of oral tolerance been so disappointing? It could well be that oral tolerance to self-antigens is not as easy to generate as first thought. Essentially, there are at least three mechanisms or oral tolerance. The Weiner group has shown that high dose of protein leads to the induction of anergy or deletion in the Lewis rat model of EAE. Low-dose administration, however, generated regulatory cells of the Th2/Th3 phenotype. Our own studies have shown that it is relatively difficult to induce oral tolerance in the H-2^u mouse model of EAE [38]. Even a low dose of antigen failed to generate tolerance. Further work by Meyer et al. confirmed the difficulty in inducing tolerance in the H-2^u model. Tolerance was achieved only by feeding vast quantities of protein [39] at levels that could never be achieved in humans on a milligram per kilogram basis. What was more disturbing from the Meyer study was the observation that low-dose oral feeding of self-antigen led to exacerbation of the clinical course of disease. We have to conclude from these studies that the induction of oral tolerance to whole self-antigens is not straightforward. The pioneering work by Weiner [36] and Meyer et al. has revealed a variety of mechanisms by which oral tolerance can be

achieved. At this point, however, it is impossible to predict how oral tolerance with complex mixtures of intact antigens could be achieved safely and reliably in humans. More work is required to investigate dosing effects, the nature of the autoantigen and the use of mucosal adjuvants [40,41] designed to enhance tolerance induction.

C. The Danger of Antigen-Specific Therapy with Intact Antigen

The obvious danger of administering an intact antigen into an individual prone to autoimmunity is that the treatment might exacerbate disease by (1) priming T cells and (2) mounting an antibody response to the self-protein by activating autoreactive B cells (Table 3). In an experimental model of multiple sclerosis induced by myelin oligodendrocyte glycoprotein (MOG), marmosets tolerized to MOG were protected against acute disease, but after treatment a lethal demyelinating disorder emerged [42]. In these animals, MOG-specific T-cell proliferative responses were transiently suppressed, cytokine production was shifted from a Th1 to a Th2 pattern, and titers of autoantibodies to MOG were enhanced. In this case, immune deviation produced by an apparently tolerogenic immunization schedule led to enhanced immune pathology.

A further danger arises from injection of intact antigens. This is that such soluble antigens can prime cytotoxic T (Tc) cells. Blanas and colleagues demonstrated that oral administration of ovalbumin (Ova) led to the induction of Ova-specific Tc cells [43]. In their model, in which Ova was expressed as a self-antigen in the pancreas, the induction of such Tc cells accelerated the onset of type 1 diabetes. More recently, Hanninen and colleagues have compared different mucosal routes for their ability to induce Tc cells and exacerbate autoimmune diabetes [44]. In their mouse model, delivery of Ova by either oral or nasal routes primed for Ova-specific Tc cells whether the protein was delivered in a high- or low-dose regimen. Ova delivered by either route triggered diabetes in a model in which mice expressed the protein in the pancreas.

The danger of delivering intact self-antigens to the body is therefore twofold. First, there is the possibility that the protein could trigger autoreactive T and B cells leading to the

Table 3 Potential Danger Associated with Antigen-Specific Therapy

Induction of	Associated danger
Autoreactive B cells and antibodies	Late complications of immune deviation therapy in a nonhuman primate: induction of TH2 cells in marmoset EAE can exacerbate disease by increasing levels of pathogenic antibodies [42]
Autoreactive CD8 "cytotoxic" T cells	Induction of autoimmune diabetes by oral administration of autoantigen: induction of CD8 cytotoxic T cells can trigger disease [43]

Here are two examples of problems arising from the administration of intact protein antigens in therapeutic protocols. In the first, administration of myelin oligodendrocyte glycoprotein led to the induction of a strong Th2 response and pathogenic antibodies. In the second, oral administration of intact protein induced CD8 positive cytotoxic T cells that caused diabetes in an animal model.

production of pathogenic antibodies. Second, intact proteins may prime antigen-specific Tc cells with devastating consequences. We must conclude from the preceding discussion that administration of intact antigens in an autoimmune setting can be highly dangerous.

D. The Case for Peptide Antigens

The dangers associated with delivery of intact proteins can be overcome by the use of peptide antigens. The objective here is to use peptides based on the structure of the major class II restricted T-cell epitopes associated with a disease. By inducing tolerance among pathogenic Th cells one would effectively remove help for both pathogenic B and Tc cells. The first advantage of this approach is that peptides are generally poorly immunogenic for B cells (1) because they usually do not retain the three-dimensional conformation of the intact antigen and (2) because well-defined T-cell epitopes rarely contain both the major Th and B-cell determinants required to prime for such a response. The second advantage is that peptide determinants can be selected such that they do not contain known pathogenic Tc epitopes, although knowledge of this is currently limited. Furthermore, there is yet no evidence that the delivery of soluble peptides leads to the induction of autoreactive Tc cells.

E. The Pros and Cons of Altered Peptide Ligands

Triggering a T cell is not the same as switching on a light. There are numerous states of activation between resting/ inactive and fully activated. Some of these states, whether they represent anergy or an altered state of cytokine production, have been associated with self-tolerance and can be generated by the use of T-cell receptor antagonists. Such antagonists are based on peptide ligands that are altered at residues interacting with the TCR. T-cell antagonism is defined as a specific and dose-dependent downmodulation of agonist-induced T-cell proliferation when both agonist and altered peptide ligand (APL) are presented to the T cell simultaneously [45]. It has been proposed that it might be safer to base antigen-specific treatment of autoimmune disease on the use of such peptides since APL should fail to activate autoreactive T cells and should be inherently safer [46]. Initial studies of APL treatment in well-defined animal models were indeed extremely promising [47–51]. Recently, however, clinical trials of APL treatment have been undertaken in MS and have been less encouraging. A common target for MBP specific T cells in HLA DR2 positive MS patients is an epitope within the 83–99 region. Two trials of peptide therapy with an APL based on MBP 83–99 were recently reported in *Nature Medicine*. The first Phase II trial using this APL had to be curtailed because of side effects [52]. Some patients developed signs of urticaria because of the Th2 response to the APL that developed following repeated administration. In a second open-label trial two patients were reported to have suffered treatment-related exacerbations of MS [53]. This disturbing observation was supported by evidence arising from *in* vitro studies of the patient's lymphocytes. Results from this trial showed (1) that a high dose (50 mg per treatment) of the peptide was highly im-

munogenic and induced APL-specific T cells in each individual, (b) three of eight patients suffered exacerbations, and (c) in two of the three patients the exacerbations were linked to the expansion of APL-specific cells that were able to cross-react with the wild-type MBP 83–99 epitope.

Why should a peptide that behaves as a TCR antagonist in vitro cause disease in vivo and why only in certain individuals? This most probably reflects the fact that an APL will function as a TCR antagonist for a T-cell clone expressing receptor A but may equally work as an agonist for a distinct clone expressing receptor B. This likelihood had previously been raised through the work of Anderton and colleagues using a well-defined mouse model and the N-terminal nonamer peptide of MBP [54]. This might be expected to be a straightforward model to study because there is limited heterogeneity of TCR usage in the H-2^u restricted response to this peptide with the majority of T-cell clones expressing similar TCRs [55]. Altered peptide ligands with appropriate substitutions at the primary TCR contact residue were prepared and shown to be effective antagonists of one specific T-cell clone (Tg4). As expected, these APLs failed to induce EAE in the Tg4 TCR-transgenic mouse and yet were found to induce disease in susceptible, nontransgenic H-2^u strains of mice. This proves that one T cell's antagonist can be the next cell's agonist and emphasizes just how diverse and flexible the TCR repertoire can be, even in a simple mouse model. Extrapolate this to the likely diversity of the TCR repertoire in an outbred population such as man and you have to conclude that the use of TCR antagonists loses its appeal as a therapeutic approach. The remainder of this chapter will therefore concentrate on the use of natural peptides as vaccines for the treatment of autoimmune diseases.

IV. RULES GOVERNING THE USE OF PEPTIDES FOR THERAPY OF AUTOIMMUNE DISEASE

Various laboratories have now tested peptide therapy as an approach to the prevention and treatment of autoimmune and allergic conditions. The favored route of administration has been mucosal. This is not to say that other routes of administration including intraperitoneal, subcutaneous, and intradermal may not be equally effective for certain peptide antigens. It is believed, however, that the mucosal immune system has evolved to tolerate encounter with antigens when they are not associated with infectious agents (see above). A logical step was therefore to test mucosal delivery of soluble antigens derived from self-antigens or allergens.

A. Peptide Therapy Is Effective in a Wide Range of Disease Models

Peptide therapy has proven effective in a wide range of disease models. Fragments of MBP were found to be as effective as the intact protein in prevention of EAE [56]. The 139–151 peptide of PLP has been shown to prevent EAE when administered by either the oral [57] or intranasal [58] route. Furthermore, Liu and colleagues revealed the synergistic effect of different MBP peptides in the rat model of EAE [59].

The nasal route of administration has proven effective for prevention of various models of arthritis. Staines et al. [60], Myers et al. [61], and Chu and Londei [62] have all demonstrated the efficacy of peptides derived from collagen in models of collagen-induced arthritis. Most interestingly, Prakken and colleagues demonstrated that a single peptide, derived from the heat shock protein HSP60 and given by the intranasal route, would protect rats from arthritis induced by either *Mycobacterium* or avridine [63]. Peptides derived from a variety of pancreatic islet antigens have been used to suppress diabetes in the NOD mouse model [64-66] and more recently in man [67]. The fact that a single peptide can prevent arthritis induced by different antigens [63] would imply a bystander suppressive mechanism. This is further supported by observations in diabetes whereby peptides derived from diverse antigens, including glutamate decarboxylase [64], insulin [65], and HSP60 [66], would equally suppress disease in the same animal model. Peptides derived from the S-antigen have been used to prevent experimental autoimmune uveitis [68], peptides from the acetylcholine receptor models of autoimmune myasthenia gravis [69] and peptides from the P2 antigen models of experimental allergic neuritis [70]. A number of groups have also described the use of the peptides to suppress the immune response to allergens. Hoyne and colleagues first described the use of nasal peptides to suppress the immune response to the major house dust mite antigen [71]. More recent work has demonstrated inhibition of mucosal and systemic Th2-type immune responses by intranasal peptide therapy in the Der P1 model [72].

B. Route of Administration

Some years ago, our laboratory compared oral and intranasal routes of peptide therapy. The nasal route proved far more effective than the oral route for tolerance to the N-terminal peptide of MBP [73]. This peptide is, however, a relatively weak antigen [74], and there is no reason why the oral route should not be equally effective for more potent antigenic epitopes. Others have compared oral and nasal routes for prevention of collagen-induced arthritis. Results have been varied with some groups demonstrating improved efficacy by the nasal route [75] and others observing no significant difference [60]. Furthermore, Jung and colleagues could show no difference between oral and nasal administration of the P2 peptide in a model of experimental autoimmune neuritis [75]. Most probably, the nasal route of administration is more sensitive than the oral route for weaker antigens because they are less likely to be destroyed before they can exert their tolerogenic or suppressive function.

C. Duration of the Effect of Peptide Therapy

The longevity of suppression mediated by a single dose of tolerogenic peptide was measured in the mouse model [76]. The N-terminal peptide of MBP had been previously shown to induce tolerance in the H-2^u mouse model of EAE [73]. This peptide was administered intranasally to either euthymic or thymectomized animals. A single dose of peptide induced permanent tolerance in thymectomized animals.

Euthymic animals, however, recovered responsiveness over an 8- to 16-week period. A single dose of intranasal peptide could therefore induce long-lasting thymus-independent, peripheral T-cell unresponsiveness, the recovery of which relied entirely on new T cells being exported from the thymus.

D. The Mechanism of Peptide Therapy

Several studies have compared the mechanism of tolerance induced by either systemic or mucosal antigen administration. High doses of antigen may induce apoptosis among antigen-specific cells. Critchfield and colleagues were able to detect apoptosis following high-dose administration of antigen in the EAE model [77]. Similarly, Kearney and colleagues described activation-induced cell death as a mechanism involved in antigen-specific tolerance induction [78]. Similarly, several investigators have shown a significant amount of deletion after repeated antigen injection or feeding [79,80]. Deletion of CD-4 T cells in the periphery, however, is never complete and usually leaves a small population of residual T cells.

Although there seems little doubt that some activation-induced cell death occurs in response to antigen in almost any setting, there is now strong evidence that induced tolerance involves alteration in cytokine production. The type of cytokines involved will depend on several conditions: (1) route of administration, (2) genetic background of the recipient, and (3) nature of the antigen. As mentioned above, the response to intact antigen encountered at mucosal surfaces tends to be dominated by Th2 and Th3 cytokines. Most notably, Th3 cells producing TGF-β have been implicated in oral tolerance to intact protein antigen. One might imagine that long peptides would mimic intact protein antigens in their mechanism of tolerance induction. A recent study by Astori and colleagues showed, however, that long peptides based on the structure of phospholipase A2 tended to induce a shift from a Th2 toward a Th1 cytokine profile [81]. Notably, however, IL-10 secretion was not measured in this study.

A detailed study by the Weiner group has compared the administration of either intact antigen or short peptides given orally or intranasally. Despite previous evidence to suggest that administration of protein or peptides in the NOD mouse would drive Th2 responses [64,65] this study showed a clear distinction between protein and peptide. Mucosal administration of intact protein primed for TGF-β, whereas mucosal peptides primed for IL-10-secreting T cells [26].

It appears then that a hierarchy of responses to mucosally administered antigen exists and this depends on the nature of the antigen. The response to intact protein is generally dominated by Th3 cells, whereas long peptides have been reported, in one strain of mouse, to induce Th1 cells. The evidence to date implies that administration of short peptides may induce IL-10-secreting cells. Our own laboratory has provided strong support for the role of IL-10 in peptide-induced tolerance. Studies in the Tg4 TCR transgenic mouse did not provide evidence for apoptosis as a tolerance mechanism following intranasal peptide administration [25]. Repeated doses of intranasal peptide nevertheless completely protected the transgenic mice from EAE induction (Table 4). Such treatment also resulted in downregulation of the capacity of antigen-specific CD-4 T cells to proliferate or to produce IL-2, interferon gamma, and IL-4 but increased the production of IL-10. The role of IL-10 in suppression of EAE was confirmed in vivo by neutralization of IL-10. This completely restored susceptibility to EAE in mice previously protected by intranasal peptide.

Interleukin-10 has been associated with the induction of long-lasting anergy in human CD-4 T cells [27], and Sundstedt et al. have described superantigen-induced unresponsiveness correlating with the downregulation of IL-4 and upregulation of IL-10 [23]. Furthermore, CD-4 T cells producing high levels of IL-10 but low levels of IL-2 and IL-4 had the capacity to prevent colitis induced in SCID mice by pathogenic CD-4 cells [29]. Moreover, transfected T-cell clones expressing antigen-inducible IL-10 were able both to inhibit the onset of EAE and to treat animals therapeutically after onset of neurological signs of disease [82].

Recent work from our laboratory has shown that it is possible to induce tolerance in H-2^b mice by intranasal administration of the MOG 35–55 peptide. Tolerance was associated with IL-10 production from spleen cells and could be transferred to naïve recipient mice by adoptive transfer (82a). Most importantly, it was not possible to induce tolerance with intranasal peptide in H-2^b mice rendered IL-10$^{-/-}$ by homologous recombination.

E. The Function of Regulatory T Cells

The IL-10-producing regulatory T cells described above resemble Tr-1 cells previously described by Groux and colleagues [27]. Tr-1 cells and Th3 cells share one common property although they produce distinct types of cytokine. Both cell types mediate bystander suppression. Bystander suppression was first described by Miller and colleagues in oral tolerance. Thus, Th3 cells specific for antigen A will inhibit responses to antigen B so long as both antigens are presented at the same site [83]. Similar work from our laboratory has shown that peptide-induced regulatory cells specific for an epitope of proteolipid protein would suppress

both PLP- and MBP-induced disease in the H-2^{uxs} model of EAE 58. IL-10 downregulates the antigen-presenting capacity of many antigen-presenting cells, including bone-marrow-derived dendritic cells and Langerhans cells, by downregulating MHC class II and a number of costimulatory molecules, including CD-80, CD-86, and CD-154 [84]. Similarly, TGF-β downregulates MHC class II and prevents upregulation of CD-80 and CD-86 [85,86]. It is likely that both peptide-induced Tr-1 cells and protein-induced Th3 cells mediate bystander suppression by suppressing the function of APC.

V. FUNCTION OF ANTIGEN-PRESENTING CELLS IN INDUCTION OF REGULATORY T CELLS

Why should short peptides induce Tr-1 cells, long peptides Th1 cells, and intact proteins Th3 cells? It seems likely that B cells play a role in the induction of Th3 responses. The mucosal immune system is designed to produce IgA in response to foreign antigen. It is therefore logical that helper T cells for IgA-secreting B cells should secrete the obligatory cytokine for IgA class switching, namely, TGF-β. Mucosal B cells will be involved in T–B collaboration and would logically respond to intact antigen. It therefore seems appropriate that the immune response to intact antigen at mucosal surfaces should involve Th3 cells providing help for the production of IgA. Peptide antigens, on the other hand, may not fold into a sufficiently stable confirmation for recognition by B cells. Long peptides would nevertheless require antigen processing. It is therefore likely that long peptides are handled by other antigen-presenting cells, including dendritic cells and macrophages. This might explain why mucosal delivery of long peptides fails to induce Th3 cells. Our working hypothesis is that short peptides may be presented to T cells by immature dendritic cells. Short peptides can bind directly to empty MHC at the surface of such cells [87] and hence induce the differentiation of regulatory T cells. Recent reports have shown that CD-4 regulatory T cells, induced by immature dendritic cells, resemble Tr-1 cells in that they secrete high levels of IL-10 but no IL-4 or IL-2 [88,89].

Table 4 Induction of Tolerance in TCR-Transgenic T Cells Following Intranasal Administration of Peptide

Pretreatment	In vitro response to antigen				
	Proliferation	IFN-γ	IL-2	IL-4	IL-10
PBS IN	+	+ +	+ +	−	−
1 × [4Y]IN	+ + +	+ +	+ +	+ +	+ +
5 × [4Y]IN	−	−	−	−	+ +
10 × [4Y]IN	−	−	−	−	+ +

Transgenic mice expressing the TCR specific for peptide Ac1-9 of MBP were treated with intranasal (IN) peptide (Ac1-9[4Y]) or PBS prior to antigenic challenge with Ac1-9 in vitro. Mice received either a single dose of peptide 24 hr or alternatively 5 or 10 doses of peptide every third or fourth day before challenge in vitro. Cervical lymph node cells were challenged in vitro with Ac1-9 and assessed for proliferation by [^{3}H]thymidine incorporation or cytokine production by ELISA.

VI. EVIDENCE FOR ANTIGEN-SPECIFIC REGULATORY T CELLS IN MAN

Although the oral tolerance trial in MS failed to provide significant evidence of clinical benefit, the laboratory studies associated with this trial demonstrated a clear effect of the treatment. A comparison of cell lines from individuals fed bovine myelin with those from nonfed patients demonstrated a marked increase in the frequency of TGF-β secreting lines specific for myelin antigens. This increase was antigen specific and highly significant [90].

Antigen-specific immunotherapy in allergy to bee venom has been associated with downregulation of allergen-specific T-cell proliferation and Th2 cytokine secretion. Recent work by Akdis and colleagues has shown that antigen-specific cells appear anergic and yet continue to secrete IL-10 [91]. Proliferative and cytokine responses to the allergen in question could be reconstituted by neutralization of IL-10 in vitro. Interestingly, the same anergic phenotype was found in T cells derived from healthy bee-keepers, all of whom had previously been stung repeatedly [92]. These naturally tolerant individuals showed similar raised levels of IL-10-secreting cells when compared with patients rendered tolerant by specific immunotherapy. Similar observations have arisen from peptide immunotherapy experiments in patients suffering from allergy to cat dander [93]. Inhibition of the late asthmatic reaction to allergen, following peptide therapy, was associated with a decrease in proinflammatory cytokines and a marked increase in IL-10.

Taken together, these observations indicate that antigen-induced regulatory cells similar to those identified in numerous experiments in animal models also exist in man. They can be induced by antigen administration and therefore constitute targets for therapeutic vaccination in man.

REFERENCES

1. Mims C, et al. Pathogenesis of Infectious Disease. London: Academic Press, 2001.
2. Kishimoto H, Sprent J. Strong TCR ligation without co-stimulation causes rapid onset of Fas-dependent apoptosis of naive murine CD4(+) T cells. J Immunol 1999; 163:1817–1826.
3. Li YS, et al. Blocking both signal 1 and signal 2 of T-cell activation prevents apoptosis of alloreactive T cells and induction of peripheral allograft tolerance. Nat Med 1999; 5:1298–1302.
4. Coutinho A, et al. Natural autoantibodies. Curr Opin Immunol 1995; 7:812–818.
5. Wraith DC. Immunological tolerance. In: Roitt BaM, ed. Immunology. Edinburgh: Mosby, 2001:191–209.
6. Willcox N, et al. Approaches for studying the pathogenic T cells in autoimmune patients. Ann N Y Acad Sci 1993; 681: 219–237.
7. Kerlero de Rosbo N, Ben Nun A. T-cell responses to myelin antigens in multiple sclerosis; relevance of the predominant autoimmune reactivity to myelin oligodendrocyte glycoprotein. J Autoimmun 1998; 11:287–299.
8. Singh RR. The potential use of peptides and vaccination to treat systemic lupus erythematosus. Curr Opin Rheumatol 2000; 12:399–406.
9. Dakin R. Remarks on a cutaneous affection produced by certain poisonous vegetables. Am J Med Sci 1829; 4:98–100.
10. Besredka A. De l'anaphylaxie. Sixieme memoire de l'anaphylaxie lactique. Ann Inst Pasteur 1909; 23:166–174.
11. Chase M. Proc Soc Exp Biol Med 1946; 61.
12. Kappler JW, et al. T cell tolerance by clonal elimination in the thymus. Cell 1987; 49, 273–280.
13. Liu GY, et al. Low avidity recognition of self-antigen by T cells permits escape from central tolerance. Immunity 1995; 3:407–415.
14. Derbinski J, et al. Promiscuous gene statement in medullary thymic epithelial cells mirrors the peripheral self. Nat Immunol 2001; 2:1032–1039.
15. Ponsford M, et al. Differential responses of CD45 + ve T cell subsets to MBP in multiple sclerosis. Clin Exp Immunol 2001; 124:315–322.
16. Schluesener HJ, Wekerle H. Autoaggressive T lymphocyte lines recognizing the encephalitogenic region of myelin basic protein: in vitro selection from unprimed rat T lymphocyte populations. J Immunol 1985; 135:3128–3133.
17. Anderton S, et al. Mechanisms of central and peripheral T-cell tolerance: lessons from experimental models of multiple sclerosis. Immunol Rev 1999; 169:123–137.
18. Theofilopoulos AN, et al. T cell homeostasis and systemic autoimmunity. J Clin Invest 2001; 108:335–340.
19. Shevach EM. Certified professionals: CD4$^+$CD25$^+$ suppressor T cells. J Exp Med 2001; 193:41–45.
20. Sakaguchi S, et al. Study on cellular events in post-thymectomy autoimmune oophoritis in mice. II. Requirement of Lyt-1 cells in normal female mice for the prevention of oophoritis. J Exp Med 1982; 156:1577–1586.
21. Faria AM, Weiner HL. Oral tolerance: mechanisms and therapeutic applications. Adv Immunol 1999; 73:153–264.
22. Burkhart C, et al. Modulation of cytokine production following intranasal administration of antigenic peptide. Transplant Proc 1998; 30:4186–4187.
23. Sundstedt A, et al. Immunoregulatory role of IL-10 during superantigen-induced hyporesponsiveness in vivo. J. Immunol 1997; 158:180–186.
24. Chen Y, et al. Regulatory T cell clones induced by oral tolerance: suppression of autoimmune encephalomyelitis. Science 1994; 265:1237–1240.
25. Burkhart C, et al. Peptide-induced T cell regulation of experimental autoimmune encephalomyelitis: a role for interleukin-10. Int Immunol 1999; 11:1625–1634.
26. Maron R, et al. Regulatory Th2-type T cell lines against insulin and GAD peptides derived from orally- and nasally-treated NOD mice suppress diabetes. J Autoimmun 1999; 12:251–258.
27. Groux H, et al. Interleukin-10 induces a long-term antigen-specific anergic state in human CD4 + T cells. J Exp Med 1996; 184:19–29.
28. Cottrez F, et al. T regulatory cells 1 inhibit a Th2-specific response in vivo. J. Immunol 2000; 165:4848–4853.
29. Groux H, et al. A CD4 + T-cell subset inhibits antigen-specific T-cell responses and prevents colitis. Nature 1997; 389:737–742.
30. Sawcer S, et al. A genome screen in multiple sclerosis reveals susceptibility loci on chromosome 6p21 and 17q22. Nat Genet 1996; 13:464–468.
31. Dyment DA, et al. Genetics of multiple sclerosis. Hum Mol Genet 1997; 6:1693–1698.
32. Bali D, et al. Genetic analysis of multiplex rheumatoid arthritis families. Genes Immun 1999; 1:28–36.
33. Herr M, et al. Evaluation of fine mapping strategies for a multifactorial disease locus: systematic linkage and association analysis of IDDM1 in the HLA region on chromosome 6p21. Hum Mol Genet 2000; 9:1291–1301.
34. Martin R, McFarland HF. Immunological aspects of experimental allergic encephalomyelitis and multiple sclerosis. Crit Rev Clin Lab Sci 1995; 32:121–182.

35. Tuohy VK, et al. Spontaneous regression of primary auto-reactivity during chronic progression of experimental autoimmune encephalomyelitis and multiple sclerosis. J Exp Med 1999; 189:1033–1042.

36. Weiner HL. Oral tolerance: immune mechanisms and treatment of autoimmune diseases. Immunol Today 1997; 18:335–343. Review. No abstract available.

37. Nussenblatt RB, et al. Treatment of uveitis by oral administration of retinal antigens: results of a phase I/II randomized masked trial. Am J Ophthalmol 1997; 123:583–592.

38. Metzler B, Wraith DC. Mucosal tolerance in a murine model of experimental autoimmune encephalomyelitis. Ann N Y Acad Sci 1996; 778:228–243.

39. Meyer AL, et al. Suppression of murine chronic relapsing experimental autoimmune encephalomyelitis by the oral administration of myelin basic protein. J Immunol 1996; 157:4230–4238.

40. Sun JB, et al. Treatment of experimental autoimmune encephalomyelitis by feeding myelin basic protein conjugated to cholera toxin B subunit. Proc Natl Acad Sci USA 1996; 93: 7196–7201.

41. Williams NA, et al. Immune modulation by the cholera-like enterotoxins: from adjuvant to therapeutic. Immunol Today 1999; 20:95–101.

42. Genain CP, et al. Late complications of immune deviation therapy in nonhuman primate. Science 1996; 274:2054–2057.

43. Blanas E, et al. Induction of autoimmune diabetes by oral administration of autoantigen. Science 1996; 274:1707–1709.

44. Hanninen A, et al. Mucosal antigen primes diabetogenic cytotoxic T-lymphocytes regardless of dose or delivery route. Diabetes 2001; 50:771–775.

45. Sloan-Lancaster J, Alleen PM. Altered peptide ligand-induced partial T cell activation: molecular mechanisms and role in T cell biology. Annu Rev Immunol 1996; 14:1–27.

46. Steinman L. Development of antigen-specific therapies for autoimmune disease. Mol Biol Med 1990; 7:333–339.

47. Franco A, et al. T cell receptor antagonist peptides are highly effective inhibitors of experimental allergic encephalomyelitis. Eur J Immunol 1994; 24:940–946.

48. Karin N, et al. Reversal of experimental autoimmune encephalomyelitis by a soluble peptide variant of myelin basic protein epitope: T cell receptor antagonism and reduction of interferon gamma and tumor necrosis factor alpha production. J Exp Med 1994; 180:2227–2237.

49. Kuchroo VK, et al. A single TCR antagonist peptide inhibits experimental allergic encephalomyelitis mediated by a diverse T-cell repertoire. J Immunol 1994; 153:3326–3336.

50. Nicholson LB, et al. A T cell receptor antagonist peptide induces T cells that mediate bystander suppression and prevent autoimmune encephalomyelitis induced with multiple myelin antigens. Proc Natl Acad Sci USA 1997; 94:9279–9284.

51. Brocke S, et al. Treatment of experimental encephalomyelitis with a peptide analogues of myelin basic protein. Nature 1996; 379:343–346.

52. Kappos L, et al. Induction of a non-encephalitogenic type 2 T helper-cell autoimmune response in multiple sclerosis after administration of an altered peptide ligand in a placebo-controlled, randomized phase II trial. Nat Med 2000; 6:1176–1182.

53. Bielekova B, et al. Encephalitogenic potential of the myelin basic protein peptide (amino acids 83–99) in multiple sclerosis: results of a phase II clinical trial with an altered peptide ligand. Nat Med 2000; 6:1167–1175.

54. Anderton SM, et al. Fine-specificity of the myelin-reactive T cell repertoire: implications for TCR antagonism in autoimmunity. J Immunol 1998; 161:3357–3364.

55. Acha-Orbea H, et al. Limited heterogeneity of T cell receptors from lymphocytes mediating autoimmune encephalomyelitis allows specific immune intervention. Cell 1988; 54:263–273.

56. Higgins PJ, Weiner HL. Suppression of experimental autoimmuneencephalomyelitis by oral administration of myelin basic protein and its fragments. J Immunol 1988; 140:440–445.

57. Al-Sabbagh A, et al. Antigen-driven tissue-specific suppression following oral tolerance: orally administered myelin basic protein suppresses proteolipid protein-induced experimental autoimmune encephalomyelitis in the SJL mouse. Eur J Immunol 1994; 24:2104–2109.

58. Anderton SM, Wraith DC. Hierarchy in the ability of T cell epitopes to induce peripheral tolerance to antigens from myelin. Eur J Immunol 1998; 28:1251–1261.

59. Liu JQ, et al. Inhibition of experimental autoimmune encephalomyelitis in Lewis rats by nasal administration of encephalitogenic MBP peptides: synergistic effects of MBP 68–86 and 87–99. Int Immunol 1998; 10:1139–1148.

60. Staines NA, et al. Mucosal tolerance and suppression of collagen-induced arthritis induced by nasal inhalation of synthetic peptide 184–198 of bovine type II collagen expressing a dominant T cell epitope. Clin Exp Immunol 1996; 103:368–375.

61. Myers LK, et al. Suppression of murine collagen-induced arthritis by nasal administration of collagen. Immunology 1997; 90:161–164.

62. Chu CQ, Londei M. Differential activities of immunogenic collagen type II peptides in the induction of nasal tolerance to collagen-induced arthritis. J Autoimmun 1999; 12:35–42.

63. Prakken BJ, et al. Peptide induced nasal tolerance for a mycobacterial hsp60 T cell epitope in rats suppresses both adjuvant arthritis and non-microbially induced experimental arthritis. Proc Natl Acad Sci USA 1997; 94:3284–3289.

64. Tian J, et al. Nasal administration of glutamate decarboxylase (GAD 65) peptides induces Th2 responses and prevents murine insulin-dependent diabetes. J Exp Med 1996; 183:1561–1567.

65. Daniel D, Wegmann DR. Protection of nonobese diabetic mice from diabetes by intranasal or subcutaneous administration of insulin peptide B-(9–23). Proc Natl Acad Sci USA 1996; 93:956–960.

66. Elias D, et al. Hsp60 peptide therapy of NOD mouse diabetes induces a Th2 cytokine burst and downregulates autoimmunity to various beta-cell antigens. Diabetes 1997; 46: 758–764.

67. Raz I, et al. Beta-cell function in new-onset type 1 diabetes and immunomodulation with a heat-shock protein peptide (DiaPep277): a randomised, double-blind, phase II trial. Lancet 2001; 358:1749–1753.

68. Thurau SR, et al. Induction of oral tolerance to S-antigen induced experimental autoimmune uveitis by a uveitogenic 20mer peptide. J Autoimmun 1991; 4:507–516.

69. Karachunski PI, et al. Prevention of experimental myasthenia gravis by nasal administration of synthetic acetylcholine receptor T epitope sequences. J Clin Invest 1997; 100:3027–3035.

70. Zou LP, et al. Antigen-specific immunosuppression: nasal tolerance to P0 protein peptides for the prevention and treatment of experimental autoimmune neuritis in Lewis rats. J Neuroimmunol 1999; 94:109–121.

71. Hoyne GF, et al. Inhibition of T cell and antibody responses to house dust mite allergen by inhalation of the dominant T cell epitope in naive and sensitized mice. J Exp Med 1993; 178:1783–1788.

72. Jarnicki AG, et al. Inhibition of mucosal and systemic Th2-type immune responses by intranasal peptides containing a dominant T cells epitope of the allergen Der p1. Int Immunol 2001; 13:1223–1231.

73. Metzler B, Wraith DC. Inhibition of experimental autoimmune encephalomyelitis by inhalation but not oral administration of the encephalitogenic peptide: influence of MHC binding affinity. Int Immunol 1993; 5:1159–1165.

74. Fairchild PJ, et al. An autoantigenic T cell epitope forms unstable complexes with class II MHC: a novel route for escape from tolerance induction. Int Immunol 1993; 5:1151–1158.

75. Jung S, et al. Oral tolerance in experimental autoimmune neuritis (EAN) of the Lewis rat. II. Adjuvant effects and bystander suppression in P2 peptide-induced EAN. J Neuroimmunol 2001; 116:21–28.

76. Metzler B, Wraith DC. Inhibition of T cell responsiveness by nasal peptide administration: Influence of the thymus and differential recovery of T cell-dependent functions. Immunology 1999; 97:257–263.

77. Critchfield JM, et al. T cell deletion in high antigen dose therapy of autoimmune encephalomyelitis. Science 1994; 263: 1139–1143.

78. Kearney ER, et al. Visualization of peptide-specific T cell immunity and peripheral tolerance induction in vivo. Immunity 1994; 1:327–339.

79. Lanoue A, et al. Conditions that induce tolerance in mature CD4+ T cells. J Exp Med 1997; 185:405–414.

80. Chen Y, et al. Peripheral deletion of antigen-reactive T cells in oral tolerance. Nature 1995; 376:177–180.

81. Astori M, et al. Inducing tolerance by intranasal administration of long peptides in naive and primed CBA/J mice. J Immunol 2000; 165:3497–3505.

82. Mathisen PM, et al. Treatment of experimental autoimmune encephalomyelitis with genetically modified memory T cells. J Exp Med 1997; 186:159–164.

82a. Massey EJ, et al. Intranasal peptide-induced peripheral tolerance: the role of IL-10 in regulatory T cell function within the context of experimental autoimmune encephalomyelitis. Vet Immunol Immunopathol 2002; 87:357–372.

83. Miller A, et al. Antigen-driven bystander suppression after oral administration of antigens. J Exp Med 1991; 174:791–798.

84. Moore KW, et al. Interleukin-10 and the interleukin-10 receptor. Annu Rev Immunol 2001; 19:683–765.

85. Geissmann F, et al. TGF-beta 1 prevents the noncognate maturation of human dendritic Langerhans cells. J Immunol 1999; 162:4567–4575.

86. Strobl H, Knapp W. TGF-beta 1 regulation of dendritic cells. Microbes Infect 1999; 1:1283–1290.

87. Santambrogio L, et al. Abundant empty class II MHC molecules on the surface of immature dendritic cells. Proc Natl Acad Sci U S A 1999; 96:15050–15055.

88. Roncarolo M-G, et al. Differentiation of T regulatory cells by immature dendritic cells. J Exp Med 2001; 193:5–9.

89. Jonuliet H, et al. Induction of interleukin 10-producing, nonproliferating CD4+ T cells with regulatory properties by repetitive stimulation with allogeneic immature human dendritic cells. J Exp Med 2000; 192:1213–1222.

90. Fukaura H, et al. Induction of circulating myelin basic protein and proteolipid protein-specific transforming growth factor-beta1-secreting Th3 T cells by oral administration of myelin in multiple sclerosis patients. J Clin Invest 1996; 98:70–77.

91. Akdis CA, et al. Role of interleukin 10 in specific immunotherapy. J Clin Invest 1998; 102:98–106.

92. Akdis CA, Blaser K. Mechanisms of interleukin-10-mediated immune suppression. Immunology 2001; 103:131–136.

93. Larche M. Inhibition of human T-cell responses by allergen peptides. Immunology 2001; 104:377–382.

87

Vaccines to Treat Drug Addiction

Paul R. Pentel and Dan E. Keyler
University of Minnesota Medical School, Minneapolis, Minnesota, U.S.A.

I. RATIONALE

Drugs of abuse produce their addictive effects by acting on neural pathways in the brain. Currently available medications for drug addiction act by targeting these pathways and altering their response to the addictive drug (Table 1). The challenge posed by this treatment strategy is that the neural pathways that are important in drug abuse are also important in mediating a myriad of other normal functions ranging from cognition to emotion. In altering these pathways to treat drug abuse, medications alter normal functions as well as lead to side effects and limitations on the dose of medication that can be administered.

Vaccines offer an alternative strategy for the treatment of drug abuse in which *the drug itself is the target rather than the brain*. Vaccines directed against these drugs elicit the production of drug-specific antibodies, which bind and sequester drug, and reduce its distribution to the brain. By virtue of acting outside the brain, vaccines appear to circumvent the central nervous system side effects that limit the usefulness of other therapies. The specificity of vaccination in binding only the drug of interest and the generally excellent safety profile of vaccination suggest that side effects outside of the central nervous system should also be minimal. Practical features of vaccination, such as an anticipated long-lasting effect and avoidance of the need for daily medication, could also prove helpful.

The concept of vaccination to treat drug abuse is not new. A vaccine against heroin was studied more than 25 years ago in monkeys [1,2], but further investigation was not pursued because of the development of other promising therapies for heroin addiction at the time. Interest in this area was rekindled in the 1990s with reports that cocaine vaccines could block a variety of cocaine effects in rats [3–6]. Vaccines are currently being investigated for the treatment of cocaine, nicotine, phencyclidine (PCP), and methamphetamine abuse. Only a cocaine vaccine has so far reached Phase I clinical trials, and efficacy studies have not yet been reported. This chapter will consider the mechanistic basis for using vaccines to treat drug addiction and their applica-

tion to specific drugs. Issues regarding the potential clinical use of these vaccines are also discussed.

II. MECHANISM OF ACTION

The vaccines discussed below act by producing antibodies that bind drugs and alter their tissue distribution or elimination. Both *active* immunization of the animals being studied (herein referred to as vaccination) and *passive* immunization (administration of exogenously produced antibodies) have been studied and will be discussed. An alternative approach involving the generation of catalytic antibodies that act by enhancing drug metabolism has also been applied to cocaine, and will be considered separately.

A. Relationship Between Addiction and Drug Concentration in Brain

A hallmark of drug abuse is the high rate with which the drug is self-administered. All addictive drugs serve as positive reinforcers (e.g., are rewarding) in that their effects on the brain increase the frequency of drug seeking and drug self-administration. The extent to which an addictive drug is reinforcing or rewarding is critically dependent on the dose reaching the brain [7]. Below a threshold dose, drug self-administration is not observed. Above that dose, drug self-administration in both animals and humans increases up to a point at which either satiation or adverse effect occurs [8]. An intervention that decreases the amount of drugs reaching the brain might, therefore, reduce or abolish its rewarding properties and lead to a reduction or cessation of self-administration. This is the primary goal of vaccination as a strategy for treating drug addiction.

B. Vaccination Effects on Drug Distribution to Brain

When an addictive drug is administered, it enters blood and distributes to tissues throughout the body, including the

Table 1 Some Medications Currently Available or Under Investigation for the Treatment of Drug Addiction

Medication	Addiction
Receptor agonists	
Nicotine	Tobacco
Methadone, L-α-acetyl methadol (LAAM)	Opiates
Receptor antagonists	
Naltrexone	Opiates
Mecamylamine	Tobacco
Neurotransmitter effect modifiers	
Bupropion, nortriptyline	Tobacco
Desipramine	Cocaine

brain (Figure 1). In a vaccinated animal, drug-specific antibody is present in the blood and extracellular fluid. Antibody is largely excluded from the brain by the blood–brain barrier, owing to its large size. Drug-specific antibody presents a potential reservoir for binding drugs outside the central nervous system and before it enters the brain. When a vaccinated animal receives the drug in question, it is bound to antibody and sequestered in the blood and extracellular fluid. If a sufficient binding capacity is available, the concentration of the unbound drug is reduced. Because only unbound drugs can enter the brain, the concentration of the drug in the brain is correspondingly reduced. The binding of

drug by the antibody can also alter its rate of entry and exit from tissues.

Altered drug distribution is illustrated in Figure 2, in which vaccinated rats received a single nicotine dose equivalent on a weight basis to the nicotine absorbed from two cigarettes by a smoker [9]. The blood nicotine concentration was increased in vaccinated animals, reflecting the binding and sequestration of nicotine in the blood. Brain nicotine concentration was decreased by two-thirds compared to nonvaccinated controls. Brain nicotine concentration was lowest in those animals with the highest nicotine-specific serum antibody titers (Figure 3), suggesting that the ratio of the antibody-binding capacity to the drug dose is an important determinant of efficacy [10]. The increased concentration of nicotine in the blood in vaccinated rats does not result in increased peripheral effects of nicotine because the antibody-bound drug is pharmacologically inactive [9].

C. Stoichiometry of Drug Binding: How Much Antibody Is Needed to Effectively Bind the Drug?

In the study illustrated in Figure 2, the estimated total body nicotine-specific antibody content of vaccinated rats (2.7×10^{-7} mol of binding sites) was approximately equal to the moles of nicotine administered. Smokers take in considerably greater nicotine doses throughout the day [11], raising the question of whether the antibodies will become saturated and therefore ineffective in a regular smoker. Surprisingly, the ability of vaccination to reduce drug distribution to the brain persists even when single nicotine doses

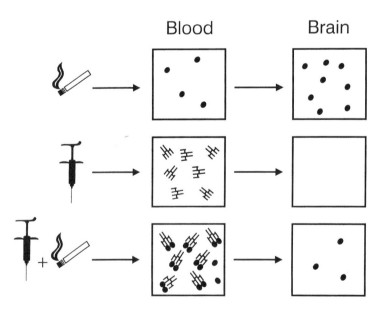

Figure 1 Effects of vaccination on drug distribution, illustrated for nicotine. Top panel: When a smoker or experimental animal is exposed to nicotine, the drug distributes first to the blood and subsequently to tissues, including the brain. Middle panel: Vaccination elicits nicotine-specific antibodies, which are located largely in the blood and extracellular fluid and which are largely excluded from the brain by the blood–brain barrier, owing to their size. Bottom panel: In a vaccinated animal, nicotine binds to nicotine-specific antibodies in the blood (and extracellular fluid), the unbound nicotine concentration is reduced, and drug distribution to the brain is reduced.

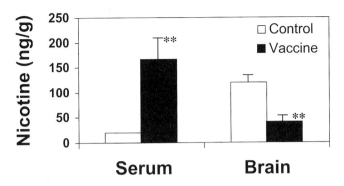

Figure 2 Vaccination reduces nicotine distribution to the brain. Rats were vaccinated with nicotine immunogen or control immunogen over a period of 7 weeks. One week after the vaccination schedule was completed, 0.03 mg/kg nicotine was administered intravenously. This dose is equivalent on a weight basis to the nicotine absorbed by a smoker from two cigarettes. Serum and brain were sampled 3 min after the injection. The serum nicotine concentration was markedly increased in vaccinated rats due to the binding of nicotine to antibody in the serum. Brain nicotine concentration was reduced by 60%. (From Ref. 9.)

Table 2 Typical Drug Doses Generally Exceed the Anticipated Binding Capacity of Drug-Specific Antibody in a Vaccinated Human

Drug dose	Ratio of drug to estimated binding capacity
Nicotine	
Single dose, 0.015 mg/kg (9.3×10^{-8} mol/kg)	0.3
Daily dose, 0.3 mg/kg (1.9×10^{-6} mol/kg)	7
Phencyclidine	
Single dose, 0.14 mg/kg (5.6×10^{-7} mol/kg)	2.1
Daily dose, 0.7 mg/kg (2.8×10^{-6} mol/kg)	10
Cocaine	
Single dose, 0.5 mg/kg (1.6×10^{-6} mol/kg)	6
Daily dose, 5 mg/kg (1.6×10^{-5} mol/kg)	59
Methamphetamine	
Single dose, 0.1 mg/kg (5×10^{-7} mol/kg)	1.9
Daily dose, 10 mg/kg (5×10^{-5} mol/kg)	190

The calculated binding capacity of 2.7×10^{-7} mol/kg is extrapolated from animal studies and assumes that 1% of total antibody (IgG) is specific for the drug in question and that there are two drug-binding sites per molecule of IgG.
Source: Ref. 9.

exceed the estimated binding capacity of antibody by up to 67-fold [12], or in the presence of a continuous infusion of nicotine at rates equivalent to two to three packs of cigarettes daily [13]. A similar unexpected efficacy in the face of very large drug doses has also been observed for cocaine [14] and phencyclidine [15] antibodies, and appears to be a general feature of vaccination for drugs of abuse. The basis for this unanticipated pharmacokinetic efficacy is not well understood, but is clearly critical for the successful clinical use of vaccination because both the single and daily doses of most addictive drugs equal or exceed the calculated binding ca-

pacity that can be provided by vaccination (Table 2). Possibly, vaccination reduces nicotine distribution to the brain to a greater extent than to other organs, as has been shown for phencyclidine [15].

D. Other Potentially Beneficial Pharmacokinetic Effects of Vaccination

The *rate* of distribution of drugs to the brain is also an important determinant of its reinforcing potency. For example, inhaled nicotine that reaches the brain in 10–20 sec is far more addictive than nicotine gum, which produces peak levels in 15–30 min [16]. Slowing drug distribution to the brain could make it less reinforcing. Limited data suggest that vaccination may slow nicotine distribution to the brain. The distribution of nicotine to the brain in vaccinated rats is reduced by 64% 1 min after a single nicotine dose, but by only 24% at steady state after a chronic nicotine infusion (unpublished data). Thus vaccination may have its greatest effect on the early distribution of nicotine to the brain, during the time when the reinforcing effects of nicotine are greatest.

The effects of vaccination on drug metabolism differ among drugs. The binding of nicotine by an antibody makes it less available for metabolism and markedly slows its elimination half-life [17]. This could be a detrimental effect in that slower elimination would favor the accumulation of

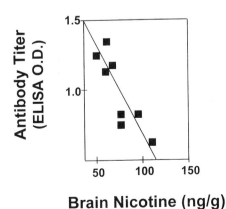

Figure 3 Effects of serum antibody titers on nicotine distribution to the brain (protocol as in Figure 2). Brain nicotine concentrations in vaccinated rats were lowest in animals with the highest serum antibody titers (a measure of antibody concentrations). (From Ref. 10.)

nicotine and the saturation of an antibody. On the other hand, slowing nicotine metabolism with a metabolical inhibitor has been shown to reduce ad libitum smoking in humans, perhaps by prolonging nicotine's effects and by delaying the onset of craving [18]. Understanding the role of altered nicotine metabolism due to vaccination will require further study. In contrast, cocaine's elimination half-life does not appear to be altered by vaccination [14].

III. VACCINE FORMULATION AND VACCINATION SCHEDULES

A. Overview

There are three principal requirements of vaccines used to treat drug addiction. First, the antibodies elicited by vaccination must have a high-enough affinity to effectively bind the drug. Second, because high ratios of antibody to drug are most effective, a vaccine must elicit and maintain high concentrations of antibody throughout the period of clinical interest. Third, antibodies must be highly specific for the drug of interest. If antibodies cross-react with drug metabolites, those metabolites could compete for binding capacity.

B. Linker

Drugs of abuse (molecular weights 150–300) are too small to elicit an immune response. Regular users of tobacco (nicotine) or cocaine do not normally have antibodies against these drugs [19] (A. Fattom, personal communication). Drugs of abuse can be rendered immunogenic by linking the drug itself or a structurally related compound (hapten) to an immunogenic carrier protein to form a complete immunogen. After initial (primary) vaccination, periodical booster doses with the complete immunogen are needed to maintain satisfactory antibody titers: exposure to the drug by itself would not be expected to elicit an anamnestic or booster response. The conjugation or linking of drug to carrier protein has generally been accomplished using five to six atom linkers of various composition [6,9,20]. The binding of linker to carrier protein lysine residues can be accomplished via succinylation. Although some linkers anecdotally seem to produce better immunogens than others, no structural rule has emerged to predict which linkers are most effective. Few published data comparing linkers, linker strategies, or haptenation ratios (drug/carrier protein molar ratio) are available. A haptenation ratio of 20:1 was used for conjugating phencyclidine to bovine serum albumin [21].

Linker position is critical to antibody specificity. Linkers that are distant from the predominant sites of drug metabolism (and which do not cover them up) allow the elicited antibodies to recognize parent compounds in preference to metabolites [6,9,20,21]. An alternative strategy has been used for cocaine, which can spontaneously hydrolyze in vitro to one of its major metabolites and potentially allow the metabolite to act as an immunogen. A linker attached at the site of potential hydrolysis was used to stabilize this site, while preserving its structure so that the resulting antibodies were specific for the parent compound [4,22].

C. Carrier Protein

A variety of carrier proteins have been used for these vaccines, including bovine albumin [6,21], keyhole limpet hemocyanin [10], cholera toxin B subunit [19], and recombinant Pseudomonas aeruginosa exoprotein A [9]. The latter two proteins have the advantage of previous use in vaccines administered to humans.

D. Vaccination Schedules

Vaccination schedules in rats have generally involved two to four doses of vaccine over a period of 4–10 weeks. Comparative data are not available to suggest an optimal vaccination schedule. The only human data available are for a cocaine vaccine, which was administered as three monthly injections of 13, 82, or 709 µg of a cholera toxin B subunit conjugate vaccine with alum adjuvant. Maximal antibody titers were reached 1 week after the third injection, titers decreased by about 50% two months later, and were nearly back to baseline 10 months after the final injection [19].

For some clinical applications, it may be desirable to vaccinate individuals before they stop their drug use, in preparation for quitting. Rat studies with nicotine [13], methamphetamine [23], and cocaine [24] vaccines have shown that vaccination during concurrent drug administration is as effective in eliciting drug-specific antibody titers as vaccination in the absence of the drug. Thus vaccination during ongoing drug use seems feasible.

E. Antibody Concentrations in Serum

In rats, a cocaine-specific antibody serum concentration of 0.05 mg/mL represents a threshold for efficacy as measured by the suppression of cocaine self-administration [24,25]. This concentration is higher than those achieved in the first clinical trial of a cocaine vaccine (mean 0.003 mg/mL) [19]. Thresholds for other drugs are not known, but serum drug-specific antibody concentrations of 0.1–0.2 mg/mL were effective in altering nicotine pharmacokinetics and effects in rats, and the magnitude of effect was related to antibody titer. Antibody titers in humans given vaccines for infectious diseases are generally lower than those achieved in experimental animals, perhaps in part because only the alum adjuvant and the intramuscular route have been used in humans (rather than Freund's adjuvant administered intraperitoneally or by other routes in animals). Nevertheless, hapten-specific antibody concentrations of up to 0.1 mg/mL in serum have been reported in humans [26,27]. Achieving adequate antibody concentration will be a key issue in determining the efficacy of vaccines for drugs of abuse, and may require additional studies of vaccination strategies.

IV. SPECIFIC DRUGS

A. Nicotine

1. Overview

Cigarette smoking kills 400,000 people each year in the United States (one of five deaths) and 10 times that many worldwide [28]. New medications and counseling have helped many smokers quit, but the majority of those who try are still unsuccessful [29]. Addiction to nicotine is the primary reason that people smoke [28]. An intervention that could reduce the reinforcing effects of nicotine and render it less addictive is therefore of interest [30].

As discussed above, nicotine distribution to the brain is substantially reduced by vaccination after clinically relevant single doses of nicotine alone or against a background of chronic nicotine dosing. The magnitude of effect is related to antibody titer or concentration in the blood [9,10,13]. In assessing the potential clinical usefulness of vaccination to treat nicotine addiction, key questions are: (a) Does vaccination reduce the reinforcing effects of nicotine? (b) Can beneficial effects be attained with antibody titers that are achievable in humans. (c) Will vaccinated animals or humans try to compensate for reduced nicotine distribution to the brain by simply taking in more nicotine, thereby overcoming the effects of vaccination? Additionally, it is possible that vaccination might affect various aspects of nicotine addiction differentially. Smokers who quit and then relapse to smoking typically do so by starting with a few puffs or a few cigarettes, a relatively small nicotine dose. Vaccination could block the reinforcing effects of those first few puffs and make them less enjoyable, thus making relapse less likely. By contrast, using vaccination to help initiate smoking cessation would involve the larger nicotine dose associated with regular daily smoking. Because the ratio of antibody to drug is important in determining vaccine efficacy, vaccination might be more effective for relapse prevention than for initiating smoking cessation.

2. Active Versus Passive Immunization

Studies of vaccine efficacy have used either active immunization (vaccination) of rats prior to nicotine challenge, or passive immunization (the transfer of antibodies produced in rabbits and then administered to rats prior to nicotine challenge). Vaccination of smokers is perhaps more attractive as a potential clinical intervention because it is less expensive and longer-lasting than passive immunization. Passive immunization has been used experimentally primarily as a methodological expedient, a means of controlling antibody dose or producing immediate effects without having to wait for the 1–2 months required for vaccination. However, the rapid onset of effect and the control of dose could also be useful in treating patients, and a clinical role for passive immunization alone or as an adjunct to vaccination is possible [30].

3. Vaccines

Two nicotine immunogens have been studied: 6-[carboxymethylureido]nicotine and 3′-[aminomethyl]nicotine [9,20]. Vaccination with either immunogen produces marked effects on nicotine distribution in rats, but the latter vaccine appears somewhat more effective. Both are linked to carrier protein (keyhole limpet hemocyanin or recombinant *Pseudomonas* exoprotein A, respectively) through a five-atom linker placed remote from the major sites of nicotine metabolism, and both show high specificity for nicotine (<3% cross-reactivity with the major nicotine metabolites cotinine and nicotine-N-oxide). Cross-reactivity with acetylcholine, the endogenous ligand for nicotinic receptors, was negligible. The K_d of elicited antibodies for nicotine has ranged from 20 to 40 nM [9,10,13,20]. Typical serum nicotine concentrations in smokers are higher than the K_d (50–500 nM), suggesting that the saturation of nicotine-specific antibodies in smokers should be high and most of the binding capacity will be utilized. Serum antibody concentrations in vaccinated rats range from 0.05 to 0.2 mg/mL, or from 0.5% to 2% of the total IgG.

4. Efficacy Studies

Passive immunization of rats with nicotine-specific IgG blocked the pressor effect (elevation of blood pressure) from nicotine in a dose-related manner [9]. Because this effect is largely mediated by peripheral autonomic ganglia, these data confirm that nicotine bound to antibody in serum is inactive.

Passive immunization of rats blocked locomotor activation following a single nicotine dose, a nicotine effect mediated in the brain [9]. Passive immunization also affects behaviors in rats that are pertinent to nicotine addiction. Rats can be made dependent on nicotine by a 1- week subcutaneous (s.c.) nicotine infusion, such that the removal of the s.c. pump results in a withdrawal or abstinence syndrome 1 day later [31]. When rats experience nicotine withdrawal, this can be relieved by again administering nicotine. However, if rats experiencing withdrawal are given nicotine-specific IgG, additional nicotine is no longer able to relieve the withdrawal [32] (Figure 4). This paradigm is analogous to a smoker relieving withdrawal symptoms and craving by smoking. Relief of withdrawal is an important reason why people fail to quit smoking: when they are uncomfortable from withdrawal, smoking a cigarette will relieve their discomfort. If it failed to do so, relapse might not occur. Thus vaccination could make relapse to smoking less likely after a quit attempt by virtue of rendering cigarettes less effective for relieving withdrawal. Vaccination also suppresses nicotine-induced dopamine release in the rat nucleus accumbens, providing evidence that an important neurochemical effect associated with nicotine dependence is altered by this intervention (T. Svennson, personal communication).

Rats can be taught to self-administer nicotine by pressing a lever to receive a nicotine dose through an indwelling intravenous (i.v.) cannula. Such a preparation serves as an animal model of smoking. If rats are first vaccinated over several months and then given access to nicotine, the acquisition of nicotine self-administration is impaired. Vaccinated rats, on average, self-administer 40% less nicotine [33]. Vaccination also impairs the reinstatement of nicotine responding, a model of relapse. In this model, rats are taught to self-administer nicotine and then responding is extinguished by substituting saline for nicotine. Responding can be reinitiated by providing a single dose of nicotine as a cue. This reinstatement of responding is blocked when rats are vaccinated during the period of extinction (T. Svennson, personal communication). Taken together with the effects of vaccination on nicotine withdrawal, these data support a

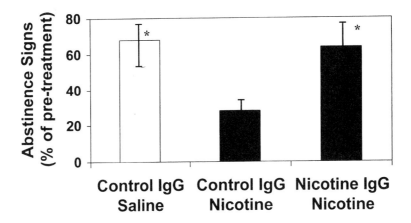

Figure 4 Passive immunization with Nic-IgG prevents the relief of nicotine withdrawal by nicotine. Rats were made dependent on nicotine with a 1-week infusion of nicotine via a s.c. pump. One day after the pump was removed, controls showed measurable withdrawal signs (left bar). Withdrawal was relieved by a single s.c. dose of nicotine (middle bar). The ability of nicotine to relieve withdrawal was blocked when nicotine-specific IgG was administered just prior to the single nicotine dose (right bar). (From Ref. 32.)

potential therapeutic or preventive role for vaccination. However, each of these behavioral models differs from human smoking behavior in important ways, including route of administration, doses, schedules, and behavioral environments. Further studies using additional models will be useful in assessing the clinical relevance of these findings.

B. Cocaine

1. Overview

Approximately 2 million people in the United States abused cocaine in 1998 [34]. Behavioral interventions are helpful in treating cocaine addiction, but there are currently no approved medications for this disorder [35].

Single and daily cocaine doses are considerably higher than those of nicotine. Even with a single dose, the calculated binding capacity of antibodies in vaccinated animals is greatly exceeded (Table 2). Nevertheless, the studies outlined below demonstrate a considerable efficacy of vaccination in reducing cocaine effects, illustrating the general principle that drug-specific antibodies can alter drug distribution even when the binding capacity is greatly exceeded.

2. Vaccines

Linkers for cocaine immunogens have been placed either distant from major sites of metabolism (norcocaine derivatives) [6], or at the methyl ester group to protect it from spontaneous degradation and the generation of the major metabolite benzoyl ecgonine [4,22]. Both strategies elicit antibodies with high specificity for cocaine compared to its metabolites. Serum antibody K_d for cocaine from a norcocaine derivative vaccine was reported as 4×10^7 to 2×10^9 M^{-1}. A vaccine has also been developed using an anti-idiotype antibody, which mimics the configuration of the cocaine molecule as the immunogen [36]. It is not clear whether this approach offers any advantage over the use of a conjugate vaccine. Vaccines studied in animals have used

bovine serum albumin or keyhole limpet hemocyanin as carrier proteins. A cocaine vaccine in clinical trials used cholera toxin B subunit as the carrier protein [19].

3. Efficacy

Passive immunization with cocaine-specific antibodies reduced early cocaine distribution to the brain in rats by 25–70%, and reduced locomotor activity and stereotypical behavior following a single cocaine dose [4,6]. Vaccination

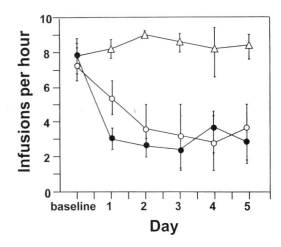

Figure 5 Passive immunization blocks cocaine self-administration in rats. Rats were trained to self-administer cocaine as 1 mg/kg i.v. bolus doses during a 2-hr daily session. Control group daily responding is stable over time (triangle). The substitution of saline for cocaine (open circle) resulted in a marked reduction in responding. The infusion of monoclonal anti-cocaine antibodies in rats that continued to receive cocaine (filled circle) resulted in a similar reduction in responding. (From Ref. 6.)

also reduced cocaine self-administration in a variety of models [6,25,37,38]. When animals had access to cocaine for 2 hr/day, cocaine self-administration was immediately reduced to control levels after passive immunization with cocaine-specific monoclonal antibodies (Figure 5). Vaccination also reduced the reacquisition [25] and reinstatement [38] of cocaine self-administration in rats, which had been previously taught to self-administer the drug, a model of relapse prevention. Self-administration in vaccinated animals is closely related to serum antibody concentrations. In rats, a serum antibody concentration of 0.05 mg/mL appears to represent a threshold for efficacy [25]. Surprisingly, increasing the cocaine dose did not reliably overcome the suppression of self-administration. In aggregate, these data provide strong evidence that vaccination reduces cocaine self-administration to a quantitatively important extent and in a manner related to serum antibody concentration.

In contrast to vaccination against nicotine, vaccination does not appear to alter cocaine's elimination half-life [6]. The accumulation of the drug with resulting saturation of antibodies may therefore be less of a problem with cocaine than with nicotine. It is possible that continued rapid cocaine elimination contributes to the high efficacy of vaccination in suppressing ongoing cocaine self-administration. A cocaine vaccine has begun Phase I clinical trials of immunogenicity and safety (see "Vaccine Formulation and Vaccination Schedules" above). No important adverse effects have been found.

C. Phencyclidine

1. Overview

Phencyclidine is structurally and pharmacologically related to the dissociative anesthetic, ketamine. Abuse is uncommon but important in particular geographical areas. Adverse effects generally consist of acute toxicity from inadvertent overdose and may be severe, but addiction may also occur. Apart from its medical importance, the study of phencyclidine abuse has shed light on the potential role of passive immunization as a treatment strategy.

2. Vaccines

A phencyclidine vaccine consisting of PCP conjugated to bovine serum albumin [21] has been used for the production of monoclonal antibodies. In contrast to vaccines for nicotine or cocaine, which aim to produce highly specific antibodies, the intent of this PCP vaccine was to elicit polyspecific antibodies that would also bind structurally related drugs that might be abused in place of phencyclidine. This was accomplished by placing the linker distant from the structural features that are conserved among the phencyclidine analogues of interest [39,40]. The monoclonal antibody most extensively studied has a K_d of 1.3 nM for phencyclidine.

3. Efficacy

The passive infusion of monoclonal phencyclidine antibodies or antibody Fab fragment (the 50-kDa antigen-binding fragment of IgG) to rats after acute or chronic phencyclidine

doses markedly reduces the phencyclidine concentration in the brain [15,41]. The protection of the brain is remarkably long-lasting, persisting for a month after a single IgG dose despite continuous infusion of phencyclidine at a daily rate that exceeds the antibody's binding capacity for drug (Figure 6). The protection of another organ (the testes) from phencyclidine distribution was not as persistent, suggesting that the distribution of phencyclidine to the brain is differentially affected. These observations are consistent with those regarding nicotine and cocaine, suggesting that drug distribution to the brain may be affected more than the distribution to other organs, and that protection occurs even when drug dose is substantially larger than the antibody's drug-binding capacity.

Monoclonal phencyclidine antibody also reduces the behavioral toxicity (changes in locomotor activity and posturing) of phencyclidine [39,42]. Like the pharmacokinetic effects, behavioral protection is long-lasting and is observed up to several weeks after a single passive infusion of antibody (M. Owens, personal communication). Phencyclidine antibodies also reverse overt phencyclidine toxicity when they are administered after a toxic phencyclidine dose [39,43]. The

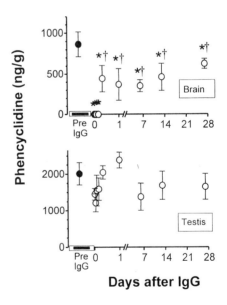

Figure 6 Phencyclidine-specific IgG produces a long-lasting decrease in brain phencyclidine concentrations. Phencyclidine was administered by continuous s.c. infusion. Monoclonal antiphencyclidine antibody was administered just once on day 2, after the initial distribution of PCP to tissues. The antibody dose was equimolar to the estimated body burden of PCP at the time. The subsequent PCP infused each day exceeded the antibody-binding capacity for the drug by more than threefold. Brain phencyclidine concentrations remained significantly reduced in the passively immunized rats for up to 1 month. Effects on phencyclidine distribution to the testes were smaller and less persistent. These data support the hypothesis that immunization preferentially reduces drug distribution to the brain. (From Ref. 15.)

considerable monoclonal antibody doses used (up to 0.4g/kg) have shown no adverse effects.

These data support a potential clinical role for passive immunization in the treatment of drug addiction. The ability to control the antibody dose and administer as large a dose as necessary may offer advantages over vaccination, particularly if the titers produced by vaccination are inadequate in some individuals. The ability to produce an immediate effect might also be helpful for initiating therapy when a patient is motivated to quit rather than having to wait months for adequate titers to develop after vaccination. The cost of producing large quantities of antibody is a factor, but improved large-scale methods for the production of monoclonal or recombinant antibodies have made this increasingly feasible.

D. Catalytic Antibodies for Cocaine

In contrast to drug-binding antibodies, catalytic antibodies are intended to hasten drug metabolism and thereby blunt the drug's effects. Enhanced metabolism could, if rapid enough, reduce initial drug distribution to the brain and could also prevent the accumulation of drug with repeated dosing. This approach is best suited to drugs that can be inactivated by one-step metabolical processes to an inactive metabolite, such as the hydrolysis of cocaine [44]. It is less well suited to drugs such as nicotine or phencyclidine, which are metabolized through multistep process by cytochrome *P*450 enzymes.

Cocaine is metabolized in humans primarily to two major metabolites that are not addictive. One of these, ecgonine methyl ester, also appears to be relatively free of toxic effects. Cocaine hydrolysis to ecgonine methyl ester is catalyzed by the plasma enzyme, pseudocholinesterase, and proceeds via a short-lived transition state, which is stabilized by the enzyme. An antibody to this transition state could similarly stabilize the transition state and serve as a catalyst [44]. Because the transition state is short-lived, it cannot be used as an immunogen, but a stable transition state analog used in this manner can elicit antibodies that markedly speed the degradation of cocaine [45–47]. One such monoclonal antibody has been shown to reduce acute cocaine toxicity and cocaine self-administration in rats [37,47]. The relative merits of this approach compared to cocaine-binding antibodies are not yet clear. Conceivably, a combination of binding antibodies to reduce initial cocaine distribution to the brain and catalytic antibodies to prevent cocaine accumulation would be advantageous.

V. CLINICAL ISSUES

A. Importance of Antibody Concentration in Serum

Vaccination is effective only insofar as sufficient antibody is present to bind drugs. For all of the drugs discussed above, antibody dose or concentration is a critical determinant of efficacy. Antibody concentrations elicited in experimental animal studies of drug abuse vaccines (0.05–2% of total IgG) have been higher than those typically elicited in humans after vaccines for infectious diseases (≤1% of total IgG, and often much less) [26,27]. Developing suitable immunogens, adjuvants, and vaccination schedules will therefore be important to the success of this approach. Passive immunization, where antibody dose can be controlled, may prove helpful as an adjunct to vaccination.

B. Onset and Duration of Effect

Vaccination will likely require multiple injections of immunogen over several months to achieve maximal titers. Vaccination can be initiated while drug use continues, with the cessation of drug use attempted once titers are adequate. Passive immunization may find application when a delay of several months is not clinically acceptable.

C. Compensation

It is likely that addicts will be able to overcome the effects of vaccination, if they are determined to do so, by using higher drug doses. Thus vaccination, like all other medications for drug abuse, will be most successful in highly motivated patients. Fortunately, most cigarette smokers want to quit and are unlikely to purposely sabotage their own efforts. Cocaine addicts who enter treatment are also motivated to quit, as illustrated by the substantial abstinence rates achieved with behavioral counseling alone.

D. Vaccination as an Adjunct to Behavioral Treatment

As a general rule, drug therapies for addictions are successful only when used in conjunction with behavioral counseling and any necessary psychiatrical or social services. It is likely that vaccination, even if effective, will be similar in this regard and should be viewed as an adjunct to counseling.

E. Combination of Vaccination with Other Therapies

Because its mechanism of action is distinct, it is possible that vaccination will have additive effects with other medications for drug abuse. It is also possible that vaccination will target some aspects of addiction better than others and will benefit from medications that complement its actions.

F. Safety

No important adverse effects have been observed in animals to date with either passive or active immunization for drug addiction. However, such vaccines have not previously been used or tested in humans. It will be important, in particular, to confirm the specificity of the antibodies elicited to assure that they do not bind endogenous compounds.

VI. SUMMARY

Vaccines to treat drug abuse are being studied for several major classes of addictive drugs. Animal data are encouraging, but none of these vaccines has yet been tested for efficacy in humans. The main action of vaccines is to elicit antibodies that bind drugs and reduce their distribution to the target organ, the brain. Vaccination reduces or blocks some of the behavioral effects of nicotine, cocaine, or phencyclidine even when drug doses substantially exceed the antibody's drug-binding capacity. Efficacy is closely correlated with antibody titer or concentration in serum, and achieving and maintaining adequate titers will be a major factor determining whether these vaccines are clinically useful. It is likely that addicts can overcome the effects of vaccination by using larger drug doses, so that vaccination will be most effective for individuals who are highly motivated to quit, and when used in conjunction with counseling. Vaccines have proven safe in animals, but their safety in humans is largely untested. The use of vaccination in combination with other medications for drug addiction, to enhance efficacy or achieve a greater spectrum of effects, may be possible.

REFERENCES

1. Bonese KF, et al. Changes in heroin self-administration by a rhesus monkey after morphine immunization. Nature 1974; 252:708–710.
2. Killian A, et al. Effects of passive immunization against morphine on heroin self-administration. Pharmacol Biochem Behav 1978; 9:347–352.
3. Bagasra O, et al. A potential vaccine for cocaine abuse prophylaxis. Immunopharmacology 1992; 23:173–179.
4. Carrera MR, et al. Suppression of psychoactive effects of cocaine by active immunization. Nature 1995; 378:727–730.
5. Ettinger RH, et al. Active immunization with cocaine–protein conjugate attenuates cocaine effects. Pharmacol Biochem Behav 1997; 58(1):215–220.
6. Fox BS, et al. Efficacy of a therapeutic cocaine vaccine in rodent models. Nat Med 1996; 2:1129–1132.
7. Carroll ME, Mattox AJ. Drug reinforcement in animals. In: Johnson BA, Roache JD, eds. Drug Addiction and Its Treatment: Nexus of Neuroscience and Behavior. Philadelphia: Lippincott-Raven, 1997:3–37.
8. Lynch WJ, Carroll ME. Regulation of drug intake. Exp Clin Psychopharmacol 2001; 9:131–143.
9. Pentel PR, et al. A nicotine conjugate vaccine reduces nicotine distribution to brain and attenuates its behavioral and cardiovascular effects in rats. Pharmacol Biochem Behav 2000; 65:191–198.
10. Hieda Y, et al. Immunization of rats reduces nicotine distribution to brain. Psychopharmacology 1999; 143:150–157.
11. Benowitz NL, Jacob P. Daily intake of nicotine during cigarette smoking. Clin Pharmacol Ther 1984; 35:499–504.
12. Tuncok Y, et al. Inhibition of nicotine-induced seizures in rats by combining vaccination against nicotine with chronic nicotine infusion. Exp Clin Psychopharmacol 2001; 9:228–234.
13. Hieda Y, et al. Vaccination against nicotine during continued nicotine administration in rats: immunogenicity of the vaccine and effects on nicotine distribution to brain. Int J Immunopharmacol 2000; 22:809–819.
14. Fox BS. Development of a therapeutic vaccine for the treatment of cocaine addiction. Drug Alcohol Depend 1997; 48: 153–158.
15. Proksch JW, et al. Anti-phencyclidine monoclonal antibodies provide long-term reductions in brain phencyclidine concentrations during chronic phencyclidine administration in rats. J Pharmacol Exp Ther 2000; 292:831–837.
16. Hatsukami DK, et al. Signs and symptoms from nicotine gum abstinence. Psychopharmacology 1991; 104:496–504.
17. Keyler DE, et al. Altered disposition of repeated nicotine doses in rats immunized against nicotine. Nicotine Tob Res 1999; 1:241–249.
18. Pianezza ML, et al. Nicotine metabolism defect reduces smoking [letter]. Nature 1998; 393:750.
19. Kosten TR, et al. Human therapeutic cocaine vaccine: safety and immunogenicity. Vaccine 2002; 20:1196–1204.
20. Hieda Y, et al. Active immunization alters the plasma nicotine concentration in rats. J Pharmacol Exp Ther 1997; 283: 1076–1081.
21. Owens SM, Mayersohn M. Phencyclidine-specific Fab fragments alter phencyclidine disposition in dogs. Drug Metab Dispos 1986; 14:52–58.
22. Carrera MR, et al. A second-generation vaccine protects against the psychoactive effects of cocaine. Proc Natl Acad Sci USA 2001; 98:1988–1992.
23. Byrnes-Blake KA, et al. Generation of anti-(+)methamphetamine antibodies is not impeded by (+)methamphetamine administration during active immunization of rats. Int Immunopharmacol 2001; 1:329–338.
24. Kantak KM, et al. Time course of changes in cocaine self-administration behavior in rats during immunization with the cocaine vaccine IPC-1010. Psychopharmacology (Berlin) 2001; 153:334–340.
25. Kantak KM, et al. Evaluation of anti-cocaine antibodies and a cocaine vaccine in a rat self-administration model. Psychopharmacology (Berlin) 2000; 148:251–562.
26. Janoff EN, et al. Humoral recall responses in HIV infection: levels, specificity, and affinity of antigen-specific IgG. J Immunol 1991; 147:2130–2135.
27. Weiss PJ, et al. Response of recent human immunodeficiency virus seroconverters to the pneumococcal polysaccharide vaccine and Haemophilus influenzae type b conjugate vaccine. J Infect Dis 1995; 171:1217–1222.
28. US Department of Health and Human Services. Nicotine Addiction: Health Consequences of Smoking. Washington, DC: DHHS, 1999.
29. Fiore M, et al. Treating Tobacco Use and Dependence. Clinical Practice Guideline: US Department of Health and Human Services. Public Health Service, 2000.
30. Vocci FJ, Chiang CN. Vaccines against nicotine: how effective are they likely to be in preventing smoking? CNS Drugs 2001; 15:505–514.
31. Malin DH, et al. A rodent model of nicotine abstinence syndrome. Pharmacol Biochem Behav 1992; 43:779–784.
32. Malin DH, et al. Passive immunization against nicotine prevents nicotine alleviation of nicotine abstinence syndrome. Pharmacol Biochem Behav 2001; 68:87–92.
33. LeSage MG, et al. Effects of a nicotine conjugate vaccine on the acquisition of nicotine self-administration in rats. Poster presented at the Seventh Annual Meeting of the Society for Research on Nicotine and Tobacco, Seattle, WA, 2001.
34. Anonymous. Summary of Finding from the 1998 National Household Survey on Drug Abuse. Washington, DC: Department of Health and Human Services, 1999.
35. Gottschalk PC, et al. Current concepts in pharmacotherapy of substance abuse. Curr Psychiatry Rep 1999; 1:172–178.
36. Schabacker DS, et al. Exploring the feasibility of an anti-idiotypic cocaine vaccine: analysis of the specificity of anticocaine antibodies (Ab1) capable of inducing Ab2beta anti-idiotypic antibodies. Immunology 2000; 100:48–56.
37. Baird TJ, et al. Natural and artificial enzymes against cocaine: I. Monoclonal antibody 15A10 and the reinforcing effects of cocaine in rats. J Pharmacol Exp Ther 2000; 295: 1127–1134.
38. Carrera MR, et al. Cocaine vaccines: antibody protection against relapse in a rat model. Proc Natl Acad Sci USA 2000; 97:6202–6206.
39. Hardin JS, et al. Pharmacodynamics of a monoclonal anti-

phencyclidine Fab with broad selectivity for phencyclidine-like drugs. J Pharmacol Exp Ther 1998; 285:1113–1122.

40. Owens SM, et al. Antibodies against arylcyclohexylamines and their similarities in binding specificity with the phencyclidine receptor. J Pharmacol Exp Ther 1988; 246:472–478.

41. Valentine JL, Owens SM. Anti-phencyclidine monoclonal antibodies significantly changes phencyclidine concentrations in brain and other tissues in rats. J Pharmacol Exp Ther 1996; 278:717–724.

42. Valentine JL, et al. Anti-phencyclidine monoclonal Fab fragments reverse PCP-induced behavioral effects and ataxia in rats. J Pharmacol Exp Ther 1996; 278:709–716.

43. Valentine JD, et al. Self-administration in rats allowed un-

limited access to nicotine. Psychopharmacology 1997; 133: 300–304.

44. De Prada P, et al. Application of artificial enzymes to the problem of cocaine. Ann NY Acad Sci 2000; 909:159–169.

45. Cashman JR, et al. Catalytic antibodies that hydrolyze (–)-cocaine obtained by a high-throughput procedure. J Pharmacol Exp Ther 2000; 293:952–961.

46. Matsushita M, et al. Cocaine catalytic antibodies: the primary importance of linker effects. Bioorg Med Chem Lett 2001; 11:87–90.

47. Mets B, et al. A catalytic antibody against cocaine prevents cocaine's reinforcing and toxic effects in rats. Proc Natl Acad Sci USA 1998; 95:10176–10181.

88

Vaccines Against Agents of Bioterrorism

Theodore J. Cieslak
San Antonio Military Pediatric Center, San Antonio, Texas, U.S.A.

Mark G. Kortepeter and Edward M. Eitzen, Jr.
United States Army Medical Research Institute of Infectious Diseases, Fort Detrick, Maryland, U.S.A.

Recent events have called enormous attention to the twin threats of biological warfare and bioterrorism. The tragedy of September 11, 2001 and the subsequent outbreak of anthrax cases associated with contaminated mail have made anthrax and smallpox household words. Nonetheless, public health, policy, and law enforcement officials have been planning a defense against potential agents of terrorism for some time now. A component of that defense has included, and is likely to continue to include, immunization. In this chapter, we discuss currently available vaccines against potential agents of biowarfare and bioterrorism. In addition, we discuss prospects for new generation vaccines against these same agents.

In 1999, a group of experts gathered at the Centers for Disease Control and Prevention (CDC) in Atlanta to develop a list of those agents most likely to constitute viable terrorist weapons. These experts soon concluded that, because terrorist's motives were often unclear, it was difficult to ascertain which agents were most likely to be employed. Rather, the group elected to consider which agents, *if employed*, constituted the gravest threats to public health and safety. Moreover, they also took into account current public health preparedness, prioritizing those agents for which a more substantial gap in preparedness was felt to exist. In the end, they divided potential agents of bioterrorism into three categories, with those in category A thought to represent the greatest threats [1]. The list developed at the CDC is provided in Table 1. We discuss here various immunization strategies against anthrax, smallpox, and three of the four remaining agents in category A. The final agent in Category A (actually multiple agents causing viral hemorrhagic fevers, considered collectively) is considered in a separate chapter ("Vaccines for Hantaviruses, Lassa Fever, and Filoviruses"). We also discuss select agents in

category B for which vaccine research appears somewhat promising.

I. CATEGORY A AGENTS

A. Anthrax

Anthrax is caused by infection with the gram-positive spore-forming rod, *Bacillus anthracis*. Although naturally occurring anthrax has become a rarity in the western world, due to changes in animal husbandry practices and, in part, to veterinary vaccination, anthrax has reemerged as the ultimate biological weapon. The ability of the dry spore form of this organism to resist environmental degradation and its behavior as a gas when disseminated in the proper particle size, combined with its rapid lethality, make it an attractive weapon in the eyes of some.

Pasteur first developed an anthrax vaccine (a "duplex vaccine," consisting of two doses prepared by significantly different methods) in 1881. His preparation, the first bacterial vaccine (Jenner's smallpox vaccine predated it by 75 years), was intended for use in cattle and sheep, and arrived just 5 years after anthrax became the first disease for which a microbial etiology was proven by Koch's postulates. Significant modifications to Pasteur's original preparation led to Sterne's live spore vaccine in 1937, and derivatives of this attenuated spore vaccine are used extensively in livestock to this day. A thorough review of the history of early anthrax vaccines has been published [2].

Significant vaccine-associated morbidity makes the use of live spore anthrax vaccines problematic in humans. Nonetheless, a live spore vaccine derived from a Sterne strain of *B. anthracis* has been widely used in humans in Russia and the former Soviet Union [3]. In the 1950s and

Table 1 Critical Agents for Health Preparedness

Category A	Category B	Category C
Variola virus	*Coxiella burnetii*	Other biological agents that
Bacillus anthracis	*Brucellae*	may emerge as future threats
Yersinia pestis	*Burkholderia mallei*	to public health, such as:
Botulinum toxin	Alphaviruses	Nipah virus
Francisella tularensis	Certain toxins (Ricin, SEB)	Hantaviruses
Filoviruses and	Food safety threat agents	Yellow fever virus
Arenaviruses	(*Salmonellae, E. coli* O157:H7)	Drug-resistant tuberculosis
	Water safety threat agents	Tick-borne encephalitis
	(*Vibrio cholerae*, etc.)	

Category A—Agents with high public health impact requiring intensive public health preparedness and intervention; Category B—Agents with a somewhat lesser need for public health preparedness. (From Ref. 1.)

1960s, development of a new generation of vaccines was made possible by an understanding of the three principal protein virulence factors in *B. anthracis,* namely protective antigen (PA), lethal factor (LF), and edema factor (EF) [4,5]. Pathogenesis of tissue edema and necrosis seen in anthrax cases is attributable to the effects of LF and/or EF, which form the "A" chain of anthrax toxins according to the A–B model of dichain toxins [6]. Protective antigen serves as the "B" chain transport protein, which binds to receptors on target cell membranes and initiates toxin uptake.

Since the appreciation of the role of PA in immunity, vaccines prepared in the United Kingdom in the 1950s and in the United States in the 1960s have employed cell-free filtrates that optimize the content of PA. A vaccine in use in Britain derives from the Sterne strain, and is prepared in a manner very similar to that used in production of the U.S. vaccine. The vaccine currently available for human use in the United States was licensed in 1970, and is derived from strain V770, a PA-rich organism originating from a case of bovine disease. Although the V770-based vaccine [licensed as "Anthrax Vaccine Adsorbed" (AVA)] was used sporadically from 1970 through 1990 to immunize select veterinary personnel, textile workers, and abattoir workers in the United States, it was not until Operations Desert Shield and Desert Storm (ODS/S) in 1990–1991 that widespread and systematic use by the U.S. military spurred a number of controversies surrounding AVA. During ODS/S, approximately 150,000 doses of AVA were administered to U.S. military personnel. The rapid victory achieved during that conflict resulted in very few individuals receiving more than two doses of the usual six-dose series of injections (normally spread over 18 months). Several years later, in 1998, Department of Defense officials resurrected the AVA-associated controversies with a phased program [the Anthrax Vaccine Immunization Program (AVIP)] mandating vaccine for all men and women serving in all branches of the U.S. Armed Forces. In general, these controversies involve questions of: (1) safety, (2) efficacy, and (3) programmatics.

To date, at least 18 studies (summarized in Table 2) have assessed, to varying degrees, the safety of AVA. While many of these studies involve exceedingly small numbers of vaccine recipients, and while several were conducted for reasons other than a direct assessment of vaccine safety per se, collectively they provide fairly convincing evidence of, at least, the short-term safety of AVA.

The first data available on the safety of AVA comes from the pivotal study of Brachman and colleagues [7] that led to licensure of the vaccine. In this study, published in 1962, employees at four goat-hair processing plants in the northeastern United States during the late 1950s were offered enrollment in a placebo-controlled trial of an anthrax vaccine developed at the U.S. Army's biological defense facility at Fort Detrick, MD. Among the 379 vaccine recipients involved in this study, approximately 30% experienced mild local reactions (typically 1–2 cm of erythema), while 4% experienced moderate local reactions (defined as erythema >5 cm in diameter). Three individuals developed large local reactions, while two experienced malaise of 24-hr duration. Of note, this study is the sole examination of data performed using only the original Fort Detrick-developed preparation (sometimes referred to as the "Merck Vaccine").

Shortly after the Brachman study was completed, minor modifications were made to the anthrax vaccine preparation that resulted in a higher concentration of PA and decreased amounts of LF and EF. This modified preparation, sometimes referred to as the "Lansing Vaccine," is the one that was ultimately licensed by the National Institutes of Health in 1970 [the Food and Drug Administration (FDA) assumed responsibility for vaccine licensure in 1972], and is the one which remains in use today. The fact that the initial safety and efficacy study leading to licensure was performed using a slightly different formulation is a source of some controversy.

Prior to the decision by military officials to mandate immunization against anthrax, further data regarding the safety of anthrax vaccine was available from at least two additional sources. First, the CDC collected data on 6985 persons at risk for occupational exposure [8]. These persons received 16,435 doses of vaccine under an Investigational New Drug (IND) permit during the years between publication of the Brachman study and ultimate vaccine licensure. In addition, investigators at Fort Detrick collected data on at-risk laboratory workers given vaccine over a 26-year period from 1973 to 1999. In their study [9], 1583 persons received 10,722 doses of vaccine. Although each of these studies showed similar low rates of reaction (moderate reactions in 1–4% and severe reactions in <1%), the former is complicated by the fact that early enrollees received the Merck vaccine while later enrollees received the Lansing preparation and the latter is limited by a passive system for the reporting of vaccine side effects. It was on the basis of the three aforementioned studies that the Department of Defense, in 1998, embarked on its plan to require universal immunization of all U.S. Armed Forces.

Since the AVIP was initially implemented in March of 1998, considerable experience with AVA has accumulated. As of January of 2002, 526,146 service members had received 2,113,155 doses of vaccine [10]. This large number of vaccine recipients has enabled a clearer picture of the problem of vaccine side effects, which have been formally studied in multiple subsets of this total patient population. Most of these studies (Table 2) are, individually, rather small, and would not detect rare untoward vaccine reactions. Moreover, as all of the experience is quite recent, vaccine-related conditions that might conceivably arise years after vaccination would not be detected. Nonetheless, taken together, these studies lead to an emerging picture of a vaccine at least as safe as most conventional vaccines.

In addition to safety, concerns have also been raised regarding the efficacy of AVA in protecting against the bioweapons threat that concerns the military. Such a threat would presumably involve aerosolized anthrax spores and would lead to inhalational anthrax, a disease of significantly different pathology than the cutaneous anthrax that had constituted the more common occupational hazard of textile workers. Although naturally occurring inhalational anthrax is too rare to permit an efficacy trial in humans, vaccine efficacy data is nonetheless available through two separate avenues of research. First, the original Brachman study saw an unexpected five cases of inhalational anthrax occur, although the aim of the study was to examine vaccine efficacy against cutaneous disease. Of these five cases, two occurred in placebo recipients and three occurred in persons who had declined to participate in the study; none occurred in vaccine recipients. While this was not statistically powerful enough to lead to a conclusion regarding efficacy, it is in line with subsequent data collected by the CDC from 1962 to 1974, wherein 24 cases of inhalational anthrax occurred among unvaccinated textile mill employees, while none occurred among employees who had elected vaccination [11].

A second source of efficacy data derives from animal trials involving nonhuman primates. In several small studies conducted at Fort Detrick's U.S. Army Medical Research Institute of Infectious Diseases (USAMRIID), adult rhesus monkeys were given one or two injections of AVA and then challenged with varying doses of aerosolized Ames-strain anthrax spores at varying intervals after immunization. In all, 62 of 65 animals survived challenge, compared with none of the 18 control animals. These studies have recently been summarized [11].

Finally, some controversy surrounds the "programmatics" of the AVIP and of anthrax immunization in general. Undoubtedly, the prospects of immunizing large numbers of individuals against anthrax are made less palatable by the unwieldy vaccine schedule. Currently, AVA is licensed as a six-dose series, with doses at 0, 2, and 4 weeks, and 6, 12, and 18 months. Moreover, annual boosters are advised for personnel at ongoing risk of contracting anthrax. In the military especially, given the mobility of its personnel and the attendant difficulties in record keeping, this presents a formidable obstacle. In fact, ongoing studies are examining the feasibility of AVA dose reduction (i.e., eliminating doses of vaccine). A preliminary study [12] comparing recipients of three doses (at 0, 2, and 4 weeks) with those who received only two doses 4 weeks apart demonstrated comparable peak anti-PA IgG antibody titers in both groups. Efforts are underway to expand on this preliminary work in anticipation of a petition to the FDA for dosing adjustment.

Another area of concern deals with vaccine employment strategy. The vaccine was initially licensed for pre-exposure prophylaxis against anthrax in those persons "who may come in contact with animal products." In fact, it was previously noted that "if a person has not previously been immunized against anthrax, injection of this product (AVA) following exposure to anthrax bacilli will not protect against infection [13]." Nonetheless, some authorities now see a potential role for AVA as a postexposure adjuvant to chemoprophylaxis. Such recommendations are based on findings that a percentage of nonhuman primates succumb to experimental inhalational anthrax following withdrawal of antibiotics after a 30-day course. Such studies were recently summarized by the CDC, which noted a "possible benefit of postexposure combination of antibiotics with vaccination [14]." Based on these same studies, the Defense Department has also acknowledged a role for postexposure immunization [15].

Finally, concern surrounds modernization efforts at AVA's manufacturer, the BioPort Corporation (Lansing, MI). BioPort acquired the assets of the Michigan Biologic Products Institute (MBPI) in September of 1998. It was MBPI that had been initially awarded a contract to provide AVA to the Department of Defense. In August of 1999, BioPort applied to the FDA for a license supplement for a renovated vaccine production facility and was asked to cease production of AVA until process validation work could be accomplished to the satisfaction of the FDA. These delays resulted in phased slowdowns of the Defense Department's AVIP in July 2000, November 2000, and June 2001. These slowdowns led to an erosion of confidence among some potential vaccine recipients and their advocates. On January 31, 2002, however, the FDA approved BioPort's Biologics License Application supplement, and full-scale resumption of the AVIP, as of this writing, awaits only the approval of the Secretary of Defense. On March 6, 2002, The National Academy of Sciences, through its Institute of Medicine, concluded that AVA was effective at protecting humans against anthrax "including inhalational anthrax" [16]. Moreover, they also noted that that AVA had a side-effect profile comparable to other vaccines commonly employed in the United States.

Prompted by the safety, efficacy, and programmatic concerns surrounding AVA, however, interest in the development of new anthrax vaccines has increased in recent years. Several approaches have been employed in the search

Table 2 Studies of Safety of Anthrax Vaccine Adsorbed (AVA)

Study	Subjects	Vaccinees[a]	Purpose of Study	Findings	Reference
Brachman, 1955–1959	Textile Workers; Original licensure study	379 (D)	Pivotal safety and efficacy trial	~30% "mild" reactions; 4% moderate (>5cm) reactions	7
CDC, 1962–1972	Occupationally At-Risk	6985 (M)	Postlicensure monitoring	3–20% mild (<3 cm); 1–3% moderate (3–12 cm) reactions	8
Ft Detrick Multidose, 1944–1971	Laboratory Workers; Hyper-Immunized	97 (M)	Evaluate effects of "hyper-immunization" with large numbers of various vaccines	No unusual disease attributed to receipt of large numbers of vaccines (including AVA)	89
Ft Detrick SIP, 1973–1999	Laboratory Workers	1583 (L)	Cohort safety study (passive surveillance) of vaccinated lab workers	3.6% local reactions; ~1% systemic reactions	9
Ft Bragg, 1992–1994	Special Forces Soldiers	495 (L)	Assess safety of AVA booster doses among those immunized during ODS/S	16–28% mild (<5 cm); 4.7–9.3% moderate; 26–45% systemic reactions	90
USAMRIID Dose Reduction, 1998	Adult Volunteers	173 (L)	Pilot study evaluating reduced dosing schedule for AVA	Induration in 3–19% of males, 38–75% of females	12
Canadian Forces Safety Survey, 1998	Military Personnel	576 (L)	Active surveillance for AVA-associated adverse reactions	Mild (<5cm) reactions in 4.4% of doses/12.7% of recipients; moderate in 0.2/0.5%	91
Tripler Survey, 1998–2000	Military Personnel	601 (L)	Self-reporting of reactions to AVA among medical personnel	2.1–2.7% reported systemic symptoms limiting activity	92
U.S. Forces Korea, 1998–1999	Military Personnel	4348 (L)	Self-reporting of reactions to AVA among military personnel	1.9% of recipients reported limitations on work performance	92

Study, Year	Population	Sample Size[a]	Objective	Findings	Ref
VAERS Reports, 1990–2000	All Vaccinees (presumably military)	1563 (L)	Collection of reports to FDA regarding adverse events	No unexpected findings in side-effect profile of AVA	92
Ft Lewis, 2000	ROTC Cadets	73 (L)	Assess reactions among those inadvertently receiving a double dose of AVA	Erythema: 39% in double group vs. 19% in standard. Lump: 44/29%; Swelling 50/19%	93
Langley AFB, 1998–1999	Air Force Personnel	4045 (L)	Study link between AVA and ambulatory diagnoses among SW Asia veterans	No link between AVA receipt and any specific ambulatory diagnosis	94
Ft Stewart, 2000–2001	Female Military Personnel	3136 (L)	Evaluate reproductive health among AVA recipient females	No link between AVA receipt and rates of conception, birth, or birth defects	95
Reproductive Outcomes Study, 1998–2000	Wives of Military Vaccinees	68,267 (L)	Evaluate reproductive outcomes of wives & neonates of vaccinees	No increase in hospitalization rates or adverse pregnancy outcomes in wives of vaccinees	96
USAF Vision Study, 1998–1999	USAF Air Crew Members	(L)	Evaluate causes of visual deterioration	No link between AVA and visual deterioration	96
Army Aviator Study, 1998–2000	Army Aviators	3356 (L)	Evaluate relationship between AVA and hearing loss	No link between AVA and hearing loss	96
Defense Medical Surveillance, 1998–2001	Military Personnel	757,540 person-years (L)	Examine hospitalization rates of vaccinated and unvaccinated individuals over time	No increase in rates of hospitalization among vaccinated for all 14 disease categories	96
Naval Health Research Center, 1998–2000	Military Personnel	(L)	Examine hospitalization rates of vaccinated and unvaccinated individuals over time	Lower hospitalization rates among vaccinated individuals compared to nonvaccinated	96

[a] Vaccine preparation utilized (see text for explanation).

ODS/S—Operations Desert Shield/Storm.

D = Ft Detrick; L = Lansing; M = Mixture of recipients of each vaccine.

for a new anthrax vaccine [17]. First, the PA gene has been cloned into *Bacillus subtilis*, a taxonomic relative of *B. anthracis* lacking virulence for humans, and into other expression vectors. Second, mutant-strain vaccines have been created from the Sterne strain which depend on aromatic compounds not found in human tissue. Finally, purified PA preparations have been combined with various adjuvants. All three approaches have led to the development of experimental vaccines which are protective against aerosolized spore challenge in guinea pigs [18–20]. In particular, a vaccine candidate composed of purified PA combined with monophosphoryl lipid A appears promising. In guinea pigs, this vaccine proved superior in efficacy to the currently available human vaccine. Moreover, lyophilization appeared to have no effect on vaccine potency—a potential advantage over the current preparation, which requires a cold storage chain. Finally, a DNA plasmid vaccine which incorporates the immunogenic and biologically active portion of PA has demonstrated protection in mice against lethal challenge with a preparation of PA + LF [21]. A concise review of the prospects for development of new generation anthrax vaccines has recently been published [22].

B. Smallpox

Smallpox, a disease limited to humans in the natural setting, was caused by infection with variola virus, a member of the *Orthopoxvirus* genus. A closely related cross-protective Orthopoxvirus, vaccinia, has long been, and remains, the basis of vaccination efforts. The global eradication of endemic smallpox, accomplished in 1977 and formally acknowledged by the World Health Organization (WHO) in 1980, stands as one of the great triumphs of public health. Unfortunately, the subsequent discontinuation of vaccination opened the door for this agent to be used as a weapon of warfare or terrorism. Currently, there exist only two WHO-authorized repositories of the virus: at the CDC in Atlanta and Koltsovo in Russia. However, concerns persist that other clandestine stocks may exist and that these stocks could find their way into the hands of terrorists. Moreover, there are concerns that other orthopoxviruses could be genetically manipulated to produce virulent organisms similar to variola.

Over the years, the numerous, often poorly characterized, strains of vaccinia virus previously employed in vaccination were abandoned under the auspices of the WHO. Ultimately, derivatives of three strains remained available: the Lister–Elstree strain, the EM63 strain (used in the Soviet Union), and the New York City Board of Health (NYC-BOH) strain, an isolate of low pathogenicity [23] used in vaccine production by Wyeth Laboratories. A fourth strain, the "Temple of Heaven" strain, remained in widespread use in the People's Republic of China. The Wyeth product, Dryvax®, is currently available through the CDC, which has approximately 15.4 million doses on hand [24]. It is administered by scarification with a bifurcated needle dipped in vaccine; further guidelines for its use are published [25]. The effectiveness of vaccinia vaccine is attested to by its success in smallpox eradication; however, future availability of the vaccine has, until recently, been a concern. Wyeth

discontinued the manufacture of Dryvax® in 1982, the existing doses are undergoing a gradual loss of potency, and all will ultimately expire. Moreover, recent testing of the product diluent revealed that the phenol level did not meet specifications. Therefore a new diluent (lacking brilliant green) has been manufactured and the vaccine must thus be administered under the CDC's IND with informed consent.

In light of these issues, three different approaches have been taken to improve the country's preparedness for an outbreak of smallpox. First, collaborative work has been undertaken by investigators at USAMRIID and the CDC to develop a nonhuman primate model for smallpox in order to test new compounds (such as cidofovir) for therapeutic efficacy. Second, clinical trials have been conducted at several universities in cooperation with the National Institute of Allergy and Infectious Diseases to evaluate whether the existing Dryvax stocks could be diluted 5-, 10-, or 100-fold and still produce an effective "take." This would provide an immediate method of expanding the existing vaccine stockpile. In a pilot study using 20 subjects per group, previously unimmunized individuals given undiluted vaccine and vaccine diluted 10- or 100-fold, 95%, 70%, and 15%, respectively, had evidence of a take [26]. The results of a larger follow-up study with 5- and 10-fold dilutions were more promising, with 232/234 (99.1%) being successfully vaccinated with a 5-fold dilution and 330/340 (97.1%) successfully vaccinated with a 10-fold dilution [27]. The mean titer of the diluted vaccine in the 10-fold dilution arm was $10^{7.0}$ PF compared with $10^{6.5}$ PFU/mL in the pilot study, indicating that a titer of approximately $10^{7.0}$ PFU/mL is needed for a higher take rate. The third approach has been to launch a large-scale effort to produce a new cell-culture-derived vaccine. Investigators at USAMRIID first developed a new vaccine at the request of the Defense Department. This cell culture preparation derives from a Connaught (NYCBOH) vaccine strain in use until the early 1970s, and recently underwent Phase II testing in human volunteers. In this study, vaccinees receiving the cell culture vaccine intradermally, with subsequent development of cutaneous pox lesions, had immune responses comparable to those receiving Dryvax® by scarification. Those recipients who failed to develop pox lesions, or who received intramuscular vaccine, experienced humoral immune responses inferior to those elicited in the Dryvax® group [28]. From this study, it is clear that administration by scarification remains necessary. An expanded trial, comparing Dryvax® and the cell-culture-derived preparation, both administered by scarification, has been completed and is pending publication. There are two additional cell-culture-derived products being evaluated. The master virus and cell banks from the USAMRIID preparation were subsequently rederived and an IND request for the new product filed by the Defense Department's Joint Vaccine Acquisition Program (JVAP) in March, 2002. The first clinical trial of this product is scheduled to begin in the near future. A second cell-culture-derived product was manufactured by Acambis Corporation, under contract with the CDC to produce 155 million doses. This product is a plaque-purified clone from Dryvax. A Phase I trial has been executed but final results are still pending. This product, like the JVAP product, is propagated in MRC5 cells.

Fortuitously, in March, 2002, Aventis Pharmaceuticals [29] revealed that they had discovered 85 million doses of frozen liquid smallpox vaccine produced in the late 1950s. Therefore, the existing U.S. stockpile of vaccine has jumped from 15 million to 100 million doses even without dilution of existing stocks or new cell-cultured vaccine production. The recently discovered product appears to be potent and clinical studies are planned.

C. Plague

Plague is caused by infection with *Yersinis pestis*, a bipolar-staining gram-negative facultative intracellular bacillus. Human plague occurs rarely in the western world, but remains endemic in India, Burma, Vietnam, Madagascar, and elsewhere. Of the three typical presentations of illness—bubonic, pneumonic, and septicemic plague—bubonic continues to be the most common, and until recently, vaccine development efforts targeted this form of the disease.

In 1897, Haffkine [30] developed a "plague prophylactic fluid," which was a killed vaccine preparation used to combat the disease in India, where it was hyperendemic. Although the preparation was apparently efficacious in preventing the bubonic form of the disease, clinicians rejected it because of the high rate of adverse reactions [31] caused by the injection of up to 12 mL of vaccine. (It was erroneously believed that doses sufficient to cause systemic febrile reactions were necessary to induce protective immunity.) Prior to World War II, a new-generation, formalin-killed modification of the original Haffkine vaccine was prepared from *Y. pestis* strain 195/P, a virulent clinical isolate from India. Ultimately, the National Research Council Committee on Medical Research recommended the use of such killed vaccines in military personnel. During World War II, approximately 12,000 troops were immunized with a two-dose vaccine series of Plague Vaccine, USP, an Army version of the formalin-killed preparation. Despite potential exposures from deployments into areas of high endemicity, none of the soldiers contracted plague, providing circumstantial evidence of efficacy [31].

Only eight cases of plague were reported among U.S. service members during the Vietnam War, where the vaccine was routinely administered. The success of the vaccine is attested to by comparing rates of the disease among the U.S. personnel and the unvaccinated South Vietnamese civilian population. U.S. personnel had a rate of approximately 1 case per million person-years of exposure [32], compared with a 330-fold greater incidence of plague among the unvaccinated South Vietnamese civilian population [33]. The relatively high incidence among U.S. troops of murine typhus, another disease transmitted in Vietnam by the same vector, *Xenopsylla cheopis*, implies that the U.S. troops likely had exposure to plague, despite the low disease rates [34].

Even though the plague vaccine appears to protect soldiers against endemic plague, the preparation most recently used is not considered protective against infection by the aerosol route [35,36], which is the route of most concern in the context of a biological attack. In addition, local reaction rates to the plague vaccine are high, with reaction

rates increasing with successive doses. Hence the initial dose is 1.0 mL, but the second and third doses of the primary series (at 1–3 and 5–6 months, respectively) are reduced to 0.2 mL [35]. In addition, 20% of vaccine recipients reported systemic reactions [37]. Moreover, 7% of vaccinees failed to respond serologically, while many others required the full three-dose series to achieve hemagglutination titers similar to those protective in mice [38]. Finally, the short duration of immunity elicited by this vaccine necessitated booster doses as often as every 6 months [35]. These difficulties, as well as supply and manufacturing problems and limited commercial demand outside the military, led to a discontinuation of production in 1999. The fact that no licensed plague vaccine is currently available, and that previous vaccines were not effective against plague transmitted by aerosol, drives an interest in new generation vaccines.

One theory guiding the search for an improved vaccine suggests that mucosal immunity in the tracheobronchial tree may be important in the defense against pneumonic plague [39]. Oral immunization of vervets with a live-attenuated *Y. pestis* vaccine, EV76, afforded some protection against inhalational challenge [40]. However, EV76 and similar live plague vaccines produced a significant number of side effects when administered subcutaneously to humans. Moreover, approximately 1% of mice given EV76 succumbed to fatal infection [41].

A more recent approach to vaccine development involves the use of recombinant subunit vaccines. The F1 ("fraction 1") and V ("virulence") antigens of *Y. pestis* have both been shown to be individually immunogenic. Moreover, their protective effects in combination appear additive [42]. Furthermore, although antibody against F1 alone protects against plague, F1 is not critical for virulence, and virulent F1-negative *Y. pestis* strains have been described [43], adding theoretical support to the case for a multiantigen vaccine. Single-dose immunization with a subunit vaccine containing F1 and V antigens has been shown to protect mice against pneumonic disease [44]. Studies are ongoing to evaluate these vaccine candidates further.

D. Tularemia

Tularemia, a plague-like illness, is caused by infection with the gram-negative coccobacillus, *Francisella tularensis*. Two biotypes of *F. tularensis* are known; *F. tularensis tularensis*, the causative agent of "Type A" tularemia, is found only in temperate areas of North America. It is an organism of extraordinarily high virulence, with as few as 10 cells representing the rabbit lethal dose (LD_{50}) and human infectious dose (ID_{50}). *Francisella tularensis palearctica*, the agent of "Type B" tularemia, on the other hand, is a low-virulence organism found in Europe and the former Soviet Union. The rabbit LD_{50} of this organism is of the order of 10 million cells. These differences have potential implications in vaccine development, although immunity against one biotype appears to be cross-protective. Current tularemia vaccines derive, by and large, from seed stocks of the "live vaccine strain" (LVS), which, in turn derives from "strain 15," biotype *palearctica*, an organism attenuated by repeated subculture. The fact that *F. tularensis* occupied a prominent position in the Cold War-era biological arsenals of both the United States and the Soviet Union is made more intriguing, considering that "strain 15" was given to U.S. investigators in 1956 by colleagues at the USSR's Gamaleya Institute. An LVS-based investigational vaccine has been sporadically used in the United States since that time to immunize laboratory workers in select settings. Multiple studies attest to its efficacy in preventing inhalational tularemia among human volunteers [45,46].

Despite their apparent efficacy, several considerations limit the potential employment of LVS-based vaccines [47]. First, knowledge of factors responsible for virulence in *F. tularensis* remains incomplete. Second, concerns persist regarding the genetic stability of the vaccine strain, namely that LVS might revert to a more virulent or, alternatively, a less protective, state. Precedent for the latter exists among *F. tularensis* vaccine strains previously employed in the Soviet Union. Third, LVS preparations consist of two colony types, only one of which appears immunogenic. Combined, these factors dictate that each new lot of tularemia vaccine is evaluated for immunogenicity prior to use [48]. Moreover, any LVS immunization strategy is potentially hampered by the need to administer the vaccine by scarification, wherein a 0.1-mL dose is applied to the skin, which is then punctured by 16 stabs of a bifurcated needle. These microbiologic and clinical concerns, the ill-defined nature of the vaccine strain, and cases of clinical tularemia among vaccinees receiving larger inocula would seem to argue for the need for an improved vaccine.

However, the search for new tularemia vaccine candidates is hampered by uncertainty over the nature of antigens required for protective cell-mediated immunity and a failure of killed vaccines to produce such immunity. In fact, few significant developments have occurred in the search for improved tularemia vaccines over the past half-century. In addition to the problems of antigenic characterization, this is likely due, in part, to the rather low incidence of endemic tularemia in the west, as well as to the lesser perceived threat posed by weaponized tularemia when compared, for example, to weaponized anthrax, smallpox, or plague. In fact, the JVAP has taken on responsibility for shepherding the current LVS vaccine through to FDA licensure.

E. Botulism

Botulism is caused by exposure to any of seven related neurotoxins (types A–G) produced by the obligately anaerobic gram-positive bacterium, *Clostridium botulinum*. While only toxin types A, B, and E appear to be significant causes of naturally occurring botulism, other toxin types have the potential to produce disease. Although a licensed antitoxin designed to treat endemic disease thus contains antibody against only types A, B, and E, defense planners anticipate that vaccines against an intentional botulism release should optimally induce immunity against a broader array of toxin types.

The relatively low incidence of naturally occurring botulism has hindered vaccine development, and no licensed product exists today. A pentavalent (types A–E) toxoid, prepared by combining separate aliquots of the five inacti-

vated toxins was originally produced by Parke-Davis. A second, less-reactogenic, pentavalent product, with a decrease in the amount of residual formaldehyde, but otherwise little changed from the original, has been produced for the U.S. Army by the Michigan Biologic Products Institute. Several thousand volunteers and at-risk laboratory workers have received this toxoid on an investigational basis. The vaccine regimen consists of a three-dose series, involving 0.5-mL subcutaneous doses at 0, 2, and 12 weeks, with annual boosters, a strategy hampered by an increasing rate of local reactions to each subsequent booster. A separate inactivated monovalent type F vaccine of similar construct has also been available on a very limited investigational basis.

Local reactions to current investigational preparations, coupled with cold-storage requirements, less than desirable antibody titers to types B and D toxin, and high cost, have spurred efforts to develop improved botulinum toxoids. Several avenues of research appear to hold promise in this regard. First, recombinant technology has been used to express a fragment of the heavy chain of type A toxin in *Escherichia coli* [49]. Mice immunized with this preparation are protected against intraperitoneal challenge with type A botulinum toxin. Second, a Venezuelan Equine Encephalitis (VEE) virus replicon vector has been employed to produce toxin antigens in vivo [50] (see also section on VEE). Finally, *C. botulinum* carboxy-terminal-fragment-coding genes have been synthesized and the nontoxic gene products expressed in yeast [51]. The resultant product induces immunity against high-level challenge in both mice and nonhuman primates.

II. SELECT CATEGORY B AGENTS

A. Brucellosis

Brucellosis is caused by infection with one of several species of the genus *Brucella*, a group of gram-negative facultative intracellular coccobacillary bacteria. Brucellosis is a major veterinary problem in many areas of the world and naturally occurring human brucellosis is not uncommon in some locales, especially in the Middle East. In addition, despite its long incubation period and low lethality, many experts consider brucellosis, because of its extraordinary infectivity, a viable terrorist threat.

Veterinary vaccines against brucellosis have long been studied and widely employed. The vaccination of livestock to reduce enzootic disease load, in combination with the slaughter of infected animals, is largely responsible for the declining incidence of human brucellosis in the United States. In fact, the decline of human brucellosis cases reported to the Centers for Disease Control has paralleled the control of *Brucella abortus* infections in cattle [52]. Most veterinary vaccines in use until recently derived from *B. abortus* strain 19, an attenuated organism with stable virulence, or from Rev 1, a live, virulence-stable *B. melitensis* strain. In 1996, a new generation vaccine, derived from strain RB51, a stable mutant of *B. abortus*, was conditionally licensed for use in cattle. This mutant strain, which lacks a polysaccharide O-chain, fails to induce antibody detectable by current veterinary screening assays. Bovine brucellosis eradication campaigns make use of such antibody detection to detect infection and institute quarantine procedures among cattle herds. RB51 has the advantage of not interfering with such campaigns.

Although live *Brucella* vaccines have been employed in humans at various times and in various developing nations [53], none are licensed in most of the Western world, including the United States. Most preparations studied in humans in the past derived from *B. abortus* strain 19, reflecting the cross-immunity among *Brucella* species, and diminished human virulence of *B. abortus* when compared with other species. Despite their relatively low virulence, however, administration of either live preparation to humans is hampered by frequent hypersensitivity reactions and by a modest but notable incidence of clinical infection. Such problems were noted in the former Soviet Union, where human vaccination is still widely employed, and in a U.S. trial of strain 19 and Rev 1 vaccines conducted 35 years ago [54]. More recently, human infections have resulted from inadvertent exposure to veterinary RB51 vaccines as well [55].

Several attempts have been made to develop fractional component vaccines derived from various *Brucella* strains. An acetic-acid extract of a variant of strain 19 *B. abortus*, yielding a complex known as "brucellosis protective antigen," was tested in the USSR [56]; immunity elicited in guinea pigs failed to persist. A "phenol-insoluble fraction" vaccine consisting primarily of delipidated strain 19 components protected mice and guinea pigs from challenge, and has been used on a small scale in humans [57]. While this latter preparation was apparently efficacious at protecting high-risk recipients, immunity was not lasting, and boosting appeared necessary every 2 years. Moreover, any strategy for immunization (and especially for reimmunization) was further complicated by the need for skin testing of potential recipients, as skin-test-positive patients react strongly to vaccine. More recently, the outer membrane protein (OMP) of *Neisseria meningitidis* has been shown to be a useful adjuvant to intranasal *B. melitensis* immunization in mice and guinea pigs [58], and a mucosal vaccine combining OMP with purified lipopolysaccharide of *B. melitensis* is under study.

B. Q-Fever

Q-fever is caused by infection with *Coxiella burnetii*, a pleomorphic gram-negative coccobacillary organism. Like brucellosis, Q-fever has a long incubation period but an extraordinary degree of infectivity. In fact, a single bacterial cell likely represents a human ID_{50}. This high degree of infectivity, combined with a resistance to heat and dessication, explain the consideration given Q-fever as a potential weapon.

Effective vaccines against *C. burnetii* have existed for over half a century. The Smadel vaccine [59] was a highly immunogenic, formalin-inactivated preparation derived from the Henzerling strain of *C. burnetii*. The history of this and related early vaccines has been reviewed [60]. Although apparently effective, early vaccines occasionally resulted in significant morbidity, with sterile abscess and sinus forma-

tion frequently occurring at inoculation sites [61]. Q-fever vaccines with improved immunogenicity followed the discovery of the phenomenon of phase variation among *C. burnetii*. The organism is pathogenic and immunogenic in its Phase I form, but reverts to an avirulent, nonimmunogenic Phase II form after serial passage in yolk sac cultures. Awareness of this phase shift permitted the manufacture of more potent vaccines formulated entirely of Phase I organisms.

A formalin-inactivated, purified, Henzerling strain, Phase I whole-cell Q-fever vaccine has been licensed for many years in Australia as Q-Vax®. While Q-Vax® has been shown to be highly efficacious at preventing clinical Q-fever in humans [62], concerns exist regarding the potential for severe local reactions in patients with pre-existing immunity to *C. burnetii*. Use of a skin test, consisting of 0.1 mL of vaccine (intradermally administered), to identify these patients, can reduce the incidence of local reactions, but adds to the cost and complexity of immunization efforts. An analogous vaccine, administered in a one-time 0.5-mL subcutaneous dose, has been used on an investigational basis for many years in the United States.

The morbidity and skin testing requirements associated with whole cell vaccines might be eliminated with the development of a chloroform–methanol residue (CMR) preparation. The CMR vaccine contains Phase I antigens, and in animal studies, is less reactogenic than Q-Vax®, with comparable efficacy [63]. In humans, CMR vaccine was safe and immunogenic in nonimmune volunteers [64] and is currently being examined for reactogenicity in Q-fever immune individuals.

C. Venezuelan Equine Encephalitis

Venezuelan Equine Encephalitis (VEE) is caused by infection with the new-world alphavirus of the same name. Despite a natural transmission cycle requiring a mosquito vector, the disease is nonetheless transmissable artificially via aerosol, accounting for its inclusion among the list of terrorist and warfare threats.

A live-attenuated vaccine against Venezuelan Equine Encephalitis, TC-83 (so called because of its 83 passages in cell culture) was first developed in 1961 [65,66]. Evidence for the efficacy of this vaccine is largely anecdotal, relying on an observed marked decline in laboratory-acquired VEE infections among vaccine recipients. Despite its apparent efficacy, however, TC-83 vaccination is complicated by a high systemic reaction rate [65]. Moreover, a substantial number of primary TC-83 vaccine recipients fail to mount an adequate serologic response [67]. A tissue culture of TC-83 vaccine, inactivated with formalin, led to a less reactogenic preparation, C-84 [68]. Unfortunately, however, when given alone, this preparation afforded inadequate protection against aerosol challenge in hamsters [69]. Moreover, in human volunteers, one or two doses of C-84 alone (as compared to a dose of TC-83 with and without C-84 boosting) led to a particularly deficient IgA antibody response [70]. It has been postulated that IgA is the dominant immunologic entity responsible for protection against VEE. In practice, select laboratory workers are now given C-84 as a booster immunization following priming with TC-83 [67].

Driven by the high systemic reaction rate and incomplete protection afforded by TC-83, new approaches to immunization against VEE are actively being explored. One strategy involves a recombinant attenuated VEE vaccine, V3526, which features mutations at two loci. These mutations minimize the risk of reversion to virulence and result in a vaccine potentially less reactogenic than TC-83. In preliminary studies, V3526 protected mice against intranasal challenge with fully virulent VEE virus [71]. A second strategy involves incorporation of TC-83 virus, inactivated by radiation, into DL-lactide-co-glycolide microspheres. In one study [72], mice immunized with this microsphere preparation experienced greater protection against systemic challenge than those immunized with free virus.

Of interest, a considerable amount of ongoing work with VEE virus involves its potential use as a vector for the delivery of other recombinant vaccines. These vaccine vectors, or replicons, are developed by substituting genes coding for a protein of interest (for example, an immunizing epitope of a different virus or bacteria) for those coding for VEE structural proteins. The result is a viral genome that encodes its own replicases and transcriptases, enabling the synthesis of abundant quantities of mRNA coding for the protein of interest. The replicon genomes can be encapsidated into virus-like particles by cotransfecting replicon RNA along with helper RNAs coding the VEE nucleocapsid and capsid proteins. These virus-like particles contain the recombinant RNA genome. Following inoculation, the particles are taken up by immune effector cells; heterologous antigens are expressed, and protective immunity results. Because the replicon genome lacks the genes for VEE structural proteins, no viral progeny are produced. Consequently, the infection is limited to one cycle; viremia does not develop, and immunity to VEE structural proteins does not develop [73]. This approach has been successful in immunizing rodents against Ebola and Marburg viruses [74], as well as against type A botulinum toxin [50] and many other agents. Replicons could theoretically be developed to encode multiple antigens, conferring immunity against numerous pathogens. Because immunity to VEE structural proteins does not result, VEE replicons could theoretically be used repeatedly for booster immunizations, or for sequential immunizations against numerous pathogens, without being inactivated by host immunity. This offers a potential advantage over vaccinia- and adenovirus-vectored recombinant vaccines [75].

Currently, laboratories employing VEE vaccines to protect those studying the virus or utilizing VEE virus as a vector in replicon work offer an initial 0.5-mL subcutaneous dose of TC-83, followed 28 days later by an assessment of plaque-reduction neutralization titers. Recipients with titers <1:20 are given a 0.5-mL subcutaneous dose of C-84. Typically, subsequent titer checks would be performed annually on recipients at ongoing risk; C-84 boosters would be administered when titers fall below 1:20.

VEE is only one of a group of alphaviruses occasionally mentioned in a bioweapons context. However, despite the fact that they tend to cause more severe disease in humans, the closely related agents of Eastern (EEE) and Western (WEE) Equine Encephalitis, are generally felt to represent less of a threat than VEE. This is principally due to the high proportion of asymptomatic infections associated with these viruses. Whereas the disease to infection ratio of VEE is on the order of 1:1, that of EEE [76] is 1:23 and of WEE [77], 1:1150. Nonetheless, investigational inactivated vaccines have been developed against EEE and WEE, employing technology analogous to that used in the production of C-84. Similarly, a live vaccine candidate against the Old World alphavirus, Chikungunya, has been developed and evaluated in Phase II human trials [78]. Currently, usage of these vaccines is limited to a small number of laboratory investigators working with the viruses. The Department of Defense's JVAP has contract options for the development of a trivalent VEE/EEE/WEE vaccine.

D. Staphylococcal Enterotoxin B Intoxication

Staphylococcal enterotoxin B (SEB) is one of several pyrogenic exotoxins produced by *Staphylococcus aureus*. A familiar cause of naturally occurring food-borne disease, SEB (and other staphylococcal enterotoxins) might be employed by terrorists to contaminate food and water. In addition, however, SEB lends itself to aerosolization, producing a systemic febrile illness accompanied by pulmonary symptoms when encountered via this route. In a recent report [79], a laboratory accident resulted in nine workers developing inhalational SEB disease. Fever was prominent in all subjects, reaching as high as 106°F. All had cough, in most cases accompanied by dyspnea and chest pain.

No SEB vaccine is currently available for human administration, although several approaches to immunization against SEB intoxication have been explored. Formaldehyde-inactivated SEB toxoid, prepared as an alum precipitate, has been incorporated into microspheres and proteosomes. Microspheres containing SEB toxoid administered intramuscularly with an intratracheal booster protect rhesus monkeys against aerosol challenge [80]. In another approach, mutations were induced in the SEB molecule which render it nontoxic yet leave its three-dimensional antigenic structure intact. Using such a preparation with three-point mutations, investigators demonstrated immunogenicity in rhesus monkeys without apparent toxicity [81]. More recently, this attenuated SEB protein has been expressed in *E. coli* and the resultant recombinant product shown to protect mice against SEB intoxication when administered nasally or orally. Moreover, protection was afforded against both inhalational and parenteral (intraperitoneal) challenge [82].

E. Ricin Intoxication

Ricin is a toxic glycoprotein derived from the castor bean. Its ease of extraction from the by-products of castor oil production and its worldwide availability combine to make it an attractive candidate agent to would-be terrorists and biocriminals. Moreover, ricin is extremely toxic by oral, respiratory, and percutaneous routes, further enhancing its potential attractiveness. In fact, ricin has been used percutaneously in multiple assassination attempts [83].

There is no effective human vaccine against ricin intoxication. Both a formalin-inactivated toxoid [84] and a deglycosylated A-chain subunit vaccine [85] have been shown capable of protecting mice against aerosol challenge. Encapsulation of toxoid in Poly(lactide-co-glycolide) microspheres resulted in mouse protection following both intramuscular [86] and oral [87] administration. A separate preparation of toxoid encapsulated within liposomes was likewise effective at protecting mice when administered intratracheally [88].

It seems clear in the aftermath of September 11 that terrorism concerns are likely to remain with us for some time. Paramount among these threats in the eyes of many planners, the biological threat has been likened to the "poor man's atomic bomb." Effective strategies must be developed to combat this threat. Immunizations are likely to play a prominent role in any comprehensive defense strategy. As our understanding of the heretofore largely obscure pathogens that constitute viable threats increases, effective vaccines against these pathogens will likely become a reality.

REFERENCES

1. Khan AS, et al. Public-health preparedness for biological terrorism in the USA. Lancet 2000; 356:1179–1182.
2. Turnbull PCB. Anthrax vaccines: past, present and future. Vaccine 1991; 9:533–539.
3. Shlyakhov EN, Rubinstein E. Human live anthrax vaccine in the former USSR. Vaccine 1994; 12:727–730.
4. Stanley JL, Smith H. Purification of factor I and recognition of a third factor of the anthrax toxin. J Gen Microbiol 1961; 26:49–66.
5. Stanley JL, Smith H. The three factors of anthrax toxin: their immunogenicity and lack of demonstrable enzymic activity. J Gen Microbiol 1963; 31:329–337.
6. Gill DM. Seven toxic peptides that cross cell membranes. In: Jeljaszewicz J, Wadstrom T, eds. Bacterial Toxins and Cell Membranes. New York: Academic Press, 1978:291–332.
7. Brachman PS, et al. Field evaluation of a human anthrax vaccine. Am J Public Health 1962; 52:632–645.
8. National Communicable Disease Center. Investigational new drug application for anthrax protective antigen, aluminum hydroxide adsorbed. FDA no. DBS-IND 180, 1970.
9. Pittman PR, et al. Anthrax vaccine: short-term safety experience in humans. Vaccine 2002; 20:972–978.
10. Personal Communication, JD Grabenstein PhD, Anthrax Vaccine Immunization Program Agency, US Army Medical Command, Falls Church VA.
11. Friedlander AM, et al. Anthrax vaccine: evidence for safety and efficacy against inhalational anthrax. J Am Med Assoc 1999; 282:2104–2106.
12. Pittman PR, et al. Anthrax vaccine: immunogenicity and safety of a dose-reduction, route-change comparison study in humans. Vaccine 2002; 20:1412–1420.
13. Package insert, Anthrax Vaccine Adsorbed, October 1987.
14. Centers for Disease Control. Use of anthrax vaccine in the United States: recommendations of the Advisory Committee on Immunization Practices (ACIP). MMWR Morb Mortal Wkly Rep 2000; 49(RR-15):1–20.
15. Headquarters, Departments of the Army, the Navy, and the Air Force, and Commandant, Marine Corps. Treatment of biological warfare agent casualties. 17 July 2000.
16. Institute of Medicine, National Institutes of Health. The anthrax vaccine: Is it safe? Does it work? National Institutes of Health Report, March 2002.
17. Ivins BE, Welkos SL. Recent advances in the development of an improved human anthrax vaccine. Eur J Epidemiol 1988; 4:12–419.
18. Ivins BE, Welkos SL. Cloning and expression of the *Bacillus anthracis* protective antigen gene in *Bacillus subtilis*. Infect Immun 1986; 54:537–542.
19. Ivins BE, et al. Immunization against anthrax with aromatic compound-dependent (Aro-) mutants of *Bacillus anthracis* and with recombinant strains of *Bacillus subtilis* that produce anthrax protective antigen. Infect Immun 1990; 58:303–308.
20. Ivins B, et al. Experimental anthrax vaccines: efficacy of adjuvants combined with protective antigen against an aerosol *Bacillus anthracis* spore challenge in guinea pigs. Vaccine 1995; 13:1779–1784.
21. Gu ML, et al. Protection against anthrax toxin by vaccination with a DNA plasmid encoding anthrax protective antigen. Vaccine 1999; 17:340–344.
22. Baillie L. The development of new vaccines against *Bacillus anthracis*. J Appl Microbiol 2001; 91:609–613.
23. Fenner F, Henderson DA, Arita I, Jezek Z, Ladnyi ID, eds. (1988). Smallpox and Its Eradication. Geneva, Switzerland: World Health Organization, 1988:581–583.
24. LeDuc JW, Becher J. Current status of smallpox vaccine. [Letter]. Emerg Infect Dis 1999; 5:593–594.
25. Centers for Disease Control. Vaccinia (smallpox) vaccine. Recommendations of the Advisory Committee of Immunization Practices (ACIP), 2001. MMWR Morb Mortal Wkly Rep 2001; 50(RR-10):1–25.
26. Frey SE, et al. Dose-related effects of smallpox vaccine. N Engl J Med 2002; 346:1275–1280.
27. Frey SE, et al. Clinical responses to undiluted and diluted smallpox vaccine. N Engl J Med 2002; 346:1265–1274.
28. McClain DJ, et al. Immunologic responses to vaccinia vaccines administered by different parenteral routes. J Infect Dis 1997; 175:756–763.
29. Weiss R. Smallpox vaccine turns up. Wash Post, March 28, 2002, A01.
30. Haffkine WM. Remarks on the plague prophylactic fluid. Br Med J 1897; 1:1461.
31. Meyer KF, et al. Plague immunization: I. Past and present trends. J Infect Dis 1974; 29(suppl):S13–S18.
32. Reports of US Army Medical Research Team. Walter Reed Army Institute of Research, Saigon, Vietnam, 1963–1971.
33. Cavanaugh DC, et al. Some observations on the current plague outbreak in the Republic of Vietnam. Am J Public Health 1968; 58:742–752.
34. Cavanaugh DC, et al. Plague immunization V. Indirect evidence for the efficacy of plague vaccine. J Infect Dis 1974; 129(suppl):S37–S40.
35. Centers for Disease Control and Prevention. Prevention of plague: recommendations of the advisory committee on immnization practices. MMWR Morb Mortal Wkly Rep 1996; 45(RR-14):1–15.
36. Williams JE, Cavanaugh DC. Measuring the efficacy of vaccination in affording protection against plague. Bull WHO 1979; 57:309–313.
37. Marshall JD Jr, et al. Plague immunization: II. Relation of adverse clinical reactions to multiple immunizations with killed vaccine. J Infect Dis 1974; 129(suppl):S19–S25.
38. Bartelloni PJ, et al. Clinical and serological responses to Plague Vaccine, USP. Mil Med 1973; 138:720–722.
39. Butler T. Plague and Other Yersinia Infections. New York: Plenum, 1983:205.
40. Chen TH, et al. Immunity in plague: protection of the vervet (*cercopithecus aethiops*) against pneumonic plague by the oral administration of live attenuated *Yersinis pestis*. J Infect Dis 1977; 135:720–722.
41. Russell P, et al. A comparison of plague vaccine, USP and EV76 vaccine induced protection against *Yersinia pestis* in a murine model. Vaccine 1995; 13:1551–1556.
42. Williamson ED. Plague vaccine research and development. J Appl Microbiol 2001; 91:606–608.

43. Friedlander AM, et al. Relationship between virulence and immunity as revealed in recent studies of the F1 capsule of *Yersinia pestis*. Clin Infect Dis 1995; 21(suppl 2):S178–S181.

44. Williamson ED, et al. A single dose subunit vaccine protects against pneumonic plague. Vaccine 2000; 19:566–571.

45. McCrumb FR. Aerosol infection of man with *Pasteurella tularensis*. Bacteriol Rev 1961; 25:262–267.

46. Saslaw S, et al. Tularemia vaccine study: II. Respiratory challenge. Arch Intern Med 1961; 107:134–146.

47. Sandstrom G. The tularemia vaccine. J Chem Tech Biotechnol 1994; 59:315–320.

48. Waag DM, et al. Cell-mediated and humoral immune response induced by scarification vaccination of human volunteers with a new lot of the live vaccine strain of *Francisella tularensis*. J Clin Microbiol 1992; 30:2256–2264.

49. Clayton MA, et al. Protective vaccination with a recombinant fragment of *Clostridium botulinum* neurotoxin serotype A expressed from a synthetic gene in *Escherichia coli*. Infect Immun 1995; 63:2738–2742.

50. Lee JS, et al. Candidate vaccine against botulinum neurotoxin serotype A derived from a Venezuelan equine encephalitis virus vector system. Infect Immun 2001; 69:5709–5715.

51. Byrne MP, Smith LA. Development of vaccines for prevention of botulism. Biochemie 2000; 82:955–966.

52. Young EJ. An overview of human brucellosis. Clin Infect Dis 1995; 21:283–290.

53. Roux J. Brucella vaccines in humans. In: Madkour MM, ed. Brucellosis. London: Butterworths, 1989:244–249.

54. Spink WW, et al. Immunization with viable *Brucella* organisms. Bull WHO 1962; 26:409–419.

55. Centers for Disease Control and Prevention. Human exposure to *Brucella abortus* strain RB51—Kansas, 1997. MMWR Morb Mortal Wkly Rep 1998; 47:172–175.

56. Vershilova PA, et al. Experimental study of *Brucella* chemical vaccine. Dev Biol Stand 1984; 56:553–554.

57. Roux J. La vacination humaine contre les brucelloses. Bull Acad Natl Med 1986; 170:289–292.

58. VanDeVerg LL, et al. Outer membrane protein of *Neisseria meningitidis* as a mucosal adjuvant for lipopolysaccharide of *Brucella melitensis* in mouse and guinea pig intranasal immunization models. Infect Immun 1996; 64:5263–5268.

59. Smadel JE, et al. Vaccination against Q fever. Am J Hyg 1948; 47:71–81.

60. Ormsbee RA, Marmion BP. Prevention of *Coxiella burnetii* infection: vaccines and guidelines for those at risk. In: Marrie TJ, ed. Q-Fever, Volume I: The Disease. Boca Raton, FL: CRC Press, 1990:225–248.

61. Stoker MGP. Q fever down the drain. Brit Med J 1957; 1: 425–427.

62. Marmion BP, et al. Vaccine prophylaxis of abattoir-associated Q fever. Lancet 1984; 2:1411–1414.

63. Waag DM, et al. Comparative efficacy of a *Coxiella burnetii* chloroform:methanol residue (CMR) vaccine and a licensed cellular vaccine (Q-Vax) in rodents challenged by aerosol. Vaccine 1997; 15:1779–1789.

64. Fries LF, et al. Safety and immunogenicity in human volunteers of a chloroform–methanol residue vaccine for Q-fever. Infect Immun 1993; 61:1251–1258.

65. McKinney RW. Inactivated and live VEE vaccines—a review. Proceedings of the Workshop Symposium on Venezuelan encephalitis. PAHO, 1972:369–389.

66. Berge TO, et al. Attenuation of Venezuelan equine encephalomyelitis virus by in vitro cultivation in guinea pig heart cells. Am J Hyg 1961; 73:209–218.

67. Pittman PR, et al. Long-term duration of detectable neutralizing antibodies after administration of live-attenuated VEE vaccine and following booster vaccination with inactivated VEE vaccine. Vaccine 1996; 14:337–343.

68. Edelman R, et al. Evaluation in humans of a new, inactivated vaccine for Venezuelan equine encephalitis virus (C-84). J Infect Dis 1979; 140:708–715.

69. Jahrling PB, Stephenson EH. Protective efficacies of live-attenuated and formaldehyde-inactivated Venezuelan equine encephalitis virus vaccines against aerosol challenge in hamsters. J Clin Microbiol 1984; 19:429–431.

70. Engler RJM, et al. Venezuelan equine encephalitis-specific immunoglobulin responses: live attenuated TC 83 versus inactivated C-84 vaccine. J Med Virol 1992; 38:305–310.

71. Davis NL, et al. Attenuated mutants of Venezuelan equine encephalitis virus containing lethal mutations in the PE2 cleavage signal combined with a second-site suppressor mutation in E1. Virology 1995; 215:102–110.

72. Greenway TE, et al. Enhancement of protective immune responses to Venezuelan equine encephalitis (VEE) virus with microencapsulated vaccine. Vaccine 1995; 13:1411–1420.

73. Pushko P, et al. Replicon–helper systems from attenuated Venezuelan equine encephalitis virus: expression of heterologous genes in vitro an immunization against heterologous pathogens in vivo. Virology 1997; 239:389–401.

74. Hevey M, et al. Marburg virus vaccines based upon alphavirus replicons protect guinea pigs and non-human primates. Virology 1998; 251:28–37.

75. Leiden JM. Gene therapy—promises, pitfalls, and prognosis. N Engl J Med 1995; 333:871–873.

76. Goldfield M, et al. The 1959 outbreak of eastern encephalitis in New Jersey: V. The inapparent infection:disease ratio. Am J Epidemiol 1968; 87:32–38.

77. Reeves WC, Hammon WM. Epidemiology of the arthropod-borne viral encephalitides in Kern County, California, 1943–52. Univ Calif Pub Health 1962; 4:257.

78. Edelman R, et al. Phase II safety and immunogenicity study of live chikungunya virus vaccine TSI-GSD-218. Am J Trop Med Hyg 2000; 62:681–685.

79. Ulrich RG, et al. Staphylococcal enterotoxin B and related pyrogenic toxins. In: Sidell FR, Takafuji ET, Franz DR, eds. Medical Aspects of Chemical and Biological Warfare. Washington: Borden Institute, 1997:621–630.

80. Tseng J, et al. Humoral immunity to aerosolized staphylococcal enterotoxin B (SEB), a superantigen, in monkeys vaccinated with SEB toxoid-containing microspheres. Infect Immun 1995; 63:2880–2885.

81. Bavari S, et al. Engineered bacterial superantigen vaccines. Vaccines 96. Cold Spring Harbor, NY: Cold Spring Harbor Press, 1996:135–141.

82. Stiles BG, et al. Mucosal vaccination with recombinantly attenuated staphylococcal enterotoxin B and protection in a murine model. Infect Immun 2001; 69:2031–2036.

83. Livingstone NC, Douglass JDJ. CBW: The Poor Man's Atom Bomb. Cambridge MA: Institute for Foreign Policy Analysis, 1984.

84. Hewetson JF, et al. Protection of mice from inhaled ricin by vaccination with formalinized ricin toxoid abstract. Toxicon 1993; 31:138–139.

85. Unpublished data, US Army Medical Research Institute of Infectious Diseases.

86. Yan C, et al. Dependence of ricin toxoid vaccine efficacy on the structure of poly(lactide-co-glycolide) microparticle carriers. Vaccine 1995; 13:645–651.

87. Kende M, et al. Oral immunization of mice with ricin toxoid vaccine encapsulated in olymeric microspheres against aerosol challenge. Vaccine 2002; 20:1681–1691.

88. Griffiths GD, et al. Liposomally-encapsulated ricin toxoid vaccine delivered intratracheally elicits a good immune response and protects against a lethal pulmonary dose of ricin toxin. Vaccine 1997; 15:1933–1939.

89. White CS, et al. Repeated immunization: possible adverse

effects: reevaluation of human subjects at 25 years. Ann Intern Med 1974; 81:594–600.

90. Pittman PR, et al. Antibody response to a delayed booster dose of anthrax vaccine and botulinum toxoid. Vaccine 2002; 20:2107–2115.

91. Canadian Forces Medical Group. Letter from Assistant Chief of Staff Operations to Canadian Clinical Trials and Special Access Programme, 15 October 1999.

92. Centers for Disease Control. Surveillance for adverse events associated with anthrax vaccination—US Department of Defense, 1998–2000. MMWR Morb Mortal Wkly Rep 2000; 49:341–345.

93. Gunzenhauser JD, et al. Acute side effects of anthrax vaccine in ROTC cadets participating in advanced camp, Fort Lewis, 2000. Surveill Med Rep Monthly 2001; 7:9–11.

94. Rehme PA, et al. Ambulatory medical visits among anthrax-vaccinated and unvaccinated personnel after return from southwest Asia. Mil Med 2002; 167:205–210.

95. Wiesen AR, Littell CT. Relationship between prepregnancy anthrax vaccination and pregnancy and birth outcomes among US Army women. J Am Med Assoc 2002;2871556–1560.

96. Anthrax Vaccine Immunization Program Agency. Detailed safety review of anthrax vaccine adsorbed. 15 November 2001. Accessed at http://www.anthrax.osd.mil/Site_Files/articles/INDEXclinical/safety_reviews.htm.

89

A Primer on Large-Scale Manufacture of Modern Vaccines

Julie B. Milstien
University of Maryland School of Medicine, Baltimore, Maryland, U.S.A.

Jean Stéphenne
GSK Biologicals, Rixensart, Belgium

Lance Gordon
VaxGen, Brisbane, California, U.S.A.

I. DIFFERENT VACCINE TYPES AND THEIR MAJOR PRODUCTION STEPS

The major vaccines licensed and used in the United States, by manufacturer, and their primary manufacturing technology are shown in Appendix A. Similar vaccines are on the market in many other countries. Table 1 divides the most commonly used vaccines into product classes and summarizes the basic techniques involved in their bulk manufacture, with examples of each. Section II outlines the basic production process and defines in more detail what is involved in each of these steps.

II. MANUFACTURING PHASES AND CRITICAL ISSUES FOR EACH

The access to manufacturing capacity includes:

- The receipt and control of raw materials to be used in the production process
- The production of purified bulk antigen from various expression systems or directly from live, possibly attenuated strains of the agents
- Aseptic filling and final packaging of stable proteins or live infectious agents
- Analytical capacity to evaluate the products using standard biochemical or physiochemical methods or specialized biological tests
- Appropriate storage and distribution

These steps will be considered in more detail below. The entire process may take from 1 to 2 years to manufacture and release a vaccine [1], although production can be fast-tracked, for example, for biodefense products or the annual formulation of influenza vaccines. This is illustrated in Figure 1. Production flowcharts to illustrate the process for oral polio vaccine and for *Haemophilus influenzae* type b conjugate vaccine (tetanus conjugate) are included in Appendix B.

A. Raw Materials

All raw materials must come from reliable sources and be shown to meet specifications. Most manufacturers use supplier qualification coupled with some quarantine release tests to assure the quality of the raw materials. Raw materials must be kept under quarantine until released from the Quality Control department. However, the primary raw materials for biological products, seeds, cells, and biological fluids, are subject to intense documentation and testing measures, which will be covered more thoroughly in Section II.B. Recently, there has been particular concern with some specific raw materials commonly used for vaccine production.

- Bovine material, most commonly fetal calf serum, is used in growth media for most cell culture-produced viral vaccines. To avoid the potential risk of transmission of bovine spongiform encephalopathy (BSE), any bovine materials must be sourced from geographic locations shown to be BSE-free and from parts of the animal shown to be at low risk for transmitting BSE. For new vaccines, avoiding bovine material is an objective, and serum-free media have now been developed.
- Human albumin has been used in formulating many vaccines, but the trend is to replace it with other products or to eliminate it.

Table 1 Process of Bulk Manufacture for Selected Vaccine Types

Vaccine type	Process	Examples
Attenuated microbial cells	Growth and purification of microbial cells adapted or engineered to delete pathogenicity, retaining immunogenicity. Steps include fermentation and purification	BCG, oral typhoid, oral cholera
Killed microbial cells	Growth, inactivation, and purification of microbial cells. Steps include fermentation, inactivation, and purification	Whole cell pertussis, anthrax, cholera/typhoid
Live attenuated viruses	Growth of cells (from cell banks of continuous cells or primary cells from animal/egg tissue), infection with attenuated virus, isolation, and purification of virus. Cells are propagated in bioreactors, roller bottles, hollow fiber, cell cubes, flasks, or microcarrier culture with various types of feeding. The medium is generally entirely synthetic but may contain blood proteins to enhance growth. Cells are infected with the vaccine virus; removal of cell or cell debris by centrifugation or ultrafiltration methodology; purification of virus if required, concentration	Yellow fever, measles–mumps–rubella, OPV, varicella
Killed viruses	Growth of cells (from cell banks of continuous cells or primary cells from animal/egg tissue), infection with virus, isolation, inactivation, and purification of virus. Cells are propagated in bioreactors, roller bottles, hollow fiber, cell cubes, flasks, or microcarrier culture with various types of feeding. The medium is generally entirely synthetic, but may contain blood proteins to enhance growth. Cells are infected with the vaccine virus; removal of cell or cell debris by centrifugation or ultrafiltration methodology; purification of virus if required, concentration; inactivation may occur before or after purification, testing for inactivation	IPV, rabies, hepatitis A, Japanese encephalitis B, influenza
Purified polysaccharides	Growth of bacterial culture, extraction, and purification of capsular polysaccharides by centrifugation or filtration; chemical extraction and, in some cases, chromatography; chemical characterization of the polysaccharide; concentration and, in some cases, drying of bulk	Meningitis polysaccharide (ACW135Y), pneumococcal polysaccharides
Conjugated polysaccharides	Growth of bacterial culture, extraction, and purification of capsular polysaccharides, preparation and purification of carrier protein. Chemical modification of polysaccharide; linker if required; chemical processing of carrier if required; conjugation; separation of conjugated from unconjugated species by chromatography; concentration of bulk conjugate if required	Meningitis C, Hib conjugate, pneumococcal 7-valent conjugate
Purified protein, excreted or cell-associated	Growth of bacteria, yeast, or cell culture where cells are expressing a recombinant protein, cell lysis (for cell-associated proteins), isolation and purification of the protein by ultrafiltration methodology; protein purification by chromatography, concentration, buffer exchange, sterile filtration	Hepatitis B (recombinant or plasma-derived), bacterial toxoids, acellular pertussis, split influenza
Live microbial vector	Fermentation in defined media; recovery of whole microbial cells by centrifugation/washing or ultrafiltration methodology	BCG-vectored HIV, Salmonella vectors
Live viral vectors	Growth of cells, infection with genetically engineered replicating nonpathogenic viruses containing added gene of interest, isolation, and purification of virus. Cell culturing in bioreactors, roller bottles, hollow fiber, cell cubes, flasks, or microcarrier culture with various types of feeding; virus infection; cell controls; removal of cell or cell debris by centrifugation or ultrafiltration methodology; purification of virus if required	MVA, canary pox, adeno, AAV vectors for an assortment of antigens
DNA vaccine	Extraction and purification of plasmid DNA from bacterial cells containing desired gene in the plasmid. Fermentation in defined media; recovery of whole microbial cells by centrifugation/washing or ultrafiltration methodology; cell lysis and removal of cell debris (filtration, centrifugation, or expanded bed chromatography); removal of host impurities, RNA, genomic DNA, proteins and endotoxins (salting out, PEG precipitation); concentration (ultrafiltration methodology, PEG precipitation); purification of plasmid DNA by IEC and/or SEC; concentration and buffer exchange; sterile filtration of final bulk	HIV candidates in DNA plasmids, other candidates

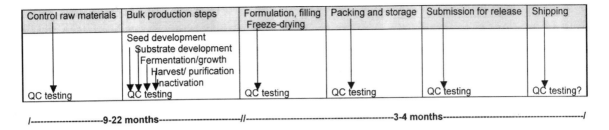

Control raw materials	Bulk production steps	Formulation, filling Freeze-drying	Packing and storage	Submission for release	Shipping
	Seed development Substrate development Fermentation/growth Harvest/ purification Inactivation				
QC testing	QC testing	QC testing	QC testing	QC testing	QC testing?

/----------------------9-22 months-----------------------//--3-4 months--/

Figure 1 Time frames for major bulk production steps.

- Manufacturers are seeking substitutes for aluminum salts used as adjuvants because of possible injection site reactions, but aluminum remains the best-documented adjuvant.
- The most commonly used preservative, thimerosal, contains mercury, and its use has been required to be minimized in many countries, making the manufacture of multidose vials of vaccine impossible in those countries. Phenoxyethanol is the second preservative widely used having bacteriocidal or bacteriostatic properties, but is less potent than thimerosal.

B. Bulk Manufacture

Production should occur in dedicated laboratory suites as per current Good Manufacturing Practices (cGMP) guidelines. It is recommended that laboratory areas for generating "clean" (prior to infection with the seed vaccine virus) cultures be segregated from production areas; this can be accomplished by physical barriers and pressurized air locks to prevent cross-contamination. Segregation of upstream (production) and downstream (purification) areas, although recommended, may not be always practical given the design and cost considerations. Release of viruses or bacteria into the environment is a concern for both air and effluents.

1. Viral Seed Preparation

Master Viral Banks (MVB) are generally used to initiate manufacture of viral vaccines and viral vectors. Virus seed stocks generated by amplifying the virus/vector in a compatible cell line are typically used to generate the MVB. The use of plaque-purified seed virus stocks aids in reducing the number of defective viral particles in the MVB.

2. Bacterial Fermentation

Fermentation generally refers to the process of growing bacteria in large-volume closed systems. In some cases, fermentation technology has been used for eukaryotic cell culture. This will be covered in Section II.B.3. To develop vaccines based on bacteria, the principle of a Master Seed Bank is used as well. The bacterial seed is obtained with a well-documented history and is stored in an appropriate manner. To initiate culture, aliquots of the bacteria are first grown in a small volume, and the culture is incubated at in-

creasingly larger volumes until the volume of the final production scale fermenter is reached. Modern fermenters control and document environmental variables such as temperature, oxygen pressure, and pH, enabling standardized production methods to be used. Because these systems are computer-driven, their validation is not trivial.

3. Cell Culture

The history of cell lines should include good documentation of their origin and their passage histories. This documentation should include the number of passages since origination, storage, and cell culture conditions. A Master Cell Bank (MCB) is produced according to cGMP guidelines and consists of frozen vials of a cell line (generally kept in liquid nitrogen) manufactured at as low a passage number as reasonably possible. Continuous cell lines are usually cloned from a single cell before a MCB is generated to assure purity of the cell line. The term MCB is used to designate stock cultures from which a second set of vials is usually generated; this second set of vials is termed the Working Cell Bank (WCB). The WCB is then extensively tested. Tests on human cell banks include those for microbial contaminants, tumor-igenicity, identification, adventitious and endogenous viruses, and specific viruses. Frozen vials of the cell line chosen for production are used for culture buildup. The cell expansion can occur in standard tissue culture plasticware, shaker/spinner flasks, Roller Bottles, Nunc™ Cell Factories, CellCube™ systems, and, in some cases, even in stirred tank bioreactors. The expansion can progress from tissue culture flasks to 1–10 L spinner cultures and for large-scale production to 50–10,000 L bioreactor systems. Unlike fermentation, mammalian cell culture split ratios range from 1:2 to a maximum of 1:10.

When large-scale production is desired, vials of MCB are used to generate the WCB at the appropriate cell density and at the desired life span of the cell line. Since vials of the WCB are typically used for commercial production, it is recommended that the WCB be generated only after all aspects of cell culture have been worked out and no changes to cell culture medium or inoculation density are expected.

4. Animals and Eggs

When animal systems or eggs (chick or duck embryos) are used, they should be from controlled herds or flocks and should be routinely tested to assure freedom from contaminating microorganisms that could impact the vaccines (specific pathogen-free—SPF).

5. Harvest

The mode and the method of harvest depend on the product being grown. Generally, a synthetic medium different from that used during cell growth is used during virus growth containing no biological or protein products. For lytic viruses, the virus can be intracellular or lysed into the cell culture medium. For viruses secreted into the cell culture medium, rather than harvesting the entire culture, the cell culture supernatant is collected at different time points during production. Perfusion systems where the spent culture supernatant is continuously harvested are popular. Depending on the type of virus, harvest may continue for a few days. Optimization of virus titer is critical during this step.

6. Purification

Once the production culture has been harvested, the antigen typically needs to be concentrated and purified. For extracellular viruses or for bacteria, the product is typically only concentrated using standard techniques such as centrifugation or ultrafiltration and often no purification step is performed. For intracellular viruses, clarification is first performed to separate the cells from the culture medium. This clarification is performed via centrifugation in small-scale systems and ultrafiltration when larger volumes are involved. The cells are then lysed to release the virus. Cell lysis can be achieved by intermittently freezing and thawing, using chemical disruption (with the help of a surfactant) or by mechanical lysis using a microfluidization system or sonication.

For large-scale production systems, the virus can be concentrated using ultrafiltration methods. Several ultrafiltration systems are available such as hollow fiber or plate and frame systems. In some cases, viruses are purified by cesium chloride gradient systems or by column chromatography for larger systems.

In the case of protein or polysaccharide antigens, these must be purified from the appropriate starting material, cell lysate, purified organism, or biological fluid, using column chromatography, ultrafiltration, or centrifugation procedures, as defined above. A sterile filtration step follows to ensure the sterility of the bulk antigen.

7. Inactivation

Inactivation of purified virus or bacterial antigens is generally done chemically using reagents such as formaldehyde or peroxide, combined in some cases with heat. Inactivation parameters must be standardized and validated to ensure that the process completely and consistently inactivates the antigen. A sterile filtration step on the bulk concentrated antigen is generally applicable before or after inactivation.

C. Formulation and Filling

A high level of control is needed to assure a consistent product including the amount of antigen, stabilizers, adjuvants, pH, volume, etc. The acceptable limits of variation in each of these factors are ultimately related to the safety and the efficacy demonstrated in clinical studies. The sterile process must be tightly controlled for these three steps: formulation, filling, and freeze-drying. This is the most sterile part of the entire production process because most vaccines, especially those based on whole organisms or those incorporating adjuvants such as alum, cannot be terminally sterilized, in contrast to the majority of drugs and large-volume parenteral solutions. The length of time that the filling process (for example, over the course of several hours or several days) can continue must be validated. In general, not more than 16 hr are allowed for filling operations in order to clean and prepare the room for the following day.

The definition of a lot, "doses that are at the same risk of contamination," depends on the size of the filling process. For some products, the filled vials are then lyophilized for better long-term stability.

D. Packing

Packaging of a vaccine product may vary depending on the market. All packaging operations must also be under strict control, and the processes must be documented.

E. Testing

It is critical that biological materials used to generate products for human use are properly qualified. Qualification can include testing for identity, presence of any adventitious viruses, microbial contamination, and mycoplasma. Safety assessments are also necessary and routine to demonstrate that the product itself remains safe. This has traditionally been performed by demonstration of lack of reversion of an attenuated virus product to a virulent state or of an inactivated bacteria or toxoid to toxicity. Figure 1 schematically indicates the multiple steps in the production process where testing is done. All tests must be standardized and validated to ensure that the test results actually reflect the presence or absence of the quality being tested for.

F. Submission for Lot Release to Regulatory Authorities

Besides testing and quality assurance procedures being performed by the manufacturer on a lot-by-lot basis, the regulatory authorities must also release the products. In some cases, this is done on bulk products, and, in other cases, on the final container vaccine. The manufacturer must program into the production process the time for lot release by the relevant regulatory authorities before the product can be shipped.

G. Storage and Shipping

Storage and shipping are also subject to documentation and validation. The temperatures, storage, and shipping conditions must be such that the product is stable, and these conditions must be reproducible. Generally, vaccines are stored and shipped using a "cold chain" to maintain temperatures close to or below freezing, depending on the product. Manufacturers often use temperature-monitoring devices to ensure that these temperatures are maintained, and real-time data on the shipping process must be obtained to ensure the integrity of the process. For products that cannot sustain freezing, it is critical to closely monitor the cold chain, as inadvertent freezing can damage the integrity of the vaccine.

III. FACILITIES DESIGN, MAINTENANCE, AND USE

There are two general types of production facilities: pilot lots for the manufacture of clinical trial material and the commercial manufacturing facility for large-scale production. Even if the large-scale production facility is used for the manufacture of clinical trial lots, it is rare that this is done at the same scale as for commercial production. Thus all processes must be established and documented to ensure consistency of the product, and these facilities and operations must all be established, operated, and maintained to assure regulatory compliance and approval of the produced product. Validation at each scale has to be established by preclinical or clinical data, depending on the changes introduced.

One of the critical strategic issues facing any developer of vaccines for human use is how to minimize the risks attendant in scaling up from pilot production to commercial operations. Often, there are technical, procedural, and/or equipment differences between the production of a few hundred or thousand doses to support clinical trials and the tens or hundreds of millions of doses that may be necessary to supply the U.S. or global markets. Some companies have elected to build, equip, and validate facilities capable of commercial-scale manufacture midway through clinical development to minimize the risk of product changes prior to entering time-consuming and expensive Phase 3 field trials. While this strategy may be the most direct and quickest route to achieving license and market launch, it can be financially devastating. Commercial manufacturing facilities can easily cost $100–600 million by the time approval is received. Product failures or even delays in the timing of product approvals can turn this investment into financial ruin. Strategies used to avoid such exposure include the use of pilot manufacturing facilities or contract manufacture organizations. The U.S. Food and Drug Administration (FDA) has provided specific guidance to manufacturers regarding the use of both contract manufacturing arrangements [2] and the use of pilot manufacturing facilities [3]. The use of consistent manufacturing technologies between small- and large-scale facilities and modest (<10-fold) differences in production scale are most probable of success. When larger scale-up strategies are necessary to manage risk or due to resource constraints, the use of consistent technologies is highly desirable. Where differences in product are unavoidable, it may be necessary to do bridging clinical studies to demonstrate that the product from the final commercial manufacturing facility is acceptably consistent with that used in the clinical studies supporting licensure.

For the longer term, investing in new manufacturing equipment or facilities is also not a simple exercise and can take anywhere between 2 years for a new packaging line (studying, ordering, installing, and validating), 5 years for a new facility, and 7 years for a new site, assuming no major complications. In practical terms for the vaccine manufacturer, this means having to take a major financial risk without knowing whether the candidate product will receive regulatory approval and market acceptance. These time and cost elements have become even more critical given the fact that manufacturing capacities have been saturated for the last few years.

As reported in the J.P. Morgan H&Q report "The State of Biologics Manufacturing" [4], the manufacturing capacity for bulk biological products is not projected to meet the demand brought by new product introductions. Due to the long life cycle of approved biologics, and the rapid evolution of manufacturing technologies, there is virtually no churning or turnover of manufacturing capacity for obsolete products into capacity to support new product introductions. The traditional vaccine business used a "one product/one building" approach for capacity into the mid-1980s. However, with the dramatic escalation in facility cost, the long lead time for facility readiness, the introduction of recombinant expression systems for vaccine antigens, and the desired flexibility for late-stage clinical manufacturing and launch plants, a multiproduct concept has evolved and matured. The multiproduct facility concept has allowed for the development of a contract manufacturing organization (CMO) industry to share risk and to provide expertise and flexible capacity to meet short-term needs (see Ref. 2 for FDA guidance on this). The economics for CMOs to establish new capacity has been less supported through growth of the market overall rather than the needs of a single product.

Multinational vaccine companies, smaller biotechnology companies developing vaccines, and even CMOs have looked conservatively at the risk/reward scenario of preinvestment in capacity prior to product approval and balked. Very recently, this has changed as evidenced by the announcements of major new investments by several CMOs, e.g., BioReliance Corporation's investment in larger-scale viral therapeutic manufacture (including vaccines), DSM Biologics's announced commitment to invest in engineering a large-scale expansion in Quebec, Cambrex's announcement to invest $18,000,000 in capacity expansion for biological product contract production, VaxGen, Inc.'s construction of a manufacturing facility in California, and announcement of a significant strategic partnership for commissioning of a large-scale (47,000 L) contract biological production facility in South Korea.

Access to manufacturing capacity thus poses a gap that may place timely approval of products at risk. The manufacturing of more traditional vaccines such as the anthrax vaccine by BioPort has demonstrated the continuing challenges to meet ever-stricter regulatory standards, with challenges to financial return and a very limited capability for immediate response to a dramatic increase in market demand. Therefore the development of new vaccines not only requires good science, efficient development, and application of current technologies, but also the long-term commitment to invest in the physical capacity to deliver these new products to a healthcare system in need of cost-effective preventative medicines.

IV. BASIC COMPONENTS OF GOOD MANUFACTURING PRACTICE

Compliance with the principles and guidelines of Good Manufacturing Practice (GMP) is a statutory requirement. The Good Manufacturing Practice regulations govern that part of quality assurance that ensures medicinal products are consistently produced and controlled to the quality standards appropriate to their intended use. Simply stated, production operations must follow clearly defined procedures. The general aspects of GMP are covered in more detail below. In addition, GMP requires evidence of prevention of cross-contamination in production, the performance of validation studies supporting the facilities, systems, processes, and equipment, control of starting materials, control of packaging materials, and handling of finished products. All aspects of these measures and methods of control are specifically defined by local regulations.

It is the primary responsibility of the Regulatory Affairs/Quality Assurance department in a manufacturing facility to ensure that all manufacturing operations performed for clinical production of human vaccines are in compliance with current GMP guidelines and follow all regulatory and safety procedures. Some specific responsibilities of this department could include review of standard operating procedures (SOPs) and batch/production records, investigation into any procedural or operational error and deviations from SOPs and/or batch/production records, system inspections/audits, validation of facilities, equipment, and testing procedures, and regular cGMP training to personnel.

A. Facilities

Facility design should provide for unidirectional flow of materials, product, and personnel. Production suites should be on separate heat, vacuum, and air conditioning (HVAC) systems that provide classified, preferably HEPA-filtered air. Airflows need to be balanced within the production areas to maintain the classification. There should be designated "clean" corridors for entry into production areas. Personnel are then made to gown in pressurized entry air locks before accessing the production suites. Exit from production areas should also be through dedicated air locks, where degowning can occur prior to exiting to the return corridor. If possible, separate personnel and equipment air locks should provide access to the production areas. Standard operating procedures should describe the use of all facilities, and all systems must be validated to ensure that they function to specifications. Containment of microorganisms must also be achieved to avoid their release into the environment. Biological wastes require special equipment for decontamination prior to release.

B. Equipment

Equipment used in production should be installed, operated, and maintained as per cGMP guidelines. Where appropriate, Installation/Operational/Performance Qualification Protocols (IQ/OQ/PQ), calibration, and validation studies need to be designed and executed. As appropriate, all equipment should be maintained on current calibration and preventive maintenance scheduled and performed as recommended by the manufacturers.

C. Documentation

All operations in GMP manufacturing whether dealing with facility, equipment, material usage, manufacturing, or product release have to be performed as outlined in the SOPs. This ensures that the manufacture of clinical material is performed in strict accordance with established manufacturing, regulatory, and safety procedures. Any deviation from SOPs has to be reported and its effect on the clinical product has to be documented. Standard operating procedures are critical documents and usually maintained by Document Control, a separate functioning department. Document Control is usually responsible for organizing, distributing, and revising SOPs as appropriate. Each SOP is uniquely identified and usually stored in both electronic and paper formats.

Production or batch records are used to document all manufacturing operations that are performed in the production of human vaccines. These records are established in accordance with appropriate SOPs and are distributed and controlled by the Document Control Department. Any deviations from manufacturing operations outlined in the SOPs are documented in the appropriate batch records. Batch records are especially important when it becomes necessary to revisit the manufacturing operations if some inconsistency or deficiency is discovered in the clinical product.

Validation is another important function performed by the Quality Assurance group in a manufacturing facility. Validation is the demonstration that a piece of equipment, process, or test performs according to specification so that the data or the products generated are credible. Validation protocols must be maintained on file as part of the documented record of a production process. Process and quality control validation are becoming more important to confirm the robustness of the methods employed. For a biological product, consistent quality is ensured by strict process application during manufacturing operations.

D. Materials Receipt and Quarantine

The primary responsibility of the Materials Management Group is to ensure that all materials (raw, in-process, and final) are properly received, uniquely identified, stored, released, documented, and inventoried. Generally, incoming products are released by the Quality Control Department from quarantine once tested or the accompanying documentation is reviewed. Standard operating procedures will describe how the receipt and quarantine process is implemented.

E. Animal House and Laboratory Testing

The Quality Control group is responsible for environmental monitoring and testing of all materials (raw, in-process, and final). Testing is performed before release to manufacturing and before release of final product. Environmental monitoring includes monitoring of plant water systems, depending on whether any or all of the following sources—city water, potable water, water for injection, etc.—are used, tracking and trending particulates in manufacturing areas, and microbial identification of environmental isolates. The animal house is for holding and, in some cases, breeding of animals used for test purposes or in cases where vaccines are produced in animal tissues (for example, Japanese Encephalitis B vaccine produced in suckling mouse brain). The animal house is subject to similar kinds of environmental monitoring and control, as well as restricted access, as the production areas. All work done in the animal house and in the quality control laboratories is covered by SOPs, and all tests must be validated.

F. Human Resources

cGMP requirements dictate that personnel performing manufacturing operations are adequately qualified and trained. Apart from having to pass physical and laboratory examinations, newly hired personnel are required to undergo intensive training in operational techniques, personal and product hygiene, before being cleared for work. These training sessions are required to be repeated on an annual or semi-annual basis. The Manufacturing department should be organized to have an adequate number of trained and qualified personnel to execute all GMP operations satisfactorily.

V. STEPS IN PRODUCT LICENSURE

For timing for product licensure, 10 years is now considered as a minimum as shown in Figure 2. In the United States, vaccines are regulated as biological products. A single set of basic regulatory approval criteria applies to vaccines, regardless of the technology used to produce the vaccine (see Ref. 5). General regulations for product manufacture are covered in the parts of the U.S. Code of Federal Regulations (CFR), and other guidelines and points to consider are tabulated in Appendix C. Specific products are not covered by guidelines, but rather the license application contains the production and testing methods that will be in use. Similar procedures are in use in other parts of the world, and Appendix C summarizes some of the relevant documentation.

A. Facilities License

In many countries, the production facility is approved as well as the product as part of the licensing process. Until recently, the United States separately licensed the vaccine (PLA or Product License Application) and the production facility in which it was manufactured (ELA or Establishment License Application). In the United States, these are now combined in a Biologics License Application (BLA). In either case, the proposed manufacturing facility undergoes a prelicensing inspection by experts in GMP and in the particular type of product to be produced, which reviews the entire production process as well as the equipment, utility (HVAC) systems, human resources, and production records of specific batches or lots of product.

B. Product License

When a potential candidate vaccine is ready to move toward the licensing pathway, the process for manufacturing the vaccine at a research scale or for clinical study must be developed into a process that is appropriate for the manufacture of large-scale commercial material (scale-up). This includes all steps of bulk production, purification, and testing. Thus all steps in the process as well as the facility must be validated, demonstrating consistency of manufacture from lot to lot. The licensing file will contain all the information related to the production of the product including documentation, a preclinical package that includes especially data on safety testing in animals, as well as results of all other quality control tests, and documentation of the consistency of production. This file is used as a basis for approval of testing in humans. All human trial results, along with the above information, comprise the license application file.

C. Phases of Clinical Trials

The clinical development of vaccines is generally carried out in four phases. Initial Phase 1 studies are intended to evaluate safety and are generally performed in a small number of healthy adults; Phase 2 studies usually include dose-ranging studies and may provide an early indication of efficacy. On the basis of Phase 1 and 2 trials, the manufacturer might choose to scale-up the production facility in preparation for Phase 3 trials, which provide the pivotal efficacy and safety data that are required for licensure. Phase 1 and 2 studies should provide the support for product dose and study the immune response and biological activity, while Phase 3 studies are larger trials to establish efficacy in the target population at the expected dose range and formula-

Discovery and preclinical	Clinical study and consistency lots			File review	
	Phase 1	Phase 2	Phase 3		File review
			Lot preparation phase 3		
				File preparation	
	1-1.5 years	1-1.5 years	0.5-1.5 years	1 year	
2.5 years	6-8 years				2 years

Figure 2 Vaccine development phases and time frames (adapted from Ref. 1).

tion. Serological correlates of efficacy are developed, if possible, in this phase, which may include hundreds to tens of thousands of subjects. Where possible, Phase 3 trials should be randomized, double-blinded, and placebo-controlled. Illustrative time frames are indicated in Figure 2.

D. Postlicensure Activities

Postlicensing, the manufacturer is still required to work with the regulatory authority in a number of areas to continue to assure the safety, potency, and consistent quality of the product. This may include monitoring of the product by lot release testing and monitoring of the production facility through periodic facility inspections, which continue as long as the manufacturer holds the license to the product. Phase 4 studies are generally large-scale postmarketing studies conducted to obtain additional data on adverse events focusing primarily on events that may occur at a very low frequency. In addition, significant adverse events occurring in routine use of the product must be reported to the regulatory authority and must be analyzed to determine if they are an indication of compromised product safety. Finally, any changes to the production of the product must be covered by SOPs and validation documentation and must be reported to the regulatory authority. Significant changes must be approved prior to their implementation. Variations may be classified into the following three categories:

- Type IA variations that for biologicals are limited to administrative modifications. These variations are submitted as notifications and are not reviewed by the authority.
- Type IB, considered as minor variations that do not modify the quality, safety, and efficacy of the product. The authority starts a 30-day evaluation and, in practice, the timescale for such variations lies between 35 and 95 days.
- Type II, major variations that require extensive data submission. For biologicals, any modification to the manufacturing process, for example, falls within this category. In practice, the approval of Type II variations is granted after 155–250 days.
- In addition to modifications within the scope of these three types, major changes to the product (e.g., new Master Cell Bank, additional dosage forms) require a full registration dossier to be submitted. The assessment may then take up to 1 year.

VI. THE SPECIAL CASE OF COMBINATION VACCINES

Combination vaccines, many of which are based on additions to the diphtheria, tetanus, and pertussis (DTP) combination, are becoming very popular as a means to reduce

injections and to minimize delivery issues even if they may be more expensive than the separate products [6]. They are being used in both the industrialized world and the developing countries, in both public and private sectors, and are being produced by a range of manufacturers, both multinational and local. They present a special issue in manufacture, as the producer must make and control up to seven antigens at the same time and have them ready for formulation: any delay in any of the components impacts the final product. Allocation issues can become very important and often antigens can become limiting.

Combination vaccines pose special issues in GMP compliance as the new use of an established antigen will require a new review of its manufacture and control protocols that may no longer meet licensing requirements. Often, each antigen must be relicensed for use in the production of the combination product, and the relicense may require renovation of production facilities or changes in process. Combination vaccines also pose special issues in regulation because of the complications to quality control of each component while in combination and the difficulties of attributing adverse events to an individual component. Finally, if serological correlates of immunity do not exist, the combination may need extensive clinical efficacy trials for licensing.

VII. THE FUTURE

Given the experience of the past, it is clear that the future will hold new technological developments for vaccine production in the form of new vaccine types, such as multiple antigen peptide vaccines, virus-like particles, and transgenic plant vaccines, and new delivery platforms, including aerosol and transcutaneous delivery systems. All of these innovations will bring with them the need for assuring their safety and consistency; thus process and testing validation criteria and cGMP compliance will become even more demanding.

REFERENCES

1. Greco M. Development and supply of vaccines: an industry perspective. In: Levine MM, Kaper JB, Rappuoli R, Liu M, Good M, eds. New Generation Vaccines. 3d ed. 2004. Chapter 7, 75–87.
2. http://www.fda.gov/cber/gdlns/coopmfr.htm.
3. http://www.fda.gov/cber/gdlns/pilot.txt.
4. Molowa David P. The State of Biologics Manufacturing. New York: JP Morgan H&Q, March 12, 2001.
5. Baylor N, et al. The role of the Food and Drug Administration in vaccine testing and licensure. In: Levine MM, Kaper JB, Rappuoli R, Liu M, Good M, eds. New Generation Vaccines. 3d ed. 2004. Chapter 11, 117–125.
6. Milstien J, et al. Issues in selection of DTwP-based combination vaccines. Vaccine 2003; 21:1658–1664.
7. http://www.who.int/vaccines-documents.
8. http://www.who.int/biologicals/Guidelines/Vaccines.htm.
9. http://www.ich.org/ich5q.html#Correction%202.
10. http://www.emea.eu.int.

Appendix A Vaccines Licensed by the U.S. Center for Biologics Evaluation and Research and Marketed in the United States

Manufacturer of record	Produce description	Primary manufacturing technology
Aventis Pasteur Inc.	Diphtheria and tetanus toxoids and acellular pertussis vaccines	Bacterial fermentation, extracted, toxoided proteins
	Influenza virus vaccine	Killed virus grown in embryonated eggs
	Meningococcal polysaccharide vaccines (ACYW135)	Bacterial fermentation, extracted capsular polysaccharide
	Yellow fever vaccine	Live virus grown in embryonated eggs
	Haemophilus influenzae type b conjugate vaccine	Bacterial fermentation, protein–polysaccharide conjugate
	Poliovirus vaccine inactivated	Killed virus grown in mammalian cell culture
	Rabies vaccine	Killed virus grown in mammalian cell culture
	Typhoid Vi polysaccharide vaccine	Bacterial fermentation, extracted capsular polysaccharide
Merck and Co., Inc.	Haemophilus influenzae type b conjugate vaccine	Bacterial fermentation, protein–polysaccharide conjugate
	Hepatitis A vaccine inactivated	Killed virus grown in mammalian cell culture
	Hepatitis B vaccine (recombinant)	Recombinant protein expressed in yeast
	Measles, mumps, and rubella live virus vaccines	Avian/avian/mammalian cell culture
	23-Valent pneumococcal polysaccharide vaccine	Bacterial fermentation, extracted capsular polysaccharide
	Varicella virus vaccine live	Virus grown in mammalian cell culture
Wyeth Pharmaceuticals	*Haemophilus influenzae* type b conjugate vaccine	Bacterial fermentation, protein–polysaccharide conjugate
	Influenza virus vaccine	Killed virus grown in embryonated eggs
	7-Valent pneumococcal conjugate vaccine	Bacterial fermentation, protein–polysaccharide conjugate
	23-Valent pneumococcal polysaccharide vaccine	Bacterial fermentation, extracted capsular polysaccharide
GlaxoSmithKline Biologicals	Diphtheria and tetanus toxoids and acellular pertussis vaccines	Bacterial fermentation (pathogenic)
	Hepatitis A vaccine inactivated	Killed virus grown in mammalian cell culture
	Hepatitis B vaccine (recombinant)	Recombinant protein expressed in yeast
	Hepatitis A + B	Hepatitis A and B vaccines combined (see above)
	DTaP-IPV-Hepatitis B	Combination of products of bacterial fermentation (inactivated), killed virus, and recombinant proteins
PowderJect Pharmaceuticals Plc	Influenza virus vaccine	Killed virus grown in embryonated eggs
Chiron Corporation	Rabies vaccine	Killed virus grown in avian cell culture
University of Massachusetts Biologic Laboratory	Tetanus and diphtheria toxoids	Bacterial fermentation (pathogenic)
BioPort Corporation	Anthrax vaccine adsorbed	Bacterial fermentation, soluble filtrate
Berna Biotech	Typhoid vaccine live oral Ty21a	Live attenuated bacteria, bacterial fermentation
Biken	Japanese encephalitis virus vaccine inactivated	Killed virus, isolated from the brain of intracerebrally infected mice

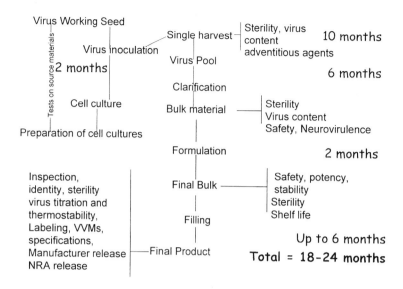

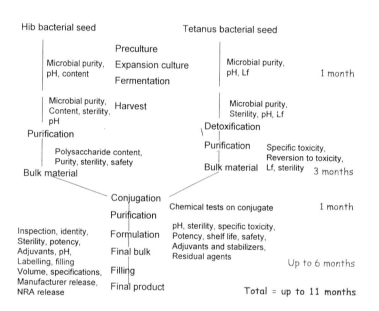

Appendix B Typical production flow charts, oral polio vaccine (top), and *Haemophilus influenzae* type b conjugate vaccine (tetanus conjugate) (bottom).

APPENDIX C. GUIDELINES RELEVANT TO LARGE-SCALE VACCINE MANUFACTURE

WHO Guidelines (see Refs. 7 and 8)

- A WHO guide to good manufacturing practice requirements, Part 1: Standard operating procedures and master formulae. Ordering code: WHO/VSQ/97.01
- A WHO guide to good manufacturing practice requirements, Part 2: Validation. Ordering code: WHO/ VSQ/97.02
- Guide for inspection of manufacturers of biological products. Ordering code: WHO/VSQ/97.03 [1170]
- Guidelines on clinical evaluation of vaccines: regulatory expectations. Adopted 2001, TRS, in press, Annex 1
- Guidelines for assuring the quality of DNA vaccines. Adopted 1996, TRS No 878, Annex 3
- Guidelines for the production and quality control of synthetic peptide vaccines. Adopted 1997, TRS No 889, Annex 1
- Requirements for the use of animal cells as in vitro substrates for the production of biologicals. Revised 1996, TRS *No 878*, Annex 1
- Good Manufacturing Practices for biological products. Adopted 1991, TRS *No 822*, Annex 1
- Guidelines for national authorities on quality assurance for biological products. TRS *No 822*, Annex 2
- Biological products prepared by recombinant DNA technology. TRS *No 814*, Annex 3
- General requirements for the sterility of biological substances. Revised 1973, TRS *No 530*, Annex 4; Amendment 1995, TRS No 872, Annex 3

FDA Guidelines (see also Ref. 5)

- Points to Consider in the Manufacture and Testing of Monoclonal Antibody Products for Human Use (1997)
- Guidance for Industry for the Evaluation of Combination Vaccines for Preventable Diseases: Production, Testing, and Clinical Studies (1997)
- Content and Format of Chemistry, Manufacturing, and Controls (CMC) Information and Establishment Description Information for a Vaccine or Related Product (1999)
- IND Meetings for Human Drugs and Biologics—Chemistry, Manufacturing, and Controls Information (2001)
- 21 CFR 25 Environmental Impact Considerations
- 21 CFR 210 Current good manufacturing practice in manufacturing, processing, packing, or holding of drugs; general

- 21 CFR 211 Current good manufacturing practice for finished pharmaceuticals
- 21 CFR 600 Biological products: general
- 21 CFR 610 General biological products standards

ICH Guidelines (see Ref. 9)

- Quality of Biotechnological Products: Viral Safety Evaluation of Biotechnology Products Derived from Cell Lines of Human or Animal Origin
- ICH Stability Guideline
- Derivation and Characterisation of Cell Substrates Used for Production of Biotechnological/Biological Products
- Analysis of the Expression Construct in Cells Used for Production of r-DNA Derived Protein Products

EMEA Guidelines (see Ref. 10)

- CPMP/BWP/2289/01 Points to Consider on the Development of Live Attenuated Influenza Vaccines
- CPMP/BWP/2517/00 Points to Consider on the Reduction, Elimination, or Substitution of Thiomersal in Vaccines
- CPMP/BWP/3354/99 Note for Guidance on the Production and Quality Control of Animal Immunoglobins and Immunosera for Human Use
- CPMP/BWP/2490/00 Note for Guidance on Cell Culture Inactivated Influenza Vaccines—Annex to Note for Guidance on Harmonisation of Requirements for Influenza Vaccines CPMP/BWP/214/96
- CPMP/BWP/3207/00 Note for Guidance on Comparability of Medicinal Products Containing Biotechnology-Derived Proteins as Drug Substance
- EMEA/410/01 *Rev. 1* Note for Guidance on Minimising the Risk of Transmitting Animal Spongiform Encephalopathy Agents via Human and Veterinary Medicinal Products
- CPMP/BWP/3088/99 Note for Guidance on the Quality, Preclinical and Clinical Aspects of Gene Transfer Medicinal Products
- CPMP/BWP/328/99 Development Pharmaceutics for Biotechnological and Biological Products—Annex to Note for Guidance on Development Pharmaceutics (CPMP/QWP/155/96)
- CPMP/BWP/477/97 Note for Guidance on Pharmaceutical and Biological Aspects of Combined Vaccines
- CPMP/BWP/268/95 Note for Guidance on Virus Validation Studies: The Design, Contribution, and Interpretation of Studies validating the Inactivation and Removal of Viruses

90

Heterogeneity of Pediatric Immunization Schedules in Industrialized Countries

James D. Campbell
University of Maryland School of Medicine, Baltimore, Maryland, U.S.A.

Margaret Burgess
Children's Hospital at Westmead, Westmead, New South Wales, Australia

I. INTRODUCTION

Many factors influence the selection of vaccines that are administered to infants and toddlers in a particular country and the immunization schedule that is followed. These include epidemiological (e.g., past and present burden and prevalence of specific infectious diseases), economic (e.g., relative cost of vaccines, including various combination vaccines), sociological (e.g., the public perception of the risk and severity of specific infectious diseases and of the safety and efficacy of specific vaccines), logistics (e.g., population dispersion, mobility, and access to health services), immunological (e.g., differences in the immune responses to specific vaccine antigens depending on age and spacing of doses), and historical factors. For infant immunizations, the national schedule for diphtheria/pertussis/tetanus (DPT) vaccine largely drives the overall infant immunization schedule. Interestingly, in most of the developing world, the Expanded Program on Immunization (as described by Bruce Aylward et al. in the chapter entitled "Reaching Every Child—Achieving Equity in Global Immunization") administers infant DPT immunizations according to only two main schedules. In the least developed countries, where the risk of pertussis in early life is a particular danger, doses of DPT are administered at 6, 10, and 14 weeks of age. Because of economic and logistical constraints in these countries, a booster immunization in the second year of life is generally not practiced. In contrast, in many newly developing and middle-income countries, where the incidence of pertussis is lower and immunization coverage is higher, such as in Latin America and parts of Asia, infant DPT immunizations are typically administered at 2, 4, and 6 months of age; these countries usually also give boosters in the second year of life (often at 18 months of age). Thus, among the nonindustrialized countries there exists an extraordi-

nary degree of harmonization of pediatric immunization schedules with most countries following one of two schedules, although the array of specific vaccines administered at these times varies greatly (largely driven by economic considerations).

In contrast, among the industrialized countries of the world one finds a remarkable heterogeneity of infant and toddler immunization schedules. This is particularly notable in Europe where neighboring countries of similar wealth and epidemiologic situation (with respect to the incidence of infections such as pertussis, diphtheria, *Haemophilus influenzae* type b, and hepatitis B) often use distinct immunization schedules. Table 1 provides some examples, limiting the comparison to DTP. Multiple distinct schedules are readily apparent. Spain and Portugal follow an infant and toddler schedule similar to that used in North America and most of Latin America (although the specific array of vaccines differs in individual countries). Ireland also immunizes its infants at 2, 4, and 6 months of age but does not give a booster to toddlers in the second year of life. Across the Irish Sea, in the United Kingdom, a completely distinct schedule is followed as infants are immunized at 2, 3, and 4 months of age; in the U.K., no booster is given to toddlers although one is given somewhat later to preschool children. Crossing the English Channel one finds that France, Belgium, Germany, and Luxembourg also immunize their infants at 2, 3, and 4 months of age, but these countries show heterogeneity in the age when a booster is administered.

The Scandinavian countries (Denmark, Norway, Sweden, and Iceland) and Italy immunize infants at 3 and 5 months with a third dose at 11–12 months of age. Meanwhile, Austria, Finland, and the Netherlands give their infants primary immunization at 3, 4, and 5 months of age with a booster at either 11 (Netherlands), 13–15 (Austria), or 20 (Finland) months.

Table 1 Examples of the Heterogeneity Among the DPT Immunization Schedules Practiced in Various Industrialized Countries

Country	1.5 mo	2 mo	3 mo	4 mo	5 mo	6 mo	7 mo	8 mo	11 mo	12 mo	13–15 mo	15–18 mo	20 mo
United States		DaPT		DaPT		DaPT						DaPT	
Canada		DaPT		DaPT		DaPT						DaPT	
Australia		DaPT		DaPT		DaPT						DaPT	
New Zealand	DaPT		DaPT		DaPT								
UK		DwPT or DaPT	DwPT or DaPT	DwPT or DaPT							DaPT		
Germany		DaPT	DaPT	DaPT						DaPT			
Ireland		DaPT	DaPT	DaPT									
Belgium and Luxembourg		DaPT	DaPT	DaPT							DaPT		
France		DwPT	DwPT	DwPT								DaPT	
Spain		DaPT		DaPT		DaPT						DaPT	
Portugal		DwPT	DwPT	DwPT		DwPT						DwPT	
Austria			DaPT	DaPT	DaPT						DaPT		
Finland			DwPT	DwPT	DwPT								
Netherlands		DwPT	DwPT	DwPT					DaPT				DaPT
Italy			DaPT		DaPT				DaPT				
Denmark			DaPT		DaPT					DaPT			
Norway			DaPT		DaPT					DaPT			
Sweden			DaPT		DaPT					DaPT			
Iceland			DaPT		DaPT					DaPT			
Japan						DaPT	DaPT	DaPT				DaPT	

aP = acellular pertussis vaccine; wP = whole-cell pertussis vaccine.

Table 2 Recommended Immunizations During the First 18 Months of Life, U.S.A.

Birth	1 mo	2 mo	4 mo	6 mo	12 mo	15 mo	18 mo
HBV1[a]		HBV2 DaPT Hib IPV	DaPT Hib IPV	HBV3 DaPT Hib[c] IPV	Hib Measles/mumps/rubella1 Varicella		DaPT[b]
		Pneumo	Pneumo	Pneumo	Pneumo		

[a] All infants should receive the first dose of HBV in the perinatal period and before hospital discharge. However, the first dose may also be given by age 2 months if the infant's mother is HB surface antigen-negative. Only monovalent vaccine can be used for the birth dose. Either monovalent or combination vaccine can be used to complete the series. Four doses may be given if a birth dose was administered. The second dose of HBV must be given at least 4 weeks after the first dose, except for combination vaccines, which cannot be administered before age 6 weeks. The third dose should be given at least 16 weeks after the first dose and at least 8 weeks after the second dose. The last dose in the vaccination series (third or fourth dose) should not be administered before 6 months age.

[b] The fourth dose of DaPT may be given as early as 12 months of age as long as at least 6 months have passed since the third dose.

[c] If PRP-OMP was given as the Hib conjugate in either monovalent or combination formulation, a third dose at age 6 months does not have to be given.

II. COMBINATION VACCINES

The different industrialized countries utilize an array of DTP-based combination vaccines, which include combinations of four vaccines (e.g., DaPT plus hepatitis B [HBV] or *Haemophilus influenzae* type b conjugate [Hib] or inactivated polio vaccine [IPV]), five vaccines (e.g., DaPT plus Hib and IPV; DaPT plus HBV and IPV; DwPT plus HBV and Hib), or six vaccines (DaPT plus HBV, Hib and IPV). (For more on infant combination vaccines see the chapter by Margaret Rennels on this subject.)

III. CONCOMITANT VACCINES

Depending on the industrialized country, various additional noncombination vaccines are concomitantly administered at the same visits when DPT is given. In a few countries oral polio vaccine is still given. Several countries routinely recommend seven-valent pneumococcal conjugate vaccine along with the first doses of DPT. A few (e.g., United Kingdom) give meningococcal C conjugate, and Japan gives

Japanese B encephalitis vaccine. As an example to illustrate the complexity of an immunization schedule in an industrialized country, the 2003 schedule for U.S. children 0–18 months of age is shown in Table 2.

IV. CONSEQUENCES OF HETEROGENEITY

The staggering array of distinct infant immunization schedules practiced by the industrialized countries (Table 1) affects the price and supply of vaccines. As new vaccines become developed with the intention that they will enter the infant/toddler immunization schedule, their safety and immunogenicity must be shown for each distinct schedule and in conjunction with the concomitant vaccines ordinarily administered at those visits. The greater the array of immunization schedules, the more separate regimens must be validated. A perusal of the examples shown in Table 1 suggests that with a relatively few modifications in just a few countries the number of regimens can be reduced. Undoubtedly, this will be difficult to achieve and will take time. Nevertheless, it is a worthy objective.

Index

ABOUT THE EDITORS

MYRON M. LEVINE is Director of the Center for Vaccine Development, Professor of Medicine, and Head of the Division of Geographic Medicine, as well as Professor of Pediatrics and Head of the Division of Infectious Diseases and Tropical Pediatrics, University of Maryland School of Medicine, Baltimore. He received the M.D. degree (1967) from the Medical College of Virginia, Richmond, and the D.T.P.H. degree (1974) from the London School of Hygiene and Tropical Medicine, England.

JAMES B. KAPER is Associate Director for Laboratory Research at the Center for Vaccine Development, and Professor of Medicine, Microbiology and Immunology, University of Maryland School of Medicine, Baltimore. He received the Ph.D. degree (1979) from the University of Maryland at College Park.

RINO RAPPUOLI is Vice President for Vaccines Research, Chiron S.r.l., Siena, Italy. He received the Ph.D. degree (1976) from the University of Siena, Italy.

MARGARET A. LIU is Visiting Professor at the Karolinska Institute, Stockholm, Sweden, and Vice-Chairman of Transgene, Inc., Strasbourg, France. She was formerly Senior Advisor for Vaccinology, Bill & Melinda Gates Foundation, Seattle, Washington. She received the M.D. degree (1981) from Harvard Medical School, Boston, Massachusetts.

MICHAEL F. GOOD is Director, Queensland Institute of Medical Research, Australia. He is a former Director of the Cooperative Research Centre for Vaccine Technology. He received the M.D. degree from the University of Queensland, Australia, and the Ph.D. degree from the Walter and Eliza Hall Institute of Medical Research, Melbourne, Australia.

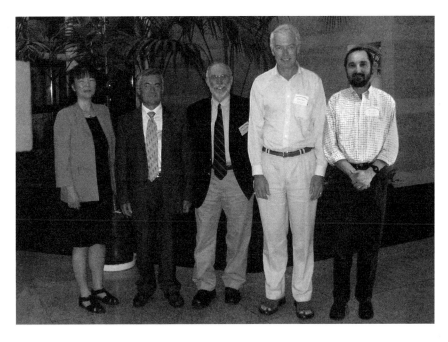

Left to right: Margaret A. Liu, M.D., Transgene, Inc.; Rino Rappuoli, Ph.D., Chiron S.r.l.; Myron M. Levine, M.D., D.T.P.H., University of Maryland School of Medicine; Michael F. Good, M.D., Ph.D., Queensland Institute of Medical Research; James B. Kaper, Ph.D., University of Maryland School of Medicine.

ISBN 0-8247-4071-8

90000